P9-CAA-909

a **LANGE** medical book

CURRENT

Pediatric Diagnosis & Treatment

Twelfth Edition

Edited by

WILLIAM W. HAY, JR., MD
Professor, Department of Pediatrics
Director, Training Program in Neonatal-Perinatal
  Medicine
Director, Neonatal Clinical Research Center
Section of Neonatology and the Division of
  Perinatal Medicine and Research
University of Colorado School of Medicine and
  The Children's Hospital, Denver

JESSIE R. GROOTHUIS, MD
Associate Professor, Department of Pediatrics
Director, Neonatal High Risk Followup Program
Section of Neonatology
University of Colorado School of Medicine and
  The Children's Hospital, Denver

ANTHONY R. HAYWARD, MD, PhD
Professor, Departments of Pediatrics and Immunology
Head, Section of Pediatric Allergy and Immunology
University of Colorado School of Medicine and
  The Children's Hospital, Denver

MYRON J. LEVIN, MD
Professor, Departments of Pediatrics and Medicine
Chief, Section of Pediatric Infectious Diseases
University of Colorado School of Medicine and
  The Children's Hospital, Denver

and Associate Authors

The Department of Pediatrics at the University of Colorado School of Medicine is affiliated with
The Children's Hospital of Denver, Colorado

APPLETON & LANGE
Norwalk, Connecticut

Copyright © 1995 by Appleton & Lange
A Simon & Schuster Company
Previous edition copyright © 1991, 1987 by Appleton & Lange

95 96 97 98 99 / 10 9 8 7 6 5 4 3 2

Prentice Hall International (UK) Limited, *London*
Prentice Hall of Australia Pty. Limited, *Sydney*
Prentice Hall Canada, Inc., *Toronto*
Prentice Hall Hispanoamericana, S. A., *Mexico*
Prentice Hall of India Private Limited, *New Delhi*
Prentice Hall of Japan, Inc., *Tokyo*
Simon & Schuster Asia Pte., Ltd., *Singapore*
Editora Prentice Hall do Brasil Ltda., *Rio de Janeiro*
Prentice Hall, *Englewood Cliffs, New Jersey*

ISBN: 0-8385-1446-4
ISSN: 0093-8556

ISBN 0-8385-1446-4

90000

9 780838 514467

Acquisitions Editor: Shelley Reinhardt
Production Editor: Christine Langan

PRINTED IN THE UNITED STATES OF AMERICA

Table of Contents

24. Kidney & Urinary Tract 683

Gary M. Lum, MD

25. Neurologic & Muscular Disorders 710

Paul G. Moe, MD, & Alan R. Seay, MD

26. Orthopedics 786

Robert E. Eilert, MD, & Gaia Georgopoulos, MD

27. Rheumatic Diseases 807

J. Roger Hollister, MD

28. Hematologic Disorders 815

Peter A. Lane, MD, Rachelle Nuss, MD, & Daniel R. Ambruso, MD

Contributors

Steven H. Abman, MD
Respiratory Tract & Mediastinum
Associate Professor, Department of Pediatrics, Section of Pediatric Pulmonary Medicine, University of Colorado School of Medicine and The Children's Hospital, Denver.

R.B. Abrams, DDS
Oral Medicine & Dentistry
Assistant Clinical Professor, Department of Growth and Development, University of Colorado School of Dentistry; and Assistant Chief of Dentistry, The Children's Hospital, Denver.

Frank J. Accurso, MD
Respiratory Tract & Mediastinum
Associate Professor, Department of Pediatrics, Section of Pediatric Pulmonary Medicine, University of Colorado School of Medicine and The Children's Hospital, Denver.

Edythe Albano, MD
Neoplastic Diseases
Assistant Professor, Department of Pediatrics, Section of Hematology/Oncology, University of Colorado School of Medicine and The Children's Hospital, Denver.

Daniel R. Ambruso, MD
Hematologic Disorders
Professor, Department of Pediatrics, Section of Pediatric Hematology and Oncology; Associate Medical Director, Belle Bonfils Blood Center, University of Colorado School of Medicine and The Children's Hospital, Denver.

Trina Menden Anglin, MD, PhD
Adolescent Substance Abuse
Associate Professor, Department of Pediatrics; Associate Chief, Section of Adolescent Medicine, University University of Colorado School of Medicine and The Children's Hospital, Denver.

F. Keith Battan, MD
Emergencies & Accidents
Assistant Professor, Department of Pediatrics, Section of Emergency and General Pediatrics, University of Colorado School of Medicine; Director, Pre-Hospital Care Program; Director, Pediatric Emergency Medicine Fellowship Program, The Children's Hospital, Denver.

Stephen Berman, MD
Ear, Nose, & Throat
Professor, Department of Pediatrics, University of Colorado School of Medicine and The Children's Hospital, Denver; Director of Health Policy, University of Colorado Health Sciences Center.

Mark M. Boucek, MD
Cardiovascular Diseases
Professor, Department of Pediatrics; Head, Section of Pediatric Cardiology, University of Colorado School of Medicine and The Children's Hospital, Denver.

Bonnie W. Camp, MD, PhD
Developmental Disorders
Professor, Departments of Pediatrics and Psychiatry, Section of Developmental and Behavioral Pediatrics, University of Colorado School of Medicine and The Children's Hospital, Denver; Director, John F. Kennedy Child Development Center, University of Colorado Health Sciences Center, Denver.

H. Peter Chase, MD
Diabetes Mellitus
Professor, Department of Pediatrics, and Clinical Director, Barbara Davis Center for Childhood Diabetes, University of Colorado School of Medicine, Denver.

R. Barkley Clark, MD
Psychosocial Aspects of Pediatrics & Psychiatric Disorders
Assistant Clinical Professor, Department of Psychiatry, Division of Child Psychiatry, University of Colorado Health Sciences Center, Denver.

Carolyn R. Comer, MD
Allergic Disorders
Clinical Instructors, Department of Pediatrics, University of Colorado School of Medicine;

Staff Physician, National Jewish Center for Immunology and Respiratory Medicine, Denver.

Richard C. Dart, MD, PhD
Poisoning
Director, Rocky Mountain Poison and Drug Center, Denver, Assistant Professor of Surgery, University of Colorado School of Medicine, Denver.

Emily M. Dobyns, MD
Critical Care
Assistant Professor, Department of Pediatrics, Section of Pediatric Critical Care Medicine, University of Colorado School of Medicine and The Children's Hospital, Denver.

Anthony G. Durmowicz, MD
Critical Care
Assistant Professor, Department of Pediatric, Section of Pediatric Critical Care Medicine, University of Colorado School of Medicine and The Children's Hospital, Denver.

Robert E. Eilert, MD
Orthopedics
Clinical Professor, Department of Orthopedic Surgery, University of Colorado School of Medicine; Chairman, Department of Orthopedic Surgery, The Children' Hospital, Denver.

George Eisenbarth, MD, PhD
Endocrine Disorders
Professor, Department of Pediatrics, and Executive Director of the Barbara Davis Center for Childhood Diabetes, University of Colorado School of Medicine, Denver.

Philip P. Ellis, MD
Eye
Professor and Chairman, Department of Ophthalmology, University of Colorado School of Medicine, Denver.

Leland L. Fan, MD
Respiratory Tract & Mediastinum
Professor, Department of Pediatrics, Section of Pediatric Pulmonary Medicine, University of Colorado School of Medicine and The Children's Hospital, Denver; Senior Staff Physician, National Jewish Center for Immunology and Respiratory Medicine, Denver.

Erwin W. Gelfand, MD
Immunodeficiency
Professor, Department of Pediatrics and Microbiology/Immunology, University of Colorado School of Medicine; Chairman, Department of

Pediatrics, National Jewish Center for Immunology and Respiratory Medicine, Denver.

Cynthia R. Gelman, BS Pharm
Drug Therapy
Consultant, Rocky Mountain Poison & Drug Center, Denver.

Gaia Georgopoulous, MD
Orthopedics
Assistant Clinical Professor, Department of Orthopedics, University of Colorado School of Medicine and the Children's Hospital, Denver.

Edward Goldson, MD
Behavioral Disorders & Developmental Variations
Associate Professor, Department of Pediatrics, Section of Developmental and Behavioral Pediatrics, University of Colorado School of Medicine and The Children's Hospital, Denver.

Stephen I. Goodman, MD
Inborn Errors of Metabolism
Professor, Department of Pediatrics, and Head, Section of Genetics, Metabolism and Birth Defects, University of Colorado School of Medicine and The Children's Hospital, Denver.

Ronald W. Gotlin, MD
Endocrine Disorders
Professor, Department of Pediatrics, Section of Endocrinology, University of Colorado School of Medicine and The Children's Hospital, Denver.

Carol L. Greene, MD
Inborn Errors of Metabolism
Associate Professor, Department of Pediatrics, Section of Genetics, Metabolism and Birth Defects, University of Colorado School of Medicine and The Children's Hospital, Denver.

Brian S. Greffe, MD
Neoplastic Diseases
Assistant Professor, Department of Pediatrics, Section of Hematology and Oncology, University of Colorado School of Medicine and The Children's Hospital, Denver.

K. Michael Hambridge, M.B., B. Chir., ScD, FRCP (Edin)
Normal Childhood Nutrition & Its Disorders
Professor, Department of Pediatrics, Director, University of Colorado Center for Human Nutrition, University of Colorado School of Medicine and The Children's Hospital, Denver.

Keith B. Hammond, MS, FIMLS
Normal Biochemical & Hematologic Values
Senior Instructor, Departments of Pediatrics and Pathology, and Director, Pediatric Clinical Research Center Laboratory, University of Colorado School of Medicine, Denver.

Randi Jenssen Hagerman, MD
Growth & Development
Professor, Department of Pediatrics, Head, Section of Developmental and Behavioral Pediatrics, University of Colorado School of Medicine and The Children's Hospital, Denver.

Anthony R. Hayward, MD, PhD
Immunodeficiency
Professor, Departments of Pediatrics and Immunology; Head, Section of Pediatric Allergy and Immunology, University of Colorado School of Medicine and The Children's Hospital, Denver.

Roxann M. Headley, MD
Ambulatory Pediatrics
Assistant Professor, Department of Pediatrics, University of Colorado School of Medicine; Medical Director, Child Health Clinic, The Children's Hospital, Denver.

Desmond B. Henry, MD
Critical Care
Clinical Instructor, Departments of Anesthesiology and Pediatrics, University of Colorado School of Medicine; Medical Director Pediatric Care Unit and Director of Children's Emergency Transport Services, Inc., The Children's Hospital, Denver.

J. Roger Hollister, MD
Rheumatic Diseases
Professor, Departments of Pediatrics and Medicine; Head, Section of Pediatric Rheumatology, University of Colorado School of Medicine and The Children's Hospital; Senior Staff Physician, National Jewish Center for Immunology and Respiratory Medicine, Denver.

David W. Kaplan, MD, MH
Adolescence
Professor, Department of Pediatrics, and Head, Section of Adolescent Medicine, University of Colorado School of Medicine and The Children's Hospital, Denver.

Michael Kappy, MD, PhD
Endocrine Disorders
Professor, Department of Pediatrics, and Head, Section of Endocrinology, University of Colorado School of Medicine and The Children's Hospital, Denver.

Elizabeth B. Kozleski, EdD
Developmental Disorders
Assistant Professor, School of Education, Division of Educational Psychology and Special Education, University of Colorado, Denver.

Nancy F. Krebs, MD, MS
Normal Childhood Nutrition
Assistant Professor, Department of Pediatrics, Section of Gastroenterology and Nutrition, and Associate Director, University of Colorado Center for Human Nutrition, University of Colorado School of Medicine and The Children's Hospital, Denver.

Richard D. Krugman, MD
Child Abuse & Neglect
Professor, Department of Pediatrics, and Dean, University of Colorado School of Medicine, Denver.

Peter A. Lane, MD
Hematologic Disorders
Associate Professor, Department of Pediatrics, Section of Pediatric Hematology and Oncology, and Director, Colorado Sickle Cell Treatment and Research Center, University of Colorado School of Medicine and The Children's Hospital, Denver.

Gary L. Larsen, MD
Respiratory Tract & Mediastinum
Professor, Department of Pediatrics, and Head, Section of Pediatric Pulmonary Medicine, University of Colorado School of Medicine and The Children's Hospital, Denver; Senior Staff Physician, National Jewish Center for Immunology and Respiratory Medicine, Denver.

Myron J. Levin, MD
Infections: Viral & Rickettsial; Infections: Mycotic & Parasitic
Professor, Departments of Pediatrics and Medicine; Chief, Section of Pediatric Infectious Diseases, University of Colorado School of Medicine and The Children's Hospital, Denver.

Stanley L. Loftness, MD
Critical Care
Assistant Clinical Professor, Departments of Pediatrics ataff Anesthesiologist and Intensivist, The Children's Hospital, Denver.

Gary M. Lum, MD
Kidney & Urinary Tract
Professor, Departments of Pediatrics and Medicine, and Head, Section of Pediatric Renal Medicine, University of Colorado School of Medicine and The Children's Hospital, Denver.

James V. Lustig, MD
Approaching the Pediatric Patient; Fluid & Electrolyte Therapy
Professor, Department of Pediatrics, University of Colorado School of Medicine, Denver.

Kathleen A. Mammel, MD
Adolescence; Sexually Transmitted Diseases
Assistant Professor, Department of Pediatrics; Section of Adolescent Medicine, University of Colorado School of Medicine and The Children's Hospital, Denver.

David K. Manchester, MD
Genetics & Dysmorphology
Associate Professor, Departments of Pediatrics and Pharmacology, Section of Genetics, Metabolism and Birth Defects, University of Colorado School of Medicine; Co-Director, Division of Genetic Services, The Children's Hospital, Denver.

Paul G. Moe, MD
Neurologic & Muscular Disorders
Professor, Departments of Pediatrics and Neurology, Division of Child Neurology, University of Colorado School of Medicine and The Children's Hospital, Denver.

Joseph G. Morelli, MD
Skin
Assistant Professor, Departments of Dermatology and Pediatrics, University of Colorado School of Medicine, Denver.

W. A. Mueller, DMD
Oral Medicine & Dentistry
Associate Clinical Professor, Department of Growth and Development, University of Colorado School of Dentistry; and Chief of Dentistry, The Children's Hospital, Denver.

Michael R. Narkewicz, MD
Liver & Pancreas
Assistant Professor, Department of Pediatrics, Section of Pediatric Gastroenterology and Nutrition and The Pediatric Liver Center, University of Colorado School of Medicine and The Children's Hospital, Denver.

Rachelle Nuss, MD
Hematologic Disorders
Assistant Professor, Department of Pediatrics, Section of Pediatric Hematology and Oncology, University of Colorado School of Medicine and The Children's Hospital, Denver.

Lorrie F. Odom MD
Neoplastic Diseases
Professor, Department of Pediatrics, Section of Pediatric Hematology and Oncology, University of Colorado School of Medicine, Clinical Director of Oncology, The Children's Hospital, Denver.

John W. Ogle, MD
Infections: Bacterial & Spirochetal
Associate Professor, Department of Pediatrics, Section of Pediatric Infectious Diseases, University of Colorado School of Medicine and The Children's Hospital, Denver; Director, Department of Pediatrics, Denver General Hospital.

David S. Pearlman, MD
Allergic Disorders
Clinical Professor, Department of Pediatrics, University of Colorado School of Medicine, and Senior Staff Physician, National Jewish Center for Immunology and Respiratory Medicine, Denver.

Robert G. Peterson, MD, PhD
Drug Therapy
Professor and Chairman, Department of Pediatrics, and Professor of Pharmacology, University of Ottawa; Children's Hospital of Eastern Ontario, Ottawa.

José R. Romero, MD
Infections: Viral & Rickettsial
Assistant Professor, Department of Pediatrics, Section of Pediatric Infectious Diseases, Creighton University, Omaha, NE.

Adam A. Rosenberg, MD
The Newborn Infant
Associate Professor, Department of Pediatrics; Medical Director, Perinatal Research, The Children's Hospital; and Medical Director of the Newborn Service, University Hospital, University of Colorado Health Sciences Center, Denver.

Harley A. Rotbart, MD
Infections: Parasitic & Mycotic
Associate Professor, Departments of Pediatrics and Microbiology/Immunology, Section of Pediatric Infectious Diseases, University of Colorado School of Medicine and The Children's Hospital, Denver.

Barry H. Rumack, MD
Poisoning; Drug Therapy
Clinical Professor, Department of Pediatrics, University of Colorado School of Medicine, and

President and Chief Executive Officer of Micromedex, Denver.

Michael S. Schaffer, MD
Cardiovascular Diseases
Associate Professor, Department of Pediatrics, Section of Pediatric Cardiology, University of Colorado School of Medicine and The Children's Hospital, Denver.

Barton D. Schmitt, MD
Ambulatory Pediatrics; Ear, Nose, & Throat
Professor, Department of Pediatrics, and Director of Pediatric Consultative Services, University of Colorado School of Medicine and The Children's Hospital, Denver.

Alan R. Seay, MD
Neurologic & Muscular Disorders
Associate Professor, Departments of Neurology and Pediatrics; Chief, Division of Child Neurology, University of Colorado School of Medicine and The Children's Hospital, Denver.

Arnold Silverman, MD
Gastrointestinal Tract; Liver & Pancreas
Professor, Department of Pediatrics, Section of Pediatric Gastroenterology and Nutrition, University of Colorado School of Medicine and The Children's Hospital, Denver.

Eric A. F. Simoes, MD, DCH
Immunization
Assistant Professor, Department of Pediatrics, Section of Pediatric Infectious Diseases, University of Colorado School of Medicine and The Children's Hospital, Denver.

Ronald J. Sokol, MD
Liver & Pancreas
Associate Professor, Department of Pediatrics, Section of Pediatric Gastroenterology and Nutrition and The Pediatric Liver Center, University of Colorado School of Medicine and The Children's Hospital, Denver.

Judith M. Sondheimer, MD
Gastrointestinal Tract
Professor, Department of Pediatrics; Head, Section of Pediatric Gastroenterology and Nutrition University of Colorado School of Medicine and The Children's Hospital, Denver.

Kurt R. Stenmark, MD
Critical Care
Professor, Department of Pediatrics; Head, Section of Pediatric Critical Care Medicine; Univer-

sity of Colorado School of Medicine; University of Colorado School of Medicine and The Children's Hospital, Denver.

Janet M. Stewart, MD
Genetics & Dysmorphology
Associate Professor, Department of Pediatrics, Section of Genetics, Metabolism and Birth Defects, University of Colorado School of Medicine and The Children's Hospital, Denver.

Linda C. Stork, MD
Neoplastic Diseases
Associated Professor, Department of Pediatrics, Section of Hematology and Oncology, University of Colorado School of Medicine and The Children's Hospital, Denver.

Eva Sujansky, MD
Genetics & Dysmorphology
Associate Professor, Departments of Pediatrics and Biochemistry, Biophysics and Genetics, Section of Genetics, Metabolism and Birth Defects, University of Colorado School of Medicine and The Children's Hospital, Denver

Elizabeth H. Thilo, MD
The Newborn Infant
Assistant Professor, Department of Pediatrics, Section of Neonatology, University of Colorado School of Medicine and The Children's Hospital; Medical Director, Care by Children's Nurseries at St. Anthony's Central, Denver.

James K. Todd, MD
Antimicrobial Therapy of Pediatric Infections
Professor, Department of Pediatrics; Head, Section of Epidemiology, University of Colorado School of Medicine and The Children's Hospital, Denver.

William L. Weston, MD
Skin
Professor and Chairman, Department of Dermatology, and Professor, Department of Pediatrics, University of Colorado School of Medicine, Denver.

Carl W. White, MD
Respiratory Tract & Mediastinum
Associated Professor, Department of Pediatrics, Section of Pediatric Pulmonary Medicine, University of Colorado School of Medicine and The Children's Hospital, Denver; Senior Staff Physician, National Jewish Center for Immunology and Respiratory Medicine, Denver.

James W. Wiggins, Jr., MD
Cardiovascular Diseases
Associate Professor, Department of Pediatrics, Section of Pediatric Cardiology, University of Colorado School of Medicine and The Children's Hospital, Denver.

Robert R. Wolfe, MD
Cardiovascular Diseases
Professor, Department of Pediatrics, Section of Pediatric Cardiology, University of Colorado School of Medicine and The Children's Hospital, Denver.

Preface

The **12th edition** of *Current Pediatric Diagnosis & Treatment* features practical, up-to-date, well-referenced information on the care of children from birth through infancy and adolescence. *CPDT* emphasizes the clinical aspects of pediatric care while also covering the important underlying principles. Its goal is to provide a guide to diagnosis, understanding, and treatment of the medical problems of all pediatric patients in an easy to use and readable format.

INTENDED AUDIENCE

Like all Lange medical books, *CPDT* provides a concise yet comprehensive source of current information. Students will find *CPDT* an authoritative introduction to pediatrics and an excellent source for reference and review. Residents in pediatrics (and other specialties) will appreciate the concise yet detailed descriptions of diseases and diagnostic and therapeutic procedures. Pediatricians, family practitioners, nurses, and other health care providers who work with infants and children also will find *CPDT* a useful reference on management aspects of pediatric medicine.

COVERAGE

Forty-two chapters cover a wide range of topics, including normal growth and development, neonatal medicine, emergency and critical care medicine, and diagnosis and treatment of specific disorders according to major problems and organ systems. A wealth of tables and figures summarizes such important information as acute and critical care procedures in the delivery room, the office, the emergency room, and the critical care unit, anti-infective agents, drug dosages, immunization schedules, differential diagnosis, and the development screening tests. The final chapter is a handy guide to normal laboratory values.

NEW TO THE EDITION

The 12th edition of *CPDT* remains an up-to-date, comprehensive pediatric treatise but this edition is the *the most comprehensive revision to date* and significantly improves this classic book. The editors and contributing authors have continued to substantially revise the book, providing recent medical advances, and increasing the book's emphasis on ambulatory care, acute critical care, and the practical approach to pediatric disorders. As editors and practicing pediatricians, we have tried to ensure that each chapter reflects the needs and realities of day-to-day practice.

New Editors: Dr. William Hay is the new Senior Editor, assisted by Dr. Jessie Groothuis. Dr. Anthony Hayward and Dr. Myron Levin have been added as Editors, replacing Dr. William Hathaway (who has retired) and Dr. John Paisley (who has moved to Emmanuel Children's Hospital, Portland, Oregon).

New Chapters: The *four new chapters* deal with the most important and timely subjects in pediatric medicine today:

Behavioral Disorders and Development Variations (7)
Child Abuse (8)
Substance Abuse (9)
Sexually Transmitted Diseases (38)

New authors have rewritten the chapters on:

Teeth and Periodontium (18)
Neoplastic Diseases (39)

Chapter Revisions: Eight chapters have been extensively revised, with new authors added in several cases, reflecting substantial new information in each of their areas of pediatric medicine:

Endocrine Disorders (30)
Cardiovascular Disorders (21)
Liver and Pancreas (23)
Critical Care (15)
Genetics and Dysmorphology (32)
Infections: Viral and Rickettsial (35)
Infections: Bacterial and Spirochetal (36)
Infections: Parasitic and Mycotic (37)

HIV has been updated completely in Chapter 35. All other chapters are substantially revised and the references updated.

ACKNOWLEDGMENTS

The editors and contributing authors wish to thank Judy Lee, Administrative Assistant, Section of Neonatology and the Department of Pediatrics, for organizational support and secretarial assistance.

June, 1994

William W. Hay, Jr., MD
Jessie R. Groothuis, MD
Anthony R. Hayward, MD, PhD
Myron J. Levin, MD

Approaching the Pediatric Patient 1

James V. Lustig, MD

PEDIATRIC HISTORY

The emphasis placed on anticipatory guidance and prevention of disease makes pediatrics unique among medical disciplines. To achieve disease prevention and provide anticipatory guidance, the pediatrician must have a comprehensive longitudinal data base depicting the child's progress to the present moment and pointing toward problems the physician should anticipate. This emphasis results in certain unique aspects of the pediatric history. Addressing growth and development is a major goal in pediatrics, because children's ability to take their place in society is critical. The future of a child who fails to develop is clearly jeopardized. This must be recognized and treated early and effectively. Children's diets reflect much about their environment and growth. It is essential to obtain data about the child's diet, especially the present diet.

Everyone is familiar with the importance of immunization, yet the number of children who have not received a complete set of immunizations remains disappointingly high. This reflects not only the expense of immunization and the concerns of parents regarding the safety of immunizations but also our need to improve both our record-keeping systems and our effectiveness in getting children into our offices to receive these important treatments.

The history must include information about the family's structure and the environment in which a child is reared. Children need a supportive, nurturing, and enabling environment. It is the physician's responsibility to help the family provide appropriate stimulation that simultaneously challenges children to develop and supports their success in development. An understanding of the social structure of a child's family is helpful because it facilitates the physician's ability to interpret information elicited from the family of a child who develops an acute problem.

Over the past few decades, pediatricians have been successful in making a broad spectrum of preventive services available to children. The next step in the development of pediatric preventive services should be a systematic study of the impact of preventive services and the development of intervention and treatment strategies for those conditions discovered through screening programs. Standard evaluations for new services such as new metabolic screening tests also need to be established. The Canadian government supported a systematic study of the efficacy of preventive services and screening procedures in the 1970s. The publication of this work stimulated the United States Department of Health and Human Services to examine the effectiveness of preventive services in the United States. The publication in 1989 of the *Guide to Clinical Preventive Services* underscored the need for a systematic longitudinal prospective study of preventive services and screening procedures.*

Often, patients do not provide their own history. Usually one or both parents interpret the child's actions to the physician, who then reinterprets the parents' summary. The problems inherent in not obtaining the history directly from the patient are aggravated by the sometimes vague exposition of the complaints offered by parents who bring children to the office. These vague complaints are often really statements of the parents' own concerns about the child's progress. Instead of hearing that Andy has had a "warm, red, tender, swollen knee for two days," the pediatrician is more likely to hear that Andy has not played well this week or that he no longer wants to play on the soccer team. Many visits are precipitated by problems at school, such as poor grades or poor peer relationships. To distinguish organic from nonorganic illness and to intervene appropriately without subjecting the child to inappropriate testing, the physician must understand the family and its hopes and concerns for the child. It is often necessary to ask specifically what problems the parent wishes to address and to determine what really precipitated the office visit. It is essential to elicit as much of the history as possible directly from the patient. Direct histories not only provide firsthand information but also reinforce the child's sense of self, give the child a degree of

---

*Report of the US Preventive Services Task Force: *Guide to Clinical Preventive Services*. Williams & Wilkins, 1989.

control over a potentially threatening situation, and may reveal familial dysfunction.

Ideally, a family's first trip to a pediatrician's office should occur before birth of the baby. A prenatal visit goes a long way toward establishing rapport and helping the family to enjoy good, structured interaction with the physician. Families who know that a physician employs an extensive anticipatory guidance program are more confident that their concerns regarding growth, development, diet, and environment will be addressed. This practice also provides a natural framework for anticipating and preventing problems. Anticipating the information needed for each type of patient encounter helps the pediatrician structure inquiries, obtain data efficiently, and provide consistent patient care.

A child's medical record can be considered a longitudinal comprehensive data base. For this reason, different types of office visits need to be documented to provide comprehensive information—in a way that does not make data collection and maintenance of records burdensome to the physician or the office staff. The components of a comprehensive pediatric history are listed in Table 1–1. Specific data elements are not included; rather, the goals of each component are set forth.

TYPES OF VISITS

Prenatal Visits

A prenatal visit can greatly enhance a physician's relationship with the family. It enables the physician to learn about a family's desires, concerns, and fears regarding the anticipated birth of a child. Furthermore, this visit fosters the development of trust in the pediatrician. If the child develops a problem during the neonatal period, the physician who has not already met the family may have difficulty establishing rapport. Prenatal visits need not take a long time. They should be conducted in a relaxed atmosphere, with both parents present whenever possible. This is often a good time to elicit a family's medical history. The position (role) of the anticipated child in the family should be determined if possible. At this time, the physician should elicit information about any problems that have occurred during the pregnancy.

If the family is new to a practice, the prenatal visit provides an easy way to acquaint them with the way in which the practice is conducted. Parents want to know to whom they will speak when they call the office, when they may bring in children for acute care visits, and how their concerns regarding a child's developmental progress will be met. At the termination of the interview, the physician should have some un-

derstanding of the family's health care needs and should also be aware of the support systems available to aid the family through times of stress.

The family should understand the mechanics of the office, including not only appointment scheduling but telephone communication and bill procedures as well. The office manager or support staff should help educate parents about the administrative aspects of the office.

Although the prenatal visit is traditionally thought of in regard to new patients, it is often desirable to schedule such visits also before all subsequent births in a family. This provides a relaxed forum in which the family can update and refocus their concerns and needs.

Acute Care Visits

Owing to the episodic nature of pediatric practice and the demands on a pediatrician's time, the acute care visit must be an efficient, structured part of the office routine. Office support personnel should have elicited the reason for the visit and provided the physician with a brief synopsis of the child's symptoms. Support personnel should list known drug allergies on the encounter form, which the physician should review in anticipation of the need to use medication. The historian should document the chronology of events related to the present problem and call attention to pertinent parts of the comprehensive record, such as immunization status, past illnesses, and related problems.

The physical examination should be carefully detailed. The physician's diagnostic impression must be clearly shown in the medical record. The record should include supporting laboratory data and should document treatments rendered and anticipatory guidance given, such as when to return to the office if the problem is not ameliorated.

Hospital Visits

Fortunately, in modern pediatric practice, hospitalization is less common than in the past. When hospitalization is necessary, it is inevitably a time of stress for patient and family. The physician must put aside time not only to answer questions about the immediate problem but also to give support and reassurance. Whenever possible, the patient must be included in discussions of anticipated treatment and progress. Because the history of a child's progress during hospitalization is often derived from nurses, technicians, house staff, and colleagues, the physician needs to interpret data not derived firsthand. Knowledge of the child's immunization status, history of past illnesses, allergy history, and problem list is important in the successful treatment of the hospitalized child with an acute problem.

Health Maintenance Visits

Because of the emphasis pediatricians place on

Table 1–1. Components of the pediatric historical data base.[1]

Demographic data	Name, date of birth, social security number, sex, race, parents' names (first and last), siblings' names, and the patient's nickname. This should facilitate office management of the child's record and establish any unusual issues related to the socioeconomic-economic environment.
Problem list	The list of all of the child's major or significant problems should be displayed in a prominent place in the chart, including the date a problem became manifest, treatments employed, and the date of resolution.
Drug allergies	Any drug allergies are prominently displayed, including the drug precipitating the reaction, the nature of the reaction, the treatment needed, and the date. (A medical alert bracelet should be obtained for all children with a significant reaction.)
Current medications	The drug dose, vehicle, and frequency of medications currently employed by children who require chronic administration of medications.
Reasons for visit	The patient's or parents' concerns, stated in their own words whenever possible should serve as a focus for the visit. A traditional "chief complaint" may be misleading.
Present illness	A crisp, chronologic summary of the problems necessitating a visit, including the duration, progression, exacerbating factors, ameliorating interventions, and associations. The reactions of the historian, the patient, and the family to the problem are important in understanding the reason for the visit.
Past history General state of health	A statement regarding the child's functionality and general well-being, including a summary record of past significant illnesses, injuries, hospitalizations, and procedures, as well as decisions made about them, eg, the prophylactic use of penicillin due to the presence of rheumatic carditis.
Screening procedures	The results of and actions taken in response to all screening procedures should be maintained as a distinct part of the medical record, including newborn screening, vision and hearing screening, any health screens, or screening labs. (Developmental screening results are maintained in the development section.)
Birth history	**Mother:** Health during pregnancy, including illnesses, medications, drugs used, complications of pregnancy; duration and ease of labor; form of delivery; analgesics/anesthetics used; need for monitoring; and labor complications. **Child:** The birth weight, estimated gestational age, Apgar scores, and problems in the neonatal period. (These data may predict a child's subsequent development.)
Diet	Eating patterns, likes and dislikes, use of vitamins, parental assessment of eating, estimate of calories ingested, and relative amounts of carbohydrate, fat, and protein in the diet. (These data provide important insights not only into the nutritional adequacy of the diet but also familial interactions, attitudes, and concerns.)
Immunizations	The date of each immunization administered, the vaccine lot number, any reaction, and any contraindication to immunization, eg, immunodeficiency or an evolving neurologic problem.
Family history	Should include information about the illnesses of relatives (and the patient's involvement with those relatives), preferably in the form of a family tree.
Socioeconomic profile	Should identify the family constellation, relationships, parents' educational background, religious preference, and the role of the child in the family. Should also provide up-to-date information regarding the socioeconomic profile of the family to identify resources available to the child, services which may be needed, and anticipated stressors.
Development	In three sections: (1) attainment of developmental milestones (including developmental testing results); (2) social habits and milestones (toilet habits, play, major activities, sleep patterns, discipline, development of relationships); (3) school progress and documentation of specific achievements and grades.
Sexual history	Familial sexual attitudes, sex education, sexual development, sexual activity, sexually transmitted diseases, and birth control measures.
Review of systems (ROS)	This area tends to be overlooked because of the work required to obtain a complete ROS and integrate data into the patient's problems list and care plan. A focused ROS is essential if any problem is to be addressed adequately. For example, if a child is wheezing, it is important to know if ventilatory support was required in a newborn period, whether there is an antecedent or concurrent illness, chronic diarrhea, or whether the patient demonstrated failure to thrive. In such a case, it is also important for the examiner to determine whether an atopic diathesis is present, there is evidence of cardiac disease, chronic or nighttime cough is present, and symptoms are precipitated or exacerbated by exercise.

[1]The components of this table should be included in a child's medical record. The medical record should be structured to allow easy review and updating of all data needed longitudinally. Acute care visits should be recorded concisely and efficiently. Items requiring follow-up should be entered into the longitudinal section of the record.

prevention of disease and anticipatory guidance, the health maintenance visit has become a standard part of practice. The goal of these visits is not only to provide anticipatory guidance but also to promote the health of the patient by ensuring that immunizations are up to date, no significant health problems have developed, growth continues to be normal, and development is progressing as expected.

The American Academy of Pediatrics (AAP), through its Committee on Practice and Ambulatory Medicine, has developed recommendations for preventive pediatric health care. These recommendations offer general guidelines for the objectives of scheduled visits for children of different ages (Figure 1–1). As implied previously, preventive health services require further study. At the present time, the United States government is supporting a major initiative, the Bright Futures project, to reassess the need for pediatric preventive services. Specific recommendations may change significantly in the near future. Examples of specific issues to be addressed at different ages are presented in Table 1–2, which is derived from the AAP's Guidelines for Health Supervision II.

Preschool Visits

A trip to the physician's office before the child starts school represents a special health maintenance visit. During the preschool visit, it is important for the physician to assess development, elimination patterns, social behaviors, and diet. Attention to the progress of development and social behavior helps the family anticipate problems the child may have at school and allows the family to ease the child's transition from home life to school. Control of bladder and bowel functions is important to successful school entry. If there is a problem, it should be addressed before the child enters school.

Traditionally, immunizations are given at the preschool visit. Screening of vision and hearing is also important at this time. Topics addressed during subsequent visits should include assessment of the school performance, anticipated problems, and a critical review of both growth and development.

Sports Physicals

A physical examination is often needed before participation in organized sports programs. Time should be allotted not only to perform the physical but also to ask questions about the safety of the activities. What kind of protective equipment is provided? Are the supervisors and coaches trained to instruct children? What health care facilities are available? Will the patient require medication during competition (eg, beta-agonists for the patient with exercise-induced asthma)? Will the patient be exposed to unnecessary hazards, such as taking a turn at bat without a safety helmet or performing on the balance beam without a spotter? Does the program emphasize learning teamwork and skills, or is competition more important? Answering these questions can protect the child during an important part of childhood and ensure the child a joyful learning experience.

Comprehensive Pediatric History

Given the time constraints of most pediatric offices, obtaining a comprehensive pediatric history is a major undertaking. Many offices use questionnaires to facilitate the development of the comprehensive history. Such questionnaires, which are filled out prior to a patient's visit, enable the physician to anticipate problems and to learn about the patient before the visit takes place. They make office time more productive, allowing the physician to address problems in detail, while reviewing and dismissing areas that are not a problem. If reviewed prior to seeing the patient, historical questionnaires can greatly facilitate the development of rapport with new patients as the pediatrician enters the encounter with a significant amount of knowledge about the patient. Failure to study such questionnaires prior to the encounter may generate some resentment, because the family will feel their time has been wasted. The longitudinally important elements of the comprehensive data base must be maintained in the medical record so that they will be readily accessible as the child grows. In many practices, the front page of the medical record includes some demographic data, a problem list, known drug allergies, current medications, and the current immunization status.

The Physical Examination

Detailed analysis of the pediatric examination is beyond the scope of this chapter. However, the approach to the examination and certain elements of the examination will be emphasized. Table 1–3 illustrates how the examination can be focused to provide information about key issues at different ages.

A. Approaching the Child: Adequate time must be allotted to allow the child to become familiar with the examiner. Care must be taken to ensure that interactions are appropriate for the patient's age and developmental level. A gentle approach, friendly manner, and a quiet voice help establish a setting that yields a productive physical examination and does not unduly threaten the patient. A physician who cannot establish rapport with the patient should proceed to perform the examination efficiently, quickly, and systematically. In any pediatric examination, invasive or painful procedures or those perceived as such by the child (eg, examining the ears of a toddler) should be done at the end of the examination.

Because the history is often incomplete and because young children may perceive the examination as threatening and become fussy, inspection is very important. The examiner should make observations throughout the visit, paying special attention to how the child interacts with the environment. Observation

RECOMMENDATIONS FOR PREVENTIVE PEDIATRIC HEALTH CARE
Committee on Practice and Ambulatory Medicine

Each child and family is unique; therefore, these **Recommendations for Preventive Pediatric Health Care** are designed for the care of children who are receiving competent parenting, have no manifestations of any important health problems, and are growing and developing in satisfactory fashion. **Additional visits may become necessary** if circumstances suggest variations from normal. These guidelines represent a consensus by the Committee on Practice and Ambulatory Medicine in consultation with the membership of the American Academy of Pediatrics through the Chapter Presidents. The Committee emphasizes the great importance of **continuity of care** in comprehensive health supervision and the need to avoid **fragmentation of care.**

A **prenatal visit** by first-time parents and/or those who are at high risk is recommended and should include anticipatory guidance and pertinent medical history.

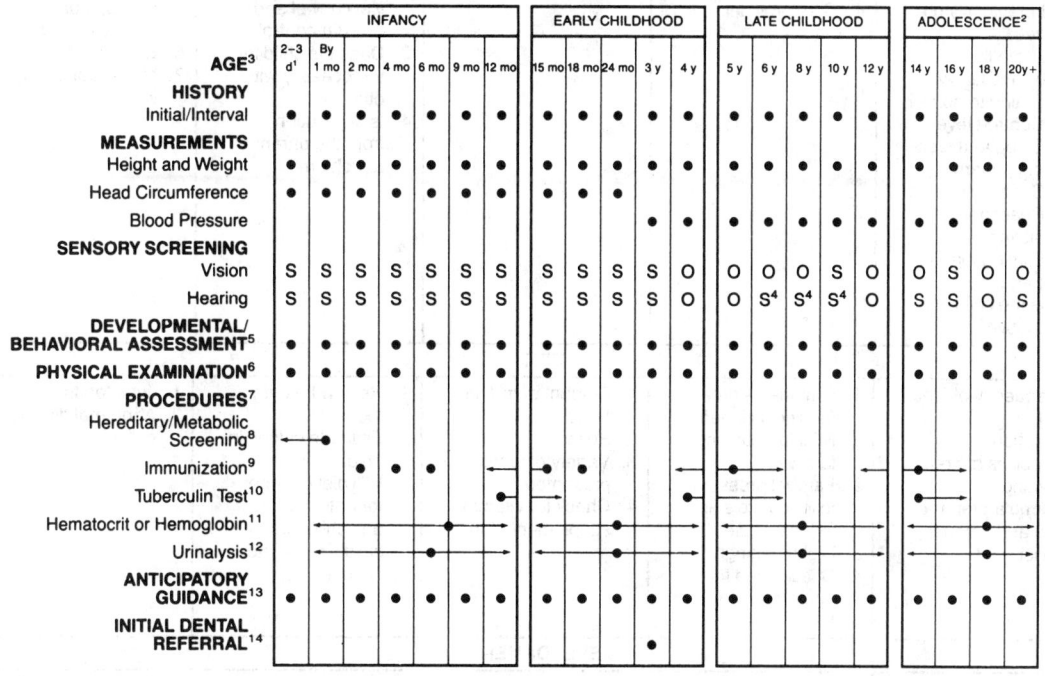

	INFANCY							EARLY CHILDHOOD					LATE CHILDHOOD					ADOLESCENCE[2]			
AGE[3]	2–3 d[1]	By 1 mo	2 mo	4 mo	6 mo	9 mo	12 mo	15 mo	18 mo	24 mo	3 y	4 y	5 y	6 y	8 y	10 y	12 y	14 y	16 y	18 y	20y+
HISTORY Initial/Interval	●	●	●	●	●	●	●	●	●	●	●	●	●	●	●	●	●	●	●	●	●
MEASUREMENTS Height and Weight	●	●	●	●	●	●	●	●	●	●	●	●	●	●	●	●	●	●	●	●	●
Head Circumference	●	●	●	●	●	●	●	●	●	●											
Blood Pressure											●	●	●	●	●	●	●	●	●	●	●
SENSORY SCREENING Vision	S	S	S	S	S	S	S	S	S	S	S	O	O	O	O	S	O	O	S	O	O
Hearing	S	S	S	S	S	S	S	S	S	S	S	O	O	S[4]	S[4]	S[4]	O	S	S	O	S
DEVELOPMENTAL/ BEHAVIORAL ASSESSMENT[5]	●	●	●	●	●	●	●	●	●	●	●	●	●	●	●	●	●	●	●	●	●
PHYSICAL EXAMINATION[6]	●	●	●	●	●	●	●	●	●	●	●	●	●	●	●	●	●	●	●	●	●
PROCEDURES[7] Hereditary/Metabolic Screening[8]	←—●																				
Immunization[9]			●	●	●			←—	●—	●			←——●					←——	●		
Tuberculin Test[10]					●—→					←——●								←—●—→			
Hematocrit or Hemoglobin[11]		←————●————→						←———●———→					←—————————●—————————→					←—————●—————→			
Urinalysis[12]		←————●————→						←———●———→					←—————————●—————————→					←—————●—————→			
ANTICIPATORY GUIDANCE[13]	●	●	●	●	●	●	●	●	●	●	●	●	●	●	●	●	●	●	●	●	●
INITIAL DENTAL REFERRAL[14]											●										

1. For newborns discharged in 24 hours or less after delivery.
2. Adolescent-related issues (eg, psychosocial, emotional, substance usage, and reproductive health) may necessitate more frequent health supervision.
3. If a child comes under care for the first time at any point on the schedule, or if any items are not accomplished at the suggested age, the schedule should be brought up to date at the earliest possible time.
4. At these points, history may suffice: if problem suggested, a standard testing method should be employed.
5. By history and appropriate physical examination: if suspicious, by specific objective developmental testing.
6. At each visit, a complete physical examination is essential, with infant totally unclothed, older child undressed and suitably draped.
7. These may be modified, depending upon entry point into schedule and individual need.
8. Metabolic screening (eg, thyroid, PKU, galactosemia) should be done according to state law.
9. Schedule(s) per *Report of the Committee on Infectious Diseases,* 1991 Red Book, and current AAP Committee statements.
10. For high-risk groups, the Committee on Infectious Diseases recommends annual TB skin testing.
11. Present medical evidence suggests the need for reevaluation of the frequency and timing of hemoglobin or hematocrit tests. One determination is therefore suggested during each time period. Performance of additional tests is left to the individual practice experience.
12. Present medical evidence suggests the need for reevaluation of the frequency and timing of urinalyses. One determination is therefore suggested during each time period. Performance of additional tests is left to the individual practice experience.
13. Appropriate discussion and counseling should be an integral part of each visit for care.
14. Subsequent examinations as prescribed by dentist.

NB: **Special chemical, immunologic, and endocrine testing** is usually carried out upon specific indications. Testing other than newborn (eg, inborn errors of metabolism, sickle disease, lead) is discretionary with the physician.

Key: ● = to be performed   S = subjective, by history   O = objective, by a standard testing method

The recommendations in this publication do not indicate an exclusive course of treatment or serve as a standard of medical care. Variations, taking into account individual circumstances, may be appropriate.

AAP News, July 1991   RE9224

American Academy of Pediatrics

Figure 1–1. Recommendations for preventive pediatric health care. (Committee on Practice and Ambulatory Medicine, American Academy of Pediatrics.)

Table 1–2. Specific goals of selected health maintenance visits.

Initial Office Visit	Two-Month Visit	Fifteen-Month Visit	Five-Year Visit	Fourteen-Year Visit
HISTORY				

1. Pregnancy, delivery, and neonatal history if not previously obtained.
2. Family history if not previously obtained.
3. How are the baby and family adjusting to home?
  a. Comfort level.
  b. Sleep and feeding patterns.
  c. Support systems.
  d. Reactions of siblings.
  e. Elimination patterns.
  f. Is the child disruptive?
	1. Interim history (new problems).
	2. Daily routine.
	3. Feeding schedule.
	4. Care provider.
		1. Interim history.
		2. Care provider.
		3. Assess pace of development.
			1. Is the family ready for the child to go to school?
			2. Be careful to review bowel and bladder control.
			3. Does the child interact easily with others?
			4. Is separation from the parents a problem?
				1. Interim history.
				2. School activities.
				3. Jobs.
				4. Relationships.
				5. Drugs: alcohol, tobacco, marihuana, others.
				6. Sexual activity.
				7. Menstrual history in girls.

DIET				
1. Frequency of feeding. 2. Duration. 3. Specifics of breast feeding. 4. Formula preparation and amount consumed.	1. If mother is breast feeding, is it beneficial to baby and family? 2. Familial pressure to introduce solid foods into diet. 3. Night feedings. 4. Check need for vitamin supplementation.	1. Amount of milk intake. 2. Solids. 3. Variety of foods presented. 4. Check for vitamin supplementation.	1. Review favorite foods. 2. Estimate caloric intake. 3. Will diet change for both mother and child due to child's entry into school?	1. Junk foods. 2. Abnormal dieting or "bulking up."
DEVELOPMENT				
1. Regards face. 2. Smiles. 3. Moves all extremities. 4. Responds to noise. 5. Vocalizes. 6. Lifts head.	1. Smiles spontaneously. 2. Grasps rattle? 3. Follows object trajectory through 180 degrees. 4. Laughs. 5. Lifts head.	1. Drinks from cup. 2. Walks well. 3. Stoops and recovers. 4. Words other than "mama" and "dada." 5. Indicates wants. 6. Tower of Z cubes.	1. Copies a rectangle. 2. Draws a man with 6 identifiable parts. 3. Recognizes 6 colors. 4. Defines opposites. 5. Capable of backward heel-to-toe walk. 6. Knows letters of the alphabet. 7. Knows name, address, phone number. 8. Dresses without supervision.	1. Grades. Be specific. 2. Self-esteem. 3. Depression. 4. Relationships.
SCREENING				
1. Subjective assessment of hearing and vision. 2. Response to noise, light.	1. Same as initial visit. 2. Informal vision screening.	1. Subjective assessment of vision and hearing.	1. Hearing. 2. Vision.	1. Vision screening. 2. Subjective hearing.
PHYSICAL EXAMINTATION: See Table 1–3.				
PROCEDURES				
1. Review newborn screening test. 2. Collect specimens for screening tests if there was early discharge from the nursery.	1. Hemoglobin. 2. Urinalysis.	1. TB testing depending on risk.		

(continued)

Table 1–2. Specific goals of selected health maintenance visits. (continued)

Initial Office Visit	Two-Month Visit	Fifteen-Month Visit	Five-Year Visit	Fourteen-Year Visit
IMMUNIZATIONS				
1. Hepatitis B	1. DTP. 2. OPV. 3. HIB. 4. Hepatitis B.	1. MMR. 2. HIB.	1. DTP. 2. OPV.	1. Td (10 years after last dose).
ANTICIPATORY GUIDANCE				

1. Stress need for car seat if not obtained.
2. Review normal infant behavior patterns.
3. Anticipate adjustment of siblings to new baby if not already addressed.
4. Review symptoms of colic or food intolerance.
5. Give information about appropriate diet for age.
	1. Immunization reactions.
	2. Check family history for immunization prior to OPV.
	3. Infant stimulation.
		1. Immunization reactions.
		2. Accident prevention.
		  a. Car seat.
		  b. Ipecac.
		3. Night bottle.
		4. Toilet training.
		5. Discipline.
			1. Review accident prevention measures.
			2. Anticipate school problems.
				1. Relationships.
				2. Trials of adolescence.
				3. Interacting with parents.
				4. Safe sex.
				5. Sexually transmitted disease.
				6. Car safety.
				7. Drugs.
				8. Sports.
				9. Motorcycle safety helmets.

also affords the examiner a chance to assess parent-child interactions.

Clothing should be removed slowly and gently to avoid chilling or threatening the child. Modesty, whenever a child exhibits it, should be respected, and drapes should be provided. The child should be offered a chaperone whenever a painful or stressful procedure is performed. Both boys and girls should be afforded chaperones. Certainly any examination of an adolescent's genitalia should be done in the presence of a chaperone. The age at which chaperones become important varies with each child. The pediatrician must be sensitive to personal, family, and cultural attitudes as they relate to this process.

The sequence of the examination is important. Those areas in which the child's cooperation is needed should be addressed first. Painful or unpleasant procedures should be postponed until the end of the examination.

Examination tables are convenient, but a parent's lap is a safe haven for a toddler or young child. An adequate examination can be conducted on a "table" formed by the parent's and examiner's legs as they sit facing each other.

B. The Growth Chart: After carefully measuring a child's height, weight, and—in children 2 years of age or younger—head circumference, the examiner can compare a child's growth to normative val-

Table 1–3. Focusing the physical examination during health supervision visits.

Initial Examination	Two-Month Visit	Fifteen-Month Visit	Five-Year Visit	Fourteen-Year Visit
1. Length, weight, OFC 2. Congenital anomalies 3. Birthmarks, rashes 4. Shape of head, fontanelles 5. Red reflex, tear ducts 6. Palate 7. Pulses, color, murmurs 8. Umbilicus 9. Genitalia 10. Neurologic competency 11. Hips	1. Length, weight, OFC 2. Congenital anomalies 3. Shape of head, fontanelles 4. Murmurs, pulses 5. Urinary stream 6. Neurologic maturity	1. Length, weight, OFC 2. Shape of head, hair 3. EOMs, cover test 4. Tympanic membranes 5. Number of teeth 6. Posture, body habitus 7. Hernias 8. Gait 9. Feet	1. Height, weight 2. EOMs, fundi 3. Teeth 4. Coordination movement 5. Interactive skills	1. Length, weight 2. Tanner stage 3. Thyroid 4. Acne 5. Breast development 6. Genitalia (as indicated) 7. Muscular development 8. Neuromuscular assessment

OFC = occipitofront circumference; EOM = extraocular muscles.

ues by plotting the data on a growth chart. Normal growth is one of the most reassuring pieces of information a physician can find. Normal growth suggests the adequacy of genetic material, diet, and environment and at the same time implies the absence of major chronic disease. When a growth record is abnormal, the pattern of abnormality can help the physician establish a differential diagnosis. The approach to a child with failure to thrive can be established by examination of the growth record. A pediatric evaluation simply is not complete if the growth chart is not plotted and reviewed.

Examination of the Newborn

The examination of the newborn is unique in that the examiner must rapidly assess the adequacy of transition from the womb to extrauterine life, discover and evaluate any congenital anomalies, and interact extensively with the family. This process is completed via a series of examinations starting in the delivery room and often culminating with a physical examination of the child in front of the child's parents to demonstrate the child's normality or explain any unusual findings. Although this is usually a joyous occasion, it is also a time of stress and anxiety as the parents grapple with their concerns about the normal development of the child.

Screening & Developmental Testing

The incidence of hypertension in an open pediatric population is not high. The AAP Committee on School Health no longer suggests screening school-age children for hypertension because of the low yield of patients who ultimately require treatment. However, this recommendation is made in a societal setting in which blood pressure readings are routinely determined when a child is examined. Blood pressure determinations during physical examinations should continue to be recorded, and physicians should routinely measure blood pressures in all infants and children for whom they provide care. Similarly, the United States Preventive Services Expert Panel has indicated that mass screenings for scoliosis are neither effective nor indicated. Again, this does not mean that an individual physician should not examine an individual patient in such a manner as to establish the presence or absence of scoliosis.

To assess development properly, the physician must know the level of the child's physiologic maturity. For this reason, the physician must pay careful attention to Tanner sexual staging (see Chapter 4). Similarly, in young children, physical development must be monitored (eg, the time at which teeth appear).

Finally, the only way to assess a child's development is to do developmental testing. Time must be set aside for this testing, and both resources and personnel must be available at all times. The practicing pediatrician soon realizes how essential developmental assessment is to the provision of care. Novices may be overwhelmed by the sophistication and meticulousness this assessment requires. Once practitioners become proficient, however, they realize they have mastered an essential set of techniques that are of great usefulness to physicians and their patients.

REFERENCES

Barness LA: *Manual of Pediatric Physical Diagnosis,* 6th ed. Year Book, 1991.

Bates B: *A Guide to Physical Diagnosis,* 4th ed. Lippincott, 1987.

Committee on Practice and Ambulatory Medicine: *Management of Pediatric Practice.* American Academy of Pediatrics, 1991.

Committee on Psychosocial Aspects of Child and Family Health: *Guidelines for Health Supervision II,* 2nd ed. American Academy of Pediatrics, 1988.

DeGowin El, DeGowin RL: *Bedside Diagnostic Examination,* 5th ed. Macmillan, 1987.

Frankenburg W et al: *Denver Developmental Screening Test Reference Manual,* rev ed. LADOCA Project & Publishing Foundation, 1975.

Green M: *Pediatric Diagnosis,* 5th ed. Saunders, 1992.

Morgan WL, Engel GL: *The Clinical Approach to the Patient.* Saunders, 1969.

Report of the US Preventive Services Task Force: *Guide to Clinical Preventive Services.* Williams & Wilkins, 1989.

Zitelli BJ, Davis HW (editors): *Atlas of Pediatric Physical Diagnosis,* Mosby, 1987.

The Newborn Infant

2

Adam A. Rosenberg, MD, & Elizabeth H. Thilo, MD

Neonatology is a discipline that encompasses all aspects of care for newborn infants. By tradition, the first 28 days of life has been considered the newborn period. Practically, however, neonatal care includes all of the care provided until discharge from the nursery, ranging from a 24-hour stay for term, healthy infants to many months of care for sick, very immature infants. Follow-up care for most newborn infants is usually provided by family physicians and pediatricians. Neonatologists or other physicians skilled in developmental pediatrics, however, may provide special follow-up services for infants discharged from intensive care nurseries. Table 2–1 summarizes the levels of nursery care commonly encountered.

NEONATAL BIRTH WEIGHT & GESTATIONAL AGE DISTRIBUTION

The mortality rates have decreased steadily for infants in all birth weight and gestational age groups. Smaller and more immature infants survive each year with aggressive delivery room management, improved neonatal stabilization, and intensive care technology. Figure 2–1 presents a recent survey of neonatal survival rates by birth weight for infants weighing less than 1500 g at seven neonatal centers in the USA from November 1987 to October 1988. Note that there is an approximately 30% survival rate for infants weighing 600–700 g and that survival rates are over 80% for infants weighing over 1000 g. A few other points should be emphasized. There is no longer a difference between survival rates for term infants who are large for gestational age (LGA) and those who are appropriate for gestational age (AGA). This development is due in large part to better obstetric management of gestational and insulin-dependent diabetic patients. Furthermore, the use of ultrasound allows obstetricians to anticipate delivery of an LGA infant and, if necessary, perform cesarean section, avoiding much of the birth trauma associated with LGA infants in the past. However, the small-for-gestational-age (SGA) infant born very prematurely is not doing very well; that is, mortality rates of these infants are comparable to those of premature babies of the same size. The same cannot be said, of course, for larger and more mature SGA infants, whose survival rate is much better than that of preterm infants of comparable size.

The birth weight and gestational age of all infants must be plotted on some appropriate standard. Birth weight-gestational age distributions vary from one population to the next. Table 2–2 lists some of the factors that affect these distributions. For these reasons, the standards should be prepared from data collected on the local population. When these are not available, any regional standard may be used: The birth weight-gestational age distribution of an infant is simply a screening tool that should always be supplemented by clinical data confirming a tentative diagnosis of intrauterine growth retardation or excessive fetal growth. These clinical data include not only the clinical features of the infant determined during the physical examination but also such factors as the size of each parent and the birth weight-gestational age distribution of infants previously born to the parents.

Table 2–3 lists causes of variations in neonatal size in relation to gestational age. An important distinction to be made, particularly in SGA infants, is whether the growth disorder is symmetric (weight, height, and occipitofrontal circumference [OFC]; ≤ 10%) or asymmetric (sparing of growth in length and OFC). Asymmetric growth retardation implies a problem late in the pregnancy, such as pregnancy-induced hypertension or placental insufficiency of any cause. Symmetric growth retardation implies an event of early pregnancy: chromosomal abnormality, drug or alcohol use, congenital viral infections.

Knowledge of a baby's birth weight in relation to gestational age is also helpful in anticipating neonatal problems. LGA babies are at risk for birth trauma, hypoglycemia, polycythemia, congenital anomalies, cardiomyopathy, hyperbilirubinemia, and hypocalcemia. SGA babies are at risk for fetal distress during labor and delivery, polycythemia, hypoglycemia, and hypocalcemia.

Table 2–1. Levels of nursery care.

Level 1 nurseries:

These nurseries care for infants presumed healthy. In such units, screening and surveillance are primary responsibilities. "Rooming-in" units are encouraged, with emphasis on support of breast feeding and assessment of parenting skills.

Level 2 nurseries:

These nurseries care for infants > 30 weeks of gestation and ≥ 1200 g who require special attention short of the need for circulatory or ventilator support and major surgical procedures. Because they address the greatest diversity of neonatal disorders, these nurseries present perhaps the greatest challenge to health care providers. A high percentage of the problems in such nurseries relates to obstetric complications (eg, birth trauma, fetal distress, obstetric anesthesia).

Level 3 nurseries:

These nurseries are staffed and equipped to care for all newborn infants who are critically ill, regardless of the level of support required. They are regional institutions serving as referral centers for other nurseries and for this reason are often linked with transport services. Optimally, these nurseries should be part of a perinatal center.

Perinatal center:

A perinatal center provides services both to high-risk mothers and to infants requiring level 3 nursery care. Ample data now clearly demonstrate a higher neonatal survival rate for high-risk pregnancies cared for in such centers. The transport of high-risk mothers to perinatal centers is preferred, therefore, to the transport of a critically ill infant following delivery.

American Academy of Pediatrics: *Guidelines for Perinatal Care,* 3rd ed. American Academy of Pediatrics, 1992.

Hack M et al: Very low birth weight outcomes of the National Institute of Child Health and Human Development Neonatal Network. Pediatrics 1991;87:587.

Kempe A et al: Clinical determinants of the racial disparity in very low birth weight. N Engl J Med 1992;327:969.

Miller E et al: Elevated maternal hemoglobin A_{1c} in early pregnancy and major congenital anomalies in infants of diabetic mothers. N Engl J Med 1981;304:1331.

Mills JL et al: Lack of relation of increased malformation

Table 2–2. Factors affecting birth weight–gestational age distributions.

1. Socioeconomic factors that affect nutritional level and access to health care
2. Altitude
3. Incidence of environmental factors that affect birth weight, eg, smoking
4. Racial distribution

rates in infants of diabetic mothers to glycemic control during organogenesis. N Engl J Med 1988;318:671.

Phelps DL et al: 28-day survival rates of 6676 neonates with birth weighs of 1250 grams or less. Pediatrics 1991;87:7.

Sibai B, Anderson G: Pregnancy outcome of intensive therapy in severe hypertension in first trimester. Obstet Gynecol 1986;67:517.

Whyte HE et al: Extreme immaturity: Outcome of 568 pregnancies of 23–26 weeks gestation. Obstet Gynecol 1993; 82:1

EVALUATION OF THE NEWBORN INFANT

HISTORY

Taking the history in newborn medicine involves three key areas: (1) the medical history of the mother and father, including a relevant genetic history; (2) the previous obstetric history of the mother; and (3) the history of the current pregnancy.

Illnesses with genetic implications and all chronic illness in the mother known to effect intrauterine development are of particular importance. The past and current obstetric history must be as detailed as possible, including documentation of such procedures as

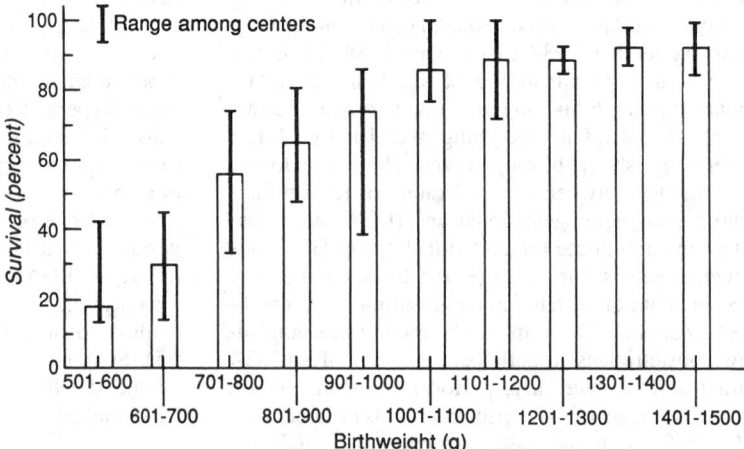

Figure 2–1. Percent survival by 100 g birth weight groups. (Reproduced, with permission, from Hack M et al: Very low birth weight outcomes of the National Institute of Child Health and Human Development Neonatal Network. Pediatrics 1991;87:587.)

Table 2–3. Etiology of variations in neonatal size in relation to gestational age.

Infants large for gestational age
Infant of a diabetic mother
Infants small for gestational age
Asymmetric
Placental insufficiency due to pregnancy-induced hypertension or other maternal vascular disease
Maternal age > 35
Poor weight gain during pregnancy
Multiple gestation
Symmetric
Maternal drug use
Narcotics
Cocaine
Alcohol
Chromosomal abnormalities
Intrauterine viral infection, eg, cytomegalovirus

ultrasound examinations, amniocentesis, screening tests, and biophysical profiles. The biophysical profile is the prenatal equivalent of an Apgar score, in which five or six indices of fetal well-being are assessed. If chorionic villus biopsy or cordocentesis (umbilical cord blood sampling) has been done, it should be documented together with the information obtained. An unusual dietary history, drug intake, smoking history, and potential exposure to infectious agents associated with congenital infection should be noted, as well as weight gain during pregnancy, the work place of the mother, and exercise level. The social history may assist the clinician in assessing parenting skills and the risks of child abuse. Acute problems in the mother, such as urinary tract infection, pregnancy-induced hypertension, bleeding, fetal distress, and meconium in the amniotic fluid should be noted. Knowledge of duration of ruptured membranes and chorioamnionitis should be obtained. In high-risk groups, the presence of HIV (human immunodeficiency virus) and HBsAg (hepatitis B surface antigen) must be determined.

PHYSICAL EXAMINATION

The extent of the physical examination of a newborn infant depends on the condition of the infant and the environment in which it is being performed. If the pediatrician is in attendance in the delivery room for a normal delivery, a physical examination is largely based upon observation coupled with auscultation of the chest and examination for congenital anomalies. Because the infant is recovering from "birth shock," the examination should not be extensive. The examination should include collecting sufficient information for an Apgar score (see Table 2–4) at 1 and 5 minutes of age. In the case of severely depressed infants, a 10-minute score should also be recorded. Serial Apgar scores provide a form of "bioassay" re-

flecting the severity of intrauterine distress or the quality of the resuscitative efforts made.

The color of the neonate's skin is a very useful indicator. Because there is normally a high blood flow to the skin, any stress that triggers a catecholamine response produces fairly dramatic changes in skin color secondary to changes in the distribution of cardiac output and perfusion of the skin. Cyanosis and pallor are two signs that are evaluated both as an index of oxygenation and as a reflection of changes in skin blood flow. In infants of very low birthweight, tissues are fragile and easily bruised. Thus, bruised areas should be considered an indication of deep tissue bleeding that may involve fairly extensive hemorrhage. The bruising not only produces problems with hyperbilirubinemia over the next few days but also can represent acute, significant blood loss that must be treated with volume expansion.

The skeletal examination immediately after delivery serves two purposes: (1) to detect any obvious congenital anomalies, and (2) to detect signs of birth trauma, particularly in LGA infants or infants in which there has been a prolonged second stage of labor.

The umbilical cord and the placenta should also be examined. The principal feature noted in the cord is the number of vessels. Normally, there are two arteries and one vein. In 1% of deliveries (5–6% of twin deliveries) the cord has only two vessels: an artery and a vein. The latter may be considered a vascular anomaly and, as is the case with other minor anomalies, carries with it a slightly increased risk of associated anomalies. The placenta is usually examined by the physician delivering it. Small placentas are always associated with small infants. The placental examination centers around the identification of membranes and vessels, particularly in multiple ges-

Table 2–4. Infant evaluation at birth (Apgar score).[1,2]

	Score		
	0	1	2
Heart rate	Absent	Slow (< 100)	> 100
Respiratory effort	Absent	Slow, irregular	Good, crying
Muscle tone	Limp	Some flexion	Active motion
Response to catheter in nostril[3]	No response	Grimace	Cough or sneeze
Color	Blue or pale	Body pink; extremities blue	Completely pink

[1]Reproduced, with permission, from Apgar V et al: Evaluation of the newborn infant—second report. JAMA 1958;168:1985. © 1958 American Medical Association.
[2]One minute and 5 minutes after complete birth of infant (disregarding cord and placenta), the following objective signs should be observed and recorded.
[3]Tested after oropharynx is clear.

tations. A single chorion always represents monozygotic twining, whereas a full set of double membranes, amnion and chorion, can be either mono- or dizygotic. The placenta is also examined for the frequency and severity of placental infarcts and for evidence of clot (placental abruption) on the maternal side.

General Examination

Heart rate should range from 120 to 160 (beats/min), and the respiratory rate is 30–60; blood pressure norms are a function of birth weight and gestational age (Figure 2–2). *Note:* an irregularly irregular heart rate, usually due to premature atrial contractions, is a common finding. This irregularity should resolve in the first days of life and is not of pathologic significance.

Plot length, weight, and head circumference on appropriate standards for percentiles.

Gestational Age Estimation

Accurate maternal dates remain the best indicator of gestational age. Other obstetric observations, such as fundal height, auscultation of fetal heartbeat with a stethoscope, and early ultrasound examination, provide supporting information. A postnatal examination (Table 2–5) can also be used, because fetal physical characteristics and neurologic development progress in predictable fashion. Table 2–5 itemizes the physical and neurologic criteria to be examined. The upper panel is the neuromuscular examination assessing primarily muscle tone and strength. The lower panel catalogs a variety of physical characteristics.

Disappearance of the anterior vascular capsule of the lens is also helpful in determining gestational age. At 27–28 weeks of gestation, the lens capsule is covered by vessels; by 34 weeks, this vasculature is completely atrophied.

Skin

Check for bruising, petechiae (common over presenting part), meconium staining, and jaundice. Peripheral cyanosis is commonly present when the extremities are cool or the infant is polycythemic. Generalized cyanosis merits immediate evaluation. Pallor may be due to acute or chronic blood loss. Plethora suggests polycythemia. Note vernix caseosa (a whitish, greasy material covering the body that decreases as term approaches) and lanugo (the fine hair covering the preterm infant's skin). Dry skin with cracking and peeling of the superficial layers is common in postterm infants. Edema may be generalized (hydrops) or localized (eg, on dorsum of the foot in Turner's syndrome). Check for birthmarks, eg, capillary hemangiomas (lower occiput, eyelids, forehead) and mongolian spot (bluish-black pigmentation over the back and buttocks). Milia (small white papules over the nose and face) are due to blocked ducts of sebaceous glands. Miliaria (pustules without a red base) are due to blocked ducts of sweat glands. Erythema toxicum is characterized by erythematous raised areas with pustules filled with eosinophils. Pustular melanosis is a pustular rash that leaves a pigmented base when the pustule ruptures. The pustules are noninfectious but contain neutrophils. Jaundice presenting in the first 24 hours of life should be considered abnormal.

Head

Check for cephalhematoma (contained within suture lines) and caput succedaneum (edema over presenting part that crosses suture lines). Subgaleal (beneath the scalp) hemorrhages are seen infrequently but are not limited by sutures, so that blood loss can be extensive. Skull fractures may be linear or depressed and may be associated with a cephalhematoma. Check size and presence of fontanelles. The anterior fontanelle varies from 1 to 4 cm in any direction, whereas the posterior fontanelle should be less than 1 cm. The third fontanelle is a bony defect along the sagittal suture in the parietal bones. Sutures

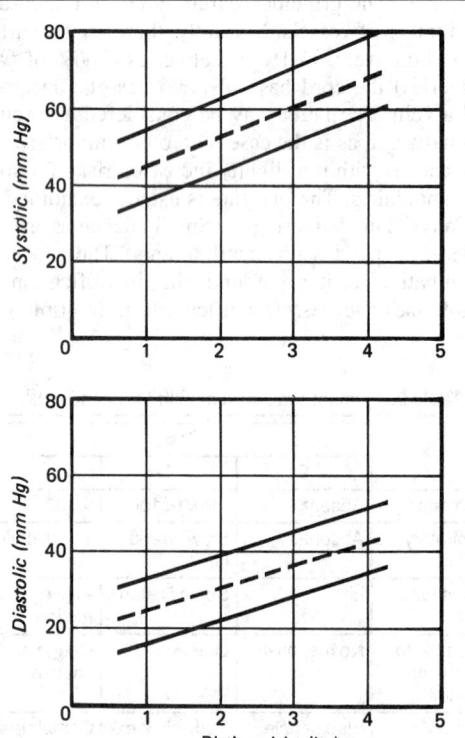

Figure 2–2. Aortic blood pressure during the first 12 hours of life in infants with birth weights of 610–4220 g. (Reproduced, with permission, from Versmold HT et al: Aortic blood pressure during the first 12 hours of life in infants with birth weight 610 to 4,220 g. Pediatrics 1981;67:607.)

Table 2–5. New Ballard Score for assessment of fetal maturation of newly born infants.[1,2]

Neuromuscular Maturity

Neuromuscular Maturity Sign	Score							Record Score Here
	−1	0	1	2	3	4	5	
Posture								
Square Window (wrist)	>90°	90°	60°	45°	30°	0°		
Arm Recoil	180°	180°	140°-180°	110°-140°	90°-110°	<90°		
Popliteal Angle		160°	140°	120°	100°	90°	<90°	
Scarf Sign								
Heal to Ear								

Total Neuromuscular Maturity Score

Physical Maturity

Physical Maturity Sign	Score							Record Score Here
	−1	0	1	2	3	4	5	
Skin	sticky, friable, transparent	gelatinous, red, translucent	smooth, pink, visible veins	superficial peeling &/or rash, few veins	cracking, pale areas rare veins	parchment, deep cracking; no vessels	leathery, cracked, wrinkled	
Lanugo	none	sparse	abundant	thinning	bald areas	mostly bald		
Plantar Surface	heel-toe 40–50 mm: −1 <40 mm: −2	>50 mm no crease	faint red marks	anterior transverse crease only	creases ant. 2/3	creases over entire sole		
Breast	imperceptible	barely perceptible	flat areola no bud	stippled areola 1–2 mm bud	raised areola 3–4 mm bud	full areola 5–10 mm bud		
Eye/Ear	lids fused loosely: −1 tightly: −2	lids open pinna flat stays folded	sl. curved pinna; soft; slow recoil	well-curved pinna; soft but ready recoil	formed & firm instant recoil	thick cartilage; ear stiff		
Genitals (male)	scrotum flat, smooth	scrotum empty faint rugae	testes in upper canal rare rugae	testes descending few rugae	testes down good rugae	testes pendulous deep rugae		
Genitals (female)	clitoris prominent & labia flat	prominent clitoris & small labia minora	prominent clitoris & enlarging minora	majora & minora equally prominent	majora large minora small	majora cover clitoris & minora		

Total Physical Maturity Score

Maturity Rating	Score	−10	−5	0	5	10	15	20	25	30	35	40	45	50
	Weeks	20	22	24	26	28	30	32	34	36	38	40	42	44

[1]Reproduced, with permission, from Ballard JL et al: New Ballard Score, expanded to include extremely premature infants. J Pediatr 1991;119:417.
[2]See text for a description of the clinical gestational age examination.

should be freely mobile. Craniosynostosis is a prematurely fused suture.

Face

Odd facies may be associated with a specific syndrome. Bruising from birth trauma (especially with face presentation) and forceps marks should be identified. Facial nerve palsy is observed when the infant cries; the unaffected side of the mouth moves normally, giving a distorted facial grimace. Face presentations may have considerable soft tissue swelling around the nose and mouth, causing transient airway obstruction.

Eyes

Subconjunctival hemorrhages are seen frequently as a result of the birth process. Extraocular movements should be assessed. Occasional uncoordinated eye movements are common, but persistent irregular movements are abnormal. The iris should be inspected for abnormalities such as Brushfield's spots (trisomy 21) and colobomas. Examine for the red reflex of the retina. Leukocoria can be caused by glaucoma (cloudy cornea), cataract, or tumor (retinoblastoma). Infants at risk for chorioretinitis (congenital viral infection) should have the retina examined while the pupil is dilated.

Nose

Examine size and shape. In utero compression can cause deformities. Babies are obligate nose breathers; any nasal obstruction (eg, bilateral choanal atresia) can cause respiratory distress. Unilateral choanal atresia can be checked for by occluding each naris. Purulent nasal discharge suggests congenital syphilis.

Ears

Malformed or malpositioned (low-set or posteriorly rotated) ears are often associated with other congenital anomalies. The tympanic membranes should be visualized.

Mouth

Epithelial (Ebstein's) pearls are retention cysts along the gum margins and at the junction of hard and soft palates. Natal teeth may be present and need to be removed to avoid the risk of aspiration. Check integrity and shape of the palate; rule out cleft lip and palate. Small mandibles may be seen with Pierre Robin syndrome. This feature can result in respiratory difficulty as the tongue occludes the airway. A prominent tongue can be seen in trisomy 21 and Beckwith-Wiedemann syndrome. Excessive drooling suggests esophageal atresia.

Neck

Webbing is seen in Turner's syndrome. Sinus tracts may be seen as remnants of branchial clefts. Check for masses: midline (thyroid), anterior to the sternocleidomastoids (branchial cleft cysts), within the sternocleidomastoid (hematoma, torticollis), and posterior to the sternocleidomastoid (cystic hygroma).

Chest & Lungs

Check for fractured clavicles (crepitus, bruising). Increased anteroposterior diameter (barrel chest) can be seen with aspiration syndromes. Check air entry bilaterally. Diminished breath sounds suggest pneumothorax or a space-occupying lesion (eg, diaphragmatic hernia). Check the position of the mediastinum. A shift is seen with pneumothorax (tension) or with a space-occupying lesion. With pneumomediastinum, heart sounds are usually muffled. Expiratory grunting and decreased air entry are seen with hyaline membrane disease. Rales are not diagnostic of disease.

Heart

Examination of the heart is described in detail in Chapter 21. *Note:* murmurs are most often benign and are not necessarily present in serious congenital heart disease in the newborn. The two most common presentations of heart disease in the newborn are cyanosis and congestive heart failure with abnormalities of pulses. In hypoplastic left heart and critical aortic stenosis, pulses are diminished throughout. In coarctation, pulses are diminished in the lower extremities.

Abdomen

Check for softness, absence of distention, and good bowel sounds. Palpate for kidneys—most abdominal masses in the newborn are associated with the kidneys (multicystic-dysplastic, hydronephrosis, etc). When the abdomen is relaxed, normal-sized kidneys can be appreciated. A markedly scaphoid abdomen plus respiratory distress suggests diaphragmatic hernia. Absence of abdominal musculature (prune-belly) may occur in association with renal abnormalities. Check the size of the liver and spleen. The outline of a distended bladder may be seen and palpated above the symphysis pubica.

Genitalia & Anus

Male and female genitals show characteristics according to gestational age (Table 2–5). In the female, an imperforate hymen may be visible. During the first few days a whitish discharge with or without blood is normal. Rule out ambiguous genitals and abnormal anal openings or fissures. Check patency and location of anus.

Skeleton

Check for obvious anomalies, eg, absence of a bone, clubfoot, and fusion or webbing of digits. Check for extra digits. Examine for hip dislocation by attempting to dislocate the femur posteriorly and then abducting the legs to relocate the femur. Examine for extremity fractures and for palsies (especially brachial plexus injuries). Rule out myelomeningoceles and other spinal deformities (eg, scoliosis). Arthrogryposis (limited joint movement) is seen with in utero limitation of movement due to lack of amniotic fluid or from a congenital muscle disease.

Neurologic Examination

Observe resting tone (normal, term newborns should exhibit flexion of the upper and lower extremities) and spontaneous movements. Look for asymmetry of movements. Extension of extremities should result in spontaneous recoil to the flexed position. Assess character of cry; a high-pitched cry may be indicative of disease of the central nervous system (eg, hemorrhage). Hypotonia and a weak cry are indicative of systemic disease or a congenital muscle disorder. Check for newborn reflexes:

(1) **Rooting reflex**—Head turns to the side of a facial stimulus.
(2) **Sucking reflex.**
(3) **Traction response**—Infant is pulled by the arms to sitting. Initially the head lags, then with active flexion comes to midline for a few seconds before falling forward.
(4) **Palmar grasp.**
(5) **Deep tendon reflexes.**
(6) **Placing**—Rub the dorsum of one foot on the underside of a surface. Then, the infant will flex the knee and bring the foot up.
(7) **Moro (startle) reflex**—Hold the infant, and support the head. Allow the head to drop 1–2 cm suddenly. The arms will abduct at the shoulder and extend at the elbow. Adduction will follow. The hands show a prominent spreading or extension of the fingers. *Note:* Several beats of ankle clonus and an upgoing Babinski reflex are normal.

American Academy of Pediatrics: Guidelines for Perinatal Care, 3rd ed. American Academy of Pediatrics, 1992.
Ballard JL et al: New Ballard score, expanded to include extremely premature infants. J Pediatr 1991;119:417.

CARE OF THE NORMAL NEWBORN

CARE IMMEDIATELY AFTER DELIVERY

Gently suction the oropharynx. Obtain Apgar scores. Support body temperature by drying the skin, then swaddle or place the infant beneath a radiant heat source. If polyhydramnios is present at delivery or if excessive oral secretions are noted, pass a soft catheter into the stomach to rule out esophageal atre-

sia. Routine eye prophylaxis must be done as defined by local health codes (eg, silver nitrate, 1%, or erythromycin ointment) to prevent gonorrheal conjunctivitis. Place identification-bands, and obtain footprint.

CORD BLOOD

Cord blood is used for blood typing, Coombs testing, and serology. Another tube is saved. Cord blood is also useful for other tests, eg, electrolytes, glucose, total protein, and toxicology screen. Blood from doubly clamped cord can also be used in testing for pH, base deficit, and lactate concentrations, if needed.

CARE IN TRANSITIONAL NURSERY

Check temperature stabilization. Give vitamin K, 1 mg intramuscularly, to prevent hemorrhagic disease of the newborn. Review pertinent history. Calculate birth weight and gestational age to assess risk for certain problems, eg, hypoglycemia. Indications that the baby is ready for feeding include the following: (1) alertness and vigor, (2) absence of abdominal distention, (3) good bowel sounds, and (4) normal hunger cry. All of these usually occur 2–6 hours after birth, but fetal distress or traumatic delivery may prolong this period. Check that all neonatal screening tests are completed.

CONTINUED CARE IN LEVEL ONE

The primary responsibilities of the Level 1 nursery are care of the well infant, enhancing successful mother-infant bonding, feeding, and teaching the techniques of newborn care. However, surveillance is a key function of the staff; they must be alert for signs and symptoms of illness.

Admission

The prenatal history and immediate postnatal events should be reviewed so that as many problems as possible are anticipated. The determination of birth weight for gestational age is very helpful in this regard. The baby's initial physical examination should be performed within the first 12 hours of life.

Temperature Control

After delivery, body temperature may be labile until the infant has stabilized. Cooling should be avoided, because it can delay normal cardiovascular adjustments and predispose the infant to persistent pulmonary hypertension. Drying the skin is absolutely essential, and radiant heating devices are excellent adjuncts, allowing both heating of the infant and adequate observation.

Observation

The infant should be observed for signs of illness, including temperature instability, change in activity, refusal to feed, pallor, cyanosis, jaundice, tachypnea and respiratory distress, delayed (beyond 24 hours) passage of first stool or void, and bilious vomiting.

Screening Laboratory

Infants born to mothers with type O or Rh-negative blood should have a blood type and direct and indirect Coombs tests performed on cord blood. The indirect Coombs test is particularly important in the diagnosis of ABO incompatibility. Dextrostix or Chemstrip testing should be performed in the infants at risk for hypoglycemia. Values of less than 40 mg/dL should be confirmed with a blood glucose. Hematocrit should be measured at 3–6 hours of age in infants at risk for or with symptoms of polycythemia or anemia. Other tests include the serologic test for syphilis and state-sponsored screens for inborn errors of metabolism. These latter screens include tests for phenylketonuria, maple syrup urine disease, homocystinuria, galactosemia, sickle cell disease, hypothyroidism, and cystic fibrosis. In well newborns, these metabolic screens are performed just prior to discharge after the infant has received milk feedings. In hospitals with early discharge policies (ie, blood obtained at < 24 hours of age), a repeat screening at 1 week of age is required. In infants with prolonged hospital stays, the test should be performed at 1 week of age.

Duration of Stay

The trend over the last several years has been toward shorter hospital stays for well mothers and infants. Criteria for early discharge (< 24 hours) at the University of Colorado are presented in Table 2–6. These criteria have been adapted from those determined by the American Academy of Pediatrics (AAP). Early discharge has proved to be safe in indigent as well as middle-income populations provided that criteria such as those in Table 2–6 are met. Of considerable importance is the fact that most infants who manifest serious cardiorespiratory and infectious problems do so in the first 6 hours of life. Other problems, such as jaundice and difficulties in breast feeding, typically occur later but can usually be handled on an outpatient basis provided that good follow-up has been arranged. The physician must order a more extended period of observation if there is any question about the hospital course and must realize that many infants will require a return appointment or a home health visit a few days after discharge rather than the customary 2 weeks.

Adapting Nursery Care to Meet the Needs of Mother

The life situation of the mother and family is important in their adaptation to the newly born infant.

Table 2–6. Criteria for early discharge.[1]

1. Delivery is vertex, single, sterile, and vaginal.
2. Apgar scores of > 7 at 1 and 5 minutes.
3. Gestational age of 38–42 weeks and weight of 2700–4000 g.
4. Minimum length of stay of 20 hours; a transition to normal thermoregulation in an open crib, completion of 2 successful feedings, evidence of stool and void, completion of neonatal screening for metabolic disease and blood type and Coombs' test (Rh-negative and O mothers) prior to discharge.
5. Vital signs within normal ranges at discharge:
Axillary temperature	36.1–37.2 °C
Heart rate	110–150/min
Respiratory rate	30–60/min
6. A normal neonatal hospital course with no signs or symptoms that require continuous observation:
   Blood dextrose maintained > 45 mg/dL
   Hematocrit 45–65%
   ABO-incompatible infants must be held until 48 hours and released only if they do not require therapy for hemolysis.
7. Physical examination completed by the physician or a trained assistant.
8. Demonstration of mother's understanding and ability to provide adequate care for her newborn; infant care education provided on a one-to-one or classroom basis by the nursing staff prior to discharge.
9. Signed documentation by mother that states her obligation to participate in follow-up care.

[1]Adapted, with permission, from Conrad PD, Wilkening RB, Rosenberg AA: Safety of newborn discharge in less than 36 hours in an indigent population. Am J Dis Child 1989;143:98. Copyright © 1989, American Medical Association.

The caretaker needs to be aware of emotional support available to the mother (spouse or other family members), financial security, maturity of the mother, and past psychiatric, drug, or alcohol problems. To provide appropriate assistance, the nursery staff needs to get to know the family. The family should receive assistance with basic care skills such as feeding, bathing, and cord and circumcision care and information on common newborn problems. One-on-one teaching is the desired means of communication, supplemented on a busy service with videotapes and printed material. If the mother's condition permits, the baby should room-in with the mother as soon as possible. The mother and infant are then supervised by the nursery staff.

Circumcision

Circumcision is an elective procedure to be performed only in healthy, stable infants. The procedure has potential medical benefits, including prevention of phimosis, paraphimosis, and balanoposthitis. In addition, circumcision has been shown to decrease the incidence of cancer of the penis and may result in a decreased incidence of urinary tract infection. The risks of the procedure include local infection, bleeding, removal of too much skin, and urethral injury. Local anesthesia (dorsal penile nerve block) may reduce physiologic and behavioral responses of the infant to the procedure but carries its own inherent risks. Circumcision is contraindicated in infants with genital abnormalities (eg, hypospadias). Appropriate laboratory evaluation should be performed prior to the procedure in infants with a family history of bleeding.

Discharge Preparation

1. Perform a physical examination.
2. Discuss cord and circumcision care.
3. Make sure the mother has mastered the essentials of newborn care.
4. Review signs and symptoms that cause concern:
   a. Increasing jaundice
   b. Poor feeding
   c. Lethargy: increased sleeping
   d. Vomiting
   e. Fever
5. Review feeding instructions.
6. Arrange follow-up.
7. Verify the identification of the infant and the person accepting the infant at discharge.
8. Check on all screening procedures.

American Academy of Pediatrics Task Force on Circumcision: Report of the Task Force on Circumcision. Pediatrics 1989;84:388.

American Academy of Pediatrics, Committee on Genetics: Issues in newborn screening. Pediatrics 1992;89:345.

American Academy of Pediatrics, Section on Endocrinology and Committee on Genetics, and American Thyroid Association Committee on Public Health: Newborn screening for congenital hypothyroidism: Recommended guidelines. Pediatrics 1993;91:1203.

American Academy of Pediatrics: *Guidelines for Perinatal Care,* 3rd ed. American Academy of Pediatrics, 1992.

American Academy of Pediatrics, Committee on Fetus and Newborn: Routine evaluation of blood pressure, hematocrit and glucose in newborns. Pediatrics 1993;92:474.

Conrad PD et al: Safety of newborn discharge in less than 36 hours in an indigent population. Am J Dis Child 1989; 143:98.

Lane PA, Hathaway WE: Vitamin K in infancy. J Pediatr 1985;106:351.

Newborn screening for sickle cell disease and other hemoglobinopathies. Pediatrics 1989;83(Suppl):813.

Pearson HA: Neonatal testing for hemoglobinopathies. Semin Perinatol 1991;15(Suppl 2):9.

Report of the 100th Ross Conference on Pediatric Research: *The Term Newborn Infant: A Current Outlook.* Ross Laboratories, 1991.

Vichinsky E et al: Newborn screening for sickle cell disease: Effect on mortality. Pediatrics 1988;81:749.

Wiswell TE, Roscelli JD: Corroborative evidence for the decreased incidence of urinary tract infections in circumcised male infants. Pediatrics 1986;78:96.

PARENT-INFANT RELATIONSHIP

Interest in parent-infant bonding has grown in the last 20 years in part due to the observation of an excessive incidence of child abuse and nonorganic failure to thrive in infants who experienced a prolonged postdelivery separation from parents. This separation had its origin in the historical approach to neonatal care, which emphasized infant isolation for the prevention of infection. On the basis of this human experience and studies of mother-infant bonding in other species, the pendulum has now shifted to permit liberal nursery-visiting policies.

DEVELOPMENT OF PARENT-INFANT BONDING

The steps in maternal attachment can be outlined as follows: (1) planning the pregnancy, (2) confirming the pregnancy, (3) accepting the pregnancy, (4) feeling fetal movement, (5) accepting the fetus as an individual, (6) experiencing birth, (7) hearing and seeing the baby, (8) touching and holding the baby, and (9) caretaking. Numerous influences can affect this process. The actions and responses of the mother and father are a function of their own genetic endowment, intrafamily relationships, cultural practices, past experiences with this or previous pregnancies, and, most important, the child-rearing practices of his or her own parents. Also critical is the in-hospital experience surrounding the birth—the behavior of doctors and nurses, separation from the baby, and hospital practices. It is particularly important for medical staff to recognize that many different parental approaches to the child are within the realm of good family interaction. Otherwise, needless and unfounded guilt and anxiety may be conveyed to the parents.

The first 1½ hours of life are an important time in the process of mother-infant bonding. The infant is alert and able to follow with the eyes, a response prompting meaningful interaction with mother. The infant's array of sensory and motor abilities evokes responses from the mother and initiates communication that may facilitate attachment and induction of reciprocal actions. Whether a critical time period for these initial interactions exists is not clear, but increased contact over the first 3 postpartum days is associated with improved parenting behavior. For these reasons, labor and delivery should pose as little anxiety to the mother as possible, and parents and baby should have time together immediately after delivery if the baby's medical condition permits. Prophylactic treatment of the eyes for gonococcal ophthalmitis should be withheld until after the initial bonding has taken place. It can be performed safely within 1 hour of birth.

THE SICK INFANT

Mothers with high-risk pregnancies are at increased risk for subsequent parenting problems. The involvement of both obstetrician and pediatrician alike before the child's birth enables the family to prepare for anticipated aspects of the baby's care and provides reassurance that the odds are heavily in favor of a live baby who will ultimately be healthy. If the need for neonatal intensive care is anticipated before birth (known congenital anomaly, refractory premature labor), *maternal* transport to the proper facility should be planned. In this way, a mother can be with her baby during critical care. In addition, repeated studies have confirmed better survival rates for high-risk infants whose mothers were transported to perinatal centers for delivery compared to infants transported after birth to neonatal intensive care units. It is also very helpful to allow the parents to tour the unit their baby will occupy before delivery. This practice greatly reduces parental anxiety after the birth.

The single basic principle in dealing with parents of a sick infant is to provide essential information clearly and accurately to both parents, preferably when they are together. Survival rates have improved, especially for premature babies; most do well. In most circumstances, one can be reasonably positive about the outcome. There is also no reason to emphasize problems that might occur in the future or to deal with individual worries of the physician. Questions, if asked, need to be answered honestly, but the tendency to overestimate the complications and handicaps should be avoided.

Before the parents' initial visit to the unit, a physician or nurse should describe what the baby and the equipment look like. When they arrive in the nursery, these details can again be reviewed. If the baby must be moved to another hospital, the mother should be given time to see and touch her infant before the transfer. The father should be encouraged to meet the baby at the receiving hospital so that he can become comfortable with the intensive care unit. He can serve as a link between baby and mother, providing information and photographs.

As a baby's course proceeds, the nursery staff can help the parents become comfortable with their infant. It is also important for the staff to discuss among themselves any problems that parents may be having and to keep a record of visits and telephone calls. This approach allows early intervention in dealing with potential problems.

CONGENITAL MALFORMATIONS

The birth of an infant with a congenital malformation is another situation in which staff support is essential. Parental reactions to the birth of a malformed infant follow a predictable course. For most parents, initial shock and denial are followed by a period of sadness and anger, gradual adaptation, and, finally, an increased satisfaction with and ability to care for the baby. The parents must be allowed to pass through these stages and, in effect, mourn the loss of the anticipated normal child. Again, information, including the prognosis for the particular problem, must be provided clearly and accurately to both parents in words they can understand, and with compassion.

DEATH OF AN INFANT

A stillbirth or the death of an infant is a highly stressful family event; there is a significant incidence of psychiatric disorders within 2 years of the death of a neonate. One of the major predispositions is a breakdown of communication between parents. The health care staff needs to encourage the parents to talk with each other, discuss their feelings, and display emotion. The staff should talk with the parents at the time of death and then several months later review the findings of the autopsy, answer questions, and see how the family is doing.

Committee on Bioethics, American Academy of Pediatrics: Treatment of critically ill newborns. Pediatrics 1983; 72:565.

Infant Bioethics Task Force and Consultants, American Academy of Pediatrics: Guidelines for infant bioethics committees. Pediatrics 1984;74:306.

Klaus MN, Kennell JH: Care of the parents. In: *Care of the High-Risk Neonate*, 4th ed. Klaus MN, Fanaroff AA (editors). Saunders, 1993.

Klein M et al: Low birth weight and the battered child syndrome. Am J Dis Child 1971;122:15.

Mahowald MB: Baby Doe committees: A critical evaluation. Clin Perinatol 1988;15:789.

Nance S: *Premature Babies: A Handbook for Parents.* Priam Books, 1982.

FEEDING OF THE NEWBORN INFANT

WHAT, WHEN, & HOW MUCH TO FEED

The healthy, term infant should be allowed to feed every 2–5 hours on demand. The first feeding usually occurs at 2–6 hours of life. Breast-feeding can start as early as in the delivery room. Although there is a trend toward earlier institution of feedings, evidence that the infant is prepared for feedings should always be present—soft, nondistended abdomen, good bowel sounds, and a strong, rhythmic suck. Breast milk or formula (20 kcal/oz) can be given. Generally, the volume increases from 0.5–1 ounce per feeding initially up to above 1.5–2 ounces per feeding on day 3. By day 3, the average term newborn takes in about 100 mL/kg/d of milk.

METHODS OF FEEDING

Bottle Feeding

Most commercial bottles and nipples are satisfactory. The preterm infant usually requires a softer nipple with a larger hole.

Breast Feeding

Although a wide range of infant formulas satisfy the nutritional needs of most neonates, breast milk is the standard on which formulas are based. The distribution of calories in human milk is 7% protein, 55% fat, and 38% carbohydrate. The ratio of whey to casein is 60:40. This allows ease of protein digestion, while fat digestion is aided by lipase in the milk. Despite low levels of several vitamins and minerals, bioavailability is high. Infants of mothers who are strict vegetarians should receive supplemental iron, folate, and vitamin B_{12}. Along with nutritional features, other advantages of breast milk include the following: (1) the presence of host resistance factors, including IgA and cellular components thought to decrease the incidence of upper respiratory and gastrointestinal infections in infancy; (2) the possibility that breast feeding may decrease the frequency and severity of childhood eczema and asthma; and (3) promotion of mother-infant bonding.

The nursery staff must be cognizant of problems associated with breast feeding and be able to provide help and support for mothers in the hospital. Feeding should be fairly frequent in early stages (every 2–3 hours) so that production of milk is stimulated. Initially, nursing time is limited to 5 minutes on each side, then increased to 10 minutes on each side. Care of the nipples should also be reviewed in hospital.

Gavage Feeding

Intermittent gavage feeding can be used for infants with a weak suck and swallow or for infants who tire easily, including preterm infants and those with medical conditions (eg, respiratory distress or congenital heart disease) precluding nipple feedings. An orogastric tube can be inserted for each feeding, or a soft, indwelling orogastric or nasogastric tube can be used. The position of the tube in the stomach should be checked prior to each feeding. The infant should be fed every 2–3 hours, depending on the age and size of patient. Generally, infants weighing less than 1200 g require 2-hour feedings, whereas larger infants are fed at 3-hour intervals. Feedings are started at 10–25% of the child's nutritional needs and advanced to full requirements (100–120 kcal/kg/d) over 3–7 days. The more rapid advancement is used in infants weighing more than 1500 g and the slowest in infants weighing less than 1000 g.

Gastrostomy

Gastrostomy feedings are indicated for infants requiring indefinite tube feedings (eg, those with neurologic disease) and for those with certain surgical conditions (eg, some cases of esophageal atresia).

Parenteral Alimentation

Nutrition can effectively be provided with hyperalimentation solutions given either through peripheral or central venous lines. Table 2–7 illustrates the use of hyperalimentation in newborns. Parenteral nutrition is indicated for infants with gastrointestinal anomalies after surgical correction, for preterm infants with necrotizing enterocolitis and other forms of feeding intolerance, and for infants too sick for any reason to tolerate enteral feedings. Central hyperalimentation has now been facilitated by Silastic lines that can be placed in the nursery under local anesthesia percutaneously or through a basilic vein cutdown.

Committee on Nutrition, American Academy of Pediatrics: Nutritional needs of low birthweight infants. Pediatrics 1985;75:976.

Dunn L et al: Beneficial effects of early hypocaloric enteral feeding on neonatal gastrointestinal function: Preliminary report of a randomized trial. J Pediatr 1988;112:622.

Gilhooly J et al: Central venous silicone elastomer catheter placement by basilic vein cutdown in neonates. Pediatrics 1986;78:636.

Greene HL et al: Guidelines for the use of vitamins, trace elements, calcium, magnesium and phosphorus in infants and children receiving total parenteral nutrition. Am J Clin Nutr 1988;48:1324.

Hay WW Jr (editor): *Neonatal Nutrition and Metabolism.* Mosby, 1991.

Heird WC, Kashyap S, Gomez MR: Parenteral alimentation of the neonate. Semin Perinatol 1991;15:493.

Lawrence R: Breastfeeding. Clin Perinatol 1987;14:1.

Tsang RC et al (editors): *Nutritional Needs of the Preterm Infant.* Williams & Wilkins, 1993.

Table 2–7. Use of parenteral alimentation solutions.

	Volume (mL/kg/d)	Carbohydrate (g/dL)	Protein (g/kg)	Lipid (g/kg)	Calories (kcal/kg)
Peripheral: Short-term (7–10 days)					
Starting solution	100–150	$D_{10}W$	1	1	46–64
Target solution	150	$D_{12.5}W$	2.5	3	102
Central: Long-term (> 10 days)					
Starting solution	100–150	$D_{10}W$	1	1	46–64
Target solution	130	$D_{20}W$	3–3.5	3	123

Notes:
1. Protein calories should be no more than 10% of total calories.
2. Advance dextrose in central hyperalimentation as tolerated by 2.5% per day as long as blood glucose remains normal.
3. Advance lipids by 0.5 g/kg/d as long as triglycerides are normal.
4. Total water should be 100–150 mL/kg/d, depending on the child's fluid tolerance.

Monitoring:
1. Chemstrips or blood glucose two or three times a day when changing dextrose concentration, then daily.
2. Electrolytes daily, then twice a week when the child is receiving a stable solution.
3. Weekly BUN and serum creatinine; total protein and serum albumin; serum calcium, phosphate, magnesium, direct bilirubin, and alkaline phosphatase; and CBC with platelet counts.

NEONATAL INTENSIVE CARE

GENERAL APPROACH

Neonatal intensive care should always have an anticipatory component; ie, obstetricians managing high-risk pregnancies should anticipate delivery as often as possible and discuss specific features of the pregnancy likely to affect the infant immediately after birth. In this way, the course of the labor and the condition of the infant during delivery are known to the baby's caregiver. A pediatrician or neonatologist should be in attendance at high-risk deliveries to provide prompt resuscitation of the infant, when needed. Furthermore, the pediatrician can request that blood tests be made on cord blood obtained at delivery, as appropriate.

TRANSPORTATION

Whenever possible, high-risk mothers should be delivered at perinatal centers so that transport of the infant after delivery can be avoided. In such circumstances, the infant is simply moved from the delivery room to the level 2 or 3 nursery. The transport unit should be easily movable and be equipped to provide ventilatory assistance and oxygen therapy to the infant and to maintain body temperature. In transports from one hospital to another, equipment for intravenous infusions should be available, together with appropriate solutions to support circulating blood volume and extracellular fluid volume. Equipment should be on hand to monitor the infant (heart rate, respirations, blood pressure, oxygen saturation, and transcutaneous PO_2). All emergency equipment necessary to resuscitate an infant should be available. The infant should be stabilized prior to transport.

PERINATAL RESUSCITATION

Perinatal resuscitation involves the steps taken by the obstetrician during labor and delivery to support the infant, as well as the traditional resuscitative steps taken by the pediatrician after delivery of the infant. Intrapartum steps to support the infant include the following: maintaining maternal blood pressure with volume expanders if needed, administering maternal oxygen therapy, positioning the mother to improve placental perfusion, readjusting oxytocin infusions if appropriate, minimizing trauma to the infant (particularly important in infants of very low birth weight), suctioning the nasopharynx if meconium is present in amniotic fluid, obtaining all necessary cord blood samples, and completing an examination of the placenta.

Steps taken by the pediatrician or neonatologist center around support of the following physiologic areas: maintenance of perfusion, maintenance of effective ventilation, temperature support, and hydration and glucose regulation. These are generally accomplished as discussed in the following paragraphs.

Resuscitation of the Newborn Infant

A number of conditions of pregnancy, labor, and delivery place the infant at risk for birth asphyxia: (1) maternal diseases such as diabetes, pregnancy-induced hypertension, heart and renal disease, and collagen-vascular disease; (2) fetal conditions such as prematurity, multiple births, growth retardation, and fetal anomalies; and (3) labor and delivery conditions, including fetal distress with or without meconium in the amniotic fluid and administration of anesthetics and narcotic analgesics.

Physiology of Birth Asphyxia

Birth asphyxia can be the result of several mechanisms: (1) acute interruption of umbilical blood flow (eg, prolapsed cord with cord compression), (2) premature placental separation, (3) maternal hypotension or hypoxia, (4) chronic placental insufficiency, and (5) failure to execute a proper newborn resuscitation.

The neonatal response to asphyxia follows a predictable pattern that has been demonstrated in a variety of species (Figure 2–3). The initial response to hypoxia is an increase in frequency of respiration and a rise in heart rate and blood pressure. Respirations then cease (primary apnea) as heart rate and blood

pressure begin to fall. This initial period of apnea lasts 30–60 seconds. Gasping respirations (3–6/min) then begin, while heart rate and blood pressure continue to decline. Secondary or terminal apnea then ensues, with further decline in heart rate and blood pressure. The longer the duration of secondary apnea, the greater the risk for hypoxic organ injury. A cardinal feature of the defense against hypoxia is the sacrifice, ie, underperfusion, of certain tissue beds (eg, skin, muscle, and gastrointestinal tract), which allows the perfusion of core organs (ie, heart and brain) to be maintained.

The response to resuscitation also follows a predictable pattern. During the period of primary apnea, almost any physical or chemical stimulus causes the baby to initiate respirations. Infants in the stage of secondary apnea require positive pressure ventilation. The first sign of recovery is an increase in heart rate, followed by an increase in blood pressure with improved perfusion. The time period required for rhythmic, spontaneous respirations to occur is related to the duration of the secondary apnea. As a rough rule, for each 1 minute past the last gasp, 2 minutes of positive pressure breathing are required before gasping begins, and 4 minutes are required to reach rhythmic breathing. However, these time periods can vary, depending on the degree and duration of intrauterine asphyxia. Not until sometime later do spinal and corneal reflexes return. Muscle tone gradually improves over the course of several hours.

Delivery Room Management

When asphyxia is anticipated, a resuscitation team of two persons, one to manage the airway and one to monitor heartbeat and provide assistance, should be present. The necessary equipment and drugs are listed in Table 2–8.

A. Steps in the Resuscitation: (Figure 2–4.)

1. Dry the infant well, and place the baby under the radiant heat source.

2. Gently apply suction to the oropharynx and nose.

3. Quickly assess the infant's condition. The best criteria are the infant's respiratory effort (apneic, gasping, regular) and heart rate (> 100 or < 100). A depressed heart rate indicative of hypoxic myocardial depression is the single most reliable indicator of the need for resuscitation.

4. Generally, infants with heart rates over 100 beats/min require no further intervention. Infants with heart rates less than 100/min and apnea or irregular respiratory efforts should be vigorously stimulated. The baby's back should be rubbed with a towel while oxygen is blown over the baby's face.

5. If the baby fails to respond rapidly to tactile stimulation, apply bag and mask ventilation, using a soft mask that seals well around the mouth and nose. For the initial inflations, pressures of 30–40 cm H_2O may be necessary to overcome surface-active forces

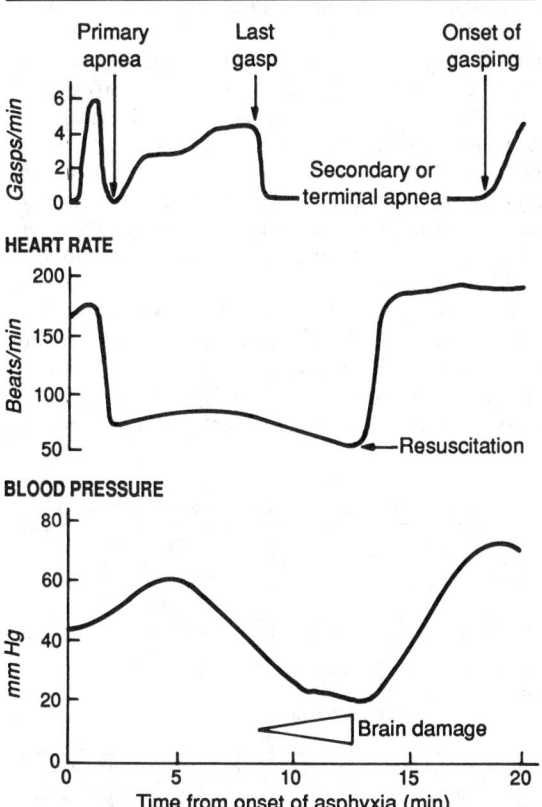

Figure 2–3. Schematic depiction of changes in rhesus monkeys during asphyxia and on resuscitation by positive pressure ventilation. (Adapted and reproduced, with permission, from Dawes GS: *Fetal and Neonatal Physiology.* Year Book, 1968.)

Table 2–8. Equipment for neonatal resuscitation.[1]

Clinical Needs	Equipment
Thermoregulation	Radiant heat source with platform, mattress covered with warm sterile blankets, servo control heating, temperature probe.
Airway management	**Suction:** Bulb suction, DeLee suction apparatus, wall vaccum suction with sterile catheters. **Ventilation:** Manual infant resuscitation bag connected to pressure manometer capable of delivering 100% oxygen, appropriate masks for term and preterm infants. **Intubation:** Neonatal laryngoscope with No. 0 and No. 1 blades; endotracheal tubes (2.5, 3.0, 3.5 mm OD with stylet).
Gastric decompression	Nasogastric tubes: 5F and 8F.
Administration of drugs and volume replacement	Sterile umbilical catheterization tray, umbilical catheters (3.5F and 5F), volume expanders (Ringer's lactate, 5% albumin), drug box with appropriate neonatal vials and dilutions, sterile syringes, and needles.
Transport	Warmed transport Isolette with oxygen source.

[1]Modified, with permission, from Rosenberg AA: Neonatal adaptation. In: *Obstetrics: Normal and Problem Pregnancies.* Gabbe SG, Niebyl JR, Simpson JL (editors). Churchill Livingstone, 1986.

in the lungs. An inspiratory time of 1–2 seconds may be helpful as well. In the premature infant, even higher pressures (40–60 cm H_2O) may be needed. Adequacy of ventilation is assessed by observing expansion of the infant's chest with bagging and a gradual improvement in color, perfusion, and heart rate. After the first few breaths, attempts should be made to lower the peak pressure. Rate of bagging should not exceed 40–60 breaths per minute.

6. Most neonates can be effectively resuscitated with a bag and mask. However, if the infant does not respond favorably in 30–40 seconds, the physician must proceed to intubation:

a. Make sure that the head is stable with the nose in the sniffing position (pointing straight upward).

b. Insert the laryngoscope blade, and sweep the tongue to the left.

c. Advance the blade to the base of the tongue, and identify the epiglottis.

d. Pick up the endotracheal tube with the right hand.

e. Slide the laryngoscope anterior to the epiglottis, and gently lift along the angle of the handle of the laryngoscope.

f. Identify the vocal cords.

g. Insert the tube in the right side of the mouth, and visualize the tube passing through the vocal cords.

h. Ventilate as described above.

i. Failure to respond to intubation and ventilation can result from (1) mechanical difficulties (Table 2–9), (2) profound asphyxia with myocardial depression, and (3) inadequate circulating blood volume.

j. Quickly rule out the mechanical causes in Table 2–9. Check to be sure the endotracheal tube passes through the vocal cords. Occlusion of the tube should be suspected when there is resistance to bagging and no chest wall movement. It is very unusual for a neonate to require either cardiac massage or drugs during resuscitation. Almost all newborns respond to ventilation with 100% oxygen.

k. If mechanical causes are ruled out, external cardiac massage should be performed for a heart rate persistently less than 100/min. Compression of 1–1.5 cm should be performed. Ventilation is of primary importance in neonatal resuscitation, and simultaneous delivery of chest compressions and positive-pressure ventilation is likely to decrease the efficiency of ventilation. Therefore, chest compressions should be interspersed with ventilation at a 3:1 ratio (90 compressions and 30 breaths per minute).

l. If drugs are needed (rarely), the drug of choice is 0.1–0.3 mL/kg of epinephrine, 1:10,000 solution (0.01–0.03 mg/kg), through the endotracheal tube or preferably an umbilical venous line. Some children and adults who do not respond to standard doses will respond to 0.2 mg/kg, but the safety and efficacy of such a dose has not been adequately evaluated in the newborn. Sodium bicarbonate, 1–2 meq/kg of the neonatal dilution, can be used for an infant with *documented* metabolic acidosis. If volume loss is suspected, 10 mL/kg of a volume expander (5% albumin, Plasmanate) should be administered through an umbilical venous line.

B. Continued Resuscitative Measures: The appropriateness of continued resuscitative efforts should be reevaluated in an infant who fails to respond to the above efforts. Today, resuscitative efforts are made even in "apparent stillbirths," ie, in-

Table 2–9. Mechanical causes of failed resuscitation.[1]

Etiology	Examples
Equipment failure	Malfunctioning bag; oxygen not connected or running
Endotracheal tube malposition	Esophagus, right main stem bronchus
Occluded endotracheal tube; insufficient inflation pressure to expand lungs	
Space-occupying lesions in the thorax	Pneumothorax, pleural effusions, diaphragmatic hernia
Pulmonary hypoplasia	Extreme prematurity, oligohydramnios

[1]Reproduced, with permission, from Rosenberg AA: Neonatal adaptation. In: *Obstetrics: Normal and Problem Pregnancies.* Gabbe SG, Niebyl JR, Simpson JL (editors). Churchill Livingstone, 1986.

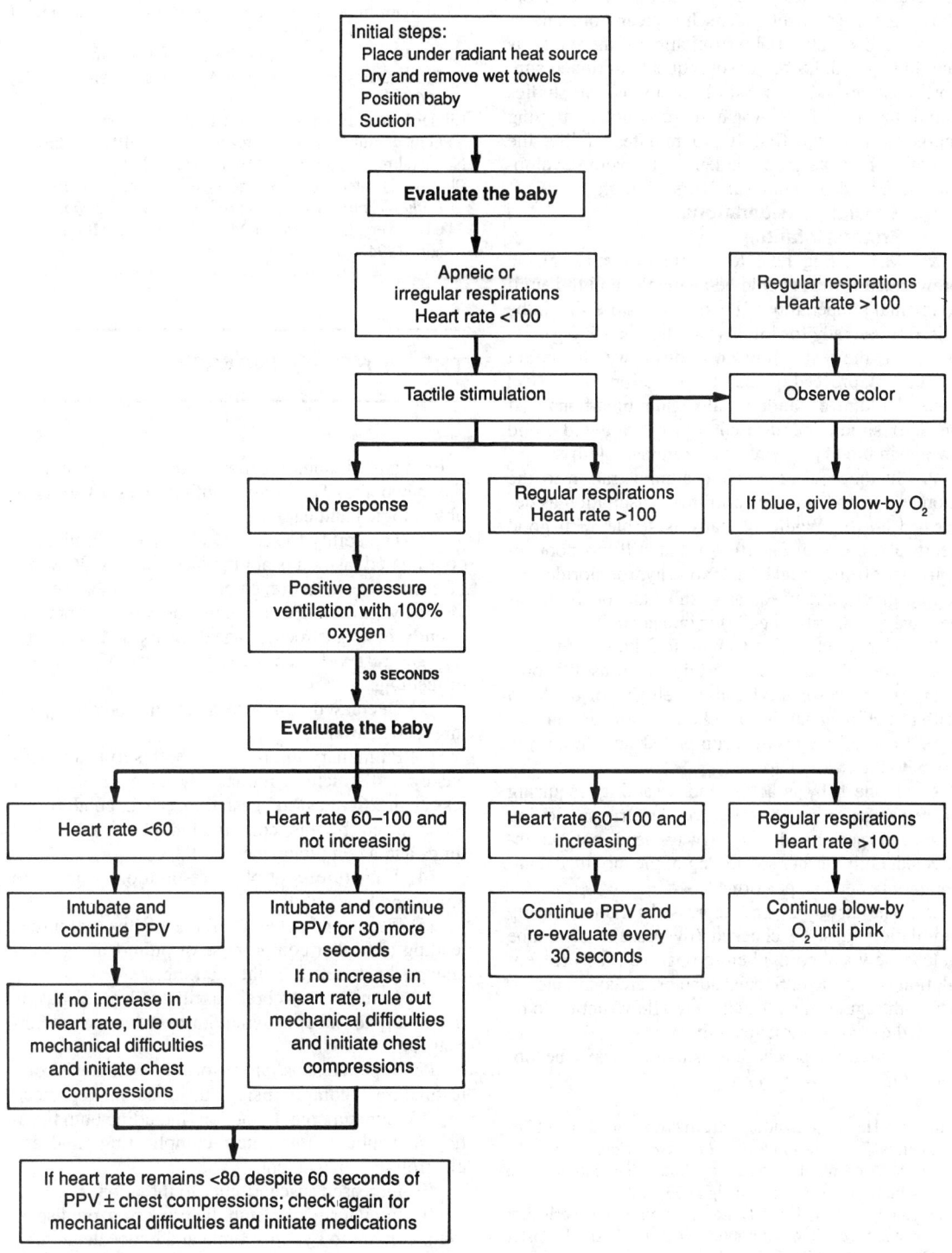

Figure 2–4. Delivery room management.

fants whose Apgar scores at 1 minute are 0–1. Modern resuscitative techniques have led to an increasing survival rate for these infants, with 60% of survivors showing normal development. It is clear from a number of studies that initial resuscitation of these infants should proceed; however, subsequent continued support must depend on serial observations. All studies emphasize that if the Apgar score is not improving markedly over the first 10–15 minutes of life, the mortality rates and the incidence of severe developmental handicap among survivors are high.

C. Special Considerations:

1. Preterm infants–

a. Minimizing heat loss improves survival, so prewarmed towels should be available, and the environmental temperature of the delivery suite should be raised (especially for infants weighing < 1500 g).

b. In the extremely low birth weight infant (< 1000 g), proceed quickly to intubation.

c. Volume expanders and sodium bicarbonate (if needed) should be infused slowly to avoid rapid swings in blood pressure and serum osmolality.

2. In the case of narcotic administration to the mother during labor, perform the resuscitation as described above. When the baby is stable with good heart rate, color, and perfusion but still has poor respiratory effort, a trial of naloxone hydrochloride (0.1 mg/kg given intramuscularly, subcutaneously, intravenously, or intratracheally) is indicated.

3. Meconium-stained amniotic fluid–

a. The obstetrician carefully suctions the oropharynx and nasopharynx after delivery of the head with a suction apparatus attached to wall suction.

b. The delivery is then completed, and the baby is given to the resuscitator.

c. If the baby is active and breathing, requiring no resuscitation, and if effective obstetric suctioning has been performed, the airway need not be inspected. Only further suctioning of the mouth and nasopharynx need be performed.

d. The airway of any depressed infant requiring ventilation must be checked (by passage of a tube below the vocal cords) before positive-pressure ventilation is instituted. Special adapters are available for use with regulated wall suction to allow suction to be applied to the endotracheal tube.

4. Universal precautions should always be observed in the delivery room.

American Heart Association and American Academy of Pediatrics: *Textbook of Neonatal Resuscitation,* 1993.

Apgar V: A proposal for a new method of evaluation of the newborn infant. Anesth Analg 1953;32:260.

Falciglia HS et al: Does DeLee suction at the perineum prevent meconium aspiration syndrome? Am J Obstet Gynecol 1992;167:1243.

Gupta JM et al: The sequence of events in neonatal apnea. Lancet 1967;2:55.

Holtzman RB et al: Perinatal management of meconium staining of the amniotic fluid. Clin Perinatol 1989;16: 825.

Jain L et al: Cardiopulmonary resuscitation of apparently stillborn infants: Survival and long-term outcome. J Pediatr 1991;118:778.

Katz VL, Bowes WA: Meconium aspiration syndrome; reflections on a murky subject. Am J Obstet Gynecol 1992; 166:171.

Linder L et al: Need for endotracheal intubation and suction in meconium stained neonates. J Pediatr 1988;112:613.

Neonatal resuscitation. JAMA 1992;268:2276.

Phibbs RH: Delivery room management. In: *Neonatology: Pathophysiology and Management of the Newborn* (4th ed). Avery GB, Fletcher MA, MacDonald MG. Lippincott, 1994.

THE PRETERM INFANT

Premature infants account for the majority of high-risk newborns. The preterm infant faces a variety of physiologic handicaps:

(1) The ability to suck, swallow, and breathe in a coordinated fashion is not in place until 34–36 weeks of gestation. Therefore, enteral feedings must be provided by gavage. Furthermore, preterm infants frequently have gastroesophageal influx and an immature gag reflex, which increase the risk of aspiration of feedings.

(2) Decreased ability to maintain body temperature (see below).

(3) Pulmonary immaturity—both surfactant deficiency and structural immaturity in those infants of less than 26 weeks of gestation. Their condition is complicated by the combination of noncompliant lungs and a compliant chest wall.

(4) Immature control of respiration, leading to apnea and bradycardia.

(5) Persistent patency of the ductus arteriosus, leading to further compromise of pulmonary gas exchange due to left-to-right shunting.

(6) Immature cerebral vasculature, predisposing the infant to subependymal/intraventricular hemorrhage.

(7) Impaired substrate absorption by the gastrointestinal tract, compromising nutritional management.

(8) Immature renal function (including both filtration and tubular functions), complicating fluid and electrolyte management.

(9) Increased susceptibility to infection.

(10) Immaturity of metabolic processes, predisposing the infant to hypoglycemia and hypocalcemia.

CARE OF THE PRETERM INFANT

Delivery Room

See Perinatal Resuscitation.

Care in the Nursery

Some general principles, eg, thermoregulation, nutrition, and fluid and electrolyte management, are covered here. Other conditions unique to the preterm infant are discussed under specific headings in the chapter.

A. Thermoregulation: Maintaining a stable body temperature is a function of heat production and conservation balanced against heat loss. Heat is produced at the rate of 4.8 kcal/L O_2 consumed. Heat production in response to cold stress can occur through voluntary muscle activity, involuntary muscle activity (shivering), and thermogenesis not due to shivering. Newborns produce heat mainly through the last of these three mechanisms. This metabolic heat production depends on the quantity of brown fat present, which is very limited in the preterm infant. Heat loss to the environment can occur through the following mechanisms: (1) Radiation—transfer of heat from a warmer to cooler object not in contact. (2) Convection—transfer of heat to the surrounding gaseous environment. This is influenced by air movement and temperature. (3) Conduction—transfer of heat to a cooler object in contact. (4) Evaporation—cooling secondary to water loss through the skin.

Heat loss in the preterm newborn is accelerated because of a large ratio of surface area to body mass and reduced insulation of subcutaneous tissue. Furthermore, water loss through the skin is accelerated because of the immaturity of the skin (especially in infants < 27–28 weeks' gestation) and because of the limited ability of skin blood vessels to constrict in response to cold.

For these reasons, the thermal environment of the preterm neonate must be carefully regulated. The infant can be kept warm in an isolette in which the air is heated and convective heat loss minimized. Alternatively, the infant can be kept warm on an open bed with a radiant heat source. Although evaporative and convective heat losses are greater when the radiant warmer is used, this system allows easy access to a critically ill neonate. Ideally, the infant should be kept in a neutral thermal environment (Figure 2–5). The neutral thermal environment allows the infant to maintain a stable core body temperature with a minimum of metabolic heat production through oxygen consumption. In other words, heat losses have been minimized. This is a desirable goal in an infant that may be at risk for hypoxia due to cardiorespiratory disease. Furthermore, the infant is able to utilize calories for growth instead of heat production. The neutral thermal environment for a given infant depends on size, gestational age, and postnatal age. The optimal environment for infants (both dressed and undressed) in isolettes has been determined (Figure

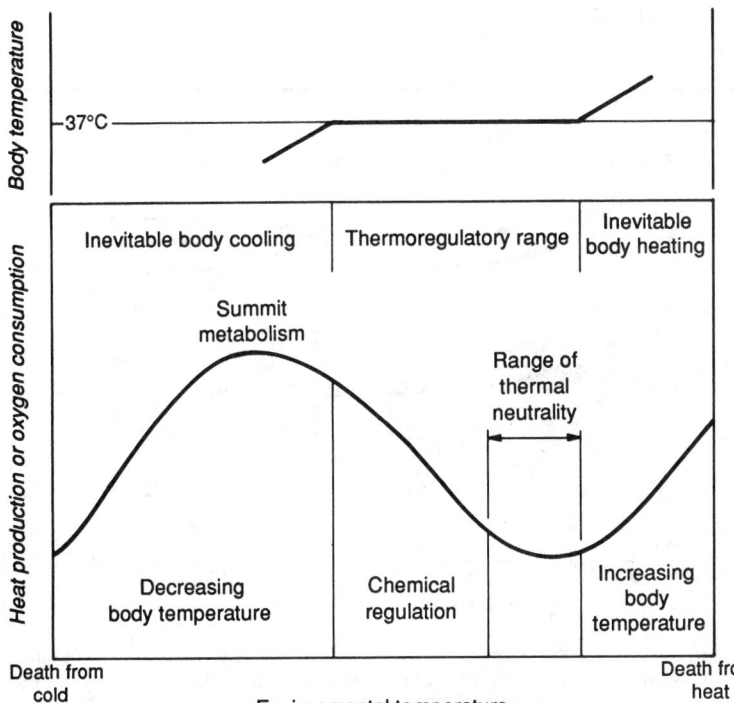

Figure 2–5. Effect of environmental temperature on oxygen consumption and body temperature. (Adapted and reproduced, with permission, from Klaus M, Fanaroff A, Martin RJ: The physical environment. In: *Care of the High-Risk Neonate,* 3rd ed. Klaus MH, Fanaroff AA [editors]. Saunders, 1986.)

2–6). Alternatively (for either isolette or radiant warmer care), the neutral thermal environment can be obtained by maintaining an abdominal skin temperature of 36.5 °C.

Temperature can be regulated in either isolettes or radiant warmers by manual or servo control adjustments. In manual control, skin temperature is regulated by manually adjusting the environmental temperature of an isolette or the heat output from a radiant warmer so that the infant maintains the desired skin temperature. In servo control, the heating equipment is adjusted automatically to maintain the desired skin temperature. The core temperature of the infant can be estimated from axillary temperatures. Although rectal temperatures provide a slightly better estimation of core temperature, they are discouraged because of the risk of rectal perforation. In infants weighing more than 1200 g, skin temperature is less than core temperature; however, in infants of very low birth weight, core temperature is lower than skin temperature and invariably below normal in the first few hours of life. Generally, when infants reach 1800–2000 g, they can maintain temperature while bundled in a bassinet.

B. Monitoring the High-Risk Infant: Care of the high-risk preterm infant requires sophisticated monitoring techniques. At a minimum, equipment to monitor heart rate, respirations, and blood pressure should be available. The ideal monitor has memory capabilities to assess episodes of apnea and bradycardia. Oxygen saturation can be assessed continuously using pulse oximetry. This determination can be correlated with arterial oxygen tension (PaO_2) as needed. Transcutaneous PO_2 and PCO_2 can also be utilized to assess oxygenation and ventilation. Finally, arterial blood gases, electrolytes, glucose, calcium, bilirubin, and other chemistries must be measured on small volumes of blood. Early in the care of a sick preterm infant, the most efficient way to sample blood for tests as well as provide fluids and monitor blood pressure is through an umbilical arterial line. Once the infant is stable and the need for frequent blood samples reduced (usually 4–7 days), the umbilical line should be removed. All indwelling lines are associated with morbidity from thrombosis/embolus, infection, and bleeding.

C. Fluid and Electrolyte Therapy: Fluid requirements in preterm infants are a function of (1) insensible losses (skin and respiratory), (2) urine output, (3) stool output (less than 5% of total), and (4) others, eg, nasogastric losses.

In most circumstances, the majority of the fluid requirement is determined by insensible losses and urine losses. The major contribution to insensible water loss is evaporative skin loss. The rate of water loss is a function of gestational age (body weight), environment (losses are greater under a radiant warmer than in an isolette), and the use of phototherapy. Respiratory losses are minimal when infants are breathing humidified oxygen. The renal contribution to water requirement is influenced by the decreased ability of the preterm neonate to concentrate the urine and conserve water.

Electrolyte requirements are minimal for the initial 24–48 hours until there is excretion in the urine. Basal requirements are as follows:

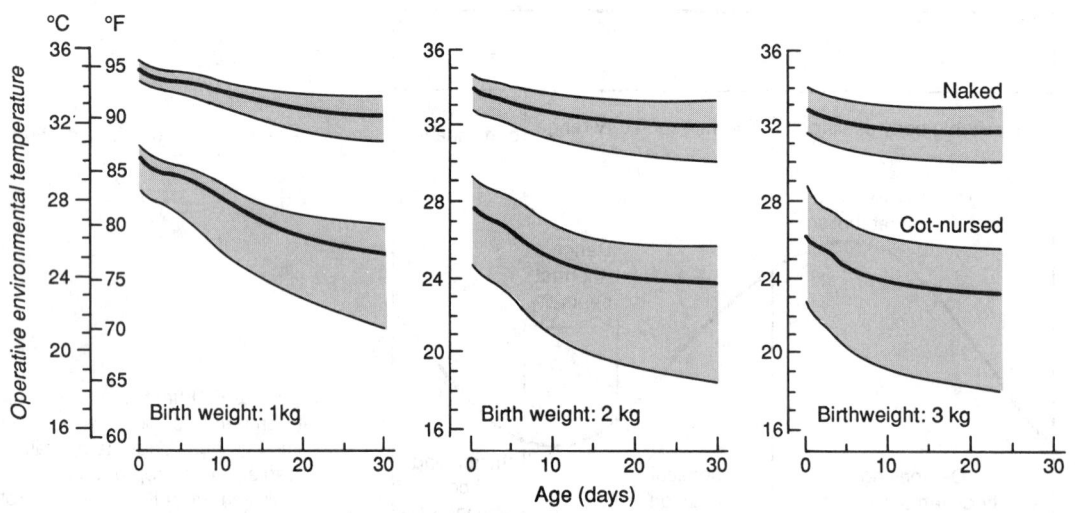

Figure 2–6. Range of environmental temperatures to maintain naked or dressed infants of 1, 2, or 3 kg in a neutral thermal environment. (Reproduced, with permission, from Hey E: The care of babies in incubators. In: *Recent Advances in Paediatrics*, 4th ed. Gairdner D, Hull D [editors]. Churchill Livingstone, 1971.)

Sodium	**3 meq/kg/d**
Potassium	**2 meq/kg/d**
Chloride	**2–3 meq/kg/d**
Bicarbonate	**2–3 meq/kg/d**

In the infant of gestational age less than 30 weeks, sodium and bicarbonate losses in the urine are frequently excessive.

Initial fluid management after birth is determined by the infant's size. Infants weighing more than 1500 g should start at 80–100 mL/kg/d of 10% dextrose in water ($D_{10}W$), whereas those weighing less should start at 100–120 mL/kg/d of either $D_{10}W$ or 5% dextrose in water (D_5W) (infants < 800 g and < 26 weeks often become hyperglycemic on $D_{10}W$). The most critical issue in fluid management is monitoring. Measurements of body weight, urine output, fluid and electrolyte intake, serum and urine electrolytes, and glucose (using Chemstrips) allow fairly precise determinations of the infant's water, glucose, and electrolyte needs. Once an infant has stabilized (usually by day 2 or 3), hyperalimentation solutions can be started to meet nutritional as well as water and electrolyte requirements.

Baumgart S: Reduction of oxygen consumption, insensible water loss, and radiant heat demand with use of a plastic blanket for low-birth-weight infants under radiant warmers. Pediatrics 1984;74:1022.

Hay WW Jr, Thilo E, Curlander JB: Pulse oximetry in neonatal medicine. Clin Perinatol 1991;18:441.

Klaus MH, Fanaroff AA, Martin RJ: The physical environment. In: *Care of the High-Risk Neonate,* 4th ed. Klaus MH, Fanaroff AA (editors). Saunders, 1993.

LeBlanc MH: Thermoregulation: Incubators, radiant warmers, artificial skins, and body hoods. Clin Perinatol 1991; 18:403.

Raj JU, Franco G: Acid-base, fluid, and electrolyte management. In: *Diseases of the Newborn.* Taeusch HW, Ballard RA, Avery ME (editors). Saunders, 1991.

Ramanathan R et al: Pulse oximetry in very low birth weight infants with acute and chronic lung disease. Pediatrics 1987;79:612.

Scopes JW: Metabolic rate and temperature control in the human body. Br Med Bull 1966;22:88.

Shaffer SG, Weismann DN: Fluid requirements in the preterm infant. Clin Perinatol 1992: 19:233.

NUTRITION OF THE HIGH-RISK INFANT

This section addresses a nutritional approach to the very immature infant, for whom nutritional problems are most difficult. The end result of good nutrition is a steady weight gain. The daily weight of an infant should, therefore, be charted against one of the standard postnatal growth curves. It is helpful to include in this weight chart the total water intake (mL/kg/d) and total caloric intake (kcal/kg/d), as shown in Figure 2–7. This practice is particularly helpful in infants who have long nursery stays: it is relatively easy to distinguish infants who are not growing because of inadequate food intake from those not growing despite adequate caloric intake. Expected weight gain for the adequately nourished preterm infant is 10–30 g per day or a minimum of 1% of the infant's weight.

In general, the long-term nutritional support for infants of very low birth weight consists of either breast milk supplemented to increase protein and caloric density or infant formulas modified for preterm infants. In all of these formulas, protein concentrations (approximately 2 g/dL) and caloric concentrations (approximately 24 kcal/oz) are relatively high. How-

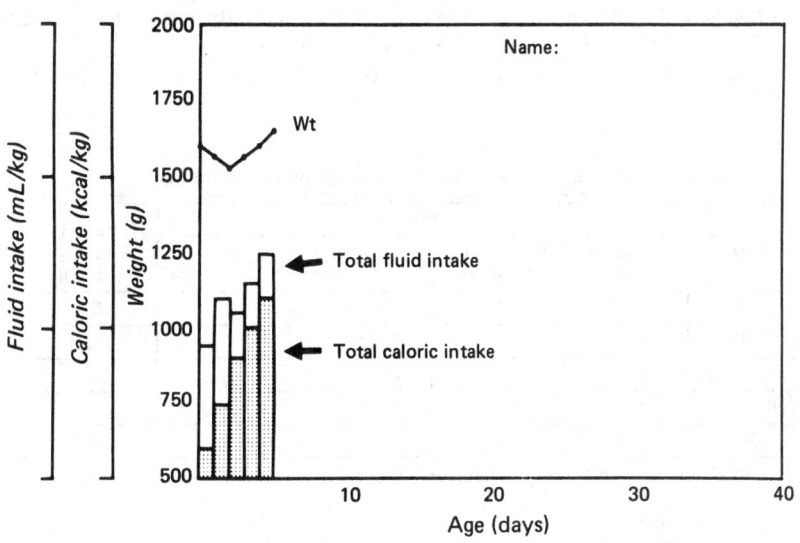

Figure 2–7. A convenient method of presenting a summary of hydration, nutrition, and body weight in newborn infants.

ever, these feedings should not be started immediately. The infant should be gradually advanced to feedings of higher caloric density after the full volume of either breast milk or formula (20 kcal/oz) is tolerated.

Initial Feedings

Infants initially require intravenous glucose infusions to maintain blood glucose concentration in the range of 60–100 mg/dL. Infusions of 5–7 mg/kg/min (approximately 80–100 mL/kg/d of a 10% dextrose solution) are usually required. After stabilization, amino acids are added to the solution to provide nitrogen intakes of 1–2 g/kg/d. It is important to emphasize that the introduction of amino acids (as well as the introduction of intravenous lipids or milk feedings) is a decision predicated on the condition of the infant. The critically ill infant may receive only glucose and sodium salts until stabilization occurs.

The infant's first milk feedings ideally consist of colostrum, or early breast milk of the mother, unsupplemented. Alternatively, formulas for preterm infants at caloric concentrations of 20 kcal/oz can be used. Each of the first few feedings should be written as an order until it is clear that the infant is managing them without distention, respiratory difficulties, or other problems. Intermittent bolus feedings (if tolerated) are preferred, because these appear to stimulate the release of gut-related hormones and may speed the maturation of the gastrointestinal tract. A suggested schedule for feedings is presented in Table 2–10.

Carbohydrates

Glucose is the only carbohydrate provided initially; once milk feedings are begun, however, the lactose in the milk provides galactose, an important carbohydrate for the newborn. It is important to measure blood glucose levels during the transition from intravenous to milk feedings (decreasing the reliance on intravenous glucose infusions), because infants fed only milk cannot sustain blood glucose concentrations unless gluconeogenesis is well-established.

Amino Acids

The amino acid composition of solutions available for intravenous use has been altered to provide a more readily usable form of nitrogen. TrophAmine is the preferred mixture for neonates since its amino acid profiles are most similar to those seen in infants on breast milk. The same principle—breast milk as the gold standard—has been applied to the design of formulas for premature infants. The increase in protein concentration in these formulas can lead to nitrogen intakes of 3–3.5 g/kg/d. These high intakes can be well utilized if caloric intake is also high.

Fats

Milk, whether breast milk or formula, constitutes a high-fat diet. A relatively high fat intake is important in establishing normal postnatal liver and gastrointestinal function. Deficiencies in essential fatty acids can develop quickly in the infant of very low birth weight, who has little body stores of essential fatty acids at the time of birth. Thus, it is important to make sure these babies receive an adequate amount of essential fatty acids, provided either intravenously or through milk feedings. Fatty acids are also required for oxidation, which in turn supports gluconeogenesis.

Vitamins

Vitamins are initially provided intravenously and later through milk feedings. It has been customary to supplement the vitamins provided in feedings with an oral multivitamin preparation because of the prolonged period before infants of very low birth weight consume enough milk to provide the necessary vitamins. However, fortified breast milk and the formulas for premature infants now provide adequate amounts of vitamins, with the possible exception of vitamin E. Although formulas designed for the preterm infant

Table 2–10. Suggested feeding regimen for preterm infants.

| Weight (g) | Initial | | | Time to Full Feedings (days) |
	Feeding (mL)	Frequency (hourly)	Advancement (mL/feeding)	
500–800	1	2[1]	1 every 12–24 h	6
800–1000	2	2[1]	1 every 12 h	4–6
1000–1200	2–3	2	1 every 12 h	4
1200–1500	4	2–3	1 every 6–8 h	4
> 1500	5–10	3	1 every other feeding	3–4

[1]Second and subsequent feedings offered only after examination of the infant show the following:

    (1) No distention
    (2) Normal bowel sounds
    (3) No residuals or vomiting

are said now to contain enough vitamin E, many practitioners still supplement with 25 IU per day in the infant weighing less than 1500 g for a period of 3 weeks to build up stores of this vitamin. This dose is adequate to prevent vitamin E deficiency hemolytic anemia. Vitamin K, 1 mg intramuscularly, is given once to all newborns immediately after delivery.

Minerals

Formulas for premature infants contain increased concentrations of calcium and phosphorus. Any premature infant receiving an adequate intake of either fortified breast milk or one of these formulas receives adequate amounts of calcium and phosphorus for bone mineralization. Osteopenia and occasionally rickets are still seen in infants receiving long-term parenteral nutrition or the calciuric diuretic furosemide. Iron supplementation (2 mg/kg/d) is recommended for premature infants, beginning at about the first 2 months of life or at 36–39 weeks postconception. This can be provided by iron-supplemented formulas. Trace elements are discussed in Chapter 11.

DISCHARGE

Discharge policies are more flexible today. Term, healthy newborns may be discharged in 24 hours. Very immature infants are usually discharged when they reach 2000–2500 g, but weight or postconceptual age alone no longer determines the time of discharge; a careful assessment of the infant's progress and the home environment also influences the decision. Factors such as the support for the mother at home and the stability of the family situation play a part in timing of discharge. The infant must at the very least be stable, eating well, and showing steady weight gain at the time of discharge. In addition, staff should observe the parents caring for the infant to confirm that the parents are capable of managing whatever special care the infant requires. Infants with special requirements, eg, oxygen therapy, may be discharged if the family clearly can manage to provide the additional support to the infant at home. The availability of a social worker or visiting nurse makes such discharge decisions easier.

FOLLOW-UP CARE

This term refers to follow-up visits to an ambulatory setting, for the purpose of tracking the achievement of behavioral and developmental landmarks in infants who have received neonatal intensive care. For infants discharged from level 2 nurseries, follow-up care can be provided by the pediatrician, with consultative visits at special care facilities as required. Infants discharged from level 3 nurseries require specialized follow-up care, because many families need

help with physical or neurologic problems and management of home oxygen therapy. In addition, the family needs ongoing support during the first few years of the child's life. The frequency of repeated hospitalizations in many infants who have experienced complications (eg, chronic lung disease and the attendant growth disturbances) after neonatal intensive care underscores the need for such support.

Allen MC, Capute AJ: Neonatal neurodevelopmental examination as a predictor of neuromotor outcome in premature infants. Pediatrics 1989;83:498.

Ballard RA (editor): *Pediatric Care of the ICN Graduate.* Saunders, 1988.

Committee on Nutrition, American Academy of Pediatrics: Nutritional needs of low birthweight infants. Pediatrics 1985;75:976.

Ellenberg JH, Nelson KB: Cluster of perinatal events identifying infants at high risk for death or disability. J Pediatr 1988;113:546.

Filer LJ (editor): Assessment of bone mineralization in infants. J Pediatr 1988;113(Suppl):165.

Georgieff MK et al: Effect of neonatal caloric deprivation on head growth and 1-year developmental status in preterm infants. J Pediatr 1987;107:581.

Gross SJ, Slagle TA: Feeding the low birthweight infant. Clin Perinatol 1993;20:193.

Hack M, Fanaroff AA: How small is too small? Consideration in evaluating the outcome of the tiny infant. Clin Perinatol 1988;15:773.

Halsey CL, Collin MF, Anderson CL: Extremely low birth weight children and their peers: A comparison of preschool performance. Pediatrics 1993;91:807.

Hay WW (editor): *Neonatal Nutrition and Metabolism.* Mosby, 1991.

Nelson KB, Ellenberg JH: Antecedents of cerebral palsy. N Engl J Med 1986;315:81.

Teplin S et al: Neurodevelopmental, health and growth status at age 6 years of children with birth weights less than 1001 grams. J Pediatr 1991;118:768.

Tsang RC et al (editors): *Nutritional Needs of the Preterm Infant.* Williams & Wilkins. 1993.

Victorian Infant Collaborative Study Group: Eight-year outcome in infants with birth weight of 500 to 999 grams: Continuing regional study of 1979 and 1980 births. J Pediatr 1991;118:761.

Victorian Infant Collaborative Study Group: Improvement of outcome for infants of birth weight under 1000 g. Arch Dis Child 1991;66:765.

MULTIPLE BIRTHS

Multiple births represent an important area in perinatal medicine. Twinning occurs in one of every 80 pregnancies. A clear distinction should be made between dizygotic (fraternal) and monozygotic (identical) twins. Race, maternal parity, and maternal age are associated only with the incidence of dizygotic twinning. Drugs that induce ovulation, such as clomiphene citrate or gonadotrophin therapy, increase the incidence of dizygotic twinning quite strikingly.

Examination of the placenta can help establish the type of twinning: two amnionic membranes and two chorionic membranes are found in all cases of dizygotic twins and in one-third of cases of monozygotic twins; two amnionic membranes and one chorionic membrane or one amnionic and one chorionic membrane always indicate monozygotic twins.

COMPLICATIONS OF MULTIPLE BIRTHS

Intrauterine Growth Retardation

There is some degree of intrauterine growth retardation in most multiple pregnancies of 36 or more weeks. If prenatal care is good, however, the growth retardation is rarely clinically significant. There are two exceptions; the first is the monozygotic twin pregnancy in which there is an arterial venous shunt from one twin's circulation to that of the other. The infant with the venous connection becomes plethoric and considerably larger than the other twin. Neonatal morbidity is more common in the larger of the two infants, in part due to the hypervolemia and hyperviscosity. Discordance in twins, that is, birth weights that are significantly different, can also occur when there are separate placentas; one placenta develops poorly, presumably because of a poor implantation site. In this instance there is no fetal exchange of blood, but there is a striking difference in the growth rate of the two infants.

Preterm Delivery

Gestation length tends to be inversely related to the number of fetuses. It is the prematurity that tends to increase the mortality or morbidity of twin pregnancies.

OBSTETRIC COMPLICATIONS

Obstetric complications, including polyhydramnios, pregnancy-induced hypertension, premature rupture of membranes, abnormal fetal presentations, and prolapsed umbilical cord, occur more frequently in women with multiple fetuses. In general, most of the complications can be avoided or minimized in terms of their impact on the infant by good obstetric management. Multiple pregnancy should always be identified prenatally with ultrasound examinations; doing so allows the obstetrician and pediatrician or neonatologist to plan their management jointly. The neonatal complications are usually related to prematurity. Prolongation of pregnancy, therefore, leads to a significant reduction in neonatal morbidity.

Follow-up studies of twin pregnancies have yielded conflicting results. In general, the studies do not suggest that twinning has a significant effect on the child's later development, especially if prematurity is excluded as a separate risk factor.

Chitkara U, Berkowitz RL: Multiple gestations. In: *Obstetrics: Normal and Problem Pregnancies,* 2nd ed. Gabbe SG, Niebyl JR, Simpson JL (editors). Churchill Livingstone, 1991.

Naeye RL, Tafari N: Twin gestations. In: *Risk Factors in Pregnancy and Diseases of the Fetus and Newborn.* Naeye RL, Tafari N (editors). Williams & Wilkins, 1983.

Warenski JC, Kochenour NK: Intrapartum management of twin gestation. Clin Perinatol 1989;16:889.

SPECIFIC DISEASES OF THE NEWBORN INFANT

RESPIRATORY DISEASES

1. APNEA

Diagnosis

In preterm infants, recurrent apneic episodes are an important clinical problem. Significant apnea is defined as a respiratory pause lasting more than 20 seconds accompanied by cyanosis and bradycardia. Shorter respiratory pauses associated with cyanosis or bradycardia also qualify as significant apnea but must be differentiated from periodic breathing, which is common in term as well as preterm infants. Periodic breathing is defined as regularly recurring ventilatory cycles interrupted by short pauses not associated with bradycardia or color change. Apnea can be a response of the preterm infant's respiratory regulatory center to various peripheral stimuli. Causes for apnea in the preterm infant are listed in Table 2–11. The items listed in Table 2–11 require some comment. Both gastroesophageal reflux and apnea are common in preterm infants. The presence of gastroesophageal reflux, therefore, does not prove that gastroesophageal reflux is the cause of the apnea. The most precise diagnostic technique is to place an esophageal pH probe for 12 hours and correlate changes in esophageal pH with apneic episodes. Anemia is another difficult diagnostic entity. Recent work does suggest that frequency of periodic breathing and apnea can be decreased by giving the anemic child blood transfusions. This treatment for apnea, however, must always be weighed against the risk of transfusions.

Apnea of prematurity is the most frequent cause of apnea. Most apnea of prematurity is the so-called

Table 2–11. Causes of apnea in the preterm infant.

Temperature instability–both cold and heat stress
Response to passage of a feeding tube
Gastroesophageal reflux
Hypoxemia
    Pulmonary parenchymal disease
    Patent ductus arteriosus
    ?Anemia
Infection
    Sepsis (viral or bacterial)
    Necrotizing enterocolitis
Metabolic causes
    Hypoglycemia
    Hyponatremia
Intracranial hemorrhage
Posthemorrhagic hydrocephalus
Seizures
Drugs, eg, morphine
Apnea of prematurity

mixed apnea characterized by a centrally (brain stem) mediated respiratory pause preceded or followed by airway obstruction. Less common is pure central or pure obstructive apnea. Apnea of prematurity is due to immaturity of both the central respiratory regulatory centers and of protective mechanisms that aid in maintaining airway patency. Onset, typically during the first 2 weeks of life, is gradual, with the frequency of spells increasing over time. Pathologic apnea can be suspected in an infant with a sudden onset of frequent apneic spells or a sudden onset of very severe spells. Apnea presenting from birth or on the first day of life is unusual, but it can occur especially in the preterm infant who does not require mechanical ventilation for respiratory distress syndrome. This presentation suggests the presence of an acute (asphyxia or birth trauma) or chronic (congenital hypotonia, structural central nervous system lesion, etc) neuromuscular abnormality.

The workup is directed by the clinical presentation of the apnea. All infants, regardless of severity and frequency of apnea, require a minimum screening evaluation, including a general assessment of the infant's well-being (eg, tolerance of feedings, stable temperature, normal physical examination), a check of the association of spells to feeding, hematocrit, measurement of PaO_2 or SaO_2, glucose Chemstrip, and a review of drug history. Infants with sudden onset of severe apnea may require a more extensive evaluation, including a workup for infection. Other specific tests are dictated by signs in the infant, eg, evaluation for necrotizing enterocolitis in an infant with apnea and abdominal distention.

Treatment

The physician treating apnea should first address any underlying cause. If the apnea is due simply to prematurity, treatment is dictated by the frequency and severity of apneic spells. Simple measures include prophylactic cutaneous stimulation and use of a water bed. Apneic spells frequent enough to interfere with other aspects of care (eg, feeding) or severe enough to necessitate bag and mask ventilation to relieve cyanosis and bradycardia require more aggressive treatment. Intubation and ventilation can eliminate apneic spells but carry the attendant risks of long-term endotracheal intubation. Conclusive evidence that methylxanthines (theophylline and caffeine) are effective in the treatment of apnea have led to their widespread use. Theophylline can be used, with a loading dose of 5 mg/kg and maintenance dose of 1–2 mg/kg every 6–12 hours. The loading dose of caffeine is 20 mg/kg (caffeine citrate); the maintenance dose is 5–10 mg/kg every 24 hours. These agents appear to work as central stimulants. Side effects include tachycardia, feeding intolerance, and (with overdosing) seizures. The minimum dose necessary to decrease the frequency of apnea and eliminate severe spells should be used. Desired drug levels are usually in the range of 5–10 µg/mL for both drugs.

Prognosis

In the majority of premature infants, apneic and bradycardiac spells cease by 34–36 weeks postconception. Occasionally the episodes last longer, and outpatient therapy with methylxanthines may be indicated. Whether to provide home monitoring for such infants is controversial. Apneic and bradycardiac episodes in the nursery are not precise predictors of later sudden infant death syndrome (SIDS). However, home monitoring in infants still experiencing apnea and bradycardia at the time of hospital discharge is probably a prudent measure. The incidence of SIDS is slightly increased in the preterm infant. Recent work in term infants has shown an increased incidence of SIDS in infants who sleep in the prone position. Whether or not this can be extrapolated to the preterm infant (in particular those with gastroesophageal reflux or persistent respiratory symptoms) is unclear. When possible, a sleeping position on the side with the right side down or supine seems prudent unless contraindicated by reflux or respiratory symptoms.

American Academy of Pediatrics Task Force on Infant Positioning and SIDS: Positioning and SIDS. Pediatrics 1992;89:1120.

Brazy JE et al: Central nervous system structural lesions causing apnea at birth. J Pediatr 1987;111:163.

DeMaio JG et al: Effect of blood transfusion on apnea frequency in growing premature infants. J Pediatr 1989; 114:1039.

Gerhardt T, Bancalari E: Apnea of prematurity. (Two parts.) Pediatrics 1984;74:58,63.

Krongrad E: Infants at high risk for sudden infant death syndrome: Have they been identified? A Commentary. Pediatrics 1991;88:1274.

Martin RJ et al: Pathogenesis of apnea in preterm infants. J Pediatr 1986;109:733.

Miller MJ, Martin RJ: Apnea of prematurity. Clin Perinatol 1992;19:789.

NIH Consensus: Developmental Conference on Infantile Apnea and Home Monitoring. Pediatrics 1987;79:292.

Ponsonby A-L et al: Factors potentiating the risk of sudden infant death syndrome associated with the prone position. N Engl J Med 1993;329:377.

Ruggins NR et al: Site of upper airway obstruction in preterm infants with problematical apnea. Arch Dis Child 1991;66:787.

Ruggins NR: Pathophysiology of apnea in preterm infants. Arch Dis Child 1991;66:70.

2. RESPIRATORY DISTRESS IN THE NEWBORN

Diagnosis

Respiratory distress is among the most common symptom complexes seen in the newborn. Respiratory distress may be due to both noncardiopulmonary and cardiopulmonary causes (Table 2–12). The cardinal clinical features include a respiratory rate of more than 60 per minute with or without associated cyanosis, nasal flaring, intercostal and sternal retractions, and expiratory grunting. It is important to consider the noncardiopulmonary causes listed in Table 2–12, because the natural tendency is to focus on the heart and lungs. Most of the noncardiopulmonary causes can be ruled out by the history, physical examination, and a few simple laboratory tests. The evaluation of cardiovascular disorders is discussed in the next section.

The physician attempting diagnosis of pulmonary disorders must consider the following major concerns in the term infant: transient tachypnea, aspiration syndromes, and congenital pneumonia.

A. Transient Tachypnea: The syndrome of transient tachypnea presents as respiratory distress in nonasphyxiated term infants (often delivered by cesarian section) or slightly preterm infants. The clini-

cal features include tachypnea, cyanosis, grunting, flaring, and retractions presenting in the first hours of life. The chest x-ray film indicating prominent perihilar streaking and fluid in the interlobar fissures is the key to diagnosis. The symptoms generally abate within 12–24 hours, although they can persist longer. The cause of the disorder is thought to be delayed resorption of fetal lung fluid.

B. Clear Fluid Aspiration: At or before delivery, the infant can aspirate clear amniotic fluid or fluid mixed with blood. The clinical presentation is much like that of transient tachypnea, with the following differences: these infants usually require higher FiO_2 to be noncyanotic (30–60% versus 25–40% in infants with transient tachypnea), and the course is more protracted (4–7 days). The chest x-ray film reveals hyperexpansion with a more patchy infiltrate pattern than that seen with transient tachypnea.

C. Meconium Aspiration Syndrome: The perinatal course in these infants is often marked by fetal distress, low Apgar scores, and meconium in the amniotic fluid. These infants exhibit tachypnea, retractions, cyanosis, an overdistended, barrel-shaped chest, and coarse breath sounds. The chest x-ray film reveals coarse, irregular infiltrates and hyperexpansion. There is a high incidence of air leaks and, in severe cases, a high rate of persistent pulmonary hypertension (see Cardiovascular Diseases).

D. Congenital Pneumonia: The lungs are the most common site of infection in the neonate. Both bacterial and viral infections can be acquired before, during, or after birth. Most commonly, infections ascend from the genital tract before or during labor. The rupture of membranes more than 12–18 hours prior to delivery is a major predisposing factor. The presence of chorioamnionitis in the mother further increases the risk. Infants with congenital pneumonia present with respiratory symptoms as early as in the delivery room, with the majority symptomatic by 6–12 hours of age. The chest x-ray is not helpful in distinguishing

Table 2–12. Causes of respiratory distress in the newborn.[1]

Noncardiopulmonary	Cardiovascular	Pulmonary
Hypothermia or hyperthermia	Left-sided outflow tract obstruction	Upper airway obstruction
Hypoglycemia	Hypoplastic left heart	Choanal atresia
Polycythemia	Aortic stenosis	Vocal cord paralysis
Metabolic acidosis	Coarctation of the aorta	Lingual thyroid
Drug intoxications or withdrawal	Cyanotic lesions	Meconium aspiration
Insult to the CNS	Transposition of the great vessels	Clear fluid aspiration
Asphyxia	Total anomalous pulmonary venous	Transient tachypnea
Hemorrhage	return	Pneumonia
Neuromuscular disease	Tricuspid atresia	Pulmonary hypoplasia
Phrenic nerve injury	Right-sided outflow obstruction	Hyaline membrane disease
Asphyxiating thoracic dystrophy		Pneumothorax
		Pleural effusions
		Mass lesions
		Lobar emphysema
		Cystic adenomatoid malformation

[1]Reproduced, with permission, from Rosenberg AA: Neonatal adaptation. In: *Obstetrics: Normal and Problem Pregnancies.* Gabbe SG, Niebyl JR, Simpson JL (editors): Churchill Livingstone, 1986.

congenital pneumonia from other forms of neonatal lung disease. The presence of shock, poor perfusion, and absolute neutropenia on blood count provide corroborating evidence for pneumonia.

E. Spontaneous Pneumothorax: This entity occurs in 1% of all deliveries. Risk is increased by manipulations such as bag and mask ventilation in the delivery room. Clinically, the infants are tachypneic with a small oxygen requirement (25–40% FiO_2). Breath sounds may be asymmetric, and if the pneumothorax is under tension, the mediastinum may be shifted. The diagnosis can be confirmed on x-ray studies. There is a small increased risk of renal abnormalities associated with spontaneous pneumothorax. Therefore, a careful physical examination of the kidneys and observation of urine output are indicated.

F. Other Pulmonary Causes: Many of the other pulmonary causes of respiratory distress are fairly rare. Bilateral choanal atresia should be suspected if there is no air movement when the infant breathes through the nose. These infants present in the delivery room with good color and heart rate while crying. When they quiet down and resume normal breathing, they become cyanotic and bradycardic. Other causes of airway obstruction are usually characterized by some degree of stridor or poor air movement despite good respiratory effort. Pleural effusions can be suspected in hydropic infants (eg, those with erythroblastosis fetalis). Space-occupying lesions cause a shift of the mediastinum and asymmetric breath sounds.

G. Hyaline Membrane Disease: The most common cause of respiratory distress in the preterm infant is hyaline membrane disease. The incidence of this disorder increases from 5% at 35–36 weeks to 65% at 29–30 weeks of gestation. This condition is due to a deficiency of surfactant. Surfactant decreases surface tension in the alveolus during expiration, allowing the alveolus to remain partly expanded, thereby maintaining a functional residual capacity. The absence of surfactant results in poor lung compliance and atelectasis. The infant must expend a great deal of effort to expand the lungs with each breath, and respiratory failure ensues. Infants with hyaline membrane disease demonstrate all the clinical signs of respiratory distress. On auscultation, air movement is diminished despite vigorous respiratory effort. The chest x-ray film demonstrates diffuse bilateral atelectasis causing a "ground-glass" appearance. Major airways are highlighted by the atelectatic air sacs creating air bronchograms. In the unintubated child, there is doming of the diaphragms and hypoexpansion.

Treatment

The cornerstone of treatment of neonatal respiratory distress is the provision of adequate supplemental oxygen to maintain a PaO_2 of 60–70 mm Hg and an arterial saturation of 92–95%. PaO_2 levels less than 50 mm Hg are associated with pulmonary vascular vasoconstriction, and those greater than 100 mm Hg may increase the risk of retinopathy of prematurity. Oxygen should be warmed, humidified, and given through an air blender. Concentration should be measured with a calibrated oxygen analyzer. An umbilical arterial line should be placed in any infant requiring more than 45% FiO_2 by 4–6 hours of life to allow frequent blood gas determinations. Noninvasive monitoring with a transcutaneous O_2 monitor or pulse oximeter can provide continuous information.

Other supportive treatment includes intravenous provision of glucose and water if the infant is in too much distress to eat. Unless infection can be absolutely ruled out, blood cultures should be obtained and broad-spectrum antibiotics started. Colloid solutions (eg, 5% albumin) can be given in infusions of 10 mL/kg over 30 minutes for low blood pressure, poor perfusion, and metabolic acidosis. Sodium bicarbonate (1–2 meq/kg) is indicated for treatment of a documented metabolic acidosis that has not responded to oxygen, ventilation, and volume. While therapy is instituted, specific workup should be pursued as indicated by history and physical findings. In most cases, a chest x-ray study, blood gas, complete blood count, and glucose Chemstrip allow a diagnosis.

Intubation and ventilation should be undertaken for signs of respiratory failure ($PaO_2 < 60$ mm Hg in 70–80% FiO_2 or $PaCO_2 > 50$ mm Hg). These guidelines, however, do not apply to infants with hyaline membrane disease. Indication for further respiratory support in these infants is a need for 50% FiO_2 to keep PaO_2 greater than 60 mm Hg. In infants greater than 30 weeks of gestation and 1500 g, a trial of continuous positive airway pressure (4–8 cm H_2O) administered either nasally or by endotracheal tube can be attempted. If this fails to provide the desired result, the infant should be ventilated. Peak pressures should be adequate to produce chest wall expansion (usually 18–24 cm H_2O). Positive end-expiratory pressure (4–6 cm H_2O) should also be used. Ventilation rates of 20–50 are usually required. The goal is to maintain PaO_2 of 60–70 mm Hg and $PaCO_2$ of 40–50 mm Hg.

Two exogenous surfactants (colfosceril palmitate [Exosurf Neonatal] and beractant [Survanta]) have been approved in the United States by the Food and Drug Administration for use in infants with hyaline membrane disease. Surfactant replacement therapy, used both in the delivery room as prophylaxis and with established hyaline membrane disease as rescue, has been shown to decrease the mortality rate in preterm infants and to decrease air leak complications of the disease. Ventilator settings and oxygen requirements are significantly less in surfactant-treated infants than controls during the acute course. Although the acute course of respiratory disease is improved, the incidence of other complications of prematurity such as intracranial hemorrhage, patent ductus arteriosus, and necrotizing enterocolitis has not been altered by surfactant replacement therapy. In addition, the incidence of chronic lung disease among survivors has not decreased. However, the severity of chronic lung disease is less in surfactant-treated newborns because of the lower inspired oxygen concentrations and ventilator settings made possible during the acute stages of respiratory distress syndrome. The dose of the artificial surfactant Exosurf is 5 mL/kg intratracheally, while that of the bovine-derived Survanta is 4 mL/kg. The usual dosing schedule when the first dose is given in the delivery room to prevent hyaline membrane disease is a total of three doses given 8–12 hours apart as long as the infant remains ventilated on greater than 30–40% inspired oxygen concentration. Rescue surfactant is given as two doses 8–12 hours apart. The first dose is optimally administered as soon as possible after birth, preferably prior to 4 hours of age. As the disease process evolves, proteins that inhibit surfactant function leak into the air spaces, making surfactant replacement less effective. The second dose should be administered to infants who continue to require ventilation and more than 40% inspired oxygen concentration. The decision to use prophylactic versus an early rescue strategy remains unresolved.

The approach to infants who go on to develop chronic lung disease has been aided by the use of dexamethasone (0.5 mg/kg) to decrease lung inflammation. Dexamethasone is most effective when started in chronically ventilated infants at 10 days to 3 weeks of age. Dosing schedules used have varied from a brief 5-day course to an initial 3–5 days at full dose followed by a gradual wean in dosage over 4–6 weeks.

Prognosis

Most of the conditions described in the term infant are acute and resolve in the first several days of life. Meconium aspiration syndrome and congenital pneumonia do have a significant rate of associated pulmonary morbidity (chronic lung disease) and mortality (approximately 10–20%). Mortality rates in these disorders have recently been reduced by use of high-frequency ventilation, inhaled nitric oxide (NO) and extracorporeal membrane oxygenation (ECMO). Mortality rates have decreased dramatically in infants with hyaline membrane disease through the use of continuous positive airway pressure, positive pressure ventilation, and, more recently, surfactant replacement therapy. Mortality rates associated with hyaline membrane disease are less than 10% for infants of greater than 28 weeks' gestation. The major long-term sequela is the development of chronic lung disease (defined as the need for oxygen or ventilation after 1 month of age), which occurs in 20% of the survivors of hyaline membrane disease. The incidence is highest at lower gestational ages. The development of chronic lung disease is a function of lung immaturity at birth and exposure to high oxygen concentrations and ventilator barotrauma. Although the use of exogenous surfactants has not decreased the incidence of chronic lung disease, the condition is not as severe in surfactant-treated infants. Up to 10% of infants who develop chronic lung disease will die in the first 2 years of life because of respiratory failure, pulmonary infection, or sudden death. However, most infants with chronic lung disease do well clinically, though abnormalities in pulmonary function persist. Some infants with chronic lung disease require home oxygen therapy. This can be monitored with pulse oximetry, with SaO_2 kept at 92–95%. Systemic hypertension can be seen in these patients; frequent blood pressure determinations, therefore, are indicated, as are ECGs and echocardiograms to monitor for left and right ventricular hypertrophy.

Avery ME et al: Transient tachypnea of the newborn. Am J Dis Child 1966;111:380.

Avery ME, Mead J: Surface properties in relation to atelectasis and hyaline membrane disease. Am J Dis Child 1959;97:517.

Blayney M et al: Bronchopulmonary dysplasia: Improvement in lung function between 7 and 10 years of age. J Pediatr 1991;118:201.

Collaborative Dexamethasone Trial Group: Dexamethasone therapy in neonatal chronic lung disease: An international placebo-controlled trial. Pediatrics 1991;88:421

Corbet A et al: Decreased mortality rate among small premature infants treated at birth with a single dose of synthetic surfactant: A multicenter controlled trial. J Pediatr 1991;118:277.

Dunn MS et al: Single versus multiple dose surfactant replacement therapy in neonates of 30–36 weeks gestation with respiratory distress syndrome. Pediatrics 1990;86:564.

Goldsmith JP, Karotkin EH (editors): *Assisted Ventilation of the Neonate.* Saunders, 1988.

Holtzman RB, Frank L (editors): Bronchopulmonary dysplasia. Clin Perinatol 1992; 19:3.

Horbar JD et al: A multicenter randomized, placebo-controlled trial of surfactant therapy for respiratory distress syndrome. N Engl J Med 1989;320:959.

Jobe AH: Pulmonary surfactant therapy. N Engl J Med 1993;328:861.

Kattwinkel J et al: Prophylactic administration of calf lung surfactant extract is more effective than early treatment of respiratory distress syndrome in neonates of 29 through 32 weeks' gestation. Pediatrics 1993;92:90.

Kendig JW et al: A comparison of surfactant as immediate prophylaxis and as rescue therapy in newborns of less than 30 weeks gestation. N Engl J Med 1991;324:864.

Long W et al: Effects of two rescue doses of a synthetic surfactant on mortality rate and survival without bronchopulmonary dysplasia in 700 to 1350 gram infants with respiratory distress syndrome. J Pediatr 1991;118:595.

Northway WH et al: Late pulmonary sequelae of bronchopulmonary dysplasia. N Engl J Med 1990;323:1793.

Northway WH Jr et al: Pulmonary disease following respirator therapy of hyaline membrane disease. N Engl J Med 1967;276:357.

O'Brodovich HM, Mellins RB: Bronchopulmonary dysplasia: Unresolved neonatal acute lung injury. Am Rev Respir Dis 1985;132:694.

Soll RF et al: Multicenter trial of single dose modified bovine surfactant extract (Survanta) for prevention of respiratory distress syndrome. Pediatrics 1990;85:1092.

Weaver TE, Whitsett JA: Structure and function of pulmonary surfactant proteins. Semin Perinatol 1989;12:213.

CARDIOVASCULAR DISEASES

Diagnosis

Cardiovascular causes of respiratory distress in the neonatal period can be divided into two major groups—structural heart disease and a structurally normal heart with shunting through fetal pathways.

A. Structural Heart Disease: The central presenting features of symptomatic congenital heart disease in the first week of life include cyanosis and congestive heart failure. Cyanotic heart disease can be due to transposition of the great vessels, tricuspid atresia, certain types of truncus arteriosus, total anomalous pulmonary venous return, and right heart obstruction (eg, pulmonary and tricuspid atresia). Infants with these disorders present with early cyanosis. The hallmark of many of these lesions is cyanosis in an infant without associated respiratory distress. Although early cyanosis is the central feature in these disorders, tachypnea develops over time in many infants either because of increased pulmonary blood flow or secondary to metabolic acidosis from hypoxia. Infants with total anomalous venous return below the diaphragm present early with tachypnea, because the pulmonary venous return is obstructed and pulmonary edema develops. Diagnostic aids include comparing a blood gas obtained while the infant breathes 100% oxygen to one obtained while the child breathes room air. Failure of the PaO_2 to increase when 100% oxygen is breathed suggests cyanotic congenital heart disease. A chest x-ray film with decreased pulmonary markings is consistent with right heart obstruction, and an ECG with left-sided predominance suggests the small right heart seen with tricuspid atresia and other forms of right heart obstruction. Diagnosis can be confirmed with echocardiography.

Infants with congestive heart failure generally have some form of left-sided outflow tract obstruction. Infants with left-to-right shunt lesions, such as ventricular septal defect, may have murmurs in the newborn period, but clinical symptoms do not occur until pulmonary vascular resistance drops enough to cause significant shunting and subsequent failure (usually 3–4 weeks of age). Infants with left-sided outflow obstruction generally do well the first day or two until the source of all or some of the systemic flow, the ductus arteriosus, closes. With ductal closure, tachypnea, tachycardia, congestive heart failure, and metabolic acidosis develop. On examination, all of these infants have abnormalities of the pulses. In aortic atresia and stenosis, pulses are all diminished, whereas in coarctation syndromes, differential pulses (diminished in the lower extremities) are evident. Chest x-ray films in these infants show a large heart and pulmonary edema. Arterial blood gases are remarkable for profound metabolic acidosis.

B. Shunting Through Fetal Pathways: The syndrome of persistent pulmonary hypertension occurs when the normal decrease in pulmonary vascular resistance after birth does not occur. Most infants with persistent pulmonary hypertension are full term or postterm and have experienced perinatal asphyxia. Other clinical associations include hypothermia, meconium aspiration syndrome, hyaline membrane disease, polycythemia, neonatal sepsis, chronic intrauterine hypoxia, and pulmonary hypoplasia.

There are three causes of persistent pulmonary hypertension: (1) acute vasoconstriction due to perinatal hypoxia, (2) prenatal increase in pulmonary vascular smooth muscle development, and (3) decreased cross-sectional area of the pulmonary vascular bed due to inadequate vessel number. In the first, an acute perinatal event leads to hypoxia and failure of the pulmonary vascular resistance to drop. In the second, abnormal muscularization of the pulmonary resistance vessels results in persistent hypertension after birth. Finally, the third includes infants with pulmonary hypoplasia (eg, diaphragmatic hernia).

Clinically, the syndrome is characterized by onset on the first day of life, usually from birth. Respiratory distress is prominent, and PaO_2 is usually poorly responsive to high concentrations of inspired oxygen. Many of the infants have associated myocardial depression with resulting systemic hypotension. Echocardiography reveals right-to-left shunting at the level of the ductus arteriosus or foramen ovale (or both).

C. Patent Ductus Arteriosus: Patent ductus arteriosus is the most common cardiovascular disorder seen in the preterm infant. Clinically, significant patent ductus arteriosus usually presents on day 3–7 of life as the respiratory distress from hyaline membrane disease is improving. Presentation can be on day 1 or 2, especially in those infants of less than 28 weeks' gestation and in infants treated with surfactant replacement therapy. The signs include a hyperdynamic precordium, increased peripheral pulses, and a widened pulse pressure, with or without a systolic heart murmur. Early presentations are not uncommonly manifested by systemic hypotension without a murmur or hyperdynamic circulation. These signs are often accompanied by an increase in respiratory support. The presence of significant patent ductus arteriosus can be confirmed by echocardiography. Before undertaking medical or surgical ligation, other structural heart disease must be ruled out.

Treatment

For congenital heart disease, early stabilization includes supportive therapy as needed (eg, intravenous glucose, oxygen, and ventilation for respiratory failure). Specific therapy includes infusions of prostaglandin E_1, 0.025–0.1 µg/kg/min, to maintain ductal patency. In some cyanotic lesions (eg, pulmonary atresia), this improves pulmonary blood flow and PaO_2 by allowing shunting through the ductus to the pulmonary artery. In left-sided outflow tract obstruction, systemic blood flow is ductal dependent; prostaglandins improve systemic perfusion and resolve the baby's acidosis. Further specific management, including palliative surgical and cardiac catheterization procedures, is discussed in Chapter 21.

Therapy for persistent pulmonary hypertension involves supportive therapy for other postasphyxia problems (eg, anticonvulsants for seizures, careful fluid and electrolyte management for renal failure). Intravenous glucose should be provided to maintain normal blood sugar, and antibiotics should be administered for possible infection. Specific therapy is aimed at both increasing systemic arterial pressure and decreasing pulmonary arterial pressure to reverse the right-to-left shunting through fetal pathways. First-line therapy includes oxygen and ventilation (to lower pulmonary vascular resistance) and colloid infusions (10 mL/kg, up to 30 mL/kg) to improve systemic pressure. Ideally, systolic pressure should be greater than 60 mm Hg. With compromised cardiac function, systemic pressors can be used as second-line therapy (eg, dopamine 5–20 µg/kg/min or dobutamine 5–20 µg/kg/min, or both). If oxygenation is still not adequate (PaO_2 < 55 mm Hg), a trial of alkalosis by hyperventilation is indicated. Many babies improve as the pH rises above 7.55–7.6. Since alkalosis seems to be helpful, any base deficit should be corrected with sodium bicarbonate to allow less vigorous hyperventilation. The use of systemically infused vasodilators (eg, tolazoline hydrochloride, 1–2 mg/kg by intravenous push followed by an infusion of 0.2 mg/kg/h) to decrease pulmonary pressure has had variable and overall disappointing results due to a lack of specificity for the pulmonary vascular bed. Recent studies using the inhaled gas nitric oxide (NO), which is identical with or very similar to endogenous endothelium-derived relaxing factor, have shown it to be a very promising and specific pulmonary vasodilator. Multicenter clinical trials are currently under way to evaluate this new therapy. In addition, use of high frequency oscillatory ventilation has proved effective in many of these infants, particularly those with severe associated lung disease.

Infants for whom conventional therapy is failing (poor oxygenation despite maximum support) may require extracorporeal membrane oxygenation (ECMO). The infants are placed on bypass with blood exiting the baby from the right atrium and returning to the aortic arch after passing through a membrane oxygenator. The lungs are essentially at rest during the procedure, and with resolution of the pulmonary hypertension, the infants are weaned from ECMO back to conventional ventilator therapy. This therapy can save infants who might otherwise die but has major side effects that must be considered prior to its institution. Neurodevelopmental outcome among survivors of ECMO is similar to that of infants with persistent pulmonary hypertension managed without the procedure.

The ductus arteriosus is managed by medical or surgical ligation. A clinically significant ductus causing compromise in the infant can be closed with indomethacin (0.2 mg/kg) given intravenously. The schedule of three doses is dependent on the infant's age. In about two-thirds of the cases, indomethacin is successful in closing the ductus. If the ductus reopens, a second course of drug may be utilized. If indomethacin fails to close the ductus or if a ductus reopens a second time, surgical ligation should be pursued. In some cases, a more prolonged course of indomethacin is being utilized to prevent recurrences. The major side effect of indomethacin is a transient oliguria, which can be treated by fluid restriction until urine output improves. Indomethacin does not increase the incidence and severity of intracranial hemorrhage. The drug should not be used if the infant is hyperkalemic, if the creatinine is greater than 2 mg/dL, or if the platelet count is less than 50,000/µL.

Prognosis

The prognosis for the congenital heart lesions, which depends on the type of lesion, is reviewed in Chapter 21. With persistent pulmonary hypertension, the mortality rate remains approximately 10–15%. Long-term neurologic morbidity occurs in approximately 10% of survivors. Recently, an increased incidence of hearing loss has been identified following hyperventilation and alkalosis in this group of infants. The other major long-term morbidity is chronic lung disease secondary to the extensive ventilator support that many of these infants require.

Clyman RI: Indomethacin therapy for patent ductus arteriosus: When is prophylaxis not prophylactic? J Pediatr 1987;111:718.

Clyman RI: Medical treatment of patent ductus arteriosus. In: *Fetal and Neonatal Cardiology.* Long WA (editor). Saunders, 1990.

Cotton RB: The relationship of symptomatic patent ductus arteriosus to respiratory distress in premature newborn infants. Clin Perinatol 1987;14:621.

Gerstmann DR, deLemos RA, Clark RH: High-frequency ventilation: Issues of strategy. Clin Perinatol 1991;18:563.

Hammerman C, Aramburo MJ: Prolonged indomethacin treatment for the prevention of recurrences of patent ductus arteriosus. J Pediatr 1990;117:771.

Henricks-Munoz KD, Walton JP: Hearing loss in infants with persistent fetal circulation. Pediatrics 1988;81:650.

HiFO Study Group: Randomized study of high frequency

oscillatory ventilation in infants with severe respiratory distress syndrome. J Pediatr 1993;122:609.

Hofkosh D et al: Ten years of extracorporeal membrane oxygenation: Neurodevelopmental outcome. Pediatrics 1991;87:549.

Kelley SR, Bohn DJ: The use of inotropic and afterload-reducing agents in neonates. Clin Perinatol 1988;15: 467.

Kinsella JP et al: Clinical responses to prolonged treatment of persistent pulmonary hypertension of the newborn with low doses of inhaled nitric oxide. J Pediatr 1993; 123:103.

Long WA: Persistent pulmonary hypertension of the newborn syndrome. In: *Fetal and Neonatal Cardiology.* Long WA (editor). Saunders, 1990.

O'Rourke PP et al: Extracorporeal membrane oxygenation and conventional medical therapy in neonates with persistent pulmonary hypertension of the newborn: A prospective randomized study. Pediatrics 1989;84:957.

Roberts JD et al: Inhaled nitric oxide in persistent pulmonary hypertension of the newborn. Lancet 1992;340:818.

Schumacher RE et al: Follow-up of infants treated with extracorporeal membrane oxygenation for newborn respiratory failure. Pediatrics 1991;87:451.

Short BL et al: Extracorporeal membrane oxygenation on the management of respiratory failure in the newborn. Clin Perinatol 1987;14:737.

Snider AR: Two-dimensional and Doppler echocardiographic evaluation of heart disease in the neonate and fetus. Clin Perinatol 1988;15:523.

Walsh-Sukys MC: Persistent pulmonary hypertension of the newborn: The black box revisited. Clin Perinatol 1993; 20:127.

Wung J-T et al: Management of infants with severe respiratory failure and persistence of the fetal circulation, without hyperventilation. Pediatrics 1985;76:488.

Zahka KG, Spector M, Hanisch D : Hypoplastic left-heart syndrome: Norwood operation, transplantation, or compassionate care. Clin Perinatol 1993: 20:145.

JAUNDICE SECONDARY TO UNCONJUGATED HYPERBILIRUBINEMIA

Jaundice is a common neonatal problem, particularly in level 1 and 2 nurseries. Because many hospitals now implement early discharge policies, a proper approach is essential.

To understand neonatal jaundice, a brief description of the pathways of normal bilirubin metabolism is necessary. The normal destruction of circulating red cells accounts for about 75% of the newborn's daily bilirubin production. The remaining sources include ineffective erythropoiesis and tissue heme proteins. Heme is converted to bilirubin in the reticuloendothelial system. The lipid-soluble unconjugated bilirubin is transported bound to albumin, which enters the liver cells by dissociation from albumin in the hepatic sinusoids. Once in the liver cell, bilirubin is conjugated with glucuronic acid in a reaction catalyzed by glucuronyl transferase. The water-soluble conjugated bilirubin is secreted into the biliary tree for excretion via the gastrointestinal tract. The en-

zyme β-glucuronidase is present in the small bowel and hydrolyzes some of the conjugated bilirubin. This unconjugated bilirubin can then be reabsorbed into the circulation, adding to the total load of unconjugated bilirubin (enterohepatic circulation).

Diagnosis

Almost every newborn develops a serum unconjugated bilirubin of greater than 2 mg/dL (average of 5–7 mg/dL) during the first week of life. This transient hyperbilirubinemia has been called physiologic jaundice. Major predisposing factors are (1) increased bilirubin load due to increased red cell volume with decreased cell survival, increased ineffective erythropoiesis, and the enterohepatic circulation; and (2) low levels of glucuronyl transferase leading to slower hepatic conjugation of bilirubin.

The clinical manifestations of physiologic jaundice are as follows: (1) jaundice does not present on day 1; (2) total bilirubin rises by less than 5 mg/dL/d, peaking at less than 14–15 mg/dL on days 3–4; (3) the conjugated fraction is less than 2 mg/dL; and (4) jaundice persists no longer than 1 week in the term infant and 2 weeks in the preterm infant. If criteria for a diagnosis of physiologic jaundice are not met, the cause of the jaundice needs to be investigated. The routine minimum laboratory evaluation for hyperbilirubinemia in the first week of life should include a blood type and Coombs testing and a hematocrit. If jaundice persists after the first week of life, a conjugated bilirubin determination is indicated. Table 2–13 lists the differential diagnoses of pathologic jaundice in two categories: overproduction of bilirubin and decrease reate of bilirubin conjugation.

Bilirubin Toxicity

Unconjugated bilirubin can enter nerve cells and produce cell death, causing a clinical syndrome of kernicterus. Kernicterus is the staining of certain areas of the brain (basal ganglia and hippocampus predominantly) by bilirubin. The factors that appear to determine bilirubin toxicity include the level of serum bilirubin as well as the integrity of the blood-brain barrier. Severe kernicterus has a high mortality rate and in term infants is manifested by lethargy, refusal to feed, a high-pitched cry, hypertonicity, opisthotonos, seizures, and apnea. Survivors usually suffer sequelae, including athetoid cerebral palsy, high-frequency hearing loss, paralysis of upward gaze, and dental dysplasia. Fortunately, kernicterus is very rare with today's neonatal management in term and preterm infants. The risk of kernicterus in a given infant is not well defined. The only group in which a specific bilirubin level (20 mg/dL) has been associated with an increased risk of kernicterus is babies with Rh hemolytic disease. This observation has been extended to the management of other neonates with hemolytic disease, although no definitive data exist for these infants. The risk is likely negligible for term

Table 2–13. Etiology of jaundice secondary to unconjugated hyperbilirubinemia.

OVERPRODUCTION OF BILIRUBIN
1. Increased rate of hemolysis
   a. Patients with a positive Coombs test
      Rh incompatibility
      ABO incompatibility
      Other blood group sensitizations
   b. Patients with a negative Coombs test
      Abnormal red cell shapes
         Spherocytosis
         Elliptocytosis
         Pyknocytosis
         Stomatocytosis
      Red cell enzyme abnormalities
         Glucose 6-phosphate dehydrogenase deficiency
         Pyruvate kinase deficiency
         Hexokinase deficiency
         Other metabolic defects
   c. Patients with bacterial or viral sepsis
2. Nonhemolytic causes of increased bilirubin load:
Unconjugated bilirubin elevated, reticulocyte count normal.
   a. Extravascular hemorrhage
      Cephalhematoma
      Extensive bruising
      Central nervous system hemorrhage
   b. Polycythemia
   c. Exaggerated enterohepatic circulation of bilirubin
      Gastrointestinal tract obstruction
      Functional ileus
DECREASED RATE OF CONJUGATION
   (Unconjugated bilirubin elevated, reticulocyte count normal.)
   "Physiologic" jaundice
   Crigler-Najjar syndrome (type I glucuronyl transferase deficiency, autosomal recessive).
   Type II glucuronyl transferase deficiency, autosomal dominant.
   Gilbert's syndrome.
   ?Galactosemia.
   ?Hypothyroidism.

---

infants without hemolytic disease, even at levels as high as 25 mg/dL. Prematures of 32–38 weeks' gestation are probably safe up to levels of 20 mg/dL, but meaningful data for infants of less than 32 weeks of gestation are not available. Finally, auditory evoked potential studies have clearly identified a reversible entry of bilirubin into the central nervous system. The relevance of this finding to long-term outcome is unknown at this time.

Treatment

A. Phototherapy: Phototherapy is used most commonly, because it is relatively noninvasive and safe. Light at a wavelength absorbed by bilirubin (blue or white light) is used. The unconjugated bilirubin in the skin is converted to a water-soluble photoisomer excreted in bile, enhancing bilirubin excretion. Phototherapy is used in term and near term babies when bilirubin concentrations are still well below the level at which an exchange transfusion would be required (approximately 5 mg/dL below exchange level). In babies with hemolytic disease, phototherapy can be instituted earlier, at a level of 10 mg/dL on day 1 and 13 mg/dL on day 2. In very immature babies, many centers use phototherapy prophylactically. Alternatively, it may be begun at unconjugated bilirubin concentrations greater than 5 mg/dL. The use of phototherapy in this way has resulted in a decrease in the frequency of exchange transfusions for hyperbilirubinemia. However, no influence on neurologic or developmental outcome has been demonstrated. When phototherapy is used, the infant's eyes should be shielded and extra water provided to compensate for increased evaporative losses. Other side effects of phototherapy include loose stools secondary to more rapid intestinal transit, skin rashes, and problems with thermoregulation. Finally, any baby placed under phototherapy requires a history, physical examination, and screening laboratory evaluation for pathologic hyperbilirubinemia (blood type, direct and indirect Coombs, hematocrit, fractionated bilirubin).

B. Exchange Transfusions: This procedure is used as the definitive treatment when bilirubin concentrations are approaching toxic levels. As discussed above, it is difficult in most circumstances to specify a precise bilirubin level at which exchange transfusion should be performed. Term infants with erythroblastosis should be exchanged as the bilirubin level approaches 20 mg/dL. This level can also be extrapolated to the management of infants with other hemolytic diseases, though definitive data for this practice do not exist. Well term infants without hemolytic disease are probably safe with levels as high as 25–30 mg/dL. In well preterm infants of more than 32 weeks' gestational age, a level of 20 mg/dL can be used as an indication for exchange, whereas sick infants (including those with hemolytic disease) in this age range are usually exchanged at lower levels, ie, 15–18 mg/dL. In infants of less than 32 weeks' gestational age, exchange transfusions are performed for bilirubin levels of 10–15 mg/dL in most settings.

Ionized calcium levels should be followed when CPD blood is used because of the binding of calcium by citrate. Two-volume exchanges should be done; a blood volume of 80 mL/kg of body weight should be assumed. This procedure will replace more than 80% of the red cells and lower bilirubin concentrations substantially. The procedure is associated with significant mortality and morbidity rates, especially in the very immature infant. It should be carried out cautiously with full intensive care monitoring over a period of approximately 1–2 hours.

Exchange transfusions can be done in two other circumstances unrelated to the bilirubin level in the infant. The first is in the markedly hydropic erythroblastotic (Rh-sensitized) infant, in whom a partial exchange transfusion with packed red blood cells (approximately 35 mL/kg) may be carried out immediately after birth to correct anemia and adjust circulating blood volume and, thus, ease the high output failure. Fortunately, this indication is becoming rare because of better management of Rh-sensitized pregnancies, including direct intrauterine transfusion of severely sensitized infants.

The second indication for exchange transfusion not determined by bilirubin levels is in the severely sensitized erythroblastotic infant. A two-volume exchange is carried out as shortly after delivery as possible after stabilization. The purpose of this exchange is to remove affected red cells and replace them with Rh-negative donor cells. This procedure is very effective in preventing a need for multiple exchange transfusions; sensitized red cells are removed prior to hemolysis and the potential bilirubin load for the infant is thus reduced. Again, good obstetric management has decreased the need for the procedure. Severely affected infants will have had in utero transfusions; consequently, when they are born, the majority of their red cells are donor Rh-negative cells. If more than 50% of cells are already donor cells, the exchange transfusion immediately after birth is not indicated.

C. Protoporphyrins: The heme oxygenase inhibitor tin protoporphyrin has been used in animal models and some human studies to decrease bilirubin production. At this time, this remains an experimental therapy.

1. BREAST MILK JAUNDICE

The key features of this disease are (1) jaundice that peaks late (within the first 3 weeks, usually between 6 and 14 days), (2) a well baby who is thriving, and (3) a peak bilirubin of 12–20. The jaundice is secondary to unconjugated hyperbilirubinemia. Breast milk jaundice can be distinguished from jaundice due to other causes by the prompt reduction in bilirubin concentration that occurs when formula is substituted for breast milk over a 2- or 3-day period. Thereafter, breast milk feedings can usually be resumed without difficulty. This entity is to be distinguished from jaundice in the breast-fed infant during the first week of life. Breast-fed infants have higher bilirubins than formula-fed infants. This phenomenon is due to decreased intake over the first several days of life. The treatment is not to stop breast feeding but to increase the frequency of feedings.

2. ABO INCOMPATIBILITY

This incompatibility is most commonly seen in type O mothers with babies of type A or B. Naturally occurring IgG anti-A or anti-B in the mother crosses the placenta into the fetal circulation. The amount of these naturally occurring antibodies is variable; the disease picture is, therefore, also variable. This dis-

ease can be difficult to manage, because cord blood levels and early bilirubin levels provide no firm basis for predicting which infants will require therapy. These infants can have anemia with or without jaundice, jaundice with or without anemia, or neither. The peripheral smear (microspherocytes are indicative), a reticulocyte count, and a Coombs test (*Note:* direct Coombs may be negative, but indirect Coombs will be positive) identify infants at risk, but management relies on phototherapy and serial bilirubin measurements to identify the occasional infant in whom an exchange transfusion is required. Phototherapy in term infants should be started if the bilirubin level is greater than 10 mg/dL on day 1; if it is greater than 13 mg/dL on day 2; and if it is 15 mg/dL or more on day 3 and beyond. An exchange transfusion is performed for a level at or greater than 20 mg/dL. Finally, after hospital discharge these infants should have serial hematocrits because of the possibility of late anemia.

3. ERYTHROBLASTOSIS

Isoimmunization to Rh antigens (D, C, E, d, c, or e), Kell, Duffy, Lutheran, and Kidd may cause erythroblastosis. Most commonly, it is due to sensitization from D. The involved red cell antigen is always absent from the mother's red cells. Therefore, if fetal red cells enter the maternal circulation (usually at delivery), the mother produces antibody to the foreign antigen. The antibody (IgG) enters the fetal circulation, causing hemolysis. The process is usually worse in successive at-risk pregnancies.

Obstetric Management of Erythroblastosis

Serial antibody screening of Rh (D-negative) mothers is performed during pregnancy. Sensitization to other antigens can be detected by a single antibody screen (performed in all pregnant women). Significant sensitization to these other antigens is rare if the initial screen is negative. If the screen is positive, titers should be performed to assess significant sensitization.

Amniocentesis to measure bilirubin (ΔOD 450) by absorbance is done to assess severity of sensitization. Further obstetric management (eg, fetal transfusions) is based on this determination and on fetal hemoglobin determined by cordocentesis and evidence of hydrops fetalis on ultrasound.

Current obstetric practice aims at the prevention of this disease by passive immunization of pregnant women with high-titer $Rh_o(D)$ immune globulin. This is given to nonsensitized women during pregnancy as well as immediately after delivery. The $Rh_o(D)IgG$ is also given for invasive procedures during the pregnancy, such as chorionic villus biopsy and amniocentesis. An Rh-negative woman should also receive prophylaxis after any miscarriage or abortion.

Pediatric Management of Erythroblastosis

The key pediatric decisions relate to the following:

(1) The degree of cardiovascular and pulmonary compromise must be assessed. Where high output failure is severe, a partial exchange transfusion with packed red blood cells (35 mL/kg) for adjustment of blood volume and correction of anemia is used. Hydropic infants generally require ventilatory support, paracentesis of large volumes of ascitic fluid, and evacuation of pleural effusions, if present. Because many of these infants are delivered early, their course is also complicated by hyaline membrane disease.

(2) Where intrauterine transfusions have not been done (either intra-abdominally or directly into the umbilical vein), the immediate poststabilization period is used for a two-volume exchange transfusion to remove affected cells. Indications for this procedure are a cord blood hematocrit less than 40 or unconjugated bilirubin greater than 6 mg/dL (or both). This procedure is performed after initial cardiovascular and respiratory stabilization.

(3) Blood glucose concentration should be immediately supported (erythroblastotic infants have islet cell hyperplasia and are prone to hypoglycemia secondary to hyperinsulinemia), and water and electrolyte balance should be provided.

(4) The rate of rise of bilirubin concentrations should be graphically depicted to allow anticipation of the need for a two-volume exchange transfusion. An increase in serum bilirubin greater than 1.5 mg/dL per hour indicates the need for an exchange transfusion. This procedure is used in infants who did not have the initial early double volume exchange.

(5) Subsequent exchange transfusions are performed for bilirubins reaching a given infant's exchange level.

(6) Infants who have had repeated exchange transfusions should be followed closely for signs of coagulation disorders, severe anemia, or the development of a cholestatic syndrome.

(7) Recent data indicate that high-dose IVIG infusion may also be helpful in decreasing hemolysis by an unknown mechanism.

(8) All Rh-sensitized infants should be followed for development of late anemia following hospital discharge.

4. EXTRAVASCULAR HEMORRHAGE

Bleeding within the body (eg, cephalhematoma, bruising, central nervous system hemorrhage) may result in unconjugated hyperbilirubinemia by creating an extra bilirubin load for the liver. Peak of jaundice tends to be at 3–4 days of age.

5. GASTROINTESTINAL TRACT OBSTRUCTION

Either functional or structural obstruction of the gastrointestinal tract can result in unconjugated hyperbilirubinemia due to enhanced enterohepatic circulation of bilirubin.

6. PROLONGED UNCONJUGATED HYPERBILIRUBINEMIA

Causes of unconjugated hyperbilirubinemia after the first week of life are presented in Table 2–14.

Committee on Fetus and Newborn: Home phototherapy. Pediatrics 1985;76:136.

Maisels MJ: Light versus tin. Pediatrics 1988;81:882.

Maisels MJ: Jaundice. In: *Neonatology: Pathophysiology and Management of the Newborn,* 4th ed. Avery GB, Fletcher MA, MacDonald MG (editors). Lippincott, 1994.

McDonagh AF: Is bilirubin good for you? Clin Perinatol 1990;17:359.

National Institute of Child Health and Human Development: Randomized, controlled trial of phototherapy for neonatal hyperbilirubinemia. Pediatrics 1985;75 (Suppl): 381.

Newman TB et al: Laboratory evaluation of jaundiced newborns: Frequency, cost and yield. Am J Dis Child 1990; 144:364.

Newman TB, Maisels MJ: Does hyperbilirubinemia damage the brain of healthy full term infants? Clin Perinatol 1990;17:331.

Newman TB, Maisels MJ: Evaluation and treatment of jaundice in the term newborn: A kinder, gentler approach. Pediatrics 1992;89:809.

Perlman M, Frank JW: Bilirubin beyond the blood-brain barrier. Pediatrics 1988;81:304.

Poland RL, Ostrea EM: Neonatal hyperbilirubinemia. In: Klaus MH, Fanaroff AA (editors). *Care of the High-Risk Neonate,* 4th ed. Saunders, 1993.

Rubo J et al: High-dose intravenous immune globulin therapy for hyperbilirubinemia caused by Rh hemolytic disease. J Pediatr 1992;121:93.

Scheidt PC et al: Intelligence at 6 years in relation to neonatal bilirubin level: Follow-up of the National Institute of Child Health and Human Development trial of phototherapy. Pediatrics 1991;87:797.

Scheidt PC et al: Phototherapy for neonatal hyperbilirubinemia: Six-year follow-up of the National Institute of Child Health and Human Development trial. Pediatrics 1990; 85:455.

Seidman DS et al: Neonatal hyperbilirubinemia and physi-

Table 2–14. Causes of prolonged unconjugated hyperbilirubinemia.

1. Hemolytic jaundice
2. Breast milk jaundice
3. Crigler-Najjar syndrome
4. Gastrointestinal tract obstruction
5. Hypothyroidism (can produce either unconjugated or mixed hyperbilirubinemia)

cal and cognitive performance at 17 years of age. Pediatrics 1991;88:828.

Stevenson DK, Vremen HJ: SN-protoporphyrin: A consideration of the first clinical trial in human neonates. Pediatrics 1988;81:880.

Tan KL: Phototherapy for neonatal jaundice. Clin Perinatol 1991;18:423.

Watchko JF, Oski FA: Bilirubin 20 mg/dL = vigintiphobia. Pediatrics 1983;71:660.

Watchko JF, Oski FA: Kernicterus in preterm newborns: past, present, and future. Pediatrics 1992;90:707.

INFECTIONS OF THE NEWBORN

GENERAL APPROACH

The fetus and newborn infant are very susceptible to infections. There are three major routes of perinatal infection:

(1) Blood-borne transplacental infection of the fetus (eg, cytomegalovirus, rubella, syphilis).

(2) Ascending infection with a disruption of the barrier provided by the amniotic membranes (eg, bacterial infections after 12–18 hours of ruptured membranes).

(3) Infection upon passage through an infected birth canal or exposure to infected blood at delivery (eg, herpes simplex, hepatitis B, bacterial infections).

The susceptibility of the newborn is related to immaturity of both the cellular and humoral immune system at birth. This feature is particularly evident in the preterm neonate. Passive protection against some organisms is provided by transfer of IgG across the placenta during the third trimester of pregnancy. Preterm infants, especially those born at less than 30 weeks, do not have the benefit of the full amount of this passively acquired antibody.

Diagnosis

A. History: Maternal and obstetric histories are very important in the diagnosis of neonatal infections. The overall incidence of early onset (< 5 days) neonatal bacterial infection is 4–5:1000 live births. Rupture of membranes more than 24 hours prior to delivery is associated with an infection rate of 1:100, and rupture of membranes with chorioamnionitis with a rate of neonatal infection of 10:100. Irrespective of rupture of membranes, infection rates are five times higher in preterm infants. Other important historical points include immunization of the mother against rubella, a prior history of genital herpes, or viral illness around the time of delivery.

B. Symptoms and Signs: Early-onset bacterial infection is related to perinatal risk factors and presents most commonly on day 1 of life, with the majority of cases at less than 12 hours. Respiratory distress is the most common presenting sign. Other features include low Apgar scores without fetal distress, poor perfusion, and hypotension. Late-onset (presentation at > 5 days of age) bacterial infection presents in a more subtle manner, with poor feeding, lethargy, hypotonia, temperature instability, altered perfusion, new or increased oxygen requirement, and apnea. Signs suggestive of congenital viral infections include small size for gestational age, microcephaly, petechiae, jaundice, and hepatosplenomegaly.

C. Laboratory Findings: Low total white counts, absolute neutropenia (< 1000/μL), and elevated ratios of immature to mature neutrophils are suggestive of neonatal bacterial infection. Thrombocytopenia is also a common feature. Other laboratory aids are hyperglycemia with no change in glucose administration and unexplained metabolic acidosis. In early-onset bacterial infection, pneumonia is invariably present; chest x-ray films show infiltrates, but these infiltrates cannot be distinguished from infiltrates due to other causes of neonatal lung disease. Antigen detection in urine or other body fluids has been helpful in the rapid identification of some bacteria (especially group B streptococcus). Definitive diagnosis is made by positive cultures from blood, cerebrospinal fluid, etc. Serologies and cultures are useful in the diagnosis of congenital viral infections.

Treatment

A high index of suspicion is important in the diagnosis and treatment of neonatal infection. Table 2–15 presents some guidelines for the evaluation and management of *term* infants with risk factors or clinical signs of infection. Because the risk of infection is greater in the preterm infant and because respiratory disease is a common sign of infection, any preterm infant with respiratory disease requires blood cultures and broad-spectrum therapy for 48–72 hours pending the results of cultures. An examination of cerebrospinal fluid should be performed in those infants in whom infection is highly suspected on a clinical basis (eg, associated hypotension, persistent metabolic acidosis, neutropenia). Other specific therapy includes the administration of intravenous gamma globulin (500–750 mg/kg) to infants with known infection or clinical signs very suggestive of true infection. Granulocyte transfusions have been used in neutropenic patients and exchange transfusions performed in sick infants unresponsive to other therapies. In sick infants, the essentials of good supportive therapy should be provided: intravenous glucose and water, colloid volume support, use of pressors as needed, and oxygen and ventilator support.

Prognosis

The prognosis for neonatal infection depends on the specific agent and type of infection. This issue is addressed in the discussion of specific infections.

Table 2–15. Guidelines for evaluation of neonatal bacterial infection in the term infant.

Risk Factor	Clinical Signs[1]	Evaluation and Treatment
12–18 hours after rupture of membranes	None	Observation.
>12–18 hours after rupture of membranes, chorioamnionitis	None	CBC, blood cultures, broad-spectrum antibiotics for 48–72 hours.
> 12–18 hours after rupture of membranes, chorioamnionitis, maternal antibiotics	None	CBC, blood cultures, urine antigen test for group B streptococci, broad-spectrum antibiotics for 48–72 hours.
None or present	Present	CBC, blood and CSF culture, perhaps urine culture (see below); broad-spectrum antibiotics.[2]

[1]If clinical signs consistent with infection are absent, close observation without treatment may be sufficient.
[2]Irrespective of age at presentation, any infant who appears infected by clinical criteria should undergo CSF examination. Urine culture is indicated in the evaluation of infants who were initially well but have developed symptoms after 2–3 days of age.

SPECIFIC INFECTIONS

1. BACTERIAL SEPSIS

The most common organisms causing bacterial sepsis in the newborn are group B β-hemolytic streptococcus and gram-negative enterics (especially *E coli*). Other organisms to consider are *Staphylococcus aureus, Listeria monocytogenes, Enterococcus,* and *Staphylococcus epidermidis* (most common in infants with indwelling central venous lines). Early-onset bacterial sepsis is usually acquired in utero (ascending) or by passage through an infected birth canal. Late-onset bacterial sepsis is more often associated with infection of cerebrospinal fluid or other local infections (eg, osteomyelitis). Clinical signs, laboratory aids, and evaluation have been noted (see above and Table 2–15).

Antibiotic coverage should be directed initially towards suspected organisms. Early-onset sepsis is usually caused by group B streptococcus or gram-negative enterics; broad-spectrum coverage, therefore, should include ampicillin plus an aminoglycoside or third-generation cephalosporin. Specific doses and schedules are given in Chapter 34. Late-onset infections can also be caused by the same organisms, but coverage may need to be expanded to include staphylococci. In particular, the preterm infant with indwelling lines is at risk for *S epidermidis,* for which vancomycin is the drug of choice.

In the last several years, strategies for the prevention of bacterial infections in newborns have been de-

veloped. Intrapartum treatment with ampicillin or penicillin to colonized women with high-risk factors (eg, premature labor, prolonged rupture of membranes, or maternal fever) has proved effective in interrupting the transmission of group B streptococcal infections. In the nursery, administration of intravenous gamma globulin has been shown in some centers to decrease the incidence of late-onset sepsis in at-risk preterm infants.

2. FUNGAL SEPSIS

With more aggressive neonatal care associated with the survival of smaller infants, infection with *Candida* species has become more common. Infants of low birth weight with central lines who have had repeated exposures to broad-spectrum antibiotics are at highest risk. For infants less than 1500 g, colonization rates of 27% have been demonstrated, with many of these infants developing cutaneous lesions. A much smaller percentage develops systemic disease. Many infants with systemic candidiasis will have associated skin lesions. Other clinical features are indistinguishable from bacterial sepsis. Treatment is the antifungal amphotericin B. In addition, *Malassezia furfur* is also seen in infants with central lines receiving intravenous fat emulsion. To clear this organism, it is necessary to remove the inciting indwelling line.

3. MENINGITIS

Any newborn with bacterial sepsis is also at risk for meningitis. The incidence is low in infants with early-onset sepsis but is much higher in infants with late-onset infection. The workup for any infant with signs consistent with infection should include a spinal tap. Diagnosis is suggested by a protein greater than 250 mg/dL, glucose less than 30 mg/dL, more than 25 wbc/µL, and a positive Gram stain. The diagnosis is confirmed by culture. Most common organisms are group B streptococcus and gram-negative enterics. While sepsis can be treated with 10–14 days of antibiotics, meningitis should be treated for 21 days with appropriate antibiotics. The mortality rate for neonatal meningitis is approximately 25%, with significant neurologic morbidity present in one-third of the survivors. Use of dexamethasone has not been studied in neonates.

4. PNEUMONIA

The respiratory system can be infected in utero or upon passage through the birth canal. Early-onset neonatal infection is usually associated with pneumonia. Pneumonia should also be suspected in older neonates with a recent onset of tachypnea, retractions, and cyanosis. In infants already receiving respiratory support, an increase in oxygen requirement or ventilator settings may indicate pneumonia. Not only bacteria but also viruses (cytomegalovirus, respiratory syncytial virus, adenovirus, influenza, herpes simplex, parainfluenza), *Chlamydia,* and *Ureaplasma* can cause the disease. In infants with preexisting respiratory disease, intercurrent pulmonary infections may contribute to the ultimate severity of chronic lung disease.

5. URINARY TRACT INFECTION

Infection of the urine is uncommon with early-onset infection. Urinary tract infection in the newborn is seen most commonly in association with genitourinary anomalies and is caused by gram-negative enterics. Urine should be evaluated as part of the workup for late-onset infection. Culture should be obtained either by suprapubic aspiration or bladder catheterization. Antibiotic therapy is continued for 10–14 days intravenously. Subsequently, evaluation for genitourinary anomalies, starting with ultrasound examination and a voiding cystourethrogram, should be undertaken.

6. OSTEOMYELITIS

Osteomyelitis is an uncommon infection in the newborn. It is seen in association with late-onset septicemia, usually with *S aureus* or group B streptococcus. More detailed discussion of osteomyelitis can be found in Chapter 36.

7. OTITIS MEDIA

Otitis media may be present in a significant number of long-term nursery residents. It is particularly common in infants who have had prolonged endotracheal intubation. An evaluation for infection in such an infant is not complete without an ear examination. Gram-negative enterics are more common infecting agents in nursery residents than in outpatients.

8. OMPHALITIS

A normal umbilical cord stump will atrophy and separate at skin level. A small amount of purulent material at the base of the cord is common but can be minimized by keeping the cord open to air and cleaning the base with alcohol several times each day. The cord can become colonized with streptococci, staphylococci, or gram-negative organisms that can cause local infection. Infections are more common in cords manipulated for venous or arterial lines. Omphalitis is diagnosed when redness and edema are evident in the soft tissues around the stump. Local and systemic cultures should be obtained. Treatment is broad-spectrum intravenous antibiotics. Complications are determined by the degree of infection of the cord vessels and include septic thrombophlebitis, hepatic abscess, necrotizing fasciitis, and portal vein thrombosis.

9. CONGENITAL VIRAL & PARASITIC INFECTIONS
(See also Chapters 35 and 37.)

Cytomegalovirus

Cytomegalovirus (CMV) is the most common virus known to be transmitted in utero. The incidence of congenital infection ranges from 0.2–2.2% among live births. Transmission of CMV can take place as a consequence of either primary or reactivated infection in the mother. The mother is usually asymptomatic from her illness, but CMV should be suspected in the face of a heterophil negative mononucleosis-like illness. Primary infection in pregnancy is more common in high than low socioeconomic groups. An important source of infection is children (especially those in day care setting), who transmit the virus to parents and workers. The incidence of primary infection in pregnancy is 1–4%, with a 40% transmission rate to the fetus. Of these infants, 85–90% are asymptomatic at birth, whereas 10–15% have clinically apparent disease—hepatosplenomegaly, petechiae, small size for gestational age, direct hyperbilirubinemia, thrombocytopenia. The risk of neonatal disease is higher when the mother acquires the infection in the first half of pregnancy. The incidence of reactivated infection in pregnancy is less than 1%, with a 0–1% incidence of clinically apparent disease. Diagnosis in a suspected infant should be confirmed with culture of the virus (blood, cerebrospinal fluid, urine, throat, placenta, amniotic fluid). Pregnant caretakers should not take care of a child excreting CMV. Although experimental, ganciclovir has been used in some severely ill neonates, and a multicenter trial is ongoing.

The mortality rate in patients with symptomatic congenital CMV may be as high as 20%. Sequelae, including hearing loss, mental retardation, delayed motor development, chorioretinitis and optic atrophy, seizures, language delays, and learning disability, occur in 90% of symptomatic survivors. The incidence is 5–15% in asymptomatic infants; the most frequent finding is hearing loss.

Perinatal infection can also occur with acquisition of virus around the time of delivery. These infections are generally asymptomatic and without sequelae. Postnatal infection is usually asymptomatic but can cause hepatitis, pneumonitis, and neurologic illness in compromised seronegative prematures. The virus is usually acquired through transfusions, but the risk can be minimized by using frozen, washed red cells.

Rubella

Congenital rubella infection occurs as a result of rubella infection in the mother during pregnancy. The frequency of infection in the infant is as high as 80% in mothers infected during the first trimester. Infection rates then decline but increase again in the last month of pregnancy. A high incidence of defects can be attributed to infection acquired during the first trimester but declines with later infection. Clinical features of congenital rubella include adenopathy, bone radiolucencies, encephalitis, cardiac defects (pulmonary arterial hypoplasia and patent ductus arteriosus), cataracts, retinopathy, growth retardation, hepatosplenomegaly, thrombocytopenia, and purpura. The diagnosis should be suspected in cases of a characteristic clinical illness in the mother (rash, adenopathy, arthritis). Maternal illness can be confirmed with serologies. IgG titers in the infant can be compared to those in the mother, and specific IgM may be looked for in the baby. Diagnosis can be confirmed by culture of pharyngeal secretions.

There is no treatment for congenital rubella. Prevention, however, is possible with immunization. Nonimmune patients of childbearing age should be immunized prior to conception. Inadvertent immunization during pregnancy does not seem to carry a risk of causing significant illness in the fetus. Congenital rubella does cause significant, long-term sequelae, including mental retardation and hearing loss. Sequelae are most severe in infections acquired during the first trimester. Infants infected late in gestation do not suffer long-term sequelae.

Varicella

Congenital varicella is rare (5% after infection acquired during the first or second trimester) but does cause a recognizable constellation of findings, including limb hypoplasia, cutaneous scars, microcephaly, cortical atrophy, chorioretinitis, and cataracts. Perinatal exposure (5 days before to 2 days after delivery) can cause severe to fatal disseminated varicella. Diagnosis can be confirmed with a rise in maternal IgG titers, evidence of specific IgM in the neonate, or viral culture from vesicles. Prophylaxis and therapy are available for perinatal varicella. If maternal varicella develops within the perinatal risk period, 1.25 mL of varicella immune globulin should be given. If this has not been done, the illness can be treated with intravenous acyclovir. (See Chapter 35.)

Very premature infants (< 28 weeks' gestation) who are exposed postnatally should receive varicella immune globulin because of poor antibody transfer across the placenta early in pregnancy.

Toxoplasmosis

Toxoplasmosis is caused by the parasite *Toxoplasma gondii*. When infection occurs during pregnancy, up to 40% of the children become infected, of whom 15% have severe clinical damage. The means of acquisition include exposure to cat feces or ingestion of raw meat. Fetal damage is most likely to occur when the infection occurs in the second to sixth month of gestation. Clinical findings include growth retardation, chorioretinitis, seizures, jaundice, hydrocephalus, microcephaly, hepatosplenomegaly, adenopathy, cataracts, rash, thrombocytopenia, and pneumonia. The majority of affected infants are asymptomatic at birth but show evidence of damage (chorioretinitis, blindness, low IQ) at a later time. Serologies, first for IgG and then the specific IgM antibody, make the diagnosis.

10. PERINATALLY ACQUIRED VIRAL INFECTIONS (See also Chapter 38.)

Herpes Simplex

Herpes simplex infection is most commonly acquired at the time of birth with passage through an infected birth canal. A mother can have either a primary or a reactivated secondary infection. Primary maternal infection, due to both high titer of organism and no maternal antibodies, poses the greatest risk to the infant. The risk of neonatal infection with vaginal delivery in this setting is 30–40%. Seventy percent of mothers with primary herpes at the time of delivery are asymptomatic. They tend to be young and to deliver prematurely. Time of presentation of localized (skin, eye, mouth) or disseminated disease (pneumonia, shock, hepatitis) in the infant is usually 5–14 days of age. Central nervous system disease usually presents at 14–28 days of age with lethargy and seizures. In about one third of patients, localized skin, eye, and mouth disease is the first indication of infection. In another third, disseminated or central nervous system disease precedes skin, eye, and mouth findings, while the remaining third have disseminated or central nervous system disease in the absence of skin, eye, and mouth disease. Preliminary diagnosis can be made by scraping the base of a vesicle and finding multinucleated giant cells. Viral culture, usually positive in 24–72 hours, makes the definitive diagnosis. In some cases, newer polymerase chain reaction DNA technology may assist in diagnosis. Risk to the infant from secondary maternal infection is low (probably less than 1–2%).

Therapy for neonatal herpes is available with adenosine arabinoside or acyclovir. Acyclovir has fewer side effects and is the drug of choice. Both agents are effective in improving survival with central nervous system and disseminated disease and in preventing the spread of localized disease. Prevention is possible by not allowing delivery through an infected birth canal (eg, by cesarean section). However, antepartum cervical cultures are poor predictors of the presence of virus at the time of delivery. Furthermore, given the low incidence of infection in the newborn in secondary maternal infection (nil to 8%), cesarean section is not indicated for asymptomatic mothers with a history of herpes. In most settings, cesarean sections are still performed in mothers with active lesions (either primary or secondary) at the time of delivery. If there is a history of recurrent herpes in the mother, both mother (cervix) at delivery and infant (eye, oropharynx, umbilicus, rectum) 24 hours after delivery should be cultured. This should be done after vaginal delivery in an asymptomatic mother and after either vaginal or cesarean deliveries in mothers with active lesions. If the infant is colonized (positive cultures), treatment with acyclovir should be considered. In cases of documented primary infection at the time of delivery, the infant should be cultured and started on acyclovir pending the results of cultures. Neonates with documented herpes infection or a likely exposure should be managed with contact isolation. The major problem facing perinatologists is the high percentage of asymptomatic primary maternal infection. In those cases, infection in the neonate is currently not preventable. Therefore, any infant who presents at the right age with symptoms consistent with neonatal herpes should be cultured and started on acyclovir pending the results of those cultures.

Prognosis is good for localized skin and mucosal disease that does not progress. The mortality rate for both disseminated and central nervous system herpes is high, with significant rates of morbidity among survivors despite treatment.

Hepatitis B

Infants can be infected with hepatitis B at the time of birth. Clinical illness is rare in the neonatal period, but exposed infants are at risk to become chronic HBsAg carriers and to develop chronic active hepatitis and are at increased risk for hepatic carcinoma. The presence of HBsAg should be determined in all pregnant women. If the result is positive, the infant should receive hepatitis B immunoglobulin (HBIG) and hepatitis B vaccine as soon as possible after birth, followed by two subsequent vaccine doses at 1 and 6 months of age. If an HBsAg has not been sent prior to birth in a mother at risk, the test should be sent after delivery, and hepatitis B vaccine should be given within 12 hours of birth. If the mother is subsequently found to be positive, HBIG should be given as soon as possible (preferably within 48 hours, but not later than 1 week after birth). Subsequent vaccine doses should be given at 1 and 6 months of age. Recently, the Centers for Disease Control and Prevention and the American Academy of Pediatrics have recommended universal immunization of all newborns with hepatitis B vaccine at birth, at 1–2 months, and at 6–18 months. *Note:* In low-birth-weight infants, the initial vaccine should be given when the infant reaches a weight of 2000 g.

Enteroviral Infection

Enteroviral infections occur with greatest frequency in the late summer and early fall. Infection is usually acquired in the perinatal period. There is often a history of a maternal illness (fever, diarrhea, rash) in the week prior to delivery. The illness presents in the infant in the first 2 weeks of life. Most commonly, the illness is characterized by fevers, lethargy, irritability, diarrhea, and rash but is not severe. Other symptom complexes include meningoencephalitis and myocarditis, as well as a severe disseminated illness with hepatitis, pneumonia, shock, and disseminated intravascular coagulation. Diagnosis can be confirmed by culture (rectum, cerebrospinal fluid, blood). There is no therapy of proved efficacy. Prognosis is good for all symptom complexes except severe disseminated disease, which carries a high mortality rate.

HIV Infection

Human immunodeficiency virus (HIV) can pass transplacentally or be acquired at the time of delivery. The prevalence of HIV infection among women of childbearing age is 1.5:1000. Transmission of virus occurs in about 30% of births. Use of AZT during pregnancy may decrease the incidence of transmission. The risk of transmission is increased in mothers with low CD4 counts and p24 antigenemia and in infants born at less than 34 weeks of gestation. The longest documented incubation period prior to presentation of illness has been 7 years. However, the majority present within 2 years of birth. Diagnosis (discussed in detail in Chapter 38) is based upon clinical, immunologic, and serologic findings. The presence of maternal antibody acquired transplacentally confuses diagnosis in the neonate. An infant who is not infected should remain healthy, and the titer of antibody should decline during the first year of life. Techniques are being developed to allow earlier definitive diagnosis in newborns with an eye toward therapeutic intervention. Protocols are under way looking at treatment during pregnancy and prior to development of AIDS symptomatology in the infant.

Protection of health care workers is also an important issue to consider. Testing should be performed in the obstetric population at risk (intravenous drug abusers, those with multiple sexual partners). Because such testing will still fail to identify some infected patients, however, universal precautions should be used. Gloves should be worn during all procedures involving blood and blood-contaminated fluids, intubation, and any invasive procedures using needles. When a splash exposure is possible (eg, in the delivery room), a mask and eye covers should be used.

11. OTHER INFECTIONS

Congenital Syphilis

The infant is usually infected in utero by transplacental passage of the *Treponema pallidum*. Findings consistent with congenital syphilis include mucocutaneous lesions, lymphadenopathy, hepatitis, bony changes, and hydrops. However, in the newborn period, infants are most often asymptomatic, so that diagnosis is based on maternal and infant serologic testing and is only presumptive. A definitive diagnosis can be made on those rare occasions when the organism is identified by darkfield or pathologic examination. Guidelines for therapy are presented in Table 2–16. It is important to note that as of January 1988, owing to the difficulty in diagnosing silent neurosyphilis, the recommended therapy for all cases of congenital syphilis is 10 days of crystalline penicillin G or procaine penicillin G. A single dose of benzathine penicillin G is no longer felt to be acceptable therapy.

Tuberculosis

Congenital tuberculosis is rare (seen only in the infant of a mother with hematogenously spread tuberculosis). Women with pulmonary tuberculosis are not likely to infect the fetus until after delivery. Management is based upon the mother's situation:

(1) Mother with a positive skin test and negative chest x-ray—the mother is treated with isoniazid, and the infant is followed with skin tests.

(2) Mother with active disease—the mother should be separated from the infant until adequate treatment has been administered to render the mother noncontagious. The infant should be followed with skin tests.

Conjunctivitis

Neisseria gonorrhoeae may colonize an infant during passage through an infected birth canal. Gonococcal ophthalmitis presents at 3–7 days with very purulent conjunctivitis. Diagnosis can be suspected when gram-negative intracellular diplococci are seen on Gram's strain and confirmed by culture (see Chapter 36 for treatment). Current therapy is aimed at prophylaxis with silver nitrate drops or erythromycin ointment at birth.

Chlamydia trachomatis is another important cause of conjunctivitis, presenting at 5 days to several weeks of age with congestion, edema, and minimal discharge. The organism is acquired at birth after passage through an infected birth canal. Acquisition occurs in 50% of infants born to infected women, with a 25–50% risk of conjunctivitis. Prevalence in pregnancy is over 10% in some populations. Diagnosis is by isolation of the organism or by rapid antigen detection tests. Treatment is oral erythromycin. Topical treatment alone will not eradicate nasopharyngeal carriage, leaving the infant at risk for the development of pneumonitis. Diagnosis in the infant requires therapy of the mother and her sexual partners.

INFECTION CONTROL

The single most important principle in nursery infection control is good hand washing. Hands should be washed with a germicidal soap for 3 minutes prior to entering the nursery to handle patients. This procedure should be repeated between patient visits. Personnel with upper respiratory tract infections should

Table 2–16. Recommended treatment of congenital syphilis.[1]

Clinical Status	Antibiotic Therapy
Proved or Highly Probable Disease	
Age ≤ 4 weeks	Aqueous crystalline penicillin G, IV or IM, for 10–14 days.[2]
Age > 4 weeks	Aqueous crystalline penicillin G, IV or IM, for 10–14 days.[3]
Asymptomatic Infant With Normal Cerebrospinal Fluid and Radiographic Examinations	
Maternal treatment None, inadequate, undocumented, or with erythromycin	Aqueous crystalline penicillin G, IV or IM, for 10 days.[2,4]
Adequate therapy given in last month before delivery	Aqueous crystalline penicillin G, IV or IM, for 10 days,[2] or benzathine penicillin G, IM, as single dose.
Adequate therapy given > 1 month before delivery	Clinical and serologic follow-up only, *or–* If follow-up cannot be ensured, benzathine penicillin G, IM, as single dose, or aqueous crystalline penicillin G, IV or IM, for 10 days.[2]

[1]Reproduced, with permission, from the American Academy of Pediatrics: *Report of the Committee on Infectious Diseases,* 22nd ed. AAP, 1991.

[2]Some experts recommend aqueous procaine penicillin G, IM, for 10–14 days.

[3]For those with late (> 1 year of age) congenital syphilis in whom cerebrospinal fluid findings exclude neurosyphilis, some experts recommend benzathine penicillin G IM weekly for 3 weeks.

[4]Alternatively, for the infant for whom adequate maternal treatment cannot be documented, some experts recommend single-dose therapy with benzathine penicillin G.

wear masks; those with gastrointestinal tract infections must be rigorous about hand washing. Wounds or herpetic lesions should be covered.

An infected infant with a communicable disease (eg, viral respiratory infection or necrotizing enterocolitis) should be isolated. Ideally, the infant should be placed in a separate room, but if one is not available, a remote site in the nursery and perhaps an isolette should be used. The number of staff caring for the infant and their exposure to other infants should be limited. Gown, gloves, and mask should be worn as indicated for type of infection, and exposed materials should be disposed of separately.

Nursery staff should also take precautions against acquiring HIV infection. Newborns should be handled with gloves prior to initial bathing to remove blood. Gloves should be worn when drawing blood and starting intravenous therapy. Aspiration of meconium from an infant's airway should be performed with wall suction.

Alkalay AL et al: Fetal varicella syndrome. J Pediatr 1987; 111:320.

American Academy of Pediatrics, Committee on Infectious Diseases and Committee on Fetus and Newborn: Guidelines for prevention of Group B streptococcal (GBS) infection by chemoprophylaxis. Pediatrics 1992;90:775.

American Academy of Pediatrics, Committee on Infectious Diseases: Universal hepatitis B immunization. Pediatrics 1992;89:795.

American Academy of Pediatrics: *Guidelines for Perinatal Care.* American Academy of Pediatrics, 1992.

American Academy of Pediatrics: *Report of the Committee on Infectious Diseases.* American Academy of Pediatrics, 1991.

Arvin AM et al: Failure of antepartum maternal cultures to predict the infant's risk of exposure to herpes simplex virus at delivery. N Engl J Med 1986;315:796.

Baker CJ et al: Intravenous immunoglobulin for the prevention of nosocomial infection in low birth-weight neonates. N Engl J Med 1992;327:213.

Baley JE: Neonatal candidiasis: The current challenge. Clin Perinatol 1991;18:263.

Boyer KM, Gotoff SP: Antimicrobial prophylaxis of neonatal group B streptococcal sepsis. Clin Perinatol 1988;15:831.

Brown ZA et al: Effects on infants of a first episode of genital herpes during pregnancy. N Engl J Med 1987;317:1246.

Brown ZA et al: Neonatal herpes simplex virus infection in relation to asymptomatic maternal infection at the time of labor. N Engl J Med 1991;324:1247.

Burgard M et al: The use of viral culture and p24 antigen testing to diagnose human immunodeficiency virus infection in neonates. N Engl J Med 1992;327:1192.

Cassell GH et al: Perinatal mycoplasmal infections. Clin Perinatol 1991;18:241.

Conboy TJ et al: Early clinical manifestations and intellectual outcome in children with symptomatic congenital cytomegalovirus infection. J Pediatr 1987;111:343.

Fowler KB et al: The outcome of congenital cytomegalovirus infection in relation to maternal antibody status. N Engl J Med 1992;326:663.

Gibbs RS, Amstey MS, Lezotte DC: Role of Cesarean delivery in preventing neonatal herpes virus infection. JAMA 1993;270:94.

Hill HR: The role of intravenous immunoglobulin in the treatment and prevention of neonatal bacterial infection. Semin Perinatol 1991;15(Suppl 2):41.

Ikeda MK, Jenson HB: Evaluation and treatment of congenital syphilis. J Pediatr 1990;117:843.

Kliegman RM, Clapp DW: Rational principles for immunoglobulin prophylaxis and therapy of neonatal infections. Clin Perinatol 1991;18:303.

Kulhanjian JA et al: Identification of women at unsuspected risk of primary infection with HSV type 2 during pregnancy. N Engl J Med 1992;326:916.

Miles SA et al: Rapid serologic testing with immune-complex-dissociated HIV p24 antigen for early detection in neonates. N Engl J Med 1993;328:297.

Nicholas SW et al: Human immunodeficiency virus infection in childhood, adolescence, and pregnancy: A status report and national research agenda. Pediatrics 1989;83:293.

Pass RF et al: Young children as a probable source of maternal and congenital cytomegalovirus infection. N Engl J Med 1987;316:1366.

Pitt J: Perinatal human immunodeficiency virus infection. Clin Perinatol 1991;18:227.

Prober CG et al: Low risk of herpes simplex infections in neonates exposed to the virus at the time of vaginal delivery to mothers with recurrent genital herpes simplex virus infection. N Engl J Med 1987;316:240.

Prober CG et al: Use of routine viral cultures at delivery to identify neonates exposed to herpes simplex virus. N Engl J Med 1988;318:887.

Remington JS, Klein JO (editors): *Infectious Diseases of the Fetus and Newborn Infant,* 3rd ed. Saunders, 1989.

Risk factors for mother-to-child transmission of HIV-1. European Collaborative Study. Lancet 1992;339:1007.

Sever JL et al: Toxoplasmosis: Maternal and pediatric findings in 23,000 pregnancies. Pediatrics 1988;82:181.

St. Geme JW, Harris MG; Coagulase-negative staphylococcal infection in the neonate. Clin Perinatol 1991;18:281.

Task Force on Pediatric AIDS: Pediatric guidelines for infection control of human immunodeficiency virus (acquired immunodeficiency virus) in hospitals, medical offices, schools, and other settings. Pediatrics 1988;82:801.

Task Force on Pediatric AIDS: Perinatal human immunodeficiency virus (HIV) testing. Pediatrics 1992;89:791.

Toltzis P: Current issues in neonatal herpes simplex virus infection. Clin Perinatol 1991;18:193.

Weisman LE et al: Early onset group B streptococcal sepsis: A current assessment. J Pediatr 1992;121:428.

Whitley R et al: A controlled trial comparing vidarabine with acyclovir in neonatal herpes simplex virus infection. N Engl J Med 1991;324:444.

Whitley RJ: Neonatal herpes simplex virus infections. Clin Perinatol 1988;15:903.

Williamson WD et al: Asymptomatic congenital cytomegalovirus infection. Am J Dis Child 1990;144:1365.

GASTROINTESTINAL & ABDOMINAL SURGICAL CONDITIONS
(See also Chapter 22.)

CONGENITAL CONDITIONS

1. TRACHEOESOPHAGEAL FISTULA & ESOPHAGEAL ATRESIA

Diagnosis

These associated conditions are characterized by a blind esophageal pouch and a fistulous connection between either the proximal or distal esophagus and the airway. In 85% of infants with this condition, the fistula is between the distal esophagus and the airway. Polyhydramnios is common because of the high level of gastrointestinal obstruction. Infants present in the first hours of life with copious secretions, choking, cyanosis, and respiratory distress. Diagnosis can be confirmed with chest x-ray after careful placement of a nasogastric tube to the point at which resistance is met. On chest x-ray, the tube will be seen in the blind pouch. If a tracheoesophageal fistula is present to the distal esophagus, gas will be present in the abdomen.

Treatment

The tube in the proximal pouch should be placed on continuous suction to drain secretions and prevent aspiration. The head of the bed should be elevated to prevent reflux of gastric contents through the distal fistula into the lungs. Intravenous glucose and fluids should be provided and oxygen administered as needed. Definitive treatment is surgical and depends on the distance between the segments of esophagus. If the distance is not too great, the fistula can be ligated, gastrostomy (for feeding and decompression) performed, and the ends of the esophagus anastomosed. In instances where the end of the esophagus cannot be anastomosed, the initial surgery entails fistula ligation and a gastrostomy. Antibiotics are usually used postoperatively.

Prognosis

Prognosis is determined primarily by the presence or absence of associated anomalies. Vertebral, cardiac, renal, limb, and anal anomalies are also seen. Evaluation for other anomalies should be done early in the infant's course.

2. HIGH INTESTINAL OBSTRUCTION

Diagnosis

Infants with high intestinal obstruction present early with vomiting. A history of polyhydramnios is also common. In cases of duodenal atresia, vomitus may or may not contain bile; in cases of malrotation and midgut volvulus and high jejunal atresia, vomitus is bilious. Midgut volvulus is seen with malrotation and involves torsion of the intestine around the superior mesenteric artery that causes occlusion of the vascular supply of most of the small intestine. If not treated promptly, the infant can lose most of the small bowel to ischemic injury. Therefore, *bilious vomiting* in the neonate demands immediate attention and evaluation. Diagnosis of high intestinal obstruction can be confirmed with x-rays. Duodenal atresia is characterized by a double bubble sign (stomach and dilated duodenum). In cases of midgut volvulus, the plain abdominal x-ray may not be definitive. Occasionally, air is present, stopping at the level of the ligament of Treitz (level of obstruction). However, air can also be present elsewhere, precluding accurate diagnosis on plain film. Diagnosis can be confirmed with an upper gastrointestinal series to determine whether contrast material passes the ligament of Treitz.

Treatment

A nasogastric tube should be placed to suction for decompression, an intravenous needle should be placed for administering glucose and fluids, and supportive respiratory treatment should be given. The definitive treatment is surgery. Midgut volvulus is an indication for emergency surgery. Other conditions can be handled promptly but need not be done in an emergency fashion. Antibiotics are usually used for these conditions.

Prognosis

Duodenal atresia is associated with trisomy 21. Prognosis in that circumstance is related to other associated conditions (eg, cardiac). Infants with other high intestinal obstructions do well after surgical correction, except those with midgut volvulus who suffer loss of considerable amounts of ischemic small bowel.

3. DISTAL INTESTINAL OBSTRUCTION

Diagnosis

Low intestinal obstruction presents with an increasing intolerance of feedings (spitting progressing to vomiting), abdominal distention, and decreased or absent stooling. Imperforate anus should be diagnosed on initial physical examination prior to onset of symptoms. In the case of a high rectal atresia, however, the obstruction can be missed on the initial examination. Other diagnostic clues to imperforate anus include the presence of perineal fistulas with meconium or the presence of meconium in the urine (rectovesical fistula). Other causes of distal intestinal obstruction include meconium ileus, Hirschsprung's disease, meconium plug syndrome, small left colon syndrome, ileal atresia, and colonic atresia. Plain film of the abdomen shows gaseous distention with air through a considerable portion of the bowel and air-fluid levels. Diagnosis of meconium ileus, meconium plug, and small left colon syndrome can be made by appearance on contrast enema. In cases of meconium plug syndrome, osmotic contrast material (eg, meglumine diatrizoate [Gastrografin]) has a therapeutic as well as a diagnostic use: it induces passage of the plug. Rectal biopsy showing absence of ganglion cells confirms the diagnosis of Hirschsprung's disease.

Treatment

Nasogastric suction to decompress the abdomen, intravenous glucose, fluid and electrotype replacement, and respiratory support as necessary should be instituted. Antibiotics are usually indicated. The definitive treatment for all these conditions (with the exception of meconium plug syndrome and small left colon syndrome) is surgery.

Prognosis

Up to 10% of infants with meconium plug syndrome are found to have cystic fibrosis, whereas all infants with meconium ileus have cystic fibrosis. In addition, meconium plug syndrome is associated with Hirschsprung's disease. Small left colon syndrome is seen in infants of diabetic mothers. Once the child develops a normal stooling pattern, feedings will usually be tolerated and no further problems noted. Imperforate anus is associated (like tracheoesophageal fistula) with other anomalies—vertebral, renal, cardiac, limb. The other conditions usually carry an excellent prognosis after surgical repair.

4. ABDOMINAL WALL DEFECTS

Omphalocele

Omphaloceles are formed by the incomplete closure of the anterior abdominal wall after return of the midgut to the abdominal cavity. The size of the defect is variable, but usually the omphalocele sac contains some intestine, stomach, liver, and spleen. The abdominal cavity is small and underdeveloped. The umbilical cord can be seen to insert onto the center of the omphalocele sac. There is a high incidence of associated anomalies, including cardiac, other gastrointestinal anomalies, and chromosomal syndromes (trisomy 13). Acute treatment involves covering the defect with sterile warm saline to prevent fluid loss, nasogastric tube decompression, intravenous fluids and glucose, and antibiotics. If the abdominal contents will fit, a primary surgical closure is done. If not, a staged closure is performed, with gradual reduction of the omphalocele into the abdominal cavity and a secondary closure. Postoperatively, third-space fluid losses may be extensive; fluid and electrolyte therapy, therefore, must be carefully monitored.

Gastroschisis

Gastroschisis is a defect in the anterior abdominal wall *lateral* to the umbilicus; there is no covering sac, and the herniated viscera is usually limited to intestine. Furthermore, the intestine has been exposed to amniotic fluid and has a thickened, beefy-red appearance. The herniation is thought to occur as a rupture through an ischemic portion of the abdominal wall. Other than intestinal atresia, associated anomalies are uncommon. Therapy is as described for omphalocele; however, primary closures can be successfully performed more frequently.

Diaphragmatic Hernia

This congenital malformation consists of herniation of abdominal organs into the hemithorax (usually left) due to a posterolateral defect in the diaphragm. Infants usually present in the delivery room with respiratory distress, cyanosis, decreased breath sounds on the side of the hernia, and shift of the mediastinum to the side opposite the hernia. The infants are often difficult to resuscitate and require early intubation. The rapidity and severity of presentation with respiratory distress is dependent on the degree of pulmonary hypoplasia. The ipsilateral and, to some extent, the contralateral lung are compressed in utero due to the hernia. Treatment is to intubate and ventilate and to decompress the gastrointestinal tract with a nasogastric tube. An intravenous needle should be placed to administer fluids and glucose. A chest x-ray confirms the diagnosis. Surgery is performed after the infant is stabilized to remove abdominal contents from the thorax and to close the diaphragmatic defect. The postoperative course is often complicated by pulmonary hypertension. The mortality rate for this condition is 50%, with survival dependent on the degree of pulmonary hypoplasia in the contralateral lung.

NECROTIZING ENTEROCOLITIS

Necrotizing enterocolitis is the most common acquired gastrointestinal emergency in the newborn; it most often affects preterm infants. In term infants, it is seen in association with polycythemia, congenital heart disease, and birth asphyxia. The pathogenesis of the disease is multifactorial, related to previous intestinal ischemia, bacterial or viral infection, and immunologic immaturity of the gut. These three factors likely contribute to different degrees in different infants. Many infants have well-defined risk factors for gut ischemia (eg, asphyxia, difficult respiratory course, presence of an umbilical arterial line). However, in up to 20% of patients, no risk factors for gut ischemia are present. The role of infection is supported by the epidemic nature of the disease.

Diagnosis

The most common presenting sign is abdominal distention. Other signs include vomiting or increased gastric residuals, heme-positive stools, abdominal tenderness, temperature instability, increased apnea and bradycardia, decreased urine output, and poor perfusion. The complete blood count may show increased white blood cell count with an increased band count or, as the disease progresses, an absolute neutropenia. Thrombocytopenia is often seen along with stress-induced hyperglycemia and metabolic acidosis. Diagnosis is confirmed by the presence of pneumatosis intestinalis (air in the bowel wall) on x-ray. There is a spectrum of disease, and milder cases may exhibit only distention of bowel loops with bowel wall edema.

Prevention

Oral aminoglycosides and systemic antibiotics given prophylactically do not alter the incidence of necrotizing enterocolitis. Type of feedings and the method of advancing feedings also do not significantly alter the incidence of disease, although a delay in instituting feeds will delay the onset. The possibility that the administration of oral IgA may decrease the incidence of disease requires more detailed studies. Epidemics can be interrupted by careful measures to control infection.

Treatment

A. Medical Treatment:

1. Decompression of gut by nasogastric tube.

2. Maintenance of oxygenation; ventilation if necessary.

3. Intravenous fluids (colloid and normal saline) to replace third-space gastrointestinal losses. Enough fluid should be given to restore a good urine output.

4. Broad-spectrum antibiotics.

5. Close monitoring of vital signs, physical examination, laboratory data (blood gases, white blood cell count, platelet count, and x-rays).

B. Surgical Treatment: Indications for surgery are evidence of perforation (free air present on a left lateral decubitus film), a fixed dilated loop of bowel on serial x-rays, abdominal wall cellulitis, and progressive deterioration despite maximal medical support. All these signs are indicative of necrotic bowel. In surgery, necrotic bowel is removed and ostomies are created. Reanastomosis is performed after the disease is resolved and the infant is bigger (usually > 2 kg). Infants managed either medically or surgically should not be refed until the disease is resolved—normal abdominal examination, resolution of pneumato-

sis on x-ray—usually a time period of 10–14 days. Nutritional support during this time should be provided by total parenteral nutrition.

Prognosis

Death occurs in 10% of cases. Surgery is needed in less than 25% of cases. Long-term prognosis is determined by the amount of intestine lost. Infants with short bowel require long-term support with intravenous nutrition and, therefore, have very long hospitalizations. Even for those infants, however, the outcome is favorable because of improved parenteral nutrition formulations. Late strictures occur in 8% of patients whether treated medically or surgically about 3–6 weeks after initial diagnosis. Some of these strictures are severe enough to require surgical intervention.

PERFORATIONS OF THE GASTROINTESTINAL TRACT

Prenatal intestinal perforation causes sterile meconium peritonitis. The perforation most often occurs as a result of meconium ileus, but it can occur with intestinal atresia, volvulus, internal hernias, congenital peritoneal bands, intussception, and gastroschisis. Abdominal x-ray films reveal intraperitoneal calcifications. In most cases, surgical exploration is necessary.

Postnatal intestinal perforation most often occurs in association with necrotizing enterocolitis and causes bacterial peritonitis. Other causes include perforated peptic ulcers (associated with chronic steroid administration), Hirschsprung's disease, intestinal atresia, gastroschisis, and malrotation with volvulus. Left lateral decubitus abdominal plain films will demonstrate free air over the liver.

Gastric perforation in the newborn occurs most often during the first 5 days of life and is associated with perinatal stress. Perforation is associated with marked abdominal distention and massive pneumoperitoneum on abdominal x-ray.

Postnatal gastrointestinal perforation is a surgical emergency. Vigorous fluid and electrolyte resuscitation, nasogastric suction, and antibiotic coverage are necessary supportive measures.

THE MECONIUM PLUG SYNDROME

Low intestinal obstruction occurs on the second day of life. Little or no meconium is passed, and abdominal distention is followed by bile-stained vomiting and dehydration. On rectal examination, the anal canal may be abnormally small. Occasionally, after the rectal examination, the meconium plug may be passed with large amounts of gas and meconium.

In addition to air distention seen on x-ray film, fluid levels are observed in half of the patients. A contrast enema performed under low pressure with a soft-tipped catheter is not only diagnostic, because it reveals a change in the caliber of the colon at the site of obstruction, but can also be therapeutic in dislodging the meconium plug. The finding of a microcolon distal to the plug makes the differentiation from Hirschsprung's disease difficult. Indeed, 10–20% of neonates with meconium plug have Hirschsprung's disease (30–50% of male patients). Rectal biopsy may be necessary to rule out Hirschsprung's disease if bowel function does not normalize after passage of the meconium plug. The presence of a rubbery meconium plug sometimes indicates the presence of cystic fibrosis, but meconium obstruction of the terminal ileum is a more common problem.

SMALL LEFT COLON SYNDROME

This condition is most often seen in infants of diabetic mothers, infants delivered by cesarean section, premature infants, and twins. It presents with failure to pass meconium in the first 24–48 hours. Plain abdominal x-ray films show air-fluid levels and a dilated colon proximal to the splenic flexure. Meconium is easily evacuated with barium or meglumine diatrizoate (Gastrografin) enema, which is both therapeutic and diagnostic. The descending colon and rectosigmoid are narrow. Hirschsprung's disease must be ruled out, but the outlook for normal colon function is good. Immaturity of the neural plexus with self-limited abnormality of colon motor function may be the cause.

Eibl MM et al: Prevention of necrotizing enterocolitis in low-birth-weight infants by IgA-IgG feeding. N. Engl J Med 1988;319:1.

Emanuel B et al: Perforation of the gastrointestinal tract in infancy and childhood. Surg Gynecol Obstet 1978;146: 926.

Hendren WH, Lillahei CW: Pediatric surgery. N Engl J Med 1988;319:86.

Kliegman RM, Fanaroff AA: Necrotizing enterocolitis. N Engl J Med 1984;310:1093.

Kosloske AM, Musemeche CA: Necrotizing enterocolitis of the neonate. Clin Perinatol 1989;16:97.

McClead RE Jr (editor): Neonatal necrotizing enterocolitis: Current concepts and controversies. J Pediatr 1990; 117:S1.

McKeown RE: Role of delayed feeding and of feeding increments in necrotizing enterocolitis. J Pediatr 1992;121: 764.

Torfs C, Curry C, Roeper P: Gastroschisis. J Pediatr 1990; 116:1.

Vidyasagar D, Reyes H: Neonatal surgery. Clin Perinatol 1989;16:1.

HEMATOLOGIC DISORDERS
(See also Chapter 28.)

BLEEDING DISORDERS

Neonatal coagulation is discussed in detail elsewhere in the text. Bleeding in the newborn may result from inherited clotting deficiencies (eg, factor VIII deficiency) or acquired disorders—hemorrhagic disease of the newborn, disseminated intravascular coagulation (DIC), liver failure, and thrombocytopenia.

Hemorrhagic Disease of the Newborn

This disorder is due to the deficiency of the vitamin K-dependent clotting factors (II, VII, IX, X). Bleeding can occur on day 1 but usually occurs on day 2–3 in an otherwise well infant. Sites of bleeding include the gastrointestinal tract, umbilical cord, circumcision site, and nose. Bleeding from vitamin K deficiency is more likely to occur in infants of mothers taking anticonvulsants or sodium warfarin. Table 2–17 distinguishes clinical and laboratory features of hemorrhagic disease, DIC, and bleeding due to hepatic failure. Hemorrhagic disease of the newborn is treated by administering 1 mg of vitamin K. DIC and liver failure are treated by addressing the underlying condition and replacing clotting factors.

Table 2–17. Features of infants bleeding from hemorrhagic disease of the newborn (HDN), disseminated intravascular coagulation (DIC), or liver failures.

	HDN	DIC	Liver Failure
Clinical	Well infant; no prophylactic vitamin K	Sick infant; hypoxia, sepsis, etc	Sick infant; hepatitis, inborn errors of metabolism, shock liver
Bleeding	Gastrointestinal tract, umbilical cord, circumcision, nose	Generalized	Generalized
Onset	2–3 days	Any time	Any time
Platelet count	Normal	Decreased	Normal or decreased
Prothrombin time (PT)	Prolonged	Prolonged	Prolonged
Partial thromboplastin time (PTT)	Prolonged	Prolonged	Prolonged
Fibrinogen	Normal	Decreased	Decreased
Factor V	Normal	Decreased	Decreased

Thrombocytopenia

Neonatal thrombocytopenia can be isolated or occur in association with a deficiency of clotting factors (see Table 2–17). The differential diagnosis for thrombocytopenia with distinguishing clinical features is presented in Table 2–18. Treatment of neonatal thrombocytopenia is transfusion of platelets (10 mL/kg of platelets increases the platelet count by approximately 70,000/μL). Indication for transfusion in the term infant is clinical bleeding or a total count less than 10,000–20,000/μL. In the preterm infant at risk for intraventricular hemorrhage, transfusion is indicated for counts less than 40,000–50,000/μL. Isoimmune thrombocytopenia requires transfusion of maternal platelets. In infants born to mothers with idiopathic thrombocytopenic purpura, corticosteroids have improved platelet counts. Treatment with IVIG has also been successful, both antenatally and postnatally.

Anemia

Anemia can be caused by hemorrhage, hemolysis, or failure to produce red cells. Anemia presenting in the first 24–48 hours of life is due to hemorrhage or hemolysis. Hemorrhage can occur in utero (fetoplacental, fetomaternal, or twin-to-twin), perinatally (cord rupture, placenta previa, incision through placenta at cesarean section), or internally (intracranial hemorrhage, cephalohematoma, ruptured liver or

Table 2–18. Differential diagnosis of neonatal thrombocytopenia.

Disorder	Clinical Tips
Immune Passively acquired antibody: idiopathic thrombocytopenic purpura, systemic lupus erythematosus, drug-induced	Proper history, maternal thrombocytopenia
Isoimmune sensitization to PLA-1 antigen	Positive antiplatelet antibodies in baby's serum, sustained rise in platelets by transfusion of mother's platelets

Infections
  Bacterial
  Congenital viral infections
	Sick infants with other signs consistent with infections

Syndromes
  Absent radii
  Fanconi's anemia
	Congenital anomalies, associated pancytopenia

Disseminated intravascular coagulation (DIC)	Sick infants, abnormalities of clotting factors
Giant hemangioma	
Thrombosis	Hyperviscous infants, vascular catheters
High risk infant with respiratory distress syndrome, pulmonary hypertension, etc	Isolated decrease in platelets is not uncommon in sick infants even in the absence of DIC

spleen). When the bleeding has been of a chronic nature in utero (eg, fetomaternal), infants are pale at birth but well-compensated, without signs of volume loss. The initial hematocrit is low. Acute bleeding presents with signs of hypovolemia (tachycardia, poor perfusion, hypotension). The hematocrit initially may be normal or decreased but after several hours of equilibration will be decreased. Hemolysis is caused by blood group incompatibilities, enzyme/membrane abnormalities, infection, and DIC. Initial evaluation should include a review of the perinatal history, a determination of the infant's volume status, and a complete physical examination. A Kleihaur Betke test for fetal cells in the mother's circulation should be done on maternal blood. A complete blood count, blood smear, reticulocyte count, and a direct and indirect Coombs should be performed. This simple evaluation should suggest a diagnosis in most infants.

ANEMIA IN THE PREMATURE INFANT

In the premature, the hemoglobin reaches its nadir at approximately 6 weeks and is 2–3 g/dL lower than that in the term infant. The lower nadir in the premature appears to be the result of a decreased erythropoietin response to the low red cell mass. Symptoms of anemia include poor feeding, lethargy, increased heart rate, poor weight gain, and possibly apnea. The decision to transfuse is based on the presence of clinical symptoms. Transfusion is not indicated in an asymptomatic infant simply because of an arbitrary hematocrit number. Most infants become symptomatic as the hematocrit drops below 25%. Because of the observed role of depressed erythropoietin response to anemia in the premature, trials are under way assessing recombinant erythropoietin therapy (epoetin alfa) for this condition. Preliminary data indicate that 100 IU/kg of erythropoietin (epoetin alfa) given subcutaneously three times per week along with iron supplementation can decrease the need for transfusions in convalescing preterm infants.

Premature infants are also at risk for a vitamin E deficiency hemolytic anemia. The syndrome presents at 4–6 weeks with a hemoglobin of 7–10 mg/dL, an increased reticulocyte count, thrombocytosis, and pedal edema. Infants at risk for this syndrome are those who have received a diet high in polyunsaturated fats, supplemental iron, and no supplemental vitamin E. Prevention is possible through the administration of 25 IU of vitamin E per day, though current formulas for premature infants contain adequate vitamin E and sufficient polyunsaturated fats to usually avoid this problem.

Supplemental iron should be started in preterm infants at 2–4 months after birth to prevent iron deficiency anemia.

POLYCYTHEMIA

Elevated hematocrits occur in 2–5% of live births. Although 50% of polycythemic infants are appropriate for gestational age, the proportion of polycythemic infants is greater in the SGA and LGA populations. Causes of increased hematocrit include (1) twin-twin transfusion, (2) maternal-fetal transfusion, (3) intrapartum transfusion from the placenta, associated with fetal distress, and (4) chronic intrauterine hypoxia (SGA infants, LGA infants of diabetic mothers).

The consequence of polycythemia is hyperviscosity since the major factor influencing blood viscosity in infants is red cell mass. Hyperviscosity decreases effective perfusion of the capillary beds of the microcirculation. Clinical symptomatology can be related to any organ system (Table 2–19). Diagnostic screening can be done by measuring a capillary (heel stick) hematocrit. If the value is greater than 70%, a peripheral venous hematocrit should be measured. Values greater than 70% at less than 12 hours of age should be considered consistent with hyperviscosity. After 12 hours of age, values greater than 65% should be considered diagnostic.

Treatment for the acute symptoms is recommended for symptomatic infants. Treatment for asymptomatic infants based strictly on hematocrit is controversial. Definitive treatment is accomplished by an isovolemic partial exchange with 5% albumin. The amount to exchange (in milliliters) is calculated using the following formula:

$$\frac{[\text{PVH (\%)} - \text{DH (\%)}] \times \text{BV (mL/kg)} \times \text{Wt (kg)}}{\text{PVH (\%)}}$$

where PVH = peripheral venous hematocrit, DH = desired hematocrit, BV = blood volume, and Wt = weight.

Blood is withdrawn at a steady rate from an umbilical venous line while the replacement solution is infused at the same rate through a peripheral intravenous line over 30–40 minutes. Desired hematocrit value is 50–55%; assumed blood volume is 80 mL/kg.

Follow-up studies in infants with hyperviscosity show that at one and 2 years of age they demonstrate more motor problems, more abnormalities on neurologic examination, and more speech delays than do controls, with subtle deficits persisting through early school age. Partial exchange transfusions may slightly decrease the rate of neurologic sequelae, but the procedure does seem to increase the risk of necrotizing enterocolitis and other gastrointestinal symptoms acutely.

Andrew M, Kelton J: Neonatal thrombocytopenia. Clin Perinatol 1984;11:359.

Black VD et al: Neonatal hyperviscosity: Association with lower achievement and IQ scores at school age. Pediatrics 1989;83:662.

Black VD et al: Neonatal hyperviscosity: Randomized study of effect of partial plasma exchange transfusion on long-term outcome. Pediatrics 1985;75:1048.

Bussell JB et al: Antenatal treatment of neonatal alloimmune thrombocytopenia. N Engl J Med 1988;319:1374.

Carnielli V et al: Effect of high doses of human recombinant erythropoietin on the need for blood transfusions in preterm infants. J Pediatr 1992: 121:98.

Erslev AJ: Erythropoietin. N Engl J Med 1991;324:1339.

Gallagher PG, Ehrenkranz RA: Erythropoietin therapy for anemia of prematurity. Clin Perinatol 1993;20:167.

Halperin DS et al: Effects of recombinant human erythropoietin in infants with the anemia of prematurity: A pilot study. J. Pediatr 1990;116:779.

Keyes WG et al: Assessing the need for transfusion of premature infants and role of hematocrit, clinical signs, and erythropoietin level. Pediatrics 1989;84:808.

Lane PA, Hathaway WE: Vitamin K in infancy. J Pediatr 1985;106:351.

Massey GV et al: Intravenous immunoglobulin in treatment of neonatal isoimmune thrombocytopenia. J Pediatr 1987;111:133.

Ohls RK, Christensen RD: Recombinant erythropoietin compared with erythrocyte transfusion in the treatment of anemia of prematurity. J Pediatr 1991;119:781.

Pearson HA: Anemia in the newborn: A diagnostic approach and challenge. Semin Perinatol 1991;15(Suppl 2):2.

Ramamurthy RS, Berlanga M: Postnatal alteration in hematocrit and viscosity in normal and polycythemic infants. J Pediatr 1987;110:929.

Schmidt B et al: Neonatal thrombotic disease: Prevention, diagnosis, and treatment. J Pediatr 1988;113:407.

Shannon KM et al: Circulating erythroid progenitors in the anemia of prematurity. N Engl J Med 1987;317:728.

Wiswell TE et al: Neonatal polycythemia: Frequency of clinical manifestations and other associated findings. Pediatrics 1986;78:26.

Table 2–19. Organ-related symptoms of hyperviscosity.

Central nervous system	Irritability, jitteriness, seizures, lethargy
Cardiopulmonary	Respiratory distress, secondary to congestive heart failure, or persistent pulmonary hypertension
Gastrointestinal	Vomiting, heme-positive stools, distention, necrotizing enterocolitis
Renal	Decreased urinary output, renal vein thrombosis
Metabolic	Hypoglycemia
Hematologic	Hyperbilirubinemia, thrombocytopenia

METABOLIC DISORDERS

HYPOGLYCEMIA

The glucose concentration of the newborn infant at birth reflects maternal glucose concentration. The cord blood glucose concentration is approximately 15 mg/dL less than the maternal glucose concentration over a very wide range of maternal glucose concentrations. The cord blood glucose measurement is useful in all infants who are at risk for neonatal hypoglycemia: infants of diabetic mothers, SGA infants, erythroblastotic infants, and infants "stressed" by birth asphyxia, hypoxia, etc. The cord blood glucose allows a more precise interpretation of the first glucose concentration obtained in the nursery, because the clinician can then estimate the glucose clearance and arrive at a more precise estimate of the glucose intake required by the infant.

Glucose concentration normally decreases in all infants in the immediate postnatal period. Although a small number of term, normal newborns have glucose concentrations below 30–40 mg/dL, this phenomenon is quite rare; the range of 30–40 mg/dL is usually used for definition of hypoglycemia. By 3 hours of age, the glucose concentration in normal, term babies stabilizes between 50 and 80 mg/dL. After the first few hours of life, concentrations below 40 mg/dL should be considered abnormal.

The two most commonly encountered groups of newborn infants at high risk for neonatal hypoglycemia are infants of diabetic mothers (IDM) and infants with intrauterine growth retardation (IUGR).

Infant of a Diabetic Mother

The IDM baby represents an example of an infant with abundant carbon stores in the form of glycogen and fat who develops hypoglycemia because of an imbalance in insulin-glucagon secretion due to hyperinsulinemia from islet cell hyperplasia. In addition, there are other tissue sites that grow abnormally in utero, probably as a consequence of increased flow of nutrients (carbohydrates, amino acids, and fats) from the maternal circulation. The result is a macrosomic infant who is at increased risk for trauma (bruising, fractures, nerve root injuries, etc) during delivery. Other problems related to the in utero metabolic environment include a cardiomyopathy (asymmetric septal hypertrophy), which can present either as cardiac failure or as respiratory distress, and, more rarely, microcolon, which presents as a low intestinal obstruction. IDMs are also at increased risk for congenital anomalies likely related to first-trimester glucose control. Other neonatal problems include a hypercoagulable state and an increased risk for poly-cythemia, a combination that predisposes the infant to large venous thromboses. Finally, these infants are somewhat immature for their gestational age and are at increased risk for hyaline membrane disease, hypocalcemia, and hyperbilirubinemia.

Intrauterine Growth Retardation

The infant with intrauterine growth retardation (IUGR) has very little carbon stores in the form of glycogen and body fat and, therefore, is prone to hypoglycemia despite relatively appropriate endocrine adjustments to birth. In addition to problems with hypoglycemia (particularly in the very preterm SGA infant), marked hyperglycemia and a transient diabetes mellitus-like syndrome occasionally may develop. These problems can usually be handled by adjusting glucose intake, although insulin is sometimes needed transiently.

Other Causes of Hypoglycemia

In addition, hypoglycemia can be found with other disorders associated with islet cell hyperplasia (Beckwith's syndrome [macroglossia, omphalocele, macrosomia], erythroblastosis fetalis, nesidioblastosis), inborn errors of metabolism (leucine sensitivity, glycogen storage disease, and galactosemia), and endocrine disorders (panhypopituitarism and other deficiencies of counterregulatory hormones). It may also occur as a complication of birth asphyxia, hypoxia secondary to cardiorespiratory disease, or other stresses, including bacterial and viral sepsis.

Diagnosis

Infants can present with a variety of clinical signs of neonatal hypoglycemia. Unfortunately, they are relatively nonspecific and are usually quite mild, including lethargy, irritability, poor feeding, and regurgitation. More severe symptoms are cardiorespiratory distress, apnea, and seizures. As the symptoms become more severe, one may find more signs associated with catecholamine release, including pallor, sweating, cool extremities, and an increased heart rate. Cardiac failure has been found when hypoglycemia has been severe, particularly in IDM babies with a cardiomyopathy. Infants with hyperinsulinemic states can also experience the onset of hypoglycemia very early (within the first 30–60 minutes of life).

Glucose concentration can be measured by one of the commercially available screening techniques that rely on a test strip method done on a drop of peripheral blood obtained by heel stick. All infants at risk should be screened, including IDMs who are not macrosomic and whose mothers have maintained good control of diabetes. In addition, all low or borderline values should be supplemented by direct measurement of blood glucose concentration determined with a glucose analyzer. There is far too great a variance in results obtained by the test strip methods to rely upon these alone in following the high-risk groups. It is important to continue surveillance of glucose concentration until the baby has been on full milk feedings for a 24-hour period. Relapse of hypoglycemia thereafter is very unlikely, but milk feedings constitute a low-glucose, high-fat intake; therefore, babies moving to full milk feedings are sustaining glucose concentration by a relatively high rate of gluconeogenesis. Because it is not certain that individual infants in the high-risk groups are capable of sustaining such a rate of gluconeogenesis, glucose surveillance must continue in this weaning period.

Infants with persistent hypoglycemia requiring intravenous glucose infusions for more than 5 days should be evaluated for less common causes of hypoglycemia. This workup should include evaluation for inborn errors of metabolism, hyperinsulinemic states, and deficiencies of counterregulatory hormones.

Treatment

Therapy is based on provision of glucose either enterally or intravenously. Suggested guidelines for treatment are presented in Table 2–20. It is also important to note that in hyperinsulinemic states rapid boluses of glucose are to be avoided. After initial correction with a bolus of $D_{10}W$, 2 mL/kg, glucose infusion should be gradually increased as needed from a starting rate of 6 mg/kg/min. Finally, in both IDM and SGA babies, those with high hematocrits and hypoglycemia are most likely to show clinical signs of hypoglycemia. In such infants, both the hypoglycemia and polycythemia should be treated.

Table 2–20. Hypoglycemia: suggested therapeutic regimens.

Screening Test	Presence of Symptoms	Action
Test strip 20–40 mg/dL	None	Confirm with blood glucose; if the infant is alert and vigorous, feed; follow with frequent test strips. If the baby continues after 1 or 2 feeds to have test strips < 40 mg/dL, provide intravenous glucose at 6 mg/kg/min.
Test strip < 40 mg/dL	Present	Confirm with blood glucose; provide bolus[1] of 10% dextrose in water ($D_{10}W$) followed by an infusion of 6 mg/kg/min.
Test strip < 20 mg/dL	None or present	Confirm with blood glucose; provide bolus[1] of $D_{10}W$ followed by an infusion of 6 mg/kg/min. If IV access cannot be obtained immediately, an umbilical venous line should be utilized.

Prognosis

Prognosis of hypoglycemia is good if therapy is prompt. Central nervous system sequelae are seen in infants with neonatal seizures due to hypoglycemia.

HYPERGLYCEMIA

Hyperglycemia may develop in preterm infants, particularly those of very low birth weight who are also SGA. Glucose concentrations may exceed 200–250 mg/dL, particularly in the first few weeks of life. This transient diabetes-like syndrome usually lasts approximately 1–2 weeks. Management may include simply reducing glucose intake while continuing to provide supplemental calories with intravenous amino acids and lipids, coupled with small milk feedings by gavage. Insulin infusions intravenously have also been used to permit a larger intravenous glucose intake without hyperglycemia. This is usually reserved for those infants in whom it has not been possible to begin any gavage milk feedings and in whom caloric intake in the form of amino acids and lipids is small. However, this approach requires careful monitoring of blood glucose concentrations directly. The errors in estimation of blood sugar using screening techniques are far too large to avoid significant hypoglycemic episodes. Since the problem is a transient one, it is usually possible to maintain adequate intake with intermittent gavage feedings plus peripheral alimentation without resorting to intravenous insulin administration.

Binder ND et al: Insulin infusion with parenteral nutrition in extremely low birth weight infants with hyperglycemia. J Pediatr 1989;114:223.

Collins et al: Insulin infusion and parenteral nutrition in low birth weight infants with glucose intolerance. J Pediatr 1991;118:921.

Conrad PD et al: Clinical application of a new glucose analyzer in the neonatal intensive care unit: Comparison with other methods. J Pediatr 1989;114:281.

Lucas A et al: Adverse neurodevelopmental outcome of moderate neonatal hypoglycemia. Br Med J 1988;297:1304.

Ogata ES: Carbohydrate homeostasis. In: Neonatology: Pathophsiology and Management of the Newborn. 4th ed. Avery GB, Flatcher MR, MacDonald MG (editors) Lippincott, 1994.

Pildes RS, Pyati S: Hypoglycemia and hyperglycemia in < 1000 gm infants. Clin Perinatol 1986;13:351.

Pildes RS: Neonatal hyperglycemia. J Pediatr 1986;109:905.

Srinivasan G et al: Plasma glucose values in normal neonates: A new look. J Pediatr 1986;109:114.

HYPOCALCEMIA

Calcium concentration in the immediate newborn period decreases in all newborn infants. The concentration in fetal plasma is higher than that of the neonate or adult. Hypocalcemia is usually defined as a total serum concentration less than 7–8 mg/dL (equivalent to a calcium activity of 3–3.5 meq/L). In general, the higher range of 8 mg/dL is used as a cutoff for term infants and the lower of 7 mg/dL in preterm infants. In most circumstances, it is useful to measure the physiologically important ionized fraction of calcium, since this is frequently normal even in the face of a low total calcium. An ionized calcium of greater than 0.9 mmol/L (1.8 meq/L; 3.6 mg/dL) is not likely to be detrimental in any way.

Diagnosis

The clinical signs of hypocalcemia and hypocalcemic tetany include a high-pitched cry, jitteriness, tremulousness (repetitive movement of the peripheral muscles), and seizures. ECG signs are primarily directed at recognition of an increased QT interval.

Hypocalcemia tends to occur at two different times in the neonatal period. The first peak occurs during the first 2 days of life, and the second toward the end of the first or early in the second week of life. Early-onset hypocalcemia has been associated with infants of diabetic mothers, sepsis of the newborn, perinatal asphyxia, prematurity, and maternal hyperparathyroidism. Late-onset hypocalcemia has been reported in children receiving modified cow's milk, which has a high content of phosphorus. Mothers in third-world countries often suffer from vitamin D deficiency, which can also contribute to late-onset hypocalcemia.

Treatment

A. Oral Calcium Therapy: The oral administration of calcium salts is a preferred method of treatment because it avoids the potential complications of a slough from calcium solutions that infiltrate subcutaneously. In most infants with early-onset hypocalcemia who do not have frank tetany or seizures, oral administration can be successfully carried out. Calcium in the form of calcium gluconate can be given either as a dilute solution or added to formula feedings several times a day. A dose of 0.5–1 g/kg/d provides approximately 45–90 mg of elemental calcium per kilogram per day. If a 10% solution of calcium gluconate is used, the dose is 5–10 mL/kg/d given in divided doses every 4 or every 6 hours.

B. Intravenous Calcium Therapy: Intravenous calcium therapy is usually needed for infants with frank "tetany of the newborn" and certainly for infants with seizures associated with hypocalcemia. A number of precautions must be observed when calcium gluconate is given intravenously. The infusion must be given slowly, and it is helpful to dilute with an equal volume of 5% glucose. The infusion is administered slowly so that there is no sudden increase in calcium concentration in blood entering the right atrium, which would otherwise cause severe bradycardia and even cardiac arrest. Furthermore, the clinician must observe very carefully and terminate infu-

sion if there is any infiltrate of the intravenous infusions: calcium in the soft tissues can cause a necrosis of the skin and underlying tissues. The intravenous administration of 10% calcium gluconate is usually given as a bolus of 100–200 mg/kg over approximately 10–20 minutes, followed by a continuous infusion (0.5–1 gm/kg/d) that is slowly tapered over a number of days. Recent evidence suggests that 10% calcium chloride (35–70 mg/kg/dose) results in a larger increment in ionized calcium and greater improvement in mean arterial blood pressure in sick hypocalcemic infants and thus may have a role in the newborn. (*Note:* Calcium salts cannot be added to intravenous solutions that contain sodium bicarbonate because they precipitate as calcium carbonate.)

Prognosis

The prognosis is good for neonatal seizures entirely caused by hypocalcemia that is promptly treated.

Broner CW et al: A prospective, randomized, double-blind comparison of calcium chloride and calcium gluconate therapies for hypocalcemia in critically ill children. J Pediatr 1990;117:986.

Itani O, Tsang RC: Calcium, phosphorus, and magnesium in the newborn: Pathophysiology and management. In: Hay WW (editor). *Neonatal Nutrition and Metabolism.* Mosby, 1991.

Longhead JL et al: Serum ionized calcium concentrations in normal neonates. Am J Dis Child 1988;142:516.

Lynch RE: Ionized calcium: pediatric perspective. Pediatr Clin North Am 1990;37:373.

Venkataraman PS et al: Early neonatal hypocalcemia in very low birth weight infants: High incidence, early onset and refractoriness to supraphysiologic doses of 1,25-dihydroxyvitamin D_3. Am J Dis Child 1986;140:1004.

INFANTS OF MOTHERS WHO ABUSE DRUGS

The problem of newborn infants born to mothers abusing drugs is increasing in all parts of the country. The most common forms of abuse include smoking and its repercussions upon fetal growth and alcohol, marihuana, narcotic, and cocaine abuse. Because these mothers frequently abuse many drugs during pregnancy, it is often difficult to pinpoint which drug may be causing the morbidity seen in a newborn infant. In addition, the history of drug abuse is unreliable.

NARCOTICS

Diagnosis

The withdrawal signs in infants born to mothers who are addicted to heroin or who have been on maintenance methadone programs are similar. Clinical manifestations begin early, usually within the first day or two of life. Symptoms are quite characteristic: irritability and hyperactivity, increased tremors, a high-pitched cry, excessive hunger and salivation, sweating, yawning, sneezing, nasal stuffiness, fist sucking, temperature instability, and regurgitation. More severely affected infants may have seizures, vomiting, and diarrhea, as well as respiratory distress in the form of tachypnea. The clinical picture characterized by excessive activity and irritability is typical enough to suggest a diagnosis even if the maternal history of drug abuse has not been obtained. The infants are often small for gestational age. Confirmation should be attempted with urine toxicology, but results will be negative unless the last drug dose was within a few days of delivery. The clinical findings in infants born to methadone-maintained mothers seem to be, if anything, more severe and prolonged.

Treatment

Careful observation of the infant is a requirement. Supportive treatment includes swaddling the infant and providing a quiet, low-light environment. In general, specific treatment should be avoided unless the symptoms and morbidity in the infant warrant it. There is no single drug that has been uniformly effective, and the first choice varies among nurseries. The drugs that have been used include phenobarbital at an initial loading dose of 15–20 mg/kg intramuscularly, followed by a maintenance dose of 5 mg/kg/d in two divided doses usually given orally. Paregoric and diazepam have also been used, although these authors prefer phenobarbital because of its safety and predictability of effect. Phenobarbital blood levels should be obtained in the more severely affected infants to ensure that the concentration of the drug remains within the therapeutic range. The treatment can then be tapered over some days, although some treatment may be necessary for weeks following delivery. Both handling and procedures in the nursery should be kept to a minimum. As an alternative, methadone has been used, particularly in the babies born to methadone-maintained mothers.

Prognosis

The prognosis is reasonably good in the immediate newborn period, although there is still a mortality rate in the more severe cases. Careful evaluation of the family situation must be made in each case. The long-term outcome in these children has not been encouraging, although it is not clear that the effects of the drug or drug withdrawal are directly responsible. Rather, the disorganized family and social situation in which drug abuse occurs is thought to play a greater role.

Infants of narcotic abusers have an increased risk of sudden infant death syndrome.

ALCOHOL

Diagnosis

Alcohol abuse, a common problem in the United States, unfortunately occurs in teenagers as well as in older women. The effects on the fetus and newborn are roughly proportionate to the degree of ethanol abuse. Fetal growth and development are adversely affected (intrauterine growth retardation and various dysmorphic features), and infants suffer withdrawal similar to that caused by narcotic abuse. The dysmorphic features include intrauterine growth retardation, short palpebral fissures, microcephaly, and a variety of anomalies, including cardiac anomalies and joint defects. The quoted congenital anomaly rate based on an alcohol intake equivalent to the consumption of two mixed drinks per day is 10%, rising to as high as 40% with much larger alcohol intakes per day.

Treatment

In addition to management of withdrawal, which should follow the treatment prescribed for narcotic withdrawal, it is imperative that the mother be encouraged to enter a program designed to cope with alcoholism. The infants themselves also commonly have the typical problems of infants who are small for gestational age, ie, hypoglycemia, polycythemia, and difficulty in maintaining body temperature.

Prognosis

The postnatal growth of infants with fetal alcohol syndrome has been shown to be delayed. There is evidence of significant mental retardation in those most severely affected and hyperactivity, which contributes to school problems.

TOBACCO SMOKING

Smoking has been shown to have a significant impact on the growth rate of the fetus. The more the mother smokes, the greater the degree of intrauterine growth retardation. This is the only well-established complication of maternal smoking, and, of course, there is no treatment other than that prescribed for problems of IUGR infants in general. Prevention by education of expectant mothers is the key. Some studies have suggested an increase in obstetric complications such as abruptio placentae, placenta previa, and prematurity, although those issues remain controversial. It is important to recognize that multiple drug abuse applies to this category as well; that is, smokers tend to use alcohol and caffeine more than nonsmokers, and the potential interaction of these three factors on fetal growth and development must be considered.

COCAINE

Cocaine abuse is a growing problem in medicine. Its use has increased greatly; moreover, cocaine is often used in association with other drugs. Specific consequences of cocaine abuse are not yet well defined, but a number of associations have been noted. The most catastrophic effects include abruptio placentae in the mother and central nervous system infarcts in the baby. Other described complications include premature labor, intrauterine growth retardation, anomalies of the genitourinary system, and irritability of the central nervous system. In the presence of a maternal history of cocaine, a toxicology screen on the infant should be done, and the infant should be observed closely for drug effect and neurologic signs suggestive of an infarct (eg, seizures). Urine toxicology screens are indicative of recent drug abuse. Recently, analysis of meconium has been utilized to document cocaine use well prior to delivery. As with the abuse of any drug, it is important to evaluate the social situation and the ability of parents to care for the child properly on discharge from the hospital.

OTHER DRUGS

There are two categories under which drugs and their effects on the newborn should be considered. In the first category are drugs to which the fetus is exposed because of exposure to the mother. Many times, these are drugs prescribed for therapy of maternal conditions. The human placenta is relatively permeable, particularly to lipophilic solutes. Thus, most drugs cross the placenta fairly rapidly. The effects on the fetus depend on the drug used. General anesthetics by and large cross the placenta rapidly, and if effective anesthesia is achieved in the mother, the baby will, in fact, be anesthetized and show these effects at birth. Generally, however, the anesthesia does not present much of a management problem if it is recognized. The babies are sleepy but recover quickly as the drug is excreted.

In the second category are drugs that the infant acquires from the mother during breast feeding. Generally, most drugs taken by the mother either inadvertently or for therapy achieve appreciable concentrations in breast milk. In most instances, however, they do not present a problem to the infant. If the drug is one that could have adverse effects on the baby, timing breast feeding to coincide with trough concentrations in the mother may be useful.

American Academy of Pediatrics, Committee on Substance Abuse: Drug-exposed infants. Pediatrics 1990;86:639.

Chasnoff IJ (editor): Chemical dependency and pregnancy. Clin Perinatol 1991;18:1.

Chasnoff IJ et al: Temporal patterns of cocaine use in pregnancy. JAMA 1989;261:1741.

Clarren SK, Smith DW: The fetal alcohol syndrome. N Engl J Med 1978;298:1063.

Doberczak TM et al: Neonatal neurologic and electroencephalographic effects of intrauterine cocaine exposure. J Pediatr 1988;113:354.

Frank DA: Cocaine use during pregnancy: Prevalence and correlates. Pediatrics 1988;82:888.

Ostrea EM, Welch RA: Detection of prenatal drug exposure in the pregnant woman and her newborn infant. Clin Perinatol 1991;18:629.

Zuckerman B et al: Effects of maternal marijuana and cocaine use on fetal growth. N Engl J Med 1989;320:762.

RENAL DISORDERS

Renal function is dependent on postconceptual age. The glomerular filtration rate (GFR) is 20 mL/min/1.73 m^2 in term neonates and 10–13 mL/min/1.73 m^2 in infants 28–30 weeks of gestation. The velocity of maturation after birth is also dependent on postconceptual age. Creatinine can be used as a clinical marker of GFR. Values over the first month of life are shown in Table 2–21. The ability to concentrate urine and retain sodium is also dependent on gestational age. Infants less than 28–30 weeks of gestation are particularly compromised in this respect and, if not observed carefully, can become quite dehydrated and hyponatremic. Preterm infants also have an increased bicarbonate excretion and have a low tubular maximum for glucose (approximately 120 mg/dL).

RENAL FAILURE

Renal failure is most commonly seen in the setting of birth asphyxia, hypovolemic shock, and bacterial sepsis. The normal rate of urine flow is 1–3 mL/kg/h. After a hypoxic or ischemic insult, acute tubular necrosis may ensue. Typically, there are 2–3 days of an-

Table 2–21. Normal values of serum creatinine (mg/dL).

Gestational Age at Birth (weeks)	Postnatal Age (days)	
	0–2	28
< 28	1.2	0.7
29–32	1.1	0.6
33–36	1.1	0.45
33–42	0.8	0.3

uria or oliguria associated with hematuria, proteinuria, and a rise in serum creatinine. The period of anuria is followed by a period of polyuria and then gradual recovery. During the polyuric phase, excessive urine sodium and bicarbonate losses may be seen. The initial step in management is restoration of the infant's volume status with colloid as needed. Then, restriction of fluids to insensible water loss (40–60 mL/kg/d) without added electrolytes, plus milliliter-for-milliliter urine replacement, should be instituted. Serum and urine electrolytes and body weights should be followed frequently. These measures should be continued through the polyuric phase. After urine output has been reestablished, urine replacement should be decreased to a ratio of between three-fourths and one-half milliliter for each milliliter of urine output to see if the infant has regained normal function. If so, the infant can be returned to maintenance fluids. Finally, many of these infants do experience fluid overload and should be allowed to diurese back to birthweight. Hyperkalemia, which may lead to a dysrhythmia, may occur in this situation despite the lack of added intravenous potassium. When the serum potassium reaches 7–7.5, an infusion of insulin and glucose (1 unit of insulin for every 3 g of glucose administered) should be started. If an arrhythmia occurs, calcium gluconate (100 mg/kg), followed by a glucose and insulin infusion, should be administered. Sodium bicarbonate (1–2 meq/kg) can also be used to lower serum potassium acutely. Peritoneal dialysis is rarely needed for the management of neonatal acute renal failure.

URINARY TRACT ANOMALIES

Abdominal masses in the newborn are most frequently due to renal enlargement. Most common is a multicystic/dysplastic kidney; congenital hydronephrosis is second in frequency. An ultrasound examination is the first step in diagnosis. In pregnancies with oligohydramnios, renal agenesis or obstruction due to posterior urethral values should be considered. Syndromes with multiple anomalies or chromosomal abnormalities frequently include renal abnormalities.

RENAL VEIN THROMBOSIS

Renal vein thrombosis is seen most frequently in infants of diabetic mothers and in the context of dehydration and polycythemia. Of particular concern is the IDM infant, prone to hypercoagulability, who is also polycythemic. If fetal distress is superimposed on these problems, prompt reduction in blood viscosity is indicated. Thrombosis usually begins in intrarenal venules and can extend into larger veins. Clinically, there is evidence of a new renal mass, usually unilateral, and blood and protein in the urine. With

bilateral renal vein thrombosis, anuria ensues. Diagnosis can be confirmed with an ultrasound examination of the kidneys. Treatment involves correcting the predisposing condition and systemic heparinization for the thrombosis. Prognosis is usually good with return of normal renal function. However, some infants will develop systemic hypertension.

Downing GJ et al: Kidney function in very low birth weight infants with furosemide-related renal calcifications at ages 1 to 2 years. J Pediatr 1992;120:599.

Fine RN: Diagnosis and treatment of fetal urinary tract abnormalities. J Pediatr 1992;121:333.

Guignard J-P, John EG: Renal function in the tiny, premature infant. Clin Perinatol 1986;13:377.

Karlowicz MG, Adelman RD: Acute renal failure in the neonate. Clin Perinatol 1992;19:139.

Robillard JE et al: Renal hemodynamics and functional adjustments to postnatal life. Semin Perinatol 1988;12:143.

Schmidt B et al: Neonatal thrombotic disease: Prevention, diagnosis, and treatment. J Pediatr 1988;113:407.

Vanpie M et al: Postnatal development of renal function in very low birthweight infants. Acta Paediatr Scand 1988;77:191.

BRAIN AND NEUROLOGIC DISORDERS

HYPOXIC ISCHEMIA ENCEPHALOPATHY

Hypoxic ischemic brain injury is an important neurologic problem in the perinatal period for both term and preterm infants. In the premature, this encephalopathy is often associated with intraventricular hemorrhage; for this reason, it is difficult in many cases to determine whether neurologic morbidity is due to one or the other cause.

Diagnosis

Prenatal history, including abnormalities in antepartum testing, fetal distress with or without passage of meconium during labor, and low scalp pH (< 7.2) are important in identifying infants at risk for hypoxic ischemic encephalopathy. Apgar scores, the rapidity of the response of the infant to resuscitation, the amount of resuscitation needed, and cord acid-base status are other important features to note. Clinical features of hypoxic ischemic encephalopathy progress over time:

(1) Birth to 12 hours: decreased level of consciousness, poor tone, decreased spontaneous movement, periodic breathing or apnea, and possible seizures.

(2) 12–24 hours: more seizures, apneic spells, jitteriness and weakness.

(3) After 24 hours: decreased level of conscious-

ness, further respiratory abnormalities (progressive apnea), onset of brain stem signs (oculomotor and pupillary disturbances), poor feeding, and hypotonia.

The severity of clinical signs and the length of time the signs persist correlate with the severity of the insult. Other evaluations helpful in assessing severity in the term infant include EEG, technetium scan, CT scan, and evoked responses. As experience in the use of magnetic resonance imaging is gained, this technique may also prove useful. Markedly abnormal EEGs with voltage suppression and slowing evolving into a burst-suppression pattern are seen with severe clinical symptomatology. On technetium scans, increased uptake of the radionuclide on delayed (2–4 hours) images is suggestive of tissue injury. A CT scan early in the course may demonstrate diffuse hypodensity, whereas later scans may demonstrate brain atrophy and focal ischemic lesions. Visual and somatosensory evoked potentials provide information about function. In most instances, it is not necessary to use all these tests, but some are obtained to confirm an ominous prognosis.

Treatment

The critical management issue in infants with hypoxic-ischemic encephalopathy is to maintain adequate delivery of oxygen to the already injured brain by supporting a normal PaO_2 and blood pressure. Glucose should be administered to maintain a normal serum glucose. Modest fluid restriction should be maintained to avoid exacerbating cerebral edema, and seizures should be controlled with phenobarbital and other anticonvulsants as needed. No other specific therapy (eg, steroids or osmotic agents) has been shown to be helpful in improving the outcome in hypoxic ischemic encephalopathy. However, many new therapies, including oxygen-free radical inhibitors and scavengers, excitatory amino acid antagonists, and calcium channel blockers, are currently under investigation.

Prognosis

Fetal heart rate tracings, cord pH, and 1- and 5-minute Apgar scores are not very precise predictors of long term outcome. Apgar scores of 0–3 at 5 minutes in term infants result in an 8% risk of death in the first year of life and a 1% risk of cerebral palsy among survivors. A 10-minute Apgar of 0–3 predicts death in the first year in 18% of cases and cerebral palsy among survivors in 5%; at 15 minutes, 48% and 9%, respectively; at 20 minutes, 59% and 57%, respectively. The single best predictor of outcome is the severity of clinical hypoxic ischemic encephalopathy (severe symptomatology carries a 75% chance of death and 100% rate of neurologic sequelae among survivors). The major sequela of hypoxic ischemic encephalopathy is cerebral palsy with or without associated mental retardation and epilepsy. Other prognostic features include prolonged seizures refractory to therapy, markedly abnormal EEGs, and CT scans with evidence of major ischemic injury.

INTRACRANIAL HEMORRHAGE

1. SUBDURAL HEMORRHAGE

Subdural hemorrhage is related to birth trauma; the bleeding is caused by tears in the veins that bridge the subdural space. Prospective studies relating incidence to specific obstetric complications are not available.

Three types of hemorrhage occur:

(1) Tentorial laceration with rupture of the straight sinus, vein of Galen, or lateral sinus. This results in an infratentorial bleed and lethal brain stem compression. The only treatment is immediate surgical drainage.

(2) Falx laceration with rupture of the inferior sinus. This hemorrhage is asymptomatic until the blood extends infratentorially, at which time immediate surgical drainage is the only treatment.

(3) The most common site is rupture of superficial cerebral veins with blood over the cerebral convexities. These hemorrhages can be asymptomatic or cause seizures with onset on day 2–3 of life, vomiting, irritability, and lethargy. Associated findings include retinal hemorrhages and a full fontanelle. Diagnosis is confirmed by CT scan. Specific treatment entailing needle drainage of the subdural space is rarely necessary.

The prognosis for the two rare types of bleeding is poor; the morbidity rate is high. In the third, more common type of bleeding, most infants survive, with 75% normal on follow-up. Fortunately, because of improved obstetric care, subdural hemorrhages in neonates have become rare altogether.

2. PRIMARY SUBARACHNOID HEMORRHAGE

Primary subarachnoid hemorrhage is the most common type of neonatal intracranial hemorrhage. In the term infant, it can be related to trauma of delivery, whereas subarachnoid hemorrhage in the preterm infant is seen in association with germinal matrix hemorrhage. Clinically, these hemorrhages can be asymptomatic or present with seizures and irritability on day 2 or, rarely, a massive hemorrhage with rapid downhill course. The seizures associated with subarachnoid hemorrhage are very characteristic—usually brief, with a normal examination interictally. Diagnosis can be suspected on a spinal tap and confirmed with CT scan. Long term follow-up is uniformly good.

3. PERIVENTRICULAR-INTRAVENTRICULAR HEMORRHAGE

Periventricular-intraventricular hemorrhage is a lesion seen almost exclusively in premature infants. The incidence is 20–30% in infants of less than 31 weeks of gestation and 1500 g. Bleeding is most commonly seen in the subependymal germinal matrix (a region of developing glial cells). Bleeding can extend into the ventricular cavity and can also be seen in other areas of the cerebral hemispheres. In addition to prematurity, birth asphyxia, severe respiratory disease, and pneumothorax are also risk factors. The proposed pathogenesis of bleeding is presented in Figure 2–8. The critical event is likely ischemia/reperfusion injury to the capillaries in the germinal matrix or other brain regions.

Diagnosis

Up to 50% of hemorrhages occur at less than 24 hours of age, and virtually all occur by the fourth day. The clinical syndrome ranges from rapid deterioration (coma, hypoventilation, decerebrate posturing, fixed pupils, bulging fontanelle, hypotension, acidosis, acute drop in hematocrit) to a more gradual deterioration with more subtle neurologic changes to absence of any specific physiologic or neurologic signs.

Diagnosis can be confirmed by real-time ultrasound scan. This can be performed whenever bleeding is clinically suspected. If symptoms are absent, routine scanning should be done at 4–7 days in all infants of less than 31 weeks of gestation or in any "sick" infant of 31–35 weeks of gestation. Hemorrhages are graded as follows: (1) Grade I: germinal matrix hemorrhage only (60% of bleeds), (2) Grade II: intraventricular bleeding without ventricular enlargement, (3) Grade III: intraventricular bleeding with ventricular enlargement, and (4) Grade IV: any of the above plus intracerebral hemorrhage.

Follow-up ultrasounds, performed to follow for ventricular enlargement, should be done in infants with small bleeds on the initial scan at 2 weeks of age. In infants with grade III and IV hemorrhages, a follow-up scan should be done within a week of the initial scan. Further scans are dictated by the progression of ventricular enlargement. Scans should also be used in seeking evidence of another ischemic injury, periventricular leukomalacia (cystic changes in the periventricular white matter). This is usually evident by 17–21 days.

Treatment

During the acute hemorrhage, supportive treatment—restoration of volume and hematocrit, oxygenation, and ventilation—should be provided to avoid further cerebral ischemia. Progressive posthemorrhagic hydrocephalus (if it develops) can sometimes be controlled by decreasing the production of cerebrospinal fluid (furosemide 1 mg/kg/d, plus acetazolamide, increasing doses from 25–100 mg/kg/d) or by removal of cerebrospinal fluid (daily lumbar punctures). The process is usually self-limited

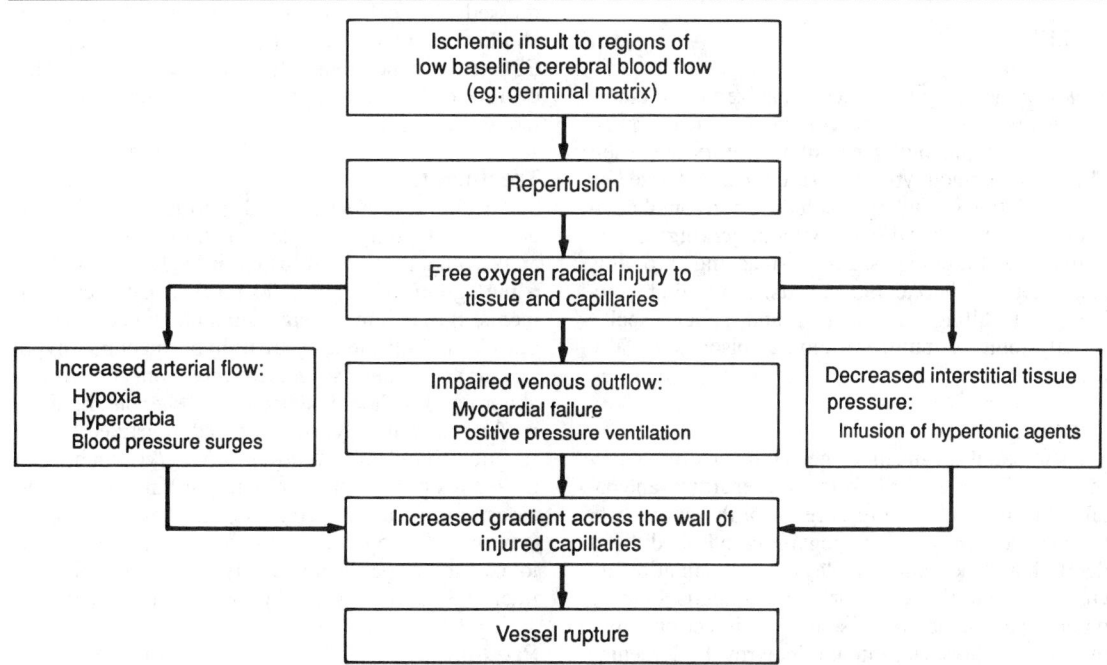

Figure 2–8. Pathogenesis of periventricular-intraventricular hemorrhage.

and spontaneously resolves; the placement of a ventriculoperitoneal shunt is usually not needed.

Interest in the last several years has focused on prevention of this complication of prematurity. Improved obstetric and neonatal care resulting in less asphyxia, improved fluid management, and improved ventilator therapy have decreased the incidence in infants of less than 31 weeks of gestation from 40–50% to 20–30%. The incidence of grade II–IV hemorrhages has also decreased; these formerly constituted 80% of all hemorrhages but now constitute only 40%. Other, less well proved treatments address the initial ischemia reperfusion injury. Agents that appear promising include postnatal vitamin E or indomethacin administration and antenatal phenobarbital.

Prognosis

There is no mortality due to grade I and II hemorrhages, whereas grade III and IV hemorrhages carry a mortality rate of 10–20%. Ventriculomegaly is rarely seen with grade I hemorrhages but is seen in 54–87% of grade II–IV hemorrhages. Very few of these infants will require a ventriculoperitoneal shunt. Long-term neurologic sequelae are seen no more frequently in infants with grade I and II hemorrhages than in preterm infants without bleeding. In infants with grade III and IV hemorrhages, severe sequelae occur in 20–25% of cases, mild sequelae in 35% of cases, and no sequelae in 40% of cases. The presence of severe periventricular leukomalacia, large parenchymal bleeds, and progressive ventriculomegaly greatly increases the risk of neurologic sequelae.

SEIZURES

Newborns rarely have well-organized tonic-clonic seizures because of their incomplete cortical organization and a preponderance of inhibitory synapses. The most common type of seizure is characterized by a constellation of findings, including horizontal deviation of the eyes with or without jerking; eyelid blinking or fluttering; sucking, smacking, drooling, and other oral-buccal movements; swimming, rowing, or paddling movements; and apneic spells. Strictly tonic or multifocal clonic episodes are also seen.

Diagnosis

Differential diagnosis of neonatal seizures is presented in Table 2–22. Information regarding antenatal drug use and the presence of birth asphyxia or trauma and family history (regarding inherited disorders) should be obtained. Physical examination focuses on neurologic features, other signs of drug withdrawal, concurrent signs of infection, dysmorphic features, and intrauterine growth. Screening workup should include blood glucose, calcium, and electrolytes in all cases. Further workup is dependent

Table 2–22. Differential diagnosis of neonatal seizures.

Diagnosis	Comment
Hypoxic-ischemic encephalopathy	Most common cause (60%); onset in first 24 hours
Intracranial hemorrhage	Up to 15% of cases; peri-ventricular-intraventricular hemorrhage, subdural or subarachnoid bleeding
Infection	12% of cases
Hypoglycemia	Small for gestational age, infant of a diabetic mother (IDM)
Hypocalcemia, hypomagnesemia	Infant of low birth weight, IDM
Hyponatremia	Rare, seen with syndrome of inappropriate secretion of anti-diuretic hormone (SIADH)
Disorders of amino and organic acid metabolism, hyperammonemia	Associated acidosis, altered level of consciousness
Pyridoxine dependency	Seizures refractory to routine therapy; cessation of seizures after administration of pyridoxine
Developmental defects	Other anomalies, chromosomal syndromes
Drug withdrawal	
No cause found	10% of cases

on diagnoses suggested by the history and physical examination. If there is any evidence of infection, a spinal tap should be done. Hemorrhages and structural disease of the central nervous system can be addressed with real-time ultrasound and CT scan. Metabolic workup should be pursued when appropriate. EEG should be done; the presence of spike discharges must be noted and the background wave pattern evaluated.

Treatment

Adequate ventilation and perfusion should be ensured. Hypoglycemia should be treated immediately with a 2 mL/kg infusion of $D_{10}W$, followed by 6 mg/kg/min of $D_{10}W$ (100 mL/kg/d). Other treatments, eg, calcium or magnesium infusion and antibiotics, are indicated to treat hypocalcemia, hypomagnesemia, and suspected infection. Electrolyte abnormalities should be corrected. Phenobarbital, 20 mg/kg intravenously, should be administered to stop seizures. Supplemental doses of 5 mg/kg can be used if seizures persist, up to a total of 40 mg/kg. In most cases, phenobarbital controls seizures. If seizures continue, therapy with phenytoin, sodium valproate, lorazepam, or paraldehyde may be indicated. For refractory seizures, a trial of pyridoxine is indicated.

Prognosis

Outcome is related to the underlying cause of the seizure. The outcomes for hypoxic-ischemic encephalopathy and intracranial hemorrhage have been discussed. In these settings, seizures that are difficult to control carry a poor prognosis for normal development. Seizures due to hypoglycemia, infection of the central nervous system, some inborn errors of metabolism, and developmental defects also have a high rate of poor outcome. Seizures due to hypocalcemia or isolated subarachnoid hemorrhage generally resolve without sequelae.

Bada HS et al: Indomethacin reduces the risk of severe intraventricular hemorrhage. J Pediatr 1989;115:631.

Fish WH et al: Effects of intramuscular vitamin E on mortality and intracranial hemorrhage in neonates of 1000 grams or less. Pediatrics 1990;85:578.

Freeman JM, Nelson KB: Intrapartum asphyxia and cerebral palsy. Pediatrics 1988;82:240.

Guzzetta F et al: Periventricular intraparenchymal echodensities in the premature newborn: Critical determinant of neurologic outcome. Pediatrics 1986;78:995.

Kaempf JW et al: Antenatal phenobarbital for the prevention of periventricular and intraventricular hemorrhage: A double-blind, randomized, placebo-controlled, multihospital trial. J Pediatr 1990;117:933.

Palmer C, Vannucci RC: Potential new therapies for perinatal cerebral hypoxia-ischemia. Clin Perinatol 1993;20:411.

Papile LA et al: Incidence and evaluation of subependymal and intraventricular hemorrhage: A study of infants with birth weights less than 1500 grams. J Pediatr 1978;92:529.

Philip AGS et al: Intraventricular hemorrhage in preterm infants: Declining incidence in the 1980's. Pediatrics 1989;84:797.

Robertson CMT, Finer NM: Long-term follow-up of term neonates with perinatal asphyxia. Clin Perinatol 1993;20:483.

Scher MS, Painter MJ: Controversies concerning neonatal seizures. Pediatr Clin North Am 1989;36:281.

Shankaran S et al: Outcome after posthemorrhagic ventriculomegaly in comparison with mild hemorrhage without ventriculomegaly. J Pediatr 1989;114:109.

Volpe JJ: *Neurology of the Newborn.* Saunders, 1987.

Volpe JJ: Brain injury in the premature infant: Is it preventable? Pediatr Res 1990;27:528.

Volpe JJ: Intraventricular hemorrhage in the premature infant: Current concepts. Ann Neurol 1989;25:3,109.

Volpe JJ: Neonatal seizures: current concepts and revised classification. Pediatrics 1989;84:422.

CONGENITAL ANOMALIES

Major congenital malformations are seen in 1.5% of live births and account for 22% of perinatal deaths, 18% of stillbirths, and 27% of neonatal deaths. This topic is discussed in detail in Chapter 32.

The individual **inborn errors of metabolism** are rare, but collectively all such disorders create significant clinical problems. The diseases are considered in detail in Chapter 31, but the diagnoses should be entertained in infants that present with sepsis-like syndromes, recurrent hypoglycemia, neurologic syndromes (seizures, altered levels of consciousness), and unexplained acidosis.

Burton BK et al: Inborn errors of metabolism: The clinical diagnosis in early infancy. Pediatrics 1987;79:359.

Czeizel AE: Prevention of congenital abnormalities by periconceptional multivitamin supplementation. Br Med J 1993;306:1645.

Goodman SI, Greene CL: Inborn errors as causes of acute disease in infancy. Semin Perinatol 1991;15(Suppl 1):31.

Graham JM Jr (editor): Fetal clinical genetics. Clin Perinatol 1990;17:4.

Graham JM Jr (editor): Fetal dysmorphology. Clin Perinatol 1990;17:3.

Graham JM: Clinical approach to human structural defects. Semin Perinatol 1991;15(Suppl 1):2.

Hudak ML et al: Differentiation of transient hyperammonemia of the newborn and urea cycle enzyme defects by clinical presentation. J Pediatr 1985;107:712.

Jones KL (editor): *Smith's Recognizable Patterns of Human Malformation,* 4th ed. Saunders, 1988.

Maestri NE et al: Prospective treatment of urea cycle disorders. J Pediatr 1991;119:923.

REFERENCES

American Academy of Pediatrics: *Guidelines for Perinatal Care,* 3rd ed. American Academy of Pediatrics, 1992.

Avery GB, Fletcher MA, MacDonald MG (editors): *Neonatology: Pathophysiology and Management of the Newborn,* 4th ed. Lippincott, 1994.

Ballard RA (editor): *Pediatric Care of the ICN Graduate.* Saunders, 1988.

Battaglia FC, Meschia G: *An Introduction to Fetal Physiology.* Academic Press, 1988.

Fanaroff AA, Martin RJ (editors): *Neonatal-Perinatal Medicine, Diseases of the Fetus and Infant,* 5th Ed. Mosby, 1991.

Gabbe SG, Niebyl JR, Simpson JL (editors): *Obstetrics: Normal and Problem Pregnancies,* 2nd ed. Churchill Livingstone, 1991.

Goldsmith JP, Karotkin EH (editors): *Assisted Ventilation of the Neonate,* 2nd ed. Saunders, 1988.

Jones KL (editor): *Smith's Recognizable Patterns of Human Malformation,* 4th ed. Saunders, 1988.

Jones MD Jr, Gleason CA, Lipstein SN (editors): *Hospital*

Care of the Recovering NICU Infant. Williams and Wilkins, 1991.

Long WA (editor): *Fetal and Neonatal Cardiology.* Saunders, 1990.

Merritt TA, Northway WH, Boynton BR (editors): *Bronchopulmonary Dysplasia.* Blackwell, 1988.

Remington JS, Klein JO (editors): *Infectious Diseases of the Fetus and Newborn Infant,* 3rd ed. Saunders, 1989.

Taeusch HW, Ballard RA, Avery ME (editors): *Diseases of the Newborn.* Saunders, 1991.

Tsang RC et al (editors): *Nutritional Needs of the Preterm Infant.* Williams & Wilkins, 1993.

Vidyasagar D (editor): The tiny baby. Clin Perinatol 1986; 13:2.

Volpe JJ (editor): *Neurology of the Newborn,* 2nd ed. Saunders, 1987.

Young TE, Mangum OB (editors): *Neofax 93. A Manual of Drugs Used in Neonatal Care,* 6th ed. Ross Laboratories, 1993.

Growth & Development

3

Randi Jenssen Hagerman, MD

This chapter outlines the continuous and dynamic process of growth and development in children. It emphasizes the interactive aspects of physical, cognitive, social, and emotional development so that the reader can appreciate the impact of each of these domains throughout the span of development.

Our understanding of development has undergone major shifts in this century as we have assimilated new information. Freud emphasized how early emotional experiences determined by the environment shape personality and psychopathology. Piaget focused on the predetermined unfolding of cognitive abilities over time in a specific progression that is innate to the child and relatively independent of the environment. In past decades, however, the influence of the environment has assumed an all-powerful role as people have appreciated how greatly the trauma of dysfunctional families and socioeconomic status affect optimal developmental outcomes. We have now reached a stage of regarding the environmental influences in a context that also takes into account the genetic components of temperament and cognitive abilities in a neurobiologic format. We can now understand development through the interaction of these forces so that the relative importance of any single factor is not inflated unless significant trauma or pathologic circumstances exist.

This chapter is divided into sections according to age so that the interactions of central nervous system maturation; physical, cognitive, and emotional growth; genetic variation; and environmental influences can be discussed at critical age levels. Major development theories are reviewed, and longitudinal changes are summarized in charts and tables to give readers an organizational framework by which to remember trends in development. Development occurs at a variable pace in each child. The developmental milestones cited refer to an average child or to group means, and the variability from child to child must be remembered.

THE NEWBORN

Normal newborns are endowed with a set of reflexes to facilitate survival, including rooting and sucking reflexes, and remarkable sensory abilities. The newborn is no longer considered a blank slate—a totally unformed being who gradually gains abilities according to environmental influences. Instead, the newborn is seen as having genetic strengths and weaknesses in neurocognitive organization that are reflected in temperament, adaptability, responsiveness, and general interaction with the environment. These responses should in turn prompt reciprocal interactions from the parents, which further shape development. The Neonatal Behavioral Assessment scale by Brazelton was developed to measure many of the newborn's characteristics of temperament, including social behavior, orienting responses to stimuli, ability to deal with disturbing stimuli, state of arousal, and motor skills. When these abilities are described to the mother, this assessment can further sensitize her to the unique aspects of her child's behavior and responsiveness. This knowledge may in turn improve their interactions.

The newborn has significant sensory abilities, which have been better identified in the last decade. Hearing is well developed at birth, and speech sounds are preferred. The infant becomes alert and oriented to a female voice with high-pitched tones more readily than to a low-pitched male voice. The lower frequency tones of a male voice are more likely to soothe an infant. High-pitched crying is distressing not only to the newborn but also to adults. Infants can shut out loud or aversive stimuli and simply not respond. Within the first few weeks of life, they learn to recognize the mother's voice and differentiate it from other female voices.

Smell is well developed at birth and plays a significant role in how infants orient themselves to the environment. Infants turn away from aversive smells and respond positively to pleasant ones. By 1 week of age, breast-fed infants recognize and discriminate the smell of their mother's breast pads. They recognize the smell of their mother, not the smell of milk alone. The infant has definite taste preferences at birth, preferring sweet tastes. Infants have more taste buds than adults do and avoid bitter or aversive tastes.

At birth, the retina is well developed, but the lens is rather immobile. Fixation and tracking through the visual field are well developed by 2 months of age.

Infants prefer to gaze at a human face rather than geometric designs, and they also prefer curved lines, bright colors, and high contrast. The length of time that an infant fixates on a paired visual stimulus has been interpreted as visual preference and has also been correlated with later cognitive development. Visual fixation tasks are the basis of the "infant IQ" tests marketed recently. Although visual acuity is poor at birth (approximately 20/400), it improves rapidly in the first 6 months of life to 20/40. Strabismus is common after birth but usually resolves by 3 months of age. If it persists, referral to an ophthalmologist is appropriate at 6 months of age.

Brazelton TB: *Neonatal Behavioral Assessment Scale,* 2nd ed. Lippincott, 1984.
Brazelton TB, Yogman MW (editors): *Affective Development in Infancy.* Ablex, 1986.
Dixon SD, Stein MT: *Encounters with Children: Pediatric Behavior and Development,* 2nd ed. Mosby Year Book, 1992. (An exceptional review of development with an emphasis on incorporating development issues into general pediatric care.)
Haith MM, Campos J: *Infancy and Developmental Psychobiology.* Vol 2 of: *Handbook of Child Psychology.* Mussen PH (editor). Wiley, 1983.
Yogman MW, Cook KV, Gersten M: Infant and toddler development: Active organization of the social world. Curr Probl Pediatr (May) 1988;18:259. (A detailed assessment of early cognitive and emotional development.)

THE FIRST YEAR

One of the most distressing features of infants is the amount of time they spend crying in the first few weeks of life. Crying gradually increases during the first 6–12 weeks of age because it is the main modality by which infants express responses to stimuli, both aversive and nonaversive. Crying can be a response to a variety of stimuli, including hunger, a wet diaper, fear, fatigue, and overstimulation. Crying gradually decreases after 12 weeks of age, as the infant develops other responses, such as smiling or reaching, or becomes more adept at self-soothing, such as by sucking the fingers or thumb. In the first weeks of life, however, crying can become a distressing problem for the parents, and crying associated with irritability is often labeled as colic. Particularly sensitive infants with a low tolerance for stimuli can be irritable and difficult to deal with at home. It is useful to help parents understand their infant's temperament and to teach them techniques for avoiding excessive stimuli (because parents often respond to excessive crying by creating excessive stimuli). Parents should be taught ways to calm the child, such as offering nonnutritive sucking, rocking the child, singing to the child, and walking while holding the child. Perhaps most important for the parents is an understanding of the developmental aspects of crying and

the emergence of improved coping skills in the baby after 12 weeks of age.

Piaget describes the first 2 years of life as the sensorimotor period, during which infants learn with increasing sophistication how to link the sensory input from the environment with a motor response. Infants build on primitive reflex patterns of behavior (termed *schema;* sucking is an example) and constantly incorporate or assimilate new experiences to further elaborate their schema. The schema evolve over time as infants accommodate new experiences and as new levels of cognitive ability unfold in a rather orderly sequence. In the first year of life, infants' perception of reality revolves around themselves and what they can see or touch. They follow the trajectory of an object through the field of vision, but prior to 6 months, the object does not exist for them once it leaves the field of vision. At 9–12 months, infants gradually develop the concept of object permanence, or the understanding that objects exist even when they are not seen. They first apply the concept of object permanence to the image of the mother because of her emotional importance; this realization is a critical part of attachment behavior, discussed below. In the second year, children extend their ability to manipulate objects by using instruments, first by imitation and later by trial and error (Table 3–1).

Freud describes the first year of life as the oral stage because so many of the infant's needs are fulfilled by oral means. Nutrition is obtained through sucking on the breast or bottle, and self-soothing also occurs through sucking on fingers or a pacifier. As Mahler emphasizes, this is a stage of symbiosis with the mother, during which the boundaries between mother and infant are blurred. The baby's needs are totally met by the mother, and the mother has been described as manifesting "narcissistic possessiveness" of the infant. This is a very positive and critical interaction in the bidirectional attachment process known as bonding. The parents learn to be aware of and read their infant's cues, which reflect needs. However, a more sensitive emotional interaction process develops, which can be seen in the mirroring of facial expressions by mother and infant and in their mutual engagement in cycles of attention and inattention, which further develops into social play. A mother who is depressed or cannot respond to the baby's expressions and cues has a profound effect on the infant's future development and attachment. Erickson's terms of basic trust versus mistrust are another way of describing the reciprocal interaction that characterizes this stage (Table 3–1).

Turn-taking games, which occur between 3 and 6 months of age, are a pleasure for both the parents and the infant and are an extension of mirroring behavior. They also represent an early form of imitative behavior, which is important in later social and cognitive development. More sophisticated games, such as peek-a-boo, occur at approximately 9 months. The

Table 3–1. Perspectives of human behavior.[1]

Age	Theories of Development			Skill Areas		Psychopathology
	Freud	Erikson	Piaget	Language	Motor	
Birth–18 mo	Oral	Basic trust vs. mistrust	Sensorimotor	Body actions; crying; naming; pointing	Reflex sitting, reaching, grasping, walking	Autism; anaclitic depression, colic; disorders of attachment; feeding, sleeping problems
18 mo–3 yr	Anal	Autonomy vs. shame, doubt	Symbolic (preoperational)	Sentences; telegraph jargon	Climbing, running	Separation issues; negativism; fearfulness; constipation; shyness, withdrawal
3–6 yr	Oedipal	Initiative vs. guilt	Intuition (preoperational)	Connective words; can be readily understood	Increased coordination; tricycle; jumping	Enuresis; encopresis; anxiety; aggressive acting out; phobias; nightmares
6–11 yr	Latency	Industry vs. inferiority	Concrete operational	Subordinate sentences; reading and writing; language reasoning	Increased skills; sports, recreational cooperative games	School phobias; obsessive reactions; conversion reactions; depressive equivalents
12–17 yr	Adolescence (genital)	Identity vs. role confusion	Formal operational	Reason abstract; using language; abstract manipulation	Refinement of skills	Delinquency; promiscuity; schizophrenia; anorexia nervosa; suicide
17–30 yr	Young adulthood	Intimacy vs. isolation	Formal operational	Reason abstract; using language; abstract manipulation	Refinement of skills	Schizophrenia; borderline personality; adjustment disorders; development of intimate relationship and difficulties with relationships
30–60 yr	Adulthood	Generativity vs. stagnation	Formal operational	Reason abstract; using language; abstract manipulation	Refinement of skills	Depression; self-doubts; career development issues; family, social network; neuroses
60 yr and over	Old age	Ego integration vs. despair	Formal operational		Loss of functions (?)	Involutional depression; anxiety; anger; increased dependency

[1]Adapted and reproduced, with permission, from Dixon S: Setting the stage: Theories and concepts of child development. In: *Encounters With Children.* Dixon S, Stein M (editors). Year Book, 1987.

infant's thrill at the reappearance of the face that vanished momentarily demonstrates the emerging understanding of object permanence.

Eight to nine months is also a critical time in the attachment process because separation anxiety and stranger anxiety become marked. Kagan describes the infant at this stage as able to appreciate discrepant events that match previously known schema only partially. These new events cause uncertainty and subsequently fear and anxiety. Cognitively, the infant must be able to retrieve the memory of previous schema and integrate the new information to previous knowledge over an extended time. These abilities are developed by 8 months of age and lead to the fears that

subsequently develop: stranger anxiety and separation anxiety. In stranger anxiety, the infant analyzes the face of a stranger, detects the mismatch with previous schema, and may subsequently respond with fear or anxiety, leading to crying. In separation anxiety, the child perceives the difference between the mother's presence and absence by remembering the schema of her presence. Perceiving the inconsistency, the child becomes uncertain and subsequently anxious and fearful. This begins at 8 months, reaches a peak at 15 months, and disappears by the end of 2 years in a relatively orderly progression because central nervous system maturation facilitates the development of new skills. A parent can put the child's understanding of object permanence to good use by placing a picture of the mother near the child or by leaving an object where the child can see it during her absence. A visual substitute for her actual presence may comfort the child.

Brazelton TB, Yogman MW (editors): *Affective Development in Infancy.* Ablex, 1986.

Dixon SD, Stein MT: *Encounters with Children: Pediatric Behavior and Development,* 2nd ed. Mosby Year Book, 1992.

Dworkin PH: The preschool child: Developmental themes and clinical issues. Curr Probl Pediatr (Feb) 1988;18:79.

Freud A: *Normality and Pathology in Childhood: Assessments of Development.* International Universities Press, 1965.

Ginsberg H, Opper S: *Piaget's Theory of Intellectual Development.* Prentice-Hall, 1969. (A readable review of Piaget's work.)

Kagan J: Canalization of early psychological development. Pediatrics 1982;70:474.

Levine MD, Carey WB, Crocker AC (editors): *Developmental-Behavioral Pediatrics,* 2nd ed. Saunders, 1992.

Piaget J: *The Origins of Intelligence in Children.* Norton, 1952.

Yogman MW, Cook KV, Gersten M: Infant and toddler development: Active organization of the social world. Curr Probl Pediatr (May) 1988;18:259.

GROWTH IN THE FIRST THREE YEARS

Fetal growth in length is most rapid at 4–6 months' gestation. However, adipose tissue begins to develop at 7 months, and weight gain accelerates, causing fetal weight to double during the last 2 months in utero. The rate of growth of males in late fetal development and during the first 6 months postnatally is more rapid than the growth rate of females because of a higher level of testosterone. The birth weight of the newborn correlates with the size, nutritional state, and general health of the mother and represents the influence of uterine constraints on ultimate size. Newborns may lose up to 10% of their birth weight in the first few days of life, but with normal nutrition birth weight is regained in approximately 10 days. The infant subsequently gains approximately 30 g per day for the first several months.

After the first 6 months of life, genetic factors influencing ultimate height begin to exert their effect. The growth percentile, therefore, may shift significantly in the first 4–18 months of life. This shift can be either up or down. An infant who is small for gestational age and has a genetic predisposition to larger stature usually experiences accelerated growth in the first 6 months, and by 18 months a relatively stable new growth percentile is established. The downward shift is seen in large infants who have a genetic predisposition to short stature. A fall-off in their growth percentiles may often be misconstrued as failure to thrive, although a stable growth percentile should be achieved by 18 months of age.

By 1 year of age, infants weigh three times as much as they did at birth and are 1½ times as long. By 2 years of age, the growth velocity curve has stabilized into the rate for mid childhood, which is a weight gain of 2–3 kg/yr and a height gain of 5–7.5 cm/yr (Figures 3–1 to 3–9). At the second birthday, a child attains approximately one-half of adult height.

The energy requirement during growth also changes dramatically in the first few years of life. Approximately 110 kcal/kg/d is necessary in early infancy because up to 40% of this total energy requirement is used for growth. The percentage used for growth gradually decreases to 3% at 2 years of age and remains at this level even during adolescence. After 2 years of age, the overall energy requirement gradually decreases from 90 kcal/kg/d to 60 kcal/kg/d during middle childhood, and the majority of the energy expenditure is accounted for by activity and basal metabolic rate of the tissues. The gradual decrease is secondary to a decline in the relative mass of organs, such as the brain and liver, that have a high requirement for energy compared to resting muscle. The relative energy expended during activity increases in adolescence, particularly for males. The percentage of body weight that is muscle increases from 22% at 3 months to 35% at 5 years and 40% at maturity in males. In contrast, organ weight is 17% of body weight in the infant, with 75% of organ weight accounted for by the brain. By maturity, only 5.1% of body weight is organ weight. Fat increases during the first year of life from 12% of body weight at birth. After the infant begins to walk and explore, however, the proportion of fat decreases and remains stable throughout childhood. In adolescence, the proportion of body weight that is fat increases with sexual maturation in girls but not in boys. For further information, see Chapter 11.

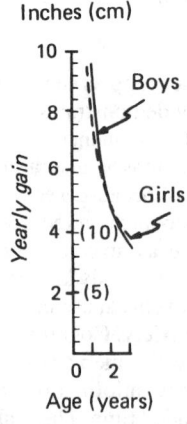

Figure 3–1. Growth rate from birth to age 3 (both sexes).

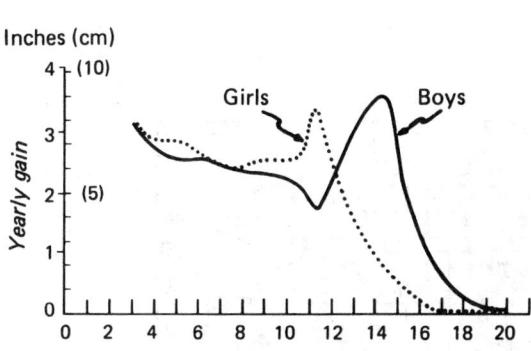

Figure 3–2. Growth rate from age 3 to age 20 (both sexes).

Falkner F, Tanner JM (editors): *Developmental Biology: Prenatal Growth.* Vol 1 of: *Human Growth: A Comprehensive Treatise,* 2nd ed. Plenum Press, 1986.

Falkner F, Tanner JM (editors): *Postnatal Growth Neurobiology.* Vol 2 of: *Human Growth: A Comprehensive Treatise,* 2nd ed. Plenum Press, 1986. (A detailed analysis of current research in physical growth and brain development.)

Jelliffe DB, Jelliffe EF: *Growth Monitoring and Promotion in Young Children.* Oxford Univ Press, 1990. (A review of growth monitoring methods.)

Lowrey GH: *Growth and Development of Children,* 8th ed. Year Book, 1986. (A detailed analysis of physical growth and development in children.)

Smith DW: *Growth and Its Disorders: Major Problems in Clinical Pediatrics,* Vol 25. Saunders, 1977. (A classic review of linear growth through childhood and adolescence.)

Tanner JM, Whitehouse RH, Takaishi M: Standards from birth to maturity for height, weight, height velocity: British children. Arch Dis Child 1965;41:454.

Brain Growth

Approximately 100 billion neurons are present in the fully developed brain, and replication of neurons is completed before birth. Most of this growth occurs in the first 3 months of gestation. Cell density subsequently decreases rapidly until birth. After birth, the decrease is slower, and ceases at 15 months. At birth, the head is three-fourths of its adult size and makes up one-fourth of the baby's length. This ratio changes dramatically in time so that by 25 years of age, the head measures one-eighth of the body length. Postnatally, the brain continues to grow rapidly, completing half of its lifetime growth by the end of the first year. The postnatal growth is due to an increase in white matter and a proliferation of synaptic connections. After 2 years of age, the head circumference increases only 2 cm/yr during middle childhood (Figures 3–8 and 3–9). By 7 years of age, nine-tenths of brain growth is completed, and many 10-year-olds have the brain weight of an adult.

The cerebellum is the area of the gray matter that develops last. It begins its growth at 30 weeks of gestation and ends at approximately 1 year of age. It is, therefore, particularly vulnerable to trauma, which may occur in late gestation or at birth. The spinal cord extends through the length of the neural canal until the third month of gestation. After this time, the torso of the fetus grows faster than the spinal cord, which is fixed in position superiorly by the brain. The lower end of the spinal cord subsequently rests at a gradually higher vertebral level through later fetal life and, by birth, is located at the third lumbar vertebra. The spinal cord doubles its weight in the first year of life and has increased eightfold by adulthood.

Myelinization begins in the spinal cord by the fourth month of gestation and begins in the brain during the last trimester. At birth, the autonomic system is matured and myelinated. The cranial nerves, except for the optic and olfactory nerves, are also myelinated. The cortex and most of its connection to the thalamus and basal ganglia are incompletely myelinated. It takes at least 2 years for myelinization of these areas and the spinal cord to be complete.

Newborn Reflexes

Reflex movement begins in fetal development as early as 9 weeks' gestation. However, most of the reflexes associated with the newborn develop between 20 and 38 weeks' gestation. Sucking, a basic reflex critical to survival, can first be seen in utero as early as 14 weeks' gestation. The rooting reflex begins by 28 weeks' gestation and is evidenced by the infant's pursing the lips and sucking after turning toward a touch to the cheek. The tonic neck reflex is elicited by forcibly turning the infant's head. In response, the infant extends the arm and leg on the side toward which the head is turned and flexes the opposite side (fencing position stance). This reflex disappears by 8 months of age unless myelinization or brain development is pathologic. The Moro embrace reflex (an em-

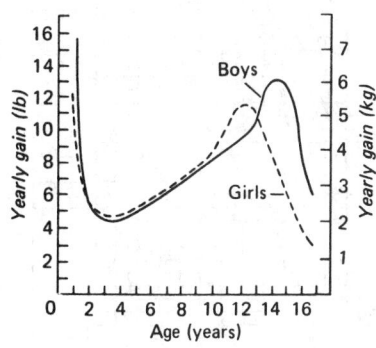

Figure 3–3. Yearly gain in weight. (Redrawn and reproduced, with permission, from Barnett HL: *Pediatrics,* 14th ed. Appleton-Century-Crofts, 1968.)

GIRLS: BIRTH TO 36 MONTHS
PHYSICAL GROWTH NCHS PERCENTILES*

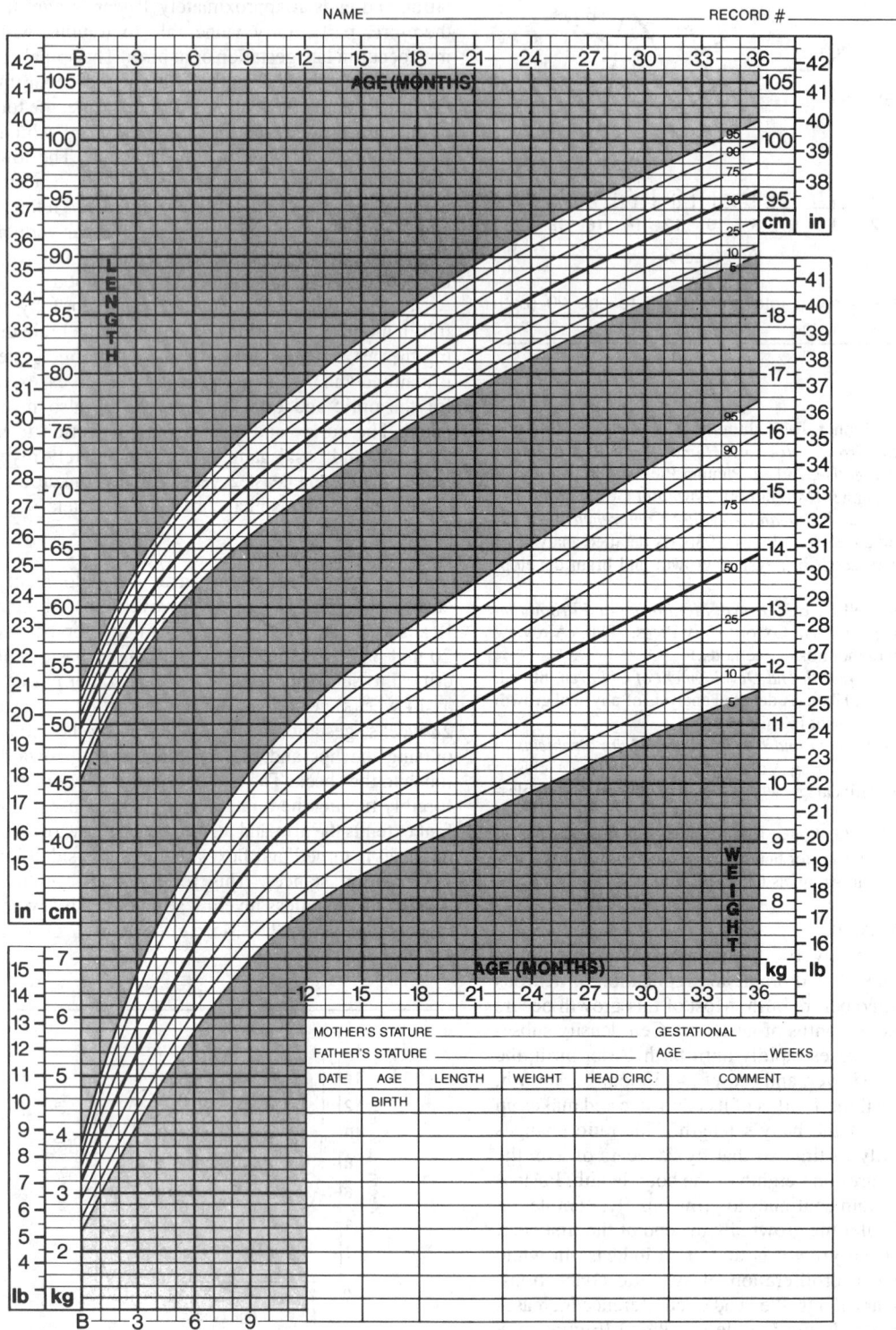

Figure 3–4. Percentile standards for weight and height in girls 0–3 years. (Reproduced, with permission, from Ross Laboratories, Columbus, OH. © 1982 Ross Laboratories.)

BOYS: BIRTH TO 36 MONTHS
PHYSICAL GROWTH NCHS PERCENTILES*

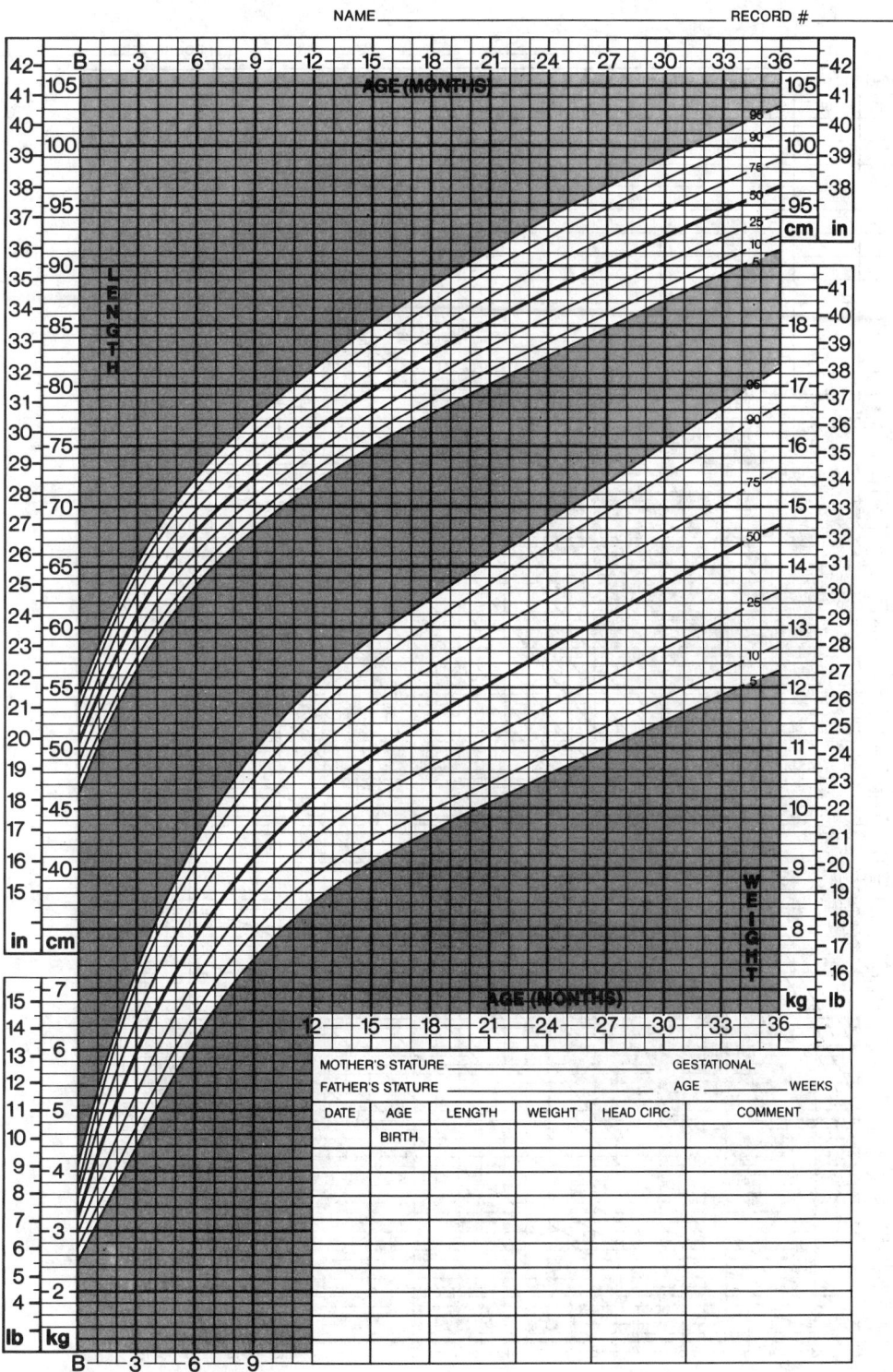

Figure 3–5. Percentile standards for weight and height in boys 0–3 years. (Reproduced, with permission, from Ross Laboratories, Columbus, OH. © 1982 Ross Laboratories.)

GIRLS: 2 TO 18 YEARS
PHYSICAL GROWTH
NCHS PERCENTILES*

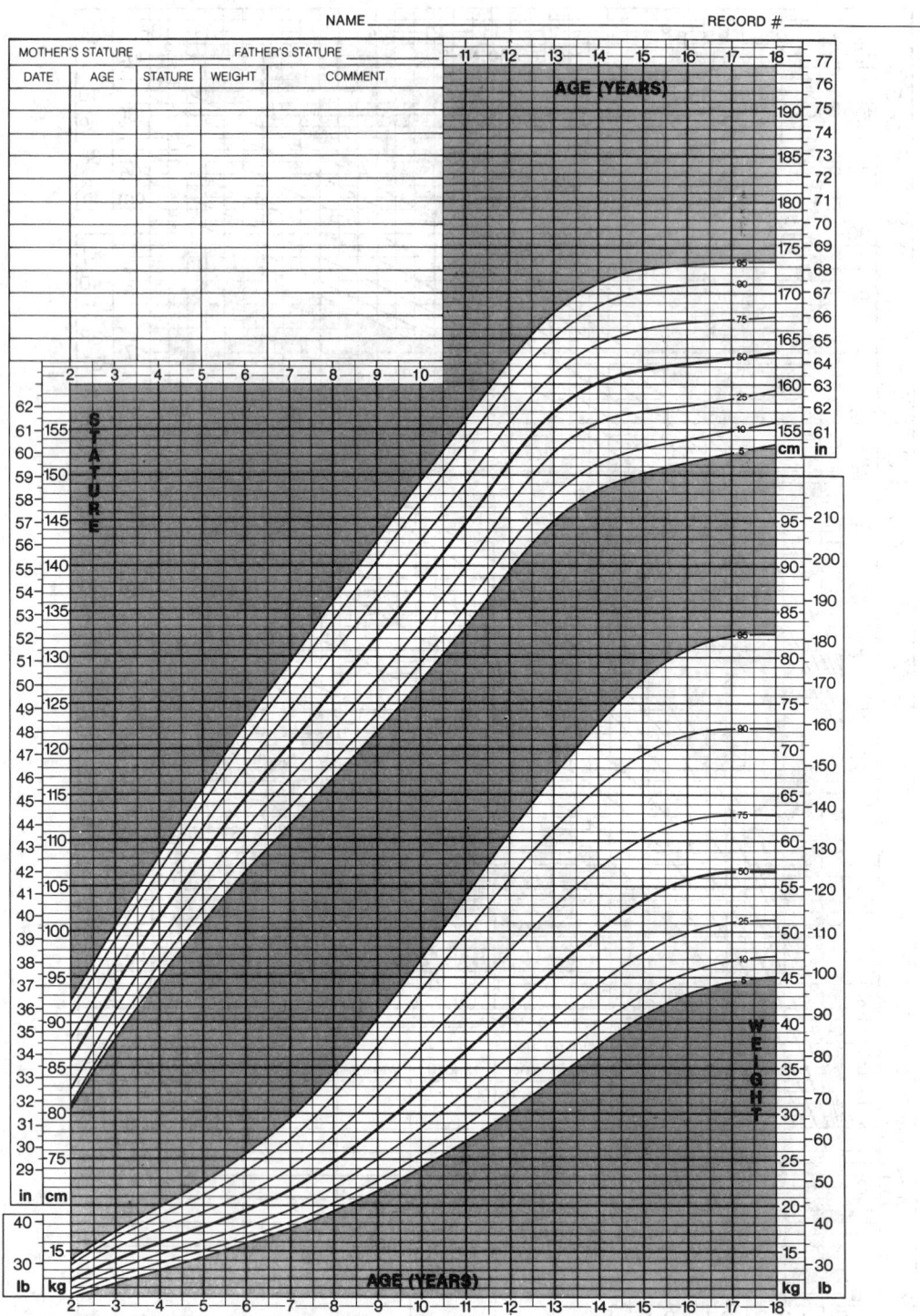

Figure 3–6. Percentile standards for weight and height in girls 2–18 years. (Reproduced, with permission, from Ross Laboratories, Columbus, OH. © 1982 Ross Laboratories.)

BOYS: 2 TO 18 YEARS
PHYSICAL GROWTH
NCHS PERCENTILES*

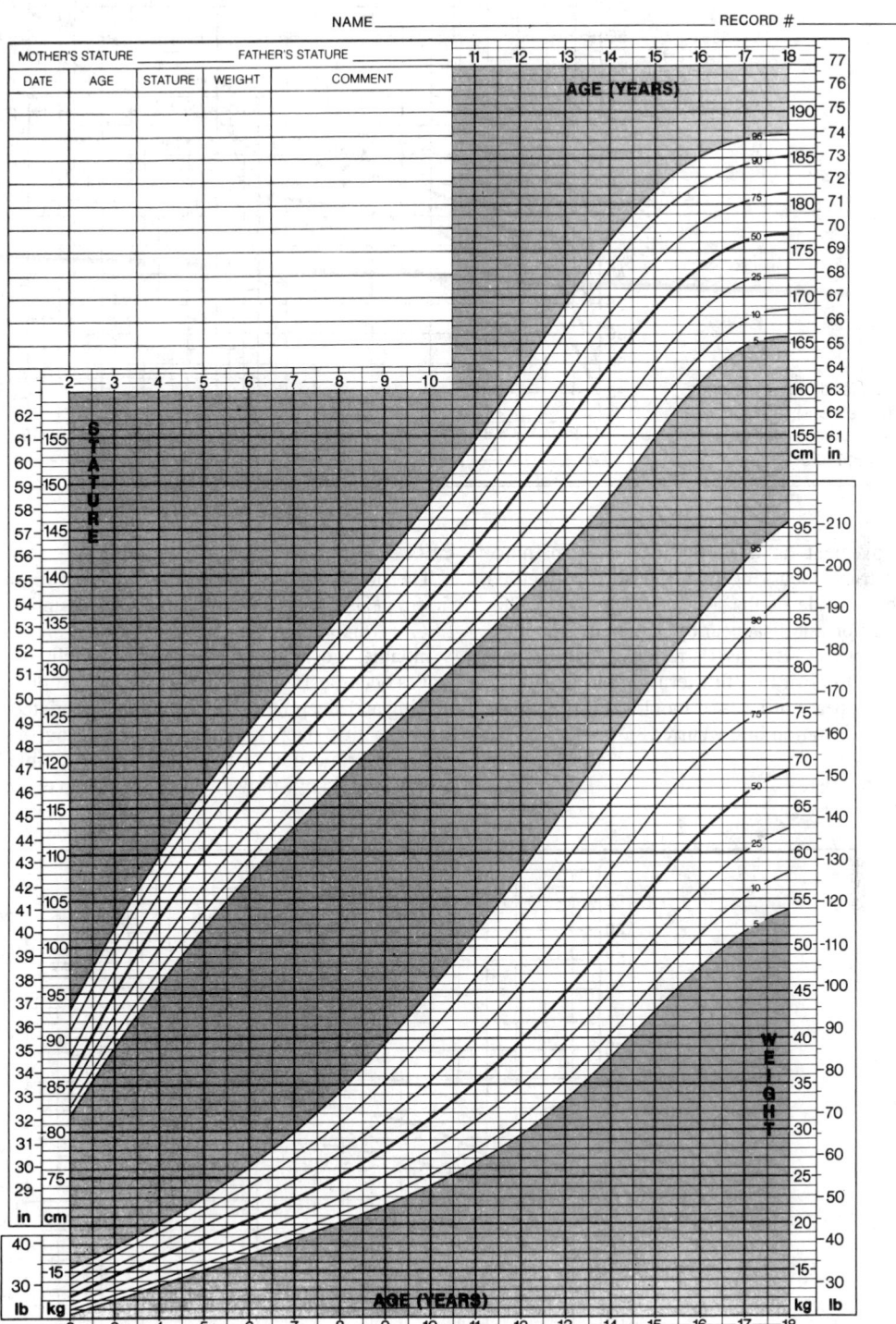

Figure 3–7. Percentile standards for weight and height in boys 2–18 years. (Reproduced, with permission, from Ross Laboratories, Columbus, OH. © 1982 Ross Laboratories.)

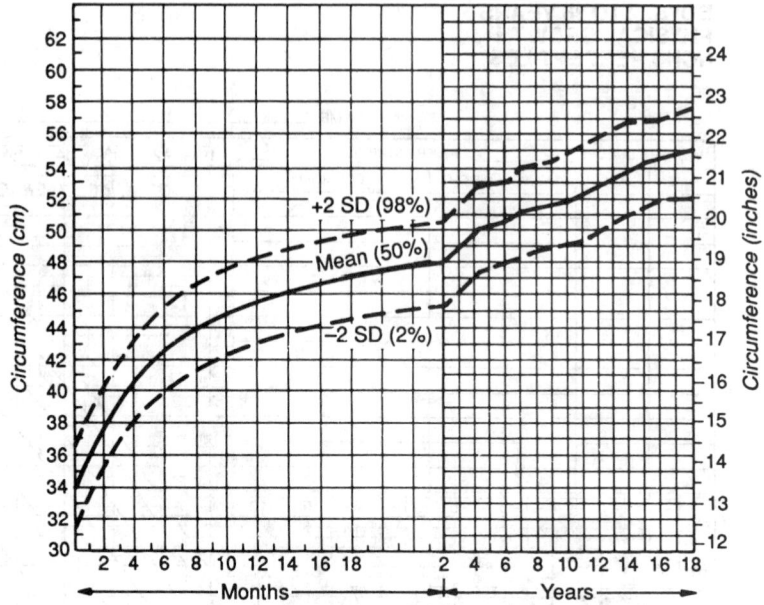

Figure 3–8. Head circumference of girls. (Modified and reproduced, with permission, from Nellhaus G: Pediatrics 1968;41:106.)

bracing movement as a startle response), palmar grasp, and trunk incurving in response to a tactile stimulus to the side of the trunk all develop by 28 weeks' gestation but disappear by 3, 4, and 5 months of age, respectively. Babinski's reflex, which develops just prior to birth in a full-term infant, does not normally disappear until 12–16 months of age, when adequate myelinization has occurred.

EEG & Sleep

The brain also undergoes rapid maturation in the first 2 years of life. Prior to 26 weeks' gestation, the EEG is disorganized and without periodicity. By 8 months' gestation, however, low-amplitude fast waves occur at 16–18 cycles per second. At birth, the waking and sleeping cycles can be differentiated, and by 4 months, sleep spindles appear. During this period, the proportion of total sleep time occupied by active or rapid eye movement (REM) sleep decreases

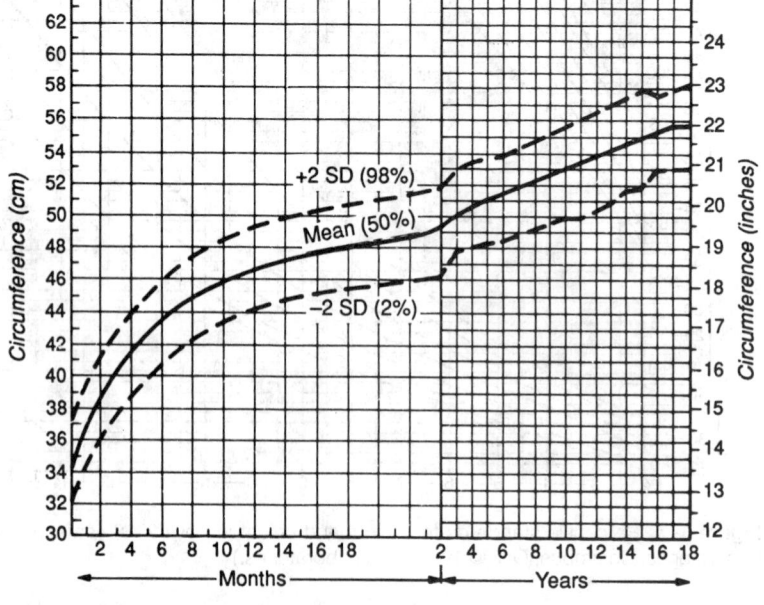

Figure 3–9. Head circumference of boys. (Modified and reproduced, with permission, from Nellhaus G: Pediatrics 1968;41:106.)

from 50% to 20%. The infant's sleep pattern at the onset of sleep also shifts from REM sleep to quiet sleep. The amount of quiet sleep also gradually increases to a maximum of 70–80% of total sleep time. These changes are a reflection of significant brain maturation, which has occurred by 4 months. Infantile reflexes, as previously mentioned, are disappearing, and the infant is becoming more alert and interactive with the environment. The infant is now reaching for and grasping objects, smiling and laughing out loud, anticipating food on sight, and sitting with support.

Motor Dexterity

The developmental progression of the grasp through the first year illustrates the gradual improvement in motor dexterity. The grasp begins as a raking motion involving mainly the ulnar aspect of the hand at 3–4 months. The thumb is used in the grasp just before 5 months, as the focus shifts to the radial side of the hand. The thumb opposes the finger for picking up a cube just before 7 months, but the neat pincer grasp used for smaller objects, such as a pellet, does not develop until approximately 9 months.

The changes in gross motor skills have a significant impact on the child's exploration of the environment. Sitting alone occurs at 6 months of age, but the onset of walking at 12 months (with a range of 9–17 months in the normal child) introduces the major theme of the second year of life, autonomy.

THE SECOND YEAR

Once children can walk independently, they can move away from the mother and explore the environment on their own. Although they use the mother as a home base and return to her frequently to reassure themselves that she is still there and available for them, they have definitely taken a quantum jump in independence and autonomy. These new themes are closely tied to the child's beginning sense of mastery over the environment and an emerging sense of self. These issues lead to the "terrible twos" and the frequent verbalizations "no" as children struggle to develop a better idea of what is under their control. This is a fragile time of ego development. Parents should not crush emerging autonomy but develop appropriate limits that foster independent exploration.

As children develop a sense of self, they begin to understand the feelings of others and develop empathy. They hug another who is in distress or become concerned when another is hurt. They begin to understand how another child feels when he or she is hit or hurt, and this realization helps them to inhibit their own aggressive behavior. They also begin to understand right and wrong and parental expectations. They realize when they have done something "bad" and may signify that awareness with "uh oh!" or distress. They also take pleasure in their accomplishments and become more aware of their bodies.

The development of these cognitive, emotional, and physical abilities is related to significant brain maturation, which occurs by 2 years of age. Myelinization is reaching its completion and, according to Rabinowicz, all the layers of the cortex reach a similar state of maturation between 15 and 24 months. Before this time, differences exist in the maturation level between cortical layers. These changes set the stage for toilet training after 18 months of age. Toddlers have developed the sensory abilities to be aware of a full rectum or bladder and are physically able to control their rectal sphincter. They also take great pleasure in their accomplishments, particularly in appropriate elimination, if it is positively reinforced. Children must be given some control over when elimination occurs. If severe restrictions are imposed, the accomplishment of this developmental milestone can become a battle between parent and child, and long-term struggles of control predisposing to encopresis may develop later. Freud terms this period the anal stage because the development issue of bowel control is the major task requiring mastery. It basically represents a more generalized theme of socialized behavior and overall body cleanliness, which is begun to be taught or imposed on the child at this age. The child is encouraged to control impulsive and aggressive behavior by acting in socially appropriate ways. Although Freud describes the by-products of anal regularity on personality development, including punctuality, reliability, cleanliness, and conscientiousness, these themes simply represent abilities emerging at the time that toilet-training is also being mastered. See Chapter 6.

Dixon SD, Stein MT: *Encounters with Children: Pediatric Behavior and Development,* 2nd ed. Mosby Year Book, 1992.

Egan DF: *Developmental Examination of Infants and Preschool Children.* Clinics in Developmental Medicine No. 112. MacKeith Press, 1990.

Falkner F, Tanner JM (editors): *Postnatal Growth Neurobiology.* Vol 2 of: *Human Growth: A Comprehensive Treatise,* 2nd ed. Plenum Press, 1986.

Lowrey GH: *Growth and Development of Children,* 8th ed. Year Book, 1986.

Rabinowicz T: The differential maturation of the cerebral cortex. In: *Postnatal Growth Neurobiology.* Vol 2 of: *Human Growth: A Comprehensive Treatise,* 2nd ed. Falkner F, Tanner JM (editors). Plenum Press, 1986.

Yogman MW, Cook KV, Gersten M: Infant and toddler development: Active organization of the social world. Curr Probl Pediatr (May) 1988;18:259.

LANGUAGE DEVELOPMENT:
1–4 YEARS

Communication is important from birth, particularly the nonverbal reciprocal interactions between the infant and caretaker, which have already been described. By 2 months of age, these interactions begin to include vocalizations that involve cooing and reciprocal vocal play between the mother and child. Babbling begins by 6–10 months of age, and the repetition of sounds, such as "da-da-da-da," is facilitated by increasing oral muscular control. Babbling reaches a peak at 12 months. The child then moves into a stage of having needs met by using individual words to represent objects or actions. It is common for children of this age to express wants and needs by pointing to objects. There is significant variability in the number of words acquired by 18 months, with an average of 20–50 words. The failure of parents or siblings to encourage vocalization and their overuse of nonverbal communication, such as pointing, slows the development of expressive vocabulary. Recurrent otitis media, which causes a fluctuating conductive hearing loss, may also have a significant impact on the achievement of early language milestones.

Receptive language usually develops more rapidly than expressive language. Word comprehension begins at 9 months; by 13 months, the receptive vocabulary may be as high as 20–100 words. After 18 months, there is a dramatic increase in expressive and receptive vocabulary, and by the end of the second year, a quantum leap occurs in language development. This leap represents a major change in cognitive development. The child begins to put words and phrases together and begins to use language to represent a new world, the symbolic world. Although the infant begins to use single words to represent objects or people in the latter part of the first year, it is not until the end of the second year that language ability begins to blossom. Children now begin to put verbs into their phrases and focus much of their language on describing their new abilities, often while they are doing them, eg, "I go out." They incorporate prepositions into speech and ask why and what questions more frequently. They also begin to appreciate time factors and to understand and use this concept in their speech (Table 3–2).

The Early Language Milestones Scale (ELM) (Figure 3–10) is a simple tool for assessing early language development in the pediatric office setting. It is

Table 3–2. Normal speech and language development.

Age	Speech	Language	Articulation[1]
1 month	Throaty sounds		Vowels: \ah\, \uh\, \ee\
2 months	Vowel sounds ("eh"), coos		
2½ months	Squeals		
3 months	Babbles, initial vowels		
4 months	Gutteral sounds ("ah," "go")		Consonants, m, p, b
5 months			Vowels: \o\, \u\
7 months	Imitates speech sounds		
8 months			Syllables: da, ba, ka
10 months		"Dada" or "mama" nonspecifically	Approximates names: baba/bottle
12 months	Jargon begins (own language)	One word other than "mama" or "dada"	Understandable: 2–3 words
13 months		Three words	
16 months		Six words	Consonants; t, d, w, n, h
18–24 months		Two-word phrases	Understandable 2-word phrases
24–30 months		Three-word phrases	Understandable 3-word phrases
2 years	Vowels uttered correctly	Approximately 270 words; uses pronouns	Approximately 270 words; uses phrases
3 years	Some degree of hesitancy and uncertainty common	Approximately 900 words; intelligible 4-word phrases	Approximately 900 words; intelligible 4-word phrases
4 years		Approximately 1540 words; intelligible 5-word phrases or sentences	Approximately 1540 words; intelligible 5-word phrases
6 years		Approximately 2560 words; intelligible 6- or 7-word sentences	Approximately 2560 words; intelligible 6- or 7-word sentences
7–8 years	Adult proficiency		

[1]Data on articulation from Berry MF:d *Language Disorders of Children*. Appleton-Century-Crofts, 1969; and from Bzoch K, League R: *Receptive-Expressive Emergent Language Scale*. University Park Press, 1970.

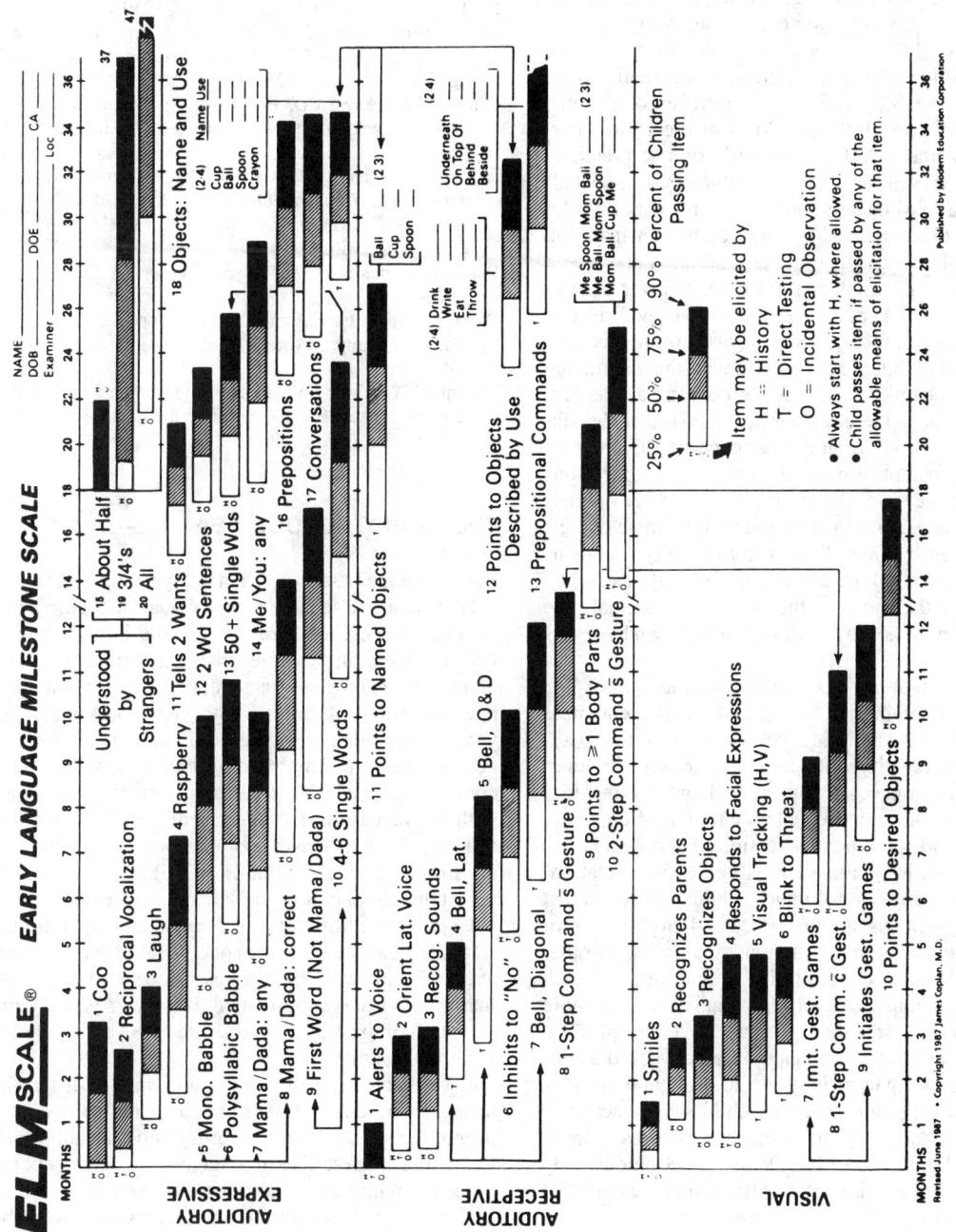

Figure 3-10. Early Language Milestone Scale. (Reproduced, with permission, from Coplan J: *Early Language Milestone Scale.* Pro Ed, Austin, TX. 1987.)

scored in the same fashion as the Denver II (Figure 3–11) but tests both receptive and expressive language areas in greater depth.

Piaget describes the 2- to 6-year-old stage as preoperational. This stage begins when language has facilitated the creation of mental images in the symbolic sense. The child begins to learn to manipulate the symbolic world. The child sorts out reality from fantasy imperfectly and may be terrified of dreams, wishes, and foolish threats. Most of the child's perception of the world is egocentric or interpreted in reference to wants, needs, or influence. Cause-and-effect relationships are confused with temporal relationships or interpreted egocentrically. For instance, children often focus their understanding of divorce on themselves; eg, "my father left because I was bad" or "my father left because he didn't love me." Illness and the need for medical care are also commonly misinterpreted at this age. The child may make a mental connection between a sibling's illness and a recent argument, a negative comment, or a wish that the sibling be ill. The child may experience significant guilt unless the parents are aware of these misperceptions and take time to sort them out.

At this age, children also endow inanimate objects with human feelings. They also assume that humans cause or create all natural events. For instance, when asked why the sun sets, they may respond that "the sun goes to his house" or "it is pushed down by someone else."

Magical thinking blossoms during the ages of 3–5 as symbolic thinking incorporates more elaborate fantasy. Fantasy facilitates development of role playing, sexual identity, and emotional growth. Children test new experiences in fantasy, both in their imagination and in play. In their play, children often create magical stories and novel situations that reflect issues they are dealing with, such as aggression, relationships, fears, and control issues. Children often invent imaginary friends at this time, and nightmares or fears of monsters are common. At this stage, other children become important in facilitating play, such as in a preschool group. Play gradually becomes more cooperative; shared fantasy leads to game playing. Freud describes the Oedipal phase between the ages of 3 and 6, when there is strong attachment to the parent of the opposite sex. The child's fantasies may focus on play acting the adult role with that parent, although by 6 years of age Oedipal issues are usually resolved, and attachment is redirected to the parent of the same sex.

Bayley N (editor): *Bayley Scales of Infant Development,* 2nd ed. Psychological Corp, 1993.

Billeaud FP: *Communication Disorders in Infants and Toddlers.* Andover Medical, 1993. (This text reviews normal language development and assessment techniques and measures as well as intervention strategies in communication disorders.)

Coplan J: *Early Language Milestone Scale,* Pro Ed, 1987.

Dixon SD, Stein MT: *Encounters with Children: Pediatric Behavior and Development,* 2nd ed. Mosby Year Book, 1992.

Erikson EH: *Childhood and Society,* 2nd ed. Norton, 1963.

Fraiberg S: *The Magic Years.* Scribner, 1959.

Frankenberg WK et al: The Denver II: A major revision and restandardization of the Denver Developmental Screening Test. Pediatrics 1991;89:91.

Glascoe FP, Martin ED, Humphrey S: A comparative review of developmental screening tests. Pediatrics 1990; 86:547.

Levine MD, Carey WB, Crocker AC (editors): *Developmental-Behavioral Pediatrics.* Saunders, 1992.

Lowrey GH: *Growth and Development of Children,* 8th ed. Year Book, 1986.

Piaget J, Inyhelder B: *The Psychology of the Child.* Basic Books, 1969.

Walker D et al: Early Language Milestone Scale and language screening of young children. Pediatrics 1989;83: 284.

Yogman MW, Cook KV, Gersten M: Infant and toddler development: Active organization of the social world. Curr Probl Pediatr (May) 1988;18:259.

THE EARLY SCHOOL YEARS: 5–7

Attendance in kindergarten at 5 years marks an acceleration in the separation/individuation theme initiated in the preschool years. The child is ready to relate to peers in a more interactive manner than demonstrated by previous parallel play. The brain has reached 90% of its adult weight. At approximately 6 years, a remodeling of the cortex occurs. The Betz cells decrease in length and increase in width. The cortex, in general, shows a decrease in total thickness, with an increase in the number of nerve cells in the different layers. Sensor-motor coordination abilities are maturing and facilitating pencil-and-paper tasks and sports, both part of the school experience.

Cognitive abilities are still at the preoperational stage, and children focus on one variable in a problem at a time. However, by $5\frac{1}{2}$ years, most children have mastered conservation of length; by $6\frac{1}{2}$ years, conservation of mass and weight; and by 8 years, conservation of volume.

By first grade, there is more pressure on the child to master academic tasks, including the recognition of numbers, letters, and words, and the ability to write. Piaget describes the stage of concrete operations beginning after age 6, when the child is able to perform mental operations concerning concrete objects that involve the manipulation of more than one variable. The child is able to order, number, and classify because these activities are related to concrete objects in the environment and because these activities are stressed in early schooling. Magical thinking diminishes greatly at this time, and the reality of cause-and-effect relationships is better understood. Fantasy and imagination are still strong and are re-

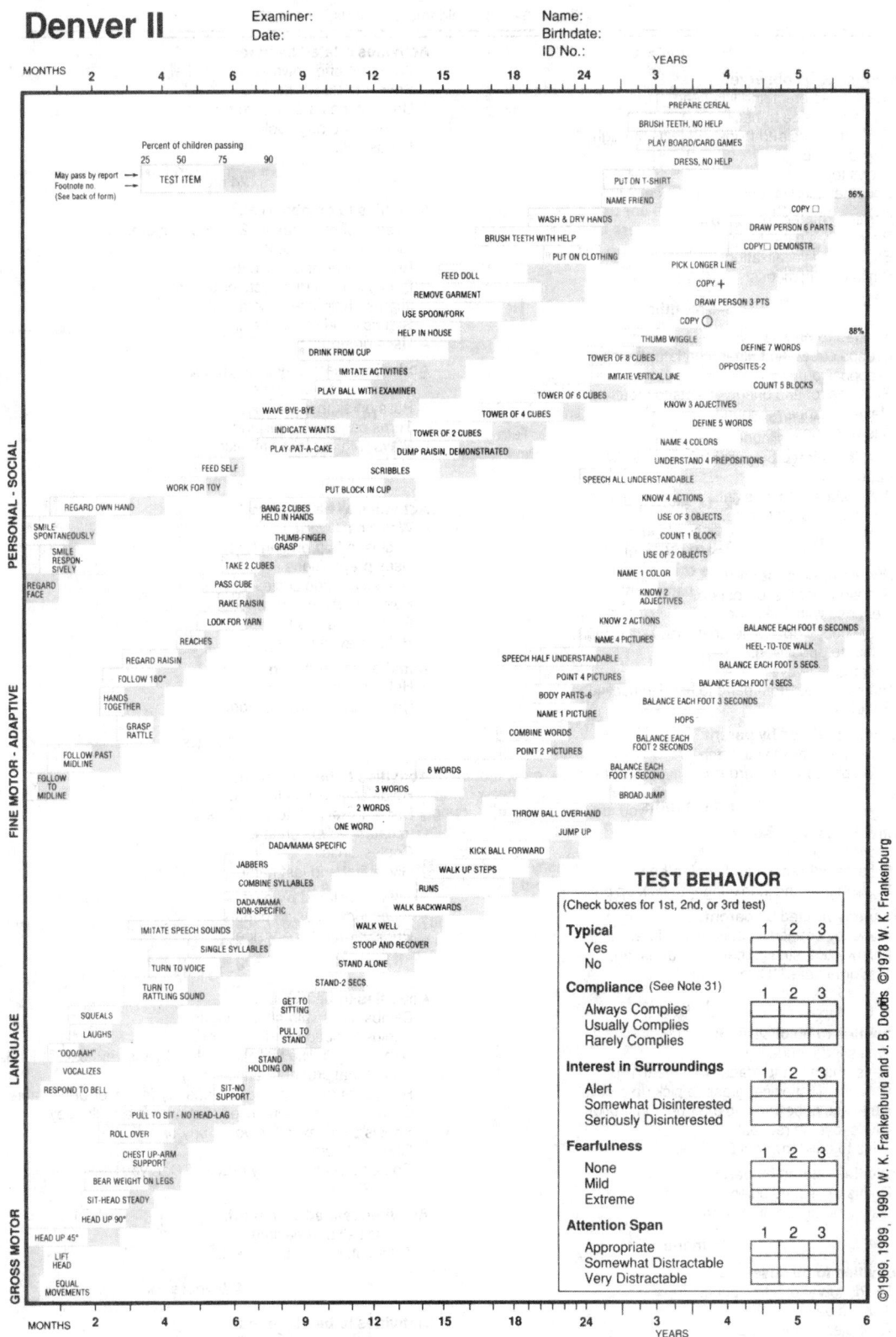

Figure 3–11. Denver II.

Table 3–3. Developmental charts.[1]

1–2 months

Activities to be observed:
Holds head erect and lifts head.
Turns from side to back.
Regards faces and follows objects through
visual field.
Drops toys.
Becomes alert in response to voice.

Activities related by parent:
Recognizes parents.
Engages in vocalizations.
Smiles spontaneously.

3–5 months

Activities to be observed:
Grasps cube—first ulnar then later thumb
opposition.
Reaches for and brings objects to mouth.
Makes "raspberry" sound.
Sits with support.

Activities related by parent:
Laughs.
Anticipates food on sight.
Turns from back to side.

6–8 months

Activites to be observed:
Sits alone for a short period.
Reaches with one hand.
First scoops up a pellet then grasps it using
thumb opposition.
Imitates "bye-bye."
Passes object from hand to hand in midline.
Babbles.

Activities related by parent:
Rolls from back to stomach.
Is inhibited by the word *no.*

9–11 months

Activities to be observed:
Stands alone.
Imitates pat-a-cake and peek-a-boo.
Uses thumb and index finger to pick up pellet.

Activities related by parent:
Walks by supporting self on furniture.
Follows one-step verbal commands, eg,
"Come here," "Give it to me."

1 year

Activities to be observed:
Walks independently.
Says "mama" and "dada" with meaning.
Can use neat pincer grasp to pick up a pellet.
Releases cube into cup after demonstration.
Gives toys on request.
Tries to build tower of 2 cubes.

Activities related by parent:
Points to desired objects.
Says one or two other words.

18 months

Activities to be observed:
Builds tower of 3 to 4 cubes.
Throws ball.
Scribbles spontaneously.
Seats self in chair.
Dumps pellet from bottle.

Activities related by parent:
Walks up and down stairs with help.
Says 4 to 20 words.
Understands a 2-step command.
Carries and hugs doll.
Feeds self.

24 months

Activities to be observed:
Speaks short phrases, 2 words or more.
Kicks ball on request.
Builds tower of 6 to 7 cubes.
Points to named objects or pictures.
Jumps off floor with both feet.
Stands on either foot alone.
Uses pronouns.

Activities related by parent:
Verbalizes toilet needs.
Pulls on simple garment.
Turns pages of book singly.
Plays with domestic mimicry.

30 months

Activities to be observed:
Walks backward.
Begins to hop on one foot.
Uses prepositions.
Copies a crude circle.
Points to objects described by use.
Refers to self as I.
Holds crayon in fist.

Activites related by parent:
Helps put things away.
Carries on a conversation.

3 years

Activities to be observed:
Holds crayon with fingers.
Builds tower of 9 to 10 cubes.
Imitates 3-cube bridge.
Copies circle.
Gives first and last name.

Activities related by parent:
Rides tricycle using pedals.
Dresses with supervision.

3–4 years

Activities to be observed:
Climbs stairs with alternating feet.
Begins to button and unbutton.
"What do you like to do that's fun?" (Answers using plurals,
personal pronoun, and verbs.)
Responds to command to place toy *in, on,* or *under* table.
Draws a circle when asked to draw a man (girl, boy).
Knows own sex. ("Are you a boy or a girl?")
Gives full name.
Copies a circle already drawn. ("Can you make one like
this?")

Activities related by parent:
Feeds self at mealtime.
Takes off shoes and jacket.

4–5 years

Activities to be observed:
Runs and turns without losing balance.
May stand on one leg for at least 10 seconds.

(continued)

Table 3–3. Developmental charts. (continued)

Buttons clothes and laces shoes. (Does not tie.)
Counts to 4 by rote.
"Give me 2 sticks." (Able to do so from pile of 4 tongue depressors.)
Draws a man. (Head, 2 appendages, and possibly 2 eyes. No torso yet.)
Knows the days of the week. ("What day comes after Tuesday?")
Gives appropriate answers to: "What must you do if you are sleepy? Hungry? Cold?"
Copies + in imitation.

Activities related by parent:
Self care at toilet. (May need help with wiping.)
Plays outside for at least 30 minutes.
Dresses self except for tying.

5–6 years

Activities to be observed:
Can catch ball.
Skips smoothly.
Copies a + already drawn.
Tells age.
Concept of 10 (eg, counts 10 tongue depressors). May recite to higher number by rote.
Knows right and left hand.
Draws recognizable man with at least 8 details.
Can describe favorite television program in some detail.

Activities related by parent:
Does simple chores at home. (Taking out garbage, drying silverware, etc.)
Goes to school unattended or meets school bus.
Good motor ability but little awareness of dangers.

6–7 years

Activities to be observed:
Copies a △.
Defines words by use. ("What is an orange?" "To eat.")
Knows if morning or afternoon.
Draws a man with 12 details.
Reads several one-syllable printed words. (My, dog, see, boy.)
Uses pencil for printing name.

7–8 years

Activities to be observed:
Counts by 2s and 5s.
Ties shoes.
Copies a ◇.
Knows what day of the week it is. (Not date or year.)
Reads paragraph # 1 Durrell:

Reading:
Muff is a little yellow kitten. She drinks milk. She sleeps on a chair. She does not like to get wet.

Corresponding arithmetic:

$$\begin{array}{cccc} 7 & 6 & 6 & 8 \\ +4 & +7 & -4 & -3 \end{array}$$

No evidence of sound substitution in speech (eg, *fr* for *thr*).
Adds and subtracts one-digit numbers.
Draws a man with 16 details.

8–9 years

Activities to be observed:
Defines words better than by use. ("What is an orange?" "A fruit.")
Can give an appropriate answer to the following:

"What is the thing for you to do if . . .
—you've broken something that belongs to someone else?"
—a playmate hits you without meaning to do so?"
Reads paragraph # 2 Durrell:

Reading:
A little black dog ran away from home. He played with two big dogs. They ran away from him. It began to rain. He went under a tree. He wanted to go home, but he did not know the way. He saw a boy he knew. The boy took him home.

Corresponding arithmetic:

$$\begin{array}{cccc} & 45 & & \\ 67 & 16 & 14 & 84 \\ + 4 & +27 & - 8 & -36 \end{array}$$

Is learning borrowing and carrying processes in addition and subtraction.

9–10 years

Activities to be observed:
Knows the month, day, and year.
Names the months in order. (Fifteen seconds, one error.)
Makes a sentence with these 3 words in it: (One of 2. Can use words orally in proper context.)
    1. work . . . money . . . men
    2. boy . . . river . . . ball
Reads paragraph # 3 Durrell:

Reading:
Six boys put up a tent by the side of a river. They took things to eat with them. When the sun went down, they went into the tent to sleep. In the night, a cow came and began to eat grass around the tent. The boys were afraid. They thought it was a bear.

Corresponding arithmetic:

$$\begin{array}{ccc} 5204 & 23 & 837 \\ - 530 & \times 3 & \times 7 \end{array}$$

Should comprehend and answer question: "What was the cow doing?"
Learning simple multiplication.

10–12 years

Activities to be observed:
Should read and comprehend paragraph # 5 Durrell:

Reading:
In 1807, Robert Fulton took the first long trip in a steamboat. He went one hundred and fifty miles up the Hudson River. The boat went five miles an hour. This was faster than a steamboat had ever gone before. Crowds gathered on both banks of the river to see this new kind of boat. They were afraid that its noise and splashing would drive away all the fish.

Corresponding arithmetic:

$$\begin{array}{ccc} 420 & & \\ \times\ 29 & 9\overline{)72} & 31\overline{)62} \end{array}$$

Answer: "What river was the trip made on?"
Ask to write the sentence: "The fishermen did not like the boat."
Should do multiplication and simple division.

12–15 years

Activities to be observed:
Reads paragraph # 7 Durrell:

(continued)

Table 3–3. Developmental charts. (continued)

Reading:
  Golf originated in Holland as a game played on ice. The game in its present form first appeared in Scotland. It became unusually popular and kings found it so enjoyable that it was known as "the royal game." James IV, however, thought that people neglected their work to indulge in this fascinating sport so that it was forbidden in 1457. James relented when he found how attractive the game was, and it immediately regained its former popularity. Golf spread gradually to other countries, being introduced in America in 1890. It has grown in favor until there is hardly a town that does not boast of a private or public course.

Corresponding arithmetic:

$$536\overline{)4762} \qquad \frac{1}{3} \qquad 7\,\frac{1}{6}$$
$$+\,\frac{1}{3} \qquad -\,\frac{3}{4}$$

Reduce fractions to lowest forms.

Ask to write sentence: "Golf originated in Holland as a game played on ice."
Answers questions:
  "Why was golf forbidden by James IV?"
  "Why did he change his mind?"
Does long division, adds and subtracts fractions.

[1]Modified from Leavitt SR, Goodman H, Harvin D: Pediatrics 1963;31:499.

flected in the themes of play. Table 3–3 lists specific developmental abilities through middle childhood and adolescence.

THE MIDDLE CHILDHOOD YEARS: 7–11

Freud terms these the latency years, during which children are not bothered by significant aggressive or sexual drives but instead devote most of their energies to school and peer group interactions. In reality, throughout this period there is a gradual increase in sexual drives, which is manifested by increasingly aggressive play and interactions with the opposite sex. Fantasy still has an active role in dealing with sexuality before adolescence, and fantasies often focus on movie stars and rock heroes. Organized sports, clubs, and other activities are other modalities that permit preadolescent children to display socially acceptable forms of aggression and sexual interest.

For the 7-year-old, the major developmental task focuses on achievement in school and acceptance by peers. Academic expectations have intensified and require the child to concentrate, attend, and process increasingly complex auditory and visual information. Children with significant learning disabilities or problems of attention may have difficulty in these tasks and subsequently may receive significant negative reinforcement from teachers and even parents. Such children may develop a poor self-image, which may be manifested as behavioral difficulties. The pediatrician must evaluate potential learning disabilities in any child who is not developing adequately at this stage or who presents with emotional or behavioral problems. Their abilities are not as easily documented as milestones in early development. In the school-age child, the quality of the response, the attentional abilities, and the child's emotional approach to the task can make a dramatic difference in how successful the child is at school. The clinician must consider all of these aspects to appropriately diagnose learning disabilities. See Chapter 5.

Hagerman RJ: Pediatric assessment of the learning disabled child. J Develop Pediatr 1984;5:274.
Levine MD et al (editors): *Developmental-Behavioral Pediatrics.* Saunders, 1983.
Piaget J, Inyhelder B: *The Psychology of the Child.* Basic Books, 1969.
Vaughan VC, Litt IF: *Child and Adolescent Development: Clinical Implications.* Saunders, 1990. (A thorough review of physical, cognitive, and behavioral development from infancy through adolescence.)

PREPUBERTAL & PUBERTAL GROWTH

The pubertal growth spurt occurs at approximately 10 years in females and 12.5 years in males. The speed of growth increases, reaching a peak of approximately 9 cm/yr in females and 10.3 cm/yr in males. Different areas of the skeleton attain their peak growth at different times. This is seen most dramatically in the feet, which first experience a growth spurt. This is followed by a rapid increase in leg length and subsequently by trunk growth. Facial growth occurs after peak height velocity. The mandible changes most remarkably, demonstrating a 25% increase in height between 12 and 20 years of age, compared to only a 6–7% increase in the size of the cranial base.

Boys have just over 2 more years of preadolescent growth than girls do; during this time leg growth increases more dramatically than trunk growth. Girls have a greater spurt in hip width, related to stature, than boys do, although boys exceed girls in most other areas of bone growth.

The Hypothalamic-Pituitary-Gonadal Axis & Puberty

Gonadal development is initiated in the fetus by 10 weeks' gestation, and it is almost complete by age 3 months in the male. This process occurs without significant input from gonadotropins, although placental hCG plays a significant role in migration of germ cells and differentiation of Leydig's cells. By the 21st week of gestation, the hypothalamus secretes gonadotropin-releasing hormone (GnRH), and the anterior pituitary releases follicle-stimulating hormone (FSH) and luteinizing hormone (LH). Their levels reach a peak by the 23rd to 24th week of gestation, which coincides with oocyte maturation in utero, including the development of primary follicles.

In the newborn period, GnRH is secreted in a pulsatile fashion, causing episodic elevations of both FSH and LH. In females, FSH predominates, and in males LH predominates; they stimulate elevations in testosterone and estrogen in the first few months of life. After this period of significant neuroendocrine activity, a quiescent period, with almost undetectable levels of gonadotropins, sets in and lasts through childhood. Hypothalamic secretion of GnRH is suppressed until puberty.

The large fetal adrenal gland regresses significantly after birth until adrenarche at 6–9 years of age. Adrenarche refers to the regrowth of the zona reticularis and the activation of its enzyme systems to produce adrenal steroids such as dehydroepiandrosterone sulfate and 17-ketosteroids. These steroids are partially responsible for body odor, the development of pubic and axillary hair, and stimulation of linear growth. Adrenarche occurs before gonadarche and is probably under the control of ACTH.

Gonadarche is initiated by the pulsatile secretion of GnRH from the hypothalamus, which in turn stimulates the release of gonadotropins. In early puberty, FSH and LH are secreted during sleep, and there is an increasing amplitude in its pulses as puberty progresses. The efficacy of FSH and LH also changes in that biopotency of these hormones improves as puberty progresses.

In conjunction with adrenal steroids and growth hormone, testosterone, stimulated from Leydig's cells, promotes a relatively specific pattern of pubertal development. The testes increase in size before 10 years of age, and pubic hair subsequently develops at the base of the penis in the first stage of puberty. The scrotum becomes more pendulous, the penis increases in size, and a mild degree of gynecomastia develops in 70% of males in the second stage of puberty. In the third and fourth stages of puberty, the voice deepens because of laryngeal growth, and there is an increase in sebaceous and sweat gland activity, often accompanied by acne. Growth hormone potentiates the action of sex steroids in males and facilitates the pubertal growth spurt. Muscle mass increases; boys gain particularly in shoulder width.

Sex steroids have some effect on bone growth but a more dramatic effect on bone maturation. They promote the fusion of epiphysial plates in a predictable order. For instance, the plate at the head of the femur fuses between 15 and 17 years in boys and between 14 and 16 years in girls. The distal epiphyses of the radius, ulna, tibia, fibula, and femur fuse at 18–20 years in boys and 17–19 years in girls. The stage of osseous development correlates better with sexual maturation than does chronologic age or any other growth parameter. Most females begin menarche when skeletal maturation is between 13 and 13.5 years.

In females, breast buds begin between 8 and 13 years, with an average onset at 11 years. Usually the growth spurt has already begun at 10 years, and pubic hair usually develops soon after 11 years. Within the next 3–4 years, the pubic hair increases, the breasts, areola, and nipples enlarge further, and the hip width increases. Growth in the breasts is initially due to elongation and thickening of the ducts secondary to estrogen stimulation. After ovulation, progesterone from the corpus luteum stimulates the distal ends of the ducts to form lobules and alveoli, further enlarging the breasts.

Menarche usually occurs approximately 2 years after the onset of breast development. However, approximately 50–90% of cycles are anovulatory during the first 2 years after menarche. Although the average age for menarche is 13 years, this age has decreased significantly over the last century. Malnutrition, a low socioeconomic level, and excessive exercise can all delay menarche. After menarche, the final stage of neuroendocrine regulation occurs, with a biphasic effect of estrogen on the hypothalamus. Estrogens initially suppress secretion of gonadotropins, but subsequently a positive feedback system develops. A critical concentration of estrogen causes a surge of FSH and LH secretion in mid cycle, which stimulates ovulation.

In late puberty and adulthood, the nighttime predominance of gonadotropin pulses ceases, and pulsatile secretion occurs throughout the day and night. After menarche, the average increase in height is 3 inches, with a range of 1–7 inches, in American girls. For further information on adolescent development, see Chapter 4.

Falkner F, Tanner JM (editors): *Postnatal Growth Neurobiology.* Vol 2 of: *Human Growth, a Comprehensive Treatise,* 2nd ed. Plenum Press, 1986.

Lowrey GH: *Growth and Development of Children,* 8th ed. Year Book, 1986.

Orr DP, Ingersoll GM: Adolescent development: A biopsychosocial review. Curr Probl Pediatr (Aug) 1988;18:447.

Vaughan VC, Litt IF: *Child and Adolescent Development: Clinical Implications.* Saunders, 1990.

ADOLESCENT COGNITIVE & SOCIAL DEVELOPMENT

Adolescence is a difficult time because of the rehashing of earlier developmental issues, such as individuation and separation, but now in a context of a rapidly growing and maturing body and changing cognitive abilities. Piaget describes the development of formal operations in cognitive development at age 12. At this stage, abstract reasoning predominates in problem solving and understanding cause-and-effect relationships. Adolescents at this stage can better appreciate the relationship between current behavior and its long-term consequences. Egocentrism diminishes, and individuals are able to empathize and understand another's viewpoint.

The reality of the situation, however, is that very few young adolescents are in the stage of formal operations, and a substantial proportion of adolescents and adults never attain formal operational thinking. The thinking of early adolescents tends to be rigid and egocentric, with an overemphasis on concrete and physical aspects of social interaction. Some adolescents do not relate present actions to future consequences and cannot conceptualize. In an interview, they often give one-word answers and may not discuss a concept at length. It is best to ask very concrete, specific questions to facilitate communication.

In mid adolescence, they begin to think abstractly, but the development of abstract thinking is a gradual process. It begins with introspection, which exacerbates the egocentrism of adolescence. Adolescents think about their own thinking and actions and develop pride in themselves, but often disdain for others, particularly adults, as they become critical of the thought processes of others. Their moral thinking advances, and they begin accepting the moral standards of the family and community rather than acting in certain ways for fear of punishment. Rules become more important, and dependence on and conformity to these rules dominate their lives, particularly at school. If they have difficulty succeeding in school, they may seek situations in which they can be successful, such as in a peer group that promotes antisocial behavior.

By mid to late adolescence, adult morality usually develops. It is marked by the development of moral principles that are autonomous and have validity apart from group rules. An individual is able to think abstractly about right and wrong and sort each problem out individually. Social cognitive growth, by late adolescence, is characterized by a lack of egocentrism and a true empathy for others. Rigidity is replaced by flexibility, and individuals become more accepting of those who are different from themselves. A lack of impulsiveness, an appropriate compliance, and an appreciation of long-term consequences facilitate the provision of health care at this stage. Some individuals do not reach this stage until adulthood, and some never achieve it. For further information, see Chapter 6.

Dixon SD, Stein MT: *Encounters with Children: Pediatric Behavior and Development,* 2nd ed. Mosby Year Book, 1992.

Felice ME: Adolescence. In: Levine MD et al (editors). *Developmental-Behavioral Pediatrics,* 2nd ed. Saunders, 1992.

Orr DP, Ingersoll GM: Adolescent development: A biopsychosocial review. Curr Probl Pediatr (Aug) 1988;18:447.

Adolescence

David W. Kaplan, MD, MPH, & Kathleen A. Mammel, MD

Adolescence is a unique period of rapid physical, emotional, cognitive, and social growth and development bridging childhood and adulthood. Generally, adolescence begins at age 11–12 years and ends between ages 18 and 21. Most teenagers complete puberty by ages 16–18 years; in Western society, however, for educational and cultural reasons, the adolescent period is prolonged to allow for further psychosocial development before the young person assumes adult responsibilities.

The developmental passage from childhood to adulthood encompasses the following steps: (1) completing puberty and somatic growth; (2) developing socially, emotionally, and cognitively—moving from concrete to abstract thinking; (3) establishing an independent identity and separating from the family; and (4) preparing for a career or vocation.

DEMOGRAPHY

In the United States in 1990, there were 17.9 million adolescents between the ages of 15 and 19 years and 19.1 million between 20 and 24 years of age. Adolescents and young adults (15–24 years of age) constitute 15% of the United States population.

MORTALITY DATA

As with all age groups in the United States, there has been a remarkable decrease in the mortality rate among 15- to 24-year-olds during this century. Deaths due to infectious diseases such as tuberculosis, influenza, and pneumonia, which were common at the beginning of the century, are rare events today. During the last 20 years, there have been changes not only in the major causes of death in the adolescent and young adult population but also in disease-specific mortality rates. Deaths due to motor vehicle crashes, suicide, and homicide have increased 300–400%. For the adolescent population, cultural and environmental rather than organic factors pose the greatest threats of death. For every 15- to 19-year-old who dies of cancer, ten die as a result of an unintentional injury.* For every teenager who dies of heart disease, 6.7 die as a result of homicide; and for every teenager who dies of kidney disease, 62 commit suicide.

The three leading causes of death (Figure 4–1) in the adolescent population (ages 15–19 years) in 1990 were unintentional injuries (48.1–78% of all unintentional injuries were caused by motor vehicle crashes), suicides (12.6%), and homicides (19.3%). These three causes of violent death accounted for 80.1% of all adolescent deaths among 15- to 19-year-olds. Examination of causes of death by ethnic grouping emphasizes how strongly socioeconomic factors contribute to adolescent mortality statistics. The unintentional injury rate among white teenagers aged 15–19 years (45.3:100,000) is almost one and one-half time higher than among blacks (29.7:100,000). This difference reflects the high rate of mortality due to motor vehicle accidents among white males. By contrast, the homicide rate among black teenagers (66.1:100,000) is eight times greater than that among white teenagers (8.2:100,000). Homicide is the leading cause of death for black male teenagers, and has increased 270% since 1983. Suicide is 1.7 times more prevalent among white teenagers (11.9:100,000) than black teenagers (6.7:100,000). Although deaths from automobile crashes have decreased over the last few years, alcohol use remains the underlying cause of most teenage motor vehicle deaths. Almost two-thirds of motor vehicle deaths involving young drinking drivers occur on Friday, Saturday, or Sunday, and 70% occur between 8:00 PM and 4:00 AM.

Deaths due to unintentional injury, homicide, and suicide among adolescents and young adults are distressing not only because of their violent nature but also because they are largely preventable.

---

*The term "injury" is preferable to "accidents," which implies "an act of God" or "bad luck." Injuries during this period most commonly are related to motor vehicle accidents, drownings, falls, and fires. Injuries comprise three elements: the host (who is affected), the agent (the direct cause), and the environment (where, when, and under what conditions).

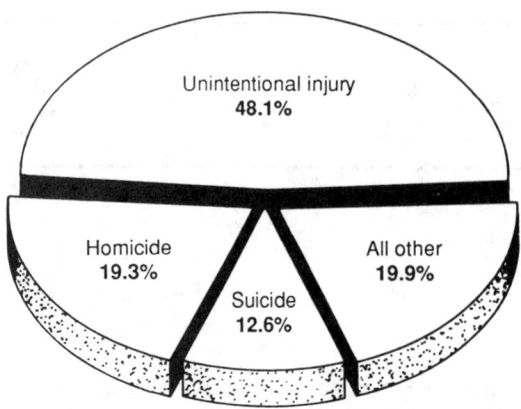

Figure 4–1. Percent mortality, ages 15–19 years, 1990.

MORBIDITY DATA

During the mid 1970s and 1980s, demographic and economic changes in the American family have had a profound effect on many children and adolescents. Between 1955 and 1980, the divorce rate rose from about 400,000 to nearly 1,200,000 a year. Between 1960 and 1984, the number of children involved in divorce each year increased from 460,000 to 1,100,000. In 1990, 25% of children were living in single-parent homes, compared with 12% in 1970. In

that year, 40% of children with only one parent were in families with an annual income of less than $10,000 per year. Forty-one percent of black, 28% of Hispanic, and 11% of white children under the age of 18 years were living in poverty.

The major causes of morbidity during adolescence are primarily psychosocial: unintended pregnancy, sexually transmitted disease, substance abuse, smoking, dropping out of school, depression, running away from home, physical violence, and juvenile delinquency. Early identification of the teenager at risk for these problems is important to prevent the immediate complications and future associated problems. High-risk behavior in one area is often associated with or may lead to problems in another area (Figure 4–2). For example, teenagers who live in a dysfunctional family (eg, having problems related to parental alcoholism or perhaps physical or sexual abuse) are much more likely than other teenagers to have emotional problems, such as depression. A depressed teenager is at greater risk for abusing drugs or alcohol, having academic difficulties, running away from home, getting involved sexually as a means of seeking the attention and affection they are not receiving at home, acquiring a sexually transmitted disease, committing suicide, and having an unintended pregnancy.

The early indicators of an adolescent at high risk for problems related to depression include the following:

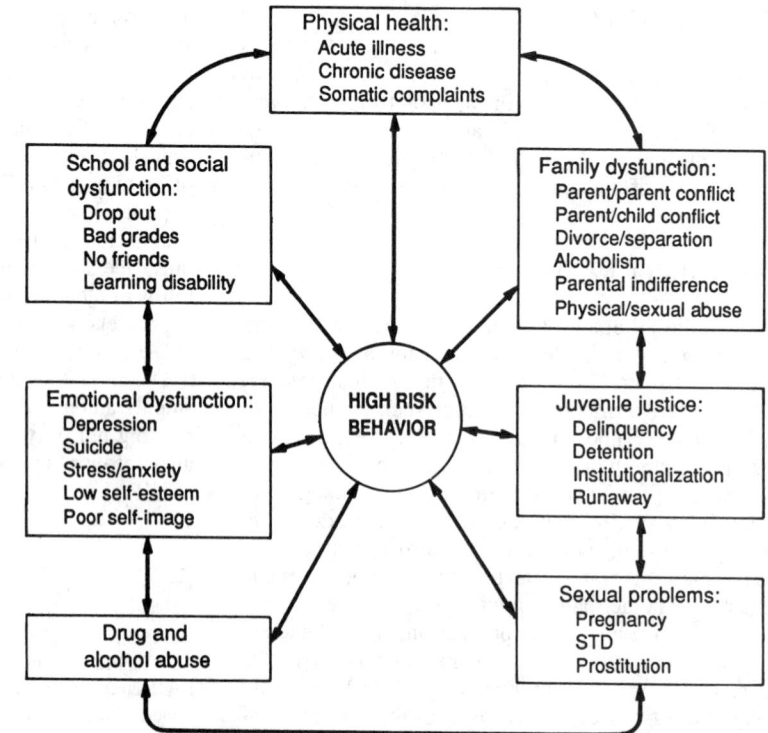

Figure 4–2. Interrelation of high-risk adolescent behavior.

(1) Decline in school performance.

(2) Excessive school absences or cutting class.

(3) Frequent or persistent psychosomatic complaints.

(4) Changes in sleeping or eating habits.

(5) Difficulty in concentrating or persistent boredom.

(6) Signs or symptoms of depression, extreme stress, or anxiety.

(7) Withdrawal from friends or family, or change to a new group of friends.

(8) Unusually severe violent or rebellious behavior, or radical personality change.

(9) Conflict with parents.

(10) Sexual acting out.

(11) Conflicts with the law.

(12) Suicidal thoughts or preoccupation with themes of death.

(13) Drug and alcohol abuse.

(14) Running away from home.

Committee on Adolescence, American Academy of Pediatrics: Firearms and adolescents. Pediatrics 1992;89:784.

Dryfoos JG: *Adolescents at Risk: Prevalence and Prevention.* Oxford Univ Press, 1990.

Haggerty RJ. Care of the poor and underserved in America. Older adolescents: A group at special risk. Am J Dis Child 1991;145:569.

Hechinger FM: *Fateful Choices: Healthy Youth for the 21st Century.* Carnegie Corporation of New York, 1992.

Irwin CE, Ryan SA: Problem behavior of adolescents. Pediatr Rev 1989;10:235.

Jessor R, Donovan JE, Costa FM: *Beyond Adolescence: Problem Behavior and Young Adult Development.* Cambridge Univ Press, 1991.

McManus MA, Newacheck PW, Greaney AM: Young adults with special health care needs: Prevalence, severity and access to health services. Pediatrics 1990;86:674.

McManus M et al: Hospital use by adolescents and young adults. J Adolesc Health 1991;12:10.

Millstein SG, Petersen AC, Nightingale EO: *Promoting the Health of Adolescents: New Directions for the Twenty-First Century.* Oxford Univ Press, 1993.

Newacheck PW, McManus MA, Fox HB: Prevalence and impact of chronic illness among adolescents. Am J Dis Child 1991;145:1367.

Rogers DE (editor). Cornell Health Policy Conference: Adolescents at risk. J Adolesc Health 1991;12:585.

Wood DL et al: Access to medical care for children and adolescents in the United States. Pediatrics 1990;86:666.

DELIVERY OF HEALTH SERVICES

How, where, why, and when adolescents seek health care depend on a number of factors: ability to pay for care, distance to health care facilities, availability of transportation, accessibility of services, time out of school, and privacy. Many common teenage health problems—eg, unintended pregnancy, sexually transmitted disease, the need for contraception, substance abuse, and depression and other emotional problems—have moral or ethical implications. Teenagers are often reluctant to confide in their parents for fear of punishment or disapproval. For example, a 15-year-old boy who thinks he has gonorrhea might be reluctant to ask his mother to take him to the doctor. Recognizing this reality, health care providers have set up many specialized programs, eg, teenage family planning clinics, drop-in centers, sexually transmitted disease clinics, hot lines, and adolescent clinics. For the physician, establishing a trusting and confidential relationship is basic to meeting an adolescent patient's health care needs. A patient who senses the physician will inform the parents about a confidential problem may lie or fail to disclose information essential for proper diagnosis and treatment.

RELATING TO THE ADOLESCENT PATIENT

Adolescence is one of the physically healthiest periods in an individual's life. The challenge of caring for adolescents does not lie in managing complex organic disease but in accommodating to the changing and developing cognitive, emotional, and psychosocial growth that influences health behavior.

How the physician initially approaches the adolescent may determine the success or failure of the visit. The physician should behave simply and honestly, without an authoritarian or excessively "professional" manner. Because the self-esteem of many young adolescents is fragile, the physician must be careful not to overpower and intimidate the patient. To establish a comfortable and trusting relationship, the physician should strive to present the image of an ordinary person who has special training and skills.

Because onset and termination of puberty may vary considerably from individual to individual, chronologic age may be a poor indicator of expected physical, physiologic, and emotional development. In communicating with an adolescent, the physician must be especially sensitive to the patient's developmental level, recognizing that physical appearance and chronologic age may not give an accurate assessment of cognitive development. Talking to a teenager as a child or, at the other extreme, as an adult, may interfere with communication and cause the patient to lose confidence in the provider.

Working with teenagers can be quite draining emotionally. Adolescents have a unique ability to identify hidden emotional vulnerabilities. The physician who has a personal need to control patients or foster dependency may be disappointed in caring for teenagers. Because teenagers are consumed with their own emotional needs, they rarely provide the physician with the ego rewards that younger or older patients do.

The physician should be sensitive to the issue of countertransference, the emotional reaction elicited in the physician by the adolescent. How the physician relates to the adolescent patient often depends on personal characteristics of the physician. This is especially true of physicians treating families with parent-adolescent conflicts. It is common for young physicians to overidentify with the teenage patient and for older physicians to see the conflict from the parents' perspective. Older physicians with adolescent children may carry over many of their own parenting conflicts, dealing with the adolescent patient as they would with their own children. Over-identification with the parents is readily sensed by the teenager, who is likely to view the physician as just another authority figure who cannot understand the problems of being a teenager. Assuming a parental-authoritarian role as a physician and lecturing the adolescent not only is counterproductive but also may seriously jeopardize establishing a working relationship with the patient. In the case of the young physician, overidentification with the teenager may cause the parents to become extremely defensive about their parenting role and discount the experience and ability of the physician.

Meeks JE: *The Fragile Alliance.* Krieger, 1980.

THE SETTING

Adolescents respond positively to a setting and services that communicate a sensitivity to their age. For instance, a pediatrician's waiting room scattered with toddler's toys and examination tables too short for a young adult make adolescent patients feel that they have outgrown the practice. Similarly, a waiting room filled with geriatric or pregnant patients can make a teenager feel out of place. An examination room designed with adolescents in mind and special appointment times may be useful in engaging this age group.

It is not uncommon to see a new teenage patient who has absolutely no interest in being there, especially when the teenager is brought in for evaluation of drug and alcohol use, parent-adolescent conflict, school failure, depression, or a suspected eating disorder. Even in cases of acute physical illness, the adolescent may feel anxiety about having a physical examination, especially if the teenager is overly modest, is worried about having blood drawn, or simply fears the unknown. If future visits are to be successful, the physician must spend time on the first visit to give the teenager a sense of trust and an opportunity to feel comfortable.

CONFIDENTIALITY

It is helpful at the beginning of the visit to talk with the adolescent and the parents about what to expect. The physician should address the issue of confidentiality, telling the parents that two meetings—one with the teenager alone and one only with the parents—will take place. Adequate time must be spent with both the patient and the parents, or important information may be missed. At the beginning of the interview with the patient, it is useful to say, "I am likely to ask you some personal questions. This is not because I am trying to snoop into your private life, but because these questions may be important to your health. I want to assure you that what we talk about is confidential, just between the two of us. If there is something I feel we should discuss with your parents, I will ask your permission first, unless I feel it is life-threatening."

THE STRUCTURE OF THE VISIT

Caring for adolescents is a time-intensive process. In many adolescent practices, a 40–50% no-show rate is not unusual, making scheduling complex. In addition, it is not uncommon for an adolescent to come in without an appointment because of a seemingly minor complaint. Because of issues related to confidentiality, teenagers may initially conceal their real concern. For example, a healthy-appearing 15-year-old girl may walk in with the chief complaint of a sore throat but actually be worried about being pregnant. What initially appeared to be a 10-minute visit for a throat culture may turn into a 1-hour visit spent counseling an anxious pregnant teenager.

By the age of 11 or 12, patients should be seen alone, without a parent. This gives them an opportunity to ask questions they may be embarrassed to ask in front of a parent. Because of the physical changes that take place in early puberty, some adolescents are too self-conscious to undress in front of a parent (and sometimes the physician). If an adolescent comes in willingly, either for an acute illness or a routine physical examination, it may be helpful to meet with the adolescent and parent together to obtain the history. In the case of angry adolescents who are brought in against their will, it is useful to meet with the parents and adolescent just long enough to have the parents describe the conflict and state their concerns. This meeting should last no longer than 3–5 minutes, and then the adolescent should be seen alone. This approach conveys that the physician is primarily interested in the adolescent patient, yet gives the physician an opportunity to acknowledge the parents' anger and the fact that the patient probably didn't want to come in the first place.

The Interview

The first few minutes of the interview may dictate the success of the visit—whether or not a trusting relationship can be established. Taking a few minutes getting to know the patient is time well spent. For example, immediately asking a teenager who is brought in for suspected marihuana use "Do you smoke marihuana?" confirms the adolescent's negative preconceptions about the physician and the purpose of the visit.

It is preferable to spend a few minutes asking nonthreatening questions. Examples are: "Tell me a little bit about yourself so I can get to know you." "What do you like to do most?" "Least?" "What are your friends like?" Neutral questions help defuse some of the patient's anger and anxiety. Examples are: "How has your health been?" "What kinds of serious accidents or injuries have you had?" Toward the end of the interview, the physician can ask more directed questions about psychosocial concerns.

Medical history questionnaires for the patient and the parents are very useful in collecting the necessary historical data and making the visit as efficient as possible (Figure 4–3). Although the history questionnaire is helpful, the physician must spend sufficient time to get to know the patient and establish a meaningful relationship.

The history should include an assessment of progress with psychodevelopmental tasks and of behaviors that are potentially detrimental to health. The review of systems should include questions about the following:

(1) Nutrition: number and balance of meals; calcium, iron, cholesterol intake.
(2) Sleep: number of hours, problems with insomnia or frequent waking.
(3) Seat belt or helmet: regularity of use.
(4) Self-care: knowledge of testicular or breast self-examination, dental hygiene, and exercise.
(5) Family relationships: parents, siblings, relatives.
(6) Peers: best friend, involvement in group activities, boyfriends, girlfriends.
(7) School: attendance, grades, activities.
(8) Educational and vocational interests: college, career, short- and long-term vocational plans.
(9) Tobacco: use of cigarettes, snuff, chewing tobacco.
(10) Substance abuse: frequency, extent, and history of alcohol and drug use.
(11) Sexuality: sexual activity, contraceptive use, pregnancies, history of sexually transmitted disease, number of sexual partners, risk for HIV infection.
(12) Emotional health: signs of depression and excessive stress.

The physician's personal attention and interest is likely to be a new experience for the teenager, who has probably received medical care only through a parent. The teenager should leave the visit with a sense of having a personal physician.

Physical Examination

During early adolescence, many teenagers may be quite shy and modest, especially if examined by a physician of the opposite sex. The examiner should address this concern directly, because it can be allayed by acknowledging the uneasiness verbally and explaining the purpose of the examination–eg, "Many boys that I see who are your age are embarrassed to have their penis and testes (balls) examined. This is an important part of the examination for a couple of reasons. First, I want to make sure that there aren't any physical problems, and second, it helps me determine if your development is proceeding normally." This also introduces the subject of sexual development for discussion.

A pictorial chart of sexual development (Figures 4–4 and 4–5) is extremely useful in showing the patient how development is proceeding and what changes to expect in the future. The chart shows the relationship between height, breast development, menstruation, and pubic hair growth in the female and between height, penis and testes development, and pubic hair growth in the male. Although many teenagers do not openly admit that they are interested in this subject, they are usually quite attentive during the discussion. This discussion is useful in counseling teenagers who lag behind their peers in physical development.

Because teenagers are especially sensitive about their changing bodies, it is useful to comment on the findings during the physical examination—eg, "Your heart sounds fine. I am examining your breasts and feel a small lump under your right breast. This is very common during puberty in boys. It is called gynecomastia and should disappear in 6 months to a year. Don't worry, you are not turning into a girl."

The question of the appropriate age for the first pelvic examination often arises. The following are indications for a pelvic examination in a teenage girl:

(1) Sexual intercourse. (The pelvic examination should be done for purposes of contraceptive counseling and to rule out sexually transmitted disease.)
(2) Abnormal vaginal discharge.
(3) Menstrual irregularities, eg, amenorrhea, hypermenorrhea, dysmenorrhea.
(4) Suspicion of anatomic abnormalities, eg, diethylstilbestrol exposure, imperforate hymen.
(5) Pelvic pain.
(6) Patient request of an examination.

If a teenage girl has not been sexually active and has no gynecologic complaints or abnormalities, a

TEEN HEALTH HISTORY

This information is *strictly confidential.* Its purpose is to help your caregiver give you better care. We request that you fill out the form completely, but you may skip any question that you do not wish to answer.

NAME _____ DATE _____
         FIRST   MIDDLE INITIAL   LAST

BIRTHDATE_____AGE_____GRADE_____Name that you like to be called_____

1. Why did you come to the clinic today? _____
_____
_____

Medical History   **STRICTLY CONFIDENTIAL**

2. Are you allergic to any medicines? . . . . YES NO
Name of medicine _____
3. Are you taking any medicines now? . . . . YES NO
Name of medicine _____
4. Do you have any longterm health conditions? . . . . YES NO
Condition _____
5. Date or age at your last tetanus (or dT) shot) _____

School Information

6. What grade do you usually make in English? _____
(Example: A, B, C, D, E, F)
7. What grade do you usually make in Math? _____
8. How many days were you absent from school last semester?_____
9. How many days were you absent last semester due to illness?_____
10. How do you get along at school? _____

1	2	3	4	5	6	7
TERRIBLE						GREAT

11. Have you ever been suspended? . . . . YES NO
12. Have you ever dropped out of school? . . . . YES NO
13. Do you plan to graduate from high school? . . . . YES NO

Job/Career Information

14. Are you working? . . . . YES NO
If YES, What is your job?_____
How many hours do you work per week? _____
15. What are your future plans or career goals? _____

Family Information

16. Who do you live with? (Check all that apply.)
_____Both natural parents _____Stepmother _____Brother(s)-ages:__
_____Mother _____Stepfather _____Sister(s)-ages: __
_____Father _____Guardian _____Other: explain ___
_____Adoptive parents _____Alone

17. Have there been any changes in your family such as: (Check all the changes that apply.)
_____a. Marriage _____d. Serious illness _____g. Births
_____b. Separation _____e. Loss of job _____h. Deaths
_____c. Divorce _____f. Move to a new house _____i. Other

18. Father's/stepfather's occupation or job: _____
Mother's/stepmother's occupation or job: _____

Figure 4–3. Adolescent medical history questionnaire.

STRICTLY CONFIDENTIAL

19. How do you get along at home?

1	2	3	4	5	6	7
TERRIBLE						GREAT

20. Have you ever run away from home? .... YES NO
21. Have you ever lived in foster care or an institution? .... YES NO

Self Information

22. On the whole, how do you like yourself?

1	2	3	4	5	6	7
NOT VERY MUCH						A LOT

23. What do you do best? _____
24. If you could, what would you like to change about your life or yourself?_____

25. List any habits you would like to break. _____

26. Do you feel people expect too much of you? .... YES NO
27. How do you get along with your friends/peers?

1	2	3	4	5	6	7
TERRIBLE						GREAT

28. Do you feel you have any friends you can count on? .... YES NO
29. Have you ever felt really sad or depressed for more than 3 days in a row? . YES NO
30. Have you ever thought of suicide as a solution to your problems? ...... YES NO
31. Have you gotten into any trouble because of your anger/temper? ...... YES NO

Health Concern

32. On a scale of 1–7, how would you rate your general health?

1	2	3	4	5	6	7
TERRIBLE						GREAT

33. Do you have questions or concerns about any of the following? (Check those that apply.)

___Height/Weight	___Skin rash	___Family violence/physical
___Blood pressure	___Arms, legs/muscle or	abuse
___Head/headaches	joint pain	___Feeling down or depressed
___Dizziness/passing out	___Frequent or painful	___Dating
___Eyes/vision	urination	___Sex
___Ears/hearing/earaches	___Wetting the bed	___Worried about VD/STD
___Nose/frequent colds	___Sexual organs/genitals	___Masturbation
___Mouth/teeth	___Trouble sleeping	___Sexual abuse/rape
___Neck/Back	___Tiredness	___Having children/parenting/
___Chest/breathing/coughing	___Diet food/appetite	adoption
___Breasts	___Eating disorder	___Cancer or dying
___Heart	___Smoking, drugs, alcohol	___Other (explain) _____
___Stomach/pain/vomiting	___Future plans/jobs	_____
___Diarrhea/constipation	___Worried about parents	

Health Behavior Information

34. Do you ever drive after drinking or when high?......................... YES NO
35. Do you ever smoke cigarettes? .... YES NO
36. Do you ever smoke marijuana? .... YES NO
37. Do you ever drink alcoholic beverages? .... YES NO
38. Do you ever use street drugs (speed, cocaine, acid, crack, etc.)? .... YES NO
39. Does anyone in your household smoke? .... YES NO
40. Does anyone in your family have a problem with drugs or alcohol? .... YES NO
41. Have you ecer been in trouble with the law? .... YES NO
42. Have you begun dating? .... YES NO

Figure 4–3. Adolescent medical history questionnaire. (continued)

STRICTLY CONFIDENTIAL

43. Do you currently have a boyfriend or girlfriend? . . . . YES NO
    If YES, how old is he/she?. . . . . YES NO
44. Do you think you might be gay/lesbian/homosexual)? . . . . YES NO
45. Have you ever had sex (sexual intercourse)? . . . . YES NO
46. Are you interested in receiving information on preventing pregnancy? . . . . YES NO
47. If you have had sex, are you (or your partner) using any kind of birth control? . YES NO
48. If you have had sex, have you ever been treated for gonorrhea or chlamydia
    or other sexually transmitted disease? . . . . YES NO

For males only
49. Have you been taught how to use a condom correctly? . . . . YES NO
50. If you have had sex, do you use a condom every time or almost every time?. . YES NO
51. Have you ever fathered a child? . . . . YES NO

For females only
52. How old were you when your periods began? . . . . _____
53. What date did your last period start? . . . . _____
54. Are your periods regular (once a month)? . . . . YES NO
55. Do you have painful or excessively heavy periods? . . . . YES NO
56. Have you ever had a vaginal infection or been treated for a female disorder? . YES NO
57. Do you think you might be pregnant? . . . . YES NO
58. Have you ever been pregnant? . . . . YES NO

Everyone
59. Do you have any other problems you would like to discuss with the caregiver? YES NO

Past Medical History
60. Were you born prematurely or did you have any serious problems as an infant? YES NO
61. Are you allergic to any medicines? vs Do you have any allergies? . . . . YES NO
    If YES, what? _____
    _____

62. List any medications that you are taking and the problems for which the
    medication was given:
    MEDICATION   REASON   HOW LONG

63. Have you ever been hospitalized? . . . . YES NO
    If YES, describe the problem and your age at the time.
    AGE   PROBLEM

64. Have you had any injuries? . . . . YES NO
    If YES, describe the injury and your age when it occurred.
    AGE   KIND OF INJURY

65. Have you had any serious illnesses? . . . . YES NO
    If YES, State the kind of illness and your age when it started.
    AGE   ILLNESS

Figure 4–3. Adolescent medical history questionnaire. (continued)

STRICTLY CONFIDENTIAL

Family History

Have any members of your family, alive or dead, (parents, grandparents, uncles, aunts, brothers or sisters) had any of the following problems? If the answer is YES, please state the age of the person when the condition occurred and this person's relationship to you.

PROBLEM	YES	NO	DON'T KNOW	AGE	RELATIONSHIP
A. Seizure disorder Epilepsy					
B. Mental retardation Birth defects					
C. Migraine headaches					
D. High blood pressure High cholesterol					
E. Heart attack or stroke at less than age 60					
F. Lung disease Tuberculosis					
G. Liver or intestinal disease					
H. Kidney disease					
I. Allergies, Asthma, Eczema					
J. Arthritis					
K. Diabetes					
L. Endocrine-Gland					
M. Obesity					
N. Cancer					
O. Blood disorders Sickle cell anemia					
P. Emotional problems Suicide					
Q. Alcoholism Drug problems					

Figure 4–3. Adolescent medical history questionnaire. (continued)

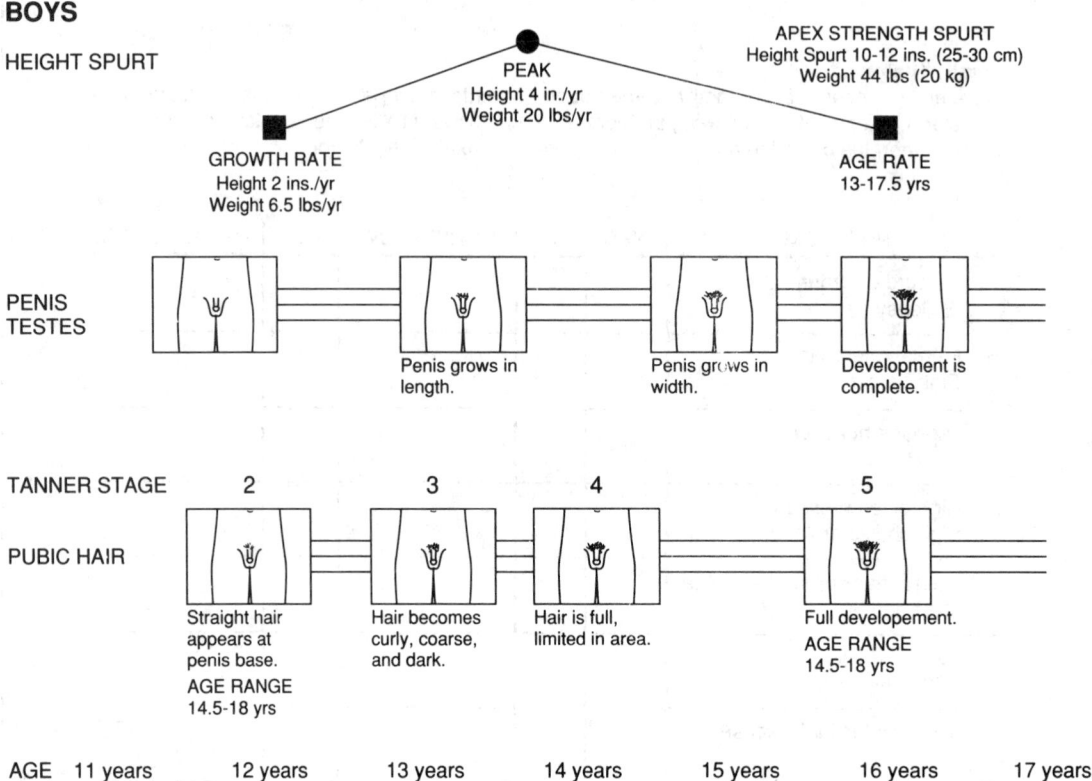

Figure 4–4. Adolescent male sexual maturation and growth. (Adapted and reproduced, with permission, from Tanner JM: *Growth at Adolescence.* Blackwell, 1962.)

pelvic examination is usually not necessary until about age 18.

Elster AB, Kuznets NJ: AMA Guidelines for Adolescent Preventive Services. Williams & Wilkins, 1994.

English A: Treating adolescents: Legal and ethical considerations. Med Clin North Am 1990;74:1097.

Marks A, Fisher M: Health assessment and screening during adolescence. Pediatrics 1987;80(Suppl):135.

GROWTH & DEVELOPMENT

PUBERTY

Pubertal growth and physical development are a result of activation of the hypothalamic-pituitary gonadal axis in late childhood. Before the onset of puberty, pituitary and gonadal hormones remain at very low levels. With the onset of puberty, the inhibition of gonadotropin-releasing hormone (GnRH) in the hypothalamus is removed, allowing pulsatile produc-

tion and release of the gonadotropins, luteinizing hormone (LH) and follicle-stimulating hormone (FSH). In early to middle adolescence, there is an increase in pulse frequency and amplitude of LH and FSH secretion, which stimulates the gonads to produce sex steroids (estrogen or testosterone). In the female, FSH stimulates ovarian maturation, granulosa cell function, and estradiol secretion. LH is important in ovulation and is also involved in corpus luteum formation and progesterone secretion. Initially, estradiol has an inhibitory effect on the release of LH and FSH. Eventually, estradiol becomes stimulatory, and the secretions of LH and FSH become cyclic. There is a progressive increase in estradiol, resulting in maturation of the female genital tract and breast development.

In the male, LH stimulates the interstitial cells of the testes, which produce testosterone. FSH stimulates the production of spermatocytes in the presence of testosterone. The testes also produce inhibin, a Sertoli cell protein that also inhibits the secretion of FSH. During puberty, circulating testosterone increases more than 20-fold. Levels of testosterone correlate with the physical stages of puberty and the degree of skeletal maturation.

GIRLS

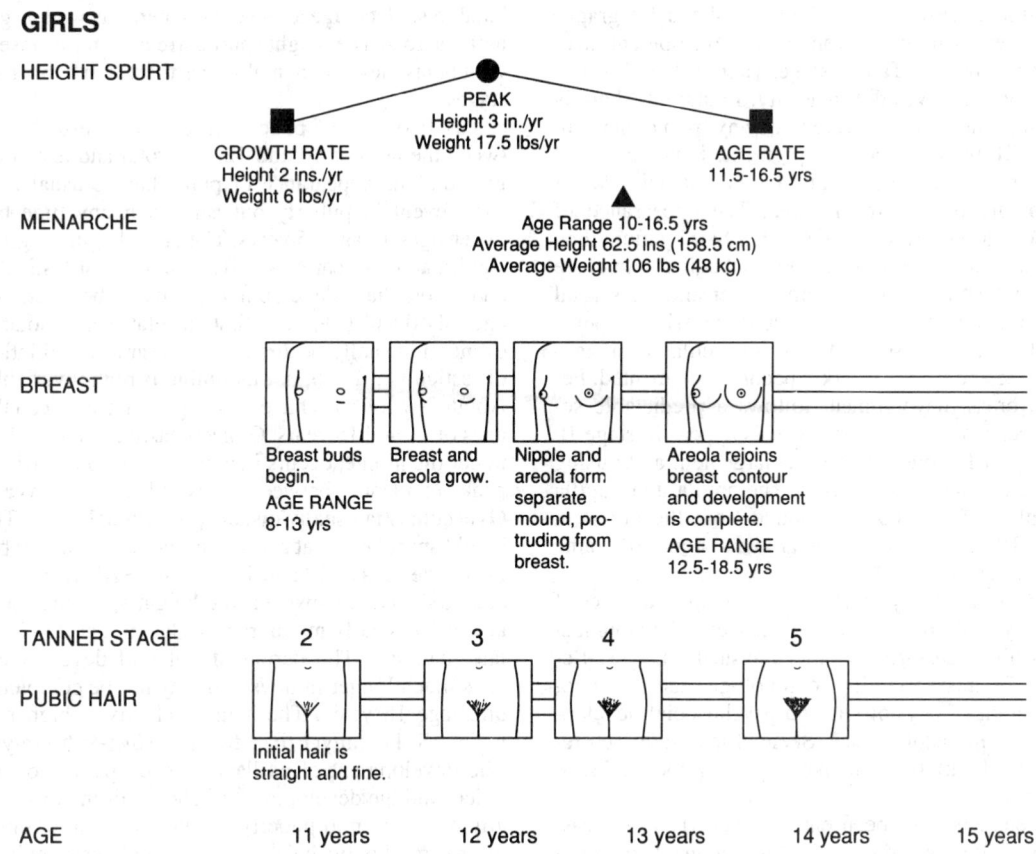

Figure 4–5. Adult female sexual maturation and growth. (Adapted and reproduced, with permission, from Tanner JM: *Growth at Adolescence.* Blackwell, 1962.)

PHYSICAL GROWTH

During adolescence, a teenager's weight doubles, and height increases by 15–20%. During puberty, major organs double in size, with the exception of lymphoid tissue, which decreases in mass. Before puberty, there is little difference in muscular strength between boys and girls. The body's musculature increases both in size and strength during puberty, with maximal strength lagging behind the increase in size by many months. Boys attain greater strength and mass, and strength continues to increase into late puberty. Although motor coordination lags behind growth in stature and musculature, it continues to improve as strength develops.

The pubertal growth spurt begins nearly 2 years earlier in girls than in boys. Girls reach their peak height velocity (PHV) between 11½ and 12 years of age; boys, between 13½ and 14 years of age. Linear growth at peak velocity is 9.5 cm/yr ± 1.5 cm for boys and 8.3 cm/yr ± 1.2 cm for girls. Pubertal growth usually takes 2–4 years and continues longer in boys than in girls. By age 11 years in girls and age 12 in boys,

83–89% of ultimate height has been attained. An additional 18–23 cm (7–9 inches) in females and 25–30 cm (10–12 inches) in males will be achieved during further pubertal growth. Following menarche, growth is rarely more than 5–7.5 cm (2–3 inches).

Boys increase the quantity of body fat before beginning the height spurt. They then lose fat until the growth spurt has finished and then gradually again increase in fat. Muscle mass doubles between ages 10 and 17 years. Girls, by contrast, gradually store fat from about age 6 and do not decrease the quantity of fat, although its location changes, with an increase of subcutaneous fat in the region of the pelvis, breasts, and upper back.

SEXUAL MATURATION

Tanner's scale of sexual maturation is useful clinically to categorize genital development. Tanner staging includes age ranges of normal development and specific descriptions for each stage of pubic hair growth, penis and testis development in boys, and breast maturation in girls. Figures 4–4 and 4–5 graphically represent this chronologic development with reference to each Tanner stage. Tanner stage I is prepuberty; stage V, adult maturity. In stage II there is sparse, fine, nonpigmented, downy pubic hair; in stage III, the hair becomes pigmented and curly and increases in amount; and in stage IV, the hair is adult in texture but limited in area. The appearance of pubic hair precedes that of axillary hair by more than a year. Male genital development begins with stage II, in which the testes become larger and the scrotal skin reddens and coarsens. In stage III, the penis lengthens; and in stage IV, the penis enlarges in general size and the scrotal skin becomes pigmented. Female breast development follows a predictable sequence. Small, raised breast buds appear in stage II. In stage III, there is general enlargement and raising of breast and areolar tissue. The areola and papilla (nipple) form a separate mound from the breast in stage IV, and in stage V the areola assumes the same contour as the breast.

Great variability exists in the timing and onset of puberty and growth, and psychosocial development does not necessarily parallel physical changes. Because of this variability, chronologic age is a poor indication of physiologic and psychosocial development during adolescence. Skeletal maturation correlates well with biologic maturity and pubertal development.

Teenagers have been entering puberty at increasingly earlier ages during the last century because of better nutrition and improved socioeconomic conditions. The age at menarche has decreased by about 4 months per decade during the last century. In the United States, the average age at menarche is 12¾ years. Frisch has shown that among girls reaching menarche, the average weight is 48 kg (106 lb), and the average height is 158.5 cm (62.5 inches). However, menarche may be delayed until age 16 or begin as early as age 10. Although the first measurable sign of puberty in girls is the beginning of the height spurt, the first conspicuous sign usually is development of breast buds between the ages of 8 and 11 years. Although breast development usually antedates the growth of pubic hair, in some normal girls the reverse may occur. A common concern for girls at this time is whether the breasts will be of the right size and shape, especially since it is not unusual for one breast to grow faster than the other. Among girls, the growth spurt starts at about age 9 years and reaches a peak at age 11½, usually at stage III–IV breast development and stage III pubic hair development. However, the height spurt may start as early as age 8 years in early maturers or as late as age 11½ in late maturers. The spurt usually ends by age 14. Girls who mature early will reach their PHV sooner and attain their final height earlier. Girls who mature late will attain a greater ultimate height due to the longer period of growth before the growth spurt. Final height is related to skeletal age at onset of puberty as well as genetic factors. The height spurt correlates more closely with breast developmental stages than with pubic hair stages.

The first sign of puberty in the male, usually between the ages of 10 and 12, is scrotal and testicular growth. The appearance of pubic hair is usually an early event in puberty but can occur any time between ages 10 and 15 years. The penis begins to grow significantly a year or so after the onset of testicular and pubic hair development, usually between the ages of 10 and 13½. The first ejaculation is a notable event and usually occurs about a year after initiation of testicular growth, but its timing is highly variable. About 90% of boys have this experience between the ages of 11 and 15 years. Gynecomastia, a hard nodule under the nipple, occurs in a majority of boys, with a peak incidence between ages 14 and 15 years. Gynecomastia usually disappears within 2 years. The height spurt begins at age 11 but increases rapidly between the ages of 12 and 13, with the PHV reached at age 13½ years. However, the height spurt may start at age 10 in early maturers or as late as age 13–14 in late maturers. The period of pubertal development lasts much longer in boys and may not be completed until age 18 years. The height velocity is higher in males (8–11 cm/yr) than females (6½–9½ cm/yr). The development of axillary hair, deepening of the voice, and the development of chest hair in boys usually occurs in mid puberty, about 2 years after onset of growth of pubic hair. Facial and body hair begin to increase at ages 16–17 years.

Rosenfeld RG: Evaluation of growth and maturation in adolescence. Pediatr Rev 1982;4:175.

Tanner JM: *Growth at Adolescence*. Blackwell, 1962.

Tanner JM, Davies PW: Clinical longitudinal standards for height and height velocity for North American children. J Pediatr 1985;107:317.

PSYCHOSOCIAL DEVELOPMENT

Adolescents are struggling to find out who they are, what they want to do in the future, and, in relation to that goal, what their personal strengths and weaknesses are. These questions arise primarily because teenagers are in the process of establishing their own identity. Adolescence is a period of progressive individuation and separation from the family. Because of the rapid physical, emotional, cognitive, and social growth occurring during adolescence, it is useful to divide the period into three sequential phases of development. Early adolescence occurs roughly between ages 10 and 13; middle adolescence, between ages 14 and 16; and late adolescence, at age 17 and later.

Early Adolescence

Early adolescence (ages 10–13) is characterized by rapid growth and development of secondary sex characteristics. Young adolescents are often preoccupied with the physical changes taking place in their bodies. Because of these rapid physical changes, body image, self-concept, and self-esteem fluctuate dramatically. Concerns about how their growth and development deviate from that of their friends may be a great worry, especially short stature in boys and delayed breast development or delayed menarche in girls. Although there is a certain curiosity about sexuality, young adolescents tend to feel much more comfortable with members of the same sex. As the young teenager begins to become more independent and family ties loosen, allegiance shifts from parents to peers, who become much more important. Young teenagers still think concretely and cannot easily conceptualize about the future. They may have vague and unrealistic professional goals, such as becoming a lead singer in a rock group or a famous movie star. Only through the experiences encountered in later adolescence do they become more realistic.

Middle Adolescence

During middle adolescence (14–16 years), as the rapid pubertal growth of early adolescence decreases, teenagers begin to adjust and become more comfortable with their "new" bodies. Intense emotions and wide swings in mood are typical. Although some teenagers go through this experience relatively peacefully, others struggle desperately. Cognitively, teenagers move from concrete thinking to formal operations and develop the ability to think abstractly. With this new mental power comes a sense of omnipotence and a belief that the world can be changed by merely thinking about it. Sexually active teenagers may believe they do not need to worry about using contraception because they "can't get pregnant—it won't happen to me." Sixteen-year-old drivers believe that they are the best drivers in the world and think the insurance industry is conspiring against them by charging such high rates for automobile insurance. With the onset of the ability to think abstractly, teenagers begin to see themselves as others see them and may become extremely self-centered. Because they are establishing their own identities, relationships with other people, including peers, are primarily narcissistic, and experimenting with different images is quite common. Peers determine the standards for identification, behavior, activities, and fashion and provide emotional support, intimacy, empathy, and the sharing of guilt and anxiety during the struggle for autonomy. The struggle for independence and autonomy is often a difficult and stressful period for both the teenager and the parents.

As sexuality increases in importance, mid-adolescents may begin dating and experimenting with sex. Relationships usually tend to be one-sided and narcissistic. By age 18, nearly half of American females and two-thirds of males have had intercourse.

Late Adolescence

Late adolescents (17 years and older) are much less self-centered and begin caring much more about others. Social relationships shift from the peer group to the individual. Dating becomes much more intimate. The older adolescent becomes more independent from the family. The ability to think abstractly allows older adolescents to think more realistically in terms of future plans, actions, and careers. Older adolescents have very rigid concepts of what is right and what is wrong. This is a period of idealism.

Homosexuality in Adolescence

Homosexual characteristics appear to be established before adolescence. Sexual orientation develops during early childhood. One's gender identity is established by age 2, and a sense of masculinity or femininity usually solidifies by age 5 or 6. Homosexual adults describe homosexual feelings during late childhood and early adolescence, years before engaging in overt homosexual acts.

Although only 5–10% of American young people acknowledge having had homosexual experiences and only 5% feel that they are or could be gay, homosexual experimentation is common, especially during early and middle adolescence. Experimentation may include mutual masturbation and fondling the genitals and does not by itself cause or lead to adult homosexuality. Theories about the etiology of homosexuality include genetic, hormonal, environmental, and psychologic models; however, there is no definitive explanation for the development of homosexual behavior.

The development of homosexual identity in adolescence commonly progresses through three stages. The adolescent feels "different," develops a crush on a person of the same sex without clear self-awareness of a gay identity, and then goes through a "coming-out" phase in which the homosexual identity is defined for the individual and revealed to others. The coming-out phase may be a very difficult period for the young person and the family. The young adolescent is afraid of society's bias and seeks to reject homosexual feelings. This struggle with identity may include episodes of both homosexual and heterosexual promiscuity, sexually transmitted disease, depression, substance abuse, attempted suicide, school avoidance and failure, running away from home, and other crises.

In a clinical setting, the issue of homosexual identity most often surfaces as a result of a teenager being seen for a sexually transmitted disease, family conflict, school problem, attempted suicide, or substance abuse rather than as a result of a consultation about sexual orientation. Pediatricians should be aware of the psychosocial and medical implications of homosexual identity and be sensitive to the possibility of these problems in gay adolescents. The successful management of these problems depends on the physician's ability to gain the trust of the gay adolescent and on a knowledge of the wide range of medical and psychologic problems for which gay adolescents may be at risk. Pediatricians must be nonjudgmental in posing sexual questions if they are to be effective in encouraging the teenager to share concerns. Physicians who for religious or other personal reasons cannot be objective must refer the patient to another professional for treatment and counseling.

Adams GR et al (editors): *Biology of Adolescent Behavior and Development.* Sage, 1989.

Kreipe RE, McAnarney ER: Psychosocial aspects of adolescent medicine. Semin Adolesc Med 1985;1:33.

Levine M et al (editors): *Developmental Behavioral Pediatrics,* 2nd ed. Saunders, 1992.

Orr DP, Ingersoll GM: Adolescent development: A biopsychosocial review. Curr Probl Pediatr 1988;18:441.

Remafedi G et al: Demography of sexual orientation in adolescents. Pediatrics 1992 89:714.

Remafedi G: Fundamental issues in the care of homosexual youth. Med Clin North Am 1990;74:1169.

Sussman EJ et al: Hormonal influences on aspects of psychological development during adolescence. J Adolesc Health Care 1987;8:492.

Vaughan VC, Litt IF: *Child and Adolescent Development: Clinical Implications.* Saunders, 1990.

BEHAVIOR & PSYCHOLOGIC HEALTH

It is not unusual for adolescents to seek medical attention for seemingly minor complaints. During early adolescence, teenagers may worry about normal developmental changes such as gynecomastia. Teenagers may present with vague symptoms—the hidden agenda may be concerns about pregnancy or a sexually transmitted disease. Adolescents with emotional disorders often present with somatic symptoms—eg, abdominal pain, headaches, dizziness or syncope, fatigue, sleep problems, chest pain—that appear to have no biologic cause. The emotional basis of such a complaint may be varied: somatoform disorder, depression, or stress and anxiety.

PSYCHOPHYSIOLOGIC SYMPTOMS & CONVERSION REACTIONS

The most common somatoform disorders during adolescence are conversion disorders or conversion reactions. (A conversion reaction is a psychophysiologic process in which unpleasant feelings, especially anxiety, depression, and guilt, are communicated through a physical symptom.) Psychophysiologic symptoms result when anxiety activates the autonomic nervous system, resulting in tachycardia, hyperventilation, and vasoconstriction. The emotional feeling may be threatening or unacceptable to the individual, who expresses it as a physical symptom rather than verbally. This process is unconscious, and the anxiety or unpleasant feeling is dissipated by the somatic symptom. The degree to which the conversion symptom lessens anxiety, depression, or the unpleasant feeling is referred to as "primary gain." Conversion symptoms not only diminish unpleasant feelings but also remove the adolescent from conflict or an uncomfortable situation. This removal is referred to as "secondary gain." Secondary gain may intensify the symptoms, especially with increased attention from concerned parents and friends. Adolescents with conversion symptoms tend to have overprotective parents and become increasingly dependent on their parents as the symptom becomes the major focus of both the parents' and the adolescent's life.

Clinical Findings

The symptom may appear at times of stress, eg, parental conflict, serious illness in a parent or grandparent, or change in school. Nervous, gastrointestinal, and cardiovascular systems are frequently involved, eg, paresthesias, anesthesia, paralysis, dizziness, syncope, hyperventilation, abdominal pain, nausea, and vomiting. Specific symptoms may reflect existing or previous illness (eg, pseudoseizures in adolescents with epilepsy) or modeling of a close relative's symptom (eg, chest pain in a boy whose grandfather died of a heart attack).

Conversion symptoms tend to be more common in girls than boys. They occur in children and adolescents from all socioeconomic levels; however, the complexity of the symptom may vary with the sophistication and cognitive level of the patient.

Differential Diagnosis

In cases of suspected conversion reaction, history and physical findings are usually inconsistent with anatomic and physiologic concepts. Conversion symptoms are exhibited most frequently at times of stress and in the presence of individuals meaningful to the patient. The patient often exhibits a characteristic personality pattern, including egocentricity, labile emotional states, and dramatic and attention-seeking behaviors.

Conversion reactions are differentiated from hypochondriasis, which is a preoccupation with the fear of developing—or the belief that one has—a serious illness. In hypochondriacal patients, despite medical reassurance that there is no evidence of disease, the patient's (or parents') fear persists. Although adolescents generally regard their symptoms (even minor complaints) with great concern, adolescents with hypochondriasis cannot be reassured that they are healthy. Over time, the fear of one disease may be replaced with concern about another. In contrast to patients with conversion symptoms, who seem relieved if an organic cause is considered, patients with hypochondriasis become more anxious when such a cause is considered.

Malingering is uncommon during adolescence. The malingering patient consciously and intentionally produces false or exaggerated physical or psychologic symptoms. Such patients are motivated by external incentives, such as avoiding work, evading criminal prosecution, obtaining drugs, or obtaining financial compensation. These patients may be hostile and aloof. Parents of patients with conversion disorders and malingering have a similar reaction to illness. They have an unconscious psychologic need to have sick children and reinforce their child's behavior.

Somatic delusions are physical symptoms that accompany other signs of mental illness. Examples are visual or auditory hallucinations, delusions, incoherence or loosening of associations, rapid shifts of affect, and confusion. The symptoms are often peculiar or unusual.

Treatment

Because the symptom is perceived as being physical, pediatricians are often the most appropriate professionals to care for a patient with a conversion symptom. The physician must plan what further tests need to be done to complete the physical evaluation. It is critical from the onset for the physician to emphasize to the patient and the family that both physical and emotional causes of the symptom need to be considered. The relationship between physical causes of emotional pain and emotional causes of physical pain needs to be described to the family, using examples such as stress causing an ulcer or making a severe headache worse. The patient should be encouraged to understand that the symptom may persist and that at least a short-term goal is to continue normal daily activities in school and with friends. Medication is rarely helpful in relieving or resolving the symptom. If the family is accepting of psychologic referral as part of the evaluation, this is often the initial step for psychotherapy. If the family resists psychiatric or psychologic referral, the pediatrician may need to begin to deal with some of the emotional factors responsible for the persistent symptom while building rapport with the patient and family so that they may accept psychologic referral in the future. Regular weekly appointments should be set up with the patient and parents. During the sessions, the teenager should be seen first and encouraged to talk about school, friends, the relationship with the parents, and the stresses and pressures of life. Discussion of the

symptom itself should be minimized; however, the physician should be supportive and never suggest that the pain is not real. As the parents gain further insight into the cause of the symptom, they will become less indulgent of the complaints, facilitating the resumption of normal activities. If management is successful, the adolescent will acquire increased coping skills and become more independent, with decreasing secondary gain.

If the symptom continues to interfere with daily activities, school attendance, participation in extracurricular activities, and involvement with peers and if the patient and parents feel that no progress is being made, psychologic referral is definitely indicated. A psychotherapist experienced in treating adolescents with conversion reactions is in the best position to establish a strong therapeutic relationship with the patient and family. After referral is made, the pediatrician should continue to follow the patient to ensure compliance with psychotherapy.

American Psychiatric Association: *Diagnostic and Statistical Manual of Mental Disorders,* 3rd rev ed. American Psychiatric Association, 1987.

Orr D: Adolescence, stress and psychosomatic issues. J Adolesc Health Care 1986;7(Suppl):97.

Prazer G: Conversion reactions in adolescents. Pediatr Rev 1987;8:279.

DEPRESSION
(See also Chapter 6.)

Symptoms of clinical depression—eg, lethargy, loss of interest, sleep disturbances, decreased energy, feelings of worthlessness, and difficulty concentrating—can be quite common during the normal emotional mood swings of adolescence. The intensity of feelings—often in response to seemingly trivial events such as a poor grade on an examination or not being invited to a party—makes it difficult to differentiate a serious depression from normal sadness or dejection. In a less serious depression, sadness or unhappiness associated with problems of everyday life is generally short-lived. The symptoms usually result in only minor impairment in school, social activities, and relationships with others. With reassurance the teenager should return to a normal affect within a few days.

Clinical Findings

Serious depression in adolescents may present in several ways. The presentation may be similar to that in adults, with vegetative signs such as depressed mood nearly every day, crying spells or inability to cry, discouragement, irritability, a sense of emptiness and meaninglessness, negative expectations of oneself and the environment, low self-esteem, isolation, a feeling of helplessness, markedly diminished interest or pleasure in most activities, significant weight loss or weight gain, insomnia or hypersomnia, fatigue or loss of energy, feelings of worthlessness, and diminished ability to think or concentrate. However, it is not unusual for a serious depression to be masked because the teenager cannot tolerate the severe feelings of sadness. Such a teenager may present with recurrent or persistent psychosomatic complaints, such as abdominal pain, chest pain, headache, lethargy, weight loss, dizziness and syncope, or other nonspecific symptoms. Other behavioral manifestations of masked depression include truancy, running away from home, defiance of authorities, self-destructive behavior, vandalism, drug and alcohol abuse, sexual acting out, and delinquency.

Differential Diagnosis

The pediatrician must first recognize that the teenager may be suffering from an affective disorder. A complete history and physical examination, including a careful review of the patient's past medical and psychosocial history, should be performed. The family history should be explored for psychiatric problems.

The teenager should be questioned directly about any specific symptoms of depression, such as extreme lethargy, decreased energy, feelings of worthlessness, problems sleeping, changes in eating habits, difficulty concentrating, periods of uncontrollable crying, prolonged sadness and unhappiness, suicidal thoughts, or preoccupation with death. The history should include an assessment of the student's school performance. The physician looks for signs of academic deterioration, excessive absences or cutting class, changes in work or other outside activities, and changes in the family (eg, separation, divorce, serious illness, loss of employment by a parent, a recent move to a new school, increasing quarrels or fights with parents, or death of a close relative). The teenager may have withdrawn from friends or family or switched allegiance to a new group of friends. The physician should seek to develop a history of drug and alcohol abuse, conflicts with the law, sexual acting out, running away from home, unusually violent or rebellious behavior, or radical personality change. Patients with vague somatic complaints (eg, headaches, abdominal pain, dizzy spells, chest pain, joint pains, concerns about having a fatal illness, or a "positive review of systems") often have an underlying affective disorder.

Because a number of physical disorders can mimic, cause, or exacerbate major depression, adolescents presenting with significant symptoms of depression deserve a thorough medical evaluation to rule out any contributing or underlying medical illness. Among the medical conditions associated with affective disorders are eating disorders (anorexia nervosa and bulimia), organic disorders of the central nervous system (tumors, vascular lesions, closed head trauma, and subdural hematomas), metabolic and endocrino-

logic disorders (systemic lupus erythematosus, hypothyroidism, hyperthyroidism, Wilson's disease, hyperparathyroidism, Cushing's syndrome, Addison's disease, premenstrual syndrome), infections (infectious mononucleosis, syphilis), and mitral valve prolapse. In addition, over 200 drugs have been reported to cause depressive symptoms. Marihuana use, phencyclidine abuse, amphetamine withdrawal, and excessive caffeine intake can cause symptoms of depression. Common prescription medications used by this age group (eg, birth control pills) and anticonvulsants may be responsible for depressive symptoms.

The majority of physical disorders presenting with symptoms of depression are usually evident by the presenting history, the past medical history, and the physical examination. However, some routine laboratory studies are indicated, including a complete blood count and determination of sedimentation rate, urinalysis, serum electrolytes, BUN, serum calcium; thyroxine and thyroid-stimulating hormone, VDRL or RPR, and liver enzymes. Although metabolic markers such as abnormal secretion of cortisol, growth hormone, and thyrotropin-releasing hormone have been useful in confirming major depression in adults, these neurobiologic markers are less reliable in adolescents.

The risk of depression appears to be greatest in families with a history of depression of early onset and a chronicity of depressive symptoms. Depression of early onset and bipolar illness are more likely to occur in families with a strong multigenerational history of depression. The lifetime risk of depressive illness in first-degree relatives of adult depressed patients has been estimated to be between 18% and 30%.

Treatment

The primary care physician may be able to counsel adolescents and parents if an underlying depression is mild or seems to be the result of an acute identifiable personal loss or frustration and if the patient is not contemplating suicide or at risk for other life-threatening behaviors. If there is evidence of a long-standing depressive disorder, suicidal thoughts, or psychotic thinking, or if the physician does not feel competent or has no interest in counseling the patient, a psychologic referral should be made. In uncomplicated depressions that are a reaction to life stresses or interpersonal conflicts, helping the adolescent put things in proper perspective may be enormously beneficial. Encouraging the adolescent to verbalize thoughts, understand emotional responses, and examine unrealistic attitudes and beliefs can help the patient find an appropriate solution to the problem that led to the depression.

Counseling involves establishing and maintaining a positive supportive relationship; following the patient at least weekly; remaining accessible to the patient at all times; encouraging the patient to express emotions openly, defining the problem and clarifying negative feelings, thoughts, and expectations; setting realistic goals; helping to negotiate interpersonal crises; teaching assertiveness and social skills; reassessing the depression as it is expressed; and staying alert to the possibility of suicide.

Patients with a clinical course consistent with bipolar disease or who have a significant depression which is unresponsive to supportive counseling, should be referred to a psychiatrist for evaluation of antidepressant medication.

Brent, DA: Depression and suicide in children and adolescents. Pediatr Rev 1993;14:380.

Hodgman CH, McAnarney ER: Adolescent depression and suicide: Rising problems. Hosp Pract (Off Ed) 1992;27;73.

Jensen PS, Ryan ND, Prien R: Psychopharmacology of child and adolescent major depression: Present status and future directions. J Child Adolesc Psychopharmacol 1992;2:31.

ADOLESCENT SUICIDE
(See also Chapter 6.)

In 1990, there were over 4900 suicides among people 15–24 years of age: 2000 suicides among those 15–19 and 2900 among those 20–24. In the younger group, males had a rate 4.9 times higher than females, and white males had the highest rate, 19.3 per 100,000. The incidence of unsuccessful suicide attempts is three times higher in females than in males. The estimated ratio of attempted suicides to actual suicides is estimated to be 100:1–50:1. Among actual suicides, firearms are the leading cause of death for both males and females, used in over 67% of suicides.

With the normal mood swings of adolescence, short periods of depression are common. At some time, a teenager may have thoughts of suicide. Normal depressive mood swings during this period rarely interfere with sleeping, eating, or participating in normal activities. Acute depressive reactions (transient grief responses) to the loss (death or separation) of a close family member or friend may result in depression lasting for weeks or even months. An adolescent who is unable to work through this grief can become increasingly depressed. A teenager who is unable to keep up with schoolwork, does not participate in normal social activities, withdraws socially, has sleep and appetite disturbances, and has feelings of hopelessness and helplessness should be considered to be at increased risk for suicide. These are signs of major depression.

Another group of suicidal adolescents is composed of angry teenagers attempting to influence others by their actions, usually the parents. They may be only mildly depressed and may not have a long-standing wish to die. Teenagers in this group, usually females, may "attempt suicide" or make a "suicidal gesture" as a way to get back at someone or gain attention by scaring another person.

The last group of adolescents at risk for suicide is made up of teenagers with a serious psychiatric problem such as acute schizophrenia or a true psychotic depressive disorder.

Risk Assessment

The physician must determine the extent of the teenager's depression and risk of inflicting self-harm. The evaluation should include interviews with both the teenager and the family. The history should include the medical, social, emotional, and academic background. (See Table 6–18, Clinical Interview to Assess Suicide Risk.) The physician should inquire about (1) common signs of depression; (2) recent events that could be at the root of an underlying depression; (3) evidence of long-standing problems in the home, at school, or with peers; (4) drug or substance use and abuse; (5) signs of psychotic thinking, such as delusions or hallucinations; and (6) evidence of masked depression, such as rebellious behavior, running away from home, reckless driving, or other acting out behavior. When seeing depressed patients, the physician should always inquire about thoughts of suicide: "Are things ever so bad that life doesn't seem worth living?" If the response is positive, a more specific question should be asked: "Have you thought of taking your life?" If the patient has thoughts of suicide, the immediacy of risk can be assessed by determining if there is a concrete, feasible plan. Although patients who are at greatest risk have a concrete plan that can be carried out in the near future—especially if they have rehearsed the plan—the physician should not dismiss the potential risk of suicide in the adolescent who does not describe a specific plan. The physician should pay attention to "gut feelings." There may be subtle nonverbal signs that the patient is at greater risk than is apparent on the surface.

Treatment

The primary care physician is often in a unique position to identify an adolescent at risk for suicide, because many teenagers who attempt suicide seek medical attention in the weeks preceding the attempt. These visits are often for vague somatic complaints or subtle signs of depression. If there is evidence of depression, the physician must assess the severity of the depression and suicidal risk. The pediatrician should always seek emergency psychologic consultation for any teenager who is severely depressed, psychotic, or acutely suicidal. It is the psychologist's or psychiatrist's responsibility to assess the seriousness of suicidal ideation and decide whether hospitalization or outpatient treatment is most appropriate. Adolescents with mild depression and at low risk for suicide should be followed closely, and the extent of the depression should be assessed on an ongoing basis. If at any point it appears that the patient is worsening or the teenager is not responding to supportive counseling, referral should be made.

Blumenthal SJ. Youth suicide: The physician's role in suicide prevention. JAMA 1990;264:3194.

Committee on School Health, American Academy of Pediatrics: The potentially suicidal student in the school setting. Pediatrics 1990;86:481.

Crumley FE. Substance abuse and adolescent suicidal behavior. JAMA 1990;263:3051.

Shaffer D et al: Preventing teenage suicide: A critical review. J Am Acad Child Adolesc Psychiatry 1988;27:675.

SUBSTANCE ABUSE

Substance abuse is a complex problem for adolescents and the broader society. See Chapter 9 for an in-depth look at this issue.

EATING DISORDERS
(See also Chapter 6.)

It is estimated that 5–10% of adolescent girls and young women have an eating disorder. Although eating disorders may occur in males, 90–95% of patients are female. Most are middle or upper-middle class, but this trend appears to be changing.

The incidence of anorexia nervosa has doubled over the past 2 decades, and the mortality rate is as high as 9%, excluding suicide. The prevalence of the symptom bulimia ranges from 4.5% to 18% among female high school and college students. The causes of eating disorders remain unclear. There are contributing psychosocial and cultural factors, eg, the current emphasis on thinness and the "superwoman" image in today's society. The genetic component and the neuroendocrine/hypothalamic role is being investigated.

A teenager with anorexia is unlikely to present to the physician of her own accord, because denial of illness is one of the components of the syndrome. Often a school nurse or coach becomes suspicious after observing weight loss, excessive concern with weight, or unusual eating and exercise behaviors. Parents, too, have become knowledgeable about eating disorders from the lay press. But often, the patient presents with abdominal pain, nausea, fainting spells, hair loss, or amenorrhea, and it is the clinician who discovers the true diagnosis. Bulimics, however, may present on their own and may feel relieved to share their burden with someone.

Clinical Findings

A. Symptoms and Signs: The diagnosis of anorexia nervosa or bulimia nervosa is largely based on history; specific diagnostic criteria are given in Table 4–1. The history needs to include the presenting

Table 4–1. Diagnostic criteria for eating disorders.[1]

Anorexia nervosa
Weight loss or failure to gain weight during growth such that weight is 15% below that expected for age and height.
Fear of weight gain or fatness despite being underweight.
Distorted body image—feels all or part of the body is fat even when severely underweight.
For females, interruption of menstrual cycles for at least 3 months (secondary amenorrhea) or failure to menstruate when expected (primary amenorrhea).
Bulimia nervosa
Repeated binge eating (large number of calories in short period of time) with a frequency of at least twice a week for 3 or more months.
Perception by patient that eating behavior is out of control.
Recurrent purging behavior to prevent weight gain (self-induced emesis; use of laxatives, diuretics, or emetics; excessive exercise, or severely restricted intake).
Excessive preoccupation with body image.

[1]Modified and reproduced from American Psychiatric Association: *Diagnostic and Statistical Manual of Mental Disorders,* 3rd rev ed. American Psychiatric Association, 1987.

symptoms; weight history, including desired weight; dietary intake, unusual eating behaviors, or avoided foods; history of any purging behaviors, eg, vomiting, excessive exercise, or use of diet pills, diuretics, emetics, or laxatives; and menstrual history for irregular cycles, secondary amenorrhea, or delay in anticipated menarche. The social history may provide clues to a perfectionistic drive in anorexics, impulsiveness in bulimics (eg, substance abuse or sexual promiscuity), or family dysfunction. Review of systems should focus on symptoms of possible complications of the above behaviors and on symptoms of other diseases in the differential diagnosis. Table 4–2 lists associated features of eating disorders. The use of the Eating Attitudes Test (EAT) and the Eating Disorder Inventory (EDI) may aid in diagnosis.

The physical examination is most often normal, but this does not rule out the diagnosis of an eating disorder. The anorexic may hide under layers of bulky clothing, but the loss of subcutaneous tissue becomes apparent when the patient disrobes. The anorexic's weight is the indicator of actual loss; however, bulimics are usually of normal weight or within 10 lb of normal (under or over). Hypothermia, bradycardia, or hypotension may be evident when the anorexic's vital signs are assessed. Other findings in anorexia include dry skin, presence of fine, downy hair on the body or an increase in pigmentation of body hair, limpness and loss of sheen in the scalp hair, excoriation over the sacral spine from excessive sit-ups, prominent ribs, atrophied breasts, scaphoid abdomen, palpable hard stool in the rectal vault, cold extremities, squaring off of the convergence of the thighs, or edema of the extremities. In patients with self-induced emesis, there may be loss of tooth enamel, particularly on the posterior aspect of the front teeth, or calluses on the dorsum of the fingers.

Table 4–2. Associated features of eating disorders.

Anorexia Nervosa	Bulimia Nervosa
Onset at age 12 to mid 30s; bimodal 13–14, 17–18	Onset at age 17–25, but may not present for many years
Extreme weight loss, refusal to maintain minimal normal weight for age	Weight fluctuations
Intense fear of becoming obese	Possible fear of fatness but a greater fear of loss of control of eating
Distorted body image	Overconcern with body shape/weight
Amenorrhea (in females)	Possible menstrual irregularities
Intense preoccupation with food	Intense preoccupation with food
Severe caloric restriction (restrictive anorexia nervosa) or severe restriction alternating with binging/purging (bulimic anorexia nervosa)	Secretive binge-eating episodes, high-carbohydrate foods
	Self-induced vomiting, purging (laxatives, diuretics, emetics), vigorous exercise
Excessive physical activity	Other impulsive behaviors (alcohol/drug use)
Isolation, asexuality	Outgoing personality, heterosexual relationships
Denial of illness	Distress, willingness to accept help

B. Laboratory Findings: The goal of laboratory tests is to exclude other diagnoses and assess the patient's status. Most laboratory studies do not change until late in the disease. It is useful to obtain a complete blood count to assess nutritional status, a sedimentation rate to help exclude inflammatory bowel disease or collagen vascular disease, and electrolyte studies to detect the presence of hypochloremic alkalosis and hypokalemia due to vomiting or of metabolic acidosis due to laxative abuse. A urinalysis may show concentrated urine or, late in anorexia nervosa, loss of urine concentrating ability. Serum total protein and albumin are usually normal until late. Serum calcium, phosphorus, and magnesium should be closely followed during refeeding, since they may quickly become depleted resulting in a medical emergency. Other laboratory studies, such as thyroid function tests, chest x-ray, upper gastrointestinal series, or CT scan of the head need only be done as indicated by the presentation.

Differential Diagnosis

The causes of weight loss are legion. Causes such as cancer, collagen vascular disease, diabetes mellitus, hyperthyroidism, malabsorptive syndromes, inflammatory bowel disease, or chronic renal, pulmonary, or cardiac disease warrant consideration in the suspected anorexic; however, in patients with these disorders there may be weight loss but no associated disturbance of body image or fear of obesity. Several psychiatric disturbances, including depression, may be associated with loss of appetite and weight loss. Some unusual central nervous system disorders may

present like bulimia, but again there is no distorted body image or overconcern with body shape or weight.

Complications

Eating disorders can result in severe consequences to nearly every system of the body (Table 4–3). The most common complications, however, are fluid and electrolyte abnormalities or constipation. In addition, there may be long-term difficulties with eating and weight management.

Treatment

First, the diagnosis must be discussed with the patient and her parents. The patient needs to know that the clinician appreciates her struggle, aims to restore her to health, will not let her become fat, and will help her to regain control. The parents need to understand that eating disorders are symptoms of underlying issues, often a family problem, and that the family is very important to the solution. They need to see that although the presenting symptoms are physical, eating disorders are psychiatric disorders and require the intervention of mental health practitioners. With this age group, it is important to have a mental health practitioner who is skilled in family therapy and has experience with adolescents (see Chapter 6).

Restoration of the nutritional and physiologic state is an early goal of treatment, because the patient may need to gain weight before she can deal effectively

Table 4–3. Complications of eating disorders.

Central nervous system	Gastrointestinal
↓REM and slow-wave sleep	Dental erosion
Cortical atrophy	Parotid swelling
Thermoregulatory abnormalities, eg, hypothermia	Esophagitis, esophageal tears
Endocrine	Delayed gastric emptying
↓LH, FSH	Gastric dilatation (rarely rupture)
↓T_3, ↑rT_3; normal T_4, TSH	Pancreatitis
Irregular menses	Constipation
Amenorrhea (primary or secondary)	Diarrhea (laxative abuse)
Metabolic	Superior mesenteric artery syndrome
Dehydration	Hypercholesterolemia
Acidosis	Mild ↑ liver function tests
Hypokalemia	**Renal**
Hypochloremia	Hematuria
Hypochloremic alkalosis	Proteinuria
Hypocalcemia	↓Renal concentrating ability
Hypophosphatemia	**Hematologic**
Hypomagnesemia	Leukopenia
Osteoporosis	Anemia
Hypercarotenemia	Thrombocytopenia
Cardiovascular	
Bradycardia	
Postural hypotension	
Dysrhythmia, sudden death	
Congestive heart failure (during refeeding)	

with her fear of fatness or other issues. A dietitian is helpful in establishing a refeeding program. The patient may not be in any metabolic danger at the time of presentation, and provided the weight can be stabilized, she may not require hospitalization but rather regular outpatient visits with medical and mental health professionals. An individualized contract can be drawn up and signed by the patient. This contract addresses such issues as long-term weight goals, rate of weight gain, amount of exercise, frequency of visits and of laboratory tests, minimal weight signaling the need for hospitalization, and consequences of failed weight goals. At each medical visit, the patient should be weighed in a gown only after she voids. The long-term goal is to achieve a weight at which menstruation can take place (Figure 4–6); however, it may be less than ideal body weight. Vital signs and chest and abdominal examinations should also be conducted at each visit, and the height and the triceps skinfold should be monitored over time.

Most often, the patient can eat sufficient amounts to replace nutrient deficits and to gain weight. High-calorie fluid supplements may be added if weekly weight goals are missed. It is best not to tell the patient that she must take in a certain number of calories, because she is already fixated on calories. Rather, plans can be developed with the assistance of the dietitian; the planned diets contain sufficient calories for weight gain. In extremely malnourished and noncompliant hospitalized patients, nasogastric tube feedings or hyperalimentation may be necessary initially. With severe anorexics, one must be on the watch for congestive heart failure caused by refeeding too rapidly. In addition, serum phosphate levels should be followed, because there may be a shift from serum to cells during conversion to anabolic metabolism.

Drug therapy—including appetite stimulants or suppressants, antidepressants, anxiolytics, and anticonvulsants—has been investigated in a number of studies, but the results to date are equivocal. Antidepressants may be helpful in select patients but need to be carefully monitored in cachectic patients. There is some evidence that drugs acting on the serotonin system, such as fluoxetine, may be useful.

Hospitalization may become necessary for medical or psychiatric reasons (Table 4–4). In addition, the patient may require hospitalization not because she is medically unstable or in emotional crisis but because she is out of control or making no progress as an outpatient and thus requires more intensive treatment.

Prognosis

Outcome is difficult to predict because there have been few long-term studies and there is little standardization of criteria and variables. It appears that 40–60% of significantly ill anorexics will make a good physical and psychosocial recovery and that

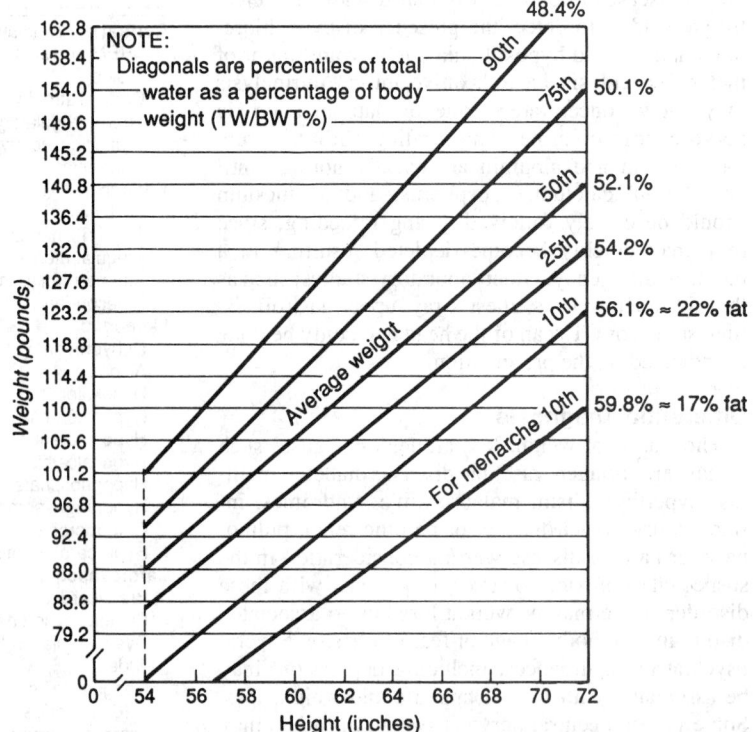

Figure 4–6. Modified Frisch nomogram for minimum weight necessary for normal menstrual cycles. The bottom line shows the minimum weight necessary for menarche. The 10th percentile line shows the minimum weight for correcting secondary amenorrhea in a mature woman. For example, according to the nomogram, an amenorrheic woman 65 inches tall would have to reach at least 103 lb before menstruation would resume. The top five diagonal lines indicate percentiles of total water as a percentage of body weight—which is an index of fatness—for fully grown, mature women in a normal sample. The bottom line represents the 10th percentile for the same sample at menarche. The 50th percentile line indicates the normal weight for height of mature women who are from 18 to 25 years old. (Reproduced, with permission, from Frisch RE: Fatness and fertility. Sci Am [March] 1988;258:88.)

Table 4–4. Criteria for hospitalization of eating disorder patients.

Medical
  Weight loss >30% of body weight over 3 months
  Severe metabolic disturbance
    Heart rate <40 beats/min
    Temperature <36 °C
    Systolic blood pressure <70 mm Hg
    Serum K⁺ <2.5 meq/L despite oral K⁺ replacement
    Severe dehydration
  Severe binging and purging
Psychiatric
  Severe depression or risk of suicide
  Psychosis
  Family crisis
  Failure to comply with a therapeutic contract, or inadequate response to outpatient treatment

75% will gain weight. The mortality rate ranges from 0–19% and is at least 5% in those receiving therapy. For bulimia, the literature is even younger, and the outcome appears less favorable. As few as 40–50% of treated bulimics are felt to be cured, and there is a greater likelihood of serious medical complications, death, and risk of suicide than for anorexics who do not manifest bulimic behavior. Recently, however, more attention has focused on eating disorders, and the lay public is becoming more aware of them. For this reason, the disease is being recognized earlier than before.

American Psychiatric Association: *Diagnostic and Statistical Manual of Mental Disorders,* 3rd rev ed. American Psychiatric Association, 1987.

Commerci GD: Eating disorders in adolescents. Pediatr Rev 1988;10:37.

Joffe A: Too little, too much: Eating disorders in adolescents. Contemp Pediatr 1990;7:114.

Kreipe RE, Uphoff M: Treatment and outcome of adolescents with anorexia nervosa. Adolescent Medicine: State of the Art Reviews 1992;3:519.

Palla B, Litt IF: Medical complications of eating disorders in adolescents. Pediatrics 1988;81:613.

Williams RL: Use of the Eating Attitudes Test and Eating Disorder Inventory in adolescents. J Adolesc Health Care 1987;8:266.

EXOGENOUS OBESITY

Obesity is the presence of excessive body fat, or weight 20% above desirable weight if the excess weight is due to fat. Body weight is most commonly used to quantitate obesity; however, this is a function of age, sex, height, frame, and Tanner stage. In children under 6–7 years of age, body weight tends to underestimate fatness, and in adolescents it overestimates fatness. Weight index, the ratio of actual to ideal weight, may also be used, and an index greater than 1.2 is considered to signal obesity. Although underwater weights may be the most accurate measure

of lean body mass, this weighing procedure is not frequently available. Triceps skinfold thickness is the most practical way to measure obesity in children and teenagers, but reproducibility is in question. A triceps skinfold measurement more than 1 SD above the mean (85th percentile) defines obesity, and one at the 95th percentile indicates superobesity (Figure 4–7). The body mass index (weight [kg] divided by height squared [m²]), used to assess obesity in adults correlates less well with the percentage of body fat in children and adolescents than skinfold thickness.

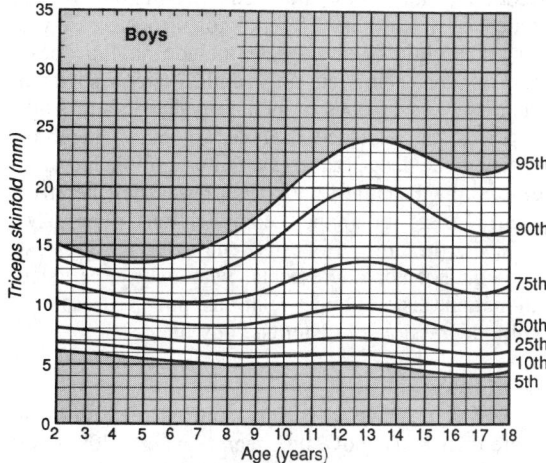

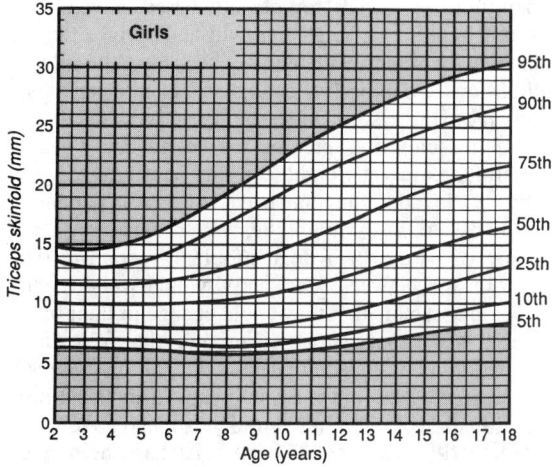

Figure 4–7. Triceps skinfold thickness in boys and girls 2–18 years. (Reproduced, with permission, from Ross Laboratories. Adapted from Johnson CL et al: Basic data on anthropometric measurements and angular measurements of the hip and knee joints for selected age groups, 1–74 years of age, United States, 1971–1975. *Vital and Health Statistics* Series 11, No. 219. [PHS] 81-1669, 1981. © 1983 Ross Laboratories, Columbus, OH 43216. May be copied for individual patient use.)

Background

Obesity is the most common nutritional disorder of children in the United States, and the prevalence of obesity increases significantly between the elementary and high school years. If a child enters adolescence obese, the odds are 4:1 against later achievement of normal weight; but if a child leaves adolescence obese, the odds are 28:1 against later normal weight. The National Children and Youth Fitness Study, parts I and II, completed in 1987, demonstrated a decline in fitness of fifth through twelfth graders and first through fourth graders, respectively. When these results were compared to those of a 1960s National Center for Health Statistics study, an increase in skinfold measurements was found. The reduction in fitness has paralleled a rise in hours of TV watched by children. Factors known to increase the risk of a child's being obese include having obese parents and being an only child. The associated medical risks of obesity include pediatric and adult hypertension, elevated triglyceride levels, cerebrovascular accidents, diabetes mellitus, gallbladder disease, slipped capital-femoral epiphyses, degenerative arthritis, and pregnancy complications. The psychosocial hazards of obesity tend to be the greatest consequence for adolescents, who may experience alienation, distorted peer relations, poor self-esteem, guilt, depression, or distorted body image.

Diagnosis

As stated above, a triceps skinfold measurement more than 1 SD above the mean or weight 20% over ideal body weight indicates obesity. Patients can be identified as at risk for obesity based on current weight relative to height, growth and weight trend, and weight of family members. The history should include onset of obesity, eating and exercise habits, amount of time spent in sedentary activities such as watching television, previous successful and unsuccessful attempts at weight loss, and family history of obesity. In addition, one needs to assess patients' readiness to lose weight, ie, whether patients are aware of or deny a weight problem; recognize the relationship between food, activity, and weight; and recognize factors that they could change in their own lives. When obesity is diagnosed, the following database can be collected: height; weight; blood pressure; triceps skinfold measurement; fat distribution; examination of the skin, thyroid, heart, and abdomen; hematocrit; and urinalysis. This database helps the physician assess the patient's status and exclude endocrine causes of obesity. Endocrine causes, eg, hypothyroidism or Cushing's disease, can generally be excluded on the basis of history and physical examination. If an adolescent is healthy and has no delay of growth or sexual maturation, an underlying endocrinologic, neurologic, or genetic cause is unlikely.

Treatment

For poorly motivated patients, it is probably best to provide some basic information about weight control and make oneself available for future visits, so as not to set the patient up for failure. For the more highly motivated patient, treatment should be appropriate to age and developmental level and should produce a significant reduction in body weight. The adolescent should be taught appropriate eating and exercise habits to maintain a weight reduction yet meet nutrition needs for growth and development.

Anorectic drugs, fasting, and bypass surgery do not have a role in the management of obese adolescents. An age-appropriate behavior modification program incorporating good dietary counseling and exercise is optimal (Table 4–5). Diet or exercise alone is not nearly as effective. Guidelines that group foods in categories according to their caloric density may be appreciated by adolescents who hate to count calories. Life-style activity, such as walking and taking the stairs, may be more effective in the long run than regimented exercise programs. Behavior modification components—-eg, recording one's eating and activity in a notebook, receiving systematic reinforcement for behavior changes, and restructuring how one sees oneself or plans for success—are especially helpful. Behavioral treatment involving parents has been shown to improve long-term maintenance of weight loss in children. One must recognize, however, that no program has the high success rate desired and that the problem of adolescent obesity must be examined further.

Arden MA: Obesity. In: *Textbook of Adolescent Medicine.* McAnarney ER et al (editors). Saunders, 1992.

Bandini LG: Obesity in the adolescent. Adolescent Medicine: State of the Art Reviews 1992;3:459.

Epstein LH et al: Ten-year follow-up of behavioral, family-based treatment for obese children. JAMA 1990;264:2519.

Raithel KS: Are American children really unfit? Physician Sports Med 1988;16:146.

Rees JM: Management of obesity in adolescence. Med Clin North Am 1990;74:1275.

SCHOOL AVOIDANCE

Any teenager who has missed more than 1 week of school for a physical illness or symptom—and whose clinical picture is inconsistent with a serious illness—should be suspected of harboring primary or secondary emotional factors that contribute to the absence. Investigation of absences may show a pattern, eg, missing morning classes or missing the same days at the beginning or end of the week. Emotional factors for school absenteeism are usually attributed to physical symptoms in this age group.

School avoidance should be suspected in children who are consistently absent in spite of parents' and

Table 4–5. Program components for weight control interventions.[1]

Component	Specific Aspects
Physical activity 1. Cardiovascular fitness 2. High-calorie equivalent	Frequency: 3 or 4 times a week. Intensity: 50–60% maximal ability (55–65% maximum heart rate). Duration: 15 minutes at start of program, building to 30–40 minutes. Mode: Use of large muscle activity, eg, walking, jogging, swimming, cycling. Interests: Encourage a wide variety of recreational activities. Enjoyment: Focus on the fun of movement and the enjoyment of being physically active.
Nutrition education	Teach critical aspects of quality nutrition, ie, food groups, serving requirements, and variety. Develop an understanding of caloric balance; calories in versus calories out. Alert children to resist the pressures of media advertising. Instruct on role of snacks and ideas for "good" snacking. Assist children with balancing fast-food eating and caloric intake. Teach children to reduce intake of high-calorie, low-nutrition foods.
Behavior modification 1. Change eating habits 2. Increase habitual physical activity	Identify those cues that affect eating, eg, location of meals, size of plates, food in easy-to-see places. Identify behavior that negatively affects weight control: speed of eating, chronic second portions, high-calorie food choices, "pickiness." Contract for increased levels of activity, using record cards or activity contracts. Develop strategies to encourage more functional activity, eg, walking to school, taking stairs, sitting rather than lying. Develop interests in a variety of recreational areas: tennis, dancing, skating. Identify cues that lead to inactivity: frequent TV watching, lying down after school or meals, friends who do not like active play.

[1]Modified and reproduced, with permission, from Ward DS, Bar-Or O: Role of the physician and physical education teacher in the treatment of obesity at school. Pediatrician 1986:13:44.

professionals' attempts to encourage school attendance. Adolescents with school avoidance problems often have a history of excessive absences or separation difficulties as a younger child. There may also be a record of recurrent somatic complaints. Parents of a school avoider often feel at a loss about how to compel their adolescent to attend school, may lack the sophistication to distinguish malingering from illness, or may have an underlying need to keep the teenager at home.

A complete history and physical should be performed, reviewing the past medical, educational, and psychiatric history. Signs of emotional problems should be explored. After obtaining permission from the patient and parents, the physician may find it helpful to speak directly with school officials and some key teachers. There may be problems with particular teachers or subjects; environmental factors at the school (eg, fears of physical violence, or problems with intimidation). Some students get so far behind academically that they see no way of catching up and feel overwhelmed. The adolescent may have a long history of separation anxiety, dating back to a traumatic separation from the mother. Separation anxiety may persist and be manifested in subconscious worries that something may happen to the mother while the teenager is at school.

The school nurse may give useful information, including the number of visits to the nurse during the last school year. An important part of the history is how the parents respond to the absences and somatic complaint. There may be a subconscious attempt to keep the adolescent at home, which may be coupled with secondary gains (increased parental attention) for remaining at home.

Treatment

The importance of going back to school in the next 2 or 3 days needs to be emphasized. The pediatrician should facilitate this process by offering to speak with school officials to excuse missed examinations, homework, and papers. The pediatrician should speak directly with teachers who are punitive. The objective is to make the transition back to school as easy as possible. The longer adolescents stay out of school, the more anxious they may become about returning, and the more difficult the return becomes. If an illness or symptoms become so severe that an adolescent cannot go to school, both the patient and the parents must be informed that a visit to the doctor's office is necessary. The physician focuses visits on the parents as much as on the adolescent to alleviate any parental guilt about sending the child to school. If the adolescent cannot stay in school, hospitalization should be recommended for an in-depth medical and psychiatric evaluation. Parents should be cautioned about the possibility of relapse after school holidays, summer vacation, or an acute illness.

Klerman LV: School absence: A health perspective. Pediatr Clin North Am 1988;35:1253.

SCHOOL FAILURE

When children graduate from grade school to middle school or junior high school, the amount and complexity of course work increase significantly. This occurs at about the same time as the rapid physical, social, and emotional changes of puberty. To perform well academically, young adolescents must have the needed cognitive ability, study habits, concentration, motivation, interest, and emotional focus. Academic failure presenting at adolescence has a broad differential: (1) limited intellectual abilities, (2) specific learning disabilities, (3) depression or emotional problems, (4) physical causes such as visual or hearing problems, (5) excessive school absenteeism secondary to chronic disease such as asthma or neurologic dysfunction, (6) lack of ability to concentrate, (7) attention deficit disorder, (8) lack of motivation,

and (9) drug and alcohol problems. Each of these possible causes must be explored in depth (Table 4–6).

A thorough history, physical examination, appropriate laboratory studies, and educational and psychologic testing should be performed. A detailed medical history is taken to look for the presence of chronic disease or sensory deficits. School avoidance (see above) should be ruled out. A history of an attention deficit disorder or use of stimulant medication in the past may be an indication of ongoing problems with concentration. Educational records, including previous educational and intelligence testing, are important background information. The emotional history may reveal past episodes of counseling for depression or other significant psychiatric problems. The presence of conflict in the family, eg, divorce or alcoholism, may play an important role, distracting the adolescent from academic responsibilities. There

Table 4–6. A classification of common developmental dysfunctions in adolescence.[1]

Dysfunction	Subtypes	Frequent Manifestations[2]
1. Attention deficits	a. Primary b. Secondary (to anxiety or poor information processing) c. Situational (only evident in certain settings)	Weak attention to detail; distractibility; impulsivity, restlessness; task impersistence; performance inconsistency; organizational problems; reduced working capacity
2. Memory impairments	a. Generalized retrieval problems b. Modality-specific retrieval problems c. Attention-retention deficiencies	Deficient, undependable, or slow recall of data from long- or short-term memory Problems with revisualization or auditory, motor, or sequential recall Poor recall associated with superficial initial registration
3. Language disorders	a. Receptive b. Expressive	Poor verbal and reading comprehension; poor listening; trouble following directions and explanations Problems with word finding, sentence formulation Difficulty with written expression
4. Higher order cognitive disabilities	a. Inferential weakness b. Poor verbal reasoning c. Poor nonverbal reasoning d. Difficulty with abstraction, symbolization e. Weak generalization and rule application	Problems understanding and assimilating new concepts; tendency to think "concretely" delays in mathematics, reading comprehension, science, social studies
5. Fine motor incoordination	a. Eye:hand coordination problems b. Impaired propriokinesthetic feedback c. Dyspraxia d. Motor memory impairment	Slow, labored, sometimes illegible writing; awkward pencil grip; dyssynchrony between cognitive tempo and writing speed; output failure —reduced productivity
6. Organizational deficiencies	a. Temporal-sequential disorientation b. Material disarray c. Integrative dysfunction d. Resynthesis problems e. Attentional disorganization	Problems with time allocation, schedules, planning, arranging ideas in writing Tendency to lose, misplace, forget books, papers; trouble organizing notebook Varying inability to integrate data from multiple sources or sensory modalities Trouble extracting most salient details, retelling and adapting data to current demands Impulsivity, erratic tempo, poor self-monitoring, careless errors
7. Socialization disabilities	a. Wide range of subtypes, including conduct disorder, social impulsivity, impaired social cognition or feedback, egocentricity	Antisocial behaviors; delinquency; withdrawal; excessive dependency on peer support

[1]Modified and reproduced, with permission, from Levine MD, Zallen BG: Learning disorders of adolescence. Pediatr Clin North Am 1984;31:2.
[2]Manifestations are likely to vary somewhat depending upon compensatory strengths, quality of educational experience, and motivation.

may be a history of school problems in other siblings or family members.

Treatment

Treatment depends on the cause. Management must be individualized to address specific needs, foster strengths, and implement a feasible program. For children with specific learning disabilities, an individual prescription for regular and special educational courses, teachers, and extracurricular activities is important. Counseling helps these adolescents gain coping skills, raise self-esteem, and develop socialization skills. If there is a history of hyperactivity or attention deficit disorder along with poor ability to concentrate, a trial of stimulant medication (eg, methylphenidate hydrochloride or dextroamphetamine sulfate) may be useful. If the teenager appears to be depressed or if other serious emotional problems are uncovered, further psychologic evaluation should be recommended.

Lerner JW: Eductional interventions in learning disabilities. J Am Acad Child Adolesc Psychiatry 28:326, 1989.

Levine M: *Keeping a Head in School: A Student's Book about Learning Abilities and Learning Disorders.* Educators Publishing Service, 1990.

Levine MD, Zallen BG: The learning disorders of adolescence: Organic and nonorganic failure to strive. Pediatr Clin North Am 1984;31:345.

Pelham WE et al: Relative efficacy of long acting stimulants on children with attention deficit-hyperactivity disorder. Pediatrics 86:226, 1990.

BREAST DISORDERS

The breast examination should become part of the routine physical examination in females as soon as breast budding occurs. The preadolescent comes to see breast examination as a routine part of health care, and it provides an opportunity to reassure her about any concerns she may have. The breast examination begins with inspection of the breasts for symmetry and Tanner stage. Asymmetric breast development is common in adolescents, who need reassurance that the asymmetry usually becomes less apparent as development progresses. Unusual causes of breast asymmetry that may require further intervention include unilateral breast hypoplasia, amastia, or absence of the pectoralis major muscle. In addition, unilateral virginal hypertrophy (massive enlargement of the breast during puberty) may result in significant asymmetry.

Palpation of the breasts can be performed with the patient in the supine position and the patient's ipsilateral arm placed behind her head. The examiner palpates the breast tissue with the flat of the fingers in widening circles from the areola out to the sternum, clavicle, and axilla. The areola should be gently compressed to check for discharge.

Instructions for breast self-examination and its purpose can be given to older adolescents during this portion of the physical examination, and the patient should be encouraged to begin monthly self-examination after each menstrual flow.

BREAST MASSES

Most breast masses in adolescents are benign (Table 4–7); however, approximately 150 cases of adenocarcinoma are reported each year in the USA in women under 25 years of age. Fibroadenomas account for 90% of breast lumps in teenagers seen in referral clinics; the remainder are cysts. In practice, cysts may account for as many as 60% of breast masses in adolescents, but they are readily diagnosed, and many resolve spontaneously.

Fibroadenoma

Fibroadenoma presents as a rubbery, well-demarcated, slowly growing, nontender mass that may occur in any quadrant but is most commonly found in the upper outer quadrant of the breast. Most are less than 5 cm in diameter. In 25% of cases, there are multiple or recurrent lesions. Quiescence can be expected after the teenage years.

Cysts

Breast cysts are generally tender and spongy, with exacerbation of symptoms premenstrually and abatement just after. Often they are multiple. Spontaneous regression occurs over two or three menstrual cycles in about half of cases.

It is reasonable to follow breast masses that are

Table 4–7. Diagnoses of female patients seen for a breast-related complaint in an adolescent medicine clinic.[1]

Clinical Diagnosis	Patients (n = 130)	Total (%)
Fibrocystic disease	66	50.8
Fibroadenoma	19	14.6
Normal breasts	17	13.1
Mastalgia	6	4.6
Unknown	6	4.6
Abscess/mastitis	5	3.9
Breast asymmetry	3	2.3
Breast hypertrophy	2	1.5
Early pregnancy	2	1.5
Hematoma	2	1.5
Granular cell myoblastoma	1	0.8
Lymphadenopathy	1	0.8
Carcinoma	0	0

[1]Modified and reproduced, with permission, from Diebl T, Kaplan DW: Breast masses in adolescent females. Sexually Active Teenagers 1988;2:151.

consistent with fibroadenoma or cyst in adolescents for two or three menstrual cycles. About one-fourth of fibroadenomas become smaller, and about one-half of cysts resolve. If there is no change in a presumed fibroadenoma after this time, an ultrasound study will differentiate a solid tumor from a cyst. Patients with solid tumors over 2.5 cm in diameter should be referred for excisional biopsy. Those with tumors less than 2.5 cm in diameter may be followed every 3–6 months, since as many will shrink or remain the same. Persistent cystic lesions may be drained by needle aspiration. Patients with suspicious lesions should be referred immediately to a breast surgeon (Table 4–8).

Fibrocystic Breasts

Fibrocystic breasts (or fibrocystic breast disease) is sometimes seen in older adolescents but is more common in women in their third and fourth decades. It is characterized by cyclic tenderness and nodularity bilaterally and is believed to be influenced by the estrogen-progesterone balance.

Reassuring the young woman about the benign nature of the process and emphasizing the importance of breast self-examination may be all that is needed. Oral contraceptives reduce the risk of fibrocystic

Table 4–8. Breast lesions.

Adenocarcinoma	Hard, nonmobile, well-circumscribed, painless mass. Generally indolent clinical course. Occurs also in males but less frequently.
Cystosarcoma phyllodes	Firm, rubbery mass that may suddenly enlarge. Associated skin necrosis. Most often benign.
Giant juvenile fibroadenoma	Remarkably large fibroadenoma with overlying dilated superficial veins. Accounts for 5–10% of fibroadenomas in adolescents. Benign but requires excision to prevent breast atrophy and for cosmetic reasons.
Intraductal papilloma	A cylindrical tumor arising from the ductal epithelium. Often subareolar but may be in the periphery of the breast in adolescents, with associated nipple discharge. Most are benign but require excision for cytologic diagnosis.
Fat necrosis	Localized inflammatory process in one breast. Follows trauma in about half of cases. Subsequent scarring may be confused with cancer.
Virginal or juvenile hypertrophy	Massive enlargement of both breasts or, less often, one breast. Attributed to end-organ hypersensitivity to normal hormonal levels just before or within a few years after menarche.
Miscellaneous	Fibroma, galactocele, hemangioma, intraductal granuloma, interstitial fibrosis, keratoma, lipoma, granular cell myoblastoma, papilloma, sclerosing adenosis.

breast disease and may be appropriate for the sexually active female with a personal history of breast cyst or family history of fibrocystic breasts. Recent studies have shown no association between methylxanthines and fibrocystic breasts; however, some women report reduced symptoms when they discontinue caffeine intake. The efficacy of vitamin E also remains unknown.

Breast Abscess

The female with a breast abscess usually complains of unilateral breast pain, and examination reveals overlying inflammatory changes. Often the examination is misleading in that the infection may extend much deeper than suspected. A palpable mass is found only late in the course. Although breast feeding is the most common cause of mastitis, trauma and eczema involving the areola are frequent factors in teenagers. *Staphylococcus aureus* is the most common cause, but other aerobic and anaerobic organisms have also been implicated.

Cyclic mastodynia, fibrocystic disease, or chest wall pain may also be causes of breast pain, but there should be no associated inflammatory signs.

Fluctuant abscesses should be surgically incised and drained. Oral antibiotics with appropriate coverage (dicloxacillin or a cephalosporin) should be given for 2–4 weeks. In addition, ice packs for the first 24 hours and heat thereafter may relieve symptoms.

GALACTORRHEA

In teenagers, galactorrhea, or inappropriate nipple discharge, is most often benign; however, a careful history and workup are necessary. Prolactinomas are the most common pathologic cause of galactorrhea in adolescents of both sexes and generally present as failure of sexual maturation. Hypothyroidism is the second most common cause in the adolescent years but has only been reported in girls, usually prepubertal.

Galactorrhea may be present after spontaneous or induced abortions as well as postpartum. Numerous prescribed and illicit drugs are associated with galactorrhea (Table 4–9). In addition, stimulation of the intercostal nerves (following surgery or due to herpes zoster), stimulation of the nipples, endocrine disorders (hypothyroidism, pituitary prolactinoma), central nervous system disorders (hypothalamic injury), or significant emotional distress may produce galactorrhea (Table 4–10).

Clinical Findings

If there is no history of pregnancy or drug use, thyroid-stimulating hormone (TSH) and prolactin levels should be determined. An elevated TSH confirms the diagnosis of hypothyroidism. An elevated prolactin and normal TSH, often accompanied by amenorrhea,

Table 4–9. Drugs associated with breast symptoms (galactorrhea, gynecomastia, pain, mass).[1]

Street drugs (illicit or abused)
Amphetamines
Marihuana
Mebrobamate
Opiates
  Codeine
  Heroin
  Morphine
Hormones or related drugs
Bromocriptine withdrawal
Estrogens
Human chorionic gonadotropin
Methyltestosterone
Oral contraceptives
Tamoxifen
Cancer drugs
Busulfan
Vincristine
Prescription medications
Amitriptyline
Chlordiazepoxide
Chlorpromazine
Cimetidine
Diazepam
Digoxin
Fluphenazine
Haloperidol
Imipramine
Isoniazid
Mesoridazine
Methyldopa
Perphenazine
Phenothiazines
Reserpine
Spironolactone
Thiethylperazine
Thioxanthines
Tricyclic antidepressants
Trifluoperazine
Trimeprazine

[1]Modified and reproduced, with permission, from Beach RK: Routine breast exams: A chance to reassure, guide, and protect. Contemp Pediatr 1987;4:70.

Table 4–10. Causes of galactorrhea.[1]

Hypothalamic disorders
Functional
  Postpartum
  Without pregnancy
Pathologic
  Infiltrative
    Sarcoid
    Histiocytosis X
    Hypothalamic tumors
  Section of pituitary stalk
Drug therapy
Tranquilizers
Tricyclic antidepressants
Methyldopa
Rauwolfia alkaloids
Oral contraceptives
Estrogens
Neoplasms
Pituitary tumors
  Prolactin secretion only
  Prolactin and ACTH secretion (Cushing's disease)
  Growth hormone secretion with or without prolactin secretion (acromegaly)
Ectopic prolactin-secreting tumors
Hypothyroidism
Neurogenic stimulation
Breast stimulation
Chest wall lesions (herpes zoster, thoracotomy)

[1]Modified and reproduced, with permission, from Fraser WM, Blackard WG: Medical conditions that affect the breast and lactation. Clin Obstet Gynecol 1975;18:51.

Treatment

Treatment of galactorrhea depends on the underlying cause. Prolactinomas may be surgically removed or suppressed with bromocriptine. Bromocriptine may also be beneficial to some amenorrheic females with normal prolactin levels.

GYNECOMASTIA

Gynecomastia is a common concern of male adolescents, the majority of whom (60–70%) develop transient subareolar breast tissue during Tanner stages II and III. Proposed causes include testosterone-estrogen imbalance, increased prolactin level, or abnormal serum binding protein levels.

Clinical Findings

In type I idiopathic gynecomastia, the adolescent presents with a unilateral (20% bilateral), tender, firm mass beneath the areola. More generalized breast enlargement is classified as type II. Pseudogynecomastia refers to excessive fat tissue or prominent pectoralis muscles.

Differential Diagnosis

Gynecomastia may be drug-induced (see Table 4–9). Klinefelter's syndrome; testicular, adrenal, or pituitary tumors; or thyroid or hepatic dysfunction

suggest a hypothalamic or pituitary tumor, and CT scan or MRI is indicated. When the prolactin level is normal, uncommon causes such as adrenal, renal, or ovarian tumors should be considered. The female with a negative workup and persistent galactorrhea may be followed with menstrual history and prolactin level every 6–12 months. In many cases, symptoms resolve spontaneously, and no diagnosis is made. The female with an elevated prolactin but negative prolactinoma workup may be treated with bromocriptine if her symptoms are bothersome or may be observed with CT scan or MRI every 18 months for several years. Males with a negative workup and normal puberty need to be intensively followed. Males with elevated prolactin levels deserve a CT scan or MRI every 12–18 months even if the galactorrhea resolves, as there is a significant risk of harboring a pituitary adenoma.

Table 4–11. Disorders associated with gynecomastia.

Klinefelter's syndrome
Traumatic paraplegia
Male pseudohermaphroditism
Testicular feminization syndrome
Reifenstein's syndrome
17-Ketosteroid reductase deficiency
Endocrine tumors (seminoma, Leydig cell tumor, teratoma,
    feminizing adrenal tumor, hepatoma, leukemia, hemo-
    philia, bronchogenic carcinoma, leprosy, etc)
Hypothyroidism
Hyperthyroidism
Cirrhosis
Herpes zoster
Friedreich's ataxia

may also be associated with gynecomastia (Table 4–11).

Treatment

If gynecomastia is idiopathic, reassurance of the common and benign nature of the process is given. Resolution may take several months to 2 years. Medical reduction has been achieved with pharmacotherapeutic agents, eg, dihydrotestosterone heptanoate, danazol, clomiphene citrate, and tamoxifen citrate, but these should be reserved for those with no decrease in breast size after 2 years. Surgery is reserved for those with significant psychologic trauma or severe breast enlargement.

Beach RK: Routine breast exams: A chance to reassure, guide, and protect. Contemp Pediatr (Oct) 1987;4:70.

Diehl T, Kaplan DW: Breast masses in adolescent females. Sexually Active Teenagers 1988;2:151.

Mahoney CP: Adolescent gynecomastia: Differential diagnosis and management. Pediatr Clin North Am 1990;37:1389.

Neinstein LS, Atkinson J, Diament M: Prevalence and longitudinal study of breast masses in adolescents. J Adolesc Health 1993;13:277.

Rohn RD: Galactorrhea in the adolescent. J Adolesc Health Care 1984;5:37.

GYNECOLOGIC DISORDERS IN ADOLESCENCE

MENSTRUAL PHYSIOLOGY

The menstrual cycle is divided into three phases: follicular, ovulatory, and luteal. During the follicular phase, pulsatile gonadotropin-releasing hormone (GnRH) stimulates anterior pituitary secretion of follicle-stimulating hormone (FSH) and luteinizing hormone (LH). Under the influence of FSH and LH, a dominant follicle emerges by day 5–7 of the menstrual cycle, and the others become atretic. Rising estradiol levels cause proliferation of the endometrium. By midfollicular phase, FSH is beginning to decline secondary to estradiol-mediated negative feedback, while LH continues to rise as a result of estradiol-mediated positive feedback.

There has been a proliferation of LH receptors on the follicle, and it secretes more estradiol in the periovulatory phase, resulting in further proliferation of the endometrium. The rising LH initiates progesterone secretion and the luteinization of the granulosa cells of the follicle. Progesterone in turn stimulates LH and FSH further. This leads to the LH surge, which causes the follicle to rupture and expel the oocyte.

During the luteal phase, the pulsatile release of GnRH occurs less frequently, and LH and FSH gradually decline. The corpus luteum secretes progesterone and 17-hydroxyprogesterone. The endometrium enters the secretory phase in response to rising levels of estrogen and progesterone, with maturation 8–9 days after ovulation. If there is no pregnancy or placental human chorionic gonadotropin (hCG), luteolysis begins; estrogen and progesterone levels decline; and the endometrial lining is shed as menstrual flow (Figure 4–8).

PELVIC EXAMINATION

A pelvic examination may be indicated to evaluate abdominal pain or menstrual disorders or to detect a suspected sexually transmitted disease in the adolescent. In addition, by approximately 16–18 years of age, a pelvic examination should be performed to obtain the first Papanicolaou smear and ensure normal reproductive anatomy if annual pelvic examination has not yet been initiated. The adolescent may be apprehensive about the first examination. It should not be rushed, and an explanation of the procedure and its purpose should precede it. The patient can be encouraged to relax by slow, deep breathing and by relaxation of her lower abdominal and inner thigh muscles. A young adolescent may wish to have her mother present during the examination, but the history should be taken privately. A female chaperone should be present for male examiners.

The pelvic examination begins by placing the patient in the dorsal lithotomy position after equipment and supplies are ready (Table 4–12). The examiner inspects the external genitalia, noting the pubic hair maturity rating, the size of the clitoris (2–5 mm is normal), Skene's glands just inside the urethral meatus, and Bartholin's glands at 4 o'clock and 8 o'clock outside the hymenal ring. In cases of alleged sexual abuse or assault, the horizontal measurement of the relaxed prepubertal hymenal opening should be taken, and the presence of any lacerations,

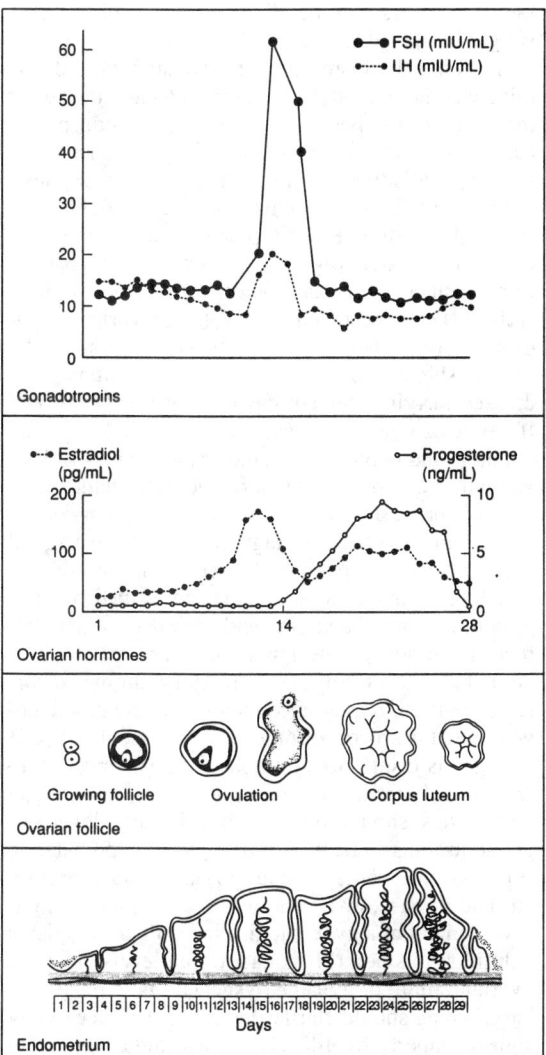

Figure 4–8. Physiology of the normal ovulatory menstrual cycle; gonadotropin secretion, ovarian hormone production, follicular maturation, and endometrial changes during one cycle. FSH = follicle-stimulating hormone; LH = luteinizing hormone. (Reproduced, with permission, from Emans SJH, Goldstein DP: *Pediatric & Adolescent Gynecology,* 2nd ed. Little, Brown, 1982.)

Table 4–12. Items for pelvic exam tray.

Medium and virginal speculums (warm)
Gloves
Applicator sticks, sterile
Sigmoidoscopy swabs to remove excess discharge
Cervical spatulas, cervical brushes
Microscope slides and cover slips (frosted and labeled)
Centrifuge tube or test tube (if swab is to be placed in drop of saline and slide prepared later)
NaCl dropper bottle
KOH dropper bottle
Slide container to send to lab
Gonorrhea culture plate (room temperature)
Chlamydia culture tube or antigen detection kit
Lubricant
Kleenex
Hemoccult cards
pH paper

olescents; the columnar epithelium extends outside the cervical os onto the face of the cervix until later adolescence, when it recedes.

At this time, specimens are obtained, including a wet preparation for leukocytes, trichomonads, and "clue cells"; potassium hydroxide preparation for yeast; cervical swab for gonorrhea culture; endocervical and cervical (transition zone from columnar to squamous epithelium) samples for Papanicolaou smear; and, lastly, a cervical swab for *Chlamydia* antigen detection testing. A cervical brush provides a higher yield of cells for the endocervical Papanicolaou slide. Papanicolaou smears should be interpreted by a cytopathologist at a laboratory employing the Bethesda system of classification.

The speculum is then removed, and the bimanual examination is performed to assess uterine size and position, adnexal enlargement or tenderness, or cervical motion tenderness. Rectovaginal examination may be helpful in assessing uterine size or detecting beading from endometriosis.

MENSTRUAL DISORDERS

1. AMENORRHEA

Amenorrhea is the lack of menses when normally anticipated. **Primary amenorrhea** is delay in menarche such that there are no menstrual periods or secondary sex characteristics by 14 years of age or no menses in the presence of secondary sex characteristics by 16 years of age. **Secondary amenorrhea** is defined as the absence of menses for at least three cycles after regular cycles have been present. In some instances, evaluation should begin immediately, without waiting for the specified age or duration of lapsed periods, eg, in patients with suspected pregnancy, short stature with the stigmas of Turner's syndrome, or an anatomic defect.

bruises, scarring, or synechiae about the hymen, vulva, or anus should be noted.

A vaginal speculum of the appropriate size is then inserted at a 45-degree twist and angled 45 degrees downward. (A medium Pedersen speculum is most often used in sexually experienced patients; a narrow Pedersen is used for virginal patients. A pediatric speculum may be necessary in examining children.) The vaginal walls are inspected for estrinization, inflammation, or lesions. The cervix should be dull pink, and cervical ectropion is commonly seen in ad-

Evaluation for Primary Amenorrhea

Primary amenorrhea may be the result of anatomic abnormalities (imperforate hymen, transverse vaginal septum, vaginal agenesis, agenesis of the cervix, absent uterus), chromosomal deviations (Turner's syndrome XO, mosaicism, testicular feminization), or physiologic delay (hypogonadotropic hypogonadism,

Table 4–13. Causes of amenorrhea.

Hypothalamic pituitary axis
  Hypothalamic repression
    Emotional stress
    Depression
    Chronic disease
    Weight loss
    Obesity
    Severe dieting
    Strenuous athletics
    Drugs (post birth control pills, phenothiazines)
  CNS lesion
    Pituitary lesion: adenoma, prolactinoma
    Craniopharyngioma and other brainstem, parasellar
      tumors
    Head injury with hypothalamic contusion
    Infiltrative process (sarcoidosis)
    Vascular disease (hypothalamic vasculitis)
  Congenital conditions[1]
    Kallmann's syndrome
Ovaries
  Gonadal dysgenesis[1]
    Turner's syndrome (XO)
    Mosaic (XX/XO)
  Injury to ovary
    Autoimmune disease (may include thyroid, adrenal,
      islet cells)
    Infection (mumps, oophoritis)
    Toxins (alkylating chemotherapetic agents)
    Irradiation
    Trauma, torsion (rare)
  Polycystic ovary syndrome (Stein-Leventhal) (virilization
    may be present)
  Ovarian failure
    Premature menopause (may result from causes of
      ovarian injury)
    Resistant ovary
    Variant of gonadal dysgenesis (mosaic)
Uterovaginal outflow tract
  Müllerian dysgenesis[1]
    Congenital deformity or absence of uterus, uterine
      tubes, or vagina
    Imperforate hymen, transverse vaginal septum, vaginal
      agenesis, agenesis of the cervix[1]
    Testicular feminization (absent uterus)[1]
  Uterine lining defect
    Asherman's syndrome (intrauterine synechiae
      postcurettage or endometritis)
    TB, brucellosis
**Defect in hormone synthesis or action (virilization may
  be present)**
  Adrenal hyperplasia[1]
  Cushing's disease
  Adrenal tumor
  Ovarian tumor (rare)
  Drugs (steroids, ACTH)

[1]Indicates condition that usually presents as primary amenorrhea.

familial delay, chronic disease, stress, obesity, or weight loss) (Table 4–13).

In taking the history, the physician should determine whether puberty has commenced and the age at menarche of the patient's relatives. A careful physical examination should be done. The examiner keeps in mind that adrenal androgens are largely responsible for axillary and pubic hair and that estrogen is responsible for breast development; maturation of the external genitalia, vagina, and uterus; and menstruation. Tanner stage and percentage of ideal body weight should be noted. The signs of Turner's syndrome should also be looked for: height less than 60 inches, shield-like chest, widely spaced nipples, increased carrying angle of the arms, webbed neck, etc. If pelvic examination reveals normal female external genitalia and pelvic organs, the physician may order a vaginal smear for estrogen influence or a challenge of medroxyprogesterone acetate (Provera), 10 mg orally twice daily for 5 days (Figure 4–9). If the vaginal smear shows estrogen influence or if withdrawal bleeding occurs after administration of medroxyprogesterone, normal anatomy and adequate estrogen effect are implied. Determination of serum LH level helps to rule out polycystic ovary syndrome; if this test is normal, reassurance may be given and the developmental process followed every few months. If estrogen is insufficient (atrophic vaginal smear or no withdrawal bleeding), serum gonadotropin (FSH and LH) levels should be determined. Low levels of gonadotropins indicate a more severe hypothalamic suppression, perhaps due to anorexia nervosa, chronic disease, or a central nervous system tumor. Involvement of a gynecologist and endocrinologist is helpful at this point. If gonadotropin levels are high, ovarian failure or gonadal dysgenesis is implied, and karyotyping should clarify the cause. Absence of any sign of puberty by 14 years of age indicates inadequate estrogen, and the physician should check FSH, LH, and karyotype first before testing for estrogen effect.

If signs of virilization are present (Figure 4–10), the first step is to determine the LH level to rule out polycystic ovaries. If the LH level is low in the presence of virilization, an adrenal disorder is the most likely diagnosis. Endocrinologic and gynecologic consultations may assist in determining the diagnosis.

If physical examination reveals an absent uterus (see Figure 4–9), karyotyping should be performed to differentiate testicular feminization from müllerian duct defect, because these two entities are managed differently.

Evaluation & Treatment of Secondary Amenorrhea

Secondary amenorrhea results when there is unopposed estrogen, maintaining the endometrium in the proliferative phase. The most common causes are

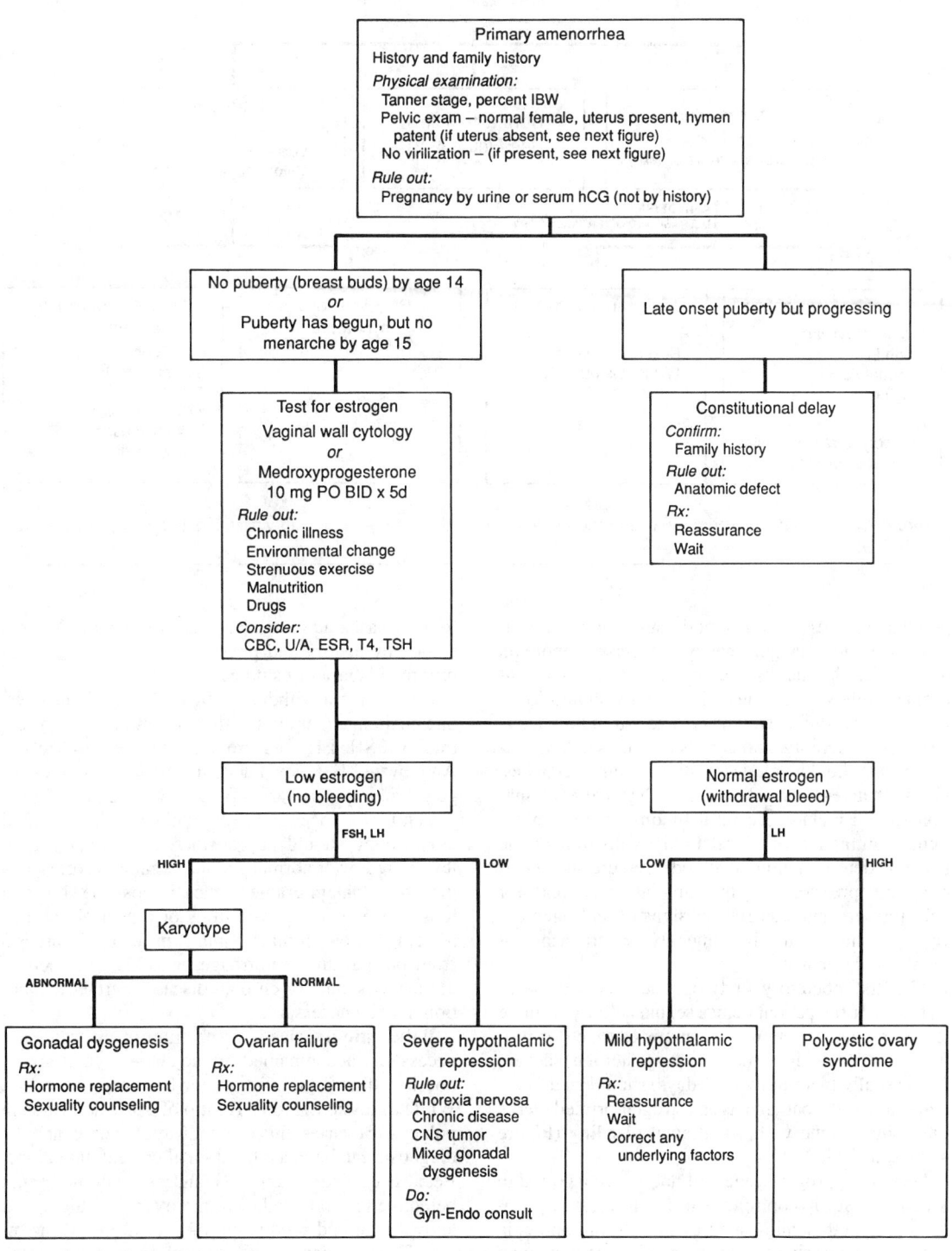

Figure 4–9. Evaluation of primary amenorrhea in a normal female. (Courtesy of Roberta K Beach, MD.)

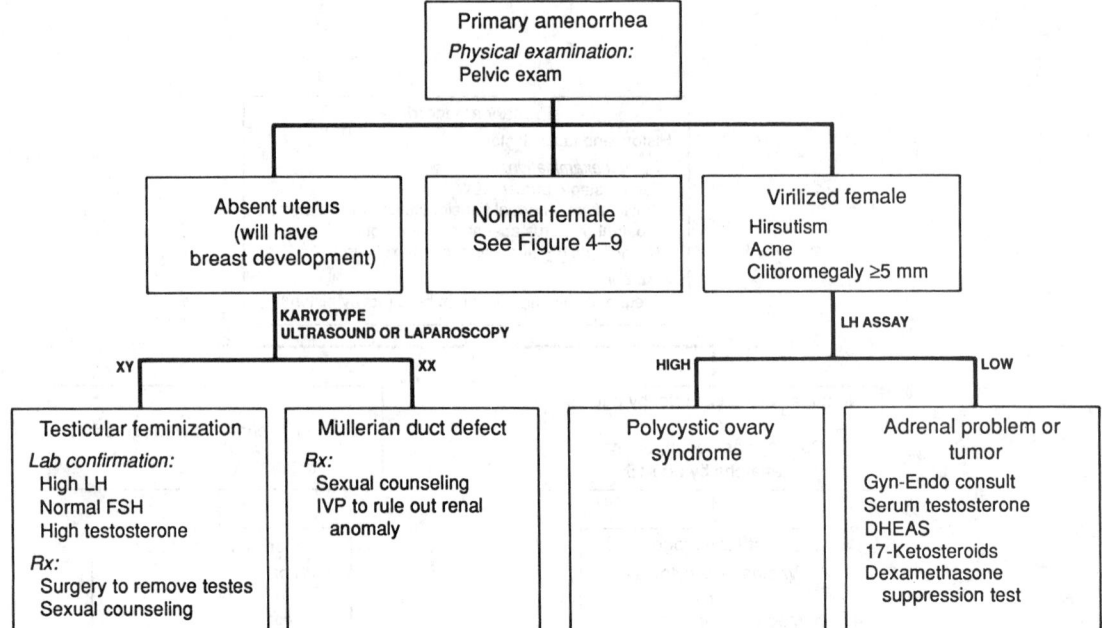

Figure 4–10. Evaluation of primary amenorrhea in a female without a uterus or with virilization. (Courtesy of Roberta K Beach, MD.)

pregnancy, stress (fever, emotional turmoil, significant weight change, heavy exercise, anorexia nervosa, or chronic disease), or Stein-Leventhal syndrome (polycystic ovaries). The history should focus on issues of stress, weight change, strenuous exercise, sexual activity, and contraceptive use. A review of systems should include questions about headaches, visual changes, and galactorrhea. Physical examination should include a careful funduscopic examination, examination of visual fields, palpation of the thyroid, determination of blood pressure and heart rate, compression of the areola to check for galactorrhea, and a search for signs of androgen excess (eg, hirsutism, clitoromegaly, severe acne, or ovarian enlargement).

The first laboratory study obtained is a pregnancy test, even if the patient denies sexual activity. If there is no pregnancy, vaginal smear for estrogen or progesterone challenge (medroxyprogesterone acetate, 10 mg orally twice daily for 5 days) should be done to determine if the patient has an estrogen-primed uterus that will respond with withdrawal bleeding (Figure 4–11 and Table 4–14).

Generally, progesterone will not induce a period in a patient with hypopituitarism due to a tumor, profound hypothalamic suppression from anorexia nervosa, or massive weight gain. Most patients who have withdrawal flow to progesterone have hypothalamic amenorrhea due to weight change, athletics, stress, or illness; however, disorders such as polycystic ovaries, adrenal disorders, ovarian tumors, thy-

roid disease, and diabetes mellitus should be excluded by history and physical examination and appropriate laboratory studies.

If there is no withdrawal flow after the progesterone challenge (see Figure 4–11), serum levels of estradiol, FSH, LH, and prolactin should be checked. An elevated FSH level accompanied by a low estrogen level implies ovarian failure, in which case blood for anti-ovarian antibodies should be obtained and laparoscopy should be considered. If gonadotropin levels are low or normal and the estradiol level is normal, hypothalamic amenorrhea is possible, but one must consider the possibilities of a central nervous system tumor (prolactinoma), pituitary infarction from postpartum hemorrhage or sickle cell anemia, uterine synechia, or chronic disease. Further evaluation may be necessary.

Polycystic ovaries is a spectrum of disorders not necessarily accompanied by the classic symptoms of obesity, hirsutism, oligomenorrhea, and infertility. While a classic LH to FSH ratio of 3:1 is described in polycystic ovaries, this is not always the case, and the diagnosis can be made by clinical presentation alone. Because of insufficient FSH, androstenedione cannot be converted to estradiol in the ovarian follicle, and anovulation and production of excess androgens result. These patients can be given progesterone each month to allow withdrawal flow if there is no evidence of progressive hirsutism and the ovaries are normal in size. Oral contraceptive pills, containing a less androgenic progestin, are an alternative treat-

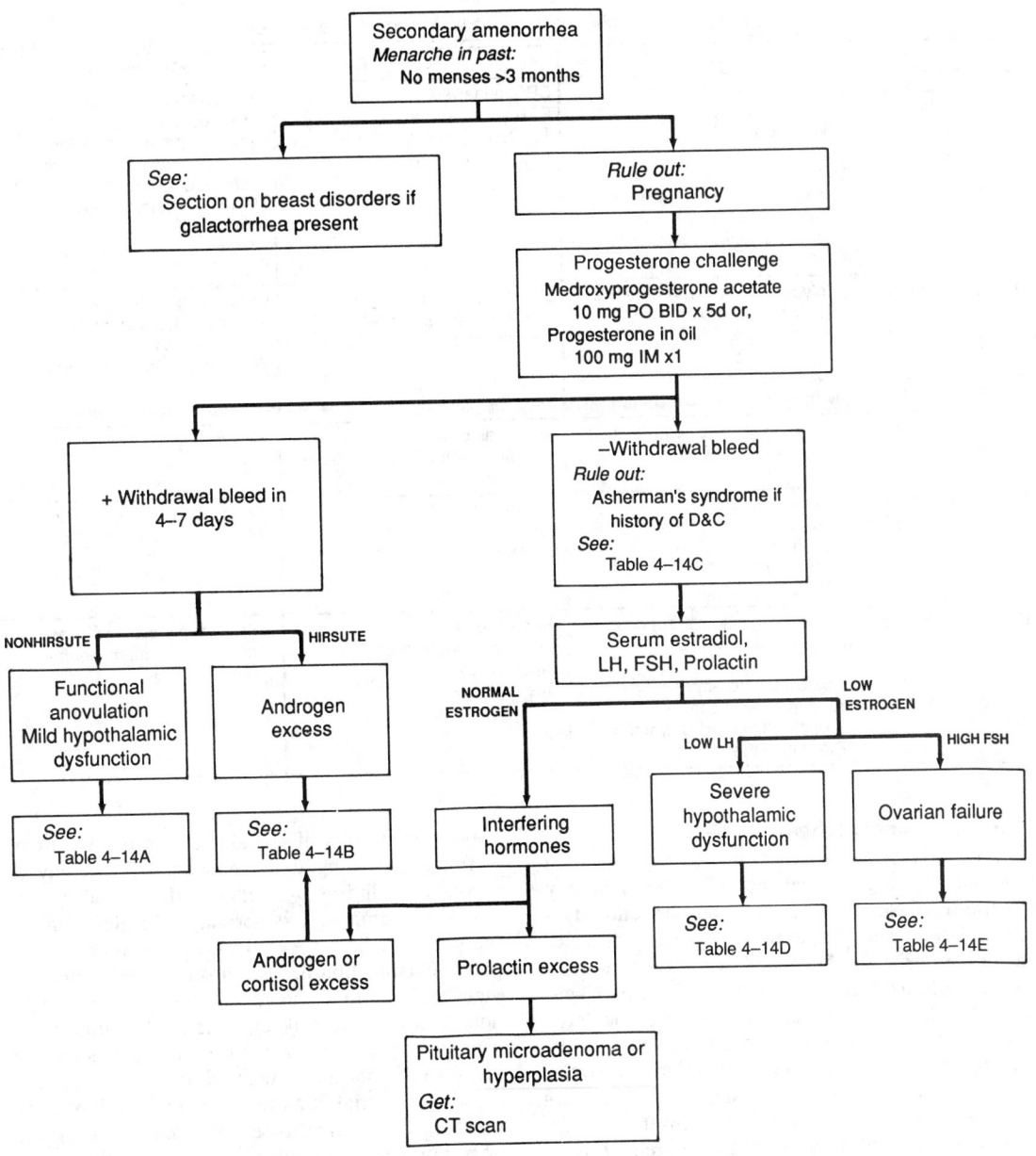

Figure 4–11. Evaluation of secondary amenorrhea. (Courtesy of Roberta K Beach, MD.)

ment. If hirsutism is present, an androgen-producing tumor should be ruled out by obtaining serum testosterone and DHEAS levels. The lipid profile should also be obtained in hirsute patients. If the patient wishes to become pregnant, she should be referred to a gynecologist for clomiphene citrate or menotropins.

2. DYSMENORRHEA

Dysmenorrhea is the most common gynecologic complaint of adolescent girls, with an incidence of about 60%. Yet many teenage girls will not seek help from a physician, relying instead on female relatives, friends, and the media for advice. Therefore, the physician should ask about "menstrual cramps" when taking a review of systems. In this era of prostaglandin inhibitors, much can be done to alleviate suffering.

Dysmenorrhea can be divided into primary and secondary dysmenorrhea on the basis of whether or not there is underlying pelvic disease.

Table 4–14. Management of secondary amenorrhea by cause.

	Cause	Lab	Management
A. Mild hypothalamic dysfunction	Recent pregnancy Physical illness Weight loss Obesity Emotional stress Environmental change Strenuous athletics Drugs (post birth control pills, phenothiazines)	CBC, urinalysis ESR T_4, TSH, etc (as indicated)	Reassurance: assessment of birth control needs Repeat of progesterone test every 3 months (after ruling out pregnancy) LH, FSH, prolactin if no menses for 1 year
B. Androgen excess	Polycystic ovary syndrome (PCO) Cushing's syndrome Adrenal hyperplasia Adrenal tumor Ovarian tumor Drugs (steroids, ACTH)	LH, FSH (high LH suggests PCO); consultation with endocrinologist to help evaluate adrenals	If PCO, birth control pills (Demulen) to control hirsutism and menses Treatment of underlying problem
C. Asherman's syndrome	Uterine synechiae posttherapeutic abortion or D&C	No bleeding after 1 cycle of combination oral contraceptive (Ovulen)	Referral to gynecologist
D. Severe hypothalamic dysfunction	Anorexia nervosa Severe emotional stress Chronic systemic disease CNS tumor Pituitary infarction	Low estrogen Low LH Check T_4, TSH, ESR, neurologic exam	Treatment of cause; slow hormone recovery expected
E. Ovarian failure	Variant of gonadal dysgenesis (mosaicism XX/XO) Postirradiation Postchemotherapy Autoimmune oophoritis Resistant ovarian syndrome Premature menopause	Chromosomes Antiovarian antibodies Laparoscopy Ovarian biopsy	Referral to gynecologist; hormone replacement therapy

Primary Dysmenorrhea

Primary dysmenorrhea, in which no pelvic disease is detectable, can be further subdivided into **primary spasmodic dysmenorrhea** and **psychogenic dysmenorrhea.** Primary spasmodic dysmenorrhea accounts for 80% of cases of adolescent dysmenorrhea and most often affects women under 25 years of age. It results from the release of excessive amounts of prostaglandin $F_{2\alpha}$, which attaches to myometrial receptor sites, causing uterine contractions, hypoxia, and ischemia. In addition, prostaglandins also directly sensitize pain receptors and lower the pain threshold. As most of the prostaglandin release is in the first 48 hours of menses, the pain generally starts with the onset of flow or just before and lasts 1–2 days. Primary spasmodic dysmenorrhea does not typically begin until 6–18 months after menarche, when the cycles become ovulatory; endometrial production of prostaglandins is higher in the luteal phase, which does not exist unless ovulation occurs. Symptoms consist of lower abdominal cramps, which may radiate to the lower back and thighs. Associated symptoms of nausea, vomiting, diarrhea, and urinary frequency may be present and are also due to prostaglandin release.

Psychogenic dysmenorrhea typically starts at menarche. Pain begins with anticipation of menses and lasts throughout the duration of flow. These patients may have a history of sexual abuse or may be having difficulty adjusting to womanhood. There may be secondary gain from school or work avoidance.

Pelvic examination is normal in females with primary spasmodic or psychogenic dysmenorrhea. The pelvic examination has diagnostic benefits and provides an opportunity to educate and reassure the patient about her normal reproductive function. However, if the patient has never been sexually active and the history is consistent with primary spasmodic dysmenorrhea, a trial of a prostaglandin inhibitor is reasonable. If the patient is sexually active or if there is no response to a prostaglandin inhibitor, pelvic examination is indicated.

The patient should be educated about normal menstrual function and reassured that the pain does not indicate disease. Exercise and positive feelings about her body can be encouraged. Relaxation techniques and biofeedback may be helpful for patients with psychogenic dysmenorrhea, but counseling may be necessary to clarify underlying issues. Application of a heating pad, warm baths, and nonprescription analgesics may be sufficient for mild primary spasmodic dysmenorrhea. For moderate to severe spasmodic dysmenorrhea, prostaglandin inhibitors—or oral contraceptive pills in sexually active patients—are appropriate. Either of these medications will relieve symptoms in about 90% of patients. The patient

Table 4–15. Prostaglandin inhibitors used for dysmenorrhea.

Generic Name	Trade Name	Preparations Available (mg)[1]
Aspirin	Many	325, 500
Ibuprofen	Motrin Rufen Advil, Nupren, Medipren	200, 300, 400, 600, 800 400, 600, 800 200
Mefenamic acid	Ponstel	250
Naproxen	Naprosyn Aleve	250, 375, 500 200
Naproxen sodium	Anaprox	275, 550

[1]Take as directed at onset of menstrual cramps or flow, then every 6–8 hours thereafter.

rate should be done. Gynecologic consultation is indicated to look for endometriosis or congenital problems by ultrasound, hysteroscopy, or laparoscopy.

Treatment depends on the cause. Infections can be treated with appropriate antibiotics (see sections on sexually transmitted disease and pelvic inflammatory disease). Hormonal suppression can be achieved with the use of estrogen or danazol in endometriosis, but surgery may be necessary for extensive disease. Prostaglandin inhibitors may be used for the menstrual cramps caused by intrauterine devices once infection is ruled out; mefenamic acid may be the drug of choice for these patients, since it also reduces menorrhagia. Complications of pregnancy require immediate gynecologic consultation.

should be instructed to begin prostaglandin inhibitors (Table 4–15) with the first sign of pain or menstrual flow. Side effects are rare, since prostaglandin inhibitors are used for only 1–4 days but may include epigastric pain, nausea, vomiting, headache, dizziness, tinnitus, or pruritus. They may decrease renal function. Relative contraindications include chronic gastrointestinal inflammation, reactive airways disease, hypersensitivity, or a bleeding diathesis.

Secondary Dysmenorrhea

Secondary dysmenorrhea is menstrual pain due to an underlying pelvic lesion. Although uncommon in adolescents, when present it is most often due to infection or **endometriosis.** In the patient with infection, there may be pelvic cramps of recent onset, excessive bleeding or intermenstrual spotting, or vaginal discharge. The patient is generally sexually active. The pain of endometriosis generally starts more than 2 years after menarche. Two-thirds of those with endometriosis will feel tenderness on examination, particularly during the late luteal phase. This disease is not limited to adults, as once thought; in one study of adolescent females with chronic pelvic pain, more than 40% who had not received a definitive diagnosis by the third visit were found to have endometriosis. If the patient has a delay in menses, a complication of pregnancy (eg, spontaneous abortion or ectopic pregnancy) should be suspected. If menstrual cramps start at menarche, congenital anomalies (eg, a transverse vaginal septum, septate uterus, or cervical stenosis) should be suspected. Intrauterine devices may cause dysmenorrhea or may increase the risk of pelvic infections and thereby cause pain. Lastly, pelvic adhesions may be responsible for pelvic pain; a history of abdominal surgery should, therefore, be elicited.

The clinician evaluating a patient with secondary dysmenorrhea should take a sexual history and conduct a pelvic examination even if the patient is not sexually active. Culture for gonococci, a complement fixation test for *Chlamydia,* a complete blood count, and determination of the erythrocyte sedimentation

3. DYSFUNCTIONAL UTERINE BLEEDING

Dysfunctional uterine bleeding may consist of hypermenorrhea or polymenorrhea. It results when an endometrium that has proliferated under unopposed estrogen stimulation finally begins to slough, but incompletely, causing irregular, painless bleeding. The unopposed estrogen stimulation occurs during anovulatory cycles, commonly in younger adolescents who have not been menstruating for long but occurring also seen in older adolescents during times of stress or illness.

Clinical Findings

Typically, the adolescent has had several years of regular cycles and then begins to have menses every 2 weeks, or complains of bleeding for 2–3 weeks after 2–3 months of amenorrhea. A past history of painless, irregular periods at intervals of less than 3 weeks may also be elicited. Bleeding for more than 10 days should be considered abnormal.

Differential Diagnosis

Dysfunctional uterine bleeding must be considered a diagnosis of exclusion. The possibility of pelvic inflammatory disease or a complication of pregnancy, eg, ectopic pregnancy or threatened, incomplete, or missed abortion, must be considered in sexually active teenagers. In patients taking birth control pills, breakthrough bleeding is a consideration. Blood dyscrasias such as iron deficiency anemia, thrombocytopenia, coagulopathy, von Willebrand's disease, or leukemia should also be considered. In addition, endocrine disorders such as hypothyroidism, hyperthyroidism, diabetes mellitus, adrenal disease, or hyperprolactinemia are also in the differential diagnosis. Trauma and foreign body insertion are also possible causes and can be ruled out by the history and physical examination. Uterine, vaginal, or ovarian abnormalities (eg, carcinoma, fibroids, adenosis secondary to diethylstilbestrol use, or premature menopause) are less likely causes in teenagers.

Treatment

A pregnancy test and pelvic examination with appropriate cultures should be performed in sexually active patients. A complete blood count, including a platelet count, should also be obtained. The history and physical findings may suggest the need for additional coagulation or hormonal studies. Management depends on the severity of the problem. If the patient has a history of shortened intervals between cycles or somewhat heavier flow and normal hemoglobin levels, she can be asked to keep a menstrual calendar, and reassurance can be given. Mefenamic acid (500 mg three times a day during menstruation) may be beneficial for the patient's heavy flow, and an iron supplement may be considered, since anemia can both contribute to and result from dysfunctional uterine bleeding.

For the patient with moderate dysfunctional uterine bleeding, mild anemia, moderately heavy and prolonged cycles, or persistently short intervals between menses, medroxyprogesterone acetate (10 mg once or twice a day for 10 days starting day 14 of the cycle) may be used for 3–6 months. To stop bleeding in progress, begin oral contraceptive pills (1/35) up to four pills per day and taper over 2–3 weeks. Bleeding generally stops in a few days. Withdrawal flow should be expected several days after the last dose. After withdrawal flow ceases, the patient can be cycled for 3–6 months on oral contraceptive pills (1/35) or medroxyprogesterone acetate. Iron supplements should also be given.

Patients with severe dysfunctional bleeding, a low hemoglobin count, and orthostatic symptoms in conjunction with heavy vaginal bleeding and disruption of menstrual cycles require hospitalization. Clotting studies should be obtained. Conjugated estrogens such as Premarin (25 mg intravenously every 4–6 hours for 24 hours) may be given for its hemostatic effect. Oral contraceptives (1/35) should be given every 6 hours until bleeding stops and then tapered over 2–3 weeks. After withdrawal flow ceases, the patient should be cycled on an oral contraceptive containing 50 μg ethinyl estradiol for 3 months, followed by a 30–35 μg monophasic or triphasic pill for another 3 months. Iron therapy should be instituted and the iron status monitored. Gynecologic consultation should be obtained, because hysteroscopy or dilation and curettage may be necessary if there is no improvement in 24 hours.

4. MITTELSCHMERZ

Mittelschmerz is the name given to the pain caused by irritation of the peritoneum due to spillage of fluid from the ruptured follicular cyst at the time of ovulation. The patient presents with a history of midcycle, unilateral dull or aching abdominal pain lasting a few minutes or as long as 8 hours. This pain rarely mimics the acute abdominal findings of appendicitis, torsion or rupture of an ovarian cyst, or ectopic pregnancy. The patient should be reassured and treated symptomatically. If the findings are severe enough to warrant consideration of the above diagnoses, laparoscopy may be done to rule them out.

5. PREMENSTRUAL SYNDROME

Premenstrual syndrome (PMS) has received much attention in the lay press. The term is applied to a cluster of physical and psychologic symptoms that are temporally related to the week preceding menstruation and are alleviated by the onset of menses. While there are no established diagnostic criteria, and the symptoms may vary from patient to patient—or from month to month in the same patient–some researchers suggest that PMS consists of several different physcial and emotional syndromes. Premenstrual symptoms most commonly cited include weight gain, edema, bloating, breast tenderness, fatigue, headache, backache, depression, emotional lability, and increased thirst or appetite. Previously thought to be a disorder limited to adult women, recent studies indicate that adolescents experience the same premenstrual symptoms as adults. Although a number of causes have been proposed (progesterone deficiency, hyperprolactinemia, estrogen excess or imbalance of the estrogen:progesterone ratio, vitamin B_{12} deficiency, fluid retention, endorphins, hypoglycemia, and psychosomatic factors), none have been proved. There may be some hormonal role; women who have undergone hysterectomy but not oophorectomy may have cyclic symptoms resembling PMS, whereas postmenopausal women have no such symptoms. Several treatments have been advocated, but none have conferred consistent benefits. Education is the most useful measure at this time. The patient can keep a calendar of symptoms for several months, and proper eating, exercise, and sleep can be stressed. Salt restriction or mild diuretics can be prescribed for patients with fluid retention. Oral contraceptives or prostaglandin inhibitors may be beneficial for some women. Tricyclic antidepressants do not have a role in the treatment of this disorder.

6. OVARIAN CYSTS

Functional cysts account for 20–50% of ovarian tumors in adolescents and are a variation of the normal physiologic process. They may be asymptomatic or may cause menstrual irregularity, constipation, or urinary frequency. Functional cysts, unless large, rarely cause abdominal pain; however, torsion or hemorrhage of an ovarian cyst may present as an acute or subacute abdomen. **Follicular cysts** account for the majority of ovarian cysts. They are produced every cycle but occasionally are not resorbed. Follicular cysts are unilateral, usually not larger than 4 cm in diameter, and resolve spontaneously. If the patient is asymptomatic, she can be given oral contraceptives containing 50 μg of estrogen for suppression and examined monthly. The patient should be referred to a gynecologist for laparoscopy if she is premenarcheal; if the cyst has a solid component or is larger than 5 cm by ultrasound; if there are symptoms or signs suggestive of hemorrhage or torsion; or if the cyst fails to regress after two or three menstrual cycles. **Lutein cysts** occur less commonly and may be 5–10 cm in diameter. The patient may have associated amenorrhea or, as the cyst becomes atretic, heavy vaginal bleeding. The patient may be monitored on suppression with oral contraceptives for 3 months but should have a laparoscopy if the cyst is larger than 5 cm or if there is pain or bleeding from the cyst.

7. ENDOMETRIOSIS

See Secondary Dysmenorrhea, above.

Beach RK: Relieving the pain of menstrual cramps. Contemp Pediatr 1986;3:115.

Blythe M: Common menstrual problems. Part 3: Abnormal uterine bleeding. Adolescent Health Update 1992;4:1.

Davis GD, Thillet E, Lindemann J: Clinical characteristics of adolescent endometriosis J Adolesc Health 1993;14:362.

Emans SJH, Goldstein DP: *Pediatric and Adolescent Gynecology,*. Little, Brown, 1990.

Fisher M, Trieller K, Napolitano B: Premenstrual symptoms in adolescents, J Adolesc Health Care 1989;10:369.

Grumbach MM: The neuroendocrinology of puberty. Hosp Pract (March) 1980;15:51.

Mansfield MJ, Emans SJ: Anorexia nervosa, athletics, and amenorrhea. Pediatr Clin North Am 1989;36:533.

National Cancer Institute Workshop: The 1988 Bethesda system for reporting cervical/vaginal cytological diagnoses. JAMA 1989;262:931.

Neinstein LS: Menstrual problems in adolescents. Med Clin North Am 1990;74:1181.

Polaneczky MM, Slap GB: Menstrual disorders in the adolescent: Amenorrhea. Pediatr Rev 1992;13:43.

Speroff L, Glass RH, Kase NG (editors): *Clinical Gynecologic Endocrinology and Infertility,* 4th ed. Williams & Wilkins, 1989.

Strasburger VC (editor): Adolescent gynecology. Pediatr Clin North Am 1989;38:3.

CONTRACEPTION

Sexually active adolescent females wait an average of one year before seeking contraception; however, one-half of teen pregnancies in the United States occur in the first 6 months after sexual activity begins. Sexuality, contraception, and pregnancy prevention are areas with which the pediatrician has become familiar out of necessity.

Abstinence & Decision Making

Adolescents may have poorly formulated skills for making decisions of any kind and often benefit from a decision-making framework that can be applied to a variety of situations, particularly those involving peer pressure. For younger adolescents, this framework can be made more concrete by providing written materials on which the adolescent fills in alternatives and their consequences.

Many adolescents have given little thought to how they feel about their developing sexuality or how they would handle sexual situations. As a result, sexual intercourse may be initiated because the individuals are ill-prepared to handle a situation. By talking with teenagers about their alternatives to sexual intercourse and its implications (unintended pregnancy; sexually transmitted diseases; possible emotional trauma; effects on education, career, and income; and responsibilities if a pregnancy occurs), physicians can help them make informed decisions before they find themselves in a dilemma.

Teenagers need to be aware that half of all teenagers have not engaged in sexual intercourse. Abstinence is the most commonly used method of birth control. If an adolescent chooses to remain abstinent, the clinician should reinforce the decision. It is also prudent to encourage adolescents to use contraception at the time they do initiate sexual intercourse.

Barrier Methods

Barrier methods of contraception have gained popularity—even among adolescents—as a result of the educational and marketing efforts driven by the AIDS epidemic. In 1988, 55% of sexually active 15- to 19-year-old males reported using a condom at first intercourse, and 57% at last intercourse—compared with about 20% of 17- to 19-year-old males in 1979. Regardless of whether another method is used, all sexually active adolescents should be counseled to use condoms. Condoms also offer protection against sexually transmitted diseases by preventing the transmission of gonococci, chlamydiae, spirochetes, hepatitis virion particles, and possibly HIV. Spermicides containing nonoxynol-9 have virucidal and bactericidal effects. Aside from the diaphragm and cervical cap, barrier methods do not require a medical visit or prescription and are widely available (Table 4–16). The polyurethane vaginal pouch, or "female condom," may soon be available. This device is associated with a failure rate and STD prevention properties similar to those of the condom, but it has the advantage of placing greater control in the hands of the female partner.

Table 4–16. Lowest expected, typical, and lowest reported failure rates during the first year of use of a method of contraception, United States. Percentage of women experiencing an accidental pregnancy in the first year of use.[1]

Method	Lowest Expected[2]	Typical[3]	Lowest Reported[4]
Chance	85	85	43.1
Spermicides[5]	3	21	0
Sponge			
Parous women	9	28	27.7
Nulliparous women		18	133.9
Cervical cap[6]	6	18	8
Diaphragm	6	18	2.1
Condom[7]	2	12	4.2
Pill			
Combined	0.1		0
Progestogen only	0.5		1.1
Depot medroxyprogesterone acetate	0.3	0.3	0
Levonorgestrel implants (Norplant System)	0.04	0.04	0

[1]Modified and reproduced, with permission, from Hatcher RA et al: *Contraceptive Technology 1990–1992*, 15th rev ed. Irvington, 1990.

[2]Among couples who initiate use of a method (not necessarily for the first time) and who use it *perfectly* (both consistently and correctly); the authors' best guess of the percentage expected to experience an accidental pregnancy during the first year if they do not stop use for any other reason.

[3]Among *typical* couples who initiate use of a method (not necessarily for the first time), the percentage who experience an accidental pregnancy during the first year if they do not stop use for any other reason.

[4]In the literature on contraceptive failure, the *lowest* reported percentage who experienced an accidental pregnancy during the first year following initiation of use (not necessarily for the first time) if they did not stop use for any other reason.

[5]Foams and vaginal suppositories.

[6]With spermicidal cream or jelly.

[7]Without spermicides.

Oral Contraceptives

Oral contraceptives have a three-pronged mechanism of action: (1) suppression of ovulation; (2) thickening of the cervical mucus, thereby making sperm penetration more difficult; and (3) atrophy of the endometrium, which diminishes the chance of implantation. The latter two actions are progestin effects.

A. Combination Oral Contraceptives: Combination oral contraceptives are birth control pills containing both estrogen and progestin. Ethinyl estradiol and mestranol (which is converted to ethinyl estradiol by the liver before it is pharmacologically active) are the two estrogens currently used in oral contraceptives in the USA. An oral contraceptive containing 30–35 μg of ethinyl estradiol is most often prescribed to adolescents beginning to take birth control pills. A number of different progestins are used in oral contraceptives and differ in their estrogenic, antiestrogenic, and androgenic effects. Triphasic oral contraceptives were introduced in the USA in 1984. Their main advantage is a 35–39% lower progestin dose over the course of the month, resulting in fewer progestin-related metabolic effects such as those on lipids, blood pressure, and carbohydrate metabolism. Disadvantages include confusion due to the multiple pill colors and a breakthrough bleeding rate that is comparable to or somewhat greater than that of low-dose biphasic counterparts. As estrogen doses decreased in oral contraceptives, the androgenic side effects of progestins became more apparent, leading to the development of three progestins (desogestrel, gestodene, and norgestimate). These "new" progestins in combination with ethinyl estradiol or mestranol are now being introduced in the United States (after about 10 years of use in Europe). To date, clinical evaluations show virtually identical efficacy rates in pregnancy prevention, very similar metabolic and side effects, and the same noncontraceptive benefits as previous combination pills.

B. Minipill: Minipills contain progestins found in combination oral contraceptives—but in smaller doses—and no estrogen. Their chief use is in women who experience unacceptable estrogen-related side effects with combination oral contraceptives. Their lack of estrogen, however, is also responsible for the main side effect, that of less predictable menstrual patterns. For this reason, and because minipills are not quite as effective as combination oral contraceptives, they are a poor choice for adolescents. Their mechanism of action relies on the progestin-mediated actions, and ovulation is suppressed in only 15–40% of cycles.

C. Indications and Contraindications: Combined oral contraceptives may be the method of choice for sexually active adolescents, who frequently have unplanned intercourse; however, the patient must be able to comply with a daily dosing regimen. Most states allow oral contraceptives to be prescribed to minors confidentially. Ideally, it is best to wait until 6–12 regular menstrual cycles have occurred before beginning oral contraceptives; however, if the teenager is already sexually active, the medical and social risks of pregnancy probably outweigh the risks of oral contraceptives.

Oral contraceptives may also be used to treat dysmenorrhea (see above).

Contraindications to combined oral contraceptives can be categorized as absolute and relative (Table 4–17). When use of estrogenic agents is contraindicated, progestin-only pills are an alternative.

D. Beginning Birth Control Pills and Follow-Up: Before a patient begins taking oral contraceptives, a careful menstrual history, medical history, and family medical history should be taken. In addition, baseline weight and blood pressure should be established, breast and pelvic examination should be performed, and specimens for urinalysis, Papanicolaou smear, gonorrhea culture, and chlamydial culture or antigen detection test obtained.

If there are no contraindications (see Table 4–17), the patient may begin her first pack of pills with her next menstrual period (either the first Sunday after flow begins or the first day of flow, depending on the brand). A triphasic or a low-dose combined oral contraceptive is used for those without contraindications to use of estrogen. With adolescents, it is wise to use 28-day packs rather than 21-day packs to reduce the chance of missing pills. The patient should be instructed on the use of her type of pills and on the pos-

sible risks and side effects and their warning signs. To ensure protection, she should use a back-up method, such as condoms and foam, for the first 2 weeks. A follow-up visit in 1 month and then every 2–3 months for the first year may improve compliance, since teenagers often discontinue birth control pills because of nonmedical reasons or minor side effects.

E. Management of Side Effects: A different type of combined oral contraceptive should be tried if a patient has a persistent minor side effect for more than the first 2–3 months. Adjustments should be made on the basis of hormonal effects (Table 4–18). Changes are most often made for persistent breakthrough bleeding not related to missed pills.

Intrauterine Devices

Because of the liability costs associated with intrauterine devices (IUDs) in recent years, most have been withdrawn from the market. Because of the risk of sexually transmitted diseases and pelvic inflammatory disease and its serious sequelae (infertility, ectopic pregnancy), IUDs are not a good method for teenagers, who frequently have multiple partners and have their childbearing years ahead of them.

A number of mechanisms of action have been suggested for IUDs, including prevention of implantation through a local inflammatory response and local production of prostaglandins.

IUDs must be inserted and removed by a physician trained in the procedure.

Injectable Hormonal Contraceptives

The depot form of medroxyprogesterone acetate (DMPA) was approved by the FDA as a long-acting injectable progestational contraceptive in 1992. It is given as 150 mg injections every 3 months. DMPA works chiefly by blocking the LH surge, thereby suppressing ovulation, but it also thickens cervical mucus and alters the endometrium to inhibit ovum implantation. With a failure rate of less than 1%, minimal compliance issues, long-acting nature, reversibility, lack of interference with intercourse, and lack of estrogen-related side effects, it may be an attractive contraceptive for many adolescents, particularly for those who consider its 50% rate of amenorrhea at 1 year of use a desirable side effect or for whom estrogens are contraindicated. DMPA may reduce intravascular sickling and increase hemoglobin and red cell survival in patients with sickle cell disease. A recent World Health Organization case-control study concluded that there was no increased risk of liver cancer or invasive squamous cell cervical cancer among users of DMPA, and the risk of endometrial and ovarian cancers was reduced. While the overall relative risk for breast cancer in long-term users of DMPA was 1.2, it is elevated in short-term users (1.7) (≤ 3 months of use) and in women under age 35 (1.4). It has been suggested that this increased risk in young

---

Table 4–17. Contraindications to combined birth control pills.[1]

Absolute contraindications
  History of thrombophlebitis, thromboembolic disorder, cerebrovascular disorder, ischemic heart disease
  Known or suspected carcinoma of the breast or estrogen-dependent neoplasia
  Known or suspected pregnancy
  History of benign or malignant liver tumor
  Undiagnosed abnormal vaginal bleeding
Strong relative contraindications
  Severe vascular or migraine headaches
  Hypertension
  Diabetes
  Active gallbladder disease
  Mononucleosis, acute phase
  Sickle cell disease or sickle C disease
  Upcoming major surgery
  Long leg cast or major injury to lower leg
  Known impaired liver function at present time
  Completion of term pregnancy within past 10–14 days

[1]Modified and reproduced, with permission, from Breedlove B, Judy B, Martin N (editors): *Contraceptive Technology 1988–1989*, 14th rev ed. Irvington Publishers, 1988.

Table 4–18. Pill side effects: hormone etiology.[1]

Estrogen Excess	Progestin Excess	Androgen Excess	Estrogen Deficiency	Progestin Deficiency
1. Nausea, dizziness	1. Increased appetite and weight gain (noncyclic)	1. Increased appetite and weight gain (noncyclic)	1. Irritability, nervousness	1. Late breakthrough bleeding and spotting
2. Edema and abdominal or leg pain with cyclic weight gain, bloating	2. Tiredness, fatigue, and weakness	2. Hirsutism	2. Hot flushes, vasomotor symptoms	2. Heavy menstrual flow and clots
3. Leukorrhea	3. Depression	3. Acne	3. Uterine prolapse, pelvic relaxation symptoms	3. Delayed onset of menses
4. Increased leiomyoma size	4. Decreased libido	4. Oily skin, rash	4. Early and midcycle spotting	4. Dysmenorrhea
5. Chloasma	5. Oily scalp, acne	5. Increased libido	5. Decreased amount of menstrual flow	5. Weight loss
6. Uterine cramps	6. Loss of hair	6. Cholestatic jaundice	6. No withdrawal bleeding	
7. Irritability, depression	7. Cholestatic jaundice	7. Pruritus	7. Decreased libido	
8. Increased fat deposition	8. Decreased length of menstrual flow		8. Diminished breast size	
9. Cervical extrophia	9. Hypertension?		9. Dry vaginal mucosa, atrophic vaginitis, and dyspareunia	
10. Poor contact lens fit	10. Headaches between Pill packages		10. Headaches	
11. Telangiectasia	11. Candidal vaginitis/cervicitis		11. Depression	
12. Vascular-type headache	12. Increased breast size (alveolar tissue)			
13. Hypertension?	13. Breast tenderness			
14. Lactation suppression	14. Decreased carbohydrate tolerance			
15. Headaches while taking the Pill	15. Dilated leg veins			
16. Cystic breast changes	16. Pelvic congestion syndrome			
17. Breast tenderness				
18. Increased breast size (ductal and fatty tissue and fluid retention)				
19. Thrombophlebitis				
20. Cerebrovascular accidents				
21. Myocardial infarction				
22. Hepatic adenoma				
23. Cyclic weight gain				

[1]Adapted and reproduced, with permission, from: Dickey RP: Medical approaches to reproductive regulation: The pill. ACOG Semin Fam Plan 1974; Table II:21; Dickey RP: *Managing Contraceptive Pill Patients,* 4th ed. Creative Infomatics, 1984; and Hatcher RA et al: *Contraceptive Technology, 1986–1987,* 13th rev ed. Irvington, 1987.

and short-term users may be related to stimulation of existing tumors rather than formation of new ones.

The levonorgestrel-containing nonbiodegradable subdermal implant (Norplant), which is inserted under the skin of the upper arm using a trocar, became available for contraception in the USA in 1991. It is highly effective for 5 years, with pregnancy rates ranging from 0.04 per 100 woman-years in the first year of use to 1.1 per 100 woman-years in the fifth year. It acts through ovulation inhibition and thickening of the cervical mucus. Menstrual irregularities (including prolonged bleeding, intermenstrual spotting, and amenorrhea) are the most common side effects, though headache, acne, weight gain or loss, and depression may occur as well. Its ease of use, lack of compliance issues, high efficacy, and long-term protection make the subdermal implant an ideal contra-

ceptive for adolescents who can tolerate the menstrual irregularities.

Miscellaneous Methods

Adolescents should understand the menstrual cycle and be taught either that there is no "safe" period or that ovulation occurs 2 weeks before the next menstrual period and may be difficult to predict. Because teenagers frequently have irregular cycles and because sexual intercourse is often spontaneous and unplanned, the rhythm or calendar method is not effective for them. Adolescents also need to be educated that withdrawal is not a reliable method of contraception. Sterilization should be viewed as a permanent method of contraception and therefore is not suitable for teenagers.

American Academy of Pediatrics, Committee on Adolescence: Contraception and adolescents. Pediatrics 1990;86:134.

Cromer BA: Depo-provera: Wherefore art thou? Adolesc Pediatr Gynecol 1992;5:155.

Dickey RP: *Managing Contraceptive Pill Patients.* Creative Infomatics, 1993.

Grimes D (editor): Subdermal implants: A new approach to contraception. Contraception Rep 1991;2:4, 10.

Grimes D (editor): Depot medroxyprogesterone acetate: An overview of DMPA and its FDA approval. Contraception Rep 1992;3:4.

Hatcher RE et al: The pill: Combined oral contraceptives. In: *Contraceptive Technology 1990–1992.* Irvington, 1990.

Sikand A, Fisher M: The role of barrier contraceptives in prevention of pregnancy and disease in adolescents. AM:STARS 1992;3:223.

PREGNANCY

More than 1 million teenage girls become pregnant in the USA each year. The overall teen pregnancy rate remained steady at 11% of US females aged 15–19 throughout the 1980s, although the birth rate increased from a low of 50.2 per 1000 females 15–19 years old in 1986 to 59.9 per 1000 in 1990. About 45% of 15- to 19-year-old females are sexually active, and more than one-third of these become pregnant within 2 years after onset of sexual activity. More than 80% of these pregnancies are unintended, and about 68% of pregnancies in women under 20 years of age are out of wedlock.

Young maternal age and associated maternal risk factors have been linked to adverse neonatal outcome, including higher rates of low birth weight babies (< 2500 g) and neonatal mortality. The psychosocial consequences for the teenage mother and her infant are listed in Table 4–19. Teenagers who are pregnant require additional support from their caregivers, and clinics for young mothers may be the best providers.

Presentation

Adolescents may present with delayed or missed menses or may even request a pregnancy test, but often they present with an unrelated concern or have a hidden agenda. Because of the high level of denial, they may come in with complaints of abdominal pain, urinary frequency, dizziness, or other nonspecific symptoms and have no concern about pregnancy. A history of symptoms such as weight gain, engorged breasts, an unusually light or mistimed period, and urinary frequency can be sought, but the adolescent may not have noted these signs of pregnancy. Denial also contributes to the delay in seeking prenatal care. Only about one-third of adolescents receive prenatal care in the first trimester. Clinicians need to have a low threshold for suspicion of pregnancy. If there is

Table 4–19. Psychosocial consequences of pregnancy for the adolescent mother and her infant.

Mother	Infant
Increased morbidity related to pregnancy	Greater health risks
Greater risk of toxemia, anemia, prolonged labor, premature labor	Increased chance of low birth weight or prematurity
Increased chance of miscarriages, stillbirths	Increased risk of infant death
Increased chance of maternal mortality	Increased risk of injury and hospitalization by age 5
Decreased educational attainment	Decreased academic achievement
Less likely to get high school diploma, go to college, or graduate	Lower cognitive scores
	Decreased development
Lower occupational attainment and prestige	Greater chance of being behind grade or needing remedial help
Less chance of stable employment (some resolution over time)	Lower chance of advanced academics
Lower job satisfaction	Lower academic aptitude as a teenager and perhaps a higher probability of dropping out of school
Lower income/wages	
Greater dependence on public assistance	
Less stable marital relationships	Psychosocial consequences
Higher rates of single parenthood	Greater risk of behavior problems
Earlier marriage (though less common than in the past)	Poverty
Accelerated pace of marriage, separation, divorce, and remarriage	Higher probability of living in a nonintact home while in high school
Faster pace of subsequent childbearing	Greater risk of adolescent pregnancy
High rate of repeat unintended pregnancy	
More births out of marriage	
Closer spacing of births	
Larger families	

any suspicion, a urine pregnancy test should be obtained.

Diagnosis

History, as above, and physical examination may assist in making the diagnosis of pregnancy. Bluish coloring and softening of the cervix may be noted on speculum examination. The uterine fundus may be palpable on abdominal examination if sufficient time has elapsed. If uterine size on bimanual examination does not correspond to dates, one must consider ectopic pregnancy, incomplete or missed abortion, twin gestation, or inaccurate dates.

Laboratory tests for human chorionic gonadotropin (hCG) are simple to perform and are usually diagnostic. Enzyme-linked immunoassay test kits specific for the β-hCG subunit and sensitive to < 50 mIU/mL of hCG can be performed on urine (preferably the first morning voided specimen, because it is more concentrated) in less than 5 minutes, and are accurate within

12 days after conception. Serum radioimmunoassay is also specific for the beta subunit, is accurate within 7 days after conception, and is helpful in ruling out ectopic pregnancy or threatened abortion. Serum radioreceptor assay may cross-react with LH, is accurate within 14 days after conception, and may be used to confirm a normal pregnancy. Slide agglutination tests are more difficult to read, less sensitive than the above tests, and cross-react with LH. Home pregnancy tests are relatively accurate, particularly when positive; however, they are expensive and have fairly complex instructions that many teenagers have difficulty following. Also, they may preclude obtaining counseling, early entry into prenatal care, or detection of ectopic pregnancy or threatened abortion.

The timing of pregnancy tests is important, since hCG levels initially rise after conception, peak at about 60–70 days, then drop to levels not detected by routine office slide tests after 16–20 weeks.

Special Issues in Management

When an adolescent presents for pregnancy testing, it is wise to find out what she hopes the results will be and what she thinks she will do before performing the test. If she wants to be pregnant and the test is negative, further counseling about the implications of teen pregnancy should be undertaken. For those who do not wish to be pregnant, this is a good time to begin contraception because teens who present for a pregnancy test that is negative have a high risk of pregnancy in the next 2 years.

If the adolescent is pregnant, the physician must discuss her support systems and her options with her (abortion, adoption, raising the baby). Many teenagers need help in telling and involving their parents. It is important to remain available for further assistance with decision making. If the patient knows what she wants to do, she should be referred to the appropriate resources. Since teenagers are often ambivalent about their plans and may have a high level of denial, it is prudent to follow up in a week to be certain that a decision has been made and to help the patient obtain prenatal care if she has chosen to continue the pregnancy.

Maternal age alone is not responsible for low birth weight and poor fetal outcome; rather, low maternal prepregnancy weight, poor weight gain, delay in prenatal care, low socioeconomic status, and black race are contributing factors. The poor nutritional status of some teenagers and their erratic diets, smoking, drinking, or substance abuse, and high prevalence of sexually transmitted diseases play a role. Teenagers are also at greater risk of eclampsia-preeclampsia, iron deficiency anemia, cephalopelvic disproportion, prolonged labor, premature labor, and maternal death. Early prenatal care and good nutrition can make a difference with a number of these problems.

Because of the high risk of a second unintended pregnancy within the next 2 years, postpartum contraceptive counseling and follow-up are imperative. Pregnancy prevention is the most cost-effective means of reducing the consequences of teenage pregnancy. Sexual decision making, contraceptive counseling, and close follow-up of sexually active adolescents of both sexes can make a difference. Adolescents who receive sexuality and contraceptive education are not more likely to have intercourse but are less likely to become pregnant than their counterparts who do not receive such instruction.

Ammerman S, Shafer MA, Snyder D: Ectopic pregnancy in adolescents: A clinical review for pediatricians. J Pediatr 1990;117:677.

Klerman LV, Horwitz SM: Reducing the adverse consequences of adolesent pregnancy and parenting: The role of service programs. AM:STARS, 1992;3:299.

McAnarney ER, Hendee WR: Adolescent pregnancy and its consequences. JAMA 1989;262:74.

Stevens-Simon C, Fullar SA, McAnarney ER: Teenage pregnancy: Caring for adolescent mothers with their infants in pediatric settings. Clin Pediatr 1989;28:282.

Teenage pregnancy: An advocate's guide to the numbers. Children's Defense Fund, Jan/March 1988.

VULVOVAGINITIS

Vaginitis may be due to pathogens or to indigenous flora after a change in milieu of the vagina. *Candida* vulvovaginitis and bacterial vaginosis (formerly called *Gardnerella, Haemophilus,* or nonspecific vaginitis) may be found in patients who are not sexually active. These are examples of indigenous flora that may cause infection. Bacterial vaginosis, however, is more prevalent in those who are sexually active. In sexually active patients, *Trichomonas* infection or cervicitis due to sexually transmitted pathogens must be considered (see section on sexually transmitted diseases, below). For this reason, sexually active patients or suspected victims of sexual abuse should have appropriate specimens taken to detect sexually transmitted disease even if yeast forms are present or bacterial vaginosis is identified.

1. PHYSIOLOGIC LEUKORRHEA

This refers to the normal vaginal discharge that begins around the time of menarche. The discharge is typically clear or whitish, and its consistency may vary according to cyclic hormonal influences. There should be no odor. Girls in early adolescence may have concerns about such a discharge and need reassurance that it is normal. This may be a good time to tell girls that there is no need for douching. If a vaginal wet preparation is examined, a few squamous epithelial cells may be revealed, but there should be fewer than five polymorphonuclear cells per high-power field.

2. CANDIDAL VULVOVAGINITIS

Candidal vulvovaginitis is caused by yeast. It typically occurs after a course of antibiotics, after which the normal perineal flora are altered and yeast is allowed to proliferate. Diabetics, patients with compromised immune systems, and those who are pregnant or receiving oral contraceptives are more prone to develop candidal infections.

Clinical Findings

The patient usually complains of vulvar pruritus or dyspareunia and a cheesy vaginal discharge, frequently beginning the week prior to menses. Examination of the vulva reveals an erythematous mucosa, sometimes with excoriation, and a thick, white, cheesy discharge. The discharge may be adherent to the walls of the vagina, which will also be inflamed if the infection is internal. Leukocytes may be seen on a wet preparation, and potassium hydroxide preparation may reveal budding yeast or mycelia. No "clue cells" should be seen. Often the vaginal preparations are unhelpful, and the patient should be treated on the basis of the clinical examination. Vaginal culture for yeasts is usually unnecessary.

Treatment

Nystatin, clotrimazole, or terconazole vaginal creams or suppositories designed for three or seven nightly doses are effective in the majority of patients. Some patients require a longer course of treatment and a vinegar douche at the conclusion of treatment to restore the vaginal pH. Patients with recurrent episodes should be given prophylactic treatment whenever they take antibiotics. It may be helpful to simultaneously treat the partners of sexually active patients with recurrent candidal infections.

3. BACTERIAL VAGINOSIS

Bacterial vaginosis may be caused by any of the indigenous vaginal flora, eg, *Gardnerella, Bacteroides, Peptococcus,* or lactobacilli.

Clinical Findings

The patient generally complains of malodorous mild discharge. On examination, a thin, homogeneous, grayish-white discharge is found adherent to the vaginal wall with diffuse vaginal erythema. A whiff test, in which a drop of potassium hydroxide is added to a smear of the discharge on a slide, results in the release of amines, causing a fishy odor. Wet preparation reveals an abundance of "clue cells" (vaginal epithelial cells stippled with adherent bacteria) and small pleomorphic rods.

Treatment

Treatment is with metronidazole (500 mg orally twice a day for 7 days) or clindamycin (300 mg orally twice a day for 7 days). Ampicillin (500 mg orally four times a day for 7 days) is the alternative for pregnant patients.

4. OTHER CAUSES OF VULVOVAGINITIS

Sexually Transmitted Diseases

Sexually transmitted diseases are an important cause of vaginal discharge in adolescents. (See chapter Sexually Transmitted Diseases.) One should obtain appropriate cultures whenever an adolescent complains of vaginal discharge, even when the cervix appears normal.

Foreign Body Vaginitis

Foreign bodies—most commonly retained tampons—cause extremely malodorous vaginal discharges. Treatment consists of removal, for which ring forceps may be useful. Further treatment is generally not necessary.

Allergic or Contact Vaginitis

Bubble baths, feminine hygiene sprays, or vaginal contraceptive foams or suppositories may cause chemical irritation of the vaginal mucosa. Discontinuing use of the offending agent is indicated.

REFERENCES

Adams GR et al (editors): *Biology of Adolescent Behavior and Development.* Sage, 1989.

Adolescent Medicine: State of the Art Reviews. Hanley & Belfus. [Series.]

Blos P: *The Adolescent Passage: Developmental Issues.* International Universities Press, 1979.

Blum RW (editor): *Chronic Illness and Disabilities in Childhood and Adolescence.* Grune & Stratton, 1984.

Blumenthal SJ, Kupfer DJ: *Suicide Over the Life Cycle: Risk Factors, Assessment, and Treatment of Suicidal Patients.* American Psychiatric Press, 1990.

Christophersen ER, Levine MD (editors): Development and behavior: Older children and adolescents. Pediatr Clin North Am 1992;39:3.

Dickey RP: *Managing Contraceptive Pill Patients.* Creative Infomatics, 1993.

Dryfoos JG: *Adolescents at Risk: Prevalence and Prevention.* Oxford University Press, 1990.

Emans SJH, Goldstein DP: *Pediatric and Adolescent Gynecology.* Little, Brown, 1990.

Erickson EH: *Identity: Youth and Crisis.* Norton, 1968.

Farrow JA (editor): Adolescent medicine. Med Clin North Am 1990;74:5.

Friedman SB, Fisher M, Schonberg SK (editors): *Comprehensive Adolescent Health Care.* Quality Medical Publishing, 1992.

Furstenberg FF Jr, Brooks-Gunn J, Morgan SP: *Adolescent Mothers in Later Life.* Cambridge Univ Press, 1987.

Greydanus DE: *Caring for Your Adolescent, Ages 12 to 21.* Bantam, 1991.

Guidelines for Adolescent Preventive Services: American Medical Association, 1992

Hatcher RA et al: *Contraceptive Technology,* 15th ed, Irvington, 1990.

Hechinger FM: *Fateful Choices, Health Youth for the 21st Century.* Carnegie, 1992.

Hendee WR (editor): *The Health of Adolescents: Understanding and Facilitating Biological, Behavioral, and Social Development.* Jossey-Bass, 1991.

Hergenroeder AC, Garrick JG (editors): Sports medicine. Pediatr Clin North Am 1990;37:5.

Hoffman A: *Adolescent Medicine.* Appleton & Lange, 1989.

Holder AR: *Legal Issues in Pediatrics and Adolescent Medicine.* Yale Univ Press, 1985.

Holmes KK et al (editors): *Sexually Transmitted Diseases,* 2nd ed. McGraw-Hill, 1990.

Jessor R, Donovan JE, Costa FM: *Beyond Adolescence: Problem Behavior and Young Adult Development.* Cambridge, 1991.

Jones RL: *Black Adolescents.* Cobb & Henry, 1989.

Journal of Adolescent Health. Official Publication of the Society for Adolescent Medicine. Litt IF (editor-in-chief). Elsevier Science Publishing Co. [Series.]

Kagan J, Coles R: *Twelve to Sixteen: Early Adolescence.* Norton, 1972.

Katchadourian H: *The Biology of Adolescence.* Freeman, 1977.

Lerner RM et al (editors): *Encyclopedia of Adolescence.* Garland, 1991.

Lerner JW: Eductional interventions in learning disabilities. J Am Acad Child Adolesc Psychiatry 1989;28:326.

Levine M: *Keeping a Head in School: A Student's Book about Learning Abilities and Learning Disorders.* Educators Publishing Service, 1990.

Levine M et al (editors): *Developmental Behavioral Pediatrics,* 2nd ed. Saunders, 1992.

Levine MD: *Developmental Variation and Learning Disorders.* Educators Publishing Service, 1987.

Litt IF: *Evaluation of the Adolescent Patient.* Hanley & Belfus, 1990.

McAnarney ER et al (editors): *Textbook of Adolescent Medicine.* Saunders, 1992.

Meeks JE: *The Fragile Alliance.* Krieger, 1980.

Miller D: *The Age Between: Adolescence and Therapy.* Aronson, 1983.

Millstein SG, Petersen AC, Nightingale EO: *Promoting the Health of Adolescents: New Directions for the Twenty-First Century.* Oxford Univ Press, 1993.

Muuss RE: *Theories of Adolescence,* 3rd ed. Random House, 1975.

Neinstein LS: *Adolescent Health Care: A Practical Guide,* 2nd ed. Urban & Schwarzenberg, 1991.

Speroff L, Glass RH, Kase NG: *Clinical Gynecologic Endocrinology and Infertility.* Williams & Wilkins, 1989.

Tanner JM: *Growth at Adolescence.* Blackwell, 1962.

Vaughan VC, Litt IF: *Child and Adolescent Development: Clinical Implications.* Saunders, 1990.

Developmental Disorders

5

Bonnie W. Camp, MD, PhD, & Elizabeth B. Kozleski, EdD

This chapter considers problems in development of cognitive and social competence. Competence is usually defined by comparing performance levels of an individual child with some norm derived from evaluating many children of the same age. Other standards of competence include comparison of the child's performance level with that of the adult norm and comparison of the child's present skills with skills needed to accomplish a given task or engage in a specific activity. Functional problems of children with mental retardation are discussed in this chapter; however, the main emphasis is on the larger group of children with learning and behavior problems that may or may not be associated with mental retardation.

Measurement of developmental competence is patterned on concepts of measuring intelligence. Although there is continued controversy over the extent to which heredity and environment determine intelligence, assessment of competence can be more usefully discussed independently of this issue. Assessment of competence hinges on the recognition that (1) children are able to perform increasingly more complex and difficult tasks as they get older; and (2) when tested at ages fairly close together, individual children tend to have a similar standing in relation to other children from one age to the next. By evaluating a child's performance on a variety of tasks requiring skills such as reasoning, abstract thinking, judgment, and planning and by determining how the child compares with other children of the same age, it is usually possible to predict school performance. Such assessments provide the basis for deriving an intelligence quotient and also may have implications for social behavior.

Measures of intelligence may be thought of as measures of general competence that attempt to determine what a child has learned in the process of exposure to an environment that provides unsystematic opportunities for learning that are grossly similar within a given culture. Anything that limits the breadth, variety, and depth of exposure or the ability of a child to profit from such exposure may place limits on the learning a given child will achieve in a given period. Anything that increases systematic exposure or increases breadth, variety, and depth of exposure potentially enhances learning.

Both biologic and psychosocial factors can increase or interfere with the growth-promoting effect of a child's performance. Assessment of a child's general developmental or intellectual standing relative to other children sheds no light on the cause of the child's performance; consequently, it is important to determine whether an intelligence test gives a representative estimate of the child's usual functioning and whether other information might provide an explanation for low scores. Differences in experiential background often account for low scores of children from nondominant cultures given standard intelligence tests. Such explanations, however, do not necessarily alter the predictive value of scores from intelligence tests.

A variety of delays or deficiencies in the development of specific cognitive competence have also been identified and may or may not be associated with deficiencies in general competence. The most significant of these are associated with failure to acquire basic academic skills such as reading, writing, and arithmetic. Specific measures of competence are usually measures of achievement in areas where systematic instruction has been given (eg, music lessons, arithmetic lessons). Here again, both biologic and psychosocial factors (eg, "musical talent" or "math aptitude") may facilitate or interfere with development of competence in these specific areas. Measures of relative standing in specific areas of achievement correlate well with measures of intelligence. This correlation provides the basis for determining a child's expected level of achievement, whereas the discrepancy between expected and actual levels of achievement is a key factor for differential diagnosis in children with developmental problems.

Traditionally, social and emotional aspects of development have not been conceptualized as a dimension of competence. However, it is increasingly recognized that social competence is an important concept for assessing some aspects of social and emotional development. This is particularly true for aspects of behavior and social interaction such as empathy, distractibility, activity level, and aggression, which show strong, regular progression with age and which are associated with what has traditionally been termed cognitive development.

129

The Role of Special Education

Federal law mandates that all children with disabilities, ages 3–21, are entitled to a free and appropriate public school education. Federal funding assists local educational agencies in meeting the specifics of the law. Although educational opportunities for persons with some types of disabilities have been available in this country for over 100 years, it was not until the passage of PL 94–142 in 1975 that all children with disabilities were guaranteed access to a free and appropriate public school education. In 1990, this bill was reauthorized and renamed as the Individuals With Disabilities Education Act (IDEA). Under this law, special education students are to receive an education based on a curriculum that can be modified and adapted to meet their unique needs. These needs are presumed to vary based on student age, preferences, ethnicity, family values, learning characteristics, physical capabilities, student motivation, and the demands of subsequent environments in which the student will be expected to perform. IDEA incorporates seven key elements: (1) access to free and appropriate public education; (2) individualization of the educational experience; (3) the right to be educated in the least restrictive environment; (4) the provision of related services; (5) guidelines for the determination of a disability; (6) protection of student and parent rights; and (7) the principles of state and local responsibilities (Overton, 1992). Under IDEA, students may receive one of the following labels: specific learning disability, seriously emotionally disturbed, deaf, deaf-blind, hard of hearing, mentally retarded, multi-handicapped, orthopedically impaired, other health impaired, speech impaired, or visually handicapped.

The due process component of the law allows parents to participate in and to challenge educational decisions made regarding their children. Multidisciplinary teams of professionals along with parents are required to determine placement in programs and to determine the types and amounts of educational services. Within the identification and assessment component, local school districts have developed policies and procedures that result in services such as Child Find, prereferral building level teams, multidisciplinary assessments, and staffings. In general, children tend to be overreferred for assessment and staffing into special education at the elementary level and underreferred at the secondary level.

Child Find, mandated by PL 94–142, requires that each district locate and assess all children and other young people from birth through age 21 who may have a disability. Child Find is typically implemented as an outreach program both within the school and in the community. Advertisements in local media encourage parents of children with perceived problems to come to local screening clinics. As a result of the screening, some children are referred for full assessments. If, as a result of a complete assessment, a multidisciplinary team concludes that the child has a disability according to federal and state guidelines and the child is age 3–21, services deemed necessary by the team must be provided by the local school system even if the child is enrolled in a private school.

Passage of PL 99–457

PL 99–457, passed in 1986, extends all rights and protections of PL 94–142 to children with disabilities through age 5 (Widerstrom, Mowder, and Sandall, 1991). This law has embraced the notion of families as a focus of intervention rather than children alone (eg, the development of an individualized educational plan [IEP] that includes a family component). Rather than focus on the child, an IFSP (individualized family service plan) has been mandated that places an emphasis on working with the family's needs rather than developing a treatment plan for the child only. Since this bill was passed, much attention has been paid to family involvement and the development of integrated preschool programs. Furthermore, this law has encouraged school systems to focus on early intervention.

Overton T: *Assessment in Special Education: An Applied Approach.* Macmillan. 1992.

Widerstrom AH, Mowder BA, Sandall S: *At Risk and Handicapped Newborns and Infants: Developmental Assessment and Intervention.* Prentice-Hall, 1991.

GENERAL PRINCIPLES IN EVALUATING COGNITIVE & SOCIAL COMPETENCE

Developmental evaluation should include (1) data that demonstrate a child's level of cognitive and social competence in both general and specific areas; (2) data that will assist in making an etiologic diagnosis; and (3) data relevant to management planning. An interdisciplinary team is often employed to develop the data base and a plan for management; this is the most thorough and effective approach. In addition to the pediatrician, the team usually includes a psychologist, social worker, educational specialist, and speech and language specialist. Assistance is also often needed from health care specialists in nursing, physical therapy, occupational therapy, ophthalmology, audiology, nutrition, and dentistry. Where an organized, functioning team is not available, the primary care physician can achieve similar results by requesting consultations from various professionals and obtaining information from other sources such as school personnel. It is also possible for the primary care physician to develop the minimal data base needed for initial assessment with only limited reliance on outside sources. The following discussion presents suggestions to assist the primary care physician in developing this data base through use of questionnaires and screening tests when assistance from other professionals is limited or unavailable.

History

A. Medical History: The medical history should focus on aspects of pregnancy, labor, and delivery that are likely to produce damage to the child's central nervous system (eg, use of drugs or x-rays during pregnancy; neonatal infections, asphyxia, and elevated bilirubin levels). Later evidence of central nervous system insults or injury, failure to thrive, chronic illnesses, hospitalizations, or abuse may also contribute significantly to a child's performance at school age. Neonatal records are often an important source of information, since they may reveal information forgotten by or unknown to parents. Recent studies have also focused on ways of combining psychosocial information about families from birth certificates to assess the risk for later problems in development.

B. Developmental History: The developmental history should include information about the age at which various milestones were passed, especially those pertaining to speech and language. Inability to use meaningful words other than "dada," "mama," "bye-bye," and "hello" by 18 months and inability to speak in short phrases by 24 months have been reported in association with specific learning disability as well as general slow learning and mental retardation. Development of motor skills is also important, particularly in assessing mental retardation, but deviance or delay in motor development may also be present in other conditions such as cerebral palsy and neuromuscular disorders. Information about sleep patterns, problems of temperament such as excessive crying or hyperactivity, and general problems may also be helpful.

C. Family History: Specific information regarding central nervous system disorders, mental retardation, epilepsy, or evidence of school problems or specific learning disabilities in other family members should be included. Details of the mother's pregnancy history, including stillbirths, deaths, and other problems, may also be helpful.

D. Educational and Learning History: In preschool children, considerable information can be obtained from a description of something the child has learned in an informal setting. If the child has been placed in a formal preschool setting, information should be obtained regarding the type of preschool and the child's relationships with other children and with teachers. Teachers can often give an excellent description of the child's performance and behavior in the classroom environment, and such assessments, even in the preschool period, are often as good as tests in predicting later problems.

Once a child has reached school age, the educational history should include details of grade placement, special education evaluations and placement, repetition of grades, and other details of academic performance and participation in special programs. Most school systems routinely test students at specific grade levels using standardized group-administered tests. These tests, which are typically administered to whole classes in the spring of the academic year, measure academic progress in reading, math, science, and social studies. Student performance is then compared with a representative sample of peers across the country who are enrolled at the same grade. Achievement scores are reported in terms of grade level attainment. For example, a 3.2 grade level means that a student is working at the third grade, second month level in a particular curriculum area. Achievement scores may also be reported as percentiles, where a student's performance is measured against other students of the same age or grade level. As a hypothetical example, suppose that Eric earned a percentile of 50. This means that 50% of the students of the same age or grade level as Eric who took the same test scored at or below Eric's score. Thus, percentile scores show only the student's performance relative to other students who took the same test. Usually, percentiles are based on the performance of a large number of students representing a national sample. When using percentiles, it is critical to make sure that the student in question is similar to those students in the standardization sample.

While group-administered, standardized tests measure student skills in academic areas, they are rarely of great value in determining a student's specific areas of academic strength and weakness. When group-administered achievement scores differ more than 1 year from a student's grade placement—or where achievement scores show a scatter of more than 1 year between scores—it may be advisable to refer that child to the child study team at the student's school to determine whether further testing is necessary to investigate the possibility that a disability is interfering with the student's ability to perform effectively.

Although a child's achievement scores can help to identify that a problem in school is occurring, it does not necessarily imply that the child has a disability that is compromising the ability to perform. Issues such as how instruction is being provided, whether the instructional delivery is appropriate for the child's learning needs, and whether the content of instruction fits the context of the student's experience must be addressed in order to determine what course of action should be taken to support the child. Information about the child's academic achievement should provide information regarding learning patterns, ability to attend to tasks, motivation to attend to new material, interest areas, and preferences for learning activities. Furthermore, when test scores are available, it is critical to determine whether the test was group-administered or individually administered. Information regarding the student's emotional reactions to school situations should focus on whether the student's behavior is appropriate to the social as well as academic contexts of school. Responses to corrections and failures reveal a great deal about one's perception of oneself as a capable learner. In the absence of a psychologist or educational specialist to provide this information, direct contact with school personnel is imperative for the primary care physician. Telephone conversations with the school nurse, teacher, social worker, or other professionals are very helpful in obtaining a clear picture of the child's school performance and behavior. Written reports from teachers using questionnaires that systematically address the most common types of learning problems can be of great assistance.

E. Psychosocial History: Family problems and parental characteristics often interfere with development of both cognitive and social competence and foster deviant behavior in the child. Children of hostile, rejecting, highly authoritarian parents tend to be the most severely affected; these children often show advanced competence at 1 year of age but a progressive decline in competence beginning around 4 years of age. Children of nurturing parents with highly authoritarian parenting practices often do better; however, children of nurturing parents who are firm and verbal in providing guidance and setting standards without being rigidly authoritarian show advanced competence that increases with age. Parents who provide little nurturance or sense of belonging, who are too lax or too harsh in punishment, or who fail to supervise their children tend to have children who show early evidence of aggressive behavior problems that persist into adolescence and adulthood.

Because developmental and behavior problems in the child are often provoked by and associated with problems within the family or seem to be associated with a lack of family support for developing new skills, a good psychosocial history is an essential part of any developmental evaluation. Ideally, this should include assessment of the family's ability to promote cognitive and social development, which includes, as a minimum, information regarding the parents' linguistic and cultural background, quality of verbal interaction, disciplinary practices (use of positive reinforcement to shape behavior, reliance on physical punishment or limited use of reasoning or verbal explanations in discipline), ability to set standards, neglect, reliance on parenting practices that interfere with or inhibit development, family instability, marital discord, a hostile attitude toward the child, limitations in cognitive and social competence, depression, signs of maladjustment (eg, alcoholism, chronic unemployment, criminal or psychiatric problems), and general stress in the parents and chaos in the family that may contribute to and intensify developmental problems in the child.

In examining only the child, it is often difficult to distinguish behavior disorders associated with family problems from developmental disorders due to immaturity or alteration in development of the neurologic system. This difficulty has resulted in diagnosis by exclusion—ie, psychosocial assessment is used to determine whether there are social or emotional factors in the child's environment that can account for the observed learning or behavior problems. This is a practical approach in middle-class families, since it is often possible to ascertain that the family is reasonably stable and able to provide adequate support and stimulation to the child. Diagnosis by exclusion is, however, a very unsatisfactory approach for dealing with children from lower socioeconomic families, ie, the majority of children with behavior problems. The need for better assessment of these children is particularly acute, since they often have delays in both social and cognitive development and combinations of developmental delay and behavior problems. Ninety percent of the children who later show mental or emotional disorders are normal at birth and appear to be casualties of inadequate or pathologic environments.

At present, the most commonly used approach to family assessment is a global, clinical social history. Some of this information is usually included in the history obtained by the primary care physician. In most instances, however, a social worker will provide the most thorough and complete analysis. In preschool children, it is often helpful to supplement the usual clinical social history with the HOME (*home observation for measurement of the environment*) interview assessment of Bradley and Caldwell (see references, below). This is the most thoroughly studied approach to the systematic evaluation of the growth-promoting aspects of the child's environment. This interview, which requires a home visit, is used to identify economically disadvantaged families unlikely to support development in their children. It may be performed by any trained person but is usually done by a social worker or nurse. A shorter, questionnaire version of the HOME interview, the Home Screening Questionnaire (HSQ), provides most of the information obtained from the longer interview version and can be administered and scored by the pediatrician during a clinic or office visit. Although it has not yet been studied widely enough to determine its clinical usefulness, the HSQ appears to be a promising tool for use by the primary care physician. Neither scale is expected to be useful in evaluating children from middle or upper socioeconomic families.

Badger E, Burne D, Vietze P: Maternal risk factors as predictors of development outcome in early childhood. Infant Ment Health J 1981;2:33.

Bradley RH, Caldwell BM: Pediatric usefulness of home assessment. In: *Advances in Behavioral Pediatrics,* vol 2. Camp BW (editor). JAI Press, 1981.

Coons CE et al: *The Home Screening Questionnaire Reference Manual.* LADOCA, 1981.

Physical & Neurologic Examination

It is essential that a thorough physical and neurologic examination be performed. A number of children will demonstrate neurologic "soft signs," eg, clumsiness, right-left confusion, disordered temporal orientation, overflow phenomena, choreiform movements, and finger agnosia. Although "soft signs" are commonly associated with school learning and behavior problems, the significance of these signs is controversial because they are also found in children who have no other problems and because most appear to represent delay in maturation rather than dysfunction. PANESS (*physical and neurologic examination for soft signs*), a standardized neurologic examination, has been studied and shows promising results for systematic evaluation of "soft signs."

In addition, recent studies linking minor physical anomalies with behavior disorders in childhood have prompted physicians to examine for the presence of dysmorphic features such as abnormal palmar creases, syndactyly, unruly hair, malformed ears, skin tags, and facial abnormalities. Although these features are commonly seen in children with mental retardation, the implications of their presence in nonretarded children are not fully understood.

Holden EW, Tarnowski KJ, Prinz RJ: Reliability of neurobiological soft signs in children: Reevaluation of the PANESS. J Abnorm Child Psychol 1982;10:163.

Sensory Function

All children in whom developmental delay or mental retardation is suspected should be examined for visual and auditory problems. In infants and young children, sensory deficits may be mistaken for retardation. Retarded children often have sensory deficits in addition to their retardation, and this increases the complexity of their problem. In most nonretarded, school-aged children, vision and hearing can be satisfactorily evaluated by the usual screening methods and referral made to a specialist for further evaluation of children with abnormal screening results.

A variety of vision problems have been proposed as causes of reading problems, most without substantial research support. Learning to read can be accomplished quite satisfactorily with limited visual acuity. Although it is important that visual defects be corrected to improve the child's overall functioning, it is generally agreed that learning problems are seldom linked to refractive errors. Difficulty with convergence at near point, however, may interfere significantly with the process of reading and should receive careful evaluation.

Hearing loss has a significant impact on language development and may be associated with severe learning and behavior problems. Intermittent hearing loss, such as that due to otitis media, has been implicated in learning disabilities. In the past, deaf children have often been mistakenly labeled retarded. Losses in the high-frequency range may be associated with problems in discriminating speech sounds necessary for school learning. Others may have problems differentiating speech sounds despite normal hearing.

Emotional & Social Behavior

Although some information can be obtained directly from the child through interviews, play, and projective testing, typically one must rely on interviews with parents and reports from school personnel to obtain a picture of the child's social competence. Much of this information is obtained by social workers, psychologists, or psychiatrists. In evaluating reports of problem behavior at home and at school, it is helpful to assess the degree of deviance by comparing an individual child's behavior with children in general. Large studies of normal children indicate that most children show a few signs of deviant behavior. The truly deviant child, however, usually demonstrates this in a variety of ways. It is especially important to seek information about positive attributes, because these appear to be more powerful indicators of later mental health than negative attributes are of later maladjustment. Three of the most important positive attributes are school attendance (irrespective of performance), positive peer relations, and nondelinquency.

General adaptation and development of self-help are often included in developmental assessments of preschool children. Beginning around age 4 years (when abstract reasoning becomes the dominant factor in measures of cognitive development), it becomes increasingly important to include some assessment of general adaptation in the differential diagnosis of mental retardation. Children from minority cultures who perform poorly on IQ tests often appear less retarded when general adaptation is evaluated.

Rating scales of behavior, such as the ACTeRS scale (ADD-H: Comprehensive Teachers Rating Scale) (Table 5–1) for identifying children with attention deficit disorder, are important tools for assessing school behavior. The ACTeRS scale has been designed to identify clusters of problems in the areas of attention, hyperactivity, social skills, and oppositional behavior. Norms to assess the degree of deviance are available. The ACTeRS scale is readily acceptable to teachers and can be used by primary care physicians to assess the need for and response to stimulant medication.

A scale for obtaining teacher ratings of general behavior is also useful for identifying children with deviant behavior other than distractibility and hyperactivity and for assessing the degree and amount of prosocial behavior. Several such scales are available for assessing children as early as the preschool period, and some include rating scales to be completed by parents as well as the teacher. The Behavior Problem Checklist (Quay and Peterson, 1983) and the Walker Behavior Problem Identification Checklist

Table 5–1.

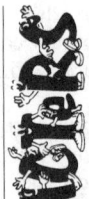

2nd Edition

Rina K. Ullmann, M.Ed.
Esther K. Sleator, M.D.
Robert L. Sprague, Ph.D.

Below are descriptions of behavior. Please read each item and compare the child's behavior with that of his or her classmates. Circle the number that most closely corresponds with your evaluation. Transfer the total raw score for each of the four sections to the profile sheet to determine normative percentile scores.

Child's Name: Elaine Sample
Rater: Mrs. Betsy J. Smith
ID #: 892772
Date: 11-15-93

ATTENTION

	Almost Never				Almost Always
1. Works well independently	①	2	3	4	5
2. Persists with task for reasonable amount of time	①	2	3	4	5
3. Completes assigned task satisfactorily with little additional assistance	①	2	3	4	5
4. Follows simple directions accurately	1	②	3	4	5
5. Follows a sequence of instructions	1	②	3	4	5
6. Functions well in the classroom	①	2	3	4	5

ADD ITEMS 1-6 AND PLACE TOTAL HERE **8**

HYPERACTIVITY

	Almost Never				Almost Always
7. Extremely overactive (out of seat, "on the go")	1	2	3	④	5
8. Overreacts	1	2	3	④	5
9. Fidgety (hands always busy)	1	2	3	④	5
10. Impulsive (acts or talks without thinking)	1	2	3	④	5
11. Restless (squirms in seat)	1	2	3	④	5

ADD ITEMS 7-11 AND PLACE TOTAL HERE **20**

SOCIAL SKILLS

	Almost Never				Almost Always
12. Behaves positively with peers/classmates	1	2	③	4	5
13. Verbal communication clear and "connected"	1	2	3	4	⑤
14. Nonverbal communication accurate	1	2	3	④	5
15. Follows group norms and social rules	1	2	③	4	5
16. Cites general rule when criticizing ("We aren't supposed to do that")	1	2	3	④	5
17. Skillful at making new friends	1	②	3	4	5
18. Approaches situations confidently	1	②	3	4	5

ADD ITEMS 12-18 AND PLACE TOTAL HERE **23**

OPPOSITIONAL

	Almost Never				Almost Always
19. Tries to get others into trouble	1	②	3	4	5
20. Starts fights over nothing	1	②	3	4	5
21. Makes malicious fun of people	1	②	3	4	5
22. Defies authority	1	②	3	4	5
23. Picks on others	1	②	3	4	5
24. Mean and cruel to other children	1	②	3	4	5

ADD ITEMS 19-24 AND PLACE TOTAL HERE **12**

MetriTech, Inc.

Table 5–1. (continued)

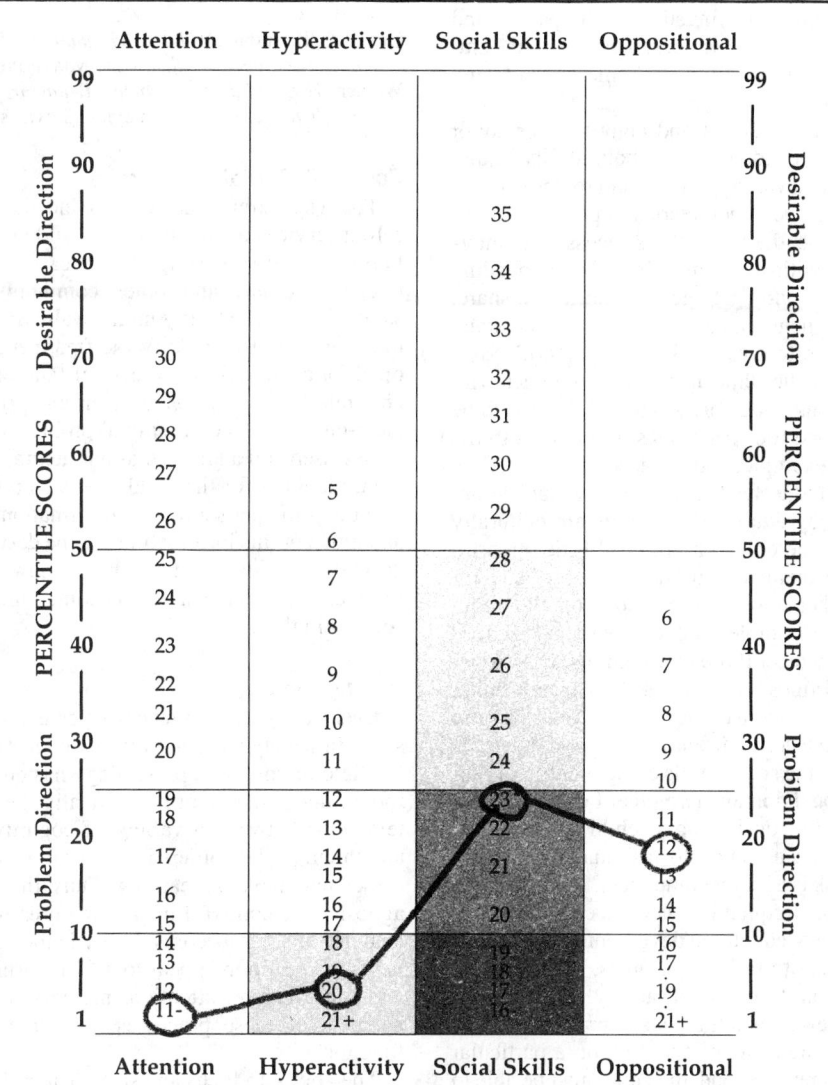

ACTeRS PROFILE—Girls' Form

Circle the raw scores in each of the four middle columns and determine percentile equivalents in the far left or right (boldface) columns. Note that some raw scores represent a range of percentiles (e.g., for Hyperactivity, the perfect score of 5 represents the range from the 56th percentile up).

Copyright © 1986, 1988, 1991 by MetriTech, Inc., Champaign, Illinois

(Walker, 1983) are rating scales that require teachers or other school personnel to rate students on a series of maladaptive behaviors. The Behavior Rating Profile (Brown and Hammill, 1983) is also based on a rating system; however, in addition to parent and teacher completion of the scale, self-rating by the student is included in three areas: home, school, and peer relationships.

Information about social and emotional behavior should include anecdotal details about ability to discriminate among a variety of roles and to perform socially within the social boundaries imposed by those roles. For instance, the social skills necessary to interact effectively with peers may include—depending on the child's chronologic age—the ability to share, to take turns, to negotiate conflict, and to understand and use humor effectively. These social skills shift somewhat when the child is asked to interact with adults in positions of authority. The child needs to be able to understand the social rules for conduct in the classroom, for example, and to respond to direction, to time limits, and to feedback within the social context prescribed by adults. These skills are culturally influenced, and the child who has had little opportunity to acquire them may be labeled as a behavior problem. The behavioral expectations of classroom environments are complex and require repeated exposures in order to meet those expectations. Classroom procedures and rules vary dramatically from teacher to teacher, and the consistency with which they are followed is also teacher-dependent.

In addition to the social skills component of the social and emotional domain, two other factors must be accounted for in considering a child's social and emotional profile: attention to task and motivation. Attention to task is a major component of information processing and is frequently related to cognitive ability. However, inadequate or developmental atypical capacity to attend to task may suggest emotional lability rather than cognitive disability. Attention to task may be viewed as a three-stage process. First, a child must be able to focus attention on a particular set of salient stimuli; second, the child must be able to sustain that attention over a span of time; and last, the child must be able to complete tasks. The inability of a child to perform any one of these components of attention to task may result from stress and anxiety imposed by a lack of predictability and routine in the classroom or home environment. Since children vary in their ability to handle disruption and multiple environments, information about the number of environments in which they are expected to participate daily or over the course of the week may suggest the need to restructure either the quantity or the quality of the environment. Children's responses to success, correction, and failure often assist teachers in understanding how to motivate children to perform successively more difficult tasks. It is advisable to gather information about performance in more than the

school environment in order to form a complete picture of social competence.

Brown L, Hammill D: *The Behavior Rating Profile.* Pro-Ed, 1983.
Quay HC, Peterson DR: *Interim Manual for the Revised Behavior Problem Checklist.* Univ Miami Press, 1983.
Walker HM: *Walker Problem Behavior Identification Checklist.* Western Psychological Services, 1983.

Family & Social Resources

The type, extent, and cost of educational and counseling services available to the child and family, the family's ability to support and carry through with treatment plans, and other community resources should be assessed early in the evaluation. These factors often limit or modify the treatment plan developed for a child. Sixty percent of families presenting children for evaluation of learning problems have clear-cut social and emotional problems that need to be assessed and addressed as an integral part of treatment planning for the child. Social services are usually the principal sources of information in this area, and much of this information will be derived from the psychosocial history. In addition, however, the primary care physician should become familiar with resources in the community.

Intelligence

Even though intelligence is perceived and understood in widely variable ways by education theorists, the field of cognitive psychology has enabled educators to understand more specifically the complex interactions between a variety of cognitive processes and the impact disorders in one or more of these processes may have on learning. Thus, the complete diagnosis of cognitive function requires more than an analysis of subtest scores. In particular, three components of cognition appear to affect learning potential and achievement: attention, memory, and the management of these processes through the executive function.

The ability to focus and sustain attention over time on events or tasks that are prescribed in school is a fundamental academic skill. While some children may fail to focus or sustain attention because of interfering emotional factors, another group appears unable to manage this cognitive function for other reasons. For this group of children, failure to attend successfully appears to be related to an inability to determine the salient features of a task, ie, what, when, and how a task needs to be accomplished and what procedures must be brought to bear to complete it. In other words, these children lack the ability to think about their thinking and to contrive or activate problem-solving procedures that will guide their performance of a given task. In the problem-solving sequence, these children have a tendency to break down in any one of several areas: (1) problem identification

("What is it I need to do here?"); (2) organization of strategies; (3) generalization from other, similar situations; (4) attainment of logical solutions; and (5) critical analysis and evaluation. Furthermore, in the problem-solving task, an inability to attend simultaneously to the task as well as monitor their performance and differentially allot attention to various elements of the task plagues many of these learners.

Another group of learners fail to perform adequately on tests of intelligence because their ability to store or retrieve information is limited. Cognitive psychologists discuss this problem in terms of storage capacity or how much information an individual can maintain in either short-term or long-term memory banks. Where capacity is not at issue, retrieval poses a second stumbling block. Children may lack a complex semantic retrieval system that enables them to access stored information from multiple avenues. Teachers often report anecdotally about these learners in terms somewhat as follows: "I know he knows it—he could do it all last week, but this week it's as if he never learned it." The complex relationship among attention, processing, retrieval, and the conscious execution of these processes is thought to be measured by intelligence tests.

These tests present an increasingly difficult set of problems. The questions tend to tap general knowledge, reasoning, judgment, and organization of analytic skills that are expected to develop in the course of experiences encountered by most children in the process of growing up. Where children have grossly different experiences from those in the standard population, their scores may be expected to vary upward or downward. Originally, the IQ score obtained from such tests represented the percentage of expected growth a child had reached at a given age. This was derived by the following equation:

(Mental age ÷ Chronologic age) × 100

Scores on most modern tests can still be reported in terms of mental age ÷ chronologic age, but the most widely used tests yield IQ scores that represent a child's relative distance from the average child in standard score units.

In the preschool period, the principal diagnostic tests in general use are the Bayley Scales of Infant Development (for children under 30 months of age), the Stanford-Binet Intelligence Scale, the McCarthy Scales of Children's Abilities (for children 3 years of age and older), and the Kaufman Assessment Battery for Children (K-ABC). These are all individually administered tests, given by trained personnel. The screening tests used most commonly in the preschool period are the Revised Denver Developmental Screening Test (Frankenberg); the Revised Developmental Screening Inventory (Knobloch et al); and, among older preschool children, the Early Screening Inventory (Meisels and Wiske). (See Table 5–2 for a summary of the screening tests discussed in this chapter.)

In recent years, several new assessment methods have been developed to capitalize on the caretaker's knowledge of the infant and preschool child. Procedures such as the Kent Infant Development Scale (KIDS) for children under 12 months of age and the Minnesota Child Development Inventory for children over 12 months of age use the caretaker's report to assess the child's general development, including cognitive, gross motor, fine motor, expressive language, self-help, and personal/social development. These procedures have several advantages: They provide for the inclusion of a large number of items at each age, are based on behavior readily observable at home, do not require extensive training for their administration, and can be used to plan and monitor appropriate intervention at home. Disadvantages include potential inaccuracy in the caretaker's reply and bias in reporting.

The Wechsler scales (Wechsler Adult Intelligence Scale [WAIS], Wechsler Intelligence Scale for Children III, and Wechsler Preschool and Primary Scale of Intelligence [WPPSI]) and the Stanford-Binet Intelligence Scale are the most widely used individual intelligence tests for school-age and older children. The Kaufman Assessment Battery for Children (K-ABC) is a relatively new test that is also gaining wide acceptance. The Stanford-Binet test is a highly verbal test with nonverbal items intermingled; results are reported as a single IQ score. The Wechsler scales are subdivided into six verbal and six nonverbal tests so that a verbal IQ and performance IQ can both be obtained as well as an IQ based on the full test (full-scale IQ). The Kaufman Battery is designed to assess differences in simultaneous and sequential processing of information as well as differences between aptitude and achievement. It is commonly thought that intelligence tests can reveal the potential for higher functioning, especially when scatter (the pattern of high and low scores) is examined carefully, and both the K-ABC and the Wechsler scales lend themselves particularly well to this task.

The standardized, individually administered tests of intelligence discussed above require extensive training for proper administration and are usually administered by trained psychologists. The Slosson Intelligence Test, however, is an abbreviated version of the Stanford-Binet test and is designed for use by nonprofessionals, including office assistants and primary care physicians. It is probably the most suitable screening test for estimating intelligence in children over 4½ years of age. More recently, the Kaufman Brief Intelligence Scale (K-Bit) has been introduced for the same purpose.

A number of briefer screening tests, such as the Peabody Picture Vocabulary Test and the Quick Test, are also suitable for use in office settings. These measure vocabulary skills alone, based on the fact

Table 5–2. Recommendations for use of assessment procedures.

Name	Type of Test	Age Range	Administered By
Wide Range Achievement Test	Achievement: reading, spelling, math, visual-perceptual	5 y–adult	Trained screener
Woodcock-Johnson Psych-Educational Battery	Aptitude and achievement	3 y–adult	Professional
Scales of Independent Behavior	Adaptive behavior	All ages	Professional
Vineland Adaptive Behavior Scales	Adaptive behavior	All ages	Professional
Bayley Scales of Infant Development	Development	3–30 mo	Professional
Revised Denver Developmental Screening Test (DDST)	Development	3 mo–6 y	Trained screener
Developmental Profile II (DPII)	Development	0–9 y	Trained screener
Early Screening Inventory	Development	4–6 y	Trained screener
Kent Infant Development Scale (KIDS)	Development	0–1 y	Caretaker response
Minnesota Child Development Inventory (MCDI)	Development	1–6 y	Caretaker response
Kaufmann Assessment Battery for Children (K-ABC)	Intelligence and achievement	2.5–12.5 y	Professional
McCarthy Scales of Children's Abilities	Intelligence	2.5–8.5 y	Professional
Slossen Intelligence Test	Intelligence	4.5 y–adult	Trained screener
Stanford-Binet Intelligence Scale	Intelligence	2 y–adult	Professional
Wechsler Intelligence Scale for Children-Revised (WISC-R)	Intelligence	6–16 y	Professional
Wechsler Preschool & Primary Scale of Intelligence (WPPSI)	Intelligence	4–6 y	Professional
Beery Test of Visual-Motor Integration	Visual-motor	2–15 y	Professional

that vocabulary has the best correlation with overall estimates of intelligence. A variety of other short screening tools are available, some of which rely on parent reporting or a combination of parent reporting and observation, but these often suffer from limited information regarding standardization data.

Achievement

Achievement usually refers to performance in specific school-related areas where a child has received instruction. In the preschool period, achievement is seldom distinguished from general development. By the time the child enters kindergarten, however, a variety of procedures are available for assessing readiness. In a child with a mental age of 6 years, two of the best predictors for readiness to enter the first grade are the ability to engage in sustained task-oriented behavior and the knowledge of letter names and sounds. A number of procedures are available to assess school readiness, and in recent years, testing programs have been specifically designed for early identification of children with learning disabilities. Although results of these programs appear to be about as accurate as teacher assessments of kindergarten performance, many feel that the programs represent an important advance. Most of the early identification testing programs are designed for use in

schools or by psychologists. Several procedures are also available for use by primary care physicians in screening for school readiness at the time of well-child visits in the 4½- to 5½-year age range. These include the developmental screening tests described previously and the preschool portions of the Wide Range Achievement Test (WRAT; see below).

For school-age children, scores on a variety of achievement tests are often available through routine classroom testing done at school, and results of such testing should be included in the educational history. Where low scores are obtained, individual testing should be performed before accepting the results as representative of the child's ability. Many school systems with special education services can administer individual tests of achievement and, with permission from the parents, give the test scores to the primary care physician. However, test scores in and of themselves do not constitute evidence of the presence of developmental disorders unless the test scores have been interpreted carefully by a trained educational specialist or school psychologist. Individually administered achievement tests such as the Woodcock-Johnson Psychoeducational Battery–Revised (Woodcock, 1990) are used to analyze more closely a learner's performance. The use of complex and lengthy tools such as the Woodcock-Johnson and the validity of the results of such an assessment rest heavily on the skills and abilities of the examiner to interpret test performance and scores on as many as 27 subtests. Analysis of discrepancies between subtests on this assessment tool assist the educational diagnostician in determining whether, for instance, discrepancies between orally identifying sight words and comprehending text are indicative of a disability or reflective of the developmental nature of these different skills. Furthermore, patterns of performance on tests that assess cognitive abilities such as memory functions or problem-solving capacities may indicate that the child has a specific learning disability in one or more cognitive functions. Individually administered achievement tests, in conjunction with measures of intelligence such as the Wechsler Intelligence Scale for Children III, are used to look at whether discrepancies between academic achievement and individual potential exist and whether these discrepancies may be attributable to some form of learning disability.

Academic achievement is additionally dependent on environmental factors that are not necessarily measured through achievement tests. These factors include cultural background and experience, motivation to achieve, expectancy for success, and instruction that accounts for these variables. A thorough diagnostic evaluation should address these concerns. Unfortunately, many children who are referred to a pediatrician for evaluation have no current achievement test scores in their school records. This is particularly true for children referred because of behavior problems. When an educational specialist or psychologist is unavailable to provide this information, the primary care physician may wish to test patients through the use of a screening test such as the Wide Range Achievement Test 3 (Williamson, 1991). Level I of this test is designed for children ages 5–12, and level II is designed for use with individuals aged 12 through adulthood. Because of the limited number of test items on this screening device, the validity of the results is somewhat questionable. However, by using this screening device, physicians can determine if further testing is desirable to determine whether a child is having difficulties in school due to cognitive or behavioral disorders.

Frankenburg WK et al: The Denver II: A major revision and restandardization of the Denver Developmental Screening Test. Pediatrics 1992;89:91.

Jastak S, Wilkinson G: *Wide Range Achievement Test 3.* Jastak, 1991.

Woodcock R: *Woodcock-Johnson Psychoeducational Battery-Revised.* Teaching Resources, 1990.

Adaptive Behavior

Assessment of adaptive behavior is seldom addressed directly in children unless a child is suspected of being mentally retarded. Because poor performance on a cognitive test may result from many factors, it is essential that the accuracy of low scores be confirmed by assessment of functional level in everyday living. Scales such as the Vineland Adaptive Behavior Scales and the Scales of Independent Behavior are questionnaire/structured interview methods for assessing the child's developmental level in areas such as social interaction, communication, personal living, and community living.

Perceptual-Motor Function

In the early school years, a number of children with delays in copying and drawing skills will also demonstrate problems in learning to read. These problems have been variously termed visual-perceptual and visual-motor problems, and their presence in children beyond 7–9 years of age has often been thought to indicate the existence of central nervous system dysfunction, although this inference is controversial. There is a relationship between visual-perceptual problems and reading problems in the early school years; as children get older, however, reading achievement becomes more and more related to intelligence, even when the perceptual problems persist. Furthermore, perceptual problems are common among children from families in lower socioeconomic groups and even among children whose only history is confinement to bed for more than 2 months during the preschool years.

Because performance on tests of copying skills is highly correlated with intelligence, such tests are most useful when there is a discrepancy between the developmental level demonstrated on visual-perceptual tests and general intelligence. Methods for assessing the degree of this discrepancy are not as well developed as for assessing the discrepancy between IQ and achievement. At a practical level, however, these problems may be severe enough to interfere with learning the skills of printing and writing. In this latter case, it is usually more helpful to analyze the child's writing, but several visual-perceptual tests, such as the Beery Test of Visual-Motor Integration, are commonly used to examine copying skills per se.

Speech & Language

Speech and language delays are common in mentally retarded children but may also occur in children with average or above-average intelligence. A number of children who appear to have specific learning problems will, on closer evaluation, show evidence of delay in language development or an articulation problem (or both). These problems can limit academic achievement in areas that depend on verbal skills (eg, reading). Speech and language delays in preschool children and methods for evaluating them have been discussed previously (see Chapter 3).

Most children should reach the adult proficiency level in language by 7–8 years of age, at which time evaluation of language skills typically becomes merged with evaluation of verbal intelligence. Scores on tests such as the Wechsler scale, the Stanford-Binet test, or the Slosson test will reflect language skills as well as intelligence. Specialized tests for assessing components of receptive and expressive language and language-processing skills are also available.

Motivation

Clinical assessment of motivation has received little attention despite mounting evidence that motivation is a key factor in determining how a child will use whatever time and help are provided for learning new skills. Studies of achievement motivation have suggested that two main motivational types can be identified, ie, those who are challenged by moderately difficult tasks and respond to success and those who are primarily motivated to avoid failure and will only attempt very easy tasks, where failure is unlikely, or very difficult ones, where failure carries no stigma. One of the major shifts that occurs in the age range of 5–7 years is from motivational dependence on social and external rewards to internal motivation for mastery of skills. Some children make this shift poorly or not at all and will fail to learn in the usual academic climate, which emphasizes mastery and competition. Often these are the children who seem primarily motivated to avoid failure and who need liberal support from external sources (praise, concrete incentives) just for trying. While motivational immaturity is seldom the principal problem, it is often a major determinant of how well a child will respond or progress in an educational program.

Beery KE: *Revised Administration, Scoring, and Teaching Manual for the Developmental Test of Visual-Motor Integration.* Modern Curriculum Press, 1982.

Bruininks RH et al: *Scales of Independent Behavior.* DLM Teaching Resources, 1984.

Frankenburg WK: *Denver Developmental Screening Test Reference Manual* (*Revised*). LADOCA, 1975.

Knobloch H, Steven F, Malone AF: *Manual of Developmental Diagnosis.* Harper, 1980.

Meisels SJ, Wiske MS: *Early Screening Inventory.* Teachers College, 1983.

Slosson RL, Nicholson CL, Hibpshman TL: *Slosson Intelligence Test-Revised.* Slosson Educational Publications, 1991.

Sparrow SS et al: *Vineland Adaptive Behavior Scales: Interview Edition, Survey Form Manual.* American Guidance Service, 1984.

Wilkinson GS: *Wide Range Achievement Test 3.* Jastak, 1993.

EVALUATING THE DISCREPANCY BETWEEN INTELLIGENCE & ACHIEVEMENT

The differential diagnosis of competence problems necessitates an evaluation of the significance of the discrepancy between expected achievement based on measures of general competence (intelligence) and actual achievement in specific areas of academic performance. The following material presents two methods of calculating the degree of discrepancy between IQ and achievement, based on grade equivalents and standard scores.

The United States Office of Education defines the discrepancy between achievement and IQ as significant when achievement is below 50% of expected grade level. The lowest level of achievement commensurate with age and intelligence is calculated by the following formula:

$$\text{Age } [(\text{IQ}/300) + 0.17] - 2.5 = \text{Lowest grade}$$

For an 8-year-old child with an IQ of 100, this formula indicates that a grade level of 1.5 is the lowest score that would be commensurate with age and intelligence. If this child's achievement test scores are below grade level 1.5, then there is a significant discrepancy. If they are at grade level 1.5 or higher, the discrepancy is not significant.

The following formula utilizes the direct correlation between intelligence test and achievement test scores to calculate the smallest difference between IQ and achievement test score needed to represent a significant discrepancy (D):

$$D = 1.96 \text{ SD } (1 - r^2)^{1/2}$$
$$\text{where SD} = \text{Standard deviation of}$$
$$\text{scores on achievement test}$$
$$r = \text{correlation between IQ}$$
$$\text{and achievement test scores}$$

This formula can be used to compare an IQ obtained from a test such as the Slosson test with a standard score obtained from the WRAT. The Slosson test manual provides the information that the correlation coefficient with the WRAT is 0.72, and the WRAT manual provides the information that the standard deviation of scores on the WRAT is 15. According to this calculation, a difference of 20 points between IQ and achievement test score is needed before a difference between these two tests is significant at the $p = 0.05$ level of confidence or better.

Both of these approaches call attention to the fact that some difference between expected and actual achievement represents normal variation, while a significant discrepancy is defined in terms of an unusual degree of difference. Individual school districts are free to adopt their own criteria in determining the extent of this discrepancy that must exist for a child to qualify for special services.

TEMPERAMENTAL TRAITS & REACTIONS TO DEVELOPMENTAL CRISES

During the ages of 5–7 years and 10–13 years, major developmental changes occur in most children. In the 5- to 7-year period, children enter school, begin to develop operational thought, and shift from associative thinking to use of verbal mediation activity in learning and thinking. The 10- to 13-year period heralds the onset of puberty, entrance into junior high school, and development of formal operational thought. Inflections in the growth curve for intelligence occur during both periods, and there is a dramatic increase in a cluster of behavior problems that appear to be phase-specific reactions to the developmental changes occurring during these periods. These problems include restless sleep, disturbing dreams, physical timidity, irritability, overdependence, and jealousy. Emotional turbulence during one of these periods may or may not be associated with turbulence during the other period, and its occurrence in either does not seem to be indicative of serious long-term problems.

Often there is overlap between these phase-specific reactions and temperamental traits, which include characteristics such as shyness, oversensitiveness, somberness, and reserve. Both phase-specific reactions and temperamental traits may be a source of conflict between parents and children, but they do not in themselves indicate the presence of serious emotional disturbance. They usually resolve with support, and the child does not need treatment.

Kohlberg, L, LaCrosse J, Ricks D: The predictability of adult mental health from childhood behavior. In: *Manual of Child Psychopathology.* Wolman BB (editor). McGraw-Hill, 1972.

DISORDERS IN DEVELOPMENT OF COGNITIVE COMPETENCE (See Table 5–3.)

SPECIFIC LEARNING DISORDERS

Essentials of Diagnosis

- Significant discrepancy between estimated intelligence (usually verbal) and achievement in one or more areas.
- Achievement commensurate with intelligence in one or more academic areas.
- No evidence of sensory deficits.
- Either presence or absence (often absence) of behavior problems.

General Considerations

Specific problems may be experienced in any area of academic achievement, but the most common problems involve reading or spelling (dyslexia). Frequent but less common problems are specific to arithmetic (dyscalculia) or writing (dysgraphia). Intelligence is usually average or above average, but the key element in making the diagnosis is demonstrating a discrepancy between actual achievement and expected achievement in a specific area. (See previous section on discrepancy.)

Descriptive Classification

A. Reading and Spelling Disorders (Developmental Dyslexia): Dyslexia is the most common type of specific learning disorder. It occurs more frequently in boys than in girls (3:1), and in 34% of cases there is a strong family history, especially among the male relatives. Speech and language problems and problems in sequencing are the most common developmental problems associated with specific reading disorders. A variety of developmental problems such as clumsiness and incoordination, directional confusion, right-left confusion, disordered temporal orientation, and difficulties in naming colors and in recognizing the meaning of pictures have been reported in children with specific reading problems. These are of lesser importance than the speech and language problems and may be more related to intelligence than to reading disorder per se. A history of delays in speech and language development is present in at least one-third of cases. This involves delays such as failure to use meaningful words other than "mama," "dada," "hello," and "bye-bye" until after 18 months of age and failure to use two-word phrases by 24 months of age. Although evidence of associated neurologic deficit or differential use of the right versus the left hemisphere can be demonstrated in some children, such results of neurologic investigations have generally contributed little to treatment or prognosis.

Traditionally, the definition of specific reading disorder (dyslexia) included failure to learn to read despite adequate sensory apparatus, conventional instruction, average intelligence, and sociocultural opportunity. Such diagnosis by exclusion was an attempt to distinguish between "unexpected" reading failure and reading failure that could be explained by a more general or pervasive factor, such as mental subnormality, cultural or educational deprivation, sensory defects, or emotional disturbance. With this approach, most children with reading problems tend to be excluded from the diagnosis of specific reading disorder—ie, their reading problems are attributed to the fact that they are slightly below average in intelligence, come from economically disadvantaged homes, or have emotional and behavior problems. Yet many in this large group show reading achievement below expectancy for their mental age; and in

Table 5–3. Differential diagnosis of learning problems.

Type of Learning Problem	Characteristics	Treatment Issues
Disorders with IQ-achievement discrepancy Specific learning disorders: Reading/spelling (dyslexia)	Achievement is below IQ in an isolated area. The disorder is not due to sensory impairment. Other areas are at levels of expectancy. Achievement is below expectancy only in reading/spelling.	Individualized instruction (often tutoring) in area of weakness should be provided. Normalized educational experiences in other areas are indicated. Specific instruction in reading/spelling/language arts is indicated. The child often exhibits generalized deficits in language processing. The child may have problems in math because of reading.
Arithmetic (dyscalculia)	Achievement is below expectancy only in arithmetic.	Specific instruction in math is indicated. Dyscalculia may be difficult to separate from a reading or writing disorder.
Writing (dysgraphia)	Achievement is below expectancy in written work.	Status of visual functioning must be clarified. Specific treatment for handwriting skill is indicated. Dysgraphia is often difficult to separate from dyslexia.
Hyperflexia	The child begins reading at a very early age (eg, 2 y). The child may appear autistic or show unusual discrepancies in abilities.	Comprehensive assessment and treatment in several areas of weakness is necessary. The prognosis for the autistic child is relatively good.
Nonspecific learning disorders: Underachievement	Achievement is below IQ in several areas. Underachievement may be due to environmental, behavioral (eg, ADHD), motivational, or situational problems, or to school absence.	The child often has emotional/behavior problems as well.
Generalized learning disability	Achievement is below IQ in several areas. The disability is not due to sensory impairment. The disability is often accompanied by evidence of visual/perceptual/motor difficulties. Associated environmental, emotional/behavioral, or motivational problems are often present.	Unusual combinations of discrepant functioning may be a reflection of abnormal brain functioning.
Disorders without IQ-achievement discrepancy Slow learner	IQ and achievement are commensurate but at low-normal to below normal levels.	Learning is slow but steady with appropriate programming.
Mental retardation	Both IQ and achievement are more than 2 SD below average.	
Educable	IQ is usually 50–70.	The child is capable of achieving rudiments of literacy.
Trainable	IQ is usually below 50.	The child is capable of acquiring preacademic and vocational skills.

neurologic status, cognitive functioning, and other areas of achievement they are indistinguishable from the group defined in the traditional sense as having specific reading disorder. In addition, the presence of a significant discrepancy between actual and expected achievement is the only characteristic that is common to members of highly specific etiologic groups such as those with genetic dyslexia diagnosed on the basis of linkage studies.

Consequently, current thinking endorses the concept that subtypes of reading disability should first be described in terms of clear-cut characteristics irrespective of etiologic considerations. There have been two major approaches to this subtyping. One approach attempts to distinguish among different problems on the basis of analysis of reading and spelling errors; this has led to subtyping into two groups based on whether performance indicates heavier reliance on auditory-sequential-phonologic skills (auditory reader) or on visual-spatial-imagery (visual reader).

The other approach uses associated disabilities such as those in language, perceptual-motor skills, and memory to distinguish the following probable subtypes: (1) a language disorder group with defects in understanding and expression of oral language; (2) a dyscoordination group with defects in speech articulation, copying skills, and understanding of oral language; (3) a visual-spatial-perceptual disorder group with visual, perceptual, and visual-constructive problems but intact oral language; and (4) a group with dysphonemic sequencing disorder.

B. Mathematics Disorders (Developmental Dyscalculia): Mathematics disorders have been studied primarily in relation to the developmental Gerstmann syndrome (dyscalculia, right-left disorientation, and finger agnosia) and often have been considered to be part of a reading disorder. However, limited studies of school children who demonstrate a significant discrepancy between actual and expected achievement in arithmetic suggest that a specific syndrome of mathematical disability does exist and affects approximately 6% of the population. Developmental disorder is distinguished from acquired disorder by the absence of clearly defined brain damage and neurologic findings in the former.

Several forms have been described and are characterized by difficulty in verbalizing, writing, reading, manipulating, or understanding mathematical operations. In individuals whose difficulties are confined to performance on numerical tests, signs of neurologic abnormalities tend to be few. In those who are unable to read or write numbers, the disorder may be associated with general disorders in reading and writing as well as mathematics, so that a learning disorder specific to mathematics may be difficult to demonstrate.

C. Writing Disorders (Developmental Dysgraphia): Children with reading problems often have illegible handwriting as well as spelling problems. In younger children, problems due to immature perceptual-motor development (eg, mirror writing, reversal of letters, and poor construction of letters) are common. Some children will have problems confined to illegible handwriting, inaccurate copying, or inability to transmit sequences of verbal information to paper. In some of these instances, illegibility is associated with mild cerebral palsy or general problems in fine motor coordination. Whether encountered alone or in combination with reading or math disability, specific training is often required to correct the penmanship problems.

A common syndrome seen in students during late elementary and junior high school involves not only elements of poor handwriting (slow, illegible, poor spatial organization) but also deficits in memory, expressive language, organization of ideas, and fluency. This has been termed "developmental output failure"; it is usually manifested by overall reduced productivity, with refusals to complete work, failure to submit assignments, and "forgetting" to do homework.

Left-handed children deserve special attention because they have frequently had poor instruction. In most instances, their problems in penmanship will improve with appropriate instruction. Despite common belief to the contrary, there is little evidence associating left-handedness with any kind of deficiency.

Etiologic Classification

Both psychobiologic and sociopsychologic factors appear to play a major causative role in specific learning disabilities. The group of children who fail to learn despite conventional instruction, adequate familial-cultural opportunity, and adequate intelligence have generally been thought to represent an idiopathic or genetically based syndrome. This group has been distinguished from children with emotionally, educationally, or culturally based limitations on the one hand and those with disorders secondary to sensory defects, brain damage, or mental retardation on the other.

In the idiopathic group, the term minimal brain dysfunction (MBD) has often been applied when neurologic "soft signs," poor motor coordination, and distractibility are present along with learning problems in children of average or above-average intelligence. The term has also been applied indiscriminately to children who show any one of these features alone, but the clinical picture of children with the full picture described above provides the most convincing evidence for attributing the problem to some type of neurologic handicap. However, because extensive research has failed to provide substantial evidence of dysfunction and because many of the characteristics are common in preschool children and tend to be present only in younger learning-disabled children, many have abandoned the concept of minimal brain damage altogether in favor of the view that the neurologic problem is one of immaturity.

Clinical Findings

A family history often reveals affected family members, especially among the males. Findings on physical examination are usually normal, and those on neurologic examination are normal except for the presence of "soft signs." Behavior problems may or may not be present. Intelligence test results often indicate average or above-average intelligence on nonverbal tests and may or may not show some decrease in verbal IQ. In contrast, achievement in the affected area of learning is significantly below nonverbal intelligence and sometimes below verbal intelligence. Achievement in nonaffected areas tends to progress normally. Vision and hearing are usually normal, although deficits in processing auditory sequential information are often noted on extensive testing.

Although reading disorders are common among brain-injured children (18–40%), a reading disorder is not necessarily associated with other evidence of altered cortical functioning. Furthermore, educational, language, and other psychometric tests are often of no help in distinguishing poor readers who are brain-injured from poor readers who are not brain-injured. Electroencephalography, CT scanning, and a variety of other procedures have been used in the past with little or no success.

Differential Diagnosis

The term "specific learning disability" is primarily a descriptive one that distinguishes between specific learning disorder, general learning disorder (slow learner), or mental retardation. Etiologic diagnosis is more difficult. The most important distinction is whether there is a strong family history, inadequate educational background, sociocultural disadvantage, or evidence of brain damage.

Treatment

There have been many claims that instruction should be tailored to the subtype of reading disorder, but research has generally failed to support this claim. In part, this may result from the fact that discussions of reading instruction often deal only with questions of content. In this regard, there are basically three approaches to teaching children to read. First, many special educators use a bottom-up approach to developing reading skills. That is, children learn to identify letters, to match sounds and letters, to develop a basic sight word vocabulary, to apply sound/letter matches to novel words, and finally to read words in text. Variations of this model include the use of syllabary (or rebus) systems to begin to decode meaning and to learn to read from left to right. With children who seem to need additional cues to discriminate between letters and words, initial, modified alphabets may be used or words may be colorcoded. This task analytic approach has been favored by special educators based on the presumption that breaking down reading into simpler discrimination tasks that lend themselves to routinized practice drills would increase the learner's success rate.

A second approach to teaching reading is based on the notion that learning to read is essentially a language development task and therefore follows the same developmental sequence that occurs when young children learn to speak. Thus, reading is taught from a holistic perspective in which teachers help children to link words that describe the world around them to print. Children are exposed to repeated readings of simple books and encouraged to read along with the teacher. Comprehension rather than word recall is stressed. This approach to reading also stresses the concurrent development of writing, since writing is the expressive aspect of the reading process. Rather than focus on the mechanics of spelling, children are urged to write using invented spelling to understand the notion of words as visual referents to the language we speak.

In a recent meta-analysis of research that analyzed the effectiveness of these two approaches to reading, Stahl and Miller (1989) found little evidence that favored either the bottom-up or the whole language approach to reading. These researchers concluded, as have many other reading and learning disabilities specialists, that careful assessment of individual learner needs should dictate the types of strategies used to help a child learn to read. There is evidence that a third approach based on an interactive model that combines attention to the graphophonemic elements of text (phonics) as well as to the semantic and experiential elements of comprehension may be the most efficient means of teaching a child to read.

It is evident from considering the various structures of the reading programs and strategies used in teaching that the number of possible approaches to reading instruction is quite large. With the variety of approaches available, selection of the best approach for a particular child may require a series of learning trials. Most children will begin to demonstrate learning after 4–6 lessons. General principles for promoting progress, however, include introduction of some phonics or word attack skills at some level of teaching; mastery of early, less difficult material before proceeding to more difficult material; and continuation of instruction over a long enough period for results to be long-lasting. Approximately 40 lessons are required before most children will register a substantial and enduring gain in reading skills. More rapid increases are sometimes reported, but these can often be attributed to spuriously depressed initial scores.

A minority of children will fail to learn to read or perform successfully in academic subjects despite individual instruction. For these children, a focus on goals that will ensure the maximum amount of independence as adults is vital even in the primary grades. Special education efficacy studies (eg, Kavale, 1982; Shepard, 1983) suggest that much of special education has not adequately addressed outcomes for the community (ie, employment and independent living), or for individuals (ie, heightened self-esteem, community membership status), or for schools (ie, efficient delivery of service). In seven statewide studies, less than 50% of the graduates of special education programs were employed full time. More than half of each sample earned less than minimum wage, and more than 60% of the graduates continued to live at home after graduation. Thus, outcome data from graduates of special programs suggest that the special education programs need to incorporate content and experiences to prepare young people to access employment and independent living opportunities in their own communities.

Several approaches to drug therapy for children with reading disability have been proposed, but none have yet received adequate study to warrant their recommendation. Furthermore, drug therapy prescribed for attention deficit disorder, if successful, may be expected to alter impulsive and distractible behavior but typically does not "cure" the learning problems if these are present. At best, the climate for learning is improved, but educational progress will still depend primarily on the quality and amount of instruction provided to the child.

Prognosis

With or without individual instruction, only a minority of children remain nonreaders into adulthood. There are, however, many adolescents and adults who read poorly. Ultimate level of skill usually depends on the child's intelligence, the type and amount of individual instruction provided, the severity of retardation, the age at which remediation is begun, motivation, and several other factors including the child's general emotional state. In some adults, poor spelling may be the only stigma of a childhood reading problem, whereas other adults may continue to show evidence of problems in reading and general language skills as well. Even with individual instruction, progress is often slow, sometimes slower than progress being made by children described as slow learners. In children with specific learning disorder, however, progress in nonaffected areas of achievement tends to proceed at a normal pace.

Kavale KA, Glass GV: The efficacy of special education interventions and practices: A compendium of meta-analysis findings. Focus Except Child 1982;15:1.

Kosc L: Developmental dyscalculia. J Learn Disab 1974; 7:164.

Myklebust HR (editor): *Progress in Learning Disabilities,* vols 1–5. Grune & Stratton, 1983.

Rutter M (editor): *Developmental Neuropsychiatry.* Guilford, 1983.

Schain RJ: *Neurology of Childhood Learning Disorders.* Williams & Wilkins, 1972.

Shepard LA, Smith LA, Vojir CP: Characteristics of pupils identified as learning disabled. J Spec Educ 1983;16:73.

Stahl S, Miller P: Whole language and language experience: Approaches for beginning reading: A quantitative research synthesis. Rev Educ Res 1989;59:87.

SLOW LEARNER

Essentials of Diagnosis

- Achievement below average.
- No mental retardation but IQ often below average.
- No significant discrepancy between IQ and achievement.
- Performance usually poor in all subjects.
- School progress at a slower rate than average but nevertheless continuous.

General Considerations

The average IQ of children in this group tends to be in the 80s. Approximately 11% have definite evidence of neurologic dysfunction, 25% show question-able neurologic findings, and 60% have difficulty in copying forms. Clumsiness, motor impersistence, and right-left confusion are twice as common in this group as in children with specific learning disorders. Forty percent tend to have at least one sign of language delay (eg, first phrases after 24 months). The frequency of neurodevelopmental problems increases in children with lower IQs.

Clinical Findings

The most important characteristic is the lack of a significant discrepancy between intelligence and achievement. These children are often low-average to borderline in intelligence, and achievement is slow but commensurate with mental age. Usually the child is slow in all areas of achievement, but achievement in one area may be slower than in others. The lower the child's intelligence, the more one is likely to find evidence of neurodevelopmental problems and associated behavior problems. The history often reveals evidence of developmental delays, especially in the language area. A family history of school problems may or may not be present. In the absence of a positive family history, problems during the pregnancy, advanced maternal age, or difficulties in the newborn period are often cited as possible causes of early brain damage that might explain the appearance of such a child in a well-educated family. In many instances, however, the mother's educational and cognitive level will be consistent with that of the child whether signs of neurodevelopmental delay are present or not.

Treatment

Educational programming that uses community, school, work, and family as the conceptual organizers for planning curriculum often makes more sense for this group of learners than the traditional academic curriculum. Families are frequently asked to participate in curriculum planning by reporting what they would like their child to be able to do 3 years from now in terms of accessing and participating in community activities, developing effective job habits, and participating in family recreational activities. By including the family in educational planning, recognition and acceptance of the child's capacities is made easier. Counseling or short-term psychotherapy can assist the family in dealing with feelings of denial or guilt. Often the school has developed an appropriate educational plan for the child, and treatment needs to be directed toward helping the family accept the school's plan.

Prognosis

Given an appropriate educational opportunity to progress at their own rate, slow learners tend to make steady progress commensurate with their mental age. In many instances, long-term follow-up may show that these children actually make better progress in their areas of deficiency than do children with specific learning disorders.

NONSPECIFIC & EMOTIONALLY BASED LEARNING DISORDERS

Essentials of Diagnosis

- Usually, average or above-average intelligence.
- Significant discrepancy between intelligence and achievement, often in more than one academic area.
- Frequent association with emotional or behavior problems.
- Frequent incidence among children from culturally disadvantaged homes and large families.

General Considerations

Included in this group are the large numbers of children with learning disorders in association with psychiatric disorders and familial-cultural problems of motivation. A significant discrepancy between intelligence and achievement may exist in one or more areas, or the child may be generally slow. Family problems are usually apparent, and children frequently come from culturally disadvantaged homes and large families. These children have many of the same educational needs as children with more specific problems—and often more—but they have, unfortunately, been excluded from federal funding for education of the learning disabled.

This group also includes children with wide discrepancies in functioning that result from or appear to result from altered brain function, with or without attendant emotional or behavior problems. Reduced functioning in several areas without significant IQ impairment is frequently observed in children with documented neurologic disorders (eg, epilepsy, structural lesions, head injury).

Differential Diagnosis

Differentiation from specific learning disabilities is made primarily on the basis of motivational and emotional problems and a lack of specificity of learning problems in children with average or above-average intelligence. Slow learners or mentally retarded children with emotional problems may be indistinguishable. The most difficult differential diagnosis is between specific reading disabilities in an emotionally disturbed child and an emotionally based learning disability concentrated in the language area.

Children with documented head injury or brain damage may not present a diagnostic problem. Often, however, the pattern of performance on psychologic tests, particularly those that are sensitive to disturbance in cortical functioning, may be the only available evidence pointing to brain dysfunction. Neurologic tests such as EEGs or CT scans are seldom beneficial in making a diagnosis.

Treatment

School systems are required by federal law to provide services to students who, through school-based diagnostic procedures, are labeled as emotionally disturbed. Services range from the development and implementation of behavior modification programs to full-day classes that serve students with these disorders. Curriculum components generally include manipulations of the instructional environment such as shortened or simplified academic tasks, cooperative learning groups, and contingency management strategies. A second curriculum component focus is on the management of aggressive or out-of-control behaviors through cognitive behavior modification and behavior control training. Additionally, curriculum that addresses the development of social and affective skills should be a component of programming. A final ingredient in programs for students with emotional problems is counseling. The effectiveness of these programs is generally related to the skills of the multidisciplinary team assigned to the program. Services should reflect the needs of the student rather than a generic approach that treats all children with emotional disturbance in a similar fashion.

MENTAL RETARDATION

Essentials of Diagnosis

- Significantly limited intelligence ($\geq$ 2 SD below average [IQ < 70]).
- Adaptation significantly below age level.
- Possible presence of sensory defects not responsible for delay.
- Onset in the developmental period.

General Considerations

Mental retardation is a descriptive term defined as significantly subaverage intellectual functioning existing concurrently with deficits of adaptive behavior and manifested during the developmental period. Significantly subaverage intelligence is defined as 2 SD or more below average (IQ below 70 on the Wechsler scales or below 69 on the Stanford-Binet test) and by definition affects approximately 2–3% of the general population. An additional 6% are considered borderline in intelligence (IQ of 70–79). Adaptive deficiency is less easily evaluated.

About 10% of the retarded population are identified during infancy and early childhood. The majority fall in the moderate to profound retardation group (IQ below 50), and most of them have clear-cut evidence of brain damage, genetic disorder, or other pathologic conditions. Moderate to profound retardation is distributed equally among different socioeconomic groups but is more common in males than in females.

The remaining 90% of the retarded population tend to be mildly retarded (IQ of 50–69), and most are not identified before entering school, partly because limited efforts are made at earlier identification. The great majority of those with mild handicaps are diagnosed as cultural-familial retardates. They entral nervous system injury, and they come from families characterized by low intelligence and low socioeconomic status. Many who are mildly handicapped and identified primarily during the school years eventually blend into society and become at least marginally adequate citizens. There is a preponderance of males at all levels of retardation, except for those with organic disorders that are diagnosed after age 5 years.

Mildly retarded children (IQ 50–69) usually are considered educable and in many instances are able to blend into society with minimal or no protective custody. Moderately retarded children (IQ 30–49) are considered trainable but require protective care (sheltered workshop, guardian, group home). More recently, the public schools have been required to provide services to members of this group. Severely to profoundly retarded children (IQ < 30) usually require continuous care, and this group often includes the most severely deformed, nonambulatory, and minimally communicative individuals. Educational programs at all levels of disability stress providing an appropriate education in the least restricted, most normalized environment.

Etiologic Considerations

Mental retardation is a descriptive diagnosis with a wide variety of causes. Many of the causative factors that can be identified are essentially untreatable. The basic data base will be helpful in deciding how far to pursue an etiologic diagnosis.

A. Genetic:

1. Inborn errors of metabolism–Aminoacidopathies, cerebral lipidoses,mucopolysaccharidoses, disorders of carbohydrate metabolism.

2. Chromosome disorders–Autosomal disorders, sex chromosome disorders such as fragile X syndrome.

B. Intrauterine: Congenital infections, placental-fetal malfunction, complications of pregnancy (maternal malnutrition, preeclampsia-eclampsia, use of drugs or radiation, intrauterine growth retardation).

C. Perinatal: Prematurity, postmaturity, metabolic disorders (hypoglycemia, hyperbilirubinemia).

D. Postnatal: Endocrinopathies, metabolic disorders, trauma, infections, poisoning, abuse.

E. Cultural-Familial: Low family intelligence, low socioeconomic status, environmental deprivation.

Clinical Findings

A. History: In infants and preschool children with developmental delays, there may be evidence of a genetic syndrome or factors in the prenatal or perinatal period that can account for delay. Often, however, there will also be evidence of maternal deprivation or neglect, particularly among children who are only mildly or moderately delayed. The older the child at the time of diagnosis, the more likely that retardation will be explained by deficiencies in early experience or by familial-cultural factors. Even when there are other family members with similar problems, a genetic basis for the retardation cannot be established unequivocally. Children who are not diagnosed until after entering school will often have a history of normal development in the first 2 years, and siblings may show a similar decline in relative competency as they get older. Children who come from nondominant cultural backgrounds will often show adequate functioning on measures of adaptation despite poor performance on standard intelligence tests. If behavior problems, especially disruptive and antisocial behavior, are absent, children who show relatively better adaptability than intelligence tend to blend into society after leaving school.

B. Symptoms and Signs: In mental retardation, the developmental or intellectual performance is at least 2 SD below the mean, and there is accompanying evidence of significant limitations in adaptability. In preschool children, developmental delay on screening tests may be the principal presenting finding. Sensory defects are also common, as are speech and language problems, motor handicaps, neurodevelopmental delays, seizure disorders, and behavior problems. Serious family problems are also common, and frequently the mentally retarded child merely appears to be enough slower than other members of the family to be identified as retarded rather than borderline or dull normal. If the child is examined adequately, signs of significant developmental delay including deficiencies in adaptation will often be evident by age 2 years.

Once the child reaches school age, general adaptation and achievement in all areas tend to be low but commensurate with mental age. Children with low IQs who are not retarded on measures of adaptation should not be diagnosed as mentally retarded. Occasionally, a mildly retarded or borderline child will show a significant discrepancy between actual and expected achievement in one academic area more than in others. This may technically represent a specific learning disability; however, if the child's overall intelligence is low enough (IQ below 70), special education will be indicated anyway. Idiot savants have been described as showing extraordinary ability in a circumscribed area while functioning on a mentally retarded level in all other ways. Neglect, abuse, and other family experiences damaging to growth may result in bizarre forms of behavior and emotional disturbance that are difficult to distinguish from autistic or psychotic behavior. Mentally retarded children are often transparent mirrors of disturbances going on within the family. The appearance of unusual behavior, sexual acting out, or bizarre activity in an otherwise stable retarded child is often an indication of a disturbance in the family.

C. Special Studies: General rules for ordering tests include (1) laboratory testing for treatable conditions when an etiologic diagnosis is unknown, eg, use of an amino acid or organic acid screen; and (2) ordering other tests such as electroencephalography, skull films, and chromosome studies only if clinical findings suggest specific syndromes or problems.

Differential Diagnosis

Once a descriptive diagnosis is made, the basic data base should provide enough information so that a decision can be made on how far to pursue an etiologic diagnosis. It is particularly important to distinguish the deaf, blind, and orthopedically handicapped from the mentally retarded. This is often difficult, since many retarded children also have sensory and orthopedic handicaps. It is also often difficult to differentiate between autism and retardation in very young children, particularly when family and social background indicates deprivation or neglect. Usually, however, the young retarded child shows delay in all areas of development, whereas the autistic child may be quite normal in motor development but show bizarre behavior and serious delays in language development.

Management

Mental retardation usually is diagnosed only after a significant period of developmental delay has been observed. The older the child at the time of diagnosis, the less the likelihood of reversing the signs of retardation even when a treatable cause can be identified. Prevention is therefore the only significant approach to treatment at present. A screening program for early detection of inborn errors of metabolism and institution of treatment before significant damage to the nervous system can occur represents the model approach to the problem of mental retardation. This same model has been used in developing preventive programs for children at risk for familial-cultural retardation. Controlled studies of stimulation programs for infants in sociocultural groups with high rates of mental retardation have shown significant long-range results after termination of the program when (1) parents have been involved in the program, (2) the infant participated in the program frequently (once every 2 weeks or more), and (3) the program continued for at least 2 years. Head Start has also been shown to decrease the number of children in special education classes and to increase the number of children from high-risk populations who remain in school.

In most instances, however, management of the retarded child does not involve treatment of the retardation per se but must be directed toward (1) assessing the impact on the family and providing support and psychotherapy, (2) providing protection for the child, (3) providing education and rehabilitation to maximize the child's potential, and (4) providing treatment of associated medical, emotional, and behavior problems.

A. Impact on the Family: The diagnosis of mental retardation is an event for which few families are prepared. Often parents can assess the mental age of their child within a few months but still refuse to accept the implications of this information. The tact and sensitivity with which the initial discussion of developmental delay is broached can determine how early the family will allow appropriate treatment, education, and rehabilitation to be started; thus, the primary care physician should be alert to parents' initial questions about developmental delay. A second opinion or repeated evaluation is almost mandatory when the impression of significant developmental delay arises unexpectedly from screening tests or school observations. Once the diagnosis is confirmed, the family will need continued assistance and support in adjusting to the diagnosis and in making contact with community resources.

Retarded children and adults can successfully remain within the family in most instances, but they usually require a host of family and community support services. These often include social services, infant education programs, and occupational and physical therapy programs and services for handicapped infants that begin as early as the newborn period. In school-age children, most services are organized through the public school systems, but the primary care physician may be called on to assist in difficult situations.

Once a severely handicapped child is "accepted" by the family, family resources may be totally consumed by care of the child, often to the detriment of normal siblings. Professionals involved with these families should provide help in developing priorities and alleviating parental guilt at being unable to do everything everyone suggests for the child. Less severely handicapped children are often less acceptable to the family, with resulting conflict and emotional disturbance as parents attempt to deny or seek more ego-syntonic diagnoses and explanations for the child's delays. Parental difficulty in accepting evidence of mild retardation often leads them to seek more than one evaluation as they pass through a mourning process and eventually develop more realistic expectations for the child. Parent support groups have been particularly helpful to families with retarded children.

B. Protection, Education, and Rehabilitation: The schools have responsibility for providing educational services to students with mental retardation ages 3–21 in the least restrictive, most normalized environment in which the student can be reasonably expected to receive educational benefit. Regardless of the extent of the individual's disability, the judicial system has interpreted the provisions of PL 94–142 to mean that *all* children—even those with the most profound mental retardation—must be served through the local public school system. Students with disabilities who are enrolled in private or parochial schools are also entitled to receive services through the local public school system. As a result, most metropolitan, suburban, and small school districts provide services for these students in their local public schools. In communities where regional or state residential services for individuals with mental retardation are provided, children living in these institutions are generally transported to classrooms located in public school buildings. Multidisciplinary teams trained to work with these individuals have responsibility for such health care procedures as catheterization, tube feeding, etc. Motor and language therapists work in concert with special education teachers to provide functional educational programs that focus on increasing levels of personal care, daily living skills, social interaction, and communication. Many schools provide opportunities for interaction with nondisabled peers to increase the quality of life and natural supports for individuals with profound disabilities as well as increase the capacity of children without disabilities to understand and appreciate the full spectrum of human diversity. Where children with mental retardation have additional cognitive capacities, the opportunities for interaction with typical peers are increased. However, the curriculum continues to focus on functional, independent living skills.

As children with mental retardation become adolescents, educational personnel are mandated by law to focus on the transition from school to adult life. Thus, multidisciplinary teams must write specific goals that address support or independent work and residential needs into individualized educational plans. Adult human service agencies must be involved in these transition plans by the time the student reaches the age of 16. Passed in 1990, the Americans With Disabilities Act (ADA) ensures that employers must make accommodations for workers with disabilities, including individuals with mental retardation. Furthermore, ADA specifies that transportation systems and businesses that serve the public must provide access and services to individuals with all types of disabilities. Human service agencies funded to provide resources and services to adults with developmental disabilities, including mental retardation, continue to serve more and more profoundly disabled individuals in nonsheltered environments. Although many adults with developmental disabilities will continue to require individual support and training throughout their lives, these supports will most likely be provided in typical rather than sheltered environments.

C. Treatment of Associated Medical, Emotional, and Behavior Problems: Sensory, motor, and orthopedic handicaps and other medical problems should be treated appropriately. The most controversial area of management concerns the use of psychotropic medication for treatment of emotional and behavior problems, especially in institutionalized retarded children. Although most of these medications are approved primarily for use in treatment of psychotic conditions, the phenothiazines in particular have been employed extensively in behavioral management of retarded persons.

Psychotropic medication practices have often resulted in too much being given for too long a time to too many institutionalized children. Frequently, several psychotropic drugs are given at the same time. Some children may be so heavily drugged that they are unable to respond maximally to educational and rehabilitative programs. These practices are often based on claims that the response to neuroleptic and psychotropic medications is altered in retarded children, but other evidence supports the interpretation that psychotropic medication often represents a "chemical straitjacket" that is used as a substitute for adequate personnel to provide more appropriate care. It is uncertain whether attention deficit disorder in mentally retarded children should be treated with stimulant medication. Some children appear to become worse with treatment (as do many psychotic children), whereas stimulant medication appears to be the treatment of choice for others. As children are withdrawn from heavy medication with phenothiazines and other major psychotropic drugs, symptoms such as dyskinesia may emerge, ie, withdrawal emergent symptoms, which require diagnosis and treatment in themselves. The most serious of these is tardive dyskinesia, which may also appear during treatment.

To avoid misuse of psychotropic medication in the mentally retarded, (1) a diagnosis of the emotional or behavior problem should be made and an appropriate drug and dosage selected on the basis of the diagnosis; and (2) the patient's response to the medication should be carefully monitored by the physician through direct evaluation and observation as well as review of reports provided by caretakers.

MOTOR HANDICAPS

A variety of nonspecific problems in development of motor coordination has been observed in children with learning disorders and also as isolated problems. Mental retardation, cerebral palsy, or a neuromuscular disorder is also present in many cases. A larger group, estimated at about 6–7% of the population, shows clumsiness, awkwardness, choreiform movements, or generally poor coordination but no signs of systemic disease except for an increased incidence of other "soft signs" on neurologic examination. Many of the children in this group also show evidence of learning problems, and the motor problems have been cited as evidence of a neurologic basis for the learning problems. However, as with "soft signs" in general, this interpretation is controversial.

Clumsiness and awkwardness have also been reported in association with attention deficit disorder. In this instance, treatment with stimulant medications has frequently been accompanied by improvement in motor coordination. Occupational and physical therapy are often recommended for these children, though there are no adequately controlled studies with data to support the efficacy of these approaches for improving educational achievement. There is clear evidence that instruction in reading is better than perceptual-motor training in improving reading ability irrespective of the child's motor status. The whole area of mild motor disability has received so little formal scrutiny, however, that much is yet to be learned about ways of identifying and ameliorating developmental impairments in motor skills.

Connolly K: Motor development and motor disability. In: *Developmental Psychiatry.* Rutter M (editor). Heinemann, 1980.
Henderson A: Research in occupational therapy and physical therapy with children. In: *Advances in Behavioral Pediatrics,* vol 2. Camp BW (editor). JAI Press, 1981.

DEVELOPMENTAL-ADAPTATIONAL PROBLEMS

Developmental-adaptational problems are behavior problems that in normal children decline steadily with age either from infancy or from their appearance in the preschool years. Manifestations include fears, distractibility, hyperactivity, destructiveness, lying, negativism, temper tantrums, enuresis, and thumbsucking. Children with these manifestations often show no maladjustment later in life; absence of these manifestations does not rule out later maladjustment. The gradual decline in these behavior problems is associated with maturation of cognitive competence, including not only intelligence but moral maturity and ego development as well. When deficiencies in social character and cognitive adaptability persist in children beyond the early school years, they are more likely to have a poor prognosis.

ATTENTION DEFICIT HYPERACTIVITY DISORDER

Essentials of Diagnosis

- Distractibility, short attention span, hyperactivity, impulsivity.
- Duration of longer than 6 months.
- No association with psychosis.

- Association with aggressive behavior, sometimes but not always present.
- Onset before age 7 years.

General Considerations

Attention deficit hyperactivity disorder is characterized by heightened distractibility, short attention span, and impulsiveness. The rate of incidence is about 5%, and the disorder is more common in boys than in girls. Most of the children previously labeled hyperactive or said to have minimal brain dysfunction are children with attention deficit hyperactivity disorder. In normal children, attention span and ability to concentrate on cognitive tasks increase throughout childhood. Ability of preschool children to engage in sustained task-oriented behavior is one of the most reliable predictors of later school performance. Some evidence suggests that even in infants, attention span may be an early indication of later cognitive performance. In older children, attentiveness is one of the major characteristics of competent children with good peer relations.

The child who persists in immature forms of attentional behavior after age mates have matured is noticeably out of phase in cognitively stressful situations such as school. In these circumstances, children may appear driven to aimless, purposeless activity. Some children also show hyperactive behavior at home, on the playground, and in the physician's office, as well as in the classroom; others may only show problems under cognitive stress. Some children with attention deficit hyperactivity disorder have also been described as hypoactive rather than hyperactive.

In evaluating behavior problems, it is important to determine whether aggressive behavior problems or conduct disorders are also present. This mixture of behavior problems is common. It is not clear whether the presence of aggressive behavior alters the short-term response to treatment. However, long-term prognosis is poorer in those who have a mixed disorder than in those whose behavior problems are confined to distractibility, impulsiveness, and short attention span.

The causes of attention deficit hyperactivity disorder are not well understood, although there is evidence of a genetic or constitutional basis for the problem in many children. The diagnosis is largely descriptive, but it carries the implication that specific causes of distractibility and short attention span (eg, neurologic insult or injury, emotional trauma, psychosis, depression) have been eliminated. Immaturity in development of the central nervous system is one of the most likely underlying causes of the problem. However, children who show the functional disorder may or may not have evidence of "soft signs" on neurologic examination or abnormal findings on electroencephalography. The presence of neurodevelopmental signs has not been consistently related to treatment outcome.

Clinical Findings

A. History: The most important diagnostic information comes from a description of behavior in the classroom and teacher ratings on a scale such as the ACTeRS (Table 5–1). Ratings on this scale that fall below the 10th percentile on attention, hyperactivity, or both, regardless of ratings on the other scales, are usually indicative of attention deficit hyperactivity disorder. If problems with attention or hyperactivity are not evident at school, it is very unlikely that the child has attention deficit hyperactivity disorder. Physicians worried about teacher bias in completing the rating will often find that ratings obtained from several teachers will show similar results. However, ratings completed by parents may or may not show deviance. It is useful to review information about oppositional behavior and social skills and obtain information about intelligence and academic performance, because many children will also show other behavior or learning problems. The most common other behavior problem encountered among children with attention deficit disorder is aggressive behavior or conduct disorder. The family history is often positive for similar problems in childhood, particularly among male relatives. Children with attention deficit disorder are frequently described as active, colicky infants, and typically parents can recall many incidents indicating distractibility and hyperactivity in the preschool period. Attention deficit hyperactivity disorder is usually first recognized as a problem after a child enters school. The diagnosis can sometimes be made with great confidence in preschool children, but many of these children are primarily in need of improved parental management.

B. Symptoms and Signs: The neurologic examination may or may not show signs of neurologic immaturity. There are usually no sensory impairments. A significant number of children also have learning problems that may be general or specific, usually depending on the child's level of intelligence. Attention deficit hyperactivity disorder occurs at all intellectual levels, but among children of average intelligence with behavior problems confined to the attention deficit hyperactivity disorder syndrome, achievement is often adequate despite teacher complaints that the child is "not learning." When a learning problem accompanies a behavior problem, the problems should be addressed separately.

Family problems may contribute to attention deficit hyperactivity disorder and increase the difficulty of treatment, especially in children who show aggressive behavior. Attention deficit disorder is excluded when a diagnosis of childhood psychotic disorder has been made, but the diagnosis may be made in mentally retarded children.

C. Special Studies: Tests measuring continuous performance or vigilance have been widely used in research on attention deficit hyperactivity disorder. These tests usually require that the child look for occurrences of one specified design among many, either on a page or sequentially flashing on a screen. One such system with norms is commercially available for electronic administration of a vigilance test; nevertheless, the clinical application of these procedures is incompletely worked out. No other special tests aid in diagnosis. If there is a question of seizure disorder or clear-cut evidence of neurologic disorder, investigation of these conditions is indicated.

Treatment

Two major effective forms of treatment are behavior modification programs in the classroom and stimulant drugs (methylphenidate [Ritalin], dextroamphetamine [Dexedrine; many others], and pemoline [Cylert]). Drug treatment, if effective, tends to have more dramatic results than behavior modification.

Approximately 50–80% of children with attention deficit hyperactivity disorder are responsive to stimulant drug therapy. Dose-response studies on methylphenidate suggest that a dose of 0.3 mg/kg produces optimal cognitive improvement (concentration) as well as significant improvement in social behavior. Greater improvement in social behavior can be achieved with higher doses, but this occurs at the expense of some loss in concentration. Peak action usually occurs 2 hours after ingestion, and most effects have dissipated after 6 hours. The usual regimen is to start with an early morning dose, followed by a dose at noon if needed. Morning activities often require the most concentration, and the noon dose may be unnecessary. If problems at home are also severe, a third dose may be given in the late afternoon. Medication on weekends and during school holidays should be tailored to the needs of the child and family. Dextroamphetamine and methylphenidate are quite similar in onset and duration of action, and most children who respond to one will respond to the other. Pemoline appears to be somewhat different in onset of action, and doses often require adjustment over a longer period of time.

Drug "holidays" are an important part of chronic drug therapy with psychotropic drugs. Medication should be withdrawn for at least 2 weeks of each year to determine whether therapy needs to be continued. Two convenient times for this are summer vacations and spring holidays. In the latter case, a week at home without medication can precede a week at school without medication.

The most common adverse reactions are decreased appetite, headache, stomach ache, increased emotional lability, and insomnia. When these side effects appear early in the course of treatment, they are often transient or respond to dosage reduction. It is sometimes difficult to determine whether or not they are indeed medication-related; however, when in doubt, the best approach is to stop or change the medication. All of the stimulants have the potential for exacerbating motor and phonic tics and Tourette's syndrome.

Dextroamphetamine is contraindicated in the presence of moderate to severe hypertension, and methylphenidate (Ritalin) should be used cautiously in the presence of hypertension. Pemoline (Cylert) is contraindicated in patients with impaired hepatic function. Methylphenidate has been implicated as lowering the threshold for seizures, though a prospective study of a small number of seizure patients did not show this effect. Pemoline has also been associated with development of seizures and elevation of liver enzymes. Decrements in predicted growth have been reported with long-term administration of stimulants, and though a causal relationship has not been established, growth should be carefully monitored.

"Rebound" effects—the appearance of symptoms in exaggerated form when "the medicine wears off"—is a common experience. This is often especially marked in children who have a dramatic response to medication. These effects can frequently be modified by use of a sustained-release form of medication or addition of a small dose of medication after school. In most cases, the family may or may not choose to give medication on the weekend; however, it is usually most beneficial to give medication on weekends in patients who have significant rebound effects.

Monitoring for side effects should be continuous. Weekly teacher reports (ACTeRS scale) during the first month are helpful for monitoring and evaluating treatment. The child should be reevaluated at 1 month to determine if the response is sufficient to justify continuing with medication.

Behavior modification programs are often tailored to an individual child's situation. Planning an individualized program usually involves the services of a psychologist or educational specialist. Think Aloud, a general cognitive behavior modification program for improving self-control in children 6–8 years of age, can be used in an office setting. Typically, it has been carried out by special teachers, psychologists, social workers, or other mental health workers but can be used by an intelligent parent or interested physician.

Prognosis

With or without treatment, the long-term outcome is better in the more intelligent children with stable families and uncomplicated attention deficit hyperactivity disorder. These children often require only short-term treatment (usually 2 years or less).

Camp BW, Bash MAS: *Think Aloud: Increasing Social and Cognitive Skills—A Problem Solving Program for Children.* Research Press, 1981.

Ingersoll B: *Your Hyperactive Child: A Parent's Guide to Coping With Attention Deficit Disorders.* Doubleday, 1988.

Wender PH: *The Hyperactive Child, Adolescent, and Adult.* Oxford Univ Press, 1987.

AGGRESSIVE ANTISOCIAL BEHAVIOR PROBLEMS

Essentials of Diagnosis

- Fighting and physically attacking other children or adults.
- Behavior often boisterous, disruptive, and argumentative, with a "chip on the shoulder" attitude.
- Probable evidence of family disturbance or disharmony.
- Frequent coexistence of poor achievement in children over 10 years of age.
- Incidence more common among less intelligent children.

General Considerations

Destructive, aggressive behavior is common in preschool children but declines significantly with the developmental shift at 5–7 years of age. Nevertheless, it is one of the most malignant behavior problems of childhood. It is more common in boys than in girls. By age 6–8, most normal children have shown a marked decrease in aggressive behavior. A significant number of those who continue to show aggressive behavior after 8 years of age will be aggressive in adolescence. Aggressive behavior is less likely to persist in children who identify with the values of one or both parents. Family disharmony and disturbance are the most important contemporaneous instigators of aggressive behavior problems at school.

Clinical Findings

A. History: Active destructive behavior is often seen at an early age and is frequently accompanied by risk-taking and other forms of behavior that make the child difficult to manage. The parents are often characterized as too strict or too lax, providing the child with little supervision or sense of belonging, and often openly rejecting the child. Aggressive behavior by the parents often complicates the diagnosis, since the child may be merely imitating the parents' behavior. Aggressive children of aggressive parents, however, often reject the parents' values even as they imitate the parents' behavior.

B. Symptoms and Signs: The most important information is from teacher, parent, and other reports of aggressive, antisocial, or disruptive behavior. Because some aggressive behavior is present in most children, only teacher and parent rating scales for general behavior that show increases of at least 1.5 SD above normal in amount of aggressive behavior should be considered significant. Neurologic examination usually shows normal results. Intelligence may be average or above average, but aggressive problems occur more frequently in children with lower IQs. Achievement may be average in the first few years of school but shows a steady decline after third grade, frequently accompanied by truancy. Learning delays in all areas are common in the aggressive delinquent adolescent, but 26% show evidence of specific learning disorders. (Most children with specific learning disability are not aggressive, however.) In early school years, the cognitive pattern of aggressive boys tends to show more impulsiveness and less verbal mediation activity than that of normal boys. By adolescence, the typical antisocial, aggressive boy shows a characteristic pattern of decreased verbal intelligence relative to nonverbal, impulsive stereotyped thinking and immaturity in ego development.

Treatment

Large-scale delinquency prevention programs for young aggressive boys have been unsuccessful even when they provided remedial reading instruction as well as counseling and family support. Small-scale behavior modification programs have had some success in normalizing cognitive and social behavior or slowing the increase in delinquent behavior. Psychotherapy and other methods of treatment have met with more modest success.

Behavior modification or other treatment programs are typically designed and monitored by psychologists or child psychiatrists. For younger children (6–8 years of age), the Think Aloud program has been used successfully by teachers, psychologists, social workers, and other mental health workers to help normalize both cognitive and social behavior at school.

When attention deficit disorder accompanies aggressive behavior problems, stimulant medication is sometimes helpful in decreasing general disruptive behavior as well as impulsiveness and distractibility, but the response may be quite variable.

Camp BW, Ray RS: Aggression. In: *Cognitive Behavior Therapy for Children.* Meyers A, Craighead LW (editors). Plenum Press, 1984.

Lefkowitz MM et al: *Growing Up to Be Violent.* Pergamon Press, 1977.

REFERENCES

Levine MD et al: *Developmental and Behavioral Pediatrics.* Saunders, 1983.

Mussen PH (editor): *Carmichael's Manual of Child Psychology,* vols 1–4. Wiley, 1983.

Reynolds CR, Mann L (editors): *Encyclopedia of Special Education,* vols 1–3. Wiley, 1987.

Rubin IL, Crocker AC: *Developmental Disabilities: Delivery of Medical Care for Children and Adults.* Lea & Febiger, 1989.

Thompson RJ Jr, O'Quinn AN: *Developmental Disabilities: Etiologies, Manifestations, Diagnoses, and Treatments.* Oxford Univ Press, 1979.

6 Psychosocial Aspects of Pediatrics & Psychiatric Disorders

R. Barkley Clark, MD

HIGHLIGHTS OF CHILD & FAMILY DEVELOPMENT

DEVELOPMENTAL STAGES

Anyone who provides for the medical or emotional needs of children understands that children change dramatically throughout the process of growing up. Each period of development offers a characteristic set of challenges and problems for children and parents alike. The manifestations of stress and of disease also change as the child changes over time. The planning of interventions by health care providers must therefore be in tune with the developmental level of the child and the corresponding needs of the parents. For these reasons, the chapter begins with a review of some of the highlights of child development that relate particularly to the psychosocial care of children. The struggles that caregivers face in providing a nurturing environment for their children are also noted. (See also Table 6–1.)

The Infant

The central developmental challenge of infancy is the emergence of specific emotional attachments, or bonds, between the infant and its caregivers. Those attachment bonds, in turn, form the basis for all meaningful and rewarding human relationships throughout the life span.

This period of forming emotional attachments is now recognized as a time of great reciprocal interaction between the child and the caregivers, with the child being an active participant in the attachment process. Shortly after birth, the child begins to display a powerful attachment behavior—the innate capacity to smile, particularly in response to the visual presentation of the human face. By the age of 2 or 3 months, the child is already beginning to smile preferentially in response to the face and voice of the primary caregivers, and by 6 months of age, a substantial bond has already been formed.

In assessing the process of attachment, one can learn much from observing the reciprocally reinforced smiles that pass between the 3- to 6-month-old infant and the primary attachment figure (typically, but not necessarily, the mother). If this process is progressing normally, the infant and the mother experience an obvious mutual pleasure in the interaction of smiling and "talking softly" to one another. In fact, the mutual pleasure in the interaction encourages further smiling and talking, which in turn further strengthens the emotional attachment bonds. Infants aged 3–4 months who do not smile interactively in response to the slow approach of a smiling, nodding, and cooing human face should be considered at risk for a primary disorder of attachment (eg, a pervasive developmental disorder). Likewise, infants at 4–6 months of age who do not smile preferentially and enthusiastically at their primary caregiver's smiling and nodding face should be considered at risk for a reactive attachment disorder (eg, maternal deprivation or disabilities in mothering).

By 6–8 months of age, the infant can clearly differentiate the primary attachment figure from other individuals. This ability is manifest even before 6 months in the wariness of infants around "strangers" (even fathers), and by 6–8 months of age, overt distress in the presence of strangers is usually apparent. This developmental landmark of stranger distress heralds the onset of the infant's capacity to recognize and distinguish the mother's face from the faces of other human beings. At the same time, beginning at 8–10 months of age, the inability of the infant to evoke a memory of the mother explains in part the separation anxiety that is seen with the threatened absence of the mother.

An understanding of these developmental landmarks can assist in the clinical assessment of the attachment process; the physician can use information about a child's distress at strangers and the onset of separation anxiety as early as 7–8 months of age. The infant who is normally attached is at ease and smiling while on the mother's lap and while looking at her face. As the physician approaches the infant and mother, and as the baby notices the physician, the face sobers; the infant then turns to face the mother.

Table 6–1. Highlights of child and family development.

Stage (Age)	Developmental Tasks	Developmental Landmarks	Developmental Concerns	Pitfall for Caregivers
Infancy (birth to 1 year)	Emotional attachment	2–3 months: responsive social smile. 7–9 months: distress in the presence of "strangers."	Temperamental variations (including colic)	Exhaustion. Lack of emotional support. Unexpected temperament. Unfulfilled expectations and fantasies.
Toddler (1–3 years)	Beginning of the separation-individuation process	8–24 months: separation anxiety. 12 months: locomotion. 15 months: "no." 24–36 months: bowel training.	Sleep disturbances (separation or over-stimulation). Breath holding and temper tantrums. "Terrible twos," ie, oppositional behavior, accident proneness.	Exhaustion. Autonomous strivings of child seen as rejection or adversarial relationship. Need for parents to set limits seen as parental failure. "Permissiveness" seen as good parent-child interaction.
Preschooler (3–6 years)	Taming of the internal world of fantasy	Symbolic play	Childhood fears: bedtime, darkness, ghosts, and monsters.	Competitive strivings of child seen as personal challenge. Egocentricity of child seen as selfishness.
School age (6–11 years)	Skills development	7 years: logical thought processes (cause-and-effect thinking); games and organizations with rules.	Continued childhood fears. School avoidance. Learning disabilities. Primary nocturnal enuresis.	Parental discomfort with separation from child. High expectations for child's performance, which is perceived as necessary for parent's own self-esteem.
Adolescence (11–20 years)	Continuation of the separation-individuation process. Identity formation ("Who am I?"). Gaining independence.			
Early (11–15 years)		Puberty: "best friends" of same sex. Self-absorption. Painful concerns about appearance.	Adolescent "turmoil"	Child's attachment to peer group seen as rejection. Self-absorption seen as irresponsible disregard for others. Exasperation with the child's changing moods.
Middle (15–17 years)		Heterosexual interests. Beginning of a truce with parents.	Adolescent sexuality	Prudish indignation. Sexual stimulation of the opposite-sex parent. Envy and anger at child's youthful energy and appearance. Rivalry and competition with suitors.
Late (17–20 years)		Orientation toward future. Pursuit of an adult work-role identity.	Will the young adult "make it"?	"Empty nest syndrome." Sense of loss and grief.

The child may cry vigorously when taken off the mother's lap for examination. The child's distress at seeing a strange face approaching and further distress when separated from the mother are signs that the attachment process is proceeding satisfactorily.

By 12 months of age, strong attachment bonds are firmly in place with primary caregivers and, to a somewhat lesser degree, with other prominent persons involved in caring for the child. By 12 months, prolonged separation from attachment figures, particularly in the context of unfamiliar surroundings, such as a hospital, can lead to a predictable series of reactions (described by John Bowlby) involving stages of protest, despair, and, ultimately, emotional detachment.

Bowlby J: Childhood mourning and its implications for psychiatry. Am J Psychiatry 1961;118:481.

Metcalf AW: Child, adolescent, and adult development. In: *Review of General Psychiatry*, 3rd ed. Goldman HH (editor). Appleton & Lange, 1992.

Minde K & Benoit D: Infant Psychiatry: It's Relevance for the General Psychiatrist. Brit J Psychiatry 1991; 159:173.

The Toddler

The toddler stage of development begins at about 1 year of age with the onset of locomotion and the use of a pincer grasp. These two developmental milestones allow children first to begin to move away from their caregivers to explore the world and second to begin to provide for themselves by self-feeding.

These landmarks herald the onset of the child's innate thrust toward independence that will become more vigorous during childhood, adolescence, and early adult life. This beginning process of developing independence during the toddler years is referred to as separation-individuation.

The developmental challenge of the separation-individuation phase is the child's development of a sense of personal mastery and autonomy, particularly in relation to a sense of control over the child's own body. This stage of development provides children with a deep sense of pride in the experience of their own activities and accomplishments and, finally, in the achievement of bowel control.

The young toddler has a love affair with the world. Children at this age are enamored of their own activities and excited by all they find in the world around them. At the same time, they are encouraged and reinforced by the delight they perceive in the expressions of caregivers regarding their wonderful new skills.

It is important at this point to stress the development of good self-esteem. A central concept is "mirroring," namely, the information children gather about themselves, over time, from the facial expressions of those around them—particularly those to whom they are emotionally attached. The earliest underpinnings of good self-esteem arise in the reciprocal and interactive smiling that occurs between the infant and the caregivers and then continue in the delight the caregivers feel in the toddler's emerging skills of independence. The personal pleasure the caregiver experiences in being with the child and observing its newly found skills of independence is reflected back to the child as information about the self. Over many years, the facial expressions of caregivers become internalized within children as deep-seated feelings and convictions about their own positive self-worth. In short, children learn much about themselves from what the world reflects back.

While the toddler is having its love affair with the world (in the form of physical activity, exploration, and beginning independence), the developmental process is complicated, at least for caregivers, by three conflicting developmental problems: willfulness, poor judgment, and separation anxiety. Regarding willfulness, Rene Spitz pointed out the importance of the child's acquisition and use of the word "no." After "mama" and "dada," "no" is frequently the first word in a child's vocabulary. Children's use of "no," either in verbal expression or in action through behavioral opposition, signifies the powerful wish on their part to be in control of themselves. This drive for self-control and self-determination is strong and should ultimately result in responsible, self-directed behavior in the future, but in the meantime it is responsible for the temper tantrums, the breath holding, and the oppositional behavior that characterize many toddlers. Because of this strong-mindedness

(and in particular the use of "no"), this period is often called "the terrible twos."

One of the biggest problems associated with children's exuberance and striving for self-determination is that their judgment is poor at this time. For example, running into the street, thrusting fingers into electrical outlets, and rummaging in medicine cabinets are clear dangers. These impulses elicit in caregivers a sense of duty to limit the child's behavior—ie, the parents must say "no" themselves. The first noticeable conflict between caregiver and child now surfaces, and that state of conflict, though absolutely necessary, is experienced as unpleasant by both child and caregiver. It portends disagreements in the future, and it places the caregiver in the sometimes difficult position of "the heavy." An important key to child rearing (in relation to the child's innate thrust toward independent functioning) is to strike a balance: autonomous behavior is enthusiastically rewarded and supported, while dangerous, destructive, or disruptive behavior is consistently and calmly limited.

The child's delight with activity and exploration is further complicated by the presence of separation anxiety. Separation anxiety begins as early as 8–10 months of age, generally peaks during the middle of the second year of life, and then gradually subsides in the latter part of the second and the beginning of the third year of life. Separation anxiety becomes manifest when the toddler perceives the threatened loss of support of the primary attachment figures. Signs typically include a distressed expression, with or without crying, and active behavioral attempts on the part of the toddler to become reunited with the parenting figures. Separation anxiety is thought by Bowlby to represent a genetically determined adaptive mechanism that promotes the safety of young children by increasing physical proximity with caregivers. Mahler refers to the need of toddlers to be "emotionally refueled" by intermittent contact with their primary attachment figures during times of exploration of the environment. Depending on the intensity of the separation anxiety, the toddler may need only brief visual contact with the parent, or the child may need physical contact and even comfort from that parent. Although remnants of separation anxiety can be seen in young school-age children—particularly in times of stress such as the start of school—the intensity and frequency of separation anxiety are thought to wane in the third year of life as children become able to calm themselves by evoking the image of their attachment figures or, at least, the feelings of safety associated with them.

The development of bowel control can be viewed as a prototype for the development of self-control in a more general sense. First, adults need to remind themselves that feces is not an inherently unpleasant or disgusting substance to toddlers. Young children play happily while soiled or will even play with feces as they might with clay. In fact, 2- and 3-year-olds often express pleasure in the "wonderful" bowel movement they have produced. The importance of this concept lies in the fact that the child must accept and take on the caregiver's view that a bowel movement is something that belongs only in certain places (ie, in the potty) and not in public (eg, in one's pants).

To incorporate the caregivers' point of view about bowel movement, the child must have the desire to please them. This desire implies a strong and positive attachment to caregivers and that the child's needs are being met—eg, appropriate care, emotional responsiveness, and positive mirroring responses from the parents. In short, the relationship between the child and caregiver is not tinged with the anger that exhausted and disillusioned caregivers feel when dealing with demanding and frustrated children.

Finally, the wish to please the responsive parent must then be reconciled with the toddler's powerful wish for control over the self. If the child's wish for self-determination is not adequately respected and if playful explorations are not encouraged, the child then feels overly controlled or coerced by too many "no's" from caregivers. The child can then develop an attitude that reflects, in effect, this view: "One thing that you cannot control is where I put my bowel movement." And in this case, the child is correct.

If, however, the child's developmental thrust toward exploration and independence has not been thwarted by too many stifling parental "noes" and if the parent-child relationship is such that the child wishes to please the parents, the child will then internalize the parents' attitude about where to put bowel movements (ie, how to behave); such children experience the personal pleasure and pride associated with *their own* proper use of the potty for its intended purpose. In the end, children who voluntarily to use the toilet not only experience positive reinforcement from their caregivers but at the same time feel pride in a personal accomplishment. An important step toward socially appropriate autonomous functioning has thus been taken.

Bowlby J: Childhood mourning and its implications for psychiatry. Am J Psychiatry 1961;118:481.

Lieberman AF: *The Emotional Life of the Toddler.* The Free Press. 1993.

Metcalf AW: Child, adolescent, and adult development. In: *Review of General Psychiatry,* 3rd ed. Goldman HH (editor). Appleton & Lange, 1992.

The Preschool Child

By the time children reach 3 years of age, an important developmental shift is already occurring: the child no longer behaves simply in relation to caregivers. The focus turns to the mental world of thoughts and feelings within the child. This shift was described by Piaget as movement from a plane of action (the sensory-motor stage of cognitive development) to the plane of thought (the preoperational stage of cognitive development). While the behavior of the infant is directed primarily toward facilitating and maintaining attachment with primary caregivers and that of the toddler toward expressing the beginning of independence from the parents, the preschool child is mentally aware of thoughts and feelings regarding the caregivers. The 3- and 4-year-old child can begin to think (albeit illogically), and with that developmental achievement a tremendous new world of thought, fantasy, and worry confronts the child.

The central developmental task of the preschool child is essentially to sort out the wondrous and sometimes frightening world that comes with thought. This new cognizance includes awareness of such exciting issues as the perception of differences between the sexes and the ensuing curiosity and worry about those differences. It includes the boastful wish to be big and powerful and the fantasy of being on a par with one's parents and even being able to displace them from their perceived positions of power and privilege.

Because preschoolers perceive themselves as being at the center of the universe, they come to believe that everyone around them must also be aware of their thoughts and motives. This perceived exposure fills the mental world of the preschool child with unspeakable dangers, leading to worries about caregivers' withdrawal of their love and admiration and even their angry physical retaliation. Preschool children are caught between wondrous fantasies on the one hand and prohibitions, dangers, and worries on the other.

The outward behavioral manifestations of this wondrous world of thought and fantasy include "showing off" behaviors, exhibiting the genitalia, sexual curiosity (exploration and comparison with other children), and competitive struggles for the parents' affection. At the same time, children display the content of their mental worlds in symbolic play. The little girl may act out coming home to favored status with daddy, and the little boy may become "superboy" slaying dragons or flying through the air.

The frightening and worrisome aspects of the child's mental world become manifest in fears (particularly at night) about ghosts, monsters, dangerous animals, and the dark. Children may even develop transient phobic symptoms that represent the displacement of internal worries onto objects in the outside world. Finally, preschool children are usually greatly concerned about bodily injury; thus, everyday "ouchies" need special care, and trips to the doctor for shots, stitches, and throat cultures are associated with considerable anxiety.

The preschool stage of mental development comes to a close as the child learns to moderate—and in a sense give up—fantasies of power and privilege by identifying with the rules for self-control represented by the observed behavior of the child's own loved ones. The internalization of parental rules and values means that children no longer have to worry so much about angering people they love and depend on. Furthermore, despite all the emotional turmoil, the child remains the object of the parents' love and attention. Recognizing this fact ultimately leaves the child in a calmer mental state. Generally, the child clearly identifies with an adult model of the same sex and is now ready to focus mental energies on adapting to the challenges to be found at school and in the social community away from the home.

Shonkoff JP: Preschool. In: *Developmental-Behavioral Pediatrics.* Levine MD et al (editors). Saunders, 1992.

Sours JA: The Oedipal and latency years. In: *Handbook of Clinical Assessment of Children and Adolescents.* Kestenbaum CH, Williams DT (editors). New York Univ Press, 1988.

The School-Age Child

Although the child of grade school age may still show residual evidence of earlier developmental challenges in the form of stress-induced separation anxiety (eg, with the start of school) and persistent nighttime fears, most children by this time should be prepared to expend mental energy to the tasks of learning and to expand their range of social interactions beyond the family. The developmental challenge of this age is to acquire confidence in mastering skills—athletic, academic, and social.

By the age of 7–8 years, the school-age child has developed the more logical and coherent thought processes that are necessary for formal academic learning (Piaget's stage of concrete mental operations, during which logical relationships of cause and effect are first perceived). The school-age child becomes involved with organized peer group activities (clubs, teams) where the rules of the game and acceptable codes of conduct become important. The child begins to devote time and energy to the development of skills, whether on the athletic field, in hobbies, or in schoolwork. Girls at this age are frequently more advanced than boys, particularly in academic endeavors. Kindergarten and first-grade boys are much more apt to be "developmentally immature" (ie, lacking in impulse control) than are girls of the same age.

Children of this age begin to experience pleasure in their ability to organize and categorize information. One may see a preoccupation with collections (eg, stamps, baseball cards, dolls) and, at the same time, they begin to exclude other children from certain activities because they are in some way perceived as different from the rest of the peer group.

During the school-age years, children should develop a sense of confidence about their abilities. The development of skills (whether athletic, academic, or social) is an important source of enhancement to self-esteem. Children with learning disorders, developmental disabilities, or problems of temperament (at-

tention, self-control) are at risk for low self-esteem. Families should avoid unrealistically high expectations of their children's performance to avoid the emotional burden of failure to "measure up."

Combrinck-Graham L: *Development of School-Age Children. In: Child and Adolescent Psychiatry: A Comprehensive Textbook.* Lewis M (editor). Williams & Wilkins, 1991.

The Adolescent

Adolescence is a stage of transition between childhood, when more emotional and physical dependence on caregivers is the rule, and adulthood, when independent and autonomous functioning is sustained without the continuous support of the family of origin. The stage of adolescence is relatively long in Western society, lasting from the onset of puberty (roughly, 11 years of age) to just beyond the high school years (roughly, age 18–20), when the individual sets out to fashion an adult identity in the working world. Developmentalists call this the second period of separation and individuation, a reliving of aspects of the "terrible twos." Parents may dread what they expect to be a period of turmoil and rebellion, but in fact the developmental tasks of adolescence are quite noble: to achieve a unique identity (answering the question, "Who am I?") and leave behind childhood dependency on the primary caregivers. Furthermore, for the vast majority of adolescents, the journey is not a tumultuous one. Four-fifths of adolescents characterize themselves as happy and enjoying life, with positive feelings about their parents (Offer, 1990). Emotional turmoil during this time is not a psychologic norm but is apt to be a sign of significant pathology.

Adolescence can be divided into early, mid, and late periods.

For most parents, **early adolescence** (roughly, ages 11–15) is the most difficult. This is when young people turn their interests away from the family and form attachments with peers of the same sex. The shift to an emotional investment outside the family may be coupled with an active distancing and pushing away from the family, a transition that is frequently painful to parents. In addition, early adolescents are notoriously inconsistent and somewhat volatile in their frequently anxious moods. They are egocentrically self-absorbed and painfully concerned about outward appearances and often question parental authority.

Mid adolescence (roughly, ages 15–17) tends to be a less difficult time for parents. Although young people begin to focus their attention on relationships with members of the opposite sex (a source of concern for many parents), mid-adolescents have typically become less emotionally labile, less anxious about their physical appearance, and with a less urgent need for conformity with the peer group. The result is a relative truce with parents and a calmer approach to the tasks of daily life. In addition, by mid adolescence, 30–50% of teens have achieved the capacity for abstract thought processes associated with Piaget's stage of **formal mental operations.** For this reason, the adolescent now takes a more thoughtful approach to situations that once provoked impulsive action.

In **late adolescence** (roughly, ages 17–20), the individual is looking toward the future. This shift in focus coincides with high school graduation and plans for leaving home. Patterns of behavior are strongly resemble what the individual has learned from the parents. The young person is, in effect, coming full circle from the initial rejection of parental values in early adolescence to a partial internalization of those values by late adolescence. Late adolescence is a time to work toward the goal of emotional and economic independence from the family of origin.

Metcalf AW: Child, adolescent, and adult development. In: *Review of General Psychiatry,* 3rd ed. Goldman HH (editor). Appleton & Lange, 1992.

Offer D, Boxer AM: Normal Adolescent Development: Empirical Research Findings. In: *Child & Adolescent Psychiatry: A Comprehensive Textbook.* Lewis M (editor). Williams & Wilkins, 1991.

Offer D et al: Normality and adolescence. Psychiatr Clin North Am 1990;13:377.

FAMILY LIFE

Family Functions

The structure of families has changed in recent years with the increase in the number of single-parent homes and reconstituted families and the decline in extended families. Despite these changes, the nuclear family continues to play a vital role in meeting the needs of society and of individual family members. The family serves the following functions: (1) the rearing of offspring to become autonomous adults, and eventually competent parents, within the context of societal expectations; and (2) meeting the needs of individual family members for nurturing, protection, feedback, recognition (mirroring), promoting adaptive behaviors, and emotional closeness and support.

The Parental Unit

The cornerstone of family functioning is the parental unit. Whether this parental unit consists of a marriage relationship, a single parent, or other family members, it must serve as the source of leadership and power in the family. The parental unit must meet the emotional and physical needs of other, more dependent family members while at the same time defining the norms of behavior that will lead to adaptive, independent functioning in the future. In short, the ways in which the parental unit exercises its leadership roles determine in large part the health or sickness of the family and its individual members.

Parenthood, as defined above, is emotionally and physically draining. In order for the parental unit to fulfill its vital role as provider and setter of limits for the family, the parties must have their own source of adult support and nurturance. In the case of a healthy marriage, the marital partners provide the necessary emotional support, respite, problem-solving advice, and adult companionship. Finding this support is more difficult for single parents, who have no "in-house" source of adult support; in such cases, unfortunately, the child is at risk of becoming a pseudo-adult companion to the single parent.

The lack of a solid marital relationship can be an important factor in virtually any child-centered problem. To function successfully as a parental unit, the couple must find the marriage mutually satisfying in the following ways: (1) the partners nurture and affirm each other; (2) the partners trust and respect each other; (3) the partners are able to recognize and resolve conflict within the marriage; and (4) the partners' needs for intimacy and sexuality are met satisfactorily within the marriage.

When the parental unit is weakened by marital dissatisfaction or by persistent marital conflict, children are at risk of becoming the focus of parental conflict. In effect, the child becomes the focus of parental attention and concern, thus "detouring" the conflict within the marriage unit onto the child. The parental concern about the child distracts the parents from their own marital problems, and the child ends up functioning as a buffer between the parents. Questions designed to screen the quality of the marital and parental relationship are outlined in the section on screening for psychosocial problems and disorders.

Barker P: Healthy families and their development. In: *Basic Family Therapy.* Oxford Univ Press, 1992.

Pruett KD: Family development and the roles of mothers and fathers in child rearing. In: *Child & Adolescent Psychiatry: A Comprehensive Textbook.* Lewis M (editor), Williams & Wilkins, 1991.

Issues in Parenthood

In rearing children, parents undertake a potentially rewarding but often tiring and frustrating task. The greatest pitfalls in parenting involve (1) physical and emotional exhaustion, and (2) unfulfilled expectations about having children. All of these can be provided in part by a mate who shares in the parenting responsibilities. In this regard, the "women's movement" has helped men broaden their parental roles and personal identities to include more nurturing activities. At the same time, single parents are at a relative disadvantage regarding the availability of a built-in support system.

In addition to the physical and emotional support derived from a mate or "significant other" (eg, a relative, a roommate, or an adult child care provider), primary caregivers are partly replenished emotionally by their child's responsiveness (in the form of smiles and excitement in the presence of the parent) and by memories of the care they received from their own parents. Children who are developmentally disabled or temperamentally difficult consume more parental energy and may not be as emotionally responsive and rewarding. The parent who had inadequate care as a child can call on fewer positive memories to help replenish energy stores.

Parental exhaustion decreases the parent's emotional and physical responsiveness toward the child and brings about a state of anger and frustration. A mild consequence may be a state of tension—a more extreme one, child abuse and neglect.

The second major pitfall in parenting involves the disappointment that comes when expectations are unfulfilled. Parents want their children to be healthy, competent, and happy. They hope that they themselves will be able to meet the child's needs and in doing so feel a sense of accomplishment and fulfillment.

Parents may also have unrealistic fantasies about their children that may serve to satisfy their own unmet needs for admiration and respect. Such fantasies may include basking in the glow of a child's exceptional achievements. Parents may fantasize that their children will thank them for all of their hard work in parenting and may even hope they will feel loved by their children in ways that will relieve the pain and loneliness they feel in their own lives.

Parents who have children with illnesses, disabilities, and temperamental difficulties have to adjust their expectations so that they can realistically meet the child's special needs. That adjustment involves grieving over the loss of the child that was hoped for but did not materialize.

For the individual whose hope was to compensate for personal unhappiness through parenthood, raising children can become an exercise in futility and a burden to the child unable to meet the parent's needs.

Each new phase of child development presents unique challenges. In infancy, irregular sleep-wake cycles and the necessity for constant care become physically exhausting, especially to a single parent. The physical demands are even greater if the child is not easily soothed.

During the toddler years, the child's striving for autonomy and independence can be misunderstood. To parents, the behavioral opposition and verbal "noes" of toddlers can seem like a rejection of parental caretaking. The resulting pain and anger can manifest itself either in irritation with the child or in attempts to smooth the relationship by giving in to the child's demands. In the former case, the child's autonomous strivings are met with parental displeasure; in the latter, the child becomes a tyrant.

In the later preschool years, parents are faced with competitive challenges from their children. A sense of humor and perspective, combined with a solid marital relationship, allows parents to balance respect for the child's wishes to be "big" with the ability to set firm limits that maintain boundaries between the private lives of the parents (eg, the parents' bedroom) and their children.

During the elementary school years, parents must come to grips with allowing their children to experience the challenges that await them outside the home and family. Parental support of skill development must be balanced with realistic definitions of success. Persistent separation anxiety on the part of parents and unrealistic standards of performance can contribute to a child's anxiety during school years.

Adolescence presents a number of challenges to parents. The early adolescent presents unpredictable changes of mood, intense attachment to peers, and a self-centered point of view, all of which deprive parents of the positive feedback they once enjoyed from the child who wanted to please the parents. Not since infancy and the toddler years have parents received so little gratitude for their efforts. And, as in toddler years, parents must remind themselves that what may seem to be a rebuff is in fact a further step along the child's road to independence. Again, like parents of toddlers, the parents of young adolescents need to support autonomy while preventing tyranny and disaster.

The sexual interests of the middle adolescent can elicit a variety of parental reactions related to parents' own concerns about sexuality. Parental reactions range from pride to fear to envy to sexual stimulation.

Finally, as the late adolescent prepares to leave home, parents face the sense of loss and grief associated with the launching of offspring into the world. Parents need to mourn the loss and, at the same time, begin to recommit to the primary importance of the marriage once the offspring leave the nest.

Pruett KD: Family development and the roles of mothers and fathers in child rearing. In: *Child & Adolescent Psychiatry: A Comprehensive Textbook.* Lewis M (editor). Williams & Wilkins, 1991.

PSYCHOSOCIAL ASSESSMENT OF CHILDREN & FAMILIES

Five to 15 percent of children in the USA are affected by psychiatric disorders, and nearly 50% of pediatric office visits are related to psychosocial or developmental problems. These statistics underscore the importance of being able to screen for and recognize psychosocial problems in children and their families.

SCREENING FOR PSYCHOSOCIAL PROBLEMS & PSYCHIATRIC DISORDERS WITHIN THE CONTEXT OF HEALTH MAINTENANCE

Although important information about psychosocial problems is obtained by interviewing children and observing the interaction of parents and their children, most authorities agree that the most efficient indicator in screening for psychosocial problems is the history provided by caregivers. Psychosocial screening with a focus on the caregiver can lead to information from three sources of data found in the pediatric office: checklists of specific symptoms completed by caregivers, general questioning of parents about psychosocial functioning, and physician-parent discussions of normal and expected child behavior at different developmental levels.

Murphy et al (1992) have devised a 35-item pediatric symptom checklist (Table 6–2) designed to screen children 6–12 years of age for psychosocial dysfunction. The checklist is to be completed in the waiting room by a parent or other caregiver. Each item is rated by the parents as "often" (two points), "sometimes" (one point), or "never" present (no points). The information can be used in two ways: first, as a psychosocial review of symptoms and point of departure for the discussion of problems that "often" or "sometimes" occur; and second, as a general screening device, with a total score of 28 or higher indicating a need for in-depth psychosocial evaluation of the child. Pediatricians find the checklist a helpful instrument for psychosocial screening (Bishop, 1991).

Jellinek has also suggested five questions to be addressed to parents as a means of uncovering areas of concern. These same questions can be slightly rephrased and then directed to children as well. The mnemonic device "PSYCH" can facilitate the five questions:

(1) *P*arent-child interaction: How are things going with you and your child?

(2) *S*chool: How are things going in school? (Academically and behaviorally.)

(3) *Y*outh: How are things with peer relationships?

(4) *C*asa: How are things going at home? (Including siblings, the marriage, and parents as individuals.)

(5) *H*appiness: Describe your child's mood? (Comfortable and happy, versus tense and unhappy.)

Finally, by way of anticipatory guidance, age-appropriate behavior norms (Table 6–1) can be reviewed. Concerns about infant attachment, "the terrible twos," childhood fears, school problems, and adolescent behavioral problems can in this way be brought in the open for further discussion.

ASSESSMENT OF PSYCHOSOCIAL SIGNS & SYMPTOMS

When an emotional or behavioral sign or symptom is presented for evaluation, a more thorough psychosocial evaluation is indicated. Data must be collected from caregivers, from the child, and sometimes from school personnel and others acquainted with the child's functioning. At least 30 minutes should be scheduled for this purpose.

It is useful to see the parents and the patient first together, then the parents alone, and then the child alone. The physician thus is able to observe interactions among family members and give the parents and the child an opportunity to speak confidentially about their concerns. Parents and children often feel shame and guilt about some personal inadequacy they perceive to be causing the problem. The physician can ease that burden and facilitate the assessment by acknowledging that the family is trying to cope and that the ultimate task of assessment is to seek solutions and not to assign blame. An attitude of nonjudgmental inquiry can be captured in supportive statements such as, "Let's see if we can figure out what might be happening."

Obtaining Data

Psychosocial information obtained from the parties can be organized into the format that follows, which is offered as a framework but not as a "cookbook" recipe to be followed in rigid sequence.

A. History of the Presenting Problem: First, the physician should obtain a detailed description of the problem. When did it start? Were there unusual stresses at that time? How is the child's life and the family's functioning affected? What does the child say about the problem? What attempts have been made to alleviate the problem? Do the parties have any theories or opinions about the cause of the problem?

B. Review of Other Psychosocial Symptoms: The techniques used in screening for psychosocial problems that were described above can be used as a guide (Table 6–3).

THE CHILD INTERVIEW

Interviewing the Preschool Child

Because preschool children frequently experience significant distress when separated from their parents in a physician's office and because they lack the capacity to describe their problems in much detail, the physician can frequently gather more information by interviewing the parents and the child together. As the parents discuss their concerns, the physician can look for the following behaviors:

(1) Does the child use the parent as a source of security and support appropriately?

Table 6–2. Pediatric symptom checklist.[1] Parents are asked to indicate which category–Never, Sometimes, or Often–best fits their child, with 0, 1, or 2 points assigned to each answer, respectively. For interpretation of scores, see text.

	Never	Sometimes	Often
1. Complains of aches or pains			
2. Spends more time alone			
3. Tires easily, little energy			
4. Fidgets, is unable to sit still			
5. Has trouble with a teacher			
6. Is less interested in school			
7. Acts as if driven by a motor			
8. Daydreams too much			
9. Is distracted easily			
10. Is afraid of new situations			
11. Feels sad, unhappy			
12. Is irritable, angry			
13. Feels hopeless			
14. Has trouble concentrating			
15. Has less interest in friends			
16. Fights with other children			
17. Is absent from school			
18. Experiences a drop in school grades			
19. Is down on himself or herself			
20. Visits doctor, with doctor finding nothing wrong			
21. Has trouble with sleeping			
22. Worries a lot			
23. Wants to be with you more than before			
24. Feels he or she is bad			
25. Takes unnecessary risks			
26. Gets hurt frequently			
27. Seems to be having less fun			
28. Acts younger than children the same age			
29. Does not listen to rules			
30. Does not show feelings			
31. Does not understand other people's feelings			
32. Teases others			
33. Blames others for his or her troubles			
34. Takes things that belong to others			
35. Refuses to share			

[1]Modified and reproduced, with permission, from Murphy JM, Jellinek M: Screening for psychosocial dysfunction in economically disadvantaged and minority children: Further validation of the pediatric symptom checklist. Am J Orthopsychiatry 1988;58:450. Copyright © 1988 by the American Orthopsychiatric Association.

(2) Does the 2- to 5-year-old warm up to the strange environment and begin to explore the room and even interact with the physician from a distance?

(3) How does the child relate to toys that are offered?

(4) What is the child's activity level?

(5) Does the child display unusual mannerisms (eg, intense clinging, stereotypical motor behaviors)?

(6) Does the child disrupt or control the interview session?

(7) Does the parent attempt to place appropriate limits on behavior? How does the child respond?

It is helpful to have in the office toy figures the child can use to portray emotional states and interpersonal interactions. After hearing the history from the

Table 6–3. Screening for psychosocial problems.

Developmental history	Observation of parents

1. Review the landmarks of psychosocial development (Table 6–1)
2. Summarize the child's temperamental traits
3. Review stressful life events and the child's reactions to them
   a. Separations
   b. Losses
   c. Marital conflict
   d. Illnesses, injuries, and hospitalizations
4. Obtain details of past mental health problems and their treatment
Family history
1. Marital history
   a. Overall satisfaction with the marriage
   b. Conflicts or disagreements within the relationship
   c. Quantity and quality of time together away from children
   d. Whether the child comes between or is a source of conflict between the parents
   e. Marital history prior to having children
2. Parenting history
   a. Feelings about parenthood
   b. Whether parents feel united in dealing with the child
   c. "Division of labor" in parenting
   d. Parental energy or stress level
   e. Sleeping arrangements
   f. Privacy
   g. Attitudes about discipline
   h. Interference with discipline from outside the family (eg, ex-spouses, grandparents)
3. Stresses on the family
   a. Problems with employment
   b. Financial problems
   c. Changes of residence
   d. Illnesses/injuries/deaths
4. Family history of mental health problems
   a. Depression? Who?
   b. Suicide attempts? Who?
   c. Psychiatric hospitalizations? Who?
   d. "Nervous breakdowns"? Who?
   e. Substance abuse problems? Who?
   f. Nervousness or anxiety? Who?
	1. Do they agree on the existence of the problem or concern?
	2. Are they uncooperative or antagonistic about the evaluation?
	3. Does the parent appear depressed or overwhelmed?
	4. Can the parents present a coherent picture of the problem and their family life?
	5. Do the parents accept some responsibility for the child's problems, or do they blame forces outside the family and beyond their control?
	6. Do they appear burdened with guilt about the child's problem?
	Observation of the child
	1. Does the child acknowledge the existence of a problem or concern?
	2. Does the child want help?
	3. Is the child uncooperative or antagonistic about the assessment?
	4. What is the child's predominant mood or attitude?
	5. What does the child wish could be different (eg, "three wishes")?
	6. Does the child display unusual behavior (activity level, mannerisms, fearfulness)?
	7. What is the child's apparent cognitive level?
	Observation of parent-child interaction
	1. Do the parents show concern about the child's feelings?
	2. Does the child control or disrupt the joint interview?
	3. Does the child respond to parental limits and control?
	4. Do the parents inappropriately answer questions addressed to the child?
	5. Is there obvious tension between family members?
	Data from other sources
	1. Waiting room observations by office staff
	2. School (teacher, nurse, social worker, counselor)
	3. Department of social services

parents and after observing the child's activities, play, and affect, the physician may question the 3- to 5-year-old child about toy figures who appear to be feeling sad, worried, angry, or bossy. Children aged 3–5 are frequently able to confirm important interpersonal relationships and attitudes in their symbolic play activities.

Interviewing the School-Age Child

Most school-age children have mastered separation anxiety sufficiently to tolerate at least a brief interview with the physician. In addition, they have important information to share about their own worries, concerns, and problems.

The child should be told beforehand by the parents or physician (or both) that the doctor wishes to talk only to the child today about how he or she is feeling. School-age children understand and even appreciate parental concern about unhappiness, worries, and dif-

ficulty in getting along with people, and they are usually willing to discuss their perceptions of these problems.

At the outset, it is useful to restate the purpose of the interview, which is to explore the child's own opinions about certain issues raised by the parents. Rapport can be enhanced by asking if the child has ever talked with anyone before about how he or she feels. If the answer is yes, the child may explain more about what he or she liked or did not like about that discussion. If the child has never before talked about personal feelings with a professional, the physician can acknowledge that it is often not easy to talk with "a stranger" about some kinds of problems.

The physician should then ascertain whether the child agrees a problem exists (eg, unhappiness, worry, "not getting along"). If that is so, the physician should ask what the child can say about the magnitude of the problem, how it affects the child and the family, and what seems to be the cause.

Asking directly about how mom and dad get along can yield significant information about parental conflicts. A kinetic family drawing—"Draw your family and have everyone doing and saying something"—can provide clues to how the child fits into the family and how members of the family interact. Questions about school can yield information about life outside the home and with peers. Questions about worries, unhappy feelings, and what makes the child angry can develop unsuspected clues to the child's emotional life. Asking a child to make "three wishes" can help to uncover important concerns that may not have been apparent from the history of overt problems or symptoms. ("Let's pretend you could have anything or change anything. What would you wish for and why?")

At the end of the child interview, it is important to share or reiterate the salient points derived from the interview and to state that the next step is to talk further with the parents about trying to find ways to make things better for the child. At that time, it is good to discuss any concerns or misgivings that the child might have about sharing information with parents so that the child's right to privacy is not arbitrarily violated. Most children want and appreciate help to make things better and therefore will allow the physician to share appropriate concerns with the parents.

Interviewing the Adolescent

Because the developmental task of adolescence is to fashion an identity separate from that of the parents, the physician must show respect for the patient's point of view. That process begins with letting the patient from the outset participate in decisions about a format for the evaluation—meeting first alone with the physician, together with the parents, or after the physician has talked further with the parents. The parents need to be told why this is necessary, and the patient is then informed of the parents' expressed concern and the physician's wish to help the family determine whether a problem does in fact exist.

The issue of confidentiality must be approached forthrightly at the first interview. A good policy is to say, "What we talk about today is between you and me unless we decide someone should know or unless it appears to me that you might be in some danger."

The interview might then start with a restatement of the parents' concern. The patient is then encouraged to describe the situation in his or her own words. It can be helpful then to sum up the salient elements of the adolescent's account, thus confirming that the physician has been listening and understands the young person's point of view.

The physician should then ask questions designed to obtain information about the following areas of concern:

(1) Predominant mood state.
(2) Nature of relationships with family members.

(3) Level of satisfaction with school and peer relationships.
(4) Plans for the future.
(5) Drug and alcohol use.
(6) Worries or concerns.
(7) Biggest "stumbling block" in the adolescent's life.
(8) What the adolescent would like to be different.

In closing the interview, it is important that the physician review the salient points and discuss a plan either for further investigation or ways of dealing with the problem.

Bishop S et al: Psychosocial screening in pediatric practice: A survey of interested physicians. Clin Pediatr (Phila) 1991;30:142.

Lewis M: Psychiatric assessment of infants, children, and adolescents. In: *Child & Adolescent Psychiatry: A Comprehensive Textbook*. Lewis M (editor), Williams & Wilkins, 1991.

Murphy JM et al.: Screening for psychosocial dysfunction in pediatric practice. Clin Pediatr 1992;31:660.

Simmons JE: *Psychiatric Examination of the Child*. Lea & Febiger, 1987.

DIAGNOSTIC FORMULATION & INTERPRETATION OF FINDINGS

The diagnostic process starts with a description of the presenting problem. The presenting problems or symptoms are then scrutinized in the context of the child's age, developmental needs and tasks, temperament, the stresses and strains on the child and the family, and the functioning of the family system. The physician develops a diagnostic hypothesis, and when all is considered, the presenting problem is understood from one or more of the following perspectives:

(1) The behavior as described is within the range of normal, given the child's developmental level.
(2) The behavior is a temperamental variation.
(3) The behavior is the result of nervous system dysfunction.
(4) The behavior is a normal reaction to stressful circumstances (eg, medical illness, change in family structure, loss of a loved one).
(5) The problem is primarily due to family dysfunction.
(6) The problem is a manifestation of a psychiatric disorder.
(7) Some combination of the above.

The physician's interpretation of the findings is then presented to the family. The interpretive process includes the following components: (1) an explanation of how the presenting problem or symptom is a reflection of a hypothesized cause (eg, children frequently display a disturbance in conduct in the wake of stressful circumstances or become bossy or demanding when parent and child roles are not defined clearly enough); and (2) a suggested plan of interaction that is based on the hypothesized mechanism.

A joint plan—physician, parents, and child—is then formulated to address the developmental needs of the child in light of the family structure and current stresses. If a plan cannot be developed with a reasonable amount of effort by the parties, the question of referral to a mental health practitioner should be raised.

DEVELOPMENTAL DISTURBANCES & CONCERNS

Developmental disturbances represent variations in normal development; they are associated with symptoms in children that cause distress or concern on the part of their adult caregivers. As a result, parents frequently contact their health care providers with questions about the "terrible twos," childhood fears and anxieties, and adolescent rebellion. In these circumstances, the health care provider is faced with making the correct diagnosis, educating the concerned parents about normal developmental variations, and then (when needed) finding strategies to help the distressed parents facilitate normal parent-child interaction.

THE PUSHY PRESCHOOLER

The push for independence and autonomy that begins in the second year of life can pose problems for parents who are uncertain or insecure about their own role as parents when faced with setting limits on a child's behavior. Preschool children typically want to have their way even when it poses a danger or breaches generational boundaries. Many children try to decide when and what the family eats, what time they go to bed, and who sleeps in which bed. In short, preschool children can be quite demanding, pushy, and bossy—all as part of their rudimentary push to become independent.

The formidable task for parents is to respect the child's wish for self-determination while setting limits and providing guidance so that the child does not become tyrannical or out of control. Parents who are having difficulty placing limits on their child's behavior will present with one of the following types of complaints:

(1) "Discipline won't work with this child."

(2) "I can't get her to do what I ask without getting mad."

(3) "He says, 'I don't have to do it if I don't want to.'"

(4) "She won't sleep in her own bed."

(5) "Other children his age don't like him. He always wants his way."

(6) "Is this child hyperactive?"

Parents who have difficulty saying "no" calmly and yet firmly and convincingly frequently have one of two problems in parenting: (1) They are emotionally drained and do not have the energy to say "no" effectively, or (2) they believe that conflicts and disagreements in interpersonal relationships must be avoided. In the former case, parental depression or emotional exhaustion from working and single parenthood is common. In the latter case, the parent typically overidentifies with the frustrated child's distress and is then reminded of painful conflicts or unhappiness in his or her own life. Keeping the child "happy," ie, avoiding conflict, keeps the parent from feeling distressed and unhappy.

In planning interventions, the physician must educate the parents about the sometimes pushy nature of children who are "feeling their oats." With that explanation comes the need for external limits, because a child's judgment and self-control are as yet underdeveloped. Parents need to know that a child's disappointment and frustration with limits does not mean poor parenting or an unhappy child.

Parents who are emotionally depleted or depressed need to be cared for themselves, either through rest, emotional support, and assistance with parenting or through professional care for their depression.

In the case of a parent who avoids conflict, the physician should suggest addressing one or two discipline problems. For example, if toys are not picked up after a reminder, they are put away out of the child's reach for some announced period of time. Likewise, if a meal is not eaten within a reasonable and specified time limit, the food is taken away and snacks are withheld until the next meal. As the parent begins to feel more comfortably in control, the child's behavior typically becomes less oppositional; at this point, the parent should use positive reinforcement, eg, "I like the way you picked up your toys—let's read a story together."

Lieberman AF: The challenges of being (and raising) a toddler. In: *The Emotional Life of the Toddler.* Free Press, 1993.

CHILDHOOD FEARS & ANXIETIES

The mental world of the child is filled with magical wonders and, at the same time, threatening dangers. The result is that childhood is a time of both excitement and worry—the latter manifested by fears and anxieties.

In a study of nearly 500 randomly selected families, mothers reported that about 43% of their children had displayed at least seven fears or worries between 6 and 12 years of age. The vast majority of childhood fears are not associated with psychologic disorders; in fact, the fearful stimuli tend to evolve and change with age in a developmental sequence (see Table 6–4) and, overall, tend to decrease in frequency with age (Spence, 1993).

Although the manifestations of many developmental anxieties, such as separation distress and fear of the dark, may wax and wane over months or years, most specific childhood fears are transient (days to weeks in duration) and not associated with significant interference with daily life. In most cases, all that is needed is to reassure the parents about the developmental nature of fears; the parents, in turn, can then reassure their children that they will be fine even though they feel frightened at times. Fears become a source of greater concern to health care providers when they appear outside the normal developmental sequence of fears, when they are persistent, when they cause severe distress, or when they interfere with adaptive functioning, such as poor attendance at school or avoidance of peer relationships. Approximately 2–3% of children have fears significant enough to require specific mental health interventions.

Childhood fears and anxieties. Harvard Medical School Ment Hlth Lett (Aug) 1988;5:1.

Lapouse R, Monk MA: Fears and worries in a representative sample of children. Am J Orthopsychiatry 1959;29:803.

Spence SH, McCathie H: The stability of fears in children: A two-year prospective study: A research note. J Child Psychol Psychiatry 1993;34:579.

ADOLESCENT REBELLION & TURMOIL

Surveys of large adolescent populations confirm that adolescence is not the turbulent state depicted in individual clinical case studies. General theoretic impressions and sampling bias at one time tended to exaggerate the turmoil of normal adolescence.

Offer's (1969) longitudinal study of a sample of normal suburban middle class boys through their high school years identified only 21% as experiencing tumultuous unrest. On closer inspection, this population was distinguished from the remainder of the sample by lower socioeconomic status, more overt marital conflicts in the family, and a higher than normal incidence of mental illness in the family. Overall, approximately 20% of normal adolescents have a stormy course; another 20% progress continuously and smoothly through adolescence; and the remainder show normal overall adjustment but have had temporary difficulty during times of stress. Eighty percent of adolescents adjust successfully with no signs and symptoms of emotional disturbances unless confronted with clear socioenvironmental stressors.

When behavioral deviance or a clearly psychopathologic disorder is identified in adolescence, those problems tend not to remit with time. In short, adolescents with significant problems do not outgrow them. Continuity does therefore seem to exist between adolescent and adult psychopathology.

Offer D et al: Normality and adolescence. Psychiatr Clin North Am 1990;13:377.

Table 6–4. Sequence of developmental anxieties.

Age at First Appearance	Source of Anxieties
Early infancy	Sudden loud noises, unpredictable stimuli, loss of postural support, heights.
1 year	Stranger, unfamiliar situations and objects. Beginning of separation distress.
2–6 years	Animals, darkness, imaginary creatures (ghosts and monsters).
School age	Bodily injury, physical danger. Fear of loss of loved one.
Teens and adulthood	Fear of failure (eg, test anxiety), concerns about social acceptance, loss of a loved one, physical danger, natural disasters.

PSYCHIATRIC DISORDERS

Since the publication of the third edition of the American Psychiatric Association's *Diagnostic and Statistical Manual of Mental Disorders* in 1980, psychiatric disturbances have been classified on the basis of descriptive and phenomenologic data rather than presumed or hypothesized etiologic mechanisms. That trend continued in the revised edition published in 1987.

A psychiatric disorder is defined as a cluster of symptoms (ie, emotions, behaviors, psychologic states) that occur with statistically significant frequency within the identified population; furthermore, the symptoms are associated with subjective distress or maladaptive behavior. This definition presumes that the individual's symptoms are of such intensity, persistence, and duration that the ability to adapt to life's challenges is compromised.

About 10% of children and adolescents are personally affected by psychiatric disorders. As a general rule, these children will benefit from treatment by professionals experienced in the treatment of psychiatric disturbances.

American Psychiatric Association: *Diagnostic and Statistical Manual of Mental Disorders,* 3rd rev ed. American Psychiatric Press, 1987.

DISTURBANCES IN PARENT-INFANT INTERACTION

(Primary Caregiver Dysfunction)

Primary caregiver dysfunction can be defined as a failure to provide parenting functions (usually, but not necessarily, by the mother) because of parental vulnerability or disability, with the result that the parent is unable to meet the caretaking or developmental needs of the child. Although these parents have no single psychiatric diagnosis (in fact, they may not be formally diagnosable at all), they can manifest anxiety, distress, exhaustion, anger, or indifference in relation to the tasks of child care. Caregiver dysfunction can result in a number of symptoms that are presented to the health care provider, usually within the first 6 months of life (Table 6–5).

These individuals frequently have difficult psychosocial histories, find themselves currently without emotional or physical support, and have many unmet personal needs of their own (see Table 6–6). Characteristics of the child may also contribute to the parent's failure to "tune in and turn on" to the child's needs. These characteristics frequently define the child as different, defective, or disappointing in the parent's eyes (see Table 6–7).

Clinical Findings

The diagnosis of caregiver dysfunction is arrived at chiefly by interviewing the parents and in observing the interaction between parent and child. The child should be evaluated for organic disorders that could explain the presenting symptoms.

A history directed toward identification of specific parental risk factors should be obtained directly from the parent (Table 6–6), with particular reference to feelings of stress or being overwhelmed by the caretaking needs of the child or by the demands of daily life. Attention should be paid to the parents' description of the child and to parental symptoms of anxiety or depression manifest by tenseness, irritability, fatigability, tearfulness, sleep disturbance, and a wish to avoid or withdraw from daily activities.

Table 6–5. Signs and symptoms suggesting primary caregiver dysfunction.

Failure to thrive
Feeding problems
Delays in development
Signs of abuse
Frequent physician visits, especially for nonspecific concerns
Excessive parental worry about illness in the child
Inadequate physical care
Child perceived as "difficult to deal with"
Sleep problems

Table 6–6. Parental risk factors contributing to primary caregiver dysfunction.

Personal history of inadequate relations with own mothering figure
Isolation from an adult support system (eg, single parenthood)
Psychiatric disorders (particularly acute or chronic depression)
Chronic psychosocial or cognitive dysfunctions (eg, unstable relationships, school problems, legal problems, employment problems)
Unresolved grief over past losses
Marital discord
Poverty/financial problems
Personal or family illnesses
Unwanted or difficult pregnancy
Current life stresses (eg, loss of a relationship, recent illness, job loss)

In observing the parent-child interaction, the physician should look for the presence of reciprocity and mutual enthusiasm and enjoyment in the relationship, as opposed to pathologic signs of tension, irritability, or apathy on either side of the relationship.

Differential Diagnosis

Physical disorders that may explain the presenting symptoms must be ruled out, but it should also be noted that caregiver dysfunction and organic disease not infrequently coexist.

Complications

Unrecognized parental dysfunction can result in nonorganic failure to thrive, child abuse, later behavioral problems in the child, and another generation of children who will themselves probably display caregiver dysfunction as parents.

Treatment

Treatment is focused primarily on supporting and educating the parents. The physician should empathize, explaining that being a parent is difficult and tiring work and that it requires health, energy, and emotional support. The task is to help the parent feel well physically and emotionally and then to facilitate the development of appropriate child care skills. Any underlying medical or psychiatric disorder the parent may have should be treated, and a social support system for the parent should be found. Parenting skills are taught and positively reinforced over time.

Table 6–7. Characteristics of the child contributing to primary caregiver dysfunction.

Prematurity
Perinatal complications
Illness in the newborn
Birth defects
Multiple births
Difficult temperament (eg, unresponsive, irritable, difficult to soothe)

Prognosis

The prognosis depends greatly on the ability of the parent to view professional support and education as helpful rather than critical or indifferent.

Green M: Mothering disabilities. In: *Ambulatory Pediatrics.* Green M, Haggerty R (editors). Saunders, 1984.
Pruett KD: Disorders of the parent/child relationship. In: *Child Psychiatry,* vol 6. Solnit AJ et al (editors). Basic Books, 1986.

PERVASIVE DEVELOPMENTAL DISORDERS & SCHIZOPHRENIA

Pervasive developmental disorders and childhood schizophrenia are a group of early-onset, severe neuropsychiatric disorders that were once referred to as childhood psychoses. Today, pervasive developmental disorders (including autism) are categorized separately from childhood schizophrenia on the basis of clinical differences and family histories. "Pervasive developmental disorder" is a term that actually denotes a spectrum from autistic disorder (most severe) to language-related disorders (least severe).

1. AUTISTIC DISORDER

Essentials of Diagnosis

- Profound deficits in social responsiveness and interpersonal relatedness.
- Abnormal speech and language development.
- Behavioral peculiarities.
- Onset in infancy or early childhood.

General Considerations

Autism is uncommon, with an incidence of approximately 4:10,000 school-age children. More boys than girls are affected (3–4:1).

Although the cause of autism remains unknown, central nervous system dysfunction is suggested by the increased incidence of autism in populations affected by perinatal problems: rubella, phenylketonuria, tuberous sclerosis, infantile spasms, encephalitis, and fragile X syndrome. In addition, studies of twins reveal over 90% concordance for autism in monozygotic twins compared to 24% in dizygotic twins. No consistent psychopathologic pattern is seen in the parents of autistic children, though 25% of families with an autistic child have other family members with language-related disorders.

Clinical Findings

Profound deficits in reciprocal social interaction—eg, delayed or absent social smile, failure to anticipate interaction with caregivers, and a lack of attention to a primary caregiver's face—are often evident even in the first year of life. In toddlers, findings include deficiencies in imitative play and a relative lack of interest in interpersonal interactions. Language development is often quite delayed. In fact, children are often first referred for evaluation because they appear to lack responsiveness to spoken language and are presumed to be hearing-impaired. When speech does begin to develop, it frequently is not used for meaningful symbolic communication but is instead echolalic and nonsensical.

Autistic children often display peculiar interests, bizarre responses to sensory stimuli, repetitive, stereotypic motor behaviors (eg, twirling and hand flapping), odd posturing, self-injurious behavior, abnormal patterns of eating and sleeping, and unpredictable mood changes. About 70% have IQs of less than 70.

Differential Diagnosis

Although autism and mental retardation often coexist, the vast majority of mentally retarded children do not show the essential characteristics of autism. A hearing or visual impairment must be ruled out with appropriate screening. Children with developmental speech and language disorders typically show an interest in interpersonal interaction that is not seen in autistic children. Youngsters should be investigated for metabolic disorders and for the fragile X syndrome.

Complications

Approximately 25% of autistic individuals eventually develop a seizure disorder. Some autistic adolescents who have higher cognitive skills become depressed as they become partially aware of their deficits.

Treatment

Behaviorally oriented special education or day treatment programs are vital in helping the autistic child acquire more appropriate social, linguistic, self-care, and cognitive skills. The goal is to normalize the child's behavior and adaptive social skills.

Antipsychotic medications (particularly haloperidol in doses of 0.5–4 mg/d) can modify a variety of disruptive symptoms, including hyperactivity, aggressiveness, and negativism, thus making the child more accessible to education (Sloman, 1991). Fenfluramine may be helpful for a few autistic children (those with elevated serotonin), but stimulants can sometimes make the symptoms of autism more severe. Naltrexone may help control self-injurious behavior (Sandman, 1990/91).

Parents and families need strong support as well as education in coping with the disorder.

Prognosis

Autism is a lifelong disorder with an overall poor prognosis. Approximately one-sixth of autistic children become gainfully employed as adults, and another one-sixth are able function in sheltered workshops and halfway houses. Two-thirds need ongoing supervision and support. The best prognosis is seen in children who have normal, testable intelligence and who have developed significant symbolic language skills by the age of 5 years.

Mauk JE: Autism and pervasive developmental disorders. Pediatr Clin North Am 1993;40:567.

Sandman C: The opiate hypothesis in autism and self injury. J Child Adolesc Psychopharmacol 1990/91;1:237.

Sloman L: Use of medication in pervasive developmental disorders. Psychiatr Clin North Am 1991;14:165.

Wolff S: Childhood autism: Its diagnosis, nature, and treatment. Arch Dis Childhood 1991;66:737.

2. LESS SEVERE PERVASIVE DEVELOPMENTAL DISORDERS

Essentials of Diagnosis

- Social impairment, delayed language development, and behavioral peculiarities.
- Much less severe than autism.
- Onset by early childhood.

General Considerations

At the less severe end of the spectrum of pervasive developmental disorder are children who display a wide range of deficits in social and language skills but who are not so severely affected that they are identified as autistic. This group includes children with Asperger's syndrome (autistic-like children with normal intelligence [Szatmari, 1991]). In the past, many of these children would have been classed in the group manifesting "atypical development." Children with less severe forms of pervasive developmental disorders probably outnumber autistic children by as much as 2–3:1.

Clinical Findings

Despite having traits similar to those of autism, these children are generally much less severely affected and therefore have a greater ability to develop more appropriate social relationships, though they may be viewed by their peers as odd or eccentric. They frequently have delays in speech and language, particularly in understanding the nuances of communication. They generally tend to be concrete, rote thinkers. Many are able to control their behavioral peculiarities and are socially acceptable.

Differential Diagnosis

Specific developmental speech and language disorders should be distinguished. Hearing impairment should be ruled out with appropriate screening.

Treatment

The backbone of treatment is special education services designed to inculcate more appropriate social and language skills. Family education and support are important.

Some children may benefit from mental health treatment for depression as they become aware of their deficiencies. Psychoactive medications may be helpful for specific target symptoms.

Prognosis

The prognosis is variable, depending on the severity of social and language deficits.

Ozonoff S et al: Asperger's syndrome: Evidence of an empirical distinction from high functioning autism. J Child Psychol Psychiatry 1991; 32:1107.

Szatmari P: Asperger's syndrome: Diagnosis, treatment, and outcome. Psychiatr Clin North Am 1991;14:81.

Wolff S: Asperger's syndrome. Arch Dis Childhood 1991; 66:178.

3. CHILDHOOD SCHIZOPHRENIA

Essentials of Diagnosis

- Rambling or illogical speech patterns.
- Bizarre thought content.
- Hallucinations, delusions, or both.

General Considerations

Childhood schizophrenia probably represents a more severe form of the spectrum of schizophrenic disorders. It is rare, affecting only one or two children in every 10,000 of the population under 15 years of age. The onset is usually after 5 years of age, and approximately equal numbers of boys and girls are affected. Childhood schizophrenia appears to be genetically related to the adult type of schizophrenia.

Clinical Findings

Affected children display many of the same clinical symptoms of adults with schizophrenia. Hallucinations or delusions, bizarre and morbid thought content, or rambling and illogical speech are hallmarks of the disorder. These children tend to withdraw into an internal world of fantasy and may then behave as though the fantasy were in fact external reality. These children generally have difficulty with schoolwork and with peer relationships. The vast majority of childhood schizophrenics have had nonspecific psychiatric symptoms or symptoms of delayed development for months or years prior to the onset of their overtly psychotic symptoms (Russel, 1989; Fish, 1992).

Differential Diagnosis

Psychotic symptoms in young children (< 8 years of age) must be differentiated from the normal vivid fantasy life. Rambling speech and bizarre thought content can be helpful distinguishing factors. Learning disabilities should also be identified. In psychotic adolescents, mania is differentiated by observation of high levels of energy, excitement, and irritability. Any youngster presenting with new psychotic symptoms requires a medical evaluation that includes a physical and neurologic examination; drug screen; metabolic screen for endocrinopathies, Wilson's disease, and delirium; and an MRI and EEG.

Treatment

The treatment of childhood schizophrenia focuses on four main areas: (1) ameliorating active psychotic symptoms, (2) teaching appropriate social and cognitive skills, (3) reducing the risk of relapse of psychotic symptoms, and (4) providing support and education to parents and family members. Antipsychotic medications and a supportive, reality-oriented focus in relationships can help in reducing hallucinations, delusions, frightening thoughts, and social withdrawal. Teaching appropriate life skills is probably best accomplished in a special education program or a day treatment setting. Support for the family emphasizes the importance of clear, focused communication and an emotionally calm climate in preventing recurrences of overtly psychotic symptoms in schizophrenic individuals.

Prognosis

Childhood schizophrenia is generally considered a chronic disorder with exacerbations and remissions in active psychotic symptoms. It is generally believed that earlier onset (prior to age 13 years) and poor premorbid functioning (oddness or eccentricity) predict a poorer prognosis.

Fish B et al: Infants at risk for schizophrenia: Sequelae of a genetic neurointegrative defect. Arch Gen Psychiatry 1992; 49:221.

McClellan JM, Werry JS: Schizophrenia. Psychiatr Clin North Am 1992;15:131.

Russel A et al: The phenomenology of schizophrenia occurring in childhood. J Am Acad Child Adolesc Psychiatry 1989;28:399.

Werry JS, McClellan JM: Predicting outcome in child and adolescent (early onset) schizophrenia and bipolar disorder. J Am Acad Child Adolesc Psychiatry 1992; 31:147.

MOOD DISORDERS

1. DEPRESSION IN CHILDREN & ADOLESCENTS

Essentials of Diagnosis

- Dysphoric mood or depressed appearance, persisting for days to weeks at a time.

General Considerations

The term "depression" can denote an emotional state, a symptom, or a clinical syndrome. All three are now well-recognized entities in children and adolescents.

The clinical syndrome of depression probably occurs about as frequently among boys as among girls. Estimates of the incidence of depression within the general pediatric population reveals a pattern of increasing occurrence with increasing age. One to three percent of prepubertal children meet diagnostic criteria for major depression, whereas 3–6% of adolescents meet those criteria (McCracken, 1992). The incidence of depression in children is significantly higher when other family members have been affected by depressive disorders.

Clinical Findings

Clinical depression can be defined as an intense, persistent state of unhappiness and misery that interferes with pleasure or productivity. The signs and symptoms of depression are surprisingly constant across the age range from early childhood to adolescence and adulthood (Table 6–8). Various combinations of these signs and symptoms are seen in individual children and adolescents with depression.

Typically, a child or adolescent with depression begins to look unhappy and may make comments such as, "I have no friends . . . life is boring . . . there is nothing I can do to make things better . . . I wish I were dead." There is usually a change in behavior patterns that includes social isolation, deterioration in schoolwork, loss of interest in usual activities, and flashes of intense anger and irritability. Sleep and appetite patterns frequently change, and the child may complain of tiredness and somatic pain.

Differential Diagnosis

Youngsters with clinical depression can be identified by actively questioning them about depressive symptoms. Children are often more accurate in as-

Table 6–8. Clinical manifestations of depression in children and adolescents.

Depressive Symptom	Clinical Manifestations
Dysphoric mood	Tearfulness; sad, downturned expression; unhappiness; slumped posture; quick temper; irritability; anger.
Anhedonia	Loss of interest and enthusiasm in play, socializing, school, and usual activities; boredom; loss of pleasure.
Fatigability	Lethargy and tiredness; no play after school.
Morbid ideation	Self-deprecating thoughts, statements; thoughts of disaster, abandonment, death, suicide, or hopelessness.
Somatic symptoms	Changes in sleep or appetite patterns; difficulty in concentrating; bodily complaints, particularly headache and stomach ache.

sessing their own mood state than are their caretakers. When symptoms are numerous, persistent, and intense, a diagnosis of major depressive disorder is appropriate. When symptoms are fewer and of less intensity but have persisted for months, a diagnosis of dysthymic disorder is made. When depressive symptoms are milder and of relatively short duration and clearly follow some stressful life event, a diagnosis of adjustment disorder with depressed mood is proper.

Children with attention deficit disorders, conduct disorders, and developmental disabilities can become quite "demoralized" or "reactively depressed" by their chronic difficulties in life. There are also substantial rates of comorbidity of depression with attention deficit hyperactivity disorder, conduct disorder, anxiety disorders, eating disorders, and substance abuse disorders (McCauley, 1993). Medically ill patients also have an increased incidence of depression. Every child and adolescent with a depressed mood state should be questioned about victimization by child abuse. Depressed adolescents should be screened for hypothyroidism and substance abuse.

Complications

Because the emotional pain associated with severe depression can be intensely distressing, suicide may become an option. In addition, adolescents have a propensity to avoid the pain of depression through substance abuse or excitement-seeking behaviors (eg, "partying," negativism and defiance, and reckless behavior).

Treatment

The treatment of depression focuses on two issues: (1) helping those in the environment to respond more effectively to the child's emotional needs, and (2) ameliorating the child's depressive symptoms. Within the context of the family, efforts are made to resolve conflicts between family members and to increase the opportunity for enjoyable time together. Attitudes, expectations, and disciplinary methods are evaluated. The child is encouraged to become involved in activities and to pursue opportunities for maximizing skills and talents.

Individual psychotherapy can increase the patient's awareness of care and concern on the part of adults. It also helps the young person to identify, label, and verbalize feelings and misperceptions.

When the symptoms of depression are severe, persistent, and disabling, antidepressant medication can be of help, especially when there is a family history of depressive disorder responding to these drugs. However, controlled studies have not shown tricyclic antidepressants to be superior to placebo in children and adolescents with major depression (Ambrosini, 1993).

Prognosis

Although there are few follow-up studies on depressed children, evidence to date suggests that clinical depression tends to be a chronically recurring disorder in children (Warner, 1992). That possibility must certainly be kept in mind when monitoring previously depressed children over time.

Ambrosini PJ et al: Antidepressant Treatments in children and adolescents: Affective disorders. J Am Acad Child Adolesc Psychiatry 1993;32:1.

Carlson GA, Kashani JH: Phenomenology of major depression from childhood through adulthood: Analysis of three studies. Am J Psychiatry 1988;145:1222.

McCauley E et al: Depression in young people: Initial presentation and clinical course. J Am Acad Child Adolesc Psychiatry 1993; 32:714.

McCracken JT: The epidemiology of child and adolescent mood disorders. Psychiatr Clin North Am 1992;1:53.

Mood disorders in children and adolescence. The Harvard Mental Health Letter 1993;10:Nos. 4 and 5.

Warner V et al: The course of major depression in the offspring of depressed parents. Arch Gen Psychiatry 1992;49:795.

2. BIPOLAR DISORDER

Essentials of Diagnosis

- Periods of abnormally and persistently elevated, expansive, or irritable mood and heightened levels of energy and activity.
- Not due to prescribed or illicit drugs.

General Considerations

Bipolar disorder (previously referred to as manic-depressive disease) is classically thought of as an episodic mood disorder manifested by distinct periods of both manic and depressive episodes or, less commonly, manic episodes alone. In children and adolescents, a clearly episodic course is not as discernible; children and adolescents more often present with a variable course of mood instability combined with problems with conduct and impulse control, with or without substance abuse. At least 20% of bipolar patients experience the onset of symptoms before the age of 20 years. The onset of bipolar disorder before puberty is thought to be infrequent.

Clinical Findings

In 70% of patients, the first symptoms are primarily those of depression; in the remainder, manic, hypomanic, or mixed states dominate the symptom presentation. Manic patients present a variable pattern of elevated, expansive, or irritable mood, along with more rapid speech, higher energy levels, some difficulty in sustaining concentration, and a decreased need for sleep. Patients often do not recognize that there is any problem with their mood or behavior. The clinical picture can be quite dramatic, with florid psychotic symptoms of delusions and hallucinations (a full-blown manic psychosis) or may consist of more subtle changes in mood or behavior (cyclothymia).

Differential Diagnosis

Diagnostic considerations must include an acute organic process, particularly substance abuse disorder. Hyperthyroidism should be ruled out. In prepubescent children, mania may be difficult to differentiate from attention deficit hypersensitivity disorder (ADHD; see below) and other disruptive behavior disorders. Intense and prolonged rages or dysphoria and some periodicity of symptom activity suggest bipolar disorder. Table 6–9 further defines points of differentiation between bipolar disorder, ADHD, and conduct disorder.

Complications

The poor judgment associated with manic episodes predisposes to dangerous, impulsive, and sometimes criminal activities. Affective disorders are associated with a 30-fold greater incidence of successful suicide.

Treatment & Prognosis

Most patients with bipolar disease respond to treatment with lithium carbonate, supportive psychotherapy, and education about the recurrent nature of the illness.

Carlson GA: Bipolar disorders in children and adolescents. In: *Psychiatric Disorders in Children and Adolescents.* Garfinkel BD et al (editors). Saunders, 1990.

Fristad MA et al: Bipolar disorder in children and adolescents. Child Adolesc Psychiatr Clin North Am 1992;1: 13.

Isaac G: Misdiagnosed bipolar disorder in adolescents in a special education and treatment program. J Clin Psychiatry 1992;52:133.

DISRUPTIVE BEHAVIOR DISORDERS

1. ATTENTION DEFICIT HYPERACTIVITY DISORDER

Essentials of Diagnosis

- Pattern of behaviors related to the following: excessive motor activity, impulsivity, distractibility.
- Developmentally excessive and inappropriate behaviors.
- Behaviors that are persistent over time and not primarily reactive to life stressors.

General Considerations

Attention deficit hyperactivity disorder (ADHD) is not a single etiologically, pathophysiologically, or clinically distinct disorder but rather a clinical syndrome with two major clusters of symptoms: symptoms of inattention (being off task) and symptoms of behavioral disinhibition (impulsivity). Within this heterogeneous population are many subgroups: ADD without hyperactivity; ADHD with comorbid learning disability; ADHD with comorbid speech and language disorders; ADHD comorbid with a variety of other psychiatric disorders; and ADHD comorbid with other disorders of brain function (eg, mental retardation, seizure disorders, fetal alcohol syndrome). The history of ADHD is reflected in the many names it has taken over the years: minimal brain damage, minimal brain dysfunction, hyperkinetic syndrome, and attention deficit disorder. When careful diagnostic criteria are applied, the incidence of the syndrome is found to be approximately 3% of school-age children, with boys outnumbering girls by a ratio of 5–9:1. Although the behavioral syndrome has been statistically associated with perinatal problems, brain

Table 6–9. Differentiating conduct behavior disorders.

	ADHD	Conduct Disorder	Bipolar Disorder
School problems	Yes	Yes	Yes
Behavior problems	Yes	Yes	Yes
Defiant attitude	Occasional	Constant	Episodic
Motor restlessness	Constant	May be present	May wax and wane
Impulsivity	Constant	May be present	May wax and wane
Distractibility	Constant	May be present	May wax and wane
Anger expression	Short-lived (minutes)	Plans revenge	Intense rages (minutes to hours)
Thought content	May be immature	Blames others	Morbid or grandiose ideas
Sleep disturbance	May be present	No	May wax and wane
Self-deprecation	Briefly, with criticism	No	Prolonged, with or without suicidal ideation
Obsessed with ideas	No	No	Yes
Hallucinations	No	No	Diagnostic if present
Family history	May be a history of school problems	May be a history of antisocial behavior	May be a history of mood disorders

injury and dysfunction, and a family history of learning disability and behavior disorders, no etiologic or structural abnormality can be identified in the affected child in the vast majority of cases. It does appear that there is approximately a 15–25% risk of ADHD among relatives of ADHD probands (Biederman, 1992). A recent review of research suggested the importance of noradrenergic-mediated inhibitory processes in the pathogenesis of the disorder (Shenker, 1992).

Clinical Findings

There are two common clinical presentations: In the first, the "difficult child," the history of a fussy, hard to soothe, overactive, behaviorally impulsive child goes as far back as the family can remember. The child is frequently described as having been "a handful" since birth.

The second common clinical presentation is that of the "immature child" whose silliness, distractibility, and motor restlessness and clumsiness become apparent upon entry into school, when problems of behavioral self-control, the focusing of attention, and relating to peers become harder to ignore. In either case, with time, these children have difficulty completing schoolwork because of their distractibility and short attention span; they also have difficulty with interpersonal relationships because of their intrusiveness, excitability, and motor restlessness.

The diagnosis is a clinical one, based largely on the history of a persistent behavioral pattern that interferes both with the development of relationships and with academic performance commensurate with the child's intellectual capacity. The symptoms are typically most noticeable in group settings. These children are almost always academic underachievers, and in perhaps 40% of cases a specific learning disability is associated with the attention deficit disorder. Symptoms of anxiety, depression, aggression, resistance to authority, or learning problems are present in 25–50% of cases (Biederman, 1992).

Differential Diagnosis

The differential diagnosis includes reactive behavioral disorders, in which a precipitating stressful event is associated with the onset of behavioral symptoms that represent a change in usual behavior patterns. In addition, children from chaotic, disorganized home environments may display behavioral dyscontrol. The symptoms of ADHD can also occur early in the course of Tourette's syndrome, with attention deficits frequently preceding the onset of tics. Symptoms of ADHD are also associated with mental retardation, pervasive developmental disorders, fragile X syndrome, fetal alcohol syndrome, and lead toxicity. Not infrequently, mood disorders can present with psychomotor agitation (see bipolar disorder). Vision and hearing abnormalities should be ruled out as a cause of social and academic dysfunction.

Complications

Many children with ADHD have coexisting psychiatric disorders such as depressive and anxiety disorders. Others go on to develop reactively depressed mood states and a significant syndrome of "demoralization" due to the difficulties they experience in getting along socially and academically. Perhaps 40–50% of these children have or later develop coexisting conduct disorders (Klein, 1991). Learning disabilities are associated with academic failure and alienation from school.

Treatment
(See also Chapter 5.)

Attention deficit hyperactivity disorder is a chronic disorder that requires multidisciplinary management over many years. In school, children do best in small, quiet, structured classrooms with teachers who are nonjudgmental yet have firm and consistent behavioral expectations. Extra tutoring in small groups can be helpful; a self-contained special education classroom may be necessary for the very distractible and impulsive child.

Positive reinforcement programs that reward socially appropriate behavior and successful task performance can be helpful both at school and at home. Cognitive and behavioral training programs such as Think Aloud can reduce impulsivity. When specific learning disabilities are present, special educational assistance is indicated.

The families of children with ADHD need to understand the nature of the problem, and they need support in structuring discipline at home so that the disciplinary techniques do not become inconsistent, overly harsh, or loaded with interpersonal conflict.

Individual psychotherapy can be helpful when depression or disorders of conduct coexist with ADHD.

The psychostimulants (dextroamphetamine, methylphenidate, pemoline), the tricyclic antidepressants, and clonidine can provide symptomatic relief in about 70% of cases (see p 188). Psychoactive medications alone are never sufficient treatment.

Prognosis

It was at one time thought that children with ADHD would outgrow the problem once they reached puberty. It is now believed that nearly 70% of these patients have problems with short attention span, impulsivity, and emotional immaturity into mid adolescence (Klein, 1991). In addition, significant numbers are chronically unhappy, repeat grades, drop out of school, and develop conduct disorders (including substance abuse disorders) that bring them into conflict with the legal authorities. Only about a third of children with ADHD reach mid adolescence with no diagnosable psychiatric disorder. Although ADHD is clearly not a benign disorder, comprehensive treatment does lead to better social skills, higher self-esteem, and less difficulty in dealing with aggression.

Barkley RA: *Attention Deficit Hyperactivity Disorder: A Handbook for Diagnosis and Treatment.* Gilford Press, 1990.

Biederman J et al: Comorbidity of attention deficit hyperactivity disorder with conduct, depressive, anxiety, and other disorders. Am J Psychiatry 1991;148:564.

Biederman J et al: Further evidence for family-genetic risk factors in attention deficit hyperactivity disorder. Arch Gen Psychiatry 1992;49:728.

Camp BW, Bash MS: *Think Aloud.* Research Press, 1981.

Klein R, Mannuzza S: Long-term outcome of hyperactive children: A review. J Am Acad Child Adolesc Psychiatry 1991;30:383.

Shenker A: The mechanism of action of drugs used to treat ADHD: Focus on catecholamine receptor pharmacology. Adv Pediatr 1992;39:337.

Weiss G (editor): Attention deficit hyperactivity disorder. Child Adolesc Psychiatr Clin North Am 1992;1:No 2.

2. CONDUCT DISORDERS

Essentials of Diagnosis

A persistent pattern of behavior that includes the following:

- Defiance of authority.
- Violating the rights of others or society's norms.
- Aggressive behavior toward others.

General Considerations

Disorders of conduct affect approximately 9% of males and 2% of females under the age of 18 years. This is a very heterogeneous population, with significant overlap among attention deficit hyperactivity disorder, learning disabilities, and family dysfunction. Many of these individuals have "difficult temperaments" and come from broken homes where domestic violence, child abuse, drug abuse, shifting parental figures, and poverty are environmental risk factors. Harsh parental discipline with physical punishment appears to lead to more aggressive behavior in children and adolescents (Weiss, 1992).

Clinical Findings

The typical child with conduct disorder is a boy with tempestuous social and academic difficulties. Defiance of authority, fighting, tantrums, running away, school failure, and destruction of property are common symptoms. With increasing age, fire setting and stealing may occur, followed in adolescence by truancy, vandalism, and substance abuse. Hyperactive, aggressive, and uncooperative behavior patterns in the preschool and early school years tend to predict conduct disorder in adolescence with a high degree of accuracy. The risk for conduct disorder increases with inconsistent and severe parental disciplinary techniques, parental alcoholism, and parental antisocial behavior.

Differential Diagnosis

Young people with conduct disorders—especially those with more violent histories—have an increased incidence of neurologic signs and symptoms, psychomotor seizures, psychotic symptoms, mood disorders, attention deficit hyperactivity disorder, and learning disabilities. Efforts should be made to identify these associated disorders (Table 6–9).

Treatment

Treatment is difficult and not very effective. Efforts should be made to stabilize the environment and improve functioning within the home, particularly as it relates to disciplinary techniques. Any associated neurologic, psychiatric, or educational disorders should be treated specifically. In severe cases, residential treatment may be needed.

Prognosis

The prognosis is poor, especially for children who present with onset before age 10 years, who display a diversity of antisocial behaviors across multiple settings, and who are raised in an environment characterized by parental antisocial behavior, alcoholism, and conflict. Nearly half of such children become antisocial as adults. Antisocial behavior in childhood tends to predict a diagnosable psychiatric disorder in adulthood with a high degree of accuracy.

Kazdin AE: *Conduct Disorders in Children and Adolescence.* Sage, 1987.

Robins LN: Conduct disorder. J Child Psychol Psychiatry 1991;32:193.

Weiss B et al: Some consequences of early harsh discipline: Child aggression and a maladaptive social information processing style. Child Dev 1992;63:1321.

ANXIETY DISORDERS

1. ANXIETY-BASED SCHOOL REFUSAL (School Avoidance)

Essentials of Diagnosis

- A persistent pattern of school avoidance related to symptoms of anxiety.
- Prominent somatic symptoms of anxiety on school mornings, with the symptoms resolving if the child is allowed to remain at home.
- No organic medical disorder that accounts for the child's symptoms.

General Considerations

Anxiety-based school refusal, or school phobia, is a clinical syndrome rather than a diagnostic entity. It refers to a pattern of school nonattendance due to symptoms of anxiety. The anxiety may be related to a dread of leaving home (ie, separation anxiety), a fear of some aspect of school (ie, "true" school phobia), or a fear of feeling exposed or embarrassed at school (ie, social phobia). In most cases, anxiety-based school refusal represents a prototype of persistent, developmentally inappropriate separation anxiety where the child feels anxious being away from primary caregivers. It affects boys and girls with approximately equal frequency, and there appear to be peaks in the incidence at the ages of 6 and 7 years, again at 10–11 years of age, and finally in early adolescence.

Clinical Findings

In preadolescent children, school refusal often begins after some clear precipitating stress, such as an illness in the child or a parent or the birth of a sibling. The child's anxiety is then manifested either as somatic symptoms or in displacement of the child's anxiety onto some aspect of the school environment that the child perceives as frightening.

The symptoms often represent somatic manifestations of anxiety, such as dizziness, nausea, and stomach distress. Characteristically, the somatic symptoms become more prominent as the time to leave for school approaches and then remit if the child is allowed to remain at home for the day. In older children, the onset of school refusal is more insidious and is often associated with symptoms of social withdrawal and depression. There is an increased incidence of anxiety and mood disorders in these families.

Differential Diagnosis

The differential diagnosis of school nonattendance is set forth in Table 6–10. Medical disorders that may be causing the somatic symptoms must be ruled out. One should investigate the possibility of "good reasons" for staying home, eg, in the case of a child who is being intimidated by bullying students or an abusive teacher. Children with learning disabilities may wish to stay home to avoid the sense of failure they experience at school. Normal children may also have very transient episodes of wanting to stay at home while they struggle with some internal conflict. Finally, truants are to be differentiated on the basis of their chronic noncompliance with adult authority and their preference for being with peers rather than at home.

Complications

The longer a child remains out of school, the more difficult it is to return and the more strained the relationship between child and parent becomes. Many parents of nonattending children feel tyrannized by their defiant, clinging child. Children often feel accused of "making up" their symptoms, leading to further antagonism between the child, parents, and medical caregivers.

Table 6–10. Differential diagnosis of school nonattendance.[1]

I. **Emotional or anxiety-based school refusal[2]**
   A. Separation anxiety disorder (50–80% of anxious refusers)
   B. Overanxious disorder
   C. Mood/depressive disorder (with or without comorbid anxiety)
   D. Social anxiety
   E. Simple phobia
   F. Panic disorder
   G. Psychosis ("voices" say not to attend)

II. **Truancy[3] behavior disorders**
   A. Oppositional defiant disorder, conduct disorder
   B. Substance abuse disorders

III. **"Realistic" school refusal**
   A. Learning disability, unaddressed or undetected
   B. Marauding students (including gangs)
   C. Psychologically abusive teacher
   D. Family-sanctioned nonattendance
      1. For companionship
      2. For child care
      3. To supplement family income
   E. Socioculturally sanctioned nonattendance (school is not valued)
   F. Homosexual attraction, gender identity concerns

IV. **Undiagnosed medical condition (including pregnancy)**

[1]Medically unexplained absence of more than 2 weeks.
[2]Subjectively distressed child who generally stays at home.
[3]Not subjectively distressed and not at home.

Treatment

The cornerstone of treatment is helping the child to confront anxiety and overcome it by returning to school. This requires development of a strong alliance between the parents and the health care provider that is built on trust. The parent must understand that no underlying medical disorder exists, that the child's symptoms are a manifestation of anxiety, and that the basic problem is anxiety that must be faced to be overcome. Parents must be reminded that being good parents in this case means helping a child to face a distressing experience. Children must be reassured that their symptoms are due to "worry" and that they will be overcome upon return to school.

A plan for returning the child to school is then developed with parents and school personnel. The child is brought to school by someone not likely to waver in the face of the child's distress—eg, the father or an older sibling. If significant symptoms develop at school, the child should be checked by the school nurse and then returned to class after a brief rest. The parents must be reassured that school staff will handle the situation at school and that school personnel can reach the child's primary health care provider if any questions arise.

In cases where parents are unable to enter into that kind of treatment contract, more in-depth mental health assistance must be provided as a way of supporting autonomy in family members. For children with more severe symptoms of separation or panic anxiety or major depression, tricyclic antidepressants or a brief course of a high-potency benzodiazepine may be an important adjunct to the behavioral treatment.

Prognosis

Although the vast majority of preadolescent children can be effectively returned to school, the long-term prognosis is more questionable. Recent studies suggest that a history of school refusal is significantly more frequent in adults with "neuroticism," panic anxiety, and agoraphobia than in the general population. Thus, there may be some correlation between symptoms of school refusal in childhood and the development of psychiatric disorders in adulthood.

Bell-Dolan D, Brazeal T: Separation anxiety disorder, overanxious disorder, and school refusal. Child Adolesc Psychiatr Clin North Am 1993;2:563.

Berg I: Absence from school and mental health. Br J Psychiatry 1992;161:154.

Berstein GA et al: Comparative studies of pharmacotherapy for school refusal. J Am Acad Child Adolesc Psychiatry 1990;29:773.

Klein RG, Last CG: *Anxiety Disorders in Children*. Sage, 1989.

2. THE OVERLY ANXIOUS CHILD

Transient developmental fears are common in early childhood. Therefore, the person evaluating the clinical significance of anxiety symptoms in children must consider the age of the child, the developmental fears that can normally be expected at that age, the form of the symptoms and their duration, and the degree to which the symptoms disrupt the child's life.

Anxiety can be manifested either directly or indirectly, as shown in Table 6–11. The characteristics of anxiety disorders in childhood are listed in Table 6–12. Community-based studies of samples of school-aged children and adolescents suggest that nearly 10% of children qualify for a diagnosis of some type of anxiety disorder (Bernstein, 1991). The differential diagnosis of symptoms of anxiety is presented in Table 6–13.

The treatment of the overanxious child frequently involves interventions at more than one level. Of greatest importance, the child's environment (ie, the family and school environment) should be evaluated for anxiety-producing circumstances, eg, marital discord, family violence, harsh or inappropriate disciplinary methods, or emotional overstimulation. The child's experience of anxiety and its relationship to life events are explored, and the child is taught specific cognitive and behavioral techniques needed to confront the anxiety. Finally, when severe separation or panic anxiety appears to play a prominent role in the child's anxiety disorder or when the child has persistent obsessive compulsive disorder, psychopharmacologic agents may be helpful (Popper, 1993). The

Table 6–11. Signs and symptoms of anxiety in children.

Direct manifestations of anxiety
  Psychologic manifestations:
    Fears and worries
    Uneasiness and apprehension
    Frightening themes in play and fantasy
  Psychomotor manifestations:
    Motoric restlessness and hyperactivity
    Sleep disturbances
    Decreased concentration
  Psychophysiologic manifestations:
    Autonomic hyperarousal
      Dizziness and light-headedness
      Palpitations
      Shortness of breath
      Flushing, sweating, dry mouth
      Nausea and vomiting
      Panic
      Headaches and stomach aches
Indirect manifestations of anxiety
  Increased dependence on home and parents
  Avoidance of social interaction outside the family
  Avoidance of anxiety-producing stimuli
  Decreased school performance
  Increased self-doubt and irritability
  Ritualistic behaviors (eg, washing and counting)

long-term prognosis for these disorders is largely unknown.

Bernstein GA, Borchardt CM: Anxiety disorder of childhood and adolescence: A critical review. J Am Acad Child Adolesc Psychiatry 1991;30:519.

Leonard HL (editor): Anxiety Disorders. Child Adolesc Psychiatr Clin North Am 1993;2:No. 4.

Popper CW: Psychopharmacologic treatment of anxiety disorders in adolescents and children. J Clin Psychiatry 1993;54 (Suppl):52.

Table 6–12. Anxiety disorders in children and adolescents.

Disorder	Major Clinical Manifestations
Separation anxiety disorder	Developmentally inappropriate wish to maintain proximity with caretakers; morbid worry of threats to family integrity; intense homesickness
Overanxious disorder (generalized anxiety)	Intense worry, often about future events
Avoidant disorder (social phobia)	Painful shyness or self-consciousness; fear of humiliation with public scrutiny
Simple phobia	Avoidance of specific feared stimuli
Panic disorder	Unprovoked, intense fear with sympathetic hyperarousal, and often palpitations and/or hyperventilation
Posttraumatic stress disorder	Fear of a recurrence of an intense, anxiety provoking experience, causing sympathetic hyperarousal, avoidance or reminders, and the reexperiencing of aspects of the traumatic event

Table 6–13. Differential diagnosis of symptoms of anxiety.

I. **Normal developmental anxiety**
  A. Stranger anxiety (5 months to 2½ years, with peak at 6–12 months)
  B. Separation anxiety (7 months to 4 years, with peak at 18–36 months)
  C. The child fearful or even phobic of the dark and monsters (3–6 years)
II. **"Appropriate" anxiety**
  A. Anticipating a painful or frightening experience
  B. Avoidance of a reminder of a painful or frightening experience
  C. Child abuse
III. **Anxiety disorder (see Table 6–12),** with or without other comorbid psychiatric disorders
IV. **Substance abuse**
V. **Medications and recreational drugs**
  A. Caffeinism (including colas and chocolate)
  B. Sympathomimetic agents
  C. Idiosyncratic drug reactions
VI. **Hypermetabolic or hyperarousal states**
  A. Hyperthyroidism
  B. Pheochromocytoma
  C. Anemia
  D. Hypoglycemia
  E. Hypoxemia
VII. **Cardiac abnormality**
  A. Dysrhythmia
  B. High-output state
  C. Mitral valve prolapse

3. POSTTRAUMATIC STRESS DISORDER

Essentials of Diagnosis

- Signs and symptoms of autonomic hyperarousal.
- Avoidant behaviors.
- Flashbacks to a traumatic event.
- All of the above following the occurrence of traumatic events such as natural disasters, unexpected personal tragedies, and ongoing interpersonal violence.

General Considerations

Interest in posttraumatic stress disorder in children really began in 1979 with Terr's classic study of the kidnapped children of Chowchilla. Since then, the field has mushroomed; at present, great interest is focused on the developing body of knowledge connecting child physical and sexual abuse with symptoms of chronic posttraumatic stress disorder.

Clinical Findings

Children who have been psychically traumatized show persistent evidence of fear and anxiety. They are hypervigilant to the possibility of recurrence of a traumatic event. In addition, they regress developmentally and experience fears of strangers, of the dark, and of being alone. They avoid reminders of the traumatic event.

In addition, children frequently reexperience elements of the traumatic events in frightening dreams and intrusive daytime flashbacks. In their symbolic play, one can often notice a monotonous repetition of some aspect of the traumatic event.

Treatment

The cornerstone of treatment for posttraumatic stress disorder is the intense education of the child and family regarding the nature of posttraumatic stress disorder so that the child's emotional reactions and regressive behavior are not mistakenly viewed as "crazy" or "manipulative." Support, reassurance, repeated explanations, and understanding are all needed. "Tincture of time" and behavioral desensitization are helpful to combat specific fears. A supportive relationship with a caretaking adult is essential. For children with more severe symptoms, a variety of psychoactive medications, including mood stabilizers, clonidine, propranolol, and antidepressants—singly or in combination—can be helpful in ameliorating symptoms of autonomic hyperarousal.

Prognosis

Children who have experienced psychic trauma often harbor significant emotional scars. At 4- to 5-year follow-ups, many children continue to have vivid and frightening memories and dreams and a pessimistic view of the future. Evidence is growing to support a connection between victimization in childhood and unstable personality and mood disorders in later life.

Pynoos RS: Post-traumatic stress disorder in children and adolescents. In: *Psychiatric Disorders in Children and Adolescents.* Garfinkel BD et al (editors). Saunders, 1990.

Pynoos RS: Traumatic stress and developmental psychopathology in children and adolescents. Rev Psychiatry 1993;12:205.

Terr LC: The children of Chowchilla. Psychoanal Study Child 1979;34:52.

Terr LC: Childhood traumas: An outline and overview. Am J Psychiatry 1991;148:10.

SOMATOFORM DISORDERS

Essentials of Diagnosis

- A symptom suggesting physical dysfunction.
- No known physical disorder accounting for the symptom.
- Symptoms cause distressor dysfunction.
- Symptoms are not voluntarily maintained.

Clinical Findings

Somatoform disorders are a group of conditions that suggest the presence of physical illness or disability for which no organic cause can be ascertained though neither the patient nor the caretaker is consciously fabricating the symptoms. The category includes conversion disorder, hypochondriasis, somatization disorder, somatoform pain disorder, and body dysmorphic disorder (see Table 6–14).

Table 6–14. Somatoform disorders in children and adolescents.

Disorder	Major Clinical Manifestations
Conversion disorder	Symptom onset follows psychologically stressful event; symptoms express unconscious feelings and result in secondary gain.
Hypochondriasis	Preoccupation with worry that physical symptoms manifest an unrecognized and threatening condition; medical assurance does not provide relief from worry.
Somatization disorder	Long-standing preoccupation with multiple somatic symptoms.
Somatoform pain disorder	Preoccupation with pain that results in distress or impairment beyond what would be expected from physical findings.
Body dysmorphic disorder	Preoccupation with an imagined defect in personal appearance.

Conversion symptoms most frequently occur in school-age children and adolescents. Their exact incidence is unclear, but in pediatric practice they are probably more often seen as transient symptoms rather than as chronic disorders requiring help from mental health practitioners. The appearance of the conversion symptom is thought to be an expression of underlying psychologic conflict or stress. Although children can present with a variety of symptoms, many presentations initially suggest a disorder of neurologic or sensory origin. Symptoms include unusual sensory phenomena, paralysis, and movement or seizure-like disorders.

In the classic case of conversion disorder, the child's symptom complex and examination are not consistent with the clinical manifestations of any organic disease process. In addition, the symptoms frequently begin as an intercurrent illness within the context of a family experiencing significant stress, eg, serious illness, a death, or family discord. On closer examination, the child's symptoms are often found to resemble symptoms present in other significant family members. Children with conversion symptoms often but not always have some secondary gain associated with their symptoms.

A number of reports have pointed to the increased association of conversion symptoms with sexual overstimulation or sexual abuse. Health care providers should always keep that possibility in mind.

Differential Diagnosis

It is sometimes not possible to be sure that the symptoms are not due to an underlying disease process. In such cases, follow-up observation is required to see whether further symptoms evolve.

Somatic symptoms can be prominent in children with anxiety and depressive disorders (Table 6–14). The child's mood state and associated symptoms of avoidance are helpful indicators in determining whether such disorders are present. Occasionally, psychotic children present with somatic preoccupations and even somatic delusions.

Treatment

In most cases, conversion symptoms resolve quickly when the child and family are reassured that the symptom is a way of reacting to identifiable stresses in the child's life. The child is encouraged to continue with daily activities as normally as possible, knowing that the symptom will resolve when the stress is resolved.

If identifiable stresses are not clearly understood or if the symptom does not resolve with reassurance, further investigation by a mental health professional is indicated. When the more chronic somatoform disorders evolve in children and adolescents, treatment with appropriate psychopharmacologic agents may be helpful (Hollander, 1993).

Hollander E: Pharmacologic treatment of obsessive-compulsive spectrum disorders. The Psychiatric Times 1993;10:36.

Nemzer ED: Somatoform disorders. In: *Child and Adolescent Psychiatry: A Comprehensive Textbook.* Lewis M (editor). Williams & Wilkins, 1991.

EATING DISORDERS

1. ANOREXIA NERVOSA
(See also Chapter 4.)

Essentials of Diagnosis

- Intense fear of becoming fat.
- Distorted view of self as overweight.
- Refusal to keep weight at a reasonable minimum.
- Amenorrhea.
- No known physical illness causing weight loss.

General Considerations

Anorexia nervosa is a disorder characterized by the relentless pursuit of thinness. It affects 0.5–1% of females between the ages of 12 and 18 years. Females account for 90–95% of all cases. The incidence of the disorder has increased significantly in recent years, presumably related in part to the high premium society places on the thin female figure. The disorder is found more frequently in families with histories of eating disorders or affective disorders.

Clinical Findings

There is a bimodal distribution to the onset of symptoms in anorexia nervosa at ages 13–14 and again at ages 17–18. Typically, the disorder begins in an overly compliant and highly achievement-oriented girl who perceives herself as overweight and therefore starts dieting. Over a period of weeks to months, the diet evolves into an obsessive preoccupation with being thin. This pathologic pursuit of thinness is manifested primarily in restriction of caloric intake but may also include excessive exercising and purging behaviors (induced vomiting and the use of laxatives and diuretics). About 40–50% of anorectics also have a history of binge eating. Although amenorrhea typically follows the onset of weight loss, cessation of menses precedes significant weight loss in about 20% of cases.

As the disorder progresses, most anorectics curtail their social relationships and become anxious, irritable, or depressed. Their thoughts increasingly focus on food and weight loss; all the while, anorectics deny that any problems exist. Physical and psychologic symptoms of starvation then ensue. In some cases, the pursuit of thinness runs a constant course toward emaciation; in others, the course is more episodic, with exacerbations and partial remissions.

Differential Diagnosis

The diagnosis is based on the characteristic findings of fear of fatness and the distorted perception of self as overweight. In bulimia, weight loss is not as pronounced as in anorexia nervosa. Other psychiatric disorders associated with weight loss or bizarre behaviors include depressive disorders, phobic reactions to food, and psychotic disorders, but these do not present with the same fear of fatness that is characteristic of patients with eating disorders.

Physical disorders to be ruled out include tumors of the hypothalamus or third ventricle, hyperthyroidism, diabetes mellitus, panhypopituitarism, inflammatory bowel disease, and peptic ulcer disease.

Complications

The complications of anorexia nervosa are frequent and numerous. The most frequent complications reflect the effects of starvation (Table 6–15). In fact, the physical and psychologic effects of starvation are thought to be prominent in perpetuating many symptoms associated with anorexia nervosa.

Dehydration, hypokalemia (particularly in patients who purge), cardiac irregularity, and gastric fullness secondary to delayed gastric emptying are not uncommon.

As many as 50% of anorectics have an associated major depressive syndrome.

Mortality rates for anorexia nervosa range from 5% to 10%, with 2–5% of chronic anorectics eventually committing suicide.

Treatment

The treatment of anorectic patients is at best difficult. A multidimensional approach to treatment is needed. Three major areas need attention: (1) the management of medical dangers, including metabolic problems (particularly hypokalemia), cardiac irregularities, hypotension, and dehydration; (2) the restora-

Table 6–15. Effects of starvation states.

Physical effects
Dry skin
Hair loss
Lanugo hair
Paresthesias
Sensitivity to noise
Hypothermia
Cold intolerance
Psychologic effects
Anxiety states
Depressed mood
Labile moods
Irritability and anger
Fatigue
Loss of motivation
Feelings of inadequacy
Decreased concentration
Social withdrawal
Intense hunger, even after eating
Preoccupation with food, including food fads

tion of normal nutrition and eating patterns; and (3) the psychiatric treatment needs of the patient and family. Because anorectics usually deny their illness, it is important to be direct and firm in addressing the problem. Treatment often begins with an open acknowledgment to the patient and family that although the striving for thinness and control is obviously very important to the patient, it has serious dangers, including physical illness, psychologic morbidity, and even death. It is helpful to relate the patient's weight to norms for age and to relate the effects of starvation to the symptoms. One should emphasize that the purpose of treatment is both to restore physical and nutritional health and to help the patient find more effective ways to feel good about herself and in control of her life.

In about half of cases, treatment is begun in the hospital. Indications for hospitalization include the following: (1) Rapid weight loss—30% or more of body weight loss within 3 months. (2) Medical complications—heart rate 40/min or less, body temperature less than 36 °C, systolic blood pressure less than 70 mm Hg, serum potassium less than 2.5 meq/L. (3) Unwavering denial of the illness. (4) Failure to agree to or comply with a contract for weight gain and ongoing treatment. (5) Severe depression, particularly with risk of suicide. (6) Severe binging and purging.

Treatment focuses on identifying a target weight to be achieved. Small, frequent meals are eaten to attain weekly weight increments of 2–3 lb. The nutritionist can often be of great help in planning such a program.

The psychiatric treatment of the child and family goes hand in hand with the nutritional rehabilitation. Individual treatment is based on the assumption that the preoccupation with food and weight is a screen for underlying problems of inadequacy and self-doubt. Patients are therefore encouraged to express their feelings and needs, to get to know themselves, and to feel more comfortable with the range of feelings they are so desperately trying to control and deny. The core cognitive distortion in anorexia nervosa is the patient's belief that the only way to feel good about her own competence is to be in rigid control of her body weight. In the course of psychiatric treatment, many issues surface: the need to behave perfectly, self-doubt, the perception that self-worth depends on the approval of others, and fear of the turbulent emotions so characteristic of a normal adolescent's inner life.

Because most families of anorectic patients have dysfunctional structures, family treatment often must accompany individual psychiatric care. The focus is often on fortifying intergenerational boundaries, decreasing parental overprotectiveness, and freeing the anorectic child from the role of peacemaker between silently warring parents.

Finally, attention must be paid to the major depression that is present in up to 50% of anorectic patients. Antidepressant medications, particularly selective serotonin reuptake inhibitors (SSRIs), can be of help in medically stable anorectics (Kaye, 1991).

Prognosis

The course and outcome of anorexia nervosa are highly variable. In general, the younger the age at onset, the better the prognosis. At 5-year follow-up, approximately 40% of anorectics are asymptomatic, 30% are significantly improved, 25% are actively symptomatic, and 5% have died as a result of medical complications or suicide. More than 50% of patients whose weight returns to normal continue to experience depression, anxiety, social maladjustment, pathologic eating patterns, or difficult relationships with family members.

American Psychiatric Association Workgroup on Eating Disorders: Practice guidelines for eating disorders. Am J Psychiatry 1993; 150:207.

Beumont PJV et al: Treatment of anorexia nervosa. Lancet 1993;341:1635.

Garner DM: Pathogenesis of anorexia nervosa. Lancet 1993;341:1631.

Hsu LKG: *Eating Disorders.* Guilford Press, 1990.

Kaye WH: An open trial of fluoxetine in patients with anorexia nervosa. J Clin Psychiatry 1991; 52:464.

2. BULIMIA

Essentials of Diagnosis

- Recurrent episodes of binge eating.
- Lack of control of eating during binges.
- Efforts to prevent weight gain.
- Overconcern with body weight and shape.

General Considerations

Binge eating is defined as the rapid consumption of large amounts of food in a brief period. It is quite common, particularly among college-age women. Up to 50% of college-age students admit to some binge eating at some time, and about 5–10% of females of high school and college age admit to binging weekly. When clinical bulimia is defined as binging at least two times a week with active attempts to prevent weight gain, 1–4% of college females meet the diagnostic criteria. As is the case with anorexia nervosa, over 95% of bulimics are female.

Clinical Findings

Bulimia is an episodic eating disorder that typically begins in later adolescence and frequently persists for years before it comes to medical attention. During an episode of binge eating, bulimics frequently consume 5000–20,000 kcal of high-carbohydrate foods. About 50–60% practice binge eating daily. The binging is followed by attempts to control weight gain by means of strict dietary measures, excessive exercising, or purging by self-induced vomiting or the use of laxatives or diuretics. These patients know that their eating behavior is abnormal, and they feel ashamed and uncomfortable about being out of control. Episodes of binging are frequently associated with stressful life events, and depression, guilt, and self-deprecation frequently follow an episode of binge eating. Most commonly, bulimics are of normal weight, but bulimia is also associated with anorexia nervosa and even with being overweight.

Differential Diagnosis

The major diagnostic question is whether the eating behavior and the resultant attempts to control weight are associated with the severe weight loss and denial of symptoms found in anorexia nervosa. Very rarely, tumors of the central nervous system or seizure-like states can result in binge eating.

Complications

Serious medical complications can result from the purging behaviors commonly seen in bulimics. The complications include the following: hypokalemia, metabolic alkalosis, dehydration, cardiac arrhythmias, dental erosion, esophageal tears, esophagitis, gastric rupture, abraded knuckles, parotid hypertrophy, and myocardial dysfunction secondary to ipecac poisoning.

The psychiatric complications of bulimia are likewise frequent. Major depression is found in up to 80% of cases, and impulse control disorders, such as substance abuse and sexual promiscuity, are not uncommon.

Treatment

After medical safety is ensured, treatment often focuses on improving the patient's self-monitoring techniques (including an understanding of precipitating life stressors, alternative strategies in dealing with the urge to eat, and relaxation training) and on working with the distorted self-image and the quality of interpersonal relationships (Fairburn, 1993). This type of psychotherapeutic work lends itself to group therapy.

Antidepressant medications (see p 189) are helpful for the frequently associated depressive symptoms and have been shown to decrease the frequency of binges in about 70% of bulimic patients (Walsch, 1991).

Prognosis

Although the long-term prognosis is uncertain, bulimics of normal weight generally do much better than patients with anorexia nervosa. In one follow-up study of 225 bulimics at 1 year after treatment, approximately 50% were judged to be symptom-free (Herzog, 1993). Many probably continue to have episodes of bulimic behavior associated with stressful life events.

American Psychiatric Association Workgroup on Eating Disorders: Practice guidelines for eating disorders. Am J Psychiatry 1993;150:207.
Fairburn CG et al: Psychotherapy and bulimia nervosa. Arch Gen Psychiatry 1993;50:419.
Herzog DB et al: Patterns and predictors of recovery in anorexia nervosa and bulimia nervosa. J Am Acad Child Adolesc Psychiatry 1993;32:835.
Hsu LKG: *Eating Disorders.* Guilford Press, 1990.
Walsch BT: Psychopharmacologic treatment of bulimia nervosa. J Clin Psychiatry 1991;52(Suppl):34.

ADJUSTMENT DISORDERS

Children's lives are filled with stresses and changes, most of which are not of their choosing. The list is endless, but the most frequent and most disturbing stresses for children and adolescents include marital discord or dissolution, family illness, the loss of a loved one, or a change of residence.

When faced with stress, children can manifest many different symptoms, including changes in mood, changes in behavior, and physical complaints. Key findings include the following: (1) the precipitating event or circumstance is identifiable; (2) the symptoms have appeared since the occurrence of the stressful event; (3) the intensity of the child's reaction is not severe and disabling; and (4) the reaction does not persist beyond a few months. The range of symptoms of patients with adjustment disorders are listed in Table 6–16.

Differential Diagnosis

When symptoms are clearly a reaction to an identifiable stressor but are severe, persistent, or disabling, depressive, anxiety, and conduct disorders must be considered.

Table 6–16. Signs and symptoms of adjustment reactions.

Irritable, angry mood
Anxious, worried mood
Unhappy, depressed mood
Angry resistance to authority
Fatigue
Aches and pains
Decreased school performance
Social withdrawal
Any combination of the above

Treatment

The mainstay of treatment is the doctor's assurance that the emotional or behavioral change is a predictable consequence of the stressful events. Such a statement serves both to validate the child's reaction and to encourage the child to talk about feelings associated with the stressful occurrence and its aftermath. Parents are asked to understand the child's reaction and encourage the appropriate verbal expression of feelings but at the same time to set out clear boundaries for behavior that prevent the child from feeling out of control.

Prognosis

The duration of symptoms in adjustment reactions depends on the severity of the stress, the child's personal sensitivity to stress, and the support system available to the child. The prognosis is generally good when these children feel understood by someone to whom they can express their feelings. Nonetheless, the loss of a parent or the breakup of a marriage can lead to years of intermittent distress in normal children. In addition, the precipitating stressful event may uncover a more chronic vulnerability to anxiety or depression.

Tomb DA: Adjustment disorder. In: *Child and Adolescent Psychiatry: A Comprehensive Textbook.* Lewis M (editor). Williams & Wilkins, 1991.

ELIMINATION DISORDERS

1. ENURESIS

Essentials of Diagnosis

- Involuntary urinary incontinence in a child 5 years of age or older.
- No physical abnormality causing the urinary incontinence.

General Considerations

Enuresis is the involuntary passage of urine into bedclothes or undergarments. At least 90% of enuretic children have primary nocturnal enuresis—ie, they wet only at night during sleep, and they have never had a sustained period of dryness. Diurnal enuresis (daytime wetting) is much less common, as is secondary enuresis, which develops after a child has had a sustained period of bladder control. The latter two varieties are much more frequently associated with emotional stress, anxiety, and psychiatric disorders. Primary nocturnal enuresis is generally viewed as a developmental disorder or maturational lag that is infrequently associated with a significant psychopathologic disorder.

Clinical Findings

Primary nocturnal enuresis is common (Table 6–17). The incidence is three times higher in boys than in girls. With each year that passes, a proportion of nighttime wetters stop wetting without any form of treatment. The family history in such cases frequently reveals other members—especially fathers—who have had prolonged nighttime bed wetting problems.

Although the cause of primary nocturnal enuresis is not established, it appears to be related to maturational delay of sleep and arousal mechanisms or to delay in development of increased bladder capacity.

Daytime wetting most often occurs in timid and shy children or in children with temperamental differences characteristic of attention deficit disorder. It occurs with about equal frequency in boys and girls, and 60–80% of daytime wetters also wet at night.

Secondary enuresis typically follows a stressful event, such as the birth of a sibling, a significant loss, or discord within the family. The symptom can be seen as the result of regression in response to stress or as a more symbolic expression of the child's feelings.

Differential Diagnosis

The differential diagnosis includes neurologic abnormalities, seizure disorders, diabetes mellitus, and abnormalities of the urinary tract. Obtaining a urinalysis and urine culture and observing the child's urinary stream can essentially rule out the vast majority of organic causes of enuresis. Some children with daytime wetting can have "difficult" temperamental variations or overt depression.

Complications

The most common complication of enuresis is low self-esteem in response to harsh criticism from caregivers.

Table 6–17. Incidence of enuresis in children.

Age (Years)	Primary Nocturnal Enuresis (%)	Occasional Daytime Enuresis (%)
5	15	8
7–8	7	—
10	3–5	—
12	2–3	1
14	1	—

Treatment

The most important aspect of treatment for children with primary nocturnal enuresis is reassuring the family and child that the symptom is a developmental lag and not indicative of emotional problems or "bad" behavior. Treatment can then be pursued if this largely "cosmetic" problem is a source of concern for the child. If the child chooses to pursue treatment, positive motivation is an important precondition to successful intervention.

Treatment can begin with a program of bladder exercises such as holding urine as long as possible during the day and then starting and stopping the urine stream during micturition. In addition, the child is instructed to practice getting up from bed and going to the bathroom at bedtime. The child lies down, counts to 50, gets up, goes to the bathroom, and tries to urinate. The child repeats this procedure 10–20 times each night before retiring. The combination of these procedures is helpful in perhaps 30–40% of children with nighttime wetting. For the remainder, an alerting buzzer that sounds early in the bed-wetting process is helpful to about 70% of children. The child is instructed to get up and go to the bathroom and finish emptying the bladder if the alarm goes off.

For others, a trial of imipramine is worthwhile at dosages of 25–50 mg at bedtime for children under 12 years of age and 50–75 mg for older children. Imipramine generally provides satisfactory results in about 70% of children. Unfortunately, many patients relapse once the drug is stopped; thus, its primary use is for camp or overnight visits, where a temporary period of dryness is important. Scharf et al (1987) have described an even more elaborate training program for children with primary nocturnal enuresis.

Mental health treatment is more often needed for children with daytime wetting or secondary enuresis. The focus is on the verbal expression of feelings that may be associated with perpetuation of the symptom.

Garfinkel BD: The elimination disorders. In: *Psychiatric Disorders in Children and Adolescents.* Garfinkel BD et al (editors). Saunders, 1990.

Howe AC, Walker CE: Behavioral management of toilet training, enuresis, and encopresis. Pediatr Clin North Am 1992;39:413.

Jarvelin MR et al: Etiologic and precipitating factors for childhood enuresis. Acta Paediatr Scand 1991;80:361.

2. FUNCTIONAL ENCOPRESIS

Essentials of Diagnosis

- Fecal incontinence in a child 4 years of age or older.
- Not due to physical abnormality.

General Considerations

Functional encopresis is defined as the repeated,

usually involuntary passage of feces in inappropriate places in a child at least 4 years of age. It affects approximately 1–1.5% of school-age children—boys four times as commonly as girls. Functional fecal incontinence is rare in adolescence.

Clinical Findings

Functional encopresis can be divided into four types: retentive, continuous, discontinuous, and "toilet phobia."

In **retentive encopresis**—also called psychogenic megacolon—the child withholds bowel movement, leading to the development of constipation, fecal impaction, and the seepage of soft or liquid feces into the underclothing. Marked constipation and painful defecation often contribute to a vicious cycle of withholding → larger impaction → further seepage. These children often have a history of crossing their legs to resist the urge to defecate and of infrequent bowel movements large enough to stop up the toilet, and they are found on examination to have large fecal masses in their rectal vaults. Most of these children are distressed by the soiling that occurs.

Children with **continuous encopresis** have never gained primary control of bowel function. Usually, the bowel movement is randomly deposited in underclothing without regard to social norms. Typically, the family structure does not encourage organization and skill training, and for that reason the child has never had adequate consistent bowel training. These children and their parents are more apt to be socially or intellectually disadvantaged.

Children with **discontinuous encopresis** have a clear history of having attained an extended period of normal bowel control. Loss of control often occurs in response to a stressful event, such as the birth of a sibling, a separation, family illness, or marital disharmony. These children then begin to put feces in "irritating places" as an expression of anger or of a wish to be perceived as younger. Typically, these children display relative indifference to the symptom.

In the infrequent case of "toilet phobia," a relatively young child views the toilet as a frightening structure to be avoided. These children may view the bowel movement as an extension of themselves, which is then swept away in a frightening manner. They may have the thought that they too may be swept away "down the toilet."

Differential Diagnosis

The main differential diagnosis involves the medical causes of constipation and retentive encopresis. Hirschsprung's disease can be ruled out with reasonable certainty by the history of passing large-caliber bowel movements in the past. Neurologic disorders, hypothyroidism, hypercalcemia, and diseases of smooth muscle must be considered as well. The child should be examined for anal fissures, which tend to encourage the withholding of bowel movement.

In addition, fecal soiling can be a presenting symptom in childhood depression and is sometimes a concomitant finding in children with attention deficit hyperactivity disorder.

Treatment

Identifying the type of encopresis is important in treatment planning. Another important variable is the child's own concern and level of distress about the symptom. Children who display denial or indifference about their symptoms are much harder to treat. Children with coexisting depression or attention deficit hyperactivity disorder need to be treated for those conditions prior to focusing treatment on the symptom of soiling.

With the most common type of encopresis—the retentive type—efforts are made to soften stool so that constipation and painful defecation do not perpetuate the behavior. These children are then taught to overcome the problem by adopting a regular schedule of postprandial sessions on the toilet. A system of positive reinforcement can be added in which the child is rewarded for each day with no soiled underclothes. The responsibility for rinsing own soiled clothing and depositing it in the appropriate receptacle rests with the child. In the case of continuous fecal soiling, the family is taught to train the child. For toilet phobia, a progressive series of rewarded desensitization steps is necessary.

Children with discontinuous soiling that persists over a number of weeks often need psychotherapy to help them recognize and express their anger and wish to be dependent verbally rather than by fecal soiling.

Prognosis

While the ultimate prognosis is excellent, parental distress and parent-child conflict may be great prior to the cessation of symptoms. The natural history of soiling is that it resolves by adolescence in all but the most severely disturbed teenagers.

Howe AC, Walker CE: Behavioral management of toilet training, enuresis, and encopresis. Pediatr Clin North Am 1992;39:413.

Mikkelson EJ: Modern approaches to enuresis and encopresis. In: *Child and Adolescent Psychiatry: A Comprehensive Textbook.* Lewis M (editor). Williams & Wilkins, 1991.

SUICIDE IN CHILDREN & ADOLESCENTS

Suicide has become the second leading cause of death among people 15–24 years of age. The suicide rate among adolescents 15–19 years of age quadru-pled—from approximately 2.7 to 11.3 per 100,000 over the last 40 years. For children 14 years of age and younger, the rate of completed suicide is low (0.7:100,000), but even that rate has doubled over a similar time period.

Adolescent girls make three to four times the num-ber of suicide attempts as do boys of the same age. On the other hand, suicide attempts of adolescent males are more lethal—the number of completed suicides is three to four times greater in males than in females. Firearms are the most commonly used method in suc-cessful suicides, accounting for 40–60% of cases; hanging, carbon monoxide poisoning, and drug over-doses each account for approximately 10–15% of completed suicides. Among young people, there are perhaps 50–100 suicide attempts for every completed suicide. Recent epidemiologic data suggest that among high school students during a 1-year period, approximately 25% seriously consider suicide, 15% make a plan, 8% make some type of attempt, and 2% come to medical attention because of a suicide at-tempt (MMWR, 1991).

Suicide is associated with psychopathologic disor-der and should not be viewed as a philosophic choice about life or death. Over 50% of suicides occur in young people who are sad, despairing, or depressed; another 20% are described as angry, with the sui-cide attempt occurring rather impulsively. Substance abuse is implicated in at least 20% of suicides.

The vast majority of young people who commit suicide give some clue to their distress or their tenta-tive plans to commit suicide. Most show signs of de-pression, such as social withdrawal, loss of interest in activities, and an irritable or depressed mood. Over 60% make comments such as "I wish I were dead" or "I just can't deal with this any longer" within the 24 hours prior to death. In one study, nearly 70% of sub-jects experienced a crisis event, such as a loss, a fail-ure, or an arrest prior to completed suicide.

Assessment of Suicide Risk

The best assessment of suicide risk comes from a high index of suspicion and a direct interview with the patient and "significant others" such as family members, peers, and teachers. A format for the inter-view for the adolescent is provided in Table 6–18.

The highest risk of suicide is associated with older white adolescent boys who express an intention to die, especially when they are away from other family members. Previous suicide attempts, a written note, and a viable plan for suicide with the availability of lethal means are high-risk factors. Signs and symptoms of major depression, a family history of suicide, a recent death in the family, and a view of death as a relief from the pain in their lives are further risk factors. Persons who have little or no family support, are fac-ing a crisis in their lives at work or school, or refuse to agree not to commit suicide are also at high risk.

Table 6–18. Clinical interview to assess suicide risk.

1. An observation or change has been noted.
2. How have you been feeling (inside/emotionally)?
3. Have you had periods of feeling down or discouraged?
   a. How often?
   b. How long?
   c. How severe?
4. Do they interfere with your life?
   a. Daily activities?
   b. School or work?
   c. Sleep or appetite (or both)?
   d. Family life?
5. Do you have feelings of
   a. Self-criticism or worthlessness?
   b. Helplessness?
   c. Hopelessness?
   d. Wanting to give up?
6. Are the feelings ever so strong that life does not seem worth living? Have you had thoughts of suicide?
   a. Are you having thought of suicide now?
   b. How persistent are they?
   c. How much effort does it take to resist?
   d. Can you tolerate the pain you are feeling?
7. Have you made any plans to carry out suicide?
   a. What are the plans?
   b. Have you taken any tentative action (eg, obtaining a gun or rope; stockpiling pills)?
   c. As you have thought about suicide, how have you viewed the idea of death?
8. What deters you from trying suicide?
9. If the suicidal feelings are subsiding, could you resist the feelings if they returned?
10. Is there someone you can turn to for help at those times? Who?
11. Has the idea of suicide come up inthe past?
    a. How often?
    b. When and under what circumstances?
    c. What has happened at those times?
12. Can you tolerate the pain that you are feeling right now?

Principles of Intervention

Intervention in cases of potential teen suicide must follow certain principles. The health care provider (1) must consider any suicide attempt a serious matter; (2) must not allow the patient to be left alone; (3) must make an effort to understand the young person's pain and convey a desire to help; (4) must meet with the patient and the family, both alone and together, and listen carefully to their problems and percep-tions; and (5) must let these patients know that their pain and feelings of hopelessness are understood. At the same time, the health care provider should ex-press the firm conviction that with the assistance of mental health professionals, solutions can be found.

These patients should be hospitalized if there ap-pears to be a high potential for suicide, if they are se-verely depressed or intoxicated, if the family does not appear properly concerned, or if there are practical limitations to providing supervision and support and ensuring safety. Doubts about the necessity for hospi-talization should be resolved in favor of that decision.

Any decision to send the patient home without hos-pitalization should be made only after consultation with a mental health expert. The decision should rest on a decrease in the risk of suicide and the family's ability to provide 24-hour supervision. The patient's home must be "sterilized" of guns, pills, knives, and razor blades, and the patient should be restricted from driving for at least the first 24 hours. The focus is on providing support and easing the emotional strain. Phone contact must be available, and the family must be committed to a plan for mental health treatment.

Finally, the physician should be aware of his or her own emotional reactions to dealing with potentially suicidal adolescents and their families. Because the assessment takes considerable time and energy, the physician should be on guard against becoming tired, irritable, or angry. The parents should not be blamed. The physician need not be afraid of precipitating suicide by direct, open, and frank discussions of suicidal risk.

Attempted suicide among high school students—United States, 1990. MMWR Morb Mortal Wkly Rep 1991;40: 633.

Blumenthal SJ: Youth suicide: The physician's role in suicide prevention. JAMA 1990;264:3194.

Hendin H: Psychodynamics of suicide, with particular reference to the young. Am J Psychiatry 1991;148:1150.

THE CHRONICALLY ILL CHILD

Reactions to Chronic Illness or Disability

Five to 10 percent of children experience a prolonged period of illness or disability during childhood, and the psychosocial effects of that illness are often profound for the child and the family. Although the specific impact of illness on children and their families depends on the characteristics of the illness, the age of the child, and premorbid functioning, it can be expected that both the child and the parents will go through predictable stages toward eventual acceptance of the disease state. Shock and disbelief at the time of diagnosis give way in time to anger and to mourning the loss of the normal, healthy child. Finally, after many months, the family reaches a level of realistic acceptance of the disease and becomes better able to cope with the stresses imposed by the illness and to resume normal life to the extent possible. These stages are, in fact, the stages of grief that one goes through with the loss of a loved one. When the stages are mastered successfully, the illness (ie, loss of the healthy child) is painfully accepted, and life proceeds with a new set of ground rules that take into account the needs of the sick child and the other members of the family. On the other hand, when anxiety and guilt remain prominent within the family, a pattern of overprotection can evolve. Likewise, when the illness is not accepted as a reality to be dealt with, a pattern of denial may become prominent. The clinical manifestations of these patterns of behavior are set forth in Table 6–19.

Assistance From Health Care Providers

Health care providers can do much to promote more effective coping in families struggling with chronic illness:

A. Educating the Patient and Family: Children and their families should be given information about the illness at frequent intervals, including its course and treatment. Factual, open discussions minimize the anxieties that are created by family secrets about the illness. The explanation should be comprehensible to all, and time should be set aside for questions and answers. The setting can be created with the invitation, "Let's take some time together to review the situation again."

B. Preparing the Child for Changes and Procedures: The physician should explain what can be expected with a new turn in the illness or with upcoming medical procedures. This explanation enables the child to anticipate and in turn to master the new development and promotes trust between the patient and the health care providers.

C. Encouraging the Normalization of Activities: The child should attend school and play with peers as much as the illness allows. At the same time, parents should be encouraged to apply the same rules of discipline and behavior to the ill child as are applied to normal siblings.

D. Encouraging Compensatory Activities, Interests, and Skill Development: For example, a child whose athletic development has been interrupted by the disability might pursue the acquisition of computer skills.

E. Promoting Self-Reliance: The health care provider should guide and encourage parents in helping ill children assume responsibility for some aspects of their medical care.

Table 6–19. Patterns of coping with chronic illness.

Overprotection
  Persistent anxiety or guilt
  Few friends and peer activities
  Poor school attendance
  Overconcern with somatic symptoms
  Secondary gain from the illness

Effective coping
  Realistic acceptance of limits imposed by illness
  Normalization of daily activities with peers, play, and school

Denial
  Lack of acceptance of the illness
  Poor medical compliance
  Risk-taking behaviors
  Lack of parental follow-through with medical instructions
  General pattern of acting-out behavior

F. Periodically Reviewing Family Coping:
From time to time, the physician should ask, "How is everyone doing with this?" The feelings of the patient, the parents, and other children in the family are explored as well as concerns about finances and the status of the marriage. Feelings of fear, guilt, anger, and grief should be watched for and accepted as normal reactions to difficult circumstances.

G. Recommending Support Groups: Lay support groups for the patient and family should be used to the fullest extent.

Long-Term Coping

The process of coping with a chronic illness is an ongoing one. Each change in the course of the illness and each new developmental stage for the child presents new challenges. With each step comes the need for new and painful acceptance of the disease and its limitations.

Garrison WT, McQuiston S: Chronic illness during childhood and adolescence: Psychological perspectives. Sage Publications, 1989.

Lavigne JV, Faier-Routman J: Psychological adjustment to pediatric physical disorders: A meta-analytic review. J Pediatr Psychol 1992;17:133.

McGrath PJ, McAlpine L: Psychological perspectives on pediatric pain. J Pediatr 1993;122(Suppl):2.

THE TERMINALLY ILL CHILD

The diagnosis of fatal illness in a child is a severe blow, even to families who have reason to suspect that outcome. Most parents face the news of a fatal illness as the worst experience of their lives, and although parents want and need to know the truth, they are best told in piecemeal fashion beginning with temporizing phrases such as, "The news is not good—it's a life-threatening illness." The parents' reactions and questions can then be scrutinized for clues to how much they want to be told at any one time. Parents' reactions then proceed in a sequence of grief, including initial shock and disbelief lasting days to weeks, followed by anger, despair, and guilt over weeks to months, ending in acceptance of the loss.

Although children probably do not fully understand the permanency of death until about 8 years of age, most ill children experience a sense of danger and doom that is associated with death before that age. Even so, the question whether to tell a child about the fatal nature of a disease should in most cases be answered in the affirmative unless the parents object. Refusal of the adults to tell the child—

especially when the adults themselves are very sad—leads to a "conspiracy of silence" that increases fear of the unknown in the child and leads to feelings of loneliness and isolation at the time of greatest need. In fact, children who are able to discuss their illness with family members are less depressed, have fewer behavior problems, have higher self-esteem, feel closer to their families, and adapt better to the rigors of their disease and its treatment.

Children are very observant and intuitive when it comes to understanding their illness and its general prognosis. At the same time, their primary concerns are the effects of the illness on everyday life, feeling sick, and limitations on normal activities. Children are also keenly aware of the family's reactions and are reluctant to bring up issues they know are upsetting to their parents. Whenever possible, parents should be encouraged to discuss the child's illness and to answer questions openly and honestly, including exploration of the child's fears and fantasies. Such interactions promote closeness and relieve the child's sense of isolation. Even with these active attempts to promote effective sharing between the child and the family, ill children frequently experience fear, anxiety, irritability, and anger over their illness and guilt over causing family distress. Sleep disturbances, tears, and clingy, dependent behavior are not infrequent or abnormal.

The siblings of dying children are also significantly affected by the stress thus imposed on the family. They feel neglected and deprived because of the time their parents must spend with the sick child. Anger and jealousy then give rise to feelings of guilt over having such "bad" feelings about their sick sibling.

After the child dies, the period of bereavement may last up to 3 years. Family members may need outside help in dealing with their grief through supportive counseling services.

Grollman EA: Talking About Death: A Dialogue Between Parent and Child. Beacon Press, 1990.

Leach P: Will I die? Parenting (April) 1993, page 105.

EFFECTS OF MARITAL DISSOLUTION

Currently, about 40% of families are destined to experience divorce. Seventy-five percent of divorced parents remarry, and another 50% divorce a second time. Approximately 90% of single parents are mothers, and about 50% of their children have little or no contact with the father.

Clinical Effects of Divorce

The adverse emotional effects of divorce are far-reaching for both adults and children. Many women who have been through a divorce report that it takes 3 years for a sense of order and stability to return to their lives.

There are significant effects on the parent-child relationship. First, there is a decrease in parenting capacity, which is manifested in irregularity of daily schedules, flares of temper, decreased emotional sensitivity and support of the child, inconsistent discipline, and decreased pleasure in the parent-child relationship. A tendency exists for the divorced parent to look to the child as a source of emotional support. Younger children become inappropriately close to their parents by acting as "little helpers" and parental advisors. Adolescents, on the other hand, may rebel in order to distance themselves from the emotional needs of their distressed parents.

The effects of divorce on children are most dramatically seen in the 2 years following dissolution of the marriage. Few children experience the dissolution of even turbulent marriages as a relief, because the breakup of the nuclear family is perceived as a loss of the structure that provides for their safety and support. Children would rarely choose divorce as a solution for their parents' problems.

The effects of divorce on children vary with the child's age and developmental level. Most preschoolers display a behavioral regression, experiencing fears of separation at night and when they are with baby-sitters. In addition, sleep disturbances and irritability toward parents, peers, and siblings are common. In children aged 5–8, grief, sadness, and tears predominate. These children are heartbroken and wish for reconciliation of the parents. Approximately 50% experience a decrease in school performance. In children aged 9–12, anger is the predominant affect, with the child blaming and taking sides against one or another parent. At the same time, a child at this age is at greatest risk of becoming a surrogate companion. In adolescence, anger and depression go hand in hand. In addition, teenagers are at risk of developing a sense of pessimism about their own future involvement in intimate relationships because of what they have been through in their own families.

Outcome

The most favorable outcome is for the parents to put aside old conflicts and resume caretaking relationships with their children. Younger children actually fare best, particularly when they have a support network (eg, siblings or grandparents) during the time when parents are preoccupied with their own problems. When the parents have their own adult support network, the children are not so apt to be burdened with the responsibility of caring for the parents.

At 5-year follow-up, nearly 33% of children of divorced parents are moderately depressed. At 10-year follow-up, 40% of such children report worry, underachievement, self-deprecation, and lingering anger. Upon reaching adulthood, most survivors of divorce fear repeating their parents' unhappy marriages.

Wallerstein JS: The long-term effects of divorce on children: A review. J Am Acad Child Adolesc Psychiatry 1991;30:349.

OVERVIEW OF PEDIATRIC PSYCHOPHARMACOLOGY

In recent years, psychopharmacologic agents have played an increased role in the treatment of psychiatric disorders in children and adolescents. The greater specificity of diagnostic criteria has allowed for more precise treatment planning based on diagnostic classification rather than on vague clinical impressions. Despite the therapeutic optimism that has evolved, one must remember that psychopharmacologic agents are never the only treatment for any psychiatric disorder.

As with any medication, the risks versus the benefits of administering psychoactive medications must be carefully considered with the child's guardian. Not only should a diagnosable psychiatric disorder be present, but that disorder must be significantly interfering with psychosocial development, interpersonal relationships, or the patient's sense of personal well-being before intervention with psychoactive drugs can be justified. Informed consent should be given by the guardian, and noted in the record.

A few rules of thumb apply to the use of psychoactive medications in children and adolescents. First, identify target symptoms that can be followed to evaluate the efficacy of the treatment. When initiating treatment, start with low doses and increase slowly, monitoring the side effects along with effects of the medication on the target symptoms. Divided daily doses are the rule with children and adolescents. When psychoactive medications are to be discontinued, dosages should be tapered over 2–4 weeks in order to minimize withdrawal effects.

Table 6–20 presents an overview of the clinical conditions for which psychopharmacologic agents might be considered as part of a treatment plan. In the column of "probable" indications are listed those agents whose efficacy has been established in controlled drug trials or after substantial clinical experience. The column of "possible" indications consists of agents for which uncontrolled, preliminary clinical investigations have suggested some therapeutic efficacy.

In the text that follows, the major classes of psy-

Table 6–20. Indications for psychopharmacologic interventions in children and adolescents.

Condition	Probable	Possible[1]
ADHD	Psychostimulants, tricyclics, clonidine	Bupropion, neuroleptics
ADD without H		Psychostimulants
Anorexia nervosa		SSRIs
Autistic disorder	Haloperidol, clomipramine, clonidine	Other neuroleptics, naltrexone
Bipolar disorder	Lithium, neuroleptics	Carbamazepine, valproate
Bulimia nervosa	SSRIs, tricyclics	
Major depressive disorder		SSRIs, tricyclics, buproprion, lithium
Nonspecific sedation	Diphenhydramine, fluoxetine	
Panic disorder	Tricyclics	High-potency benzodiazepine, SSRIs
Posttraumatic stress disorder		SSRIs, beta-blockers, clonidine, lithium, carbamazepine, high-potency benzodiazepines, tricyclics
Schizophrenia	Neuroleptics	
Self-injurious behavior	Naltrexone	Neuroleptics, SSRIs
Separation anxiety disorder	Tricyclics	High-potency benzodiazepines
Severely aggressive behavior	Neuroleptics, lithium, carbamazepine	Beta-blockers, clonidine
Tourette's disorder	Haloperidol	Clonidine, tricyclics, clomipramine, SSRIs

[1]SSRIs = selective serotonin reuptake inhibitors.

chopharmacologic agents with probable clinical indications in child and adolescent psychiatric practice are represented. The more commonly prescribed drugs from each class are reviewed with reference to indications, relative contraindications, initial medical screening procedures (in addition to a general pediatric examination), dosage, adverse effects, drug interactions, and medical follow-up recommendations.

PSYCHOSTIMULANTS

Methylphenidate

A. Indications: Psychostimulants are the drugs of first choice for treating attention deficit and hyperactivity disorder (ADHD) in children and adolescents. Approximately 75% of ADHD children exhibit improved attention span, decreased hyperactivity, and decreased impulsivity when given stimulant medications. Up to 75% of children with ADHD who do not respond favorably to one stimulant will respond to another. Attention deficit disorder (ADD) without hyperactivity appears to be somewhat responsive to the stimulant medications also.

B. Relative Contraindications: Methylphenidate is contraindicated in individuals with a personal or family history of motor tics or Tourette's syndrome. It is also contraindicated if other members of the family have known and untreated substance abuse disorders.

C. Initial Medical Screening: One should search for a history of personal or family motor tics or Tourette's syndrome. The child should be observed

for involuntary movements. Height, weight, pulse, and blood pressure should be recorded.

D. Dosage: 0.2–0.5 mg/kg/dose (usually 5–20 mg), administered before school and at noon, with or without another dose at 4 PM. The dose is titrated upward weekly, checking for clinical effects. Administration on weekends and during vacations is determined by the need at those times. The duration of action is approximately 3–4 hours. The sustained-release preparation (Ritalin-SR) is not as effective in some children, and the duration of action may not be as long as the purported equivalent of 10 mg of methylphenidate in the morning and at noon.

E. Adverse Effects: (Often dose-related and time-limited.)

1. Common adverse effects–Anorexia, weight loss, abdominal distress, headache, insomnia, dysphoria and tearfulness, irritability, lethargy or "zombie-like" appearance, mild tachycardia, mild elevation in blood pressure.

2. Less common effects–Interdose rebound of ADHD symptoms, emergence of motor tics or Tourette's syndrome, behavioral stereotypy, seizures, significant tachycardia or hypertension, depression, mania, psychotic symptoms. Reduced growth velocity is seen only during active administration. Growth rebound occurs during periods of discontinuation. There is usually no significant compromise of ultimate height. Psychostimulants do not appear to predispose to future substance abuse.

F. Drug Interactions: Additive stimulant effects are seen with sympathomimetic amines (ephedrine and pseudoephedrine).

G. Medical Follow-Up: Pulse, blood pressure, height, and weight should be recorded every 3–4 months and at times of dosage increases. Assess for abnormal movements at each visit.

Dextroamphetamine Sulfate

Indications, contraindications, medical screening and follow-up procedures, adverse effects, and drug interactions are the same as for methylphenidate (see above). The dosage is 2.5–10 mg/dose administered twice daily before school and at noon, with or without another dose at 4 PM. A sustained-release preparation (Dexedrine Spansules) may have clinical effects for up to 8 hours.

Pemoline

A. Indications: Indication are as for methylphenidate and dextroamphetamine. The onset of effect may occur more gradually over 2–4 weeks.

B. Relative Contraindications: As for methylphenidate, plus history of hepatic dysfunction or disease.

C. Initial Medical Screening: As for methylphenidate, plus liver function tests.

D. Dosage: The longer half-life of pemoline allows for the administration of a single dose each morning. The usual starting dose of 37.5 mg is increased weekly by 18.75 mg to the desired clinical effect or to a maximum daily dose of 112.5 mg.

E. Adverse Effects: Generally as for methylphenidate, but with fewer cardiovascular effects and less interdose rebound. Elevated liver enzymes occur in 1–3% of children receiving pemoline; hepatotoxic effects appear to be reversible with drug discontinuation.

F. Drug Interactions: As for methylphenidate.

G. Medical Follow-Up: As for methylphenidate, plus liver function tests every 6 months.

TRICYCLIC ANTIDEPRESSANTS

Imipramine

A. Indications: Imipramine is the most frequently prescribed antidepressant in children and adolescents. It has clinical efficacy in the treatment of ADHD, panic disorder, anxiety-based school refusal, separation anxiety disorder, bulimia, primary nocturnal enuresis, night terrors, and sleepwalking. It may be helpful in major depression in children and adolescents.

B. Relative Contraindications: Known cardiac disease or arrhythmia, undiagnosed syncope, known seizure disorder, family history of sudden cardiac death or cardiomyopathy, known electrolyte abnormality (with binging and purging).

C. Initial Medical Screening: The family history should be searched for sudden cardiac death and the patient's history for cardiac disease, arrhythmias, syncope, seizure disorder, or congenital hearing loss (associated with prolonged QT interval). Other screening procedures include serum electrolytes and BUN (with patients who have eating disorders), cardiac examination, and a baseline ECG.

D. Dosage: Daily dosage requirements vary considerably with different clinical disorders. Enuresis and sleep disorders can generally be treated with 25–75 mg of imipramine at bedtime, depending on the size of the child. Treatment for ADHD often requires 1–3 mg/kg/d in two divided doses. The treatment of major depressive disorder and the anxiety disorders in children and adolescents frequently requires 3–5 mg/kg/d in two divided doses. The onset of clinical effect may take 4–6 weeks to occur.

The starting dose is 1 mg/kg/d. Dosage increases of 25% are made every 4 or 5 days as tolerated to 3 mg/kg/d. Regular cardiovascular and electrocardiographic monitoring are required with each dosage increase above 3 mg/kg/d. Therapeutic antidepressant effect is most clearly associated with steady-state plasma levels of imipramine plus desipramine (see below) ranging between 150 and 300 ng/mL.

E. Adverse Effects:

1. Cardiotoxic effects–The cardiotoxic effects of tricyclic antidepressants appear to be more frequent in children and adolescents than in adults. In addition to anticholinergic effects, tricyclic antidepressants have quinidine-like effects that result in slowing of cardiac conduction. Increased plasma levels appear to be weakly associated with an increased risk of cardiac conduction abnormalities. Steady-state plasma levels of desipramine or of desipramine plus imipramine should therefore not exceed 300 ng/mL. In addition, each dosage increase above 3 mg/kg/d must be carefully monitored with pulse, blood pressure, and repeat ECGs. The cardiovascular parameters that are thought to represent the upper limits of safety when administering tricyclic antidepressants to children and adolescents are presented in Table 6–21.

2. Anticholinergic effects–Tachycardia, dry mouth, stuffy nose, blurred vision, constipation, sweating, vasomotor instability, withdrawal syndrome (gastrointestinal distress and psychomotor activation).

Table 6–21. Upper limits of cardiovascular parameters with tricyclic antidepressants.

Heart rate	≤ 130/min
Systolic blood pressure	≤ 130 mm Hg
Diastolic blood pressure	≤ 85 mm Hg
PR interval	≤ 0.20 s
QRS interval	≤ 0.12 s, or no more than 30% over baseline
QT corrected	≤ 0.45 s

3. Other effects–Orthostatic hypotension, lowered seizure threshold, increased appetite and weight gain, sedation, irritability and psychomotor agitation, rash (often associated with yellow dye No. 5), headache, abdominal complaints, sleep disturbance and nightmares, mania.

F. Drug Interactions: Tricyclic antidepressants may potentiate the effects of central nervous system depressants and stimulants; barbiturates and cigarette smoking may decrease plasma levels; phenothiazines, methylphenidate, and oral contraceptives may increase plasma levels; tachycardia may be more pronounced with marihuana.

G. Medical Follow-Up: Pulse and blood pressure with each dosage increase up to 3 mg/kg/d; pulse, blood pressure, and ECG with each dosage increase above 3 mg/kg/d; height, weight, pulse, blood pressure, and ECG every 3–4 months at steady state.

Desipramine

A. Indications: As for imipramine, but often preferred over that drug because of fewer anticholinergic side effects.

B. Relative Contraindications: As for imipramine.

C. Initial Medical Screening: As for imipramine.

D. Drug Dosage: As for imipramine. Steady-state plasma levels of desipramine should be between 150 and 300 ng/mL. Plasma levels above 300 ng/mL or total doses greater than 5 mg/kg/d should be avoided. As with imipramine, careful attention must be paid to pulse, blood pressure, and ECG with dosage increases above 3 mg/kg/d.

E. Adverse Effects: As for imipramine, except less prominent anticholinergic effects.

F. Drug Interactions: As for imipramine.

G. Medical Follow-Up: As for imipramine.

Nortriptyline

Indications, contraindications, initial medical screening procedures, and drug interactions are as listed above for imipramine.

A. Dosage: Daily dosage for major depressive disorder ranges from 0.5 to 2 mg/kg/d in two divided doses. Therapeutic antidepressant effects appear to be associated with plasma levels between 60 and 100 ng/mL in children.

B. Adverse Effects: As for imipramine, but with fewer anticholinergic effects. Daily doses should not exceed 2 mg/kg/d, and plasma levels should not exceed 150 ng/mL.

C. Medical Follow-Up: Careful cardiac monitoring with dosage increases.

Clomipramine

A. Indications: Clomipramine has been shown to be effective in the treatment of obsessive compulsive disorder in children and adolescents, resulting in moderate to marked symptomatic improvement in 75% of individuals by week 5 of treatment. The effects of clomipramine in management of obsessive compulsive disorder appear to be independent of the drug's antidepressant effect. Clomipramine also appears to be helpful in reducing the repetitive, ritualized behaviors of some autistic children (Gordon, 1993).

B. Relative Contraindications: As for imipramine.

C. Initial Medical Screening: As for imipramine, plus liver function tests.

D. Dosage: The initial daily dose of 1 mg/kg/d is advanced gradually to a target dose of approximately 3 mg/kg/d (with a maximum daily dose of 200 mg/d). Therapeutic blood levels are not yet established. In prepubertal children, daily doses are given in two divided doses.

E. Adverse Effects: As for imipramine. Some hepatotoxicity has been noted. Clomipramine appears to be as well tolerated as desipramine or imipramine.

F. Drug Interactions: As for imipramine.

G. Medical Follow-up: As for imipramine.

SELECTIVE SEROTONIN REUPTAKE INHIBITORS (SSRIs)

Fluoxetine

A. Clinical Indications: Fluoxetine is a nontricyclic, selective serotonin reuptake inhibitor that is receiving great clinical attention because of its favorable side effect profile, its relative lack of cardiotoxicity, and its wide margin of safety in overdose situations. It is probably indicated in the treatment of major depressive disorder in adolescents, particularly when there may be a greater risk of drug overdose. Fluoxetine also appears to be helpful in adolescents with anorexia and obsessive compulsive disorder.

B. Relative Contraindications: None known.

C. Initial Medical Screening: General medical examination only.

D. Dosage: The major metabolites of fluoxetine have half-lives of approximately 1 week. This allows for once-daily or even alternate-day dosing. The initial daily dose of 5–10 mg is increased by 5–10 mg every 1–2 weeks as tolerated to a maximum dose of 40 mg/d. Antidepressant response is generally achieved in adolescents on daily doses of 20–40 mg by the sixth week of treatment. Fluoxetine is usually administered as a single morning dose but may be divided into morning and noon doses if side effects so dictate.

E. Adverse Effects:

1. Common effects–(Often dose-related and time-limited.) Psychomotor activation (excitable or restless), gastrointestinal distress, nausea, headache, tremulousness, anorexia and weight loss, insomnia.

2. Uncommon effects–Behavioral disinhibition or impulsivity, possible activation of suicidal behavior (King, 1991), precipitation of mania.

F. Drug Interactions: All SSRIs inhibit the efficiency of the hepatic P450 microsomal enzyme system. This can lead to higher than expected blood levels of other coadministered medications, including other antidepressants (Crewe, 1992). Tryptophan may result in a serotonergic syndrome of psychomotor agitation and gastrointestinal distress.

G. Medical Follow-Up: General medical examination with weight and blood pressure.

Sertraline & Paroxetine

A. Indications: As for fluoxetine.

B. Relative Contraindications: None known.

C. Initial Medical Screening: General medical examination.

D. Dosage: Both sertraline and paroxetine have shorter half-lives (approximately 1–2 days) than fluoxetine (approximately 1 week). This still generally allows for once-daily dosing, usually in the morning. Therapeutic doses of sertraline range from 50 mg to 150 mg per day, while therapeutic doses of paroxetine range from 10 mg to 40 mg per day.

E. Adverse Effects: As for fluoxetine.

F. Drug Interactions: As for fluoxetine.

G. Medical Follow-Up: As for fluoxetine.

OTHER ANTIDEPRESSANTS

Bupropion

A. Indications: Bupropion is a nontricyclic antidepressant that is receiving favorable attention for its therapeutic effects with major depressive disorder in adolescents and with ADHD in children and adolescents (Casat, 1989). Like the SSRIs, bupropion has very few anticholinergic or cardiotoxic effects.

B. Relative Contraindications: History of seizure disorder. Teratogenic effects are uncertain.

C. Initial Medical Screening: General medical examination if there is a history of seizures.

D. Dosage: The dosage is not well established, but the range is thought to be from 150 to 375 mg/d in two divided doses. The maximum daily dosage in adolescents should be less than 450 mg.

E. Adverse Effects: Psychomotor activation (agitation or restlessness), headache, gastrointestinal distress, nausea, anorexia with weight loss, insomnia, tremulousness, precipitation of mania, and the induction of seizures with doses above 450 mg/d.

F. Drug Interactions: Uncertain.

G. Medical Follow-Up: General medical examination.

NEUROLEPTICS

As a class, the neuroleptics—also known as antipsychotics—are most clearly indicated for control of psychotic symptoms in schizophrenia. They are utilized also in the management of acute mania and as an adjunct to antidepressants in the treatment of psychotic depression (with delusions or hallucinations). They can be used very cautiously in refractory ADHD and in individuals with markedly aggressive behavioral problems.

Haloperidol

A. Indications: Haloperidol in particular has also demonstrated efficacy in the suppression of tics in Tourette's syndrome and specific target symptoms in autistic disorder.

B. Relative Contraindications: Haloperidol is contraindicated in patients with a history of poorly controlled seizures, cardiac arrhythmias, or agranulocytosis, previous neuroleptic malignant syndrome, or tardive dyskinesia.

C. Initial Medical Screening: One should observe and examine for abnormal movements and establish baseline complete blood count and liver function tests. An ECG should be taken if there is a history of cardiac disease or arrhythmia.

D. Dosage: Conservative treatment with haloperidol generally starts with a beginning dose of 0.5–1 mg/d, increasing by 0.5 mg every 3–5 days to clinical effect, side effects, or a maximum daily dose of 4 mg. Daily doses above 4 mg should be reserved for the most disturbed and refractory patients. Antipsychotic effects may take 2–3 weeks to become fully apparent. The drug is usually given in two daily doses.

E. Adverse Effects: While neuroleptic medications can produce a variety of adverse effects, the two most troublesome are cognitive slowing due to sedation and one or another of the extrapyramidal syndromes. The high-potency neuroleptics (eg, haloperidol) cause less sedation but have a greater frequency of extrapyramidal effects. The low-potency neuroleptics (eg, thioridazine) can cause greater sedation but fewer extrapyramidal effects. In any case, sedation, cognitive slowing, and extrapyramidal effects all tend to be dose-related. Because of the risk of tardive dyskinesia, neuroleptic medications should be reserved for children and adolescents for whom less harmful treatments are not available.

1. Extrapyramidal syndromes–Acute dystonic reactions are tonic muscle spasms, often of the tongue, jaw, or neck, which may result in such dramatically distressing symptoms as oculogyric crisis, torticollis, and even opisthotonos. The onset usually occurs within days after a dosage change and may occur in up to 25% of children treated with neuroleptics. Thioridazine is much less frequently associated with dystonic reactions. Acute neuroleptic-induced dystonias are quickly relieved by anticholinergics such as diphenhydramine.

2. Pseudoparkinsonism–Pseudoparkinsonism is usually manifested 1–4 weeks after the start of treatment. It presents as muscle stiffness, cogwheel rigidity, masked facies, bradykinesia, drooling, and occasionally pill-rolling tremor. Anticholinergic medications or dosage reductions are helpful.

3. Akathisia–Akathisia is usually manifested after 1–6 weeks of treatment. It presents as a very unpleasant feeling of driven motor restlessness that ranges from vague muscular discomfort to a markedly dysphoric agitation with frantic pacing. Anticholinergic agents or beta-blockers are sometimes helpful.

4. Neuroleptic malignant syndrome–This is a medical emergency manifested by severe muscular rigidity, altered sensorium, hyperpyrexia, autonomic lability, and myoglobinemia. Mortality rates have been reported as high as 30%.

5. "Rabbit syndrome"–This is a rare parkinsonian-like tremor of the mouth that develops late, presenting as rapid chewing-like movements similar to what is observed in rabbits.

6. Withdrawal symptoms–Dyskinesias are reversible movement disorders that appear following the withdrawal of neuroleptic drugs. They occur in up to 25% of children exposed to neuroleptics for 1 year and in approximately 50% of those exposed to neuroleptics for 2½ years. After withdrawal of the drug, dyskinetic movements develop within 1–4 weeks and may then persist for months before resolving.

7. Tardive dyskinesias–Tardive dyskinesias are the dreaded late-developing, irreversible movement disorders that appear after long-term use of neuroleptic medications. They most often present as choreoathetoid movements of the tongue and mouth but may also involve the extremities and trunk. The risk of tardive dyskinesia is thought to be small in patients exposed to neuroleptics for less than 6 months. There is no effective treatment.

8. Other adverse effects of neuroleptics–Orthostatic hypotension, cardiac arrhythmias, anticholinergic effects, weight gain, irregular menses, gynecomastia (even galactorrhea), sexual dysfunction, photosensitivity, rashes, lowered seizure threshold, hepatic dysfunction, blood dyscrasias.

F. Drug Interactions: Potentiation of central nervous system depressant effects or the anticholinergic effects of other drugs may occur, as well as increased plasma levels of antidepressants.

G. Medical Follow-Up: One should examine the patient at least every 3 months for signs of tardive dyskinesia.

Thioridazine

A. Indications: Thioridazine is effective in the treatment of psychotic disorders and severely aggressive disorders. It is not helpful for Tourette's syndrome.

B. Relative Contraindications: As for haloperidol.

C. Initial Medical Screening: As for haloperidol.

D. Dosage: Therapeutic doses generally range from 20 to 200 mg/d given in two divided doses.

E. Adverse Effects: Generally as for haloperidol, though thioridazine is considered less likely to cause acute dystonic reactions and pseudoparkinsonian effects. In doses above 800 mg/d, thioridazine is associated with retinitis pigmentosa.

F. Drug Interactions: As for haloperidol.

G. Medical Follow-Up: As for haloperidol.

MOOD STABILIZERS

Lithium Carbonate

A. Indications: Lithium remains the treatment of choice for bipolar mood disorder. It may be helpful also in the treatment of patients with severely aggressive symptoms, emotionally unstable behavior disorders, and behaviorally disturbed children whose parents are known lithium responders. Lithium has sometimes been shown to have an augmenting effect when combined with SSRIs in individuals with treatment-resistant depression and obsessive compulsive disorder.

B. Relative Contraindications: Lithium is contraindicated in patients with known renal, thyroid, or cardiac disease, those at high risk for dehydration and electrolyte imbalance (with binging and purging), and those at risk of pregnancy (teratogenic effects).

C. Initial Medical Screening: General medical screening with pulse, blood pressure, height, and weight; complete blood count; serum electrolytes, BUN, and creatinine; and thyroid function tests with TSH.

D. Dosage: Oral doses of lithium up to 1800 mg/d are frequently necessary to maintain therapeutic blood levels of 1–1.5 meq/L. Occasionally, blood levels must be increased to 1.8 meq/L in adolescents and 2 meq/L in preadolescents in order to achieve therapeutic effects (Popper, 1991). Daily dosage is generally given in three divided doses—or two doses with sustained-release lithium preparations. Lithium blood level samples should be drawn 12 hours after the last dose.

E. Adverse Effects:

1. Lithium toxicity–Lithium has a low therapeutic index–ie, blood levels required for therapeutic effects are close to blood levels that produce toxic symptoms. Mild symptoms of toxicity include increased tremor, gastrointestinal distress, neuromuscular irritability, and altered consciousness that can be seen with blood levels above 1.5 meq/L. Moderate to severe symptoms of lithium toxicity are associated with blood levels above 2 meq/L.

2. Common lithium side effects–Intention tremor, gastrointestinal distress (including nausea and vomiting and sometimes diarrhea), polyuria and polydipsia, drowsiness, malaise, weight gain, acne, and granulocytosis.

3. Uncommon lithium side effects–Lithium-induced hypothyroidism, chronic renal disease, unknown effects on developing bone.

F. Drug Interactions: Excessive salt intake and salt restriction should be avoided. Thiazide diuretics and nonsteroidal anti-inflammatory agents (except aspirin and acetaminophen) lead to increased lithium levels. Precautions against dehydration are required in hot weather and with vigorous exercise.

G. Medical Follow-Up: Serum lithium levels should be measured 5–7 days following a change in dosage and then monthly at steady state; serum creatinine and TSH concentrations should be determined every 3–4 months.

ALPHA-ADRENERGIC AGONIST

Clonidine

A. Indications: Clonidine has been found to be clinically useful in decreasing states of hyperarousal. It seems to be particularly helpful as an adjunct to methylphenidate in children with ADHD when the history is of very early onset of marked hyperactivity, aggression, and oppositional behavior. It is also frequently effective in the treatment of ADHD and tics in Tourette's syndrome (Leckman, 1991) and in states of hyperarousal associated with posttraumatic stress disorder. Clonidine also appears helpful with ADHD-like symptoms in some autistic children (Frankhauser, 1992).

B. Relative Contraindications: Clonidine is contraindicated in patients with known renal or cardiovascular disease and those with a family or personal history of depression.

C. Initial Medical Screening: The pulse and blood pressure should be recorded and a baseline ECG taken.

D. Dosage: Initial dosage of clonidine is 0.05 mg at bedtime; that dose is increased after 3–5 days by giving 0.05 mg also in the morning; and further dosage increases are made by adding 0.05 mg alternating in the morning, at noon, or in the evening every 3–5 days to a maximum total daily dose of 0.3 mg (3–5 μg/kg/d) in three divided doses. Although a clinical response generally becomes apparent by about 4 weeks, treatment effects may increase over 2–3 months. Therapeutic doses of methylphenidate can frequently be decreased by 30–50% when used in conjunction with clonidine.

Transdermal administration of clonidine using a skin patch can be quite effective but may result in significant skin irritation in 40% of cases.

E. Adverse Effects: Sedation can be promi-

nent. Other side effects include fatigability, mild hypotension, increased appetite and weight gain, headache, sleep disturbance, gastrointestinal distress, skin irritation with transdermal administration, and rebound hypertension with abrupt withdrawal. Cardiac arrhythmia is a rare side effect.

F. Drug Interactions: Increased sedation with central nervous system depressants; possible cardiotoxicity with cocaine; increased anticholinergic toxicity.

G. Medical Follow-Up: Pulse and blood pressure should be recorded every 2 weeks for 2 months and then every 3 months.

BETA-ADRENERGIC BLOCKERS

Propranolol

A. Indications: Propranolol is a nonselective beta-adrenoceptor blocking agent that reduces peripheral autonomic tone and in that way ameliorates the somatic symptoms of anxiety, including palpitations, tremulousness, sweating, and blushing. Propranolol appears to have clinical efficacy in the treatment of performance anxiety (stage fright), posttraumatic stress disorder, episodic outbursts of rage, lithium-induced tremor, and neuroleptic-induced akathisia.

B. Relative Contraindications: Propranolol should not be given to patients with a history of diabetes, cardiovascular disease, reactive airway disease, and depression.

C. Initial Medical Screening: Pulse and blood pressure should be recorded, and the fasting blood sugar in patients with a family history of diabetes.

D. Dosage: Daily doses for prepubertal children range from 10 to 120 mg/d and for adolescents from 20 to 300 mg/d. Blood pressure should be kept above 90/60 mm Hg in adolescents, and the pulse should be kept above 60/min. The drug is usually given in three divided daily doses.

E. Adverse Effects: Sedation, fatigue, bradycardia, hypotension, bronchospasm, depression, sleep disturbance, hypoglycemia in diabetics, sexual dysfunction.

F. Drug Interactions: Propranolol may inhibit the action of sympathomimetics and xanthines.

G. Medical Follow-Up: Pulse and blood pressure must be closely monitored.

OPIOID ANTAGONIST

Naltrexone

A. Indications: Naltrexone is helpful in some cases of autistic disorder and in the management of self-injurious behavior in autistic and mentally retarded individuals (Sandman, 1990/91).

B. Dosage: A single oral daily dose of 0.5–1.5

mg/kg has been found to decrease self-injurious behavior, social withdrawal, hyperactivity, and stereotypy.

C. Adverse Effects: Sedation.

Barrickman L et al: Treatment of ADHD with fluoxetine: A preliminary trial. J Am Acad Child Adolesc Psychiatry 1991;30:762.

Biederman J: Sudden death in children treated with a tricyclic antidepressant. J Am Acad Child Adolesc Psychiatry 1991;30:495.

Casat CD: Bupropion in children with attention deficit disorder. Psychopharmacol Bull 1989;25:198.

Coffey BJ: Anxiolytics for children and adolescents: Traditional and new drugs. J Child Adolesc Psychopharmacol 1990;1:57.

Crewe HK et al: The effects of SSRI's on cytochrome P4502D6 (CYP2D6) activity in human liver microenzymes. Br J Clin Pharmacol 1992;34:262.

Dulcan MK: Using psychostimulants to treat behavioral disorders in children and adolescents. J Child Adolesc Psychopharmacol 1990;1:7.

Elliot G, Popper C: Tricyclic antidepressants: The QT interval and other cardiovascular parameters. J Child Adolesc Psychopharmacol 1990/91;1:187.

Frankhauser MP et al: A double-blind, placebo controlled study of the efficacy of transdermal clonidine in autism. J Clin Psychiatry 1992;53:77.

Gordon CT et al: A double-blind comparison of clomipramine, desipramine, and placebo in the treatment of autistic disorder. Arch Gen Psychiatry 1993;50:441.

Green WH: Principles of psychopharmacotherapy and specific drug treatments. In: *Child and Adolescent Psychiatry: A Comprehensive Textbook.* Williams & Wilkins, 1991.

Hunt RD et al: Clonidine in child and adolescent psychiatry. J Child Adolesc Psychopharmacol 1990;1:87.

King RA et al: Emergence of self-destructive phenomena in children and adolescents during fluoxetine treatment. J Am Acad Child Adolesc Psychiatry 1991;30:176.

Leckman JF et al: Clonidine treatment of Gilles de la Tourette's syndrome. Arch Gen Psychiatry 1991;48:324.

Leonard HL, Rapoport JL: Psychopharmacotherapy of childhood obsessive compulsive disorder. Psychiatr Clin North Am 1989;12:963.

Popper CW: Therapeutic use of lithium in adolescents and children. Presented at AACAP Annual Meeting Institute on Changing Practices in Child and Adolescent Psychopharmacology, October 15, 1991.

Riddle M et al: Behavioral side effects of fluoxetine in children and adolescents. J Child Adolesc Psychopharmacol 1990/91;1:193.

Ryan ND: Heterocyclic antidepressants in children and adolescents. J Child Adolesc Psychopharmacol 1990;1:21.

Sandman CA: The opiate hypothesis in autism and self injury. J Child Adolesc Psychopharmacol 1990/91;1:237.

Settle EC: Bupropion: Update 1993. Int Drug Ther Newsl 1993;28:29.

Sloman L: Use of medication in pervasive developmental disorders. Psychiatr Clin North Am 1991;14:165.

Teicher MH, Glod CA: Neuroleptic drugs: Indications and guidelines for their rational use in children and adolescents. J Child Adolesc Psychopharmacol 1990;1:33.

Wilens T et al: Nortriptyline in the treatment of ADHD: A chart review of 58 Cases. J Am Acad Child Adolesc Psychiatry 1993;32:343.

REFERENCES

Garfinkel BD, Carlson GA, Well EG: *Psychiatric Disorders in Children and Adolescents.* Saunders, 1990.

Lewis M (editor): *Child and Adolescent Psychiatry: A Comprehensive Textbook.* Williams & Wilkins, 1991.

Behavioral Disorders & Developmental Variations

7

Edward Goldson, MD

Behavioral disorders and concerns about variations in behavior encompass a wide range of issues concerning the growth and development of children. Most recently, disorders and variations in behavior and development have emerged as significant problems in pediatric practice. Most of the issues discussed below are not new to the practitioner. However, with increasing knowledge of neurologic and behavioral organization of children, newer concepts of these disorders are evolving, and different approaches to diagnosis and management are emerging.

The prevailing view of variations in behavior is that they reflect a blend of intrinsic biologic characteristics of the child and the environment with which the child interacts. This chapter will first review behavior and temperament. It will then focus on those variations in development which frequently are of concern to parents. The discussion will be organized in the following manner: colic, feeding disorders; nonepileptic paroxysmal events, sleep disturbances, and temper tantrums and associated behaviors.

Greydanus DE, Wolraich ML: *Behavioral Pediatrics.* Springer, 1992.
Jenkins S et al: Continuities of common behaviour problems in preschool children. J Child Psychol Psychiatry 1984; 25:75.

NORMALITY & TEMPERAMENT

In considering each of the behaviors listed above, one is immediately confronted by what is considered "normal." What is the relationship between the parent and child? What are the parents' expectations, and what does the child bring, intrinsically, to this relationship? Critical to understanding these behaviors is an understanding of what is meant by "normal" and an understanding of childhood temperament. The physician confronted by a disturbance in physiologic function is usually able to define what is normal from a physiologic viewpoint and what is clearly abnormal. In contrast, such an all-or-none, yes/no approach is counterproductive in dealing with the problems we are concerned with in this chapter. By labeling many

of these behaviors as "disorders," we imply *abnormality* and may give rise to a behavior disorder where none previously existed. The approach of this chapter is to view the behaviors described here as encompassing a continuum of responses by the child to a variety of internal and external experiences.

The goal, for example, is not to "cure" crying or nightmares (once underlying disease has been excluded) but rather to help the parent and child understand what is wrong and to facilitate a functional approach to management in the specific context in which crying or nightmares occur. In other words, the approach should be to adjust to the child as the child adapts to his or her environment and to avoid pharmacologic management whenever possible.

An associated phenomenon to be considered when addressing variations in behavior is **temperament.** The concept of temperament has been of interest to philosophers and writers since ancient times. The Greeks proposed four temperament types: choleric, sanguine, melancholic, and phlegmatic. In more recent times, accepted folk wisdom defined temperament as being a genetically influenced behavioral disposition that is stable over time. Although there are a number of proposed models of temperament, the current debate revolves around four approaches.

Thomas & Chess Model

Thomas and Chess describe temperament as being the "how" of behavior, as distinguished from motivation, the "why," and the abilities, the "what" of behavior. Temperament is an independent psychologic attribute that is expressed as a response to some external stimulus and must always be considered in terms of the social context in which it is expressed. Moreover, the influence of temperament is bidirectional— ie, the effect of a particular experience will be influenced by the child's temperament. and the child's temperament will affect the responses of those in the child's environment. Temperament is therefore the style with which the child interacts with the environment.

Since the Thomas and Chess model is an interactive one, the perceptions and expectations of parents must always be taken into consideration when a child is evaluated. A child that one parent might describe as being hyperactive would not be so for another parent. This can be expanded to include all the temperament dimensions. Thus, the concept of "goodness of fit" comes into play. For example, if the parents want and expect their child to be predictable and that is not the child's temperament (behavioral style), what emerges is a lack of "goodness of fit" and a potential source of tension. This may be expressed as the parents' perceiving the child as being "bad" or having a "behavioral disorder" rather then as a variation of development that must be addressed both in terms of the child and of the child's environment. An appreciation of this phenomenon is important, since the physician may be able to enhance the parents' understanding of the child and beneficially influence their responses to the child's behavior. When there is a "goodness of fit," there will be less tension and stress, more harmony, and the potential for enhanced development not only of the child but also for the family. When there is not a "goodness of fit," the stage is set for tension and stress that can result in parental anger, disappointment, and frustration and conflict with the child.

Rothbart Model

A second approach to temperament is that proposed by Rothbart. This model is based primarily on behavioral observations of infants in the laboratory. Rothbart considers temperament to be relatively stable—primarily biologically based individual differences in reactivity and self-regulation. Self-regulation encompasses processes such as attention, reactivity, inhibition, and avoidance. Rothbart seems to view temperament as being subsumed under "personality" while providing the biologic basis for the developing personality. This view differs from that held by Thomas and Chess.

Buss & Plomin Model

Buss and Plomin view temperament as a set of inherited personality traits that appear early in life. Their premise is that the traits are genetic in origin, becoming observable in the first year of life and remaining relatively stable over the life span. They are distinguished from other acquired personality traits. These authors have identified three traits as constituting temperament: emotionality (distress and arousal), activity (tempo and vigor, which are measured by assessing the rate and amplitude of movement and speaking), and sociability (preference for being with others or being alone).

Goldsmith & Campos Model

Goldsmith and Campos define temperament in terms of individual differences in the expression of primary emotions and emotional arousability. They acknowledge that their view may be somewhat narrow but argue that other theorists' temperament traits or dimensions can be reconceptualized within their emotion-based framework.

In reviewing these four different conceptualizations (see Table 7–1), it is important to recognize that all seek to identify those characteristics in the child's behavior that are intrinsic to the child and lead him or her to respond to the world in a unique manner. One child may be highly emotional another less so ("calmer") in response to a variety of stressful or pleasant experiences. One child may be perceived as being hyperactive by one parent but not by the other. One child may tolerate change easily, while another has great difficulty in adapting to change. One child may tolerate discomfort more easily than another. One child may be quite sociable, while another may be more retiring and reticent. What is important for the clinician is to recognize that each child brings some intrinsic, biologically based traits to his environment and that they are neither good nor bad, right nor wrong, normal nor abnormal. Instead, they are part of the child and must be recognized and respected as such. Thus, as one looks at variations in development, one should move away from the illness model and use this construct as a means of understanding the nature of the child's behavior and its influence on the parent-child relationship.

Barr RG: Normality—a clinically useless concept: The case of infant crying and colic. J Dev Behav Pediatr 1993; 14:264.

Prior, M: Childhood temperament. J Child Psychol Psychiatry 1992;33:249.

Goldsmith HH, Buss AH, Plomin R, Rothbart MK, Thomas A, Chess S, Hinde R, McCall RB: Roundtable: What is temperament? Four approaches. Child Dev 1987;58:505.

Thomas A, Chess S: *Temperament and Development*. Brunner/Mazel, 1977.

Table 7–1. Theories of temperament.

Thomas and Chess	Temperament is an independent psychologic attribute, biologically determined, which is expressed as a response to an external stimulus. It is the child's behavioral style: an interactive model.
Rothbart	Temperament is a function of biologically based individual differences in reactivity and self-regulation. It is subsumed under the concept of "personality" and goes beyond mere "behavioral style."
Russ and Plomin	Temperament is a set of genetically determined personality traits that appear early in life and are different from other inherited and acquired personality traits.
Goldsmith and Campos	Temperament is the individual's differences in the probability of experiencing and expressing the primary emotions and arousal.

COMMON DEVELOPMENTAL CONCERNS

COLIC

The "syndrome" of colic is described as severe and paroxysmal crying that occurs mainly in the late afternoon. The infant's knees are abducted to the abdomen, with expulsion of flatus; the abdomen is distended, the facies "pained," the fists clenched, and there is minimal response to attempts at soothing. Among the difficulties for all concerned is the definition of this variation from normal behavior, its cause and, its treatment. Much of the problem lies in the name itself. The word "colic" is derived from Greek *kolikos* ("pertaining to the colon"). Thus, while colic has been attributed to a disturbance of the gastrointestinal tract, this has never been proved. Colic is a behavioral sign or symptom that begins in the first few weeks of life and usually peaks at 2 or 3 months. However, in about 30–40% of cases, colic continues into the fourth and fifth month.

Crying is considered a normal phenomenon of infancy and is present in all racial and ethnic groups around the world. Studies in the United States have reported that among most middle class infants, crying increases in duration until 6 weeks of age and gradually declines at about 4 months to baseline. At about 2 weeks of age, crying lasts an average of about 2 hours per day, increases to about 3 hours per day by 6 weeks, and gradually decreases to about 1 hour per day by 3 months. It is noted that normal crying can be modulated somewhat by a sensitive caretaker's intervention.

Excessive crying—or colic—in the absence of any physical disorder has a similar pattern, but the duration and intensity of crying are more prolonged. The most common definition of colic is the one used by Wessel; a colicky infant is one who is healthy and well fed but cries for more than 3 hours a day, for more than 3 days a week, and for more than 3 weeks—commonly referred to as the "rule of threes." A "healthy child" is the operative concept. The infant with colic has no definable physiologic disorder. Thus, before the "diagnosis" of colic can be made, the pediatrician needs to rule out diseases that might be causing the symptom.

Among the myriad suggested causes of colic are intolerance to cow's milk proteins, intestinal gas, gastrointestinal motility, immaturity of the gastrointestinal and neurologic systems, or the caretaker's style of feeding. With the exception of the relatively few infants who respond to elimination of cow's milk from the infant's or the mother's diet, there has been little firm evidence of an association with gastrointes-tinal disorders. There have been pharmacological attempts to eliminate gas with simethicone and to slow gut motility with the use dicyclomine. Simethicone has not been shown to ameliorate the behavior. Dicyclomine has been associated with apnea in infants and is contraindicated.

This then leaves characteristics intrinsic to the child, such as temperament, and parental caretaking patterns as contributing to colic. Behavioral states have three features: (1) they are self-organizing—ie, they are maintained until it is necessary to shift to another one; (2) they are stable over several minutes; and (3) the same stimulus elicits a state-specific response that is different from other states. There is a crying state, a quiet alert state, an active alert state, a transitional state, and a state of deep sleep, among others. The states of importance with respect to colic are the crying state and transitional states. During transition from one state to another, infant behavior may be more easily influenced. Once an infant is in a stable state, ie, crying, it becomes more difficult to bring about a change, ie, soothe. How these transitions are accomplished is probably influenced by the infant's temperament as well as his neurologic maturity. Some infants move from one state to another easily and can be easily diverted, while other infants will sustain a particular state and may be resistant to change.

The other component that needs to be considered with the colicky infant is the feeding and handling behavior of the caretaker. Colic is a behavioral phenomenon that involves interaction between the infant and the caretaker. Different caretakers perceive, interpret, and respond to crying behavior quite differently. If the caretaker perceives the crying infant as being spoiled and demanding and is not sensitive or knowledgeable of the infant's cues and rhythms, or is hurried, or is somewhat "rough" with the baby, the infant's ability to organize himself, soothe himself, or respond to the caretaker's attempts at soothing may be compromised. On the other hand, if the temperament of an infant with colic is understood and the rhythms and cues can be deciphered, the crying can be anticipated and the caretaker should be able to intervene appropriately before the behavior becomes "organized" in the crying state and more difficult to extinguish.

Management of Colic

There are a number of approaches that can be taken toward management of the infant with colic.

(1) The parent needs to be educated about the normal developmental characteristics of crying behavior and made aware that crying increases normally into the second month and abates usually by the third to fourth months.

(2) The pediatrician needs to reassure the parent, after having taken a complete history and performed a physical examination, that the infant is not "sick."

While these behaviors are stressful they are a normal variant of crying and are usually self-limited. This discussion can be facilitated by having the parent keep a diary of crying and weight gain. If there is a diurnal pattern and adequate weight gain, an underlying disease process is less likely to be present. Parental anxiety must be relieved, as it may be a factor contributing to the problem.

(3) In order for the parents to be able to soothe and comfort the infant, they need to learn and interpret the baby's cues. The pediatrician can be helpful in this process while observing and monitoring the infant's behavior and devising interventions aimed at calming both the infant and the parents. The clinician can suggest changes in the parents' behavior to include creation of a quiet environment without excessive handling. Rhythmic stimulation such as a gentle swing or gentle rocking, music, drives in the car, or walks in the stroller may be particularly helpful, especially if the parents are able to anticipate the onset of the crying before it becomes fixed. Another approach is to change the feeding technique so that the infant is not rushed, has ample opportunity to burp, and, if necessary, to be fed more frequently so as to decrease gastric distention if that seems to be contributing to the problem.

(4) In the past, medications such as phenobarbital elixir and dicyclomine have been used and found to be somewhat helpful. Presently however, they have been discontinued.

(5) For colicky babies refractory to behavioral management, a trial of changing the feedings by eliminating cow's milk from the formula or from the mother's diet if she is nursing may be indicated.

Barr RG: Colic and gas. In: *Pediatric Gastrointestinal Disease: Pathophysiology, Diagnosis, and Management.* Walker WA et al (editors). BC Decker, 1991.

Barr RG, Geertsma MA: Colic: The pain perplex. In: *Pain in Infants, Children and Adolescents.* Schechter NL, Berde CB, Yaster M (editors). Williams & Williams, 1993.

Carey WB: "Colic": Primary excessive crying as an infant-environmental interaction. Pediatr Clin North Am 1984; 31:993.

Miller AR, Barr RG: Infantile colic: Is it a gut issue? Pediatr Clin North Am 1991;38:1407.

FEEDING DISORDERS

This cluster of behaviors occurs in two forms: overeating, leading to obesity; and undereating, leading to inadequate weight gain. Eating disorders are not uncommon in adolescents, where one may encounter marked obesity or anorexia nervosa and bulimia. Concerns about poor feeding and failure to gain weight in infants and young children are also among the more common complaints brought to the pediatrician. A healthy-appearing infant who is well nourished is a source of pride to most parents and in our society is the mark of good parenting. The focus of this section will be on the infant who does not eat. Eating disorders of adolescence are covered elsewhere.

The reasons why children have feeding problems are quite varied. The common denominator, however, is usually food refusal. Infants and young children may refuse to eat because they find eating aversive (eg, it hurts or is frightening); they may have had unpleasant experiences (emotional or physiologic) associated with eating; they may be depressed; or they may be engaged in a developmental conflict with their caretaker which is being played out in the arena of feeding. The child—more commonly the infant—may also refuse to eat if the rhythm of the feeding experience with the caretaker is not harmonious.

The child who has had an esophageal atresia repair and has a stricture—or even a mild narrowing of the esophagus—may find eating uncomfortable or even painful. The very young infant with severe oral candidiasis will refuse to eat because it hurts. The child who has had a choking experience associated with feeding may be terrified to eat (oral motor dysfunction or aspiration). The child who is forced to eat by a maltreating parent or an overzealous caretaker may come to refuse feeds, as may the child who is threatened. The child who may have tasted foods that he or she does not like or which were associated with some discomfort will refuse to eat those foods or foods in general.

Children who are depressed express this psychologic state in a variety of ways, one of which may be through food refusal. Food refusal may develop when the infant's cues around feeding are not correctly interpreted by the parent. The baby who needs to burp more frequently or the one who needs time between bites but instead is rushed will often passively refuse to eat. On the other hand, some will be more active refusers and will turn their heads away to avoid the feeder, may spit out food, or push food away.

Chatoor and coworkers have adopted a developmental and interactive view of the feeding experience. They consider the various stages through which the child normally progresses: establishment of homeostasis (0–2 months), attachment (2–6 months), and separation and individuation (6 months to 3 years). During the establishment of homeostasis, feeding can be most easily accomplished when the parent allows the infant to determine the timing, amount, pacing, and preference of food intake. During the attachment phase, allowing the infant to control the feeding permits the parent to effectively engage the infant in a positive manner. This provides the basis for the separation and individuation phase.

When there is a disturbance in the parent-child relationship at any of these developmental levels, there may ensue difficulty in feeding, with both the parent and the child contributing to the dysfunctional interaction. One of the most striking manifestations of food refusal occurs during the stage of separation and individuation. If the parent seeks to impose his or her will on the child through intrusive and controlling feeding behavior while at the same time the child is striving to achieve autonomy, conflict may arise. The scenario then observed is of the parent forcing food on the child while the child refuses to eat. This often leads to extreme parental frustration and anger at the child. At the same time, the child may be inadequately nourished and developmentally and emotionally thwarted.

When the pediatrician is attempting to sort out the factors contributing to the complaint of food refusal (feeding disorder), it is essential to obtain a complete history, including a social history. This should include information concerning the parents' perception of the child's behaviors and their expectations of the child. Second, a complete physical examination needs to be performed, with considerable emphasis on oral-motor behavior and the pursuit of other findings suggesting neurologic dysfunction or anatomic or physiologic abnormality that could make feeding difficult. As part of this evaluation, the child's emotional state and developmental level must be determined. This is particularly important if there is concern about depression or if there is a history of developmental delays. If there is evidence for these disturbances, a more complete behavioral evaluation needs to be obtained. If there is evidence for oral-motor difficulty, evaluation by an occupational therapist is warranted. Third, the feeding interaction needs to be observed. Finally, the physician needs to help the parent understand that in the face of a normal examination, infants and children may indeed have different styles of eating and food preferences and may refuse foods they do not like. This is not necessarily abnormal but rather reflects temperamental differences and variations in the child's way of processing olfactory, gustatory, and tactile stimuli.

Management of Feeding Disorder

The goal of intervention is to identify factors contributing to the disturbance and to work with the parent and child to alter the circumstances leading to the difficulty. This may mean that the parents must learn to view the child's behavior differently and not impose their expectations and desires on an unwilling child. On the other hand, the child's behavior may need to be modified in order for the parent to be able to appropriately nourish and nurture the baby.

When the chief complaint is failure to gain weight or failure to thrive, a somewhat different approach should be taken. A child who is failing to gain weight is one whose weight is falling across the percentile curves of weight by 2 SD or has a persistent deviation below the expected or established weight curve. The differential diagnosis should include food refusal as contributing to the problem but must take into consideration also medical disturbances and issues of maltreatment. The essential reason children do not gain weight is that they are not being adequately nourished for whatever reason. They may have excessive losses as a result of vomiting or diarrhea; they may not be given adequate food or the amount they receive may not meet their physiologic needs; or they may not be efficiently utilizing the nutrients they are receiving. Failure to gain weight is usually due to a combination of several of these factors. As with case of the food-refusing child, a complete history and physical examination must be performed. A comprehensive psychosocial and developmental history should be obtained along with observation of the feeding experience.

Basic laboratory studies include a complete blood count, erythrocyte sedimentation rate, urinalysis and urine culture, blood urea nitrogen, serum electrolytes and creatinine, and stool for ova and parasites and to look for evidence of malabsorption. Some practitioners also include liver and thyroid profiles.

Recognizing that the cause of failure to gain weight is multifactorial, the approach toward diagnosis and treatment needs to be broad-based and multidisciplinary. Because of its complexity, no one discipline has sufficient skills to comprehensively evaluate the child and family. Thus, a team should be utilized that consists of a physician, a nurse, a social worker, and a dietitian as well as occupational and physical therapists, developmentalists, and psychologists as required. In this way, a diagnosis can be arrived at and a comprehensive treatment and monitoring plan developed.

The overall goals for the management of the child with poor weight gain are to establish a normal pattern of weight gain and to facilitate improved family functioning. Guidelines to accomplishing these goals include the following:

(1) Establishing a comprehensive diagnosis that considers all the factors contributing to the poor weight gain.

(2) Monitoring the feeding interaction and assuring appropriate weight gain.

(3) Monitoring the developmental progress of the child and changes in the family dynamics that facilitate optimal weight gain and psychosocial development.

(4) Provision of support to the family as they seek to help the child.

Frank D, Zeisel SH: Failure to thrive. Pediatr Clin North Am 1988;35:1187.

Goldbloom RR: Failure to thrive. Pediatr Clin North Am 1982;29:151.

Goldson E: Failure to thrive/failure to gain weight. In: *APSAC Handbook on Child Abuse.* Briere J et al (editors). Sage Publications. [In press, 1994.]

Macht J: *Poor Eaters.* Plenum Press, 1990.

Stevenson RD: Failure to thrive. In: *Behavioral Pediatrics.* Greydanus DE, Wolraich ML (editors). Springer, 1992.

SLEEP DISORDERS

It is estimated that 20–30% of children experience sleep problems severe enough to cause concern to their families. These problems are usually divided into three groups: (1) nighttime attacks (parasomnias), (2) sleeplessness (insomnias or dyssomnias), and (3) excessive sleepiness during the day. We will discuss parasomnias and dyssomnias here. Research and clinical experience during the last 3 decades have added greatly to our understanding of sleep problems, many of which can be explained in terms of the physiology of sleep and individual circadian rhythms. Sleep is a complex physiologic process that is influenced by intrinsic biologic properties, individual temperamental characteristics, cultural norms and expectations, and environmental conditions.

Normal sleep is made up of two cycling, distinctly different states that have been identified clinically and with the use of **polysomnography,** which consists of electroencephalography, electro-oculography, and electromyelography. The two states are rapid eye movement (REM) sleep and non-rapid eye movement (NREM) sleep. REM sleep is a very active state physiologically and mentally and is characterized by both deep and light sleep. Muscle tone is reduced, though the sleeper may twitch and grimace. The regulation of temperature, blood pressure, heart rate, and respirations has increased variability, while higher cortical functions appear active. Dreaming is closely associated with REM sleep. REM cycles last about 90 minutes at intervals during the night but are most frequent during the latter half of the night.

NREM sleep is what we think of as sleep and is divided into four stages. In the process of falling asleep, the individual enters stage 1, light sleep, which is characterized by reduced bodily movements, eye rolling, and sometimes opening and closing of the eyelids. Stage 2 sleep is characterized by slowing of eye movements, slowing of respirations and heart rate, and weakening of the muscles but with repositioning of the body. Some dreaming may occur in this stage. Most mature sleepers spend about half of their sleeping time in this stage. Stages 3 and 4 (also called delta or slow-wave sleep) are quite similar. They are the deepest NREM sleep stages during which time the sleeper's body is relaxed, breathing is slow and shallow, and the heart rate is slow. Nighttime sleep consists of repeated alternating episodes of NREM and REM sleep.

The onset of sleep occurs when the individual enters NREM stage 1 sleep. The individual then progresses to NREM stage 2 and on to NREM stages 3 and 4. The deepest NREM sleep occurs during the first 1–3 hours after going to sleep, with transitions to NREM stage 2 sleep and brief awakenings. REM and NREM stage 2 sleep cycles occur during the latter part of the night and are also interspersed with brief awakenings. The importance of understanding these patterns is that during NREM deep sleep, parasomnias occur; and during REM sleep, dreaming and nightmares occur.

1. PARASOMNIAS

Parasomnias are undesirable physical nighttime attacks that are disorders of arousal from deep NREM sleep. Of all the sleep disorders, they are probably the most frightening for parents. The parasomnias include night terrors (pavor nocturnus), sleepwalking (somnambulism), nocturnal seizures, and nightmares.

Night terrors commonly occur within 2 hours after falling asleep during the deepest stage of sleep and are often associated with sleepwalking. They are reported in about 3% of children. During a night terror, the child may sit up in bed screaming and thrashing about, with rapid breathing, tachycardia, and sweating. The child often has a glazed look in his eyes and is essentially incoherent. During the episode the child seems not to be helped by and may even resist parental attempts at comforting. The attack may last for several minutes to half an hour, after which the child goes back to sleep and has no memory of the event the next day. What is critical for parents is that they be reassured that the child is not in pain and that they should let the episode run its course. However, there is an association between fatigue and emotional and psychosocial stress. Therefore, maintaining adequate sleep and decreasing daytime stresses become critical. In this context, behavioral approaches have been found to be most helpful. Although the condition is benign, treatment is important, first to allay parents' fears and second to prevent sleepwalking, which can result in injury. The parents should determine when the episode usually occurs and awaken him to full arousal about 15 minutes before that time. After 4 or 5 minutes, the child is allowed to return to sleep. The waking is discontinued once the terrors stop, which in most circumstances is usually within a week. It should be remembered that sleepwalking can occur independently of night terrors and is another disorder of arousal. Under all of these conditions, the parents need to create an environment such that the child will not endanger himself or others. In the most severe cases, pharmacologic interventions have been used and only on a temporary basis. Dahl suggests 25–50 mg of imipramine at bedtime as a window for more long-lasting behavioral approaches which are used to increase the total amount of sleep, to identify the causes of sleep disruption, and to address the sources of anxiety and stress.

Nightmares, in contrast to night terrors, are frightening dreams that typically are followed by awakening and occur during REM sleep, usually in the latter part of the night. The peak occurrence is in the age group from 3 to 5 years, with an incidence between 25% and 50%. A child who awakens during these episodes is usually alert. He or she can often can describe the frightening images, recall the dream, and talk about it during the day. The child seeks and will respond positively to parental reassurance. Moreover, the child will often have difficulty going back to sleep and will want to stay with the parents. By and large, nightmares are self-limited and need little treatment. However, if the child has recurrent nightmares, the pediatrician may have to make a more extensive investigation. Nightmares are often associated with stressful or frightening daytime events or anxieties that may include frightening television programs, traumatic life events, and chronic stresses in the family such as discord between the mother and father. These may need to be addressed if the child is to be helped. In more severe cases, a psychologist or psychiatrist may need to be consulted.

2. DYSSOMNIAS

The second group of disturbances are the insomnias or dyssomnias, namely, problems of going to sleep and nighttime awakenings. While the parasomnias are quite frightening to most parents, this group of behaviors tends to be annoying and frustrating. Among other things, they can result in daytime fatigue of both the parents and the child, parental discord about management, and family disruption. There are a number of factors that contribute to disturbances of sleep. First, there is the influence of infant feeding. The quantity and timing of feeds in the first years of life will influence nighttime awakening. Most infants beyond 6 months of age can go through the night without being fed. Thus, it must be considered that under normal circumstances night waking for feeds is a learned behavior and is a function of the child's arousal and the parents' response to that arousal. Second, co-sleeping can play a role in night waking. In many cultures, co-sleeping is an accepted behavior. However, when it intrudes on the parents' rest and their sexual relationship, it can be a problem. Third, child rearing approaches and the practices by which bedtime is initiated can influence settling in for the night as well as awakening and staying awake at night. If the child learns that going to sleep is always associated with a pleasant parental behavior such as rocking, singing, or nursing, if and when he arouses at night and the parent is not available, going back to sleep can be difficult. Fourth, the child's temperament is another factor contributing to sleep. It has been reported that children with low sensory thresholds and less rhythmicity are more prone to night waking. Fifth, children who have had perinatal difficulties have a greater incidence of night waking and difficulties returning to sleep. Finally, psychosocial stressors can play a role in night waking.

Management

There are a variety of approaches to the management of children with dyssomnias, but there is general agreement that it is not acceptable to allow the child to "cry it out." Basic to all the strategies is obtaining a detailed sleep history and diary to which both parents contribute. Problems often arise when parents try to get the child to sleep at a time when the child is not biologically ready for sleep. For example, if they put the child down too early, he will lie awake and cry (late sleep phase), or the parents may wait too long to put him down, resulting in crankiness and early awakening and disrupted nap times (early sleep phase). Second, a complete medical and psychosocial history should be obtained and a physical examination performed. If these data do not provide adequate information, some clinicians employ polysomnography for diagnostic purposes.

A helpful developmental approach to management of these sleep difficulties is suggested by Largo (see references for other approaches). He advocates that the child's individual sleep behavior characteristics have to be taken into account and parental expectations and fears need to be identified and addressed. Counseling is then provided on the following premises:

(1) Sleep is a highly active and organized process that matures during the first years of life. One-week-old infants sleep about 16½ hours a day, with 10 of those hours being at night, whereas a 2-year-old sleeps a total of 13 hours a day, with only one of those hours being during the day.

(2) Individual circadian rhythms do not change immediately and require consistency and regularity over a period of time before change will occur.

(3) The duration of sleep for a given individual does not vary significantly, but there are large variations among different children.

(4) The duration of nighttime sleep is negatively correlated with daytime sleep, and bedtimes and awakening times are positively correlated with each other.

(5) Night waking occurs in 40–60% of infants and young children. If the child does not cry or wake up the parents, such behavior should not be considered a sleep disturbance.

In working with parents, it is important to point out unrealistic expectations with regard to sleep behavior and identify and seek to correct inconsistencies in parental behavior around sleep. The inadvertent behaviors that parents use to reinforce the undesired sleep and waking behavior need to be identified and the parents educated. Parents need to set distinct limits for the child while acknowledging the child's individual biologic rhythms. At the same time, they need to be sure not to get caught up in the child's attempts to prolong bedtime or his attempts to engage them during nighttime awakenings. Putting a child to bed after prolonged rocking, feeding, or when the child has already fallen asleep frequently results in disturbances of settling down at night or going back to sleep after a nighttime awakening. The establishment of clear bedtime rituals, placing the child in bed before he is asleep, and creating a quiet, secure bedtime environment are essential if sleep problems are to be avoided and can also be used in treating them if they arise.

For the child who has a delayed sleep phase—difficulty in both falling asleep and waking at desired times but no difficulty at later times—a regular schedule and consistent, nonstimulating bedtime rituals must be provided. Approaches used to alter the child's behavior include having the parents withdraw the attention elicited by the wakeful child and by positive reinforcement of the desired behavior. Another strategy to alter this sleep pattern is to gradually move the bedtime hour up and awaken the child earlier in the morning. However, it must be remembered that there is nothing intrinsically normal or abnormal in this pattern. It only becomes a problem when it differs from what the parents want.

Some children are afraid to go to sleep. The parent needs to help the child identify what is frightening about going to sleep and may need to stay near the child as he goes to sleep, reassuring him that he is safe and that mommy and daddy will not let anything happen to him. Over a period of time, the child can be reassured and the parent may not need to be so involved. This also applies to nighttime awakenings.

The key to management of children who have difficulty going to sleep or who awaken during the night and disturb others is to recognize that both the child and the parent play significant roles in initiating and sustaining what may be an undesirable behavior. Thus, it becomes important for the physician and parents to understand normal sleep patterns, the parents' responses that inadvertently reinforce undesirable sleep behavior, and the child's individual temperament traits.

Adair RH, Bauchner H: Sleep problems in childhood. Curr Probl Pediatr 1993;23:147.

Dahl RE: The pharmacologic treatment of sleep disorders. Psychiatr Clin North Am 1992;15:161.

Ferber R: Sleeplessness, night awakening, and night crying in the infant and toddler. Pediatr Rev 1987;9:69.

Lozoff B, Zuckerman B: Sleep problems in children. Pediatr Rev 1988;10:17.

Mahowald MW, Rosen GM: Parasomnias in children. Pediatrician 1990;17:21.

Richman N: Recent progress in understanding and treatment of sleep disorders. Adv Develop Behav Pediatr 1986;7:45.

Sladkin K, Brown LW: Sleep disorders in children and adolescents. In: *Behavioral Pediatrics*. Greydanus DE, Wolraich ML (editors). Springer, 1992.

TEMPER TANTRUMS & BREATH-HOLDING SPELLS

1. TEMPER TANTRUMS

Temper tantrums as an expression of anger and frustration are common between 12 months and 4 years of age, occurring about once a week in 50–80% of children in this age group. The behavior is characterized by the child lying or throwing himself down, kicking and screaming, on occasion throwing things or hitting and occasionally holding his breath. These behaviors can usually be considered normal as the young child seeks to achieve mastery over his environment and autonomy in his actions. They are often a reflection of immaturity as the child strives to accomplish age-appropriate developmental tasks and meets with difficulty because of a lack of fine and gross motor skills, language development, impulsiveness, or restrictions placed on him by his parents. In the home, these behaviors can be annoying for parents, but they can be managed. In public, they serve as an embarrassment.

It is not clear why some children have tantrums while others do not. Under normal circumstances, this is probably related to the child's temperament. Some children tolerate frustration well, are able to persevere at tasks, and cope with difficulties relatively easily, while others have a much greater problem dealing with experiences they may not understand and are still too immature to cope with. Tantrums can be minimized with an understanding of the child's temperament and what the child is trying to communicate as well as a commitment to supporting the child's drive to master his feelings. Appropriate intervention can also provide an opportunity for enhancing the child's growth. It should be remembered that the tantrum is a loss of control on the child's part and a blow to his self-image which is quite frightening for the child. Therefore, the parent and physician need to view these behaviors within the child's developmental context rather than from a negative, adversarial, angry viewpoint.

Management

Several suggestions can be offered for parents and physicians in managing these normal responses to frustrations and anger:

(1) Minimize the need to say no by "child-proofing" the environment such that fewer restrictions need to be placed on the child and thus less chance for conflict to arise.

(2) Use distraction when frustration increases, direct the child to other less frustrating activities, and reward the child's positive response.

(3) Present choices and options within the limits of what is acceptable so that the child does have a chance to practice mastery and autonomy.

(4) Fight only those battles that clearly need to be

won and avoid those that set up an unnecessary conflict that may serve no significant purpose and may create more problems.

(5) Do not abandon the preschool child when a tantrum occurs, and stay in close proximity during the episode without intruding on him. At times the child may need to be contained in order to gain control, and the parent should be willing and able to help. For the older child, suggest that he go to his room until he settles down. No threats or arguments should be used, since they serve no purpose.

(6) Do not use negative terms when the tantrum is occurring. Instead, point out that the child is out of control and praise him when he regains control.

(7) Never let a child hurt himself or others.

(8) Do not "hold a grudge" after the tantrum is over. However, the child's demands leading to the tantrum should not be granted.

(9) Seek to maintain an environment that provides positive reinforcement for desired behavior. Do not overreact to undesired behavior, but set reasonable limits and provide responsible direction for the child.

Approximately 5–20% of young children have severe temper tantrums that go beyond what is considered normal. Tantrums become a problem that must be dealt with when they are very frequent and disrupt the family or when the child uses them as more than an expression of frustration. Such tantrums are often the result of a disturbance in the parent-child interaction. They may have their origin in poor parenting skills, with a lack of limit-setting and permissiveness, or may be part of a larger behavioral or developmental disorder. They may also emerge under adverse socioeconomic conditions, in circumstances of maternal depression and family dysfunction, or when the child is in poor health. The pediatrician can serve an important role by helping the parents identify the underlying conditions leading to the behavioral outburst and by acknowledging the parent's feelings of anger, shame, and frustration. The parent can then help develop strategies to extinguish the behavior. If there are significant disturbances in the family, referral to psychologist or psychiatrist is appropriate while the pediatrician continues to support and work with the family.

2. BREATH-HOLDING SPELLS

While temper tantrums can be frustrating and annoying to parents, breath-holding spells can be terrifying. DiMario maintains that the name for this behavior is a misnomer in that it connotes volitional behavior resulting in prolonged inspiration. Instead, it occurs during expiration and is reflexive in nature. This is a paroxysmal event occurring in 0.1–5% of healthy children ages 6 months to 6 years. The spells usually start during the first year of life, often in response to anger or a mild injury. The child is provoked, starts to cry—briefly or for a considerable time—and then becomes noiseless. This is followed by a color change. Spells have been described as either pallid (acyanotic) or cyanotic, with the latter usually associated with anger and the former usually with an injury such as a fall. Following the period of noiselessness, the spell may resolve, the child may lose consciousness, or, in severe cases, may become limp and progress to opisthotonos and body jerks and urinary incontinence. Only rarely does a spell proceed to asystole or a seizure.

For the child with frequent spells, disorders such as seizures, orthostatic hypotension, obstructive sleep apnea, abnormalities of the central nervous system, tumors, familial dysautonomia, and Rett's syndrome need to be considered. There is also an association between breath-holding spells, pica, and iron deficiency anemia. These conditions can be ruled out on the basis of the history, the physical examination, and appropriate laboratory studies. Once it has been determined that the child is essentially healthy, the primary form of treatment is for the pediatrician to reassure the parents that the problem will spontaneously resolve with time. There are no prophylactic medications. However, atropine, 0.01 mg/kg/ dose, has been used to prevent spells accompanied by bradycardia or asystole.

Thus, the focus of treatment is behavioral. Parents should be taught to handle the spells in a matter-of-fact manner and monitor them for any untoward events. The reality is that parents cannot completely protect their child from upsetting and frustrating events and probably should not try to do so. Instead, as in the case of temper tantrums, parents need to help the child control his responses to frustrating and difficult events, using some of the techniques previously described. Moreover, they need to be careful not to be too permissive and submit to the child's every whim for fear he might have a "spell." Such behavior can hamper the child's emotional and cognitive development and may be harmful to the parent-child relationship. If a syncopal event should occur, the child should be placed in a lateral, supine position to protect his head from injury and to avoid aspiration. Cardiopulmonary resuscitation should be avoided although maintaining a patent oral airway is essential.

Needlman R, Howard B, Zuckerman B: Temper tantrums: When to worry. Contemp Pediatr 1989;6:12.

Needlman R, Stevenson J, Zuckerman B: Psychosocial correlates of severe temper tantrums. J Dev Behav Pediatr 1991;12:77.

DiMario FJ Jr: Breath-holding spells in childhood. Am J Dis Child 1992;146:125.

SUMMARY

This chapter has focused on several of the more common complaints about behavior encountered by those who care for children. It is important to understand that these behavioral "disorders" are, by and large, normal variations in behavior. They are a reflection of each child's individual biologic and temperament traits and the parental response to these characteristics as they are behaviorally expressed. The health provider should recognize there are no "cures" but that there are strategies which can enhance the parental understanding of the child and his or her relationship to the environment. Thus, diagnosis and management of these conditions requires a comprehensive and often transdisciplinary approach. The health provider can play a major role in diagnosis and, when possible, in coordinating the child's evaluation, interpreting the results to the family and providing reassurance and ongoing support.

Child Abuse & Neglect

8

Richard D. Krugman, MD

The problem of child abuse and neglect, barely recognized as a significant problem in the earliest editions of this textbook, has grown to a problem of such serious proportions that the United States Advisory Board on Child Abuse and Neglect called the present state of the nation's ability to protect children a "national emergency." What Kempe and his colleagues called "battered child syndrome" was thought to affect 749 children in the United States in 1960. The best data now suggest that 2–2.5% of American children are abused or neglected annually. In 1992, there were just under 3 million reports of abuse and neglect, with 1.2 million of these substantiated by child protective service agencies. This dramatic increase in cases has resulted from significantly increased recognition of the problem by professionals, in part from the influence of mandatory reporting statutes; a broadening of the definition of abuse and neglect from the original "battered child" concept; and changes in the demography and social structure of families and neighborhoods over the past several decades. Abuse and neglect of children is best considered in an ecologic perspective that recognizes the individual, family, social, and psychologic influences that come together to contribute to the problem. For most pediatric health care professionals, however, their involvement will be limited to individual cases. This chapter, therefore, will focus on the knowledge necessary for the recognition, intervention, and follow-up of the more common forms of child maltreatment and to highlight the role of pediatric professionals in prevention.

FORMS OF CHILD MALTREATMENT

It should be noted that the forms of maltreatment briefly described below may occur either within or outside the family. The proportion of intrafamilial to extrafamilial cases varies with the type of abuse as well as the gender and age of the child.

Physical Abuse

Physical abuse, or nonaccidental trauma, occurs when injury is inflicted on children, most often by a caretaker but occasionally by strangers. The most common manifestations of physical abuse include bruises, burns, fractures, and head and abdominal injuries. A small but significant number of unexpected deaths of infants and children are related to physical abuse.

Sexual Abuse

Sexual abuse is defined as the engaging of dependent, developmentally immature children in sexual activities they do not fully comprehend and to which they cannot give informed consent or which violate the laws and taboos of a society. It includes pedophilia and all forms of incest, and rape. It also involves fondling, oral-genital contact, and all forms of intercourse, exhibitionism, voyeurism, and the involvement of children in the production of pornography.

Emotional Abuse

Emotional abuse—or, more broadly, "psychologic abuse" has been defined as the rejection, ignoring, criticizing, isolation, or terrorizing of children, all of which have the effect of eroding their self-esteem. The most common form is verbal abuse or denigration.

Physical Neglect

Physical neglect is the failure to provide the necessities of food, clothing, shelter, and a safe environment in which children can grow and develop normally. Although associated with poverty, these cases involve a more serious problem than just absence of financial resources. There is often a component of emotional neglect and an inability to recognize and respond to the needs of the child.

Emotional Neglect

The most common feature of emotional neglect is the absence of normal parent-child attachment and a subsequent inability to recognize and respond to an infant's or child's needs. The most common manifestation of emotional neglect in infancy is nutritional (nonorganic) failure to thrive.

Medical Care Neglect

Medical care neglect is failure to provide needed

treatment to infants or children who have generally life-threatening or other serious medical conditions.

Munchausen Syndrome by Proxy

This is a relatively unusual disorder in which a caretaker, usually the mother, either simulates or creates the symptoms or signs of illness in the child.

RECOGNITION OF ABUSE & NEGLECT

Recognition of abuse and neglect of children can only occur if the possibility is entertained in the differential diagnosis of the condition for which the child is brought for care. The approach to the family should be supportive, empathic, and nonaccusatory. The individual who brings the child for care may not have any involvement in the abuse. Approximately one-third of the incidents of child abuse occur in extrafamilial settings. Nevertheless, the assumption that the caretaker is "nice" combined with failure to raise the possibility of abuse can be costly, even fatal. In 1993, nearly 95% of the American public was aware of the existence of child abuse and neglect. Raising the possibility that a child has been abused in a neutral, calm manner is *not* the same as accusing the caretaker of being the abuser. The health professional who is examining the child can explain to the family that there are several reasons that might explain the injuries or abuse-related symptoms the child has. If the family (or whoever brings the child in for evaluation) is not involved, they will welcome a report and investigation.

History

The medical diagnosis of **physical abuse** is based on the presence of a "discrepant history." The history offered by the caretaker does not accord with the clinical findings. The "discrepancy" may exist because there is no history, a partial history, changing histories over time, or simply an illogical or improbable history. The presence of a discrepant history should lead to a request for consultation with a multidisciplinary child protection team or a report to the child protective services agency mandated by state law to receive and investigate reports of suspected child abuse and neglect. It may take a social services or law enforcement investigation and home visit to sort out the circumstances of the child's injuries. Other features that are present in many abuse cases are listed in Table 8–1.

Sexual abuse may present in three different ways. (1) The child may be brought in for routine care or for an acute problem and sexual abuse may be suspected by the examining professional as a result of the history obtained or physical findings found. (2) The parent or other caretaker may bring the child to the pediatric health care provider because of a suspicion that the child may have been sexually abused, asking for

Table 8–1. Common historical features in abuse cases.

Discrepant history
Delay in seeking care
Stressed caretaker
Behavior by child that triggered assault
History of abuse in caretaker's childhood
Unrealistic expectations of caretaker for child
Social isolation of caretaker
Pattern of increased severity of injury if no intervention
Use of multiple hospitals or caretakers for injuries to child

an examination to "rule in or rule out" the possibility. (3) The child may be referred by child protective services or law enforcement personnel for an evidentiary examination following disclosure by the child or an allegation by a parent or third party. Table 8–2 lists the numerous ways sexual abuse may present in children. It should be emphasized that with the exception of certain sexually transmitted diseases and forensic laboratory findings, none of these presentations are specific. They should, however, raise the possibility of abuse and lead the practitioner to ask about the possibility of abuse—again, in a compassionate, nonaccusatory way. The American Academy of Pediatrics has recently published guidelines for the evaluation of child sexual abuse by primary care physicians.

Emotional abuse may cause nonspecific symptoms in children. Loss of self-esteem or self-confidence, sleep disturbances, somatic symptoms (eg, headaches, stomach aches), hypervigilance, or avoidant or phobic behaviors (eg, refusal to go to school or running away) may be presenting symptoms or complaints. Emotional abuse can occur in the home or in day care, school, sports team or other settings.

Neglect of children is not easily documented on history. **Physical neglect**—which must be differentiated from the effects of poverty—will be present

Table 8–2. Presentations of sexual abuse.

General or direct statements about sexual abuse
Sexualized play in developmentally immature children
Medical conditions
Recurrent abdominal pain
Genital, urethral, or anal trauma
Sexually transmitted diseases
Recurrent urinary tract infections
Enuresis or encopresis
Pregnancy
Behavioral changes
Sleep disturbances (eg, nightmares and night terrors)
Appetite disturbances (eg, anorexia, bulimia)
Neurotic or conduct disorders
Withdrawal, guilt or depression
Temper tantrums, aggressive behavior
Suicidal or runaway threats or behaviors
Hysterical or conversion reactions
Excessive masturbation
School problems
Substance abuse
Promiscuity, prostitution
Sexual abuse of other children by the victim

even after the provision of adequate social services to families in financial need. Neglectful parents appear to have an inability to recognize the physical or emotional states of their children. Emotionally neglectful parents respond differently to their children than their nurturing parent counterparts. A baby's cry may be perceived as an expression of anger at the parent, which can then be ignored. If hunger cries are misinterpreted in this way, the infant may not get adequate food, leading to failure to thrive.

The history offered in cases of **failure to thrive** is often discrepant with the findings as well. Infants who have dropped below the third percentile or who have experienced a significant deceleration in the growth curve are probably not receiving adequate amounts and appropriate types of food, in spite of a history that the infant takes adequate amounts of formula daily. In such cases, out-of-home placement is usually followed by a dramatic weight gain.

The hallmark of cases of **Munchausen syndrome by proxy** is that children have repeated visits to health care providers for unexplained illnesses. When the physician begins to think that the child he is seeing is a possible subject for a "case report," it may be time to think of this possibility.

Physical Findings

The physical findings of **physically abused** children include bruises, burns, lacerations, scars, bony deformities, alopecia, dental trauma, and, in the case of head or abdominal trauma, findings consistent with these injuries. The bruises of physically abused children are sometimes patterned (eg, belt marks, looped electric cord, or oval grab marks), and are usually found over the soft tissue areas of the body. Toddlers or older children who sustain accidental bruising usually do so over bony prominences. *Any* bruise in an infant not yet developmentally able to be mobile should be viewed with concern. Lacerations of the frenulum and bruising of the lips are associated with forced feeding. Burns may also exhibit pathognomonic features. Scald burns in stocking or glove distribution, immersion burns of the buttocks, sometimes with a "doughnut hole" area of sparing, and cigarette burns are most common. The absence of splash marks or a pattern consistent with a spillage are helpful in differentiating accidental from non-accidental burns.

The physical findings of **sexually abused children** have been reviewed recently in two atlases. It is important to realize that children who are victims of sexual abuse may have no physical findings attributable to the abuse. Similarly, there are abnormalities of the genital and rectal regions that are nonspecific and, in the absence of a history, mean little or nothing. Children who present to the practitioner with the symptoms and signs of sexually transmitted diseases should be strongly suspected of having been sexually abused. The presence of gonorrhea or syphilis in chil-

dren after the perinatal period is diagnostic of sexual abuse. Chlamydial infection, HSV-2 infections, trichomoniasis, and venereal warts in children are all probably sexually transmitted, though the course and duration of these perinatally acquired infections may be protracted. This possibility must be considered as part of the evaluation.

Children with nonorganic **failure to thrive** have an absence of subcutaneous fat in the cheeks, buttocks, and extremities. If the condition has persisted for some time, they may also appear and act depressed. Older children who have been emotionally neglected for long periods may also have short stature ("deprivation dwarfism"). The head circumference in children with emotional neglect and failure to thrive is usually normal, giving these children the appearance of relative macrocephaly. If the head circumference has also decreased in its relative percentiles, the likelihood of more serious and possibly permanent developmental delay is greater.

Children with Munchausen syndrome by proxy present, if they are ill, with the physical findings of whatever illness is factitiously induced. Among reported presentations are children with dehydration resulting from induced diarrhea or vomiting, the signs of sepsis when contaminated material is injected into the child, or signs of poisoning.

Radiologic & Laboratory Findings

Certain radiologic findings are strong indicators of **physical abuse:** Metaphysial "corner" or "bucket handle" fractures of the long bones in infants, spiral fractures of the long bones in nonambulatory infants, and multiple fractures of the ribs or long bones at different stages of healing are examples. These findings should trigger a search for an explanation. Skeletal surveys are particularly useful in preverbal children who are suspected of being abused. CT or MRI findings of subdural hemorrhage in infants is highly correlated with abuse, especially after the advent of infant seat restraint laws, which have dramatically reduced the incidence of head trauma in infants. Ultrasound is useful in the delineation of abdominal injuries in children, but it is not useful in the diagnosis of subdural hematomas.

Coagulation studies are useful in children who have many bruises at different ages. Various types of coagulopathy may confuse the diagnostic picture, but abuse and coagulopathy are independent entities. There is as much abuse seen in hemophilia clinics as in the general population.

Several recent reviews have discussed the differentiation of physical abuse from **osteogenesis imperfecta.** The radiologic findings are different in most cases, but there may be variants that are difficult to diagnose. If the approach to these cases—as in all cases of suspected abuse—is compassionate, empathic, and nonaccusatory, the potential harm of "mislabeling" a parent as abusive when in fact the child has another physical disorder that allows signs of trauma with normal childhood activity, will be avoided.

The **forensic evaluation** of sexually abused children requires a setting that permits the evaluation to be done in a way that will prevent further trauma to the child. If there is a history that the child has been involved in abuse that included the possibility of ejaculation within 72 hours, an examination looking for semen, acid phosphatase, or other forensic evidence should be performed according to published protocols. If there is no recent evidence of an acute sexual encounter, the laboratory findings would be limited to a search for sexually transmitted diseases. Chlamydial infection and gonorrhea are the most common examples. Syphilis, trichomoniasis, herpetic infection, and venereal warts are also noted as sequelae of sexual abuse. HIV infection has also been reported. The laboratory evaluation of sexually abused children should be modified depending on the history of the type of contact and the epidemiology of these infectious agents in the community.

Children with **failure to thrive** should not have an extensive workup. A CBC, urinalysis, and serum electrolyte panel are sufficient screening tests. A skeletal survey may be helpful in diagnosing the minority of these children who are also physically abused. The best "test" for the condition, however, is placement in a setting in which the child can be fed "ad lib" and the weight monitored. Hospital or foster care management may be appropriate. Weight gain may not occur for several days to a week in severe cases.

Any child with polymicrobial sepsis, recurrent apnea, chronic dehydration of unknown cause, or other highly unusual laboratory findings should be suspected of having Munchausen syndrome by proxy.

MANAGEMENT & REPORTING OF ABUSE & NEGLECT

Physical injuries should of course be treated. If the child has a **sexually transmitted disease,** this should be treated immediately. Children with **failure to thrive** on the basis of emotional neglect need to be placed in a setting where they can be fed. If weight gain does not occur within a reasonable time, further evaluation for the myriad of organic causes of failure to thrive can be instituted.

In every state in the United States, practitioners (and many other professionals who come in contact with children) are "mandated reporters." If abuse or neglect is suspected, a report must be made to the local or state agency designated to take and investigate these reports. In most cases, this will be a child protective services agency. Law enforcement personnel may also receive reports. The purpose of the report is to permit professionals to gather enough information to assess whether the environment in which the child is placed is safe. Many hospitals and communities have child protection teams available for consultation when there are questions about diagnosis or management. A listing of pediatric consultants in child abuse is available from the American Academy of Pediatrics.

The reporting of **emotional abuse,** except in extreme cases, is not likely to be responded to by most child protection agencies. Practitioners can encourage parents to get involved with parent effectiveness training programs (eg, Parents as First Teachers, Parents Anonymous) or seek mental health consultation to help them in this area.

If **Munchausen syndrome by proxy** is suspected, judicial involvement is usually required, either to obtain permission for video surveillance of the parent-child interaction in the hospital or to place the child out of the home environment to see if the "illness" resolves.

PREVENTION OF ABUSE & NEGLECT

Physical abuse is preventable in many cases. Extensive experience and evaluation of high-risk families has shown that the provision of "home visitor" services to families at risk can prevent physical abuse of children. These services can be provided by public health nurses or trained paraprofessionals. This makes it as easy for the family to pick up the telephone and ask for help *before* they abuse a child as it is for a neighbor or the physician to report an episode of abuse after it has occurred. Parent education and anticipatory guidance, particularly with respect to handling of situations that stress parents (eg, crying, toilet training), may also be helpful.

The prevention of **sexual abuse** is more difficult. Most efforts in this area involve training children to protect themselves and their "private parts" from harm. These programs are useful in individual cases but in general are not as efficacious as necessary. More rational approaches to prevention will place the responsibility for prevention on the adults who supervise children than on the children themselves.

Efforts to prevent **emotional abuse** of children have been undertaken through extensive media campaigns. No data are available to assess the effectiveness of this approach.

REFERENCES

American Academy of Pediatrics: Guidelines for the evaluation of sexual abuse of children. Pediatrics 1991;87:254.

Giardino AP et al: *A Practical Guide to the Evaluation of Sexual Abuse in the Prepubertal Child.* Sage, 1992.

Helfer RE: The neglect of our children, Pediatr Clin North Am 1990;37:923.

Johnson CF: Inflicted injury versus accidental injury. Pediatr Clin North Am 1990;37:791.

Ludwig S, Kornberg AE (editors): *Child Abuse: A Medical Reference,* 2nd ed. Churchill Livingstone, 1992.

Olds D: Home visitation for pregnant women and parents of young children. Am J Dis Child 1992;146: 704.

Rosenberg DA: Web of deceit: A literature review of Munchausen syndrome by proxy. Child Abuse Negl 1987;11:547.

9 Adolescent Substance Abuse

Trina Menden Anglin, MD, PhD*

INTRODUCTION

Definitions

The term **"substance abuse"** connotes a social definition; it implies that a drug or alcohol is used in a way that deviates from a culture's approved medical or social pattern. The American Psychiatric Association defines **psychoactive substance abuse** as a maladaptive pattern of use that is (1) continued despite knowledge of having a persistent or recurrent social, occupational, psychologic, or physical problem that is caused or exacerbated by use of the substance; or (2) recurrent in situations that are physically hazardous.

"Dependence" is a general term for a behavioral syndrome in which use of the substance is given a high priority which outranks other behaviors that once had a higher value. Dependence is frequently associated with **tolerance** (over time, the need to consume a larger dose to obtain the effects observed with the original dose of a substance), and with the development of physical (biologic) dependence, or neuroadaptation (an altered physiologic state produced by the repeated administration of a substance that necessitates its ongoing consumption in order to prevent the development of a withdrawal or abstinence syndrome). Based on these concepts, the American Psychiatric Association defines **psychoactive substance dependence** as exhibiting at least three of the following eight characteristics: (1) substance taken in larger amounts or over a longer period than intended; (2) persistent desire or at least one unsuccessful attempt to decrease or control substance use; (3) a great deal of time spent in obtaining the substance, taking it, or recovering from its effects; (4) frequent intoxication or symptoms of withdrawal when expected to fulfill role obligations or when substance use is physically hazardous; (5) important social, occupational, or recreational activities given up or reduced because of substance use; (6) continued substance use despite knowledge that its use is causing or exacerbating a social, psychologic, or physical problem; (7) characteristic withdrawal symptoms that are substance-specific; (8) substance often taken to relieve or avoid withdrawal symptoms.

The term **"drug addiction"** connotes a severe degree of drug dependence. Use of the drug affects every life domain and activity of the user. It represents the extreme set of circumstances in which use of a drug controls the user's behavior.

American Psychiatric Association: *Diagnostic and Statistical Manual of Mental Disorders,* 3rd ed rev. APA, 1987.
Jaffe JH: Drug addiction and drug abuse. In: *Goodman and Gilman's The Pharmacological Basis of Therapeutics,* 8th ed. Gilman A et al (editors). Pergamon, 1990.

Problems Linked With Substance Abuse

Most adolescents who have used alcohol and drugs do not develop dependency. In fact, experimental use of alcohol and even marijuana may be considered normative experiences for teenagers living in the United States, because such large numbers of young people have tried these substances at least once. Youngsters who experiment with substances but who do not use them on a regular basis have been found to demonstrate better psychologic adjustment than adolescents who by the age of 18 have never experimented with any drugs. Predictably, however, it has been found that teenagers who use drugs frequently are not well adjusted and demonstrate emotional distress, a sense of alienation from others, and poor impulse control.

The pediatrician needs to recognize that many other serious adolescent problems are linked to the use of alcohol and drugs. Non-intentional trauma—including motor vehicle accidents, drownings, and falls—is clearly associated with the use of alcohol and drugs. Interpersonal violence, including fights between peers and among family members, as well as homicide, is strongly linked to the use of drugs and alcohol. It has also been demonstrated that teenagers who have been victimized by physical abuse or sex-

*Portions of this chapter were adapted from a previous work by the author: Interviewing guidelines for the clinical evaluation of adolescent substance abuse. Pediatr Clin North Am 1987;34:381. Permission to adapt and to update this work for publication as a chapter in this book has been granted by W.B. Saunders Company.

ual abuse during childhood are at heightened risk for substance abuse. Certain common mental health problems, including depression, suicidal behavior, and anxiety disorders, are frequently associated with substance abuse. There is a definite relationship between conduct disorder and delinquency, and substance use. However, it is probable that adolescents with attention deficit hyperactivity disorder are *not* at higher risk for substance abuse unless they also demonstrate evidence of a conduct disorder. It should be noted, however, that covariance between sexual activity and substance abuse has not been consistently demonstrated, especially among urban African-American adolescents. However, there appear to be clear associations between sexual activity and use of tobacco, alcohol, and illicit substances among younger adolescents. Even though pregnant and parenting adolescents have been reported to be at relatively high risk for alcohol and illicit substance use, adolescents with a history of substance abuse prior to pregnancy have also been found to limit their use of alcohol, marijuana, and other illicit substances voluntarily and substantially during pregnancy.

Pediatricians also need to recognize when an adolescent's use of alcohol and drugs is causing functional impairment and is interfering with normal adolescent development. In general, a pediatrician who uncovers problems relating to inappropriate use of substances or believes that an individual youngster is at high risk for abusing chemicals should share this assessment with the adolescent and the family in order to guide them to appropriate resources for further evaluation and treatment if necessary. Most pediatricians do not have the personal expertise or resources necessary to provide ongoing counseling or treatment for adolescents harmfully engaged in substance use. As trusted advisors, however, they can help ensure that youngsters and their families do receive appropriate treatment for substance abuse as well as for underlying or coexisting problems.

Assessment of adolescent substance abuse can be difficult for the following reasons:

(1) Compared with adults, adolescents have a relatively short history of chemical use and therefore have not always experienced numerous negative consequences from it.

(2) There is normative acceptance of excessive levels of alcohol and drug use among substance-abusing young people, so that an adolescent who consumes similar quantities will not consider the behavior abnormal or deviant.

(3) The psychologic, familial, and social dysfunction that frequently accompanies a substance abuse problem may have existed prior to the chemical use or may have been caused by it.

(4) Most adolescents' cognitive skills are not yet fully developed. Self-definition and effective problem-solving skills may be limited by the adolescent's cognitive immaturity.

Abma JC, Mott FL: Substance use and prenatal care during pregnancy among young women. Fam Plann Perspect 1991;23:117.

Alcohol, Drug Abuse and Mental Health Administration: *Report of the Secretary's Task Force on Youth Suicide.* Vol 2: *Risk Factors for Youth Suicide.* DHHS Pub. No. (ADM) 89-1622. Superintendent of Documents, U.S. Government Printing Office, 1989.

Bukstein OG, Brent DA, Kaminer Y: Comorbidity of substance abuse and other psychiatric disorders in adolescents. Am J Psychiatry 1989;146:1131.

Dembo R et al: Longitudinal study of the relationships among alcohol use, marijuana/hashish use, cocaine use, and emotional/psychological functioning in a cohort of high-risk youths. Int J Addict 1990;25:1341.

Elliott DS, Huizinga D, Menard S: *Multiple Problem Youth: Delinquency, Substance Abuse, and Mental Health Problems.* Springer, 1989.

Hernandez JT: Substance abuse among sexually abused adolescents and their families. J Adolesc Health 1992;13:658.

Kokotailo PK et al: Cigarette, alcohol, and other drug use by school-age pregnant adolescents: Prevalence, detection, and associated risk factors. Pediatrics 1992;90:328.

Lohr MJ et al: Factors related to substance use by pregnant, school-age adolescents. J Adolesc Health 1992;13:475.

Millstein SG et al: Health-risk behaviors and health concerns among young adolescents. Pediatrics 1992;89:422.

Shedler J, Block J: Adolescent drug use and psychological health. A longitudinal inquiry. Am Psychol 1990;45:612.

Stanton B et al: Early initiation of sex and its lack of association with risk behaviors among adolescent African-Americans. Pediatrics 1993;92:13.

SCOPE OF & CHRONOLOGIC TRENDS IN ADOLESCENT SUBSTANCE USE

The most useful and widely cited information regarding adolescent substance use in the United States comes from a national self-reporting annual survey of high school seniors—and recently of eighth and tenth graders—conducted by the University of Michigan's Institute for Social Research.

High School Seniors

Table 9–1 summarizes trends in prevalence of substance use by successive classes of high school seniors since 1975. It has three components, which correspond to the concepts of experimental use (lifetime prevalence), probable misuse (30-day prevalence), and actual abuse of drugs and alcohol (daily prevalence). Except for cocaine and inhalants, use of illicit substances peaked in 1979. In that year, 65% of high school seniors had used an illicit drug at least once, 54% had done so within the past year, and 39% had done so within the preceding month. In contrast, use of cocaine peaked in 1985 (not shown in Table 9–1, but during that year lifetime prevalence was 17%, use during the preceding 30 days was reported by 7% of high school seniors, and daily use was reported by 0.4%). Although use of inhalants appeared to increase

Table 9–1. Trends in prevalence of substance abuse by high school seniors living in the United States.[1]

LIFETIME PREVALENCE
% Ever Used

Substance[2]	1975[3]	1979	1983	1987	1991	1992
Alcohol	90	93	93	92	88	88
Marijuana	47	60	57	50	37	33
Total cocaine[4]	9	15	16	15	8	6
Inhalants[5]	NA	18	18	19	18	17
Stimulants	22	24	27	22	15	14
Sedatives	18	15	14	9	7	6
Hallucinogens[6]	16	18	14	11	10	9
Cigarettes	74	74	71	67	63	62
Steroids	NA	NA	NA	NA	2	2

THIRTY-DAY PREVALENCE
% Used Within Last 30 Days

Substance[2]	1975[3]	1979	1983	1987	1991	1992
Alcohol	68	72	69	66	54	51
Marijuana	27	36	27	21	14	12
Total cocaine[4]	2	6	5	4	1	1
Inhalants[5]	NA	3	2	3	3	2
Stimulants	8	10	9	5	3	3
Sedatives	5	4	3	2	1	1
Hallucinogens[6]	5	5	3	3	2	2
Cigarettes	37	34	30	29	28	28
Steroids	NA	NA	NA	NA	0.8	0.6

DAILY PREVALENCE
% Used for at Least 20 Days in the Last Month

Substance[2]	1975[3]	1979	1983	1987	1991	1992
Alcohol	6	7	5	5	4	3
Marijuana	6	10	5	3	2	2
Total cocaine[4]	0.1	0.2	0.2	0.3	0.1	0.1
Inhalants[5]	NA	0.1	0.2	0.4	0.5	0.2
Stimulants	0.5	0.6	0.8	0.3	0.2	0.2
Sedatives	0.3	0.1	0.2	0.1	0.1	0.1
Hallucinogens[6]	0.1	0.2	0.2	0.2	0.1	0.1
Cigarettes	27	25	21	19	18	17
Steroids	NA	NA	NA	NA	0.1	0.1

[1]Johnston, L.D., O'Malley, P.M., & Bachman, J.G. (1993) National Survey Results on Drug Use from the Monitoring the Future Study, 1975–1992. (NIH Pub. No. 93–3597.) Washington, DC: National Institute on Drug Abuse.

[2]Selected categories of substances are presented. The actual survey addressed 16 classes and subclasses of substances, including tranquilizers, heroin, and other opioids, which are not included in the table.

[3]Although this survey has been conducted annually since 1975, the information presented in this table represents data from every fourth year. Comparison of 1991 and 1992 data yields short-term trends. Sample size for 1992 was 49,000 students.

[4]Total cocaine includes crack, though specific questions addressing use of crack were not included until 1986.

[5]The survey did not include questions about inhalants until 1976. The presented rates have been adjusted for underreporting of amyl and butyl nitrites.

[6]Starting in 1979, the presented rates have been adjusted for underreporting of PCP.

between 1980 and 1990, a more recent decline in use has been observed.

Use of alcohol has shown a different pattern. It was not until 1990 that fewer than 90% of the senior class reported any lifetime use. As recently as 1987, two-thirds of high school seniors reported alcohol use within the preceding month, although this proportion decreased to 51% by 1992. Thirty percent of the class of 1992 reported having become intoxicated within the preceding month. However, daily drinking peaked in 1979 and has declined slowly since then. It is thought that the drug education programs sponsored by many school districts in this country have helped to bring about this encouraging downward trend for high school seniors.

Eighth & Tenth Graders

In contrast to the high school seniors' general decrease in use of illicit substances, it is possible that successive classes of tenth and especially eighth graders may be experiencing increasing patterns of utilization. For example, this national survey found that 10% of students who were in eighth grade in 1991 had used marijuana at least once, 6% had used it in the preceding year, and 3.2% had used it in the past month. Corresponding rates of use of marijuana for students who were in the eighth grade in 1992 were 11%, 7%, and 3.7%. Rates of use among eighth graders also increased for the majority of other categories of illicit substances and for frequent use of alcohol. Students in the eighth grade during 1992 were less likely to disapprove of use of marijuana and cocaine compared with the 1991 class. It is thought that this discouraging reversal among younger students may reflect the declining public attention drug abuse is currently receiving in this country, as other issues have replaced it.

Pediatricians can use the national data to help estimate the prevalence of substance use and substance abuse by the teenagers they encounter. It should be remembered, however, that local communities may have patterns of substance use that differ from national averages and that different groups of teenagers may also display differing patterns of use.

The University of Michigan: *National High School Senior Drug Abuse Survey 1975–1992: Monitoring the Future Survey.* News and Information Services, The University of Michigan, 1993.

CONTEXT OF EVALUATION

Although the approach to evaluating an adolescent patient for risk of substance abuse follows the same general interviewing guidelines regardless of the context of presentation, specific circumstances require comment. All teenagers should be screened for their risk for harmful involvement with chemicals as part of health maintenance care, upon entering into mental health counseling, as part of the evaluation process for poor or deteriorating scholastic performance, and as part of the intake process into the juvenile justice system. Opportunities for health maintenance visits for adolescents include examinations for school and camp, preparticipation sports evaluations, and pre-employment examinations. A pediatrician who has known a teenager since childhood should not slip into complacency regarding evaluation of the patient's psychosocial status. All teenagers deserve periodic reassessment of their psychosocial development and functioning. Screening for substance use and abuse should be routinely included as part of an adolescent's general psychosocial assessment. Pediatricians need to screen adolescent patients for substance use and substance abuse when there are complaints of fatigue, recurrent abdominal pain, chest pain, palpitations, headache, chronic cough, persistent severe nasal congestion, and sore throat.

Concerned family members or school personnel may request that an adolescent be evaluated specifically for involvement with chemicals or to search for a medical explanation for dysfunctional behavior, deteriorating school performance, or a diffuse worry that a teenager just "doesn't seem healthy." Parents frequently turn to pediatricians in times of family trouble. Parents may request help spontaneously or under duress from school officials. Many schools' policies now mandate the suspension of adolescents who were high or intoxicated during school hours or who were found carrying or storing drugs or drug paraphernalia on school property. Readmission to school may be conditioned on an agency or physician evaluation for substance abuse.

In contrast, pediatricians are unlikely to encounter the following circumstances regarding evaluation of teenagers for substance abuse. First, it is unlikely that teenagers who are experiencing dysfunctional consequences from involvement with drugs or alcohol will directly request evaluation and intervention. It is unlikely also that youngsters will appear for scheduled appointments intoxicated or high. Even though most adolescents will not keep appointments in an intoxicated state, some youngsters enrolled in chemical dependency programs have boasted later that their physicians or counselors never recognized that they had been high during the sessions. Therefore, pediatricians need to be alert in order to detect overt and subtle signs of alcohol and drug effects.

In contrast to an office setting, teenagers are frequently brought to emergency departments either because they are acutely intoxicated from ingesting drugs or alcohol or because their friends, family, or the police have been stirred to action by observing their behavior or level of consciousness. Adolescents may also be injured while intoxicated or high and visit emergency departments for treatment. Teenagers may be arrested while intoxicated or high and brought to an emergency department for medical attention. In these circumstances, pediatricians will be able to document the substance use through interview, physical findings, and toxicologic screening of urine.

Pediatricians may also become aware of a possible substance abuse problem when they need to prescribe medication and review instructions for its use. Pharmaceuticals that interact with alcohol are good examples and include oral metronidazole for treatment of trichomoniasis and bacterial vaginosis and antihistamines available over-the-counter for allergic rhinitis. Teenagers who drink alcohol will frequently disclose this information to clinicians as part of this discussion. The pediatrician provides factual information about the disulfiram-like effect of metronidazole when used in association with alcohol—or about the risks of mixing alcohol and many antihistamines—prefatory to asking about the adolescent's personal use of alcohol. Unless there is a compelling reason to proceed more quickly, thorough assessment for risk of misuse of alcohol and other chemicals could be postponed to a follow-up visit so that clinical issues do not become confused for the adolescent patient.

INTERVIEWING TECHNIQUES

General strategies for interviewing adolescents are addressed in Chapter 4. Suggested techniques for interviewing adolescents about substance use are summarized in Table 9–2. The remainder of this section

Table 9–2. Interviewing techniques.

- Interview the adolescent privately.
- Discuss the parameters of confidentiality.
- Avoid parental subterfuge.
- Ask open-ended questions.
- Do not barrage the adolescent with questions.
- Do not lecture or moralize.
- Be sensitive to the adolescent's responsiveness to your style and to specific questions.
- Determine what types of information the adolescent would like to learn or verify, and then provide it.
- If the adolescent has no questions, offer information that is developmentally appropriate, using the technique of generalization.

focuses on strategies helpful for interviewing adolescents who are actually experiencing substance abuse.

Youngsters who abuse substances may resort to several defenses as they struggle to conceal their problem. These behaviors are not directed personally at the physician. They occur if an adolescent feels that continued substance use is being threatened. The interviewer will earn respect from the adolescent by recognizing and acknowledging these behaviors as protective strategies and returning the interview to its appropriate course. For example, a frightened or angry adolescent may show resistance by refusing to answer questions. The interviewer can frequently cut through this behavior by describing what is occurring in a warm, empathic way. "You seem quite upset [angry, unhappy] about coming here today. I can understand your not wanting to come"—allow the adolescent to respond briefly—"but even though you feel that way, we have a job to do." Angry adolescents may also use profanity or vulgar language to express themselves or in an attempt to discomfit the interviewer. Calmly accepting the language by acknowledging its use is an appropriate response.

Adolescents who abuse substances may also attempt to divert attention from themselves. One tactic is to disclose another family member's problem behavior, such as physical abuse or parental drinking. This information is obviously valuable for the clinical evaluation. However, for the time being, it must remain tangential to the interviewer's focus. It is appropriate to acknowledge receiving the information by saying, "I can understand your being upset [concerned] about that. Let's talk about it later [at our next visit]. Right now, however, I need to ask you . . ."

Adolescents who abuse substances may minimize their involvement or distort factual information. The parents frequently perceive them as liars. These behaviors are actually strategies that help the adolescent maintain the pattern of use. It is important to let the adolescent know that the attempted deception has not succeeded. During an initial assessment, however, direct confrontation is frequently counterproductive. For example, if the adolescent presents obviously inconsistent information, the pediatrician might

say, "That doesn't make sense. Earlier you said that . . . [your mother said that . . .] Now you are telling me . . . It just doesn't add up." Attempts to mislead the interviewer should be made part of the assessment record.

Friedman LS, Johnson BA, Brett AS: Evaluation of substance-abusing adolescents by primary care physicians. J Adolesc Health Care 1990;11:227.

PSYCHOSOCIAL ASSESSMENT

A general psychosocial assessment of an adolescent provides the infrastructure for addressing actual chemical use. It helps to determine: what roles if any psychoactive substance use plays in the adolescent's life. Information should be gathered that will help determine whether an adolescent is at risk for abusing substances, is making satisfactory developmental progress or has suffered impairment of adaptive functioning skills, or has experienced any negative consequences from substance abuse. Table 9–3 outlines the key substantive areas of exploration.

SUBSTANCE USE HISTORY

Order of Interview Process

Where in the interview process should more specific questions about use of drugs and alcohol be asked? The interviewer should discuss general lifestyle questions before inquiring about use of substances. There are two important reasons for this sequence. The first is that the teenager needs time to develop or renew a relationship with the pediatrician before being asked to discuss a sensitive subject. The second reason is that the pediatrician will be able to use general psychosocial information as a data base to help determine how much at risk an adolescent may be for harmful involvement with chemicals. This information will help determine how deeply the pediatrician must probe in this section of the interview.

One strategy that can provide order to the interview process and improve the quality of information gathered is to start with the least threatening and then move on to increasingly more sensitive substances. Use of tobacco products, including cigarettes and smokeless tobacco, is so common among adolescents in the United States that it can almost be considered normative behavior even though purchase of tobacco by minors is nominally illegal. (Note that some states and communities are starting to enforce the law forbidding the sale of tobacco products to minors.) Questions about use of tobacco may be considered a mildly sensitive area. Learning about use of alcohol is the next step on the continuum. Again, drinking by teenagers can almost be considered normative behavior, but the sensitivity is somewhat intensified be-

Table 9–3. Substantive areas of psychosocial assessment.

- Home and family relationships (constellation, shared activities, respect for parents, organization of family's daily life, isolation, conflict, breaking of family rules, running away)
- Family history (use by parents, sibs, and relatives)
- School (performance and classroom placement, attendance, behavior, ability to concentrate and remember, involvement in sports and extracurricular activities)
- Peers (developmental appropriateness, shared activities, fighting, substance use, involvement in gang activities and gang membership, legal involvement, motor vehicle accidents and traffic citations)
- Sexual behavior (romantic involvement, use by boyfriend/girlfriend, risk for pregnancy/fatherhood and sexually transmitted infections, number of partners, prostitution, trading sex for drugs)
- Leisure activities (fun, relaxation, preferred music and video genres, community organizations and service)
- Employment (where, position, schedule, disposition of earnings)
- Role of religion (religiosity of parents and of adolescent, any unique beliefs associated with their religion's tenets, involvement with youth group activities)
- Physical health (general health and somatic concerns, symptoms of withdrawal, toxic reactions to specific drugs and to alcohol, overdoses, blackouts, history of trauma and injuries, bulimic binging and purging)
- History of victimization by abuse (physical, sexual)
- Motor vehicle history (driving record, accidents and near misses, traffic citations)
- Access to weapons (family, peers, firearm ownership)
- Police and court involvement (probation status, history of illegal activities, incarceration, pattern of charges and offenses)
- Mental health (depression and moods, alienation, anxiety, hallucinations, suicidal ideation and attempts, anger, impulsivity, history of intervention and hospitalization)
- Aspirations and goals for the future (hopes and plans for beyond high school)
- Self-perception (self-liking and satisfaction with current life)

cause purchase of alcoholic beverages by minors carries clear legal sanctions. Inquiry about marijuana use is the next step. Use of this substance may be considered more sensitive than use of alcohol, because marijuana is an illicit substance for adults as well as for minors. Furthermore, teenagers' parents are far less likely to use marijuana than they are to drink alcoholic beverages. This gulf increases adult social (and consequently societal) disapproval. Even though 22% of 1992's senior high school class used marijuana during the preceding 12 months, this figure represents less than one-third of the proportion of high school seniors who had used alcohol during the same period. This relatively lower percentage of use is consistent with decreased social acceptability and contributes to its greater sensitivity as a topic of discussion. Finally, the interviewer should ask about the use of other illicit drugs, reviewing major techniques of use (eg, pills, smoking, sniffing or huffing, snorting, needles) as well as classes of drugs.

In summary, this organization of the interview provides a natural order of progression, moving from the socially accepted to the socially tolerated to the socially disapproved to the overtly illegal.

Initial Exploration

People who abuse chemicals tend to minimize their involvement with them. On the other hand, substance abusers will provide a valid history if they trust and respect the interviewer. In particular, most teenagers whose lifestyles do not revolve around substance use will provide sufficient information about their use of alcohol and drugs to allow the pediatrician to complete an accurate evaluation. It is critical, however, for the physician to establish an appropriate atmosphere for the interview and to convey an impression of trustworthiness and sincerity. The purpose of initial exploratory inquiries is to establish the tone of this section of the interview. During this process, the pediatrician may be tested by the adolescent patient. If the interviewer appears to register disapproval, dismay, or condescension in reaction to initial disclosure statements, it is doubtful that the adolescent will provide accurate information about substance use. The pediatrician will have failed the teenager's test and will not be deemed trustworthy or credible. The interviewer can measure the adolescent's willingness to offer information during this exploratory phase.

Exploratory issues are phenomenologic—they address the adolescent's perceptions of how widely drugs and alcohol are used by other teenagers. Specifically, the pediatrician can inquire about whether many students at the teenager's school are "into drinking or doing drugs." If someone wanted to buy marijuana, crack, or uppers, how easy would it be? What happens at parties and social occasions that the teenager has heard about? Or at parties the teenager has personally attended? This approach is less threatening because it does not ask for information about personal involvement.

Elements of a Formal Substance Use History

The goal of this set of questions is to determine the quality and depth of the relationship the adolescent has with substances. Minimal time is needed to discuss these issues with a teenage patient who is functioning well and who admits to little or no use of alcohol and drugs. These questions are very useful, however, when the pediatrician needs to explore an adolescent's use of substances more intensively. Table 9–4 summarizes the elements of a substance use history.

When asking an adolescent to discuss personal use of alcohol and drugs, it is less threatening to establish a historical perspective. Before addressing current use patterns, find out about the teenager's first experiences with alcohol and with marijuana. "Tell me about the first time you ever had anything to drink. What was it like?" "When was the first time you ever got really high?" With these questions, the interviewer is trying both to help the teenager disclose accurate information and to determine whether the adolescent is preoccupied with the experience of getting

Table 9–4. Elements of a substance use history.

- First use: age, circumstances, feeling effects
- Past substance use patterns
- Current motivation to use (perceived benefits of use)
- Current feeling effects of use (include both pleasant and negative experiences)
- Current patterns of use (substances used, frequency, binging behavior, circumstances of use)
- Current frequency of intoxication or becoming "high"
- Tolerance (how much alcohol does it take to get high now? What about 6 months ago? A year ago?)
- Substance of choice
- Personal limits to categories of substances willing to try
- How substance obtained
- Financial resources
- Dealing activities
- Perceptions of significant others about use (family members, peers, boyfriend or girlfriend)

high. Although one cannot ask specific questions that directly address the latter goal, one can frequently document this preoccupation through the adolescent's enthusiastic descriptions of what it feels like to be "high."

The pediatrician should gradually move the questions forward from their historical environment to the present time. "About how much are you drinking now compared to last fall when school started?" In identifying patterns of use, the pediatrician will need to learn how frequently the adolescent uses particular substances and how much is consumed at a time. "How many times did you get high in the last month?" Forced multiple choice answers are a useful strategy for adolescents who find it difficult to answer spontaneously. For example, one could provide the choices: "About once every month, Saturday nights only, or three times a week?" When was the last time the teenager got high? Is the adolescent using drugs or alcohol on school nights or only on weekends?

It may be less threatening to determine approximate quantities of substances consumed by using the concept of tolerance rather than asking for this information directly. Increasing tolerance for specific agents is associated with increasing use. Tolerance can be addressed historically by determining how much it takes to get a little high and how much to get really high. Have the teenager compare these amounts with what was necessary to get high 6 months ago and a year ago.

The pediatrician should learn about the circumstances of use. Does the teenager use substances only during parties or also when alone? Has the teenager ever used at school? What does the adolescent gain from the experience of becoming high? Examples of possible questions that can explore this experience follow. "What is it like to be high?" "Has anything really good ever happened while you've been high?" "What does getting high do for you?" The appetitive effects of substances serve as important motivators

for individuals to continue their use once they experience pleasurable sensations.

Another important area concerns the benefits substance use may offer the teenager. Does intoxication relieve negative pressures and enhance the ability to relax? Teenagers who have learned to use substances for anxiety relief are at special risk for developing more serious problems. These youngsters risk developing a dependent relationship with drugs and alcohol. What is more, they have not been able to learn healthy mechanisms for coping with stress or for addressing troublesome issues. A possible exploratory question is, "How do you make yourself feel better when you're really upset or nervous about something?"

The concept outlined above—that adolescents who use substances perceive benefits from their use—has been elaborated into a formal brief screening instrument. The five items that compose the empirically validated scale can be incorporated into the clinical interview by asking the teenager how much drugs and alcohol help make it easier to relax, be friendly, forget problems, and feel good about oneself. When used in this manner, these questions are meant to enrich clinical information and to help youngsters gain insight into their relationships with substances; they are not meant to serve as a formal screening instrument.

Learning how a teenager obtains drugs and alcohol may not be possible unless a trusting relationship has developed. To obtain supplies, youngsters who have become chemically dependent frequently resort to deviant and illegal behaviors, such as stealing, dealing, and prostitution. An adolescent who engages in such activities obviously has a very serious problem. (However, some adolescent dealers may not use in order to retain a sharp bussiness acumen.) There is an excellent chance that such an adolescent will exhibit dysfunctional behavior in other areas. Even though an adolescent may vociferously deny stealing from the parents, it may be this very behavior that finally forces parents to seek help. Some exploratory questions include, "How much do you spend a week on drugs?" (Try to be as specific as possible, naming drugs that you know the adolescent favors.) "Have you ever needed to borrow money or take something that didn't belong to you so you could get a supply?" "Have you ever traded sex for drugs?" "Have you ever gotten into trouble with the law trying to get drugs?" "How much do you deal?"

It is often enlightening to learn who is concerned about an adolescent's use of alcohol and drugs. Family members, friends, and boyfriends or girlfriends who worry that an adolescent may be using alcohol or drugs excessively are usually right. The pediatrician should be aware, however, that heightened media publicity about drug use may overly sensitize cautious parents about an adolescent's experimentation. A teenager who abuses substances may be able to admit that a parent is anxious about the use even while minimizing or belittling the concern. It is unusual, however, for an adolescent who is harmfully involved with chemicals to admit spontaneously that the involvement is dysfunctional even when use has caused significant problems.

Dysfunctional Consequences

Even though adolescents who are abusing alcohol and drugs may not recognize dysfunctional consequences associated with the abuse, pediatricians can play an important role by pointing out to both the family and the adolescent that use has caused problems. The impact of associating a negative consequence with use of substances is more powerful if it occurs close to the time the consequence occurred. For example, during recovery from the ill effects of an overdose or acute intoxication, the adolescent and the family may be more receptive to intervention. The need for an emergency room visit or hospitalization for chemically associated trauma, behavioral aberration, or mental status impairment is a medical consequence that a pediatrician should target. Such episodes can be helpful in convincing a family that a substance abuse problem exists—when people are frightened, they feel vulnerable and perhaps more open to offers of help. For example, most adolescents admitted to inpatient substance abuse treatment programs are in crisis. However, the parents have usually been aware of the substance abuse for 1–2 years.

In summary, substance-using teenagers and their families may be more receptive to help during times of acute crisis than they are at other times. The unfortunate corollary is that they may not seek help until a crisis erupts.

The pediatrician should look for other common consequences associated with the use of substances by focused interview questions. Table 9–5 outlines areas that should be explored.

Table 9–5. Exploration for consequences of substance use.[1]

Medical and physical
  Somatic symptoms
  Blackouts
  Trauma and accidental injury
  Visits to emergency facility for intoxication or overdose
Social
  Motor vehicle accidents and near misses
  Conflict with family
  Loss of friends
  Loss of a romantic relationship
  Fighting
  Impulsive sexual behavior
  Destruction of property
  Theft
  School failure
  Disciplinary action (DUI, other legal involvement, school suspension, dropped from sports team)

[1]Note that these common examples of consequences of substance use are embedded in the psychosocial history.

SYNTHESIZING INTERVIEW INFORMATION

The pediatrician must judge the accuracy of an adolescent's history by indirect measures. The pediatrician can compare the adolescent's individual historical use of substances with empirical information that supports the "stepping stone theory." It has been demonstrated that most adolescents follow a specific sequence of substance use. They rarely begin with an illicit drug—the usual sequence is beer or wine, tobacco, hard liquor, and then marijuana. The use of these substances precedes involvement with other drugs, such as cocaine. For example, if a youngster who admits using amphetamines denies every having used anything else, this information is not consistent with empirically described patterns. Even though a youngster may have a substance of choice, other drugs previously used on a regular basis are not usually abandoned altogether. There is more apt to be an addition of a chemical rather than a substitution. However, adolescents may avoid categories of substances that have caused unpleasant or frightening effects in prior experience.

The pediatrician must synthesize information learned during the substance use history with the general psychosocial assessment. The purpose of the psychosocial assessment is to determine whether the adolescent appears at risk for harmful involvement with drugs and alcohol and whether the adolescent's behavior is dysfunctional. Can the dysfunctional behavior be linked to use of substances? The substance use history can provide the key to explaining a set of disturbing behaviors.

Stages of Chemical Dependency

How can the physician decide whether involvement with chemicals is causing behavioral dysfunction? One hypothesized scheme regards chemical dependency as a progressive disease with four stages. It is important to remember, however, that use of substances at one stage does not necessarily mean that an adolescent will progress to a more serious stage of use.

The first stage is experimentation. The teenager experiences the positive mood effects associated with chemical use and experiments with substances in social settings. Adolescents who progress to the second stage actively seek the mood changes associated with substance use. They develop expertise in the use of chemicals for mood regulation. These youngsters may purchase their own supplies of drugs and may start to use chemicals more frequently. Although they do not perceive drugs as causing undesirable consequences, they may manifest early changes in psychosocial functioning and may use drugs to relax or to relieve anxiety. Their schoolwork may start to deteriorate; their relationships with other family members may become conflictual; and they may start to associate with others who use substances regularly.

The third stage of this conceptual scheme concerns preoccupation with drugs and alcohol. Adolescents who have slipped into this phase have lost control over the use of substances and are frequently labeled "chemically dependent." They believe that drugs and alcohol are indispensable for coping with stress. They develop tolerance and frequently use many drugs. Although their major focus appears to be attainment of drug-induced euphoria, they may actually be using drugs to prevent withdrawal symptoms. Psychosocial functioning deteriorates significantly and may include antisocial behavior.

The fourth stage is termed "burnout." Young people who have progressed to this final stage are thought to have developed a chronic brain syndrome that may be reversible. They use drugs now to prevent negative feelings rather than to seek euphoria, and if use stops they do experience withdrawal symptoms. They are no longer able to function productively. People who reach this stage are usually older adolescents or young adults.

Dusenbury L, Khuri E, Millman RB: Adolescent substance abuse: A sociodevelopmental perspective. In: *Substance Abuse: A Comprehensive Textbook,* 2nd ed. Lowinson JH et al (editors). Williams & Wilkins, 1992.

Kandel D, Yamaguchi K: From beer to crack: Developmental patterns of drug involvement. Am J Public Health 1993;83:851.

CONFIDENTIALITY

Confidentiality of patient care is a maxim of adolescent medicine. In general, clinical practitioners honor the confidentiality of adolescent patients unless there is concern that the adolescent is engaging in life-jeopardizing or seriously health-compromising behavior. Substance abuse is clearly a health-compromising behavior. Most physicians would agree that parents need to be included in the process if an adolescent is experiencing serious behavioral dysfunction from substance use or if referral to a treatment program is necessary. It should be recognized, however, that state laws vary regarding need for parental consent for treatment. Statutes in 46 states permit minors to consent to treatment of drug and alcohol abuse, but 28 states have placed various limitations on minors' ability to consent, which include age restrictions and mandated physician notification of parents. In practice, the problem of reimbursement for treatment services usually necessitates parental involvement.

Substance misuse represents a different circumstance. For example, a pediatrician may be faced with the realization that an adolescent drives while intoxicated or accepts automobile rides from an intoxicated driver. The parents do not seem to be aware of these practices. Except for this risky behavior, the teenager appears to be functioning well. How can the pediatrician intervene effectively? Should the parents be warned? In this situation, the pediatrician may well decide that directly informing the parents would be counterproductive. An alternative approach is to involve the parents and the adolescent in a discussion of prevention of unsafe driving practices and "passengership." Have the family unit decide how it would handle a request from an intoxicated adolescent for help getting home. The pediatrician can help parents and teenagers prepare to deal with risky situations that are frequently part of the maturational process in this society.

English A: Legal aspects of care. In: *Textbook of Adolescent Medicine.* McAnarney ER et al (editors). Saunders, 1992.

Gans JE (editor): *Confidential Health Services for Adolescents.* American Medical Association, 1993.

Schonberg SK: Perspective on the role of the pediatrician in the management of adolescent drug use. Pediatr Rev 1985;7:131.

CLINICAL SCREENING INSTRUMENTS

Pediatricians who lack the time to conduct more comprehensive interviews of adolescents may use formal clinical screening instruments, which include both interview and written questionnaire formats and provide a highly structured and efficient approach to screening. In contrast, the detailed clinical interview, as outlined in earlier sections, is descriptive, open-ended, and interactive. If conducted skillfully, it can also offer a contextual richness that is missing from more structured approaches. The time-honored clinical interview is generally accepted as a valid procedure. In contrast, some of the formal screening instruments have been validated against self-report written questionnaires developed for use in survey research and may be less time-consuming. In clinical settings, however, written questionnaires cannot be administered in the absence of interaction between the patient and the clinician. Both approaches to the process of assessment can help the pediatrician achieve the following goals: to describe the presenting problems clearly; to identify the pattern of behavioral, psychologic, and physiologic conditions associated with substance use; and to determine whether referral to an appropriate facility for further evaluation and intervention is indicated.

Kaminer Y, Bukstein O, Tarter RE: The teen-addiction severity index: Rationale and reliability. Int J Addict 1991; 26:219.

Mayer JE, Filstead WJ: Empirical procedures for defining adolescent alcohol misuse. In: *Adolescence and Alcohol.* Mayer JE, Filstead WJ (editors). Ballinger, 1980.

Petchers MK et al: Revalidation and expansion of an adolescent substance abuse screening measure. J Dev Behav Pediatr 1988;9:25.

Rahdert ER (editor): *The Adolescent Assessment/Referral System Manual.* US Department of Health and Human Services, Alcohol, Drug Abuse and Mental Health Administration, National Institute on Drug Abuse, DHHS Publication No. (ADM) 91-1735. Superintendent of Documents, U.S. Government Printing Office, 1991.

Riggs SG, Alario AJ: Adolescent substance use. Instructor's Guide. In: *The Project ADEPT Curriculum for Primary Care Physician Training.* Dubé CE et al (editors). Project ADEPT, Brown Univ Press, 1989.

Tarter RE: Evaluation and treatment of adolescent substance abuse: A decision tree method. Am J Drug Alcohol Abuse 1990;16:1.

Winters K: The need for improved assessment of adolescent substance involvement. J Drug Issues 1990;20:487.

PHYSICAL & PHYSIOLOGIC SCREENING OF ADOLESCENTS WHO HAVE USED SUBSTANCES

Medical Assessment

Unless an adolescent is experiencing the effects of an overdose and seeks help from a free clinic or hospital emergency department, it is unusual to be able to diagnose substance abuse by physical examination findings. Individuals suffering from acute effects, overdoses, and withdrawal from alcohol and specific classes of drugs will demonstrate recognized constellations of physical and mental status findings. (The acute medical presentations of substance abuse are summarized in Chapter 13.) Table 9–6 lists chronic or recurrent physical symptoms and mental health problems that may cause an adolescent substance user to seek medical care or that may be disclosed during a review of systems. Certain chronic symptoms are clearly linked to specific classes of substances, but others are more general and may be caused by more than one type of substance.

Some symptoms represent the acute effects of use (eg, cocaine causes tachycardia) and some represent complications of use. For example, cocaine can cause cardiac arrhythmias, which can be experienced as palpitations, as well as constriction of blood vessels supplying the heart, which can cause chest pain; and chronic use of toluene can cause cerebellar ataxia. Other symptoms, such as fatigue and disordered sleep, do not always have such straightforward explanations.

A medical evaluation, including a thorough physical and neurologic examination, is recommended as part of the assessment process for adolescent substance abusers. It has several goals: First, many teenagers who have used substances do not receive regular health care and deserve age-appropriate screening and immunizations. Second, although organ system damage is unusual among adolescent substance abusers, it can occur. Substance abusers with specific symptoms (eg, upper abdominal pain) should be evaluated carefully to ensure that complications of alcohol use (such as gastritis or pancreatitis) are not causing it. Finally, young people who abuse substances are at risk for multiple problems, largely because of their lifestyles. For example, they are at risk for sexually transmitted infections, pregnancy, and sexual assault. They also experience disproportionately high rates of non-intentional injury. Chronic users of certain classes of drugs may be at risk for malnutrition.

It is generally agreed that laboratory testing of adolescents' body fluids does not provide a valid technique for diagnosis of chronic alcohol and marijuana use. In contrast, adult alcoholics may demonstrate elevation of certain hepatic enzymes, an increased mean volume of red blood cells, and changes in high-density lipoproteins. However, none of these changes are sensitive or specific enough to serve as markers for alcoholism. No similar laboratory parameters have been identified in individuals of any age who have used other categories of substances.

For these reasons, routine laboratory testing to search for standing physiologic changes is not recommended. Adolescent substance abusers may be nutritionally deficient, however, and should be screened for aneicitymia, along with appropriate laboratory and imaging assessment of symptoms and abnormal physical findings. Adolescents who inject drugs should be screened for hepatitis B and C and for HIV infection. They are also at risk for medical complications such as cellulitis, osteomyelitis, thrombophlebitis, pneumonia, brain abscess, and chronic liver

Table 9–6. Recurrent physical symptoms and mental health problems that may be related to substance use.

General	Neurologic
Fatigue	Headaches
Poor appetite	Blackouts (amnesia)
Weight loss	Lightheadedness and vertigo
Malnutrition	Syncope
Insomnia	Ataxia
Increased sleeping	Peripheral neuropathy
Respiratory	Seizures
Cough	Head injury
Laryngitis	Cognitive dysfunction
Bronchitis	**Hormonal and reproductive**
Wheezing	Abnormal menstrual cycles
Mucous membranes and nose	Male sexual dysfunction
Conjunctival irritation	Male gynecomastia
Nasal congestion	**Skin**
Nosebleeds	Skin infections
Sinusitis	**Psychiatric**
Cardiac	Depression and suicidality
Tachycardia	Mania
Palpitations	Anxiety
Chest pain	Psychosis
Gastrointestinal	Eating disorders
Abdominal pain	Personality disorders
Vomiting	
Constipation	

disease. Debilitated and homeless adolescents should be screened for tuberculosis. Finally, substance-abusing adolescents should be screened for problems such as sexually transmitted infections and hepatitis A because their behavior enhances their risk.

Alling FA: Detoxification and treatment of acute sequelae. In: *Substance Abuse: A Comprehensive Textbook,* 2nd ed. Lowinson JH et al (editors). Williams & Wilkins, 1992.

Dackis CA, Gold MS: Psychiatric hospitals for treatment of dual diagnosis. In: *Substance Abuse: A Comprehensive Textbook,* 2nd ed. Lowinson JH et al (editors). Williams & Wilkins, 1992.

Farrow, JA, Rees JM, Worthington-Roberts BS: Health, developmental and nutritional status of adolescent alcohol and marijuana abusers. Pediatrics 1987;79:218.

Leigh G, Skinner HA: Physiologic assessment. In: *Assessment of Addictive Behavior.* Donovan DM, Marlatt GA (editors). Guilford Press, 1988.

Novick DM: The medically ill substance abuser. In: *Substance Abuse: A Comprehensive Textbook,* 2nd ed. Lowinson JH et al (editors). Williams & Wilkins, 1992.

Pharmacologic Testing

Pharmacologic or drug screening of body fluids for substances of abuse is a technologically sophisticated but controversial procedure. Public and institutional policies that mandate involuntary, obligatory, and random urine testing for substances of abuse continue to be debated. However, this section discusses the pharmacologic testing of individual teenagers for clinical purposes. It should be remembered that drug testing can only differentiate between individuals who have used a drug and those who have not. Drug tests cannot provide information about the abuse of or dependence on drugs or about any related physical or mental impairment. In contrast, blood alcohol levels are correlated with degrees of neurologic impairment even though individual variation exists. Furthermore, because most substances and their metabolic products have relatively short half-lives, the time window following exposure during which they can be detected is limited. Therefore, a negative test cannot guarantee that the adolescent does not use substances. Retention times, or ability to detect the substance after last use, vary by class of substance and range from approximately 10 hours (alcohol) to 2–4 days (cocaine metabolites), to 2–8 days (occasional use of marijuana), to 14–42 days (chronic use of marijuana).

There are several clinical circumstances that necessitate drug screening in adolescents. They include psychiatric symptoms, mental status and performance changes, acute-onset behavior states, recurrent and unexplained non-intentional trauma (eg, motor vehicle accidents and falls), recurrent respiratory symptoms, and unexplained somatic symptoms. Many physicians would obtain drug tests on adolescents in legal-social crises such as running away and engaging in delinquent behaviors. Teenagers with these

problems are considered to be at high risk for substance abuse. Finally, any adolescent who sustains trauma serious enough to warrant care at a hospital emergency department should undergo pharmacologic testing for alcohol and drugs at that time. Even trauma patients whose blood alcohol concentrations are nil are at high risk for psychoactive substance abuse disorders as defined by interview or questionnaire techniques.

Pharmacologic testing for drugs is not recommended as part of routine adolescent health care. Screening by interview has been found to be more sensitive than testing body fluids, because it also explores the possibility of use in the past.

Even though some substance-using adolescents will not accurately describe their usage patterns at a first interview, most pediatricians agree that obtaining drug tests on youngsters who show no acute behavioral problems or physical symptoms is counterproductive. Merely confronting substance abusers with objective evidence of their use (eg, positive drug tests) appears to have little impact on behavior and offers little chance in a medical setting to motivate them to stop using. Pharmacologic testing should be incorporated into a comprehensive plan of assessment rather than being conducted independently.

If an anxious parent or institutional authority requests a drug screen on an adolescent, the information outlined above should be conveyed. The pediatrician should then determine what the consequences would be if the results of the drug screen were positive and what would occur if they were negative. The intent is often to document use of illicit substances in order to take disciplinary action. A 1989 statement from the American Academy of Pediatrics reminds us that pediatricians' roles in this area should be counseling and treatment, not police work. Therefore, pediatricians in clinical practice should not perform drug testing for the primary purpose of detecting illegal use. The pediatrician must present and discuss the screening request with the adolescent and explain the reasons for the request. Assuming that the adolescent is mentally competent, informed consent should be obtained. Parental permission for testing is not sufficient for involuntary screening of a mentally competent teenager. It can be predicted that if the adolescent agrees to drug testing, the results will be negative. Refusing to submit to testing may well arouse suspicion. However, the physician will be more likely to retain the trust of the adolescent for future encounters and will have maintained the confidentiality of the medical relationship. The pediatrician should use this opportunity to encourage better communication between the teenager and parents.

If the decision is made to proceed with drug testing, the pediatrician must be cognizant of the four stages of screening. Errors at any stage can lead to inappropriate management and may have legal ramifications. The first stage, preparation of the "donor" (the adolescent), and the fourth stage, clinical application of the laboratory results, have been discussed above. The remainder of this discussion focuses on the technical aspects of drug screening.

Urine screening provides the best way of identifying illicit chemical substances in the body. Special attention must be paid to collection of the urine specimen especially if the results may have punitive or disciplinary consequences or affect employability or eligibility for participation in sports programs. In general, the specimen must be obtained under direct observation and under circumstances that minimize opportunity for tampering (eg, no sink in the room, minimal clothing and personal belongings allowed in the room, noting urine color and temperature, using a colored disinfectant in the toilet bowl water, and labeling and holding the urine specimen in a secure refrigerator).

The third stage of urine screening is the laboratory analysis. Drug testing must be conducted by an accredited laboratory, which will perform two types of tests: screening and confirmatory. Screening tests should be highly sensitive and are usually efficient and relatively inexpensive. Confirmatory tests on specimens that screen positive are more complex, labor-intensive, and expensive. Two independent test methods are often used to confirm positive screens. Several techniques are available for use by modern laboratories to analyze specimens for various compounds. In order to screen for all classes of substances of abuse, laboratories may need to use more than one method. Current techniques include enzyme immunoassay (EIA) eg, the enzyme-multiplied immunoassay test (EMIT) radioimmunoassay (RIA) fluorescent polarization immunoassay (FPIA) thin-layer chromatography (TLC) (sensitivity can be enhanced by use of high-power thin-layer chromatography [HPTLC] and gas-liquid chromatography (equipped with a nitrogen-phosphorus detector). Enzyme immunoassay is frequently used to screen for a panel of drugs; it is relatively inexpensive, does not require extraction of drugs from body fluids, is sufficiently sensitive, and is adaptable for high-volume automated screening. In contrast, some laboratories use thin-layer chromatography for routine drug screening because it is inexpensive. However, it is not sufficiently sensitive to detect such common drugs as marijuana, PCP, and LSD and may not detect low levels of cocaine, barbiturates, and opioids. Gas chromatography and mass spectrometry are used as a combined technique to confirm positive screening results. This technique is highly sensitive and specific and is the only test admissible as evidence of substance use in most courts of law.

American Medical Association, Council on Scientific Affairs: Scientific issues in drug testing. JAMA 1987;257: 3110.

MacKenzie RG, Cheng M, Haftel AJ: The clinical utility and evaluation of drug screening techniques. Pediatr Clin North Am 1987;34:423.

MacKenzie RG, Kipke MD: Substance use and abuse. In: *Comprehensive Adolescent Health Care.* Friedman SB, Fisher M, Schonberg SK (editors). Quality Medical Publishing, 1992.

Rivara FP et al: A descriptive study of trauma, alcohol, and alcoholism in young adults. J Adolesc Health 1992;13: 663.

Soderstrom CA et al: Psychoactive substance dependence among trauma center patients. JAMA 1992;267:2756.

Verebey K: Diagnostic laboratory: Screening for drug abuse. In: *Substance Abuse: A Comprehensive Textbook.* Lowinson JL et al (editors). Williams & Wilkins, 1992.

COUNSELING STRATEGIES FOR REFERRAL OF ADOLESCENTS WITH SUBSTANCE ABUSE PROBLEMS

Most pediatricians will not—and probably should not—assume the responsibility for actual treatment of substance-abusing adolescents and their families. However, they can employ counseling strategies to ensure effective communication and referral. Many substance-abusing adolescents and even their families have not previously considered substance use to be a source of concern, even though it is objectively associated with dysfunctional consequences. These teenagers and their families may be less able to accept the recommendation that treatment would be helpful. Using the "stages of change" model, these individuals may be placed in the "precontemplative" stage, which describes the substance use pattern prior to any active consideration of change. The pediatrician may need to modify the counseling goal for these youngsters and their families and may need to accept success in calling the teenager's and family's attention to substance abuse as a problem behavior, which may encourage them to proceed to the "contemplation" or "motivation and commitment" stage. Although individuals in this stage are clearly considering addressing the substance abuse problem, they may also experience motivational conflict and ambivalence. The pediatrician's goal for teenagers and their families who are at this second stage is to move them forward to the "action stage," in which they make active attempts to change. A successful counseling outcome for these adolescents and their families would be acceptance of the screening evaluation and follow-through with the recommendation for full assessment and therapeutic intervention.

Counseling strategies the pediatrician can use to help teenagers and their families make the transition to a drug abuse treatment agency are summarized in Table 9–7 and elaborated below. First, the pediatrician should permit the adolescent to describe perceptions of the substance use and the problems it may be causing. Regardless of the adolescent's perceptions, the pediatrician should then summarize the informa-

Table 9–7. Counseling strategies.

- Allow the adolescent to verbalize his or her understanding of the substance use.
- Summarize information disclosed as part of the interview and from any collateral sources, using a nonconfrontational style.
- Clarify the problem behaviors regarding the substance use.
- Provide clear information about dysfunctional consequences, including medical and psychosocial problems, that have resulted from substance use, but do not moralize.
- Communicate concern for the adolescent's well-being.
- Allow the adolescent and family to express their responses to your summary and synthesis of the problems.
- Clarify your role in the evaluation and intervention process.
- Provide concrete assistance to the adolescent and family to enhance the likelihood that successful completion of a referral to a treatment agency will occur.
  1. If necessary, assume responsibility for acting as an intermediary between the adolescent and parents.
  2. Assume responsibility for initiating the referral to a treatment agency.

tion gathered during the assessment. This approach shows respect for the adolescent and allows the pediatrician to make adjustments in communication style so as to respond most effectively to the adolescent's concerns. In addition to preparing the adolescent and family for future steps, summarization ensures that the physician understands the historical information and can communicate the problem accurately. A descriptive summary provides a clear statement of the problem behaviors to the adolescent and family. It is helpful to outline dysfunctional behavior in the context of substance use. The following example illustrates this process.

"I know that many teenagers occasionally smoke marijuana. However, since this school year started, you have been using marijuana more frequently than you did last year, and a lot of things have happened that have aroused concern. First, you haven't been feeling well—you are tired all the time, and have been coughing. Second, school isn't going well for you—you've already been suspended twice for fighting, you dropped out of the debating club and quit soccer, and your grades are down. Third, you were really shaken up last week by that traffic accident. And fourth, you have been feeling very sad, and other people see you as being angry all the time. I am very worried about you."

Following communication of concern, the next step is to provide useful information without moralizing or lecturing.

"When a person becomes really involved with drinking or doing drugs, without realizing it, or even wanting it to happen, the alcohol and drugs can take over a person's life. This is what I believe is happening to you."

At this point, the teenager may again need a chance to respond. Do not expect your assessment to be automatically accepted by either the teenager or the family even if the adolescent is experiencing serious dysfunction.

Clarify your role as you facilitate the referral process. Try not to allow the teenager and family to perceive the referral as rejection by you. Two techniques you can use to avoid this issue are commitment to continued appropriate involvement with the adolescent and personalization of the referral process:

"I believe it would really help you to feel better if you and your family learned more about chemical dependency and enrolled in a treatment program for teenagers who have problems with drugs and alcohol. I would like you to meet a friend of mine who knows a lot about teenagers, families, and the problems that drugs and alcohol can cause. I don't have the background to give you really expert help with this problem. I will continue to be here for you as your doctor, but you also need counseling help."

It may be necessary to provide concrete assistance in facilitating referral to a treatment agency. The pediatrician should be familiar with community resources and the philosophies of treatment of various programs, the actual services they provide, and their fee schedules. Establish personal contact with program staff members. Teenagers and families often feel overwhelmed and powerless when they are confronted with serious problems. Your status as their doctor will help provide the stimulus they need to complete the referral successfully. You may want the patient or family to telephone the counseling professional or treatment agency from your office. Ask the family to call you after their first appointment. Let them know that you will have the agency or counselor contact you if the adolescent misses the first appointment.

Marlatt GA: Matching clients to treatment: Treatment modules and stages of change. In: *Assessment of Addictive Behavior.* Donovan DM, Marlatt GA (editors). Guilford Press, 1988.

Riggs SG, Alario AJ: Adolescent substance use: Instructor's guide. In: *The Project ADEPT Curriculum for Primary Care Physician Training.* Dubé CE et al (editors). Brown Univ Press, 1989.

TREATMENT SERVICES

Teenagers require professional treatment for substance use if they develop physical, social, or emotional problems. Broad treatment goals include the elimination of substance abuse and any accompanying undesirable behaviors and restoration of the teenager to a healthy functional status.

There are several categories of treatment services for adolescents who abuse substances, but they are all based on the "disease" model of chemical dependency. Virtually all treatment programs in the United States share the belief that treatment begins with cessation of use and requires stable maintenance of sobriety, and have the goal of a substance-free lifestyle. Participation in self-help groups such as Alcoholics Anonymous is usually included in other treatment programs, but its efficacy as the sole treatment strategy has not been validated. Outpatient counseling programs are most appropriate for motivated teenagers during the early stages of substance abuse. They are frequently supported by public funding and are usually financially accessible to young people from families with low incomes. Residential programs include several subtypes but represent a more intensive treatment format. Adolescents frequently remain in residential programs for several months, during which time they progress through structured stages as they prepare for return to their homes. Inpatient substance abuse treatment programs represent the most intensive format. They provide short-term services that include medical care and detoxification as well as counseling and engagement in structured activities. Teenagers who require hospitalization exhibit evidence of severe chemical dependency and may have failed less intensive treatment formats.

Dual diagnosis inpatient units for teenagers are a relatively recent phenomenon. They are able to address the needs of teenagers who have both psychiatric or behavioral problems and substance abuse problems. However, because many inpatient programs only accept private insurance, teenagers from low-income families may have limited access to them.

Finally, individual programs have historically offered the same treatment package to all clients regardless of the characteristics of the adolescent, the family, the social setting, or the adolescent's functional capacity. Client-treatment matching is a relatively new concept which recognizes that treatment options should be graded to the level of intensity and should be relevant to individual teenagers' problems and needs. However, because most substance abuse treatment programs continue to provide a uniform treatment "package," little information is available to guide the clinical application of client-treatment matching.

Chatlos JC, Tufaro JB: Treatment of the dually diagnosed adolescent. In: *Dual Diagnosis in Substance Abuse.* Gold MS, Slaby AE (editors). Marcel Dekker, 1991 .

Dusenbury L, Khuri E, Millman RB: Adolescent substance abuse: A sociodevelopmental perspective. In: *Substance Abuse: A Comprehensive Textbook,* 2nd ed. Lowinson JH et al (editors). Williams & Wilkins, 1992.

Hoffman NG, Sonis WA, Halikas JA: Issues in the evaluation of chemical dependency treatment programs for adolescents. Pediatr Clin North Am 1987;34:449.

Marlatt GA: Matching clients to treatment: Treatment mod-

ules and stages of change. In: *Assessment of Addictive Behavior.* Donovan DM, Marlatt GA (editors). Guilford Press, 1988.

Moncher MS, Holden GW, Trimble JE: Substance abuse among Native-American Youth. J Consult Clin Psychol 1990;58:408.

US Congress, Office of Technology Assessment: Alcohol, tobacco and drug abuse: Prevention and services. Adolescent Health, vol II: *Background and the Effectiveness of Selected Prevention and Treatment Services.* OTA-H-468. US Government Printing Office, 1991.

Wheeler K, Malmquist J: Treatment approaches in adolescent chemical dependency. Pediatr Clin North Am 1987;34:437.

TOBACCO

Prevalence of Use

Although the proportion of adolescents who smoke cigarettes has been gradually decreasing over the past 15 years (see Table 9–1), in 1992 about 28% of high school seniors had smoked within the preceding 30 days, 17% had smoked daily, and 10% had smoked at least one-half pack per day. Smoking starts during late childhood (10 years of age or younger) for 10% of girls and 14% of boys and increases during early adolescence, peaking at ages 13–14, when 25% of females and 24% of males smoke their first full cigarette. By ages 15–16, over half of both males and females have initiated smoking. Based on empirical information, it is estimated that 20% of adolescents progress from experimental to regular smoking. It has also been found that 90% of adolescents who smoke three or four cigarettes become regular smokers.

Over the past decade, adolescent use of smokeless tobacco has also aroused concern. The national prevalence of its use was first measured in 1986. Although high school seniors' use has not been measured consistently, it is possible that more students are using smokeless tobacco now than in 1989. In 1992, almost one-third of high school seniors had used smokeless tobacco at least once, 11% had used it within the preceding 30 days, and 4% had done so on a daily basis. Regular use by younger students is also of concern. In 1992, about 7% of eighth graders and 10% of tenth graders had used smokeless tobacco within the preceding 30 days, and almost 2% of eighth graders and a full 3% of tenth graders had used it every day. White male adolescents, especially those living in rural and small communities, appear to be at highest risk for using smokeless tobacco.

Nicotine Dependence

Regular use of tobacco is now defined as nicotine dependence. Although nicotine has harmful health effects in its own right, including the promotion of atherosclerosis, coronary artery disease, and cerebrovascular and peripheral vascular disease (probably because it stimulates sympathetic ganglia, releases catecholamines, and activates chemoreceptors in the aortic and carotid bodies), multiple other physiologically active toxic substances found in cured tobacco products and tobacco smoke are chiefly responsible for the development of local cancers, chronic lung disease, susceptibility to respiratory tract infection, and exacerbation of reactive airway disease.

Adolescents may be particularly susceptible to initiating and maintaining smoking. The long latency period to the development of cardiovascular disease and malignancy makes these problems appear unreal or hypothetical to adolescents, who have not yet developed the skills of formal operational thinking (see Chapters 4 and 6). Second, smoking does not cause significant mental or motor impairment, as do all other categories of substance use; on the contrary, nicotine may actually enhance cognitive and motor performance. Finally, adolescents (and children) may be more easily entrapped than adults by tobacco companies' advertising campaigns and marketing strategies.

Although nicotine may initially cause a mild euphoria, tolerance for this pleasurable sensation develops rapidly. Nicotine has been found to release dopamine in the reinforcement areas of the brain. However, it is currently postulated that negative reinforcement is largely responsible for nicotine dependence—ie, smokers need to use nicotine for relief of withdrawal symptoms. Ritual behaviors associated with smoking (eg, smoking following a meal) are considered secondary positive reinforcers.

Nicotine is readily absorbed through the skin and all mucosal surfaces. Given the large pulmonary surface for absorption and the ability to bypass the venous circulation, inhalation of nicotine through cigarette smoking is the most efficient way to raise nicotine blood levels. Inhalation is also the most addictive form of nicotine use. Physiologically, nicotine causes release of catecholamines, with a secondary increased heart rate, peripheral vasoconstriction, and a fine tremor. Individuals unused to nicotine may develop nausea and vomiting, lightheadedness, and vertigo. Nicotine also exerts the following nervous system effects: facilitation of attention and memory, speed and accuracy of motor function, appetite suppression, and self-reported relaxation of mood.

Nicotine withdrawal causes a specific syndrome that includes mood changes and physiologic symptoms and signs. Withdrawal symptoms can start abruptly within 2 hours after the last nicotine use, which may help to explain heavy smokers' compulsive need to smoke. (The approximate half-life of nicotine is 2 hours.) Adverse changes in mood and in cognitive and motor performance peak within 1–3 days of withdrawal and gradually subside over several days to several weeks. Individuals who withdraw from nicotine also experience a decrease in heart rate, blood pressure, and measured levels of epinephrine, norepinephrine, and cortisol, and increased peripheral blood flow. Common mood changes include irritability and anxiety. Individuals also experience restlessness, difficulty concentrating, and hunger, which can result in weight gain. Individuals "crave" nicotine and have a strong urge to smoke. These symptoms of withdrawal quickly resolve with resumption of nicotine intake.

Counseling Strategies to Help Adolescents Quit Smoking

One should not assume that all teenagers who smoke want to continue. More than half of a large school-based sample of adolescents who smoked regularly had attempted to quit. In general, 75% of teenagers who had started to smoke when they were older—compared with teenagers who had started to smoke at a younger age—attempted to quit at an earlier time after starting to smoke (within a year). However, more than half of teenagers who had started to smoke during elementary school had made at least one quitting attempt in the first 3 years of regular smoking. Unfortunately, only 22% of adolescents who tried to quit smoking without help managed to abstain for 6 months. Based on data from adults, we also know that most smokers who were able to quit did so on their own, frequently using a "cold turkey" approach, rather than using an assisted approach such as a formal smoking cessation program or nicotine gum prescribed by a physician.

Although no data are available for adolescents, firm advice from a physician has been found to influence adult smokers to quit. Success rates are enhanced when physicians formalize brief protocols for themselves and their office staff for use with every patient who smokes.

In 1989, the National Cancer Institute published a manual for physicians: *How to Help Your Patients Stop Smoking*. Its strategies are based on principles of behavioral treatment. First, individuals must be motivated to quit smoking, but motivation by itself is not sufficient. Learning how to use coping skills to prevent relapse is thought to be the most important element of smoking cessation. Positive feedback is also helpful. Finally, to help prevent relapse, it is important for individuals who are trying to quit smoking to have a smoke-free environment. Table 9–8 outlines specific steps, adapted from the National Cancer Institute's recommendations, which pediatricians can follow to help their adolescent patients quit smoking.

Pharmacologic Treatment of Nicotine Dependence

At present, two types of nicotine replacement systems are available by prescription and are recommended to control symptoms of withdrawal in adults who smoke at least 20 cigarettes a day and who express a clear motivation to quit. However, these agents have not been tested for safety or efficacy in adolescents and are FDA-approved for labeling pur-

Table 9–8. Clinical steps to help adolescent patients quit smoking.

Ask all preadolescents and adolescent patients whether they or their friends smoke or use smokeless tobacco:
- How old were they when they first tried smoking?
- How old were they when they first started to smoke regularly?
- What made them start smoking?
- Why do they continue to smoke? (e.g., stress and anxiety, friends smoke bored, something to do)
- Where do they smoke? (at home, at school, at work, with friends)
- Where do they obtain their cigarettes? (Note that it is illegal for minors to purchase tobacco products, and, conversely, for vendors to sell tobacco products to minors.)
- How soon after waking do they have their first cigarette?
- How much do they enjoy smoking?
- Have they ever tried to quit? What happened?
- Do their parents or siblings smoke?
- What do their parents think about their smoking?
- Safety: Have they ever fallen asleep while smoking? Ever smoked in bed? Ever been burned?
- How interested are they in stopping smoking?
- What do they know about the health effects of tobacco use? Where did they learn this information? Have they learned about tobacco in school? Does their school provide a program that enhances teenagers' ability to handle uncomfortable social situations?

Advise all teenagers who smoke to stop: (Note that pediatricians should also advise parents who smoke to stop, regardless of their children's ages.)
- State your advice clearly but nonjudgementally.
- Personalize your message to quit, based on the adolescent's activities and developmental status.
  1. General messages for adolescents can include cosmetic reasons (bad breath, stained teeth and fingers, smelly clothes, burned clothes and furniture), cost (what they could do with money saved), lack of independence (being controlled by cigarettes), hampered sports performance through compromised respiratory function, sore throats, coughs, and more frequent respiratory infections.
  2. It is easier to stop now than it will be when they are older. The vast majority of adults who smoke wish they had never started and would like to stop smoking.
  3. Teenagers with reactive airway disease: more difficult to control.
  4. For adolescents starting oral contraceptive pills, increased risks for thromboembolic phenomena. (Such counseling should be done skillfully. The actual risk in adolescents is low, and you don't want adolescents to choose continuation of smoking over effective pregnancy prevention.).
  5. Pregnant teenagers: Risk of an unhealthy newborn with low birthweight; increased rate of fetal death; as parents, smoking provides a poor role model; exposure to smoke can harm their children's health through respiratory infections.

Assist the patient in stopping:
- Establish a quit date. Negotiate with the adolescent for a date within the next 2–4 weeks. Acknowledge that no time is ideal.
- Provide self-help materials, and review them with the adolescent. (Materials are available from the National Cancer Institute and from local chapters of the American Heart Association, the March of Dimes, and the American Respiratory Diseases Association.)
- Establish a "No Smoking" contract with the patient. It should be developed together, and personalized. Its format can be written or oral, sealed with a handshake.
- Help the adolescent to solve problems in advance
  1. Rehearse through role play how to respond to social situations where other adolescents may be smoking.
  2. How to handle irritability
  3. How to handle "cravings"
  4. How to handle hunger
  5. How to help satisfy need for oral activity
  6. How to help satisfy need for hand activity
  7. Encourage participation in activities incompatible with smoking (eg, athletic activities).
- Suggest having a friend or family member with whom to quit. (This suggestion to promote successful smoking cessation was the one made most frequently by adolescents.)
- If the parent is aware of the adolescent's smoking and the adolescent wants the parent's encouragement, involve the parent. If the adolescent and parent have a conflict-ridden relationship, the adolescent may be alienated by a parent's comments or advice.
- For adolescents who don't want to stop smoking or who deny that they might have a problem with nicotine dependence:
  1. Try not to alienate them with a "hard sell." You want them to return as your patients.
  2. Consider an independent substance abuse problem.
  3. Consider having them complete a motivational questionnaire that measures nicotine dependence. (Note that these materials were developed primarily for adults.)
  - National Cancer Institute pamphlet "Why do you smoke?" (available from 800-4-CANCER)
  - Fagerström Test for Nicotine Dependence (a six-item questionnaire with scores ranging from 0 to 10)

Arrange follow-up visits:
- Schedule a brief follow-up visit 1–2 weeks following the quit date.
  1. Provide positive reinforcement if the adolescent was successful, and encouragement if the adolescent was not successful in stopping or has relapsed.
  2. Determine circumstances of any relapse.
  3. Review strategies to help prevent future relapse.
  4. Discuss any patient concerns.
- Schedule a second brief follow-up visit within a month.
- With the patient's permission, call (or have a member of the office staff call) or write the adolescent within a week after the visit, reminding the patient of the quit date, and reinforcing the decision to stop smoking.

poses only for adults. However, in combination with counseling, selected adolescent patients may benefit from such a prescription. Almost 30% of adolescents believe that medication to make quitting easier would be useful in helping teenagers to stop smoking.

Nicotine polacrilex gum was introduced about 20 years ago. If used correctly (slow chewing followed by lodging the gum in the buccal cavity for mucosal absorption), this technique is able to produce low and slowly rising levels of nicotine for weaning. Although controlled trials with adults have demonstrated enhanced cessation rates for smoking compared with placebo, clinical use is problematic. Many patients do not use the gum correctly, and many do not receive counseling to help prevent relapse.

Transdermal nicotine patches were introduced commercially in 1992. They offer several advantages for individuals interested in smoking cessation. The constant slow transdermal absorption of nicotine produces a steady state concentration that effectively relieves the majority of withdrawal symptoms; the patches are easy to use, which enhances patient compliance; and side effects are minimal (local erythema and contact dermatitis; sleeping difficulties, which are relieved by using an intermittent patch). However, the dosing is inflexible, and a relatively long interval of 4–6 hours is necessary to reach plasma levels high enough to alleviate symptoms of nicotine withdrawal. The total duration of patch therapy is usually 6–8 weeks. In adults, controlled clinical trials yielded 6-month abstinence rates of 22–42%. Counseling, including both cognitive and behavioral strategies, remains essential in helping people to stop smoking.

A variety of pharmacologic agents have been used in adults to help reduce craving and relieve the anxiety and depression commonly associated with nicotine withdrawal. They include clonidine, anxiolytics such as buspirone, and antidepressants such as fluoxetine. However, there is either inconsistent information or little published data regarding the efficacy of these agents. Furthermore, anticholinergic drugs such as transcutaneous scopolamine have been reported to reduce nicotine craving and withdrawal symptoms. Lobeline, which is available without prescription, has been available for many years as a weak nicotine receptor agonist. (They are both ganglionic stimulators.) There is no evidence for lobeline's efficacy in helping individuals to quit smoking.

Epps RP, Manley MW: A physician's guide to preventing tobacco use during childhood and adolescence. Pediatrics 1991;88:140.

Ershler J et al: The quitting experience for smokers in sixth through twelfth grades. Addict Behav 1989;14:365.

Escobedo LG et al: Sports participation, age at smoking initiation, and the risk of smoking among U.S. high school students. JAMA 1993;269:1391.

Fiore MC et al: Tobacco dependence and the nicotine patch. JAMA 1992;268:2687.

Heatherton TF et al: The Fagerström test for nicotine dependence: A revision of the Fagerström tolerance questionnaire. Br J Addict 1991;86:1119.

Jarvik ME, Schneider NG: Nicotine. In: *Substance Abuse: A Comprehensive Textbook*, 2nd ed. Lowinson JH et al (editors). Williams & Wilkins, 1992.

Manley MW, Epps RP, Glynn TJ: The clinician's role in promoting smoking cessation among clinic patients. Med Clin North Am 1992;76:477.

Miller NS, Cocores JA: Nicotine dependence: Diagnosis, chemistry, and pharmacologic treatments. Pediatr Rev 1993;14:275.

ANABOLIC STEROIDS

Although professional athletes have used anabolic steroids for at least 4 decades, concern about adolescent use is more recent. The Monitoring the Future Study first included questions about steroid use in 1989. Table 9–1 shows that in 1992, 2% of high school seniors had used anabolic steroids, and 0.6% reported use within the preceding month. Male students (approximately 5% lifetime use) are at much higher risk than are female students (approximately 1–2% lifetime use). About half of male students who use anabolic steroids first tried them by the tenth grade. Interestingly, adolescent students who use anabolic steroids are also likely to use tobacco products and such traditional substances as alcohol, marijuana, and cocaine. Polysubstance use is well recognized among adults who use anabolic androgenic steroids.

Several forms of synthetic anabolic androgenic steroids exist. Although formulations approved by the FDA are legitimately used to replace endogenous testosterone, to enhance serum complement factors in the treatment of hereditary angioneurotic edema, and to treat endometriosis and fibrocystic breast disease, it is illegal to prescribe anabolic androgenic steroids for athletic or cosmetic purposes. The majority of individuals who use these compounds illicitly obtain them from smuggled foreign sources and from veterinary suppliers.

Both parenteral and oral formulations are available. The latter have a shorter half-life but impose a greater risk of hepatotoxicity. Users tend to take anabolic androgenic steroids in cycles of 4–18 weeks, interspersed with "drug holidays." The daily dose can range from 2 to 200 times the pharmacologic doses recommended for treatment of medical problems. Some users "stack," or use multiple compounds simultaneously. Increasing the size of the dose over time is called "pyramiding."

Medical Consequences of Use

Several medical consequences are recognized for high-dose use of anabolic androgenic steroids. However, few well-designed studies are available, so that much of our information comes from clinical series and case reports. Athletes who use anabolic steroids believe that these agents promote muscle growth and enhance muscle capacity, increase strength and endurance, and quicken recovery from exercise, which together permit individuals to engage in more frequent workouts and to exercise at a higher intensity. Although these peripheral effects on muscle function are theoretically possible, it has been difficult to distinguish them from anabolic steroids' effects on the central nervous system, which may drive individuals' motivation for heightened performance, so that observed physical changes are secondary. Small measured changes in muscle function may confer a competitive advantage. It has been observed clinically, however, that individuals who use anabolic steroids may increase their lean body mass and improve their strength if they engage in high-intensity resistance training and maintain an adequate protein intake.

Other medical effects of high-dose anabolic androgenic steroids are less desirable. High doses induce hypogonadotropic hypogonadism, which for males results in a significant decrease in testicular volume and oligospermia. These effects, though probably reversible, can persist for long periods. High circulating levels of testosterone in younger adolescents who have not yet completed longitudinal growth can promote early epiphysial closure with consequent foreshortened stature and premature virilization. Adolescent males may be susceptible to gynecomastia as a feminizing side effect, which results from the peripheral conversion of testosterone to estrogen. Virilizing effects in females are largely irreversible and include hirsutism, male pattern baldness, coarsening of the voice, and clitoral enlargement. Both males and females can develop significant acne.

Users of anabolic androgenic steroids frequently develop hepatic dysfunction. Oral agents produce cholestasis, and users may develop cholestatic jaundice. Serum levels of liver enzymes can also rise, but this phenomenon is probably transient. Individuals using androgens for long-term legitimate medical treatment appear to be at risk for peliosis hepatis (blood-filled cysts in the liver) and for hepatocellular carcinoma.

Individuals who use anabolic steroids may also be at risk for cardiovascular disease. The HDL:LDL cholesterol ratio is reversed, which may accelerate atherosclerosis. They may also be at risk for thromboembolic phenomena, partly because of increased red cell mass, potentiated platelet aggregation, and high estrogen levels. Sodium retention may cause edema and heightened blood pressure. It is also possible that use of anabolic steroids enhances the risk for cardiomyopathy, tendon rupture, and prostatic hypertrophy.

Anabolic steroids have important psychoactive effects. They can provide a sensation of euphoria and increased libido. Individuals who use anabolic steroids are also at risk for aggressive behaviors, including fighting and purposeful destruction of property. They are prone to impulsivity and impaired judgment as well as feelings of irritation and hostility with urges to harm others. Although no single psychiatric syndrome has been linked with the use of anabolic androgenic steroids, some users have met criteria for bipolar disorder and others have exhibited paranoid thoughts and delusions, grandiose delusions, auditory hallucinations, and other psychotic features. Some users have experienced anxiety, panic attacks, feelings of profound sadness, and suicidal ideation.

Users of anabolic steroids may meet psychiatric criteria for drug dependence. Over time, they take larger doses, complete more cycles of use, and are unable to stop use, even if they experience significant negative side effects or want to stop the practice. Individuals who stop use, either on a cyclical or a permanent basis, are likely to experience symptoms consistent with an abstinence syndrome, which include drug craving, dissatisfaction with body image, headaches, fatigue, depressed mood, restlessness and insomnia, anorexia, and decreased libido. It is during times of withdrawal that users of anabolic steroids appear most likely to use other illicit substances, perhaps in an attempt to ameliorate the symptoms of withdrawal.

Buckley WE et al: Estimated prevalence of anabolic steroid use among male high school seniors. JAMA 1988;260: 3441.

DuRant RH et al: Use of multiple drugs among adolescents who use anabolic steroids. N Engl J Med 1993;328:922.

Kashkin KB: Anabolic steroids. In: *Substance Abuse: A Comprehensive Textbook.* Lowinson JH et al (editors). Williams & Wilkins, 1992.

Office of Inspector General: Adolescent steroid use. Office of Evaluations and Inspections, U.S. Department of Health and Human Services, OEI-06-90-01080, 1991.

CLINICAL PREVENTION OF ADOLESCENT SUBSTANCE ABUSE

The major focus of this chapter has been the identification and counseling of substance-abusing adolescents. The pediatrician can also play an important role in helping prevent adolescent substance abuse. Physicians' health messages have been found to promote smoking cessation and sobriety in adults and condom use by sexually active adolescents. However, little information is available regarding the effectiveness of office-based interventions for the prevention of substance use and abuse by adolescents.

It is thought that pediatricians may be able to provide more effective health counseling regarding use of alcohol and drugs if they model their office-based clinical interventions after the most successful classroom-based prevention programs. A social reinforcement paradigm that specifically develops students' abilities to recognize and resist social pressures to use drugs and alcohol—as well as to identify the social and physical consequences of drug use—has been the foundation for the most successful school-based programs. Teaching methods include discussion, behavior modeling and role play, practice sessions, and a public commitment not to use. In contrast, it has been found that merely learning factual information about drugs and alcohol and attending programs that focus on self-esteem enhancement and development of general decision-making and interpersonal skills without specific attention to drugs and alcohol are not sufficient to postpone adolescents' use of substances. "Booster" sessions over time are necessary to maintain early successes.

Pediatricians should ask every adolescent about use of alcohol and drugs at every health maintenance visit. Rather than just lecturing or distributing a written brochure, the pediatrician should attempt to engage the adolescent in a relevant conversation. For example, the pediatrician can ask an adolescent going out for football, "What have you heard about steroids?" In this way, the adolescent's knowledge can be gauged and accurate cautionary information can be communicated as part of the conversation. The pediatrician can provide positive reinforcement for correct knowledge and a decision not to try steroids, and if necessary can use the opportunity to attempt to modify an adolescent's favorable attitude toward steroid use. Older adolescents with expectations of a positive outcome from substance use are more likely to use more heavily. However, it has also been found that young adults are actually able to decrease their substance use when their specific beliefs about it are challenged. Finally, as a strategy to practice decision-making and social skills, the pediatrician can engage the adolescent in role play. For example, how would he handle social pressure to try steroids? In this way, the pediatrician can help the adolescent to prepare for social situations with preformulated decisions and can help promote the patient's social competence.

Anglin TM: Life skills training for adolescent health promotion. Adolesc Health Update 1992;5:1.

Botvin GJ et al: Preventing adolescent drug abuse through a multimodal cognitive-behavioral approach: Results of a 3-year study. J Consult Clin Psychol 1990;58:437.

Bruvold WH: A meta-analysis of adolescent smoking prevention programs. Am J Public Health 1993;83:872.

Werner MJ, Walker LS, Greene JW: Alcohol expectancies, problem drinking, and adverse health consequences. J Adolesc Health 1993;14:446.

REFERENCES

American Academy of Pediatrics, Center for Advanced Health Studies: *Substance Abuse: A Guide for Health Professionals.* AAP, 1988.

Donovan DM, Marlatt GA (editors): *Assessment of Addictive Behavior.* Guilford Press, 1988.

Lowinson JL et al (editors): *Substance Abuse: A Comprehensive Textbook,* 2nd ed. Williams & Wilkins, 1992.

Newcomb MD, Bentler PM: *Consequences of Adolescent Drug Use.* Sage Publications, 1988.

Immunization

10

Eric A.F. Simoes, MD, DCH

The routine use of immunization has become an integral part of pediatric practice in the United States over the last 50 years. Despite problems arising out of complacency, increased cost, and threats of litigation, vaccinations continue to be a critical feature of well child care. Experience with smallpox has shown that complete eradication of a disease is possible when mass coverage with an effective vaccine is achieved and maintained.

Every immunization is intended to prevent either the primary manifestations of infection with a particular organism or secondary phenomena resulting from that infection. To decide which children should routinely receive a particular product, public health officials pay careful attention to the probable benefits from use of the product as well as the inherent risks. This principle guides public health strategies for mass vaccinations, and it also guides the individual practitioner's approach to each child.

The benefit of an immunization is the extent to which it eliminates the risk of a particular illness or its complications. Any calculation of benefit must take into account the likelihood that the illness will occur in a defined population or individual as well as the likelihood that the vaccination will prevent that illness. This benefit must be weighed against the risk to the individual child of using it. It is the obligation of the physician to present this information to the parents or legal guardian in lay terminology and to record their understanding of the information and their consent to immunization. Although there is no single right way for a physician to conduct such a discussion with parents—nor is it required in most jurisdictions—the responsible physician must do so. (See Legal Issues in Immunization at the end of this chapter.)

The recommendations for use of immunizations outlined in this chapter are current. However, as technology and our understanding of the epidemiology of vaccine-preventable diseases change, the recommendations will also change. The most useful sources for current information are listed below:

(1) *Morbidity and Mortality Weekly Report.* Published weekly by the Centers For Disease Control and Prevention (CDC), Atlanta 30333. *MMWR* contains recommendations of the United States Public Health Service Advisory Committee on Immunization Practices (ACIP).

(2) *Report of the Committee on Infectious Diseases.* Published at 2- to 3-year intervals by the American Academy of Pediatrics, the *"Red Book"* is available from The American Academy of Pediatrics, 141 Northwest Point Boulevard, PO Box 927, Elk Grove Village, IL 60009–0927. Updates are published in the journal *Pediatrics* as needed.

STANDARDS FOR PEDIATRIC IMMUNIZATION PRACTICES

While 97–98% of children in the United States are vaccinated by or shortly after school entry, as many as 37% to 56% of the 7.8 million 2-year-olds in this country are not fully immunized. Low immunization coverage has been attributed to difficulties in reaching certain socioeconomic groups, including the urban poor and racial and ethnic minorities. However, the health care delivery system appears to bear much of the responsibility for low immunization coverage as well. Thus, parents seeking immunization for their children face significant barriers; not all providers take advantage of opportunities to administer vaccines, and inadequate or absent third party payment for immunizations further reduces coverage. Standards for Pediatric Immunization Practices (Table 10–1) were prepared by consensus of the National Vaccine Advisory Committee and the Ad Hoc Working Group for the Development of Standards for Pediatric Immunization Practices. They constitute the most essential and desirable immunization policies and practices. Simultaneously, a guide to Contraindications and Precautions to Immunization were developed that reflect the current recommendations of the Advisory Committee on Immunization Practices and the Committee of Infectious Diseases of the American Academy of Pediatrics (Table 10–2). Copies of these published standards with explanations for each of the standards can be obtained from Information

Table 10–1. Standards for pediatric immunization practices.

1. Immunization services are readily available.
2. There are no barriers or unnecessary prerequisites to the receipt of vaccines.
3. Immunization services are available free or for a minimal fee.
4. Providers utilize all clinical encounters to screen and, when indicated, vaccinate children.
5. Providers educate parents and guardians about immunization in general terms.
6. Providers question parents or guardians about contraindications and, before vaccinating a child, inform them in specific terms about the risks and benefits of the vaccinations their child is to receive.
7. Providers follow only true contraindications.
8. Providers administer simultaneously all vaccine doses for which a child is eligible at the time of each visit.
9. Providers use accurate and complete recording procedures.
10. Providers co-schedule immunization appointments in conjunction with appointments for other child health services.
11. Providers report adverse events following vaccination promptly, accurately, and completely.
12. Providers operate a tracking system.
13. Providers adhere to appropriate procedures for vaccine management.
14. Providers conduct semiannual audits to assess immunization coverage levels and to review immunization records in patient populations they serve.
15. Providers maintain up-to-date, easily retrievable medical protocols at all locations where vaccines are administered.
16. Providers practice patient-oriented and community-based approaches.
17. Vaccines are administered by properly trained persons.
18. Providers receive ongoing education and training regarding current immunization recommendations.

Services Office, Mailstop E-06, National Center for Prevention Services, Centers for Disease Control and Prevention, Atlanta GA 30333–4018.

Standards for pediatric immunization practices. MMWR Morb Mortal Wkly Rep 1993;42(RR-5):1.

SAFETY OF IMMUNIZATION

VACCINE FACTORS

All vaccines licensed for use in the United States are subjected to routine rigorous testing for purity and uniformity of content. The safety standards are established by the Food and Drug Administration (FDA) and involve regular examination of manufacturing techniques as well as production lots of vaccine. As a result of these standards, there have been no incidents of bacterial or viral contamination of vaccines at the factory level in the United States for decades.

FACTORS RELATED TO VACCINE ADMINISTRATION

The use of disposable syringes and needles or some other form of single-dose delivery of vaccine is preferred to minimize the opportunity for contamination. If reusable glass syringes are employed, they must be thoroughly cleaned and autoclaved after each use. The American Academy of Pediatrics has recommended that the autoclave be set at 121 °C for 15 minutes at 15 lb of pressure. If autoclaving is not possible, either dry heat of 170 °C for 2 hours or boiling for 30 minutes is an acceptable alternative. A 70% solution of alcohol is appropriate for disinfection of the stopper of the vaccine container and of the skin at the injection site.

The manufacturer's recommendations for route and site of administration of injectable vaccines are critical for safety and efficacy. All vaccines containing an adjuvant must be administered intramuscularly to avoid granuloma formation or necrosis. Such injections should be given in the anterolateral thigh (not intragluteally) in infants (< 15 months of age) and may be given in the deltoid or triceps in older children. A 22-gauge needle 1–1¼ inches long is recommended for children, but a 25-gauge ⅝-inch needle may be sufficient for young infants. Aqueous vaccines may be administered intramuscularly, subcutaneously, or intradermally. For subcutaneous or intradermal injections, a 25-gauge ½- to ¾-inch needle is recommended. Good injection technique, including aspiration prior to injection, must always be practiced. In general, a separate syringe and needle should be used for each vaccine.

It is safe to administer many combinations of vaccines simultaneously without increasing the risk of adverse effects (see individual preparations below for further discussion). Inactivated vaccines (with the exception of cholera and yellow fever) can be given simultaneously or at any time after a different vaccine. Whenever possible, live-virus vaccines, if not administered on the same day, should be given at least 30 days apart. If an immunoglobulin has been administered, live-virus vaccination should ordinarily be delayed by at least 90 days to avoid interference with the immune response. Exceptions include the simultaneous administration, at different sites, of several human hyperimmune globulins along with their associated vaccines under the appropriate clinical circumstances (see below under the specific preparations). OPV and yellow fever vaccines are not affected by immunoglobulin administration.

HOST FACTORS

Healthy Children

Minor acute illnesses, with or without low-grade fever, are not contraindications to vaccination, since

Table 10–2. Guide to contraindications and precautions to vaccinations.

GENERAL FOR ALL VACCINES (DTP/DTaP, OPV, IPV, MMR, Hib, HBV)

Contraindications	Not contraindications
Anaphylactic reaction to a vaccine contraindicates further doses of that vaccine Anaphylactic reaction to a vaccine constituent contraindicates the use of vaccines containing that substance Moderate or severe illnesses with or without a fever	Mild to moderate local reaction (soreness, redness, swelling) following a dose of an injectable antigen Mild acute illness with or without low-grade fever Current antimicrobial therapy Convalescent phase of illnesses Prematurity (same dosage and indications as for normal, full-term infants) History of penicillin or other nonspecific allergies or family history of such allergies

DTP/DTaP

Contraindication	Not contraindications
Encephalopathy within 7 days of administration of previous dose of DTP **Precautions[1]** Fever of $\geq$ 40.5 °C (105 °F) within 48 hours after vaccination with a prior dose of DTP Collapse or shocklike state (hypotonic-hyporesponsive episode) within 48 hours after receving a prior dose of DTP Seizures within 3 days of receiving a prior dose of DTP (see footnote 2 regarding management of children with a personal history of seizures at any time) Persistent, inconsolable crying lasting $\geq$ 3 hours within 48 hours of receiving a prior dose of DTP	Temperature of < 40.5 °C (105 °F) following previous dose of DTP Family history of convulsions[2] Family history of sudden infant death syndrome Family history of an adverse event following DTP administration

OPV[3]

Contraindications	
Infection with HIV or a household contact with HIV Known altered immunodeficiency (hematologic and solid tumors; congenital immunodeficiency; and long-term immunosuppressive therapy) Immunodeficient household contact **Precaution[1]** Pregnancy	Not contraindications Breast feeding Current antimicrobial therapy Diarrhea

IPV

Contraindication	
Anaphylactic reaction to neomycin or streptomycin **Precaution[1]** Pregnancy	

MMR[3]

Contraindications	Not contraindications
Anaphylactic reactions to egg ingestion and to neomycin[4] Pregnancy Known immunodeficiency (hematologic and solid tumors; congenital immunodeficiency; and long-term immunosuppresive therapy) **Precaution[1]** Recent (within 3 months) immune globulin administration	Tuberculosis or positive skin test Simultaneous TB skin testing[5] Breast feeding Pregnancy of mother or recipient Immunodeficient family member or household contact Infection with HIV Nonanaphylactic reactions to eggs or neomycin

Hib

Contraindications	
None identified	

HBV

Contraindications	Not a contraindication
None identified	Pregnancy

[1]The events or conditions listed as precautions, although not contraindications, should be carefully reviewed. The benefits and risks of administering a specific vaccine to an individual under the circumstances should be considered. If the risks are believed to outweigh the benefits, the immunization should be withheld; if the benefits are believed to outweigh the risks (eg, during an outbreak or foreign travel), the immunization should be given. Whether and when to administer DTP to children with proved or suspected underlying neurologic disorders should be decided on an individual basis. It is prudent on theoretical grounds to avoid vaccinating pregnant women. However, if immediate protection against poliomyelitis is needed, OPV, not IPV, is recommended.

[2]Acetaminophen given prior to administering DTP and thereafter every 4 hours for 24 hours should be considered for children with a personal or family history of convulsions in siblings or parents.

[3]There is a theoretical risk that the administration of multiple live virus vaccines (OPV and MMR) within 30 days of one another if not given on the same day will result in a suboptimal immune response. There are no data to substantiate this.

[4]Persons with a history of anaphylactic reactions following egg ingestion should be vaccinated only with extreme caution. Protocols have been developed for vaccinating such persons and should be consulted. (J Pediatr 1983;102:196; J Pediatr 1988;113:504).

[5]Measles vaccinations may temporarily suppress tuberculin reactivity. If testing cannot be done the day of MMR vaccination, the test should be postponed for 4–6 weeks.

there is no evidence that vaccination under these conditions increases the rate of adverse effects or decreases efficacy. A moderate to severe febrile illness is reason to postpone vaccination. Routine physical examination and taking temperatures are not prerequisites for vaccinating apparently healthy infants and children.

Children With Chronic Illnesses

Most chronic diseases are not of themselves contraindications to vaccination; in fact, children with chronic diseases may be at greater risk of complications from vaccine-preventable diseases, especially influenza and pneumococcal infections. Premature infants are a good example. It is clear that they should be immunized according to their chronologic, not gestational, age. Vaccine doses should not be reduced for preterm or low-birth-weight infants. The one exception to this rule may be children with progressive central nervous system disorders. Vaccination may be deferred or avoided entirely for them, whereas children with static central nervous system diseases are candidates for vaccination.

Immunodeficient Children

Congenitally immunodeficient children should not be immunized with live-virus or live-bacteria vaccines. Depending on the nature of the immunodeficiency, other vaccines are safe and may evoke an immune response. Children with cancer and children being treated with corticosteroids or other immunosuppressive agents should not be vaccinated with live-virus or live-bacteria vaccines. This contraindication does not apply if the malignancy is in remission and chemotherapy has not been administered for at least 90 days. In addition, previously healthy children who are being treated with low to moderate doses of corticosteroids for less than 14 days, children receiving low to moderate doses of alternate-day corticosteroids, children being maintained on physiologic corticosteroid therapy without other immunodeficiency, and children using only topical or intra-articular corticosteroids may receive live vaccines safely. These guidelines apply to children with documented HIV infection, with the exception that live measles, mumps, and rubella vaccinations are recommended for these children while oral attenuated poliovirus vaccine is not. No distinction is made between children with asymptomatic HIV infection and those with symptomatic infection for the purpose of this recommendation. Siblings and household contacts of a child who is immunodeficient should not receive oral poliovirus vaccine unless the immunodeficient child has been successfully immunized against poliomyelitis. If that is not the case, the siblings should receive inactivated poliovirus vaccine. Measles, mumps, and rubella vaccines are not contraindicated under these circumstances.

Allergic or Hypersensitive Children

Hypersensitivity reactions are rare following vaccination. They are generally attributable to a trace component of the vaccine rather than to the antigen itself. Measles, mumps, and rubella vaccines and inactivated poliovirus vaccine (IPV) contain microgram quantities of neomycin, and IPV also contains trace amounts of streptomycin. Children with known anaphylactic responses to these antibiotics should not be given these vaccines. Trace quantities of egg antigens may be present in influenza vaccines, measles, mumps, and yellow fever vaccines. Children who have had anaphylactic reactions to eggs should not be given these vaccines. Children with less serious reactions to eggs may generally be safely immunized with these products. If doubt exists about the nature of a child's egg sensitivity, a skin testing procedure is outlined in the *Red Book*.

Borkowsky W et al: Cell-mediated and humoral immune responses in children infected with human immunodeficiency virus during the first few years of life. J Pediatr 1992;120:371.

General recommendations on immunization: Recommendations of the Immunization Practices Advisory Committee (ACIP). MMWR Morb Mortal Wkly Rep 1989;38:205, 219.

Immunization of children infected with human immunodeficiency virus: Supplementary ACIP statement. MMWR Morb Mortal Wkly Rep 1988;37:181.

THE COMPOSITION OF IMMUNIZING AGENTS

ACTIVE IMMUNIZATION

Although each vaccine is unique, the practitioner should be familiar with the general constituents of a vaccine. The antigenic component, or immunogen, may be a single well-defined entity, such as tetanus toxoid, or it may be a mixture of defined entities, such as the capsular polysaccharides of pneumococcal vaccine. The immunogen may be a live attenuated organism such as BCG or measles vaccine, or it may be whole killed organisms such as the IPV. The antigenic component may be a complex of killed disrupted organisms and products, as in pertussis vaccine. All antigens are not equally capable of inducing an immunologic response in all hosts. The factors influencing host responses include genetic variability in the immunogenic response, age at first exposure, and any prior experience with the antigen. A small proportion of children receiving certain antigens simply do not mount a response that is capable of conferring protection. For this reason, every vaccine has a definable failure rate.

The immunogen is suspended or dissolved in a fluid, like sterile water or saline. The fluid may also be more complex, such as tissue culture medium, and it may contain constituents from the biologic system used to produce the immunogen.

Most vaccines contain certain materials to preserve or stabilize the immunogen, particularly mercurials. In addition, trace amounts of antibiotics such as neomycin may be present to prevent bacterial overgrowth.

Some vaccines contain adjuvants—eg, alum, aluminum hydroxide, and aluminum phosphate—that are nonspecific immune stimulants. They also help to retain the immunogen in a "depot site" for a prolonged time, thus increasing the antigenic stimulation provoked by the primary immunogen.

Finally, despite rigorous testing and high standards of mechanical and biologic purity and stability, vaccines may contain unwanted and undetectable antigens and other materials. Although unlikely, vaccine administration could have unforeseen adverse consequences. Thus, vaccines should be administered where there is ready access to emergency resuscitative equipment and drugs such as epinephrine.

PASSIVE IMMUNIZATION

Immune globulin (IG) is derived from pooled donations of large numbers of individuals (more than 1000 per lot). IG is prepared by alcohol fractionation, is sterile, and will not transmit any infectious agents (including hepatitis B virus and HIV). IG is a 16.5% solution consisting primarily of immunoglobulin G with small amounts of immunoglobulins A and M.

ROUTINE CHILDHOOD IMMUNIZATIONS

See Table 10–3 for a detailed schedule of the administration of routine immunizations to normal infants and children. Even if the interval elapsed between doses in a series of immunizations is longer than recommended, that series can be resumed as if no interruption had taken place; it is not necessary to begin the series again. Children with an unknown vaccination status should be considered unprotected. Table 10–4 presents recommended schedules for children who did not start vaccination at the recommended time during the first year of life. Variations from these schedules may be necessitated by epidemiologic or individual clinical circumstances.

Safe Handling of Vaccines

The numerous vaccines and other immunologic substances, such as antibody preparations and immunoglobulins for routine use by the practitioner, vary in correct storage temperatures. Table 10–5 shows the recommended temperatures of storage for most of the commonly used vaccines after they have been shipped. The only vaccine that requires routine freezing is OPV. Yellow fever vaccine may also be stored frozen. Consult individual product package inserts for detailed information on storage conditions and shelf life.

Casto DT, Brunell PA: Safe handling of vaccines. Pediatrics 1991;87:108.

DIPHTHERIA

Diphtheria toxoid is prepared by the formaldehyde inactivation of diphtheria toxin. The toxoid content of the several available preparations varies and is measured in limit of flocculation units (Lf). The protective efficacy of diphtheria toxoid has never been measured on a mass scale but is estimated to be greater than 85%.

Preparations Available

(1) Diphtheria toxoid is used only when tetanus toxoid and pertussis vaccine are both contraindicated. It contains 10–12 Lf units per immunizing dose.

(2) Diphtheria-tetanus (DT) (pediatric) is used when pertussis vaccine is contraindicated. DT contains 6.7–12.5 Lf units of diphtheria toxoid per dose. Pediatric DT should not be used in adults because of potentially severe adverse reactions.

(3) Tetanus-diphtheria (Td) (adult) is for use in persons 7 years of age or older and contains 2 Lf units or less of diphtheria toxoid. It is less likely to produce local reactions while still eliciting a good immunogenic response in this population.

(4) Diphtheria-tetanus-pertussis (DTP) is the standard immunizing agent for healthy children and contains 6.7–12.5 Lf units of diphtheria toxoid per dose.

Dosage & Schedule of Administration

The above preparations are administered intramuscularly in a dose of 0.5 mL. Administration of these adsorbed preparations by jet injection may be associated with more local reactions. See Table 10–3 for the routine schedule and Table 10–4 for those children not appropriately immunized during the first year of life.

Adverse Effects

No significant adverse reactions have been associated with diphtheria toxoid alone.

Table 10–3. Recommended schedule for active immunization of normal infants and children.[1,2]

Recommended Age[3]	Immunizations[4]	Comments
Birth	HBV[5]	HBV should be given within 12 hours of birth to infants of HBsAg-positive mothers or those with an unknown HBsAg status; and as soon as possible after birth to infants of HBsAg-negative mothers.
1 month	HBV[5]	HBV should be given at 1 month to infants of HBSAg-positive mothers and between 1 and 2 months to all others.
2 months	DTP, HbCV,[6] OPV	DTP and OPV can be initiated as early as 4 weeks after birth in areas of high endemicity or during epidemics.
4 months	DTP, HbCV,[6] OPV	Two-month interval (minimum of 6 weeks) desired for OPV to avoid interference from previous dose.
6 months	DTP, HbCV,[6] HBV[5,7]	Third dose of OPV is not indicated in the USA but is desirable in geographic areas where polio is endemic.
15 months	MMR,[8] HbCV[9]	Tuberculin testing may be done at the same visit.
15–18 months	DTP,[10,11] (DTaP),[12] OPV[13]	(See footnotes.)
4–6 years	DTP,[14] (DTaP),[12] OPV (MMR)[15]	At or before school entry.
11–12 years	MMR	At entry to middle school or junior high school unless second dose previously given.
14–16 years	Td	Repeat every 10 years throughout life.

[1]Modified and reproduced, in part, with permission, from: *The 1991 Report of the Committee on Infectious Diseases,* 22nd ed. American Academy of Pediatrics, 1991.

[2]For all products used, consult manufacturer's package insert for instructions for storage, handling, dosage, and administration. Biologicals prepared by different manufacturers may vary, and package inserts of the same manufacturer may change from time to time. Therefore, the physician should be aware of the contents of the current package insert.

[3]These recommended ages should not be construed as absolute. For example, 2 months can be 6–10 weeks. However, MMR usually should not be given to children younger than 12 months. (If measles vaccination is indicated, monovalent measles vaccine is recommended, and MMR should be given subsequently, at 15 months.)

[4]DTP = diphtheria and tetanus toxoids with pertussis vaccine; HbCV = *Haemophilus* b conjugate vaccine; HBV = hepatitis V vaccine; HBsAg = hepatitis B surface antigen; DTaP = diphtheria and tetanus toxoids and acellular pertussis vaccine; OPV = oral poliovirus vaccine containing attenuated poliovirus types 1, 2, and 3; MMR = live measles, mumps, and rubella viruses in a combined vaccine; Td = adult tetanus toxoid (full dose) and diphtheria toxoid (reduced dose) for adult use.

[5]See section on hepatitis B virus vaccine for details.

[6]See section on *Haemophilus influenzae* vaccination for details.

[7]HBV should be given at 6 months in infants of HBsAg-positive mothers but can be given between 6 and 18 months to all others.

[8]May be given at 12 months of age in areas with recurrent measles transmission.

[9]Any licensed *Haemophilus* b conjugate vaccine may be given.

[10]Should be given 6–12 months after the third dose.

[11]May be given simultaneously with MMR at 15 months.

[12]DTaP is recommended only if 3 doses of DTP have already been administered. See section on pertussis and acellular pertussis vaccine for details.

[13]May be given simultaneously with MMR and HbCV at 15 months or at any time between 12 and 24 months; priority should be given to administering MMR at the recommended age.

[14]Can be given up to the seventh birthday.

[15]The ACIP recommends MMR at this time.

Antibody Preparations

Equine diphtheria antitoxin is available for use in the treatment of the disease. Dosage depends upon the size and location of the diphtheritic membrane and an estimation of the patient's level of intoxication. Before proceeding with the use of this preparation, the presence or absence of equine serum sensitivity must be determined using conjunctival (1:10 dilution) or intradermal (1:100 dilution) tests. If present, desensitization must be undertaken. If absent, the following doses are suggested:

Site	Duration of Lesion	Toxic?	Dose (units)
Pharyngeal or laryngeal	≤ 48 hours	...	20,000–40,000
Nasopharyngeal	...	...	40,000–60,000
Extensive or brawny swelling of neck	≥ 72 hours	Yes	80,000–100,000
Cutaneous?	...	...	20,000–40,000

Table 10–4. Recommended immunization schedules for normal children not immunized in the first year of life.[1]

Recommended Time/Age	Immunizations[2]	Comments
YOUNGER THAN 7 YEARS		
First visit	DTP, OPV, MMR HbCV[3]	MMR if child ≥ 15 months old; tuberculin testing may be done at same time. For children aged 15–59 months, can be given simultaneously with DTP and other vaccines (at separate sites).[4]
Interval after first visit		
2 months	DTP, OPV (HbCV)[5]	Second and third dose of HbCV is indicated only in children whose first dose was received when younger than 15 months.
4 months	DTP (HbCV)	Third dose of OPV is not indicated in the USA but is desirable in other geographic areas where polio is endemic.
10–16 months	DTP, (DTaP),[6] OPV	OPV is not necessary if third dose was given earlier.
4–6 years (at or before school entry)	DTP, (DTaP),[6] OPV (MMR)[5]	DTP is not necessary if the fourth dose was given after the fourth birthday; OPV is not necessary if the third dose was given after the fourth birthday.
11–12 years	MMR	At entry to middle school or junior high.
10 years later	Td	Repeat every 10 years throughout life.
7 YEARS AND OLDER[7,8]		
First visit	Td, OPV, MMR[9]	
Interval after first visit		
2 months	Td, OPV	
8–14 months	TD, OPV	
11–12 years	MMR	Repeat every 10 years throughout life.
10 years later	Td	At entry to middle school or junior high.

[1]Modified and reproduced with permission, from: *The 1991 Report of the Committee on Infectious Diseases,* 22nd ed. American Academy of Pediatrics, 1991.
[2]Abbreviations are explained in footnote 4 to Table 10–3.
[3]See *Haemophilus influenzae* vaccination section.
[4]The initial three doses of DTP can be given at 1- to 2-month intervals; hence, for the child in whom immunization is initiated at age 15 months or older, one visit could be eliminated by giving DTP, OPV, and MMR and HBV at the first visit; DTP and HbCV at the second visit (1 month later); and DTP, HBV, and OPV at the third visit (2 months after the first visit). Subsequent doses of DTP and OPV 10–16 months after the first visit are still indicated. HbCV, MMR, DTP, and HBV can be given simultaneously at separate sites if failure of the patient to return for future immunizations is a concern.
[5]Please see section on hepatitis B vaccine for discussion of recommendations by the AAP and ACIP.
[6]DTaP is recommended only if 3 prior doses of DTP have been administered.
[7]The ACIP recommends MMR at this time.
[8]If person is ≥18 years old, routine poliovirus vaccination is not indicated in the USA.
[9]Minimal interval between doses of MMR is 1 month.

TETANUS

Tetanus toxoid also is prepared by inactivating the toxin with formaldehyde. Its activity is measured in Lf and is generally 4–10 Lf per immunizing dose for adsorbed products and 4–5 Lf per dose for the fluid product. The protective efficacy of tetanus toxoid also has never been measured in any large study, but it is believed to be high.

Preparations Available

(1) Tetanus toxoid (fluid) is used rarely, only when rapid immunization is desirable.

(2) Tetanus toxoid adsorbed on aluminum phosphate is the standard single antigen "booster" toxoid.

(3) Tetanus-diphtheria (pediatric DT and adult Td) is discussed above.

(4) Diphtheria-tetanus-pertussis (DTP).

(5) Diphtheria-tetanus-acellular pertussis (DTaP).

(6) Diphtheria-tetanus-pertussis-*Haemophilus influenzae* b (DTP-Hib) is discussed below in the section on Hib.

Dosage & Schedule of Administration

The above preparations are administered intramuscularly in a dose of 0.5 mL. See Table 10–3 for the routine schedule and Table 10–4 for children not appropriately immunized during the first year of life.

Adverse Effects

Significant reactions to tetanus toxoid, historically an extremely safe preparation, are very unusual. Some older individuals who have had repeated doses may experience severe local reactions.

Antibody Preparations

Tetanus immune globulin (TIG) is indicated in the management of tetanus-prone wounds in individuals who have had an uncertain number or fewer than three tetanus immunizations. Fully immunized per-

Table 10–5. Recommended storage conditions for commonly used vaccines.[1]

Vaccine	Storage Temperature	Duration of Stability
SHOULD NOT BE FROZEN		
Diphtheria toxoid	2–8 °C	2 years
Tetanus toxoid	2–8 °C	2 years
DT, Td, DTP	2–8 °C	18 months
IPV	2–8 °C	1 year
IPV-E	2–8 °C	1 year
Haemophilus b polysaccharide conjugate vaccine (diphtheria toxoid)	2–8 °C	2 years
Haemophilus b oligosaccharide conjugate vaccine (diphtheria CRM[197] protein)	2–8 °C	2 years
Pneumococcal vaccine (polyvalent)	2–8 °C	Determined by expiration date on vial
Influenza virus vaccine (subvirion)	2–8 °C	Good only for the year for which it was manufactured
Hepatitis B virus vaccine (recombinant)	2–8 °C	2 years
Reconstituted vaccines		
Measles virus vaccine	2–8 °C	8 hours
Mumps virus vaccine	2–8 °C	8 hours
Rubella virus vaccine	2–8 °C	8 hours
Haemophilus b polysaccharide vaccine	2–8 °C	8 hours (single-dose vials); 30 days (multidose vials)
Haemophilus b conjugate vaccine (meningococcal protein)	2–8 °C	24 hours
SHOULD BE OR MAY BE FROZEN		
Oral poliovirus vaccine	<0 °C	1 year
Lyophilized measles virus vaccine	2–8 °C	1–2 years
Lyophilized mumps virus vaccine	2–8 °C	1–2 years
Lyophilized rubella virus vaccine	2–8 °C	1–2 years
Lyophilized *Haemophilus* b polysaccharide vaccine	2–8 °C	2 years

[1]Pediatrics 1991;87:108.

sons need not receive TIG regardless of the nature of their wound. The dose is 250–500 units (one or two vials) intramuscularly.

PERTUSSIS

Pertussis vaccines currently used in the United States for initial immunization are killed whole cell preparations. Recently, two acellular formulations of DTP (DTaP) have been licensed for use by the FDA for the fourth and fifth doses. Bacterial inactivation is achieved by heat or thimerosal or both. The immunogenicity of the vaccine is standardized in an indirect but reproducible assay, the mouse protection test. Currently available DTP preparations have a protective efficacy of about 80% after three doses. Further epidemiologic evidence of the efficacy of pertussis vaccine is provided by the observation of a large increase in reported pertussis cases in Great Britain and Japan after those two countries reduced or abandoned use of the vaccine.

Preparations Available

(1) Pertussis vaccine (adsorbed) is manufactured by the Division of Biologic Products, Michigan Department of Public Health, for use within that state. It may be obtained for other use by consultation with the department.

(2) Diphtheria-tetanus-pertussis (DTP).

(3) Diphtheria-tetanus-pertussis-*Haemophilus influenzae* b (DTP-Hib).

Dosage & Schedule of Administration

Each of the available preparations is administered in a dose of 0.5 mL intramuscularly. See Table 10–3 for the routine schedule and Table 10–4 for those children not appropriately immunized during the first year of life.

Adverse Effects

A large number of adverse reactions have been attributed to pertussis vaccine. These can be divided into three categories: local reactions, mild to moderate systemic reactions, and severe systemic reactions. The estimated rates of these reactions within the first

Table 10–6. Frequency of common adverse events within 48 hours after DTP.[1]

Adverse Event	Frequency:Dose
Local	
Pain	1:2
Swelling > 2.4 cm	2:5
Redness > 2.4 cm	1:3
Mild to moderate systemic	
Fever ≥ 38 °C	1:2
Fretfulness	1:2
Drowsiness	1:3
Anorexia	1:5
Vomiting	1:15
Severe	
Persistent crying (3 hours)	1:100
Fever ≥ 40.5 °C	1:330
High-pitched unusual crying	1:900
Hypotonic, hyporesponsive episodes	1:1750
Seizures	1:1750

[1]These data are derived from 15,752 DTP immunizations. Modified from: Cody CL et al: Nature and rates of adverse reactions associated with DTP and ET immunizations in infants and children. Pediatrics 1981;68:650.

48 hours after vaccination are shown in Table 10–6. The only absolute contraindications to the further use of pertussis vaccine are an anaphylactic reaction to the vaccine or a severe acute neurologic illness within 7 days after vaccination (Table 10–2). Precaution is urged for the following associations: a convulsion within 3 days; persistent, severe, inconsolable screaming or crying for over 3 hours or a high-pitched cry within 48 hours; a hypotonic-hyporesponsive episode within 48 hours; an unexplained temperature rise to 40.5 °C within 48 hours.

Controversy continues regarding the causation of serious neurologic illness by pertussis vaccine. A newly published analysis of the only large scale case-control study with enough statistical power to examine this issue—the British National Childhood Encephalopathy Study (NCES)—has led to a reappraisal of the relationship. This controversy has engendered two epidemics: In the United Kingdom and Japan, alleged DTP-associated deaths or encephalopathy caused DTP vaccination rates to fall dramatically, resulting in epidemics of pertussis; while in the United States, an epidemic of DTP-associated litigation threatens to overwhelm the National Vaccine Injury Compensation Program.

A causal relationship is almost impossible to establish for three reasons: (1) no specific clinical sign, neuropathologic change, or laboratory test has been consistently described in neurologic illnesses temporally associated with DTP vaccination; (2) any assessment of prior neurologic normality is hampered by the young age of the infants; and (3) there is no biologic plausibility—ie, there is no animal model and no convincing evidence that *Bordetella pertussis* or any of its components or products is neurotoxic. Thus, the British NCES conducted between 1976 and

1979 sought to assess the temporal relationship between DTP vaccination and permanent brain damage. Using a case-control methodology, the estimated population attributable risk for acute neurologic illness was one case per 140,000 pertussis vaccinations, and for permanent brain damage in previously normal children it was 1:330,000. A review of the NCES data indicates that only one of the 29 children who received DTP vaccination in the previous 7 days appeared to have no alternative explanation for the neurologic abnormalities. It was calculated that while the attributable risk for serious acute neurologic injury ranges from less than 1:1,000,000 to 1:140,000, the risk for permanent brain damage is even lower if indeed there is any risk at all. This reassessment, along with new studies, has led the American Academy of Pediatrics, the Canadian National Advisory Committee, and the British Pediatric Association to conclude that pertussis vaccine has not been proved to be the cause of brain damage and to reaffirm the safety and effectiveness of routine whole cell pertussis vaccine in immunization programs for infants and children.

On July 3, 1991, the National Academy of Sciences Institute of Medicine released a report entitled *Adverse Effects of Pertussis and Rubella Vaccines* in response to a congressional request to review evidence about serious adverse events and immunization with pertussis and rubella vaccines. The committee concluded that there was no experimental evidence in humans or animals that clearly proved or disproved a causal relation between pertussis vaccine and any of the 18 adverse events reviewed. The conclusions were as follows:

(1) No evidence bearing on a causal relation: Autism.

(2) Evidence is insufficient to indicate a causal relation: Aseptic meningitis, chronic neurologic damage, erythema multiform or other rash, Guillain-Barré syndrome, diabetes, learning disabilities and attention deficit disorder, peripheral mononeuropathy, and thrombocytopenia.

(3) Evidence does not indicate a causal relation: Infantile spasms, hypsarhythmia, Reye's syndrome, and sudden infant death syndrome.

(4) Evidence is consistent with a causal relation: Acute encephalopathy, shock and "unusual shock-like state."

(5) Evidence indicates a causal relation: Anaphylaxis, protracted and inconsolable crying.

The committee concluded that the vaccine caused four adverse events: acute encephalopathy, the range of excess risk being nil to 10.5 per million immunizations; shock (and unusual shock-like state), 3.5 to 291 cases per 100,000 immunizations; anaphylaxis, two cases per 100,000 injections of DTP; and protracted, inconsolable crying, 0.1–6% of recipients. Thus, while epidemiologic evidence may be consistent with a causal relation, a recent study found no evidence for a role of biologically active pertussis toxin in severe DTP reactions. Several committees in North America concur in the view that no causal relationship exists between pertussis vaccination and acute encephalopathy, though a temporal relationship may exist.

Antibody Preparations

Pertussis immune globulin, no longer available, is ineffective in either the prophylaxis or treatment of pertussis. Recently, a hyperimmune immunoglobulin has been shown to reduce the frequency of coughing spells and elevated lymphocyte count within 72 hours in adults with pertussis.

DIPHTHERIA-TETANUS-PERTUSSIS (DTP)

Diphtheria and tetanus toxoids and pertussis vaccine (DTP) is the recommended vehicle for the vaccination of healthy infants against the three diseases. It has been in wide use in the United States for more than 40 years. It has the combined clinical efficacy of the three single-dose preparations, and the efficacy of pertussis vaccine may even be enhanced by the adjuvant effect of the toxoids. It can be safely and effectively administered simultaneously either with live attenuated poliovaccine or inactivated poliovaccine, measles-mumps-rubella vaccine, and the *Haemophilus influenzae* type b vaccines.

Preparations Available

Each dose of combined diphtheria and tetanus toxoids and whole cell pertussis vaccine contains 6.7–12.5 Lf units of diphtheria toxoid, 5 Lf units of tetanus toxoid, and not more than 16 opacity units of pertussis vaccine adsorbed with one of several adjuvants (alum, aluminum phosphate, or aluminum hydroxide, depending on the manufacturer).

Dosage & Schedule of Administration

DTP is administered in a dose of 0.5 mL intramuscularly. See Table 10–3 for the routine schedule and Table 10–4 for children not appropriately immunized during the first year of life.

Adverse Effects; Antibody Preparations

See above with the individual component vaccines.

American Academy of Pediatrics, Committee on Infectious Diseases: The relationship between pertussis vaccine and brain damage: Reassessment. Pediatrics 1991;88:397.

Blumberg DA et al: Severe reactions associated with diphtheria-tetanus-pertussis vaccine: Detailed study of children with seizures, hypotonic-hyporesponsive episodes, high fevers, and persistent crying. Pediatrics 1993;91:1158.

Bruss JB, Siber G: Treatment of severe pertussis with intravenous pertussis immune globulin. ICAAC Abstract 103761, 1993.

Child Neurology Society: Report of the Therapeutics and Technology Assessment Subcommittee of the American Academy of Neurology. Assessment: DTP vaccination. Neurology 1992;42:471.

Diphtheria, tetanus, and pertussis: Recommendations for vaccine use and other preventive measures. Recommendations of the Immunization Practices Advisory Committee (ACIP). MMWR Morb Mortal Wkly Rep 1991;40(RR-10):1.

Howson CP and Fineberg HV: The ricochet of magic bullets: Summary of the institute of medicine report, *Adverse Effects of Pertussis and Rubella Vaccines.* Pediatrics 1992;89:318.

Miller DL et al: Pertussis immunization and serious acute neurologic illnesses. Vaccine 1989;7:487.

Miller DL et al: Safety of pertussis vaccine. Lancet 1990; 335:655.

Onorato IM et al: Efficacy of whole-cell pertussis vaccine in preschool children in the United States. JAMA 1992; 267:2745.

DIPHTHERIA-TETANUS & ACELLULAR PERTUSSIS VACCINE

Two basic types of acellular (DTaP) vaccines have been studied: The T type vaccines are produced by extraction and purification of *B pertussis* cultures. In contrast, the B type vaccines contain combinations of pertussis toxin (PT), filamentous hemagglutinin (FHA), pertactin (Prn), and fimbriae (Fim). It has been hypothesized that immunity against PT alone may be sufficient to protect against pertussis, but this view has been challenged, and it has been claimed that FHA, Prn, and Fim antibodies may be required for optimal protection.

Efficacy trials of various acellular pertussis vaccines in Japan and Sweden have established a two- to tenfold lesser frequency of "minor" adverse events compared with the whole cell vaccine, good immunogenicity, and a protective efficacy ranging from 54% to 95%. Drawbacks to the studies include the following: There was poor correlation between an immune response and protection; there were four deaths in the 7–9 months postvaccination and none in placebo recipients (in the Swedish study); hypotonia and "persistent and unusual crying" (neurologic events temporally related to whole-cell vaccine administration) developed in two children; and trials were conducted in children 6 months of age or older. On the basis of those trials and smaller ones in the USA, the FDA has licensed use of two DTaP vaccines for use as a fourth and fifth dose in children 15 months to 7 years of age, only after they receive three primary doses of DTP. Studies have been done in infants in the USA at 2, 4, and 6 months of age. The B type vaccines produced higher levels of PT antibody than the T type vaccines. All vaccines were less reactogenic than the whole cell vaccines. The routine licensure of acellular products for initial immunization awaits an NIH-sponsored protective efficacy trial.

Preparations Available

(1) Diphtheria-tetanus-acellular pertussis (Lederle/Takeda) contains 7.5 Lf of diphtheria toxoid, 5 Lf of tetanus toxoid, and 300 hemagglutinating units of Takeda acellular pertussis component, adsorbed to aluminum hydroxide and aluminum phosphate and preserved with 1:10,000 thimerosal.

(2) Diphtheria-tetanus-acellular pertussis (Connaught/Biken) contains 6.7 Lf of diphtheria toxoid, 5 Lf of tetanus toxoid, 23.4 µg of inactivated PT, and 23.4 µg of FHA, absorbed to aluminum potassium sulfate and preserved with 1:10,000 thimerosal.

Dosage & Schedule of Administration

DTaP is administered in a dose of 0.5 mL intramuscularly. See Table 10–3 for the routine schedule and Table 10–4 for the procedure in children not immunized during the first year.

DTaP is licensed for use only as the fourth and fifth doses for children who have received three prior doses of DTP and are between 15 months and 7 years of age.

Adverse Effects

Local reactions, fever, and other mild systemic events occur with one-fourth to two-thirds the frequency noted following whole cell DTP vaccination. Moderate to severe systemic events, including fever of 40.5 °C, persistent inconsolable crying lasting 3 hours or more, and hypotonic-hyporesponsive episodes, have rarely been reported and appear to be less frequent than with whole cell DTP. These are without sequelae. Severe neurologic events have not been temporally associated with DTaP vaccinations in limited use in the USA.

Blennow M et al: Adverse reactions and serologic response to a booster dose of acellular pertussis vaccine in children immunized with acellular or whole-cell vaccine as infants. Pediatrics 1989;84:62.

Edwards KM: Acellular pertussis vaccines: A solution to the pertussis problem? J Infect Dis 1993;168:15.

Feldman S et al: Comparison of acellular (B type) and whole-cell pertussis-component diphtheria-tetanus-pertussis vaccines as the first booster immunization in 15 to 24 month-old children. J Pediatr 1992:857.

Pertussis vaccination: Acellular pertussis vaccines for reinforcing and booster use: Supplementary ACIP statement. Recommendations of the Immunization Practices Advisory Committee (ACIP). MMWR Morb Mortal Wkly Rep 1992;41(RR-1):1.

Pichichero ME et al: Safety and immunogenicity of an acellular pertussis vaccine booster in 15 to 20 month-old children previously immunized with acellular or whole-cell pertussis vaccine as infants. Pediatrics 1993;91:756.

Storsaeter J et al: Mortality and morbidity from invasive bacterial infections during a clinical trial of acellular pertussis vaccines in Sweden. Pediatr Infect Dis J 1988; 7:637.

POLIOMYELITIS

Vaccines directed against poliovirus infections have largely eliminated the naturally occurring disease in developed countries. In the United States, the number of reported cases of paralytic poliomyelitis has fallen from more than 18,000 in 1954 to less than 13 per year during the 1970s and about nine per year in the 1980s and 1990s. Despite—or perhaps because of—this extraordinary success, controversy continues over the appropriate poliovirus vaccine for mass usage. Live attenuated oral poliovirus vaccine (OPV) (Sabin) is prepared via passage in monkey kidney cells or human diploid cells, depending on the manufacturer. Inactivated injectable poliovirus vaccine (IPV) (Salk) is currently grown in human diploid cells and then inactivated by formaldehyde. A newer preparation, injectable poliovirus vaccine of enhanced potency (IPV-E) (van Wezel), has a higher content of antigens than the old IPV, and field trials have demonstrated that fewer doses of IPV-E are required to attain immunity comparable to that achieved by OPV or IPV.

IPV is incapable of causing poliomyelitis by virtue of being inactivated, whereas OPV can cause such cases rarely. The rate of these complications in the United States is estimated to be three to five cases of paralytic disease per 10 million doses of OPV distributed. Ninety-three percent of recipient cases and 76% of all vaccine-associated paralytic poliomyelitis (VAPP) occur after administration of the first or second dose of OPV. The risk of paralysis in the immunodeficient recipient may be as much as 2000 times that in normals. IPV cannot multiply in the gut as OPV does—in theory, not protecting against intestinal infection with wild virus, as OPV does—and thus cannot produce "secondary vaccination" of close contacts of vaccinees. IPV, however, produces a much higher serologic response than OPV alone, a higher booster response at lower prevaccination levels, and an equivalent mucosal response. IPV has the practical advantage of not requiring freezing for storage, as OPV does. However, the mass administration of OPV requires no needles and syringes (a major advantage because of the new recommendations for *Haemophilus* b and hepatitis B vaccination in infancy, both administered intramuscularly. Weighing all the advantages and disadvantages of each vaccine, the Institute of Medicine, the National Academy of Sciences, and the Committee on Infectious Diseases of the American Academy of Pediatrics all continue to recommend the use of OPV under most circumstances in the United States. Exceptions include immunodeficient recipients (including HIV-positive individuals), recipients with immunodeficient persons or unimmunized adults in their households, and unvaccinated adults, all of whom should receive IPV. In addition, anyone who is informed of the risks and benefits of OPV should be permitted to elect to receive IPV if prepared to commit to a full schedule of vaccination with that preparation. This recommendation is regularly reexamined and could be changed if the epidemiology of poliomyelitis in the USA changes.

Preparations Available

(1) Inactivated injectable poliovirus vaccine of enhanced potency (IPV-E) contains 40, 8, and 32 D-antigen units, respectively, of types 1, 2, and 3 poliovirus grown in human diploid cells or Vero cells and is formaldehyde-inactivated.

(2) Trivalent live attenuated oral poliovirus vaccine (OPV) contains at least $10^{5.4}$, $10^{4.5}$, and $10^{5.2}$ $TCID_{50}$ of attenuated Sabin strains of poliovirus types 1, 2, and 3, respectively, propagated in monkey kidney cells.

Dosage & Schedule of Administration

A. IPV-E: This is the only vaccine preparation available and is administered in a dose of 0.5 mL subcutaneously. Combination vaccines DPT-IPV-E are not yet licensed in the USA.

B. OPV: A single thawed ampule is given orally for each dose. See Table 10–3 for the routine schedule and Table 10–4 for children not appropriately immunized during the first year of life.

Adverse Effects

IPV has essentially no adverse effects associated with it other than possible rare hypersensitivity reactions to trace quantities of neomycin, streptomycin, or polymyxin B. OPV carries a risk of vaccine-associated paralytic disease for immunodeficient recipients, immunodeficient contacts of recipients, and unvaccinated healthy adult contacts of recipients.

Antibody Preparations

None available.

Abraham R et al: Shedding of virulent poliovirus revertants during the immunization with oral poliovirus vaccine after prior immunization with inactivated polio vaccine. J Infect Dis 1993;168:1105.

Faden H et al: Long-term immunity to poliovirus in children immunized with live attenuated and enhanced-potency inactivated trivalent poliovirus vaccines. J Infect Dis 1993;168:453.

Onorato IM et al: Mucosal immunity induced by enhanced-potency inactivated and oral polio vaccines. J Infect Dis 1991;163:1.

Patriarca PA et al: Factors affecting the immunogenicity of oral poliovirus vaccine in developing countries: Review. Rev Infect Dis 1991;13:926.

Simoes EA, Abzug MJ: Enteroviruses: Issues in poliomyelitis immunization and perinatal enterovirus infections. Curr Opin Infect Dis 1993;6:547.

MEASLES

Routine measles vaccination was introduced in the USA in 1963. An inactivated and a live attenuated vaccine (Edmonston B strain) were initially used, the former until 1967 and the latter until 1972. The problem of atypical measles in inactivated vaccine recipients is, by virtue of their age, no longer an issue for pediatricians. A further attenuated form of the Edmonston B strain (Schwarz strain) was licensed in 1965, and another, similar preparation (Moraten strain) became available in 1968. The latter two strains are as effective as Edmonston B and have fewer adverse effects. Since 1976, only the Moraten strain vaccine has been used in the USA. In 1979, an improved stabilizer was added that made the vaccine more heat-stable.

After the introduction of measles vaccine in 1963, the annual number of reported cases in the United States decreased from about 500,000 to 1497 in 1983. The average annual incidence between 1981 and 1988 was about 3000 cases. During 1989, there was a resurgence of measles, with 18,000 cases and 41 deaths reported; that trend intensified in 1990, with more than 27,000 cases and over 60 deaths. The major reasons for the increase in cases and resulting deaths are failure to provide vaccine to preschool children 15 months of age or older where up to 65% of children may be unvaccinated; the presence in the community of susceptible children under 15 months of age, which is the age group in which outbreaks occur; and the accumulation of appropriately vaccinated but nonimmune individuals (primary vaccine failures: 2–10%) in schools and colleges. These reasons have led to recommendations for the routine revaccination of all children.

Given the efficacy rate of the current vaccine (> 95%), the elimination of indigenous measles from the United States is an attainable public health goal. (Currently, 5–7% of all cases reported each year are either acquired outside the USA or result from exposure to such a case.) Each year, about one-third of reported indigenous cases are judged to be potentially preventable. One-fourth occur in persons who would not have been immunized by virtue of age or exemption, and about 40–60% occur in persons with a history of adequate vaccination. An aggressive two-dose campaign directed at ensuring that all eligibles are immunized at the appropriate ages would certainly reduce the number of cases and might eliminate indigenous transmission completely.

Recently, alternative high-titer vaccines containing approximately 100-fold higher doses of live measles virus, such as the Edmonston-Zagreb (E-Z) vaccine and the AIK-C vaccine were found to be more immunogenic in young infants—less than 9 months of age—than the usual measles vaccines. Initial enthusiasm for these vaccines, however, has been tempered by recent reports of severe measles and a higher mortality rate in children given the E-Z vaccine in Guinea-Bissau, Senegal, and Haiti. As a result, these vaccines are no longer in use in any country. Health care providers and parents will need reassurance about the safety and benefits of standard titer measles vaccine.

Preparations Available

The Moraten strain is the only vaccine currently available in the United States. It is derived from the Edmonston B strain after multiple passages in chick embryo tissue culture and contains 1000–5000 $TCID_{50}$ of the United States Reference Measles Virus. The Moraten strain is also available in combination: with mumps vaccine (MM), with rubella vaccine (MR), and with mumps and rubella vaccines (MMR). It is equally effective alone and in each of these combinations.

Dosage & Schedule of Administration

A. Routine Vaccination: Under ordinary circumstances, the first dose of measles vaccine should be given as MMR to 15-month-old children. A dose of 0.5 mL, whether alone or in combination, should be given subcutaneously. The recommended age for the second vaccination with MMR varies: 4–6 years (ACIP) or 11–12 years (AAP). The advantages of the former recommendation are that implementation is easy, there is no extra cost for physician visits, and elementary schools have an extensive tracking system to ensure compliance. The disadvantage is the delay in impact, which will be seen in 7–13 years, as most outbreaks in vaccinated individuals occur at 12–18 years of age. The advantage of the later age of vaccination is that it has a rapid impact, since it is closer to the age when outbreaks occur. The individual practitioner can adopt either recommendation but may be preempted in this decision by laws mandating revaccination at school entry.

B. Vaccination in High-Risk Areas: A high-risk area has been defined by the ACIP as (1) a county with over five cases among preschool children during each of the last 5 years; (2) a county with a recent outbreak among preschool children; or (3) a city with a large unvaccinated population. The age at primary vaccination may be lowered to 12 months, and the second dose should be administered at 4–6 or 11–12 years of age.

C. Revaccination Under Other Circumstances: Persons entering colleges and other institutions for education beyond high school, medical personnel beginning employment, and persons traveling abroad should have documentation of immunity to measles—receipt of two doses of measles vaccine

after their first birthday *or* other evidence of measles immunity, such as birth before 1957 or a documented measles history or immunity. Children traveling to endemic areas should be dealt with as if they were in an outbreak area (see next section).

D. Outbreak Control: An outbreak exists in a community whenever a single case of measles is documented. Control depends on immediate protection of all susceptible persons (defined as persons who have no documented immunity to measles). In the case of unvaccinated individuals, the following recommendations hold: (1) 6–11 months of age: monovalent measles vaccine (or MMR) if cases are occurring in children less than 1 year old, followed by MMR at 15 months and again at 4–6 or 11–12 years; and (2) 12 months of age or older: MMR followed by revaccination at the recommended times.

A child with an unclear or unknown vaccination history should be reimmunized with MMR. Anyone with a known exposure who is not certain of receiving two doses of MMR should receive an additional dose. Measles vaccination is contraindicated in pregnant women, women intending to become pregnant within the next 90 days, immunocompromised persons (except those with HIV infection), and persons with anaphylactic egg or neomycin allergy. Children with minor acute illnesses (including febrile illnesses), nonanaphylactic egg allergy, or a history of tuberculosis should all be immunized. Monovalent measles or MMR may be safely administered simultaneously with DTP and OPV.

Adverse Effects

Between 5% and 15% of vaccinees become febrile to 39.5 °C or higher approximately a week after vaccination, and 5% may develop a transient morbilliform rash. Encephalitis and other central nervous system conditions are reported to occur at a frequency of one per 3 million doses in the United States. This rate is lower than the rate of these conditions in the general unvaccinated population, implying that the relationship between them and measles vaccination may not be causal. Recent reports have suggested that there is an increased risk of convulsions in children with a family or personal history of seizures. This risk is low, and there is no association between these seizures and brain damage.

Antibody Preparations

IG, given at a dose of 0.25 mL/kg (0.5 mL/kg in the immunocompromised) intramuscularly, is effective in preventing or modifying measles if it is given within 6 days after exposure. If a child is seen within 72 hours of exposure, vaccination is the preferred method of protection. If IG has been given for this or any other reason to an unimmunized child, vaccination should be given but must be deferred for at least 90 days provided the child is at least 12 months old. A recent study has shown that IG may inhibit the immune response for up to 9 months, and it may be advisable to defer immunization to this time. In an epidemic situation, two doses may be advised, with the second one at least 10 months after the IG.

American Academy of Pediatrics Committee on Infectious Diseases: Measles: Reassessment of the current immunization policy. Pediatrics 1989;84:1110.

Halsey NA: Increased mortality after high titer measles vaccines: Too much of a good thing. Pediatr Infect Dis J 1993;12:462.

Markowitz LE et al: Patterns of transmission in measles outbreaks in the United States, 1985–1986. N Engl J Med 1989;320:75.

National Vaccine Advisory Committee: The measles epidemic. The problems, barriers and recommendations. JAMA 1991;266:1547.

Simoes EA et al: Antibody response of children to measles vaccine mixed with diphtheria-pertussis-tetanus or diphtheria-pertussis-tetanus-poliomyelitis vaccine. Am J Dis Child 1988;142:309.

MUMPS

The use of mumps vaccine has dramatically reduced the incidence of this infection and its complications and mortality rate in the United States. Since its routine use from 1977, the incidence of mumps decreased from 152,000 cases in 1968 to a low of 2982 cases in 1985. Since then, however, the incidence has increased, with outbreaks occurring in highly vaccinated populations scattered throughout the country.

A live attenuated vaccine was first licensed in the United States in 1967. This vaccine, the Jeryl Lynn strain, is prepared from virus isolated from a child and passaged in embryonated hens' eggs and in chick embryo tissue culture. The duration of protective immunity from this vaccine is at least 19 years.

Preparations Available

The Jeryl Lynn Strain is the only preparation available as monovalent vaccine. It contains the equivalent of over 20,000 $TCID_{50}$ of the United States Reference Mumps Virus. The Jeryl Lynn vaccine is also available in combination with measles vaccine (MM), with rubella vaccine, and with measles and rubella vaccines (MMR).

Dosage & Schedule of Administration

Mumps vaccine is given to children in the combination vaccine MMR at the age of 15 months and again at 4–6 or 11–12 years of age. Despite the over 95% efficacy of the mumps vaccine, outbreaks have been reported in highly vaccinated (> 99%) populations. Most cases were attributed to primary vaccine failure. It is hoped that the two-dose schedule will prevent these outbreaks. As monovalent vaccine, it is safe and effective if given after the first birthday. The dose of either monovalent or MMR vaccines is 0.5

mL given subcutaneously. Use of the monovalent vaccine is limited to susceptibles with proved immunity to the other constituents of MMR. Revaccination with mumps vaccine or any of the vaccines in MMR is not harmful. Anyone with an unclear vaccination history should therefore be immunized. The same recommendations and contraindications apply to mumps vaccine as to measles vaccine (see above).

Adverse Effects

Illnesses after mumps vaccination are rare and include parotitis, low-grade fever, and orchitis. In 1989, a nationwide surveillance of neurologic complications after mumps vaccine was conducted in Japan. There were at least 311 cases of aseptic meningitis (96 had vaccine type mumps virus in the cerebrospinal fluid) among 630,157 recipients. Meningitis was mild, and there were no sequelae. It may be more common than was previously suspected (1–4 per 10,000 vaccinations).

Antibody Preparations

Immune globulin and mumps immune globulin have not been shown to be effective in postexposure prophylaxis.

Fujinaga T et al: A prefecture-wide survey of mumps meningitis associated with measles, mumps and rubella vaccine. Pediatr Infect Dis J 1991;10:204.

Hersh BS et al: Mumps outbreak in a highly vaccinated population. J Pediatr 1991;119:187.

King JC et al: Measles, mumps and rubella antibodies in vaccinated Baltimore children. AJDC 1993;147:558.

Mumps prevention. Recommendations of the Immunization Practices Advisory Committee (ACIP). MMWR Morb Mortal Wkly Rep 1989;38:388, 397.

Sugiura A, Yamada A: Aseptic meningitis as a complication of mumps vaccination. Pediatr Infect Dis J 1991;10:209.

RUBELLA

The use of rubella vaccine represents an important deviation from the public health philosophy underlying the other vaccines discussed in this chapter—ie, it is not intended to protect individuals from the consequences to themselves of rubella infection but rather to prevent congenital rubella syndrome. In the United States, the approach has been to vaccinate young children. The intent is to reduce transmission to women of childbearing age via a herd immunity effect and to enable girls to remain protected once they attain childbearing age. Immunity lasts for at least 15 years. Other countries, notably the United Kingdom, vaccinate pubertal girls (ages 11–14). The relative efficacy of these two strategies in the prevention of congenital rubella syndrome is not clear.

With the use of rubella vaccines since 1970, rubella incidence rates have declined more than 95% to an all-time low of 225 cases reported to the CDC in

1988. However, there has been an increase to 1093 cases in 1990, including many cases of congenital rubella syndrome, especially in California. In 1991, at least nine outbreaks with over 400 cases have been reported in Amish communities. Other outbreaks occurred in settings where adult susceptibles congregated (prisons, colleges, etc). In most cases, failure to vaccinate susceptible individuals, not vaccine failure, was implicated in causation.

Preparations Available

(1) The RA 27/3 strain is the only vaccine available in the United States. It is grown in human diploid cells. Each dose contains > 1000 $TCID_{50}$ of the United States Reference Rubella Virus. The RA 27/3 strain is available in combined preparations with measles vaccine (MR), mumps vaccine, and measles and mumps vaccines (MMR).

Dosage & Schedule of Administration

Either the monovalent or combined forms should be administered subcutaneously in a dose of 0.5 mL. Current practice is to use MMR vaccine at 15 months of age and at 4–6 or 11–12 years of age. Susceptible pubertal girls and postpubertal women identified by premarital or prenatal screening should also be immunized. All susceptible adults in certain institutional settings (including colleges), day care center personnel, military personnel, and hospital and health care personnel should be immunized. Whenever rubella vaccination is offered to a woman of childbearing age, pregnancy should be ruled out and the woman advised to prevent conception during the 90 days following vaccination.

It has been estimated that the risk of serious malformations attributable to the RA 27/3 vaccine is from nil to 1.6%. This is much less than the over 20% risk of congenital rubella syndrome after maternal infection in the first trimester of pregnancy. Because of the continuing occurrence of rubella among women of childbearing age and this low risk from the vaccine, susceptible adolescent and adult females of childbearing age should be vaccinated. A person can be considered immune only if there is documentation of either serologic immunity to rubella or vaccination with at least one dose of rubella vaccine after 1 year of age. A clinical diagnosis of rubella is unacceptable. The other contraindications to vaccination are the same as for measles (see above).

Adverse Effects

In children, adverse effects from rubella vaccination are very unusual. In adults, arthralgia and arthritis occur in 10–25% of vaccinees. The IOM member committee found sufficient evidence to determine that chronic arthritis may be causally related to RA 27/3 vaccinations and that the vaccine causes acute arthritis in 13–15% of adult women vaccines, with lower levels among children, adolescents, and adult

males. Rash occurs alone or as mild rubella in 1–4% of adults. Rare complications include peripheral neuritis and neuropathy, transverse myelitis, and diffuse myelitis.

Antibody Preparations

None available.

Best JM: Rubella vaccines: Past, present and future. Epidemiol Infect 1991;107:17.

Herrmann KL: Rubella in the United States: Toward a strategy for disease control and elimination. Epidemiol Infect 1991;107:55.

Howson CP, Fineberg HV: Adverse events following pertussis and rubella vaccines. JAMA 1992;267:392.

Increase in rubella and congenital rubella syndrome. MMWR Morb Mortal Wkly Rep 1991;40:94.

Outbreaks of rubella among the Amish. MMWR Morb Mortal Wkly Rep 1991;40:264.

Rubella prevention. Recommendations of the Immunization Practices Advisory Committee (ACIP). MMWR Morb Mortal Wkly Rep 1990;39(RR-15):1.

HAEMOPHILUS INFLUENZAE TYPE b INFECTION

The first vaccine licensed against *Haemophilus influenzae* type b in the United States was composed of the capsular polysaccharide of *H influenzae* type b polyribosylribitol phosphate (PRP). This vaccine, which became available in 1985 for children between 2 and 5 years of age, was moderately effective in preventing *H influenzae* type b disease. Conjugation of the PRP with protein carriers confers T cell-dependent characteristics on the vaccine and enhances the immunologic response to PRP. As of early 1994, four conjugate vaccines and a combination vaccine (DTP-Hib, Tetramune) are licensed for use in children. (Table 10–7)

Studies in infants aged 2–6 months demonstrated the immunogenicity of each of these vaccines. A geometric mean titer (GMT) of 1 µg/mL of anti-polysaccharide antibody 3 weeks postvaccination has correlated with long-term protection from invasive disease. After three doses at ages 2, 4, and 6 months, each of the three vaccines—HbOC, PRP-OMP, and PRP-T—produces protective levels of antibody, while the response to PRP-D is limited. Regardless of the vaccine used in the primary series, booster vaccination of children over age 12 months with any licensed vaccine elicits an adequate response. Furthermore, each vaccine is immunogenic, as a single dose given after 15 months of age. Limited information on interchangeability of different Hib vaccines (excluding PRP-D) suggests that any combination of the three doses of Hib conjugate vaccines will provide adequate protection.

Clinical trials for all three conjugate vaccines among infants 2–6 months of age have been pub-

Table 10–7. *Haemophilus influenzae* type b conjugate vaccines licensed for use in children.

Vaccine	Trade Name and Manufacturer	Polysaccharide	Linkage	Protein Carrier
PRP-D	ProHIBiT (Connaught)	Medium	6-carbon	Diphtheria toxoid
HbOC	HibTITER (Lederle-Praxis)	Small	None	CRM[197] mutant *C diphtheriae* toxin protein
PRP-OMP	PedvaxHIB (MSD)	Medium	Thioether	*N meningitidis* outer membrane protein complex
PRP-T	ActHIB OmniHIB (Pasteur Merieux Vaccines)	Large	6-carbon	Tetanus toxoid

lished. The first study from Finland using the PRP-D vaccine administered to infants at 3, 4, and 6 months of age demonstrated an efficacy of 87% (95% CI = 50–96%). Results differed, however, in a study in Alaska native infants who received the PRP-D vaccine at 2, 4, and 6 months of age. The protective efficacy was only 35% (95% CI = 57–73%). For this reason, PRP-D has not been licensed for use in the United States in infants under 15 months of age. Two large trials have examined the protective efficacy of the more recently licensed conjugate vaccines. The HbOC vaccine was tried in northern California in infants vaccinated at 2, 4, and 6 months of age. The efficacy was 100% (95% CI = 68–100%). In a trial of PRP-OMP vaccine among Navajo infants vaccinated at 2 and 4 months of age, vaccine efficacy was estimated at 93% (95% CI = 45–99%). Trials evaluating the efficacy of PRP-T were terminated prematurely, but no cases of invasive disease occurred in more than 6000 vaccinees. In Finland, no Hib diseases has been reported in over 97,000 infants who received more than two doses of PRP-T.

These studies form the basis for the FDA approval of vaccine use and new recommendations by the American Academy of Pediatrics and the Immunization Practices Advisory Committee on the use of *Haemophilus* b conjugate vaccines. Because of the differences in the immunogenic response and the dif-

ferent regimens used in these trials, the recommendations for use of HbOC/PRP-T and PRP-OMP differ and are summarized in Table 10–8. All infants should be immunized with either HbOC or PRP-T or PRP-OMP at 2 months of age or as soon as possible thereafter. The HbOC/PRP-T should be administered in a four-dose schedule, the initial three doses at 2, 4, and 6 months of age and the fourth dose at 15 months of age. The PRP-OMP should be administered in a three-dose schedule, the first and second doses at 2 and 4 months of age, and the third dose at 12 months of age. No efficacy information is available for the DTP-HbOC combination vaccine, but immunogenicity data suggest it will provide protection similar to that of its components. Other combination vaccines have been tested (PRP-D-DTaP, HbOC-DTaP, PRP-T-DTP) but are not yet licensed for use. If the exact conjugate vaccine previously administered is unknown, it is recommended that at least three doses of conjugate vaccine be administered to children between 2 and 6 months of age. Unvaccinated or partially vaccinated children younger than 24 months of age who experience invasive *H influenzae* type b disease should receive a complete series of vaccinations. Children over the age of 24 months mount an adequate immune response to invasive *H influenzae* type b disease and do not require further vaccinations. Unimmunized children 5 years of age or older with a

Table 10–8. Schedule for Hib conjugate vaccine administration.

Vaccine	Age at First Vaccination (months)	Primary Series	Booster
HbOC/PRP-T[1]	2–6	3 doses 2 months apart	12–15 months
	7–11	2 doses 2 months apart	12–18 months
	12–14	1 dose	2 months later
	15–59	1 dose	...
PRP-OMP	2–6	2 doses 2 months apart	12–15 months
	7–11	2 doses 2 months apart	12–18 months
	12–14	1 dose	2 months later
	15–59	1 dose	...
PRP-D	15–59	1 dose	...

[1]TETRAMUNE may be administered by the same schedule for primary immunization as HbOC/PRP-T (when the series begins at 2–6 months of age). A booster dose of DTP or DTaP should be administered at 4–6 years of age, before kindergarten or elementary school. This booster is not necessary if the fourth vaccinating dose was administered after the fourth birthday.

chronic illness that is known to be associated with invasive *Haemophilus influenzae* type b disease, eg, sickle cell anemia and asplenia, should be given a single dose of any of the licensed conjugate vaccines. Regardless of the regimen implemented, it is crucial to complete the series, since cases of invasive *H influenzae* type b disease have been described in partially vaccinated children.

Preparations Available
See Table 10–7.

Dosage & Schedule of Administration
Regardless of which preparation is used, 0.5 mL should be given intramuscularly.

Adverse Effects
These are the first vaccines for which the FDA requires active surveillance for adverse reactions after licensure. Accordingly, there are good early data for all three of the conjugate vaccines. Fewer than 5% of those immunized develop any minor local or systemic reaction (including fever) to the vaccine. Adverse events following the second dose of PRP-OMP are more frequent than following the first dose and more frequent following the third dose of HbOC than following the first two doses. There have been no reports of more severe reactions.

Antibody Preparations
There is no commercially available preparation. A bacterial polysaccharide immune globulin obtained from adult donors who have been immunized with PRP as well as polyvalent pneumococcal and meningococcal vaccines is being investigated at the Massachusetts Biologic Laboratory. The routine use of IGIM or IGIV in antibody-deficient children, such as those with agammaglobulinemia or HIV infection, may prevent *H influenzae* type b infections.

American Academy of Pediatrics Committee on Infectious Diseases: *Haemophilus influenzae* type b conjugate vaccines: Recommendations with recently and previously licensed vaccines. Pediatrics 1993;92:480.

Black SB et al: Safety, immunogenicity, and efficacy in infancy of oligosaccharide conjugate *Haemophilus influenzae* type b vaccine in a United States population: Possible implications for optimal use. Pediatr Infect Dis J 1992;165:S139.

Bulkow LR et al: Comparative immunogenicity of four *Haemophilus influenzae* type b conjugate vaccines in Alaska native infants. Pediatr Infect Dis J 1993;12:484.

Decker MD et al: Responses of children to booster immunization with their primary conjugate *Haemophilus influenzae* type B vaccine or with polyribosylribitol phosphate conjugated with diphtheria toxoid. J Pediatr 1993;122:410.

Paradiso PR et al: Safety and immunogenicity of a combined diphtheria, tetanus, pertussis and *Haemophilus influenzae* type b vaccine in young infants. Pediatrics 1993;92:827.

Recommendations for use of haemophilus b conjugate vaccines and a combined diphtheria, tetanus, pertussis, and *Haemophilus* b vaccine: Recommendations of the advisory committee on immunization practices (ACIP). MMWR Morb Mortal Wkly Rep 1993;42:1.

Santosham M et al: The efficacy in Navajo infants of a conjugate vaccine consisting of *Haemophilus influenzae* type b polysaccharide and *Neisseria meningitidis* outer-membrane protein complex. N Engl J Med 1991;324:1767.

Vadheim CM et al: Effectiveness and safety of an *Haemophilus influenzae* type b conjugate vaccine (PRP-T) in young infants. Pediatrics 1993;92:272.

HEPATITIS B

Hepatitis B vaccine is the first to be prepared from material derived exclusively from human donors. It was licensed in the United States in 1981. Although it was initially developed as a means of preventing infection via percutaneous and sexual exposure routes, subsequent studies have shown it to be more than 85% effective in preventing perinatally acquired infection and 80–95% effective in preventing most postnatally acquired infections.

In 1988, the American College of Obstetrics and Gynecology recommended that all pregnant women be routinely screened for hepatitis B surface antigen (HBsAg). Women with positive reactions are highly likely to transmit the infection to their offspring. Both mother and child have an increased risk of hepatocellular carcinoma and cirrhosis. Female infants are highly likely to pass the infection perinatally to their own offspring after they attain childbearing age, thus perpetuating the cycle. The use of hepatitis B vaccine, along with hepatitis B immune globulin (HBIG), has been established as an effective means of interrupting this cycle in all but the 2–3% of infants who acquire hepatitis B in utero. It is therefore imperative that pediatricians and obstetricians establish effective means of communicating the HBsAg status of every woman while she is in labor, so that appropriate preventive measures can be instituted as soon as possible after delivery.

In addition to newborns at high risk of acquiring hepatitis B, several other risk categories have been identified as target populations for preexposure vaccination. Those that are relevant to physicians caring for children include clients and staff in institutions for the developmentally delayed, clients and staff of hemodialysis units, recipients of clotting factor concentrates, homosexually active males, users of illicit injectable drugs, household contacts of chronic hepatitis B carriers, and health care personnel (including pediatricians and family physicians and their office staff). With the exception of high-risk neonates, all persons identified as high risk should be screened for markers of past infection and immunized only if they are proved susceptible. Since vaccines consist of a purified inactive subunit of the virus and are not infectious, they are not contraindicated in immunosuppressed individuals or in pregnant women.

Each year about 300,000 persons in the United States are infected with hepatitis B virus; one-half of these develop clinical hepatitis, 10,000 are hospitalized, and an estimated 20,000–30,000 become chronic carriers. The risk of carriage varies inversely with age; thus, though only 1–3% of the infections occur in children under 5 years of age, they account for 20–30% of new carriers each year. Chronic carriers are at 12–300 times greater risk than noncarriers of developing primary liver cancer, and one-fourth develop chronic active hepatitis that progresses to cirrhosis over 5–20 years.

Hepatitis B vaccine has been available since 1982. It is highly immunogenic; seroconversion rates are 95% or more, and higher titers are obtained when vaccination is begun later in infancy or childhood and with longer intervals between the second and third doses. Antibody persists longer in younger persons, and 7–61% of adults or children who seroconvert maintain good antibody levels above 10 mIU/mL for 5–8 years. Even when antibody levels fall below these levels, protection against viremia and clinical disease persists (except in some HIV-positive individuals). The protective efficacy of hepatitis B vaccine correlates well with antibody levels, and virtually all persons with 10 mIU/mL or more are protected in clinical trials.

The present strategy for hepatitis B vaccination of only high-risk groups has had little overall impact on morbidity. (In 1981, 21,152 cases were reported to the CDC; in 1991, 19,939 cases were reported.) Persons in high-risk groups are often reached after exposure has occurred; heterosexual transmission accounts for 25% of reported cases, and 30–90% of cases do not fall into any of the 12 major risk groups identified. Furthermore, the vaccine is very safe; probably confers long-term protection against disease, especially if vaccination is started at a young age; and is cost-effective. The estimated annual cost of vaccinating all infants is about $62 million in the public sector (a saving of 85% over an estimated $352 million cost of HBV disease).

Thus, the impact of universal vaccination with hepatitis B vaccine in infancy could be substantial. Universal child vaccination has recently been recommended both by the ACIP and the AAP. The recommendations are flexible, based on the need to incorporate the vaccine into routine preventive health care and on the availability of vaccine. When resources are limited, the AAP recommends giving the highest priority to immunization of high-risk infants and children, followed by all infants, adolescents in high-risk areas, and, finally, all adolescents. The AAP has recently published recommendations for the prevention of hepatitis B infections in school settings.

Since the vaccine is highly immunogenic using different schedules, this flexibility is possible. Optimally, two intramuscular doses are needed. Increasing the interval between the first and second doses has little effect on immunogenicity, but longer intervals between the last two doses (4–12 months) results in higher titers of anti-HBs. Thus, adequate responses and seroconversion rates are achieved with doses administered at birth, 1 month, and 6 months; or birth, 2 months, and 6 months; or 2 months, 4 months, and 6 months. Simultaneous administration with other vaccines at different sites is safe and efficacious.

Preparations Available

Recombinant vaccine, licensed in 1986, is the only vaccine type available. It is made by inserting a plasmid containing the gene for one subtype of HBsAg into baker's yeast *(Saccharomyces cerevisiae).* The HBsAg is harvested by lysing the yeast cells and then purified. It is immunologically indistinguishable from the HBsAg found in chronic carriers. Two vaccines, adsorbed with aluminum hydroxide and thimerosal, are licensed: Recombivax HB (Merck Sharpe & Dohme), containing 10 µg/mL; and Engerix-B (Smith Kline), containing 20 µg/mL.

Dosage & Schedule of Administration

Note: Hepatitis B vaccine should only be given in the deltoid muscle for adolescents and children and in the anterolateral thigh muscle for infants and neonates. Administration intradermally or in the buttocks has resulted in poor immune response in some individuals, and these sites are not recommended.

A. Neonatal: Infants of HBsAg-positive mothers should be cleansed of the bloody products of conception in the delivery room. Both hepatitis B vaccine (see Table 10–9) and hepatitis B immune globulin (HBIG, 0.5 mL intramuscularly) should be administered simultaneously at different sites as soon as the baby is physiologically stable, preferably in the delivery room or within 12 hours after birth. The vaccine should be repeated at 1 month and 6 months. At 12–15 months of age, immunized infants should be tested for antibody to HBsAg (anti-HBs). If the anti-HBs is positive, vaccination has been effective. If negative, HBsAg should be tested for, and if positive, immunization has failed and the infant is a chronic carrier. If both HBsAg and anti-HBs are negative, a fourth dose of vaccine should be administered, followed by the same testing sequence in another 30 days.

For infants born to HBsAg-negative mothers, the first dose should be administered in the newborn period—or, if this is not possible, at least before 2 months of age. The doses and schedule for routine vaccination of these infants are shown in Table 10–9.

Infants born to mothers with unknown HBsAg status should receive hepatitis B vaccine within 12 hours of birth in the dose for infants born to HBsAg-positive mothers. If the mother's HBsAg is positive, the

Table 10–9. Hepatitis B vaccine schedule and dosage.

	Vaccine Dose		
	Recombivax HB	**Engerix-B**	**Schedule: Doses at Ages–**
Infants of HBsAg-negative mothers[1]	0.25 mL	0.5 mL	0–2 days, 1–2 months, and 6–18 months
Older children <11 years (not vaccinated at birth)	0.25 mL	0.5 mL	1–2, 4, and 6–18 months[2]
Infants of HBsAg-positive mothers (HBIG 0.5 mL should also be given)	0.5 mL	0.5 mL	Day 0, 1 month, and 6 months
Children and adolescents aged 11–19 years	0.5 mL	1.0 mL	Day 0, 1 month, and 6 months; or day 0, 2 months, and 4 months
Immunosuppressed persons and dialysis patients	1.0 mL[3]	2.0 mL[4]	

[1]Infants of mothers with unknown HBsAg status should be tested at delivery. The infant should receive hepatitis B vaccine within 12 hours after birth in a dose appropriate for infants born to HBsAg-positive mothers.
[2]May be given along with routine vaccinations.
[3]Special formulation containing 40 µg/mL at day 0, 1 month, and 6 months.
[4]Two doses of 1 mL at one site in a four-dose schedule at day 0 and at 1, 2, and 6 months.

infant should receive HBIG as soon as possible and within 7 days after birth. (HBIG has been shown to be effective if given within 12 hours after birth.) The infant should then receive the remainder of the vaccinations as for an infant of an HBsAg-positive mother. If the mother is found to be HBsAg-negative, the infant should receive routine hepatitis B vaccinations.

If maternal screening is not possible, the infant should receive the first dose within 12 hours after birth, the second at 1–2 months of age, and the third at 6 months.

B. Older Children and Adolescents: Both the AAP and ACIP recommend vaccination of adolescents at high risk for HBV infection, ie, those with more than one sexual partner in 6 months; intravenous drug abusers and those living in areas with increased rates of intravenous drug abuse; those with teenage pregnancies or sexually transmitted diseases; and any individual in the high-risk groups described earlier. Resources permitting, the universal immunization of all adolescents is recommended. (See Table 10–9 for dosages and schedules.)

C. Immunosuppressed Persons and Dialysis Patients: Hemodialysis patients and other immunocompromised persons should be vaccinated with larger doses or increased numbers of doses (or both) (Table 10–9).

D. Younger Children Not Fitting These Categories: Neither the AAP nor the ACIP has made specific recommendations for this large group of children—the major reason probably being doubts about the availability of resources. The individual pediatrician is left to decide whether to vaccinate this large group of children. The imminent availability of combined vaccines will make the decision much easier. The major arguments for vaccinating all children can be summarized as follows:

1. Vaccination in the perinatal period could prevent 22,000 cases of acute HBV infection and a maximum of 6000 chronic HBV infections annually. However, it is estimated that 300,000 persons become infected with HBV and 20,000–30,000 become chronic carriers annually. The majority of cases occur after infancy.

2. The strategy of vaccinating targeted adolescents suffers from all the disadvantages that have prompted the move toward universal immunization in the first place (see above).

3. The dose of vaccine in children is half that of adolescents.

4. Compliance with vaccination is better in infancy than adolescence.

E. Postexposure Prophylaxis: Postexposure prophylaxis is indicated in individuals with inadvertent percutaneous or permucosal exposure to HBsAg-positive blood, sexual exposure to an HBsAg-positive individual, or household exposure of an infant under 12 months of age to a caregiver with acute hepatitis B. Unvaccinated individuals should receive HBIG (0.06 mL/kg—maximum 5 mL—within 24 hours [its value after 7 days is unknown]) and the first dose of hepatitis B vaccine at a separate site or within 7 days of exposure. Previously vaccinated persons with an unknown response or known responders should be retested for anti-HBs. If levels are adequate (≥ 10 mIU/mL), no treatment is necessary. If levels are inadequate, a booster dose is required, and in individuals with an unknown response, a dose of HBIG should be given. A known nonresponder should receive either two doses of HBIG (a month apart) or one dose of HBIG and one of vaccine. If the patient becomes a chronic carrier, all household contacts should also receive a course of vaccination.

Adverse Effects

The overall rate of adverse effects is low. Such effects have all been minor, and they include fever (1–6%) and pain at the injection site (3–29%). Despite vaccination of approximately 2.5 million persons with recombinant vaccine, no excess risk of Guillain-Barré syndrome has been observed.

Antibody Preparations

HBIG is prepared from HIV-negative donors with high titers of HBs antibody and has an anti-HBs titer of greater than 1:100,000 by radioimmunoassay. The Cohn fractionation process used to prepare this product inactivates HIV, and there is no evidence for HIV transmission by HBIG. The use of HBIG is described above.

American Academy of Pediatrics Committee on Infectious Diseases: Universal hepatitis B immunizations. Pediatrics 1992;89:745.

American Academy of Pediatrics Committee on Infectious Diseases: Prevention of hepatitis B virus infection in school setting. Pediatrics 1993;91:848.

Greenberg DP et al: Pediatric experience with recombinant hepatitis B vaccines and relevant safety and immunogenicity studies. Pediatr Infect Dis J 1993;12:438.

Halsey NA et al: Discussion of Immunization Practices Advisory Committee/American Academy Of Pediatrics recommendations for universal infant hepatitis B vaccination. Pediatr Infect Dis J 1993;12:446.

Hepatitis B virus: A comprehensive strategy for eliminating transmission in the United States through universal childhood vaccination. Recommendations of the Immunization Practices Advisory Committee (ACIP). MMWR Morb Mortal Wkly Rep 1991;40(RR-13):1.

Margolis HS et al: Prevention of acute and chronic liver disease through immunization: Hepatitis B and beyond. J Infect Dis 1993;168:9.

VACCINATIONS FOR SPECIAL SITUATIONS

INFLUENZA

Influenza occurs each winter and early spring and with equal regularity is associated with significant morbidity and mortality rates in certain high-risk individuals. This includes children with hemoglobinopathies and with chronic cardiac, pulmonary (including asthma), metabolic, renal, and immunosuppressive diseases. Children and teenagers receiving long-term aspirin therapy should also receive the vaccine. Household members (including children) of persons in high-risk groups should be vaccinated. The vaccine may be administered to any person over 6 months of age in order to reduce the chance of becoming infected with influenza. Physicians should identify high-risk children in their practices and encourage parents to seek influenza vaccination for these children each fall. In pandemic years, it may be important to advocate vaccination in all children regardless of their usual state of health. Influenza vaccination has a 65–80% efficacy in protecting against disease.

Each year, recommendations are formulated in the spring and summer regarding the constituents of influenza vaccine for the coming season. These recommendations are based on the results of surveillance in Asia and the southern hemisphere during the spring and summer. The vaccine each year is a trivalent inactivated vaccine containing antigens from one or more strains of influenza A and influenza B. Thus, the vaccine for the 1993–1994 season includes A/Texas/36/91-like (H1N1), A/Beijing/32/92-like (H3N2), and B/Panama/45/90-like hemagglutinin antigens. Influenza vaccine virus is grown in hens' eggs and then formalin-inactivated. These whole virus preparations may be further treated with a variety of detergents to produce split (subvirion) or purified-surface-antigen vaccines.

Influenza causes serious illness in very young children; however, the trivalent inactivated vaccine has limited efficacy in this age group. Protection is short-lived and often incomplete. Live attenuated influenza A and B vaccines are being produced by genetic reassortment. A live cold-adapted type A vaccine administered intranasally has been shown to be safe and immunogenic in children as young as 6 months of age. Studies are under way to determine whether combinations of live and inactivated vaccines are immunogenic in young children.

Preparations Available

Several manufacturers produce similar vaccines each year. Whole virus vaccines produce unacceptably high rates of adverse reactions in children and are therefore contraindicated. Only split virus or purified-surface-antigen preparations should be used. These are also effective in adults and adolescents.

Dosage & Schedule of Administration

Children under 6 months of age cannot be immunized. Two doses are recommended for children under 9 years of age who are receiving influenza vaccine for the first time and one dose after 9 years. The dosage for children 6–35 months of age is 0.25 mL and for older children 0.5 mL given intramuscularly. Split virus vaccine should be used for children under 12 years of age and either split or whole virus after 12 years. The recommended site of vaccination is the anterolateral aspect of the thigh for younger children and the deltoid for older children. Public health authorities should be consulted annually for proper dosage information. Since this vaccine is inactivated, pregnancy is not an absolute contraindication to its use.

Adverse Effects

A small proportion of children will experience some systemic toxicity, consisting of fever, malaise, and myalgias. These symptoms generally begin 6–12 hours after vaccination and may last 24–48 hours. Rarely, some children will have anaphylactic reactions, presumably due to egg hypersensitivity. Cases of Guillain-Barré syndrome followed the swine influenza vaccination program in 1976–1977, but careful study showed no association with that vaccine in children and young adults, nor in any age with subsequent vaccines. In patients with anaphylactic egg allergies in whom influenza vaccination is indicated, a protocol for influenza vaccination has been referenced below.

Antibody Preparations

None available.

Groothuis JR et al: Immunization of high-risk infants younger than 18 months of age with split-product influenza vaccine. Pediatrics 1991;87:823.

Gruber WC et al: Comparison of monovalent and trivalent live attenuated influenza vaccines in young children. J Infect Dis 1993;168:53.

Murphy KR, Strunk RC: Safe administration of influenza vaccine in asthmatic children sensitive to egg proteins. J Pediatr 1985;106:9313.

Prevention and control of influenza: Recommendations of the Immunization Practices Advisory Committee (ACIP). MMWR Morb Mortal Wkly Rep 1992;41(RR-9):1.

PNEUMOCOCCAL INFECTIONS

Infections with *Streptococcus pneumoniae* cause significant morbidity and mortality in certain high-risk groups of children. These include children with anatomic and functional asplenia (including sickle cell disease), nephrotic syndrome, chronic renal failure, cerebrospinal fluid leaks, and immunosuppression (including those with HIV infection and organ transplant recipients). Revaccination after 3–5 years should be considered for children with nephrotic syndrome, asplenia, or sickle cell anemia who would be under 10 years old at revaccination. The vaccine is of limited efficacy in children under 2 years of age and should therefore not be given to children in the above groups until their second birthday. It is not indicated for children having only recurrent upper respiratory tract infections such as otitis media or sinusitis. The protective efficacy of the vaccine in high-risk children has not been well studied but is presumed to be about 60%, based on extrapolation from investigations in adults. In persons over 5 years of age, the overall efficacy has been estimated to be 57% (95% CI = 45–66%). The currently used 23-valent vaccine

was licensed in 1983. Conjugate pneumococcal vaccines that may work in young children are undergoing clinical trials.

Preparations Available

The standard dose of currently available vaccines contains 25 μg each of the purified capsular polysaccharide antigen of 23 serotypes of *S pneumoniae*. These 23 types cause 88% of the bacteremic and meningitic pneumococcal disease in adults and nearly 100% in children in the United States—and nearly 85% of acute pneumococcal otitis media in children. Cross-reactive antibody responses may protect against an additional 8% of bacteremic serotypes in adults.

Dosage & Schedule of Administration

The dose is 0.5 mL given intramuscularly or subcutaneously, and the vaccine is generally given only once. If splenectomy or immunosuppression can be anticipated, the vaccine should be given at least 2 weeks previously. Routine revaccination is not indicated because of an increased risk of adverse reactions. However, some centers revaccinate children with sickle cell anemia 3–5 years after initial vaccination because of their very high risk of pneumococcal infection. Children who received their initial vaccination during chemotherapy for Hodgkin's disease should be revaccinated 3–4 months after cessation of chemotherapy. Revaccination may be considered after 3–5 years in children at high risk of fatal pneumococcal infection such as those with nephrotic syndrome, renal failure, organ transplants, or asplenia. Pregnant women should generally not be vaccinated. Vaccination is not a substitute for antibiotic prophylaxis in certain high-risk children.

Adverse Effects

Half of all vaccine recipients develop pain and redness at the injection site. Less than 1% develop systemic side effects such as fever and myalgia. Anaphylaxis is rare.

Antibody Preparations

Most authorities recommend the routine use of IGIM or IGIV in agammaglobulinemic patients and some patients with HIV infection, in part to prevent pneumococcal disease.

Butler JC et al: Pneumococcal polysaccharide vaccine efficacy: An evaluation of current recommendations. JAMA 1993;270:1826.

Jorgensen JH et al: Serotypes of respiratory isolates of *Streptococcus pneumoniae* compared with the capsular types included in the current pneumococcal vaccine. J Infect Dis 1991;163:644.

Konradsen HB, Henrichsen J: Pneumococcal infections in splenectomised children are preventable. Acta Pediatr Scand 1991;80:423.

Opravil M et al: Poor antibody response after tetanus and pneumococcal vaccination in immunocompromised, HIV-infected patients. Clin Exp Immunol 1991;84:185.

Pneumococcal polysaccharide vaccine. MMWR Morb Mortal Wkly Rep 1989;38:64, 73.

RABIES

Human rabies has been rare in the United States over the last several decades, but animal rabies persists in many feral animal species throughout the country, and domestic animals may be secondarily infected. Travelers to developing countries, where dogs are a major vector, account for about 70% of cases of human rabies in the United States, and they are therefore a high-risk group. The risk of rabies transmission is highly dependent on the nature of the animal-to-human contact (the risk of rabies after a bite is 50 times the risk of a scratch of a rabid animal), the species of animal involved (in the USA, 3–20% of bats are positive for rabies and 12–70% of raccoons, skunks, or foxes, but only 0.01% of rodents are positive), and the locale of the incident. Local public health officials are well-versed in the epidemiology of animal rabies in their jurisdictions and should be consulted before any postexposure rabies prophylaxis is undertaken. First, they can avert unnecessary vaccination. Second, they can assist in the proper handling of the animal if confinement or testing is appropriate. Third, they can supply needed biologicals that may not be routinely stocked in hospitals, offices, or pharmacies. In some jurisdictions, these biologicals are supplied at no expense to the recipient if the use is authorized by the appropriate public health official. In order to facilitate discussion, the physician should have the following information at hand: the species of animal, whether it is available for testing or confinement, the nature of the attack (provoked or unprovoked), and the nature of the exposure (bite, scratch, lick, aerosol of saliva, etc). Confinement and observation of the biting animal is *only* appropriate when that animal is either a dog or a cat and appears well.

Preexposure prophylaxis is indicated for veterinarians, animal handlers, and any persons, including children, whose work or home environment potentially places them in close contact with animal species in which rabies is endemic—bats, skunks, raccoons, and foxes. Travelers visiting foreign areas of enzootic rabies for over 30 days should also receive a primary course of vaccination.

Preparations Available

(1) Human diploid cell rabies vaccine (HDCV) is prepared from the Pitman-Moore strain of rabies virus grown in human diploid cell culture, concentrated by ultracentrifugation and inactivated with β-propionolactone. It is supplied in two forms: a single-dose vial of 1 mL, when reconstituted for intramuscular use; and a single-dose vial of 0.1 mL for intradermal use.

(2) Rabies vaccine, adsorbed (RVA), was licensed in March 1988 and is distributed by the Biologics Products Program, Michigan Department of Public Health. It is produced from the Kissling strain of rabies virus, grown on fetal rhesus lung diploid cell culture, inactivated with β-propionolactone and adsorbed to aluminum phosphate.

Dosage & Schedule of Administration

Both types are equally safe and efficacious for both preexposure and postexposure prophylaxis when given intramuscularly. Only the HDCV has been evaluated for the intradermal route.

A. Primary Preexposure Vaccination:

1. Intramuscular route–This consists of three intramuscular injections in the deltoid area of 1 mL of HDCV or RVA on days 0, 7, and 21 or 28. The intragluteal route of administration is not recommended because of a poor immunologic response.

2. Intradermal route–The intradermal route has been recommended as an alternative mode of vaccination and consists of three intradermal doses of 0.1 mL of HDCV (RVA cannot be used) in the area over the deltoid on days 0, 7, and 21 or 28. *Note:* Concomitant chloroquine phosphate use (for malaria chemoprophylaxis) interferes with the antibody response to intradermal vaccination with HDCV but not with the intramuscular mode of vaccination. Thus, when simultaneous rabies and malaria prophylaxis is indicated, the intramuscular mode of vaccination is preferred.

B. Postexposure Prophylaxis:

1. In unvaccinated individuals–The wound should be immediately and thoroughly cleansed with soap and water. As soon as possible after the exposure (and up to 7 days after the first dose of vaccine), administer 20 IU/kg of rabies immune globulin (RIG) intramuscularly (if possible, half the dose should be infiltrated around the wound and the other half given intramuscularly in the gluteal area). At a different site—also as soon as possible after exposure—administer the first dose of HDCV. Four subsequent doses of HDCV should be given on days 3, 7, 14, and 28. The WHO recommends an additional dose on day 90, based on studies in Germany and Iran, but the ACIP does not recommend this practice.

2. In previously vaccinated individuals–The wound should be cleaned with soap and water. RIG is not necessary, and only two doses of HDCV or RVA, 1 mL intramuscularly each on days 0 and 3 are needed.

C. Booster Vaccination:

1. Preexposure booster doses of vaccine– Travelers living or visiting (for more than 30 days) in areas where rabies is enzootic in dogs should have a serum sample tested for rabies antibody every 2 years. If the titer is less than 1:5 for complete neutralization by the rapid fluorescent focus inhibition test (RFFIT), a booster dose should be administered either intramuscularly or intradermally.

Adverse Effects

HDCV is relatively free of side effects. Approximately 30–74% of adults experience pain, swelling, or erythema at the injection site, 7% have headache, 5% have nausea, and 4% have fever. Children complain of side effects less frequently. Allergic reactions occur, chiefly after booster doses. The rate of anaphylaxis in this setting is estimated to be one per 10,000 doses. An immune complex-like reaction occurs in about 6% of persons 2–21 days after receiving booster doses of HDCV and is due to β-propionolactone-altered human serum albumin in the HDCV.

Travelers to countries where rabies is enzootic in dogs may need rabies vaccine immediately and may have to use indigenously available vaccines and antisera. In many developing countries, the only vaccines readily available may be nerve tissue vaccines (NTV) derived from the brains of adult animals or suckling mice, and the antirabies sera may be of equine origin. While the antisera have complication rates of only 1–6%, the NTV may induce neuroparalytic reactions in 1:2000 to 1:200 vaccinees; this is a significant risk and may motivate preexposure vaccination with the HDCV prior to travel.

Antibody Preparations

Rabies immune globulin is prepared from the plasma of human volunteers hyperimmunized with rabies vaccine. The rabies-neutralizing antibody content is 150 IU/mL and is supplied in 2 mL or 10 mL vials. It is very safe. Usage is described above.

Berlin BS: Rabies vaccine adsorbed: Neutralizing antibody titers after three-dose pre-exposure vaccination. Am J Public Health 1990;80:476.

Chutivongse S et al: Postexposure prophylaxis for rabies with antiserum and intradermal vaccination. Lancet 1990;335:896.

Fishbein DB et al: Rabies. N Engl J Med 1992;329:1632.

Rabies postexposure immunization regimens: Thailand. MMWR Morb Mortal Wkly Rep 1990;39:759.

Rabies prevention: United States, 1991. MMWR Morb Mortal Wkly Rep 1991;40(RR-3):1.

Reid-Sanden FL et al: Administration of rabies vaccine in the gluteal area: A continuing problem. Arch Intern Med 1991;151:821.

WHO expert committee on rabies. World Health Organ Tech Rep Ser 1992;824:1.

TYPHOID FEVER

Typhoid vaccine has shown variable efficacy in field trials. Protection is inversely related to inoculum size in laboratory-based volunteer studies, which may be why some field trials have been disappointing. Three vaccines are available in the United States: a heat- and phenol-inactivated whole bacterial vaccine for parenteral use; an acetone-inactivated vaccine, available only to the armed forces; and a live attenuated vaccine for oral use (Ty21a). The inactivated vaccines have been in use for many decades, and their protective efficacy ranges from 51–76% (heat- and phenol-inactivated) to 66–94% (acetone-inactivated). However, they frequently cause marked systemic and local adverse reactions. The Ty21a vaccine has demonstrated equivalent efficacy in trials in Egypt and Chile (59–94%), and the reaction rates have been low. Moderate protection against invasive *Salmonella typhi* has been demonstrated for 2–5 years following vaccination.

Routine typhoid vaccination is not recommended in the United States. It is indicated for use in children who reside in a household with a proved typhoid carrier or in children who are going to reside in an endemic area. The oral vaccine is most commonly used. However, noncompliance with dosing instructions occurs frequently (30% of patients in one study), and correct usage should be stressed. Although the vaccine is not approved for use in children under 6 years of age, a liquid formulation was found to be safe and immunogenic (70% seroconversion) in children aged 2–6 years. Travelers should be advised, however, that since neither vaccine offers total protection, careful selection of food and drink is imperative.

Preparations Available

(1) Parenteral killed vaccine is a saline suspension of heat- and phenol-inactivated *Salmonella typhi* organisms at a concentration of not less than 1000 million killed bacteria per milliliter. It is supplied in multidose vials of 5, 10, or 20 mL.

(2) Oral live attenuated vaccine is supplied as enteric-coated capsules and contains the attenuated strain *S typhi* Ty21a.

Dosage & Schedule of Administration

The parenteral vaccine is given subcutaneously in a series of two injections of 0.5 mL each (for children ≥ 10 years of age) or 0.25 mL (children < 10 years of age), given 4 weeks or more apart, with booster doses every 3 years if residence in an endemic area continues. The booster dose is 0.5 mL (age ≥ 10 years) or 0.25 mL (age < 10 years) subcutaneously or 0.1 mL intradermally.

The dose of the oral preparation is one capsule a day on alternate days to a total of four capsules, taken before meals. The capsules should be kept refrigerated. A full course of four capsules is recommended every 2–5 years if exposure continues. Vaccine is not approved for children under 6 years of age, and capsules should not be dispensed from a package that has been opened beforehand.

Adverse Reactions

The parenteral vaccine produces 1–2 days of severe discomfort at the injection site in 6–40% of vaccinees, causing missed school or work in 13–24% of vaccinated individuals. Fever and other systemic reactions occur in 15–30% of vaccinees. The only contraindication is a previous severe reaction to parenteral typhoid vaccination. It can be used in immunocompromised individuals.

The oral preparation rarely produces side effects; the most common ones are abdominal discomfort, nausea, and vomiting. This vaccine should not be used in immunocompromised individuals.

Antibody Preparations

None are available.

Black RE et al: Efficacy of one or two doses of Ty21a *Salmonella typhi* vaccine in enteric-coated capsules in a controlled field trial. Chilean Typhoid Committee. Vaccine 1990;8:81.

Cryz SJ et al: Safety and immunogenicity of *Salmonella typhi* Ty21a vaccine in young Thai children. Infect Immun 1993;61:1149.

Forrest BD et al: The human humoral immune response to *Salmonella typhi* Ty21a. J Infect Dis 1991;163:336.

Rahman S et al: Use of oral typhoid vaccine strain Ty21a in a New York state travel immunization facility. Am J Trop Med Hyg 1993;48:823.

Typhoid immunization: Recommendations of the Immunization Practices Advisory Committee (ACIP). MMWR Morb Mortal Wkly Rep 1990;39(RR-10):1.

MENINGOCOCCAL DISEASE

A quadrivalent vaccine containing 50 μg each of purified bacterial polysaccharide antigen from capsular groups A, C, Y, and W135 is available in the United States. Since meningococcal infection is not endemic in the United States, routine use of this vaccine is unnecessary. However, functionally or anatomically asplenic children should be vaccinated, and vaccination should be considered also for children deficient in the terminal components of complement. It will protect travelers to countries with hyperepidemic or endemic disease. The group A component is immunogenic in children over 3 months of age and the group C component in those over 24 months of age. The dose is 0.5 mL given once subcutaneously. In epidemic situations, children under 18 months of age have been vaccinated with two doses 3 months apart. In general, the vaccine should not be administered to such children before their second birthday. Adverse reactions are unusual, consisting of local pain and erythema at the injection site. The antibody levels decline after 5 years and are unaffected by booster doses. Sustained protection may require the development of vaccines that induces T cell memory.

Andreoni J et al: Vaccination and the role of capsular polysaccharide antibody in prevention of recurrent meningococcal disease in late complement component-deficient individuals. J Infect Dis 1993;168:227.

Ceesay SJ et al: Decline in meningococcal antibody levels in African children 5 years after vaccination and the lack of an effect of booster immunization. J Infect Dis 1993;167:1212.

Laboratory-based surveillance for meningococcal disease in selected areas, United States, 1989–1991. MMWR Morb Mortal Wkly Rep 1993;42:21.

Meningococcal vaccines. MMWR Morb Mortal Wkly Rep 1985;34:255.

Stroffolini T et al: The effect of meningococcal group A and C polysaccharide vaccine on nasopharyngeal carrier state. Microbiologica 1990;13:225.

CHOLERA

The currently available cholera vaccine is a phenol-killed whole bacterial cell preparation. Its use is limited because it has a maximum protective efficacy of only 50% with a duration of protection of only 3–6 months. Its primary importance is to satisfy the entrance requirements for travel to some countries. Vaccination frequently results in redness and pain at the injection site, and fever, malaise, and myalgia occur approximately 1% of the time. The vaccine may be administered subcutaneously or intramuscularly, and a primary series consists of two doses at least 1 week apart. Boosters may need to be given as frequently as every 6 months. For the quantity to be administered, see below. Vaccine should not be given to children under 6 months of age.

	Age at Immunization		
	6 months to 4 years	5–10 years	>10 years
Dose	0.2 mL	0.3 mL	0.5 mL

Since *Vibrio cholerae* is not invasive and secretory IgA (sIgA) is crucial, the newer vaccines are administered orally. Two oral nonliving vaccines (one consisting solely of killed whole vibrios and the other in combination with the B subunit of cholera toxin) are safe and immunogenic. In field trials in Bangladesh, the protective efficacy was only 55–60% over 2 years of follow-up. Live oral vaccines are being developed against cholera by either deleting genes coding for virulence factors or expressing the genes coding for O antigens of *V cholerae* O1 in an *S typhi* carrier vaccine strain Ty21a. These approaches show promise, and a useful vaccine may be available in the next few years. A newly described toxigenic *Vibrio cholerae* 0139 strain has been the cause of epidemics of cholera in India and Bangladesh. A case has been reported in the USA imported from India. The rapid spread of this epidemic among immune adults suggest that pre-existing immunity to *Vibrio cholerae* 01 either by natural infection or cholera vaccine does not protect against this new strain, and travelers to the Indian subcontinent should be warned.

Cholera vaccine. MMWR Morb Mortal Wkly Rep 1988; 37:617, 623.

Imported cholera associated with a newly described toxigenic *Vibrio cholerae* 0139 strain—California, 1993. MMWR Morb Mortal Wkly Rep 1993;42:501.

Quiding M et al: Intestinal immune responses in humans: Oral cholera vaccination induces strong intestinal antibody responses and interferon-gamma production and evokes local immunological memory. J Clin Invest 1991;88:143.

Ramamurthy T et al: Emergence of novel strain of *Vibrio cholerae* with epidemic potential in southern and eastern India. (Letter.) Lancet 1993;341:703.

Sack DA et al: Antibody responses after immunization with killed oral cholera vaccines during the 1985 vaccine field trial in Bangladesh. J Infect Dis 1991;164:407.

Tacket CO et al: Safety, immunogenicity, and efficacy against cholera challenge in humans of a typhoid-cholera hybrid vaccine derived from *Salmonella typhi* Ty21a. Infect Immun 1990;58:1620.

PLAGUE

Plague vaccine is composed of inactivated whole bacteria *(Yersinia pestis)*. It should be used in children who reside in or are traveling to endemic areas. It should be administered intramuscularly according to the following dosage schedule:

	Age (years)			
	<1	1–4	5–10	>10
Day 0	0.1 mL	0.2 mL	0.3 mL	0.5 mL
Day 30	0.1 mL	0.2 mL	0.3 mL	0.5 mL
Day 60–120	0.04 mL	0.08 mL	0.12 mL	0.2 mL

Booster doses in the amount of the last dose listed above should then be given at 6-month intervals until five doses have been given. Boosters should then be given at intervals of 1–2 years as long as the child resides in the endemic area.

Plague vaccine. Recommendations of the Immunization Practices Advisory Committee (ACIP). MMWR Morb Mortal Wkly Rep 1982;31:301.

TUBERCULOSIS

BCG vaccine consists of live attenuated *Mycobacterium bovis.* Several large clinical efficacy trials have been conducted with conflicting results. BCG is not currently indicated for mass use in the United States, chiefly because of doubts about its efficacy. BCG may be useful in tuberculin-negative infants or older children residing in households where untreated or poorly treated individuals with active infection with isoniazid- and rifampin-resistant *M tuberculosis* also reside. BCG may be indicated in infants or children living under constant exposure (where > 1% of the population develops new-onset tuberculosis annually) without access to prophylaxis and treatment. It is given intradermally in a dose of 0.05 mL for newborns and 0.1 mL for all other children. Mantoux testing is advised 2–3 months later, and revaccination is advised if the test is negative. Adverse effects occur in 1–10% of healthy individuals and include ulceration, regional lymph node enlargement, and lupus vulgaris. The vaccine may cause disseminated or fatal infection in immunocompromised individuals, including those with HIV infection, and is therefore contraindicated in such circumstances. BCG almost invariably causes its recipients to be tuberculin-positive. However, in a child with a history of BCG vaccination who is being investigated for tuberculosis as a case contact, a positive Mantoux test should be interpreted as indicating infection with *M tuberculosis,* essentially ignoring the history of BCG vaccination.

BCG is the most widely used vaccine in the world and has been administered to over 2.5 billion people with a low incidence of serious complications. It is cheap, can be given any time after birth, sensitizes the vaccinated individual for 5–50 years, and stimulates both B and T cell immune responses. BCG has recently been used as a novel live vaccine vehicle to express genes from different viruses, bacteria, and parasites. These recombinant BCG vaccines have been shown to induce both T and B cell responses in mice to the non-BCG antigens. It is conceivable that such vaccines may be useful vehicles for protecting individuals against multiple pathogens simultaneously, starting at a very young age.

Clarke A, Rudd P: Neonatal BCG immunisation. Arch Dis Child 1992;67:473.

Management of persons exposed to multidrug-resistant tuberculosis. MMWR Morb Mortal Wkly Rep 1992; 41(RR-11):61.

Purified protein derivative (PPD)-tuberculin anergy and HIV infection: Guidelines for anergy testing and management of anergic persons at risk of tuberculosis. MMWR Morb Mortal Wkly Rep 1991;40(RR-5):27.

Tuberculosis and human immunodeficiency virus infection: Recommendation of the Advisory Committee for the Elimination of Tuberculosis (ACET). MMWR Morb Mortal Wkly Rep 1989;38:236, 243.

Use of BCG vaccines in the control of tuberculosis: A joint statement by the ACIP and the Advisory Committee for Elimination of Tuberculosis (ACET). MMWR Morb Mortal Wkly Rep 1988;37:663, 669.

YELLOW FEVER

Immunization against yellow fever is indicated for children traveling to endemic areas or to countries that require it for entry. Public health authorities maintain updated information on these requirements and must be consulted. Yellow fever vaccine is a live vaccine made from the 17D yellow fever attenuated virus strain, grown in chick embryos. It is contraindicated in infants less than 4 months of age, in pregnant women, in persons with anaphylactic egg allergy, and in immunocompromised individuals. It can only be administered at licensed yellow fever vaccination sites (usually public health departments). The dose is standardized to 1000 mouse LD_{50} units by the WHO. The package insert must therefore be consulted to determine the appropriate volume to be administered (generally 0.5 mL). It is injected subcutaneously. The International Health Regulations require revaccination at 10-year intervals, but immunity may last 30–35 years and is probably lifelong. Adverse reactions are generally mild—consisting of fever, headache, and myalgia 5–10 days after vaccination—and are uncommon, occurring in 2–5% of vaccinees. Rarely, encephalitis occurs within 30 days following vaccination (two cases reported after more than 24 million doses have been given in the USA). Yellow fever and cholera vaccines, when given simultaneously or less than 3 weeks apart, induce a poor immune response to both. These two vaccines should be administered at least 3 weeks apart. There is no contraindication to giving other live-virus vaccines simultaneously with yellow fever vaccine.

Yellow fever vaccine: Recommendations of the Immunization Practices Advisory Committee (ACIP). MMWR Morb Mortal Wkly Rep 1990;39(RR-6):1.

INVESTIGATIONAL VACCINES

Vaccines for many common childhood pathogens are currently under investigation. Among them are rotavirus, respiratory syncytial virus, hepatitis A, adenovirus, rhinovirus, and HIV vaccines. Only varicella vaccine is discussed here.

VARICELLA

A live attenuated varicella vaccine, the Oka strain, has been developed in Japan and thoroughly field-tested both there and in the United States. The initial population studied in both countries was susceptible leukemic children whose chemotherapy was temporarily interrupted for the purpose of immunizing them. The vaccine has also been extensively evaluated in normal children in both countries. It has been shown to be safe and effective in both normal and leukemic children and normal childern. Long-term follow-up on leukemics immunized in the USA shows that the incidence of herpes zoster is less than expected in the absence of vaccination. The effective dose of vaccine virus is over 500 plaque-forming units (PFU) administered subcutaneously. Planned vaccines will contain >1500 PFU. Adverse effects in leukemic children included mild varicella rash in roughly 20% of recipients and fever in a smaller percentage. The incidence of these side effects is less than 5% in immunized healthy children. Licensure by the FDA is thought to be imminent.

Until—and very likely after—the licensure of varicella vaccine, the only effective means of preventing or modifying varicella infection in exposed, susceptible individuals will be varicella-zoster immune globulin (VZIG). The use of this preparation, obtained from pooled plasma donations from individuals known to have high titers of antivaricella antibody, is indicated in several categories of high-risk exposed susceptible individuals. These include immunocompromised individuals, some healthy persons 25 years of age or older, pregnant women, newborns whose mothers develop varicella between 5 days before and 48 hours after delivery, hospitalized premature infants of over 28 weeks of gestational age whose mothers are susceptible, and hospitalized premature infants less mature than that regardless of maternal status. Exposure is defined as household contact, playmate contact (over 1 hour a day), hospital contact (in the same contiguous room or ward), and newborn contact (as defined above). Susceptibility is defined as the absence of detectable antibody by a sensitive test. VZIG must be administered within 96 hours after exposure in order to be effective. Maximum effectiveness is achieved if VZIG is administered within 48 hours after exposure. Newborns should be given (1 vial) a dosage of 125 units intramuscularly. The dose for all others is 125 units per 10 kg of body weight intramuscularly to a maximum dose of 625 units. If more than 2 weeks has elapsed from the last dose of VZIG and a susceptible high-risk person is reexposed, VZIG should be readministered.

Arbeter AM et al: Immunization of children with acute lymphoblastic leukemia with live attenuated varicella vaccine without complete suspension of chemotherapy. Pediatrics 1990;85:338.

Diaz PS et al: Lack of transmission of the live attenuated varicella vaccine virus to immunocompromised children after immunization of their sibling. Pediatrics 1991;87:166.

Englund JA et al: Placebo-controlled trial of varicella vaccine given with or after measles-mumps-rubella vaccine. J Pediatr 1989;114:37-44.

White CJ et al: Varicella vaccine (VARIVAX) in healthy

children and adolescents: Results from clinical trials, 1987 to 1989. Pediatrics 1991;87:604.

PASSIVE IMMUNIZATION

Immune globulin (IG) is indicated as replacement therapy in antibody deficiency disorders at a dose of 0.6 mL/kg/month. It may prevent or modify infection with hepatitis A virus if administered in a dose of 0.02 mL/kg within 14 days after exposure. Measles infection may be prevented or modified in a susceptible individual if IG is given in a dose of 0.25 mL/kg within 6 days of exposure. Special forms of IG include tetanus immune globulin (TIG), hepatitis B immune globulin (HBIG), rabies immune globulin (RIG), and varicella-zoster immune globulin (VZIG). These are obtained from donors known to have high titers of antibody against the organism in question. Their use has been described in appropriate sections above. IG is administered via the intramuscular route only (IGIM). The dose varies depending on the clinical indication.

Adverse reactions include pain at the injection site, headache, chills, dyspnea, nausea, and anaphylaxis, though all but the first are rare.

There is also an immune globulin (IGIV), for intravenous use. Its primary indications are for replacement therapy in antibody-deficient individuals, for the treatment of Kawasaki disease, and for the treatment of some patients with idiopathic thrombocytopenic purpura. It may also be beneficial in some children with HIV infection. It must only be administered intravenously. Adverse reactions include headache, flushing, diaphoresis, hypotension, fever, nausea, vomiting, and anaphylaxis. Special forms of IGIV have been used in the prevention and treatment of infectious diseases: cytomegalovirus immune globulin (CMVIG) and respiratory syncytial virus immune globulin (RSVIG).

Finally, there are some immune globulins of animal origin available for use in certain specific situations. These include botulism antitoxins, diphtheria antitoxin, and snake and spider antivenins. A variety of adverse reactions, including acute febrile responses, anaphylaxis, and serum sickness, may develop as a result of the use of these products. Their use should therefore be restricted to clinical circumstances in which the need is clear. A schedule for hypersensitivity testing and desensitization for antisera of equine origin can be found in the *Red Book*.

LEGAL ISSUES IN IMMUNIZATION

The National Childhood Vaccine Injury Act of 1986 became effective as of October 1, 1988. The Act set up two programs, the National Vaccine Program (NVP) and the National Vaccine Injury Compensation Program (NVICP). The purpose was to provide "no-fault" compensation for persons found to have been injured by certain vaccines. It provides that liability claims against those who administer or manufacture vaccines must go before a federal compensation board before a civil suit may be filed. Compensation may be sought for certain events following certain immunizations within specified time intervals. Legal representatives (parents, guardians) must reject the judgment rendered by this compensation board before a civil suit may be filed in either state or federal court. The compensation system was funded by a trust fund created by an initial grant of $80 million from Congress and a continuing surcharge levied against the manufacturers for each dose of the specified vaccines.

In order to receive compensation for injury from vaccines administered after September 30, 1988, the injured person or his or her representative must (1) go through the NVICP; (2) present evidence of death or residual effects lasting longer than 6 months and expenses greater than $1000; (3) must file a claim within 3 years after onset of the first symptoms or within 2 years after death; and (4) supply medical records or sworn affidavits in support of the claim.

Following a claim, the secretary of the Department of Health and Human Services, the defendant, evaluates the petition. Compensation is recommended if there is no alternative cause and the injury is a listed reportable event (see MMWR reference, below)—or, if the injury was not a reportable event, a vaccine was the proximate cause. Claims are then heard (if contested) by "special masters" in the claims court who receive evidence from both parties, evaluate it, and make a decision. Once a decision is made, the petitioner can accept or reject it within 90 days. If petitioner accepts the decision, no claim can thereafter be filed against the manufacturer or the vaccine provider. If the claim is not accepted, civil relief is available through the tort system, but the manufacturer cannot be sued for failure to warn the vaccinee of the risks associated with the product.

The Act imposes specific record-keeping and adverse reaction reporting duties on physicians who administer vaccines. For each dose administered, the medical record of the vaccinee or some other permanent record maintained in the administrator's office must set forth (1) the date of administration; (2) the name of the manufacturer and lot number of the vaccine; and (3) the name, work address, and title of the person administering the vaccine. Physicians administering the specified vaccines are also obliged by the Act to report any of the specified reactions to the Vaccine Adverse Events Reporting System (VAERS)—call 1-800-822-7967 for forms. Compensation forms from the NVICP may be obtained by calling 1-800-338-2382. The Act provides no penalty for failure to report.

Vaccine information materials are available from the CDC to meet the requirements of the Act. They are about 1500–2000 words long, and there are separate forms for DTP, MMR, and poliovirus vaccines. Patients or parents are legally required to sign these forms if the vaccine is purchased on a federal contract. Informed consent is also needed for physicians who wish to be fully covered by the vaccine compensation program.

National Childhood Vaccine Injury Act: Requirements for permanent vaccination records and for reporting of selected events after vaccination. MMWR Morb Mortal Wkly Rep 1988;37:197.

Normal Childhood Nutrition & Its Disorders

11

K. Michael Hambidge, MB, B. Chir, ScD, & Nancy F. Krebs, MD, MS

NUTRITIONAL REQUIREMENTS

NUTRITION & GROWTH

The nutrient requirements of the child are influenced substantially by the rate of growth, body composition, and composition of new growth. These factors vary with the age of the subject and are especially important during early postnatal life. Growth rates are higher in early infancy than at any other stage of the life cycle, including the peak of the adolescent growth spurt (Table 11–1). These rates decline rapidly starting in the second month of postnatal life (proportionately later in the premature infant). Because of a more rapid rate of growth in early infancy, nutrient requirements for males are slightly higher than those for females.

Nutrient requirements also depend on body composition. In the adult, the brain, which accounts for only 2% of body weight, contributes 19% to the total basal energy expenditure. In contrast, in a term neonate, the brain accounts for 10% of body weight and for 44% of total energy needs under basal conditions. The liver accounts for a further 20% of basal energy expenditure. Thus, in the young infant, basal energy expenditure is relatively high in relation to body weight, and the brain and liver account for a relatively high percentage of basal energy requirement.

Composition of new weight gain is a third factor that influences nutrient requirements and changes the nutrient requirements with age. For example, fat accounts for about 40% of weight gain between birth and 4 months but for only 3% between 24 and 36 months. The corresponding figures for protein are 11% and 21%; for water, 45% and 68%. The high physiologic rate of fat deposition in early infancy has implications not only for energy requirements but also for the optimal composition of infant feeds.

Because of the high nutrient requirements for growth, the body composition, and the relatively large size and continued growth of the brain of the young infant, undernutrition at this stage of life has profound implications. Slowed physical growth rate is an early and prominent sign of undernutrition in the young infant. The limited fat stores of the very young infant mean that energy reserves are unusually restricted. The relatively large size and continued growth of the brain render the central nervous system especially vulnerable to the effects of malnutrition in early postnatal life.

ENERGY

The major determinants of energy expenditure are basal metabolism, metabolic response to food, physical activity, and growth. In addition, the efficiency of energy utilization may be a significant factor, and thermoregulation may contribute in extremes of ambient temperature if the body is inadequately clothed. Because adequate data on requirements for physical activity in infants and children are not available and because individual growth requirements are quite variable, recommendations have been based on calculations of actual intakes by healthy subjects. The distinct recent trend toward lower figures for infants reflects a move away from hypercaloric and possibly inappropriate feeding practices that were in vogue between 1930 and 1970, when the growth data giving rise to the National Center for Health Statistics (NCHS) standards were collected. Suggested guidelines for energy intake of infants and young children are given in Table 11–2. Also included in this table are carefully calculated energy intakes of fully breast-fed infants, which have been verified recently in a number of centers. Though the growth pattern of breast-fed infants tends to differ from that of formula-fed infants, growth velocity during the first 3 months typically equals or exceeds the 50th percentile for the NCHS grids. Calculations of energy requirements based on recent direct measurement of energy expenditure in normal infants accord well with the intakes of breast-fed infants. The recommended energy intakes of the Food and Nutrition Board, National

Table 11–1. Changes in growth rate, energy required for growth, and body composition in infants and young child.

Age (Mo)	Growth Rate (g/d)			Energy Requirements for Growth (kcal/kg/d)	Body Composition[1]		
	Male	Both	Female		Water	Protein	Fat
0–0.25		0 (See note 2.)			75	11.5	11
0.25–1	40		35	50			
1–2	35		30	25			
2–3	28		25	16			
3–6		20		10	60	11.5	26
6–9		15					
9–12		12					
12–18		8					
18–36		6		2	61	16	21

[1]Data from Fomon SJ: *Infant Nutrition,* 2nd ed. Saunders, 1974.
[2]Birth weight is regained by 10 days. Weight loss of more than 10% of birth weight indicates dehydration or malnutrition.

Academy of Sciences, National Research Council (10th edition) are not synonymous with requirements. Moreover, the RDAs to not take into account the rapid changes in requirements that occur over the course of infancy, especially in the first 6 months. For these reasons, this source cannot be recommended for calculating nutrient requirements of infants.

After the first 4 years, energy requirements expressed on a body weight basis fall progressively to 40 kcal/kg/d by the end of adolescence. Approximate energy requirements can be calculated by adding 100 kcal/yr to a base of 1000 kcal at 1 year of age. Appetite and growth are reliable indices of caloric needs of most healthy children, but intake also depends, to some extent, on the energy density of the formula. Individual energy requirements of normal infants and children vary considerably, and malnutrition and disease add enormously to this variation. Basal energy requirements for the premature infant are approximately 120 kcal/kg/d.

One method of calculating requirements for malnourished patients is to base these on the ideal body weight (IBW, ie, 50th percentile weight for patients length/height-age or 50th percentile weight-for-height) rather than actual weight. Alternatively, the extra requirement kcal/d for "catch-up" growth can be calculated as:

$$\frac{5 \times \text{weight (g) deficit below IBW}}{\text{interval (days) for correction of deficit}}$$

where 5 kcal is the energy cost of each gram of new tissue deposited.

These calculations should be adjusted on an ongoing basis according to the growth response.

Heining MJ et al: Energy and protein intakes of breast-fed and formula-fed infants during the first year of life and their association with growth velocity: The Darling Study. Am J Clin Nutr 1993;58:152.

Table 11–2. Recommendations for energy and protein intake.[1]

	Energy (kcal/kg/d)			Protein (g/kg/d)	
	Based on Measurements of Energy Expenditure	Intake From Human Milk	Guidelines for Average Replacement	Intake From Human Milk	Guidelines for Average Requirements
10 days to 1 month	...	105	120	2.05	2.5
1–2 months	110	110	115	1.75	2.25
2–3 months	95	105	105	1.36	2.25
3–4 months	95	75–85	95	1.20	2.0
4–6 months	95	75–85	95	1.05	1.7
6–12 months	85	70	90	...	1.5
1–2 years	85	...	90	...	1.2
2–3 years	85	...	90	...	1.1
3–5 years	...	...	90	...	1.1

[1]Compiled from Krebs NF et al: Krebs NF Growth and intakes of energy and zinc in infants fed fuman milk. J. Pediatr. 1994;124:32–9 and from Garza C, Butte NF: Energy intakes of human milk-fed infants during the first year. J Pediatr 1990;117:5124.

Prentice AM et al: Are current dietary guidelines for young children a prescription for overfeeding? Lancet 1988; 2:1066.

World Health Organization: *Report of a Joint FAO/WHO/ UNO Expert Consultation: Energy and Protein Requirements.* WHO Tech Rep Ser No. 724, 1985.

PROTEIN

Only amino acids and ammonium compounds are usable as sources of nitrogen in human nutrition. Amino acids are provided by dietary protein. Dietary protein is hydrolyzed by pepsin in the stomach and by pancreatic trypsin digestion in the lumen of the small intestine. This is followed by peptidase digestion by pancreatic and intestinal peptidases. Nitrogen is absorbed from the gut lumen as amino acids and via short-peptide carrier systems. Absorption of nitrogen is more efficient from synthetic diets that contain peptides in addition to amino acids. Some intact proteins can be absorbed in early postnatal life and may result in allergies to these proteins. The liver plays a central role in amino acid metabolism, including regulation of the absorbed amino acids. Excess amino acids, including essential amino acids, are degraded in the liver—except for the branched-chain amino acids, which pass into the systemic circulation and are taken up primarily by muscle. Insulin stimulates this uptake and suppresses muscle protein catabolism. Protein turnover rates far exceed intake, indicating a marked reutilization of amino acids. However, some of these amino acids released from protein turnover are degraded. After removal of the amino group, the keto acids are either utilized directly for energy or converted to carbohydrate and fat. Nitrogen is excreted primarily via the kidney as urea.

All of the body's protein plays a role in body structure or function. Because there are no true stores of body protein, a regular dietary supply is necessary, and any loss of protein decreases functional capacity. In infants and children, optimal growth depends on an adequate dietary protein supply. Relatively subtle effects of protein deficiency are now recognized—especially those affecting tissues with rapid protein turnover rates, such as the immune system and the gastrointestinal mucosa.

In relation to body weight, protein synthesis rates, protein turnover rates, and increments in body protein are exceptionally high in the infant, especially the premature infant. Eighty percent of the dietary protein requirement of the premature infant is utilized for growth, compared with only 20% in the 1-year-old child. Protein requirements expressed on a body weight basis decline rapidly across infancy as growth velocity decreases. The figures given in Table 11–2, which are derived chiefly from the report of the Joint FAO/WHO/UNO Expert Committee and are similar to those published in *Recommended Dietary Allowances* (10th edition), deliver a comfortable margin above the quantity provided in breast milk. The recommendations for premature infants weighing less than 1500 g is 3 g/kg/d or more. When this amount of nitrogen is administered to the infant of low birth weight, protein calories should not exceed 17% of total calories, or 3 g protein/100 kcal.

Protein requirements increase in the presence of unusual cutaneous or enteral losses, burns, trauma, and severe sepsis. Requirements also increase during times of catch-up growth accompanying recovery from malnutrition (approximately 0.2 g protein per gram of new tissue deposited). In a young infant during rapid recovery, this could amount to as much as 1–2 g/kg/d of extra requirement. By 1 year of age, this is unlikely to be more than 0.5 g protein/kg/d. Circumstances in which the intake of protein may be deficient include significant low-protein supplementation (eg, fruit juices) in the breast-fed infant, protein malabsorption (cystic fibrosis), or the use of a low-protein weaning food (eg, cassava) as the dietary staple.

The quality of protein depends on its amino acid composition. Infants require 43% of protein as essential amino acids, and children require 36%. Eight essential amino acids cannot be synthesized by adults: isoleucine, leucine, lysine, methionine, phenylalanine, threonine, tryptophan, and valine. Histidine may be added to this list. Cysteine and tyrosine are considered partially essential because their rates of synthesis are limited and may be inadequate in certain circumstances. During early development, rates of synthesis of cysteine, tyrosine, and perhaps taurine do not provide sufficient amounts of these substances. Taurine is a substrate in the conjugation of bile acids, and taurine supplements have been reported to improve fat absorption in preterm infants and in infants with cystic fibrosis. Taurine supplements have been reported to improve auditory brain stem-evoked potentials in preterm infants. Lack of an essential amino acid leads to weight loss within 1–2 weeks. Wheat and rice are deficient in lysine, and legumes are deficient in methionine. Appropriate mixtures of vegetable protein are therefore necessary to achieve high protein quality.

Glutamine is an important example of a nonessential amino acid whose synthesis is inadequate under certain abnormal circumstances. The integrity of the enterocyte, for example, may be dependent on addition of glutamine to parenteral nutrition in infants who cannot tolerate any enteral intake.

Because the mechanisms for removal of excess nitrogen are efficient, moderate excesses of protein are not harmful and may help to ensure an adequate supply of certain micronutrients. Adverse effects of excessive protein intakes may include increased calcium losses in urine and, over a life span, increased loss of renal mass. A gross excess of protein may cause elevated blood urea nitrogen, acidosis, hyperammonemia, and, in the premature infant, failure to thrive, lethargy, and fever.

Gaul GE: Taurine in pediatric malnutrition: Review and update. Pediatrics 1989;83:433.
Souba WW: Intestinal glutamine metabolism and nutrition. J Nutr Biochem 1993;4:2.

LIPIDS

Fats are the main dietary energy source for infants and account for up to 50% of energy in human milk. Over 98% of these fats are in the form of triglycerides, which have an energy density of 9 calories per gram. Fats can be efficiently stored in adipose tissue with a minimal energy cost of storage. This is especially important in the young infant. Fats are required for the absorption of fat-soluble vitamins and for myelination of the central nervous system. Fat also provides essential fatty acids (EFA) necessary for brain development, for phospholipids in cell membranes, and for the synthesis of prostaglandins and leukotrienes. The EFA are polyunsaturated fatty acids derived from linoleic acid (18:2ω6, ie, 18 carbons and two double bonds from the methyl [omega] end) and linolenic acid (18:3ω3) by elongation and further desaturation. Among these are arachidonic acid (20:4ω6), which can be obtained from dietary linoleic acid and is present primarily in membrane phospholipids. Oxygenation of arachidonic acid through the lipoxygenase pathway yields leukotrienes, and oxygenation through the cyclooxygenase pathway yields prostaglandins. Important derivatives of linolenic acid are eicosapentaenoic acid (20:6ω3) and docosahexaenoic acid (22:6ω3), which is found in human milk and brain lipids. Visual acuity of formula-fed premature infants is improved with the addition of 20:6ω3, which is not derived readily from 18:3ω3.

Clinical features of EFA ω6 deficiency include growth failure, abnormal scaliness, erythematous skin lesions, decreased capillary resistance, increased fragility of erythrocytes, thrombocytopenia, poor wound healing, and increased susceptibility to infection. The clinical features of deficiency of ω3 fatty acids are less well defined, but dermatitis and neurologic abnormalities—including blurred vision, peripheral neuropathy, and weakness—have been reported. Marine oil-supplemented formula improves visual acuity of preterm infants through 4 months of age by improving docosahexaenoic acid status. Fatty fish are the best dietary source of ω3 fatty acids. A high intake of fatty fish is associated with a decrease in platelet adhesiveness and decreased inflammatory response.

Up to 5–10% of fatty acids in human milk are polyunsaturated. The majority of these are ω6 series, but long-chain ω3 fatty acids are also present. Breast milk also contains about 40% of fatty acids as monounsaturates, primarily oleic acid (18:1) and up to 10% of total fatty acids as medium-chain triglycerides (MCT). In general, the percentage of calories derived from fat is a little lower in infant formulas than in human milk. Typically, these formulas contain a relatively high percentage of linoleic acid but very little long-chain ω3. The American Academy of Pediatrics recommends that infants receive a minimum of 30% of calories from fat, including a minimum of 1.7% of total calories from ω6 fatty acids and 0.5% of calories from ω3. Providing up to 40–50% of energy requirements as fats is desirable at this age. In contrast, children older than 2 years should derive a *maximum* of 30% of total calories from fat and no more than 10% of calories either from saturated fats or polyunsaturated fats.

Triglycerides are hydrolyzed to monoglycerides, free fatty acids, and glycerol in the lumen of the gut. Substantial hydrolysis of triglycerides in milk formulas occurs in the stomach by the action of lingual and gastric lipases. Pancreatic lipases and bile salt levels are relatively low in early postnatal life, but breast milk contains a bile salt-stimulated lipase that is effective in the lumen of the duodenum. Bile salts promote the formation of the colipase-lipase complex, which adheres to the triglycerides prior to hydrolysis. Bile salts also have a major role in the emulsification of fatty acids, allowing their passage through the unstirred water layer to the surface of the mucosal cell. After passage into the enterocyte, long-chain ($\geq C_{12}$) fatty acids and monoglycerides are reesterified to triglycerides and are packaged with phospholipids, cholesterol, and protein into chylomicrons, which are transported in the lymphatics to the systemic circulation. At the capillary endothelial surfaces in adipose and muscle tissue, lipoprotein lipase (LPL) hydrolyzes triglycerides from chylomicrons, releasing free fatty acids and glycerol, which are taken up by the adjacent cells. LPL also hydrolyzes triglycerides synthesized in the liver and transported to peripheral tissues as very low density lipoproteins.

β-Oxidation of fatty acids takes place in the mitochondria of muscle and liver. Carnitine is necessary for the oxidation of the fatty acids, which must cross the mitochondrial membranes as acylcarnitine. Carnitine is synthesized in the human liver and kidney from lysine and methionine. Carnitine needs of infants are met by breast milk or formulas, and carnitine has recently been added to soy-based formulas but is not present in intravenous infusates. In the liver, substantial quantities of fatty acids are converted to ketone bodies, which are then released into the circulation and provide an important source of fuel for the brain in the young infant.

Medium-chain triglycerides (MCT C_8 and C_{10}, ie, energy density 7.6 kcal/g) are sufficiently soluble that micelle formation is not required for them to diffuse through the unstirred water layer. They are much more readily absorbed than long-chain triglycerides and are then transported directly to the liver via the portal circulation. MCTs are rapidly metabolized in the liver, undergoing β-oxidation or ketogenesis. They do not require carnitine to enter the mitochondria. Ketones are formed from MCT even when provided orally. MCTs are useful for patients with luminal phase defects (eg, cirrhosis), absorptive defects (eg, short bowel syndrome), and chronic inflammatory bowel disease. The potential side effects of MCT administration include diarrhea when they are given in large quantities, high octanoic acid levels in patients with cirrhosis, and, if they are the only source of lipids, deficiency of essential fatty acids.

Carlson SE: Visual acuity development in healthy preterm infants: Effects of marine oil supplementation. Am J Clin Nutr 1993;58:35.

CARBOHYDRATES

The energy density of carbohydrate is 4 kcal/g. Approximately 40% of caloric intake in human milk is in the form of lactose, or "milk sugar." The percentage of energy from lactose in cow's milk is only 20%, but infant formulas generally provide a somewhat higher percentage of energy from carbohydrates than does human milk.

After the first 2 years of life, 60% or more of energy requirements should be derived from carbohydrates, including no more than 10% from simple sugars. These dietary guidelines are, unfortunately, not reflected in the diets of North American children, who typically derive 25% of energy from sucrose and less than 20% from complex carbohydrates. Diets high in complex carbohydrates are, however, typical for the majority of the world's population of children.

The rate at which lactase hydrolyzes lactose to glucose and galactose in the brush border determines how quickly milk carbohydrates are absorbed. Lactase levels are highest in young infants, declining by more than 50% later in the first year. Lactase levels decline further with age, especially in children who are not of Northern European descent. Many black and Hispanic children cannot consume large amounts of dairy products without some evidence of lactose intolerance, eg, flatulence and loose stools. Lactase is located predominantly at the tip of the intestinal villi, where it is especially vulnerable to the effects of gastroenteritis or malnutrition. Thus, it may be helpful to avoid giving lactose-containing foods to children recovering from gastroenteritis or malnutrition, though this is not universally necessary. Galactose is preferentially converted to glycogen in the liver prior to conversion to glucose for subsequent oxidation. Infants with galactosemia, an inborn metabolic disease caused by deficient galactose-1-phosphate uridyl-transferase, require a lactose-free diet starting in the neonatal period.

Starch is broken down in the lumen of the gut into disaccharides and oligosaccharides, which are hydrolyzed into glucose by maltase, isomaltase, and glucoamylase in the brush border. Glucoamylase, which hydrolyzes oligosaccharides of 4–9 glucose units, is located predominantly at the base of the villi, where it may be protected from partial villus atrophy. Glucose polymers of this length are used extensively in special infant formulas and for caloric supplementation. Advantages include a relatively low osmolar effect in the lumen of the intestine as well as relatively easy hydrolysis by the compromised mucosa. Glucose and galactose are absorbed actively with sodium. This provides the theoretic basis for the composition of oral rehydration solutions in the management of diarrhea. The glucose enhances the absorption of sodium (and thus of water) and also supplies some energy.

During and immediately following a meal, plasma glucose levels are maintained by glucose absorption. If less than 10% of dietary energy is provided by carbohydrate, ketosis results. Within 2–4 hours after a meal, maintenance of plasma glucose depends increasingly on utilization of hepatic glycogen stores. These provide only 100–150 g glucose in the adult and only 6 g in the neonate. Subsequently, until the next meal, there is progressive dependence on gluconeogenesis. Glucose is the principal fuel for the brain and is a necessary energy source for certain other tissues, including red and white blood cells.

Children and adolescents in North America consume large quantities of sucrose (table sugar) in such items as soft drinks, candy, syrups, and sweetened breakfast cereals. Average consumption by adolescents is 210 lb per year. A high intake of sucrose predisposes to obesity and is a major risk factor for dental caries. Sucrase hydrolyzes sucrose to glucose and fructose in the brush border of the small intestine. Fructose is absorbed more slowly than and independently of glucose by a facilitated diffusion process. This characteristic provides a distinct advantage. Neither fructose nor galactose stimulates insulin secretion. Fructose, however, is easily converted to hepatic triglycerides, which may be especially undesirable in malnourished subjects.

Dietary fiber can be classified into two major types: nondigested carbohydrate (β1–4 linkages) and noncarbohydrate (lignin). Insoluble fibers (cellulose, hemicellulose, and lignin) increase stool bulk and water content and decrease gut transit time. They may to some extent impair mineral absorption. Soluble fibers (pectins, mucilages, and oat bran) bind bile acids and reduce lipid and cholesterol absorption. Pectins also slow gastric emptying and the rate of nutrient absorption. Fiber intakes are quite low in North America. Few data regarding the fiber needs of children are available.

MAJOR MINERALS
(See Table 11–3 for recommended intakes.)

Calcium

The major dietary sources of calcium are milk and other dairy products. Although some calcium is available from other sources, including fortified cereals, it is difficult to achieve an adequate intake of calcium if dairy products are excluded from the diet. In such cases, a calcium supplement may be desirable. Average calcium absorption, which depends on calcium status and intake, is 20–30%, but calcium absorption from human milk is 60%. Absorption is enhanced by lactose, glucose, and protein and is impaired by phytate, fiber, oxalate, and unabsorbed fat. Control of calcium absorption is exerted primarily by changes in levels of 1,25-dihydroxycholecalciferol, which are increased in response to an increase in circulating parathyroid hormone (PTH). PTH, which is secreted in response to a fall in plasma ionized calcium, also increases the release of calcium from bone. The desirable ratio of dietary calcium:phosphorus is 1.5:1 or greater in the young infant and 1:1 or greater at all other ages. The low calcium:phosphorus ratio found in unmodified cow's milk can cause hypocalcemic tetany and convulsions in the neonate. Calcium is excreted primarily via the kidney. It is the most abundant mineral in the body, and more than 99% is in the skeleton. Many vital cellular processes depend on calcium, especially changes in cytosolic free calcium levels. Changes in these levels also occur in various pathologic states and can grossly disturb intracellular metabolism. A deficiency in dietary calcium can occur in premature infants and lactating adolescents as a result of a restricted milk intake and also in patients with steatorrhea. The effect is a decrease in bone density, possibly progressing to rickets. Bone density increases with increasing calcium intake up to daily intakes of more than 1000 mg in adolescents. Maximizing bone density at this stage of the life cycle has important implications for minimizing postmenopausal osteoporosis.

Chan GM: Dietary calcium and bone mineral status of children and adolescents. Am J Dis Child 1991;145:631.
Horsman A et al: Bone mineral accretion rate and calcium intake in preterm infants. Arch Dis Child 1989;64:910.
Johnston CC et al: Calcium supplementation and increases in bone mineral density in children. N Engl J Med 1992;327:82.

Phosphorus

Phosphorus is abundant in meats, eggs, dairy products, grains, legumes, and nuts. Phosphorus levels are high in processed foods and very high in colas and other soft drinks. Approximately 80% of dietary phosphorus is absorbed; the kidney is responsible for homeostatic control. PTH decreases tubular reabsorption of phosphorus. More than 85% of body phosphorus is in bone. Phosphorus is also a component of many organic compounds that have a vital role in metabolism, including ATP and 2,3-diphosphoglycerate. Many of the clinical effects of phosphorus deple-

Table 11–3. Suggested dietary intakes of minerals and trace elements.[1]

Nutrient	Premature Infant[2]	Term Infant	Children > 1 Year
Sodium		50 mg/kg/d (2 mmol/kg/d)	250–500 (10–20 mmol/d)
Potassium		80 mg/kg/d (2 mmol/kg/d)	800 (20 mmol/d)
Chloride		70 mg/kg/d (2 mmol/kg/d)	700 (20 mmol/d)
Calcium	180	400 (200) (See note 3.)	800
Phosphorus	150	300 (100) (See note 3.)	600
Magnesium	15	40	100
Iron	2 (after first 1–2 mo)	1 mg/kg/d (≤ 0.1) (See note 3.) (after 2 mo)	10 (18 in adolescence)
Zinc	1.5	$4 \rightarrow 2$ ($2 \rightarrow 0.75$)	2–10
Copper	0.12	0.2–0.4	0.5–2
Selenium	0.003	0.01–0.03	0.03–0.1
Iodine	0.01	0.05	0.07–0.15

[1] Amounts expressed in mg/d unless otherwise indicated.
[2] The figures in this column indicate mg/kg/d.
[3] Amounts in parentheses are for the fully breast-fed infant aged less than 4–6 months.

tion are attributable to cellular energy depletion from lack of ATP or to cellular anoxia secondary to impaired release of oxygen from hemoglobin. Other key compounds containing phosphorus include cell membrane phospholipids and nucleotides.

Nutritional phosphorus deficiency is rare but has been documented in very premature infants fed human milk—in whom it can cause osteoporosis and rickets—and in patients undergoing rehabilitation from protein-energy malnutrition. Nonnutritional causes of phosphorus depletion include the ingestion of phosphorus-binding antacids. Severe hypophosphatemia results from a deficiency together with an acute extracellular to intracellular shift in phosphorus. This shift can be triggered by a glucose load, by insulin, or during nutritional rehabilitation of the malnourished patient. Phosphorus deficiency affects most organ systems, including muscle (weakness progressing to rhabdomyolysis), cellular components of blood (both physiologic and functional changes), the gastrointestinal system, the central nervous system, and bone (bone pain, osteomalacia, rickets). Respiratory insufficiency may result from weakness of the diaphragm. Phosphate depletion in the premature infant can cause hypercalcemia. Phosphorus depletion can be treated with phosphorus salts, cola drinks, or skim milk. Phosphorus excess may cause neonatal tetany due to decreased calcium. Phosphorus retention in chronic renal disease leads to metabolic bone disease.

Knochel JP: The clinical status of hypophosphatemia. N Engl J Med 1985;313:447.
Sagy M et al: Phosphate-depletion syndrome in a premature infant fed human milk. J Pediatr 1980;96:683.

Magnesium

Two-thirds of dietary magnesium is derived from vegetables, cereals, and nuts. The kidney exerts very effective control of magnesium homeostasis. When intake is low, excretion is minimal, and intracellular levels are maintained very effectively. Magnesium is the second most abundant intracellular cation; 50% is in bone. Levels in the cell cytosol are ten times those of the extracellular fluids and are especially high in mitochondria. Magnesium activates many enzymes, especially phosphorus-hydrolyzing and transferring enzymes involved in energy metabolism. Magnesium also plays major roles in nucleic acid metabolism.

Dietary magnesium deficiency is not recognized except as a component of protein-energy malnutrition, but magnesium depletion may occur secondary to renal disease or intestinal malabsorption. Clinical effects include increased neuromuscular excitability, muscle fasciculation and tremors, personality changes, neurologic abnormalities, and electrocardiographic changes (depression of ST segment and T waves). Disturbances of PTH metabolism can cause secondary hypocalcemia. Acute states of magnesium

depletion can be treated with a 50% solution of $MgSO_4$ providing 0.3–0.5 meq of magnesium per kilogram (3–6 meq maximum) given intravenously over 3 hours and repeated over the remainder of a 24-hour period. Magnesium excess can cause respiratory depression, lethargy, and coma.

Zelikovic I et al: Severe renal osteodystrophy without elevated serum immunoreactive parathyroid hormone concentrations in hypomagnesemia due to renal magnesium wasting. Pediatrics 1987;79:403.

Sodium

In the USA and Western Europe, only 10% of sodium intake is derived directly from food. Fifteen percent is derived from cooking and 75% from processed foods. The 10% derived from unprocessed foods is more than adequate to meet the normal requirement. Current dietary recommendations include a reduction from the typical intakes of North Americans, in which the ratio of sodium to potassium is 2:1; this ratio is 0.25:1 in other societies and in other mammalian species. High sodium:potassium ratios have been implicated in the pathogenesis of hypertension, especially if the intake of dietary calcium is low. Fifteen percent of the population may be susceptible to adverse effects from high sodium:potassium ratios. The sodium intake of breast-fed infants, while adequate (4–6 mmol/d), is low in comparison to that of most formula-fed infants.

Excessive sweating or cystic fibrosis may increase sodium requirements. Sodium deficiency, which occurs most commonly as a result of diarrhea and vomiting, causes dehydration. Anorexia, vomiting, and mental apathy may result from chronic depletion of sodium chloride. Hyponatremic and hypernatremic dehydration are discussed in Chapter 37.

Severe malnutrition and severe stress or hypermetabolism can disturb the ionic gradient across cell membranes and lead to an excess in intracellular sodium, which can adversely affect cellular metabolism. Sodium should be administered only with great caution in these circumstances.

Chloride

The intake and homeostasis of dietary chloride are closely linked with those of sodium. However, chloride is itself important in the physiologic mechanisms of the kidney and of the gut. Active chloride transport in the ascending loop of Henle is necessary for the passive reabsorption of sodium. Thus, a deficiency of chloride leads to a decrease in the absorption of sodium in the ascending loop of Henle and an increase in the amount of sodium presented to the lumen of the distal tube. This sodium is exchanged for H^+ and K^+, which can result in hypokalemic alkalosis.

Infants fed formulas low in chloride have experienced a nutritional deficiency of chloride. Other causes of chloride deficiency include cystic fibrosis, pyloric stenosis and other causes of vomiting, familial chloride diarrhea, chronic diuretic (furosemide) therapy, and Bartter's syndrome. Chloride deficiency has been associated with failure to thrive and may especially affect head growth. Other clinical features may include anorexia, lethargy, muscle weakness, vomiting, dehydration, and hypovolemia. Laboratory features include hypochloremia, hypokalemia, metabolic alkalosis, and hyperreninemia. Urine chloride levels depend on the cause of the depletion.

Malloy MH et al: Hypochloremic metabolic alkalosis from ingestion of a chloride deficient infant formula: Outcome 9 and 10 years later. Pediatrics 1991;87:811.

Perlman JM et al: Is chloride depletion an important contributing cause of death in infants with bronchopulmonary dysplasia? Pediatrics 1986;77:212.

Potassium

Potassium is readily available in unprocessed foods, including nuts, whole grains, meats and fish, beans, bananas, and orange juice. Relatively high potassium intakes are encouraged except in the presence of renal failure. The kidneys control potassium homeostasis via the aldosterone-renin-angiotensin endocrine system. Potassium is the principal intracellular cation. The amount of total body potassium, therefore, depends on lean body mass. Potassium deficiency occurs in protein-energy malnutrition and, if not aggressively treated during the acute management stage, can be a cause of sudden death from cardiac failure. Because of loss of lean body mass, excessive potassium is excreted in the urine in any catabolic state. Again, this requires aggressive replenishment during recovery. In acidosis, intracellular potassium is exchanged for H^+. Potassium, thus shifted into the extracellular fluid, is subsequently lost in the urine, and total body potassium is depleted (eg, in diabetic ketoacidosis) despite normal or elevated levels of plasma potassium. Other prominent causes of potassium deficiency include diarrhea and the use of diuretics. The effects of potassium deficiency are muscle weakness, mental confusion, and sudden death from arrhythmias. Electrocardiographic findings include depression of the ST segment and low T waves. Hyperkalemia may result from renal insufficiency.

TRACE ELEMENTS

Trace elements that have a recognized role in human nutrition are iron, iodine, zinc, copper, selenium, manganese, molybdenum, chromium, cobalt (as a component of vitamin B_{12}), and fluoride. Dietary requirements of trace elements are summarized in Table 11–3. Iron deficiency is discussed in Chapter 25. In general, good dietary sources of trace elements include human milk, meats, shellfish, legumes, nuts,

and whole-grain cereals. Fish are a good source of selenium. Absorption of iron, zinc, copper, and probably other trace elements from human milk is especially favorable; the breast-fed infant does not normally require other sources of trace elements, including iron, for the first 4–6 months. Factors affecting the absorption of trace elements include the quantity of that trace element in the diet; dietary factors that form insoluble complexes (phytate, fiber, phosphate, oxalate); factors affecting oxidation state (ascorbic acid increases iron absorption and decreases copper absorption); chemical form (heme versus nonheme iron); competitive inhibition at mucosal cell (interactions of iron, zinc, and copper); and host factors (including nutritional status, diarrhea, impaired mucosal function). The gastrointestinal tract is the major site of homeostatic control for iron and zinc, the liver for copper, the intestinal tract and liver for manganese, and the kidneys for selenium, chromium, and iodine.

Deficiencies of iron, zinc, and possibly copper occur in the free-living population; in certain geochemical areas, the same is true of iodine and selenium. Infants fed cow's milk are at risk for deficiencies in iron and copper. Excessive losses, factors impairing absorption, or iatrogenic factors can cause deficiencies of iron, zinc, or copper. Deficiencies in these elements, as well as selenium, chromium, manganese, and molybdenum, have been associated with the use of synthetic diets, especially intravenous feeding. Protein-energy malnutrition may be complicated by deficiencies in iron, zinc, copper, selenium, or chromium. Finally, deficiencies in zinc, copper, iron, and molybdenum occur as a result of specific inborn metabolic diseases affecting the metabolism of these elements.

Hambidge KM: Trace element requirements in premature infants. In: *Textbook of Gastroenterology and Nutrition in Early Childhood*, 2nd ed. Lebenthal M (editor). Raven Press, 1988.

Zinc

Zinc is a component of many enzymes, plays multiple roles in nucleic acid metabolism and protein synthesis, and is important for membrane structure and function. Causes of zinc deficiency include diets low in available zinc during periods of rapid growth in infancy and childhood, synthetic oral or intravenous diets lacking adequate zinc supplements, diseases associated with impaired absorption (eg, regional enteritis) or excessive losses (eg, chronic diarrhea) of zinc, and one or more inborn diseases of zinc metabolism. Zinc deficiency may be a factor of secondary importance in some cases of anorexia nervosa. Clinical effects of a mild deficiency include impaired growth and poor appetite. More severe cases are characterized by changes in mood, irritability, and lethargy. Impairment of the immune system, especially T cell function, has been linked to increased susceptibility to infection. The most severe cases are characterized by an acro-orificial skin rash, usually accompanied by diarrhea and alopecia. These features occur in patients with acrodermatitis enteropathica, an inborn error of zinc metabolism; in those undergoing intravenous feeding without adequate zinc supplements; and in some premature breast-fed infants whose mothers have a defect in the secretion of zinc by the mammary gland. Plasma zinc collected before breakfast is below 6 μmol/L (40 μg/dL) in cases of severe zinc deficiency and 6–9 μmol/L (40–60 μg/dL) in cases of moderate zinc deficiency. In cases of mild zinc deficiency, plasma zinc concentrations may be within the normal range (9–15 μmol/L). Moderate hypozincemia occurs in response to release of interleukin-1 and in pregnancy even when zinc intake is adequate. Suspected dietary zinc deficiency can be treated with 1 mg/kg/d of zinc for 3 months (eg, 4.5 mg $ZnSO_4 \cdot 7H_2O$ per kilogram per day), preferably administered separately from meals and from iron supplements. Sustained clinical remissions in acrodermatitis enteropathica are usually achieved with 30–50 mg Zn^{2+} per day, but larger quantities may be required.

Hambidge KM: Zinc deficiency in the premature infant. Pediatr Rev 1985;6:209.

Walravens PA, Koepfer DM, Hambidge KM: A double-blind, controlled study of zinc supplementation in infants with a nutritional pattern of failure to thrive. Pediatrics 1989;83:532.

Copper

Copper is a vital component of several oxidative enzymes, including cytochrome c oxidase, the terminal oxidase in the electron transport chain; cytosolic and mitochondrial superoxide dismutases, which have key roles in the body defense against free radicals; lysyl oxidase, which is necessary for the cross-linking of elastin and collagen; and ferroxidases (including ceruloplasmin) necessary for the oxidation of ferrous storage iron to ferric iron prior to attachment to transferrin for transport to the red cell precursors in the bone marrow. Cu^{2+} is highly reactive and must be transported in the circulation tightly bound to ceruloplasmin so that its oxidative potential (when it is free or loosely bound) can be contained.

Copper deficiency may occur in the following circumstances: in premature infants fed milk preparations low in copper; in association with prolonged feeding with unmodified cow's milk; in association with more generalized malnutritional states; in patients maintained on prolonged total parenteral nutrition without copper supplementation; and secondary to intestinal malabsorption states or prolonged diarrhea.

Osteoporosis is an early finding. Later skeletal changes include enlargement of costochondral cartilages, cupping and flaring of long-bone metaphyses, and spontaneous fractures of the ribs. The radiologic findings must be distinguished from battering (not symmetric), rickets, and scurvy. Neutropenia and hypochromic anemia are other early manifestations. The anemia is unresponsive to iron therapy. Very severe central nervous system disease is present in Menkes' steely (kinky) hair syndrome, in which a profound copper deficiency state results from a specific X-linked inherited defect in cellular metabolism of copper.

A low plasma copper or ceruloplasmin level helps confirm the diagnosis of copper deficiency. However, these levels are normally very low in the young infant, especially the premature infant, and are higher than adult values in later infancy and early childhood. Hence, carefully age-matched normal data are necessary for comparison. Interleukin-1 grossly elevates ceruloplasmin and copper levels; these levels are also very high in pregnancy.

Copper deficiency can be treated with a 1% solution of copper sulfate (2 mg of the salt or 500 μg of elemental copper per day for infants).

Salmanpera L et al: Copper supplementation: Failure to increase plasma copper and ceruloplasmin concentrations in healthy infants. Am J Clin Nutr 1989;50:843.

Selenium

Selenium is an essential component of glutathione peroxidase, which catalyzes the reduction of hydrogen peroxide to water in the cell cytosol by the addition of reducing equivalents derived from glutathione. Hence, selenium plays an important role in the body's defenses against free radicals.

Selenium deficiency is now recognized as the major etiologic factor in Keshan disease, an often fatal cardiomyopathy affecting primarily infants, children, and young women in a large area of China where there is a severe geochemical deficiency of selenium. Similar cases have been identified in the USA in patients maintained on long-term total parenteral nutrition without adequate selenium supplements. Other patients receiving parenteral nutritional support have manifested selenium deficiency with incapacitating skeletal muscle pain and tenderness. Macrocytosis and loss of hair pigment occur in milder states of selenium deficiency. Blood levels are especially low in premature infants with bronchopulmonary dysplasia. It appears that the selenium intake of infants, especially premature infants, is suboptimal and is likely to be increased in the near future.

A plasma selenium level less than 0.5 μmol/L (less than 40 μg/L) is compatible with mild selenium deficiency; a level less than 0.12 μmol/L (less than 10 μg/L) indicates a possible severe selenium deficiency.

Litov RE, Combs GF Jr: Selenium in pediatric nutrition. Pediatrics 1991;87:339.

Iodine

Endemic goiter due to iodine deficiency has been eradicated in North America by effective prophylactic measures but continues to be a major health problem in many developing countries. Goiter occurs when iodine intake or excretion in urine is less than 20 μg/d. Most goitrous persons are clinically euthyroid. Maternal iodine deficiency causes endemic cretinism in about 5–15% of neonates who develop endemic goiters.

"Neurologic" endemic cretinism, seen clinically in most regions, is characterized by severe mental retardation, deaf-mutism, spastic diplegia, and strabismus. Clinical evidence of hypothyroidism is usually absent, and it is thought that the neurologic damage may be due to a direct effect of fetal iodine deficiency or to an imbalance between T_4 (low) and T_3 (normal or elevated). "Myxedematous" endemic cretinism predominates in some central African countries. Signs of congenital hypothyroidism are seen in this type. Milder neurologic damage occurs in many other cases of endemic neonatal goiter.

In North American countries, the use of iodized salt has been highly effective in preventing goiter. In areas where endemic goiter occurs, intramuscular depot injections of iodized oil have also been used extensively for prevention.

Fluoride Supplementation

When fluoride is incorporated into the hydroxyapatite matrix of dentin, it affords an inexpensive and effective means of helping to prevent dental caries. Fluoride is most effectively administered in the drinking water, but in infancy and childhood, fluoride in vitamin preparations or tablets serves the same purpose. Ready-made formulas provide less than 0.3 ppm. A dosage schedule as recommended by the American Academy of Pediatrics is set forth in Table 11–4. Breast-fed infants should be given fluoride supplements after 6 months of age. Earlier supplementation for the breast-fed infant, though its value has not been demonstrated conclusively, has been recommended by the American Academy of Pediatrics Committee on Nutrition.

Table 11–4. Supplemental fluoride requirements (mg/d).

Age	Concentration of Fluoride in Drinking Water		
	< 0.3 ppm	0.3–0.7 ppm	> 0.7 ppm
2 wk to 2 y	0.25	0	0
2–3 y	0.5	0.25	0
3–16 y	1	0.5	0

VITAMINS

1. FAT-SOLUBLE VITAMINS

Because they are insoluble in water, the fat-soluble vitamins require digestion and absorption of dietary fat and a carrier system for transport in the blood. Deficiencies in these vitamins develop more slowly than deficiencies in water-soluble vitamins because the body accumulates stores of fat-soluble vitamins. Excessive intakes carry a considerable potential for toxicity (Table 11–5).

Moran JR, Greene HL: Nutritional biochemistry of fat-soluble vitamins. In: *Pediatric Nutrition: Theory and Practice.* Grand RJ et al (editors). Butterworths, 1987.

Tsang RC (editor): *Vitamin and Mineral Requirements in Preterm Infants.* Marcel Dekker, 1985.

Vitamin A

Dietary sources of vitamin A include dairy products, fortified margarine, eggs, liver, meats, fish oils,

Table 11–5. Effects of vitamin toxicity.

Thiamin
(Very rare.) Anaphylaxis; respiratory depression.
Riboflavin
None.
Pyridoxine
(Very rare.) Sensory neuropathy.
Niacin
Histamine release → cutaneous vasodilation; cardiac arrythmias; cholestatic jaundice; gastrointestinal disturbance; hyperuricemia; glucose intolerance.
Pantothenic acid
Diarrhea.
Biotin
None.
Folate
May mask B_{12} deficiency, hypersensitivity.
Cobalamin
None.
Vitamin C
Interference with copper absorption; decreased tolerance to hypoxia; increased oxalic acid excretion.
Carnitine
None recognized.
Vitamin A
(> 20,000 IU/d): Vomiting increased intracranial pressure (pseudotumor cerebri); irritability; headaches; insomnia; emotional lability; dry, desquamating skin; myalgia and arthralgia; abdominal pain; hepatosplenomegaly; cortical thickening of bones of hands and feet.
Vitamin D
(> 40,000 IU/d): Hypercalcemia; vomiting; constipation; nephrocalcinosis.
Vitamin E
? 25–100 mg/kg/d IV: Necrotizing enterocolitis and liver toxicity (but probably due to polysorbate 80 used as a solubilizer).
Vitamin K
Lipid-soluble vitamin K: Very low order of toxicity. Water-soluble, synthetic vitamin K: Vomiting; porphyrinuria; albuminuria; hemolytic anemia; hemoglobinuria; hyperbilirubinemia (do not give to neonates).

and corn. The vitamin A precursor β-carotene occurs in abundance in yellow and green vegetables. Dietary retinyl palmitate requires hydrolysis by pancreatic and intestinal hydrolases. Beta-carotene is cleaved in the intestinal mucosal cells by dioxygenase to yield two molecules of retinal (retinaldehyde), which is then reduced to retinol (vitamin A alcohol). Dioxygenase is stimulated by thyroxine; thus, individuals with hypothyroidism accumulate carotene because they cannot convert it to retinol. Carotene appears to have an important physiologic role in its own right as a powerful antioxidant. Data on the in vivo role of carotene in children are quite limited.

Retinol is reesterified in the mucosal cells and transported in chylomicrons to the liver, where it is stored. From the liver, vitamin A is transported to the rest of the body attached to retinol-binding protein complexed to prealbumin. Retinol-binding protein may be decreased in liver disease or in protein-energy malnutrition. Circulating retinol-binding protein may be increased in chronic renal failure.

Vitamin A has a unique and specialized role in the photochemical basis of vision. The photosensitive pigment rhodopsin is formed from retinal and a protein called opsin. Vitamin A also modifies differentiation and proliferation of epithelial cells, especially in the respiratory tract. Vitamin A is necessary for glycoprotein synthesis and for the integrity of the immune system and may affect gene expression. Retinol can be irreversibly oxidized to retinoic acid, which is effective in glycoprotein synthesis but is ineffective for vision.

Vitamin A deficiency occurs in premature infants, in association with intravenous nutrition with inadequate vitamin A supplements, and in association with protein-energy malnutrition, when the manifestations are frequently made more severe by measles. Other causes of vitamin A deficiency are cultural factors (failure to grow vegetables even when practical, eg, in Central America and the Philippines), fat malabsorption syndromes (including biliary atresia), giardiasis, and cystic fibrosis.

The classic features of vitamin A deficiency are primarily related to the eye and vision. Night blindness progresses to xerosis (dryness of cornea and conjunctiva), xerophthalmia (extreme dryness of the conjunctiva), Bitot's spots, keratomalacia (clouding and softening of the cornea), ulceration and perforation of the cornea, prolapse of the lens and iris, and eventually blindness. Vitamin A deficiency is the leading cause of irreversible blindness in children worldwide. Other features of vitamin A deficiency can include follicular hyperkeratosis (dry, thickened, rough skin), pruritus, growth retardation, increased susceptibility to infection, anemia, and hepatosplenomegaly. Vitamin A deficiency in the neonatal period may be an etiologic factor in the onset of bronchopulmonary dysplasia in premature infants.

Serum levels of retinol below 20 μg/dL are considered low; a level below 10 μg/dL indicates deficiency. A ratio of retinol:retinol-binding protein below 0.7 is also indicative of vitamin A deficiency.

Suggested intakes of vitamin A are summarized in Table 11–6. Therapy of xerophthalmia requires 50,000–100,000 IU orally or intramuscularly. The standard maintenance dose in fat malabsorption syndromes is 2500–5000 IU (800–1600 μg). Doses as high as 25,000–50,000 IU/d may be needed, but monitoring to avoid toxicity is essential. Vitamin A can be provided in these circumstances as a water-soluble preparation, Aquasol A (1 mL = 50,000 IU). The effects of vitamin A toxicity are summarized in Table 11–5.

Fawzi WW et al: Vitamin A supplementation and child mortality: A meta-analysis. JAMA 1993;269:898.
Shenai JP et al: Plasma retinol-binding protein response to vitamin A administration in infants susceptible to bronchopulmonary dysplasia. J Pediatr 1990;116:607.

Table 11–6. Suggested intakes of vitamins.

	Premature Infants[1] (per kg/d)	Term Infants[1] (per day)	Adults[2] (per day)
Thiamin (mg)	0.35	12	1.5
Riboflavin (mg)	0.2	0.5	1.7
Pyridoxine (mg)	0.2	0.6	2.0
Niacin (mg NE)[3]	7	17 (NE)	19 (NE)
Pantothenic acid (mg)	2	5	4–7
Biotin (μg)	6	20	30–100
Folic acid (μg)	50	140	400
Cobalamin (μg)	0.3	1	2.0
Vitamin A (μg RE)[4]	500	700	1000
Vitamin C (mg)	25	80	60
Vitamin D (μg) (cholecalciferol)	4 (160 IU)	10 (400 IU)	5
Vitamin E (mg) (α-tocopherol)	3 (See note 5)	7	10
Vitamin K (μg)	80	20	80

[1]Based on recent recommendations for intravenous vitamins. (Greene HL, Hambidge KM, Schanier R, Tsang RC: Guidelines for the use of vitamins, trace elements, calcium, magnesium, and phosphorus in infants and children receiving total parenteral nutrition: Report of the Subcommittee on Pediatric Parenteral Nutrient Requirements from the Committee on Clinical Practice Issues of The American Society for Clinical Nutrition. *Am J Clin Nutr* 1988;48:1324 © *Am J Clin Nutr.* American Society for Clinical Nutrition.)

[2]Based on *Recommended Dietary Allowances,* 10th ed. National Research Council, National Academy Press, 1989 (except for folate).

[3]NE Niacin equivalents.

[4]RE Retinol equivalents (1 μg retinol or 6 mg β-carotene = 1 RE; 1 IU = 0.3 μg retinol).

[5]Oral doses up to 25 mg/d are now frequently used with the expectation that this may help to combat oxidant stress.

Zachman RD: Retinol (vitamin A) and the neonate: Special problems of the human premature neonate. Am J Clin Nutr 1989;50:413.

Vitamin D

Vitamin D requirements are normally met primarily from ultraviolet radiation of dehydrocholesterol in the skin with the formation of cholecalciferol (vitamin D_3). Similarly, vitamin D_2, or ergocalciferol, is derived from radiation of ergosterol. Vitamin D is transported from the skin to the liver attached to a specific carrier protein. The primary dietary source is vitamin D-fortified milk and formulas. Egg yolk and fatty fish contain some vitamin D. Vitamin D absorption depends on normal fat absorption. Absorbed vitamin D is transported to the liver in chylomicrons. Vitamins D_2 and D_3 undergo 25-hydroxylation in the liver and then 1α hydroxylation in kidney proximal tubules to yield 25-hydroxycholecalciferol and 1,25-dihydroxycholecalciferol, respectively. Parathyroid hormone activates the 1α-hydroxylase enzyme in the kidney. Calcifediol (25-hydroxycholecalciferol) is the major circulating form of vitamin D. Calcitriol (1,25-dihydroxycholecalciferol) is the biologically active form of vitamin D. Calcitriol stimulates the intestinal absorption of calcium and phosphate, the renal reabsorption of filtered calcium, and the mobilization of calcium and phosphorus from bone.

Vitamin D deficiency results from lack of adequate sunlight coupled with a low dietary intake. An infant requires only 30 minutes per week of total body sun exposure or 2 hours per week of head exposure to maintain adequate vitamin D status. Even without exposure to sunlight, the breast-fed infant can acquire sufficient vitamin D from human milk if the mother's vitamin D status is optimal. Otherwise, a vitamin D supplement is required to avoid risk of rickets. In the United States, cow's milk and infant formulas are routinely supplemented with vitamin D. Nutritional rickets may occur in older infants and children who are not exposed to the sun and who do not drink vitamin D-fortified milk.

Vitamin D deficiency also occurs in fat malabsorption syndromes, including small intestinal disease, cholestasis, and lymphatic obstruction. Use of P-450-stimulating drugs may decrease hydroxylated vitamin D, which can also be decreased by hepatic and renal disease and by inborn errors of metabolism. End-organ unresponsiveness to calcitriol may also occur.

The clinical effects of vitamin D deficiency are osteomalacia (adults) or rickets (children), in which there is an accumulation in bone of osteoid (matrix) with reduced calcification. Cartilage fails to mature and calcify. The effects include craniotabes, rachitic rosary, pigeon breast, bowed legs, delayed eruption of teeth and enamel defects, Harrison's groove, scoliosis, kyphosis, dwarfism, painful bones, fractures, anorexia, and weakness. X-ray findings include cupping, fraying, and flaring of metaphyses; the loss of sharp definition of bone trabeculae accounts for the general decrease in skeletal radiodensity. The diagnosis is supported by characteristic radiologic abnormalities of the skeleton, low serum phosphorus levels, high serum alkaline phosphatase levels, and high parathyroid hormone levels. The diagnosis can be confirmed by a low level of serum 25-hydroxycholecalciferol.

Rickets is treated with 1600–5000 IU/d of vitamin D_3 (1 IU = 0.25 µg). If this is poorly absorbed, 25-hydroxycholecalciferol, 2 µg/kg/d, or 1,25-dihydroxycholecalciferol, 0.05–0.2 µg/kg/d, is given. Renal osteodystrophy is treated with 1,25-dihydroxycholecalciferol (calcitriol).

Suggested dietary intakes for vitamin D are summarized in Table 11–6 and toxic effects in Table 11–5.

Hillman LS: Mineral and vitamin D adequacy in infants fed human milk or formula between 6 and 12 months of age. J Pediatr 1990;117:134.

Vitamin D: New perspectives. (Editorial.) Lancet 1987; 1:1122.

Vitamin E

Vegetable oils provide the main dietary source of vitamin E. Coconut and olive oils, however, are low in vitamin E. Some vitamin E is present in cereals, dairy products, and eggs. Activity may decrease with processing, storage, or heating. Vitamin E is a family of compounds, the tocopherols. There are four major forms: alpha, gamma, beta, and delta; α-tocopherol has the highest biologic activity. Vitamin E can donate an electron to a free radical molecule to stop oxidant reactions. Oxidized vitamin E is then reduced by ascorbic acid or glutathione. The reduced tocopherol is able to "scavenge" another free radical. The nutrients that participate in antioxidant defenses include β-carotene, vitamin C, selenium, copper, manganese, and zinc. Vitamin E is located at specific sites in the cell to protect polyunsaturated fatty acids in the membrane lipids from lipid peroxidation and to protect thiol groups and nucleic acids. Vitamin E also functions as a cell membrane stabilizer, may function in the electron transport chain, and may modulate chromosomal expression.

Vitamin E deficiency may occur in the following circumstances: in the premature infant; in cholestatic liver disease, pancreatic insufficiency (including cystic fibrosis), abetalipoproteinemia, and short bowel syndrome; as an isolated inborn error of vitamin E metabolism; and perhaps as a result of increased utilization due to oxidant stress.

Vitamin E deficiency shortens red cell half-life and may cause hemolytic anemia. Chronic vitamin E deficiency secondary to malabsorption results in a progressive neurologic disorder with loss of deep tendon reflexes, loss of coordination, loss of perception of vibration and position sensation, abnormalities in eye movements, weakness, scoliosis, and degeneration of the retina. In premature infants, vitamin E deficiency may contribute to oxidant injury of the lung, retina, and brain (brain hemorrhage). These putative adverse effects in the premature infant require confirmation.

Vitamin E nutritional status can be partially assessed with serum vitamin E (normal range for children is 3–15 µg/mL). The ratio of serum vitamin E:total serum lipid is normally more than 0.8 mg/g. Hydrogen peroxide-induced hemolysis is also used as a test of vitamin E status.

Suggested intakes are summarized in Table 11–6. Requirements increase if dietary polyunsaturated fatty acids (PUFA) increase (there is a need for 0.4–0.5 mg of vitamin E per gram of PUFA in the diet). One international unit = 1 mg of dl-α-tocopheryl acetate.

Large oral doses (up to 100 IU/kg/d) of vitamin E correct the deficiency resulting from most malabsorption syndromes. Intramuscular injections (5–7 mg/kg/week) may be necessary in some cases of cholestatic liver disease. For abetalipoproteinemia, 100–200 IU/kg/d of vitamin E are needed. Vitamin E therapy in ischemia-reperfusion injury and in the prevention of intracranial hemorrhage in the preterm infant remains experimental. Toxic effects of vitamin E are summarized in Table 11–5.

Machlin LJ, Bendich A: Free radical tissue damage: Protective role of antioxidant nutrients. FASEB J 1987; 1:441.
Sokol RJ: Vitamin E deficiency and neurologic disease. Annu Rev Nutr 1988;8:351.

Vitamin K

Vitamin K_1 (phylloquinone) is obtained from leafy vegetables, soybean oil, fruits, seeds, and cow's milk. Vitamin K_2 (menaquinone), which has 60% of the activity of K_1, is synthesized by intestinal bacteria. K_2 may be a major source of vitamin K in infants and young children, but less is produced in the intestine of the breast-fed infant.

Vitamin K is necessary for the posttranslational carboxylation of glutamic acid residues of the vitamin K-dependent coagulation proteins. Carboxylation allows these proteins to bind calcium, leading to activation of the clotting factors. Thus, vitamin K is necessary for the maintenance of normal plasma levels of coagulation factors II (prothrombin), VII, IX, and X and is also necessary for maintenance of normal levels of the anticoagulation protein C. Vitamin K deficiency occurs in newborns, especially those who are breast-fed and who do not receive vitamin K prophylaxis at delivery. This deficiency results in hemorrhagic disease of the newborn. Later, vitamin K deficiency may result from fat malabsorption syndromes and the use of nonabsorbed antibiotics and anticoagulant drugs (eg, warfarin). Clinical features are hemorrhage into the skin (purpura), gastrointestinal tract, genital urinary tract, gingiva, lungs, joints,

and central nervous system, which may be fatal. Vitamin K status can be assessed with plasma levels of protein-induced vitamin K absence or by prothrombin time.

Vitamin K requirements are summarized in Table 11–6. Newborns require prophylactic intramuscular vitamin K (0.5–1 mg). For older children with acute bleeding, 3–10 mg of vitamin K is given intramuscularly or intravenously. For chronic malabsorption syndromes, 2.5 mg twice weekly to 5 mg/d is given orally. To reverse warfarin effect, 50–100 mg of intravenous vitamin K is given. Toxic effects are summarized in Table 11–5.

2. WATER-SOLUBLE VITAMINS

Deficiencies of water-soluble vitamins are much less common in the USA because infant formulas and many foods are fortified, particularly with B vitamins. Most bread and wheat products are now routinely fortified with B vitamins. There is now conclusive evidence that folic acid supplements (400 µg/d) during the periconceptional period provide a strong protective effect for neural lobe defects. A good dietary intake of folate, which is likely to result from conformity with current dietary guidelines, also results in significant protection. A good dietary intake of folate as well as a multivitamin supplement in the periconceptional period may also afford protection against neuroectodermal brain tumors in young children.

The danger of toxicity from water-soluble vitamins is not as great because excesses can be excreted in the urine. However, deficiencies in these vitamins can also develop more quickly than deficiencies in fat-soluble vitamins because of the limited stores.

Additional salient details are summarized in Tables 11–6 to 11–11. Although dietary intake of the water-soluble vitamins on a daily basis is not necessary, these vitamins, with the exception of vitamin B_{12}, are not stored in the body.

Carnitine is synthesized in the liver and kidneys from lysine and methionine. In certain circumstances (Table 11–10), however, synthesis is inadequate, and carnitine can then be considered a vitamin. A dietary supply of other organic compounds, such as inositol, may also be required in certain circumstances.

Bunin GR et al: Relation between maternal diet and subsequent primitive neuroectodermal brain tumors in young children. N Engl J Med 1993;329:526.
Recommendations for use of folic acid to reduce number of spina bifida cases and other neural tube defects. MMWR Morb Mortal Wkly Rep 1992;41:1.

Table 11–7. Summary of biologic roles of water-soluble vitamins.

B vitamins involved in production of energy of metabolism
Thiamin (B$_1$)
  Thiamin pyrophosphate is coenzyme in oxidative decarboxylation (pyruvate dehydrogenase, alpha ketoglutarate dehydrogenase, and transketolase).
Riboflavin (B$_2$)
  Coenzyme of several flavoproteins (eg, flavin mononucleotide [FMN] and flavin adenine dinucleotide [FAD]) involved in oxidative/electron transfer enzyme systems.
Niacin
  Hydrogen-carrying coenzymes: nicotinamide-adenine dinucleotide (NAD), nicotinamide-adenine dinucleotide phosphate (NADP); decisive role in intermediary metabolism.
Pantothenic acid
  Major component of coenzyme A.
Biotin
  Component of several carboxylase enzymes involved in fat and carbohydrate metabolism.
Hematopoietic B vitamins
Folic acid
  Tetrahydrofolate has essential role in one-carbon transfers. Essential role in purine and pyramidine synthesis; deficiency → arrest of cell division (especially bone marrow and intestine).
Cobalamin (B$_{12}$)
  Methyl cobalamin (cytoplasm): synthesis of methionine with simultaneous synthesis of tetrahydrofolate (reason for megaloblastic anemia in B$_{12}$ deficiency). Adenosyl cobalamin (mitochondria) is coenzyme for mutases and dehydratases.
Other B vitamins
Pyridoxine (B$_6$)
  Prosthetic group of transaminases, etc involved in amino acid interconversions; prostaglandin and heme synthesis; central nervous system function; carbohydrate metabolism; immune development.
Other water-soluble vitamins
L-Ascorbic acid (C)
  Strong reducing agent—probably involved in all hydroxylations. Roles include collagen synthesis; phenylalanine → tyrosine; tryptophan → 5-OH tryptophan; dopamine → norepinephrine; Fe^{3+} → Fe^{2+}; folic acid → folinic acid; cholesterol → bile acids; leukocyte function; interferon production; carnitine synthesis. Copper metabolism; reduces oxidized vitamin E.
Carnitine
  Transfer of long-chain fatty acids from cytosol to mitochondria (necessary for β-oxidation).

Table 11–8. Major dietary sources of water-soluble vitamins.

Thiamin
  Whole grains, cereals (including fortification), lean pork, liver
Riboflavin
  Dairy products, meat, poultry, wheat germ, leafy vegetables
Pyridoxine
  All foods
Niacin
  Meats, poultry, fish, legumes, wheat, all foods except fats, synthesized in body from tryptophan
Pantothenic acid
  Ubiquitous
Biotin
  Yeast, liver, kidneys, legumes, nuts, egg yolks (synthesized by intestinal bacteria)
Folic acid
  Leafy vegetables (lost in cooking), fruits, whole grains, wheat germ, orange juice, beans, nuts
Cobalamin
  Eggs, dairy products, liver, meats; none in plants
Vitamin C
  Fresh fruits and vegetables
Carnitine
  Meats, dairy products, none in plants

logic factors in breast milk (including secretory IgA, lysozyme, lactoferrin, bifidus factor, and macrophages) help to provide protection against gastrointestinal and upper respiratory infections. In developing countries, lack of refrigeration and contaminated water supplies frequently make formula feeding especially hazardous. Allergic diseases are less common among infants who have been breast-fed. Although formulas have improved progressively and are made to resemble breast milk as closely as possible, it is impossible to mimic the nutritional or immune composition of human milk. Additional differences of physiologic importance continue to be identified; recently identified examples include the substantial quantities of taurine and docosahexaenoic acid found

Table 11–9. Circumstances in which the possibility of vitamin deficiencies merit particular consideration.

Circumstance	Possible Deficiency
Prematurity	All vitamins
Protein-energy malnutrition	B$_1$, B$_2$, folate, A
Synthetic diets (including TPN)	All vitamins
Inherited disorders	Folate, B$_{12}$ D, carnitine
Vitamin-drug interactions	B$_6$, biotin, folate, B$_{12}$, carnitine, fat-soluble vitamins
Fat malabsorption syndrome	Fat-soluble vitamins
Breast-feeding	B$_1$,[1] folate,[2] B$_{12}$,[3] D,[4] K[5]
Periconceptional	Folate

[1]Alcoholic or malnourished mother.
[2]Folate-deficient mother.
[3]Vegan mother.
[4]Infant not exposed to sunlight and mother's vitamin D status suboptimal.
[5]Maternal status poor; neonatal prophylaxis omitted.

INFANT FEEDING

BREAST FEEDING

Breast feeding, one of the most important influences on children's health worldwide, provides optimal nutrition for the normal infant during the early months of life. Numerous immunoactive immuno-

Table 11–10. Causes of deficiencies in water-soluble vitamins.

Thiamin
Infantile beriberi; seen in infants breast-fed by mothers with history of alcoholism or poor diet; has been described as complication of total parenteral nutrition (TPN); protein-energy malnutrition; prematurity.

Riboflavin
General undernutrition; prematurity; inactivation in TPN solutions exposed to light.

Pyridoxine
Prematurity (these infants may not convert pyridoxine → pyridoxal-5-P); B_6 dependency syndromes; drugs (Isoniazid); heat-treated formulas (historical).

Niacin
Maize or millet diets (high leucine and low tryptophan intakes); prematurity.

Pantothenic acid
None.

Biotin
Suppressed intestinal flora and impaired intestinal absorption.

Folic acid
Prematurity; seen in term breast-fed infants whose mothers are folate deficient and in term infants fed unsupplemented processed cow's milk or goat's milk; kwashiorkor; chronic overcooking; malabsorption of folate due to a congenital defect; sprue; celiac disease; drugs (phenytoin).
Increased requirements: chronic hemolytic anemias, diarrhea, malignancies, hypermatabolic states, infections, extensive skin disease, cirrhosis, pregnancy.

Cobalamin
Rare; seen in breast-fed infants of mothers with latent pernicious anemia or who are on an unsupplemented strict vegetarian diet; absence of luminal proteases; congenital malabsorption of B_{12}.

Vitamin C
Prematurity; maternal megadoses during pregnancy → deficiency in infants; lack of fresh fruits or vegetables; seen in infants fed formula and pasteurized cow's milk (historical).

Carnitine
Seen in premature infants fed unsupplemented soy formula or fed intravenously; dialysis; inherited defects in carnitine synthesis; organic acidemias; valproic acid.

transmission. Current recommendations are that HIV-infected mothers in developed countries refrain from breast feeding because of the widely available, safe alternatives. In developing countries, the risk of HIV infection via breast milk is generally considered less than the known benefits of breast feeding, particularly when alternative feeding methods may be hazardous.

The premature infant under 1500 g may benefit from the addition of a milk fortifier, particularly to increase the density of protein, energy, calcium, and phosphorus. Breast-fed infants with cystic fibrosis quite frequently need an energy and protein supplement.

Management of Breast-Feeding

Because most of today's grandmothers bottle-fed their children, the "art" of breast feeding is no longer automatically passed from mother to daughter. Hence, the role of the health professional in supporting and promoting breast feeding is of greater importance. Organizations such as the La Leche League have been effective in promoting breast feeding.

Perinatal hospital routines and follow-up pediatric care have a great impact on the successful initiation of breast feeding. Breast feeding is promoted by pre-

Table 11–11. Clinical features of deficiencies in water-soluble vitamins.

Thiamin
Infantile beriberi (cardiac; aphonic; pseudomeningitic).

Riboflavin
Cheilosis; angular stomatitis; glossitis; soreness and burning of lips and mouth; dermatitis of nasolabial fold and genitals; ± ocular signs (photophobia → indistinct vision).

Pyridoxine
Listlessness; irritability; seizures; gastrointestinal disturbance; anemia; cheilosis; glossitis.

Niacin
Pellagra (weakness; lassitude; dermatitis of exposed areas; diarrhea; dementia).

Pantothenic acid
Weakness; gastrointestinal disturbance; burning feet.

Biotin
Scaly dermatitis; alopecia; irritability; lethargy.

Folate
Megaloblastic anemia; neutropenia; thrombocytopenia; growth retardation; delayed maturation of central nervous system in infants; diarrhea (mucosal ulcerations); glossitis; jaundice; mild splenomegaly; neural tube defects.

Cobalamin
Megaloblastic anemia; neurologic degeneration.

Vitamin C
Anorexia; irritability; apathy; pallor; fever; trachycardia; diarrhea; failure to thrive; increased susceptibility to infections; hemorrhages under skin, mucous membranes, into joints and under periosteum; long-bone tenderness; costochondral beading.

Carnitine
Increased serum triglycerides and free fatty acids; decreased ketones; fatty liver; hypoglycemia; genetic: progressive muscle weakness or cardiomyopathy or hypoglycemia.

in human milk. Furthermore, the relationship developed through breast feeding can be an important part of early maternal interactions with the infant and provides a source of security and comfort to the infant.

In the last decade, breast feeding has been reestablished as the predominant mode of feeding the young infant in the United States. Unfortunately, breast feeding rates remain low among several subpopulations of women, including low-income, minority, and young mothers; many mothers face obstacles in maintaining lactation once they return to work. Skilled use of a breast pump, particularly an electric one, may help to maintain lactation in these circumstances.

Absolute contraindications to breast feeding are rare. They include tuberculosis (in the mother) and galactosemia (in the infant). Although breast milk may serve as a vehicle for transmission of HIV, preliminary evidence suggests this is not a major route of natal and postpartum education, frequent mother-baby contact after delivery, one-on-one advice about breast feeding technique, demand feeding, rooming-in, avoidance of bottle supplements, early follow-up after delivery, maternal confidence, family support, adequate maternity leave, and good advice about common problems such as sore nipples. Breast feeding is undermined by mother and baby separations, feeding babies in the nursery at night, routinely offering supplemental bottles, conflicting advice from staff, incorrect infant positioning and latch-on, scheduled feedings, lack of maternal confidence or support, delayed follow-up, early return to employment, and inaccurate advice for common breast feeding difficulties.

It is important for the mother to know that very few women are unable to nurse their babies. The newborn is generally fed ad libitum every 2–3 hours, with longer intervals (4–5 hours) at night. Thus, a newborn infant nurses eight to ten times a day, so that a generous milk supply is stimulated. This frequency is not an indication of inadequate lactation. Mothers also frequently need to be reassured about stooling pattern. In early stages, a loose stool is often passed with each feeding; later, there may be an interval of several days between stools.

Expressing milk may be indicated if the mother returns to her job or if the infant is premature, cannot suck adequately, or is hospitalized. Modern electric breast pumps are very effective and can be borrowed or rented.

Technique of Breast Feeding

Breast feeding can be started after delivery as soon as both mother and baby are stable. Correct positioning and breast feeding technique are necessary to ensure effective nipple stimulation and optimal breast emptying with minimal nipple discomfort.

If the mother wishes to nurse while sitting, the infant should be elevated to the height of the breast and turned completely to face the mother, so that their abdomens touch. The mother's arms supporting the infant should be held tightly at her side, bringing the baby's head in line with her breast. The breast should be supported by the lower fingers of her free hand, with the nipple compressed between the thumb and index fingers to make it more protractile. The infant's initial licking and mouthing of the nipple helps make it more erect. When the infant opens its mouth, the mother should rapidly insert as much nipple and areola as possible.

Some breast-fed infants fail to thrive. The most common cause of early failure to thrive is poorly managed mammary engorgement, which rapidly decreases milk supply. Unrelieved engorgement can result from inappropriately long intervals between feeding, improper infant suckling, a nondemanding infant, sore nipples, maternal or infant illness, nursing from only one breast, and latching difficulties.

The mother's ignorance of technique, inappropriate feeding routines, and inadequate amounts of fluid and rest for the mother can all be factors. Some infants are too sleepy to do well on an ad libitum regimen and, in particular, may need waking to feed at night. Primary lactation failure is rare but does occur. Some decline in weight for age percentiles after 3 months should not necessarily be interpreted as an indication of inadequate nutrition, because the commonly used percentile charts have been constructed primarily from data on infants who have been formula-fed.

Rigid time restrictions should not be imposed. Sensible guidelines are 5 minutes per breast at each feeding the first day, 10 minutes on each side at each feeding the second day, and approximately 15 minutes per side thereafter. A vigorous infant can obtain most of the available milk in 5–7 minutes, but additional sucking time ensures breast emptying and ongoing milk production and satisfies the infant's sucking urge. The side on which feeding is commenced should be alternated. The mother may break suction gently after nursing by inserting her finger between the baby's gums.

Follow-Up

Individualized assessment before discharge should identify the mothers and infants needing additional support. All cases require early follow-up after discharge. The onset of copious milk secretion between the second and fourth postpartum day is a critical time in the establishment of lactation.

Common Problems

Mild nipple tenderness requires attention to proper positioning of the infant and correct latch-on. Ancilary measures include nursing for shorter periods, beginning feedings on the less sore side, air drying the nipples well after nursing, and the application of lanolin cream. Severe nipple pain and cracking usually indicate improper infant attachment. Temporary pumping, which is well tolerated, may be needed.

Breast feeding jaundice is exaggerated physiologic jaundice associated with inadequate intake of breast milk, infrequent stooling, and unsatisfactory weight gain. If possible, the jaundice should be managed by increasing the frequency of nursing and, if necessary, augmenting the infant's sucking with regular breast pumping. Supplemental feedings may be necessary, but care should be taken not to decrease breast milk production further.

In a small percentage of breast-fed infants, breast milk jaundice is caused by an unidentified property of the milk that inhibits conjugation of bilirubin. In severe cases, interruption of breast feeding for 24–36 hours may be necessary. The mother's breast should be emptied with an electric breast pump during this period.

Maternal mastitis should be suspected when a nursing mother complains of a flu-like illness with local breast tenderness. Antibiotic therapy providing coverage against β-lactamase-producing organisms should be given for 10 days. Analgesics may be necessary, but breast feeding should be continued. Breast pumping may be a helpful adjunctive therapy.

Maternal Drug Use

Many factors play a role in determining the effects of maternal drug therapy on the nursing infant, including the route of administration, dosage, molecular weight, pH, and protein binding. In general, any drug prescribed therapeutically to newborns can be consumed via breast milk without ill effect. Very few therapeutic drugs are absolutely contraindicated; these include radioactive compounds, antimetabolites, lithium, diazepam, chloramphenicol, antithyroid drugs, and tetracycline. For up-to-date information, a regional drug center should be consulted.

Maternal use of illicit or recreational drugs is a contraindication to breast feeding. If a woman is unable to discontinue drug use, she should not breastfeed. Expression of milk for a feeding or two after use of a drug is not an acceptable compromise. The breast-fed infants of mothers taking methadone (but no alcohol or other drugs) as part of a treatment program have generally not experienced ill effects when the daily maternal methadone dose is under 40 mg.

Nutrient Composition

The nutrient composition of human milk is summarized and compared with that of cow's milk and formulas in Table 11–12. Outstanding characteristics include (1) the relatively low protein content, which is, however, quite adequate for the normal infant; (2) a generous but not excessive quantity of essential fatty acids; (3) the presence of long-chain unsaturated fatty acids of the ω3 series, of which docosahexaenoic acid is thought to be especially important; (4) a relatively low sodium and solute load; and (5) the lower concentration of calcium, iron, and zinc, which with the very favorable absorption provides adequate quantities of these nutrients to the normal breast-fed infant for 4–6 months despite the relatively low intakes.

Table 11–12. The composition of milk (per 100 kcal).

Nutrient (Unit)	Minimum Level Recommended[1]	Mature Human Milk	Typical Commercial Formula	Cow's Milk (Mean)
Protein (g)	1.8 (see note 2.)	1.3–1.6	2.3	5.1
Fat (g)	3.3 (See note 3.)	5	5.3	5.7
Carbohydrate (g)	. . .	10.3	10.8	7.3
Linoleic acid (mg)	300	560	2300	125
Vitamin A (IU)	250	250	300	216
Vitamin D (IU)	40	3	63	3
Vitamin E (IU)	0.3 FT 0.7 LBW 1 g linoleic	0.3	2	0.1
Vitamin K (μg)	4	2	9	5
Vitamin C (mg)	8	7.8	8.1	2.3
Thiamin (μg)	40	25	80	59
Riboflavin (μg)	60	60	100	252
Niacin (μg)	250	250	1200	131
Vitamin B_6 (μg)	15 μg/g protein	15	63	66
Folic acid (μg)	4	4	10	8
Pantothenic acid (μg)	300	300	450	489
Vitamin B_{12} (μg)	0.15	0.15	0.25	0.56
Biotin (μg)	1.5	1	2.5	3.1
Inositol (mg)	4	20	5.5	20
Choline (mg)	7	13	10	23
Calcium (mg)	5	50	75	186
Phosphorus (mg)	25	25	65	145
Magnesium (mg)	6	6	8	20
Iron (mg)	1	0.1	1.5 in fortified	0.08
Iodine (μg)	5	4–9	10	7
Copper (μg)	60	25–60	80	20
Zinc (mg)	0.5	0.1–0.5	0.65	0.6
Manganese (μg)	5	1.5	5–160	3
Sodium (meq)	0.9	1	1.7	3.3
Potassium (meq)	2.1	2.1	2.7	6
Chloride (meq)	1.6	1.6	2.3	4.6
Osmolarity (mosm)	. . .	11.3	16–18.4	40

[1]Committee on Nutrition, American Academy of Pediatrics.
[2]Protein of nutritional quality equal to casein.
[3]Includes 300 mg essential fatty acids.

Weaning

Weaning can take place according to the needs and desires of both infant and mother. Gradual weaning, starting typically after 4–6 months, is preferred. Bottle feedings (or cup feedings) are increased progressively over a period of several weeks as breast feedings are omitted.

Committee on Drugs, American Academy of Pediatrics: Transfer of drugs and other chemical to human milk. Pediatrics 1989;84:924.

Cunningham AS, Jelliffe DB, Jelliffe EFP: Breast-feeding and health in the 1980s: A global epidemiologic review. 1991;118:659.

Dewey KG et al: Growth of breast-fed and formula-fed infants from zero to 18 months: The Darling Study. Pediatrics 1992;89:1035.

Freed GL, Landers SC, Schanler RJ: A practical guide to successful breast-feeding management. Am J Dis Child 1991;145:917.

Krebs NF et al: Growth and intakes of energy and zinc in infants fed human milk. J Pediatr 1994;124:32–9.

Lawrence RA: *Breastfeeding: A Guide for the Medical Profession,* 3rd ed. Mosby, 1989.

Oxtoby MJ: Human immunodeficiency virus and other viruses in human milk: Placing the issues in broader perspective. Pediatr Infect Dis J 1988;7:825.

SPECIAL DIETARY PRODUCTS FOR INFANTS

Feeding During the Second Six Months

The standard (iron-fortified) infant formulas are suitable for use in the second 6 months. These formulas are preferred to unmodified cow's milk, which may be introduced cautiously after 9 months of age.

Soy Protein Formulas

The major indication for the use of soy protein formulas is lactose intolerance. For example, it is reasonable to recommend a soy protein formula during recovery from acute gastroenteritis for a period of 2–4 weeks. A lactose-free cow's milk-based formula is also available (Lactofree, Mead Johnson). Soy protein formulas are also used frequently in cases of suspected intolerance to cow's milk protein. However, infants who have true cow's milk protein intolerance may also be intolerant of soy protein. Many infants in the United States are currently fed soy protein formulas without good reason.

Semielemental Formulas

These formulas include Pregestimil (Mead Johnson), Nutramigen (Mead Johnson), and Alimentum (Ross). The major nitrogen source of each of these products is casein hydrolysate, supplemented with selected amino acids. Each contains an abundance of EFA from vegetable oil; Pregestimil and Alimentum also provide substantial amounts of medium-chain triglycerides (MCT). Pregestimil contains corn syrup solids; Nutramigen contains sucrose, which also provides part of the carbohydrate content in Alimentum.

These formulas are invaluable in a wide variety of malabsorption syndromes, including short bowel syndromes and some cases of chronic diarrhea and cystic fibrosis. They are also effective in feeding infants who cannot tolerate cow's milk and soy protein.

Formula Supplements

The most useful formula supplements are MCT oil and polycose, both of which may be used to increase the energy density of a formula. Often it is more appropriate, however, to increase the concentration of the formula and thus increase the density of all nutrients.

Special Formulas

Special formulas include those in which one component, often an amino acid, is reduced in concentration or removed for the dietary management of specific inborn metabolic diseases. Also included under this heading is Amin-Aid (American McGaw).

Complete information regarding the composition of these special formulas, the standard infant formulas, and special formulas for premature infants can be found in standard reference texts such as the Harriet Lane handbook (*A Manual for Pediatric House Officers,*)* and in the manufacturer's literature.

PRUDENT DIET

A prudent diet should be encouraged for all children 2 years of age and older: children with high cholesterol levels tend to become adults with high cholesterol levels and are likely, therefore, to have an increased risk of coronary heart disease. Nutritional habits are formed early in life; dietary intervention may, therefore, be exceptionally effective when started in early childhood.

Salient features of a prudent diet include the following:

(1) Total fat should constitute less than 30% of caloric intake, with saturated fats and polyunsaturated fats providing less than 10% each. Thus, monounsaturated fats should provide 10% or more of caloric intake from fat.

(2) Cholesterol intake should be less than 100 mg/1000 kcal/d, to a maximum of 300 mg/d.

(3) Carbohydrates should provide 60% or more of daily caloric intake, with 50% or more in the form of complex carbohydrates (ie, no more than 10% in the form of simple sugars). A high-fiber diet is also recommended.

---

*References: (1) Foman SJ et al: Formulas for older infants. J Pediatr 1990;116:690. (2) Greene MG: *The Harriet Lane Handbook,* 12th ed. Mosby Year Book, 1991.

(4) The diet should be nutritionally complete, include a variety of foods, and be adequate for optimal growth and activity.

(5) A low salt intake is advised.

The consumption of lean cuts of meats and poultry should be encouraged. Fish should be broiled or baked. Skim milk, soft margarine, and vegetable oils (especially olive oil) should be used. Consumption of egg yolks should be limited to two or three occasions per week. Whole-grain bread and cereals and plentiful amounts of fruits and vegetables are recommended. The consumption of processed foods, soft drinks, desserts, and candy should be limited.

A prudent diet should be only one component of counseling on life-styles for children. Other aspects are the maintenance of ideal body weight, a regular exercise program, avoidance of smoking, and screening for hypertension. Universal screening for total cholesterol is controversial. Current recommendations are to routinely screen those children who have a positive family history of premature cardiovascular disease, although this approach will identify only about 50% of those with significantly elevated cholesterol levels. If the result is high ($\geq$ 200 mg/dL), a lipoprotein analysis should be obtained.

Committee on Nutrition, American Academy of Pediatrics: Statement on cholesterol. Pediatrics 1992;90:469.

Lund EK et al: Dietary fat intake and plasma lipid levels in adolescents. Eur J Clin Nutr 1992;46:857.

National Cholesterol Education Program Coordinating Committee. Highlights of the report of the expert panel on blood cholesterol levels in children and adolescents. Bethesda, MD: NHLBI Information Center, 1991.

INTRAVENOUS NUTRITION

INDICATIONS

Supplemental Peripheral Nutrition

Supplemental peripheral nutrition is indicated when complete enteral feeding is not possible or desirable (eg, in the premature infant of very low birth weight during the first few days of postnatal life or in the malnourished surgical patient during the early postoperative period). Short-term partial intravenous feeding is a preferred alternative to dextrose and electrolyte solutions alone. A suitable central line, if already available, can be used, but supplemental short-term nutrition may also be administered via a peripheral vein. Because of the osmolality of the solutions required, it is usually impossible to achieve total parenteral nutrition via a peripheral vein.

Total Parenteral Nutrition

Total parenteral nutrition (TPN) should be provided only when clearly indicated. Apart from the expense, numerous risks are associated with this method of feeding (see below). In addition, the powerful homeostatic control mechanisms provided by the intestine and the liver are bypassed. Even when TPN is indicated, every effort should be made to provide at least a minimum of nutrients enterally to help preserve the integrity of the gastrointestinal mucosa and of gastrointestinal function. Such feeding helps, at least to some extent, to maintain the physiologic release of gut hormones, bile flow, and the integrity of the enterocyte.

The primary indication for TPN is the loss of function of the gastrointestinal tract that prohibits the provision of more than a small proportion of required nutrients by the enteral route. Important examples include short bowel syndrome and some congenital defects of the gastrointestinal tract.

CATHETER SELECTION & POSITION

The Broviac is the catheter of choice for long-term intravenous nutrition. For periods of up to 3–4 weeks, a percutaneous central venous catheter threaded into the superior vena cava from a peripheral vein can be used. For the infusion of dextrose concentrations higher than 12.5%, the tip of the catheter should be located in the superior vena cava or right atrium. After placement, a chest x-ray must be obtained to check this position. If the catheter is to be used for nutrition and medications, a double-line catheter should be inserted.

COMPLICATIONS

Mechanical Complications

A. Related to Catheter Insertion or to Erosion of Catheter Through Major Blood Vessel: There is an extensive list of complications involving trauma to adjacent tissues and organs, including damage to the brachial plexus, hydrothorax, pneumothorax, hemothorax, and cerebrospinal fluid penetration. The catheter may slip, especially if care is not taken at the time of dressing or tubing change. The patient may manipulate the line.

B. Clotting of the Catheter: Addition of heparin (1 unit/mL) to the solution is an effective means of preventing this complication. If a catheter does become occluded, urokinase can be administered for clot lysis.

C. Related to Composition of Infusate: Calcium phosphate precipitation is a major problem if excess amounts of calcium or phosphorus are administered. The quantities of calcium and phosphate that can be added to the infusate vary widely, depending upon the particular commercial amino acid source. Intravenous calcium boluses should not be administered through a Broviac catheter. Factors that increase the risk of calcium phosphate precipitation include increasing pH and decreasing concentrations of amino acids. Precipitation of medications incompatible with TPN or lipids can also cause clotting.

Septic Complications

Septic complications are the most common cause of nonelective catheter removal, but strict use of aseptic technique and once-daily entry into the catheter at tubing change can result in greatly reduced rates of line sepsis. *For this reason, strict adherence to the standardized nursing protocol (for nurses and physicians) is mandatory.*

Metabolic Complications

A wide variety of metabolic complications associated with total parenteral malnutrition has been documented. Many of these have been related to deficiencies or excesses of specific nutrients. The incidence of these complications has decreased as a result of improvements in amino acid solutions and lipid emulsions and a better understanding of how to achieve appropriate intakes of most nutrients. However, specific deficiencies still occur, especially in the premature infant. Avoidance of deficiencies and excesses and of metabolic disorders requires careful attention to the nutrient balance, electrolyte composition, and delivery rate of the infusate and careful monitoring, especially when the composition or delivery rate is changed.

Currently, the most challenging metabolic complication is cholestasis, particularly common in premature infants of very low birth weight. Amino acids competing for and blocking bile acid receptors at the hepatocyte appear to be one critical factor in the pathogenesis of this disorder. Complete lack of oral feeding, sepsis, free radical damage, or toxic factors present in TPN solutions may contribute to this problem. There are no amino acid solutions currently available that have been proved to decrease cholestasis. Maneuvers that *may* minimize cholestasis include administering some enteral feedings (even if very small) as soon as feasible, protecting the TPN solutions from light, and alternating relatively larger doses with lower doses of amino acids every other day (eg, 1 g/kg/d alternating with 3 g/kg/d rather than administering 2 g/kg/d).

NUTRIENT REQUIREMENTS & DELIVERY

Energy

When patients are fed intravenously, no fat and carbohydrate intakes are unabsorbed, and no energy is used in nutrient absorption. These factors account for at least 7% of energy in the diet of the enterally fed subject. The intravenously fed patient also expends less energy in physical activity because of the impediment to mobility. Average energy requirements are, therefore, at least 7% lower in children fed intravenously, and the decrease in activity probably increases this figure to a total reduction of 10–15%. Caloric guidelines for the intravenous feeding of infants and young children are as follows:

Age (months)	Requirements (kcal/kg/d)
2–4	100–110
4–36	90–100
4–36	75–80

These guidelines are averages; individuals vary considerably. Some older infants require 70 kcal/kg/d or less and on higher intravenous intakes will become obese. A multitude of factors can significantly increase the energy requirement, including exposure to a cold environment, fever, sepsis, burns, trauma, cardiac or pulmonary disease, and "catch-up" growth after malnutrition.

With few exceptions, eg, some cases of respiratory insufficiency, at least 60% of energy requirements is provided as glucose. Up to 40% of calories may be provided by intravenous fat emulsions.

Dextrose

The energy density of intravenous dextrose (monohydrate) is 3.4 kcal/g. Thus, a 10% solution of dextrose in water ($D_{10}W$) provides 0.34 kcal/mL. Dextrose is the main exogenous energy source provided by total intravenous feeding. Intravenous dextrose suppresses gluconeogenesis and provides a substrate that can be oxidized directly, especially by the brain, red and white blood cells, and wounds. Because of the high osmolality of dextrose solutions ($D_{10}W$ yields 505 mosm/kg H_2O), concentrations greater than 10–12.5% cannot be delivered via a peripheral vein or improperly positioned central line.

It is customary to think only in terms of dextrose concentrations when ordering intravenous solutions. However, the amount of glucose supplied is determined by the rate of administration as well as the dextrose concentration. Consequently, it is important to calculate the desired glucose load in planning dextrose infusions. If fluid volume is restricted, a higher dextrose concentration can be used to deliver the same quantity of dextrose per unit of time into the superior vena cava. Conversely, if unusually rapid initial flow rates are being used, a correspondingly lower dextrose concentration is indicated.

The standard initial quantity of dextrose administered is 10 g/kg/d, which provides 34 kcal/kg/d. This is typically, but not necessarily, provided as 100 mL/kg/d of $D_{10}W$. Tolerance to intravenous dextrose normally increases rapidly, primarily because hepatic production of endogenous glucose is suppressed. Dextrose can be increased by 2.5 g/kg/d. Standard final infusates for infants usually contain $D_{20}W$, but if necessary (especially at low flow rates), concentrations up to $D_{30}W$ or greater may be used. Again, these high concentrations should be delivered only into the superior vena cava or right atrium. Tolerance to intravenous dextrose loads is markedly diminished in the premature neonate and in patients in hypermetabolic states.

Problems associated with intravenous dextrose administration include hyperglycemia, hyperosmolality, and glucosuria (with osmotic diuresis and dehydration). Possible causes of unexpected hyperglycemia include the following: (1) inadvertent infusion of higher glucose concentrations than ordered; (2) uneven flow rate; (3) sepsis; (4) a stress situation; and (5) pancreatitis. Intravenous insulin reduces hyperglycemia but does not increase glucose oxidation rates; it may also decrease the oxidation of fatty acids, resulting in less energy for metabolism. Hence, insulin should be used very cautiously. A standard intravenous dose is 1 unit per 4 g of carbohydrate, but much smaller quantities may be adequate. Exogenous insulin is probably contraindicated in hypermetabolic states.

Hypoglycemia may occur after an abrupt decrease in or cessation of intravenous glucose. When cyclic intravenous nutrition is provided, the intravenous glucose load should be decreased steadily for 1–2 hours prior to discontinuing the infusate. If the central line must be removed, the intravenous dextrose should be gradually tapered over several hours.

The maximum oxidation rate of infused dextrose in infants is 18 g/kg/d (less if given with $\geq$ 3 g lipid/kg/d). The corresponding rates at 6 years, at 10 years, and in adult life are 13, 8, and 4.3 g/kg/d, respectively. The very low birth weight neonate seldom tolerates more than 8–12 g/kg/d. Quantities of exogenous dextrose in excess of maximal glucose oxidation rates are used initially to replace depleted glycogen stores; hepatic lipogenesis occurs thereafter. Excess hepatic lipogenesis may lead to a fatty liver when hepatic secretion of very low density lipoproteins fails to keep pace with lipogenesis. Lipogenesis results in release of carbon dioxide, which when added to the amount of carbon dioxide produced by glucose oxidation (which is 40% greater than that produced by lipid oxidation) may elevate the $PaCO_2$ and aggravate respiratory insufficiency or impede weaning from a respirator.

Lipids

Several commercial fat emulsions are now available for intravenous use. All consist of more than 50% linoleic acid and 4–9% linolenic acid. It is recognized that this high level of linoleic is far from ideal except when small quantities of lipid are being given to prevent a deficiency in essential fatty acids. Ultimately, improved emulsions are anticipated. The particle size is approximately that of chylomicrons (0.5 µm), but the particle contains no protein. Thus, the infused fat emulsion must acquire apolipoprotein C-II from HDL particles before it can be acted on by endothelium-bound lipoprotein lipase (LPL) or hepatic triglyceride lipase. The level of LPL activity is the rate-limiting factor in the metabolism and clearance of fat emulsions from the circulation. LPL activity is inhibited or decreased by malnutrition, leukotrienes, immaturity, growth hormone, hypercholesterolemia, hyperphospholipidemia, and theophylline. LPL activity is enhanced by glucose, insulin, lipid, catecholamines, and exercise. Heparin releases LPL from the endothelium into the circulation and enhances the rate of hydrolysis and clearance of triglycerides. In small premature infants, low-dose heparin infusions may increase tolerance to intravenous lipid emulsion. After hydrolysis of the triglycerides, the residual phospholipid forms a vesicle that acquires free cholesterol from peripheral cell membranes, forming an abnormal lipoprotein particle (LpX). This particle is metabolized only slowly by the liver and accounts for the hyperphospholipidemia and hypercholesterolemia that may occur during administration of intravenous fat emulsions. Because 10% and 20% lipid emulsions contain the same concentrations of phospholipids, a 10% solution delivers more phospholipid per gram of lipid than a 20% solution. Twenty percent lipid emulsions are preferred for all patients.

The advantages of using fat emulsions to provide up to 40% of caloric intake include the following:

(1) The energy density, which is 2 kcal/mL for 20% emulsions, allows more energy to be provided when fluid volume is restricted.

(2) The low osmolality is (280 mosm/kg H_2O) is of special value when using a peripheral line.

(3) Deficiencies in essential fatty acids can be prevented.

(4) The production of CO_2 is 40% lower per unit of energy, an important consideration in cases of pulmonary insufficiency.

(5) The energy cost of fat storage is negligible (energy does not have to be synthesized from dextrose).

(6) The risk of fatty liver is decreased because of decreased hepatic lipogenesis from dextrose.

Potential disadvantages of fat emulsions include the following:

(1) Impairment of function of lymphocytes, neutrophils, macrophages, and the reticuloendothelial system.

(2) Coagulation defects, including thrombocytopenia, elevated prothrombin time (PT), and partial thromboplastin time (PTT).

(3) Decrease in pulmonary oxygen diffusion.

(4) Competition with bilirubin and drugs for albumin-binding sites.

(5) Increase in LDL cholesterol.

In general, these adverse effects can be avoided by starting with modest quantities and advancing cautiously in light of results of triglyceride monitoring and clinical circumstances. In cases of severe sepsis, special caution is required to ensure that the lipid is effectively metabolized. Continuous monitoring with long-term use is also essential.

Start with 1 g/kg/d. Advance every 1–2 days by 0.5–1 g/kg/d up to 2.5 g/kg/d in an infant and 3.5 g/kg/d in a child. Check serum triglycerides before starting and before and after increasing dose. Request results the same day. As a general rule, do not increase dose if serum triglyceride is greater than 250 mg/dL during infusion (150 mg/dL in neonates and septic patients). Clearance 4 hours postinfusion should also be monitored (< 150 mg/dL).

Note: Linoleic acid must constitute 2–3% of caloric intake (300 mg linoleic acid per 100 kcal) so that a deficiency in essential fatty acids can be avoided. Linolenic acid (1%) is also needed and is adequately supplied when linoleic acid needs are met.

Nitrogen

One gram of nitrogen is yielded by 6.25 g of protein (1 g of protein contains 16% nitrogen). Caloric density of protein is equal to 4 kcal/g (but protein calories must *not* be included in calculations of daily caloric intake).

A. Protein Requirements: Protein requirements for intravenous feeding are the same as those for normal oral feeding (Table 11–2).

B. Protein-Energy Interactions: There are important interactions between protein and energy requirements. A positive nitrogen balance cannot be achieved on a hypocaloric diet, because protein will be catabolized for energy. When energy intakes are low, the administration of some amino acid does, however, improve the severity of the negative nitrogen balance. Conversely, when nitrogen intake is low, the provision of calories improves nitrogen balance to some extent. In infants, the energy necessary to minimize nitrogen loss associated with an amino acid-free diet is approximately 70 kcal/kg/d. At this level of energy intake, a positive nitrogen balance can be achieved to a degree that depends on the level of nitrogen intake and is independent of further increase in energy intake.

In infants receiving about 50 kcal/kg/d, increasing protein intake up to 3 g/kg/d improves the nitrogen balance. In these circumstances, therefore, a ratio of grams of nitrogen per kilocalorie as low as 1:100 can be advantageous. However, at higher levels of energy intake, ratios of 1:250 to 1:150 or more are optimal. Although these ratios provide a useful crude check, they are not usually the best means of determining protein requirements.

C. Intravenous Amino Acid Solutions: Nitrogen requirements are provided by one of the commercially available amino acid solutions. All of the standard preparations are equally good sources of amino acids. There is some preliminary evidence, however, that the use of TrophAmine in premature infants is associated with superior nitrogen retention. The putative benefits of TrophAmine are quite likely attributable in part to the cysteine that can be added to the solution immediately before use. Forty milligrams of cysteine is added for each gram of TrophAmine. Thus, 1 L of 2% solution requires an addition of 800 mg of cysteine. Cysteine (when given as Trophamine or as Aminosyn-PF) provides a good source of taurine.

Normally, the final infusate contains 2–3% amino acids, depending on the rate of infusion. In the very low birth weight or severely malnourished infant, the initial amount should be 1 g/kg/d.

Because of the high osmolality of amino acid solutions, the concentration should not be advanced beyond 2% in peripheral vein infusates.

D. Monitoring: Monitoring for tolerance of the intravenous amino acid solutions should include routine blood urea nitrogen (BUN). Blood ammonia should be assayed if clinically indicated, but the incidence of hyperammonemia has decreased since the development of the newer intravenous nitrogen preparations. More important are assays (serum alkaline phosphatase, γ-glutamyltransferase) to detect the onset of cholestatic liver disease.

E. Special Amino Acid Preparations: Some solutions are designed to provide high concentrations of branched-chain amino acids. These solutions are expensive and should not be ordered without a specific reason, which does not include their routine use in liver disease. They may be indicated in hepatic failure and are also undergoing experimental use in multisystem organ failure. In this circumstance, the branched-chain amino acids are given as a source of metabolizable energy, providing up to 25% of energy intake. Solutions containing only essential amino acids have some application in the management of patients with renal failure.

F. Albumin: Albumin (0.5–1 g/kg/dose) can be added to the infusate when clinically indicated to restore blood volume. If the pathogenetic origin of hypoalbuminemia is considered to be primarily nutritional, however, the hypoalbuminemia—even if severe—should be managed by careful nutritional rehabilitation rather than by intravenous administration of albumin. Albumin is deficient in isoleucine and tryptophan and has too long a half-life (15–20 days) to be considered a useful nutritional source of amino acids.

Minerals & Electrolytes

A. Calcium, Phosphorus, and Magnesium: The results of two recent studies have indicated that the intravenously fed premature and term infant should be given relatively high amounts of calcium and phosphorus. Although lower amounts of calcium are routinely provided in many centers, current recommendations are as follows: calcium, 500–600 mg/L; phosphorus, 400–450 mg/L; and magnesium, 50–70 mg/L. After the age of 1 year, the recommendations are as follows: calcium, 200–400 mg/L; phosphorus, 150–300 mg/L; and magnesium, 20–40 mg/L. The calcium:phosphorus ratio should be 1.3:1 by weight or 1:1 by molar ratio. These recommendations are deliberately presented on a per liter infusate basis to avoid inadvertent administration of concentrations of calcium and phosphorus that are high enough to precipitate in the tubing. During periods of fluid restriction, care must be taken not to inadvertently increase the concentration of calcium and phosphorus in the infusate. These recommendations assume an average fluid intake of 120–150 mL/kg/d and an infusate of 25 g of amino acid per liter. With lower amino acid concentrations, the concentrations of calcium and phosphorus should be decreased.

B. Electrolytes: Standard recommendations are given in Figure 11–1. After chloride requirements are met, the remainder of the anion required to balance the cation should be given as acetate to avoid the possibility of acidosis resulting from excessive chloride. The required concentrations of electrolytes depend to some extent on the flow rate of the infusate and must be modified if flow rates are unusually low or high and if there are specific indications in individual patients. Intravenous sodium should be administered very sparingly in the severely malnourished patient because of impaired membrane function and high intracellular sodium levels. Conversely, generous quantities of potassium are indicated. Replacement electrolytes and fluids should be delivered via a separate infusate.

C. Trace Elements: Recommended intravenous intakes of trace elements are given in Figure 11–1.

When intravenous nutrition is only supplemental or limited to less than 2 weeks, only zinc need routinely be added.

Intravenous copper requirements are relatively low in the young infant because of the presence of hepatic copper stores. These are significant even in the 28-week fetus. Circulating levels of copper and manganese should be monitored in the presence of cholestatic liver disease. If monitoring is not feasible, temporary withdrawal of added copper and manganese is advisable. Copper and manganese are excreted primarily in the bile, but selenium, chromium, and molybdenum are excreted primarily in the urine. These trace elements, therefore, should be administered with caution in the presence of renal failure.

For patients on long-term parenteral nutrition, a dose of 1 µg/kg/d of iodine avoids any risk of iodine deficiency and does not increase the risk of toxicity from accidental absorption of topical iodine-containing preparations.

Although low doses of iron are routinely added in some centers to the intravenous infusate for infants and children, no official recommendation has been made because of the lack of adequate published data regarding compatibility. Iron added to the infusate should be in a diluted form of iron dextran in a concentration of 1 mg/L. After 2 months of age, maintenance intravenous iron requirements for the term infant are approximately 100 µg/kg/d intravenously. After the first month, the premature infant requires up to 200 µg/kg/d intravenously. Although overload is unlikely to occur during short-term parenteral nutrition, a surreptitious accumulation of extra iron could occur if parenteral nutrition is prolonged. This risk is enhanced if the patient has received blood transfusions. A second concern is that the potential for free iron is increased in malnourished infants with low transferrin levels. Excess iron is thought to enhance the risk of gram-negative septicemia. Iron has powerful oxidant properties and can enhance the demand for antioxidants, especially vitamin E. None of these concerns appear to preclude the routine use of iron supplements during intravenous nutrition, but they do emphasize the need for a conservative attitude in determining dosage schedules.

Currently, intravenous infusates are contaminated with aluminum. In infants, aluminum accumulation in bone after 3 weeks of intravenous feeding can be marked. Aluminum intakes should be measured when possible, especially in the premature infant and in the infant or child with impaired renal function.

Vitamins

Recommendations for intravenous vitamin intakes are given in Table 11–6. MVI Pediatric (Armour) meets the guidelines for term infants. The recommended dose of MVI Pediatric for premature infants is 2 mL (40%) of a single-dose vial per kilogram per day. This formulation is not optimal (too little vitamin A, excessive amounts of water-soluble vitamins), but it is currently the best available.

Intravenous lipid preparations contain enough tocopherol to effect total blood tocopherol levels. The majority of tocopherol in soybean oil emulsion is γ-tocopherol, which has substantially less biologic activity than α-tocopherol, which is present in safflower oil emulsions. Premature infants may possibly be susceptible to liver damage from excessive intakes of vitamin E. The intravenous administration of 25–100 mg/d of α-tocopherol acetate for as little as one week has been associated with coagulopathy and progressive liver failure in several infants of very low birth weight. The toxicity may well have been due to the solubilizer, polysorbate 80, rather than to the α-tocopherol.

Recent data indicate that a dose of 40 IU/kg/d of vitamin D (maximum 400 IU/d) is adequate for both term and preterm infants. The higher dose of 160 IU/kg/d has not been associated with any complication and continues to be recommended.

PEDIATRIC PARENTERAL NUTRITION (PN) ORDER FORM

Imprint Patient Plate

_____

Weight of patient _____ kg   Central line _____   Peripheral line _____

Rate _____

	Standard Order	Modifications To Standard Order	*Adjustments for Neonates and Premature Infants (Circle these when required and cross out corresponding items* under "standard order").
Protein (as amino acid)*	g%		*Use trophamine and cysteine for patients in level II and III nurseries who have a central line or are on day 6 of peripheral therapy.
Dextrose	g%		
Na	30 meq/L		
K	25 meq/L		
Cl	20 meq/L		
Acetate	45 meq/L		
Ca (as gluconate) (10 mM Ca/L)	20 meq/L		
Mg (as sulfate)	3 meq/L		
P	10 meq/L		
MVI Pediatric	*5.0 mL/d		*2 mL/kg/d for patients < 2.5 kg
Zinc	*1.0 mg/L		*Zn: 400 µg/kg/d < 2 kg body weight
Copper	200 µg/L		250 µg/kg/d others < 3 mo old
Manganese	5.0 µg/L		
Chromium	2.0 µg/L		
Selenium	20.0 µg/L		
Iodide	10 µg/L		
Heparin	1000 Units/L		
Cysteine (40 mg/g trophamine)*	._____ mg/L		*Use only with trophamine

Pharmacy will automatically account for electrolytes provided in amino acid preparation.
Changes in Na or K to be made as: Cl only __, or Acetate only __, or Cl: Acetate 1:1 __, or other
Cl: Acetate ratio (specify _____).

Date: _____   Signature: _____ M.D.

Figure 11–1. Example of pediatric parenteral nutrition order. Standard recommendations for minerals and trace elements are indicated.

Fluid Requirements

The initial fluid volume and subsequent increments in flow rate are determined by basic fluid requirements, the clinical status of the patient, and the extent to which additional fluid administration can be tolerated and may be required to achieve adequate nutrient intake. Calculation of initial fluid volumes to be administered should be based on standard pediatric practice. Tolerance of higher flow rates must be determined on an individual basis. If replacement fluids are required for ongoing abnormal losses, these should be administered via a separate line.

Ordering

An example of a parenteral nutrition order form for pediatrics is given in Figure 11–1. Orders should be reviewed daily when changes are made and when the patient is acutely ill.

Monitoring

Vital signs should be checked at each shift.

With central catheter in situ and fever more than 38 °C, peripheral and central line blood cultures, urine cultures, complete physical examination, and examination of intravenous entry point are required. Instability of vital signs, elevated white blood cell count with left shift, and glycosuria suggest sepsis. Appropriate antibiotic therapy should be instituted after cultures and blood cultures repeated every 24 hours until results are negative. Removal of the central venous catheter should be considered if patient is toxic or unresponsive to antibiotics (the patient must be weaned of dextrose prior to removal of the catheter).

A. Physical Examination: Monitor especially for hepatomegaly (differential diagnoses include fluid overload, congestive heart failure, steatosis, and hepatitis) and edema (differential diagnoses: fluid overload, congestive heart failure, hypoalbuminemia, thrombosis of superior vena cava).

B. Intake/Output Record: Calories and volume delivered should be calculated from previous day's intake and output sheets (that which was delivered rather than that which was ordered). The following should be recorded on flow sheets: intravenous, enteral, and total fluid (mL/kg/d); dextrose (g/kg/d); protein (g/kg/d); lipids (g/kg/d); energy (kcal/kg/d).

C. Growth, Urine, and Blood: Routine monitoring guidelines given in Table 11–13 are only a guide. These are minimum requirements, except in the very long term stable patients. Individual variables should be monitored more frequently as indicated, as should additional variables or clinical indications. For example, a blood ammonia should be ordered in an infant with lethargy, pallor, poor growth, acidosis, azotemia, and elevated liver enzymes.

Fomon SJ, Heird WC (editors): *Energy and Protein Needs During Infancy.* Academic Press, 1986.

Greene HL et al: Guidelines for the use of vitamins, trace elements, calcium, magnesium, and phosphorus in infants and children receiving total parenteral nutrition: Report of the Subcommittee on Pediatric Parenteral Nutrient Requirements from the Committee on Clinical Practice Issues of the American Society for Clinical Nutrition. Am J Clin Nutr 1988;48:1324.

Heird WC et al: Amino acid mixture designed to maintain normal plasma amino acid patterns in infants and children requiring parenteral nutrition. Pediatrics 1987;80: 401.

Kerner JA (editor): *Manual of Pediatric Parenteral Nutrition.* Wiley, 1983.

INTENSIVE CARE NUTRITION

Intravenous Delivery of Nutrients

The availability of sufficient intravenous lines for nutrition in addition to other multiple needs for intravenous access is a perennial problem in the intensive care setting. In many instances, the position of these lines, frequently placed for other purposes under emergency conditions, also prevents their use for nutritional support. Double-lumen catheters, with tips

Table 11–13. Routine monitoring summary.

Variables	Acute Stage	Long-Term
Growth		
Weight	Daily	Weekly
Length	Weekly	
Head circumference	Weekly	
Urine		
Glucose (dipstick)	Void	Twice weekly
Specific gravity	Void	
Volume	Daily	
Blood		
Glucose	4 hours after changes,[1] then daily for 2 days	Twice weekly
Na+, K+, Cl−, CO_2, BUN	Daily for 2 days after changes,[1] then twice weekly	Twice weekly
Ca^{2+}, Mg^{2+}, P	Initially, then twice weekly	Weekly
Total protein, albumin, bilirubin, AST, and alkaline phosphatase	Initially, then weekly	Every other week
Zinc and copper	Initially, then weekly	Monthly
Triglycerides	Initially, 1 day after changes,[1] then weekly	Weekly
CBC	Initially, then twice weekly; according to clinical indications (see text)	Twice weekly

[1]Changes include alterations in concentration or flow rate.

located in the superior vena cava or right atrium, should be placed whenever possible so that these difficulties can be minimized. In some cases, these catheters can be placed electively prior to major procedures.

The need for fluid restriction, combined with extensive administration of fluids for nonnutritional purposes, also limits opportunities to provide adequate nutrition. This problem can be mitigated to some extent by the immediate use of more concentrated solutions of dextrose, amino acids, vitamins, and trace elements. Provided that the catheter tip is placed in the superior vena cava, the most important factor is the quantity delivered and not the concentration in the line. The only exceptions to this principle are calcium and phosphorus.

Provision of Nutrients in Hypermetabolic States

The most important principle is to continue enteral feeding whenever possible. If enteral feeding must be discontinued, it should be reintroduced as soon as possible so that the integrity of the enterocytes can be maintained. The increase in energy requirements varies according to the severity of hypermetabolism and its cause. Requirements are highest in burn patients, but major trauma and severe sepsis increase energy expenditure by 20–50%.

The uncontrolled muscle proteolysis and negative nitrogen balance, which are among the most outstanding features of hypermetabolic states, cannot be counteracted totally by aggressive nutrition support or by other known therapeutic modalities. However, optimal nutrition support does help significantly in reversing the adverse effects of hypermetabolism. Negative nitrogen balance can be improved by providing 1½ to two times the basal protein requirement for that age. Larger quantities do not further improve nitrogen balance; furthermore, they require substantial energy expenditure for their oxidation and increase CO_2 production. Additional amounts of branched-chain amino acids, however, are currently being used experimentally as an energy source to provide up to 25% of caloric needs.

Another major metabolic aberration in hypermetabolic states, compared with the metabolic response to fasting, is persistent, uncontrolled hepatic gluconeogenesis. Elevated blood glucose concentrations are one of the early laboratory indicators of hypermetabolism. Gluconeogenesis is not switched off—as would normally be expected—by the administration of intravenous dextrose. Although some exogenous dextrose will be oxidized, the amount is likely to be quite limited. Dextrose administration tends to aggravate hyperglycemia and increase hepatic lipogenesis. The aim should be to provide at least 50% of energy requirements as dextrose, but in some patients (especially those who develop multisystem organ failure), only very modest quantities will be tolerated. If severe hyperglycemia and glycosuria occur, temporary insulin therapy is necessary. However, the putative effects of insulin in hypermetabolic states are complex and not well clarified. Hypermetabolism is characterized by insulin resistance. Insulin does not reverse the uncontrolled muscle catabolism and gluconeogenesis, nor does administration of insulin increase glucose oxidation. Theoretically, insulin administration could decrease lipolysis and thus deprive the hypermetabolic patient of some of the major sources of utilizable endogenous fuel.

Lipolysis is increased in hypermetabolic states; β-oxidation of fatty acids is also increased initially. Ketogenesis, although it occurs in starvation states, does not occur in hypermetabolic states. Utilization of exogenous lipids depends on the rate of release of endogenous fatty acids versus the rate of β-oxidation. Intravenous lipids can usually be utilized quite well in early stages, and up to 50% of energy may be provided as lipid. Metabolically, lipid is the preferred fuel in patients with severe sepsis. Lipid tolerance deteriorates in advanced multisystem organ failure. Carnitine deficiency may limit utilization in some cases.

The metabolic and nutritional advantages of lipid as a fuel must be balanced against potential adverse effects in the septic child. These may include some impairment of the function of lymphocytes, neutrophils, and macrophages and possible coagulation defects. It is important to monitor these factors closely (including triglyceride, PT, PTT, and platelets) and not to administer fat emulsion in excess of quantities that can be cleared effectively from the circulation.

In summary, nutritional management of hypermetabolic states includes the administration of only modest quantities of intravenous glucose; more liberal use of intravenous fat emulsions in some cases; and the administration of 1½ to two times the basal amino acid requirement. These intakes should be tailored to the tolerance of each individual patient and should be very closely monitored. On a research basis, additional amounts of branched-chain amino acids may be given as an energy source. Sodium intake should be strictly limited because of increased intracellular levels. Enteral feeding should be recommenced at the earliest possible moment.

Hypoalbuminemia may occur in hypermetabolic states because of the direct effect of interleukin-1 and as a response to sepsis. Hence, low serum albumin does not necessarily result from protein deficiency in these circumstances.

Shaw JHF, Wolfe RR: Energy and protein metabolism in sepsis and trauma. Aust N Z J Surg 1987;57:41.

Ambulatory Pediatrics

12

Barton D. Schmitt, MD, & Roxann M. Headley, MD

This chapter offers guidelines for the conduct of four specific types of pediatric visits: (1) health supervision care, (2) acute illness care, (3) chronic disease follow-up, and (4) consultation. Each type of visit requires a specific service that is different in many ways from the others. If the pediatrician and the office staff can mentally classify each visit in this way and vary their approach accordingly, the delivery of pediatric care will become more logical and consistent.

This efficient organization of ambulatory care has three general advantages: (1) The quality of care is improved by the comprehensiveness that only a systematic approach can ensure. (2) The practice of pediatrics is made more enjoyable because the establishment of clear office guidelines and policies prevents many frustrations and much duplication of effort by the physician. (3) The cost of medical care is reduced by increasing the efficiency of health care delivery.

Special attention is paid to the problem of fever and its management at the end of the chapter.

HEALTH SUPERVISION VISITS

OBJECTIVES

Health maintenance or health supervision visits are the key to preventive pediatrics. These visits involve three people: the physician, the parent, and the child. Children should assume more active roles in their own health care with each passing year. The visit has multiple purposes: responding to the parent's or child's current concerns, presenting age-appropriate anticipatory guidance, assessing growth and development (see Chapter 3), performing a physical examination (Chapter 1), obtaining laboratory screening tests, and administering immunizations (Chapter 10). One natural outcome of these visits is a deepening of family-physician rapport.

PARENTAL CONCERNS

The first part of each well child visit should be directed toward dealing with the current concerns of the parents. Most expectant parents have many questions that should be discussed with the pediatrician several weeks prior to delivery. The most frequent concerns include arguments for and against breast-feeding and circumcision, hospital policies about rooming-in and parent-infant contact in the delivery room, essential baby equipment, separation problems affecting other children in the household during the mother's confinement, and ways of decreasing sibling jealousy. It was at one time traditional for the first newborn office visit to take place at 6 weeks. A 2-week postpartal office visit, however, is much more logical. First-time mothers who are breast feeding should bring the baby in for a feeding evaluation at 5–7 days of age.

A health supervision visit without parental concerns is uncommon. Some parents bring a list of questions: "How much should babies cry?" "How do I know he's getting enough to eat?" "Can I spoil her by picking her up too much?" "Is it all right to spank children?" "How old should Johnny be before I let him cross the street alone?" Many of the questions have no obvious answers. The experienced pediatrician usually enjoys the challenge of these discussions and the satisfaction that accompanies reassuring an anxious parent.

Charney E: Counseling of parents around the birth of a baby. Pediatr Rev 1982;4:167.

Dershewitz R: Prenatal anticipatory guidance. Clin Perinatol 1985;12:343.

Green M et al: The changing picture of well-child care. Contemporary Pediatr 1988;5(8):14.

ANTICIPATORY GUIDANCE

Anticipatory guidance usually includes advice on nutrition (see Chapter 11), injury prevention, behavior, development (Chapter 3), sex education, dental care (Chapter 18), and health promotion. Special counseling is in order for adolescents (Chapter 4). A list of suggested topics to be discussed at particular ages is found on the health supervision forms (Anticipatory Guidance Checklist) provided at the end of this chapter (Table 12–4). These topics can be covered in a variety of ways. Some physicians prefer to discuss all the items with the parents personally; others prefer to delegate the discussion of some of these issues to the office nurse; and still others use printed materials to expand upon what the physician covers personally.

Schmitt BD (editor): *The Pediatric Advisor 5.0.* Clinical Reference Systems Ltd, 1993. (Computer-generated parent handouts.)

INJURY PREVENTION

Injuries kill more children than the eight other leading causes of childhood deaths combined. Between ages 1 and 14, over 60% of deaths are due to injuries, and between ages 15 and 24, over 75% are due to injuries. Each year, 100,000 children under 15 years of age are left with permanent disabilities due to injuries. During the first 3 years of life, children have little sense of danger or self-preservation and thus are totally dependent on adult supervision for their safety.

Accident prevention advice should be an integral part of health supervision care for all infants and children. Several years ago, the American Academy of Pediatrics established The Injury Prevention Program (TIPP), which includes parent questionnaires for assessing risk and information sheets to aid parents in preventing accidents. The main thrust of the program is to advise parents of the following five preventive measures: (1) approved car restraints for children, (2) smoke detectors, (3) hot water heater set to less than 54 °C, (4) guards for windows and gates for stairways, and (5) syrup of ipecac.

TIPP materials can be obtained from the American Academy of Pediatrics, Publications Department, 141 Northwest Point Boulevard, PO Box 927, Elk Grove Village, IL 60007; phone 1-800-433-9016.

Motor Vehicle Accidents

The foremost killer and crippler of children in the United States is the motor vehicle. Proper use of car safety seats can reduce fatalities and hospitalizations by at least 70%. Laws have been passed in all 50 states requiring that children riding in cars be restrained in an approved safety seat. The child's weight determines the type of safety seat to be used. In general, the smaller seats are more protective and should be used as long as they are appropriate:

Less than 20 lb: rear-facing infant seat
20–40 lb: forward-facing toddler seat
40–60 lb: booster seat with lap belt
Over 60 lb: regular lap belt
Over 48 inches: shoulder strap with lap belt

Prevention of Firearm Injuries

The morbidity and mortality from firearms are increasing in the United States, especially among adolescents. Injuries may be unintentional or due to homicide or suicide.

(1) Store your weapons unloaded and uncocked in a securely locked container.

(2) Store your firearm and ammunition in separate locations.

(3) Do not store your handgun in a bedside table or under your pillow or mattress.

Prevention of Drowning

Children between the ages of 1 and 3 years have the highest rate of drowning. In some warm-weather states, drowning deaths exceed the number of deaths due to motor vehicle or pedestrian accidents.

(1) Never leave a child under age 3 unattended in a bathtub or wading pool.

(2) Never leave a child who cannot swim unattended near a swimming pool. (More children drown in backyard swimming pools than at beaches or in public pools.)

(3) Remember that infant water programs are for fun, not for learning how to swim. (Children cannot be made water safe before age 3.)

(4) Try to arrange swimming lessons for your child between ages 3 and 8.

(5) Fence home pools and hot tubs.

(6) Learn CPR if you have a home pool.

(7) Eliminate large buckets of water from the home.

Prevention of Burns

Scald burns are the most common type of pediatric burn. While the majority of scald burns involve food and beverages, nearly a quarter involve tap water.

(1) Never drink anything hot while holding a baby.

(2) Keep hot substances, pot handles, and curling irons away from the edge of a table or stove.

(3) Do not let a child touch the faucet handles in the bathtub.

(4) Set hot water heaters to less than 54 °C.

(5) Install smoke detectors in the home and replace batteries annually or when the "dead battery alarm" sounds.

(6) Keep cigarette lighters and matches away from children.

(7) Keep electrical cords unplugged or out of the reach of children. Use safety guards in electrical outlets.

Prevention of Choking

(1) Do not give a child any foods that are commonly aspirated into the lungs (nuts of any kind, sunflower seeds, orange seeds, cherry pits, raw carrots, raw peas, raw celery) until the child is old enough to chew or spit out such foods (usually 4 years of age).

(2) Carefully chop up any foods that might block the windpipe, such as hot dogs, grapes, caramels.

(3) Warn babysitters and siblings not to share these foods with small children.

(4) Do not allow a child with food in the mouth to run or play.

(5) Avoid toys with small detachable parts that could enter the windpipe.

(6) Be especially careful when disposing of button batteries.

Prevention of Head Trauma

(1) Never leave an infant of any age alone on a high place.

(2) Always keep the side rails on the crib up.

(3) Avoid bunk beds before age 6.

(4) Do not use baby walkers. (Over 35% of infants using them have an accident requiring emergency care. The most serious accidents occur when a child in a walker falls down a stairway. Keep a sturdy gate at the top of all stairways.)

(5) Teach children to cross the street safely at age 5 or 6.

(6) Do not teach a child to ride a bicycle until age 7 or 8.

(7) Never allow a child to ride a bicycle without a bicycle helmet. All-track vehicles and motorcycles are too unsafe to ride, even with a helmet.

(8) Forbid trampolines.

Prevention of Poisoning

(1) Remember to keep drugs and chemicals locked up and out of reach.

(2) Keep in mind that drain cleaners, furniture polish, and insecticides are the most dangerous of the common poisons (other than drugs).

(3) Keep the safety cap on all drug containers.

(4) Keep syrup of ipecac handy; use only if directed to do so.

(5) Know the telephone number of the nearest poison control center.

Greensher J: Recent advances in injury prevention. Pediatr Rev 1988;10:171.

Healthy People 2000: National Health Promotion and Disease Prevention Objectives. DHHS Publication No. (PHS) 91-50212.

Rivara F (editor): Injury control: Issues and methods for the 1980's. Pediatr Ann 1992;21:411.

PHYSICAL EXAMINATION

A complete physical examination should be performed at each health supervision visit (see Chapter 1). Height, weight, and head circumference should be measured and plotted on growth curves (see Chapter 3). During childhood, most chronic diseases will affect growth. Although these examinations are usu-

ally normal, they serve as a point of reference in evaluating future illnesses. Therefore, the extent of the examination should be carefully recorded. To save time, the checklist shown in Table 12–1 can be used. Elaboration is required only for the abnormal findings.

Some physical findings are silent—ie, they are not noticeable to parents and cause few if any symptoms. Of greatest concern are disorders that are treatable if detected early but potentially serious when not detected. A routine examination will diagnose most such conditions (eg, congenital heart disease). A few conditions are detected only by detailed examination

Table 12–1. Checklist for physical examination.

	Normal	Abnormal
1. GENERAL APPEARANCE: well-nourished, hydrated, alert		
2. SKIN: color, rash, swelling, hair, nails		
3. HEAD: shape, anterior fontanelle		
4. EYES: conjunctiva, cornea, pupils, extraocular movement		
5. EARS: pinnae, canals, tympanic membrane appearance, mobility		
6. NOSE: nares, turbinates		
7. MOUTH: tongue, teeth, oral mucosa, tonsils, pharynx		
8. NECK: thyroid, range of motion		
9. NODES: cervical, axillary, inguinal, other		
10. CHEST: symmetry, expansion, breasts		
11. LUNGS: rate, auscultation, percussion		
12. HEART: rate, rhythm, S_1, S_2, murmur, femoral pulses		
13. ABDOMEN: contour; palpation of liver, spleen, and kidney; mass; tenderness		
14. GENITALIA: ♀ external; ♂ penis, meatus, testes, hernia		
15. SPINE: curvature (scoliosis), sacral area		
16. EXTREMITIES: range of motion, tenderness, edema, clubbing, cyanosis		
17. NEUROLOGIC (SCREEN): cranial nerves 3, 4, 6, 7, and 12; gait; cerebellar function; motor system (strength, tone)		
18. NEUROLOGIC (COMPLETE): above plus other cranial nerves; sensory and motor systems (deep tendon reflexes, clonus)		

(eg, retinoblastoma [red fundus reflection test], strabismus [corneal light reflection test], congenital hip dislocation [Ortolani maneuver, or restricted abduction], scoliosis, coarctation of the aorta [femoral pulses], hypertension, lower urinary tract obstruction [inquire about urine stream], imperforate hymen, and labial adhesions). Visual deficits (eg, refractive errors or color blindness) and hearing deficits can also be missed if appropriate testing is not included. Dental caries may be overlooked by physicians who assume, not always rightly, that their patients are receiving periodic dental examinations (see Chapter 18). Baby bottle caries of the upper incisors should be looked for in any child over age 1 who still receives a bottle. Early cancer detection can be improved by teaching self-examination of the breasts or testes.

Strong WB, Linder CW: Preparticipation health evaluation for competitive sports. Pediatr Rev 1982;4:113.

THE SCHOOL READINESS EXAMINATION

The preschool examination of the 4- or 5-year-old child should answer the basic question, "Is the child ready for school?" Auscultation of the heart and lungs at this time is probably far less important than noting any abnormalities of speech, hearing, or vision and determining if developmental age is commensurate with chronologic age, if attention span is adequate for learning, and if parents have prepared the child adequately for separation when entering school. These problems should also be investigated earlier, but they are of greatest significance at the preschool examination.

Vision

Five to 10 percent of preschool children have some kind of visual impairment. The illiterate E chart, Snellen chart, STYCAR test, or Allen picture cards can be used for checking visual acuity, and each eye should be tested separately. Testing should be attempted at age 3. The 5-year-old child should have a visual acuity of 20/30 or better in both eyes, and there should be no more than a one-line difference between the two eyes. Suppression amblyopia affects 3% of children and must be detected early before permanent loss of vision occurs. Amblyopia is often secondary to strabismus, which can be detected by noting the position where light is reflected off both corneas or by the cover test (see Figure 14–4). Alignment can be tested by 6 months of age.

Hearing

Fixed hearing deficits occur in approximately 1% of young school children, and in 10% of these the loss is profound and bilateral. More children have a temporary hearing loss from recurrent purulent otitis media or serous otitis media. Although the losses are generally not too severe, if they occur at an inopportune time they may be sufficient to prevent an early school-age child from learning phonics; hence, the effect of the loss may be carried on and magnified throughout much of the school years (see Chapter 19). If such losses are detected before entry into school, some of the learning, behavior, and discipline problems that occur secondary to poor attention might be averted. Audiologic screening tests can be performed by nonprofessional technicians and should be a part of the preschool examination.

Speech

The child entering school should be able to speak distinctly and clearly without difficulty; should be able to answer questions; and, after a period of getting acquainted, should be able to carry on a conversation with the physician about recent events. Poor speech may impair performance in school. An easily administered language screening test (Early Language Milestones) and an articulation screening test (Denver Articulation Screening Exam) have been developed to identify children who should be referred to a speech pathologist for definitive evaluation (see Figure 3–10).

Emotional Development & Behavior

The assessment of emotional development and behavior is an important part of the preschool examination. In one study, 42 physicians were observed conducting 673 health supervision visits. On the average, they said fewer than two sentences per visit to the mother that were relevant to child behavior. Yet, when given the opportunity to respond to a questionnaire about behavior, 85% of mothers of preschool children (ages 1½–6 years) indicated one or more such concerns (mean of 3½ concerns per child). A simple self-administered questionnaire is an effective and efficient device which not only indicates to the parent that the physician is interested in discussing behavioral problems and emotional growth but also helps the physician to concentrate on areas of guidance most relevant to the parent's concerns. The pediatric health supervision forms (provided at the end of this chapter) stress anticipatory guidance and counseling for behavioral aspects of pediatrics.

Physical, emotional, and developmental maturation proceeds at different rates for different children. Some children are ready for school long before their fifth birthday; others are not nearly ready at that age. Some parents tend to push their children into experiences that are beyond their capacities at a given age. Children should begin their school experiences with successes; the child who starts with failure is often criticized and becomes discouraged and less interested in school, so that a pattern of failure may develop. The child may continue to lag behind and miss the early fundamentals of learning, which are the basis for further education. Many children develop behavioral disorders and truancy simply because they cannot read and so are unable to understand what is going on in the classroom. Part of the physician's role is to help parents recognize physical, emotional, and developmental lags early, so that corrective measures can be taken to prepare the child for school. A number of easily administered developmental tests are available. The Denver Developmental Screening Test (see Chapter 3) is extremely helpful in the younger age groups.

Coplan J et al: Unclear speech: Recognition and significance of unintelligible speech in preschool children. Pediatrics 1988;82:447.
Crouch E et al: Pediatric vision screening: Why? When? What? How? Contemporary Pediatr 1991;8(September Special Issue:9.
Dworkin PH: Educational readiness. Pediatrician 1986; 13:62.
Nozza R: Screening audiometry: A sound investment for your practice. Contemporary Pediatr 1986;3:71.
Palfrey et al: School placement. Pediatr Rev 1987;8:261.

LABORATORY SCREENING TESTS

A health supervision flow sheet (see example in Table 12–2) is a helpful reminder to the nurse and physician that certain procedures, laboratory tests, developmental evaluations, and immunizations need to be done. All of these items can be initiated by the nurse or aide if the physician establishes the routine to be followed.

Blood

Iron deficiency anemia (see Chapter 28) is found more often in lower socioeconomic populations and has its highest incidence in infants between 9 and 24 months of age. A routine hemoglobin or hematocrit measurement is recommended in this age group and is particularly important in the child who received a low-iron formula or whose current diet is low in iron-containing foods. The American Academy of Pediatrics (1991) continues to recommend routine hematocrits at 9 months and at 2, 8, and 18 years.

Children with sickle cell disease (see Chapter 28) must be diagnosed before 6 months of age to prevent death due to sepsis or splenic sequestration (10–20% mortality rate). Do not wait for the routine hematocrit at age 9 months. Prophylactic antibiotics should be started as soon as the diagnosis is made, preferably by age 3 months. It is strongly recommended that newborn screening include screening for sickle cell disease. For accuracy, this test must be done before any transfusion.

Screening for phenylketonuria (see Chapter 2) should be done by blood test in the hospital nursery prior to the infant's discharge, and in all states such a test is required by law. An infant with this disorder who failed to ingest sufficient milk protein may have a negative test in the first few days of life. Therefore, most centers recommend a repeat test at 10–14 days of age if the first test was performed before 24 hours of age. Screening of newborns for congenital hypothyroidism, another preventable cause of mental retardation, is also done in all 50 states. While a number of states mandate newborn screening for diseases such as galactosemia and maple syrup urine disease, mass screening for cystic fibrosis and neuroblastoma is currently not recommended.

Screening for lead poisoning (see Chapter 13) is extremely important. While severe, acute lead poisoning, characterized by encephalopathy, is rare, chronic low-level exposure is widespread and can have significant effects on the developing central nervous system. In 1984, it was estimated that more than 3 million children, ages 6 months to 5 years, had blood lead levels greater than 15 µg/dL. Most experts agree that children with lead levels greater than 10–15 µg/dL risk subtle injury to the central nervous system. The major sources of lead exposure for children in the United States are lead-based paint and contaminated dust and soil. All children should be screened by questionnaire for possible environmental risk factors at the time of health supervision visits between the ages of 6 months and 6 years. (See a sample questionnaire from the Centers for Disease Control and Prevention in Table 12–3.) If any risk factor is identified, a blood lead level should be obtained at that time. In addition, routine screening of blood lead levels should be performed on all children at 9–12 months and at 2 years of age, regardless of the presence or absence of historical risk factors. As more data are collected, low-risk communities may be identified where routine blood lead screening would be unnecessary.

Universal cholesterol testing of all children is controversial. For the present, the American Academy of Pediatrics recommends selective testing of children who have a family history of hyperlipidemia (cholesterol > 240 mg/dL) or early myocardial infarction (< 50 years of age in men and < 60 in women). Testing of these children should be performed at age 2–3 years.

Urine

Routine urinalysis has a low yield in the asymptomatic patient. In contrast to the adult population, it is unusual for a child to have asymptomatic diabetes, and proteinuria is a rare presenting sign of renal abnormality in an asymptomatic child. Transient orthostatic proteinuria is common in adolescents but is a benign condition. Although many recommend that the urine dipstick test be performed only on symptomatic children, testing once at age 3 or 4 is not unreasonable. The American Academy of Pediatrics (1991) continues to recommend routine urinalysis at 6 months and at 2, 8, and 18 years.

Table 12–2. Health Supervision Flow Sheet.

Patient's name and date of birth: _____

Directions: Record date for all immunizations
Record value for head circumference, height, weight, blood pressure, and hematocrit.
Record N (normal) or Abn (abnormal) for all other items.
Omit where shaded.

	NB	2 wk	2 mo	4 mo	6 mo	9 mo	12 mo	15 mo	18 mo	2 yr	3 yr	4 yr	5 yr	6 yr	8 yr	10 yr	12 yr	14 yr	16 yr	18 yr
Today's date																				
Head circumference (cm)											▓	▓	▓	▓	▓	▓	▓	▓	▓	▓
Height (cm)																				
Weight (kg)																				
Blood pressure	▓	▓	▓	▓	▓	▓	▓	▓	▓	▓										
Dental caries screen	▓	▓	▓	▓	▓	▓	▓	▓	▓											
DTP (Td after 7 years)	▓	▓				▓	▓	▓		▓	▓			▓	▓	▓	▓	▓		▓
Polio	▓	▓			▓	▓	▓	▓		▓	▓			▓	▓	▓	▓	▓	▓	▓
H influenzae type b[1]	▓	▓				▓		▓	▓	▓	▓	▓	▓	▓	▓	▓	▓	▓	▓	▓
Hepatitis B vaccine[2]		▓		▓	▓			▓	▓	▓	▓	▓	▓	▓	▓	▓	▓	▓	▓	▓
Measles, mumps, rubella	▓	▓	▓	▓	▓	▓			▓	▓	▓	▓	▓	▓	▓	▓		▓	▓	▓
Tuberculosis test[3]	▓	▓	▓	▓	▓	▓		▓	▓	▓	▓	▓	▓	▓	▓	▓		▓	▓	▓
Developmental screen[4]	▓	▓	▓	▓	▓			▓	▓				▓	▓	▓	▓	▓	▓	▓	▓
Speech screen[5]	▓	▓	▓	▓	▓	▓	▓	▓	▓				▓	▓	▓	▓	▓	▓	▓	▓
Hearing screen[6]		▓		▓		▓	▓	▓	▓	▓	▓		▓	▓	▓	▓	▓		▓	▓
Vision screen[7]	▓				▓	▓	▓	▓	▓	▓		▓	▓		▓	▓	▓	▓	▓	▓
Newborn metabolic screen[8]			▓	▓	▓	▓	▓	▓	▓	▓	▓	▓	▓	▓	▓	▓	▓	▓	▓	▓
Sickle cell test (black patients)[9]		▓		▓	▓	▓	▓	▓	▓	▓	▓	▓	▓	▓	▓	▓	▓	▓	▓	▓
Hematocrit	▓	▓	▓	▓	▓		▓	▓	▓	▓	▓	▓	▓	▓	▓	▓		▓	▓	▓
Lead screen[10]	▓	▓	▓	▓	▓		*	▓	▓	*	▓	▓	▓		▓	▓	▓	▓	▓	▓
Pap smear/GC/*Chlamydia*[11]																				

[1]HIB schedule depends upon the product used.

[2]If mother is hepatitis B surface antigen-positive, infant should receive vaccine and immunoglobulin at birth. The second immunization is then given at 1 month of age.

[3]Test yearly in high-risk groups.

[4]Screen with Denver II at listed intervals; more often if there are specific concerns.

[5]Screen with ELM (Early Language Milestones).

[6]High-risk inquiry (newborn); listens to soft sounds (2 months); turns to sound (6 months); audiometrics (4 years and thereafter).

[7]Red reflex (newborn or 2 weeks); regards smiling face (2 months); follows past midline (4 months); corneal light reflections test (6 months); visual acuity (3 years and thereafter; color vision once (6 years).

[8]PKU, thyroid, others according to state law; PKU retest (2 weeks) if first test done before 24 hours.

[9]If not performed in newborn, perform at 2 months of age.

[10]Lead exposure screening questionnaire (Table 12–3) at ages indicated; blood lead levels (*) at ages 9–12 months and 2 years and if questionnaire is positive.

[11]Sexually active patients.

Table 12–3. Lead exposure screening questionnaire.[1]

Does your child–

1. Live in or regularly visit a house with peeling or chipping paint built before 1960? This could include a day care center, preschool, the home of a babysitter or relative, etc.
2. Live in or regularly visit a house built before 1960 with recent, ongoing, or planned renovation or remodeling?
3. Have a brother or sister, housemate, or playmate being followed up or treated for lead poisoning (ie, blood level ≥ 15 mg/dL)?
4. Live with an adult whose job or hobby involves exposure to lead?
5. Live near an active lead smelter, battery recycling plant, or other industry likley to release lead?

[1]From the Centers for Disease Control and Prevention.

In screening for asymptomatic urinary tract infection, microscopic examination of the urinary sediment is time-consuming and not reliable. Several inexpensive methods are available to screen a first morning specimen for bacteriuria (eg, nitrite or leukocyte detection strips), followed by a urine culture if the dipstick test is positive. Since untreated asymptomatic bacteriuria usually clears spontaneously and does not lead to renal damage, screening should be reserved for high-risk groups (eg, children with diabetes). However, the clinician must not hesitate to check a specimen for bacilluria in any child with unexplained fevers, unexplained abdominal pain, enuresis, foul-smelling urine, or other vague symptoms.

Teenage girls who are sexually active will benefit from annual gonococcal and chlamydial cultures, and Papanicolaou smears. Birth control counseling and sexuality counseling can also be offered at this time.

Committee on Environmental Health, American Academy of Pediatrics: Lead poisoning: from screening to primary prevention. Pediatrics 1993;92:176.

Committee on Genetics, American Academy of Pediatrics: Issues in newborn screening. Pediatrics 1992;89:345.

Committee on Nutrition, American Academy of Pediatrics: Indications for cholesterol testing in children. Pediatrics 1989;83:141.

Hein K et al: The need for routine screening in the sexually active adolescent. J Pediatr 1977;91:123.

Kemper K et al: The case against screening urinalyses for asymptomatic bacteriuria in children. AJDC 1992;146:343.

IMMUNIZATIONS

A child's immunization status can be easily monitored on the health supervision flow sheet (Table 12–2). A record of the child's immunizations should also be given to the parents and updated by the nurse as additional immunizations are given. The details of routine immunization of children are presented in Chapter 10.

GROUP WELL CHILD CARE

The newest model for providing health supervision visits is seeing four or five patients of the same age group during a 1-hour block of office time. This model has been pioneered by Dr Lucy Osborn. The first 45 minutes are spent on health education, using lectures, videotapes, and discussion. Children are present during this time. The last 15 minutes are used to perform physical examinations on the children and to give immunizations.

For the parents, the advantages of group visits include the following: (1) Parents can benefit from a complete curriculum of anticipatory guidance topics. (2) They hear the concerns of other parents. (3) They are able to observe other infants' behaviors, and (4) they acquire a social support group. For the physician, the main advantages include (1) more contact time per parent, (2) more time to address behavior problems, (3) fewer telephone calls at later times regarding these topics, (4) a higher percentage rate of kept appointments, (5) more referrals generated by the parents, and (6) more stimulating interaction. It should be noted that this process does not save physician time or increase the overall fees generated.

Dr Osborn suggests that the 2-week visit be an individual one and that this program begin with the 2-month visit. She prefers to schedule the first hour in the morning and the first hour in the afternoon for group care. Adequate space for meeting with five or more adults is required. Any sensitive issues that the parents need to address can be covered during the physical examination. In summary, this new model was preferred by the majority of parents and physicians who followed it.

Osborn L et al: Group health supervision visits more effective than individual visits in delivering health care information. Pediatrics 1993;91:668.

ACUTE ILLNESS VISITS

The episodic office visit for the child with an acute illness places special demands on the physician.

OBJECTIVES

Diagnosis and treatment of the chief complaint is the first priority for the parents, patient, and physician. Extenuating circumstances (eg, a crowded waiting room) rarely justify an incomplete workup of an acute chief complaint. Detection of patients who have a chronic disease (eg asthma) or an undiagnosed chronic complaint (eg, recurrent abdominal pains), however, should lead to a scheduled follow-up appointment when sufficient time can be devoted to complete evaluation.

COMMON TYPES OF ACUTE ILLNESSES

The following diagnoses or conditions are the acute illnesses most commonly seen in office practice, listed in approximate order of frequency. Any health care provider who sees children must master the evaluation and management of these disorders: common colds, acute otitis media, viral pharyngitis and tonsillitis, gastroenteritis, acute tracheitis and bronchitis, influenza, conjunctivitis, streptococcal pharyngitis, sinusitis, diaper rash, thrush, impetigo, chickenpox, viral maculopapular rashes, skin trauma, head trauma, facial trauma, sprains, urinary tract infection, pneumonia, croup, bronchiolitis, cellulitis and boils, and ingestions.

ASSESSING ACUTE ILLNESS

Optimal management of an acute illness mainly includes telephone triaging, office triaging, diagnosis, assessment of the need for hospitalization, home therapy, and a follow-up plan.

1. TELEPHONE TRIAGING & ADVICE

Does the Patient Need to Be Seen?

The physician is the person best qualified to give medical advice, both in the office and over the phone. However, because talking with parents on the phone may take too much physician time, this function is usually delegated to another member of the office team. Most of the questions are routine ones that require only routine answers. An office nurse specifically trained for the role is probably the best person to take routine calls. Office policies about medical advice over the phone should be standardized. Routine instructions for handling minor infections, minor injuries, reactions to immunizations, infant feeding problems, newborn care, and prescription refills are easy to communicate to parents if they are written down in an office protocol book. The protocol book should also specify the point at which each problem requires an office visit. This decision depends on (1) the type of symptom, (2) the duration of the symptom, (3) the age of the patient, (4) whether or not the patient acts "very sick," (5) an assessment of the calling parent's anxiety, and (6) the presence of any underlying chronic disease. (For example, most patients under 1 year of age with diarrhea *and* vomiting need

to be examined.) After telephone baseline data are gathered, the nurse must be able to decide whether the child needs to be seen immediately, seen later by appointment, or can safely be cared for at home. The nurse should err on the side of seeing the patient when in doubt. For all calls, pertinent telephone data should be entered on a log sheet.

It is helpful if parents understand two general telephone rules: (1) The nurse will screen all calls during office hours except emergency ones and (2) nighttime calls should be restricted to emergencies or urgent problems that cannot wait until morning. Many routine calls come from anxious, inexperienced parents who need reassurance and acceptance, not criticism. The conversation with the nurse should help to build up a young parent's confidence. Parents can be asked what they had considered doing, and that plan of action should be strongly endorsed if possible. If parents are helped to become more confident and independent in these matters, unnecessary visits will be less frequent. However, the conversation should convey the message that telephone calls are an important aid in medical care and that the parent is free to call whenever concerned.

The physician directly accepts some calls: (1) emergency calls from parents, (2) calls from physicians and other professionals, (3) calls regarding hospitalized patients, (4) long distance calls, (5) calls from a parent who demands to talk to the physician, and (6) calls whose import the nurse is unclear about. Parents reasonably expect that their child's personal physician or a designated substitute should be readily available for emergencies, even if the "emergency" exists only from their viewpoint. The physician must be conscientious about accepting calls after midnight, for they often relate to psychosocial crises or urgent medical problems that cannot be ignored even for a few hours.

There are four other methods of dealing with telephone calls, none of which serve as an acceptable alternative to having an office nurse screen calls and give telephone advice: (1) The physician can accept calls at any time throughout the day. These interruptions are unacceptable to most physicians and parents. (2) The physician can have a telephone hour at the beginning, middle, and end of the day and accept only emergency calls at other times. The disadvantages of this approach are that some parents must then wait for answers to urgent questions, and the physician lengthens his or her day with many routine calls. (3) The physician may charge for telephone advice. This decreases the number of calls, but in the process it may discourage important calls and thus interfere with preventive pediatrics. (4) The physician can allow various nonmedical office personnel to accept telephone calls randomly themselves. This approach would result in inconsistent medical advice and could be dangerous. The physician is of course legally liable for any harm to a patient proximately caused by improper advice given over the phone by employees.

Fosarelli P, Schmitt B: Telephone dissatisfaction in pediatric practice: Denver and Baltimore. Pediatrics 1987; 80:28.

Katz HP, Wick W: Malpractice, meningitis, and the telephone. Pediatr Ann 1991;20:85.

Schmitt BD: *Pediatric Telephone Advice,* 2nd ed. Little, Brown, 1994.

When Does the Patient Need to Be Seen?

Some patients must be seen immediately (eg, for removal of an ocular foreign body). Others can be seen later the same day (eg, for a cough that kept the patient awake much of the preceding night). Other patients can be scheduled 1 or 2 days later (eg, for recurrent leg pains). The nurse can make these decisions.

Where Should the Patient Be Seen?

Most sick patients can be seen in the physician's office by appointment. The physician can keep the first and last hour of each day plus at least 15 minutes out of each hour reserved for acute problems. Most of the first-hour appointments will be given to parents who called the physician during the preceding evening.

Another facility where patients can be seen for medical care is the hospital emergency room. This routing applies to patients who are highly likely to be admitted (eg, for stridor). Some physicians also send patients with poisonings, lacerations, or possible fractures to the nearest emergency room.

A third possibility is a house call. Most physicians consider this disadvantageous to themselves financially and to the patient medically, because laboratory services are not available. A rare indication for a house call might be a contagious disease that needs confirmation (eg, varicella). The physician could occasionally see such a patient in the office parking lot.

2. OFFICE TRIAGING & PROCEDURES

How Sick Is the Patient?

The nurse should screen all sick patients as soon as possible after they arrive at the office. They can be thought of in terms of three general groups: emergency, contagious, and minor illness. Most patients have a minor illness (eg, cold, accident, earache) and can be seen at their appointed time. Some patients are contagious until proved otherwise and should quickly be moved from the waiting room to an isolated examining room (eg, febrile illnesses with rashes, lice, jaundice, possible pertussis). An attempt should be made to keep children with bronchiolitis or croup away from infants. When an office emergency (eg, fe-

brile seizures, respiratory distress) is recognized by the nurse, the physician should be notified immediately. The physician can take appropriate emergency action, stabilize the patient, and arrange for transfer to the hospital if necessary (eg, an acidotic, dehydrated infant). (See Chapter 14.)

Russo RM et al: Triage abilities of nurse practitioner vs pediatrician. Am J Dis Child 1975;129:673.

Preparation of the Patient for the Physician

The office aide can record the sick patient's temperature, height, and weight. The office nurse can record the chief complaint. Depending upon the symptom, the nurse can take vital signs and initiate the office's standing orders on laboratory procedures and symptomatic treatment listed below.

Initial Treatment & Laboratory Workup

Steps in initial management are listed below. Details of procedures are outlined elsewhere in the text.

A. Abdominal Pain: Take samples for urinalysis and urine culture; save stool specimen for occult blood testing.

B. Animal Bite: Wash out immediately with liquid soap and water for 10 minutes. Initiate the official reporting form, and call the county health department. Delay irrigation if the wound is infected and a culture is needed.

C. Cough: If present over 1 month, apply a tuberculin skin test.

D. Diarrhea: Take a sample for stool culture if the stool contains blood or mucus or if diarrhea has persisted for more than 1 week at any age. For children under age 2, give 180 mL (6 oz) of an oral electrolyte solution and record the naked weight on each visit. If a child appears dehydrated, collect urine for specific gravity determination.

E. Earache: Give acetaminophen if the child is in obvious pain. If there is a possibility of mumps, isolate the patient.

F. Eye Injury: Test visual acuity if the child is over age 3. Place eye tray in the examining room.

G. Fever Over 39 °C: Give acetaminophen at a dose of 15 mg/kg. Put the child in an examining room and assist with undressing. Give a sponge bath if temperature exceeds 40 °C despite drugs and if the child is uncomfortable. Provide a bag for urine if the child is not toilet-trained. If unexplained fever has been present over 24 hours, order a white count and differential. If the infant is under 2 months of age, notify the physician immediately.

H. Fractures: Notify the physician immediately, obtain equipment to immobilize the site, and fill out an x-ray request.

I. Head Injury: Record vital signs and level of

consciousness, and check pupils for equal size and reaction to light.

J. Hepatitis A Exposure: Record weights of persons who have had close contact with the patient, and anticipate giving immune globulin, 0.02 mL/kg intramuscularly.

K. Lacerations: Wash thoroughly (at least 10 minutes). Check date of last tetanus shot and record. Shave around the wound edges if necessary (but never shave eyebrows).

L. Nosebleed: Instruct the parent or child on how to compress the bleeding site for 10 minutes. Check blood pressure. If nosebleed is a chronic problem, perform fingerstick for hematocrit determination.

M. Painful Urination (Burning or Frequency): Take sample for urinalysis, urine culture, and nitrite dipstick.

N. Pinworms: Record the approximate weights of all family members if the infection is a recurrent one (for calculation of dosage of medication, see Chapter 37).

O. Sore Throat: Take material for throat culture (contraindicated if the patient has croup).

P. Streptococcal Sore Throat (Culture-Positive): Inquire about penicillin allergy and record. Arrange for symptomatic family contacts to have throat cultures taken.

Q. Vomiting: Record exact weight. Give patient emesis basin and sips of ice water while waiting. If patient appears dehydrated, collect urine for specific gravity.

3. THE WORKING DIAGNOSIS

The physician makes the final decision about the diagnosis and the severity of the disease. Emergency conditions (eg, shock or meningitis) may be noted upon entering the examination room and emergency intervention initiated. History taking can be modified to emphasize the chief complaint. A history of recent contact with persons with contagious diseases often points to the correct diagnosis. Severity can be partially assessed by inquiries about playfulness, energy, ability to sleep, and the parent's feelings about how sick the child is this time compared with other times. If a family of sick children is brought in, the physician should ask the mother which children she considers the sickest. The physical examination often can be directed toward the chief complaint. A patient with a dog bite does not require a complete examination, but a patient with an earache must be checked for mastoid swelling and meningeal signs in addition to otoscopic examination. A child with a fever usually requires a complete examination.

Utilizing the conventional techniques of history, physical examination, and laboratory tests, the physician will correctly diagnose most acute chief complaints. However, an alert clinical mind is necessary in order not to miss a diagnosis of septicemia. Septic children usually present with unexplained fever, but (unlike children with acute viral fevers) they often will not smile or play, even with their parents. They frequently are physically exhausted and too weak to resist the physical examination, constantly irritable and unable to sleep, and respond paradoxically to cuddling by the mother. Irritability usually stems from pain or hypoxia. A less common finding in the toxic child is constant lethargy or sleepiness. This is difficult to assess, because most sick children sleep more than normally.

McCarthy PL et al: Predictive value of abnormal physical examination findings in ill-appearing and well-appearing febrile children. Pediatrics 1985;76:167.

Nelson KG: An index of severity for acute pediatric illness. Am J Public Health 1980;70:804.

4. INDICATIONS FOR HOSPITALIZATION

For every acute problem, the physician must decide whether to treat the child at home or in the hospital. Patients are mainly admitted for treatment services not available in the home setting. Even complex diagnostic evaluations can usually be performed on an outpatient basis.

Patients whose problems fit into one of the following three groups of indications should be hospitalized:

Major Emergencies

Some examples of obvious life-threatening conditions are shock, severe dehydration, coma, meningitis (bacterial or of unknown cause), respiratory distress, congestive heart failure, cyanosis, symptomatic hypertension, acute renal failure, status epilepticus, and surgical emergencies.

Potentially Life-Threatening or Crippling Illnesses

Some patients are not in critical condition when first seen but require hospitalization because they require inpatient therapy (eg, intravenous antibotics) or their problem may be rapidly progressive during treatment. If deterioration occurs in the hospital, emergency therapy can be rapidly instituted. Most of the entities in this group are caused by infection or trauma. Endogenous diseases rarely change this rapidly. Although absolute rules cannot be formulated for every situation, the following guidelines can be applied to most cases of acute illness. Obviously, these recommendations will have some exceptions such as when the emergency room has a 8-hour observation area. Also, the list is not complete (eg, chronic diseases are not listed).

These problems are listed according to body systems:

A. Skin:

1. Cellulitis if the patient is less than 2 months old; if there is buccal involvement or the cavernous sinus drainage area is involved; if underlying sinusitis or osteomyelitis is suspected; if cellulitis is secondary to a puncture wound in the foot; or if there is no response after 2 days of therapy.

2. Erysipelas, toxic epidermal necrolysis, or acute necrotizing fasciitis. Omphalitis if the patient is less than 2 months old.

3. Suspected thrombophlebitis.

4. Burns (second- or third-degree) involving more than 10% of surface area (> 15% if the patient is more than 1 year old); burns of perineal area, hand, or face if they might need grafting; all inhalation burns; and most electrical burns.

5. Purpura or petecchiae with fever, without fever but unexplained, or without fever but progressive.

B. Eyes:

1. Gonococcal conjunctivitis or bacterial keratitis.

2. Eye injury if visual acuity is decreased.

3. Papilledema.

C. Ears, Nose, and Throat:

1. Acute otitis media if the patient is less than 1 month old with fever, systemic symptoms, or no response after 2 days of therapy.

2. Mastoiditis.

3. Sinusitis ifoverlying cellulitis, suspected central nervous system complications, or fever unresponsive to 2 days of oral antibiotics.

4. Nasal obstruction if the patient is less than 6 months old and an apneic episode has occurred.

5. Epistaxis if uncontrolled; if hypertension is present; if there is bleeding elsewhere; or if severe anemia is present.

6. Fluctuant tonsillar abscess.

7. Retropharyngeal abscess.

8. Diphtheria (any symptoms at any age).

9. Cervical adenitis if the patient is toxic, dehydrated, dysphagic, dyspneic, or less than 6 months old and needs treatment by incision and drainage.

D. Respiratory System:

1. Epiglottitis (all cases).

2. Croup if there is stridor at rest, dyspnea, or drooling; if the child has repeatedly awakened from sleep with stridor; if there is a history of a previous bout with rapid progression; if there are apneic or cyanotic episodes; or if the patient is less than 1 year old and the stridor is easily provoked (eg, occurs with any crying).

3. Pertussis if symptomatic and the patient is less than 1 year old; pertussis at any age if accompanied by apnea, respiratory distress, a whoop, or weight loss.

4. Bronchiolitis if the patient is dyspneic, has a resting respiratory rate > 60/min, has apneic or cyanotic episodes (PO_2 < 50 mm Hg), has poor fluid intake, or is unable to sleep.

5. Asthma if respiratory distress persists after two injections of epinephrine or two nebulized doses of a beta-agonist.

6. Pneumonia if the patient is less than 1 month old; if bacterial pneumonia is suspected and the patient is less than 6 months old; if there is a history of apnea, cyanosis, or choking spells; if there is dyspnea (any age); if there is pleural effusion; if staphylococcal pneumonia is suspected (any age); if aspiration pneumonia is present; if fluid intake is poor; if there is underlying cystic fibrosis or congenital heart disease; or if there is no response after 2 days of therapy.

7. Suspected foreign body of the airway.

8. Hemoptysis if unexplained, if there is bleeding elsewhere, or if anemia is present.

9. Apnea in all cases except periodic breathing, breath-holding spells, or mild choking on food.

E. Cardiovascular System:

1. Suspected subacute infective endocarditis.

2. Any myocarditis or pericarditis.

3. Acute hypertension or shock.

4. Unexplained dysrhythmias.

F. Gastrointestinal System:

1. Vomiting with dehydration, delirium, or persistent abdominal pain.

2. Hematemesis if documented and not caused by swallowed blood.

3. Diarrhea if typhoid fever is suspected in a patient of any age; if acute *Shigella* infection is suspected in a patient less than 1 year old; or in a patient who has moderate or mild dehydration with vomiting or fluid refusal.

4. Melena or unexplained bright-red blood mixed in the stools.

5. Suspected appendicitis, peritonitis, or intussusception.

6. Abdominal trauma if penetrating injury has occurred or if damage to the spleen, liver, kidneys, pancreas, or intestines is suspected.

7. Toxic ileus.

G. Urinary System:

1. Pyelonephritis if the patient is less than 2 months old, toxic, or unimproved after 2 days of therapy; if gram-negative sepsis is suspected; if underlying renal disease is present; or if recurrences have been frequent.

2. Acute edema, oliguria, or azotemia of renal origin.

3. Hematuria with symptoms listed in (2), renal colic, and unexplained or posttraumatic gross hematuria.

4. Acute urinary retention.

H. Genitalia:

1. Vaginitis if associated with salpingitis.

2. Vaginal injury with sharp object.

3. Suspected testicular torsion.

4. Priapism.

I. Skeletal System:

1. Suspected osteomyelitis.

2. Suspected septic arthritis.

3. Wringer injury if above the elbow; if a hematoma or avulsed skin is present; if a fracture or nerve injury is present; or if the peripheral pulse is diminished.

J. Nervous System:

1. Aseptic meningitis if the level of consciousness is depressed or there is a motor deficit.

2. Suspected tetanus.

3. Suspected epidural spinal abscess or brain abscess.

4. Febrile or afebrile seizures if they continue more than 30 minutes; if there are persistent neurologic signs; if the level of consciousness is decreased; or if serious underlying disease cannot be ruled out.

5. Head injury if the patient has been unconscious longer than 5 minutes; if there are persistent neurologic signs; if the level of consciousness is decreased; if a seizure has occurred; if cerebrospinal fluid rhinorrhea or otorrhea is present; if there is significant swelling over the middle meningeal artery; if there are retinal hemorrhages or progressive headaches; or if abnormal or irregular vital signs are present.

6. Skull fractures that are depressed or compound (ie, into air sinuses or overlying scalp laceration), fractures across the middle meningeal artery or venous sinus, occipital fracture into the rim of the foramen magnum, or any fracture with an underlying bleeding disorder.

7. Suspected spinal cord trauma.

8. Acute muscle weakness.

9. Acute altered mental status, or delirium that is unexplained or persists longer than 2 hours.

10. Suspected increased intracranial pressure.

K. General:

1. Fever if the patient is less than 2 months old; if toxicity is evident and serious underlying disease cannot be ruled out; or if fever is due to heat stroke.

2. Poisoning if the patient is symptomatic (eg, respirations slow or irregular, drowsiness, etc). If the agent or dosage is unknown or the dosage is a potentially fatal one, the child can usually be observed in the Emergency Department.

3. Lead poisoning.

4. Unexplained mass.

5. Failure to thrive if severe or unexplained.

6. Unexplained hypoglycemia.

7. Suspected anaphylactic reaction with laryngeal reaction, bronchospasm, hypotension, or dysrhythmias.

8. Inconsolable crying or irritability lasting several hours and unexplained after thorough evaluation.

Gururaj VJ: Short stay in an outpatient department. Am J Dis Child 1972;123:128.

Kreger BE, Restuccia JD: Assessing the need to hospitalize children: Pediatric appropriateness evaluation protocol. Pediatrics 1989;84:242.

Lovejoy FH et al: Unnecessary and preventable hospitalizations: Report on an internal audit. J Pediatr 1971;79:868.

Psychosocial Indications for Hospitalization

Temporary admission to a pediatric ward is occasionally needed for the following situations:

A. Child Problems:

1. An incapacitating emotional symptom (eg, a severe conversion reaction such as paraplegia or blindness).

2. Suicide attempt. A short hospital admission allows time for the mental health worker to make an evaluation and for the family to look seriously at their problems.

3. A destructive, dangerous child can be held on a pediatric ward pending placement. A dangerous adolescent will require a psychiatric care facility.

B. Disease Problems:

1. An incapacitating (but not life-threatening) physical disease (eg, severe Sydenham's chorea).

2. Initial diagnosis of a disease with a complex treatment regimen. The parents and patient deserve a careful, unhurried, and organized introduction to the complex home management of some chronic diseases (eg, diabetes mellitus).

3. Initial diagnosis of a life-threatening disease— This gives the family time to work through the impact phase (eg, leukemia).

4. Terminal care if the family does not want the child to die at home.

5. Chronic diseases that are exacerbated by family conflicts (eg, ulcerative colitis).

Remove from Environment Without Hospitalization

When parents are abusive, neglectful, hospitalized, overwhelmed, or intoxicated, arrangements must be made to care for the children. Often the child can stay for a short time with a relative. In most cities, a child can also be placed in an emergency receiving home. In rare cases, admission to the hospital may be required for children with the following parent problems:

(1) Child abuse (eg, physical abuse without serious injury, failure to thrive secondary to neglect, or incest).

(2) Incipient battering (eg, the parent has made a homicidal threat against a child).

(3) Absent parents (eg, abandonment, emancipated minors without caretakers, or the parents themselves are hospitalized).

(4) Physically exhausted parents (eg, no sleep for 2 or more nights).

(5) Severely overanxious parents (eg, if the parents remain immobilized and extremely anxious after a careful explanation of the child's illness).

(6) Neglectful parents who seem uninterested in the child's illness or therapy (eg, neglected eczema). This is a rare situation compared with overly anxious parents.

(7) Intellectually incompetent parents (eg, a mentally retarded mother who cannot reliably follow verbal or written instructions).

(8) Emotionally disturbed parents who need psychiatric hospitalization and treatment for their own problems (eg, a floridly psychotic mother).

(9) Parent who is intoxicated from substance abuse.

Unnecessary Hospitalization

In the USA, overhospitalization is currently a greater problem than underhospitalization. In recent studies, at least 20% of hospitalizations were judged to be unnecessary. Moreover, 25% of unnecessary patient days were due to delayed discharge because the patient was simply waiting for transportation home. Overhospitalization takes three general forms: (1) Hospitalization for an acute illness sometimes occurs because the primary physician is uncertain of the diagnosis and prognosis (eg, viral rashes). Reassurance in the face of such uncertainty can often be gained by immediate consultation with a colleague or subspecialist. (2) Hospitalization is sometimes arranged for a diagnostic evaluation and tests because the patient has no outpatient insurance (eg, urinary tract infection). Fortunately, ambulatory studies have become more reimbursable. (3) Periodic hospitalizations sometimes are ordered for routine reevaluations of a chronic disease (eg, chronic glomerulonephritis). Even if the patient travels a great distance, this reevaluation can be done on an ambulatory basis if it is carefully planned in advance. The combined costs of the special studies plus hotel accommodations will be far less than hospitalization charges. In cases of elective hospitalization, preadmission evaluations can reduce hospital stays by 2 or 3 days.

The indications for hospitalization are becoming more selective. The time has passed when every child with infectious mononucleosis, hepatitis, pneumonia, acute rheumatic fever, gross hematuria, or a urinary tract infection is automatically admitted. Fewer than 10% of patients with these acute disorders require hospitalization. In fact, in emergency departments with special observation units, children with moderate dehydration, diabetic ketoacidosis, status asthmaticus, etc, are treated and released in 3–6 hours.

Home-care programs have expedited the discharge of many acutely ill children. Infections that can be treated at home with intravenous antibiotics include osteomyelitis, septic arthritis, endocarditis, pelvic inflammatory disease, pyelonephritis, and cellulitis. Other types of home care services include phototherapy, total parenteral alimentation, continuous enteral feedings, and intravenous chemotherapy.

Unnecessary hospitalization carries five main problems or risks, the last one probably being the most serious: (1) Children under 3 years of age can experience separation problems. Children of all ages cope with their illnesses better in a nurturing home setting. (2) The parents' confidence in caring for a sick child themselves is undermined. (3) There is a danger of cross-infection to the patient and others. (4) There is a risk of medical error, such as the wrong medication or wrong dosage. (5) Society sustains an endlessly rising cost for medical care. Home care services cost approximately 20% of comparable hospital services.

An acutely ill child can be observed in the office for several hours if it is not clear whether or not hospitalization is necessary. This will allow time for any reassurance given to the mother to take effect, and it permits the physician to compare the patient at two points in time and determine whether the condition is improving or getting worse. This interval also helps one decide what to do when the mother's history and the physical examination are inconsistent (eg, "recurrent vomiting" without dehydration, "no urination" without bladder distention). If necessary, another physician can be called in for consultation during this time.

Goldbloom RB, Macleod MU: Impact of preadmission evaluations on elective hospitalization of children. Pediatrics 1984;73:656.
Kemper KJ: Medically inappropriate hospital use in a pediatric population. N Engl J Med 1988;318:1033.
Schuman AJ: Homeward bound: The explosion in pediatric home care. Contemporary Pediatr 1990;7:26.

5. TREATMENT OF THE ACUTELY ILL PATIENT

Words are as necessary as drugs in the treatment of a sick child. The parents expect to be told their child's diagnosis and its causes, prognosis, and treatment. They also need to have their special concerns acknowledged and clarified. If this communication does not take place, the parents will often be dissatisfied with the quality of care being given, and their compliance with regard to medications, advice, and follow-up will probably be less than optimal.

If the child has a mild acute illness (eg, viral nasopharyngitis), the parent would be reassured by the following general types of comment.

Diagnosis

"David has a cold." The diagnosis should be conveyed in plain English, not in medical jargon. If the physician does not specifically state the diagnosis, the parents may assume none has been arrived at. (See also Ambiguous Diagnosis, below.)

Etiology

"It's due to a virus." This means to most parents that the infection is not serious. Some parents need an added statement that there was nothing they could have done to prevent it—eg, "Lots of children are coming down with this."

Parents' Concerns

Mothers often do not listen to the physician's instructions until their own main concerns have been discussed. These concerns are easily elicited by Korsch's three questions: (1) "Why did you bring David to the clinic today?" (2) "What worried you most about him?" (3) "Why did that worry you?" After these concerns are out in the open, the physician is in a position to clarify misconceptions. Reassurance can be specific—eg, "He doesn't have meningitis . . . [appendicitis . . . dehydration . . . etc]."

Treatment

In self-limited disease, the goal of treatment is to keep the patient comfortable. A list of useful approaches to management (sometimes overlooked) is as follows: (1) Most symptoms don't need a drug. An antipyretic is not needed unless the patient's fever causes discomfort. (2) Cough and cold medicines have little if any effect. Teaching the parent how to suction the nose properly can turn a restless baby into a sleeping one. The key maneuver is loosening up the dried mucus with water or saline nose drops. (3) The patient can usually be allowed to dictate the diet during periods of illness. (4) In most cases, the patient can also be allowed to decide whether to stay in bed, to be up in pajamas watching television, etc. (5) Isolation within the family structure is rarely indicated, because exposure has usually preceded the diagnosis. (6) Parents can be reassured about temporary emotional regression during an acute illness. A return to the previous level of maturity need not be encouraged until good health returns.

Prognosis

"David will probably feel better in two or three days. This is not a serious infection. If his fever lasts over three days or if he gets worse, give me a call." Nothing is gained by mentioning all the possible complications. Without promoting anxiety, the door to additional medical evaluation is quietly left open for any new problems that might arise.

Closing

"You're doing a fine job with David. Just hold the fort and he will be his old self in a few days." The visit should close on a positive note, even a compliment if possible. If David is older, an attempt can be made to boost his morale as well—eg, "This won't keep you out of action for long."

The Ambiguous Diagnosis

An unclear diagnosis presents special problems in communication with the parents. The physician must be honest about the inconclusive diagnosis and yet not unduly alarm the parents. "David's illness is not far enough along to be diagnosed exactly. Another day or so will be needed to pinpoint the problem. I can tell you a few things for certain. He is not in any serious trouble. He doesn't have meningitis. I definitely want to see him tomorrow. Call me sooner if there are any new developments."

Symptomatic therapy should also be prescribed.

Carey WB, Sibinga MS: Avoiding pediatric pathogenesis in the management of acute minor illness. Pediatrics 1972; 49:553.

Korsch B et al: Practical implications of doctor-patient interaction analysis for pediatric practice. Am J Dis Child 1971;121:110.

Waller DA, Levitt EE: Concerns of mothers in a pediatric clinic. Pediatrics 1972;50:931.

6. FOLLOW-UP OF THE ACUTELY ILL PATIENT

Many children seen for an acute illness have conditions that require follow-up (eg, asthma, bronchiolitis, croup, pneumonia, otitis media, burns, seizures). If a child has an ambiguous diagnosis (eg, high fever of unknown origin) or an unpredictable course (eg, vomiting), daily follow-up is necessary. This protects both the patient and the physician. This follow-up can be accomplished by revisits, telephone calls, or a visiting nurse.

Revisits

Daily office visits are the best approach to the more serious problem. The weight of an infant with diarrhea and the degree of respiratory distress in a child with croup cannot be estimated over the phone. If a scheduled appointment is not kept, the office clerk should immediately notify the physician, and a phone call or home visit should be made on that same day. If transportation is a problem for the parent, a community service agency can usually help. If the late results of laboratory tests indicate that an illness is quite serious (eg, stool culture growing *Salmonella* in a 2-month-old infant) and reasonable attempts to locate the parents fail, the police may be asked to find and bring the patient to the clinic or office.

Telephone Calls

A daily telephone call will suffice for milder problems when only historical follow-up data are needed (eg, vomiting or lethargy). Since these calls are essential to proper management, the physician or nurse should make them. A daily telephone list can be kept and the charts pulled prior to calling. If the follow-up is felt to be important, parents should not be depended upon to initiate these calls. Telephone calls become the realistic choice of follow-up when long distances are a factor.

Home Visits

The evaluation of children with allergies, obesity, failure to thrive, recurrent accidents, recurrent ingestions, or behavior problems is enhanced by a home visit. The follow-up of early-discharge newborns is simplified by home visits. Dressing changes of burns or wounds can readily be done in the home. Most of these house calls are made by the public health nurse, but the office nurse or physician can also become involved. Mothers of large families who have both a baby-sitter problem and a transportation problem appreciate this type of follow-up. Mothers who have several sick children or who are themselves in poor health also benefit from home visits.

Berger LR, Samet KP: Home visits: Extending the boundaries of comprehensive pediatric care. Am J Dis Child 1981;135:812.

DeAngelis C, Fosarelli P: Assignment of follow-up appointments from an emergency room by pediatric residents. Am J Dis Child 1985;139:341.

PREVENTION OF MALPRACTICE SUITS

The management of acute illness offers the greatest potential for malpractice litigation in pediatrics. Physicians are legally liable for injuries caused not only by their own mistakes but by the mistakes of their employees as well. Errors can be made in any of the areas previously discussed. An error in telephone triaging can result in a delay in diagnosis (eg, calling meningococcemia a viral exanthem, or arranging an appointment for the next day for scrotal pain that turns out to be testicular torsion). An error in underhospitalization can lead to death (eg, epiglottitis being treated on an outpatient basis) or disability (eg, meningitis being missed in a child who receives a second antibiotic when his otitis media and fever fail to respond to the first-line antibiotic). Errors in therapy may result in sciatic nerve palsy if an injection is given into an inappropriate quadrant of the buttocks or may result in acute rheumatic fever if penicillin is not given for a streptococcal sore throat because the throat was not cultured. Errors in follow-up can result in undiagnosed abdominal pain silently progressing to ruptured appendix.

To improve patient care and decrease your risk for malpractice suits, consider the following suggestions:

(1) Stay up to date in your field. Read journals, attend conferences, and discuss cases with your colleagues. Understand the changing standards of care for the various conditions you treat.

(2) Maintain accurate, complete, and legible medical records. Consider common complications of the conditions you diagnose, and record their absence. See comments on page 154 about improving your documentation through chart reviews.

(3) Document all telephone advice. Telephone triage by office staff should be linked to written protocols.

(4) Do not prescribe prescription drugs without examining the patient first.

(5) Avoid excessive waiting time in your office, since this is a leading cause of parent dissatisfaction.

(6) Seek consultation whenever you are uncertain about what is happening with an acutely and perhaps seriously ill patient.

(7) Obtain parents' written consent (eg, for lumbar punctures) or oral consent (eg, for suturing) unless an emergency exists.

(8) Base all medical decisions on what is best for the patient.

Cohn B: Office malpractice pitfalls. Pediatr Ann 1991; 20:69.

Reynolds SL, Jaffe D, Glynn W: Professional liability in a pediatric emergency department. Pediatrics 1991;87:134.

CHRONIC DISEASE FOLLOW-UP VISITS

Chronic diseases are defined as conditions present for at least 3 months. From 10% to 15% of children in the United States have one or more chronic illnesses. From 2% to 4% of children have severe illnesses that interfere with activities of daily living and a normal childhood. Management of these patients is thus a major part of pediatric practice. Office visits for a child with known or potential chronic disease present special problems. There are five broad types of chronic disease, each being progressively more difficult to manage: (1) potential chronic disease (eg, the preterm infant, the infant with hemolytic-uremic syndrome, or the older child who has recovered from meningitis); (2) reversible chronic disease (eg, gastroesophageal reflux of infancy, eczema, or idiopathic thrombocytopenic purpura); (3) static chronic disease (eg, cerebral palsy, deafness, or mental retardation); (4) progressive chronic disease (eg, diabetes mellitus or sickle cell anemia); and (5) life-threatening disease (eg, some cancers). Children with these problems usually receive excellent care when they are hospitalized. They should also receive the same thoughtful care when they do not occupy a hospital bed.

Stein REK: Chronic physical disorders, Pediatr Rev 1992, 13:224.

COMMON TYPES OF CHRONIC DISORDERS

The following diagnoses or conditions are the chronic disorders most commonly seen in office practice: serous otitis media, hay fever, asthma, obesity, enuresis, recurrent abdominal pain, recurrent headaches, acne, developmental delays or mental retardation, seizures, learning disabilities, attention deficit disorder, menstrual problems, visual defects, hearing defects, depression, child abuse, recurrent urinary tract infections, vesico-ureteral reflux, hypertension, congenital heart disease, failure to thrive, short stature, eczema, cerebral palsy, constipation or soiling, recurrent hematuria, scoliosis, chronic diarrhea, peptic ulcer, and diabetes mellitus.

OBJECTIVES

There are three primary objectives in the management of a chronic disease. The first is to counteract the effects of the disease to the extent possible. This requires the aggressive use of every available treatment measure that could be useful for the individual patient's problems. A second objective is to screen for associated complications and, if any are detected, to provide early intervention. Examples are developmental delays in preterm children, speech delays in children with chronic otitis media, scoliosis in those with neurofibromatosis, and rapid head growth in children with myelomeningocele. The third objective is to help the patient and parents make a suitable emotional adjustment to the treatment regimen and to the effects of the disease that cannot be controlled. Except for necessary restrictions imposed by the disease, the child should be reared just like other children. The goal of management is to enable the patient to live as normal a life as possible in all positive respects.

Chronic disease management is optimal when the following receive ongoing attention: continuity of care, frequent visits, problem-oriented records, chronic disease flow sheets, personal medical identification documents, a chronic disease patient registry kept in the office, and medical passport.

1. CONTINUITY OF CARE

The patient with a chronic disease may have multiple problems that are difficult to manage. If anyone deserves continuous medical care from one physician, this person does. Discontinuous care by several physicians (eg, in emergency rooms) often results in partial treatment, conflicting treatments, and a confused patient. When the patient has a progressive or life-threatening disease, depression can occur. In such a situation, patients depend upon a single sustaining physician to help them maintain their tenuous hope for the child's survival. Fragmented medical care usually accentuates a poor psychologic adjustment. The physician who agrees to care for a patient with a chronic disease should be available by phone at all times, even when at home. If the physician cannot deal with a problem personally, arrangements can be made for the patient to be seen by another physician who has been fully briefed. If the physician must be away for any reason, a substitute physician who has been designated well in advance should be available.

American Academy of Pediatrics Task Force: The medical home. Pediatrics 1992,90:774.

Brewer EJ et al: Family-centered, community-based, coordinated care for children with special health care needs. Pediatrics 1989;83:1055.

Liptak GS, Revell GM: Community physician's role in case management of children with chronic illnesses. Pediatrics 1989;84:465.

2. FREQUENT VISITS

The patient with a chronic disease should be contacted frequently. Monitoring the patient's disease and response to therapy is impossible without periodic visits or telephone communications. If the problem is stabilized, the patient should be seen personally at least every 6 months; 3-month intervals are better for progressive diseases. If the disease is in relapse, the patient may need to be seen daily.

3. PROBLEM-ORIENTED RECORDS

In addition to a personal physician, comprehensive care of the chronically ill patient depends upon good record keeping. No physician's memory is completely reliable, and in any case the patient must have accurate office records should the physician move or die. An excellent system of record keeping has been developed and refined in a practice setting (see references, below). It has four components: the initial data base, the active problem sheet, the plan for each problem, and the progress notes that contribute to the continually expanding data base and problem list.

Initial Data Base

The conventional present illness, review of systems, past medical history, family history, psychosocial history, physical examination, and laboratory screening tests comprise the data base. Information from all accessible sources is used. (See Chapter 1.)

Active Problem Sheet

The active problem list is the keystone of this system. It lists all of the patient's significant problems, including psychosocial ones. These problems are defined from the data base currently at hand. They can be expressed as an etiologic diagnosis (eg, rheumatic heart disease), a pathophysiologic state (eg, congestive heart failure), or a sign or symptom (eg, edema). When the therapy carries medical risk, it should be listed as a problem (eg, corticosteroids or tracheostomy). An attempt is made to list the problems in order of priority. Each problem is then assigned a permanent number. Thereafter, this number should precede any entry in the chart concerning this problem. The active problem sheet should be kept in the front of the patient's chart as a table of contents. The dates should be date of onset and date of resolution. New problems are added as identified, and old problems are transferred to the "resolved or inactive" column when appropriate. Symptom problems should be reidentified as diagnosed problems when the data accumulated justify doing so. When a patient with multiple diseases is cared for by several physicians, the last column on the active problem list can be used to list the responsible physician for each problem. This technique is especially helpful for improving continuity of care in a large medical center.

The active problem list can become somewhat standardized if "1" is always used for "health maintenance care" (or well child care) and "2" is always used for "minor acute illnesses" (or temporary problems). The latter category is a convenient place to bury self-limited minor illnesses that do not warrant being given individual permanent numbers. Examples are colds, coughs, gastroenteritis, conjunctivitis, viral exanthems, impetigo, diaper rash, insect bites, minor trauma, etc. Acute illnesses that can be serious (eg, pneumonia) or recurrent (eg, otitis media) should be given different numbers. Some proponents of the active problem list suggest we include a category called "family strengths". Notations such as supportive extended family, intact family, caring older brother, and church or synagogue remind us of whom to mobilize when the family becomes stressed.

Plan for Each Problem

Each problem as listed in the active problem sheet needs an individual diagnostic, therapeutic, and educational plan. If the plans for all the problems are combined, omissions are likely to occur.

Progress Notes

Progress notes contain newly collected data, an analysis of the data, and a reassessment of the plan. These notes should always pertain to one of the problems on the active problem sheet and be so labeled both by number and by title, eg, as follows:

Seizures, grand mal

Subjective: Two seizures last week, lasting 1 minute and 5 minutes. Occurred at 7 AM and 10 AM. No precipitating events apparent. Last seizure 3 months ago. No headaches or vomiting. Not drowsy from medication.

Objective: Neurologic examination and fundi normal. No nystagmus.

Assessment: Seizures—inadequate control.

Plan: Continue carbamazepine 200 mg tid. Recheck blood level. Review and reinforce reasons for strict compliance.

Gordon IB: Office medical records. Pediatr Clin North Am 1981;28:565.

4. THE CHRONIC DISEASE FLOW SHEET

There are many variables in the management of a chronic disease. The variables can become lost in the substance of the chart and relatively unavailable for comparison and interpretation. For a patient with a chronic disease or multiple problems, critical data from the progress note should be recorded on a chronic disease flow sheet which tabulates variables so that trends and correlations can be accurately determined. The long axis of the flow sheet has time intervals. Inpatient flow sheets maintained for a critically ill child usually monitor vital signs, intake and output, blood gases, and numerous chemical determinations. Outpatient flow sheets often contain little of the above. Although a specific flow sheet is designed for each chronic disease, the following variables are commonly present in the ambulatory management of most chronic diseases.

Disease Status

One must monitor the activity level of the disease to know whether therapy is being effective or not. Such activity can be evaluated through the history, physical findings, laboratory data, consultations, and hospitalizations. Variables so determined can be tabulated on the flow sheet.

A. Symptom Data: Frequency of attacks and duration of attacks are the main determinants of the success of asthma therapy. Migraine headaches, seizure episodes, and psychogenic recurrent abdominal pain must also be monitored largely by attack rates.

B. Physical Findings: Childhood nephrosis must be followed by weighing the patient and observing the presence or absence of edema. Splenomegaly is an important variable in leukemia. Motor milestones are important in cerebral palsy.

C. Laboratory Data: Voiding cystourethrograms are important for following vesicoureteral reflux, tympanograms for chronic serous otitis media, liver enzyme levels for chronic active hepatitis, urine cultures for recurrent urinary tract infection, etc.

D. Data for Early Detection of Complications: Some chronic diseases have complications that are not preventable but respond much better to therapy if they are detected early. Warning signs of these complications should be listed on the flow sheet. Examples are (1) head circumference measurements to detect early subdural effusions or hydrocephalus after meningitis and (2) blood pressure measurements to detect early hypertension in chronic renal disease. Once hypertension is discovered, it is no longer an anticipated complication but an indicator of disease activity.

E. Consultations: One of the patient's problems may be managed by another specialist. The primary physician should record on the flow sheet, under the dates of these visits, the consultant's name and a brief note about that specialist's conclusions. The date will permit easy location of the consultation report in the chart when it is needed.

F. Hospitalizations: All hospitalizations need to be recorded under the problem they were required for. They usually represent a marker of increased activity of the disease.

G. Emotional Status: Emotional maladjustments are a frequent and often unnecessary side effect of chronic diseases. The physician can prevent them in many instances by reviewing an emotional problem checklist on every visit. Some of the more common but unspoken maladjustments are unnecessary restrictions, overprotectiveness, favoritism, school absenteeism, underdiscipline, and teasing by peers. This subject is more fully discussed in Chapter 6.

Treatment Regimen

Therapy may or may not be responsible for improvements in clinical status. Examining the temporal relationship of one to the other allows the physician to decide if treatment has been effective. A chronic disease flow sheet should supply this information.

A. Medications: All medications and dosages should be listed with the dates when started, when discontinued, and when the dosage is changed. The dosage may be increased because the patient has outgrown it or because the problem is not under optimal control (eg, increasing the dosage of digoxin in persistent congestive heart failure). New drugs should be added when other drugs have been pushed to tolerance without adequate control (eg, adding cromolyn to daily albuterol nebulizers in asthma). Any drug the patient is receiving should have at least one related variable listed under disease status that permits rapid assessment of the efficacy of the drug (eg, bowel movements per day recorded for the patient with ulcerative colitis who is taking sulfasalazine).

B. Toxicity: If drugs with side effects are being used, these problems should be anticipated. The bone marrow, kidney, or liver function tests that need monitoring should be recorded on the flow sheet, as well as the required frequency of testing. If the potential toxicity is high, the drug should also be recorded on the problem list. If suddenly discontinuing the drug could lead to a severe adverse reaction, this risk should be frequently discussed with the patient (eg, anticonvulsants).

C. Nondrug Therapy: Other methods of treatment besides drugs should be recorded on the flow sheet so that their effect on the course of the disease can be estimated. Examples are specific food avoidance in recurrent urticaria or bubble bath avoidance in recurrent urinary tract infection. In static diseases, compensatory devices (eg, braces in cerebral palsy or hearing aids in deafness) should be listed, as well as the recommended interval for routine checks of these devices. Reassurance and other forms of supportive psychotherapy will generally be given on every visit and need not be listed here.

D. Therapy for Prevention of Complications: Many chronic diseases have predictable complications that are preventable if therapy is instituted in advance. If these are listed in the flow sheet, the physician will be certain to remind the parent of them on each visit. Examples are performing daily range-of-motion exercises to prevent contractures in rheumatoid arthritis, requesting penicillin prophylaxis before dental procedures to prevent subacute bacterial endocarditis in congenital heart disease, avoidance of altitudes over 10,000 feet to prevent a crisis in sickle cell disease, and carrying an antihypoglycemic food in the pocket at all times in diabetes mellitus.

E. Compliance With Therapy: The best treatment regimen is useless unless the patient complies with it. A check on the patient's compliance can be performed by inquiring about the degree of satisfaction or dissatisfaction with the medical care received; by asking if the medications have been difficult to take; or in some cases by measuring blood or urine levels (eg, aspirin, penicillin).

F. Disease Education Reviews: Patients may not cooperate with a therapeutic plan until they are intellectually and emotionally committed to it. Unless the family fully understands what they are expected to do, they cannot do it. Unless they understand priorities, they may unknowingly discontinue some critical element in the treatment program when the program as a whole becomes frustrating. Optimal patient education is reached when patient and family know as much about the home treatment of the disease as the physician does and when they can make minor adjustments in treatment independently.

When facts regarding the disease and its treatment are reviewed, one should begin with basic information even though it has been covered many times before. After the first session, the subject is reviewed by asking the patient questions. In the early years, the facts are covered with the patient and both parents present. If the father does not share responsibility for medical care of the child, serious marital problems may develop. In the adolescent years, the review sessions should be done privately with the teenager. The patient's understanding of the problems should be explored approximately every 6 months. In the period immediately following diagnosis, it should be covered on every visit for a few months.

G. School Notification: Each fall the physician should ask the parent to notify the school nurse about any patient whose disease may become manifest or cause a problem of any sort at school. This notification will prevent emotional problems secondary to mishandling of the physical problem by the school. The patient with chronic heart or lung disease may need a gym excuse (no gym) or a modified gym status (eg, no gym on days of wheezing; no rope climbing). Both nurse and teacher need to know how to respond to a seizure or insulin reaction at school. The physician should have this listed on the flow sheet so it is never overlooked. The parents of the patient's closest friends should also have this information, as should the baby-sitters.

Schmitt BD: The chronic disease flow sheet in ambulatory pediatrics. Pediatrics 1973;51:722.

5. THE MEDICAL IDENTIFICATION CARD

The patient with a chronic disease should carry an identification card that sets forth the active problem list, medications being taken currently, the physician's telephone number, and the parents' telephone numbers at home and at work. If the disease can lead to sudden changes in consciousness (eg, insulin reaction in diabetes mellitus) or if an allergy is present that could be fatal if violated (eg, penicillin hypersensitivity), the patient should obtain a medical identification bracelet or necklace.

6. CHRONIC DISEASE PATIENT REGISTRY

Every effort should be made to keep certain patients from being "lost to follow-up." People with chronic diseases (eg, those with rheumatic heart disease receiving prophylactic penicillin) fall into this group. To prevent the disappearance of any of these patients, the physician should keep them listed in a chronic disease patient registry. Their charts should have a special mark placed on the corner of the cover to show that they are special high-risk patients. These patients should be sent a reminder card 1 week prior to appointments. If the parent cancels an appointment and promises to call back and make another one, the patient's name should be placed on a critical phone call list that automatically goes into effect if the appointment is not remade within 2 weeks. If the patient misses an appointment, the physician should be notified that same day and should call the patient. If the

parent has no phone, a letter should be sent. If there is no response to the letter, a visiting nurse referral should be sent. This usually returns the patient to the physician or shows that the family has changed physicians. If the family does not wish further medical care from anyone and the patient's disease is life-threatening but treatable (eg, tuberculosis, chronic pyelonephritis), the physician should report the case to the local child protective services. Since this is an example of medical care neglect, a court order will be issued for treatment of the child. The physician should assume personal responsibility for following any high-risk patient until transfer of care occurs.

7. THE MEDICAL PASSPORT

Every year, 20% of North American families change residences. Some of them have children with chronic diseases. Nothing is more frustrating for a physician than to take a complicated new patient with no past records. Legally, the records belong to the physician; but morally, the records belong to the patient. The patient who moves should carry a copy of the active problem list, chronic disease flow sheet, health maintenance flow sheet (including immunizations), growth charts, consultation reports, hospital discharge summaries, pertinent x-ray reports, and a covering letter. Original copies should never be sent, because they may be lost. The physician should also give the family the names of two or three pediatricians they might use in the city they are moving to. These may be personal acquaintances or selections made from the American Academy of Pediatrics *Fellowship Directory.*

CONSULTATIVE VISITS

The physician must know both how to serve as a general consultant and how to seek subspecialty consultation when it is called for. The general pediatrician is still the best consultant for many pediatric problems.

OBJECTIVES

The usual purpose of a consultation is the evaluation of an undiagnosed problem followed by therapeutic recommendations. Some referrals are for treatment advice only. A secondary goal of consultation is to provide the referring physician with a continuing medical educational experience.

THE PEDIATRICIAN IN THE ROLE OF GENERAL CONSULTANT

Referring Source

A. Self-Referral: Although not technically a consultation, some problems require the same kind of intensive approach that is needed when consulting with a colleague. A problem requiring a careful diagnostic evaluation may be detected during a well-child visit or a sick child visit. These "big" problems are often not mentioned by the parent until the end of the visit or may be detected by a screening questionnaire. The physician should arrange to see such patients again. These diagnostic evaluations can keep practice stimulating. The physician who is unsure about the workup of a particular problem can take time to review the literature beforehand.

B. Physician Referral: Family practitioners or other specialists occasionally refer patients to a pediatrician for consultation. Within the pediatric community, some pediatricians refer patients to other physicians who have a subspecialty interest or expertise in a specific disease. This is more common within a group practice.

C. Nonphysician Referral: A physician who is well thought of receives referrals from dentists, school officials, psychologists, social workers, and nurses. Not uncommonly, parents seek a second opinion. Some of these referred patients will require a consultation type of visit.

McCrindle BW Starfield B: Subspecialization within pediatric practice: A broader spectrum. Pediatrics 1992, 90:573.

Appointments

Consultations usually require 45- to 60-minute appointments. In some cases, two visits may be required to complete the evaluation. The average pediatrician will need to have two or three of these 1-hour appointments scheduled each week. The visit will be considerably more productive if a screening questionnaire is completed in advance. The questionnaire should delineate the patient's physical, intellectual, and emotional problems and serve as an initial data base.

These long appointments are easily arranged when the patient is referred by another professional, because a telephone call or letter usually precedes the patient. However, a patient with almost any problem requiring a careful evaluation can walk into a physician's office at any time. When the mother of a 10-year-old patient who is being seen for acute otitis media mentions that her child has experienced 4 years of encopresis or 6 months of "staring spells" at school, the busy physician may feel under some pressure to make a quick recommendation. The temptation may be strong to do a 5-minute workup and order some laboratory tests, or to hospitalize the patient for

evaluation at greater leisure, or even to disregard the complaint or minimize its importance. Needless to say, these responses do not serve the patient's best interests. Long-standing diagnostic dilemmas require a comprehensive assessment that takes at least an hour. Most such evaluations can be done on an ambulatory basis. Shortcuts can lead to tentative conclusions, unconvinced parents, postponement of the indicated workup, "doctor shopping," secondary gain for the patient, and an unresolved problem.

The first visit can serve a useful purpose. One can tell the parents that the child's problem is complicated and requires a complete evaluation. A few screening laboratory tests such as a blood count and erythrocyte sedimentation rate may be ordered. The parent can fill out the screening data questionnaire. A release can be signed for hospital discharge summaries, prior consultation reports, laboratory test results (especially any tests that are dangerous, painful, or expensive), school reports, and growth information. These data will make the consultation visit more meaningful and avoid duplication of effort. In these consultations (unlike hospitalized consultations), an immediate appointment is rarely needed, and the patient can be rescheduled for the following week or later if more time is needed to accumulate data.

Extent of Services

When the patient is referred by a physician, there are five possible degrees of service the consulting physician can offer. If the referring physician does not specify precisely what is needed, the consulting physician may either ask in advance or may assume that this cannot be predicted and must await the results of the evaluation.

A. Evaluation Only: The consultant can do a diagnostic evaluation on a patient and tell the parents nothing except that the findings will be discussed with their primary physician. Parents generally do not like this approach. They are paying for the consultation, and they want to hear something directly from the expert. Common courtesy suggests that they are right.

B. Evaluation and Interpretation: After the evaluation is completed, the consultant usually discusses the diagnosis and the causes of the problem with the family. Recommendations for therapy can be reviewed in general terms and with the clear understanding that the referring physician will be coordinating the therapy. A specific return appointment date with the referring physician should be given. This type of consultation may be appropriate for a patient with a chronic disease who lives at a great distance. The consultant may be called upon periodically to reassess the response to therapy and to offer revised recommendations.

C. Evaluation and Treatment of an Isolated Problem: Often the referring physician wants the consultant to assume responsibility for management of the problem that is the subject of referral. This usually happens with treatable problems that will require only two to four visits (eg, recurrent headaches, breath-holding spells, encopresis or failure to thrive). The consultant should clearly define and support the referring physician's role as the continuing provider of health supervision and acute illness care during this interval. When the problem is resolved, the patient should be returned to the referring physician for resumption of care.

D. Total Health Care: Occasionally, a physician refers a patient to a consultant for management of a specific problem plus all future medical care. This may occur when the family is moving to a new area or is unable for financial reasons to maintain the contact with a private physician.

E. Evaluation and Referral for Additional Consultation: The patient's problem may require the expertise of a subspecialist (eg, pediatric hematologist). Before this step is taken, permission must be sought from the original physician for further consultation. The pediatrician's advice about where to seek further subspecialty consultations will usually be accepted.

Communication With the Referring Source

Communication is the key to a satisfactory referral process. The consulting physician is mainly responsible for this aspect of consultation. The referring physician should not have to ask the consultant for the results. The following procedure serves as an appropriate format for completing the process diplomatically.

A. Acknowledge the Referral: As soon as a referral letter is received, the consulting physician should send the referral source a brief note acknowledging the referral. Additional information can also be requested at this time: "Thank you for your recent referral letter on David Jones. He is scheduled for an evaluation on _____. I will be in contact with you regarding the results. Best regards."

B. Send a Consultation Report: This report should be sent promptly. The content of the final report depends on the referring source. School officials do not want to know medical details; they usually just want to know if the patient is physically healthy or, if not, what their responsibility is. A referring physician expects a full report that will be helpful in treating the patient. Recommendations should therefore be specific (drugs, dosages, other forms of therapy, duration of therapy, specific laboratory tests, the frequency of these tests, etc). A copy of or reference to a recent review article on the subject will also be appreciated.

This evaluation should be typed as a formal consultation report. It should not contain personal comments. When written in this style, it can serve as an official evaluation report for anyone who might request a copy of it in the future. A copy can also be sent to the family for their records. To make this communication to the referring physician more personal, it can be accompanied by a covering letter: "It was a pleasure to see David Jones today. A complete summary of his evaluation is included. The recommendations may need to be modified in the light of your previous experience with this family. As you know, the marital situation is very stormy. It would be a privilege to see David again if you feel the need arises."

C. Call the Referring Physician Selectively: Most referring physicians prefer a consultation report to a phone call because the former can become a permanent part of the patient's record. Some cases require a brief telephone report in addition to the written report. These cases include situations where the patient needs to return to the referring physician before a consultation report can be sent, where the patient needs to be referred to an additional specialist, or where a question exists about proper disposition.

D. Arrange a Return Appointment With the Referring Physician: At the end of the consultation, the consultant should tell the parents when the patient should see the primary physician—usually in 1–2 weeks. Positive comments about the referring physician's competence and judgment should be made. The parents must feel confident that the primary physician can provide the necessary follow-up care. If the referring physician had tentatively made the correct diagnosis prior to referral, the consultant's corroboration should be made clear to the parents and recorded in the consultation report.

Fees for Services Rendered

Many pediatricians are reluctant to charge adequately for their time. This seems illogical, since an ambulatory consultation can prevent the high cost of an unnecessary hospital workup. Even if ambulatory insurance does not cover the full cost of such an evaluation, the pediatrician should bill for these evaluations as "office consultations" and charge for the time allotted. A reasonable fee is $2–3 a minute. This amounts to $120–180 for the initial evaluation and $60–90 for follow-up visits. An hour is worth the same whether it is spent with one consultation or several well or sick children.

Bailie MD et al: When the pediatrician is the consultant. Contemporary Pediatr 1988,5:137.
Stickler GB: The pediatrician as a consultant. Am J Dis Child 1989;143:73

THE PEDIATRICIAN IN THE ROLE OF REFERRING PHYSICIAN

Indications for Referral

There are generally eight indications for seeking consultation. The last two are primarily to help the parents deal with reality.

A. Uncertain Diagnosis: Referral for a diagnostic evaluation is a time-honored indication. The ambulatory consultation is preferable to hospitalization.

B. Treatment Requires Special Expertise: *Example:* Surgery.

C. Treatment Is Nonmedical: *Examples:* Services of psychiatrists, psychologists, social workers, special education teachers, speech therapists.

D. Treatment Is Complex or Multidisciplinary: The treatment of some diseases is so complex that the physician unfamiliar with it should refer those patients. *Examples:* Cystic fibrosis, muscular dystrophy, leukemia.

E. Conventional Treatment Is Not Effective: When the patient is not doing as well as expected, one must seek help. Even with diseases the physician has successfully treated many times, an atypical problem may arise that requires a fresh opinion (eg, recalcitrant seizures). Phone consultation with the appropriate subspecialist will sometimes provide new insights.

F. Medicolegal Problems: Parents bring in children with injuries that have given rise to legal action against a physician or other person. The pediatrician's main task is to decide if the alleged disability or defect is real. If the injury proves to be significant, the physician can help the family find an expert consultant whose testimony will be credible in court (eg, an orthopedist in the case of a hand injury). If it seems that the parents are exaggerating the disability for financial gain, the physician should declare the child healthy and recommend return to full activity without confronting the family with such suspicions.

G. Parents Insist on Overtreatment: The pediatrician can help the family avoid inappropriate intervention by recommending consultation with experts known to have scientifically based views. Even though there are honest differences of opinion about the indications for tonsillectomy, "corrective shoes," hyposensitization, etc, it is in the patient's best interests not to have to undergo painful or protracted procedures with little chance of substantial benefit.

H. Parents Are Thinking About a Consultation: When the parents have to ask for a consultation or obtain one without telling the physician, the pediatrician has waited too long. Such an attitude should be suspected when the parents seem angry, critical, or uncertain about following advice (eg, a child with recurrent pain or multiple symptoms). The parents' tendency for denial can be anticipated with certain diseases (eg, life-threatening diseases and mental retardation). This denial should be respected if it does not interfere with therapy.

Method of Referral

A. Obtain Permission from the Family: The family will usually agree to a referral if the reason for it is made clear. Patients sometimes feel that a referral means they are being abandoned by their physician. The referring physician's continuing availability for primary medical care must be made clear. The family should also be told in advance that the consultation will cost more than a regular visit but that it will be worth more.

B. Help the Family Choose a Consultant: The physician should maintain a file listing the best consultants locally and at the nearest medical center. The parents can be given the names of two or three competent physicians. If one is outstanding, however, the pediatrician should not be reluctant to state a preference. If the parents suggest someone they have heard of but whom the physician feels is unqualified, the pediatrician should express doubts about that person's degree of expertise in this particular kind of case. It often happens that only one subspecialist is available in the community (eg, oncologist) and that no choice exists.

C. Make an Appointment for the Family: After the family has agreed to the referral, the physician's secretary should arrange an appointment. This increases compliance. If the case is particularly complicated, a long consultation visit should be requested. At a minimum, a phone number should be provided.

D. Send a Referral Letter: A referral letter should be sent immediately so that it will arrive well in advance of the appointment with the consultant. All pertinent information, such as copies of previous evaluations, hospital discharge summaries, growth charts, and laboratory results, should be included. If time is short, the consultant can be prepared for the visit by phone or pertinent data can be sent along with the patient.

E. Specify the Service Requested: The specific questions to be answered and the future role of the referring physician should be clarified if possible in the referral letter.

Bailie MD et al: Making consultation and referrals count. Contemporary Pediatr 1988;5:96.
Survey: The pattern of pediatric referrals. Contemporary Pediatr 1988;5:20.

QUALITY IMPROVEMENT OF AMBULATORY PEDIATRIC CARE USING CHART REVIEWS

Quality assurance committees in hospitals review selected indicators such as admission criteria and length of stay. In emergency rooms and specialty clinics, the attending physician usually reviews and countersigns all charts. Care of office patients, on the other hand, usually is not reviewed systematically.

Office chart reviews can improve the quality and cost-effectiveness of pediatric care, enhance continuing education, make ambulatory practice more challenging and satisfying, and reduce the malpractice risk. Physicians can attempt to schedule 1 hour a week for chart review. Several pediatricians should be present to make this a maximal learning experience. In group practice, the participants are already available. The pediatrician in solo practice can meet with the one or two pediatricians who share the responsibility for responding to night calls. The group can focus on random charts or on selected ones that cover a specific problem. The latter method requires an office data retrieval system.

THE FOCUS OF CHART REVIEWS

Health Maintenance Chart Review

The delivery of comprehensive health maintenance care can be easily audited by reviewing the health supervision flow sheet (see Table 12–2). Because the nursing staff is primarily responsible for filling out these flow sheets, this type of review is largely a check on their ability to comply with office protocol and need not be done very often. The office protocols themselves require periodic review and revision.

Acute Illness Chart Review

Acute illness charts can be audited for completeness in diagnosis and therapy of the chief complaint. The following questions can be asked: (1) Was the diagnosis valid? Validity is substantiated if the chart contains adequate historical, physical, or laboratory data to document the diagnosis. (2) Was the therapy optimal? (3) Was the follow-up plan optimal? Charts of patients with a specific acute illness (eg, acute lymphadenitis or streptococcal pharyngitis) can be pulled and audited to test the group consensus about therapy and follow-up. The American Board of Pediatrics has prepared several guides for record review. Each guide provides criteria for assessing patient records dealing with specific problems (eg, acute gastroenteritis and closed head injury).

Chronic Disease Chart Review

Examination of the chronic disease flow sheet is an easy way to audit chronic disease management. If no such flow sheet exists for the patient, the variables recommended above for monitoring chronic disease can be assessed as one reviews the entire chart. This process could then result in the formation of a chronic disease flow sheet for that patient. Chart review sessions can be more educational if only one chronic disease is considered each time and if an "expert" on that disease is present. The expert can be an actual sub-specialist or a member of the group who has reviewed the literature or attended a workshop on this disease.

Diagnostic Problem Chart Review

An easy way to review consultations is to criticize the consultation report. The following questions can be asked: (1) Was the data base adequate? (2) Was the differential diagnosis reasonable? (3) Was the diagnostic plan for each problem optimal? (4) Were the final diagnoses valid? (5) Was the recommended therapy for each diagnosis optimal? (6) Was the role of the referring physician clarified and the patient reappointed to him or her? If these consultations are concerned with general pediatric problems, an outside consultant will usually not be required.

Bergman DA: Quality improvement: Buzz words. Pediatr Rev 1993;14:208.

Berwick DM: Measuring health care quality. Pediatr Rev 1988;10:11.

Nazarian LF: Medical record documentation of head injury. Pediatr Rev 1993,14:300.

MEDICAL CARE COMPLIANCE

Correct diagnoses and optimal therapeutic recommendations can be enhanced by the voluntary type of peer review discussed above. An aspect of the quality assurance not easy to assess by chart review but which needs to be borne in mind is patient compliance. Superb recommendations do not guarantee implementation. Medical care does not become effective until the parent accepts the diagnosis and carries out the therapeutic recommendations. Compliance is improved by providing written instructions, including the parents in treatment planning, simplifying the treatment regimen, linking medication taking with daily routines, explaining the reason for each treatment, and clarifying misconceptions. Strong parent-physician rapport also enhances compliance. The physician must make an effort to find out why appointments are not kept, medications are not given, etc; otherwise, even the best-conceived therapeutic goals will often not be achieved.

Charney E: Patient-doctor communication: Implications for clinicians. Pediatr Clin North Am 1972;19:263.

Maiman LA et al: Improving pediatricians' compliance-enhancing practices. Am J Dis Child 1988;142:773.

PRACTICAL TIPS FOR AMBULATORY CARE

FOREIGN BODIES

Metallic Foreign Body in the Soft Tissues

Tape a straight pin with the point over the site where the metallic object entered the skin. Then obtain an x-ray of the area. An exact measurement can then be obtained to locate the foreign body in relation to the straight pin. Located in this manner, the foreign body can be removed with minimal exploration.

Splinters Under the Nails

With a single-edged razor blade or a sharp thin scalpel, gently shave the nail over the distal end of the splinter until the splinter is exposed. The sliver can then be easily pulled out with a pair of fine-pointed tweezers.

Embedded Fishhook

Fishhooks can be removed (eg, from a finger) without wire cutters by bringing them back through their point of entry. For shallow wounds, cut the skin overlying the metal barb and lift the fishhook out. For deeper wounds, a technique that does not include yanking is preferred. Insert an 18-gauge needle into the wound through the point of entry. Slide the needle point along the hook until it reaches the barb. After the needle bevel is locked firmly over the barb, the fishhook and needle can be slowly withdrawn through the original wound as a unit. Local anesthesia is essential in children.

Feasting Ticks

Grasp the tick as close to the skin surface as possible with tweezers. Pull straight upward with steady, even pressure. Do not twist or jerk the tick, as this may cause the mouth parts to break off. Wash the site of the bite and the hands thoroughly after removal. While traction is uniformly effective, covering the tick with petroleum jelly, fingernail polish, or rubbing alcohol is uniformly ineffective. Applying a hot match also fails to induce detachment.

Needham GR: Evaluation of five popular methods for tick removal. Pediatrics 1985;75:997.

The Zipper-Entrapped Foreskin

A young child in a hurry to urinate can inadvertently catch his foreskin in his zipper. A zipper is composed of 2 rows of zipper teeth plus a zipper fastener in the middle. The zipper fastener is composed of an upper and a lower plate. The plates are joined by a U-shaped median bar. This U-shaped bar should be cut with bone cutters or wire cutters. After this is done, the zipper fastener will come apart, and this will usually free the skin. If the skin remains attached to the zipper teeth, these can be separated by grasping them on both sides and using a circular motion, rotating the two sides away from each other. Use local anesthesia for initial pain.

Saraf P, Rabinowitz R: Zipper injury of the foreskin. Am J Dis Child 1982;136:557.

Ring on a Swollen Finger

In most cases, an attempt is made to save the ring. The key to removing the ring is reducing finger edema. At 5-minute intervals, the patient should alternate soaking the hand in ice water and holding it (fingers extended) high in the air. At 30 minutes (after the hand has been elevated for the third time), mineral oil or cooking oil can be applied to the finger. While the hand remains elevated, steady upward pressure can be applied until the ring slides off.

A string technique may work in some resistant cases. Pass a piece of string under the ring and then wind the distal end of the string in close loops tightly from the distal edge of the ring past the knuckle. Exert a slow, firm pull on the proximal end of the string. The edema passes underneath the ring, and the ring is slowly pulled distally as the cord unwinds.

As a last resort, the ring must be cut off. If there is a dentist's office nearby, have the dentist cut it off with a Carborundum disk attached to the drill. The flesh of the finger must be protected by an inserted strip (eg, a tongue blade segment). This method has the disadvantage of destroying the ring and possibly heating the ring enough to burn the finger.

Hair Wrapped Around a Digit

A piece of fine hair wrapped about an infant's digit and left unnoticed can cause severe edema or even gangrene of the digit. Removal of the hair is usually difficult because it cannot be readily grasped. Application of a liquid hair remover (eg, Nair) will usually dissolve the hair within 15 minutes.

Douglas ED: (Correspondence.) J Pediatr 1977;91:162.

Gum in the Hair

An easy and nontraumatic way to remove gum from children's hair is by rubbing the gum with peanut butter until the hairs are freed from the gum. This technique is far superior to pulling or cutting the gum out of the hair.

Tar on the Skin

Tar can be removed by applying ice to it or soaking it in ice water for 1 or 2 minutes. The ice causes the tar to become hard and nonsticky, so that it can be easily peeled from the skin. Hydrocarbon solvents merely soften the tar and smear it around, and they are painful if a wound is present.

Fiberglass Spicules or Cactus Spines

The small glass spicules from fiberglass can be removed by applying a layer of wax depilatory (hair remover). Either let it air dry for 5 minutes or accelerate the process with a hair dryer. Then peel it off. White glue can also be tried, but it is less effective. This treatment is also helpful for some plant stickers (eg, cactus, stinging nettle). A corticosteroid cream applied twice daily for 1–2 days may be helpful after the treatment.

LACERATIONS

Wound Cleaning in a Resistant Child

TAC liquid (tetracaine, adrenaline, cocaine) applied topically for 10–15 minutes has been shown to provide complete anesthesia in over 95% of minor lacerations. This will cause only momentary discomfort. The area will then be relatively anesthetized, and vigorous wound cleaning will be tolerated. If needed, the subcutaneous injection of additional lidocaine after the wound is cleaned will also be better tolerated. Topical anesthesia with agents containing adrenaline or cocaine (vasoconstrictors) must be avoided on digits, the penis, ear pinna, or the nose. If TAC is not available, the wound can be covered with gauze saturated with 1% lidocaine for 15 minutes.

Bonadio WA, Wagner V: Efficacy of TAC topical anesthetic for repair of pediatric lacerations. Am J Dis Child 1988;142:203.

Avoiding Unwanted Tattoos

Dirty abrasions of the knee, face, and elbow can result in permanent tattooing if all particulate matter, especially carbon particles, is not meticulously removed. The area should be anesthetized as described above and then scrubbed gently with an antibacterial cleanser and a soft surgical nail brush. Tar can usually be removed by rubbing with petrolatum. Some contaminated pieces of skin may need debridement.

Laceration Closure in a Frightened Child

Wounds can often be closed without local anesthesia or sutures by using microporous adhesive tape (Steri-Strip). The skin adjacent to the laceration is made tacky with tincture of benzoin. The ⅛-inch strips of tape are applied in either a parallel or crisscross pattern. This microporous tape is a decided improvement over "butterfly" tape.

Suture Removal

There is a way to avoid having to dig embedded sutures out of the skin of a struggling child. At the time the laceration is closed, a straight needle threaded with silk can be passed under each suture used for skin closure. The ends of this silk suture can be tied together, leaving a loose loop. At the time of removal, picking up this loose loop will lift the sutures that have been used to close the wound. The scissors can then be easily slid underneath the sutures for snipping. A new, inexpensive sterile stitch cutter makes suture removal easy.

BLUNT TRAUMA

Subungual Hematomas

The painful pressure secondary to a subungual hematoma can easily be relieved by applying a disposable eye-cautery heating device or a red-hot paper clip to the nail surface. The paper clip is held by a clamp. A hole is quickly bored through the nail, and the blood is allowed to escape. This "hot iron" approach can be frightening for a child unless his head is turned away. If there is a dentist's office nearby, you may ask the dentist to bore a hole quickly through the nail with a high-speed drill. A physician can bore a hole through the nail by manually rotating an 18-gauge needle.

Traumatic Tooth Avulsion

Reimplantation of a tooth is possible only with the permanent teeth. The physician or parent should attempt to replace the avulsed tooth in its socket prior to going to the dentist. If this proves impossible, the tooth should be placed in cold milk or normal saline solution and sent with the patient to the dentist. The deadline for successful replacement is 2 hours.

MISCELLANEOUS PROCEDURES

Genital Labial Adhesions

A nontraumatic method for separating thicker labial adhesions is application of estrogen cream (eg, Premarin) twice daily to the medial line for 2–4 weeks. Introducing a probe into the opening remaining in the introitus and then separating the adhesions can be quite painful. This method is only acceptable for filmy adhesions. An ointment should be applied to the newly separated surfaces for 1–2 weeks to prevent them from resealing.

Hiccup

One teaspoonful of ordinary white granulated sugar swallowed "dry" will result in immediate cessation of hiccup in most patients. If the hiccups recur, this method will again be effective. Recalcitrant hiccups may respond to stimulation of the nasopharynx with a rubber catheter.

Inadvertent Subcutaneous Injections

When intramuscular agents are given subcutaneously by mistake, complications can result. The location of the needle point can be rapidly assessed by trying to wiggle it prior to injection. If it is in a muscle mass, the needle point will be relatively fixed. If it is in the subcutaneous fatty tissues, it can be felt to move freely.

Painful Bee Stings or Other Insect Bites

If a stinger is visible, flick it off with the edge of a knife blade or credit card. A dash of meat tenderizer (papain powder) and a drop of water massaged into the sting site for 5 minutes will quickly relieve the pain. If these ingredients are not available, an ice cube often helps.

Paraphimosis

In this condition, the foreskin has become retracted and trapped behind the corona. Manual reduction can usually be achieved by placing the tips of the index and middle fingers of one hand behind the swollen foreskin, the thumb of the other hand over the urethral meatus, and applying gradual pressure. The foreskin will usually return to its normal position after this technique has been applied continuously for 4–5 minutes. If this approach fails, a urologist should be consulted for an emergency dorsal slit.

Plastibell Circumcision Ring Paraphimosis

Sometimes the Plastibell circumcision ring slips behind the glans onto the shaft of the penis and cannot be slipped forward. Local swelling can be reduced by applying cold compresses and pressure for 10 minutes. The plastic ring can then be cut with a pair of scissors. Mineral oil can be applied to allow the scissors blade to slip easily under the ring. If the operator is worried about cutting the skin, a piece of a small feeding tube can be threaded under the ring and used as a guide for the scissors.

Postcircumcision Skin Tags

Parents occasionally bring their infant in during the first month of life because the foreskin has an irregular skin tag. A clamp can be applied along the desired line of cleavage for 1 minute. After the clamp is removed, an iris scissors can be used to cut along the crushed skin line without causing any significant bleeding.

FEVER

Definition of Fever

(1) Rectal temperature over 38 °C.
(2) Oral temperature over 37.5 °C.
(3) Axillary temperature over 37 °C.

While the body's average temperature is 37 °C orally, it normally fluctuates during the day from a low of 36.4 °C in the morning to a high of 37.5 °C in the late afternoon (normal diurnal variation). Mild elevations of 38–38.5 °C can be caused by exercise, excessive clothing, a hot bath, or hot weather. Anderson (1990) recently found that bottle or breast feedings tended to raise the infant's temperature for a half hour or more. Warm food or drink can elevate an oral temperature. If one of these causes is suspected, the temperature should be taken again in a half hour after eliminating the possible cause.

Causes of Fever

Fever is a symptom, not a disease. Fever is the body's normal response to infections, and it plays a role in fighting them. Fever turns on the body's immune system, thereby increasing the release and activity of white blood cells, interferon, and other substances. The usual fevers (37.8–40 °C) that all children have at times are not harmful. Most are due to viral illnesses; some are due to bacterial ones. Most "fevers" that stay under 38.3 °C are simply due to hot weather or overdressing. Teething does not cause fever over 38.4 °C.

Expected Course of Fever

Most fevers associated with viral illnesses range between 38.3 and 40 °C and last for 2–3 days. In general, the height of the fever does not relate to the seriousness of the illness; how sick the child acts is what matters. Fever causes no symptoms until it reaches 38.9 or 39.4 °C. Fever causes no harm (such as brain damage) until it reaches 41.7 or 42.2 °C. Fortunately, the brain's thermostat keeps untreated fevers due to infections below 40.1 or 41.1 °C. While all children have fever, only 4% develop a febrile convulsion. This type of seizure is generally harmless.

Guidelines for Evaluating Children With Fever

A. **Immediately If–**
The child is under 2 months old.
The fever is over 40.1 °C.
The child is crying inconsolably or whimpering.
The child cries when moved or otherwise touched by the parent.

The child is difficult to awaken.

The neck is stiff.

Any purple spots are present on the skin.

Breathing is difficult and no better after the nose is cleared.

The child is drooling saliva and is unable to swallow anything.

A convulsion has occurred.

The child acts or looks very sick.

B. Within 24 Hours If–

The child is 2–4 months old (unless fever occurs within 48 hours of a DPT shot and the infant has no other serious symptoms).

The fever is between 40 and 40.1 °C (especially if the child is under 2 years old).

Burning or pain occurs with urination.

The fever has been present more than 24 hours without an obvious cause or location of infection.

C. During Office Hours If–

The fever went away for more than 24 hours and then returned.

The fever has been present more than 72 hours.

The child has a history of febrile seizures.

Treatment of Fever

A. "Fever Phobia" and the Overtreatment of Fever: "Fever phobia" is a term that describes the parents' anxious response to the fevers that all children experience. Schmitt's study (1980) found that 80% of parents thought fevers between 40 and 41.1 °C cause brain damage. About 20% of parents thought that if they did not treat the fever, it would keep going higher. Neither of these statements is true. Because of these misconceptions, many parents treat low-grade fevers with unnecessary medicines and sponging.

B. Acetaminophen: Children older than 2 months of age can be given an acetaminophen product every 4–6 hours. Acetaminophen is indicated if the fever is over 39 °C, but it should be given only if the child is uncomfortable. Acetaminophen will reduce the fever by 1–2 °C within 2 hours after it is given. Antipyretics do not bring the temperature down to normal unless the fever was low-grade to begin with.

C. Liquid Ibuprofen: In 1989, ibuprofen received FDA approval for treatment of fever in children 6 months to 12 years of age. It is available only by prescription. Ibuprofen and acetaminophen are similar in safety and in their ability to lower fever. One advantage of ibuprofen over acetaminophen is that ibuprofen has a longer duration of action (6–8 hours versus 4–6 hours). When the issue is fever control, acetaminophen is still the drug of choice for most conditions. Children with special problems (eg, febrile seizures) requiring a longer period of fever control, however, may do better with ibuprofen.

D. Cautions About Aspirin: The American Academy of Pediatrics has recommended that children and adolescents (through age 21 years) not receive aspirin if they have chickenpox or influenza (any cold, cough, or sore throat symptoms). This recommendation stems from several studies that have linked aspirin to Reye's syndrome. Most pediatricians have stopped using aspirin for fevers associated with any illness.

E. Sponging for Fever: Indications for immediate sponging with lukewarm water (never alcohol) are febrile delirium, febrile seizure, or any fever over 41.1 °C. For other children, sponging is rarely necessary. Acetaminophen should always be given 30 minutes prior to sponging. Until acetaminophen has taken effect (by resetting the body's thermostat), sponging will just cause shivering. Heat stroke requires immediate cold water sponging (antipyretics are not beneficial).

F. Other Measures: Extra fluids should be encouraged but not forced. Body fluids are lost during fevers because of sweating. Clothing should be kept to a minimum, because most heat is lost through the skin. Bundling can be dangerous, especially with infants who are unable to undress themselves if they become overheated.

Types of Thermometers

A. Glass (With Mercury) Thermometers: This type of thermometer has been the standard since 1870. While these are the least expensive thermometers, they record the temperature slowly and are often hard to read. Using this thermometer, rectal temperatures are the most accurate. Oral temperatures are also accurate if done properly. No hot or cold drinks or food can be consumed in the preceding 10 minutes. Axillary temperatures are the least accurate but better than no measurement. In general, rectal temperatures are uncomfortable, embarrassing for older children, and may perforate the rectum if improperly inserted. They are usually reserved for children under age 5. Oral temperatures are usually reliably obtained in older children. The thermometer must be left in place for 2 minutes for rectal temperatures, 3 minutes for oral, and 5–6 minutes for axillary.

B. Digital Thermometers: Digital thermometers record temperatures with a heat sensor and are powered by a button battery. They measure quickly, usually in less than 30 seconds. The temperature is displayed in numbers on a small screen. A study in Consumer Reports (January 1988) found they were more accurate than glass thermometers.

C. Tympanic Thermometers: Many hospitals and medical offices now take temperature using an infrared thermometer that reads the temperature of the eardrum. In general, the eardrum temperature provides a measurement that is at least as accurate as the rectal temperature. The outstanding advantage of this instrument is that it measures temperatures in less than 2 seconds. It also requires little cooperation by the child and causes no discomfort. The equipment is expensive.

D. Temperature Strips: Liquid crystal strips applied to the forehead and temperature-sensitive pacifiers have been studied and found to be inaccurate. They miss fevers in many children. Touching the forehead also tends to miss mild fevers, but it is fairly reliable for detecting fevers over 38.9 °C, according to a 1984 study by Banco and Veltri.

Anderson ES et al: Factors influencing the body temperature of 3-4 month old infants at home during the day. Arch Dis Child 1990;65:1308.

Banco L, Veltri D: Ability of mothers to subjectively assess the presence of fever in their children. Am J Dis Child 1984;138:976.

Beach P, McCormick D: Fever and tympanic thermometry. Clin Pediatr 1991;30(Suppl):1.

Casey R et al: Fever therapy: and educational intervention for parents. Pediatrics 1984;73:600.

Doran TF et al: Acetaminophen: More harm than good for chickenpox? J Pediatr 1989;114:1045.

Norris J: Taking temperatures: The changing state of the art. Contemporary Pediatr 1985;2:22.

Schmitt BD: Fever phobia: Misconceptions of parents about fever. Am J Dis Child 1980;134:176.

EVALUATION OF THE FEBRILE INFANT AND "OUTPATIENT" BACTEREMIA*

Essentials of Diagnosis

- Infant less than 2 years old with fever.
- No focal infection found on physical examination.

General Considerations

Although fever may be due to serious infection at any age, young children are at greater risk because of their immunologic immaturity. In the first weeks of life, multiple defense mechanisms are immature (including complement, polymorphonuclear function, mucosal integrity, and immunity), and infections may be fulminant. After several months, transplacental IgG is lost, and the infant is especially susceptible to infections due to encapsulated bacteria such as pneumococcus, meningococcus, and *Haemophilus influenzae* type b.

Infants less than 2 years old with a rectal temperature over 39 °C and no focus of infection on examination have a 3–5% incidence of "occult" bacteremia. The height of the temperature does not correlate well with severity of illness. In particular, infants less than 3 months old may be bacteremic even though they have low grade fever and appear nontoxic on examination. This is one reason why more laboratory tests and hospitalization are indicated for very young infants.

Occult bacteremia is due to the pneumococcus in 50–80% of cases. *H influenzae* type b has been the next most common organism, but this will become rare in adequately immunized children. Meningococcus or *Salmonella* may also be the cause; any symptoms of enteritis or Hematest-positive stools should make the latter organism more suspect. Bacteremia with organisms such as *Escherichia coli* suggests a urinary or intestinal focus. In infants less than 3–4 months old, group B streptococcus and *Listeria* bacteremia are possible and require the inclusion of ampicillin in the antimicrobial regimen; they are very rare in older children. Herpes simplex viremia is a rare but dangerous cause of fever in infants less than 2 weeks old. A history of maternal genital herpes, suggestive cutaneous lesions, or other signs must be sought (see Chapter 35). Other viral infections that cause fever and few other symptoms include roseola and enteroviruses. Influenza and adenovirus infections are usually accompanied by respiratory symptoms.

Clinical Findings

A. History: Although bacteremia cannot be excluded by the history, many infants with viral infections have household contacts with febrile illnesses, early symptoms of respiratory or intestinal infection, or a history of exposure to a specific communicable infection such as salmonellosis. Infants with urinary tract infections, on the other hand, usually have no significant exposure history. Since infants with mild viral infections can also be bacteremic, not too much emphasis should be placed on exposure to ill contacts.

B. Symptoms and Signs: Careful examination should detect focal infections. Those that are notoriously hard to diagnose by physical examination include bacterial pneumonia, sinusitis, urinary tract infection, and meningitis. Pneumonia may present with only mild tachypnea and normal auscultation; preceding or concurrent respiratory signs (rhinitis, cough) are usually present. Significant congestion and often purulent rhinitis are common with sinusitis. Children with urinary tract infections may vomit or have mild abdominal discomfort but often have no abnormal physical findings.

Infants with meningitis may only be irritable; the younger the infant, the less reliably the physical examination excludes meningitis. The ease with which the temperature is normalized by antipyretics does not correlate with the cause of the underlying illness. Bacteremic children over 3 months of age are more likely to be lethargic and disinterested in their surroundings and more likely not to make eye contact with the examiner than nonbacteremic children. The experienced caregiver synthesizes all this information in determining the probability of serious infection and need for diagnostic tests.

*This section is contributed by John W. Paisley, MD.

Laboratory & Imaging Evaluation

The diagnostic test for bacteremia is a blood culture. If possible, obtain 3 mL of blood. A single site may be used, since contaminants are usually easy to distinguish from pathogens.

Many rapid tests have been evaluated for their ability to distinguish bacteremia from nonbacteremic infants. After the sensitivity, specificity, expense, ease of performance, and processing time have been analyzed, only the total and differential leukocyte count have practical application. The incidence of bacteremia increases as the total count increases. About two-thirds of bacteremic children will have leukocyte counts over 15,000/µL. Although a very abnormal count may be helpful (over 20,000/µL with a marked left shift, suggesting bacterial infection, or profound neutropenia, suggesting immune deficiency or overwhelming infection), recent analysis has suggested that a blood culture alone combined with expectant antimicrobial therapy is actually most cost-effective.

A lumbar puncture is advised on all infants less than 3 months old and on most infants 3–12 months old with no focal findings. The need for a lumbar puncture in older infants is based on the degree of irritability and toxicity. It is strongly recommended for children who are still febrile despite oral antibiotics regardless of findings on physical examination, since they may have partially treated bacterial meningitis.

The next most important test is urinalysis. Voided specimens, especially those obtained with a bag, are often unreliable. Contamination with leukocytes or bacteria so often leads to incorrect management that a catheterized or suprapubically aspirated specimen is preferred. Infection may be present without significant pyuria or a positive dipstick test for nitrate or leukocyte esterase. A Gram stain is the best rapid test to exclude bacteriuria.

A complete evaluation includes a chest radiograph to exclude pneumonia. The yield is higher in younger infants and in those with some evidence of respiratory infection by history or on examination.

Differential Diagnosis

An incorrectly taken temperature or unreliable thermometer must be excluded. Environmental fever (eg, the heavily wrapped neonate, recent hot baths), dehydration, drugs, normal diurnal variation, undue parental concern about low-grade fevers, and, rarely, factitious fever should be considered. True fevers are usually due to viral infections—especially enteroviruses. Other causes include missed bacterial infection (ruptured appendix, osteomyelitis), Kawasaki's disease, leukemia, lymphoma, juvenile rheumatoid arthritis, and enteric fever.

Treatment

Therapy is individualized. Treatment in the hospital is indicated for infants who are less than 2–3 months old; those with unreliable caregivers; those who are toxic, have unstable vital signs, or have poor perfusion; and those in whom meningitis cannot be excluded due to a traumatic lumbar puncture.

Experienced clinicians often perform laboratory tests on or treat only those children who appear ill. Those with temperatures under 39 °C who are nontoxic and have reliable caregivers may often be managed as outpatients with no antimicrobial therapy.

If there is enough suspicion of bacteremia to obtain a blood culture, expectant antimicrobial therapy usually should be given as follows:

(1) For hospitalized infants under 3 months old, give ampicillin (50 mg/kg intravenously every 6 hours) and ceftriaxone (50 mg/kg intravenously every 24 hours) or cefotaxime or cefuroxime (50 mg/kg intravenously every 8 hours).

(2) For hospitalized infants over 3 months old, give ceftriaxone (50 mg/kg intramuscularly or intravenously every 24 hours) for jaundiced infants, give cefotaxime or cefuroxime (50 mg/kg intravenously every 8 hours).

(3) For outpatients, give ceftriaxone (50 mg/kg intramuscularly once daily). While expensive, it ensures immediate antimicrobial activity and provides excellent antimicrobial effects for 24 hours against the common pathogens.

(4) Continue antimicrobial therapy until the cultures are negative for at least 48 hours. If the infant is doing well and no focal infection is diagnosed, discontinue medication.

(5) If the blood culture is positive for one of the encapsulated bacteria, the cerebrospinal fluid is sterile, and the infant is afebrile and clinically well when reexamined, it is usually safe to complete a 10-day course of therapy on an outpatient basis with an appropriate oral antimicrobial and follow the patient closely. Compliance must be ensured. If such an infant never had a lumbar puncture, consider performing one before determining subsequent therapy (especially if the organism is *H influenzae* type b).

Prognosis

Even without treatment, up to 80% of cases of occult pneumococcal bacteremia resolve. The remainder would persist with bacteremia or localized infection in the meninges, lungs, joints, or elsewhere. Although most children who are evaluated and treated promptly with antimicrobials are quickly cured, a few will remain febrile and require a repeat lumbar puncture and other tests to detect sites of localization.

Recurrence of bacteremia is unusual and suggests immune deficiency such as HIV infection or complement defects.

Baraff LT, Bass JW, et al: Practice guideline for the management of infants and children 0 to 36 months of age with fever without source. Pediatrics 1993,92:1

Table 12–4. Pediatric Health Maintenance Charts.

PEDIATRIC HEALTH MAINTENANCE

Birth through 3 months

Patient's concerns

Newborn data base
Birth weight ___ Gestational age ___
Pregnancy or delivery problems ___ Neonatal problems ___

Growth (comment on growth curve)

Feeding advice
Formula ___ oz/24 hours ___
Breast feeding: Frequency ___ min/feeding ___
Vitamins ___ Iron ___
Solids ___ Fluoride drops ___
Feeding problems ___
Advice: Introduce bottle in breast fed (2m) ☐ Introduce fluids other than milk (2m) ☐

Developmental status
Stimulation advice: Hold baby (2w) ☐ Talk to baby (2m) ☐

Child rearing advice
Sleep pattern ___
Crying or colic ___
Mother-child interaction ___
Sibling rivalry (2w) ___
Advice: Paternal involvement, family planning (2w) ☐ Utilize sitter (2m) ☐
Utilize sitter (sm) ☐

Family status

Accident prevention advice
Car seats, crib safety (2w) ☐ Rolling over (2m) ☐ Smoke detector ☐

Medical Advice
Demonstrate use of suction bulb for nose (2w) ☐ Foreskin or circumcision care ♂ (2w) ☐
Temperature taking, Tylenol and fever handout (2m) ☐ Discuss when to call doctor (2m) ☐

Intercurrent illness

312

PEDIATRIC HEALTH MAINTENANCE

4 months through 14 months

Parent's concerns

Growth (comment on growth curve)

Feeding advice
Formula ___ oz/24 hours ___
Breast feeding: Frequency ___ min/feeding ___
Vitamins ___ Iron ___
Solids ___ Fluoride drops ___
Feeding problems ___
Advice: No bottles in bed; introduce solids, spoon, cup (4m) ☐
Confirm intake of iron-rich solids (6m) ☐ Introduce finger foods, confirm on 3 meals/day (9m) ☐
Entirely on table foods. Phase out bottle by 18m (12m) ☐

Developmental status
Stimulation advice: Toys for reaching (4m) ☐ Avoid confining baby equipment (6m) ☐
Repeat baby's sounds (9m) ☐ Name objects and pictures for baby (12m) ☐

Child rearing advice
Sleep pattern ___
Behavior problems ___
Advice: Sleeps through the night (4m) ☐ Normal separation anxiety (6m) ☐
Discipline: Use negative voice and eye contact rather than physical punishment (9m) ☐
Don't punish for normal exploratory behavior, discuss positive strokes for good behavior (12m) ☐

Family status

Accident prevention advice
Safe toys (4m) ☐ Stairs and gates, drowning in bathtub (9m) ☐
Electrical cords (6m) ☐ Ipecac and poison talk (12m) ☐

Medical advice
Teething myths (6m) ☐ Avoid expensive shoes (9m) ☐ Use of 911 (12m) ☐

Intercurrent illness

(continued)

Table 12–4. Pediatric Health Maintenance Charts. (continued)

PEDIATRIC HEALTH MAINTENANCE
15 months through 3 years

Parent's concerns

Growth (comment on growth curve)

Diet
Milk _____ oz/24 hours
Eating problems
Advice: Entirely on table foods, off all bottles (18m) ☐
Normal decreased appetite, iron intake (2y) ☐

Developmental status
Advice: Read to child (1½, 2) ☐ Listen to child (2) ☐ TV rules (3) ☐

Child rearing advice
Sleep problems
Behavior problems
Frequency of spanking
Advice: Don't punish for normal negativism, ignore temper tantrums (1½) ☐
Discuss toilet training and readiness (1½, 2, 3) ☐ Discuss positive "strokes" for
good behavior (2) ☐
Emphasize consistency in discipline and use of time-out room (2, 3) ☐

Family status

Accident prevention advice
Scalds, aspiration foods (1½) ☐ Street/garage safety (2) ☐
Drowning in ditch and pools (3) ☐

Dental advice
Brushing frequency _____ Fluoride intake _____
Advice: Avoid snacks that cause cavities (1½) ☐ Benefits of fluoride toothpaste (2) ☐
Brushing techniques (3) ☐

Intercurrent illness

PEDIATRIC HEALTH MAINTENANCE
4 years through 5 years

To be completed by parent   Check correct answer

School readiness:
1. Does your child pay attention when being read to?   Yes   No
2. Can your child play quietly alone for over ½ hour?   Yes   No
3. Does your child mind adults and follow instructions?   Yes   No
4. Does your child speak clearly enough for others to
   understand?   Yes   No
5. Does your child object to being with a sitter?   No   Yes
6. Can your child dress without help?   Yes   No
7. Does your child ever wet or soil him/herself during the
   day?   No   Yes

To be completed by physician or nurse

Parent's concerns

Growth (comment on growth curve)

Diet

School readiness
Problems detected by above questions _____
Development: PDQ (4, 5) Score _____   Weak category _____
DDST (if fails PDQ) Result _____
Articulation: DASE (4) Score _____   Percentile _____
Advice: Preschool if any problems (4) ☐

Accident prevention advice
Adult seat belts, petting dogs (4) ☐ Crossing street, trampoline (5) ☐

Dental advice
No daytime thumb-sucking (4) ☐ No nighttime thumb-sucking (5) ☐
Frequency of brushing _____ Type of toothpaste _____ Fluoride intake _____

Intercurrent illness

(continued)

Table 12–4. Pediatric Health Maintenance Charts. (continued)

PEDIATRIC HEALTH MAINTENANCE

6 years through 11 years

Parent's concerns

Diet

School
Name of school _____ Grade _____
Academic performance _____
Attendance _____
Behavior _____
Advice: Child's responsibility for schoolwork (6) ☐ Adult at home before and after school (6, 10) ☐

Behavior
Behavior problems _____
Chores _____
Friends _____
Advice: TV less than 2 h/d (6) ☐ Understanding of death (6) ☐
One sport or club (8, 10) ☐ Smoking (10) ☐

Family status

Sex education
Discuss puberty and menarche before junior high school (10) ☐
Menstrual status (10 ♀)

Accident prevention advice
Bicycle safety (6) ☐ Swimming lessons (8) ☐
Fires, matches (10) ☐

Dental advice
Frequency of brushing _____ Type of toothpaste _____ Fluoride intake _____
Dental referral (6) ☐

Intercurrent illness

PEDIATRIC HEALTH MAINTENANCE

12 years through 18 years

Parent's concerns

Adolescent's concerns

Growth (comment on growth curve)

Diet

School
Name of school _____ Grade _____
Academic performance _____
Attendance _____
Behavior _____
Career plans _____

Behavior
Free time/friends _____
Chores/job _____
Person to confide in _____
Predominant mood _____
Advice: Discuss values of babysitting (12) ☐ Discuss drugs and alcohol (12, 16) ☐
Discuss smoking (14) ☐

Family status
Advice: Discuss independence and parent's trust (16) ☐

Sex education
Dating, masturbation (14) ☐ Marriage (18) ☐
Sexual activity, preventing pregnancy, STD (14, 16, 18)

Accident prevention advice
Firearms (12) ☐ Cycling safety (14) ☐ Driving safety, water safety (16) ☐
Motorcycles, riding with driver who drinks, seat belts (18) ☐

Dental advice
Frequency of brushing _____ Type of toothpaste _____

Medical advice
Acne ☐ Personal hygiene (14) ☐ Teach self-examination of breasts (16 ♀) ☐

Intercurrent illness

314

Downs SM et al: Management of infants at risk for occult bacteremia: A decision analysis. J Pediatr 1991;118:11.

Powell KR: Evaluation and management of febrile infants younger than 60 days of age. Pediatric Infect Dis J 1990;:153.

Wasserman GM, White CB: Evaluation of the necessity for hospitalization of the febrile infant less than three months of age. Pediatr Infect Dis J 1990;9:163.

REFERENCES

Ambulatory Pediatrics Association: *Educational Guidelines for Training in General/Ambulatory Pediatrics.* Ambulatory Pediatrics Association, 1984.

American Academy of Pediatrics: *Guidelines for Health Supervision II.* American Academy of Pediatrics, 1988.

American Academy of Pediatrics: *Management of Pediatric Practice.* American Academy of Pediatrics, 1991.

Charney E: *Well-Child Care.* Ross Roundtable, 17th Report, Ross Laboratories, 1986.

Dershewitz RA: *Ambulatory Pediatric Care,* 2nd ed. Lippincott, 1993.

Dixon SD, Stein MT: *Encounters With Children: Pediatric Behavior and Development,* 2nd ed. Year Book, 1992.

Goldbloom RB: *Pediatric Clinical Skills.* Churchill Livingstone, 1992.

Gordon IB, Paulson JA: Issues for the practicing pediatrician. Pediatr Clin North Am 1981;28:535.

Green M, Haggerty RJ (editors): *Ambulatory Pediatrics.* Vols 1, 2, 3, and 4. Saunders, 1968, 1977,1984 and 1990.

Hoekelman RA et al (editors): *Primary Pediatric Care.* Mosby, 1986.

Liptak GS, Revell GM: Community physician's role in case management of children with chronic illnesses. Pediatrics 1989;84:465.

Oski FA (editor): *Principles and Practice of Pediatrics.* Lippincott, 1990.

Schwartz NW: *Pediatric Primary Care,* 2nd ed. Year Book, 1990.

13 Poisoning

Richard C. Dart, MD, PhD & Barry H. Rumack, MD

Poisonings, the fourth most common cause of death in children, result from the complex interaction of the agent, the child, and the family environment. The peak incidence is at age 2 years, and most of these are ingestions that do not produce toxicity. Accidents occur most often in children under 5 years of age as a result of insecure storage of drugs, household chemicals, etc. Twenty-five percent of children will have a second episode of ingestion of a toxic substance within a year following the first one. Repeated poisonings may be a sign of a family problem requiring intervention on the child's behalf. Accidental poisonings are unusual after age 5 years. "Poisonings" in older children and adolescents usually represent manipulative behavior, chemical or drug abuse, or genuine suicide attempts.

Litovitz TL et al: 1991 annual report of the American Association of Poison Control Center's National Data Collection system. Am J Emerg Med 1992;10:452.

PREVENTING CHILDHOOD POISONINGS

Each year, children are accidentally poisoned by medicines, polishes, insecticides, drain cleaners, bleaches, household chemicals, and garage products. It is the responsibility of adults to make sure that children are not exposed to potentially toxic substances.

Here are some suggestions:

(1) Insist on packages with safety closures and learn how to use them properly.

(2) Keep household cleaning supplies, medicines, garage products, and insecticides out of the reach and sight of your child. Lock them up whenever possible. Remember the child's area of investigation and "reach."

(3) Never store food and cleaning products together. Store medicine and chemicals in original containers and never in food or beverage containers.

(4) Avoid taking medicine in your child's presence. Children love to imitate. Always call medicine by its proper name. Never suggest that medicine is "candy"—especially aspirin and children's vitamins.

(5) Read the label on all products and heed warnings and cautions. Never use medicine from an unlabeled or unreadable container. Never pour medicine in a darkened area where the label cannot be clearly seen.

(6) If you are interrupted while using a product, take it with you. It takes only a few seconds for your child to get into it.

(7) Know what your child can do physically. For example, if you have a crawling infant, keep household products stored above floor level, not beneath the kitchen sink.

(8) Keep the phone number of your doctor, poison center, hospital, police department, and fire department or paramedic emergency rescue squad near the phone.

PHARMACOLOGIC PRINCIPLES OF TOXICOLOGY

In the evaluation of the poisoned patient, it is important to compare the anticipated pharmacologic or toxic effects with the clinical presentation of the patient. If the history is that the patient ingested phenobarbital 30 minutes ago but the clinical examination reveals dilated pupils, tachycardia, dry mouth, absent bowel sounds, and active hallucinations—clearly anticholinergic toxicity—diagnosis and therapy should proceed accordingly.

Knowledge of the pharmacokinetics of the toxic agent helps the physician to plan a rational approach to definitive care after necessary life-supporting measures have been instituted.

LD50, MLD

Health professionals occasionally attempt to use the LD50 or MLD (minimum lethal dose) of an ingested substance to determine if the child will become ill. Unfortunately, such information is not of clinical value, since it is usually impossible to accurately determine how much the child has swallowed, how much has been absorbed, the metabolic status of the patient, or where the patient's response to the agent will fall in the normal distribution curve. Furthermore, these values are often not valid in humans even if the history is accurate.

Half-Life ($t_{1/2}$)

The $t_{1/2}$ of an agent must be interpreted carefully in the overdose situation. Most published $t_{1/2}$ values are for therapeutic dosages. The $t_{1/2}$ may increase as the quantity of the ingested substance increases for many common intoxicants such as barbiturates, salicylates, and phenytoin. One cannot rely upon the published $t_{1/2}$ for salicylate (2 hours) to assume rapid elimination of the drug with a concomitant short toxic course. In an acute salicylate overdose (> 150 mg/kg), the apparent $t_{1/2}$ is prolonged to 24–30 hours.

Volume of Distribution (V_d)

The volume of distribution (V_d) of a drug represents the volume into which a drug is distributed. It is obtained by dividing the amount of drug absorbed by the blood level. With theophylline, for example, this is roughly equivalent to the body water volume and can be expressed as 0.46 L/kg body weight, or 32 L in an adult. Ethchlorvynol, a lipophilic drug, on the other hand, distributes well beyond total body water. Because the calculation produces a volume above body weight (300 L in an adult, five times the body weight in children), this figure is frequently referred to as an **apparent volume of distribution**, a designation shared by many drugs (Table 13–1).

The V_d can be useful in predicting which drugs will be removed by dialysis or exchange transfusion. When a drug is differentially concentrated in body lipids or is heavily tissue- or protein-bound and has a high volume of distribution, only a small proportion of the drug will be in the free form and thus accessible to diuresis, dialysis, or exchange transfusion. On the other hand, a drug that is water-soluble and has a low volume of distribution may cross the dialysis membrane well and also respond to diuresis. In general, methods of extracorporeal elimination are not effective for toxic agents with a V_d greater than 1 L/kg.

Metabolism & Excretion

The route of excretion or detoxification—correlated with other information—will assist with therapeutic decisions. Methanol, for example, is metabolized to the toxic product, formic acid. This metabolic step may be blocked by the administration of ethanol. Long-acting barbiturates are metabolized chiefly in the liver but are also partially excreted in the urine, which means that forced diuresis will increase excretion. Secobarbital, a short-acting barbiturate, is poorly excreted in the urine and has a larger V_d, making forced diuresis ineffective.

Blood Levels

Care of the poisoned patient should never be guided solely by the results of laboratory measurements. Treatment should be directed first against the clinical signs and symptoms, followed by more specific therapy based on laboratory determinations. The laboratory pathologist should be given whatever information is needed regarding the history, clinical presentation, and class of the suspected toxic agent (sedative-hypnotic, opioid, amphetamine, etc), so that the specific agent can be identified as rapidly as possible.

Handling of Specimens

A. Vomitus and Gastric Lavage Fluid: Collect and send to the laboratory initial material recovered; place in separate containers. Send also an aliquot of the remainder, and make a "best guess" estimate of its volume. Include material appearing to be pill fragments.

B. Blood: After informing the pathologist of the history and current physical findings, determine specifically what type of container and anticoagulant are required before drawing the sample.

C. Urine: Collect an initial sample of 100 mL for analysis. Subsequently, timed 6- to 12-hour collections may be useful in determining the excretion rate of the agent.

Table 13–1. Some examples of pK_a and V_d.[1]

Drug	pK_a	Diuresis	Dialysis	Apparent V_d
Amobarbital	7.9	No	No	200–300% body weight
Amphetamine	9.8	No	Yes	60% body weight
Aspirin	3.5	Alkaline	Yes	15–40% body weight
Chlorpromazine	9.3	No	No	40–50 L/kg (2800–3500% body weight)
Codeine	8.2	No	No	5–10 L/kg (350–700% body weight)
Desipramine	10.2	No	No	30–40 L/kg (2100–2800% body weight)
Ethchlorvynol	8.7	No	No	5–10 L/kg (350–700% body weight)
Glutethimide	4.5	No	No	10–20 L/kg (700–1400% body weight)
Isoniazid	3.5	Alkaline	Yes	61% body weight
Methadone	8.3	No	No	5–10 L/kg (350–700% body weight)
Methicillin	2.8	No	Yes	60% body weight
Phenobarbital	7.4	Alkaline	Yes	75% body weight
Phenytoin	8.3	No	No	60–80% body weight
Tetracycline	7.7	No	No	200–300% body weight

[1]See Table 41–2 for additional V_d values.

GENERAL TREATMENT OF POISONING

The telephone is often the first contact in pediatric poisoning. Proper telephone management can reduce morbidity and prevent unwarranted or excessive treatment. After initial telephone advice has been given, the decision to refer the patient is based on the identity and dose of the ingested agent, the age of the child, the time of day, the reliability of the parent, and whether child neglect or endangerment is suspected.

Initial Telephone Contact

Evaluate the urgency of the situation and decide whether immediate emergency transportation to a health facility is indicated. Transportation of seriously poisoned patients should be by competent emergency rescue personnel who have suction, oxygen, and other equipment available.

Basic information that should be *written down* at the first telephone contact includes the patient's name, age, weight, address and telephone number, the agent and amount of agent ingested, the patient's present condition, and the time elapsed since ingestion or other exposure.

Facts Concerning the Ingestion

This information is usually given by the parent in the first few moments of the call. (*Example:* "My three-year-old just swallowed ten of the vitamin pills!") Use these and other basic facts to help decide whether the ingestion is immediately dangerous. If immediate danger does not exist, the physician should develop more details about the suspected toxic agent. It may be difficult to obtain an accurate history. For example, an empty bottle of iron tablets may have rolled out of sight under the couch, and the parent may then assume that only the vitamin capsules have been swallowed. Obtain names of drugs or ingredients, manufacturers, prescription numbers, names and phone numbers of prescribing physician and pharmacy, etc. Find out whether the substance was shared among several children, whether it had been recently purchased, who had last used it, how full it was, and how much was spilled. If one is unsure of the significance of an exposure, consultation with a certified Poison Control Center is recommended.

FIRST AID FOR POISONING
(Advice for Parents)

Treatment at home should include external and internal decontamination if appropriate.

Always keep syrup of ipecac in your home. Determine whether activated charcoal for home use is available in your area, and store it with the ipecac if obtainable. The ipecac is used to induce vomiting; the activated charcoal is used to adsorb poisons. Use them only as instructed by your Poison Control Center or doctor, and follow their directions for use.

Inhaled Poisons

If smoke, gas, or fumes have been inhaled, immediately drag or carry the patient to fresh air. Then call the poison center or your doctor. Do not enter an area where there are poisonous fumes without protection or safeguards. Too often the rescuer becomes a victim as well.

Poisons on the Skin

If the poison has been spilled on the skin or clothing, remove the clothing and flood the involved parts with water. Wash with soapy water and rinse thoroughly. Then call the Poison Control Center or your doctor.

Swallowed Poisons

If the substance swallowed is a medicine, give nothing. Milk or water should be immediately administered to any patient who has ingested a strongly acid or alkaline agent. Do not give more than 15 mL/kg (250 mL maximum in a child weighing 16 kg or more). Do not induce vomiting in patients who are comatose, convulsing, or who have lost the gag reflex. If emesis is induced on the way to the hospital, syrup of ipecac should be administered as described in the section on prevention of absorption (see p 320). *Caution:* Antidote labels on products may be incorrect. Do not give salt, vinegar, or lemon juice. Call before doing anything else.

Poisons in the Eye

Irrigation of the eye with plain water should begin before the patient arrives at the emergency room. Use plain tap water—do not try to neutralize acids or alkalies. Have the head held back over the sink and direct a gentle stream of water into the eye from the tap, or pour water into the eye from a drinking glass or pitcher. Irrigation should be continued for 15–20 minutes. Then transport the patient to the hospital for ophthalmologic examination.

Bring the Poison to the Hospital

If the patient is to be seen in the Emergency Department, everything in the vicinity of the patient that may be a cause of poisoning should be brought along.

Poison Information

Up-to-date data on ingredients of commercial products and medications can usually be obtained from a certified regional poison center. *POISINDEX Information System* offers current data about toxic ingredients based on computer contact with manufacturers. It is important to have the actual container at hand if the manufacturer is called. In some cases, the experience of the company physician may be of value in management. *Caution:* Antidote information on labels of commercial products may be incorrect or inappropriate.

Follow-Up

In over 95% of cases of ingestion of potentially toxic substances by children, a trip to the hospital is not required. If it is decided that an ingestion is not toxic or that vomiting induced at home is the only treatment required, it is important to call the parent at 1 and 4 hours after an ingestion. If the child has actually ingested an additional unknown agent and develops symptoms, a change in management may be needed, including transportation to the hospital. An additional call should be made 24 hours after the ingestion to begin the process of poison prevention.

Poison Prevention Over the Telephone

This may be instituted with a few simple questions about storage of hazardous substances in unsafe locations. The following is a partial list of potentially poisonous substances that must be stored safely if there are small children in the home: drain-cleaning crystals or liquid, dishwasher soap and cleaning supplies, paints and paint thinners, garden spray and other insecticide materials, automobile products, and all medications.

If it seems that there are problems that may lead to further episodes of poisoning, it will be useful to arrange an appointment with the parent to discuss the problems or to send a public health nurse to the home to examine storage practices and make suitable recommendations.

PREVENTION OF POISONING

A major goal of pediatricians is to reduce the number of accidental ingestions in the high-risk age group under 5 years of age. A systematic poison education effort should be part of the routine care of every patient. Parents of very young children should be encouraged to search the house and identify all hazardous substances that should be removed from the home or locked up.

The section entitled "Preventing Childhood Poisonings," reproduced on p 316, may be copied from this book and given to parents along with a bottle of syrup of ipecac at the 6-month checkup.* Reinforcement should occur at the 1-year checkup to make certain that adequate poison-proofing measures have been instituted and maintained.

---

*No request for permission to reproduce the chart is necessary provided it is done without modification.

INITIAL EMERGENCY DEPARTMENT CONTACT

If the decision has been made to see the child in the hospital—or if the patient has bypassed the initial phone call and is brought to the emergency department—the following steps should be taken.

Make Certain the Patient Is Breathing

As in all emergencies, the principles of treatment are attention to airway, breathing, and circulation. These are sometimes overlooked under the stressful conditions of a severe pediatric poisoning.

Treat Shock

Initial therapy of the hypotensive patient should consist of laying the patient flat and administering isotonic solutions. Vasopressors should be reserved for poisoned patients in shock who do not respond to these standard measures.

Treat Burns

Burns may occur following exposure to strong acid or strong alkaline agents or petroleum distillates. Burned areas should be decontaminated by flooding with sterile saline solution or water. A burn unit should be consulted if more than minimal burn damage has been sustained. Skin decontamination should be performed in a patient with cutaneous exposure. Emergency department personnel in contact with a patient who has been contaminated (with an organophosphate insecticide, for example) should themselves be decontaminated if their skin or clothing becomes contaminated.

Take a Pertinent History

The history should be taken from the parents and all individuals present at the scene. It may be crucial to determine all of the kinds of poisons in the home. These may include drugs used by family members, chemicals associated with the hobbies or occupations of family members, or the purity of the water supply. Unusual dietary or medication habits or other clues to the possible cause of poisoning should also be investigated.

Assess Coma, Hyperactivity, & Withdrawal

It is useful to determine the level of coma, the degree of hyperactivity, or the severity of withdrawal symptoms as a means of assessing the efficacy of treatment.

A. Determine the Level of Coma: Coma is graded on a scale of 0–4:

0   Asleep but can be aroused and can answer questions.
1   Comatose: withdraws from painful stimuli; reflexes intact.
2   Comatose: does not withdraw from painful stimuli; most reflexes intact; no respiratory or circulatory depression.
3   Comatose: most or all reflexes absent; no depression of respiration or circulation.
4   Comatose: reflexes absent; respiratory depression with cyanosis, circulatory failure, or shock.

B. Determine the Degree of Hyperactivity:

1+   Restlessness, irritability, insomnia, tremor, hyperflexia, sweating, mydriasis, flushing.
2+   Confusion, hyperactivity, hypertension, tachypnea, tachycardia, extrasystoles, sweating, mydriasis, flushing, mild hyperpyrexia.
3+   Delirium, mania, self-injury, marked hypertension, tachycardia, cardiac arrhythmias, hyperpyrexia.
4+   The above symptoms and signs plus convulsions, coma, circulatory collapse.

C. Determine the Severity of Narcotic Withdrawal Symptoms: Score the following findings on a scale of 0–2:

Diarrhea	Insomnia
Dilated pupils	Lacrimation
Gooseflesh	Muscle cramps
Hyperactive bowel	Restlessness
sounds	Tachycardia
Hypertension	Yawning

A score of 1–5 represents mild, 6–10 moderate, and 11–15 severe withdrawal symptoms.

Seizures, which are unusual in narcotic withdrawal, indicate severe withdrawal problems.

DEFINITIVE THERAPY OF POISONING

Antidotes

There are few specific antidotes. A few poisons that may require immediate antidotal therapy are listed here:

Poison	Antidote
Carbon monoxide	Oxygen
Cyanide	Sodium nitrite (pediatric dosage), sodium thiosulfate
Nitrites and nitrates	Treat methemoglobinemia with methylene blue
Organophosphate insecticides	Atropine, pralidoxime (2-PAM)
Anticholinergics	Physostigmine
Opioids	Naloxone
Methanol, ethylene glycol	Ethanol

Prevention of Absorption

A. Emesis: Induced vomiting is *contraindicated* in patients who are comatose, convulsing, have lost the gag reflex, or have ingested strong acids, strong bases, or some hydrocarbons. In the case of hydrocarbons, vomiting should be induced if more than 1 mL/kg has been ingested or if the substance contains heavy metals.

1. Ipecac method–Adult dose, 30 mL; pediatric dose, 15 mL. Give orally and repeat once in 20 minutes if necessary. The procedure is as follows:

a.   Give ipecac orally.

b.   Follow with up to 6 oz of water or whatever fluid the child will drink (ipecac on an empty stomach is "like squeezing an empty balloon").

c.   Keep the patient ambulatory.

d.   After 20 minutes, repeat the dose if vomiting has not occurred.

2. Other emetics–The only approved oral emetic agent is syrup of ipecac. Use of sodium chloride may lead to lethal hypernatremia. Apomorphine should not be used because its depressant effect outlasts the duration of reversal by naloxone. Other emetic agents, such as mustard and soap, are not as effective as syrup of ipecac and should be avoided.

B. Lavage: If the patient is or is becoming unconscious, is convulsing, or has lost the gag reflex, gastric lavage following endotracheal or nasotracheal intubation should be performed rather than induction of vomiting. Lavage is less effective than emesis if a small (8–16F) tube is utilized but not if the recommended 28–36F Ewald tube is used. The tube should be inserted orally, and lavage should be with warm saline solution in a small child to avoid hyponatremia or hypothermia. Save the initial aspirate for laboratory determination and lavage until the returns have been clear for 1 liter. Monitor the amount of fluid given. The amount instilled should approximate the amount removed.

Emesis and lavage recover an average of about 30% of the stomach contents. While these procedures may be helpful in reducing the amount of material available for absorption, approximately 70% of an ingested dose will remain. Additional measures such as charcoal and cathartics should be instituted to prevent further absorption.

C. Charcoal: Thirty grams of charcoal should be made into a slurry with a minimum of 240 mL of diluent. Give 1–2 g/kg (maximum, 100 g) per dose. The charcoal may be in an aqueous slurry or mixed with a saline cathartic or sorbitol.

In some poisonings, it may be advantageous to administer more than one dose of activated charcoal. Repeating the dose is particularly useful for those agents that undergo enterohepatic circulation or those that may slow passage through the gastrointestinal tract. When multiple doses of activated charcoal are given, repeated doses of sorbitol or saline cathartics should not be given. Repeated doses of cathartics may cause electrolyte imbalances and fluid loss. Charcoal dosing is repeated every 2–6 hours until charcoal is passed per rectum.

The patient may regurgitate some of the charcoal, but 70% is usually retained. Charcoal has been shown to reduce the half-life of an agent even when it is given after the intravenous administration of phenobarbital or theophylline.

D. Catharsis: *Caution:* Despite their widespread use, cathartics have not been shown to improve outcome. The use of cathartics should therefore be limited to patients in whom they can be safely used. In particular, do not give cathartics containing magnesium or phosphate to patients in renal failure. Pneumonitis may occur following aspiration of oil-based cathartics.

Acceptable cathartics include magnesium sulfate or sodium sulfate (250 mg/kg/dose orally [maximum, 30 g]); magnesium citrate (4 mL/kg/dose [maximum, 300 mL]); and sorbitol (1–1.5 g/kg/dose, of a 35% solution, for children over 1 year of age [maximum, 50 g/dose]). Sorbitol should be administered in a health care facility so that fluid and electrolyte status can be monitored, especially in children. Fleet's Phospho-Soda (15–30 mL, diluted 1:4—entire amount to adolescents and about one-fourth to children) may also be used.

E. Whole Gut Lavage: Whole bowel lavage utilizes an orally administered, nonabsorbable hypertonic solution such as Colyte or Golytely. These are being studied as an alternative method of gastrointestinal decontamination.The use of this procedure in poisoned patients is currently controversial. Preliminary recommendations for use of whole bowel irrigation include sustained-release preparations, mechanical movement of items through the bowel (eg, cocaine packets), and substances poorly absorbed by charcoal (lithium, iron). Underlying bowel pathology and functional obstruction are relative contraindications to its use.

Kulig K et al: Management of acutely poisoned patients without gastric emptying. Ann Emerg Med 1985;14:562.
Merigian KS et al: Prospective evaluation of gastric emptying in the self poisoned patient. Am J Emerg Med 1990; 8:479.
Tenenbein M, Cohen S, Sitar DS: Efficacy of ipecac-induced emesis, orogastric lavage and activated charcoal for acute drug overdose. Ann Emerg Med 1987;16:838.
Tenenbein M: Whole bowel irrigation for toxic ingestions. Clin Toxicol 1985;23:177.

Enhancement of Urinary Excretion

Urinary excretion of certain substances can be hastened by urinary alkalinization or dialysis (hemodialysis or peritoneal dialysis). In the past, forced diuresis or forced alkaline diuresis was used. While these have been abandoned because of their high complications rates, it is important to make certain that the patient is not volume-depleted. Volume-depleted patients should receive a normal saline bolus of 10–20 mL/kg, followed by sufficient intravenous fluid administration to maintain urine output at 2–3 mL/kg/h.

A. Urinary alkalinization:

1. Alkaline diuresis–Urinary alkalinization should be chosen on the basis of the substance's pK_a, so that ionized drug will be trapped in the tubular lumen and not reabsorbed. (See Table 13–1.) Thus, if the pK_a is less than 7.5, urinary alkalinization is appropriate; if it is over 8.0, this technique will not usually be beneficial. The pK_a is sometimes included along with general drug information. Urinary alkalinization can usually be achieved with sodium bicarbonate. It is well to observe for potassium depletion, caused by the shift of potassium intracellularly. Follow serum K^+ and observe for electrocardiographic evidence of hypokalemia.

B. Dialysis: Hemodialysis (or peritoneal dialysis if hemodialysis is unavailable) is useful in the poisonings listed below. Dialysis should be considered part of supportive care if the patient satisfies any of the following criteria:

1. Clinical criteria–

a. Stage 3 or 4 coma or hyperactivity that is caused by a dialyzable drug and cannot be treated by conservative means.

b. Hypotension threatening renal or hepatic function that cannot be corrected by adjusting circulating volume.

c. Apnea in a patient who cannot be ventilated.

d. Marked hyperosmolality that is not due to easily corrected fluid problems.

e. Severe acid-base disturbance not responding to therapy.

f. Severe electrolyte disturbance not responding to therapy.

g. Marked hypothermia or hyperthermia not responding to therapy.

2. Immediate dialysis–Immediate dialysis may be considered in ethylene glycol and methanol poisoning only if acidosis is refractory and blood levels of ethanol of 100 mg/dL are consistently maintained during dialysis.

3. Dialysis indicated on basis of condition of patient–(In general, dialyze if patient is in coma deeper than level 3.)

Alcohols	Bromides	Paraldehyde
Ammonia	Calcium	Potassium
Amphetamines	Chloral hydrate	Quinidine
Anilines	Fluorides	Quinine
Antibiotics	Iodides	Salicylates
Barbiturates	Isoniazid	Strychnine
(long-acting)	Meprobamate	Thiocyanates
Boric Acid		

(Other drugs may be dialyzable, but the information should be verified prior to institution of dialysis therapy.)

4. Dialysis not indicated except for support—
Therapy consists of intensive care.

Antidepressants (cyclics and MAO inhibitors)	Heroin and other opioids
Antihistamines	Methaqualone
Barbiturates (short-acting)	Methyprylon
Chlordiazepoxide	Oxazepam
Diazepam	Phenothiazines
Digitalis and related drugs	Phenytoin
Diphenoxylate with atropine	Synthetic anticholinergics and belladonna compounds

While the long-acting barbiturates (cleared by the kidneys) are more readily dialyzable than the short-acting ones (cleared by the liver), dialysis may be helpful if the patient satisfies the criteria for supportive dialysis needs as outlined above.

Salicylates generally respond very well to intensive alkaline diuretic therapy, but if complications such as renal failure or pulmonary edema develop, hemodialysis alone or with hemoperfusion may be helpful.

Peritoneal dialysis and **exchange transfusion** may be more useful in small children than hemodialysis, as much for fluid and electrolyte homeostasis as for poison removal.

Dialysis should *not* be performed as initial therapy but only when the criteria listed above are met.

Hemoperfusion

Perfusion of blood through charcoal- or resin-filled devices is gradually becoming more widely available in many centers. These techniques will probably allow rapid removal of many substances previously considered dialyzable but will not be likely to remove large quantities of agents with large V_dS.

MANAGEMENT OF SPECIFIC COMMON POISONS

Unless otherwise contraindicated, syrup of ipecac should be given to all conscious patients poisoned by the substances listed in the following section, particularly if it can be administered within 1 hour after ingestion. Whenever possible, patients should be evaluated regarding the need for emesis, which depends on the severity of the exposure. Gastric lavage is usually indicated for comatose patients after an endotracheal tube is inserted.

ACETAMINOPHEN (Paracetamol)

Acetaminophen is an analgesic antipyretic contained in numerous preparations accessible to children. In recommended doses, the drug is a safe and effective agent. In overdosage, acetaminophen can cause severe hepatotoxicity. The incidence of hepatotoxicity in adults and adolescents has been reported to be ten times higher than in young children; in the latter group, only three of 4187 patients under the age of 5 years developed transient hepatotoxicity.

Acetaminophen is normally metabolized in the liver. A small percentage of the drug goes through a pathway leading to a toxic metabolite. Normally, this nucleophilic reactant is removed harmlessly by conjugation with glutathione. In overdosage, the supply of glutathione becomes exhausted, and the metabolite may bind covalently to hepatic macromolecules to produce necrosis.

Treatment

Treatment is to supply a surrogate glutathione by giving acetylcysteine. In the USA, it may only be given orally. Consultation on difficult cases may be obtained from the Rocky Mountain Poison Center (1-800-525-6115). Blood levels should be obtained as soon as possible after 4 hours and plotted on Figure 13–1. Acetylcysteine is administered to patients whose acetaminophen levels plot in the toxic range on the nomogram (Figure 13–1). Preliminary evidence suggests that acetylcysteine may also be of use even after 24 hours post ingestion.

The dose is 140 mg/kg orally, diluted to a 5% solution in sweet fruit juice or carbonated soft drink. The primary problems associated with administration are nausea and vomiting. After this loading dose, 70 mg/kg should be administered orally every 4 hours for 72 hours. AST, ALT, serum bilirubin, and plasma prothrombin time should be followed daily.

Parker D et al: Safety of late acetylcysteine treatment in paracetamol poisoning. Hum Exp Toxicol 1990;9:25.

Peterson RG, Rumack BH: Pharmacokinetics of acetaminophen in children. Pediatrics 1978;62:877.

Rumack BH et al: Acetaminophen overdose. Arch Intern Med 1981;141:380.

Smilkstein M et al: Efficacy of oral N-acetylcysteine in the treatment of acetaminophen overdose. N Engl J Med 1988;319:1557.

ALCOHOL, ETHYL (Ethanol)

Alcoholic beverages, tinctures, cosmetics, and rubbing alcohol are common sources of poisoning in children. Concomitant exposure to other depressant drugs increases the seriousness of the intoxication.

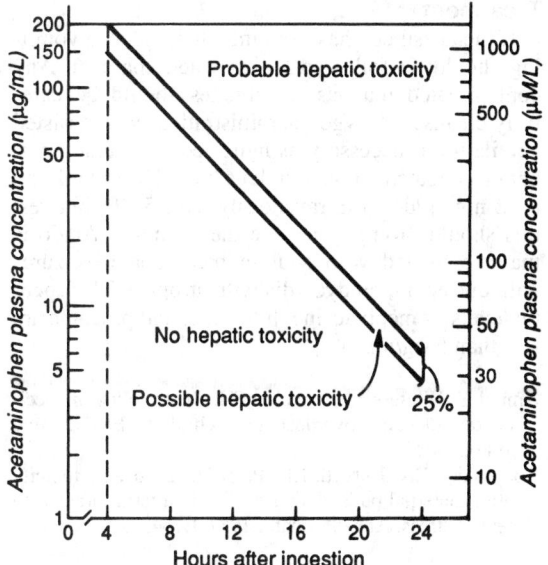

Cautions for use of this chart:
1. The time coordinates refer to time of ingestion.
2. Serum levels drawn before 4 hours may not represent peak levels.
3. The graph should be used only in relation to a single acute ingestion.
4. The lower solid line 25% below the standard nomogram is included to allow for possible errors in acetaminophen plasma assays and estimated time from ingestion of an overdose.

Figure 13–1. Semilogarithmic plot of plasma acetaminophen levels versus time. (Modified and reproduced, with permission, from Rumack BH, Matthew H: Acetaminophen poisoning and toxicity. Pediatrics 1975; 55:871.)

(Blood levels cited are for adults; comparable figures for children are not available. In most states, alcohol levels of 50–80 mg/dL are considered compatible with impaired faculties, and levels of 80–150 mg/dL are considered evidence of intoxication.)

50–150 mg/dL: Incoordination, slow reaction time, and blurred vision.

150–300 mg/dL: Visual impairment, staggering, and slurred speech. Marked hypoglycemia may be present.

300–500 mg/dL: Marked incoordination, stupor, hypoglycemia, and convulsions.

> 500 mg/dL: Coma and death, except in individuals who have developed tolerance.

Complete absorption of alcohol requires 30 minutes to 6 hours, depending upon the volume, the presence of food, the time spent in consuming the alcohol, etc. The rate of metabolic degradation is constant (about 20 mg/h in an adult). Less than 10% is excreted in the urine. Absolute ethanol, 1 mL/kg, results in a peak blood level of about 100 mg/dL in 1 hour after ingestion. Acute intoxication and chronic alcoholism increase the risk of subarachnoid hemorrhage.

Treatment

Supportive treatment, including aggressive management of hypoglycemia and acidosis, is usually the only measure required. Start an intravenous drip of D_5W or $D_{10}W$ if blood glucose is under 60 mg/dL. Fructose has been suggested as an accelerator of metabolism, but it may cause vomiting, intensify lactic acidosis, and decrease blood volume via osmotic diuresis. Glucagon does not correct the hypoglycemia, because hepatic glycogen stores are reduced. Monitoring of oxygen saturation and oxygen administration are indicated in serious overdoses because death is usually caused by respiratory failure. In severe cases, cerebral edema should be treated with dexamethasone, 0.1 mg/kg intravenously every 4–6 hours. Hemodialysis is indicated in life-threatening intoxication. Peritoneal dialysis may be used if hemodialysis is unavailable.

Amene PC: Intravenous fructose for acute alcoholism: Double-blind study. JACEP 1976;5:253.
Hammond K, Rumack B, Rodgerson D: Blood ethanol. JAMA 1973;226:63.
Leung AKC: Ethyl alcohol ingestions in children. Clin Pediatr (Phila) 1986;25:617.
Scherger DL et al: Ethyl alcohol (ethanol)-containing cologne, perfume, and aftershave ingestions in children. Am J Dis Child 1988;142:630.

AMPHETAMINES & RELATED DRUGS (Methamphetamine)

Clinical Presentation

A. Acute Poisoning: Amphetamine poisoning is common because of the widespread availability of "diet pills" and the use of "speed," "crank," "crystal," and "ice" by adolescents. (Care must be taken in the interpretation of slang terms because they have multiple meanings.) Symptoms include central nervous system stimulation, anxiety, hyperactivity, hyperpyrexia, hypertension, abdominal cramps, nausea and vomiting, and inability to void urine. Severe cases may include rhabdomyolysis. A toxic psychosis indistinguishable from paranoid schizophrenia may occur.

B. Chronic Poisoning: Chronic amphetamine users develop such a high tolerance that more than 1500 mg of intravenous methamphetamine can be used daily. Hyperactivity, disorganization, and euphoria are followed by exhaustion, depression, and coma lasting 2–3 days. Upon awakening, the patient is ravenously hungry. Heavy users, taking more than 100 mg/d, have restlessness, incoordination of thought, insomnia, nervousness, irritability, and visual hallucinations. Psychosis may be precipitated by the chronic administration of high doses. Depression, weakness, tremors, gastrointestinal complaints, and suicidal thoughts occur frequently.

Treatment

Standard decontamination procedures should be used: gastric emptying followed by charcoal in recent ingestions; activated charcoal alone if ingestion occurred hours ago. The treatment of choice is with diazepam. If this fails to reduce hyperactivity, chlorpromazine (0.5–1 mg/kg intravenously) may be given and repeated in 30 minutes. A maximum daily dose of 2.5–6 mg/kg may be used. Chlorpromazine may produce hypotension. In case of extreme agitation or hallucinations, droperidol (0.1 mg/kg/dose) or haloperidol (up to 0.1 mg/kg) parenterally has been used. When combinations of amphetamines and barbiturates (diet pills) are used, the action of the amphetamines begins first, followed by a rebound depression caused by the barbiturates. In these cases, treatment with additional barbiturates is contraindicated because of the risk of respiratory failure.

Chronic users may be withdrawn rapidly from amphetamines. On the other hand, if amphetamine-barbiturate combination tablets have been used, the barbiturates must be withdrawn gradually to prevent withdrawal seizures. Psychiatric treatment should be provided.

Jackson JG: The hazards of smokable methamphetamine. New Engl J Med 1989;321:907.

Broscoe JG et al: Pemoline-induced choreoathetosis and rhabdomyolysis. Med Toxicol 1988;3:72.

Catravas JD et al: Haloperidol for acute amphetamine poisoning: A study in dogs. JAMA 1975;231:1340.

Gary NE, Saidi P: Methamphetamine intoxication. Am J Med 1978;64:537.

ANESTHETICS, LOCAL

Intoxication from local anesthetics may be associated with central nervous system stimulation, acidosis, delirium, ataxia, shock, convulsions, and death. Methemoglobinuria has been reported following local dental analgesia.

Local anesthetics used in obstetrics cross the placental barrier and are not efficiently metabolized by the fetal liver. Mepivacaine, lidocaine, and bupivacaine can cause fetal bradycardia, neonatal depression, and death. Prilocaine causes methemoglobinemia, which should be treated if levels in the blood exceed 40% or if the patient is symptomatic.

Accidental injection of mepivacaine into the head of the fetus during paracervical anesthesia has caused neonatal asphyxia, cyanosis, acidosis, bradycardia, convulsions, and death.

Treatment

If the anesthetic has been ingested, induced vomiting should be followed by activated charcoal. Any contaminated mucous membranes should be carefully cleansed. Oxygen administration, with assisted ventilation if necessary, is indicated. Methemoglobinemia is treated with methylene blue, 1%, 0.2 mL/kg (1–2 mg/kg/dose) intravenously over 5–10 minutes; this should promptly relieve the cyanosis. Acidosis may be treated with sodium bicarbonate, seizures with diazepam, bradycardia with atropine. Therapeutic levels of mepivacaine, lidocaine, and procaine are less than 5 μg/mL.

Amitai Y, Whitesell L, Lovejoy FH: Death following accidental lidocaine overdose in a child. N Engl J Med 1986;314:181.

Bozynski MEA, Rubarth LB, Patel JA: Lidocaine toxicity after maternal pudendal anesthesia in a term infant with fetal distress. Am J Perinatol 1987;4:164.

ANTIHISTAMINES

Although antihistamines typically cause central nervous system depression, children often react paradoxically with excitement, hallucinations, delirium, ataxia, tremors, and convulsions followed by central nervous system depression, respiratory failure, or cardiovascular collapse. Anticholinergic effects such as dry mouth, fixed dilated pupils, flushed face, fever, and hallucinations may be prominent.

Antihistamines are widely available in allergy, sleep, cold, and antiemetic preparations, and many are supplied in sustained-release forms, which increases the likelihood of dangerous overdoses. They are absorbed rapidly and metabolized by the liver, lungs, and kidneys. A potentially toxic dose is 10–50 mg/kg of the most commonly used antihistamines, but toxic reactions have occurred at much lower doses.

Treatment

Activated charcoal should be used to reduce drug absorption. Emetics may be ineffective if the antihistamine is structurally related to phenothiazines. A cathartic is indicated for sustained-release preparations. Physostigmine, 0.5–2 mg slowly intravenously, dramatically reverses the central and peripheral anticholinergic effects of antihistamines, but it should be used only for diagnostic purposes. Diazepam, 0.1–0.2 mg/kg intravenously, can be used to control seizures. Forced diuresis is not helpful. Exchange transfusion was reported effective in one case.

Tobin JR et al: Astemizole-induced cardiac conduction disturbances in a child. JAMA 1991;266:2737.

Magera BE et al: Hydroxyzine intoxication in a 13-month-old child. Pediatrics 1981;67:280.

Richmond M, Seger D: Central anticholinergic syndrome in a child: A case report. J Emerg Med 1985;3:453.

Rumack BH et al: Ornade and anticholinergic toxicity, hypertension, hallucinations and arrhythmia. Clin Toxicol 1974;7:573.

ARSENIC

Clinical Presentation

A. Acute Poisoning: Abdominal pain, vomiting, watery and bloody diarrhea, cardiovascular collapse, paresthesias, neck pain, and garlic odor on breath occur. Convulsions, coma, anuria, and exfoliative dermatitis are later signs. Inhalation may cause pulmonary edema. Death is the result of cardiovascular collapse.

B. Chronic Poisoning: Anorexia, generalized weakness, giddiness, colic, abdominal pain, polyneuritis, dermatitis, nail changes, alopecia, and anemia often develop.

Arsenic is commonly used in insecticides (fruit tree or tobacco sprays), rodenticides, weed killers, and wallpaper. It is well absorbed primarily through the gastrointestinal and respiratory tracts, but skin absorption may occur. Arsenic can be found in the urine, hair, and nails by laboratory testing.

Highly toxic soluble derivatives of this compound, such as sodium arsenite, are frequently found in liquid preparations and can cause death in as many as 65% of victims. The alkyl methanearsonates found in "persistent" or "preemergence" type weed killers are relatively less soluble and less toxic. Poisonings with a liquid arsenical preparation that does not contain alkyl methanearsonate compounds should be considered potentially lethal. Patients with clinical signs other than gastroenteritis should be treated until laboratory tests indicate that treatment is no longer necessary.

Treatment

In acute poisoning, induce vomiting and administer activated charcoal. Then immediately give dimercaprol (BAL), 2.5 mg/kg intramuscularly, and follow with 2 mg/kg intramuscularly every 4 hours. The dimercaprol-arsenic complex is dialyzable. Succimer is approved for use in children. The initial dose is 10 mg/kg every 8 hours for 5 days. A third choice is penicillamine, 100 mg/kg orally to a maximum of 1 g/d in four divided doses.

Chronic arsenic intoxication should be treated with succimer or penicillamine. Collect a 24-hour baseline urine specimen and then begin chelation. If the 24-hour urine arsenic level is greater than 50 μg, continue chelation for 5 days. After 10 days, repeat the 5-day cycle once or twice depending on how soon the urine arsenic level falls below 50 μg/24 h.

Donofrio PD et al: Acute arsenic intoxication presenting as Guillain-Barré-like syndrome. Muscle Nerve 1987;10:114.

Fournier L et al: 2,3-Dimercaptosuccinic acid treatment of heavy metal poisoning in humans. Med Toxicol 1988;3:499.

Peterson RG, Rumack BH: Arsenic poisoning treated with D-penicillamine. J Pediatr 1977;91:661.

BARBITURATES

A patient who has ingested barbiturates in toxic amounts can present with a variety of findings, including confusion, poor coordination, coma, miotic or fixed dilated pupils, and increased or (more commonly) decreased respiratory effort. Respiratory acidosis is commonly associated with pulmonary atelectasis, and hypotension occurs frequently in severely poisoned patients. Ingestion of more than 6 mg/kg of long-acting or 3 mg/kg of short-acting barbiturates is usually toxic; however, chronic users of barbiturates can tolerate blood levels up to 25 mg/dL.

Treatment

If the patient is awake, vomiting should be induced and activated charcoal should be given. Careful, conservative management with emphasis on maintaining a clear airway, adequate ventilation, and control of hypotension is critical. Urinary alkalinization and the use of multiple-dose charcoal may decrease the elimination half-life of phenobarbital but have not been shown to alter the clinical course. Hemodialysis is not of significant help in the treatment of poisoning with short-acting barbiturates. Analeptics are contraindicated.

Amitai Y, Degani Y: Treatment of phenobarbital poisoning with multiple dose activated charcoal in an infant. J Emerg Med 1990;8:449.

Gröschel D, Gerstein A, Rosenbaum J: Skin lesions as a diagnostic aid in barbiturate poisoning. N Engl J Med 1970;283:409.

Zawada ET et al: Advances in the hemodialysis management of phenobarbital overdose. South Med J 1983;76:6.

BELLADONNA ALKALOIDS
(Atropine, Jimsonweed, Potato Leaves, Scopolamine, Stramonium)

Patients with atropinism have common complaints which include dry mouth; thirst; decreased sweating with hot, dry, red skin; high fever; and tachycardia that may be preceded by bradycardia. The pupils are dilated, and vision is blurred. Speech and swallowing may be impaired. Hallucinations, delirium, and coma are common. Leukocytosis may occur, confusing the diagnosis.

Atropinism has been caused by normal doses of atropine or homatropine eye drops, especially in children with Down's syndrome. Many common plants and over-the-counter sleeping medications contain belladonna alkaloids.

Treatment

Emesis or lavage should be followed by activated charcoal and cathartics. Gastric emptying is slowed by anticholinergics, so that gastric decontamination may be useful even if delayed. Physostigmine, 0.5–2 mg slowly intravenously (can be repeated every 30 minutes as needed), dramatically reverses the central and peripheral signs of atropinism but should be used only as a diagnostic agent. Neostigmine is ineffective because it does not enter the central nervous system. High fever must be controlled. Catheterization may be needed if the patient cannot void.

Beech M, Hell C, Nightingale P: Central anticholinergic syndrome. Lancet 1987;1:1089.
Fitzgerald DA et al: Seizures associated with 1% cyclopentolate eyedrops. J Paediatr Child Health 1990;26:106.

CARBON MONOXIDE

Tables which were developed correlating clinical signs with carboxyhemoglobin levels are often inaccurate, especially if taken after oxygen has been given or when there has been some time since exposure.

The degree of toxicity correlates well with the carboxyhemoglobin level after acute exposure. Onset of symptoms may be more rapid and more severe if the patient lives at a high altitude, has a high respiratory rate (ie, infants), is pregnant, or has myocardial insufficiency or lung disease. Normal blood may contain up to 5% carboxyhemoglobin.

The most prominent early symptom is headache. Proteinuria, glycosuria, elevated serum aminotransferase levels, or electrocardiographic changes may be present in the acute phase. Permanent cardiac, liver, renal, or central nervous system damage occasionally occurs. The outcome of severe poisoning may be complete recovery, vegetative state, or any degree of mental injury between these extremes. The primary mental deficits are neuropsychiatric.

Treatment

The biologic half-life of carbon monoxide on room air is approximately 200–300 minutes; on 100% oxygen, it is 60–90 minutes. Hyperbaric oxygen therapy at 2–2.5 atm of oxygen shortens the half-life to 30 minutes. After the level has been reduced to near zero, therapy is aimed at the nonspecific sequelae of anoxia. Dexamethasone, 0.1 mg/kg intravenously or intramuscularly every 4–6 hours, should be added if cerebral edema develops.

Crocker PJ, Walker JS: Pediatric carbon monoxide toxicity. J Emerg Med 1985;3:443.
Farrow JR et al: Fetal death due to nonlethal maternal carbon monoxide poisoning. J Forensic Sci 1990;35:1448.
Norkool DM, Kirkpatrick JN: Treatment of acute carbon monoxide poisoning with hyperbaric oxygen: A review of 115 cases. Ann Emerg Med 1985;14:1168.
Raphael JC et al: Trial of normobaric and hyperbaric oxygen for acute carbon monoxide intoxication. Lancet 1989;2:414.

CAUSTICS

1. ACIDS (Hydrochloric, Hydrofluoric, Nitric, & Sulfuric Acids; Sodium Bisulfate)

Strong acids are commonly found in metal and toilet bowl cleaners, batteries, etc. Hydrofluoric acid is the most toxic and hydrochloric acid the least toxic of these household substances. However, even a few drops can be fatal if aspirated into the trachea.

Painful swallowing, mucous membrane burns, bloody emesis, abdominal pain, respiratory distress due to edema of the epiglottis, thirst, shock, and renal failure can occur. Coma and convulsions sometimes are seen terminally. Residual lesions include esophageal, gastric, and pyloric strictures as well as scars of the cornea, skin, and oropharynx. Hydrofluoric acid burns may be deep and penetrating, requiring special care.

Treatment

Emetics and lavage are contraindicated. Water or milk (< 15 mL/kg) are used to dilute the ingestant, because a heat-producing chemical reaction does not occur. Take care not to induce emesis by excessive fluid administration. Alkalies should not be used. Burned areas of the skin, mucous membranes, or eyes should be washed with copious amounts of warm water. Opioids for pain may be needed. An endotracheal tube may be required to alleviate laryngeal edema. Esophagoscopy should be performed if the patient has significant burns or difficulty in swallowing. Acids are likely to produce gastric burns or esophageal burns. Evidence is not conclusive, but corticosteroids have not proved to be of use.

Hydrofluoric acid is a particularly dangerous poison. Dermal exposure creates a penetrating burn that can progress for hours or days. Large dermal exposure or ingestion may produce life-threatening hypocalcemia as well as burn reactions. Monitor closely. Dermal exposures may require application of a 10% calcium gluconate gel or calcium gluconate infusion. Severe exposure may require large doses of calcium. Therapy should be guided by calcium levels, the ECG, and clinical signs.

2. BASES
(Clinitest Tablets, Clorox, Drano, Liquid-Plumr, Purex, Sani-Clor)

Alkalies produce more severe injuries than acids. Some substances, such as Clinitest Tablets or Drano, are quite toxic, whereas the chlorinated bleaches (3–6% solutions of sodium hypochlorite) are usually not toxic. When sodium hypochlorite comes in contact with the acid pH of the stomach, hypochlorous acid, which is very irritating to the mucous membrane and skin, is formed. Rapid inactivation of this substance prevents systemic toxicity. Chlorinated beaches, when mixed with a strong acid (toilet bowl cleaners) or ammonia, may produce irritating chlorine or chloramine gas.

Alkalies can burn the skin, mucous membranes, and eyes. Respiratory distress may be due to edema of the epiglottis, pulmonary edema resulting from inhalation of fumes, or pneumonia. Mediastinitis or other intercurrent infections or shock can occur. Perforation of the esophagus or stomach is rare.

Treatment

The skin and mucous membranes should be cleansed with copious amounts of water. A local anesthetic can be instilled in the eye if necessary to alleviate blepharospasm. The eye should be irrigated for at least 20–30 minutes. Ophthalmologic consultation should be obtained for all alkaline eye burns.

Ingestions should be treated with water as a diluent. Routine esophagoscopy is no longer indicated to rule out burns of the esophagus due to chlorinated bleaches unless an unusually large amount has been ingested or the patient is symptomatic. The absence of oral lesions does not rule out the possibility of laryngeal or esophageal burns following granular alkali ingestion. The use of corticosteroids is controversial but has not been shown to improve long-term outcome. Antibiotics may be needed if mediastinitis is likely, but they should not be used prophylactically.

Gaudreault P et al: Predictability of esophageal injury from signs and symptoms: A study of caustic ingestion in 378 children. Pediatrics 1983;71:767.

Lovejoy FH Jr: Corrosive injury of the esophagus in children: Failure of corticosteroid treatment reemphasizes prevention. (Editorial.) N Engl J Med 1990;323:668.

Wijburg HA, Heymans HSA, Urbanus NAM: Caustic esophageal lesions in childhood: Prevention of stricture formation. J Pediatr Surg 1989;24:171.

COCAINE

Street names of cocaine may include "free-base, crack, rock, baseball, speedball, coke, snow, gold dust, bernice, lady, nose-candy, champagne, Dama Blanca," and "rich man's drug." Free-base is prepared by treating cocaine hydrochloride with a basic solution, such as sodium hydroxide. The precipitated alkaloid is filtered, dried, and smoked. Crack is prepared by mixing the cocaine hydrochloride with baking soda and water, then heating to form a "rock," which is then smoked. Most street cocaine is adulterated. Cocaine is absorbed intranasally or via inhalation or ingestion. Effects are noted almost immediately when the drug is taken intravenously or smoked. Peak effects are delayed for about an hour when the drug is taken orally or nasally. Cocaine prevents the reuptake of endogenous catecholamines, thereby causing an initial sympathetic discharge, followed by catechol depletion after chronic abuse.

Clinical Findings

A local anesthetic and vasoconstrictor, cocaine is also a potent stimulant to both the central nervous system and the cardiovascular system. The initial tachycardia, hyperpnea, hypertension, and stimulation of the central nervous system are often followed by coma, seizures, hypotension, and respiratory depression. In severe cases, various dysrhythmias may be seen, including sinus tachycardia, atrial arrhythmias, premature ventricular contractions, bigeminy, and ventricular fibrillation. If large doses are taken intravenously, cardiac failure, dysrhythmias, or hyperthermia may result in death.

Treatment

Testing for cocaine in blood or plasma is generally not clinically useful, but a qualitative analysis of the urine may aid in confirming the diagnosis. For severe cases, an ECG is indicated. When a teenager is suspected of being a "body packer," x-rays of the gastrointestinal tract are warranted. Cocaine is usually smoked or taken intranasally or intravenously; for this reason, decontamination is seldom possible. When cocaine is taken orally, lavage may be indicated, depending on the potential for seizures or loss of gag reflex. Activated charcoal may also be indicated. For body packers, whole bowel lavage may be useful in passing the packets quickly. Seizures may be treated with intravenous diazepam titrated to response or intravenous phenytoin (loading dose 10–15 mg/kg, maintenance 4–7 mg/kg/24 h). Hypotension may be treated with standard agents. However, because cocaine abuse may deplete norepinephrine, an indirect agent such as dopamine may be less effective than a direct agent such as norepinephrine. Agitation is best treated with diazepam.

Conway EE Jr, Mezey AP, Powers K: Status epilepticus following the oral ingestion of cocaine in an infant. Pediatr Emerg Care 1990;6:189.

Durand DJ, Espinoza AM, Nickerson BT: Association between prenatal cocaine exposure and sudden infant death syndrome. J Pediatr 1990;117:909.

Fitzmaurice LS et al: TAC use and absorption of cocaine in a pediatric emergency department. Ann Emerg Med 1990;19:515.

CONTRACEPTIVE PILLS

The only known toxic effects following acute ingestion of oral contraceptive agents are nausea, vomiting, and vaginal bleeding in girls.

COSMETICS & RELATED PRODUCTS

The relative toxicities of commonly ingested products in this group are listed in Table 13–2.

Permanent wave neutralizers may contain bromates, peroxides, or perborates. Bromates have been removed from most products because they can cause nausea, vomiting, abdominal pain, shock, hemolysis, renal failure, and convulsions. Perborate can cause boric acid poisoning. Four grams of bromate salts is potentially lethal.

Poisoning is treated by induced emesis or gastric lavage with 1% sodium thiosulfate followed by demulcents to relieve gastric irritation. Sodium bicarbonate, 2%, in the lavage fluid may reduce hydrobromic acid formation. Sodium thiosulfate, 1%, 100–500 mL, can be given intravenously, but methylene blue should not be used to treat methemoglobinemia in this situation, because it increases the toxicity of bromates. Dialysis is indicated in renal failure but does not enhance excretion of bromate.

Fingernail polish removers used to contain toluene or aliphatic acetates, which produce central nervous system irritation and depression. They now usually have an acetone base, which does not require specific treatment other than monitoring central nervous system status.

Cobalt, copper, cadmium, iron, lead, nickel, silver, bismuth, and tin are sometimes found in metallic hair dyes. In large amounts, they can cause skin sensitization, urticaria, dermatitis, eye damage, vertigo,

hypertension, asthma, methemoglobinemia, tremors, convulsions, and coma. Treatment for ingestions is to administer demulcents and, only with large amounts, the appropriate antidote for the heavy metal involved.

Home permanent wave lotions, hair straighteners, and hair removers usually contain thioglycolic acid salts, which cause alkaline irritation and perhaps central nervous system depression.

Shaving lotion, hair tonic, hair straighteners, cologne, and toilet water contain denatured alcohol, which can cause central nervous system depression and hypoglycemia.

Deodorants usually consist of an antibacterial agent in a cream base. Antiperspirants are aluminum salts, which frequently cause skin sensitization. Zirconium oxide can cause granulomas in the axilla with chronic use.

Fischer H, Caurdy-Bess L: Scalp burns from a permanent wave product. Clin Pediatr (Phila) 1990;29:53.
Lehman AJ: Health aspects of common chemicals used in hair-waving preparations. JAMA 1949;41:842.

CYCLIC ANTIDEPRESSANTS

Cyclic antidepressants (amitriptyline, imipramine, etc) have a very low toxic:therapeutic ratio, and even a moderate overdose can have serious effects. Cyclic antidepressant overdosage causes dysrhythmias, coma, convulsions, hypertension (and, later, hypotension), and hallucinations. These may be life-threatening and require rapid intervention. One agent, amoxapine, differs in that it causes fewer cardiovascular complications, but it has a higher incidence of seizures .

An ECG should be taken in all patients. If dysrhythmias are demonstrated, the patient should be admitted and monitored until free of irregularity for 24 hours. Another indication for monitoring is persistent tachycardia of more than 110 beats/min plus additional findings of anticholinergic toxicity. The onset of dysrhythmias is rare beyond 24 hours after ingestion.

Decontamination should include gastric lavage and administration of activated charcoal.

Treatment

Phenytoin or lidocaine may be used primarily for treatment of dysrhythmias. Alkalinization with sodium bicarbonate, 0.5 meq/kg intravenously, or hyperventilation may dramatically reverse *ventricular* dysrhythmias and narrow the QRS interval. Sodium bicarbonate should be administered to all patients with significant dysrhythmias to achieve a plasma pH of 7.5–7.6. Forced diuresis is contraindicated. A QRS interval greater than 100 ms specifically identifies patients at risk to develop dysrhythmias. Diazepam should be given for convulsions.

Table 13–2. Relative toxicities of cosmetics and similar products.

High toxicity	Low toxicity
Permanent wave	Perfume
neutralizers	Hair removers
	Deodorants
Modern toxicity	Bath salts
Fingernail polish	
Fingernail polish remover	**No toxicity**
Metallic hair dyes	Liquid makeup
Home permanent wave	Vegetable hair dye
lotion	Cleansing cream
Bath oil	Hair dressing
Shaving lotion	(nonalcoholic)
Hair tonic (alcoholic)	Hand lotion or cream
Cologne, toilet water	Lipstick

Hypotension is a major problem. Cyclic antidepressants block the reuptake of catecholamines, thereby producing a rebound hypotension following initial hypertension. Treatment with physostigmine is not effective. Vasopressors are generally effective. Dopamine is the agent of choice because it is readily available. If dopamine is ineffective, norepinephrine (0.1–1 μg/kg/min, titrated to response) should be added. Diuresis and hemodialysis are not effective.

Ellison DW, Pentel PR: Clinical features and consequences of seizures due to cyclic antidepressant overdose. Am J Emerg Med 1989;7:5.

Kulig K et al: Amoxapine overdose: Coma and seizures without cardiotoxic effects. JAMA 1982;248:1092.

Lavoie RW, Gansert CG, Weiss RE: Value of initial ECG findings and plasma drug levels in cyclic antidepressant overdose. Ann Emerg Med 1990;19:696.

DIGITALIS & OTHER CARDIAC GLYCOSIDES

Manifestations include nausea, vomiting, diarrhea, headache, delirium, confusion, and, occasionally, coma. Cardiac irregularities such as atrial fibrillation, paroxysmal atrial tachycardia, and atrial flutter often occur. Death usually is the result of ventricular fibrillation.

Transplacental intoxication by digitalis has been reported.

Treatment

If vomiting has not occurred, induce emesis or provide lavage followed by charcoal and cathartics. Potassium should not be given in acute overdosage unless there is laboratory evidence of hypokalemia. In acute overdosage, hyperkalemia is more common.

The patient must be monitored carefully for electrocardiographic changes. Every type of dysrhythmia has been reported in digitalis intoxication. The correction of acidosis better demonstrates the degree of potassium deficiency present. Bradycardias have been treated with atropine. Phenytoin, lidocaine, magnesium salts (not in renal failure), amiodarone, and bretylium have been used to correct arrhythmias.

Definitive treatment is with digoxin antibody fragments (digoxin immune Fab). Indications for Fab use include ventricular dysrhythmias and progressive bradydysrhythmia. Techniques of determining dosage are described in product literature.

Antman EM et al: Treatment of 150 cases of life-threatening digitalis intoxication with digoxin-specific Fab antibody fragments. Circulation 1990;81:1744.

Kaufman J et al: Use of digoxin Fab immune fragments in a seven-day-old infant. Pediatr Emerg Care 1990;6:118.

DIPHENOXYLATE HYDROCHLORIDE (Lomotil)

Lomotil contains diphenoxylate hydrochloride, a synthetic narcotic, and atropine sulfate. Early signs of Lomotil intoxication are due to its anticholinergic effect and consist of fever, facial flush, tachypnea, and lethargy. However, the miotic effect of the narcotic predominates. Later, hypothermia, increasing central nervous system depression, and loss of the facial flush occur. Seizures are probably secondary to hypoxia. Small amounts are potentially lethal in children; it is contraindicated in children under age 2 years.

Treatment

Prolonged monitoring (24 hours) with pulse oximetry is sufficient in most cases. If respiratory depression occurs, an airway should be established with an endotracheal tube. Gastric lavage and administration of activated charcoal may be useful because of the prolonged delay in gastric emptying time.

Naloxone hydrochloride (0.4–2 mg intravenously in children and adults) should be given. A transient improvement in respiration may be followed by respiratory depression. Repeated doses may be required because the duration of action of diphenoxylate is considerably longer than that of naloxone. The anticholinergic effects do not usually require treatment.

Al Ragheb et al: A case of fatal Lomotil overdosage. Med Sci Law 1982;22:210.

Rumack BH, Temple AR: Lomotil poisoning. Pediatrics 1974;53:495.

DISINFECTANTS & DEODORIZERS

1. NAPHTHALENE

Naphthalene is commonly found in mothballs, disinfectants, and deodorizers. Naphthalene's toxicity is often not fully appreciated. It is absorbed not only when ingested but also through the skin and lungs. It is potentially hazardous to store baby clothes in naphthalene, because baby oil is an excellent solvent that may increase dermal absorption.

Metabolic products of naphthalene may cause severe hemolytic anemia, similar to that due to primaquine toxicity, 2–7 days after ingestion. Other physical findings include vomiting, diarrhea, jaundice, oliguria, anuria, coma, and convulsions. The urine may contain hemoglobin, protein, and casts.

Treatment

Induced vomiting should be followed by activated charcoal and a cathartic. Urinary alkalinization may prevent blocking of the renal tubules by acid hematin crystals. Anuria may persist for 1–2 weeks and still be completely reversible.

Ostlere L, Amos R, Wass JAH: Haemolytic anaemia associated with ingestion of naphthalene-containing anointing oil. Postgrad Med J 1988;64:444.

Picchioni AL: Mothball poisoning in children. Am J Hosp Pharm 1960;17:303.

2. *p*-DICHLOROBENZENE, PHENOLIC ACIDS, & OTHERS

Disinfectants and deodorizers containing *p*-dichlorobenzene or sodium sulfate are much less toxic than those containing naphthalene. Disinfectants containing phenolic acids are highly toxic, especially if they contain a borate ion. Phenol precipitates tissue proteins and causes respiratory alkalosis followed by metabolic acidosis. Some phenols cause methemoglobinemia.

Local gangrene occurs after prolonged contact with tissue. Phenol is readily absorbed from the gastrointestinal tract, causing diffuse capillary damage and, in some cases, methemoglobinemia. Pentachlorophenol, which has been used in terminal rinsing of diapers, has caused infant fatalities.

The toxicity of alkalies, quaternary ammonium compounds, pine oil, and halogenated disinfectants varies with the concentration of active ingredients. Wick deodorizers are usually of moderate toxicity. Iodophor disinfectants are the safest. Spray deodorizers are not usually toxic, because a child is not likely to swallow a very large dose.

Manifestations of acute quaternary ammonium compound ingestion include diaphoresis, strong irritation, thirst, vomiting, diarrhea, cyanosis, hyperactivity, coma, convulsions, hypotension, abdominal pain, and pulmonary edema. Acute liver or renal failure may develop later.

Treatment

Activated charcoal may be used prior to gastric lavage. Castor oil dissolves phenol and may retard its absorption. This property of castor oil, however, has not been proved clinically. Mineral oil and alcohol are contraindicated because they increase the gastric absorption of phenol. A cathartic may be useful. The metabolic acidosis must be carefully managed. Anticonvulsants or measures to treat shock may be needed.

Because phenols are absorbed through the skin, exposed areas should be irrigated copiously with water. Undiluted polyethylene glycol may be a useful solvent as well.

Mucklow ES: Accidental feeding of dilute antiseptic solution (chlorhexidine 0.05% with cetrimide 1%) to five babies. Hum Toxicol 1988;7:567.

Pegg SP, Campbell DC: Children's burns due to cresol. Burns 1985;11:294.

Van Berkel M, de Wolff FA: Survival after acute benzalkonium chloride poisoning. Hum Toxicol 1988;7:191.

DISK BATTERY

Small, flat, smooth disk-shaped batteries measure between 10 and 25 mm in diameter. About 69% of them pass through the gastrointestinal tract in 48 hours and 85% in 72 hours. Some may become entrapped. These batteries contain caustic materials and heavy metals.

Batteries impacted in the esophagus may cause symptoms of refusal to take food, increased salivation, vomiting with or without blood, and pain or discomfort. Aspiration into the trachea may also occur. Fatalities have been reported in association with esophageal perforation.

When a history of disk battery ingestion is obtained, x-rays of the entire respiratory tract and gastrointestinal tract should be taken so that the battery can be located and the proper therapy determined.

Treatment

If the disk battery is located in the esophagus, it must be removed immediately. If the battery has been in the esophagus for more than 24 hours, the risk of caustic burn is greater, and removal by endoscopic means may be necessary.

Location of the disk battery below the esophagus has been associated with tissue damage, but the course has been benign in most cases. Perforated Meckel's diverticulum has been the major complication. It may take as long as 7 days for spontaneous passage to occur, and lack of movement in the gastrointestinal tract may not require removal in an asymptomatic patient. Some have suggested repeated x-rays and surgical intervention if passage of the battery pauses, but this approach may be excessive. Batteries that have opened in the gastrointestinal tract have been associated with some toxicity due to mercury, but the patients have recovered.

Emesis is ineffective in removal of the battery from the stomach. Asymptomatic patients may simply be observed and stools examined for passage of the battery. If the battery has not passed within 7 days or if the patient becomes symptomatic, x-rays should be repeated. If the battery has come apart or appears not to be moving, a purgative, enema, or nonabsorbable intestinal lavage solution should be administered. If these methods are not successful, surgical intervention may be required. Levels of heavy metals (mainly of mercury) should be measured in patients in whom the battery has opened or symptoms have developed.

Litovitz TL: Button battery ingestions. JAMA 1983;249:2495.

Mank TGK et al: Mercury poisoning after disc-battery ingestion. Hum Toxicol 1987;6:179.

Rumack BH, Rumack CM: Disk battery ingestion. JAMA 1983;249:2509.

Votteler TP, Nash JC, Rutledge JC: The hazard of ingested alkaline disk batteries in children. JAMA 1983;249:2504.

HYDROCARBONS
(Benzene, Charcoal Lighter Fluid, Gasoline, Kerosene, Petroleum Distillates, Turpentine)

Ingestion may cause irritation of mucous membranes, vomiting, blood-tinged diarrhea, respiratory distress, cyanosis, tachycardia, and fever. Although a small amount of certain hydrocarbons (10 mL) is potentially fatal, patients have survived ingestion of several ounces of other petroleum distillates. The more aromatic a hydrocarbon and the lower its viscosity rating, the more potentially toxic it is. Benzene, gasoline, kerosene, and red seal oil furniture polish are the most dangerous. A dose exceeding 1 mL/kg is likely to cause central nervous system depression. A history of coughing or choking, as well as vomiting, suggests aspiration with resulting hydrocarbon pneumonia. This is an acute hemorrhagic necrotizing disease that usually develops within 24 hours of the ingestion and resolves without sequelae in 3–5 days. However, several weeks may be required for full resolution of a hydrocarbon pneumonia. Pneumonia may be caused by the aspiration of a few drops of petroleum distillate into the lung or by absorption from the circulatory system. Pulmonary edema and hemorrhage, cardiac dilatation and dysrhythmias, hepatosplenomegaly, proteinuria, and hematuria can occur following large overdoses. Hypoglycemia is occasionally present. A chest film may reveal pneumonia within hours after the ingestion. An abnormal urinalysis in a child with a previously normal urinary tract suggests a large overdose.

Treatment
Both emetics and lavage should be avoided when only a small amount has been ingested. It is impossible to do a "cautious gastric lavage" unless a cuffed endotracheal tube is inserted. Under these circumstances, gastric lavage may be done using saline. Following lavage, magnesium or sodium sulfate should be left in the stomach. (Mineral oil should not be given, because it is capable of causing a low-grade lipoid pneumonia.)

Emetics are probably preferable to gastric lavage if massive ingestion has occurred. Epinephrine should not be used with halogenated hydrocarbons because it may affect an already sensitized myocardium. Analeptic drugs are contraindicated. The usefulness of corticosteroids is debated, and antibiotics should be reserved for patients with infections. Oxygen and mist are helpful. Extracorporeal membrane oxygenation has been successful in at least two cases of failure with standard therapy.

Anas N, Namasonthi V, Ginsburg C: Criteria for hospitalizing children who have ingested products containing hydrocarbons. JAMA 1981;246:840.

Jaeger RW, Scalzo AS, Thompson MW: ECMO in hydrocarbon aspiration (abstract). Vet Hum Toxicol 1987;29:485.

Kulig K, Rumack BH: Hydrocarbon ingestion. Curr Top Emerg Med 1981;3:1.

IBUPROFEN

Ibuprofen is a popular anti-inflammatory and analgesic agent. Most exposures in children do not produce symptoms in one study, for example, children ingesting up to 2.4 g remained asymptomatic. When symptoms occur, the most common are abdominal pain, vomiting, drowsiness, and lethargy. In rare cases, apnea (especially in young children), seizures, metabolic acidosis, and central nervous system depression leading to coma have occurred.

Treatment
If a child has ingested less than 100 mg/kg, dilution with water or milk may be all that is necessary to minimize the gastrointestinal upset, which occurs even with therapeutic amounts. In children, the volume of liquid used for dilution should be less than 4 oz. When the ingested amount is more than 400 mg/kg, there is a potential for seizures or central nervous system depression; therefore, gastric lavage may be preferred to emesis. If the ingested amount is between 100 and 400 mg/kg, emesis may be of equal value. Activated charcoal and a cathartic may also be of some value. Multiple doses of activated charcoal have also been suggested because of the possibility of enterohepatic circulation. There is no specific antidote. Neither alkalinization of the urine nor hemodialysis has been proved helpful.

Hall AH, Rumack BH: Treatment of patients with ibuprofen overdose. Ann Emerg Med 1988;17:185.

Hall AH et al: Ibuprofen overdose: A prospective study. West J Med 1988;148:653.

Jenkinson ML et al: The relationship between plasma ibuprofen concentrations and toxicity in acute ibuprofen overdose. Hum Toxicol 1988;7:319.

Perry SJ, Streete PJ, Volans GN: Ibuprofen overdose: The first 2 years of over-the-counter sales. Hum Toxicol 1987;6:173.

INSECT STINGS
(Bee, Wasp, & Hornet)

Insect stings are painful but not usually dangerous; however, death from anaphylaxis may occur. Bee venom, for example, has hemolytic, neurotoxic, and histamine-like activities that can on rare occasions cause hemoglobinuria and severe anaphylactoid reactions.

Treatment
The physician should remove the stinger, taking

care not to squeeze the attached venom sac. For allergic reactions, epinephrine 1:1000 solution, 0.01 mL/kg, should be administered intravenously or subcutaneously above the site of the sting. Three to four whiffs from an isoproterenol aerosol inhaler may be given at 3- to 4-minute intervals as needed. Corticosteroids (hydrocortisone), 100 mg intravenously, and diphenhydramine, 1.5 mg/kg intravenously, are useful ancillary drugs but have no immediate effect. Ephedrine or antihistamines may be used for 2 or 3 days to prevent recurrence of symptoms.

A patient who has had a potentially life-threatening insect sting should be desensitized against the Hymenoptera group, because the honey bee, wasp, hornet, and yellow jacket have common antigens in their venom.

For the more usual stings, cold compresses, aspirin, and diphenhydramine 1 mg/kg orally, are sufficient.

Barsky HE: Stinging insect allergy: Avoidance, identification, and treatment. Postgrad Med J 1987;82:157.
Reisman RE, Livingstone A: Late-onset allergic reactions, including serum sickness after insect stings. J Allergy Clin Immunol 1989;84:331.

INSECTICIDES

The petroleum distillates or other organic solvents used in these products are often as toxic as the pesticide. Unless otherwise indicated, induced vomiting or gastric lavage after insertion of an endotracheal tube is warranted.

DePalma AE, Kwalich DS, Zukerberg N: Pesticide poisoning in children. JAMA 1970;211:1979.
Rumack BH, Spoerke DG, Smolinske SC (editors): POISINDEX © Information System. Micromedex, Inc., Denver, Colorado. [Published quarterly.]

1. CHLORINATED HYDROCARBONS (Aldrin, Carbinol, Chlordane, DDT, Dieldrin, Endrin, Heptachlor, Lindane, Toxaphene, Etc)

Signs of intoxication include salivation, gastrointestinal irritability, abdominal pain, vomiting, diarrhea, central nervous system depression, and convulsions. Inhalation exposure causes irritation of the eyes, nose, and throat; blurred vision; cough; and pulmonary edema.

Chlorinated hydrocarbons are absorbed through the skin, respiratory tract, and gastrointestinal tract. Decontamination of skin (tincture of green soap) and evacuation of the stomach contents are critical. All contaminated clothing should be removed. Castor oil, milk, and other substances containing fats or oils should not be left in the stomach because they increase absorption of the chlorinated hydrocarbons. Convulsions should be treated with diazepam, 0.1–0.3 mg/kg intravenously. Epinephrine should not be used because it may cause cardiac arrhythmias.

2. ORGANOPHOSPHATE (CHOLINESTERASE-INHIBITING) INSECTICIDES (Chlorthion, Co-Ral, DFP, Diazinon, Malathion, Paraoxon, Parathion, Phosdrin, TEPP, Thio-TEPP, Etc)

Dizziness, headache, blurred vision, miosis, tearing, salivation, nausea, vomiting, diarrhea, hyperglycemia, cyanosis, sense of constriction of the chest, dyspnea, sweating, weakness, muscular twitching, convulsions, loss of reflexes and sphincter control, and coma can occur.

The clinical findings are the result of cholinesterase inhibition, which causes an accumulation of acetylcholine. The onset of symptoms occurs within 12 hours of the exposure. Red cell cholinesterase levels should be measured as soon as possible. (Some normal individuals have a low serum cholinesterase level.) Normal values vary in different laboratories. In general, a decrease of red cell cholinesterase to below 25% of normal indicates significant exposure.

Repeated low-grade exposure may result in sudden, acute toxic reactions. This syndrome usually occurs after repeated household spraying rather than agricultural exposure.

Although all organophosphates act by inhibiting cholinesterase activity, they vary greatly in their toxicity. Parathion, for example, is 100 times more toxic than malathion. The toxicity is influenced by the specific compound, the type of formulation (liquid or solid), the vehicle, and the route of absorption (lungs, skin, or gastrointestinal tract).

Treatment

Atropine plus a cholinesterase reactivator, pralidoxime, is an antidote for organophosphate insecticide poisoning. After assessment and management of the ABCs, large doses of atropine should be given and repeated every few minutes until signs of atropinism are present. An appropriate starting dose of atropine is 2–4 mg intravenously in an adult and 0.05 mg/kg in a child. The patient should receive enough atropine to stop secretions (approximately ten times the normal dose). Severe poisoning may require gram quantities of atropine per 24 hours.

Because atropine antagonizes the muscarinic parasympathetic effects of the organophosphates but does not affect the nicotinic receptor, it does not improve muscular weakness. Pralidoxime should also be given immediately in more severe cases and repeated every 6–12 hours as needed (25–50 mg/kg diluted to 5% and infused over 5–30 minutes at a rate of no more than 500 mg/min). Pralidoxime should be used in addition to—not in place of—atropine if red cell cholinesterase is less than 25% of normal. Pralidoxime is most useful within 48 hours after the exposure but has shown some effects 2–6 days later. Morphine, theophylline, aminophylline, succinylcholine, and tranquilizers of the reserpine and phenothiazine types are contraindicated. Hyperglycemia is common in severe poisonings.

Decontamination of skin, nails, hair, and clothing with soapy water is extremely important. Decontamination must be done carefully to avoid abrasions, which increase organophosphate absorption.

Bardin PG, Van Eeden SF: Organophosphate poisoning: Grading the severity and comparing treatment between atropine and glycopyrrolate. Crit Care Med 1990;8:956.

Borowitz SM: Prolonged organophosphate toxicity in a 26-month-old child. J Pediatr 1988;112:302.

Chaturvedi AK et al: Toxicological evaluation of a poisoning attributed to ingestion of malathion inspect spray and correlation with in vitro inhibition of cholinesterases. Hum Toxicol 1989;8:11.

3. CARBAMATES
(Carbaryl, Sevin, Zectran, Etc)

Carbamate insecticides are reversible inhibitors of cholinesterase. The signs and symptoms of intoxication are similar to those associated with organophosphate poisoning but are generally less severe. Atropine titrated to effect is sufficient treatment. Pralidoxime should not be used with carbaryl poisoning but is of value with other carbamates. In combined exposures to organophosphates, give atropine but reserve pralidoxime for cases in which the red cell cholinesterase is depressed below 25% of normal or marked effects of nicotinic receptor stimulation are present.

Harris LW et al: The relationship between oxime induced reactivation of carbamylated acetylcholinesterase and antidotal efficacy against carbamate intoxication. Toxicol Appl Pharmacol 1989;98:128.

4. BOTANICAL INSECTICIDES
(Black Flag Bug Killer, Black Leaf CPR Insect Killer, Flit Aerosol House & Garden Insect Killer, French's Flea Powder, Raid, Etc)

Allergic reactions, asthma-like symptoms, coma, and convulsions have been seen. Pyrethrins, allethrin, ryania, and rotenone do not commonly cause signs of toxicity. Antihistamines, short-acting barbiturates, and atropine are helpful as symptomatic treatment.

IRON

Five stages of intoxication occur following iron intoxication: (1) Hemorrhagic gastroenteritis, which occurs 30–60 minutes after ingestion and may be associated with shock, acidosis, coagulation defects, and coma. This phase usually lasts 4–6 hours. (2) Phase of improvement, lasting 2–12 hours, during which patient looks better. (3) Delayed shock, which may occur 12–48 hours after ingestion and is usually associated with a serum iron level greater than 500 μg/dL. Metabolic acidosis, fever, leukocytosis, and coma may also be present. (4) Liver damage with hepatic failure. (5) Residual pyloric stenosis, which may develop about 4 weeks after the ingestion.

Once iron is absorbed from the gastrointestinal tract, it is not normally eliminated in feces but may be partially excreted in the urine, giving it a red color prior to chelation. A reddish discoloration of the urine suggests a serum iron level greater than 350 μg/dL.

Treatment

Gastrointestinal decontamination is based on clinical assessment. Syrup of ipecac may be administered at home, with appropriate follow-up, provided the history does not warrant an emergency department visit. The patient should be referred to a health care facility if symptomatic or if the history indicates toxic amounts. Gastric lavage and whole bowel irrigation should be considered in these patients.

Shock must be treated in the usual manner. Sodium bicarbonate or Fleet's Phospho-Soda left in the stomach to form the insoluble phosphate or carbonate have not shown clinical benefit and have caused lethal hypernatremia or hyperphosphatemia. Deferoxamine, a specific chelating agent for iron, is a useful adjunct in the treatment of severe iron poisoning. It forms a soluble complex that is excreted in the urine. It is contraindicated in patients with renal failure unless dialysis can be used. Institute intravenous deferoxamine chelation therapy if the patient is symptomatic and a serum iron determination cannot be readily obtained, or if the peak serum iron exceeds 400 μg/dL (62.6 μmol/L) at 4–5 hours after ingestion.

Deferoxamine should not be delayed until serum iron levels are available in serious cases of poisoning. Intravenous administration is indicated if the patient is in shock, in which case it should be given at a dosage of 15 mg/kg/h. Infusion rates up to 35 mg/kg/h have been used in life-threatening poisonings. Rapid intravenous administration can cause hypotension, facial flushing, urticaria, tachycardia, and shock. Deferoxamine, 90 mg/kg intramuscularly every 8 hours (maximum, 1 g), may be given if intravenous access cannot be established, but the procedure is painful. The drug should not be given orally. The indications for discontinuation of deferoxamine have not been clearly delineated. Generally, it can be stopped after 12-24 hours if the acidosis has resolved and the patient is improving.

Hemodialysis, peritoneal dialysis, or exchange transfusion can be used to increase the excretion of the dialyzable complex, if necessary. Urine output should be monitored and urine sediment examined for evidence of renal tubular damage. Initial laboratory studies should include blood typing and cross-matching; total protein; serum iron, sodium, potassium, and chloride; CO_2; pH; and liver function tests. Serum iron levels fall rapidly even if deferoxamine is not given.

After the acute episode, liver function studies and an upper gastrointestinal series are indicated to rule out residual damage.

Mann KV et al: Management of acute iron overdose. Clin Pharm 1989;8:428.

Schauben JL et al: Iron poisoning: Report of three cases and a review of therapeutic intervention. J Emerg Med 1990;8:309.

Chyka DA, Butler AY: Assessment of acute iron poisoning by laboratory and clinical observations. Am J Emerg Med 1993;11:99.

LEAD

Lead poisoning causes a vague assortment of symptoms, including weakness, irritability, weight loss, vomiting, personality changes, ataxia, constipation, headache, and colicky abdominal pain. Late manifestations consist of retarded development, convulsions, and coma associated with increased intracranial pressure. The latter is a medical emergency.

Plumbism usually occurs insidiously in children under 5 years of age. The most likely sources of lead include flaking leaded paint, artist's paints, fruit tree sprays, solder, brass alloys, home-glazed pottery, and fumes from burning batteries. Only paint containing less than 1% lead is safe for interior use (furniture, toys, etc). Repetitive ingestions of small amounts of lead are far more serious than a single massive exposure. Toxic effects are likely to occur if more than 0.5 mg of lead per day is absorbed.

Blood lead levels are used to assess the severity of exposure. A complete blood count and serum ferritin concentration should be ordered; iron deficiency increases absorption of lead. Glycosuria, proteinuria, hematuria, and aminoaciduria occur frequently. Blood lead levels usually exceed 80 µg/dL in symptomatic patients. Abnormal blood lead levels should be repeated in asymptomatic patients to rule out laboratory error. Specimens must be meticulously obtained in acid-washed containers. A normocytic,

slightly hypochromic anemia with basophilic stippling of the red cells and reticulocytosis may be present in plumbism. Stippling of red blood cells is absent in cases involving only recent ingestion.

The cerebrospinal fluid protein is elevated, and the white cell count is usually less than 100 cells/mL. Cerebrospinal fluid pressure may be elevated in patients with encephalopathy; lumbar punctures must be performed cautiously to prevent herniation.

Treatment

Standard gastrointestinal decontamination is indicated if an acute ingestion has occurred or lead is noted on the abdominal x-ray. Succimer is 2,3-dimercaptosuccinic acid, an orally administered chelator approved for use in children only and reported to be as efficacious as calcium edetate. Succimer should be initiated at blood lead levels over 45 µg/dL. The initial dose is 10 mg/kg (350 mg/m^2) every 8 hours for 5 days. The same dose is then given every 12 hours for 14 days. At least 2 weeks should elapse between courses. Blood lead levels increase somewhat ("rebound") after discontinuation of therapy. Courses of dimercaprol (4 mg/kg/dose) and calcium edetate may still be used but are no longer the preferred method. Treatment for children with blood lead levels of 20–45 µg/dL has not been determined.

Anticonvulsants may be needed. Mannitol or corticosteroids are indicated in patients with encephalopathy. Fluid intake should be restricted. A high-calcium, high-phosphorus diet and large doses of vitamin D may remove lead from the blood by depositing it in the bones.

A public health team should evaluate the source of the lead. Necessary corrections should be completed before the child is returned home.

Chisholm J et al: Recognition and management of children with increased lead absorption. Arch Dis Child 1979; 54:249.

Lin-Fu J: Lead exposure among children: A reassessment. N Engl J Med 1979;300:731.

Needleman HL et al: The long term effects of exposure to low doses of lead in childhood: An 11-year follow-up report. N Engl J Med 1990;322:83.

Graziano JG et al: Controlled study of meso-2,3 dimercaptosuccinicacid for the management of childhood lead intoxication. J. Pediatr. 1992;120:133.

MUSHROOMS

Toxic mushrooms are often difficult to distinguish from edible varieties. Symptoms vary with the species ingested, time of year, stage of maturity, quantity eaten, method of preparation, and interval since ingestion. A mushroom that is toxic to one individual may not be toxic for another. Drinking alcohol and eating certain mushrooms may cause a reaction similar to that seen with disulfiram and alcohol. Cooking destroys some toxins but not the deadly one produced by *Amanita phalloides,* is responsible for 90% of deaths due to mushroom poisoning. Mushrooms toxins are absorbed relatively slowly. Onset of symptoms within 2 hours of ingestion suggests muscarinic toxin, whereas a delay of symptoms for 6–48 hours after ingestion strongly suggests *Amanita* (amatoxin) poisoning. Patients who have ingested *A phalloides* may relapse and die of hepatic or renal failure following initial improvement.

Mushroom poisoning may be manifested by muscarinic symptoms (salivation, vomiting, diarrhea, cramping abdominal pain, tenesmus, miosis, and dyspnea), coma, convulsions, hallucinations, hemolysis, and delayed hepatic and renal failure.

Treatment

Induce vomiting and follow with activated charcoal and a saline cathartic. If the patient has muscarinic signs, give atropine, 0.05 mg/kg intramuscularly (0.02 mg/kg in toddlers), and repeat as needed (usually every 30 minutes) to keep the patient atropinized. Atropine, however, is only used when there are cholinergic effects and not for all mushrooms. Hypoglycemia is most likely to occur in patients with delayed onset of symptoms. It is important, if at all possible, to identify the mushroom specifically if the patient is symptomatic. Local botanical gardens, university departments of botany, and societies of mycologists may be able to help. Supportive care is usually all that is needed except in the case of A phalloides, where penicillin, silibinin, or hemodialysis may be indicated.

Lampe KF, McCann MA: Differential diagnosis of poisoning by North American mushrooms, with particular emphasis on *Amanita phalloides*-like intoxication. Ann Emerg Med 1987;16:956.

Spoerke DG, Rumack BH (editors): *Mushroom Poisoning, Diagnosis and Treatment,* 2nd ed. CRC Press, 1994.

NITRITES, NITRATES, ANILINE, PENTACHLOROPHENOL, & DINITROPHENOL

Nausea, vertigo, vomiting, cyanosis (methemoglobinemia), cramping abdominal pain, tachycardia, cardiovascular collapse, tachypnea, coma, shock, convulsions, and death are possible manifestations of nitrite or nitrate poisoning.

Nitrite and nitrate compounds found in the home include amyl nitrite, butyl nitrates, isobutyl nitrates, nitroglycerin, pentaerythritol tetranitrate, sodium nitrite, nitrobenzene, and phenazopyridine. Pentachlorophenol and dinitrophenol, which are found in wood preservatives, produce methemoglobinemia and high fever because of uncoupling of oxidative phosphorylation. Headache, dizziness, and bradycardia have

been reported. High concentrations of nitrites in water or spinach have been the most common cause of nitrite-induced methemoglobinemia. Symptoms do not usually occur until 15–50% of the hemoglobin has been converted to methemoglobin. A rapid test is to compare a drop of normal blood with the patient's blood on a dry filter paper. Brown discoloration of the patient's blood indicates a methemoglobin level of more than 15%.

Treatment

Induce vomiting, administer activated charcoal, and follow with a cathartic. Decontaminate affected skin with soap and water. Oxygen and artificial respiration may be needed. If the blood methemoglobin level exceeds 30%, or if levels cannot be obtained and the patient is symptomatic, give a 1% solution of methylene blue, 0.2 mL/kg intravenously over 5–10 minutes. Avoid perivascular infiltration, because it causes necrosis of the skin and subcutaneous tissues. A dramatic change in the degree of cyanosis should occur. Transfusion is occasionally necessary. Epinephrine and other vasoconstrictors are contraindicated. If reflex bradycardia occurs, atropine should be used.

Bardoczky GI, Wathieu M, D'Hollander A: Prilocaine-induced methemoglobinemia evidenced by pulse oximetry. Acta Anaesthesiol Scand 1990;34:162.

Caudill L, Walbridge J, Kuhn G: Methemoglobinemia as a cause of coma. Ann Emerg Med 1990;19:677.

Kaplan A et al: Methaemoglobinaemia due to accidental sodium nitrite poisoning: Report of 10 cases. S Afr Med J 1990;77:300.

OPIOIDS*
(Codeine, Heroin, Methadone, Morphine, Propoxyphene)

Opioid-related medical problems may include drug addiction, withdrawal in a newborn infant, and accidental overdoses.

Unlike other narcotics, methadone is readily absorbed from the gastrointestinal tract. Most opioids, including heroin, methadone, meperidine, morphine, and codeine, are excreted in the urine within 24 hours and can be readily detected.

Adolescent narcotic addicts often have other medical problems, including cellulitis, abscesses, thrombophlebitis, tetanus, infective endocarditis, HIV infection, tuberculosis, hepatitis, malaria, foreign body emboli, thrombosis of pulmonary arterioles, diabetes mellitus, obstetric complications, nephropathy, and peptic ulcer.

---

*Diphenoxylate poisoning is discussed on p 329.

Treatment of Overdosage

Opioids can cause respiratory depression, stridor, coma, increased oropharyngeal secretions, sinus bradycardia, and urinary retention. Pulmonary edema rarely occurs in children; deaths usually result from aspiration of gastric contents, respiratory arrest, and cerebral edema, singly or in combination. Convulsions may occur with propoxyphene overdosage.

While suggested doses for naloxone hydrochloride range from 0.01 to 0.1 mg/kg, it is generally unnecessary to calculate the dosage on this basis. This extremely safe antidote should be given in sufficient quantity to reverse opioid binding sites. For children under 1 year of age, 1 ampule (0.4 mg) should be given initially; if there is no response, give five more ampules (2 mg) rapidly. Older children should be given 1–2 ampules, followed by 5–10 more ampules if there is no response. An improvement in respiratory status may be followed by respiratory depression, because the depressant action of narcotics may last 24–48 hours but the antagonist's duration of action is less than 1 hour. Neonates poisoned in utero may require 10–30 μg/kg to reverse the effect.

Withdrawal in the Addict

The severity of withdrawal signs should be evaluated as explained on p 337. Seizures and hallucinations are almost always associated with concomitant withdrawal from sedative-hypnotics.

Diazepam, 10 mg every 6 hours orally, has been recommended for the treatment of mild narcotic withdrawal in ambulatory adolescents. Management of withdrawal in the confirmed addict may be accomplished with the administration of clonidine, by substitution with methadone, or with reintroduction of the original addicting agent, if available through a supervised drug withdrawal program. A tapered course over 3 weeks will accomplish this goal. Death rarely, if ever, occurs. The abrupt discontinuation of narcotics (cold turkey method) is not recommended and may cause severe physical withdrawal signs.

Withdrawal in the Newborn

A newborn infant in narcotic withdrawal is usually small for gestational age and demonstrates yawning, sneezing, decreased Moro reflex, hunger but uncoordinated sucking action, jitteriness, tremor, constant movement, a shrill protracted cry, increased tendon reflexes, convulsions, vomiting, fever, watery diarrhea, cyanosis, dehydration, vasomotor instability, seizure, and collapse. The onset of symptoms commonly begins in the first 48 hours but may be delayed as long as 8 days depending upon the timing of the mother's last fix and her predelivery medication. The diagnosis can be easily confirmed by identifying the narcotic in the urine of the mother and baby.

Several methods of treatment have been suggested for narcotic withdrawal in the newborn. Phenobarbi-

tal, 8 mg/kg/d intramuscularly or orally in four doses for 4 days and then reduced by one-third every 2 days as signs decrease, may be continued for as long as 3 weeks. Methadone may be necessary in those infants with congenital methadone addiction who are not controlled in their withdrawal by large doses of phenobarbital. Dosage should be 0.5 mg/kg/d in two divided doses but can be gradually increased as needed. Slow tapering off may be necessary over 4 weeks for methadone addiction.

It is not clear whether prophylactic treatment with these drugs decreases the complication rate. The mortality rate of untreated narcotic withdrawal in the newborn may be as high as 45%.

AAP Committee on Drugs: Emergency drug doses for infants and children and naloxone use in newborns: Clarification. Pediatrics 1989;83:803.

Bradberry JC, Raebel MA: Continuous infusion of naloxone in the treatment of narcotic overdose. Drug Intell Clin Pharm 1981;15:945.

Martin WR: Naloxone. Ann Intern Med 1978;85:765.

Reddy AM, Harper RG, Stern G: Observations on heroin and methadone withdrawal in newborn. Pediatrics 1971; 48:353.

PHENOTHIAZINES
(Chlorpromazine, Prochlorperazine, Trifluoperazine)

Clinical Presentations

A. Extrapyramidal Crisis: Episodes characterized by torticollis, stiffening of the body, spasticity, poor speech, catatonia, and inability to communicate although conscious are typical manifestations. These episodes usually last a few seconds to a few minutes but have rarely caused death. Extrapyramidal crises may represent idiosyncratic reactions and are aggravated by dehydration. The signs and symptoms occur most often in children who have received prochlorperazine. They are commonly mistaken for psychotic episodes.

B. Overdose: Lethargy and deep prolonged coma commonly occur. Promazine, chlorpromazine, and prochlorperazine are the drugs most likely to cause respiratory depression and precipitous drops in blood pressure. Occasionally, paradoxic hyperactivity and extrapyramidal signs as well as hyperglycemia and acetonemia are present. Seizures are uncommon.

Treatment

Extrapyramidal signs are alleviated within minutes by the slow intravenous administration of diphenhydramine, 1–2 mg/kg (maximum, 50 mg), or benztropine mesylate, 1–2 mg intravenously (1 mg/min). No other treatment is usually indicated.

Patients with overdoses should be treated conservatively. Vomiting should be induced with ipecac followed by administration of activated charcoal. Emetics are often unsuccessful because phenothiazines are potent antiemetics; gastric lavage may be the only practical way to remove gastric contents. Hypotension may be treated with standard agents, starting with isotonic saline administration. However, because cocaine abuse may deplete norepinephrine, an indirect agent such as dopamine may be less effective than a direct agent such as norepinephrine. Agitation is best treated with diazepam. Neuroleptic malignant syndrome may be treated with dantrolene, 1 mg/kg (maximum, 50 mg) every 12 hours, or with diphenhydramine. Epinephrine should not be used, because phenothiazines reverse epinephrine's effects.

Baker PB et al: Hyperthermia, hypertension, hypertonia, and coma in massive thioridazine overdose. Am J Emerg Med 1988;6:346.

Sanders KM, Minnema AM, Murray GB: Low incidence of extrapyramidal symptoms in treatment of delirium with intravenous haloperidol and lorazepam in the intensive care unit. J Intens Care Med 1989;4:201.

PLANTS

Many common ornamental, garden, and wild plants are potentially toxic. Only in a few cases will small amounts of a plant cause severe illness or death. Effects usually involve the cardiovascular, gastrointestinal, and central nervous systems and the skin. Table 13–3 lists the most toxic plants, symptoms and signs of poisoning, and treatment.

Frohne D, Pfander HJ: A Colour Atlas of Poisonous Plants. Wolfe, 1984.

Lampe KF, McCann MA: AMA Handbook of Poisonous and Injurious Plants. American Medical Association, 1985.

PSYCHOTROPIC DRUGS

Psychotropic drugs consist of four general classes: stimulants (amphetamines, cocaine), depressants (narcotics, barbiturates, etc), antidepressants and tranquilizers, and hallucinogens (LSD, PCP, etc).

The following clinical findings are commonly seen in patients abusing drugs:

Table 13–3. Poisoning due to plants.[1]

	Symptoms and Signs	Treatment
Arum family: *Caladium, Dieffenbachia,* calla lily, dumb cane (oxalic acid)	Burning of mucous membranes and airway obstruction secondary to edema caused by calcium oxalate crystals.	Accessible areas should be thoroughly washed. Corticosteroids relieve airway obstruction. Apply cold packs to affected mucous membranes.
Castor bean plant (ricin—a toxalbumin) Jequinty bean (abrin—a toxalbumin)	Mucous membrane irritation, nausea, vomiting, bloody diarrhea, blurred vision, circulatory collapse, acute hemolytic anemia, convulsions, uremia.	Fluid and electrolyte monitoring. Saline cathartic. Forced alkaline diuresis will prevent complications due to hemagglutination and hemolysis.
Foxglove, lily of the valley, and oleander[2]	Nausea, diarrhea, visual disturbances, and cardiac irregularities (eg, heart block).	See treatment for digitalis drugs in text (p 307)
Jimsonweed: See Belladonna Alkaloids, p 304	Mydriasis, dry mouth, tachycardia, and hallucinations.	Atropine.
Larkspur (ajacine, *Delphinium,* delphinine)	Nausea and vomiting, irritability, muscular paralysis, and CNS depression.	Symptomatic. Atropine may be helpful.
Monkshood (aconite)	Numbness of mucous membranes, visual disturbances, tingling, dizziness, tinnitus, hypotension, bradycardia, and convulsions.	Activated charcoal, oxygen. Atropine is probably helpful.
Poison hemlock (coniine)	Mydriasis, trembling, dizziness, bradycardia. CNS depression, muscular paralysis, and convulsions. Death is due to respiratory paralysis.	Symptomatic. Oxygen and cardiac monitoring equipment are desirable. Assisted respiration is often necessary. Give anticonvulsants if needed.
Rhododendron (grayanotoxin)	Abdominal cramps, vomiting, severe diarrhea, muscular paralysis, CNS and circulatory depression. Hypertension with very large doses.	Atropine can prevent bradycardia. Epinephrine is contraindicated. Antihypertensives may be needed.
Yellow jessamine (active ingredient, geisemine, is related to strychnine)	Restlessness, convulsions, muscular paralysis, and respiratory depression.	Symptomatic. Because of the relation to strychnine, activated charcoal and diazepam for seizures is worth trying.

[1]Many other plants cause minor irritation but are not likely to cause serious problems unless large amounts are ingested. See Lampe KF, McCann MA: AMA Handbook of Poisonous and Injurious Plants. American Medical Association, 1985. See also Rumack BH, Spoerke DG (editors): POISINDEX® Information System. Micromedex, IAC, Denver, Colorado. [Published quarterly.]
[2]Done AK: Ornamental and deadly. Emerg Med (April) 1973;5:255.

Stimulants. Agitation, euphoria, grandiose feelings, tachycardia, fever, abdominal cramps, visual and auditory hallucinations, mydriasis, coma, convulsions, and respiratory depression.

Depressants. Emotional lability, ataxia, diplopia, nystagmus, vertigo, poor accommodation, respiratory depression, coma, apnea, and convulsions. Dilatation of conjunctival blood vessels suggests marijuana ingestion. Narcotics cause miotic pupils and, occasionally, pulmonary edema.

Antidepressants and tranquilizers. Hypotension, lethargy, respiratory depression, coma, and extrapyramidal reactions.

Hallucinogens and psychoactive drugs. Belladonna alkaloids cause mydriasis, dry mouth, nausea, vomiting, urinary retention, confusion, disorientation, paranoid delusions, hallucinations, fever, hypotension, aggressive behavior, convulsions, and coma. **Psychoactive drugs** such as LSD cause mydriasis, unexplained bizarre behavior, hallucinations, and generalized undifferentiated psychotic behavior.

See also other entries discussed in alphabetic sequence in this chapter.

Management of the Patient Who Abuses Drugs

Only a small percentage of the persons using drugs come to the attention of physicians; those who do are usually suffering from adverse reactions such as panic states, drug psychoses, homicidal or suicidal thoughts, or respiratory depression.

Even with cooperative patients, an accurate history is difficult to obtain. The user often does not really know what drug has been taken or how much. "Street drugs" are almost always adulterated with one or more other compounds. Multiple drugs are often taken together, making it impossible to clinically define the type of drug. Friends may be a useful source of information. A drug history is most easily obtained in a quiet spot by a gentle, nonthreatening, honest examiner.

The general appearance, skin, lymphatics, cardiorespiratory status, gastrointestinal tract, and central nervous system should be stressed during the physical examination, because they often provide clues suggesting drug abuse. A drug history should not be taken from an adolescent in the parents' presence.

Hallucinogens are not life-threatening unless the patient is frankly homicidal or suicidal. A specific diagnosis is usually not necessary for management; instead, the presenting signs and symptoms are treated. Does the patient appear intoxicated? In withdrawal? "Flashing back?" Is some illness or injury (eg, head trauma) being masked by a drug effect? (Remember that a known drug user may still have hallucinations from meningoencephalitis.)

The signs and symptoms in a given patient are a function of not only the drug and the dose but also the level of acquired tolerance, the "setting," the patient's physical condition and personality traits, the potentiating effects of other drugs, and many other factors.

A common drug problem is the "bad trip," which is usually a panic reaction. This is best managed by "talking the patient down" and minimizing auditory and visual stimuli. Sitting with a friend while the drug effect dissipates may be the best treatment that can be offered. This may take several hours. The physician's job is not to terminate the drug effect but to help the patient over the bad experience.

Drug therapy is often unnecessary and may complicate the clinical course of a patient with a panic reaction. Although phenothiazines have been commonly used to treat "bad trips," they should be avoided if the specific drug is not known, because they may enhance toxicity or produce unwanted side effects. Diazepam is the drug of choice if a sedative effect is required. Physical restraints are rarely indicated and usually increase the patient's panic reaction.

For treatment of life-threatening drug abuse, consult the section on the specific drug elsewhere in this chapter and the section on general management at the beginning of the chapter.

After the acute episode, the physician must decide whether psychiatric referral is indicated; in general, patients who have made suicidal gestures or attempts and adolescents who are not communicating with their families should be referred. On the other hand, adolescents who are "experimenting" with drugs may not need psychiatric referral.

Cohen S: The "angel dust" states: Phencyclidine. Pediatr Rev 1979;1:17.

Consroe PF: Treatment of acute hallucinogenic drug toxicity: Specific pharmacological intervention. Am J Hosp Pharm 1973;30:80.

Smith D et al: PCP problems and prevention. J Psychedelic Drugs 1980;12:181.

Teitelbaum DT: Poisoning with psychoactive drugs. Pediatr Clin North Am 1970;17:557.

SALICYLATES

The use of childproof containers and publicity regarding accidental poisoning have reduced the incidence of acute salicylate poisoning. Nevertheless, serious intoxication still occurs and must be regarded as an emergency.

Salicylates uncouple oxidative phosphorylation, leading to increased heat production, excessive sweating, and dehydration. They also interfere with glucose metabolism and may cause hypoglycemia or hyperglycemia. Respiratory center stimulation occurs early.

Patients usually have signs of hyperventilation, sweating, dehydration, and fever. Vomiting and diarrhea sometimes occur. In severe cases, disorientation, convulsions, and coma may develop.

The severity of acute intoxication can in some measure be judged by serum salicylate levels (Figure 13–2). High levels are always dangerous irrespective of clinical signs, and low levels may be misleading in chronic cases. Other laboratory values usually indicate metabolic acidosis despite hyperventilation; low serum K^+ values; and, often, abnormal serum glucose levels.

Salicylate poisoning is classified as mild when plasma pH is greater than 7.4 and urine pH is greater than 6.0; as moderate when plasma pH is greater than 7.4 and urine pH is less than 6.0; and as severe when plasma pH is less than 7.4 and urine pH is less than 6.0.

In mild and moderate poisoning, stimulation of the respiratory center produces respiratory alkalosis. In severe intoxication (seen in severe acute ingestion with high salicylate levels and in chronic toxicity with lower levels), respiratory response is unable to overcome the metabolic overdose.

Once the urine becomes acidic, progressively smaller amounts of salicylate are excreted. Until this process is reversed, the half-life will remain prolonged, because metabolism contributes little to the removal of salicylate.

Chronic severe poisoning may be seen as early as 3 days after a regimen of salicylate is begun. Findings usually include vomiting, diarrhea, and dehydration.

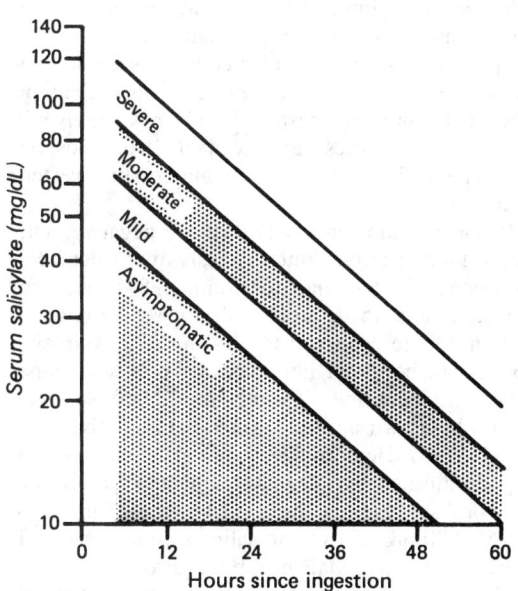

Figure 13–2. Nomogram relating serum salicylate concentration and expected severity of intoxication at varying intervals following ingestion of a single dose of salicylate. (Redrawn and reproduced, with permission, from Done AK: Salicylate intoxication. Pediatrics 1960;26:800.)

Treatment

Charcoal binds salicylates well and, after emesis or lavage, should be given on a cyclic basis every 4 hours until charcoal appears in stool.

Mild poisoning may require only the administration of oral fluids and confirmation that the salicylate level is falling.

Moderate poisoning is reflected by moderate dehydration and depletion of potassium. Fluids must be administered at a rate sufficient to correct dehydration and produce urine with a pH of greater than 7.0 at a rate of 2–3 mL/kg/h. Initial intravenous solutions should be isotonic, with sodium bicarbonate constituting half the electrolyte content. Once the patient is rehydrated, the solution can contain more free water and approximately 40 meq of potassium per liter.

Severe ingestion is marked by major dehydration in cases of chronic poisoning. Symptoms may be confused with those of Reye's syndrome, encephalopathy, and metabolic acidosis. Salicylate levels may even be in the "therapeutic range." Major fluid correction of dehydration is required. Once this has been accomplished, hypokalemia must be corrected and sodium bicarbonate given. Usual requirements are sodium bicarbonate, 1–2 meq/kg/h over the first 6–8 hours, and K^+, 20–40 meq/L. A urine flow of 2–3 mL/kg/h should be established.

Vitamin K should be administered, although hemorrhaging is rare except in severely poisoned patients. Renal failure or pulmonary edema is an indication for dialysis. Hemodialysis is most effective and peritoneal dialysis relatively ineffective. Acetazolamide should not be used.

Hill JB: Salicylate intoxication. N Engl J Med 1973;288:1110.

Keller RE, Schwab RA, Krenzelok EP: Contribution of sorbitol combined with activated charcoal in prevention of salicylate absorption. Ann Emerg Med 1990;19:654.

Snodgrass W et al: Salicylate toxicity following therapeutic doses in young children. Clin Toxicol 1981;18:247.

SCORPION STINGS

Scorpion stings are common in arid areas of the southwestern USA. Scorpion venom is more toxic than most snake venoms, but only minute amounts are injected. Although neurologic manifestations may last a week, most clinical signs subside within 24–48 hours.

The most common scorpions in the USA are members of the *Vejovis, Hadrurus, Androctonus,* and *Centruroides* species. Stings by the first three produce edema and pain. Stings by *Centruroides* cause tingling or burning paresthesias that begin at the site of the sting; other findings include hypersalivation, restlessness, muscular fasciculation, abdominal cramps, opisthotonos, convulsions, urinary incontinence, and respiratory failure.

Treatment

Sedation is the primary mode of therapy. In severe cases, the airway may become compromised by secretions and weakness of respiratory muscles. Endotracheal intubation may be required. Patients may require treatment for seizures, hypertension, or tachycardia.

The prognosis is good as long as the airway is managed appropriately.

Bond GR: Antivenom administration for *Centruroides* scorpion sting: Risks, benefits (abstract). Vet Hum Toxicol 1990;32:367.

Rachesky IJ et al: Treatments for *Centruroides exilicauda* envenomation. Am J Dis Child 1984;138:1136.

Russell RE, Madon MB: Introduction of the scorpion *Centruroides exilicauda* into California and its public health significance. Toxicon 1984;22:658.

SNAKEBITE

Despite the lethal potential of venomous snakes, human morbidity and mortality rates are surprisingly low. The outcome depends on the size of the child, the site of the bite, the degree of envenomation, the type of snake, and the effectiveness of treatment.

Children in snake-infested areas should wear boots and long trousers, should not walk barefoot, and should be cautioned not to explore under ledges or in holes.

Ninety-eight percent of poisonous snakebites in the USA are caused by pit vipers (rattlesnakes, water moccasins, and copperheads). A few are caused by elapids (coral snakes), and occasional bites occur from cobras and other nonindigenous exotic snakes kept as pets. Snake venom is a complex mixture of enzymes, peptides, and proteins that may have predominantly cytotoxic, neurotoxic, hemotoxic, or cardiotoxic effects but other effects as well. The snake seldom uses all its venom in a single bite. Up to 25% of bites by pit vipers do not result in venom injection.

Pit viper venom is predominantly cytotoxic and hemotoxic, causing a severe local reaction with pain, discoloration, and edema, as well as hemorrhagic effects. Peripheral and central neurologic abnormalities can also occur.

Swelling and pain occur soon after rattlesnake bite and are a certain indication that envenomation has occurred. During the first few hours, swelling and ecchymosis extend proximally from the bite. The bite is often obvious as a double puncture mark surrounded by ecchymosis. Hematemesis, melena, hemoptysis, and other manifestations of coagulopathy develop in severe cases. Respiratory difficulty and shock are the ultimate causes of death. Even in fatal rattlesnake bite, there is usually a period of 6–8 hours between the bite and death; there is, therefore, usually enough time to start effective treatment.

Coral snake envenomation causes little local pain, swelling, or necrosis, and systemic reactions are often delayed. The signs of coral snake envenomation include bulbar paralysis, dysphagia, and dysphoria; these may appear in 5–10 hours and may be followed by total peripheral paralysis and death in 24 hours.

Snakebites are an important hazard in many parts of the world; in India there are thought to be over 30,000 deaths per year from cobra bites. The general principles outlined here apply to any bite, but specific therapy will naturally vary between species.

Treatment

The treatment of snakebite envenomation is controversial, but the following approach seems most useful.

A. Emergency (First Aid) Treatment: The most important first aid measure is transportation to a medical facility. Splint the affected extremity and minimize the patient's motion. Tourniquets and ice packs are contraindicated.

Incision and suction are not useful for either crotalid or elapid snake bite. High vacuum suction (Extractor) has been shown to remove venom in a rabbit model. Its value in humans is unknown.

B. Definitive Medical Management: Blood should be drawn for typing and cross-matching, hematocrit, clotting time and platelet function, and serum electrolyte determinations. Close monitoring of the hematocrit and electrolytes is indicated. Establish two secure intravenous sites for the administration of antivenin and other medications.

Specific antivenin is indicated when signs of progressive envenomation are present. Polyvalent pit viper antivenin and eastern coral snake antivenin (Wyeth Laboratories) are available from hospital pharmacies. There is no antivenin for the western coral snake.

If horse serum sensitivity tests are negative, antivenin should be given intravenously over 1 hour. For pit vipers, give 5–8 vials for minimal, 8–15 vials for moderate, and 15 or more vials for severe envenomation. Dilute each vial to 50–200 mL. (Antivenin should not be given intramuscularly or subcutaneously.) Epinephrine, 0.3 mL of 1:1000 solution, should be drawn up in a syringe before antivenin is administered. Hemorrhage, pain, and shock are rapidly diminished by adequate amounts of antivenin. For coral snakes, give three to five vials of antivenin in 250–500 mL of isotonic saline solution. An additional three to five vials may be required.

Codeine, 1–1.5 mg/kg per dose orally, or meperidine, 0.6–1.5 mg/kg per dose orally or intramuscularly, is necessary to control pain. Cryotherapy is contraindicated because it commonly causes additional tissue damage. Early physiotherapy minimizes contractures. In rare cases, fasciotomy to relieve pressure within muscular compartments is required. The evaluation of function as well as of pulses will better predict the need for fasciotomy. Corticosteroids (hydrocortisone, 1–2 g intravenously every 4–6 hours) are useful in the treatment of serum sickness or anaphylactic shock. Antibiotics are not needed unless clinical signs of infection occur. Tetanus status should be evaluated and treated, if needed.

Kitchens CS, Van Mierop LHS: Envenomation by the eastern coral snake *(Micrurus fulvius fulvius)*: A study of 39 victims. JAMA 1987;258:1615.

Russell FE: *Snake Venom Poisoning.* Scholium International, 1983.

SOAPS & DETERGENTS

1. SOAPS

Soap is made from salts of fatty acids. Some toilet soap bars contain both soap and detergent. Ingestion of soap bars may cause vomiting and diarrhea, but they have a low toxicity.

Dilute with milk or water. Induced emesis is unnecessary.

2. DETERGENTS

Detergents are nonsoap synthetic products used for cleaning purposes because of their surfactant properties. Commercial products include granules, powders, and liquids. Electric dishwasher detergents are very alkaline and can cause caustic burns. Low concentrations of bleaching and antibacterial agents as well as enzymes are found in many preparations. These pure compounds are moderately toxic, but the concentration used is too small to alter the product's toxicity significantly, although occasional primary or allergic irritative phenomena have been noted in housewives and in employees manufacturing these products.

There are three general types of detergents: cationic, anionic, and nonionic.

Cationic Detergents (Ceepryn, Diaperene, Phemerol, Zephiran)

Dilute solutions (0.5%) cause mucosal irritation, but higher concentrations (10–15%) may cause caustic burns to mucosa. Clinical effects include nausea, vomiting, collapse, coma, and convulsions. As little as 2.25 g of some cationic agents have caused death in an adult. In four cases, 100–400 mg/kg of benzalkonium chloride caused death. Cationic detergents are rapidly inactivated by tissues and ordinary soap.

Because of the caustic potential and rapid onset of seizures, emesis is not recommended. Activated charcoal and a cathartic should be administered. Anticonvulsants may be needed.

Anionic Detergents

Most common household detergents are anionic. Laundry compounds have water softener (sodium phosphate) added, which is a strong irritant and may reduce ionized calcium. Anionic detergents irritate the skin by removing natural oils. Although ingestion causes diarrhea, intestinal distention, and vomiting, no fatalities have been reported.

The only treatment usually required is to discontinue use if skin irritation occurs and replace fluids and electrolytes. Induced vomiting is not indicated following ingestion of electric dishwasher detergent, because of its alkalinity. Dilute with water or milk.

Nonionic Detergents (Brij Products; Tritons X-45, X-100, X-102, & X-144)

These compounds include lauryl, stearyl, and oleyl alcohols and octyl phenol. They have a minimal irritating effect on the skin and are almost nontoxic when swallowed.

Deichmann WB, Gerarde HW: Hazards of alkaline laundry detergents. JAMA 1972;220:1014.

Enzyme detergents. (Editorial.) Br Med J 1970;1:518.

Jeven JE: Severe dermatitis and "biological" detergents. Br Med J 1970;1:299.

SPIDER BITES

Most medically important bites in the USA are caused by the black widow spider *(Latrodectus mactans)* and the North American brown recluse (violin) spider *(Loxosceles reclusa)*. Many spider venoms have common chemical and pharmacologic properties. It is helpful if positive identification of the spider can be made, since many spider bites may mimic those of the brown recluse spider.

Black Widow Spider

The black widow spider is endemic to nearly all areas of the USA. The initial bite may be hemorrhagic and associated with a sharp fleeting pain. Local and systemic muscular cramping, abdominal pain, nausea and vomiting, and shock can occur. Convulsions are more commonly seen in small children. Systemic signs of black widow spider bite may be confused with other causes of acute abdomen. Although paresthesias, nervousness, and transient muscle spasms may persist for weeks in survivors, recovery from the acute phase is generally complete within 3 days. In contrast to popular opinion, death is extremely rare.

Most authors recommend calcium gluconate as initial therapy (50 mg/kg intravenously per dose, up to 250 mg/kg/24 h), although it is often not effective and the effects are of short duration. Methocarbamol (15 mg/kg orally) or diazepam titrated to effect is useful.

Morphine or barbiturates may occasionally be needed for control of pain or restlessness, but they increase the possibility of respiratory depression. Antivenin is available but should be reserved for severe cases in which the above therapies have failed.

Local treatment of the bite is not helpful.

Brown Recluse Spider (Violin Spider)

The North American brown recluse spider is most commonly seen in the central and midwestern areas of the USA. Its bite characteristically produces a localized reaction with progressively severe pain within 24 hours. The initial bleb on an erythematous ischemic base is replaced by a black eschar within a week. This eschar separates in 2–5 weeks, leaving an ulcer that heals slowly. Systemic signs include cyanosis, morbilliform rash, fever, chills, malaise, weakness, nausea and vomiting, joint pains, hemolytic reactions with hemoglobinuria, jaundice, and delirium. Fatalities are rare. Fatal disseminated intravascular coagulation has been reported.

Although of unproved efficacy, the following therapies have been used: dexamethasone (4 mg intravenously four times a day) during the acute phase; hydroxyzine 1 mg/kg/dose intramuscularly; polymorphonuclear leukocyte inhibitors, such as dapsone or colchicine, and oxygen applied to the bite site; and total excision of the lesion to the fascial level.

Alario A et al: Cutaneous necrosis following a spider bite: A case report and review. Pediatrics 1987;79:618.
Vorse H: Disseminated intravascular coagulopathy following fatal brown spider bite. J Pediatr 1971;80:1035.
Wasserman GS, Anderson PC: Loxoscelism and necrotic arachnidism. J Tox Clin Toxicol 1984;21:451.
Yarbrough BE: Current treatment of brown recluse spider bites. Curr Concepts Wound Care 1987;Winter:4.

THYROID PREPARATIONS (Thyroid Desiccated, Sodium Levothyroxine)

Ingestion of the equivalent of 50–150 g of desiccated thyroid can cause signs of hyperthyroidism, including irritability, mydriasis, hyperpyrexia, tachycardia, and diarrhea. Maximal clinical effect occurs about 9 days after ingestion—several days after the protein-bound iodine level has fallen dramatically.

Induce vomiting. If the patient develops clinical signs of toxicity, propranolol, 0.01–0.1 mg/kg (maximum, 1 mg), is useful because of its antiadrenergic activity.

Golightly LK et al: Clinical effects of accidental levothyroxine ingestion in children. Am J Dis Child 1987;141:1025.

Gorman RL et al: High anxiety–low toxicity: A massive T_4 ingestion. Pediatrics 1988;82:666.

VITAMINS

Accidental ingestion of excessive amounts of vitamins rarely causes significant problems. Occasional cases of hypervitaminosis A and D do occur, however, particularly in patients with poor hepatic or renal function. The fluoride contained in many multivitamin preparations is not a realistic hazard, because a 2- or 3-year-old child could eat 100 tablets, containing 1 mg of sodium fluoride per tablet, without producing serious symptoms. Iron poisoning has been reported with multiple vitamin tablets containing iron. Pyridoxine abuse has caused neuropathies; nicotinic acid, myopathy.

Dalton K, Dalton MJT: Characteristics of pyridoxine overdose neuropathy syndrome. Acta Neurol Scand 1987;76:8.
Dean BS, Krenzelok EP: Multiple vitamins and vitamins with iron: Accidental poisoning in children. Vet Hum Toxicol 1988;30:23.
DiPalma JR, Ritchie DM: Vitamin toxicity. Ann Rev Pharm Tox 1977;17:133.
Litin SC, Anderson CF: Nicotinic acid-associated myopathy: A report of three cases. Am J Med 1989;86:481.

WARFARIN

Warfarin is used as a rodenticide. It causes hypoprothrombinemia and capillary injury. It is readily absorbed from the gastrointestinal tract but is absorbed poorly through the skin. A dose of 0.5 mg/kg of warfarin may be toxic in a child. A prothrombin time is helpful in establishing the severity of the poisoning.

Treatment consists of induced vomiting followed by a saline cathartic. If bleeding occurs or the prothrombin time is prolonged, give 1–5 mg of vitamin K_1 (phytonadione) intramuscularly or subcutaneously. For large ingestions with established toxicity, 0.6 mg/kg may be given.

A new group of long-acting anticoagulant rodenticides (brodifacoum, difenacoum, bromadiolone, diphacinone, pinone, valone, and coumatetralyl) have been a more serious toxicologic problem than warfarin. They also cause hypoprothrombinemia and a bleeding diathesis that responds to phytonadione, though the anticoagulant activity may persist for periods ranging from 6 weeks to several months. Treatment with vitamin K_1 may be needed for weeks.

Smolinske SC et al: Superwarfarin poisoning in children: A prospective study. Pediatrics 1989;84:490.

REFERENCES

Arena JM, Drew RH: *Poisoning: Toxicology, Symptoms, Treatments,* 5th ed. Thomas, 1986.

Baselt RC, Cravey RH: *Disposition of Toxic Drugs and Chemicals in Man,* 3rd ed. Year Book, 1989.

Bayer MJ, Rumack BH, Wanke L: *Toxicologic Emergencies: A Manual of Diagnosis and Management.* Brady-Prentice Hall, 1983.

Bresinsky A, Besl H: *A Colour Atlas of Poisonous Fungi: A Handbook for Pharmacists, Doctors, and Biologists.* Wolfe, 1990.

Clayton GD, Clayton FE: *Patty's Industrial Hygiene and Toxicology,* 4th ed. Vol 2. Wiley-Interscience, 1993.

Doull J, Klaassen C, Amdur M (editors): *Cassarett and Doull's Toxicology: The Basic Science of Poisons,* 4th ed. Macmillan, 1991.

Ellenhorn MJ, Barceloux DG: *Medical Toxicology: Diagnosis and Treatment of Human Poisoning.* Elsevier, 1988.

Finkel AJ (editor): *Hamilton & Hardy's Industrial Toxicology,* 4th ed. Publishing Sciences Group, 1983.

Goldfrank LR et al: *Goldfrank's Toxicologic Emergencies,* 4th ed. Appleton-Century-Crofts, 1990.

Grant WM: *Toxicology of the Eye,* 3rd ed. Thomas, 1986.

Haddad LM, Winchester JF: *Poisoning and Drug Overdose,* 2nd ed. Saunders, 1990.

Koren G: *Maternal-Fetal Toxicology–A Clinician's Guide.* Marcel Dekker, 1990.

Lampe KF, McCann MA: *AMA Handbook of Poisonous and Injurious Plants.* American Medical Association, 1985.

Olson KR (editor): *Poisoning and Drug Overdose.* Appleton & Lange, 1990.

Rumack BH, Spoerke DG, Smolinske SC (editors): *POISINDEX*ρ Information System. [Published quarterly.] Micromedex, Inc, Denver, Colorado.

14

Emergencies & Accidents

F. Keith Battan, MD

The primary mission of pediatric emergency departments is **resuscitation,** ie, the rapid identification and treatment of the child whose life is threatened by illness or injury. The complete spectrum of acute, less urgent problems is addressed as well. Knowledge from many subspecialties is utilized, including pediatric surgery, orthopedics, critical care, anesthesiology, neurosurgery, toxicology, and emergency medicine.

Pediatric emergency medicine as a subspecialty has developed over the past decade with the emergence of pediatricians who have experience and subspecialty training in all aspects of urgent care of infants, children, and adolescents. The body of research literature in this field is growing rapidly. Subspecialty fellowship training exists at 47 centers, and there is a subspecialty certification board. Pediatric emergency medicine relates to the entire spectrum of care that may affect a severely ill or injured child: community injury prevention, prehospital care by emergency medical technicians and paramedics, hospital-based stabilization and critical care, and rehabilitation. Emergency pediatricians are increasingly involved in the care of the severely injured child as awareness increases that trauma is the leading cause of death among children over 1 year of age.

Fleisher G: Pediatric emergency medicine on the move. Pediatr Emerg Care 1990;6:67.

Krauss BS, Harakal T, Fleisher GR: The spectrum and frequency of illness presenting to a pediatric emergency department. Pediatr Emerg Care 1991;7:67.

Li M, Baker MD, Ropp LJ: Pediatric emergency medicine: A developing subspecialty. Pediatrics 1989;84:336.

Lohr KN, Durch JS (editors): *Emergency Medical Services for Children, Report to the Nation from the Institute of Medicine, Committee on Pediatric Emergency Medical Services.* National Academy Press, 1993.

Schafermeyer RW: Pediatric trauma in the 90s. Pediatr Emerg Care 1990;6:150.

ESTIMATION FORMULAS		
Estimated body weight (kg)	=	(Age in years × 2) + 8
Median blood pressure (systolic)	=	(Age in years × 2) + 90
5th percentile systolic blood pressure (hypotension)	=	(Age in years × 2) + 70
Endotracheal tube size	=	$\dfrac{\text{(Age in years + 16)}}{4}$

ADVANCED LIFE SUPPORT FOR INFANTS & CHILDREN

Children may present in cardiopulmonary failure from a wide variety of causes, mainly respiratory disorders. Regardless of the primary origin, however, a systematic approach will allow rapid determination of the patient's physiologic status followed by initiation of resuscitative measures. The goal of rapid assessment and intervention is not necessarily to make a specific etiologic diagnosis but rather to determine the degree of physiologic derangement and then to intervene promptly to ensure adequate oxygenation, ventilation, and circulation.

Children who become apneic and pulseless have a dismal prognosis. When progressive deterioration leads to bradycardia and ultimately to asystole, sufficient hypoxic and ischemic insult to the brain and other vital organs has occurred to make neurologic recovery extremely unlikely. Children who respond to ventilation and oxygenation alone or to less than 5 minutes of advanced life support are much more likely to survive neurologically intact. Therefore, it is essential to recognize the child who is at risk for progressing to cardiopulmonary arrest and to provide timely intervention.

THE ABCs OF RESUSCITATION

In assessing a severely ill child, one must perform a rapid sequential evaluation of *a*irway patency, *b*reathing adequacy, and *c*irculation integrity. When abnormalities are detected, derangements must be corrected *before* one can proceed to the next function. Thus, if a child's airway is obstructed, one must open the airway (eg, by head positioning and the chin lift maneuver) before assessing breathing and then circulation.

A child presenting with severe illness requires rapid cardiopulmonary assessment and intervention and, concurrently—to the extent possible—initiation of appropriate monitoring and access. Monitoring and vascular access will be discussed later.

Airway

Look, listen, and feel for airway patency: (1) *Look* for signs of obstruction such as inspiratory work or suprasternal retractions. Rapidly assess the level of consciousness. A patient with significant airway obstruction will have an altered level of consciousness, eg, agitation or unresponsiveness. (2) *Listen* for adventitious breath sounds such as stridor, snoring, or gurgling. (3) *Feel* for air movement with your face near the child's mouth and nose.

The airway should be classified as **clear or patent** (no obstruction), **maintainable** (airway patency can be restored by noninvasive means, eg, chin lift, suctioning, or bag-valve-mask ventilation), or **unmaintainable** (requiring invasive maneuvers such as endotracheal intubation or cricothyroidotomy). If neck injury is suspected, the cervical spine must be immobilized. (See care of the trauma patient, below.) The following discussion assumes that basic life support techniques have been mastered. The references should be consulted for more complete discussions of advanced techniques.

Knowledge of pediatric anatomic differences will help the physician assess and manage the airway. Infants are obligate nasal breathers; therefore, secretions or blood can cause significant distress. Children's tongues are large relative to their oral cavities, and the larynx is high and anteriorly located. In unconscious children, prolapse of the tongue into the posterior pharynx is the most common cause of airway obstruction. If airway obstruction is present, take immediate measures to restore patency:

A. Place the head in the "sniffing position" (Figure 14–1). The neck should be slightly flexed and the head gently extended so as to bring the face forward. This position aligns the oral, pharyngeal, and tracheal planes (Figure 14–2). The head should be repositioned if airway obstruction persists after head tilt and jaw thrust. In an infant, the relatively large occiput puts the head in a sniffing position when supine; in an older child, more head extension is necessary. Avoid hyperextension of the neck, especially in infants.

B. Perform the chin lift or jaw thrust maneuver (Figure 14–3). Lift the chin upward while avoiding pressure on the submental triangle, or lift the jaw by traction upward on the angle of the jaw. Jaw thrust without head tilt should be done if cervical spine injury is possible.

C. Suction the mouth of secretions, blood, and foreign material.

D. Remove visible foreign bodies, using the fin-

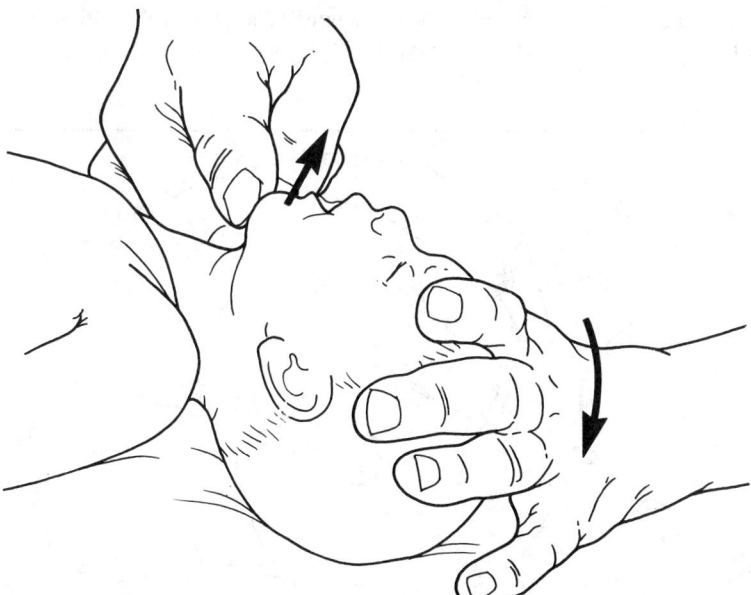

Figure 14–1. Head tilt with chin lift. (Reproduced, with permission, from: *Textbook of Pediatric Advanced Life Support.* American Heart Association/American Academy of Pediatrics, 1988.)

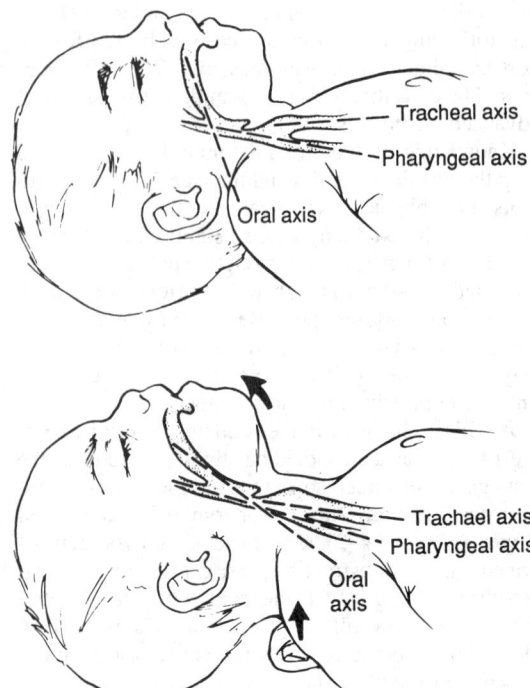

Figure 14–2. Alignment of oral, pharyngeal, and tracheal axes. (Reproduced, with permission, from: *Textbook of Pediatric Advanced Life Support.* American Heart Association/American Academy of Pediatrics, 1988.)

gers or a Magill forceps—visualizing by means of a laryngoscope if necessary. Blind finger sweeps should *not* be done.

E. Insert an oropharyngeal or, in the conscious patient, a nasopharyngeal airway (Figures 14–4 and 14–5) to relieve upper airway obstruction due to prolapse of the tongue and mandibular block of tissue

into the posterior pharynx. The correct size for an oropharyngeal airway is obtained by measuring from the central gumline to the angle of the jaw. Nasopharyngeal airways should fit snugly but not tightly within the nares and are sized from the nares to the tragus.

Breathing

Assessment of respiratory status is largely accomplished by *inspection.* To assess for adequacy of oxygenation and ventilation, look, listen, and feel: (1) *Look* for adequate and symmetric chest rise and fall, respiratory rate, increased work of breathing including retractions, flaring, and grunting, skin color, and tracheal deviation. (2) *Listen* for adventitious breath sounds, eg wheezing. Auscultate for air entry, symmetry of breath sounds, and rales. (3) *Feel* for subcutaneous crepitus. Peripheral pulses may be diminished if respiratory failure is present. Adequate minute ventilation is obtained from an adequate tidal volume and respiratory rate.

If there is no or inadequate spontaneous breathing, initiate positive-pressure ventilation with bag-valve-mask ventilation and 100% oxygen or, if that equipment is unavailable, by mouth-to-mouth rescue breathing. *Universal precautions should be maintained whenever possible during resuscitations.* If some respiratory effort is present, coordinate bagging with the patient's efforts. Adequacy of ventilation is reflected in adequate rise and fall of the chest and auscultation of good air entry bilaterally. The presence of asymmetric breath sounds in a child in cardiac arrest or in severe distress suggests pneumothorax and is an indication for needle thoracostomy. In infants, the transmission of breath sounds throughout the chest may impair the ability to auscultate the presence of a pneumothorax. If the chest does not rise and fall easily with bagging, one should reposition the airway and repeat the maneuvers in the "airway" sec-

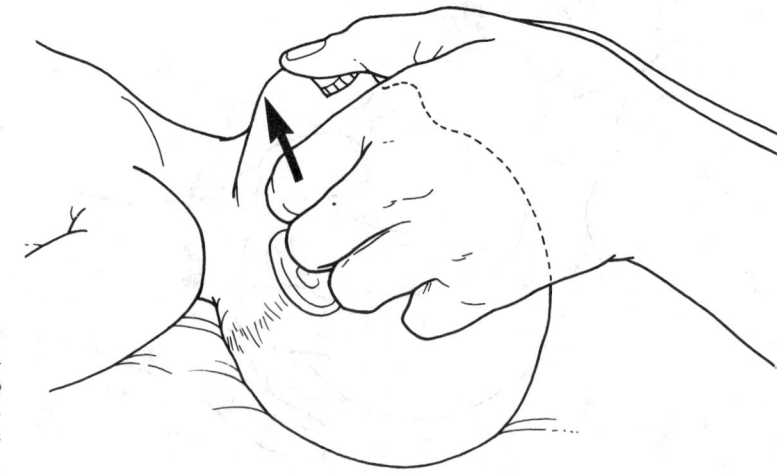

Figure 14–3. Jaw thrust. (Reproduced, with permission, from: *Textbook of Pediatric Advanced Life Support.* American Heart Association/American Academy of Pediatrics, 1988.)

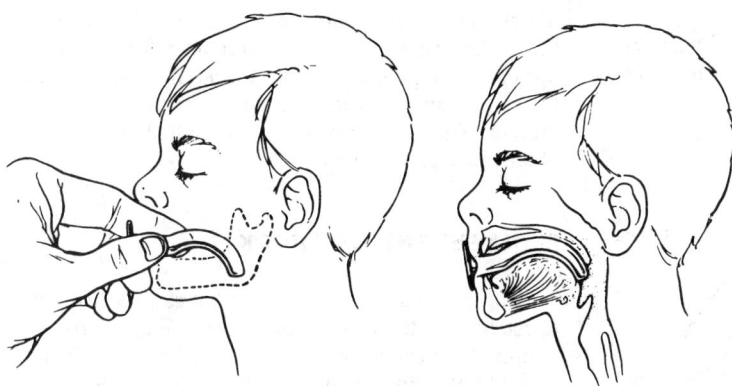

Figure 14–4. Oropharyngeal airway. (Reproduced, with permission, from: *Textbook of Pediatric Advanced Life Support.* American Heart Association/ American Academy of Pediatrics, 1988.)

tion. Perform airway foreign body maneuvers if the airway remains obstructed. *Note:* Effective oxygenation and ventilation are the keys to successful resuscitation.

Intubate the trachea with cricoid pressure (Sellick's maneuver) in patients unresponsive to bag-mask ventilation, those in coma, those who require airway protection, or those who will require prolonged ventilation. Advanced airway management techniques are described in the references accompanying this section. Cricothyroidotomy is rarely necessary. (See care of the trauma patient, below.)

Circulation

Clinical assessment of hemodynamic status can be done rapidly. The diagnosis of shock can and should be made by clinical examination before the blood pressure is measured. In contrast to respiratory assessment, the circulatory assessment is largely hands-on.

Shock is present if two of the following signs are abnormal, eg, tachycardia and delayed capillary filling time, or poor pulses and cool extremities, regardless of blood pressure.

A. Pulses: Check adequacy of peripheral pulses and heart rate. Pulses can be bounding in the early phases of septic shock, or weak and thready in hypoperfusion states. Tachycardia is a nonspecific sign of distress, whereas bradycardia for age is indicative of rapidly impending arrest and necessitates aggressive resuscitation.

B. Extremities: If distal extremities are cool, locate the proximal point at which they become warm to assess the severity of shock. For example, a child whose extremities are cool distal to the elbows and knees is severely hypoperfused.

C. Capillary Refill Time: This is an important indicator of perfusion. A refill time longer than 1.5 seconds is abnormal.

D. Mental Status: A hypoxic, hypercapnic, or ischemic state will result in altered mentation.

E. Skin Color: Cyanosis is a late finding in children owing to their relative anemia. Compromised cardiopulmonary status can be reflected in pallor or gray, mottled, or ashen skin colors.

F. Blood Pressure: Determination of blood pressure is not necessary to make the diagnosis of

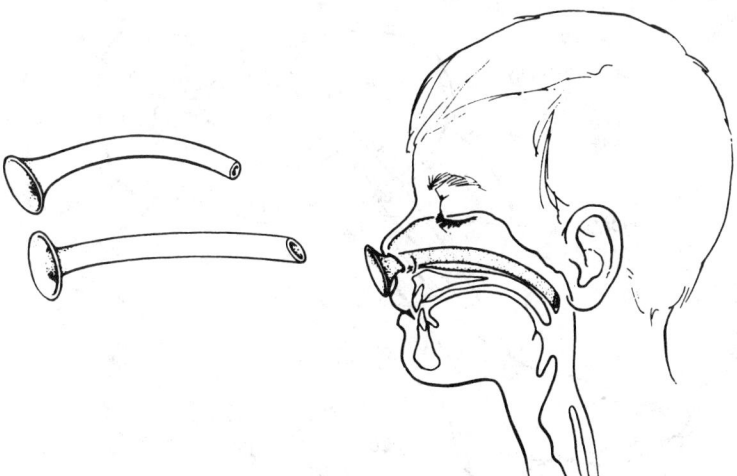

Figure 14–5. Nasopharyngeal airway. (Reproduced, with permission, from: *Textbook of Pediatric Advanced Life Support.* American Heart Association/American Academy of Pediatrics, 1988.)

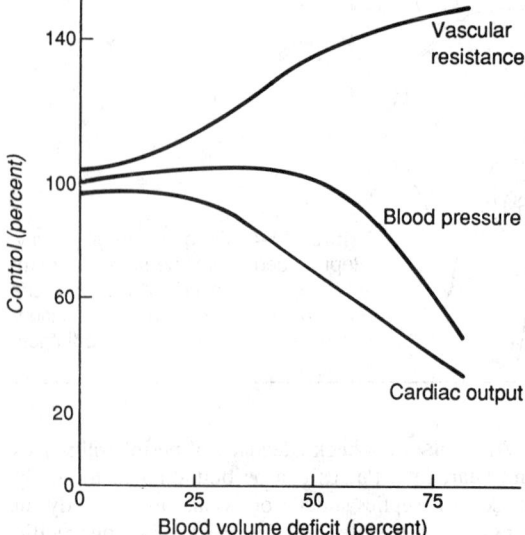

Figure 14–6. Relationship of blood pressure, systemic vascular resistance, and cardiac output to hemorrhage. Note that blood pressure doesn't begin to fall until an approximately 50% deficit in blood volume. Blood pressure declines precipitously thereafter. (Reproduced, with permission, from: *Textbook of Pediatric Advanced Life Support.* American Heart Association/American Academy of Pediatrics, 1988.)

shock. It is important to remember that shock or hypoperfusion of vital organs may be present before the blood pressure falls below normal limits for age. As intravascular volume falls, peripheral vascular resistance increases so that blood pressure is maintained until there is 25–30% depletion of blood volume—followed by a precipitous and often irreversible decrease in blood pressure. (See Figure 14–6.)

Shock that occurs with signs of decreased perfusion (eg, tachycardia and delayed capillary refill time) but normal blood pressure is **compensated shock.** When blood pressure also falls, **decompensated shock** is present. The appropriate-sized cuff must be used to obtain an accurate blood pressure.

MANAGEMENT OF SHOCK

Intravenous access is essential but can be difficult to establish in the volume-contracted patient. First attempts should be via peripheral access, especially the antecubital veins, with attempts limited to 90 seconds. Central cannulation—depending on individual preference and expertise—follows quickly. Alternatives are percutaneous cannulation of femoral, subclavian, or internal or external jugular veins; cutdown at antecubital, femoral, or saphenous sites; or intraosseous lines (Figure 14–7). Consider intraosseous needle placement in any severely ill child when venous access cannot be rapidly established. Use short, wide-bore catheters to allow maximal flow rates. Severely ill children or children in shock should have two intravenous access sites started. Consider arterial access if frequent arterial blood gas determinations or laboratory tests will be needed. In newborns, the umbilical veins may be cannulated.

Differentiation of Shock States & Initial Therapy

Therapy for inadequate circulation is based on the type of circulatory failure.

A. Hypovolemic Shock: The most common type of shock in the pediatric population is hypovolemic. Common causes include dehydration from vomiting and diarrhea, diabetes, or heat illness; hemorrhage; or loss of plasma from burns or trauma.

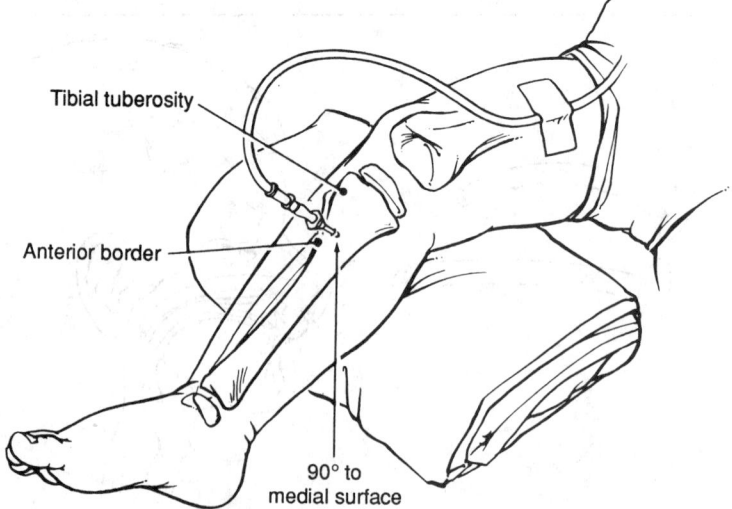

Figure 14–7. Placement of intraosseous needle. Intraosseous needle, spinal needle, or bone marrow needle inserted perpendicularly into medial tibial plateau 1–3 cm below anterior tibial tubercle. (Reproduced, with permission, from: *Textbook of Pediatric Advanced Life Support.* American Heart Association/American Academy of Pediatrics, 1988.)

Therapy is by volume replacement. Initial fluid resuscitation is with isotonic crystalloid solution—ie, lactated Ringer's solution or normal saline solution. Give 20 mL/kg body weight, repeated as necessary with frequent reassessments, until perfusion normalizes. Children tolerate large volumes of fluid replacement—up to and over the full circulating blood volume of 80 mL/kg can be given safely with appropriate monitoring. Blood product replacement may be necessary in trauma patients not responding to two boluses of crystalloid solution. Red blood cell transfusion should be guided by *repeated* hematocrit readings. Pressors are not required in simple hypovolemic states unless myocardial injury has also occurred in the unusual case.

B. Distributive Shock: Distributive shock represents relative hypovolemia from increased vascular capacitance of circulating volume. Examples include sepsis, anaphylaxis, and central nervous system injury.

Initial therapy is again by isotonic volume replacement, but pressors may be necessary if perfusion does not normalize after delivery of two 20 mL/kg boluses of fluid.

C. Cardiogenic Shock: Cardiogenic shock can occur as a complication of congenital heart disease, myocarditis, dysrhythmias, ingestions (eg, clonidine, tricyclic antidepressants), from serious infections, or as a sequela of shock due to any cause. The diagnosis is suggested by any of the following signs: abnormal cardiac rhythm, distended neck veins, abnormal heart sounds such as an S_3 or S_4, friction rub, narrow pulse pressure, or hepatomegaly. Chest radiographs will show cardiomegaly and pulmonary edema—not seen in shock due to other causes. An initial bolus of crystalloid may be given, but dopamine or other pressors, and agents to reduce afterload are necessary to improve perfusion. Full cardiopulmonary monitoring is essential.

Children in cardiogenic shock must be admitted to the pediatric intensive care unit.

Observation & Further Management

Reassess perfusion immediately after each bolus of fluid to determine additional fluid needs. Serial central venous pressure determinations or a chest radiograph will aid clinical assessments to help determine volume status. Place a Foley catheter to monitor urine output.

With shock due to any cause, caution must be exercised with volume replacement if intracranial pressure is potentially elevated, eg, in severe head injury or meningitis. Even in such situations, however, *intravascular volume must be restored to achieve adequate cerebral perfusion pressure.*

Summary of Cardiopulmonary Resuscitation

Assess the ABCs in sequential fashion, and begin interventions as soon as a derangement is detected—before assessing the next system. After each intervention, it is essential that each system be *reassessed* to ensure improvement and to avoid deterioration.

Carcillo JA, Davis AL, Zaritsky A: Role of early fluid resuscitation in pediatric septic shock. JAMA 1991;266:1242.

Chameides L (editor): *Textbook of Pediatric Advanced Life Support.* American Heart Association/American Academy of Pediatrics, 1988.

Pryor RW, Kline MW, Matson JR: Septic shock: Principles of management in the emergency department. Pediatr Emerg Care 1989;5:193.

Silverman BK (editor): *Textbook of Advanced Pediatric Life Support.* APLS Joint Task Force: American College of Emergency Physicians/American Academy of Pediatrics, 1993.

EMERGENCY PEDIATRIC DRUGS

Careful attention to airway and breathing remains the mainstay of pediatric resuscitation. Drugs should be considered only after optimal oxygenation and ventilation have been accomplished and, in general, only if hemodynamic compromise exists. Rapid delivery to the central circulation is essential. Infuse medications close to the catheter's hub and flush in with saline to achieve the most rapid systemic effects. If no intravenous access is achievable, some drugs may be given by endotracheal tube (see Table 14–1). The use of preprinted resuscitation drug charts or length/dose resuscitation tapes (Broselow tapes) speeds drug dose and equipment determinations and helps eliminate dosing errors.

Table 14–2 sets forth current recommendations for selected emergency drugs used in pediatrics. Controlled trials demonstrating improved outcomes generally have not been done.

American Heart Association, Subcommittee on Pediatric Resuscitation: *Pediatric Basic and Advanced Life Support. JAMA 1992;268:2251.*

Goetting MG, Paradis NA: High-dose epinephrine improves outcome from pediatric cardiac arrest. Ann Emerg Med 1991;20:22.

Paradis NA, Koscove EM: Epinephrine in cardiac arrest: A critical review. Ann Emerg Med 1990;19:1288.

Table 14–1. Emergency drugs that can be given by endotracheal tube.

Lidocaine
Naloxone
Epinephrine
Atropine

Table 14–2. Emergency pediatric drugs.

Drug	Indications	Dosage and Route	Comment
Atropine	1. Bradycardia, especially cardiac in origin 2. Vagally mediated bradycardia, eg, during laryngoscopy and intubation 3. Anticholinesterase poisoning 4. Asystole, after epinephrine use	0.01–0.02 mg/kg (minimum, 0.1 mg; maximum, 1–2 mg) IV, IO, ET. May repeat every 5 minutes.	Atropine may be useful in hemodynamically significant primary cardiac-based bradycardias. Because of paradoxical bradycardia sometimes seen in infants, a minimum dose of 0.1 mg is recommended by the American Heart Association. Epinephrine is the first-line drug in pediatrics for bradycardia caused by hypoxia or ischemia.
Bicarbonate	1. Documented metabolic acidosis 2. Hyperkalemia	1 meq/kg IV or IO by arterial blood gas: $3 \times$ kg $\times$ base deficit. May repeat every 5 minutes.	Infuse slowly. Sodium bicarbonate will be effective only if the patient is adequately oxygenated, ventilated, and perfused. Has some adverse side effects.
Calcium chloride 10%	1. Documented hypocalcemia 2. Calcium channel blocker overdose 3. Hyperkalemia, hypermagnesemia	10–30 mg/kg slowly IV, preferably centrally, IO	Calcium is no longer indicated for asystole. Potent tissue necrosis results if infiltration occurs. Use with caution.
Epinephrine	1. Bradycardia, especially hypoxic-ischemic 2. Hypotension (by infusion) 3. Asystole 4. Fine ventricular fibrillation refractory to initial defibrillation 5. Pulseless electrical activity 6. Anaphylaxis	Bradycardia and first dose in arrests: 0.01 mg/kg IV or IO of 1:10,000 solution. Second and subsequent doses in arrests: 0.1–0.2 mg/kg IV or IO of 1:1000 solution. Repeat every 3 minutes. ET: 0.1 mg/kg of 1:1000 solution. SC: .01 mg/kg 1:1000 solution (= 0.01 mL/kg) (anaphylactic shock). Maximum dose: 0.3–0.5 mL. Infusion: 0.1–1 µg/kg	Epinephrine is the single most important drug in pediatric resuscitation. Evidence from animal studies and small series of human subjects indicates that the present recommended dose may be insufficient and that doses of 0.1–0.3 mg/kg may be optimal. A randomized controlled trial has not been done.
Glucose	1. Hypoglycemia 2. Altered mental status (empiric) 3. With insulin, for hyperkalemia	0.5–1 g/kg IV, IO. May repeat as necessary.	Neonates: 2 mL/kg D_{10}W. Older child: 2–4 mL/kg D_{25}W, 6–10 mL/kg D_{10}W
Naloxone	1. Opiate overdose 2. Altered mental status (empiric)	< 10 kg: 0.1 mg/kg IV, IO, ET. > 10 kg: 0.01 mg/kg IV, IO, ET. May repeat as necessary.	Side effects are few. A dose of 2 mg may be given in young children, 4 mg in adolescents. Repeat as necessary, or as constant infusion in narcotic overdoses.

ET = Endotracheally   IO = Intraosseously   IV = Intravenously   SC = Subcutaneously

APPROACH TO THE SEVERELY ILL CHILD

Often a child will present in cardiorespiratory failure of unknown cause. Cardiopulmonary failure represents global derangements of oxygenation, ventilation, and perfusion. Occasionally, an unstable patient will present with a known diagnosis, eg, a known asthmatic in status asthmaticus and respiratory failure, or a child with known congenital heart disease. The initial approach is identical, however, and designed to rapidly identify and reverse life-threatening conditions.

Preparation for Emergency Management

Resuscitation of a severely ill child requires action simultaneously at two levels: a rapid cardiopulmonary assessment, with indicated stabilizing measures while initiating monitoring and venous access (sometimes called "lifelines"). A method of accomplishing these concurrent goals is outlined below.

A. If advance notice of the patient's arrival has been received from prehospital providers or via telephone, prepare a resuscitation room and summon appropriate consultants as needed, eg, neurosurgery for an unresponsive child after severe head injury, radiology technician for assessment of line and tube placement.

B. Assign team responsibilities, including a team

leader plus others designated to manage the airway, perform chest compressions, achieve vascular access, draw blood for laboratory studies, place monitors, gather additional historical data, and provide family support.

C. Age-appropriate equipment should be made ready, including a cardiorespiratory monitor, pulse oximeter, and appropriate blood pressure cuff. Age- and weight-based laryngoscope blades, endotracheal tubes, nasogastric tubes, and indwelling urinary catheter should be assembled for rapid access. (See Table 14–3 for sizes.)

Reception & Assessment

When the patient arrives, the team leader begins a rapid assessment as team members perform their pre-assigned tasks. Interventions and medications should be ordered only by the team leader to avoid confusion, and the leader should refrain from personally performing distracting procedures. A complete record should be kept of what transpires, including medications, timing of interventions, and response to intervention.

A. All Cases: In addition to cardiac compressions and ventilation, ensure that the following are instituted.

1. 100% oxygen.
2. Cardiorespiratory monitoring.
3. Pulse oximetry.
4. Intravenous (peripheral, intraosseous, or central) access within 90 seconds.
5. Blood drawn and sent.
6. Full vital signs obtained.

B. As Appropriate:

1. Immobilize neck.
2. Chest x-ray for line and tube placement.

3. Arterial line.
4. Remove clothes.
5. Insert Foley catheter and nasogastric tube.
6. Complete history.
7. Notify needed consultants.
8. Family support.

APPROACH TO THE PEDIATRIC TRAUMA PATIENT

Injuries, including motor vehicle crashes, falls, burns, and immersions, account for the greatest number of deaths among children over 1 year of age. Pediatricians must be cognizant of this sobering statistic and work with injury prevention specialists, prehospital health care providers, and emergency and critical care physicians and nurses to reduce the loss of life and limb among children.

An organized team approach to the seriously injured child, using preassigned roles, will optimize outcomes. Accurate, timed records are invaluable. A calm atmosphere in the receiving unit will contribute to thoughtful care. Compiling a problem list helps determine priorities in timing of definitive care. Assignment of a pediatric trauma score assists in triage decisions and prognosis. Conscious children are terribly frightened by serious injury; constant reassurance can help alleviate anxiety. Analgesia and sedation can and should be given to appropriately stable patients. Parents often feel angry and guilty and require ongoing support; enlist the services of social workers or

Table 14–3. Equipment sizes and estimated weight by age.

Age (years)	Weight (kg)	Endotracheal Tube Size (mm)[1]	Laryngoscope Blade	Chest Tube (F)	Foley (F)
Premature	1–2.5	2.5 uncuffed	0	8	5
Term newborn	3	3.0	0–1	10	8
1	10	3.5–4.0	1	18	8
2	12	4.5	1	18	10
3	14	4.5	1	20	10
4	16	5.0	2	22	10
5	18	5.0–5.5	2	24	10
6	20	5.5	2	26	12
7	22	5.5–6.0	2	26	12
8	24	6.0 cuffed	2	28	14
10	32	6.0–6.5 cuffed	2–3	30	14
Adolescent	50	7.0 cuffed	3	36	14
Adult	70	8.0 cuffed	3	40	14

[1]Internal diameter.

Child Life workers (therapists knowledgeable about child development) whenever possible.

The past decade has seen the emergence of designated pediatric trauma centers, where dedicated teams of *pediatric* specialists in trauma surgery, orthopedics, neurosurgery, critical care, and emergency pediatrics combine to provide optimal multidisciplinary care. Children with significant injuries to more than one organ system or with life-threatening injury to a single organ system are cared for by these teams. Because most children with severe injuries are not seen in these centers, however, pediatricians and others must be able to provide initial assessment and stabilization of the child with life-threatening injuries before transport to a referral center.

Mechanism of Injury

The mechanism of injury is important in evaluation and definitive care. One should document the time of occurrence, the type of energy transfer to the child (eg, hit by a car, rapid deceleration), secondary injury at impact if the child was thrown by the initial impact, appearance of the child at the scene according to bystanders, time and type of stabilization, and clinical condition during transport. The report of prehospital providers is invaluable. If the patient undergoes secondary transport to a referral facility, all information of this type must be communicated to the receiving facility.

Initial Assessment & Management

Children die from injuries during three distinct time periods: at the scene, usually from irreparable central nervous system injury, disruption of major vessels, or airway compromise; within minutes to hours after the injury, usually from intracranial hemorrhage, hemopneumothorax, liver or spleen injury, or bleeding from multiple sites; and much later, usually in intensive care units, from multiorgan failure. It is this middle group that can benefit most from expeditious management—hence the term "golden hour" of trauma.

The American College of Surgeons teaches a method for evaluating injured patients in a systematic way that provides a rapid assessment and stabilization phase, followed by a head-to-toe examination and definitive care phase. These are called the primary and secondary surveys, respectively. This schema can be used to care for children with the spectrum of injuries from a minor head "bonk" to major multisystem trauma.

PRIMARY SURVEY

The primary survey is designed to rapidly identify and *immediately treat* physiologic derangements. It is the *resuscitation* phase. Priorities are still *a*irway,

*b*reathing, and *c*irculation, but with important further considerations in the trauma setting:

> **A**irway, with cervical spine control
> **B**reathing
> **C**irculation, with hemorrhage control
> **D**isability (neurologic status)
> **E**xposure (undress the patient completely and examine)

Evaluation and treatment of the ABCs are as discussed previously. Modifications in the trauma setting will be added here. During resuscitation, it is worth remembering that most deaths from trauma in children are due to head injuries; therefore, principles of cerebral resuscitation are important. Trauma in children is predominantly blunt, though penetrating trauma does occur. Head and abdominal injuries are particularly important in the pediatric age group.

Airway

Effective management of airway and breathing is essential to avoid the secondary insults of hypoxia and hypercapnia. failure to manage the airway appropriately is the most common cause of preventable death. Administer 100% high-flow oxygen to all patients. During assessment and management of the airway, one should provide cervical spine protection, initially by manual in-line immobilization (not traction). A hard cervical spine collar is then applied and the head is taped to a backboard, surrounded by some means of cushioning (eg, rolled blankets) to further immobilize the head and allow log-rolling of the child in case of vomiting.

The airway is assessed for patency as before. Head positioning must avoid flexion or extension of the neck—eg, use jaw thrust rather than chin lift. The mouth and pharynx are suctioned free of blood, foreign material, or secretions, and loose teeth are removed. A nasopharyngeal or oropharyngeal airway is inserted if upper airway noises are heard or obstruction from posterior prolapse of the tongue occurs. A child with a depressed level of consciousness or a need for prolonged ventilation, hyperventilation, or operative intervention requires endotracheal intubation. Orotracheal intubation is possible without cervical spine manipulation and is the route of choice. Nasotracheal intubation may be possible in children 12 years or older with spontaneous respirations—if not contraindicated by midfacial injury with the possibility of cribriform plate disruption. Rarely, if tracheal intubation cannot be accomplished—particularly in the setting of massive midfacial trauma— cricothyroidotomy may be necessary. Needle cricothyroidotomy using a large-bore catheter through the cricothyroid membrane is the procedure of choice in the younger patient (< 12 years). Operative revision will be indicated for formal controlled tracheostomy.

Lateral, anterior-posterior, and odontoid x-rays of the cervical spine are obtained as soon as possible, keeping in mind that "normal" radiographs can miss fractures, significant ligamentous injuries, and significant spinal cord injuries.

Breathing

Most ventilatory problems are adequately resolved by the airway maneuvers described above and by positive-pressure ventilation. Breathing assessment is as described previously: One should assess for adequate and symmetric chest rise, increased work of breathing, color, tracheal deviation, deformity, or penetrating wounds. Sources of traumatic pulmonary compromise include pneumothorax, hemothorax, pulmonary contusion, flail segments, and central nervous system depression. Asymmetric breath sounds, particularly if tracheal deviation or bradycardia is present, suggest pneumothorax, probably under tension. To evacuate the pneumothorax, insert a large-bore catheter-over-needle attached to a syringe into the pleural cavity and withdraw air. If a pneumothorax or hemothorax was present, chest tube placement will follow. Insertion should be over the rib to avoid the neurovascular bundle, using the fourth intercostal space in the anterior axillary line. Open pneumothoraces can be treated temporarily by taping petrolatum-impregnated gauze on three sides over the wound, creating a flap valve.

Once airway and breathing have been stabilized, hemodynamic status may be addressed.

Circulation

Sudden, ongoing hemorrhage, external or occult, gives pediatric trauma some of its unique anxiety-provoking character. During the assessment of circulation, intravenous access should be achieved, preferably with two peripheral short, large-diameter catheters for optimal flow rates. If peripheral access is not readily available, a central line, cutdown, or intraosseous line should be established. A cardiorespiratory monitor should be applied early in the resuscitation. Blood pressure measurements should be recorded at frequent intervals. When establishing intravascular lines, samples for laboratory studies should be obtained, including hematocrit, blood type and crossmatch, liver function tests, and serum amylase.

External hemorrhage can generally be controlled by direct pressure. To avoid damage to adjoining nerves and vessels, one should avoid placing hemostats on vessels, except in the scalp.

Detection of the site of internal hemorrhage can be challenging. Sites include the chest, abdomen, retroperitoneum, pelvis, and thighs. Bleeding into the intracranial vault rarely causes shock in children except in infants. The aid of an experienced pediatric trauma surgeon and radiologic studies—principally double-contrast CT—are necessary for diagnosis of the site of internal bleeding.

Suspect cardiac tamponade after penetrating or crush injury to the chest if shock, narrowed pulse pressure, distended neck veins, hepatomegaly, or muffled heart sounds are present. Treatment is by volume infusion and pericardiocentesis.

Blood loss at the scene and ongoing losses should be replaced on a 3:1 basis with crystalloid solution. Total blood volume is 80 mL/kg; therefore, in a 10 kg child, 25% blood loss—sufficient to cause shock—is only 200 mL. Crystalloid replacement (ie, lactated Ringer's solution or normal saline) should therefore be 600 mL. Treat any signs of poor perfusion vigorously: A tachycardiac child with a capillary refill time of 3 seconds is *in shock and sustaining vital organ insults.* Remember that hypotension is a late finding. Volume replacement is initially accomplished by rapid infusion of isotonic crystalloid at 20 mL/kg of body weight, followed by 10 mL/kg of packed red blood cells if perfusion does not normalize after two crystalloid infusions.

Reassessment should be done rapidly following the initial bolus. If clinical signs of perfusion have not normalized, repeat the bolus. Lack of response or later signs of hypovolemia suggest the need for blood transfusion and possible surgical exploration.

A common problem is the brain-injured child who is at risk for cerebral edema and intracranial hypertension and who is also hypovolemic. In such cases, circulating volume must be restored to ensure adequate cerebral perfusion; therefore, fluid replacement is required until perfusion normalizes and fluid restriction may be instituted thereafter.

Disability

A brief neurologic examination is performed to assess pupillary size and reaction to light and the level of consciousness. The level of consciousness can be reproducibly characterized by the AVPU system (Table 14–4). Pediatric Glasgow Coma Scale assessments (Table 14–5) should be done as part of the secondary survey (see below). Changes in intracranial pressure or cerebral perfusion will eventually be reflected in changes in these scales.

Exposure

Significant injuries can be missed unless the child is completely undressed and examined fully, including the back, which calls for log-rolling the patient. Movement can be minimized by cutting away clothing as necessary. Because of their high ratio of surface area to body mass, infants and children cool rapidly. Because hypothermia compromises outcome, it

Table 14–4. AVPU system for evaluation of level of consciousness.

A	Alert
V	Responsive to *Voice*
P	Responsive to *Pain*
U	*Unresponsive*

Table 14–5. Glasgow Coma Scale.

Eye opening response	
Spontaneous	4
To speech	3
To pain	2
None	1
Verbal response	
Oriented	5
Confused conversation	4
Inappropriate words	3
Incomprehensible sounds	2
None	1
Best upper limb motor response	
Obeys	6
Localizes	5
Withdraws	4
Flexion in response to pain	3
Extension in response to pain	2
None	1

is necessary to monitor the body temperature and use warming techniques as necessary.

Monitoring

Cardiopulmonary monitors with pulse oximetry should be applied immediately. At the completion of the primary phase, additional "tubes" that should be placed are as follows:

A. Nasogastric or Orogastric Tube: Children's stomachs should be assumed to be full at all times, and gastric distention from positive-pressure ventilation increases the chance of vomiting and aspiration.

B. Urinary Catheter: An indwelling urinary bladder catheter should be placed to monitor urine output. Contraindications are based on the risk of urethral transection—signs include blood at the meatus or in the scrotum or a displaced prostate detected on rectal examination. Urine should be tested for blood. Urine output should exceed 1 mL/kg/h.

SECONDARY SURVEY

After the resuscitation phase, a head-to-toe examination should be performed to reveal all injuries and determine priorities for definitive care.

Skin

Search for lacerations, hematomas, swelling, and abrasions. Remove foreign material, and cleanse as necessary. Cutaneous signs may indicate underlying trauma (eg, a flank hematoma overlying a renal contusion), though surface signs may be absent with significant internal injury. Skin changes may evolve. Make certain that the child's tetanus immunization status is current.

Head

Check for hemotympanum and for clear or bloody discharge from the nares from cerebrospinal fluid leak. Battle's sign and raccoon eyes are late signs of basilar skull fracture. Explore wounds, excluding defects in galea or skull and foreign bodies. Closed head injury is most commonly encountered. CT scan of the head has become an integral part of evaluation for altered level of consciousness, seizure after trauma, or focal neurologic findings (see below).

Spine

Cervical spine injury must be ruled out in all but verbal, alert children who have no history of transient neurologic impairments, who can deny neck pain and tenderness to palpation, and who have a normal neurologic examination. Symmetric voluntary movement of the extremities must be observed. A cross-table neck radiograph is obtained initially, followed by anterior-posterior and odontoid views. "Normal" studies do not exclude significant injury, which can be bony, ligamentous, or of the spinal cord itself. The entire thoracolumbar spine must also be palpated and areas of pain or tenderness examined by radiography.

Chest

Pneumothoraces will be detected and decompressed during the primary survey. Hemothoraces can occur with rib fractures and intercostal vessel injury, large pulmonary vessel injury, or pulmonary laceration. Tracheobronchial disruption is suggested by large continued air leak despite chest tube decompression. With large energy transfer, pulmonary contusion can occur, requiring ventilatory support. Myocardial contusions are unusual in children.

Abdomen

Blunt abdominal injury is very common in multisystem injuries. Significant injury can exist without cutaneous signs or instability of vital signs. Tenderness, guarding, distention, lack of bowel sounds, or hemodynamic instability mandates immediate evaluation by a pediatric trauma surgeon. Injury to solid viscera frequently can be managed conservatively in hemodynamically stable patients; however, intestinal perforation or hypotension requires operative treatment. Serial examinations and CT scan—or, less often, diagnostic peritoneal lavage—provide diagnostic help. Elevated liver function tests have good specificity and fair sensitivity for hepatic injury.

Pelvis

Pelvic fractures are classically manifested as pain, crepitus, and abnormal motion. Pelvic fracture is a relative contraindication to urethral catheter insertion. Perform a rectal examination, noting prostate position in boys, tone, and tenderness. Stool should be tested for blood. Orthopedic consultation is indicated if pelvic fracture is suspected.

Genitourinary

If urethral transection is suspected (see above), perform a urethrogram before catheter placement. Diagnostic imaging of the child with hematuria is evolving, with CT scan becoming the modality of choice. Intravenous pyelograms are performed at some centers. Management of kidney injury is largely conservative except for renal pedicle injuries.

Extremities

Long bone fractures are common but rarely life-threatening. Test for pulses, perfusion, and sensation. Neurovascular compromise requires immediate orthopedic consultation. Careful palpation and serial examination will reveal orthopedic injuries requiring diagnostic imaging and treatment. Delayed diagnosis of fracture is not uncommon when children are comatose; reexamination is essential if one is to avoid missing previously occult fractures.

Neurologic

Because most children who die of multisystem trauma die of head injuries, the principles of neurointensive care are of primary concern in continued trauma care. Significant injuries include cerebral edema, subdural and epidural hematomas, parenchymal hemorrhages, and spinal cord injury. A full sensorimotor examination should be performed, noting pupillary size and extraocular movements. Deficits require immediate neurosurgical consultation. Extensor or flexor posturing implies intracranial hypertension (not seizure activity) until proved otherwise and should be treated with hyperventilation, adequate but not excessive volume resuscitation, and consideration of diuretics, usually mannitol. Normal peripheral perfusion must be assured before fluid restriction is started to optimize cerebral perfusion. Level of consciousness by the AVPU system or Glasgow Coma Scale (Tables 14–4 and 14–5) should be serially assessed. Seizure activity is uncommon in the child with severe injuries and warrants exclusion of significant intracranial injury. Acute spinal cord injury may benefit from high-dose methylprednisolone therapy. Steroids are not indicated in traumatic head injuries.

Aldrich EF et al: Diffuse brain swelling in severely head-injured children. J Neurosurg 1992;76:450.

Bracken MB et al: A randomized, controlled trial of methylprednisolone or naloxone in the treatment of acute spinal cord injury. N Engl J Med 1990;322:1405.

Jaffe D, Wesson D: Emergency management of blunt trauma in children. N Engl J Med 1991;324:1447.

Klem SA et al: Resource use, efficiency, and outcome prediction in pediatric intensive care of trauma patients. J Trauma 1990;30:32.

Moulton SL et al: Operative intervention for pediatric liver injuries: avoiding delays in treatment. J Pediatr Surg 1992;27:958.

Orenstein JB et al: Delayed diagnosis of pediatric cervical spine injury. Pediatrics 1992;89:1185.

Sahdev P et al: Evaluation of liver function tests in screening for intra-abdominal injuries. Ann Emerg Med 1991; 20:838.

Saladino R, Lund D, Fleisher G: The spectrum of liver and spleen injuries in children: Failure of the pediatric trauma score and clinical signs to predict isolated injuries. Ann Emerg Med 1991;20:636.

Trunkey DD (editor): Textbook of Advanced Trauma Life Support Course. American College of Surgeons Committee on Trauma, 1993.

Williams MD et al: Steroid use is associated with pneumonia in pediatric chest trauma. J Trauma 1992;32:520.

BURNS

Thermal injury is a major cause of accidental death and disfigurement in children. The pain, morbidity, association with child abuse, and the preventable nature of burns constitute an area of major concern in pediatrics. Common causes include hot water or food, appliances, flames, grills, and curling irons. Burns occur commonly in toddlers—in boys more frequently than in girls. The mortality rate for deep partial-thickness or full-thickness burns involving more than 30% of body surface area (BSA) approaches 30%.

Electrical Burns

Even brief contact with a high-voltage source will result in a contact burn. If an arc is created with passage of current through the body, the pattern of the thermal injury will depend on the path of the current; therefore, a thorough search should be made for an exit wound and intervening injuries. Extensive damage to deep tissues may occur. Current traversing the heart may cause nonperfusing dysrhythmias. Neurologic effects of electrical burns can be immediate, eg, confusion, disorientation, and peripheral nerve injury; secondary; or late, eg, impaired concentration or memory.

Electric cords are a common source of these injuries. Typically, an infant or toddler bites an electric cord, sustaining burns to the oral commissure that appear gray and necrotic, with surrounding erythema. Delayed coagulation around the mouth may occur, and as the burn heals, sloughing of eschar may lead to brisk bleeding.

Care of skin burns is as for other thermal injuries. Surgical revision may be necessary. Admission to hospital is generally indicated.

EVALUATION OF THE BURNED PATIENT

The nature of the burn, the extent and thickness of the burn, and associated injuries should be ascertained in the initial evaluation.

Classification

Burns are classified clinically according to the depth of thermal injury to the epidermis and dermis. **Superficial burns** are easily recognized and treated. They are painful, dry, red, and hypersensitive. Sunburn is a common example. Healing occurs with minimal damage to epidermis. At the other end of the spectrum are **full-thickness burns** affecting all epidermal and dermal elements, leaving avascular skin. The wound is dry, depressed, leathery in appearance, and without sensation. Unless skin grafting is provided, the scar will be hard, uneven, and fibrotic. **Partial-thickness burns** may be more difficult to recognize and treat. They are further classified as superficial or deep, depending on appearance and healing time, with each subgroup treated differently. Superficial partial-thickness burns are red and may blister. Deep partial-thickness burns are white, dry, blanch with pressure, and have decreased sensitivity to pain. This classification expands on the former system of first-, second-, and third-degree burns.

Management

Burn management depends on the depth and extent of thermal injury. Burn extent can be classified as major or minor. Minor burns are less than 10% BSA for superficial and partial-thickness burns, or less than 2% if full-thickness. Burns of the hands, feet, face, eyes, ears, and perineum are considered major.

A. Superficial and Partial-Thickness Burns: These injuries can generally be treated in the outpatient setting. Superficial burns are treated with cool compresses and analgesia. Treatment of partial-thickness burns with blisters consists of aseptic debridement, antiseptic cleansing, and topical antimicrobial coverage. Blisters appear early in deeper partial-thickness burns and if open should be debrided. After debridement, the wound should be cleansed with dilute (1–5%) povidone-iodine solution, thoroughly washed with normal saline, and covered with topical antibiotic, commonly silver sulfadiazine. The wound should be protected with a bulky dressing and reexamined within 24 hours and serially thereafter depending on the course. Wounds with a potential for causing loss of function or scarring—especially wounds of the hand or digits—should be promptly referred to a burn surgeon.

B. Full-Thickness and Deep or Extensive Partial-Thickness Burns: Major burns place particular importance on the ABCs of trauma management. Early establishment of an artificial airway is critical with oral or nasal burns because of their association with inhalation injuries and critical airway narrowing.

BURN RESUSCITATION PROTOCOL

- Secure the airway
- Administer 100% oxygen
- Assist ventilation if necessary
- Remove all clothing
- Stop the burning process
- Irrigate chemical burns
- Establish IV access
- Restore intravascular volume
- Perform complete examination

The trauma resuscitation protocol outlined on p 324 should be followed. One must not overlook the possibility of inhalation injury from carbon monoxide, cyanide, or other toxic products if flames were present. A nasogastric tube and bladder catheter should be placed. The secondary survey should ascertain if any other injuries are present, including those suggestive of abuse.

Fluid administration is based on several principles. Capillary permeability is markedly increased. Fluid needs are based on percentage of BSA burned, depth, and age. Maintaining normal intravascular pressure and replacing fluid losses are essential. Figure 14–8 shows percentages of BSA by body part in infants and children. The Parkland formula for fluid therapy is 4 mL/kg per percent BSA burned for the first 24 hours, with half in the first 8 hours, in addition to maintenance rates. Acutely, however, fluid resuscitation should be based on assessment of volume depletion as described above. Considerable literature exists concerning rates and tonicity of fluid administration, choice of crystalloid or colloid, and onset of enteral feeding.

Indications for admission include major burns as defined above; uncertainty of follow-up; suspicion of abuse; presence of upper airway injury; explosion, inhalation, electrical, or chemical burns; burns associated with fractures; or the need for parenteral pain control. Children with chronic metabolic or connective tissue diseases and infants deserve hospitalization.

Deitch EA: The management of burns. N Engl J Med 1990;323:1249.

Erickson et al: Differences in mortality from thermal injury between pediatric and adult patients. J Pediatr Surg 1991;26:821.

Gerding RL et al: Outpatient management of partial-thickness burns: Biobrane versus 1% silver sulfadiazine. Ann Emerg Med 1990;19:121

Joffe MD: Burns. In: *Textbook of Pediatric Emergency Medicine*, 3rd ed. Fleisher G, Ludwig S (editors). Williams & Wilkins, 1993.

Yamamoto LG et al: A one-year prospective ED cohort of pediatric burns: A proposal for standardizing scald burns. Pediatr Emerg Care 1991;7:80-84.

Infant Less Than One Year of Age

Name _____ Age _____ Ward _____

1st-degree erythema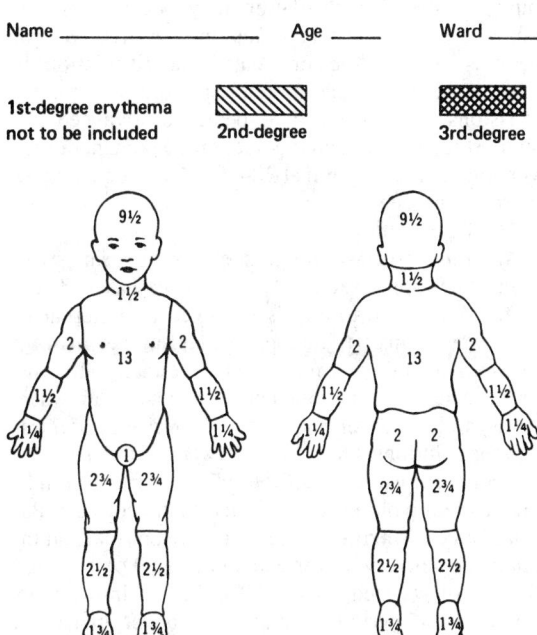
not to be included   2nd-degree   3rd-degree

Variations From Adult Distribution in Infants and Children (in Percent).

	New-born	1 Year	5 Years	10 Years
Head	19	17	13	11
Both thighs	11	13	16	17
Both lower legs	10	10	11	12
Neck	2			
Anterior trunk	13			
Posterior trunk	13			
Both upper arms	8	These percentages		
Both lower arms	6	remain constant at		
Both hands	5	all ages.		
Both buttocks	5			
Both feet	7			
Genitalia	1			
	100			

Figure 14–8. Lund and Browder modification of Berkow's scale for estimating extent of burns. (The table under the illustration is after Berkow.)

HEAT PROSTRATION

Heat injury and illness cover a spectrum from mild cramps to life-threatening heat stroke. **Heat cramps** are characterized by brief, severe cramping (not rigidity) of skeletal or abdominal muscles following exer-

tion. Heat cramps may be associated with a relative sodium deficiency. Core temperature is normal or only slightly elevated. Mild cases can be treated with oral salt-containing solutions; more severe cases require intravenous infusion of normal saline solution. **Heat exhaustion** is manifested by constitutional symptoms after exposure to heat and humidity. Patients continue to sweat, and core temperature is again normal or only slightly increased. Patients with heat exhaustion have varying proportions of salt and water depletion. Presenting symptoms and signs include weakness, fatigue, headache, disorientation, thirst, nausea and vomiting, and occasionally muscle cramps. Shock may be present. There should be no major central nervous system dysfunction. Treat with intravenous fluids, modified by measured electrolyte levels. Both heat cramps and heat exhaustion can be avoided with acclimatization and liberal water and salt intake during exercise.

Heat stroke represents failure of thermoregulation and is a life-threatening emergency. The diagnosis is based on a rectal temperature of over 40 °C with associated neurologic signs in a patient with an exposure history. Lack of sweating is *not* a necessary criterion. Symptoms are similar to those of heat exhaustion, but central nervous system dysfunction is more prominent. Patients with heat stroke are often incoherent and combative. In more severe cases, coma, seizures, nuchal rigidity, and posturing may be present. Patients can have high, low, or normal cardiac output. Cellular hypoxia, enzyme denaturation and inactivation, and disrupted cell membranes lead to global end-organ derangements: rhabdomyolysis, myocardial necrosis, acute tubular necrosis, hepatic degeneration, adult respiratory distress syndrome, and disseminated intravascular coagulation. Other complications include vomiting, shivering, sodium and potassium derangements, renal failure, and shock. *After* rapid cooling is begun (see below), consider infectious causes, malignant hyperthermia, and neuroleptic malignant syndrome in the differential diagnosis.

Heat Stroke Management

A. Remove patient from heat source and immediately cool body with cool water mist, ice, fans, etc.

B. Maintain the airway if comatose: ABCs.

C. Administer intravenous fluids: Isotonic fluid for hypotension, $D_5\frac{1}{2}NS$ for maintenance. Consider central venous pressure determination.

D. Institute monitoring and insert appropriate tubes: cardiac monitor, continuous rectal temperatures, Foley catheter, nasogastric tube, 100% oxygen.

E. Obtain laboratory tests: Complete blood count, electrolytes, glucose, creatinine, prothrombin time and partial thromboplastin time, creatine kinase, liver function tests, arterial blood gases, urinalysis, and serum calcium, magnesium, and phosphate.

F. Admit to pediatric intensive care unit.

Baker MD, et al: Household electrical injuries in children. Am J Dis Child 1989;143:59.

Thompson AE: Environmental emergencies. In: *Textbook of Pediatric Emergency Medicine,* 3rd ed. Fleisher GR, Ludwig S (editors). Williams & Wilkins, 1993.

Yarbrough B: Heat illness. In: *Emergency Medicine: Concepts and Clinical Practice,* 3rd ed. Rosen P et al (editor). Mosby, 1992.

HYPOTHERMIA

Hypothermia in children, defined as core temperature less than 35 °C, is frequently associated with cold water submersion accidents. Many other disorders cause incidental hypothermia, including sepsis, metabolic derangements, ingestions, central nervous system disorders, and endocrinopathies. Neonates, trauma victims, intoxicated patients, and the chronically disabled are particularly at risk. Diagnosis requires maintaining a high index of suspicion, particularly in temperate climates. Mortality rates are high and are related to the underlying disorder.

Core temperature normally is closely regulated and is a balance between heat loss and heat production. As core temperature falls, a variety of mechanisms begin to conserve and produce heat. Peripheral vasoconstriction allows optimal maintenance of core temperature. Heat production can be increased by a hypothalamic-mediated increase in muscle tone and metabolism. When shivering begins, heat production increases to two to four times basal levels.

Clinical Findings

Clinical manifestations of hypothermia depend on the severity of body temperature depression. Severe cases (< 28 °C) mimic death: Patients are pale or cyanotic, pupils may be fixed and dilated, muscles are rigid, and there may be no palpable pulses. Heart rates as low as 4–6/min may provide adequate perfusion, however, because of the lowered metabolic needs in severe hypothermia. If these findings are *primarily* a result of hypothermia and not postmortem changes, the fact of death cannot be ascertained until the patient has been rewarmed and remains unresponsive to resuscitative efforts. Children with a core temperature as low as 19 °C have survived neurologically intact.

Treatment

A. General Supportive Measures: Management is complex but largely supportive. One must document hypothermia by continuously monitoring with a low-reading rectal thermometer. Patients must be handled gently, since the hypothermic myocar-

dium is exquisitely sensitive and prone to dysrhythmias. Ventricular fibrillation may occur spontaneously or as a result of minor handling or invasive procedures. If asystole or ventricular fibrillation is present on the cardiac monitor, perform chest compressions and use standard pediatric advanced life support techniques and medications. Spontaneous reversion to sinus rhythm at 28–30 °C may occur as rewarming proceeds.

B. Rewarming:

1. *Passive* rewarming, such as covering with blankets, is appropriate only for mild cases (> 33 °C).

2. *Active* rewarming is achieved by external or core rewarming techniques. **External rewarming** methods include warming lights, thermal mattresses or electric warming blankets, immersion in warm baths, and hot water bottles or warmed bags of intravenous solutions. One must be aware of the potential for core temperature "afterdrop" as warmed peripheral acidemic blood is distributed to the core circulation. **Core rewarming** techniques are optimal and include the delivery of warmed, humidified oxygen and the use of warmed (to 40 °C) fluids for intravenous replacement, peritoneal dialysis, bladder irrigation, and, in severe cases, mediastinal lavage. When available and in life-threatening cases, hemodialysis and extracorporeal blood rewarming achieve controlled core rewarming, can stabilize volume and electrolyte disturbances, and are maximally effective. (See Table 14–6.)

Bolte RG et al: The use of extracorporeal rewarming in a child submerged for 66 minutes. JAMA 1988;260:377.

Gentilello LM et al: Continuous arteriovenous rewarming: Rapid reversal of hypothermia in critically ill patients. J Trauma 1992;32:316.

Table 14–6. Management of hypothermia.

General measures
- Administer warmed and humidified 100% oxygen.
- Monitor core temperature, heart and respiratory rates, and blood pressure continuously.
- Consider central venous pressure determination.

Laboratory studies
- Complete blood count.
- Serum electrolytes, glucose, creatinine, amylase.
- Prothrombin time, partial thromboplastin time.
- Arterial blood gases.
- Consider toxicology screen.

Treatment
- Correct hypoxemia, hypercapnia, pH < 7.2, clotting abnormalities, and glucose and electrolyte disturbances.
- Start rewarming techniques: passive, active (core and external), depending on degree of hypothermia.
- Replace intravascular volume with intravenous normal saline or lactated Ringer's injection at 43 ÉC.
- Treat asystole and ventricular fibrillation per ALS protocols. Cardiac massage should be continued at least until core temperature reaches 30 ÉC, when defibrillation is more likely to be effective.

Iversen RJ et al: Successful CPR in a severely hypothermic patient using continuous thoracostomy lavage. Ann Emerg Med 1990;19:1335.

Thompson AE: Environmental emergencies. In: *Textbook of Pediatric Emergency Medicine,* 3rd ed. Fleisher GR, Ludwig S:(editors). Williams & Wilkins,1993.

Weinberg AD: Hypothermia. Ann Emerg Med 1993;22:370.

HEAD INJURY

Closed head injury is a frequent cause of Emergency Department visits. Injuries range from minor asymptomatic head injuries without sequelae to intracranial hemorrhage and subsequent death. Head injury, including the shaken-baby syndrome, is common in child abuse. Most deaths following multiple trauma are from head injury. Even following minor closed head injury, many parents are concerned about neurologic sequelae.

Children may be classified clinically at the time of initial evaluation as having mild, moderate, or severe head injury (see Table 14–7).

Assessment

The considerations discussed above in the care of the trauma patient apply here. The history should include the time and mechanism of injury. How far did the child fall and onto what surface? Was there loss of consciousness? Does the child remember events preceding, during, and following the injury? What have been the levels of consciousness and activity since the injury? Has there been vomiting, headache, or diplopia?

The physical examination should be complete, keeping in mind the mechanism of injury, and should include a detailed neurologic examination. One should look for associated injuries such as mandibular fracture, scalp or skull injury, or cervical spine in-

jury. Cerebrospinal fluid leak from the ears or nose, or the two later appearing signs of periorbital hematomas (raccoon eyes) and Battle's sign imply a basilar skull fracture. Obtain vital signs and assess the level of consciousness by the AVPU system (Table 14–4) or by the Glasgow Coma scale (Table 14–5) in children over 3 years of age, noting irritability or lethargy; pupillary equality, size, and reaction to light; funduscopic examination; reflexes; body posture; and rectal tone. The injuries observed should be consistent with the history.

Radiographic studies may be indicated. Plain films are useful chiefly for assessing depressed skull fractures or penetrating head trauma. Major morbidity does not stem from skull fracture per se but rather from the associated intracranial injury. The presence of a skull fracture on plain films increases the likelihood of finding a serious intracranial injury demonstrated by CT scanning. There is no uniform agreement on indications for obtaining a CT scan. CT scan should be performed in the child with a history of significant impact or with an abnormal or lateralizing neurologic examination, including an abnormal mental status that does not quickly return to normal.

CONCUSSION

A concussion injury is defined as a brief loss or alteration of consciousness followed by a return to the normal state. There is no anatomic damage to brain tissue. There may be pallor, amnesia, or several episodes of vomiting. There are no focal findings on detailed neurologic examination. Disposition is based on the clinical course and suitability of follow-up. If the level of consciousness is normal or improving, the patient may be discharged when neurologically normal after a period of observation. Parents should assess the child at home every 3–4 hours for the first 24–36 hours, and return if the child exhibits altered level of consciousness, persistent vomiting, gait disturbances, unequal pupils, seizures, or increasing headache, or if the parents have any concerns.

CONTUSION

A bruise—which implies local hemorrhage, usually minimal—of the brain matter is a contusion. There is a decrease in level of consciousness, and focal findings are present that correspond to the area of brain injured. These patients require CT scan, admission for observation, and consideration of neurosurgical consultation.

Table 14–7. Clinical classification of head-injured patients.[1]

Mild	No loss of consciousness or amnesia. Alert and oriented. Asymptomatic or with only slight headache and dizziness.
Moderate	Possible findings: history of loss of consciousness, amnesia; posttraumatic seizures, vomiting, more than slight headache, listlessness, lethargy.
Severe	Possible findings: disoriented, unable to follow commands, decreasing level of consciousness, focal neurologic signs, penetrating skull injury or depressed skull fracture.

[1]Reproduced, with permission, from: Rosenthal BW, Bergman I: Intracranial injury after moderate head trauma in children. J Pediatr 1989;115:346.

ACUTE INTRACRANIAL HYPERTENSION

Close observation by medical and nursing personnel will detect early signs and symptoms of intracranial pressure elevation. Early recognition is essential in avoiding disastrous outcomes. Serious intracranial pathology after closed head injury includes subdural or epidural hematomas, parenchymal hemorrhage, diffuse axonal injury, and cerebral edema. In addition to traumatic causes, intracranial pressure elevation with or without herniation syndromes may be seen in spontaneous intracranial hemorrhage, central nervous system infection, hydrocephalus, ruptured arteriovenous malformation, metabolic derangement (eg, diabetic ketoacidosis), or tumor. Symptoms include headache, diplopia, vomiting, agitation, gait difficulties, and a progressively decreasing level of consciousness. Other signs include stiff neck, cranial nerve palsies, and progressive hemiparesis. Cushing's triad (bradycardia, hypertension, and irregular respirations) is a late and pre-arrest finding. Papilledema is also a *late* finding. Lumbar puncture should never be performed before CT scan if there is concern about intracranial pressure elevation because of the risk of precipitating herniation.

Therapy for intracranial pressure elevation must be swift and aggressive. Strict attention to the ABCs is paramount. Controlled rapid sequence intubation with appropriate sedation, muscle relaxation, and agents to reduce the ICP elevation that accompanies is followed by hyperventilation and avoidance of hypoxemia. These measures effectively reduce cerebral blood flow and acutely lowers ICP. (See Figure 14–9.) Normal arterial blood pressure and peripheral perfusion should be maintained by fluid infusion and pressors if necessary. Adjunctive measures include elevating the head of the bed 30 degrees, treating hyperpyrexia and pain, and maintaining the head in a midline position. Mannitol (0.5 g/kg intravenously), an osmotic diuretic, will reduce brain water, as will furosemide (1–2 mg/kg intravenously). Obtain immediate neurosurgical evaluation.

Further details about management of intracranial hypertension (cerebral edema) are presented in Chapter 12.

DISPOSITION FOR CHILDREN WITH CLOSED HEAD INJURY

Patients with mild head injury as defined in Table 14–7 may be discharged with detailed written instructions—after a period of brief observation—if the examination remains normal and parental supervision and follow-up are appropriate. Some children with moderate head injury will require admission or prolonged observation. Obtain CT scans in children with focal neurologic examinations, persistent vomiting, or those who have a persistently depressed level of consciousness. If the patient responds to voice commands and mental status is gradually improving over a period of several hours, in-hospital observation may be done without further radiographic studies. If the mental status deteriorates, however, CT scan and neurosurgical consultation are indicated. If the CT scan is normal and if the physical findings normalize, these children may also be discharged after a period of observation.

Clearly, patients with severe head injury will require cerebral resuscitation, evaluation by a neurosurgeon, and admission to hospital.

Aldrich EF et al: Diffuse brain swelling in severely head-injured children. J Neurosurg 1992;76:450.

Pigula FA et al: The effect of hypotension and hypoxia on children with severe head injuries. J Pediatr Surg 1993; 28:310.

Pons P: Head trauma. In: *Emergency Medicine: Concepts and Clinical Practice,* 3rd ed. Rosen P et al (editors). Mosby, 1992.

Rosenthal BW, Bergman I: Intracranial injury after moderate head trauma in children. J Pediatr 1989;115:346.

Tepas JJ 3rd et al: Mortality and head injury: The pediatric perspective. J Pediatr Surg 1990;25:92.

Yamamoto LG et al: Rapid sequence anesthesia for emergency intubation. Pediatr Emerg Care 1990;6:200.

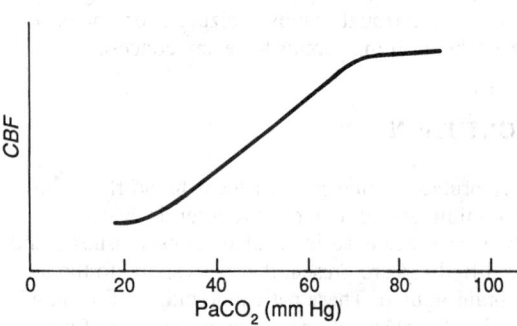

Figure 14–9. Relationship of cerebral blood flow to intracranial pressure. (Reproduced, with permission, from: Silverman BK [editor]: *Textbook of Advanced Pediatric Life Support.* APLS Joint Task Force: American College of Emergency Physicians/American Academy of Pediatrics, 1989.)

DROWNING
(See also Chapter 15.)

Drowning is the second most common cause of death by unintentional injury among children. Water hazards are ubiquitous and include lakes and streams, swimming pools, bathtubs and hot tubs, drainage ditches and culverts, construction site excavations, and even toilets, buckets, and washing machines. Risk factors include epilepsy, alcohol, intentional trauma, and lack of supervision. Males predominate in submersion deaths, as in most other accidental deaths. All pediatricians must make efforts to prevent these needless tragedies.

Submersion incidents are classified according to outcome: drowning accidents are those with death occurring within 24 hours; survival for over 24 hours constitutes near-drowning. Major morbidity stems from pulmonary and central nervous system insult. Fresh water aspiration results in pulmonary surfactant disruption and membrane leak, with subsequent pulmonary edema. Salt-water aspiration creates an osmotic gradient for the influx of water into the lungs. However, the type of water aspirated generally has little clinical significance. Not all submersion accidents lead to aspiration. Laryngospasm or breath-holding may lead to loss of consciousness and cardiovascular collapse before aspiration can occur.

Anoxia from laryngospasm or aspiration leads to irreversible central nervous system damage after only 4–6 minutes. Only if immersion hypothermia rapidly *precedes* anoxic damage is there a protective effect from cold water submersion. In practical terms, the child must fall through ice or directly into icy water for cerebral metabolism to slow quickly enough to be protective against hypoxemia.

Cardiovascular changes include myocardial depression and dysrhythmias. Electrolyte alterations are generally slight. Unless hemolysis occurs, hemoglobin concentrations also change only slightly.

Assessment & Management

Depending on the duration of submersion and any protective hypothermia effects, children may appear clinically dead or completely normal. Observation over time assists with prognosis. The normothermic apneic and pulseless child in the Emergency Department will probably not survive to discharge, or be left with severe neurologic deficits. Until a determination of brain death can be made, however, aggressive resuscitation is appropriate.

The trauma-related ABCDEs should be followed as described above. One should keep in mind possible associated injuries, such as the adolescent who dives into shallow water, sustaining neck injury. It is essential as always to ensure a patent airway. Unconscious patients should be intubated. Normal oxygenation and ventilation must be maintained and metabolic acidosis treated as appropriate. Poor perfusion should be treated with boluses of intravenous fluid, or pressors if necessary. Core temperature should be monitored continuously with a low-reading rectal thermometer.

For children who appear well initially, observation

for 12–24 hours will detect late decompensation in gas exchange. An abnormal chest radiograph, abnormal arterial blood gases, or hypoxemia by pulse oximetry indicates the need for treatment with supplemental oxygen, cardiopulmonary monitoring, and frequent reassessment. The degree of respiratory distress and the mental status must be serially assessed. Signs of pulmonary infection may appear many hours after the submersion event.

Patients who are in coma and who require mechanical ventilation have a high risk of anoxic encephalopathy. The value of therapy with hyperventilation, steroids, intentional hypothermia, and barbiturates continues to be debated.

Nichter MA, Everett PB: Childhood near-drowning: Is cardiopulmonary resuscitation always indicated? Crit Care Med 1989;17:993.

Quan L: Drowning issues in resuscitation. Ann Emerg Med 1993; 22(Part 2):366.

Quan L, Kinder D: Pediatric submersions: Prehospital predictors of outcome. Pediatrics 1992;90:909.

Yamamoto LG et al: A one-year series of pediatric ED water- related injuries: The Hawaii EMS-C project. Pediatr Emerg Care 1992;8:129.

BITES & STINGS

MAMMALIAN BITES

Bites account for a large number of Emergency Department visits. Most fatalities are due to dog bites. However, the majority of infected bite wounds are from human and cat bites.

Dog Bites

Boys are bitten more frequently than girls, and the dog is known by the victim in the vast majority of cases. Younger children have a higher incidence of head and neck wounds, whereas school-age children are bit most often on the upper extremities.

Dog bites are cared for in a similar fashion to other wounds: high-pressure, high-volume irrigation with normal saline, debridement of any devitalized tissue and removal of foreign matter, and tetanus prophylaxis. The risk of rabies is low in developed countries, but rabies prophylaxis should be considered when appropriate. Wounds should be sutured only if necessary for cosmetic reasons. Prophylactic antibiotics have not been shown to decrease rates of infection in low-risk dog bite wounds not involving the hands or feet. If a bite involves a joint, periosteum, or neurovascular bundle, prompt orthopedic surgery consultation should be obtained.

Pathogens that infect dog bites include *Pasteurella*

multocida, streptococci, staphylococci, and anaerobes. Infected dog bites can be treated with penicillin for *P multocida,* or broad-spectrum coverage can be provided by amoxicillin and clavulanic acid. Complications of dog bites include central nervous system infections, septic arthritis, osteomyelitis, endocarditis, and sepsis.

Cat Bites

Cat-inflicted wounds occur more frequently in girls, with infection being the primary form of morbidity. Wound management is similar to that for dog bites. Cat wounds should not be sutured except when absolutely necessary for cosmetic reasons. Cat bites create a puncture-wound inoculum, and prophylactic antibiotics are recommended. *P multocida* is the most common pathogen.

Infected cat bites are treated with antibiotics as mentioned for dog bites. Complications include cat scratch disease, cellulitis, septic arthritis, tenosynovitis, and osteomyelitis.

Human Bites

Most human bites occur during assaults. *P multocida* is not a known pathogen in human bites. Cultures most commonly grow streptococci, anaerobes, staphylococci, and *Eikenella corrodens.* Hand wounds and deep wounds should be treated with coverage against *E corrodens* and gram-positives by a penicillinase-resistant penicillin. Wound management is the same as for dog bites. Only severe lacerations involving the face should be sutured. Other wounds can be managed by delayed primary closure or healing by second intention.

A major complication of human bite wounds is infection of the metacarpophalangeal joints. Clenched-fist injuries from human bites (as from fistfights) should be evaluated by a hand surgeon. Operative debridement is followed in many cases by intravenous antibiotics.

Avner JR et al: Dog bites in urban children. Pediatrics 1991;88:55.

Dire DJ: Cat bite wounds: Risk factors for infection. Ann Emerg Med 1991;20:973.

Leung AKC et al: Human bites in children. Pediatr Emerg Care 1992;8:255.

Zubowicz VN et al: Management of early human bites of the hand: A prospective randomized study. Plast Reconstr Surg 1991;88:111.

INSECT STINGS & ARTHROPOD BITES

Children are frequently stung by insects, only a few of which are potentially hazardous. Most insect stings are from bees, wasps, and ants. Biting arthropods include insects, spiders, scorpions, ticks, mites, centipedes, and millipedes.

Clinical Findings

A. Insect Stings: Bee and wasp stings lead to immediate local pain, with variable redness, swelling, and later itching. Many children have pronounced local reactions with swelling. These reactions can become greater with successive stings.

The most serious sequela of sting is **anaphylaxis.** Onset of symptoms is from 15 minutes to 6 hours after the sting, with symptoms of urticaria, bronchospasm, respiratory distress, upper airway obstruction, hypotension, and vascular collapse. Treatment is described below. Delayed reactions such as serum sickness are possible.

B. Spider Bites: Serious envenomations from **spider bites** are associated with only a few species, including the black widow and brown recluse spiders, tarantulas, and other much less common species. Black widows and brown recluse spiders account for the vast majority of deaths due to spider bites.

1. Black widow spider bites–Children may not notice the bite. Mild local erythema and edema may progress to significant symptoms within 60 minutes. Ensuing pain may be severe in regional lymph nodes or local muscle groups. Classically, severe cramping pains of the abdomen, thorax, and back ensue. Pain is intense, and the patient will be quite anxious. Hypertension and other sympathomimetic symptoms may occur.

2. Brown recluse spider bites–Brown recluse spider bites characteristically occur indoors in the warmer months. Again, the victim may not be aware of the initial bite or may feel a mild pinprick sensation. A latent period presages local symptoms of itching, redness, and tenderness at the site, with a classic target lesion appearance. This may progress to an enlarging macular lesion that forms a necrotic central region covered by eschar, which may heal very slowly. Systemic symptoms may be delayed up to 72 hours and include headache, fever, chills, malaise, and other systemic symptoms. Intravascular hemolysis has been reported in children.

Treatment

A. Anaphylaxis: Regardless of the source of envenomation, **anaphylaxis** is the one life-threatening emergency that must be treated aggressively.

Anaphylaxis treatment consists initially of subcutaneous epinephrine, 0.01 mL/kg of 1:1000 solution, up to 0.5 mL. If upper airway obstruction from edema is evolving, early intubation should be performed. Volume infusion and pressor support may be necessary. Bronchospasm is treated with nebulized beta-adrenergic agents by inhalation. Give 100% oxygen. Anaphylaxis kits and referral to an allergist should be considered for children who have had systemic symptoms and are at high risk. Ensure that these patients are aware of EMS access through 911.

B. Local Treatment: The vast majority of stings can be treated with first aid measures such as cool compresses and elevation. The site of bee and wasp stings should be cleansed locally with skin disinfectant. Give tetanus prophylaxis if needed.

C. General Supportive Treatment: Oral antihistamines can be useful to control swelling and itching. Low-grade allergic symptoms should be treated with diphenhydramine, 1–2 mg/kg intramuscularly or orally. Generalized urticaria, wheezing, chest or throat tightness, syncope, or dizziness call for epinephrine subcutaneously. Establish intravenous access and give 100% oxygen. Treat hypotension with crystalloid solution or with pressors if unresponsive. Residual wheezing can be treated in the usual fashion with inhaled agents.

Patients with moderate to severe systemic symptoms should be admitted to hospital.

Spider bite therapy is supportive. Black widow antivenom is available but has significant side effects. Diazepam and calcium are sometimes used. Centipede and millipede envenomations are treated symptomatically.

Clark RF et al: Clinical presentation and treatment of black widow spider envenomation: A review of 163 cases. Ann Emerg Med 1992;21:782–787.

Eitzen EM Jr, Seward PN: Arthropod envenomations in children. Pediatr Emerg Care 1988;4:266.

Hodge D, Tecklenburg FW: Bites and stings. In: *Textbook of Pediatric Emergency Medicine.* 3rd ed. Fleisher G, Ludwig S (editors). Williams & Wilkins, 1993.

Rees R et al: The diagnosis and treatment of brown recluse spider bites. Ann Emerg Med 1987;16:9.

SNAKE BITES

About one-fourth of all snake bites are from venomous species, principally pit vipers (the Crotalidae) and coral snakes (Elapidae families). The latter have distinctive ring color sequences, with poisonous species have yellow (not black) rings adjacent to red rings, giving rise to the saying, "Red on black, friend of Jack; red on yellow, kill a fellow."

Tissue destruction from envenomation is from peptides and enzymes, leading to systemic and local signs and symptoms, including swelling, ecchymosis, severe pain, hemorrhagic blebs and bullae, paresthesias, fasciculations, and paralysis, especially of the cranial nerves. In severe cases, shock, hemolysis, and pulmonary edema may occur/

Treatment is largely supportive, but antivenom is available. Consult with regional resources such as the Tucson Poison Control Center (1-602-626-6016).

Jansen PW et al: Mojave rattlesnake envenomation: Prolonged neurotoxicity and rhabdomyolysis. Ann Emerg Med 1992;21:322–325.

15

Critical Care

Emily L. Dobyns, MD, Anthony G. Durmowicz, MD, Desmond B. Henry, MD,
Stanley Loftness, MD, and Kurt R. Stenmark, MD

INTRODUCTION

Pediatric critical care has evolved into a sub-specialty devoted to the understanding of the patho-physiology of life-threatening diseases and to the development of technical facilities for monitoring and treating these patients. It encompasses many aspects of physiology, pharmacology, and medicine as they relate to critical care issues and therefore is a multi-disciplinary and multiprofessional field. The patients often require the attention of multiple specialized services such as an emergency transport service, stabilization in the Emergency Department, operative treatment, and nutritional support. It is the high level of interdisciplinary collaboration and communication that have improved patient survival in the ICU.

Children are not small adults and have unique care requirements. They are resilient and have tremendous recovery potential. They have healthy cardiovascular systems and recover from injuries that adults would not survive. They may be nonverbal, uncooperative, and unable to understand their illness or the hospital environment, and thus may require the services provided by social workers, psychiatrists, physical therapists, and speech therapists to help their families and themselves cope with their illness. The dynamic features of continuing growth and development (unique features of pediatrics) must always be factored into the patient and family needs.

The pediatric intensive care unit provides the specialized environment, equipment, and specialists needed to evaluate, diagnose, and treat critically ill patients on a 24-hour basis. This unit permits close observation by experienced team members, thereby permitting rapid responses to changes in the patients' acuity. In many cases these changes can be anticipated and management plans altered accordingly.

American Academy of Pediatrics: Committee on Hospital Care. Guidelines and levels of care for pediatric intensive care units. Crit Care Med 1993;21:1077.

Hazinski MF: Physician-nurse interaction in the paediatric intensive care unit. In: *Textbook of Pediatric Critical Care*. Holbrook PR, editor. Saunders, 1993.

Pollack MM: Outcome analysis. In: *Textbook of Pediatric Critical Care*. Holbrook PR, editor. Saunders, 1993.

ACRONYMS USED IN THIS CHAPTER	
ARDS	Adult respiratory distress syndrome
CPAP	Constant positive airway pressure
CPR	Cardiopulmonary resuscitation
ECG	Electrocardiogram
ECMO	Extracorporeal membrane oxygenation
EEG	Electroencephalogram
FEV_1	Forced expiratory volume in 1 second
FRC	Functional residual capacity
ICP	Intracranial pressure
ICU	Intensive care unit
IMV	Intermittent mandatory ventilation
MAP	Mean arterial pressure
NSAID	Nonsteroidal anti-inflammatory drug
PDGF	Platelet-derived growth factor
PEEP	Positive end-expiratory pressure
PEFR	Peak expiratory flow rate
PICU	Pediatric intensive care unit
SIMV	Synchronized intermittent mandatory ventilation
TGF	Tumor growth factor

Pollack MM et al: Improved outcomes from tertiary center pediatric intensive care. Crit Care Med 1991;19:150.

ACUTE RESPIRATORY FAILURE

Respiratory failure is defined as inability of the respiratory system to deliver adequate oxygen or to remove CO_2 from the pulmonary circulation, thereby leading to arterial hypoxia, hypercapnia, or both. It is a relatively common problem in infants and children and accounts for approximately 50% of all deaths of children under 1 year of age. Infants are at higher risk for respiratory failure because of physiologic, anatomic, and mechanical differences between their respiratory systems and those of adults. In infants, the thoracic cage is soft and therefore provides an unstable base for the ribs. Intercostal muscles are poorly developed, and children therefore cannot achieve the classic bucket handle motion that characterizes adult breathing. Furthermore, the diaphragm is less effective in infants because it is relatively flat and short and has fewer type I muscle fibers. During REM sleep, the ventilatory movements of the rib cage become uncoordinated and out of phase with those of the diaphragm. The infant's trachea is small, only one-third the diameter of the adult trachea. Therefore, according to Poiseuille's law, a 1-mm thickening of the respiratory mucosa in an infant causes a 75% reduction in cross-sectional area in the infant airway, compared to only a 20% reduction in the adult airway. Lastly, children's alveoli are smaller and have less collateral ventilation with fewer pores of Kohn, resulting in a greater tendency for the alveolus to collapse and thus cause atelectasis.

Respiratory failure can be classified into two types, though it should be remembered that pediatric patients with respiratory failure usually display a variable combination of the two. Patients with **type I** respiratory failure generally have a low PaO_2 with a normal to low $PaCO_2$; **type II** patients have a low PaO_2 with a high $PaCO_2$. Type I is the failure of the lung to oxygenate the blood and occurs in three situations: (1) The most frequent cause is a **ventilation/perfusion defect** (V/Q mismatch), which occurs when blood flows to parts of the lung that are poorly ventilated or underventilated, ie, when blood flow and alveolar ventilation are mismatched. (2) **Diffusion defects** result from disturbances such as a thickened alveolar membrane or a buildup of interstitial fluid at the alveolar-capillary junction. (3) **Intrapulmonary shunt** occurs when blood flows through areas of the lung that are never ventilated.

Type II respiratory failure, characterized by a high $PaCO_2$ and a low PaO_2, can be viewed as respiratory "pump" failure and is generally the result of alveolar hypoventilation and not of a primary disease of the lung. Numerous disease processes can contribute to this hypoventilation (Table 15–1). It is important to remember that hypoxemia is not always related to respiratory failure. Right-to-left cardiac shunts, high al-

titude with its low ambient oxygen concentration, and the production of methemoglobin all may produce severe hypoxemia with normal respiratory function.

Clinical Findings

A. Symptoms and Signs: The clinical findings in respiratory failure are determined by the adverse effects of low oxygen and high CO_2 in arterial blood gas tensions (PaO_2 and $PaCO_2$) and pH on the function of susceptible organ systems, chiefly the lung, heart, kidneys, and brain. As respiratory failure ensues, physical findings such as tachypnea, retractions, cyanosis, restlessness, or even somnolence can be seen (Table 15–2). The hypoxemia or hypercapnia that results from ventilation/perfusion mismatch, shunt, or hypoventilation may interfere with brain metabolism, depress the myocardium, or cause pulmonary hypertension. Hypercapnia depresses the central nervous system, and the resulting acidemia depresses myocardial function. Thus, patients in respiratory failure can exhibit significant changes in central nervous system and cardiac function (Table 15–2). It is important to realize that the manifestations of respiratory failure are not always clinically evident and that some signs or symptoms may be due to nonrespiratory causes. Furthermore, a strictly clinical assessment of arterial hypoxemia or hypercapnia is not reliable. Thus, precise assessment of oxygenation and ventilatory adequacy must be based on both clinical and laboratory data.

B. Laboratory Findings: Laboratory findings are often helpful in gauging the severity and acuity of respiratory failure. The **pulse oximeter** determines arterial saturation by measuring differences in absorption of light by oxygenated and reduced hemoglobin in pulsatile blood flow. Therefore, arterial oxygen saturation can be measured continuously and noninvasively. Pulse oximetry may be affected by

Table 15–1. Types of respiratory failure.

Findings	Causes	Examples
Type I Hypoxia Decreased PaO_2 Normal $PaCO_2$	Ventilation/perfusion defect	Positional (supine in bed), ARDS, atelectasis, pneumonia, pulmonary embolus, bronchopulmonary dysplasia.
	Diffusion impairment	Pulmonary edema, ARDS, interstitial pneumonia.
	Shunt	Pulmonary arteriovenous malformation, congenital adenomatoid malformation.
Type II Hypoxia Hypercapnia Decreased PaO_2 Increased $PaCO_2$	Hypoventilation	Neuromuscular disease (polio, Guillain-Barré syndrome), head trauma, sedation, chest wall dysfunction (burns), kyphosis, severe reactive airways.

Table 15–2. Clinical criteria for respiratory failure.

Respiratory
 Wheezing
 Expiratory grunting
 Decreased or absent breath sounds
 Flaring of alae nasi
 Retractions of chest wall
 Tachypnea, bradypnea, or apnea
 Cyanosis
Cerebral
 Restlessness
 Irritability
 Headache
 Confusion
 Convulsions
 Coma
Cardiac
 Bradycardia or excessive tachycardia
 Hypotension or hypertension
General
 Fatigue
 Sweating

poor perfusion, hyperbilirubinemia, severe anemia, methemoglobinemia, and hypercapnia. It should be routinely used in the assessment and management of all patients with suspected respiratory failure. Capnography provides a continuous noninvasive measure of $PaCO_2$. End-tidal CO_2 ($ETCO_2$) approximates alveolar CO_2. $ETCO_2$ may be falsely lowered in severe respiratory disease due to increased dead space. Despite this limitation, $ETCO_2$ provides a trend for assessing the disease process over time. Owing to this discrepancy and the ongoing need to assess the acid base status of the patient, **arterial blood gas measurement** remains the best means for assessment of acute respiratory failure. Arterial blood gases give information on the acid-base status (with a measured pH and calculated bicarbonate level) as well as information on the status of oxygenation (PaO_2) and ventilation ($PaCO_2$) in the patient. The $PaCO_2$ is a sensitive measure of ventilation and is inversely related to the minute ventilation (Figure 15–1). Knowing the arterial blood gas values and the inspired oxygen concentration enables one to calculate several parameters that may be helpful in determining the efficiency of gas exchange. The difference between alveolar oxygen concentration and the arterial oxygen value is the **alveolar-arterial oxygen difference** ($AaDO_2$). The $AaDO_2$ is less than 15 mm Hg under normal conditions, and it increases with increasing inspired oxygen concentrations to about 100 mm Hg in normal patients breathing 100% oxygen. Diffusion impairment, shunts, and ventilation/perfusion mismatches all cause increased $AaDO_2$ (Table 15–3).

In addition to the calculation of the $AaDO_2$, assessment of the intrapulmonary shunting of blood may be

helpful. The intrapulmonary shunt is that percentage of pulmonary blood flow which passes through nonventilated areas of the lung. It has the same effect as a right-to-left cardiac shunt in that oxygen saturations are lowered as shunting increases. Normal individuals have less than a 5% physiologic shunt from bronchial, thebesian, and coronary circulations. Shunt fractions greater than 15% usually indicate the need for aggressive respiratory support. When intrapulmonary shunt reaches 50% of pulmonary blood flow, PaO_2 does not increase regardless of the amount of supplemental oxygen used.

Dead space ventilation is that part of the breath in the conducting air passages plus the alveolar volume which is ventilated but not perfused by the pulmonary circulation. Dead space ventilation is increased in bronchopulmonary dysplasia, V/Q mismatches, pulmonary interstitial emphysema, pulmonary embolism, and many other entities. Decreasing dead space ventilation depends on its cause, but such methods as tracheostomy in patients with chronic respiratory failure or streptokinase therapy in persons with pulmonary emboli are examples.

Treatment

A. Oxygen Supplementation: Patients with hypoxemia induced by respiratory failure may respond to supplemental oxygen administration alone (Table 15–4). Those with hypoventilation and diffusion defects respond better than patients with shunts or V/Q mismatches. Severe V/Q mismatches often do not respond to anything but aggressive airway management and mechanical ventilation. Patients with a decreased functional residual capacity (FRC)—the amount of air left in the lungs at the end of passive expiration—often respond to the delivery of continuous positive airway pressure (CPAP), 5–10 cm H_2O by either mask or endotracheal tube. This improves oxygenation by increasing FRC to above closing capacity (closing capacity is the combination of the expiratory reserve volume and closing volume and represents the volume that the FRC must exceed during tidal breathing to prevent closure of airways). Patients with severe hypoxemia, hypoventilation, or apnea require assistance with bag and mask ventilation until the airway is intubated. Ventilation may be maintained for some time with a mask of the proper size, but gastric distention, emesis, and inadequate tidal volumes are possible complications. In patients who fail to respond to simple oxygen supplementation, establishment of an artificial airway is often lifesaving.

B. Intubation: Intubation of the trachea in infants and children requires experienced personnel and the right equipment. Details of the steps involved are included in all advanced life support courses and are outlined only briefly here. A patient in respiratory failure whose airway must be stabilized requires many interventions before the actual intubation. The

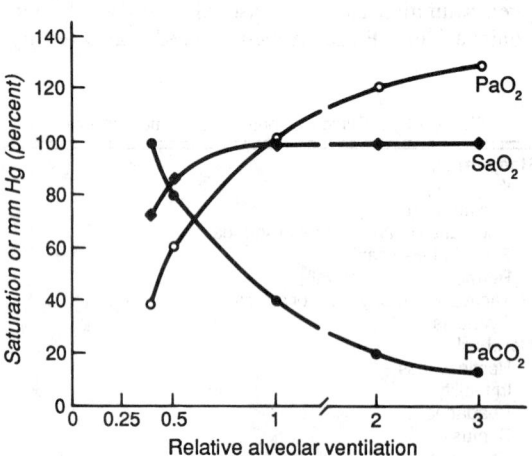

Figure 15–1. Relationship between alveolar ventilation, arterial oxygen saturation (Sao_2), and partial pressures of oxygen and CO_2 in the arterial blood (Pao_2 and $Paco_2$). (Reproduced, with permission, from Pagtakhan RD, Chernicic V: Respiratory failure in the pediatric patient. Pediatr Rev 1982;3:244.)

Table 15–3. Pulmonary status equations.

Pio_2 = (barometric pressure – 47) × % inspired oxygen concentration
$AaDO_2$ = $Pio_2 – (Paco_2/R) – Pao_2$ (Normal = 5 – 15 mm Hg)
Co_2 = (1.34 × hemoglobin × Sao_2) + (.003 × Pao_2)
Do_2 = $Cao_2 × CI × 10$ (Normal 620 ± 50 mL/min/m²)
Oxygen consumption (Vo_2) = ($Cao_2 – Cvo_2$) × CI × 10 (Normal 120 to 200 mL/min/m²)

$$\frac{Qs}{Qt} = \frac{Cco_2 – Cao_2}{Cco_2 – Cvo_2} \quad \text{(Normal < 5%)}$$

$$Vd = \frac{(Paco_2 – Peco_2)}{(Pcco_2)} \quad \text{(Normal approximately 2 mL/kg)}$$

$$Compliance = \frac{Volume\ (Tidal\ volume)}{Pressure\ (PIP – PEEP)} \quad \text{(Normals vary with age)}$$

$AaDO_2$	=	Alveolar-arterial oxygen difference (mm Hg).
Cao_2	=	Oxygen content of arterial blood (mL/dL).
Cco_2	=	Oxygen content of pulmonary capillary blood (mL/dL).
CI	=	Cardiac index (L/min).
Co_2	=	Oxygen content of the blood (mL/dL).
Cvo_2	=	Oxygen content of mixed venous blood (mL/dL).
Do_2	=	Oxygen delivery (mL/min).
$Paco_2$	=	Partial pressure of carbon dioxide in arterial blood (mm Hg).
Pao_2	=	Partial pressure of oxygen in arterial blood (mm Hg).
$Pcco_2$	=	Partial pressure of carbon dioxide in capillary blood (mm Hg).
$Peco_2$	=	Partial pressure of carbon dioxide in expired air (mm Hg).
Pio_2	=	Partial pressure of oxygen in inspired air (mm Hg).
Qs/Qt	=	Intrapulmonary shunt (in patients without cardiac shunt) (%).
R	=	Respiratory quotient (usually = 0.8).
Sao_2	=	Arterial oxygen saturation (fractional).
Vd	=	Physiologic dead space (anatomic dead space + alveolar dead space) (mL).
Ve	=	Expiratory minute volume (L/min).
Vo_2	=	Oxygen consumption per minute.

patient must be properly positioned to facilitate air exchange while supplemental oxygen is given. The sniffing position is used in infants. Head extension with jaw thrust is used in older children without neck injuries. If obstructed by secretions or vomitus, the airway must be cleared by suction. When not obstructed by a foreign body or epiglottitis, airways should open with proper positioning and placement of an oral or nasopharyngeal airway of the correct size. Nasal airways are better tolerated than oral airways by conscious patients. As each step is taken, it is imperative to monitor changes in chest movement,

Table 15–4. Supplemental oxygen therapy.

Source	Maximum % O_2	Range of Flow Rates	Advantages	Disadvantages
Nasal cannula	35–40%	0.125–4 L/min	Easily applied, relatively comfortable	Uncomfortable at higher flow rates, requires open nasal airways, easily dislodged, lower % O_2, nosebleeds
Simple mask	50–60%	5–10 L/min	Higher % O_2, good for mouth breathers	Uncomfortable, dangerous for patients with poor airway control and at risk for emesis, hard to give airway care, unsure of % O_2
Face tent	40–60%	8–10 L/min	Higher % O_2, good for mouth breathers, less restrictive	Uncomfortable, dangerous for patients with poor airway control and at risk for emesis, hard to give airway care, unsure of % O_2
Rebreathing mask	80–90%	5–10 L/min	Higher % O_2, good for mouth breathers, highest O_2 concentration	Uncomfortable, dangerous for patients with poor airway control and at risk for emesis, hard to give airway care, unsure of % O_2
Oxyhood	90–100%	5–10 L/min (mixed at wall)	Stable and accurate O_2 concentration	Temperature regulation, hard to give airway care

airway and breath sounds, skin color, and mental status. In patients with a normal airway, an intravenous anesthesia induction for intubation may be performed by those experienced with the drugs and the intubation procedure (Table 15–5). Patients with obstructed upper airways (eg, patients with croup, epiglottitis, foreign bodies, or subglottic stenosis) should be awake when intubated unless trained airway specialists decide otherwise.

Insertion of an endotracheal tube of the correct size is of critical importance in pediatrics. A tube that is too large for a pediatric patient may cause pressure necrosis of the tissues in the subglottic region. (See Table 11–3 for sizes.) (The subglottic region is the narrowest portion of the upper airway in children—in contrast to the glottis in adults.) Insertion of inappropriately large endotracheal tubes has been associated with scarring and in some cases permanent stenosis of the subglottic region, requiring tracheostomy or cricoid split for repair. Too small an endotracheal tube can result in inadequate pulmonary toilet and excessive air leak around the endotracheal tube, making optimal ventilation and oxygenation difficult. There are many ways to calculate the size of endotracheal tube that is appropriate for a child. A useful method is the following: tube size = (16 + age in years) ÷ 4. Patients under 8 years of age should have uncuffed endotracheal tubes. After placement of the endotracheal tube, breath sounds should be evaluated for bilateral equality. One should then check for a leak between the endotracheal tube and the larynx. To do this, connect a pressure-monitored anesthesia bag to the circuit and allow it to inflate, creating positive pressure. Check for the leak by auscultating over the throat, noting the pressure at which air escapes around the endotracheal tube. Leaks of 15–20 cm H_2O are acceptable. Larger leaks (> 20 cm H_2O) are acceptable

only in patients having severe lung disease and poor compliance and requiring high pressures to achieve ventilation. In this situation, one must be aware of the possible postextubation complications of subglottic stenosis in the patient. A chest x-ray is necessary for final assessment of endotracheal tube placement.

Demling RH, Knox JB: Basic concepts of lung function and dysfunction: Oxygenation, ventilation, and mechanics. New Horizons 1993;1:362.

Guiterrez G, Pohl RJ: Oxygen consumption is linearly related to O_2 supply in critically ill patients. J Crit Care 1986;1:45.

Heffner JE: Tracheal intubation in mechanically ventilated patients. Clin Chest Med 1988;9:23.

Katz R, Pollack M, Spady D: Cardiopulmonary abnormalities in severe acute respiratory failure. J Pediatr 1984;104:357.

Kelly HW: Pharmacotherapy of pediatric lung disease: Differences between children and adults. Clin Chest Med 1987;8:681.

Newth CJL: Respiratory disease and respiratory failure: Implications for the young and the old. Br J Dis Chest 1986;80:209.

Pagtakhan RD, Chernick J: Respiratory failure in the pediatric patient. Pediatr Rev 1982;3:247.

Pagtakhan RD, Pasterkamp H: Intensive care for respiratory disorders. In: *Disorders of the Respiratory Tract in Children,* 5th ed. Chernick V (editor). Saunders, 1990.

Prevoznik SJ: Intubation of the trachea. In: *Introduction to Anesthesia,* 7th ed. Dripps RD, Eckenhoff JE, Vandam LD (editors). Saunders, 1988.

Raphaely RC: Acute respiratory failure in infants and children. Pediatr Ann 1986;15:315.

Rennie JM: Transcutaneous carbon dioxide monitoring. Arch Dis Child 1990;65:345.

Schumacker PT, Samsel RW: Oxygen supply and consumption in the adult respiratory distress syndrome. Clin Chest Med 1990;11:715.

Table 15–5. Drugs commonly used for controlled intubation.

Drug	Dose (mg/kg)	Advantages	Disadvantages
Atropine	0.02; minimum of 0.1	Blocks bradycardia, dries secretions	Tachycardia, fever, histamine release, seizures, coma
Thiopental	3–5	Fast onset, short duration of action	Vascular irritant, negatively inotropic, no analgesic properties, histamine release (avoid in asthma), induces porphyria
Ketamine	1–2 IV 4–8 IM	Fast onset, positively inotropic	Increased bronchorrhea, increased pulmonary and systemic vascular resistance, increased intracranial pressure, emergence problems
Succinylcholine (depolarizing muscle relaxant)	1–2	Fast onset, short duration of action	Bradycardia (premedicate with atropine); fasciculations; contraindicated in burns, hyperkalemia, massive trauma, and various neurologic disorders
Pancuronium (nondepolarizing muscle relaxant)	0.1	Lasts 40–60 min, can be given by continuous infusion, reversible	Slow onset (2–3 min), tachycardia
Vecuronium (nondepolarizing muscle relaxant)	0.1	Lasts 20–30 min, can be given by continuous infusion, reversible	Slow onset (2–3 min)

Schumaker PT, Cain SM: The concept of a critical oxygen delivery. Intensive Care Med 1987;13:223.

Steward DJ: *Manual of Pediatric Anesthesia.* Churchill Livingston, 1985.

Steward DJ: Anesthesia in children. In: *Textbook of Pediatric Clinical Pharmacology.* MacLeod SM, Radde IC (editors). PSG Publishing, 1985.

Ward CF: Pediatric head and neck syndromes. In: *Anesthesia and Uncommon Pediatric Diseases.* Katz J, Steward DJ (editors). Saunders, 1987.

MECHANICAL VENTILATION

The increased compliance of an infant's chest wall, the increasing number of alveoli until approximately the age of 8, the small size of the airways and the lack of collateral ventilation make pediatric ventilation challenging. Mechanical ventilators are designed to facilitate movement of air into and out of the lungs and to deliver oxygen. They use either positive pressure to "pump" the lung full of gas or negative pressure to "suck" air into the lungs, much like the diaphragm does. This section will deal with the more commonly used positive-pressure mechanical ventilators that are most appropriate for acute situations. Negative-pressure ventilators are primarily used in patients with chronic respiratory failure.

Pressure Ventilators

Pressure-limited, time-cycled ventilators are usually reserved for neonates and infants weighing less than 10 kg. In pressure-limited ventilators, increased air flow is generated at the start of the inspiratory cycle and continues until a preset pressure is reached. Pressure is maintained for a preset inspiratory time usually (0.3–0.6 second), and at the end of the inspiratory time, the exhalation valve opens. Pressure ventilators provide intermittent mandatory ventilation (IMV); for example, at a setting of 15 breaths per minute, the machine delivers a breath every 4 seconds. Spontaneous respirations may interfere with the mandatory cycle when the patient's own exhalation coincides with the ventilator's inspiratory phase and causes the peak inspiratory pressure to be reached prematurely. The advantages of pressure-limited ventilators lie in their ability to support spontaneous respirations with continuous gas flow, their avoidance of barotrauma by limiting the pressure of breaths, and their relatively simple operation. The main disadvantages are the possibility of inadequate tidal volumes (especially during periods of rapidly changing lung compliance), and the possible interference with spontaneous respirations.

Volume Ventilators

With the advent of ventilators with low working volumes and low compliance ventilator tubing, volume ventilators may now be used in patients of any age. With these ventilators, a standard tidal volume is set (10–15 mL/kg), and the inspiratory time is set either to an absolute value (0.3–1.5 seconds) or to a percentage of the respiratory cycle. In contrast to pressure-limited ventilators, volume-limited ventilators always deliver a preset tidal volume. The pressure that is generated in response to a preset tidal volume may change, and this ratio of pressure to volume is an index of compliance in the lung. There is usually a dial where a preset pressure can be set above which the ventilator breath will be halted. This is a safety mechanism to avoid dangerously high lung inflation pressures. These ventilators may function in either an intermittent (IMV) or synchronized (SIMV) fashion. SIMV allows a window of time during which a patient's inspiratory effort will initiate the delivery of a tidal volume and is often helpful in patients who breathe spontaneously. Volume ventilators are volume-limited and either volume- or time-cycled. They may provide either continuous flow through the system, allowing uninterrupted access of fresh gas to the patient (which decreases the work of breathing, especially in young infants), or they may provide flow that is held in check until an inspiratory effort opens a demand valve.

Volume ventilators may have as added variables an inspiratory hold or pressure support. The advantages of volume ventilators include ensured delivery of a preset volume, compliance measurements, and availability of SIMV. Disadvantages of some volume ventilators include possible increased barotrauma from excessive delivery pressure and lack of a continuous flow system.

Positive End-Expiratory Pressure

All mechanical ventilators open their expiratory limbs at the end of inspiration until a preset pressure is achieved; this is the positive end-expiratory pressure (PEEP) value. During ventilation of normal lungs, "physiologic" PEEP is felt to be 2–4 cm H_2O pressure. In disease states, a higher PEEP may increase the functional residual capacity, open previously collapsed alveoli, increase mean airway pressure (MAP), and improve oxygenation. A higher PEEP, though often valuable, may cause CO_2 retention, barotrauma with extrapleural air leaks, decreased central venous return, decreased cardiac output, and increased intracranial pressure. Continuous positive airway pressure (CPAP) is the lowest expiratory pressure a spontaneously breathing patient achieves and for practical purposes is synonymous with PEEP. PEEP and CPAP have an optimal setting for each individual patient, maximally improving FRC and ventilation/perfusion mismatches while not causing the problems associated with excessive intrathoracic pressure (see above). Multiple parameters have been proposed with varying success to define "optimal PEEP." Variables that should be considered in determining appropriate PEEP include PaO_2, central venous pressure, cardiac output, and clinical situations such as pulmonary air leak and cerebral edema (decreased PEEP) or pneumonia, pulmonary edema, and adult respiratory distress syndrome (ARDS) (increased PEEP).

Ventilator Management

Mechanical ventilators affect both ventilation and oxygenation. Ventilation is related to alveolar minute volume. On a pressure ventilator, the minute volume is directly related to rate and peak inspiratory pressure; on a volume ventilator, it is related to rate and tidal volume. Thus, either increased rate, tidal volume, or peak inspiratory pressure will increase ventilation (decreased $PaCO_2$). Changes in oxygenation other than those due to the concentration of delivered oxygen depend in part on the variables that determine mean airway pressure (MAP), or the average of all the pressures experienced by the lung in one respiratory cycle. These include PEEP, inspiratory time, and either the set peak inspiratory pressure or that achieved using one or the other type of ventilator. By increasing any of these settings, one achieves an elevation in MAP and, up to a point, an increase in oxygenation. One must remember that increasing these settings can worsen ventilation/perfusion mismatches, decrease cardiac output, and decrease oxygen delivery to the tissue. Therefore, the changes resulting in elevated MAP do not always improve arterial oxygenation or O_2 delivery.

The intubated patient deserves attention directed toward improving comfort and decreasing anxiety. Chloral hydrate, benzodiazepines, and narcotics have been used. Continuous infusions of the short-acting benzodiazepines and opioids create a steady state of sedation. Occasionally, patients are so agitated that ventilation and oxygenation suffer. In these cases, muscle paralysis may facilitate oxygenation and ventilation. The nondepolarizing neuromuscular blocking agents pancuronium bromide and vecuronium bromide are most commonly used for this purpose. They may be given as necessary or as continuous infusions. When giving muscle relaxants, one must be prepared to provide, by mechanical means, ventilation and oxygenation to the patient who previously breathed spontaneously; in most cases, ventilatory support must be increased.

Monitoring the Ventilated Patient

Monitoring of the ventilated patient starts with a physical examination. Respiratory rate and activity, chest wall movement, and quality of breath sounds must be noted. Next, the gas exchange should be measured. Although arterial blood gases are the standard, oxygenation can also be measured by transmission oximetry with lightweight digital or earlobe probes. O_2 (PtO_2) or CO_2 ($PtCO_2$) can be measured transcutaneously with sufficient accuracy in younger patients with good skin perfusion. $PaCO_2$ may also be assessed by monitoring end-tidal CO_2 ($PetCO_2$). This is done by placing a gas sampling port on the endotracheal tube and analyzing expired gas for $PetCO_2$. This technique appears more valuable in patients with large tidal volumes, and its accuracy improves with more proximal sampling, ie, closer to the airways. $PetCO_2$ values may differ from measured $PaCO_2$ and are most useful for following relative fluctuations in $PaCO_2$.

The ventilator itself has many variables. The most common are tidal volume, minute ventilation, peak inspiratory pressure, and inspiratory and expiratory time. Mean airway pressure should be monitored in mechanically ventilated patients and maintained as low as possible to achieve adequate oxygenation and ventilation. Work of breathing and oxygen consumption may also be measured; these measurements may be helpful in making ventilator changes in chronically ventilated patients. Ways to obtain measurements by computer at the bedside and evaluate all these measurements are becoming available. These technologic advances offer more information but do not eliminate the need for good clinical judgment and instinct.

Alternative Methods of Ventilation

New techniques of ventilating the patient in respiratory failure are now available. High-frequency jet ventilation with passive expiration (300–3000/min) and high-frequency oscillation with active expiration (300–1800/min) have been used to manage select groups of neonates and older pediatric patients, including those suffering from major pulmonary barotrauma (air leaks, pulmonary interstitial emphysema), respiratory distress syndrome, and congenital diaphragmatic hernia. These techniques have also been used to manage patients who have undergone operative procedures on airway structures, so that mean airway pressure can be maintained with lower peak inspiratory pressures, thus helping prevent postoperative air leaks at the surgical site.

Pressure-controlled inverse ratio ventilation and permissive hypercapnia have also been used successfully to manage severe respiratory failure such as that seen in adult respiratory distress syndrome. These techniques allow maintenance of high mean airway pressures while reducing peak inspiratory pressure and the incidence of barotrauma to as low as a level as possible.

Betit P, H Thompson JE, Benjamin PK: Mechanical ventilation. In: *Neonatal and Pediatric Respiratory Care,* 2nd ed. Mosby Year Book, 1993.

Biondi JW, Schullman DS, Matthay RA: Effects of mechanical ventilation on right and left ventricular function. Clin Chest Med 1988;9:55.

Cogwill CJ et al: Neonatal and pediatric high frequency ventilation: Principles and practice. Respir Care 1991; 36:596.

Demling RH, Knox JB: Basic concepts of lung function and

dysfunction: Oxygenation, ventilation, and mechanics. New Horizons 1993;1:362.

Hickling KG, Henderson SJ, Jackson R: Low mortality associated with low volume pressure limited ventilation with permissive hypercapnia in severe ARDS. Intensive Care Med 1990;16:372.

Marini JJ, Ravenscraft SA: Mean airway pressure: Physiologic determinants and clinical importance: (Two parts.) Crit Care Med 1992;20:1461, 1604.

Marini JJ: Monitoring during mechanical ventilation. Clin Chest Med 1988;9:73.

Martin LD et al: Principles of respiratory support and mechanical ventilation. In: *Textbook of Pediatric Intensive Care,* 2nd ed. Williams & Wilkins, 1992.

Vyas H, Helms P, Cheriyan G: Transcutaneous oxygen monitoring beyond the neonatal period. Crit Care Med 1988;16:844.

ADULT RESPIRATORY DISTRESS SYNDROME (ARDS)

ARDS is a syndrome of acute respiratory failure characterized by increased pulmonary capillary permeability and pulmonary edema that results in refractory hypoxemia, decreased lung compliance, and bilateral diffuse alveolar infiltrates on chest radiography. Although the exact incidence in the pediatric population is unknown, ARDS accounts for approximately 1% of PICU admissions.

ARDS may be precipitated by a variety of insults or events (Table 15–6). Sepsis is the most common clinical disorder associated with the development of ARDS: 20–40% of patients with sepsis develop the syndrome. Other important causes in the pediatric patient are near-drowning, trauma, and primary lung infections, including viral, bacterial, and fungal pneumonias. Despite the diversity of causes, the clinical presentation is remarkably similar in most cases.

According to Nichols, four findings are common to all patients with ARDS: (1) a severe "event" in a patient with previously normal lungs; (2) findings of respiratory distress with hypoxemia, increased right-to-left intrapulmonary shunt, and decreased pulmonary compliance; (3) radiologic appearance of diffuse infiltrates; and (4) cardiac disease and congestive heart failure not the initiating events.

Several recent studies, however, have suggested that the clinical course and prognosis are extremely variable and have led to an expanded definition of ARDS or acute lung injury. The expanded definition attempts to better define the clinical problem. First, the severity of acute lung injury is scored through assessments of arterial oxygenation (PaO_2/FiO_2), chest radiographs, static lung compliance, and the level of PEEP required. Second, because the clinical disorder or disorders that led to the development of acute lung injury clearly influence the patient's prognosis for recovery, precise definition of the underlying problem becomes important. For instance, although the average mortality rate in this population is 45–60%, the rate is quite variable and appears dependent on the associated clinical disorder, with mortality rates of 90% in ARDS associated with sepsis and only 10% in ARDS associated with fat embolism. The third part of the definition specifies the failure of organs other than the lung. The importance of nonpulmonary organ failure is of major importance in the outcome of the ARDS patient. For instance, concomitant hepatic failure and ARDS are associated with an almost 100% mortality rate. In fact, any combination of three organs that have failed for more than 7 days carries a 98% mortality rate.

Thus, a more quantitative definition of pulmonary and nonpulmonary organ failure, including the associated clinical disorders, is critical for establishing the actual incidence of ARDS and for determining the prognosis for recovery.

Clinical Presentation & Pathophysiology

ARDS can be roughly divided into four clinical phases. In the earliest phase the patient may exhibit dyspnea and tachypnea with a relatively normal PO_2 and a hyperventilation-induced respiratory alkalosis. No significant abnormalities are noted on physical or radiologic examination of the chest. Experimental studies suggest early neutrophil sequestration into the lungs is occurring during this stage. Over the next few hours, hypoxemia increases and respiratory distress becomes clinically apparent, with cyanosis, tachycardia, irritability, and dyspnea. Radiographic evidence of early parenchymal change is noted by "fluffy" alveolar infiltrates initially appearing in dependent lung fields, indicative of pulmonary edema. The edema fluid typically has a high concentration of protein (75–95% of plasma protein concentration) which is characteristic of an increased-permeability edema and differentiates it from cardiogenic or hydrostatic pulmonary edema. In addition to endothelial damage, epithelial injury is now emerging as an important component also of the acute lung injury syndrome. Injury to the epithelium lowers the threshold for alveolar edema and results in significant deterioration in

Table 15–6. ARDS risk factors.

Direct Lung Injury	Indirect Lung Injury
Aspiration of gastric contents	Sepsis syndrome
Inhalation of toxic fumes	Multiple trauma
Near-drowning	Multiple transfusions
Oxygen toxicity	Fat embolism
Pulmonary contusion	Shock
Pneumonia: bacterial, viral, other	Pancreatitis
	Drug overdoses (especially aspirin, opioids, tricyclic antidepressants, barbiturates)
	Burns

gas exchange. If patients can reabsorb excess alveolar edema in the first 12 hours after developing pulmonary edema, alveolar epithelial function remains reasonably intact and there is an excellent chance for recovery and survival. In contrast, patients who have no change in edema fluid content or protein concentration in the first 12 hours after onset of mechanical ventilation have a much higher mortality rate. Pulmonary hypertension, decreases in lung compliance, and increases in airway resistance are also noted. Importantly, airway abnormalities are being increasingly recognized as an important component of acute lung injury. Bronchoconstriction is an important component of many gram-negative endotoxin models of lung injury. Clinical studies suggest that airway resistance may be increased in 50% of patients with ARDS. Pathologic changes demonstrate marked neutrophil infiltration, intra-alveolar protein, and fibrin strands in the airway.

The interstitium of the lung becomes involved during the subacute phase of ARDS (5–10 days after lung injury). Type II cell and fibroblast proliferation are noted. Decreased lung volumes and signs of consolidation are noted clinically and radiographically. Worsening of the hypoxemia with an increasing shunt fraction as well as a further decrease in lung compliance are noted. Some patients develop an accelerated fibrosing alveolitis in which there is a marked increase in fibroblasts and collagen formation in the interstitium. The mechanisms responsible for these changes are not clear. Current investigation centers on the role of growth and differentiation factors released by alveolar macrophages, mast cells, and other cells in the lung.

During the chronic phase of ARDS (10–14 days after lung injury), there is evidence of intense fibrosis, emphysema, and pulmonary vascular obliteration. In the chronic phase, patients usually do not have as severe an oxygenation defect as they did in the acute phase, and the requirements for PEEP may decline. Patients have large amounts of dead space and may require a high minute ventilation. During this phase of the disease, there is still decreased lung compliance that may be secondary to pulmonary fibrosis and insufficient surface-active material.

Secondary pulmonary and nonpulmonary infections are common in the subacute and chronic phases of ARDS and significantly influence the outcome. Nosocomial pneumonia is a common complicating problem, particularly during the subacute phase. The

Table 15–7. Pathophysiologic changes of modern adult respiratory distress syndrome (low-pressure pulmonary edema).[1]

Radiographic Change	Clinical Findings	Physiologic Change	Pathologic Change
Phase 1 (early changes)			
Normal radiograph	Dyspnea, tachypnea, normal chest examination	Mild pulmonary hypertension, normoxemic or mild hypoxemia, hypercapnia.	Neutrophil sequestration, no clear tissue damage.
Phase 2 (onset of parenchymal changes)[2]			
Patchy alveolar infiltrates beginning in dependent lung No perivascular cuffs (unless a component of high-pressure edema is present) Normal heart size	Dyspnea, tachypnea, cyanosis, tachycardia, course rales.	Pulmonary hypertension, normal wedge pressure, increased lung permeability, increased lung water, increasing shunt, progressive decrease in compliance, moderate to severe hypoxemia.	Neutrophil infiltration, vascular congestion, fibrin strands, platelet clumps, alveolar septal edema, intra-alveolar protein, white cells, type I epithelial drainage.
Phase 3 (acute respiratory failure with progression, 2–10 days)			
Diffuse alveolar infiltrates Air bronchograms Decreased lung volume No bronchovascular cuffs Normal heart	Tachypnea, tachycardia, hyperdynamic state, sepsis syndrome, signs of consolidation, diffuse rhonchi.	Phase 2 changes persist. Progression of symptoms, increasing shunt fraction, further decrease in compliance, increased minute ventilation, impaired oxygen extraction of hemoglobin.	Increased interstitial and alveolar inflammatory exudate with neutrophil and mononuclear cells, type II cell proliferation, beginning fibroblast proliferation, thromboembolic occlusion.
Phase 4 (pulmonary fibrosis, pneumonia with progression, >10 days)[3]			
Persistent diffuse infiltrates Superimposed new pneumonic infiltrates Recurrent pneumothorax Normal heart size Enlargement with pulmonale	Symptoms as above, recurrent sepsis, evidence of multiple organ system failure.	Phase 3 changes persist. Recurrent pneumonia, progressive lung restriction, impaired tissue oxygenation. Impaired oxygen extraction. Multiple organ system failure.	Type II cell hyperplasia, interstitial thickening; infiltration of lymphocytes, macrophages, fibroblasts; loculated pneumonia or interstitial fibrosis; medial thickening and remodeling of arterioles.

[1]Modified slightly and reproduced, with permission from _____ . . . .
[2]Process readily reversible at this stage if initiating factor is controlled.
[3]Multiple organ system failure common. Mortality rate >80% at this stage, since resolution is more difficult.

mechanisms responsible for increased host susceptibility to infection during this phase are not well understood.

The mortality rates in the late phase of ARDS exceed 80%. Death is usually due to multiple system organ failure and systemic hemodynamic instability rather than hypoxia. A large number of patients with unresolving ARDS will develop multiple organ system failure syndrome, with the liver usually being the next organ to fail.

Pathogenic Mechanisms

Infection or tissue trauma appear to initiate the ARDS process by generating a systemic inflammatory reaction. The response can be the result of intense local inflammation (eg, burns, pancreatitis), circulating factors (eg, endotoxin, microemboli), or tissue ischemia-reperfusion injury. The result is a release of cytokines and second mediators from all membranes. Activation of the coagulation, fibrinolytic, and kinin cascades occurs. Subsequent neutrophil activation, aggregation, and then adherence in the lung microcirculation occurs. As a result, the lung endothelium is exposed to an array of products that are potentially toxic to cells. Abnormal neutrophil-endothelial interactions appear particularly important in initiating this lung injury, though other cells clearly participate (Table 15–8). Discussion of the array of mediators released and apparently active during this process is beyond the scope of this chapter but has been recently reviewed (see references).

Treatment

A. Ventilatory Support: Because the hypoxemia of ARDS is related to pulmonary edema, V/Q mismatch, decreased functional residual capacity, and increased dead space, it does not respond simply

Table 15–8. Potential mediators of injury and repair in AIDS.

Circulating cells	Neutrophils Monocytes Platelets ?Lymphocytes
Resident lung cells	Alveolar and intravascular macrophages Fibroblasts Epithelial cells, type II

Mediators	Cyclooxygenase products
	Lipoxygenase products
	Platelet activating factor
	Complement activation (C5a)
	Oxygen radicals, lipid peroxides
	Neutrophil proteases
	Plasma proteolytic enzymes
	Histamine, serotonin
	Cytokines
	  Tumor necrosis factor
	  Interleukins
	Growth factors
	  PDGF
	  TGFβ

to an increase in inspired oxygen concentration. Furthermore, high concentrations of oxygen (FiO_2 greater than 50% over 24 hours) can cause additional lung injury to these patients, who have already altered barrier function. To decrease the potentially injurious effects of high oxygen concentrations, physicians may use positive-pressure ventilation and PEEP to improve oxygenation under the least injurious conditions. Ventilation is best maintained on a volume ventilator because of the rapidly changing compliance of the lungs. Because of poor compliance, high peak inspiratory pressure may result from the required preset tidal volume. PEEP is used to open collapsed alveoli, reduce shunting, and increase FRC above the closing volume. All these measures decrease dead space ventilation and may improve oxygenation. PEEPs of 15–25 cm H_2O have been used successfully in some patients. The PEEP that provides the best combination of oxygenation, lung compliance, cardiac output, and lowered intrapulmonary shunt is found by increasing the PEEP by increments (2–3 cm H_2O every 30 minutes) until pulmonary and hemodynamic measurements fit the patient's requirements. Before increasing PEEP, one should optimize conditions by making sure that the intravascular volume is appropriate, the endotracheal tube fits well and has no significant leak, and the patient is well sedated or paralyzed. A QS/QT of less than 15%, oxygen saturations greater than 90% on a FiO_2 of less than 60%, and a good cardiac output may signal the end point of PEEP adjustments.

Recently, the idea that normalization of blood gases (PaO_2 and $PaCO_2$) at the cost of injuring the lung with high pressures and high concentrations of oxygen may not be necessary and may even be detrimental. Therefore, passive hypercapnia in the face of normal blood pH is acceptable. Newer ventilator strategies (discussed above) are also being tried in an attempt to decrease lung injury. These include primarily a switch from volume-controlled to pressure-controlled modes of ventilation.

B. Hemodynamic Support: Hemodynamic support is directed toward increasing perfusion and oxygen delivery. Volume expansion is achieved by giving packed red blood cells to maintain the hematocrit between 40% and 50% and by giving either colloid or crystalloid solutions to nonanemic volume-depleted patients. There is no one recommendation on the type of fluid to give the nonanemic patient. Certainly, colloids should be used in patients with low intravascular oncotic pressures as estimated by reduced total protein or albumin concentrations. In all other ARDS patients, however, the optimal fluid resuscitation has not been well established. Use of inotropic drugs is often necessary. The most effective inotropic dosages should be determined by monitoring blood pressure, urinary output, cardiac output, pulmonary and systemic vascular resistances, and the patient's gas exchange.

C. Control of Infection: An extremely important consideration in the management of ARDS is prevention of infection or its early diagnosis and treatment. In addition to the usual steps taken to reduce the incidence of nosocomial infection, the roles of prophylactic antibiotics and decontamination regimens in patients with ARDS are currently being investigated. Immunotherapy is perhaps the most promising therapeutic option for preventing and treating infection in patients with ARDS. Active and passive immunization against gram-negative bacteria and its components is being investigated.

D. Pharmacotherapy: Drug therapies have not proved particularly successful in ARDS. Clinical research has been directed at blocking the host's inflammatory response to injury. Steroids could work by stabilizing lysosomal membranes, preventing aggregation of platelets, and inhibiting phospholipase A_2, resulting in decreased eicosanoid production. However, clinical studies have not demonstrated steroid therapy to be of any benefit in ARDS patients. Ibuprofen and indomethacin block synthesis of eicosanoids and have been tried without benefit. Vasodilators such as nitroglycerin, sodium nitroprusside, PGE_1, PGI_2, and calcium channel blockers have all been used to combat pulmonary vasoconstriction, but their use is frequently limited by the development of systemic hypotension. As yet, there is no clear evidence suggesting that these drugs have beneficial effects. Pentoxifylline, an anti-inflammatory agent, has been shown to attenuate leakage in animal models of acute lung injury. Some enthusiasm also exists for the treatment of patients with antibodies specific to circulating mediators of sepsis and lung injury. Antitumor necrosis factor antibodies are an example.

E. Monitoring: Multi-organ system monitoring is needed in patients with ARDS. Ventilation can be assessed by monitoring arterial blood gases, oxygen saturation, and end-tidal CO_2. Lung compliance should be known as increases in PEEP or tidal volume are made. Obtaining chest films daily is important for patients receiving vigorous support because severe ARDS is associated with a 40–60% incidence of air leaks. Hemodynamic monitoring should include, at a minimum, central venous monitoring to determine volume status; if PEEPs greater than 12 cm H_2O are used, a pulmonary artery catheter is recommended. Surveillance for infection or sepsis is important because secondary infections are common and increase the mortality rate strikingly. Renal, liver, and gastrointestinal function need close attention because of the great the likelihood of multiple organ dysfunction.

F. Alternative Management: New techniques have evolved in the respiratory treatment of ARDS. **High-frequency ventilation** has proved helpful only in patients with large air leaks, though more and better trials evaluating the efficacy of high-frequency oscillatory or jet ventilation are needed. Surfactant replacement therapy has been considered in patients with ARDS. Surfactant replacement could improve lung compliance and allow patients' lungs to be ventilated at a smaller FiO_2, with weaning from mechanical ventilation earlier than is currently possible. Prospective randomized trials are needed. Pediatric patients with severe ARDS who received **extracorporeal membrane oxygenation (ECMO)** have better survival rates than historical controls. There is currently a prospective study evaluating veno-venous ECMO as treatment for ARDS. The results of that study are not complete, but to date the data show no difference between the control and the ECMO-treated groups. Criteria for selecting which patients should receive these new therapies have not been established. Very recent reports have demonstrated that inhaled **nitric oxide (NO)** may be beneficial in ARDS. This effect is based on the ability of NO to reduce pulmonary artery pressure and to improve the matching of ventilation with perfusion without producing systemic vasodilation. Criteria for selecting which patients should receive these new therapies have not been established, nor has their efficacy been documented in prospective randomized clinical trials.

G. Follow-Up: The follow-up of pediatric ARDS patients is limited. One report of ten children followed 1–4 years after severe ARDS showed three still symptomatic and seven with hypoxemia at rest. Until further information is available, all patients with a history of ARDS need close follow-up of pulmonary function.

Bersten A, Sibald WJ: Acute lung injury in septic shock. Crit Care Clin 1989;5:49.

Demling RH: Adult respiratory distress syndrome: Current concepts. New Horizons 1993;1:388.

Enhorning G: Surfactant replacement in adult respiratory distress syndrome. Am Rev Respir Dis 1989;140:281.

Holcroft JW, Vassar MJ, Weber CJ: Prostaglandin E and survival in patients with the adult respiratory syndrome. Ann Surg 1986;203:371.

Katz R: Adult respiratory distress syndrome in children. Clin Chest Med 1987;8:635.

Knaus WA, Wagner DP: Multiple systems organ failure: Epidemiology and prognosis. Crit Care Clin 1989;5:221.

Luce JM et al: Ineffectiveness of high-dose methylprednisolone in preventing parenchymal lung injury and improving mortality in patients with septic shock. Am Rev Respir Dis 1988;136:62.

MacNaughton PD, Evans TW: Management of adult respiratory distress syndrome. Lancet 1992;339:469.

Murray JF et al: An expanded definition of the adult respiratory distress syndrome. Am Rev Respir Dis 1988;138:720.

Nichols DG, Rogers MC: Adult respiratory distress syndrome. In: *The Textbook of Pediatric Intensive Care.* (editor). Williams & Wilkins, 1987.

Pinsky MR: The effects of mechanical ventilation on the cardiovascular system. Crit Care Med 1990;6:660.

Potkiw RT: Effect of PEEP on right and left ventricular function in patients with the adult respiratory distress syndrome. Am Rev Respir Dis 1987;135:307.

Repine JE: Scientific perspectives on adult respiratory distress syndrome. Lancet 1992;339:466.

Rossaint R et al: Inhaled nitric oxide for the adult respiratory distress syndrome. N Engl J Med 1993;328:399.

Royal JA, Levin DL: Adult respiratory distress syndrome in pediatric patients. 1. Clinical aspects, pathophysiology, and mechanisms of lung injury. J Pediatr 1988;112:169.

Royal JA, Levin DL: Adult respiratory distress syndrome in pediatric patients. 2. Management. J Pediatr 1988;112:335.

Snyder LS et al: Failure of lung repair following acute lung injury: Regulation of the fibroproliferative response. (Two parts.) Chest 1990;98:733, 989.

Weiner-Kronish JP, Gropper MA, Matthay MA: The adult respiratory distress syndrome: Definition and prognosis, pathogenesis and treatment. Br J Anaesth 1990;65:107.

NEAR-DROWNING
(See also Chapter 14.)

Near-drowning is the survival for 24 hours or more after suffocation by submersion. Inasmuch as it is one of the leading causes of accidental death in children, it is a frequent cause of admission to the PICU.

The major sites of near-drowning episodes in children less than 2 years of age are the bathtub and large buckets of water. In children over 2 years of age, the major sites become open bodies of water—in most cases, private swimming pools.

Pathophysiology

In over 90% of near-drownings, there is fluid aspiration. This aspiration and the associated apnea result in hypoxemia. Following resuscitation, the fluid aspiration may result in atelectasis, intrapulmonary shunt, and pulmonary edema, which then leads to the persistence of hypoxemia. It is rare for fluid aspiration to be of sufficient magnitude to result in clinically important changes in serum electrolytes or hemolysis. The ultimate cause of major morbidity and mortality in near-drowning is hypoxic-ischemic injury to the brain.

Cold water near-drowning appears to provide some element of protection to the time-dependent onset of cerebral ischemic damage. Normal neurologic recovery has been reported with up to 40 minutes of submersion in water less than 5°C. This effect may be more pronounced in children as a consequence of their high body surface area to weight ratio and the relatively large surface area of their cranium.

Treatment

The initial approach to the near-drowning victim is to follow the ABCs of resuscitation. Mouth-to-mouth resuscitation should be started as soon as possible, even in the water. After removal from the water, the neck should be stabilized and mouth-to-mouth resuscitation continued. If no pulse is present, closed-chest massage should be initiated. Supplemental oxygen and positive pressure ventilation should be started as soon as possible. Unless awake and well-oxygenated, submersion victims should then be intubated and ventilated.

On arrival in the Emergency Department, the presence of respiratory insufficiency and blood gas analysis should serve as a guide to continued intubation and mechanical ventilation. Continued hypoxemia should be treated with positive end-expiratory pressure.

Fluid redistribution following resuscitation usually results in hypovolemia as a presenting symptom. Intravenous access should be established and appropriate fluid resuscitation provided. Arterial and central venous pressure monitoring may be necessary in low cardiac output states.

Neck and skull films should be obtained in all patients where the nature of the injury is unknown, since childhood near-drowning episodes are frequently associated with diving attempts.

Hypothermia should be corrected rapidly to a temperature consistent with good cardiovascular output. Once this temperature has been reached, warming should be slowed to avoid shivering and increased oxygen demand.

Water that is grossly contaminated, such as with sewage, may result in infectious pneumonia. This group of patients should be treated with antibiotics. Serial tracheal aspirates may guide in the delineation of therapy.

Neither deliberate hypothermia nor barbiturate-induced coma has improved outcome from near-drowning. In fact, none of the advanced brain preservation techniques have been shown to improve neurologic outcome. No techniques other than general physiologic supportive measures are indicated at this time.

Outcome

Predictors of poor neurologic prognosis include prolonged submersion (> 10 minutes), delay in the provision of effective CPR, severe metabolic acidosis (pH < 7.1 after correction for PCO_2), asystole, and fixed, dilated pupils on arrival in the Emergency Department, and a Glasgow coma score of < 5. None of these predictors singly or in conjunction are infallible, and good neurologic outcome has been reported with all of them. However, arrival in the Emergency Department with a temperature over 35 °C, asystole, and fixed, dilated pupils is virtually always followed by demise. Resuscitation should be discontinued if there is no return of spontaneous circulation after 25 minutes of effort.

Modell JH: Drowning. N Engl J Med 1993;328:253.

Nussbaum E, Maggi JC: Pentobarbital therapy does not improve neurologic outcome in nearly drowned, flaccid-comatose children. Pediatrics 1988;81:630.

Nichter MA, Everett PB: Childhood near-drowning: Is cardiopulmonary resuscitation always indicated? Crit Care Med 1989;17:993.

Quan L, Kinder D: Pediatric submersions: Prehospital predictors of outcome. Pediatrics 1992;90:909.

ASTHMA
(Life-Threatening)

Status asthmaticus may be defined as asthma that is refractory to sympathomimetic agents and that may progress to respiratory failure without prompt and aggressive intervention. Life-threatening asthma is caused by severe bronchospasm, excessive mucous secretion, and inflammation and edema of the airways. Reversal of these mechanisms is the key to successful treatment. Status asthmaticus remains a common diagnosis among children admitted to the ICU, and asthma continues to be associated with a surprisingly high mortality rate. Among adolescents, the mortality rate associated with asthma has actually increased over the last decade. Possible explanations for this increase include undertreatment, overtreatment, overuse of "quick fix" medications such as β_2-agonist metered dose inhalers, increased corticosteroid use, and an increase in environmental pollutants.

The physical examination helps determine the severity of illness. Respiration marked by sternocleidomastoid contractions correlates well with an FEV_1 and peak expiratory flow rates (PEFR) less than 50% of normal predicted values. Paradoxic pulse of over 22 mm Hg has been correlated with elevated $PaCO_2$ levels. The absence of wheezing may be misleading because, in order to produce a wheezing sound, the patient must take in a certain amount of air. The arterial blood gas remains the single most important laboratory determination in the evaluation of a child in severe status asthmaticus. Patients with severe respiratory distress, signs of exhaustion, alterations in consciousness, elevated $PaCO_2$, or acidosis, should be admitted to the PICU.

Treatment

Because of inadequate minute ventilation and ventilation/perfusion mismatching, severe asthmatics, are almost always hypoxemic and should receive supplemental humidified oxygen immediately.

A. Pharmacotherapy:

1. The cornerstone of treatment is β_2-agonist therapy. First-line drugs are albuterol and terbutaline, which may be delivered by nebulization with oxygen. If the patient is in severe distress and has poor inspiratory flow rates, thus preventing adequate delivery of nebulized medication, subcutaneous injection of epinephrine or terbutaline may be required. The frequency of β_2-agonist administration varies according to the severity of the patient's symptoms and the occurrence of adverse side effects. Terbutaline or albuterol can be given continuously by nebulization, usually without serious side effects. The heart rate and other vital signs of these patients must be closely monitored to keep the heart rate at less than 180/min and to detect ventricular ectopy.

2. The use of theophylline in addition to β_2-agonists offers little benefit in the first hour of treatment; however, by 24 hours it has been shown to have additional benefit over the use of steroids plus β_2-agonists alone. Besides bronchodilation, its actions include increased mucociliary clearance and ventilatory drive, inhibition of the release of inflammatory mediators, and suppression of microvascular permeability. Recent toxicity issues and behavioral side effects do not appear as significant as previously believed.

3. Systemic **corticosteroids** speed the resolution of severe asthma exacerbations refractory to bronchodilator therapy and should be given to all patients admitted to the hospital with severe asthma. The optimal dose is not known. The acute complications of corticosteroid usage include gastrointestinal bleeding and perforations.

4. Nebulized **anticholinergic agents** are also recommended, at least as a trial, in severe asthmatics. In some patients, cholinergic-related bronchoconstriction is more marked than in others, and so not all patients respond. Nebulized ipratropium bromide is the drug of choice, but the drug is currently available only in metered-dose inhaler form in the United States. Atropine has more potential side effects than ipratropium bromide, eg, tachycardia, urinary retention, and unilateral or bilateral pupillary dilation, but it can be given in a nebulizer.

5. Intravenous beta-agonists such as isoproterenol and terbutaline are used in children with severe airway obstruction and impending respiratory failure. Isoproterenol is a nonspecific beta-agonist and will cause a great increase in heart rate, which may lead to myocardial ischemia and arrhythmia. Terbutaline is more β_2 receptor-specific and usually causes fewer cardiac side effects. Patients placed on intravenous beta-agonist therapy should have indwelling arterial lines for continuous blood pressure and blood gas monitoring and have CK enzymes monitored for signs of myocardial damage.

B. Specific Drugs and Dosages:

1. Give humidified oxygen. Try to keep O_2 saturations at 90% or higher.

2. Begin beta-sympathomimetic therapy (albuterol or terbutaline) by nebulization (albuterol, 0.1 mg/kg per nebulization, up to 2.5 mg; or terbutaline, 0.1–0.2 mg/kg per nebulization, up to 4 mg). This may be given continuously.

3. Give corticosteroids (methylprednisolone, 2 mg/kg intravenously as loading dose, then 1 mg/kg intravenously every 6 hours).

4. Give aminophylline intravenously. Each mg/kg of aminophylline given as a loading dose will increase the aminophylline level by approximately 2 μg/dL. In a patient who has not previously received aminophylline or oral theophylline preparations, load with 7–8 mg/kg of aminophylline in an attempt to achieve a level of 15 μg/dL; then start a continuous infusion of aminophylline at a dosage of 0.8–1 mg/kg/h. Watch closely for toxicity (gastric upset, tachycardia, seizures) and follow levels closely, trying to maintain steady state levels of 13–16 μg/dL.

5. Institute anticholinergic therapy (atropine, 0.025–0.05 mg/kg per dose up to 2 mg every 6–8 hours) by nebulization (useful in a select group of patients).

6. Begin beta-sympathomimetic therapy (terbutaline and isoproterenol) by continuous intravenous infusion. This should be used only in patients who have not responded to the above steps and have worsening respiratory failure.

a. Terbutaline–Give 10 μg/kg over 10 minutes as loading dose, and then start an infusion at 0.1 μg/kg/min, increasing by increments of 0.1 μg/kg/min every 30 minutes until a response is achieved or side effects (tachycardia, tremor, nausea) become apparent.

b. Isoproterenol–Give 0.1 μg/kg/min, increasing by increments of 0.1 μg/kg/min to a maximum of 1 μg/kg/min, again titrating therapy to the patient's response or until side effects (tachycardia, arrhythmia) become a problem.

7. Intravenous administration of magnesium sulfate has been reported as being an effective bronchodilator in adults in severe status asthmaticus. Its smooth muscle relaxation properties are probably due to interference with calcium flux in the bronchial smooth muscle cell.

C. Mechanical Ventilation: If the above aggressive management regimen fails to result in significant improvement, mechanical ventilation may be necessary. In general, if there is steady deterioration despite intensive therapy for asthma, the patient should be intubated and mechanically ventilated. Mechanical ventilation in asthmatics is difficult and by no means simplifies treatment. The goal of mechanical ventilation in an intubated asthmatic is to maintain adequate oxygenation and ventilation with the least amount of barotrauma until other therapies have had a chance to become effective. Intubation should be done by experienced personnel once the patient is sedated and paralyzed. Airway obstruction from persistent bronchoconstriction remains a major problem because the constricted bronchus is lined with smooth muscle, and paralyzing drugs affect only skeletal muscle. The patient, once intubated, should remain paralyzed and sedated. A volume ventilator is necessary to deliver a reasonable tidal volume in patients with poor lung compliance. Expiratory time should be prolonged to avoid air trapping. The IMV rate may need to be lowered to allow proper expiration time. PEEP should be kept low. There are isolated reports of patients who require greater PEEP, but these are the exception. Aerosolized beta-agonists may be given through the ventilator circuit and should be administered as close to the endotracheal tube as possible.

Weaning the very ill asthmatic from ICU therapy should begin with ventilatory support and then with the aggressive drug therapy. Changes should be made slowly, because patients can rebound and worsen quickly.

D. Metabolic Changes in the Severe Asthmatic: Metabolic disorders may occur in the severe asthmatic. Hypercapnia, hypoxia, and poor perfusion may lead to acidosis. Slow intravenous sodium bicarbonate therapy (1 meq/kg for a pH < 7.20) in the ventilated patient is a reasonable treatment of metabolic acidosis and allows a better metabolic milieu. The physician must keep in mind that the arterial CO_2 may climb because of sodium bicarbonate therapy. Hypokalemia is also a complication of beta-agonist therapy, and serum potassium needs to be monitored, especially in patients receiving nebulized beta-agonist drugs continuously.

E. Monitoring: Monitoring the severe asthmatic should include obtaining values for oxygen saturation, arterial blood gases, and, if the patient is ventilated, end-tidal CO_2. Ventilator monitoring must be meticulous, because increases in peak inspiratory pressure or decreases in pulmonary compliance may signal worsening bronchoconstriction or an extrapleural air leak. Chest films of ventilated asthmatics must be obtained daily.

Benatar SR: Fatal asthma. N Engl J Med 1986;314:423.

Jeene JW, Murphy S: Drug therapy for asthma: Research and clinical practice. In: *Lung Biology in Health and Disease.* Vol 5: *Asthma.* Marcel Dekker, 1987.

Kelly HW et al: Safety of frequent high dose nebulized terbutaline in children with acute, severe asthma. Ann Allergy 1990;64:229.

Kelly HW, Murphy S: Should anticholinergics be used in acute severe asthma? DICP 1990;24:409.

Koff PB, Durmowicz AG: Pharmacology. In: *Neonatal and Pediatric Respiratory Care,* 2nd ed. Mosby Year Book, 1993.

Kolski GB: Hypokalemia and respiratory arrest in an infant with status asthmaticus. J Pediatr 1988;112:304.

McFadden ER Jr: Dosages of corticosteroids in asthma. Am Rev Respir Dis 1993;147:1306.

Milgram H, Bender B: Current issues in the use of theophylline. Am Rev Respir Dis 1993;147:533.

National Asthma Education Program, Expert Panel Report: *Guidelines for the Diagnosis and Management of Asthma, 1991.* National Heart, Lung, and Blood Institute, 1991.

Noppen M: Bronchodilating effect of intravenous magnesium sulfate in acute severe bronchial asthma. Chest 1990;97:373.

Schuh S et al: Nebulized albuterol in acute childhood asthma: Comparison of two doses. Pediatrics 1990;86:509.

POSTOPERATIVE CARDIAC VENTILATORY SUPPORT

The outcome for pediatric patients undergoing cardiac surgery has been improved not only by advances in surgical technique and myocardial preservation but also by better postoperative care and ventilatory management in the ICU. Recent improvements in the ability of invasive cardiologists to treat lesions in the catheterization laboratory has also led to a cohort of nonsurgically managed patients who require postprocedural care. Ventilator support of the postoperative patient is now specifically tailored for individual patients after a consideration of such variables as pulmonary hypertension, pulmonary edema, and cardiopulmonary bypass time.

Treatment

General anesthesia is associated with atelectasis and decreased functional reserve capacity, which is thought to be related to an upward shift of the diaphragm and changed chest wall compliance. Additionally, cardiopulmonary bypass results in increased alveolar-arterial oxygen difference, increased interstitial lung water, decreased pulmonary compliance, and increased work of breathing. Therefore, optimizing ventilation starts in the operating room with good anesthetic care. On arrival in the PICU, most patients are intubated, although after simple repairs, eg, repair of an atrial septal defect, stable patients may be extubated in the operating room by experienced cardiac anesthesiologists. Once in the PICU, patients are supported with a volume ventilator at a tidal volume of 12–15 mL/kg and a rate dependent on individual need. The use of PEEP is dictated not only by the pulmonary fluid status but also by the need in some cases to keep pulmonary vascular resistance as low as possible. The primary cardiac lesion often dictates the duration and method of ventilation following surgical repair. Special care should be given to patients who are sensitive to decreases in pulmonary blood flow or who are at risk for pulmonary hypertensive crises (the sudden elevation of pulmonary blood pressures to or near systemic levels). Extreme caution should be taken to avoid manipulations that cause decreases in functional residual capacity, pH, and PaO_2 or increases in $PaCO_2$, since any of these may contribute to significant elevations in pulmonary vascular resistance and lead to a worsening of their condition. Manipulations of PEEP, tidal volume, ventilation rate, and FiO_2 almost always allow one to achieve normal oxygenation ($PaO_2 > 80$ mm Hg), ventilation ($PaCO_2 \leq 40$ mm Hg), and FRC yet not increase mean airway pressure to levels that can decrease pulmonary blood flow.

Knowledge of the patient's primary lesion and recognition of postoperative pulmonary complications also dictate how aggressively the patient can be weaned from the ventilation. For example, patients with ventricular septal defects and high pulmonary-to-aortic pressure and resistance ratios require mechanical ventilation for significantly longer times than those with lower ratios. Patients with pulmonary edema, hematomas, or significant effusions after surgery require longer ventilation times.Extubation is considered when the patient is hemodynamically stable, arrhythmias are controlled, reoperation is not planned, and the patient can maintain an airway with satisfactory gas exchange. Premature extubation decreases FRC, pH, and PaO_2 and significantly increases pulmonary vascular resistance.

Close monitoring of the postoperative cardiac patient is important. Physical assessment of heart and breath sounds is helpful in detecting cardiac tamponade, pneumothorax, hemothorax, and signs of congestive heart failure. Endotracheal tube placement and pulmonary status are checked with a chest film. Knowledge of the amount, level, and direction of residual intracardiac shunt helps in deciding appropriate oxygenation values. Otherwise, low O_2 saturation values must be considered as pulmonary in origin and suggest the need for more aggressive therapy. Close monitoring of physical examination data, laboratory data, and ventilation promotes a faster and safer recovery.

Fullerton D et al: The effect of respiratory acidemia on pulmonary vascular resistance following cardiopulmonary bypass. Anesth Analg 1990;70:S1.

Matthay MA, Wiener-Kronish JP: Respiratory management after cardiac surgery. Chest 1989;95:424.

Murray JP, Lynn AM, Mansfield PB: Effect of pH and PaO_2 on pulmonary and systemic hemodynamics after surgery in children with congenital heart disease and pulmonary hypertension. J Pediatr 1988;113:474.

Valta P et al: Effects of PEEP on respiratory mechanics after open heart surgery. Chest 1992;102:227.

Wieman DS et al: Perioperative respiratory management in cardiac surgery. Clin Chest Med 1993;14:283.

SHOCK

Shock may be defined as failure of the cardiovascular system to deliver critical substrates and to remove toxic metabolites. This failure leads to anaerobic metabolism in cells and ultimately to irreversible cellular damage. Shock has been categorized into a series of recognizable stages: compensated, uncompensated, and irreversible. Patients in compensated shock have relatively normal cardiac output and normal blood pressures but have alterations in the microcirculation. Because of these alterations, certain tissue beds receive decreased flow while others receive increased flow. The pediatric patient in this state of shock exhibits several compensatory mechanisms. In infants, compensatory increases in cardiac output are achieved primarily by tachycardia rather than increases in stroke volume (cardiac output = stroke volume × heart rate). In young infants in compensated shock, heart rates of 190–210/min are not uncommon, but heart rates over 220/min raise the possibility of supraventricular tachycardia. In older patients, cardiac contractility (stroke volume) and heart rate increase to improve cardiac output. Blood pressure remains normal initially because of peripheral vasoconstriction and increased systemic vascular resistance. Thus, hypotension occurs late and is more characteristic of the uncompensated stage of shock. In the uncompensated stage, there is further deterioration of the oxygen and nutrient supply to the cells with subsequent cellular breakdown and release of toxic substances, causing further redistribution of flow. At this point, the patient is hypotensive, with poor cardiac output. Irreversible shock involving organ damage of the brain and heart is considered terminal.

The causes of shock fall into three general categories: hypovolemic, cardiogenic, and distributive. In many clinical situations, one can see a combination of two or perhaps all three categories. **Hypovolemic shock** is caused by decreased circulating blood volume. This may result from the loss of whole blood or plasma or from excess renal and intestinal fluid losses. These patients usually have intact compensatory mechanisms with increased cardiac output, normal blood pressure, and a shunting of blood away from certain organs. All these responses serve to protect blood flow to the heart and brain. Obviously, if untreated, hypovolemic shock can progress to an irreversible stage.

Cardiogenic shock is an ominous state of decreased substrate delivery secondary to "pump failure." The causes include congenital heart disease, cardiac surgery (following cardioplegia and ventriculotomy), cardiomyopathy secondary to infection or toxins, and ischemic-reperfusion injuries. The patient's compensatory efforts (eg, release of catecholamines with increases in blood pressure, heart rate, and systemic vascular resistance) often have deleterious effects on an already stressed and injured myocardium.

"Distributive shock" is a catch-all phrase for those cases that involve arterial and capillary shunting past tissue beds with an increase in venous capacitance. Examples include anaphylaxis and septic shock. Gram-negative septic shock appears to be mediated by endotoxins (lipopolysaccharides) and subsequent formation of lymphokines (eg, tumor necrosis factor), eicosanoid products, bradykinin, and endorphins. These agents can directly mediate many of the manifestations of septic shock, and they also amplify the injury by attracting granulocytes and macrophages—cells that cause further epithelial injury, activate additional cells, and release mediators. Vasodilators (PGI_2, endorphins) predominate early, causing a drop in systemic vascular resistance. Cardiac output generally is increased to compensate for

the decreased systemic vascular resistance. This phase has been described as "warm shock," since the skin remains well perfused and warm. As septic shock progresses, the heart is no longer able to maintain such a high output, and vasoconstrictors (thromboxane, leukotrienes, endothelin) predominate with resultant decreased peripheral perfusion. Extremities become cool, urine output decreases, and oxygen delivery falls. The speed with which distributive shock progresses varies according to the cause; it can be quite fast in anaphylaxis and insidious in cases associated with gram-positive cocci.

Other Organ Involvement

Organ dysfunction during and after an episode of shock is common. Systems most often affected include the kidney, the blood coagulation system, the lungs, the central nervous system, the liver, and the gastrointestinal tract. The kidney responds to hypotension by increasing plasma renin and angiotensin concentrations, causing a decrease in glomerular filtration rate and urine output. This can progress to damage of the energy-consuming renal parenchyma, causing acute tubular necrosis. Coagulopathies may exist in any type of shock but are especially common in septic shock. This is the result of the release of mediators that activate the clotting cascade, leading ultimately to a consumptive coagulopathy. The central nervous system dysfunction is related to decreased cerebral perfusion pressure and thus to decreased substrate delivery to the brain. Liver dysfunction commonly occurs after shock and may be manifested by increases in liver enzymes or a bleeding diathesis. Gastrointestinal problems include ileus, bleeding (eg, gastritis and ulcers), and necrosis with sloughing of intestinal mucosa. These organ system complications should be aggressively searched for after an episode of shock. When multiple organ system failure exists secondary to shock, the mortality rates increase dramatically. Therefore, the goal of resuscitation efforts should be not only to improve cardiac and volume status but also to maintain and preserve organ function.

Clinical Findings

Both noninvasive and invasive monitoring of the patient in shock provide information on the severity, progression, and response to treatment. The physical examination is the cornerstone of noninvasive monitoring. Extremely valuable information can be derived from examination of the cardiovascular, central nervous, renal, musculoskeletal, and mucocutaneous systems.

A. Symptoms and Signs: The physical examination can be performed quickly and will provide invaluable information on the physiologic status of the patient in shock.

1. Cardiovascular system–Heart rate and blood pressure are the easiest cardiovascular parameters to measure at the bedside. Tachycardia is an early sign, but it is nonspecific and not always present even in profound hypotension. Hypotension is a specific but late sign in pediatric shock (mean systolic blood pressure for a child over 2 years of age can be estimated by adding 90 mm Hg to twice the age in years). An important part of the cardiovascular examination is simultaneous palpation of distal and proximal pulses. An increase in the amplitude difference of pulses between proximal arteries (carotid, brachial, femoral) and distal arteries (radial, posterior tibial, dorsalis pedis) can be palpated in early shock and reflects increased systemic vascular resistance. Distal pulses may be thready or absent even in the presence of normal blood pressure due to poor stroke volume compensated by tachycardia and increased systemic vascular resistance. In uncompensated shock, hypotension is present and proximal pulses are also diminished. Early shock causes peripheral cutaneous vasoconstriction, which preserves flow to vital organs.

2. Skin–Because of peripheral vasoconstriction, the skin is gray or ashen in newborns and pale and cold in older patients. Capillary refilling after blanching is slow (> 3 seconds). Mottling of the skin may also be observed.

3. Musculoskeletal system–Decreased oxygen delivery to the musculoskeletal system produces hypotonia. Decreased spontaneous motor activity, flaccidity, and prostration are observed.

4. Urinary output–Measurement of urinary output gives important information about perfusion of an essential organ system because output is directly proportionate to renal blood flow and the glomerular filtration rate. Catheterization of the bladder is necessary to give accurate and continuous information. (Normal urine output is ≥ 1 mL/kg/h; outputs < 0.5 mL/kg/h are considered significantly decreased.)

5. Central nervous system–The patient's level of consciousness reflects the adequacy of cortical perfusion. When cortical perfusion is severely impaired, the infant or child fails to respond first to verbal stimuli, then to light touch, and finally to pain.

Lack of motor response and failure to cry in response to venipuncture or lumbar puncture should alert the clinician to the severity of the situation. In uncompensated shock in the presence of hypotension, brain stem perfusion may be decreased. Poor thalamic perfusion can result in loss of sympathetic tone. Finally, poor medullary flow produces irregular respirations followed by gasping, apnea, and respiratory arrest.

B. Invasive Monitoring: Patients identified as being significantly hypovolemic with poor cardiac output often need invasive monitoring for diagnostic and therapeutic reasons. Intravascular arterial catheters give constant blood pressure readings, and, to an experienced interpreter, the shape of the wave form is helpful in evaluating cardiac output. Central venous pressure monitoring, accomplished by placing any intravenous catheter within the thorax, gives useful information about relative changes in volume status as therapy is given. Central venous pressure monitoring does not provide information about absolute volume status because intravascular volume, which is considered preload, is most accurately inferred from left ventricular and diastolic pressures. Therefore, intravascular volume is more accurately assessed by monitoring pulmonary capillary wedge pressure or left atrial pressure. Measurements of pulmonary capillary wedge pressure can be obtained with a pulmonary artery catheter. The pulmonary artery catheter provides additional valuable information on volume and cardiac status but is associated with a higher complication rate than central venous pressure lines. This clinical tool provides other information (Table 15–9), including cardiac output, systemic and pulmonary vascular resistances, and right and left ventricular work indexes. Measurements of arterial and mixed venous oxygen saturations, along with cardiac output data, are useful in calculating oxygen delivery, consumption, and extraction. Oxygen consumption is frequently reduced long before hypotension is present. With the use of a pulmonary artery catheter, the effects of manipulating hemoglobin, oxygen saturation, and cardiac output (the determinants of oxygen

Table 15–9. Hemodynamic parameters.[1]

Parameter	Formula[2]	Normal Values	Units
Cardiac output	CO = HR × SV	Wide age-dependent range	L/min
Cardiac index	CI = CO/BSA	3.5–5.5	L/min/m^2
Stroke index	SI = SV/BSA	30–60	mL/m^2
Systemic vascular resistance	SVR = 79.9 $\frac{(MAP - CVP)}{CI}$	800–1600	dyne sec/cm^{-5}/m^2
Pulmonary vascular resistance	PVR = 79.9 $\frac{(MPAP - PCWP)}{CI}$	80–240	dyne sec/cm^{-5}/m^2

[1]Formulas and normals from Katz RW, Pollack M, Weibley R: Pulmonary artery catheterization in pediatric intensive care. Adv Pediatr 1984;30:169.
[2]HR = Heart rate, SV = Stroke volume, BSA = Body surface area.
MAP = Mean arterial pressure, CVP = Central venous pressure.
MPAP = Mean pulmonary artery pressure, PCWP = Pulmonary capillary wedge pressure.

consumption and delivery) can be followed in attempts to achieve independence of oxygen delivery and consumption. Patients receiving significant inotropic or ventilatory support may also benefit from the placement of a pulmonary artery catheter.

New developments in the monitoring of shock in adults include constant esophageal echocardiographic evaluation of cardiac contractility and volume status as well as Doppler cardiac outputs. A suprasternal Doppler method of measuring cardiac output is available for infants. In infants and children, cardiac output can be measured via thoracic bioimpedance. Along with these less invasive measurements, direct oximetry of mixed venous blood appears useful for detecting changes in oxygen consumption and delivery. These and other new tools need careful evaluation in a pediatric setting before they become part of standard care.

Treatment

A. Fluid Resuscitation: The treatment of shock should begin with a logical, stepwise, and quickly instituted plan that takes into account both physical and laboratory assessment as well as the natural history of the disease. A timely infusion of fluids may reverse the shock in patients with hypovolemic and distributive shock. Patients with cardiogenic shock, however, may worsen when given intravenous fluids unnecessarily because of the diminished ability of the left ventricle to handle volume.

Knowing the pathophysiology of the disease helps decide the proper fluid regimen. Initially, most patients tolerate crystalloid (salt solution), which is readily available and inexpensive. However, 4 hours after a crystalloid infusion, only 20% of the solution remains in the intravascular space. Patients with serious capillary leaks and ongoing plasma losses (eg, burn cases) should initially receive crystalloid, because in these cases colloid (protein and salt solution) leaks into the interstitium. The protein draws intravascular fluid into the interstitium, thus increasing ongoing losses. Patients with hypoalbuminemia or those with intact capillaries who need to retain volume in the intravascular space (eg, patients at risk for cerebral edema) probably benefit from colloid infusions. Experience with dextran (a starch compound dissolved in salt solution) is limited. The amount of fluids given should be governed by physical examination, cardiovascular status, and laboratory results. Patients with normal heart function tolerate increased volume better than those with poor function.

B. Pharmacotherapy: Pharmacologic therapy in the form of inotropic support may be needed in patients unable to meet the increased demand for cardiac output. Numerous pharmacologic agents are available, all capable of stimulating cardiac contractility but with varied effects on pulmonary and systemic vascular resistance. Dopamine provides inotropic support and can increase renal, coronary, and cerebral blood flow by its action on beta and dopaminergic receptors. At higher doses (15 μg/kg/min), alpha vasoconstrictor actions predominate. Dobutamine is often added to dopamine. Indeed, dobutamine may be the drug of choice in low cardiac output states because—unlike dopamine—it increases stroke volume and therefore cardiac output while decreasing left ventricular wall tension and myocardial oxygen consumption. Norepinephrine can be used to increase peripheral vasoconstriction, especially in septic shock. Epinephrine should be used with caution. While epinephrine does increase cardiac contractility, it also increases heart rate and afterload, neither of which may be well tolerated in the failing heart. Amrinone acts via different mechanisms (phosphodiesterase inhibitor) but exhibits actions similar to those of dobutamine, increasing cardiac output and decreasing systemic vascular resistance, right atrial pressure, pulmonary capillary wedge pressure, and pulmonary artery pressure, and is increasingly being used in shock states. Patients with increased systemic vascular resistance receiving cardiotonic drugs may benefit from a direct vasodilator to reduce the systemic vascular resistance or afterload and increase cardiac contractility (Table 15–10).

New techniques for treating shock are under trial. Infusions of endotoxin into experimental animals have demonstrated a major role for endotoxin in the pathophysiology of septic shock. As a result, antiendotoxin therapy has reduced the mortality rate in adults with proved gram-negative bacteremia. Passive immunotherapy using healthy adult serum with antiendotoxin activity (induced J5 antiserum and naturally occurring high-titer anti-lipopolysaccharide plasma) have demonstrated improved survival in patients with gram-negative shock. Recently, excess production of nitric oxide has been demonstrated to contribute to the hypotension and poor perfusion seen in shock. Analogues of L-arginine (L-NMA) have been used to block the production of nitric oxide in animal models of septic shock with some improvement in survival. Anecdotal use in adults with severe septic shock has demonstrated some success.

Corticosteroids, by virtue of their action on many mediators thought to play a role in shock—and based on positive results in animal models of septic shock—have been advocated for treatment of shock. Results of recent clinical trials, however, have shown no difference in mortality rates between steroid- and placebo-treated groups.

Extracorporeal membrane oxygenation has been considered in the treatment of shock in patients with recoverable cardiac and pulmonary function who require both pulmonary and cardiac support. This procedure was able to provide cardiopulmonary support to neonatal piglets with septic shock, but mortality rates did not improve. Eight of ten neonates with fulminant septic shock not responsive to conventional

Table 15-10. Pharmacologic support of the shock patient.

Drug	Dose	Alpha-Adrenergic Effect	Beta-Adrenergic Effect	Vasodilator Effect	Actions and Advantages	Disadvantages
Dopamine	1–20 µg/kg/min	+ to + + + (dose-related)	+ to + + + (dose-related)	At low doses, renal vasodilation occurs (dopaminergic receptors).	Moderate inotrope, wide and safe dosage range, short half-life.	May cause worsening of pulmonary vasoconstriction.
Dobutamine	1–10 µg/kg/min	0	+ + +		Moderate inotrope, less chronotropic, fewer dysrhythmias than with isoproterenol or epinephrine.	Marked variation among patients.
Amrinone	Bolus, 0.75 mg/kg over 3 minutes; infusion, 5–10 µg/kg/min	0	0	Direct smooth muscle relaxant.	Non-β-adrenergic inotrope, afterload reduction.	Arrhythmias, thrombocytopenia, gastrointestinal complaints.
Epinephrine	0.05–1 µg/kg/min	+ + to + + + (dose-related)	+ + +		Significant increases in inotropy, chronotropy, and systemic vascular resistance.	Tachycardia, dysrhythmias, renal ischemia, systemic and pulmonary vascular resistance.
Isoproterenol	0.05–1 µg/kg/min	0	+ + +	Peripheral vasodilation.	Significant increase in inotropy and chronotropy. Systemic vascular resistance can drop, and pulmonary vascular resistance should not increase and may decrease.	Significant myocardial oxygen consumption increases, tachycardia, dysrhythmia.
Norepinephrine	0.05–1 µg/kg/min	+ + +	+ + +		Powerful vasoconstrictor (systemic and pulmonary); rarely used except possibly in patients with very low systemic vascular resistance or in conjunction with vasodilator.	Reduced cardiac output if afterload is too high, renal ischemia.
Nitroprusside	0.05–8 µg/kg/min	0	0	Arterial and venous dilation (smooth muscle relaxation)	Decreases systemic and pulmonary vascular resistance, very short-acting. Blood pressure returns to previous levels within 1–10 minutes after infusion is stopped.	Toxicities (thiocyanates and cyanide), increased intracranial pressure and ventilation/perfusion mismatch, methemoglobinemia, increased intracranial pressure.

Key: 0 = no effect; + = small effect; + + = moderate effect; + + + = potent effect

treatment survived after treatment. Further data are needed to determine the role of this modality in the treatment of shock.

Anderson OA, Bensard DD, Harken AH: The role of platelet activating factor and its antagonists in shock, sepsis and multiple organ failure. Surgery 1991;172:415.

Astiz ME, Rackow EC, Weil MH: Pathophysiology and treatment of circulatory shock. Crit Care Clin 1993; 9:183.

Balk RA, Bone RC: The septic syndrome: Definition and clinical implications. Crit Care Clin 1989;5:129.

Bihari DJ, Tinker J: The therapeutic value of vasodilator prostaglandins in multiple organ failure associated with sepsis. Intensive Care Med 1988;15:2.

Bone RC: Gram-negative sepsis. Chest 1991;100:802.

Boyd JL, Stanford GC, Chernow B: The pharmacotherapy of septic shock. Crit Care Clin 1989;5:133.

Burns KM: Vasoactive drug therapy in shock. Crit Care Nurs Clin North Am 1990;2:167.

Calandra T et al: Treatment of gram-negative septic shock with human IgG antibody to *Escherichia coli* J5: J Infect Dis 1988;158:312.

Cunnion RE, Parillo JE: Myocardial dysfunction in sepsis. Crit Care Clin 1989;5:1.

Dinarello CA: The proinflammatory cytokines interleukin-1 and tumor necrosis factor and treatment of the septic shock syndrome. J Infect Dis 1991;163:1177.

Fields AI: Invasive hemodynamic monitoring in children. Clin Chest Med 1987;8:611.

Fink MP: Gastrointestinal mucosal injury in experimental models of shock, trauma, and sepsis. Crit Care Med 1991;19:627.

Griffin MP et al: Extracorporeal membrane oxygenation for gram-negative septic shock in the immature pig. Circ Shock 1991;33:195.

Hazinski MF: Shock in the pediatric patient. Crit Care Nurs Clin North Am 1990;2:309.

Introna RPS: Use of transthoracic bioimpedance to determine cardiac output in pediatric patients. Crit Care Med 1988;16:1101.

Jacobs RF, Tabor DR: Immune cellular interactions during sepsis and septic injury. Crit Care Clin 1989;5:9.

Katz RW, Pollack MM, Weibley RE: Pulmonary artery catheterization in pediatric intensive care. Adv Pediatr 1984;30:169.

Kaufman BS, Kalkow EC, Falk JL: The relationship between oxygen delivery and consumption during fluid resuscitation of hypovolemic and septic shock. Chest 1984;85:336.

Kilbourn RG et al: Reversal of endotoxin mediated shock by NG-methyl-L-arginine, an inhibitor of nitric oxide synthesis. Biochem Biophys Res Commun 1990;172:1132.

Mileski WJ: Sepsis. Surg Clin North Am 1991;71:749.

Nicholson DP: Review of corticosteroid treatment in sepsis and septic shock: Pro or con. Crit Care Clin 1989;5:123.

Perkin RM, Levin DL: Shock in pediatric patients. (Two parts.) J Pediatr 1982;101:163, 319.

Putterman C: Modern approaches to the therapy of septic shock. Am J Emerg Med 1990;8:152.

Sanford TJ: An anesthesiologist's view: The right internal jugular vein. J Clin Monit 1985;1:58.

Shoemaker WC: Relationship of oxygen transport patients to the pathophysiology and therapy of shock states. Intensive Care Med 1987;13:230.

Simpson SQ, Casey LC: The role of tumor necrosis factor in sepsis and acute lung injury. Crit Care Clin 1989;5:137.

St John RC, Dorinsky PM: Immunologic therapy of ARDS, septic shock, and multiple organ failure. Chest 1993; 103:932.

Stenzel JP: Percutaneous femoral venous catheterizations: A prospective study of complications. J Pediatr 1989; 114:411.

Stroud M, Swindell B, Bernard GR: Cellular and humoral mediators of sepsis syndrome. Crit Care Nurs Clin North Am 1990;2:151.

Summers G: The clinical and hemodynamic presentation of the shock patient. Crit Care Nurs Clin North Am 1990;2:161.

Venkataraman ST, Orr RA, Thompson AE: Percutaneous infraclavicular subclavian vein catheterization in critically ill infants and children. J Pediatr 1988;113:480.

Ward CK: An update on pediatric monitoring. J Clin Monit 1985;1:172.

Whitfield JM, Dobyns EL, Webb SA: Neonatal sepsis. In: Textbook of Critical Care. Holbrook PR, editor. Saunders, 1993.

Worthley L, Tyler P, Moran JL: A comparison of dopamine, dobutamine and isoproterenol in the treatment of shock. Intensive Care Med 1985;11:13.

Ziegler EJ et al: Treatment of gram-negative bacteremia and septic shock with HA-1A human monoclonal antibody against endotoxin. The HA-1A Sepsis Study Group. N Eng J Med 1991;324:429.

VASCULAR CATHETER PLACEMENT

Placement of catheters into the central venous circulation may be justified for purposes of assessment of volume, cardiac status, frequent laboratory testing, or administration of central hyperalimentation or drugs. The following is a description of general rules and methods for the placement of intravascular lines.

General Rules for Central Venous System

These are general rules for the placement of central venous lines using the Seldinger technique:

(1) Particularly in the awake or sedated patient, greater success can be achieved if two people perform the procedure (in addition to those occupied with restraining or positioning the patient).

(2) By restricting the variety of kits and equipment used for these procedures, you will achieve greater consistency and success.

(3) Open the kit and test all the equipment. This includes feeding the wire through the needle and filling all lines with normal saline to prevent air from entering the system.

(4) Sterilize and drape the area around the point of entry.

(5) Use local anesthetic as needed.

(6) When searching for the vessel, make straight passes and maintain slight negative pressure. Advance and withdraw needle at same speed. Frequently the blood return will occur during withdrawal.

(7) Once there is a free flow of venous blood into the syringe, take the syringe off and feed the wire into the vein. The wire should pass easily into the vein. Watch the ECG for arrhythmias since they are frequently seen when the wire touches the right side of the heart.

(8) Withdraw the needle over the wire and clean the wire of blood.

(9) Make a nick with a No. 11 blade at a point where the skin and wire meet and place the introducer and intravascular catheter over the wire.

(10) With the catheters in place, remove the wire along with the introducer.

(11) Check to make sure that blood can be drawn easily through the new line.

(12) Verify the position of the line by obtaining an x-ray film.

Points of Entry for Venous Line Placement

After placing a line through any of the following points, be sure to obtain an x-ray film to verify placement and search for complications.

A. External Jugular Vein: Place a shoulder roll beneath the patient and turn the head to the contralateral side (Figure 15–2). Valsalva, Trendelenburg, or occlusion at the clavicular level are ways of temporarily increasing jugular filling and visibility. If a cen-

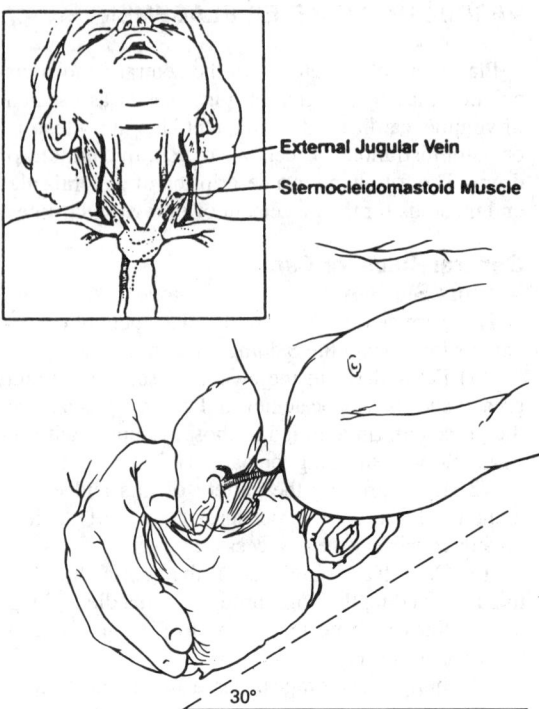

Figure 15–2. External jugular vein technique. (Reproduced, with permission, from Chameides L: *Textbook of Pediatric Advanced Life Support.* American Heart Association, 1988.)

tral venous line is attempted, use a soft J-wire to prevent perforation of the tortuous vein. For patients needing only a simple intravenous line, an intravenous catheter is appropriate.

B. Internal Jugular Vein: Once the patient has been prepared, draped, and positioned as shown Figure 15–3, feel for the trachea halfway between the angle of the jaw and the suprasternal notch and then feel lateral to the trachea for the carotid artery. At that point, at a 30-degree angle from horizontal, insert a finder needle (25 gauge) over the carotid artery, aiming for the ipsilateral nipple. Once venous return is established, remove the finder needle and repeat the procedure using the Seldinger technique.

C. Subclavian Entry: After the patient has been prepared, draped, and positioned (Figure 15–4), move the needle flat along the chest, entering along the inferior edge of the clavicle and over the first rib just lateral to the midclavicular line and aiming for the suprasternal notch. Once venous return is established, use the Seldinger technique.

D. Femoral Approach: With the patient's leg slightly abducted (Figure 15–5), find the femoral artery 3–4 cm below the inguinal ligament. The femoral vein should be found along the path of the artery but medial to it. Insert the needle at a 30- to 45-degree

angle. Once venous return is established, use the Seldinger technique.

E. Antecubital Approach: "PIC" (peripherally inserted catheter) lines (2.8–4F) are long, soft Silastic styleted catheters most commonly threaded from an antecubital vessel to the right atrium. These lines are not difficult to insert and are easy to dress and keep clean. They are suited for long-term use because they are less thrombogenic, tolerable for the patient, and good for infusion of hyperalimentation and drugs. In general they are not suitable for obtaining blood for laboratory analysis.

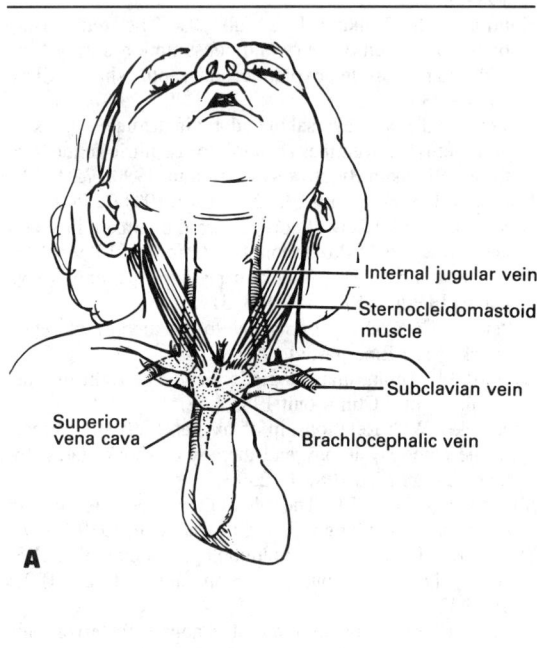

A

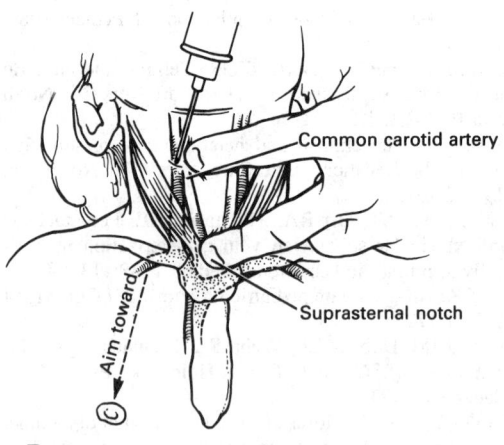

B

Figure 15–3. *A:* The internal jugular vein and its relationship to the surrounding anatomy. *B:* Technique, anterior internal jugular cannulation. (Reproduced, with permission, from Chameides L: *Textbook of Pediatric Advanced Life Support.* American Heart Association, 1988.)

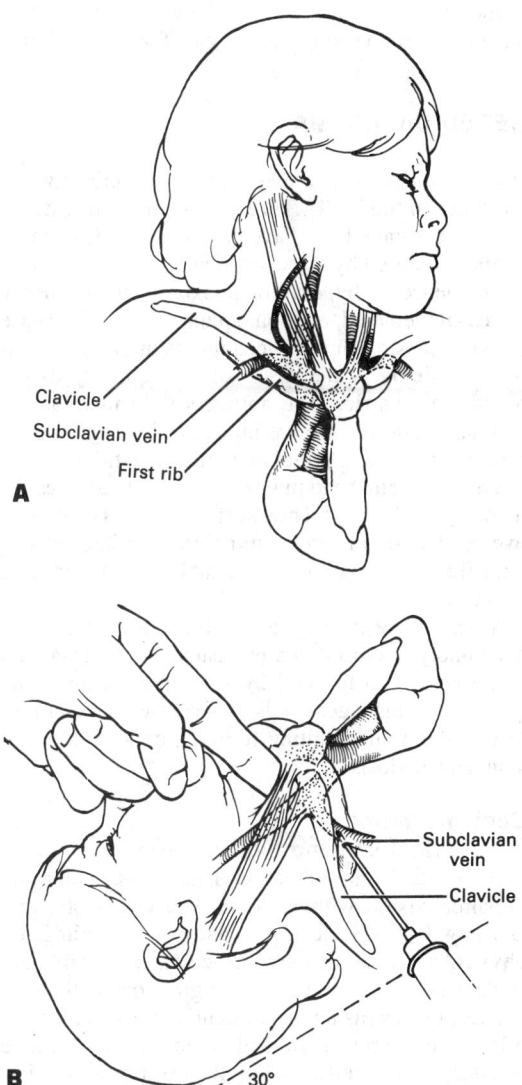

Figure 15–4. Subclavian vein. **A:** Anatomy. **B:** Technique. (Reproduced, with permission, from Chameides L: *Textbook of Pediatric Advanced Life Support.* American Heart Association, 1988.)

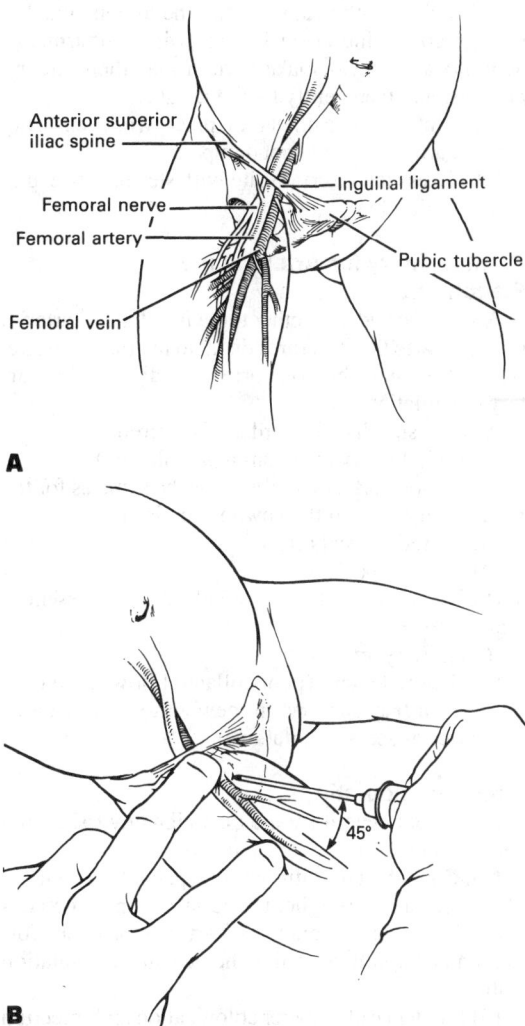

Figure 15–5. Femoral vein. **A:** Anatomy. **B:** Technique. (Reproduced, with permission, from Chameides L: *Textbook of Pediatric Advanced Life Support.* American Heart Association, 1988.)

General Rules for the Arterial System

The following are general rules for the placement of catheters into the arterial circulation:

(1) Rules 1–5 for Central Venous System apply for the arterial system as well.

(2) Seldinger technique can be applied for arterial tree cannulation.

(3) Most arteries can be cannulated percutaneously.

(4) Puncture the skin at the insertion site to eliminate any drag or resistance on the catheter advancement.

(5) Insert cannula at a 30-degree angle to the skin surface, advancing at a slow rate toward the arterial pulse. Watch the hub of the cannula for a flash of arterial blood.

(6) When arterial flash is seen, lower catheter to a 10-degree angle with the surface of the skin and advance the catheter into the lumen of the artery. If successful, pulsatile arterial flow will continue into the catheter. Advance an additional centimeter to make certain that the catheter is in the arterial lumen.

(7) Hold catheter while removing needle stylet. Arterial blood will pulse out of catheter if the tip is in the arterial lumen.

(8) Advance the catheter into the lumen; attach a syringe containing normal saline with 1 unit/mL of heparin; aspirate to make certain that there are no bubbles; and then gently flush the catheter.

(9) Suture the catheter in place while ensuring that the arterial trace is not damped.

(10) Dress the insertion site with sterile gauze, and tape it to the skin.

Point of Entry for Arterial Line Placement

Always consider whether there is collateral arterial blood flow to the structures distal to the insertion site. Allen's test must be done prior to radial or ulnar artery cannulation.

Arterial sites listed in order of preference:

(1) Radial artery (nondominant arm first)

(2) Femoral artery (morbidity is the same as for the radial artery beyond the newborn period).

(3) Posterior tibial artery.

(4) Dorsalis pedis artery.

(5) Ulnar artery (if distal radial filling is present in that hand).

(6) Axillary artery.

(7) Brachial artery (poor collateral flow, used only during cardiac surgery in newborn-sized patients with arterial access limitations).

Final Considerations

(1) Patient benefit should outweigh any risks from central venous or arterial cannulation.

(2) Coagulation status of the patient at time of placement and throughout time of use must be considered, since deep venous and arterial thrombus formation is partially related to the patient's coagulation status.

(3) Incidence of catheter colonization and infection increases if central venous and arterial lines are left in more than 6 days.

COMA*

The workup of the comatose patient is complex and needs to be carried out quickly. Patients with known causes of coma should be treated appropriately for the underlying cause. Occasionally, coma is induced in certain patients, eg, those with extreme and recalcitrant status epilepticus or intractable elevations of intracranial pressure requiring barbiturate coma therapy.

The comatose patient most often requires basic support, including maintenance of the airway by intubation and ventilation. Nutritional support is important and should be started early. Monitoring the comatose child is important, and a convenient scale, such as the Glasgow Coma Scale, should be applied

*This subject is covered in more detail in Chapter 25.

to monitor neurologic status. Many pediatric centers have adapted a version of this scale for their patients.

CEREBRAL EDEMA

Cerebral edema is a major cause of morbidity and mortality in the PICU. Three mechanisms or categories of cerebral edema have been defined. **Cytotoxic edema** is caused by direct cellular injury, usually as a consequence of hypoxia or anoxia. Cellular energy stores are depleted, and ionic pumps of the cell cease activity, causing fluid to accumulate in the cell. **Vasogenic edema** is the result of direct injury to the blood-brain barrier. The normally tight junctions of capillary endothelium are injured, allowing extravasation of water and protein into the interstitium of the brain. Traumatic head injury characteristically results in this type of edema. **Interstitial edema** is caused by overproduction of cerebrospinal fluid or interference with fluid drainage and is treatable with ventricular shunting.

Much of the damage to the brain from traumatic head injury is a result of direct damage to neurons and therefore not influenced by intensive therapy. The goal of ICU management is to decrease secondary injury to the brain resulting from hypoxia, hypoperfusion, and acidosis.

Clinical Findings

A. Symptoms and Signs: Patients with elevations in ICP may develop headaches, vomiting, impaired vision with diplopia, seizures, worsening Glasgow Coma Scale scores, and coma. Findings on physical examination may include alterations in mental status and responsiveness, bulging fontanelle, split sutures, or increasing head circumference (in infants prior to suture fusion), and alterations in muscle tone and deep tendon reflexes. Pupillary response is an important prognostic indicator, with a mortality rate of 50% associated with absent unilateral response and 90% with absent response bilaterally. Papilledema may be present but can take 8–12 hours to develop. The young patient may not demonstrate the Cushing reflex (increase in blood pressure and bradycardia). These signs and symptoms may be quite subtle, especially in patients with long-standing mild to moderate cerebral edema. A complete history and physical examination are often the most useful tools.

B. ICP Monitoring (Table 15–11): The basis for a decision to monitor ICP is not always clear-cut. Patients with acute closed head injury, acute non-communicating hydrocephalus, and Reye's syndrome appear to benefit most from monitoring. Patients with cerebral hemorrhage, meningitis, encephalitis, and cerebral mass lesions may also benefit from monitoring. Patients with hypoxic-ischemic injuries (eg, due to near-drowning or respiratory arrest) have not been shown to benefit.

Table 15–11. Comparison of intracranial pressure monitoring techniques.

Type of Monitor	Placement	Advantages	Disadvantages
External (pressure-sensitive)	Over the skin of open anterior fontanelle	Noninvasive. Useful as trending device.	Very indirect measurement. Useful in limited age group.
Epidural (fiberoptic, hydraulic, and pneumatic)	Between skull and dura	Easy placement. Low risk of infection. Difficult to occlude.	Unable to draw off CSF fluid. May create epidural bleeding.
Subarachnoid (hydraulic or fiberoptic)	Between dura and brain substance	Easy placement. Low risk of infection.	May be occluded by debris. Unable to draw off CSF fluid. May give falsely low readings.
Intraventricular (hydraulic, fiberoptic)	Inside the lateral ventricle	Most direct measurement. Therapeutic if able to draw off CSF.	Requires adequately sized lateral ventricles. Increased risk of bleeding and infection.

Treatment

It is not always necessary to know the ICP before starting treatment. The natural history of the patient's disease often gives sufficient indication to institute treatment early.

A. Traditional Approach: The following steps outline the traditional approach to treatment in increased ICP.

1. The head of the bed should be elevated to a 30-degree angle and the patient's head kept in the midline to facilitate venous drainage.

2. Ventilation should be used in maintaining the airway ($PO_2 > 80$ mm Hg and PCO_2 25–30 mm Hg) to reduce cerebral blood flow.

3. Proper circulation and blood pressure must be maintained to provide a good cerebral perfusion pressure (CPP = mean arterial pressure – intracranial pressure). This pressure, which should be 50–60 mm Hg, is maintained by volume resuscitation or by improving the cardiac status with inotropic drugs if necessary. If the patient is significantly hypertensive, a trial of short-acting hypotensive agents may be necessary to determine if the elevated blood pressure is causing a secondary elevation of ICP.

4. Patients often must be paralyzed to control ventilation and reduce the agitation induced by ICU procedures. Most relaxants need to be stopped at least once every 24 hours for reevaluation of neurologic status.

5. Sedation is controversial and if used should be tailored to each patient, realizing that many of the agents can lower blood pressure and therefore cerebral perfusion pressure. Sedatives also may mask neurologic changes that are important indicators of changing central nervous system status.

6. Fluid imbalance must be corrected early. In patients not requiring intravascular volume repletion, some restriction is helpful. In patients who can withstand a reduction of intravascular volume, administering mannitol and furosemide reduces the intravascular volume. Raising the osmolality of the blood to between 300 and 310 mosm/kg helps to keep the ICP as low as possible. Osmolality and the electrolyte status must be monitored constantly, because the syndrome of inappropriate antidiuretic hormone or diabetes insipidus may develop at any time. Nutrition needs should be addressed early to ensure adequate glucose supply. Physicians must keep in mind that certain patients have very high caloric requirements.

7. Lidocaine or thiopental loading before endotracheal tube suctioning and painful procedures is often helpful in blunting ICP elevation. More aggressive therapies, such as barbiturate coma, hypothermia, and decompressive craniotomy, may be helpful in a very limited patient group, and all have very serious complications.

B. Modified Traditional Approach: A recent study has challenged the approach outlined above. In older adolescents and adults, Rosner and Daughton (1990) were able to improve the mortality rate from 60% predicted to 22% in patients with Glasgow scores less than 5. This was accomplished without dehydration, hyperventilation, or induction of coma. Cerebral perfusion pressure was maintained at or over 70 mm Hg with the idea that doing so would decrease cerebral vasoconstriction and attendant ischemia. This study has raised interesting questions and should provide the impetus for further investigations.

Baethmann A: Mediators of brain edema and secondary brain damage. Crit Care Med 1988;16:972.

Borel C et al: Intensive management of severe head injury. Chest 1990;98:180.

Culditz PB: Fontanelle pressure and cerebral perfusion pressure: Continuous measurements in neonates. Crit Care Med 1988;16:876.

Dean JM, Rogers MC, Traystman RJ: Pathophysiology and clinical management of intracranial vault. In: *Textbook of Pediatric Intensive Care.* Rogers MC (editor). Williams & Wilkins, 1987.

Duck SC, Wyatt DT: Factors associated with brain herniation in the treatment of diabetic ketoacidosis. J Pediatr 1988;113:10.

Emergency Paediatrics Section: Management of children with head trauma. Can Med Assoc J 1990;142:949.

Guertin SR: Cerebral fluid shunts: Evaluation, complications, and crisis management. Pediatr Clin North Am 1987;34:203.

Kaner RK: Infectious complications and duration of intracranial pressure monitors. Crit Care Med 1985;13: 837.

McGillicuday JE: Cerebral protection: Pathophysiology and

treatment of increased intracranial pressure. Chest 1985;87:85.

Olshaker JS, Whye DW Jr: Head trauma. Emerg Med Clin North Am 1993;11:165.

Rosner MJ, Daughton S: Cerebral perfusion pressure management in head trauma. J Trauma 1990;30:933.

Vernon-Levett P: Head injuries in children. Crit Care Nurs Clin North Am 1991;3:411.

BRAIN RESUSCITATION

The subspecialty of neurologic intensive care has grown rapidly over the past 20 years, mainly as a result of longer survival of sicker patients and the more rapid transport of critically ill patients with head injuries. Interest in preventing and limiting hypoxic ischemic damage following primary brain injury has increased dramatically. However, attempts to reverse this damage have met with little success. The role of hypoxia and ischemia in causing damage is related both to the metabolic breakdown caused by intracellular hypoxia and by the cascade of events that follows cell reperfusion.

Initial enthusiasm for use of barbiturate coma to decrease cerebral metabolism has somewhat subsided. Barbiturates do not appear to selectively lower cerebral metabolism without lowering cerebral blood flow. They are now recommended for limited use to treat increased intracranial pressure, with close observation for potential hemodynamic instability induced by barbiturates.

Reperfusion injury in the ischemic region is believed to be related to free radical interaction with lipid membranes, DNA, and intracellular calcium, resulting in cellular damage. Animal research using free radical scavengers and calcium channel blockers show promising results, and human trials are being undertaken.

Recently, specific amino acids have been identified as excitatory neurotransmitters and are postulated to play a role in neurologic injury and seizures. Use of antagonists may be effective treatment and is being investigated.

One must keep in mind that respiratory arrest in the research setting causes more brain damage than does the global ischemia caused by circulatory arrest. This finding is worrisome, because the typical arrest in pediatrics is respiratory.

Kochanek PM: Novel pharmacologic approaches to brain resuscitation after cardiorespiratory arrest in the pediatric patient. Crit Care Clin 1988;4:661.

Krause GS: Brain cell death following ischemia and reperfusion: A proposed biochemical sequence. Crit Care Med 1988;16:714.

Rogers MC, Kirsch JR: Current concepts in brain resuscitation. JAMA 1989;261:3143.

Safar P: Resuscitation from clinical death: Pathophysiologic limits and therapeutic potentials. Crit Care Med 1988; 16:923.

Sutton-Tyrrell K et al: Brain Resuscitation Clinical Trial Study Group: Risk monitoring of randomized trials in emergency medicine: Experience of the brain resuscitation clinical trial II. Am J Emerg Med 1991;9:112.

ETHICAL CONSIDERATIONS IN INTENSIVE CARE

Patient Autonomy

Although the pediatric patient is generally a minor, respect for the patient's rights and wishes should still play a part in the decision-making process. Whenever appropriate, the child should be included in discussions concerning the clinical problem and its management.

Brain Death

The determination of brain death is of increasing importance in the intensive care setting. This is the result of improving out-of-hospital resuscitation and increased therapeutic options for sustaining physiologic functions. In addition, the limited pool of organ donation candidates and the increasing number of potential recipients has made the diagnosis of death prior to the cessation of physiologic function an imperative professional obligation. Currently, the diagnosis of brain death is fairly straightforward and accepted in all jurisdictions. It requires the following conditions:

(1) The absence of a primary remediable condition that might mimic brain death (eg, acute subdural hemorrhage). This generally requires a clear history or a CT scan.

(2) The absence of hypotension with consequent cerebral hypoperfusion that would alter cerebral activity.

(3) The absence of hypothermia, which would alter cerebral activity. Generally this requires a temperature of greater than 35 °C.

(4) The absence of exposure to drugs or toxins that would mimic brain death. This generally requires a toxicology screen. Therapeutic levels of anticonvulsants and sedatives will not mimic brain death.

Once these conditions have been met, the brain death examination can be performed. This examination is designed to guarantee the absence of any cortical or brain stem activity. The following procedures must be performed:

(1) Assessment of cranial nerve function. Test the following reflexes: optic light, oculocalorics, oculocephalics, cough, gag, and corneal. Test for pain sensation on the face.

(2) Assessment of pain response. The body should be examined for the presence of purposeful withdrawal to pain. Caution must be exercised in the interpretation of spinal reflexes.

(3) Assessment of respiratory drive. A 3-minute apnea test should be performed starting with a PCO_2 of 55 mm Hg, and with the patient on 100% oxygen during the test.

Discontinuance of Life Support

In spite of advances in medicine, ICU patients are frequently at the limits of the physician's ability to sustain life. In the interests of the quality of life for the patient and the family, it is often necessary to consider the limitation or discontinuance of life-sustaining treatments. While the topic is too complex and patient variability is too great to allow for a comprehensive discussion of this topic, certain principles underlie the majority of such decisions:

(1) The patient should be considered terminal. Generally, this implies that continuation of life in the best of possible circumstances will be less than a year. In addition, some patients with no ability to meaningfully interact with their environment may also be considered.

(2) There must be single organ system failure that is not amenable to transplant (eg, the cerebral cortex) or multiple organ system failure.

(3) There must be a medical consensus among involved health care personnel as to these diagnoses. This requires the concurrence of at least two physicians as well as of nursing and social services personnel.

(4) The burden of continued existence—pain and suffering—should outweigh any potential gain of continued therapy.

(5) The patient, if appropriate and capable, and the patient's parents and guardians must be fully informed and in agreement with the course of action.

Hospital ethics committees may be of assistance in situations where there is disagreement among health care providers.

Once the decision to limit or discontinue medical therapy has been agreed upon, a course of action that is both humane and in compliance with good medical practice must be determined. All medical therapy may be considered to be extraordinary in certain circumstances.

These decisions cannot be considered irrevocable. If at any time the family or health care providers wish to reconsider the decision, full medical therapy should be reinstituted until the situation is clarified.

Nelson LJ, Nelson RM: Ethics and the provision of futile, harmful, or burdensome treatment to children. Crit Care Med 1992;20(3):427.

Task Force on Ethics of the Society of Critical Care Medicine: Consensus report on the ethics of foregoing life-sustaining treatments in the critically ill. Crit Care Med 1990;18:1435.

Truog RD, Fackler JC: Rethinking brain death. Crit Care Med 1992;20(12):1705.

NUTRITIONAL SUPPORT AFTER INJURY

Metabolic & Physiologic Responses

Trauma, sepsis, and significant injury are associated with a variety of profound metabolic and physiologic responses (Table 15–12). Nutritional status has an impact on in-hospital morbidity rates and mortality outcomes. Inadequate nutrition can impair wound healing and immune function and prevent early weaning from mechanical ventilation. Stress in critically ill children induces more than simple starvation. The hypermetabolic response seen during severe stress results in increased energy usage and endogenous nutrient requirement, especially protein. It is associated with elevated serum catecholamines, corticosteroids, and cytokines. Children under 2 years of age and surgical patients of any age are at greatest risk for nutritional depletion.

Plasma hormone levels are generally elevated as a result of injury. Increases in insulin, glucagon, catecholamines, and glucocorticoids have been reported. Insulin causes increased synthesis of triglycerides and inhibits lipoprotein lipase, thus accounting for the low levels of free fatty acids often observed in febrile or injured patients. Reduced serum ketone bodies, often observed in the injured patient, may also be accounted for by increased insulin levels. This reduc-

Table 15–12. Metabolic and physiologic responses to severe illness.

Physiologic
  Muscle function
    Easier fatigability
    Slower relaxation
    Altered force-frequency pattern
  Respiration
    Increased minute ventilation secondary to increased
      respiratory frequency
    Inefficient gas exchange (see text)
    Increased carbon dioxide responsiveness
Metabolic
  Hormone and hormone-like levels
    Increased insulin
    Increased glucocorticoids
    Increased catecholamines
    Increased interleukin-1
    Increased tumor necrosis factor
  Carbohydrate metabolism
    Increased blood sugar
    Increased gluconeogenesis
    Increased glucose turnover
    Glucose intolerance
  Fat metabolism
    Increased lipid turnover and utilization
    Insuppressible lipolysis
    Decreased ketogenesis
  Protein metabolism
    Increased muscle protein catabolism
    Increased muscle branched-chain amino acid oxidation
    Increased serum amino acids
    Increased mitogen losses

tion in ketones is not insignificant because of the usual protein-sparing effect that ketones provide.

Glucose metabolism is significantly altered in critically ill patients. Despite elevated insulin levels, hyperglycemia and glucose intolerance are frequently observed in the critically ill. This problem is partially due to the increased secretion of counterregulatory products, such as glucagon, cortisol, and norepinephrine, which promote glycogenolysis and enhance the synthesis of glucose from noncarbohydrate compounds (ie, gluconeogenesis). Gluconeogenesis in injury is primarily due to mobilization of alanine, glutamine, and other amino acids from muscle and their biosynthesis to glucose and urea by the liver. The gluconeogenesis observed in injury, as opposed to that seen in starvation, is not easily inhibited or decreased by glucose infusions. Insulin resistance may also develop in skeletal muscle and peripheral adipose tissues in postinjury states. Decreased glucose and fatty acid uptake results, and the energy needs of skeletal muscle must be met by the increased oxidation of the branched-chain amino acids. Because branched-chain amino acids are essential amino acids, their oxidation depletes a valuable pool of precursors required for protein synthesis.

Lipids are the major energy source during periods of stress starvation. Lipolysis occurs despite high levels of insulin. During stress starvation, peripheral tissues, such as skeletal muscle, myocardium, and respiratory muscles, are able to utilize lipids as their major energy source. This is true despite high circulating levels of glucose because of the suppression of glucose use in these tissues. In the stressed patient, lipolysis is much more rapid and efficient and may cause unrelenting depletion of fat stores.

Significant changes in protein metabolism occur in stress. The contribution of protein to total caloric expenditure (protein utilization) increases from 10% in normal children to 15–20% in severely stressed children. There are also marked changes in nitrogen dynamics following injury because of increases in nitrogen excretion. Amino acid levels may be elevated in stressed patients because of the unsuppressible gluconeogenesis. Increased levels of alanine and branched chain amino acids have been correlated with survival in septic patients. Studies in burn patients and septic animal models demonstrate both increased protein synthesis and breakdown. Most critically ill patients are in negative nitrogen balance (protein degradation exceeds synthesis). This condition can be reduced or even reversed with increased nonprotein caloric and protein nutrition, and the increased nutrient intake appears to make a difference in the ability of the patient to tolerate stress.

These abnormalities in classic hormone profiles do not entirely explain the breakdown of skeletal muscle protein. Recently, peptides produced by macrophages and polymorphonuclear leukocytes have been identified as mediators in the nutritional response to injury.

Interleukin-1 (IL-1) and tumor necrosis factor (TNF) are considered the major mediators of the stress response. IL-1 induces fever, leukocytosis, and activation of B and T cells; increases gluconeogenesis; and acts directly on muscle to increase proteolysis. Furthermore, a small peptide found in septic patients' serum is thought to be a breakdown product of IL-1 and has similar effects. TNF inhibits lipoprotein lipase, thereby reducing the capacity of peripheral tissues to utilize triglycerides. All these effects ultimately result in further muscle wasting. These findings appear to link the metabolic and immunologic reactions to infection and trauma.

Besides loss of tissue mass, muscle function abnormalities are also observed during stress. Among the abnormalities reported are an altered force-frequency pattern, slower relaxation, and easier muscle fatigability. Easier fatigability could contribute to the subjective feeling of weakness that accompanies recovery from surgery or injury. Significant changes in the pattern of ventilation have been reported. These include increased minute ventilation (secondary to increases in respiratory frequency) and increases in the ratio of dead space to tidal volume ventilation.

Nutritional Assessment

The physician assessing the nutritional needs of the injured patient must address two major issues: the preexisting nutritional status of the patient and the degree of stress imposed by the disease process.

The pediatric patient is at a marked disadvantage compared to adults during periods of stress starvation. Not only is there the problem of increased proteolysis that is less responsive to carbohydrate administration alone, but there is an additional caloric requirement for growth. If this extra energy is not available, growth ceases. Furthermore, children have grater caloric requirements per weight and less caloric reserves than adults. They also have greater energy requirements because the major metabolic organs (brain, kidneys, liver, heart) make up a greater percentage of their body weight than adults.

Several methods are available for assessing nutritional status (see Chapter 8). The degree of metabolic stress accompanying the injury should also be examined. Resting energy expenditure is elevated by a minimum of about 15% in critically ill patients and may be much higher. The energy needs of a patient may be approximated by multiplying the estimated basal metabolic rate (BMR), as derived from the Harris-Benedict equation, by a factor of 1.75:

Male: BMR = 66 + (13.7 × W) + (5.0 × H) – (6.8 × A)

Female: BMR = 655 + (9.6 × X) + (1.7 × H) – (4.7 × A)

where BMR = basal metabolic rate in kilocalories, W = weight in kilograms, H = height in centimeters and A = age in years.

Another practical method of evaluating the nutritional stresses on a patient is by computing the catabolic index:

$$\text{Catabolic index} = UUN - (0.5 \times N_{in} + 3)$$

where UUN = 24-hour urine urea nitrogen in grams, N_{in} = 24-hour nitrogen intake in grams.

This equation expresses the level of dietary intake and the extent of protein degradation as a single number. Scores of –5 to 0 indicate no significant stress; 0–5, moderate stress; and 5–10, severe stress. High scores may predict which patients may benefit from amino acid solution augmented with branched-chain amino acids.

Enteral & Parenteral Alimentation

A. Enteral Alimentation: Present evidence suggests that the enteral route of feeding provides a more normal and homeostatic milieu than parenteral feeding does. Several advantages of enteral over parenteral nutrition have been demonstrated. Some reports suggest that host responses or defenses during stress starvation may be improved when the patient is fed via the gastrointestinal tract. Others have demonstrated that malnutrition increased mortality rates in laboratory animals after septic peritonitis. Furthermore, malnourished animals fed enterally had much higher survival rates after sepsis induced by *Escherichia coli* than septic animals fed parenterally. Both cellular and humoral immunity can be affected by route of feeding. Lymphocyte function is better and secretory IgA levels higher in animals fed enterally than in those fed parenterally. Lower levels of catabolic hormones (cortisol, glucagon, norepinephrine) have been found in injured animals following early institution of enteral feeding than in injured animals receiving parenteral nutrition. Thus, the hypermetabolic state may be reduced by early enteral feeding. Jejunal weight and thickness are also improved by enteral feeding. This increase has beneficial effects on gastrointestinal function, including potentially decreased translocation of bacteria across the gut, which could reduce the incidence of secondary infections in stressed patients. Enteral nutrition may also protect against stress ulceration, a serious yet not uncommon complication in severely ill patients.

Complications of enteral feeding are relatively common in critically ill children. Nausea and vomiting occur in up to 20% of patients, usually when gastric emptying time is prolonged as a result of paralytic ileus or gastrointestinal edema. Edema may occur postoperatively or in response to trauma, burns, sepsis, or malnutrition. The incidence of diarrhea is high in critically ill patients receiving enteral alimentation. Diarrhea appears to be related to lower serum albumin levels. Hypoalbuminemia is associated with the development of diffuse gastrointestinal edema, re-

sulting in impaired gastrointestinal absorptive capacity. Some patients with acute kwashiorkor-like hypoalbuminemia develop a protein-losing enteropathy. This can be diagnosed by elevated levels of fecal $\alpha 1$-antitrypsin. Tolerance to enteral alimentation in hypoalbuminemic patients may be improved by providing peptide-based rather than standard intact protein diets. These diets are composed of protein hydrolysates of varying chain lengths and of varying concentrations of peptides, free amino acids, fat, and carbohydrate. This type of enteral alimentation attenuates protein turnover in the intestine and results in a rise in serum albumin level. It has been reported that this method of feeding avoids the need for parenteral albumin and total parenteral nutrition when intervention occurs early enough to prevent the development of malnutrition. Thus, peptide-based diets could improve nitrogen retention and the nutritional status of critically ill patients.

B. Parenteral Nutrition: When the gastrointestinal tract is not functional and severe stress is present, central intravenous hyperalimentation should be instituted to provide adequate calories and nutrition during the hypermetabolic state. Carbohydrates should be provided at a rate of 2–3 mg/kg/min; proteins, at 1.5 g/kg/d; and fat, at approximately 15–33% of the total caloric demand. Rationales for these recommendations and for the provision of a balanced parenteral diet are provided in Chapter 8. Because several complications and problems occur in patients with central lines, the placement of these lines must not be taken lightly. Placement of central lines is associated with such complications as pneumothorax, arterial injury, and infection. Central venous thrombosis at the catheter site has been documented by venography in up to 24% of patients. This complication may be reduced by the addition of heparin (1–3 units/mL) to the hyperalimentation solution. Hyperglycemia, which may already be present in the stressed patient, can be aggravated by the large amounts of glucose necessary to meet caloric demands. Insulin infusions occasionally may be necessary to control high levels of blood sugar. And finally, if fever is present in a patient receiving central intravenous alimentation, a routine protocol should be followed. In the absence of frank shock or purulent drainage around the catheter site (which would necessitate immediate removal of the catheter), the catheter can be changed over a wire (Seldinger technique). At this time, cultures are obtained of blood drawn through the catheter and of the peripheral blood. Diagnosis and therapy are guided by culture results.

Balistrevi WF, Farrell MK: Enteral feeding: Scientific basis and clinical applications. Report of the Ninety-Fourth Ross Conference on Pediatric Research. Columbus Ohio, Ross Laboratories, 1988.

Ball MJ: Parenteral nutrition in the critically ill: Use of a medium chain triglyceride emulsion. Intensive Care Med 1993;19:89.

Bower RH: Nutrition during critical illness and sepsis. New Horizons 1993;1:348.

Cerra FB et al: Improvement in immune function in ICU patients by enteral nutrition supplemented with arginine, RNA, and Menhaden oil is independent of nitrogen balance. Nutrition 1991;7:193.

Christman JW, McCain RW: A sensible approach to the nutritional support of mechanically ventilated critically ill patients. Intensive Care Med 1993;19:129.

Dayl JM et al: Enteral nutrition with supplemental arginine, RNA, and omega-3 fatty acids in patients after operation: Immunologic, metabolic, and clinical outcome. Surgery 1992;112:56.

Huddleston KC, Ferraro-McDuffie A, Wolff-Small T: Nutritional support of the critically ill child. Crit Care Nursing Clin North Am 1993;5:65.

Kudsk KA et al: Enteral versus parenteral feeding: Effects on septic morbidity after blunt and penetrating trauma. Ann Surg 1992;215:503.

Pollack MM: Nutritional support of children in the intensive care unit. In: *Textbook of Pediatric Nutrition.* Suskind RM, Lewinter-Suskind L (editors). Raven Press Ltd, 1993.

Skeie B: Intravenous emulsion and lung function: A revue. Crit Care Med 1988;16:183.

PAIN & ANXIETY CONTROL
(Table 15–13)

Anxiety control and pain relief are two of the most important responsibilities of the critical care physician. Earlier perceptions that children do not require pain relief have drastically changed in response to documented proof of improved outcomes in children receiving appropriate pain relief. The anxiety of patients in the PICU is well known. These responses may interact to heighten fear and the perception of pain and may reach levels sufficient to cause deterioration in the patient's clinical condition. It is important to distinguish between anxiety and pain, since pharmacologic therapy may be directed at either one or at both of these symptoms.

Sedation

Sedative (anxiolytic) drugs are used to quiet the patient, relieve excitement, and induce calmness without producing sleep—though at high doses all anxiolytics will cause drowsiness and sleep. The five indications for use of sedative drugs are (1) to allay fear and anxiety; (2) to manage acute confusional states; (3) to facilitate treatment or diagnostic procedures; (4) to facilitate mechanical ventilation; and (5) to obtund physiologic responses to stress, ie, reduce tachycardia, hypertension, or increases in intracranial pressure. Although the "ideal" sedative does not exist, it would be a drug that provides good clinical sedation, has no effect on the cardiovascular and respiratory system, has a short elimination half-life, does not affect the metabolism of other drugs, and has no cumulative effects with repeated administration. In the ICU setting, a parenteral (intravenous bolus or infusion) preparation is essential to allow titration of clinical effects in the face of possible impaired organ dysfunction (cardiac, respiratory, hepatic, renal, etc). Sedatives fall into several classes, with the opioid and benzodiazepine classes serving as the mainstay of anxiety treatment in the ICU. The opioids possess both sedative and analgesic properties and will be discussed separately below.

Table 15–13. Pain and anxiety control.

Drug	Dose and Method of Administration[1]	Advantages	Disadvantages	Usual Duration of Effect
Morphine	IV, 0.1 mg/kg; Continuous infusion; 0.01–0.05 mg/kg/h	Excellent pain relief, reversible	Respiratory depression, hypotension, nausea, suppression of intestinal motility, histamine release	2–4 hours
Meperidine	IV, 1 mg/kg	Good pain relief, reversible	Respiratory depression, histamine release, nausea, suppression of intestinal motility	2–4 hours
Fentanyl	IV, 1–2 µg/kg; Continuous infusion; 0.5–2 µg/kg/h	Excellent pain relief, reversible, short half-life	Respiratory depression, chest wall rigidity, severe nausea and vomiting	30 min
Diazepam	IV, 0.1 mg/kg	Sedation and seizure control	Respiratory depression, jaundice, phlebitis	1–3 hours
Lorazepam	IV, 0.1 mg/kg	Longer half-life, sedation and seizure control	Nausea and vomiting, respiratory depression, phlebitis	2–4 hours
Midazolam	IV, 0.1 mg/kg	Short half-life, only benzodiazapine given as continuous infusion	Respiratory depression	30–60 min

[1]IV administration is most common in the ICU. Effects of morphine, meperidine, and fentanyl are reversible by administration of naloxone (opioid antagonist).

A. Benzodiazepines: Benzodiazepines possess anxiolytic, hypnotic, anticonvulsant, and skeletal muscle relaxant properties. Although their exact mode of action is not known, it appears to be located within the limbic system of the central nervous system and to involve the neuroinhibitory transmitter γ-aminobutyric acid. Most benzodiazepines are metabolized in the liver, with their metabolites subsequently excreted in the urine; thus, patients in liver failure are likely to have long elimination times. The benzodiazepines are not removed in appreciable amounts by hemodialysis.

Benzodiazepine overdosage results in amplification of their therapeutic effects. They can cause respiratory depression if given rapidly in high doses, and they potentiate the analgesic and respiratory depressive effects of opioids and other central nervous system depressant medications such as barbiturates.

Three benzodiazepines with differing half-lives are presently used in the intensive care unit setting.

1. Midazolam–Midazolam has the shortest half-life (1½–3½ hours) of the benzodiazepines and is the only benzodiazepine that should be administered as a continuous intravenous infusion. It produces excellent retrograde amnesia lasting for 20–40 minutes after a single intravenous dose. Therefore, it can be used either for short-term sedation or for "awake" procedures such as endoscopy or as a continuous infusion to produce anxiolysis, drowsiness, and anterograde amnesia in the anxious, restless patient. The single intravenous dose is 0.1 mg/kg, while a continuous infusion should be started at a rate of 0.1 mg/kg/h after an initial loading dose of 0.1 mg/kg. The midazolam infusion dosage must be titrated upward to achieve the desired effect. Midazolam is not an analgesic, and if very high doses are being used without the proper effect and it is felt that analgesia is also needed, the dose of midazolam can usually be lowered by the concurrent use of small doses of an appropriate analgesic such as morphine or fentanyl. When administering midazolam or any other benzodiazepine, it is important to monitor cardiorespiratory status and have everything needed available to deal with sudden unexpected decompensations such as hypotension and apnea.

2. Diazepam–Diazepam has a longer half-life than midazolam and can be given orally as well as by the intravenous route. Its disadvantage in the ICU is its intermediary metabolite, nordiazepam, which has a very long elimination half-life and may accumulate, causing prolonged sedation. It produces excellent anxiolysis and amnesia. Additionally, it is used to treat acute status epilepticus. The intravenous dose is 0.1 mg/kg and can be repeated every 15 minutes to achieve the desired effect or until undesirable side effects such as somnolence and respiratory depression occur.

3. Lorazepam–Lorazepam possesses the longest half-life of the three benzodiazepines discussed here

and can be used to achieve sedation for as long as 6–8 hours. It has less effect on the cardiovascular and respiratory systems than other benzodiazepines and can be given orally, intravenously, or intramuscularly, with the intravenous route the most effective in the ICU setting. The intravenous dosage is 0.1 mg/kg. Lorazepam can also be used to treat acute status epilepticus.

B. Other drugs:

1. Chloral hydrate–Chloral hydrate is an enteral sedative and hypnotic agent frequently used in children. After either oral or rectal administration, it is rapidly metabolized by the liver to its active form trichloroethanol, which has an 8-hour half-life. A sedative dose is 6–20 mg/kg/dose, usually given every 6–8 hours, while the hypnotic dose is up to 50 mg/kg with a maximum dose of 1 g. The hypnotic dose is frequently used to sedate young children for outpatient radiologic procedures such as CT scanning and MRI. There is little effect on respiration or blood pressure with therapeutic doses of chloral hydrate. The drug is irritating to mucus membranes, however, and may cause gastric upset if administered on an empty stomach.

2. Ketamine–Ketamine is a phencyclidine derivative that produces a trance-like state of immobility and amnesia known as "dissociative anesthesia." After intramuscular or intravenous administration, it causes central sympathetic nervous system stimulation with resultant increases in heart rate, blood pressure, and cardiac output. (In vitro, ketamine produces direct myocardial depression, emphasizing the importance of intact sympathetic nervous system for cardiac stimulating effects.) Respiration is not depressed at therapeutic doses. However, salivary and tracheobronchial mucous gland secretions are increased, leading to the recommendation that an antisialagogue be administered 20 minutes prior to the ketamine. A distinct disadvantage of its use is the occurrence of unpleasant dreams or hallucinations, though the incidence is decreased in children compared to adults and can be reduced even further by the concurrent administration of a benzodiazepine. Because of its inotropic properties, it is useful for the sedation of certain critically ill patients whose condition is unstable. It is given as an intravenous injection of 1–2 mg/kg over 60 seconds, with supplementary doses of 0.5 mg/kg being required every 10–30 minutes to maintain an adequate level of anesthesia. Alternatively, it can be administered as an intramuscular injection of 5–10 mg/kg, which usually produces the desired level of anesthesia within 3–4 minutes. If prolonged anesthesia is required, ketamine can be administered by intravenous infusion at doses of 3–20 mg/kg/h.

3. Antihistamines–The antihistamines **diphenhydramine** and **hydroxyzine** can be used as sedatives but are not felt to be as effective as the benzodiazepines. Diphenhydramine produces sedation in only 50% of those treated. It can be given intravenously, intramuscularly, or orally at a dose of 1 mg/kg. Hydroxyzine can be given either intramuscularly or orally. It is frequently used concurrently with morphine or meperidine, adding anxiolysis and potentiating the effects of the opioid. The sedative effects of both drugs can last from 4 to 6 hours following a single dose.

4. Propofol–Propofol is an anesthetic induction agent whose main advantage is a rapid recovery time and no cumulative effects due to its rapid hepatic metabolism. It has no analgesic properties, frequently causes pain on injection, and causes a dose-related fall in blood pressure because of decreases in systemic vascular resistance. There are only a few clinical reports of its use as a sedative agent in pediatric patients, and the drug is very expensive. The sedative dose is 1 mg/kg as an intravenous bolus followed by an infusion of 1 mg/kg/h.

5. Barbiturates–Barbiturates (phenobarbital, thiopental) can cause direct myocardial and respiratory depression and are, in general, poor choices for sedation of seriously ill patients. Phenobarbital has a very long half-life (up to 4 days), and recovery from thiopental, though it is a "short-acting" barbiturate, can be prolonged because remobilization of tissue stores occurs.

Analgesia

A. Opioid Analgesics: Opioid analgesics (morphine, fentanyl, codeine, meperidine) are the mainstays of therapy for most forms of acute severe pain as well as chronic cancer pain management. They possess both analgesic and dose-related sedative effects, though there is a range of plasma concentrations that produce analgesia without clouding of the sensorium. In addition, opioids can cause respiratory depression, nausea, pruritus, slowed intestinal motility, miosis, urinary retention, cough suppression, biliary spasm, and vasodilation. There is great individual variation in the dose of opioid required to produce adequate analgesia. Therefore, in the intensive care setting, a continuous infusion of morphine or fentanyl allows dosages to be easily titrated to achieve the desired effect.

In general, infants under 3 months of age are more susceptible to the respiratory depressant effects of opioids, and starting dosages for these patients should be about one-third to one-half the usual pediatric dose. Most opioids (except meperidine) have minimal cardiac depressive effects, and critically ill patients generally tolerate them well. Fentanyl does not cause the histamine release that morphine does and thus produces less vasodilation and drop in systemic blood pressure. Opioids are metabolized in the liver, with metabolites excreted in the urine. Thus, patients with hepatic or renal impairment may have a prolonged response to their administration. Patients who receive regular doses of opioids for 2 weeks or more

frequently develop a physiologic dependence with the development of withdrawal symptoms (agitation, tachypnea, tachycardia, sweating, diarrhea) upon acute termination of the drug. In these patients, gradual tapering of the opioid dosage over a 5- to 10-day period will prevent withdrawal symptoms. As with any potent sedative or analgesic used in the ICU setting, appropriate patient monitoring (pulse oximetry, cardiorespiratory monitoring, and blood pressure monitoring) should be used during the period of opioid administration, and equipment should be available to support prompt intervention if undesired side effects occur.

The ICU regimen for sedation and analgesia must be carefully modified when the patient is transferred to the ward or a lower vigilance area. Patients with baseline respiratory, hepatic, or renal insufficiencies are most predisposed to respiratory insufficiency from sedatives or opioid analgesics.

Patient-controlled analgesia (PCA) is a computer-controlled infusion pump for constant infusion or patient-controlled bolus infusion of opioid analgesics. The basal infusion mode is intended to provide a constant serum level of analgesic. The bolus mode allows the patient to self-administer, by pushing a button, additional doses for breakthrough pain. The patient is usually permitted six boluses an hour, with 10-minute blockouts. If the patient is using allotted hourly boluses, this usually means that the basal infusion rate is too low.

The patient must understand the concept of PCA in order to be a candidate for its use. There are circumstances in pediatrics where it is appropriate for the nurse or parent to administer the bolus dose.

Naloxone reverses the analgesia, sedative, and respiratory depressive effects of opioid agonists. Its administration should again be titrated to achieve the desired effect (such as reversal of respiratory depression, since full reversal using 0.01–0.02 mL/kg may cause acute anxiety, dysphoria, nausea, and vomiting). Furthermore, since the duration of effect of naloxone is shorter (30 minutes) than that of most opioids, the patient must be carefully observed for reappearance of the undesired effect.

B. Nonopioid Analgesics: Nonopioid analgesics used in the treatment of mild to moderate pain include acetaminophen, aspirin, and other nonsteroidal anti-inflammatory agents such as ibuprofen and naproxen.

1. Acetaminophen–Acetaminophen is the most commonly used analgesic in pediatrics in the United States and is the drug of choice for mild to moderate pain because of its low toxicity and lack of effect on bleeding time. It is metabolized by the liver. Suggested doses are 10–15 mg/kg orally to approximately 10–20 mg/kg rectally every 4 hours.

2. Aspirin–Aspirin is also an effective analgesic for mild to moderate pain at doses of 10–15 mg/kg orally every 4 hours. However, its prolongation of bleeding time, association with Reye's syndrome, and propensity to cause gastric irritation limit its usefulness in pediatric practice. Aspirin and other NSAIDs are still useful especially for pain of inflammatory origin, bone pain, and pain associated with rheumatic conditions.

3. Other NSAIDs–Ibuprofen and naproxen are both NSAIDs whose use has been limited in pediatrics to date. **Naproxen** is FDA-approved for children 2–12 years of age (5–7 mg/kg orally every 8–12 hours), while **ibuprofen** requires more frequent dosing intervals (4–10 mg/kg orally every 6–8 hours).

All of the NSAIDs have a therapeutic "ceiling"— ie, unlike opioids, which have a dose-related increase in potency, there is no increase in analgesic potency above the recommended dose. They all can cause gastritis and should be given with antacids or with meals. In addition, the analgesic effects of acetaminophen, aspirin, and other NSAIDs are additive to those of opioids. Thus, if additional analgesia is required, their use should be continued and an appropriate oral opi-

oid (codeine, morphine) or parenteral opioid (morphine, fentanyl) begun.

Berde C et al: Report of the Subcommittee on Disease-Related Pain in Childhood Cancer. Pediatrics 1990; 86:8180.

Crippen DW: The role of sedation in the ICU patient with pain and agitation. Crit Care Clin 1990;6:369.

Lloyd-Thomas AR: Pain management in paediatric patients. Br J Anaesth 1990;64:85.

Oh TE, Duncan AW: Sedation in the seriously ill. Med J Austr 1990;152:540.

Schecter NL, Allen DA, Hanson K: Status of pediatric pain control: A comparison of hospital analgesic usage in children and adults. Pediatrics 1986;77:11.

Shannon M, Berde CB: Pharmacologic management of pain in children and adolescents. Pediatr Clin North Am 1989;36:855.

Temme JB, Anderson JC, Matecko S: Sedation of children for CT and MRI scanning. Radiol Technol 1990;61:283.

Yaster M, Deshpande JK: Management of pediatric pain with opioid analgesics. J Pediatr 1988;113:421.

16

Skin

Joseph G. Morelli, MD, & William L. Weston, MD

GENERAL PRINCIPLES OF DIAGNOSIS

Examination of the Skin

Examination of the skin requires that the entire surface of the body be palpated and inspected in good light. The onset and duration of each symptom should be recorded, together with a description of the primary lesion and any secondary changes, using the following terminology:

A. Primary Lesions (the First to Appear):

1. Macule–Any circumscribed color change in the skin that is flat. *Examples:* White (vitiligo), brown (café au lait spot), purple (petechia).

2. Papule–A solid, elevated area < 1 cm in diameter whose top may be pointed, rounded, or flat. *Examples:* Acne, warts, small lesions of psoriasis.

3. Plaque–A solid, circumscribed area > 1 cm in diameter, usually flat-topped. *Example:* Psoriasis.

4. Vesicle–A circumscribed, elevated lesion < 1 cm in diameter and containing clear serous fluid. *Example:* Blisters of herpes simplex.

5. Bulla–A circumscribed, elevated lesion > 1 cm in diameter and containing clear serous fluid. *Example:* Bullous erythema multiforme.

6. Pustule–A vesicle containing a purulent exudate. *Examples:* Acne, folliculitis.

7. Nodule–A deep-seated mass with indistinct borders that elevates the overlying epidermis. *Examples:* Tumors, granuloma annulare. If it moves with the skin on palpation, it is intradermal; if the skin moves over the nodule, it is subcutaneous.

8. Wheal–A circumscribed, flat-topped, firm elevation of skin resulting from tense edema of the papillary dermis. *Example:* Urticaria.

B. Secondary Changes:

1. Scales–Dry, thin plates of keratinized epidermal cells (stratum corneum). *Examples:* Psoriasis, ichthyosis.

2. Lichenification–Induration of skin with exaggerated skin lines and a shiny surface resulting

from chronic rubbing of the skin. *Example:* Atopic dermatitis.

3. Erosion and oozing–A moist, circumscribed, slightly depressed area representing a blister base with the roof of the blister removed. *Examples:* Burns, bullous erythema multiforme. Most oral blisters present as erosions.

4. Crust–Dried exudate of plasma on the surface of the skin following acute dermatitis. *Examples:* Impetigo, contact dermatitis.

5. Fissure–A linear split in the skin extending through the epidermis into the dermis. *Example:* Angular cheilitis.

6. Scar–A flat, raised, or depressed area of fibrotic replacement of dermis or subcutaneous tissue. *Examples:* Acne scar, burn scar.

7. Atrophy–Depression of the skin surface due to thinning of one or more layers of skin.

C. Color: The lesion should be described as red, yellow, brown, tan, or blue. Particular attention should be given to the blanching of red or brown lesions, eg, petechiae.

D. Configuration of Lesions: Clues to diagnosis may be obtained from the characteristic morphologic arrangement of primary or secondary lesions.

1. Annular (circular)–Annular nodules represent granuloma annulare; annular papules are more apt to be due to dermatophyte infections.

2. Linear (straight line)–Linear papules represent lichen striatus; linear vesicles, incontinentia pigmenti; linear papules with burrows, scabies.

3. Grouped–Grouped vesicles occur in herpes simplex or zoster.

4. Discrete–Discrete lesions are independent of each other.

E. Distribution: It is useful to note whether the eruption is generalized, acral (hands, feet, buttocks, or face), or localized to a specific skin region.

F. Description of Skin Lesions: Skin lesions are described in reverse order from that of their identification. One begins with distribution, configuration, color, secondary changes, and then primary lesion; eg, guttate psoriasis could be described as generalized discrete, red, scaly papules.

GENERAL PRINCIPLES
OF TREATMENT OF SKIN DISORDERS

TOPICAL THERAPY

Treatment should be simple and aimed at preserving or restoring the physiologic state of the skin. It is essential to keep in mind that one is treating the child and not the anxious parent or grandparent. Topical therapy is often preferred because medication can be delivered in optimal concentrations at the exact site where it is needed.

Water is an important therapeutic agent and optimally hydrated skin is soft and smooth. This occurs at approximately 60% environmental humidity. Because water evaporates readily from the cutaneous surface, the skin (stratum corneum of the epidermis) is dependent on the water concentration in the air, and sweating contributes little. However, if sweat is prevented from evaporating (eg, in the axilla, groin), the humidity and hydration of the skin are increased. As humidity falls below 15–20%, the stratum corneum shrinks and cracks; the epidermal barrier is lost and allows irritants to enter the skin and induce an inflammatory response. Replacement of water will correct this condition if evaporation is prevented. Therefore dry and scaly skin is treated by soaking the skin in water for 5 minutes and then adding a barrier to evaporation (Table 16–1). Oils and ointments prevent evaporation for 8–12 hours so they must be applied once or twice a day. In areas already occluded (axilla, diaper area), ointments or oils will merely increase retention of water and should not be used.

Overhydration (maceration) can also occur. As environmental humidity increases to 90–100%, the number of water molecules absorbed by the stratum corneum increases and the tight lipid junctions between the cells of the stratum corneum are gradually replaced by weak hydrogen bonds; the cells eventually become widely separated, and the epidermal barrier falls apart. This occurs in immersion foot, diaper areas, axillae, etc. It is desirable to enhance evaporation of water in these areas by air drying.

WET DRESSINGS

By placing the skin in an environment where the humidity is 100% and allowing the moisture to evaporate to 60%, pruritus is relieved. Evaporation of water stimulates cold-dependent nerve fibers in the skin and this may prevent the transmission of the itching sensation via pain fibers to the central nervous system. It also is vasoconstrictive, thereby helping to

Table 16–1. Bases used for topical preparations.

Base	Combined With	Uses
Liquids		Wet dressings: relieve pruritus, vasoconstrict.
	Powder	Shake lotions, drying pastes: relieve pruritus, vasoconstrict.
	Grease and emulsifier; oil in water	Vanishing cream: penetrates quickly (10–15 minutes) and thus allows evaporation.
	Excess grease and emulsifier; water in oil	Emollient cream: penetrates more slowly and thus retains moisture on skin.
Grease		Ointments: occlusive (hold material on skin for prolonged time) and prevent evaporation of water.
Powder		Enhances evaporation.

Characteristics of bases for topical preparations:
1. Most greases are triglycerides (eg, Aquaphor, petrolatum, Eucerin).
2. Oils are fluid fats (eg, Alpha Keri, olive oil, mineral oil).
3. True fats (eg, lard, animal fats) contain free fatty acids that increase in amount upon standing and cause irritation.
4. Ointments (eg, Aquaphor, petrolatum) should not be used in intertriginous areas such as the axillae, between the toes, and in the perineum, because they increase maceration. Lotions or creams are preferred in these areas.
5. Oils and ointments hold medication on the skin for long periods of time and are therefore ideal for barriers or prophylaxis and for dried areas of skin. Medication gets into the skin more slowly from ointments.
6. Creams carry medication into skin and are preferable for intertriginous dermatitis.
7. Solutions, gels, or lotions should be used for scalp treatments.

reduce the erythema and also decreasing the inflammatory cellular response.

Gauze of 20/12 mesh is commonly used for wet dressings. Parke-Davis 4-inch gauze comes in 100-yard rolls, and 5 yards is usually sufficient for application to the extremities. Curity 18-inch gauze can be used for application to the trunk. An alternative is to use the "two long johns" technique, in which a pair of wet cotton long-sleeved and long-legged underwear is covered by a dry pair.

Warm but not hot water is used, and the gauze or long johns are soaked in the water and then wrung out until no more drops come out. The dressings are then wrapped around the extremities and fastened with a safety pin. The wet dressings are then covered with dry flannel or dry long johns, thereby slowing down the evaporation process but not completely retarding it, so that the wet dressings need only be changed every 4 to 6 hours.

TOPICAL GLUCOCORTICOIDS

Twice daily application of topical steroids is the mainstay of treatment for all forms of dermatitis (Table 16–2). Topical steroids can also be used under wet dressings. Wet dressings are removed every 4–6 hours and topical steroid applied; then the skin is covered again with wet dressings. If treatment is applied throughout the 24-hour period, maximum benefit is obtained after 72 hours; if treatment is applied only at night, maximum benefit is obtained after 7 days. When the condition has improved, the wet dressings are discontinued and a steroid ointment applied twice daily. Daily application of steroids is not to be continued for more than 1 month. Only low-potency steroids (Table 16–2) are applied to the face or intertriginous areas.

Weston WL: Use and abuse of topical steroids. Contemp Pediatr 1988;5:57.

DISORDERS OF THE SKIN IN NEWBORNS

TRANSIENT DISEASES IN THE NEWBORN

Milia

Multiple white papules 1 mm in diameter scattered over the forehead, nose, and cheeks are present in up to 40% of newborn infants. Histologically, they represent superficial epidermal cysts filled with kerati-

Table 16–2. Topical glucocorticoids.

	Concentrations (Percent)
Low potency = 1–9	
Hydrocortisone	0.5 and 1.0
Desonide	0.05
Moderate potency = 10–99	
Mometasone furoate	0.1
Hydrocortisone valerate	0.2
Fluocinolone acetonide	0.025
Triamcinolone acetonide	0.01
Amcinonide	0.1
High potency = 100–499	
Desoximetasone	0.25
Fluocinonide	0.05
Halcinonide	0.1
Super potency = 500–7500	
Betamethasone dipropionate	0.05
Clobetasol propionate	0.05

nous material associated with the developing pilosebaceous follicle. Their intraoral counterparts are called Epstein's pearls and are even more common than facial milia. All of these cystic structures spontaneously rupture and exfoliate their contents.

Sebaceous Gland Hyperplasia

Prominent yellow macules at the opening of each pilosebaceous follicle, predominantly over the nose, represent overgrowth of sebaceous glands in response to the same androgenic stimulation that occurs in adolescence.

Acne Neonatorum

Open and closed comedones, erythematous papules, and pustules identical in appearance to adolescent acne may occur in infants over the forehead, cheeks, and chin. The lesions may be present at birth but usually do not appear until 3–4 weeks of age. Spontaneous resolution occurs over a period of 6 months to a year. Rarely, neonatal acne may be a manifestation of a virilizing syndrome.

Harlequin Color Change

A cutaneous vascular phenomenon unique to neonates occurs when the infant (particularly one of low birth weight) is placed on one side. The dependent half develops an erythematous flush with a sharp demarcation at the midline, and the upper half of the body becomes pale. The color changes usually subside within a few seconds after the infant is placed supine but may persist for as long as 20 minutes.

Mottling

A lace-like pattern of dilated cutaneous vessels appears over the extremities and often the trunk of neonates exposed to lowered room temperature. This feature is transient and usually disappears completely upon rewarming.

Erythema Toxicum

Up to 50% of term infants develop erythema toxicum. Usually at 24–48 hours of age, blotchy erythematous macules 2–3 cm in diameter appear, most prominently on the chest but also on the back, face, and extremities. These are occasionally present at birth. Onset after 4–5 days of life is rare. The lesions vary in number from two or three up to as many as 100. Incidence is much higher in term infants than in premature ones. The macular erythema may fade within 24–48 hours or may progress to develop urticarial wheals in the center of the macules or, in 10% of cases, pustules. Examination of a Wright-stained smear of the lesion will reveal numerous eosinophils. This may be accompanied by peripheral blood eosinophilia of up to 20%. All of the lesions fade and disappear by 5–7 days. A similar eruption in black newborns has a neutrophilic predominance and leaves hyperpigmentation.

Sucking Blisters

Bullae, either intact or in the form of an erosion representing a blister base without inflammatory borders, may occur over the forearms, wrists, thumbs, or upper lip. These presumably result from vigorous sucking in utero. They resolve without complications.

Miliaria

Obstruction of the eccrine sweat ducts occurs often in neonates and produces one of two clinical pictures depending upon the level of obstruction. **Miliaria crystallina** is characterized by tiny (1–2 mm) superficial grouped vesicles without erythema over intertriginous areas and adjacent skin (eg, neck and upper chest). Obstruction occurs in the stratum corneum portion of the eccrine duct. More commonly, obstruction of the eccrine duct deeper in the epidermis results in erythematous grouped papules in the same areas and is called **miliaria rubra.** Rarely, these may progress to pustules. Heat and high humidity predispose to eccrine duct pore closure. Removal to a cooler environment is the treatment of choice.

Subcutaneous Fat Necrosis

Reddish or purple, sharply circumscribed, firm nodules occurring over the cheeks, buttocks, arms, and thighs and occurring between day 1 and day 7 in infants represent subcutaneous fat necrosis. Cold injury is thought to play an important role. These lesions resolve spontaneously over a period of weeks, although—as in all instances of fat necrosis—they may calcify.

Sclerema

Premature newborns, especially those who suffer metabolic alterations (eg, metabolic acidosis, hypoglycemia, hypothermia), are susceptible to a diffuse hardening of the skin that makes the skin look shiny and feel tight. Treatment consists of protecting the infant from undue exposure to cold and repairing metabolic and nutritional deficiencies.

Mallory SB: Neonatal skin disorders. Pediatr Clin North Am 1991;38:745.
Storrer J et al: Neonatal skin and skin disorders. In: *Pediatric Dermatology.* Schachner L, Hansen R (editors). Churchill Livingstone, 1988.

1. PIGMENT CELL BIRTHMARKS, NEVI, & MELANOMA

Birthmarks may involve an overgrowth of one or more of any of the normal components of skin: pigment cells, blood vessels, lymph vessels, etc. A nevus is a hamartoma of highly differentiated cells that retain their normal function.

Mongolian Spot

A blue-black macule found over the lumbosacral area in 90% of Native American, black, and Asian infants is called a mongolian spot. These spots are occasionally noted over the shoulders and back and may extend over the buttocks. Histologically, they consist of spindle-shaped pigment cells located deep in the dermis. The lesions fade somewhat with time, but some traces may persist into adult life.

Café au Lait Macule

A café au lait macule is a light brown, oval macule (dark brown on black skin) that may be found anywhere on the body. Ten percent of white and 22% of black children have café au lait spots greater than 1.5 cm in their longest diameter. These lesions persist throughout life and may increase in number with age. The presence of six or more such lesions over 1.5 cm in their longest diameter may represent a clue to neurofibromatosis-1 (NF-1). Patients with Albright's syndrome also have increased numbers of café au lait macules. Most newborns with NF-1 will acquire the macules later.

Junctional Nevus & Compound Nevus

Dark brown or black macules, usually few in number at birth but becoming more numerous with age, represent junctional nevi. Histologically, these lesions are large clones of melanocytes at the junction of the epidermis and dermis. With aging, they may become raised (papules) and contain intradermal melanocytes, creating a compound nevus. Often the surface becomes irregular and roughened.

Brown to blue solitary papules with smooth surfaces represent intradermal nevi. When pigmentation is present deeper in the dermis, the lesions appear blue or blue-black and are called blue nevi.

Spindle & Epithelioid Cell Nevus

A reddish-brown solitary nodule appearing on the face or upper arm of a child represents a spindle and epithelioid cell nevus. Histologically, it consists of pigment-producing cells of bizarre shape with numerous mitoses.

Melanoma

Pigmented lesions with variegated colors (red, white, blue), notched borders, and nonuniform, irregular surfaces should arouse a suspicion of melanoma. Ulceration and bleeding are advanced signs of melanoma. If melanoma is suspected, excisional biopsy for pathologic examination should be done as the treatment of choice.

Giant Pigmented Nevus (Bathing Trunk Nevus)

An irregular dark brown to black plaque over 10 cm in diameter represents a giant pigmented nevus. Often the lesions are of such size as to cover the entire trunk (bathing trunk nevi). Histologically, they are compound nevi. Transformation to malignant melanoma has been reported in as many as 10% of cases in some series, although the true incidence is probably much less. Malignant change may occur at birth or at any time thereafter.

Tissue expanders may be useful in excision of large lesions. The risk of melanoma and the potential for cosmetic improvement should be carefully evaluated for each patient.

Angelucci D et al: Rapid perinatal growth mimicking malignant transformation in a giant congenital melanocytic nevus. Hum Pathol 199;22:297

From L: Congenital nevi: Let's be practical. Pediatr Dermatol 1992;9:345

Mackie RM: Nevi as risk factors for melanoma. Pediatr Dermatol 1992;9:340

Ruiz-Maldanado R et al: Giant pigmented nevi: Clinical, histologic, and therapeutic considerations. J Pediatr 1992;120:906

2. VASCULAR BIRTHMARKS

Capillary Malformations

Flat vascular birthmarks can be divided into two types: those that are orange or light red (salmon patch) and those that are dark red or bluish red (port wine stain).

A. Salmon Patch: The salmon patch is a light red macule found over the nape of the neck, upper eyelids, and glabella. Fifty percent of infants have such lesions over their necks. Eyelid lesions fade completely within 3–6 months; those on the nape of the neck fade somewhat but usually persist into adult life.

B. Port Wine Stain: Port wine stains are dark red or purple macules appearing anywhere on the body. A bilateral port wine stain or one covering the entire half of the face may be a clue to **Sturge-Weber syndrome,** which is characterized by seizures, mental retardation, glaucoma, and hemiplegia. Most infants with smaller unilateral port wine stains do not have Sturge-Weber syndrome.

Similarly, a port wine stain over an extremity may be associated with hypertrophy of the soft tissue and bone of that extremity **(Klippel-Trenaunay syndrome).**

The pulsed dye laser is the treatment of choice for infants and children with port wine stains.

Talman B et al: Portwine stains and the likelihood of ophthalmologic or CNS complications. Pediatrics 1991; 87:323.

Tan OT: Lasers for vascular lesions in pediatric dermatology. Pediatr Dermatol 1992;9:358.

Hemangioma

A red, rubbery nodule with a roughened surface is a hemangioma. The lesion is often not present at birth but is represented by a permanent blanched area on the skin that is supplanted at 2–4 weeks of age by red nodules. Histologically, these are benign tumors of capillary endothelial cells. Hemangiomas may be superficial, deep, or mixed. The terms "strawberry" and "cavernous" are misleading and should not be used. The biologic behavior of a hemangioma is the same despite its location. Fifty percent resolve spontaneously by age 5, 70% by age 7, 90% by age 9, and the rest by adolescence.

Hemangiomas resolve, leaving redundant skin, hypopigmentation, and telangiectasia. Local complications include superficial ulceration and secondary pyoderma.

Complications that require immediate treatment are (1) thrombocytopenia due to platelet trapping within the lesion **(Kasabach-Merritt syndrome);** (2) airway obstruction (hemangiomas of the head and neck are often associated with subglottic hemangiomas); (3) visual obstruction (with resulting amblyopia); and (4) cardiac decompensation (high-output failure). In these instances, the treatment of choice is with prednisone, 1–2 mg/kg orally daily or every other day for 4–6 weeks. Recently, interferon alfa-2a has been used to treat serious hemangiomas unresponsive to prednisone. If the lesion is ulcerated or bleeding, pulsed dye laser treatment may be helpful.

Esterly NB: Hemangiomas in infants and children: Clinical observation. Pediatr Dermatol 1992;9:353.

Eskowitz RAB, Mulliken JB, Folkman J: Interferon alfa-2a therapy for life-threatening hemangiomas of infancy. N Engl J Med 1992;326:1456.

Garden JM, Bakus AD, Paller AS: Treatment of cutaneous hemangiomas by the flashlamp-pumped pulsed dye laser: Prospective analysis. J Pediatr 1992;120:555.

Morelli JG et al: Treatment of ulcerated and bleeding hemangiomas with pulsed dye laser. Am J Dis Child 1991;145:1052.

Lymphangioma

Lymphangiomas are rubbery, skin-colored nodules occurring in the parotid area (cystic hygromas) or on the tongue. They often result in grotesque enlargement of soft tissues. Surgical excision is the only treatment available, though the results are not satisfactory.

3. EPIDERMAL BIRTHMARKS

Epidermal Nevus

Linear or groups of linear, warty, papular, unilateral lesions represent overgrowth of epidermis since birth. These areas may range from dirty yellow to brown or may be darkly pigmented. The histologic features of the lesions include thickening of the epidermis and elongation of the rete ridges and hyperkeratosis. Clinically, widespread lesions may be associated with focal motor seizures, mental subnormality, and skeletal anomalies.

Treatment once or twice daily with topical tretinoin 0.05% (retinoic acid [Retin-A]) will keep the lesions flat.

Rogers M: Epidermal nevi and the epidermal nevus syndrome: A review of 233 cases. Pediatr Dermatol 1992; 9:342.

Nevus Comedonicus

The lesion known as nevus comedonicus consists of linear groups of widely dilated follicular openings plugged with keratin, giving the appearance of localized noninflammatory acne. The treatment of choice is surgical removal. If this is not feasible, topical retinoic acid is helpful.

Nevus Sebaceus

The nevus sebaceus of Jadassohn is a hamartoma of sebaceous glands and underlying apocrine glands that is diagnosed by the appearance at birth of a yellowish, hairless, smooth plaque in the scalp or on the face. The lesion may be contiguous with an epidermal nevus on the face and constitute part of the linear epidermal nevus syndrome.

Histologically, nevus sebaceus represents an overabundance of sebaceous glands without hair follicles. At puberty, with androgenic stimulation, the sebaceous cells in the nevus divide, expand their cellular volume, and synthesize sebum, resulting in a warty mass. Because 15% of these lesions become basal cell carcinomas after puberty, excision is recommended before puberty.

4. CONNECTIVE TISSUE BIRTHMARKS (Juvenile Elastoma, Collagenoma)

Connective tissue nevi are smooth, skin-colored papules 1–10 mm in diameter that are grouped on the trunk. A solitary, larger (5–10 cm) nodule is called a **shagreen patch** and is histologically indistinguishable from other connective tissue nevi that show thickened, abundant collagen bundles with or without associated increases of elastic tissue. Although the shagreen patch is a cutaneous clue to tuberous sclerosis, the other connective tissue nevi occur as isolated events. These nevi remain throughout life, and no treatment is necessary.

Uitto J, Santa Cruz DJ, Eisen AZ: Connective tissue nevi of the skin. J Am Acad Dermatol 1980;3:441.

HEREDITARY SKIN DISORDERS

The Ichthyoses

Ichthyosis is a term applied to several heritable diseases characterized by the presence of excessive scales on the skin. Major categories are listed in Table 16–3. X-linked ichthyosis is related to cholesterol sulfatase deficiency. Epidermolytic hyperkeratosis is caused by mutations in the genes coding for keratins 1 or 10. Treatment consists of controlling scaling with Lac-Hydrin 12% applied once daily. Restoring water to the skin is also very helpful.

Williams ML: Ichthyosis: Mechanisms of disease. Pediatr Dermatol 1982;9:365.

Epidermolysis Bullosa

The diagnostic feature of this group of diseases is the formation of blisters in response to slight trauma. They can be divided into scarring and nonscarring types (Table 16–4). The genetic abnormalities re-

Table 16–3. Four major types of ichthyosis.

Name	Age at Onset	Clinical Features	Histology	Inheritance
Ichthyosis with normal epidermal turnover				
Ichthyosis vulgaris	Childhood	Fine scales, deep palmar and plantar markings	Decreased to absent granular layer, hyperkeratosis	Autosomal dominant
X-linked ichthyosis	Birth	Palms and soles spared; thick scales that darken with age; corneal opacities in patients and carrier mothers; cholesterol deficiency	Hyperkeratosis	X-linked
Ichthyosis with increased epidermal turnover				
Epidermolytic hyperkeratosis	Birth	Verrucous, yellow scales in flexural areas and palms and soles	Hyperkeratosis, vacuolated reticular spaces in epidermis	Autosomal dominant
Lamellar ichthyosis	Birth; collodion baby	Erythroderma, ectropion, large coarse scales; thickened palms and soles	Hyperkeratosis, many mitotic figures	Autosomal recessive

Table 16–4. Types of epidermolysis bullosa.

Name	Age at Onset	Clinical Features	Histology	Inheritance
Nonscarring types Epidermolysis bullosa simplex	Birth	Hemorrhagic blisters over the lower legs; cooling prevents blisters	Disintegration of basal cells	Autosomal dominant
Recurrent bullous eruption of the hands and feet (Weber-Cockayne syndrome)	First few years of life	Blisters brought out by walking	Cytolysis of suprabasal cells; keratotic cells	Autosomal dominant
Junctional bullous dermolysis (Herlitz's disease)	Birth	Erosions on legs, oral mucosa; severe perioral involvement	Separation between plasma membrane of basal cells and PAS-positive basal lamina	Autosomal recessive
Scarring types Epidermolysis bullosa dystrophica, dominant	Infancy	Numerous blisters on hands and feet; milia formation	Separation of PAS-positive basal lamina; anchoring fibrils lost	Autosomal dominant
Epidermolysis bullosa dystrophica, recessive	Birth	Repeated episodes of blistering, secondary infection and scarring— "mitten hands and feet"	Separation below PAS-positive basal lamina; anchoring fibrils lost	Autosomal recessive

sponsible for the major types of epidermolysis bullosa have recently been identified. Epidermolysis bullosa simplex is caused by mutations in the genes coding for keratins 5 and 14; dystrophic epidermolysis bullosa is caused by mutations in the gene coding for type VII collagen;and junctional epidermolysis bullosa appears to be caused by alterations in the gene coding for epiligrin.

Treatment usually consists of systemic antibiotics for infection, protective dressings of petrolatum or zinc oxide, and cooling the skin. If hands and feet are involved, reducing skin friction with 5% glutaraldehyde every 3 days is helpful.

Incontinentia Pigmenti

Linear blisters in the newborn represent incontinentia pigmenti. These are replaced by hypertrophic, linear, warty bands within several months, followed by swirling brown hyperpigmentation. Most cases are thought to be X-linked dominant, lethal to the male. Mental retardation and seizures were reported in as many as 30% of cases in one series, but the true incidence is probably much less.

Fine JD et al: Revised clinical and laboratory criteria for subtypes of inherited epidermolysis bullosa. J Am Acad Dermatol 1991;24:119.
Lecher-Gruskay D et al: Nutritional and metabolic profile of children with epidermolysis bullosa. Pediatr Dermatol 1988;5:22.

COMMON SKIN DISEASES IN INFANTS, CHILDREN, & ADOLESCENTS

ACNE

Essentials of Diagnosis

- Seen in newborns and adolescents.
- Inflammatory papules, open and closed comedones on surface.
- Face, upper chest, and back involvement common.

Clinical Findings

The common forms of acne in pediatric patients occur at two ages: in the newborn period and in adolescence. Neonatal acne is a response to maternal androgen, first appearing at 4–6 weeks of age and lasting until 4–6 months of age. The lesions are primarily on the face, upper chest, and back, in a distribution similar to that seen in adolescent acne. It has been hypothesized but not proved that infants who have severe neonatal acne will develop severe adolescent acne.

The onset of adolescent acne is between ages 8 and 10 in 40% of children. The early lesions are usually limited to the face and are primarily closed comedones (whiteheads; see below). Eventually, 85% of adolescents will develop some form of acne.

Acne occurs in sebaceous follicles, which, unlike hair follicles, have large, abundant sebaceous glands and usually lack hair. They are located primarily on the face, upper chest, back, and penis. Obstruction of the sebaceous follicle opening produces the clinical lesion of acne. If the obstruction occurs at the follicular mouth, the clinical lesion is characterized by a wide, patulous opening filled with a plug of stratum corneum cells. This is the open comedone, or blackhead. Open comedones are the predominant clinical lesion in early adolescent acne. The black color is due not to dirt but to oxidized melanin within the stratum corneum cellular plug. Open comedones do not often progress to inflammatory lesions. Closed comedones, or whiteheads, are caused by obstruction just beneath the follicular opening in the neck of the sebaceous follicle, which produces a cystic swelling of the follicular duct directly beneath the epidermis. The stratum corneum produced accumulates continuously within the cystic cavity. The resultant lesion is an enlarging sphere just beneath the skin surface. Most authorities believe that closed comedones are precursors of inflammatory acne. If open or closed comedones are the predominant lesions on the skin in adolescent acne, it is called **comedonal acne.**

In typical adolescent acne, several different types of lesions are present simultaneously, eg, open and closed comedones and inflammatory lesions such as papules, pustules, and cysts. Inflammatory lesions may also rarely occur as interconnecting, draining sinus tracts. Adolescents with cystic acne require prompt medical attention, since ruptured cysts and sinus tracts result in severe scar formation. New acne scars are highly vascular and have a reddish or purplish hue. Such scars return to normal skin color after several years. Acne scars may be depressed beneath the skin level, raised, or flat to the skin. In adolescents with a tendency toward keloid formation, keloidal scars can occur following acne lesions, particularly over the sternal area.

Differential Diagnosis

Consider rosacea, nevus comedonicus, flat warts, the angiofibromas of tuberous sclerosis, miliaria, and molluscum contagiosum.

Pathogenesis

The primary event in acne formation is obstruction of the sebaceous follicle. Ordinarily the lining of such follicles contains one or two layers of stratum corneum cells, but in acne the stratum corneum is overproduced. This phenomenon is androgen-dependent in adolescent acne. The sebaceous follicles contain an enzyme, testosterone 5α-reductase, which converts plasma testosterone to dihydrotestosterone. This androgen is a potent stimulus for nuclear division of the follicular germinative cells and subsequently of excessive cell production. Thus, obstruction requires the presence of both circulating androgens and the converting enzyme. After the production or the administration of androgens, there is a delay until cellular proliferation occurs and follicular obstruction subsequently appears.

The pathogenesis of inflammatory acne is not well understood. Undoubtedly, physical manipulation of a closed comedo could lead to rupture of the cavity contents into the dermis with a subsequent inflammatory response. Spontaneous inflammation also occurs in obstructed follicles, but the reason for this is unclear. An attractive hypothesis is that overgrowth of gram-positive bacteria in the obstructed follicle (either *Propionibacterium acnes* or *Staphylococcus epidermidis*) might produce enzymes or other factors that initiate inflammation. Overproduction of sebum and free fatty acid formation seem unlikely as causes of inflammation in acne as presently understood.

Adolescent acne may result from several external causes. Frictional acne due to headbands, football helmets, or tight-fitting brassieres or other garments occurs predominantly underneath the area where the garment is worn. Oil-based cosmetics may be responsible for predominantly comedonal acne, and hair sprays may produce acne along the hair margin.

Drug-induced acne should be suspected in teenagers if all lesions are in the same stage at the same time and if involvement extends to the lower abdomen, lower back, arms, and legs. Drugs responsible for acne include corticotropin (ACTH), glucocorticoids, androgens, hydantoins, and isoniazid. They have the common property of elevating plasma testosterone.

Treatment

A. Topical Keratolytic Agents: The mainstay of acne therapy is the use of potent topical keratolytic agents applied to the skin to relieve follicular obstruction. Two classes of potent keratolytic agents are available: tretinoin (retinoic acid) and benzoyl peroxide gel. These have been found to be the most efficacious agents in the treatment of acne. Either agent may be used once daily, or the combination of retinoic acid cream applied to acne-bearing areas of the skin once daily in the evening and a benzoyl peroxide gel applied once daily in the morning may be used. This regimen will control 80–85% of adolescent acne.

B. Topical Antibiotics: Topical antibiotics are used to avoid the side effects caused by systemic antibiotics. Topical antibiotics are less effective than systemic antibiotics and at best are equivalent in potency to 250 mg of tetracycline orally once a day. One percent clindamycin phosphate solution is the most efficacious of all topical antibiotics. Some percutaneous absorption may occur rarely with this drug, resulting in diarrhea and colitis; 1.5% and 2% topical erythromycin solutions are effective; 1% topical tetracycline solution is minimally effective.

C. Systemic Antibiotics: Antibiotics that are concentrated in sebum, such as tetracycline and erythromycin, are very effective in inflammatory acne. The usual dose is 0.5–1 g taken once or twice daily on an empty stomach (nothing to eat 1 hour before or after the medication). Tetracycline or erythromycin should be continued for 2–3 months until the acne lesions are suppressed.

D. Oral Retinoids: An oral retinoid, 13-*cis*-retinoic acid (isotretinoin; Accutane), offers the most efficacious treatment of severe cystic acne. The precise mechanism of its action is unknown, but decreased sebum production, decreased follicular obstruction, decreased skin bacteria, and general anti-inflammatory activities have been described. The initial dosage is 40 mg once or twice daily. This drug is not effective in comedonal acne or other mild forms of acne. Side effects include dryness and scaliness of the skin, dry lips, and, occasionally, dry eyes and dry nose. Up to 10% of patients experience mild, reversible hair loss. Elevated liver enzymes and blood lipids have rarely been described. Isotretinoin is teratogenic. Use in young women of childbearing age is not recommended unless strict adherence to manufacturer's guidelines is ensured.

E. Other Acne Treatments: There is no convincing evidence that dietary management, mild drying agents, abrasive scrubs, oral vitamin A, ultraviolet light, cryotherapy, or incision and drainage have any beneficial effects in the management of acne.

F. Avoidance of Cosmetics and Hair Spray: Acne can be aggravated by a variety of external factors that result in further obstruction of partially occluded sebaceous follicles. Discontinuing the use of oil-based cosmetics, face creams, and hair sprays may alleviate the comedonal component of acne within 4–6 weeks.

Patient Education & Follow-Up Visits

It is important to explain the mechanism of acne and the treatment plan to adolescent patients. Time should be set aside at the first visit to answer the patient's questions. Explain that there will not be much improvement for 4–8 weeks. Establish guidelines for ideal control, and explain that the best the patient might achieve is one or two new pimples a month. No drug is available that will prevent an adolescent from ever having another acne lesion. A written education sheet is most useful.

Follow-up visits should be made every 4–6 weeks. The criterion for ideal control is a few lesions every 2 weeks. Explain again what medications are being used and what the treatment is intended to achieve, and question the patient to determine whether the medications are being used properly.

Winston MH, Shalita AR: Acne vulgaris. Pathogenesis and treatment. Pediatr Clin North Am 1991;38:889.

BACTERIAL INFECTIONS OF THE SKIN

Impetigo

Erosions covered by honey-colored crusts are diagnostic of impetigo. Staphylococci and group A strep-

tococci are important pathogens in this disease, which histologically consists of superficial invasion of bacteria into the upper epidermis, forming a subcorneal pustule.

Although topical antibiotics may effect a clinical cure, parenteral penicillin or oral penicillin for 10 days is necessary to eradicate streptococci. The risk of nephritogenic strains varies considerably from area to area, but active treatment of patients and contacts with systemic penicillin will significantly reduce the incidence of acute glomerulonephritis in endemic areas. Dicloxacillin or other antistaphylococcal antibiotics are used when staphylococcal infection is suspected.

Dagan R: Impetigo in childhood: Changing epidemiology and new treatments. Pediatr Ann 1993;22:235.

Ecthyma

Ecthyma is a firm, dry crust, surrounded by erythema, that exudes purulent material. It represents deep invasion by the streptococcus through the epidermis to the superficial dermis. Treatment is with systemic penicillin.

Cellulitis

Cellulitis is characterized by erythematous, hot, tender, ill-defined plaques accompanied by regional lymphadenopathy. Histologically, this disorder represents invasion of microorganisms into the lower dermis and sometimes beyond, with obstruction of local lymphatics. *Haemophilus influenzae, Streptococcus pneumoniae,* and *Streptococcus pyogenes* are the most common offending organisms. Septicemia is common, and treatment with the appropriate systemic antibiotic is indicated.

Sachs MK: Cutaneous cellulitis. Arch Dermatol 1991; 127:493.

Folliculitis

A pustule at a follicular opening represents folliculitis. If the pustule occurs at eccrine sweat orifices, it is correctly called **poritis.** Staphylococci and streptococci are the most frequent pathogens. Treatment consists of measures to remove follicular obstruction—either cool wet compresses for 24 hours or keratolytics such as are used for acne.

Abscess

An abscess occurs deep in the skin, at the bottom of a follicle or an apocrine gland, and is diagnosed as an erythematous, firm, acutely tender nodule with ill-defined borders. Staphylococci are the most common organisms. Treatment consists of incision and drainage and systemic antibiotics.

Scalded Skin Syndrome

This entity consists of the sudden onset of bright

red, acutely painful skin, most obvious periorally, periorbitally, and in the flexural areas of the neck, the axillae, the popliteal and antecubital areas, and the groin. The slightest pressure on the skin results in severe pain and separation of the epidermis, leaving a glistening layer (the stratum granulosum of the epidermis) beneath. The disease is due to a circulating toxin (exfoliatin) elaborated by phage group II staphylococci (types 71, 55, 3A, 3B, and 3C). The site of action of exfoliation is the intracellular area of the granular layer, resulting in a separation of cells.

Scalded skin syndrome includes **Ritter's disease** of the newborn, toxic shock syndrome, and the mildest form, staphylococcal scarlet fever. (See also Bullous Impetigo, below.) In all of the forms of this entity, the causative staphylococci may not be isolated from the skin but rather from the nasopharynx, an abscess, blood culture, etc. Treatment consists of systemic administration of antistaphylococcal drugs, eg, dicloxacillin, 25–50 mg/kg/d orally, or methicillin, 200–300 mg/kg/d intravenously.

Bullous Impetigo

All impetigo is bullous, with the blister forming just beneath the stratum corneum, but in "bullous impetigo" there is, in addition to the usual erosion covered by a honey-colored crust, a border filled with clear fluid. Staphylococci may be isolated from these lesions, and systemic signs of circulating exfoliatin are absent. "Bullous varicella" is a disorder that represents bullous impetigo in varicella lesions. Treatment with dicloxacillin, 25–50 mg/kg/d orally for 5–6 days, is effective. Application of cool compresses to debride crusts is a helpful symptomatic measure.

Wooldridge WE: Managing skin infections in children. Postgrad Med 1991;89:109.

FUNGAL INFECTIONS OF THE SKIN

1. DERMATOPHYTE INFECTIONS

Essentials of Diagnosis

- Red, scaly, round lesions.
- Hair loss with or without scaling in tinea capitis.

General Considerations

Dermatophytes become attached to the superficial layer of the epidermis, nails, and hair, where they proliferate. They grow mainly within the stratum corneum and do not invade the lower epidermis or dermis. Release of toxins from dermatophytes, especially those whose natural host is animals or soil, eg, *Microsporum canis* and *Trichophyton verrucosum*, results in dermatitis. Fungal infection should be suspected with any red and scaly lesion.

Classification & Diagnosis

A. Tinea Capitis: Thickened, broken-off hairs with erythema and scaling of underlying scalp are the distinguishing features (Table 16–5). In epidemic ringworm, hairs are broken off at the surface of the scalp, leaving a black dot appearance. Pustule formation and a boggy fluctuant mass on the scalp occur in *Microsporum canis* and *Trichophyton tonsurans* infections. This mass, called a **kerion,** represents an exaggerated host response to the organism. Fungal culture should be performed in all cases of suspected tinea capitis.

B. Tinea Corporis: Tinea corporis presents either as annular marginated papules with a thin scale and clear center or as an annular confluent dermatitis. The most common organisms are *Trichophyton mentagrophytes* and *M canis*. The diagnosis is made by scraping thin scales from the border of the lesion, dissolving them in 20% KOH, and examining for hyphae.

C. Tinea Cruris: Symmetric, sharply marginated lesions in inguinal areas are seen with tinea cruris. The most common organisms are *Trichophyton rubrum, T mentagrophytes,* and *Epidermophyton floccosum.*

D. Tinea Pedis: The diagnosis of tinea pedis in a prepubertal child must always be regarded with skepticism; atopic feet or contact dermatitis is a more likely diagnosis in this age group. Tinea pedis is seen most commonly in postpubertal males with blisters on the instep of the foot. Fissuring between the toes is occasionally seen.

E. Tinea Unguium (Onychomycosis): Loosening of the nail plate from the nail bed (onycholysis), giving a yellow discoloration, is the first sign of fungal invasion of the nails. Thickening of the distal nail plate then occurs, followed by scaling and a crumbly appearance of the entire nail plate surface. *T rubrum* and *T mentagrophytes* are the most common causes. The diagnosis is confirmed by KOH examination and fungal culture. Usually one or two nails are involved. If every nail is involved, psoriasis or lichen planus is a more likely diagnosis than fungal infection.

Table 16–5. Clinical features of tinea capitis.

Most Common Organisms	Clinical Appearance	Microscopic Appearance in KOH
Trichophyton tonsurans (90%)	Hairs broken off 2–3 mm from follicle; "black dot"; no fluorescence	Hyphae and spores within hair
Microsporum canis (10%)	Thickened broken-off hairs that fluoresce yellow-green with Wood's lamp[1]	Small spores outside of hair; hyphae within hair

[1]Select fluorescent hairs for examination in KOH and culture.

Treatment

The treatment of dermatophytosis is quite simple: *If hair or nails are involved, griseofulvin is the treatment of choice.* Topical antifungal agents do not enter hair or nails in sufficient concentration to clear the infection. The absorption of griseofulvin from the gastrointestinal tract is enhanced by a fatty meal; thus, whole milk or ice cream taken with the medication increases absorption. The dosage of griseofulvin is 20 mg/kg/d. With hair infections, it should be continued for a minimum of 6 weeks; in nail infections, for a minimum of 3 months. It is supplied in capsules containing 250 mg or as a suspension containing 125 mg/5 mL. The side effects are few, and the drug has even been used successfully in the newborn period.

Tinea corporis, tinea pedis, and tinea cruris can be treated effectively with topical medication after careful inspection to make certain that the hair and nails are not involved. Treatment with clotrimazole (Lotrimin), miconazole (Micatin), econazole (Spectazole), or haloprogin (Halotex) applied twice daily for 3 or 4 weeks is recommended.

Gan VN et al: Epidemiology and treatment of tinea capitis: Ketoconazole vs. griseofulvin. Pediatr Infect Dis J 1987; 6:46.

Degreef H: The treatment of superficial skin infections caused by dermatophytes. Curr Top Med Mycol 1992; 4:189.

2. TINEA VERSICOLOR

Tinea versicolor is a superficial infection caused by *Pityrosporum orbiculare* (also called *Malassezia furfur,*) a yeast-like fungus. It characteristically causes polycyclic connected hypopigmented macules and very fine scales in areas of sun-induced pigmentation. In winter, the polycyclic macules appear reddish-brown.

Treatment consists of application of selenium sulfide (Selsun), 2.5% suspension, or 25% sodium thiosulfate (Tinver). Selenium sulfide should be applied to the whole body and left on overnight. Treatment can be repeated again in a week and then monthly thereafter. It tends to be somewhat irritating, and the patient should be warned about this difficulty.

Borelli D, Jacobs PH, Nall L: Tinea versicolor: Epidemiological, clinical and therapeutic aspects. J Am Acad Dermatol 1991;25:300.

3. *CANDIDA ALBICANS* INFECTIONS

In addition to being a frequent invader in diaper dermatitis, *Candida albicans* also infects the oral mucosa, where it appears as thick white patches with an erythematous base **(thrush)**; the angles of the mouth, where it causes fissures and white exudate **(perlèche)**; and the cuticular region of the fingers, where thickening of the cuticle, dull red erythema, and distortion of growth of the nail plate suggest the diagnosis of candidal paronychia. *C albicans* is able to penetrate the stratum corneum layer and locally activate the complement system.

Nystatin (Mycostatin) is the drug of first choice for *C albicans* infections. It is supplied as an ointment or a cream, as an oral suspension, and as vaginal tablets. In diaper dermatitis, the cream form can be applied every 3–4 hours. In oral thrush, the suspension should be applied directly to the mucosa with the parent's finger or a cotton-tipped applicator, since it is not absorbed and acts topically. In candidal paronychia, nystatin is applied over the area, covered with occlusive plastic wrapping, and left on overnight after the application is made airtight. Haloprogin, miconazole, econazole nitrate, or clotrimazole are effective alternatives.

Butler KM et al: *Candida:* An increasingly important pathogen in the nursery. Pediatr Clin North Am 1988;35:543.

VIRAL INFECTIONS OF THE SKIN

Herpes Simplex

Grouped vesicles or grouped erosions suggest herpes simplex. The microscopic finding of epidermal giant cells after scraping the vesicle base with a No. 15 blade, smearing on a slide, and staining with Wright's stain (Tzanck smear) suggests herpes simplex or varicella-zoster. A rapid immunofluorescent test for HSV is now available. In infants, lesions due to herpes simplex type 1 are seen on the gingiva and lips, periorbitally, or on the thumb in thumb suckers. Recurrent erosions in the mouth are usually aphthous stomatitis in children rather than recurrent herpes simplex. Herpes simplex type 2 is seen on the genitalia and in the mouth in adolescents. Herpes simplex infection of the genitalia is now the second most common venereal disease. Cutaneous dissemination of herpes simplex occurs in patients with atopic dermatitis **(eczema herpeticum, Kaposi's varicelliform eruption).**. The treatment of this and other herpesvirus infections is discussed in the infectious diseases section. In severe disseminated infection, oral acyclovir may be helpful.

Balfour HH Jr et al: Antiviral drugs in pediatrics. Am J Dis Child 1989;143:1307.

Arbesfeld DM, Thomas I: Cutaneous herpes simplex virus infections. Am Fam Physician 1991;43:1655.

Varicella-Zoster

Grouped vesicles in a dermatome on the trunk or face suggest herpes zoster. Zoster in children is not painful and usually has a mild course. In patients with compromised host resistance, the appearance of an erythematous border around the vesicles is a good prognostic sign. Conversely, large bullae without a tendency to crusting imply a poor host response to the virus. Varicella-zoster and herpes simplex lesions undergo the same series of changes: papule, vesicle, pustule, crust, slightly depressed scar. Varicella appears in crops, and many different stages of lesions are present at the same time.

Itching is usually the only symptom, and cool baths as frequently as necessary or drying lotions such as calamine lotion are sufficient to relieve symptoms. In immunosuppressed children, intravenous or oral acyclovir should be considered.

Weller TH: Varicella and herpes zoster: A perspective and overview. J Infect Dis 1992:166(Suppl 1):1.

Whitley RJ: Therapeutic approaches to varicella-zoster virus infections. J Infect Dis 1992;166(Suppl 1):551.

HIV Infection

The average time of onset of skin lesions after perinatally acquired HIV infection is 4 months—11 months after transfusion-acquired HIV infection. Persistent oral candidiasis and recalcitrant candidal diaper rash are the most frequent cutaneous manifestations of infantile HIV infection. Severe herpetic gingivostomatitis, herpes zoster, and molluscum contagiosum are seen. Recurrent staphylococcal pyodermas, tinea of the face, and onychomycosis are also observed. A generalized dermatitis with features of seborrhea is extremely common. In general, persistent, recurrent, or extensive skin infections should make one suspicious of HIV infection.

Prose NS: Cutaneous manifestations of pediatric HIV infections. Pediatr Dermatol 1992;9:326.

Virus-Induced Tumors

A. Molluscum Contagiosum: Molluscum contagiosum consists of umbilicated, white or whitish-yellow papules in groups on the genitalia or trunk. They are common in sexually active adolescents as well as in infants and preschool children. Crushing a lesion between glass slides followed by microscopic examination after staining with Wright's stain will demonstrate epidermal cells with inclusions. Molluscum contagiosum is a poxvirus that induces the epidermis to proliferate, forming a pale papule.

Removal of the lesion with a sharp curette or knife is curative. This therapy may leave a small scar, and one must weigh the advantage of removal of lesions that will disappear in 2 or 3 years.

B. Warts: Warts are skin-colored papules with irregular (verrucous) surfaces. They are intraepidermal tumors caused by infection with human papillomavirus. This DNA virus induces the epidermal cells to proliferate, thus resulting in the warty growth.

No therapy for warts is ideal, and some types of therapy should be avoided because the recurrence rate of warts is high. Flat warts generally require no treatment. They may be considered a mild wart virus infection, and since they usually disappear within 6–9 months they are best left alone. This holds true especially for all flat warts on the face. A good response to 0.05% tretinoin (Retin-A) cream, applied once daily for 3–4 weeks, has been reported.

The best treatment for the solitary **common ("vulgaris") wart** is to freeze it with liquid nitrogen. The liquid nitrogen should be allowed to drip from the cotton-tipped applicator onto the wart without pressure. Pressure exaggerates cold injury by causing vasoconstriction and may produce a deep ulcer and scar. Liquid nitrogen is applied by drip until the wart turns completely white and stays white for 20–25 seconds. Large and painful plantar warts are treated most effectively by applying 40% salicylic acid plaster cut with a scissors to fit the lesion. The sticky brown side of the plaster is placed against the lesion, taped on securely with adhesive tape, and left on for 5 days. The plaster is then removed, and the white necrotic warty tissue can be gently rubbed off with the finger and a new salicylic acid plaster applied. This procedure is repeated every 5 days, and the patient is seen every 2 weeks. Most plantar warts resolve in 2–4 weeks when treated in this way.

Sharp scalpel excision, electrosurgery, and radiotherapy should be avoided, since the resulting scar often becomes a more difficult problem than the wart itself and there may be recurrence of the wart in the area of the scar.

Condyloma acuminatum is best treated with 25% podophyllum resin (podophyllin) in alcohol. This should be painted on the lesions and then washed off after 4 hours. Re-treatment in 7–10 days may be necessary. A condyloma not on the vulvar mucous membrane but on the adjacent skin should be treated as a common wart and frozen.

For isolated warts and periungual warts, cantharidin (Cantharone, Verr-Canth) is effective and painless in children. It causes a blister and sometimes is difficult to control. An undesirable complication is the appearance of warts along the margins of the cantharidin blister. Cantharidin is applied to the skin, allowed to dry, and covered with occlusive tape such as Blenderm for 24 hours.

No wart therapy is immediate and definitive, and recurrences are reported in 20–30% of cases even with the best care.

Beutner KR: Cutaneous viral infections. Pediatr Ann 1992;22:247.

Cobb MW: Human papilloma virus infection. J Am Acad Dermatol 1990;22:547.

INSECT INFESTATIONS

These disorders are characterized generally by discrete red papules, nodules, and S-shaped burrows on the skin. Hand and foot involvement is common.

Scabies

Scabies is suggested by the appearance of linear burrows about the wrists, ankles, finger webs, areolas, anterior axillary folds, genitalia, or face (in infants). Often, there are excoriations, honey-colored crusts, and pustules from secondary infection. Identification of the female mite or her eggs and feces is necessary to confirm the diagnosis. Slice off an unscratched papule or burrow with a No. 15 blade and examine microscopically in either immersion oil or 10% KOH to confirm the diagnosis. In a child who is often scratching, scrape under the fingernails. Examine the parents for unscratched burrows.

Lindane (gamma benzene hexachloride; Kwell) and permethrin are excellent scabicides. However, since lindane is concentrated in the central nervous system and central nervous system toxicity from systemic absorption in infants has been reported, the following restricted use of this agent is recommended: (1) For adults and older children, one treatment of lindane lotion or cream applied to the entire body and left on for 4 hours, followed by shower, is sufficient. (2) Infants tend to have more organisms and many more lesions and may have to be re-treated in 7–10 days. All family members should be treated simultaneously. Permethrin 5% cream (Elimite) may be substituted for lindane in infants.

Schultz MW et al: Comparative study of 5% permethrin cream and 1% lindane lotion for the treatment of scabies. Arch Dermatol 1990;127:167.

Pediculoses
(Louse Infestations)

Excoriated papules and pustules with a history of severe itching at night suggest infestation with the human body louse. This louse may be discovered in the seams of underwear but not on the body. In the scalp hair, the gelatinous nits of the body louse adhere tightly to the hair shaft. The pubic louse may be found crawling among pubic hairs, or blue-black macules may be found dispersed through the pubic region (maculae ceruleae). The pubic louse is often seen in the eyelashes of newborns.

Lindane (gamma benzene hexachloride; Kwell) has been the treatment of choice. Since this agent is concentrated in the central nervous system and central nervous system toxicity from systemic absorption in infants has been reported, the following modification in its use is recommended: For head lice, a shampoo preparation is left on the scalp for 5 minutes and rinsed out thoroughly. The hair is then combed with a fine-tooth comb to remove nits. This may be repeated in 7 days. Lindane cream or lotion applied to the body for 4 hours may be necessary for body lice, but washing the clothing in boiling water followed by ironing the seams with a hot iron usually eliminates the organisms. Permethrin 1% creme rinse is also efficacious for the elimination of lice.

Lindane cream or lotion applied to the pubic area for 24 hours is sufficient to treat pediculosis pubis. It may be repeated in 4–5 days.

Churge RN et al: A review of the epidemiology, public health importance, treatment and control of head lice. Can J Public Health 1991;82:196.

Hogan DJ, Schachner L, Tanglertsampan C: Diagnosis and treatment of childhood scabies and pediculosis. Pediatr Clin North Am 1991;38:941.

Papular Urticaria

Papular urticaria is characterized by grouped erythematous papules surrounded by an urticarial flare and distributed over the shoulders, upper arms, and buttocks in infants. These lesions represent delayed hypersensitivity reactions to stinging or biting insects and can be reproduced by patch testing with the offending insect. Fleas from dogs and cats are the usual offenders. Less commonly, mosquitoes, lice, scabies, and bird and grass mites are involved. The sensitivity is transient, lasting 4–6 months. The logical therapy is to remove the offending insect. Topical corticosteroids and oral antihistamines will control symptoms.

DERMATITIS*
(Eczema)

Essentials of Diagnosis

- Red skin with disruption of skin surface.
- Vesicles, crusting, or lichenification may be present.

General Considerations

The terms dermatitis and eczema are currently used interchangeably in dermatology, although the etymologic implication of eczema is "a boiling over" and the term originally denoted an acute weeping dermatosis. All forms of dermatitis, regardless of cause, may present with acute edema, erythema, and oozing with crusting, mild erythema alone, or lichenification. Lichenification is diagnosed by thickening of the skin with a shiny surface and exaggerated, deepened skin markings. It is the response of the skin to chronic rubbing or scratching.

Although the lesions of the various dermatoses are histologically indistinguishable, clinicians have nonetheless divided the disease group called dermatitis

---

*From the perspective of a dermatologist. See also the discussion of atopic dermatitis in Chapter 33.

into several categories based on known causes in some cases and differing natural histories in others.

Atopic Dermatitis

Atopic dermatitis is not a clearly defined clinical entity but a general term for chronic superficial inflammation of the skin that can be applied to a heterogeneous group of patients. Many (not all) patients go through three clinical phases. In the first, infantile eczema, the dermatitis begins on the cheeks and scalp and frequently expresses itself as oval patches on the trunk, later involving the extensor surfaces of the extremities. The usual age at onset is 2–3 months, and this phase ends at age 18 months to 2 years. Only one-third of all infants with atopic eczema progress to phase 2—childhood or flexural eczema—in which the predominant involvement is in the antecubital and popliteal fossae, the neck, the wrists, and sometimes the hands or feet. This phase lasts from age 2 years to adolescence. Some children will have involvement of the soles of their feet only, with cracking, redness, and pain—the so-called **atopic feet.** Only a third of children with typical flexural eczema will progress to adolescent eczema, which is usually manifested by hand dermatitis only. Atopic dermatitis is quite unusual after age 30.

Atopic dermatitis has no known cause, and despite the high incidence of asthma and hay fever in these patients (30%) and their families (70%), evidence for allergy beyond this hereditary association is limited to testimonials. The case for food and inhalant allergens as specific causes of atopic dermatitis is not strong.

A few patients with atopic dermatitis have immunodeficiency with recurrent pyodermas, unusual susceptibility to herpes simplex and vaccinia virus, hyperimmunoglobulinemia E, defective neutrophil and monocyte chemotaxis, and impaired T lymphocyte function.

A faulty epidermal barrier may predispose the patient with atopic dermatitis to itchy skin. Inability to hold water within the stratum corneum results in rapid evaporation of water, shrinking of the stratum corneum, and "cracks" in the epidermal barrier. Such skin forms an ineffective barrier to the entry of various irritants—and, indeed, it may be clinically useful to regard atopic dermatitis as a primary irritant contact dermatitis and simply tell the patient, "You have sensitive skin." Chronic atopic dermatitis is frequently secondarily infected with *Staphylococcus aureus* or *Streptococcus pyogenes.*

A. Treatment of Acute Stages: Application of wet dressings and topical corticosteroids is the treatment of choice for acute, weeping atopic eczema. A topical steroid preparation is applied four times daily and covered with wet dressings as outlined at the beginning of this chapter. Systemic antibiotics chosen on the basis of appropriate skin cultures may be nec-

essary, since lesions in the acute stages are often secondarily infected with *S aureus* or streptococci.

B. Treatment of Chronic Stages: Treatment is aimed at avoiding irritants and restoring water to the skin. No soaps or harsh shampoos should be used, and the patient should avoid woolen clothing or any rough clothing. Restoring water to the skin is important in atopic dermatitis. This can be accomplished by two baths daily, less than 5 minutes each, after which lubricating oils or ointments are applied. Moisturel is a useful lubricant. Plain petrolatum and lards are often too greasy and may cause considerable sweat retention. Liberal use of Cetaphil lotion as a soap substitute four or five times a day is also satisfactory as a means of lubrication. A bedroom humidifier is often helpful. Topical corticosteroids should be limited to the less potent ones (see Table 16–2). Hydrocortisone ointment, 1% twice daily, is often sufficient. There is *never* any reason to use super- or high-potency corticosteroids in atopic dermatitis. In superinfected atopic dermatitis, systemic antibiotics for 10–14 days (erythromycin, 40 mg/kg/d; dicloxacillin, 50 mg/kg/d) are necessary.

Treatment failures in chronic atopic dermatitis are most often due to patient noncompliance. This is a frustrating disease for parent and child.

de Prost Y: Atopic dermatitis: Recent therapeutic advances. Pediatr Dermatol 1992;9:386.
Morelli JG et al: Soaps and shampoos in pediatric practice. Pediatrics 1987;80:634.
Yohn J et al: Topical glucocorticosteroids. Curr Probl Dermatol 1990;2:29.

Nummular Eczema

Nummular eczema is characterized by numerous symmetrically distributed coin-shaped patches of dermatitis, principally on the extremities. These may be acute, oozing, and crusted or dry and scaling. The disease lasts 9 months to 2 years. The differential diagnosis should include tinea corporis and atopic dermatitis.

The same topical measures should be used as for atopic dermatitis, though treatment is often more difficult.

Primary Irritant Contact Dermatitis (Diaper Dermatitis)

Contact dermatitis is of two types: primary irritant and allergic eczematous. Primary irritant dermatitis develops within a few hours, reaches peak severity at 24 hours, and then disappears. Allergic eczematous contact dermatitis (see below) has a delayed onset of 18 hours, peaks at 48–72 hours, and often lasts as long as 2 or 3 weeks, even if exposure to the offending antigen is discontinued.

Diaper dermatitis, the most common form of primary irritant contact dermatitis seen in pediatric practice, is due to prolonged contact of the skin with urine and feces, which contain irritating chemicals such as urea and intestinal enzymes. The diagnosis of diaper dermatitis is based on the picture of erythema and thickening of the skin in the perineal area and the history of skin contact with urine or feces. In 80% of cases of diaper dermatitis lasting more than 3 days, the affected area is colonized with *Candida albicans* even before the classic signs of a beefy red, sharply marginated dermatitis with satellite lesions appear.

Treatment consists of changing diapers frequently. Because rubber or plastic pants serve as occlusive dressings and prevent the evaporation of the contactant and enhance its penetration into the skin, they should be avoided as much as possible. Air drying is useful. Streptococcal perianal cellulitis should be included in the differential diagnosis. Treatment of long-standing diaper dermatitis should include application of nystatin (Mycostatin) or an imidazole cream with each diaper change.

Lane AT, Rehder PA, Helm K: Evaluation of diapers containing absorbent gelling materials with conventional diapers in newborn infants. Am J Dis Child 1990;144:315.

Lichen Simplex Chronicus (Localized Neurodermatitis)

Lichen simplex chronicus is a sharply circumscribed single patch of lichenification, usually found on the back of the neck in adolescent girls. Patients produce the morphologic skin changes by chronic rubbing and scratching.

Treatment of the thickened lesions is with topical corticosteroids. Because the epidermal barrier has thickened, penetration of topical corticosteroids is poor. Penetration can be enhanced in several ways. Airtight occlusion with plastic dressings (eg, Saran Wrap) overnight over topical corticosteroids is useful, or flurandrenolide (Cordran) tape impregnated with corticosteroids will penetrate the lesion. Covering the lesion will also prevent scratching of the area.

Allergic Eczematous Contact Dermatitis (Poison Ivy Dermatitis)

Children often present with acute dermatitis with blister formation, oozing, and crusting. Blisters are often linear and of acute onset. Plants such as poison ivy, poison sumac, and poison oak cause most cases of allergic contact dermatitis in children.

Allergic contact dermatitis has all the features of delayed type (T lymphocyte-mediated) hypersensitivity. Although many substances may cause such a reaction, nickel sulfate (metals), potassium dichromate, and neomycin are the most common causes. The true incidence of allergic contact dermatitis in children is not known.

Treatment of contact dermatitis in localized areas is with topical corticosteroids. In severe generalized

involvement, prednisone, 1–2 mg/kg/d orally for 14–21 days, can be used.

Weston WL: Prevalence of positive epicutaneous tests among infants, children and adolescents. Pediatrics 1986;78:1070.

Seborrheic Dermatitis

Seborrheic dermatitis consists of an erythematous scaly dermatitis accompanied by overproduction of sebum occurring in areas rich in sebaceous glands, ie, the face, scalp, and perineum. This common condition occurs predominantly in the newborn and at puberty, the ages at which hormonal stimulation of sebum production is maximal. Although it is tempting to speculate that the overproduction of sebum causes the dermatitis, the exact relationship is unclear.

Seborrheic dermatitis on the scalp in infancy is often confused with atopic dermatitis, and only after other areas are involved or flexural involvement occurs is it clear that the diagnosis is atopic dermatitis. Psoriasis also occurs in seborrheic areas in older children and should always be considered in the differential diagnosis.

Seborrheic dermatitis responds well to topical corticosteroids; 1% hydrocortisone cream three times daily is often sufficient to control this disorder.

Dandruff

Physiologic scaling or mild seborrhea, in the form of greasy scalp scales, may be treated by medicated dandruff shampoos.

Dry Skin Dermatitis (Asteatotic Eczema, Xerosis)

Newborns and older children who live in arid climates are susceptible to dry skin, characterized by large cracked scales with erythematous borders. The stratum corneum is dependent upon environmental humidity for its water, and below 30% environmental humidity the stratum corneum loses water, shrinks, and cracks. These cracks in the epidermal barrier allow irritating substances to enter the skin, predisposing to dermatitis.

Treatment consists of increasing the water content of the skin's immediate external environment. House humidifiers are very useful. Two 5-minute baths a day with immediate application of oils or ointments (petrolatum) after the bath will allow the skin to retain water. Frequent soaping of the skin impairs its water-holding capacity and serves as an irritating alkali, and all soaps should therefore be avoided. Frequent use of emollients (eg, Cetaphil, Eucerin, Lubriderm, Moisturel) should be a major part of therapy.

Keratosis Pilaris

Follicular papules containing a white inspissated scale characterize keratosis pilaris. Individual lesions are discrete and may be red. They are prominent on the extensor surfaces of the upper arms and thighs and on the buttocks and cheeks. In severe cases, the lesions may be generalized. Such lesions are seen frequently in children with dry skin and have also been associated with atopic dermatitis and ichthyosis vulgaris.

Treatment is with keratolytics such as topical retinoic acid, lactic acid, or urea creams followed by skin hydration.

Pityriasis Alba

White, scaly macular areas with indistinct borders are seen over extensor surfaces of extremities and on the cheeks in children. Suntanning exaggerates these lesions. Histologic examination reveals a mild dermatitis. These lesions may be confused with tinea versicolor. There is no satisfactory treatment.

Polymorphous Light Eruption

The appearance of vesicular, eczematous, or urticarial lesions in sun-exposed areas (cheeks, nose, chin, dorsum of the hands and arms) in the springtime should suggest a diagnosis of polymorphous light eruption. Confirmation can be made by skin biopsy demonstrating dense lymphocytic infiltrates in the dermis or by reproducing the lesion by daily exposure to artificial ultraviolet light. In American Indians, it is inherited as an autosomal dominant. Onset is usually at age 5 or 6, and spontaneous improvement occurs at puberty. The first rays of sunlight of sufficient energy reaching the earth's surface in early spring induce the disease. As summer progresses, the skin thickens in response to sunlight, less ultraviolet energy enters the skin, and the disease subsides. The differential diagnosis includes erythropoietic protoporphyria, in which patients experience severe pain and itching after 5 or 10 minutes of exposure to the sun but do not develop significant skin lesions except for small papules over the dorsum of the hand; and photodermatitis from plants (psoralens) or drugs, eg, thiazide diuretics, antihistamines, phenothiazine tranquilizers, tetracyclines, and sulfonamides.

Treatment of the dermatitis with topical corticosteroids, eg, 1% hydrocortisone cream to the face three times daily, and daily use of a sunscreen applied at bedtime and each morning are sufficient.

Ferguson J: Investigation of the photosensitive child. Pediatr Dermatol 1992;9:348.

COMMON SKIN TUMORS

If the skin moves with the nodule on lateral palpation, the tumor is located within the dermis; if the skin moves over the nodule, it is subcutaneous. Table 16–6 lists the tumors according to these categories.

Table 16–6. Common skin tumors.

Intradermal
Epidermal inclusion cyst
Pilomatricoma
Dermatofibroma
Melanocytic nevus
Pyogenic granuloma
Neurofibroma
Hemangioma
Granuloma annulare
Subcutaneous
Lipoma
Rheumatoid nodule

Knight BJ et al: Superficial lumps in children: What, when and why? Pediatrics 1983;72:147.

Epidermal Inclusion Cysts

Epidermal inclusion cysts are smooth, dome-shaped nodules in the skin that may grow to 2 cm in diameter. In infants they may be found about the eyes and in older children and adolescents on the chest, back, or scalp. They are the most common superficial lumps in children. Treatment, if desired, is surgical excision.

Granuloma Annulare

Circles or semicircles of nontender intradermal nodules found over the lower legs and ankles, the dorsum of the hands and wrists, and the trunk, in that order, suggest granuloma annulare. Histologically, the disease appears as a central area of tissue death (necrobiosis) surrounded by macrophages and lymphocytes. No treatment is necessary. Lesions resolve spontaneously within 1 or 2 years in most children.

Pyogenic Granuloma

Rapid growth of a dark red papule with an ulcerated and crusted surface over 1–2 weeks following skin trauma suggests pyogenic granuloma. Histologically, this represents excessive new vessel formation with or without inflammation (granulation tissue). It is neither pyogenic nor granulomatous but should be regarded as an abnormal healing response. Pulsed dye laser or excision are the treatments of choice.

Keloids

Keloids are scars raised above the skin surface with many radial projections of scar tissue. They continue to enlarge over several years. They are often found on the face, earlobes, neck, chest, and back. Keloids show no racial predilection. Treatment includes intralesional injection with triamcinolone acetonide, 20 mg/mL, or excision and injection with corticosteroids.

PAPULOSQUAMOUS ERUPTIONS
(See Table 16–7.)

Pityriasis Rosea

Erythematous papules that coalesce to form oval plaques preceded by a large oval plaque with central clearing and a scaly border (the herald patch) establish the diagnosis of pityriasis rosea. The herald patch has the appearance of ringworm and is often treated as such. It appears 1–30 days before the onset of the generalized papular eruption. The oval plaques are parallel in their long axis and follow Langer's lines of skin cleavage. In whites, the lesions are primarily on the trunk, accentuated in the axillary and inguinal areas. In blacks, lesions are primarily on the extremities. This disease is common in school-age children and adolescents and is presumed to be viral in origin. It lasts 6 weeks and may be pruritic the first 7–10 days. The major differential diagnosis is secondary syphilis, and a VDRL test should be done if syphilis is suspected. A chronic variant of this disease may last 2 or 3 years and is called **chronic parapsoriasis or pityriasis lichenoides chronicus.**

Exposing the skin to sunlight until a mild sunburn occurs (slight redness) will hasten the disappearance of lesions. Ordinarily, no treatment is necessary.

Ginsburg CM: Pityriasis rosea. Pediatr Infect Dis J 1991; 10:858.

Psoriasis

Psoriasis is characterized by erythematous papules covered by thick white scales. Guttate (drop-like) psoriasis is a common form in children that often follows an episode of streptococcal pharyngitis by 2–3 weeks. The sudden onset of small (3–8 mm) papules, which are seen predominantly over the trunk and quickly become covered with thick white scales, is characteristic of guttate psoriasis. Chronic psoriasis is marked by thick, large (5–10 cm) scaly plaques over the elbows, knees, scalp, and other sites of trauma. Pinpoint pits in the nail plate are seen as well as yellow discoloration of the nail plate resulting from onycholysis. Thickening of all 20 nails is an uncommon feature. The sacral and seborrheic areas are commonly involved. Psoriasis has no known cause and demonstrates active proliferation of epidermal cells

Table 16–7. Papulosquamous eruptions in children.

Psoriasis
Pityriasis rosea
Secondary syphilis
Lichen planus
Chronic parapsoriasis
Pityriasis rubra pilaris
Tinea corporis
Dermatomyositis
Lupus erythematosus

with a turnover time of 3–4 days versus 28 days for normal skin. These rapidly proliferating epidermal cells are producing excessive stratum corneum, giving rise to thick opaque scales. Papulosquamous eruptions that present problems of differential diagnosis are listed in Table 16–7.

All therapy is aimed at diminishing epidermal turnover time. Sunlight or artificial ultraviolet light (UVL) alone will produce some improvement. Coal tar enhances the effect of UVL and hastens the disappearance of psoriatic lesions. Bathing with a bath product containing tar (eg, Balnetar) at night, followed by UVL the next day, may be sufficient in mild cases. In more severe psoriasis, 10% liquor carbonis detergens in petrolatum should be applied after the bath. The newer tar gels (Estar gel, psoriGel) cause less staining and are most efficacious. They are applied twice daily for 6–8 weeks.

Crude coal tar therapy is messy and stains bedclothes, and patients may prefer to use topical corticosteroids. Penetration of topical corticosteroids through the enlarged epidermal barrier in psoriasis requires that more potent preparations be used, eg, fluocinonide 0.05% (Lidex) or triamcinolone 0.5% (Aristocort, Kenalog) four times daily.

Anthralin therapy is also useful. Anthralin is applied to the skin for a short contact time (eg, 20 minutes once daily) and then washed off with a neutral soap (eg, Dove). A 6-week course of treatment is recommended.

Scalp care using a tar shampoo (Polytar, Zetar, many others) requires leaving the shampoo on for 5 minutes, washing it off, and then shampooing with commercial shampoo to remove scales. It may be necessary to shampoo daily until scaling is reduced.

More severe cases of psoriasis are best treated by a dermatologist.

Griffiths CE: Psoriasis: 1. Pathogenesis. J Am Acad Dermatol 1992;27:98.

Lichen Planus

Lichen planus consists of pruritic, light purple, flat-topped, many-sided papules, predominantly on the lower legs, penis, wrists, and arms. A white lacy pattern in the buccal mucosa is often seen. Pruritus may be severe.

If pruritus is mild, no treatment is necessary, and the disease will disappear in 6–12 months. With severe pruritus, a trial of antihistamines, eg, diphenhydramine, 5 mg/kg/d, or hydroxyzine, 2 mg/kg/d orally, is warranted. Rapid relief of pruritus and disappearance of the lesions can be achieved by administering prednisone, 1 mg/kg/d orally for 3–4 weeks.

Boyd AS, Neldner KH: Lichen planus. J Am Acad Dermatol 1991;25:593.

HAIR LOSS
(Alopecia)

Hair loss in children (Table 16–8) imposes great emotional stress on the parent and the patient. A 60% hair loss in a single area is necessary before hair loss can be detected clinically. Examination should begin with the scalp to determine if there are color changes or infiltrative changes. Hairs should be examined microscopically for breaking and structural defects and to see if growing or resting hairs are being shed. Placing removed hairs in mounting fluid (Permount) on a glass microscope slide makes them easy to examine. Three diseases account for most cases of hair loss in children: alopecia areata, tinea capitis, and trichotillomania.

Alopecia Areata

Loss of every hair in a localized area is called alopecia areata. This is the most common cause of hair loss in children. An immunologic pathogenic mechanism is suspected because dense infiltration of lymphocytes precedes hair loss. Ninety-five percent of children with alopecia areata completely regrow their hair within 12 months, though as many as 40% may have a relapse in 5 or 6 years. A rare and unusual form of alopecia areata begins at the occiput and proceeds along the hair margins to the frontal scalp. This variety, called **ophiasis,** often results in total scalp hair loss **(alopecia totalis).** The prognosis for regrowth in ophiasis is poor.

No treatment is indicated for alopecia areata. Systemic corticosteroids given to suppress the inflammatory response will result in hair growth, but the hair will fall out again when the drug is discontinued. In children with alopecia totalis, a wig is most helpful.

Price VH: Alopecia areata: Clinical aspects. J Invest Dermatol 1991;96:685

Table 16–8. Other causes of hair loss in children.

Hair loss with scalp changes
 Nodules and tumors:
  Nevus sebaceus
  Epidermal nevus
 Thickening:
  Linear sclerodrema (morphea) (en coup de sabre)
  Burn
 Atrophy:
  Lupus erythematosus
  Lichen planus
Hair loss with hair shaft defects (hair fails to grow out
  enough to require haircuts):
 Monilethrix—alternating bands of thin and thick areas
 Trichorrhexis nodosa—nodules with fragmented hair
 Trichorrhexis invaginata (bamboo hair)—intussusception
  of one hair into another
 Pili torti—hair twisted 180 degrees, brittle
 Pili annulati—alternating bands of light and dark
  pigmentation

Trichotillomania

Traumatic hair pulling causes the hair shafts to be broken off at different lengths, an ill-defined area of hair loss, petechiae around follicular openings, and a wrinkled hair shaft on microscopic examination. This may be merely habit or the result of severe anxiety in the child. Eyelashes and eyebrows rather than scalp hair may be pulled out. Such episodes are best considered a nervous habit. Oiling the hair to make it slippery is an aid to behavior modification.

Nail Disorders

Nail biting and *Candida* paronychia are the two most common nail disorders. Onychomycosis is uncommon. Nail pitting is seen in psoriasis and alopecia areata.

Pappert AS, Scher RK, Cohen JL: Nail disorders in children. Pediatr Clin North Am 1991;38:921.

REACTIVE ERYTHEMAS

Erythema Multiforme

Erythema multiforme begins with papules that later develop a dark center and then evolve into lesions with central blisters and the characteristic target lesions (iris lesions) with three concentric circles of color change. Primary injury is to endothelial cells, with later destruction of epidermal basal cells and blister formation. Erythema multiforme has sometimes been diagnosed in severe mucous membrane involvement, but **Stevens-Johnson syndrome** is the usual term for severe involvement of conjunctiva, oral cavity, and genital mucosa.

Many causes are suspected, particularly herpes simplex virus, sulfonamide drugs, and *Mycoplasma* infections. Recurrent erythema multiforme is usually associated with reactivation of herpes simplex virus. In the mild form, spontaneous healing occurs in 10–14 days, but Stevens-Johnson syndrome may last 6–8 weeks if untreated.

Treatment is symptomatic in uncomplicated erythema multiforme. Removal of offending drugs is an obvious necessary measure. Oral antihistamines such as hydroxyzine, 2 mg/kg/d orally, are useful. Cool compresses and wet dressings will relieve pruritus.

Brice SL et al: Erythema multiforme. Curr Probl Dermatol 1990;2:1.
Weston WL et al: Herpes simplex virus in childhood erythema multiforme. Pediatrics 1992;89:32.

Erythema Nodosum

Erythema nodosum consists of painful, erythematous nodules on the anterior lower legs. In streptococcal infections, coccidioidomycosis, histoplasmosis, and tuberculosis, the onset of erythema nodosum parallels the appearance of cell-mediated immunity.

Streptococcal infections and birth control pills are the most common causes of this panniculitis in the USA.

Treatment consists of removal of the offending drug or eradication of infection. Topical corticosteroids afford some relief, but prednisone, 1–2 mg/kg/d orally, may be necessary for 2–3 weeks.

Fox MD, Schwartz RA: Erythema nodosum. Am Fam Physician 1992;46:818.

Drug Eruptions

Drugs may produce urticarial, morbilliform, scarlatiniform, or bullous skin eruptions. Urticaria may appear within minutes after drug administration, but most reactions begin 7–14 days after the drug is first administered. Drugs commonly implicated in skin reactions are listed in Table 16–9.

MISCELLANEOUS SKIN DISORDERS ENCOUNTERED IN PEDIATRIC PRACTICE

Aphthous Stomatitis

Recurrent erosions on the gums, lips, tongue, palate, and buccal mucosa are often confused with herpes simplex. A smear of the base of such a lesion stained with Wright's stain will aid in ruling out herpes simplex by the absence of epithelial giant cells. A culture for herpes simplex is also useful in this difficult differential diagnostic problem. It has been shown that recurrence of aphthous stomatitis correlates positively with lymphocyte-mediated cytotoxicity.

There is no specific therapy for this condition. Rinsing the mouth with liquid antacids will provide relief in most patients. Topical corticosteroids in a gel base (eg, fluocinonide gel) may provide some relief. In severe cases that interfere with eating, prednisone,

Table 16–9. Common drug reactions.

Erythema multiforme/toxic epidermal necrolysis
  Sulfonamides
  Nonsteroidal anti-inflammatory drugs
  Anticonvulsants
Urticaria
  Penicillins
  Sulfonamides
  Barbiturates
  Opioids
Morbilliform eruption
  Penicillins
  Cephalosporins
  Sulfonamides
  Anticonvulsants
Photodermatitis
  Psoralens
  Tetracyclines
  Thiazides
  Sulfonamides

1 mg/kg/d orally for 3–5 days, will suffice to abort an episode.

Brice SL: Recurrent aphthous stomatitis. Curr Probl Dermatol 1991;3:109.

Vitiligo

Vitiligo is characterized clinically by the development of areas of depigmentation. These are often symmetrical and occur mainly on extensor surfaces. The depigmentation results from a destruction of melanocytes. The basis for this destruction is unknown but immunologically mediated damage is likely and vitiligo sometimes occurs in individuals with selective IgA deficiency, graft versus host disease or autoimmune endocrinopathies. Treatment is not very effective. Topical psoralens with UV irradiation are reserved for children over 12 years of age.

Corns & Calluses

Thickened areas of epidermis in response to repeated or prolonged friction or pressure are called either corns or calluses. Corns are clearly demarcated and painful, whereas calluses have ill-defined margins and are not tender. A painful corn may overlie an exostosis, and one should get an x-ray film of that digit.

Treatment begins with removing the cause of friction or pressure, if possible, such as ill-fitting shoes. Local therapy consists of paring down the lesion with a razor blade or No. 15 knife blade and covering it with a cut-to-size piece of 40% salicylic acid plaster. Cover firmly with adhesive tape to prevent loosening due to sweating. The plaster should not be allowed to get wet. It can be removed every 5 days and the dead skin gently removed. The plaster may then be put in place.

Morphea
(Linear Scleroderma)

Morphea is characterized by the appearance, anywhere on the body, of well-circumscribed, shiny, white, firmly adherent skin. It is particularly cosmetically deforming on the face. A light purple border is indicative of an early lesion or continuing activity. Skin biopsy reveals replacement of subcutaneous fat with thickened collagen fibers. The lesions tend to burn themselves out in 3–5 years. It may be difficult to differentiate morphea from lichen sclerosis et atrophicus, which has similar white patches that occur primarily on the upper back and genitalia. Histopathologic differentiation is often necessary and may be difficult. *Borrelia* infections have recently been implicated in morphea.

Necrobiosis Lipoidica
Diabeticorum

A depressed yellow area with telangiectasia surrounded by an erythematous nodular border found on the anterior lower leg is diagnostic of necrobiosis lipoidica diabeticorum. Histopathologic findings include atrophy of the epidermis and a palisading granuloma of lymphocytes and macrophages surrounding an area of homogenized devitalized dermis. Lesions are most often found in diabetics but can be seen in nondiabetic children. There is no satisfactory treatment.

REFERENCES

Schachner L, Hansen R: *Pediatric Dermatology.* Churchill Livingstone, 1988.

Weston WL, Lane, AT: *Color Textbook of Pediatric Dermatology.* Mosby Year Book, 1991.

17

Eye

Philip P. Ellis, MD

GROWTH & DEVELOPMENT OF THE EYE

Although the eye is not completely developed at birth, it is a relatively large functioning sensory organ in the newborn. The postnatal growth of the eye and the brain are comparable. By the end of the fourth year, the eye has attained about 70% of its adult volume. Subsequent growth is much slower, until about age 10–12 years, when adult proportions are reached.

The average anteroposterior diameter of the newborn infant's eye is approximately 17.3 mm (the average adult diameter of the eye is slightly over 24 mm). The cornea is comparatively large, with an average transverse diameter of 10 mm; by the second year of life, the average adult corneal diameter of 12 mm is reached. The cornea in infants is much steeper than in adults, and the iris contains little pigment and appears to have a bluish color. As pigment forms, the color of the iris becomes more distinct. By the age of 6 months, it is usually possible to determine whether the irides will become brown or remain blue.

The lens in the newborn infant's eye is more spherical than in the adult eye. This feature—and the steeper cornea—help to overcome some of the hyperopia (farsightedness) resulting from the comparative shortness of the eyeball. At birth, approximately 75–80% of children are hyperopic. Hyperopia may increase for the first 7 or 8 years of life and then frequently diminishes. This contrasts to myopia (nearsightedness), which does not usually develop until age 8–10 and then increases until 20–30 years of age.

Of all the ocular structures, the retina is the least developed functionally at birth. The macula is poorly developed, and this characteristic is a major factor in the poor vision of newborns. Full development of the macula does not occur until about 6 months of age. The periphery of the retina is not as well developed as the remainder. Peripheral vascularization is not complete until about the time of full-term delivery.

Myelinization of the optic nerve is incomplete at birth; further myelinization continues until about the fourth month of life. The sclera is relatively pliable and thin; the underlying uvea is what causes the blue color of the newborn sclera. Scleral fibers soon thicken to give a whiter appearance to the eye.

The orbit is almost round at birth. It undergoes rapid changes in size and shape; by the first year of life, orbital volume is quadrupled, and by the sixth year it is redoubled. The lacrimal gland is poorly developed at birth, which accounts for the paucity of tears when the newborn cries. Tear production does not occur until 4 weeks of life. The nasolacrimal duct is usually patent at birth, but in many infants the distal end remains plugged for several months (see discussion under lacrimal apparatus).

Coordinated movement of the eyes is not well developed for the first few months of life, although many full-term infants establish ocular alignment within 4 weeks of birth. Binocular visual responses begin to develop between the ages of 2 and 6 months and become firmly established during the second 6 months of life. Variable or intermittent ocular deviations (strabismus) are common in early infancy. Constant deviations should always be investigated by an ophthalmologist.

Visual acuity in full-term neonates is about 20/400. At the age of 5 months, it is about 20/100; at 2 years, about 20/60; and at 4–5 years, almost 20/20.

Apt L, Gaffney WL: The eyes. In: *Pediatrics,* 18th ed. Rudolph AM, Hoffman JIE (editors). Appleton & Lange, 1987.

Droste PJ, Archer SM, Helveston EM: Measurement of low vision in children and infants. Ophthalmology 1991; 98:1513.

Gallo JE, Lennerstrand G: A population based study of ocular abnormalities in premature children aged 5 to 10 years. Am J Ophthalmol 1991;111:539.

Hoyt CS, Nickel B, Billson FA: Ophthalmological examination of the infant: Developmental aspects. Surv Ophthalmol 1982;26:177.

Isenberg SJ (editor): *The Eye in Infancy.* Year Book, 1989.

Nelson LB, Calhoun JH, Harley RD (editors): *Pediatric Ophthalmology,* 3rd ed. Saunders, 1991.

Norcia AM et al: Visual acuity development in normal and abnormal preterm human infants. J Pediatr Ophthalmol Strabismus 1987;4:70.

GENERAL PRINCIPLES
OF DIAGNOSIS

A careful history is essential in establishing an accurate diagnosis of an ocular disorder. The history should include time and rate of onset of the presenting symptoms, associated symptoms, past history of eye disorders and treatment, history of prematurity, and pertinent family and social history. However, many eye problems, such as poor vision in one eye, are asymptomatic and are discovered only on testing of visual acuity or other objective diagnostic methods.

COMMON NONSPECIFIC
SYMPTOMS & SIGNS

Redness

Redness is a common finding in many ocular disorders. It is produced by dilatation of conjunctival and superficial scleral vessels in response to inflammation, infection, or irritation. The differential diagnosis of redness of the eye is presented in Table 17–1.

Tearing

In infants, tearing is usually due to nasolacrimal duct obstruction. Tearing may also be associated with local inflammatory, allergic, and viral diseases and with congenital glaucoma or corneal irritation.

Discharge

Purulent discharge is usually associated with bacterial infections. Mucoid discharge is usually associated with chemical irritations, some viral infections, or allergic conditions; it may be secondary to obstructions of the nasolacrimal duct.

Pain

Pain in or about the eye may be due to foreign bodies in the cornea or conjunctiva, corneal abrasions, acute infections of the lid, orbital cellulitis, acute dacryocystitis, acute iritis, or glaucoma. Refractive errors seldom produce headaches in young children. Large refractive errors or poor convergence may produce headaches in older children, particularly those who read a good deal.

Poor Vision
(Amblyopia)

In young infants, poor vision is usually due to a serious ophthalmologic or neurologic disorder such as congenital nystagmus, corneal or lenticular opacities, disorders of the retina, optic nerve and central nervous system abnormalities, or very high myopia. In

Table 17–1. Differential diagnosis of redness of the eye in pediatric patients.

	Acute Conjunctivitis	Acute Iritis	Acute Glaucoma[1]	Corneal Abrasion
Incidence	Very common.	Uncommon.	Rare.	Fairly common.
Etiology	Usually bacterial; may be viral, fungal, or allergic.	Usually unknown; may be associated with juvenile rheumatoid arthritis.	Developmental defects or obstruction of aqueous drainage channels.	Foreign body; abrasion.
Redness	Diffuse injection of conjunctiva; greater toward fornices.	Purple-red; circumcorneal injection.	Often diffuse injection of bulbar conjunctiva.	Diffuse injection of conjunctiva.
Discharge	Moderate to heavy; mucoid or mucopurulent.	None.	None; tearing.	Watery.
Visual acuity	Normal.	Decreased.	Decreased.	Decreased.
Corneal transparency	Clear.	Clear or some haze.	Hazy; cornea enlarged in congenital form.	Variable haze. Positive fluorescein stain.
Anterior chamber depth	Normal.	Normal; cloudy.	Shallow; deep in congenital form.	Normal.
Pupil size	Normal.	Constricted.	Dilated.	Normal.
Intraocular pressure	Normal.	Usually normal; may be low or elevated.	Elevated.	Normal.
Conjunctival smear results	Causative organisms identified; numerous polymorphonuclear neutrophils found in bacterial infection; numerous mononuclear cells found in viral infection.	Normal.	Normal.	Normal.

[1]Primary narrow-angle glaucoma is very rare in children. Congenital glaucoma may not produce redness of the eye.

older infants and children, the development of poor vision is often associated with refractive errors or strabismus.

Amblyopia is usually a unilateral reduction in vision, uncorrectable with glasses, that occurs in an eye that is normal on ophthalmoscopy; rarely is it bilateral. It is found in 2–4% of the general population. In children, most amblyopia is unilateral and secondary to strabismus. It is the result of a long, continued deviation of one eye with suppression of the retinal image in the deviating eye to avoid diplopia. Amblyopia also may occur when there is a large difference in refractive errors between the two eyes (anisometropia). Usually the eye with the greatest refractive error does not develop a clear retinal image, and as a consequence vision fails to develop fully.

Leukocoria

A white spot in the pupil is a serious finding that may be due to congenital cataract, retinopathy of prematurity, retinal dysplasia, intraocular infection, retinoblastoma, or persistence and hyperplasia of primary vitreous (see Figure 17–1).

EXAMINATION

Visual Acuity

Routine testing of visual acuity should be part of every general physical examination. It is the single most important test of visual function. Each eye should be tested separately. In children 4 years of age or older, satisfactory visual acuity tests can usually be obtained with the use of Snellen test charts. In children 2½–3 years old, vision can often be tested with

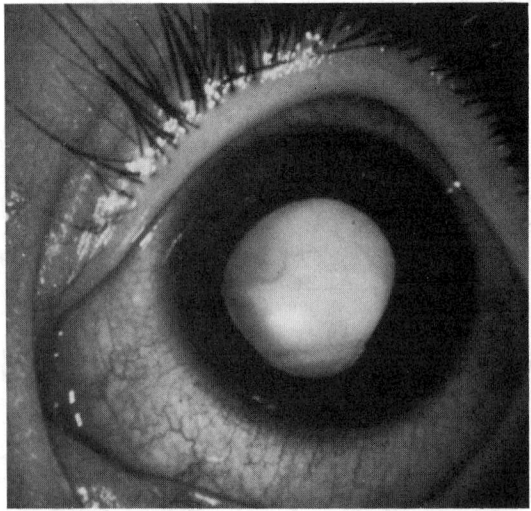

Figure 17–1. Retinoblastoma presenting with leukocoria (white reflection in pupil).

the use of Allen or E cards. Objects familiar to the child (eg, animals, trees, houses) are depicted on the Allen cards in graduated sizes. When E cards are used, the child is asked to point in the direction of the "feet" of the figure E. Because of distractions in the office, children are sometimes unable to perform this test adequately; special illiterate E cards may be sent home so that the parents can test the vision at home under better circumstances. The parent can repeat the test at leisure, and the final result is usually more accurate than that obtained from testing done in the office.

The ability to fixate on objects is the most reliable test for vision in infancy. Visual acuity is difficult to evaluate in infants. One can observe whether an infant will fixate on and follow a light or a bright attractive toy in different directions of gaze. The examiner's face is an excellent target to elicit ocular fixation and following movements. Each eye is tested separately. If the infant fails to respond to such testing, one can observe the pupillary responses for reaction to direct light stimulus. These responses depend upon a functioning retina and optic nerve. However, cortical blindness can exist with preservation of pupillary light reflexes. The demonstration of optokinetic nystagmus (slow pursuit movements in the direction of a moving stimulus and quick saccadic movements in the reverse direction or "railway nystagmus") indicates that there are functioning neural receptors in the retina and intact neural pathways.

Infants can also be tested by alternately covering each eye. If visual acuity is poor in one eye, the infant will resist actively when the good eye is covered and vision is disturbed but will be much less affected when the eye with decreased vision is covered.

Poor visual acuity due to refractive errors in older children can be differentiated from poor vision due to other diseases by a pinhole test. If the reduced visual acuity is due to a refractive error, placement of a pinhole before this eye in line with the pupil will result in improved vision.

External Examination

External examination should include general inspection of the lids and eyeballs, noting their prominence, size, and position as well as any growths, inflammations, discharge, or vascular injection. Forward protrusion (exophthalmos) or retraction (enophthalmos) of the globe should be noted. Unusual size of the globes as indicated by megalocornea or microphthalmos should be noted. The positions of the lids in relation to the globe and the coverage of the lids over the closed eyes should be observed. Normally, with the eyes open, the lower lid margin is at the lower border of the cornea in the forward position of gaze, and the upper lid should cover approximately 2 mm of the cornea. Any drooping of the upper lid (ptosis) or retraction of the eyelids should be noted. The lid margins should be inspected to see if they are in proper alignment against the globes or if there is ectropion (turning outward of the lid margins) or entropion (turning inward). The distribution of the lashes and their position should be studied. The lid margins should be inspected for inflammation, crusting, and patency of the lacrimal puncta.

If a conjunctival foreign body is suspected, the lids should be everted and the palpebral and bulbar conjunctivae inspected. Examination may be facilitated with a drop of a topical anesthetic. The upper lid may be everted by pulling the lid forward (grasping the lashes), placing a small applicator behind the tarsal area, and gently pressing down on the lid (Figure 17–2). The maneuver is facilitated if the patient looks downward. If a corneal abrasion or foreign body is suspected or if there is sudden unexplained pain in the eye, sterile fluorescein solution should be instilled into the conjunctival cul-de-sac and the cornea observed to see if there is any staining. Observation of staining is enhanced with the use of a blue light. Pupillary light reflexes should be tested for each eye, and both direct and consensual reflexes should be noted.

Corneal sensitivity may be tested by touching the cornea gently with a fine wisp of cotton. If corneal sensation is intact, a brisk blink reflex will result.

Extraocular Muscles

The position of the eyes should be observed by inspection. As a rule, there is little difficulty in telling whether gross strabismus is present. A quick estimation of the alignment of the eyes can be made by the corneal light reflection technique (Hirschberg test). The light reflection should come from corresponding parts of each cornea when a light is shone into the eyes. If there is lateral displacement of the light reflection, esotropia (internal deviation) of the eye is present (Figure 17–3). If the light reflection is dis-

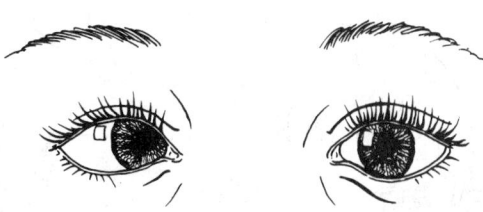

Figure 17–3. Lateral displacement of light reflection showing esotropia (internal deviation) of the right eye. Nasal displacement of the reflection would show exotropia (outward deviation).

placed nasally, exotropia (outward deviation) is present. A more refined method of judging alignment of the eyes is by means of the cover test. In this test, the patient is instructed to look at any target, and one eye is then covered. If the uncovered eye has been looking straight forward at the object, there will be no shift in movement of this eye. If, however, the eye has been turned either inward or outward, then a corresponding corrective movement will be made with this eye to align the object in the visual gaze (Figure 17–4). The other eye is then similarly tested. The eye under cover should also be observed to see whether there is inward or outward movement, indicating the presence of a phoria, or a tendency for ocular deviation. If the eye remains in the deviated position after removing the occluder, a tropia (deviation of the eyes not corrected by the fusion mechanism) rather than a phoria (deviation that is corrected by the fusion mechanism) is present.

The cardinal positions of gaze should be checked. An object or light is shown to the infant, and the ability to follow the movement of the object in different directions is tested. If marked strabismus or muscle paralysis is present, there may be limitation of movement in one direction of gaze. To determine if true paresis of an extraocular muscle is present, the nondeviating eye should be covered and the ocular movement of the uncovered eye tested in all directions of gaze. In small infants, extraocular muscle function may be checked by rapidly turning the infant in different directions and observing whether the eyes turn to the side opposite to which the head was turned (doll's head phenomenon).

Nystagmus

If nystagmus is present, its characteristics should be observed and the movements classified, first by rate or variation in rate of movement and then by direction. **Pendular (undulatory) nystagmus** consists of excursions that are equal in each direction of gaze; this type of nystagmus is usually observed in children with poor vision and is usually ocular in origin. **Jerking (rhythmic) nystagmus** is characterized by a slow component followed by a quick corrective component; it may be congenital, physiologic (at the ex-

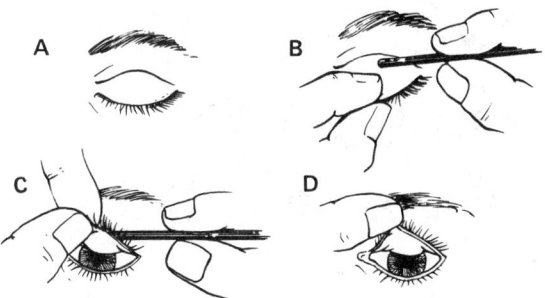

Figure 17–2. Eversion of the upper lid. **A:** The patient looks downward. **B:** The fingers pull the lid down, and a rod is placed on the upper tarsal border. **C:** The lid is pulled up over the rod. **D:** The lid is everted. (Redrawn and reproduced, with permission, from Liebman SD, Gellis SS [editors]: *The Pediatrician's Ophthalmology.* Mosby, 1966.)

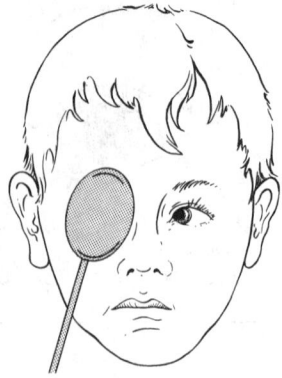 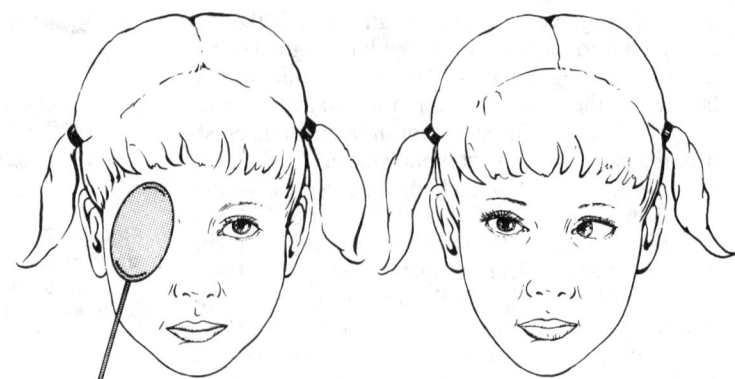

The eyes of a child with severe amblyopia may not be able to fixate an object even when the good eye is covered. Vision of such an eye is 20/200 or less.

If the child with an amblyopic eye will fixate an object only when the good eye is covered but does not hold fixation when the cover is removed, vision of the poor eye is usually from 20/100 to 20/50.

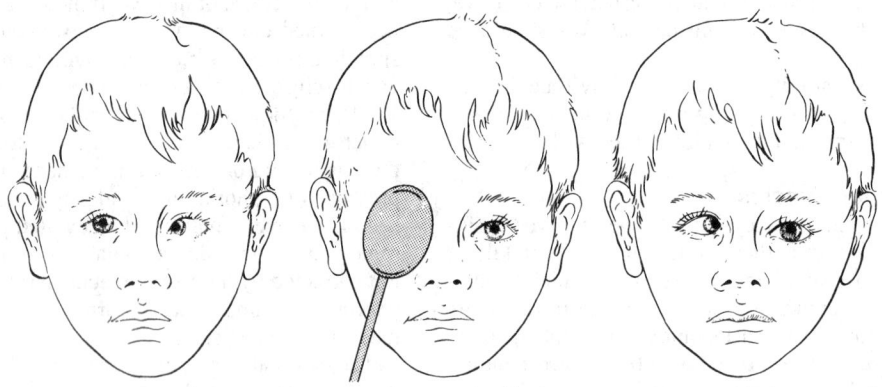

If covering the fixing eye causes fixation with the other eye, and if this second eye maintains fixation for some time even when the cover is removed, the second eye will usually have vision between 20/50 and 20/30.

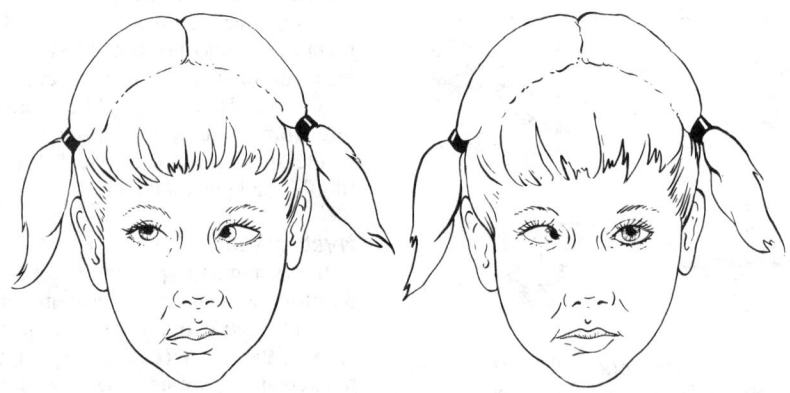

Spontaneous alternation of fixation between the 2 eyes occurs if vision is equal (no suppression amblyopia).

Figure 17–4. Estimation of visual acuity in amblyopia. (Modified slightly. Redrawn and reproduced, with permission, from Havener WH: *Synopsis of Ophthalmology,* 5th ed. Mosby, 1979.)

treme positions of gaze), due to inner ear disease, or secondary to central nervous system disease. **Congenital nystagmus** is a type of jerking nystagmus that is usually not associated with other neurologic disorders. The nystagmus is present in all directions of gaze, but it is usually minimized when the patient's eyes are turned slightly to one side or the other. This type of nystagmus usually decreases when the eyes converge. Children often assume abnormal head positions to dampen the nystagmus. **Latent nystagmus** is manifest only when one eye is covered.

Nystagmus is further classified according to the direction of movement (horizontal, rotatory, vertical, or mixed). Rotatory and vertical nystagmus result from brain stem disorders. Spasmus nutans is a rare disorder in which vertical head nodding is associated with nystagmus; the nystagmus is usually horizontal but may be vertical. An anomalous head tilt is often present. The condition occurs in small infants and usually disappears within the first 2 years of life. Rarely, spasmus nutans is associated with a central nervous system disorder, most commonly chiasmal glioma.

Measurement of Intraocular Pressure

The only satisfactory method of measuring ocular pressure is with a tonometer. Tactile tension, particularly in infants, is totally unreliable.

If glaucoma is suspected because of unexplained tearing or enlarged and hazy corneas, the patient should be referred to an ophthalmologist. Intraocular pressures should be measured with any enlarged or hazy corneas or traumatic hyphema (blood in the anterior chamber).

Ophthalmoscopic Examination

Satisfactory ophthalmoscopic examination of the infant eye can be accomplished only after pupillary dilation. The combination of 1% tropicamide or 2–5% homatropine with 2.5% phenylephrine or that of 0.2% cyclopentolate with 1% phenylephrine instilled two or three times at intervals of 10–15 minutes usually gives satisfactory pupillary dilatation. In children 2 years of age and older, 1% cyclopentolate gives good pupillary dilatation; a second dose may be necessary in children with dark irides.

When an ophthalmoscope is held 30–45 cm (12–18 inches) in front of the eye and the eye is observed through the plus 10 or 15 lens, an orange-red reflection of light (the "red reflex") is observed through the pupil. If the red reflex is not present or dark spots are noted in the reflected light, an opacity of the cornea, lens, or vitreous is probably present. If red reflexes from both eyes are different (eg, irregular or distorted), refractive errors in one or both eyes should be suspected.

Ophthalmoscopic study should include all structures of the eye, such as the cornea, lens, vitreous, optic disk, and retina. In the infant, the optic disk ap-

pears paler than in the adult. The foveal light reflection is absent. The periphery of the fundus is gray. The peripheral retinal vessels are not well developed.

Refraction Test for Glasses

Cycloplegia is necessary to perform satisfactory refractions in infants and small children. The topical instillation of 1% cyclopentolate or 5% homatropine is usually adequate. More complete cycloplegia can be obtained with 0.5–1% atropine instilled two or three times a day for 3 days, but this is seldom necessary. Retinoscopy is used to determine the refractive error in children up to 7–8 years of age. Subsequently, subjective methods of refraction are also used.

Visual Fields

It is virtually impossible to judge visual fields in infants. One can sometimes estimate gross restriction of peripheral visual fields by covering one eye and directing the infant's gaze to an object. A second object is brought in from the side, and the infant is observed to see when the direction of the gaze is first shifted to the new object. Different types of toys and colored lights can be used for the visual test objects.

Perimetry examination of visual fields in children is easier to perform than tangent screen examination. By age 6 or 7 years, satisfactory perimetry examinations can usually be performed. Attractive toys and large objects are brought in along the perimetry arm.

Abadi RV, Whittle J: The nature of head postures in congenital nystagmus. Arch Ophthalmol 1991;109:216.

Campbell LR, Charney E: Factors associated with delay in diagnosis of childhood amblyopia. Pediatrics 1991;87:178.

Dhillon B, Millar, GT: *The Child's Eye*. Oxford Univ Press, 1993.

Epelbaum M et al: The sensitive period for strabismic amblyopia in humans. Ophthalmology 1993;100:323.

Harrington DO, Drake MV: *The Visual Fields. Text and Atlas of Clinical Perimetry*, 6th ed. Mosby, 1990.

Hoyt CS, Nickel B, Billson FA: Ophthalmological examination of the infant: Developmental aspects. Surv Ophthalmol 1982;26:177.

Isenberg SJ (editor): *The Eye in Infancy*, 2nd ed., Mosby, 1993.

Kutschke PJ, Scott WE, Keech RV: Anisometropic amblyopia. Ophthalmology 1991;98:258.

Nelson LB, Calhoun JH, Harley RD (editors): *Pediatric Ophthalmology*, 3rd ed., Saunders, 1991.

Robinson CG, Jan JE: Acquired ocular visual impairment in children 1960–1989. Am J Dis Child 1993;147:325.

GENERAL PRINCIPLES OF TREATMENT OF OCULAR DISORDERS

For diseases of the anterior segment of the eye, topical medication is effective. For diseases of the posterior segment of the eye and of the orbit, systemic medication is necessary. In many instances (eg, severe intraocular infections or uveitis), a combination of topical and systemic medications is required.

The intraocular penetration of topically applied drugs depends upon their solubility in fat and water. The epithelium of the cornea presents a barrier to medications that are not fat-soluble. The alkaloids, the corticosteroids, and some of the anesthetics penetrate the eye quite easily after topical application to the cornea. Most antibiotics do not penetrate the eye in therapeutic concentrations when topically applied.

The degree of intraocular penetration of systemically administered drugs depends upon their ability to pass the blood-aqueous and blood-vitreous barriers. In the normal eye, most systemically administered antibiotics do not penetrate the barriers. In the inflamed eye, the barriers are broken down, and drugs penetrate much better. Systemically administered corticosteroids penetrate the eye quite easily. Certain drugs, such as mannitol and glycerol, do not cross the blood-aqueous barrier and therefore are valuable in the temporary treatment of acute glaucoma because an osmotic gradient is produced in which the blood is hypertonic to the aqueous and vitreous.

Solutions Versus Ointments

Topical ophthalmic preparations may be administered either as solutions or ointments. In children, ointments have several advantages over solutions: They are not washed away with the tears; they are quite comfortable upon initial instillation; there is less absorption into the lacrimal passage; and since the contact time in the eye is much longer, they can be used less frequently. The chief disadvantage of ointments is that they produce a film over the eye and interfere with vision. The advantages of solutions are that they do not interfere with vision and cause fewer contact dermatitis reactions than ointments; the chief disadvantage is that they must be instilled frequently.

Topical Corticosteroids

The corticosteroids are effective in many eye diseases, including allergic blepharitis and conjunctivitis, vernal conjunctivitis, phlyctenular keratoconjunctivitis, mucocutaneous conjunctival lesions, contact dermatitis of the eyelid and conjunctiva, interstitial keratitis, and many forms of iritis and iridocyclitis. Weaker corticosteroid preparations such as 1% med-rysone, 0.5–1.5% hydrocortisone, and 0.125% prednisolone are usually adequate for the management of allergic reactions of the conjunctiva and eyelid.

Many complications follow long- and short-term administration of topical corticosteroids. Among these are increased incidence or aggravation of herpes simplex keratitis, fungal ulcers of the cornea, decreased healing of corneal abrasions and wounds, glaucoma, and cataract formation. The incidence of complications increases with the use of the more potent corticosteroid preparations such as 0.1% dexamethasone, 1% prednisolone, 0.1% triamcinolone, and 0.1% betamethasone. The use of these agents generally should be reserved for the treatment of severe intraocular inflammation. Any eye disorder severe enough to require prolonged topical corticosteroid therapy should be treated by an ophthalmologist.

Topical Antibiotics & Chemotherapeutic Agents

Ideally, the infecting organism should be identified and its antibiotic sensitivity established before specific antibiotic therapy is started. This is often impractical, however, and topical antibiotics are in most cases instituted empirically. Topical use of antibiotics that are seldom employed systemically will decrease the risk of hypersensitivity reactions. For this reason, a mixture of neomycin, bacitracin, and polymyxin—or a mixture of trimethoprim and polymyxin B is frequently used in the treatment of conjunctivitis. Broad-spectrum antibiotics and sulfacetamide or sulfisoxazole seldom produce sensitivity. Topical penicillin therapy should be avoided.

In Tables 17–2 and 17–3 are listed the commonly used topical chemotherapeutic and antibiotic ophthalmic agents.

Mydriatics & Cycloplegics

Mydriatics are agents that dilate the pupil without paralyzing the ciliary muscle of accommodation. They are useful for ophthalmoscopic examination and in preventing and breaking posterior synechiae (adhesions of the iris to the lens). The most commonly used mydriatic is phenylephrine, 2.5–10% (the 10% should not be used in infants and small children). The duration of effect is only a few hours.

Cycloplegic drugs are agents that produce paralysis of accommodation as well as pupillary dilatation. They are used in refraction and in the treatment of acute inflammatory conditions of the iris and ciliary body. The more commonly used cycloplegics are atropine, 0.25–2%; homatropine, 2–5%; scopolamine, 0.2%; cyclopentolate, 1–2%; and tropicamide, 1%.

Atropine is the most powerful cycloplegic; its effect may last for as long as 14 days. Scopolamine has an effect that lasts 2–5 days, whereas the effects of homatropine are usually gone within 48 hours. Cyclopentolate and tropicamide produce more rapid

Table 17–2. Topical chemotherapeutic and antibiotic agents.

Drug	Trade Name	Solution	Ointment
Amphotericin B	Fungizone	0.5–1.5 mg/mL[1]	
Bacitracin	Baciguent	2000–10,000 units/mL[2]	500 units/g
Chloramphenicol	Chloromycetin, many others	1.6–5 mg/mL	10 mg/g
Ciprofloxacin	Ciloxan	3 mg/mL	
Colistin	Coly-Mycin S	1.2–5 mg/mL[1]	
Erythromycin	Ak Mycin, Ilotycin	5 mg/mL[1]	5 mg/g
Gentamicin	Garamycin, many others	3 mg/mL	3 mg/g
Neomycin	Myciguent	1.75–3.5 mg/mL[2]	5 mg/g
Norfloxacin	Chibroxin	3 mg/mL	
Polymyxin B		5000–16,250 mg/mL[2]	5000–10,000 units/g[2]
Streptomycin		50 mg/mL[1]	
Sulfacetamide sodium	Many	100–300 mg/mL	100 mg/g
Sulfisoxazole	Gantrisin	40 mg/mL	40 mg/g
Tetracycline group	Many	10 mg/mL	10 mg/g
Trimethoprim sulfamethoxazole		10 mg/mL[2]	
Tobramycin	Tobrex	3 mg/mL	3 mg/g

[1]Not commercially available.
[2]Available commercially only in combined drug preparations.

cycloplegia than the other agents, but their effect is usually gone within 24 hours.

A combination product of 0.2% cyclopentolate and 1% phenylephrine is a preferred agent in babies under 6 months of age.

Topical Anesthetics

The most commonly used local anesthetics are proparacaine, 0.5%; benoxinate, 0.4%; and tetracaine, 0.5%. Topical anesthetics may be used before the removal of a conjunctival or corneal foreign body. They may be necessary to relieve the blepharospasm induced by a chemical injury before satisfactory irrigation and examination of the eye can be accomplished. They should never be prescribed for home use, since they might mask a serious ocular disorder or result in corneal ulceration.

Table 17–3. Combinations of anti-infective drugs.

Drugs	Trade Name
Bacitracin and polymyxin B	Ak-Poly-Bac, Polysporin
Bacitracin (gramicidin), neomycin, and polymyxin B[1]	Neosporin, many others
Oxytetracycline and polymyxin B	Terramycin-Polymyxin B
Neomycin and polymyxin B	Many
Trimethoprim sulfamethoxazole and polymyxin B sulfate	Polytrim

[1]Some commercial preparations utilize gramicidin in place of bacitracin.

Sterility of Topical Medication

Any ophthalmic medication may become contaminated. This is particularly true of solutions of fluorescein, which frequently become infected with *Pseudomonas aeruginosa*. It is well to discard all old ophthalmic solutions and any container whose tip has been touched by the examiner's hand or by the patient's eyelids. In the case of fluorescein, single-use disposable solution or impregnated filter paper strips should be employed.

Systemic Absorption of Topical Medication

Since absorption of topical eye medication into the circulation may occur in sufficient quantity to produce systemic side effects, the total dosage should be carefully considered. For example, each drop of 1% atropine contains 0.5 mg of atropine. If 1% atropine drops were instilled into each eye and total absorption occurred, a toxic reaction would result in children. Other drugs most likely to produce toxicity include scopolamine, cyclopentolate, echothiophate iodide, and 10% phenylephrine (the latter should never be used in infants and small children).

When medication is instilled into the eye of an infant, pressure should be exerted over the lacrimal sac for a minute or two to prevent the drug from reaching the nasal mucosa, where it could be absorbed. Alternatively, the head may be tipped temporally to the side of the treated eye so that the excess medication will run out of the outer corner of the eye.

Fraunfelder FT, Roy FH (editors): *Current Ocular Therapy,* 3rd ed. Saunders, 1990.

Palmer EA: How safe are ocular drugs in pediatrics? Ophthalmology 1986;93:1038.

Pavan-Langston D, Dunkel EC: *Handbook of Ocular Drug Therapy and Ocular Side Effects of Systemic Drugs.* Little, Brown, 1991.

OCULAR INJURIES

FOREIGN BODIES

Conjunctival Foreign Body

A conjunctival foreign body can usually be removed with a moist cotton applicator. A common site for foreign bodies is the furrow immediately behind the margin of the upper lid. Eversion of the upper lid, as described above, is necessary to visualize these foreign bodies.

Corneal Foreign Body

Superficial corneal foreign bodies usually can be removed without difficulty. A sterile topical anesthetic should be instilled into the eye and an attempt made to wipe away the foreign body with a moist cotton applicator. If this is not successful, a blunt spud or small, sterile, dull hypodermic needle (No. 20) can be used. Care must be taken not to injure the deeper layers of the cornea; if the foreign body is deeply embedded in the stroma, the patient should be referred to an ophthalmologist. Rust rings from foreign bodies should be removed primarily. An antibiotic ointment should be instilled, and the eye should be patched until epithelialization of the cornea has occurred. The patient should be reexamined within 24 hours to make certain that infection has not occurred.

Intraocular Foreign Body

Intraocular foreign bodies are serious injuries that may not be suspected on initial examination. The usual history is that the patient was pounding on a metallic object with a hammer when something flew up into the eye. Eye injuries caused by foreign bodies projected from power lawn tools are becoming more frequent. Examination may show a perforating wound of the cornea, a hole in the iris, an irregular or "peaked" pupil, and an opaque lens. However, the foreign body may be so small that little evidence of penetration is seen. X-rays of the eye may be necessary to rule out the possibility of foreign body. If there is any question of a foreign body, the patient should be referred to an ophthalmologist because removal of these foreign bodies is extremely difficult. The visual prognosis is guarded.

Benson WE: Intraocular foreign bodies. In: *Clinical Ophthalmology,* vol 5. Duane TD (editor). Harper & Row, 1989.

Catalano RA, Belin M: *Ocular Emergencies.* Saunders, 1992.

LaRoche GR, McIntyre L, Schertzer RM: Epidemiology of severe eye injuries in childhood. Ophthalmology 1988; 95:1603.

Nelson LB, Wilson TW, Jeffers JB: Eye injuries in childhood: Demography, etiology and prevention. Pediatrics 1989;84:438.

Roper-Hall MJ: *Eye Emergencies.* Churchill Livingstone, 1987.

INJURIES OF THE EYELIDS

Ecchymosis

Severe ecchymosis of the eyelids should be treated first with cold compresses to reduce hemorrhage and swelling. After 24–48 hours, hot packs will speed absorption of extravasated blood. It is important to rule out any concurrent injury to the globe.

Lacerations

Lacerations of the eyelids should be sutured primarily. When the laceration involves the lid margin, particularly the lower lid, it is imperative that the margins be sutured as evenly as possible to prevent development of a notch. In such cases, the patient should be referred to an ophthalmologist. Lacerations involving the medial portion of the eyelids should be examined to rule out injury to the lacrimal canaliculi. If the canaliculi are cut, they should be repaired at the time of primary closure of the lid laceration, since delayed attempts to repair cut canaliculi are less successful. Patients with deeper lacerations with presentation of fat or poor levator function should be referred.

Catalano RA, Belin M: *Ocular Emergencies.* Saunders, 1992.

Deutsch TA, Feller DB: *Paton & Goldberg's Management of Ocular Injuries,* 2nd ed. Saunders, 1985.

Reifler DM: Management of canalicular laceration. Surv Ophthalmol 1991;36:113.

Roper-Hall MJ *Eye Emergencies.* Churchill Livingstone, 1987.

CORNEAL INJURIES

Corneal Abrasions

Corneal abrasions usually produce severe discomfort. The diagnosis is made by instilling fluorescein into the eye and observing the cornea for staining.

Treatment consists of the instillation of a mild cycloplegic such as 5% homatropine or 1% cyclopentolate, the application of antibiotic ointments, and firm patching of the eye for 24–48 hours or until the epithelium has healed.

Corneal Lacerations

Patients with corneal lacerations should be referred to an ophthalmologist for primary suturing. The patient should be observed for the development of intraocular infection. Systemic antibiotics and tetanus toxoid are indicated if the perforation occurred with a contaminated object.

See references under Injuries of Eyelids, above.

HYPHEMA

Hyphema (blood in the anterior chamber) is a common contusion injury in children (Figure 17–5). It is a serious injury, often requiring hospitalization. Secondary bleeding may occur, usually within 6 days after the primary bleeding. Patients with hyphema should be examined for the development of glaucoma. Ophthalmoscopy should also be attempted to ascertain whether there has been more extensive injury to the posterior part of the eye. Black children with hyphema should be tested for sickle cell disease, because if the disease is present, they are more likely to develop complications.

Treatment consists of bed rest, eye bandages, and sedatives. Binocular bandages were commonly used in the past, but recent studies have suggested that bed rest and monocular patches are as effective as binocular patches in mild or moderate hyphemas. However, in severe hyphemas, binocular patches are preferred. No pupillary dilating (mydriatic) or pupillary constricting (miotic) drops should be used initially. Topical and systemic corticosteroids have been recommended to reduce associated inflammation, but they should be prescribed only by an ophthalmologist. If glaucoma develops, the use of carbonic an-

hydrase inhibitors, intravenous urea or mannitol, or oral glycerol is indicated initially. If this does not control the glaucoma, surgical removal of the blood clot by irrigation or with a cryoprobe or vitrectomy instrument is indicated. To reduce the incidence of rebleeding, some authors have recommended the use of systemic aminocaproic acid or tranexaminc acid for 5 days after the initial hemorrhage. Aspirin should be avoided since it increases the incidence of rebleeding.

Another complication of hyphema is blood staining of the cornea. This occurs only if the hemorrhage remains for a long period; it may occur whether or not glaucoma develops.

Agapitos PJ, Leon-Paul N, Clarke WN: Traumatic hyphema in children. Ophthalmology 1987;94:1238.

Catalano RA, Belin M: *Ocular Emergencies.* Saunders, 1992.

Deutsch TA, Feller DB: *Paton & Goldberg's Management of Ocular Injuries,* 2nd ed. Saunders, 1985.

Farber MD, Fiscella R, Goldberg MF: Aminocaproic acid versus prednisone for the treatment of traumatic hyphema: A randomized clinical trial. Ophthalmology 1991;98:279.

Uusitalo RJ, Ranta-Kemppainen L, Tarkkanen A: Management of traumatic hyphema in children: An analysis of 340 cases. Arch Ophthalmol 1988;106:1207.

BURNS

Burns of the eyelids should be treated like burns of the skin elsewhere. It is important to protect the eyeballs from infection and exposure. Since burns frequently become contaminated with *Pseudomonas* organisms that can produce severe corneal ulceration, an antibiotic preparation containing either colistin, gentamicin, tobramycin, or polymyxin B should be instilled into the eyes three or four times a day. As the burns begin to heal, cicatricial ectropion with corneal exposure may develop. To prevent corneal exposure, ointments should be applied inside the eyelids. Plastic surgery often is necessary to correct cicatricial ectropion.

Chemical burns of the cornea and conjunctiva should be treated initially with thorough irrigation with any clean nonirritating fluid. This may be tap water, saline or boric acid solution, or whatever is available. In no case should a delay occur because of attempts to obtain a particular irrigating solution. It may be necessary to instill topical anesthetics into the eye to relieve blepharospasm before irrigation can be accomplished. Adequacy of the irrigation can be judged by testing the conjunctival fluid for neutrality with pH test paper. After irrigation, the eye should be inspected for retained chemical particles, which can be removed with a moist cotton applicator. The extent of the damage is then determined. If the burn involves the cornea, the pupil should be dilated with 1% atro-

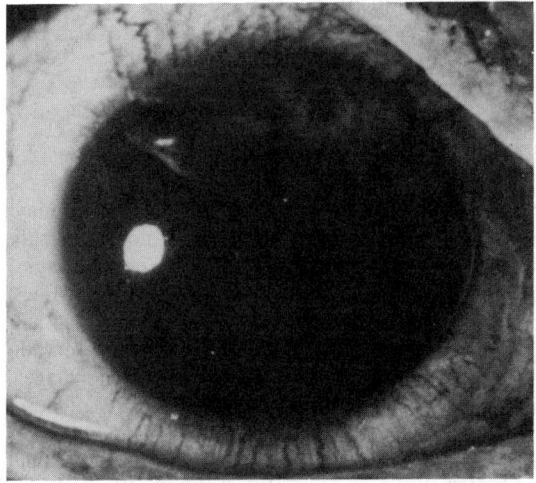

Figure 17–5. Hyphema (blood in anterior chamber).

pine or 5% homatropine after irrigation to provide comfort. An antibiotic ointment should be instilled and the eye patched. Any patient who has suffered a severe chemical burn of the eye should be hospitalized and should be seen by an ophthalmologist.

Ultraviolet burns of the cornea usually cause severe pain and tearing. There is a history of exposure to ultraviolet light (eg, a welder's arc, snow on the ski slopes, sunlamp or treatment lamp). Symptoms develop 10–12 hours after exposure. Examination shows superficial corneal edema and pinpoint areas that stain with fluorescein. Treatment consists of the application of a topical anesthetic every 5–10 minutes until the pain is relieved. After pain has subsided, an antibiotic or an antibiotic-corticosteroid ointment is instilled into the eye and the eye is patched. Systemic analgesics and sedatives are then prescribed. Recovery is usually prompt and complete within 48 hours. (*Note:* Topical anesthetics should never be sent home with the patient.)

Retinal burns with permanent loss of vision may occur as a result of exposure to strong infrared light, such as that received from observing an eclipse. If this condition is suspected, the patient should be referred to an ophthalmologist.

Catalano RA, Belin M: *Ocular Emergencies.* Saunders, 1992.

Guy RJ et al: Three-years' experience in a regional burn center with burns of the eyes and eyelids. Ophthalmic Surg 1982;13:383.

Pfister RR: Chemical injuries of the eye. Ophthalmology 1983;90:1246.

Spoor TC, Nesi FA (editors): *Management of Ocular, Orbital and Adnexal Trauma.* Raven Press, 1988.

FRACTURES OF THE ORBIT

Fractures of the orbit with any degree of displacement of the bones should be surgically reduced. The techniques of surgery depend upon the location and extent of the fracture. If the fractures are not satisfactorily reduced, complications occur that include displacement of the globe, enophthalmos, and diplopia. Any injury severe enough to cause an orbital fracture may cause further skull fractures and intracranial and intraocular damage. The patient should be studied for these possibilities.

Blowout fractures generally result from blunt injury such as a blow from a ball or fist. The bones of the orbital rim usually remain intact, but there is a blowout of the floor of the orbit (rarely, the medial wall of the orbit) with herniation of the orbital contents into the blowout site. Blowout fractures should be suspected if there is evidence of diplopia in any direction of gaze or if there is limitation of ocular movement, particularly upward. Hypesthesia of the skin in the distribution of the infraorbital nerve is present in about 30% of patients. Subcutaneous emphysema may be present. Weakness of ocular movement, particularly downward gaze, and enophthalmos may be present initially or develop later. Blowout fractures are not always seen on routine x-ray films of the orbit. CT scans are sometimes necessary to demonstrate this fracture. Surgical treatment is often required to release entrapped extraocular muscles.

Greenwald MJ et al: Orbital roof fractures in childhood. Ophthalmology 1989;96:491.

Linberg JV: *Oculoplastic and Orbital Emergencies.* Appleton & Lange, 1990.

Spoor TC, Nesi FA (editors): *Management of Ocular, Orbital and Adnexal Trauma.* Raven Press, 1988.

CONTUSIONS OF THE GLOBE

In addition to the hyphema mentioned above, contusions of the globe may result in dislocation of the lens, hemorrhage into the vitreous, retinal edema and hemorrhage, retinal detachment, choroidal hemorrhage, choroidal rupture, and rupture of the eyeball. The diagnosis of these conditions is based upon (1) changes in visual acuity and (2) direct observation with the ophthalmoscope and slit lamp. If the fundus can be visualized well and if visual acuity is good, there is little likelihood that any significant damage to the posterior part of the eye has occurred. However, complications such as retinal detachment or dislocation of the lens may not appear until weeks after the initial injury.

Cinotti AA: *Handbook of Ophthalmologic Emergencies,* 3rd ed. Medical Examination, 1985.

Eagling EM: Ocular damage after blunt trauma to the eye: Its relationship to the nature of the injury. Br J Ophthalmol 1974;58:126.

Linberg JV: *Oculoplastic and Orbital Emergencies.* Appleton & Lange, 1990.

Spoor TC, Nesi FA (editors): *Management of Ocular, Orbital and Adnexal Trauma.* Raven Press, 1988.

NONACCIDENTAL TRAUMA

A wide range of injuries to the eye and eyelids may occur in children who suffer from nonaccidental trauma (battered child syndrome, shaken baby syndrome, etc). Most common among these are lid ecchymoses, conjunctival hemorrhages, hyphema, and retinal hemorrhages. These last are often observed. The presence of unexplained retinal hemorrhages should alert the physician to the possibility of nonaccidental trauma. Careful ophthalmoscopic examination should be performed in all children suspected of suffering from nonaccidental trauma. Retinal and vitreal hemorrhages may persist long after the child has recovered from other injuries and may lead to the development of amblyopia.

Buys YM et al: Retinal findings after head trauma in infants and young children. Ophthalmology 1992;99:1718.

Han DP, Wilkinson WS: Late ophthalmic manifestations of the shaken baby syndrome. J Pediatr Ophthalmol Strabismus 1990;27:299.

Levin AV: Ocular manifestations of child abuse. Ophthalmol Clin North Am 1990;3:249.

Riffenburgh RS, Sathyavagiswaran L: Ocular findings at autopsy of child abuse victims. Ophthalmology 1991; 98:1519.

REFRACTIVE ERRORS

Myopia (nearsightedness) is easily diagnosed; distant objects are blurred. Near vision is not usually impaired except in very high myopia. Frequently, the patient squints in order to form a physiologic pinhole to improve visual acuity.

The diagnosis of **hyperopia (farsightedness)** in children is more difficult. Children are able to accommodate much more effectively than adults and thus overcome their hyperopia. Sometimes there are associated symptoms of eyestrain or headaches after prolonged periods of close work. Children with severe farsightedness may have internal deviations of the eyes (accommodative esotropia).

Astigmatism produces distorted vision. Children will attempt to overcome the blurry vision by squinting their eyes and forming a pinhole. Children with severe astigmatism may complain of eyestrain and headaches.

Anisometropia is a difference in refractive errors of the two eyes. Severe anisometropia may cause amblyopia.

Treatment of significant refractive errors consists of the proper fitting of glasses. Small degrees of hyperopia need not be corrected in children. Full correction of myopia is indicated. The use of bifocals in myopic children usually is ineffective in preventing the progressive type of myopia. Other forms of treatment such as the use of "eye exercises" or certain diets do not appear to influence the progression of myopia. Long-term use of atropine drops may reduce progression of myopia, but this therapy is impractical and not usually recommended. Amblyopia secondary to anisometropia should be treated with occlusion (patching) of the better seeing eye in addition to correction of the refractive error.

Contact lenses are seldom indicated in children. The exception is the child with unilateral aphakia (absence of the lens), severe anisometropia, corneal scarring producing an irregular astigmatism, or kerato-conus. Contact lenses have been purported to reduce the progression of myopia, but there is little evidence to support this view.

Abrahamsson M, Fabian G, Sjöstrand J: Refraction changes in children developing convergent or divergent strabismus. Br J Ophthalmol 1992;76:723.

Garcia GE: *Handbook of Refraction,* 4th ed. Little, Brown, 1989.

Michaels DD: *Basic Refraction Techniques.* Raven, 1988.

Stein HA, Slatt BJ, Stein RM: *Fitting Guide for Rigid and Soft Contact Lenses,* 3rd ed. Mosby, 1990.

STRABISMUS
(Squint)

Approximately 5% of children have strabismus. The eyes may deviate inward (esotropia), outward (exotropia), upward (hypertropia), or downward (hypotropia). Strabismus is comitant if the same degree of deviation exists in all fields of gaze and noncomitant if the angle of deviation changes in the various directions of gaze. The terms tropia and phoria are both used to describe abnormal positions of the eye; tropias are manifest deviations, which are present all of the time, whereas phorias are latent, intermittent deviations that become manifest only if fusion or binocular vision is blocked.

Nonparalytic strabismus is usually first observed either shortly after birth or at the age of 2–3 years; rarely, the onset is at a later age. Infants do not develop coordinated eye muscle movements until about 3–5 months of age. Infants often are observed to have temporary deviation of the eyes, followed by subsequent realignment. Any child who has a constant deviation that persists for several weeks or who develops a constant deviation after the age of 6 months should be investigated for the cause of the strabismus. There is often a family history of strabismus, but well-defined inheritance patterns are unusual. Strabismus is more common in prematurely born children and in developmentally disabled children with cerebral palsy.

The diagnosis of strabismus is frequently made by simple inspection. If the eyes are deviated considerably, the diagnosis is evident. If there is only a slight deviation or if there is a questionable deviation because of wide epicanthal folds (pseudostrabismus) with more of the white of the eye being exposed temporally than nasally, the diagnosis is established by the corneal light reflection technique (Figure 17–3) or the cover test (Figure 17–4), as described above. Strabismus may also be suspected on the basis of marked reduced visual acuity in one eye. Children with a persistent head tilt or face turn may have strabismus with very little apparent displacement of the eyes.

During visual development, diplopia occurs if alignment of the eyes is such that the object viewed does not fall on corresponding parts of the two retinas. To avoid diplopia, the child learns to suppress the vision in the deviating eye. If one eye continually deviates, then suppression is always in this eye, with the result that macular vision never develops. This condition is called **amblyopia ex anopsia** or **suppression amblyopia.** Visual screening examination of preschool children is important in diagnosing early suppression amblyopia.

Paralytic or noncomitant strabismus may result from central nervous system diseases or anatomic maldevelopments of the ocular muscles. The sudden onset of paralytic strabismus in any child should prompt examination for central nervous system disease.

Treatment

Children do not outgrow strabismus. Early treatment is important and should be given by an ophthalmologist. Treatment is directed toward the development of good visual acuity in each eye, realignment of the eyes in good cosmetic position, and functional cures with the establishment of binocular vision. The following steps are considered in the treatment of strabismus: (1) careful ophthalmoscopic examination to rule out an organic intraocular cause for the deviation, eg, congenital cataracts, tumors, optic nerve atrophy; (2) cycloplegic refraction and prescription of lenses; (3) occlusion of the good eye to develop macular vision in the bad eye; and (4) surgery to align the eyes if glasses are unsuccessful in correcting the deviation. Glasses may be required after surgical treatment.

Early surgery (ages 4–24 months) with alignment of the eyes is more likely to result in a functional cure than surgery performed at age 4–5 years or later.

Orthoptic exercises are of value in establishing binocular vision if the visual axes are nearly aligned. They are also of value in certain forms of intermittent strabismus, especially convergence insufficiency.

Archer SM, Sondhi N, Helveston EM: Strabismus in infancy. Ophthalmology 1989;96:133.

DelMonte MA, Archer SM: *Atlas of Pediatric Ophthalmology and Strabisumus Surgery.* Churchill Livingstone, 1993.

Helveston EM et al: Early surgery for essential infantile esotropia. J Pediatr Ophthalmol Strabismus 1990;27:115.

Nelson LB et al: Congenital esotropia. Surv Ophthalmol 1987;31:363.

Reinecke RD, Parks MM: *Strabismus: A Programmed Text,* 3rd ed. Appleton & Lange, 1987.

von Noorden GK: *Burian-von Noorden's Binocular Vision and Ocular Motility,* 4th ed. Mosby, 1990.

PTOSIS

Ptosis is a drooping of the upper eyelid. It may be congenital or acquired and unilateral or bilateral. Ptosis may be associated with anisometropia.

Congenital ptosis usually results from incomplete development of the levator muscle. Occasionally, it is associated with third cranial nerve trauma at the time of birth or congenitally misdirected third cranial nerve fibers, in which case other abnormalities of ocular movement are often present.

Acquired ptosis may be traumatic in origin, may follow inflammation or scarring of the eyelids, or may present as a sign of some neurologic disorder. When ptosis is a sign of myasthenia gravis, an injection of edrophonium chloride will produce prompt improvement. (See discussion of myasthenia gravis in Chapter 25.)

The treatment of congenital ptosis is surgical. The operation is usually performed at the age of 3–4 years. Rarely, the surgery should be done earlier if the eyelid covers the pupil completely and prevents development of normal vision. Unequal refractive errors between eyes may be associated with ptosis. The treatment of acquired ptosis depends upon the origin, but primary consideration should be directed toward treating any underlying disease.

Crawford JS, Iliff CE, Stasior OG: Symposium on congenital ptosis. J Pediatr Ophthalmol Strabismus 1982;19:245.

Hornblass A (editor): *Oculoplastic Orbital and Reconstructive Surgery,* vol 1: *Eyelids.* Williams & Wilkins, 1988.

Saunders RA, Grice CM: Early correction of severe congenital ptosis. J Pediatr Ophthalmol Strabismus 1991;28:271.

GLAUCOMA

Primary Glaucoma

Primary congenital glaucoma (hydrophthalmos) is due to an abnormal development of the aqueous drainage structures; it may be present at birth or may develop within the first 2 years of life. Diagnosis is based upon (1) enlarged corneas that are frequently edematous and show linear white opacities (breaks in Descemet's membrane; see Figure 17–6), (2) symptoms of photophobia and tearing, (3) increased intraocular pressure, and (4) enlarged cupping of the optic disk. Because the coats of the eye of an infant are not as rigid as those of an adult, increased in-

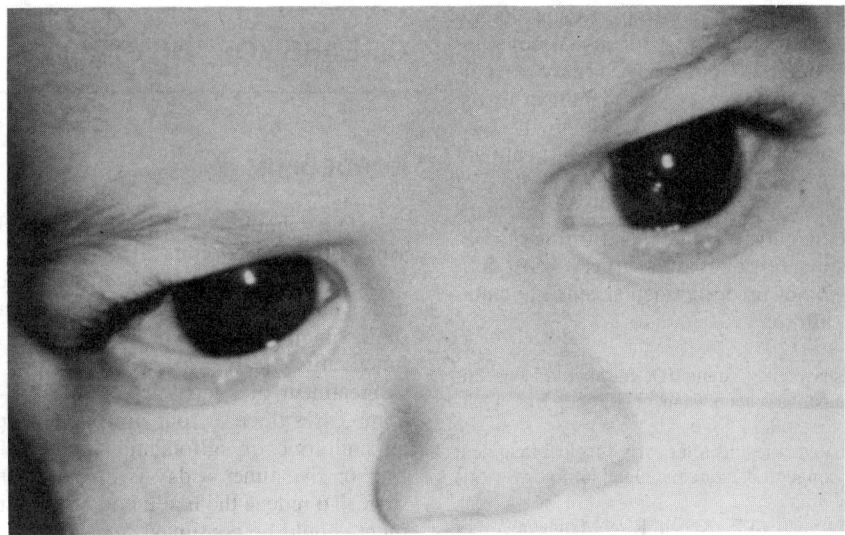

Figure 17–6. Congenital glaucoma. Enlarged, hazy corneas are present. (Reproduced, with permission, from Eichenwald HF, Stroder J [editors]: *Current Therapy in Pediatrics–2.* BC Decker, 1989.)

traocular pressure results in stretching of the corneal and scleral tissues.

Early surgery is essential. Medical therapy is of little value. Surgery is successful in controlling intraocular pressure in about 75% of cases. Without treatment, permanent blindness occurs at an early age.

Glaucoma may be associated with other developmental anomalies. These include aniridia, posterior embryotoxon (failure of reabsorption of the mesodermal tissue in the periphery of the iris and drainage angle), Sturge-Weber disease, Lowe's syndrome, Marfan's syndrome, Hurler's syndrome, Pierre Robin syndrome, Rubinstein-Taybi syndrome, neurofibromatosis, homocystinuria, congenital rubella syndrome, and trisomy 13 (D) or 18 (E_1).

Secondary Glaucoma

Secondary glaucoma may be due to many causes. The mechanism of this type of glaucoma is usually an obstruction of the aqueous outflow channels. The various causes include lens dislocation, hemorrhage into the eye, iritis, tumors (including retinoblastoma), retinopathy of prematurity, and xanthogranulomas in the iris. Treatment of these conditions is complicated, and the patient should be referred to an ophthalmologist.

Epstein DL (editor): *Chandler & Grant's Glaucoma,* 3rd ed. Lea & Febiger, 1986.

Goethals M, Missotten L: Intraocular pressure in children up to five years of age. J Pediatr Ophthalmol Strabismus 1983; 20:49.

Hoskins HD Jr, Kass M: *Becker-Shaffer's Diagnosis and Therapy of the Glaucomas,* 6th ed. Mosby, 1989.

Lewis TL, Fingeret M (editors): *Primary Care of the Glaucomas.* Appleton & Lange, 1993.

Ritch R, Shields MB, Krupin T (editors): *The Glaucomas,* vol 2. Mosby, 1989.

CATARACTS

A cataract is an opacity of the lens; it consists of precipitated lens protein. Cataracts may be unilateral or bilateral and partial or complete; considerable variation exists in the extent, position, shape, and density of cataract formation. They may be congenital and associated with other congenital anomalies. They can occur as a result of maternal rubella during the first trimester of pregnancy. Cataracts may be secondary to ocular trauma or associated with systemic diseases such as diabetes mellitus, galactosemia, atopic dermatitis, Marfan's syndrome, or Down's syndrome. They may also be due to long-term systemic corticosteroid therapy.

The symptoms vary considerably according to location and extent. Vision may be affected very slightly, or considerable reduction in vision can occur. White spots may be observed in the pupil. In a few cases, strabismus or pendular nystagmus is present.

The diagnosis is made by inspection with a flashlight or by examination with an ophthalmoscope or slit lamp. In some cases, cataracts can be observed only when the pupils are dilated.

Surgical lens extraction (within the first few weeks of life) is indicated if the cataracts are sufficiently dense so that vision cannot develop. If cataracts are not dense enough to interfere with visual development, surgery should be deferred. Surgery is indicated when visual loss is a serious handicap to the child.

In the past, the visual results of surgical treatment of unilateral congenital cataracts were poor. The prognosis for vision has improved with early surgery (as soon as the diagnosis is made) and fitting of contact lenses within a few days after surgery. Most ophthalmologists do not favor intraocular lens implantation in young children.

Burke JP, Willshaw HE, Young JD: Intraocular lens implants for uniocular cataracts in childhood. Br J Ophthalmol 1989;73:860.

Cheng KP et al: Visual results after early surgical treatment of unilateral congenital cataracts. Ophthalmology 1991; 98:903.

Drummond GT, Scott WE, Keech RV: Management of monocular congenital cataracts. Arch Ophthalmol 1989; 107:45.

Hing S, Speedwell L, Taylor D: Lens surgery in infancy and childhood. Br J Ophthalmol 1990;74:73.

Jaffe MS, Jaffe GF: *Cataract Surgery: Its Complications,* 5th ed. Mosby, 1990.

Lewis TL et al: Vision in the "good" eye of children treated for unilateral congenital cataract. Ophthalmology 1992; 99:1013.

Parks MM, Johnson DA, Reed GW: Long-term visual results and complications in children with aphakia. Ophthalmology 1993;100:826.

DISLOCATED LENS

Dislocation (luxation) or partial dislocation (subluxation) of the lens may result from blunt trauma to the eye and orbit. It may also be observed in patients with genetic dwarfism, scleroderma, Rieger's syndrome, and other hereditary disorders, including Marfan's syndrome and Marchesani's syndrome (with the lens usually dislocated superiorly) and homocystinuria (lens usually dislocated inferiorly).

Glaucoma is a common complication of dislocated lenses. All children with dislocated lenses should be evaluated by an ophthalmologist.

Isenberg SJ (editor): *The Eye in Infancy.* Year Book, 1989.

Nelson LB, Maumenee IH: Ectopia lentis. Surv Ophthalmol 1982;27:143.

Plager DA et al: Surgical treatment of subluxated lenses in children. Ophthalmology 1992;99:1018.

DISEASES OF THE EYELIDS

HORDEOLUM

External hordeolum (sty) is a staphylococcal abscess of the sebaceous glands of the lid margin. Symptoms consist of localized tenderness, redness, and swelling. Internal hordeolum is an acute infection of the meibomian glands that usually points conjunctivally.

Treatment of both types consists of warm moist compresses three or four times a day. Instillation of an antibiotic or sulfonamide ophthalmic ointment four or five times a day is useful during the acute stage. To reduce the likelihood of a recurrence, treatment should be continued for several days after the lesion has subsided.

Spontaneous rupture frequently occurs, but if it does not, the lesion should be incised when it becomes large and pointed. The removal of an eyelash may promote drainage of an external hordeolum.

Ostler HB, Ostler MW: *Disease of the External Eye and Adnexa: A text and Atlas.* Williams & Wilkins, 1993.

CHALAZION

Chalazion is a granulomatous inflammation of the meibomian glands. The cause is not known. Symptoms consist of slight discomfort in the eyelid and a slight redness and a lump on the conjunctival surface of the lid overlying the involved meibomian gland. Local excision is often necessary, but chalazia may disappear after treatment with warm moist compresses. Corticosteroid injection into the chalazion is often effective.

Epstein GA, Putterman AM: Combined excision and drainage with intralesional corticosteroid injection in the treatment of chronic chalazia Arch Ophthalmol 1988;106: 514.

Ostler HB, Ostler MW: *Disease of the External Eye and Adnexa: A text and Atlas.* Williams & Wilkins, 1993.

BLEPHARITIS
(Granulated Eyelids)

Chronic inflammation of the lid margins may be seborrheic (nonulcerative), staphylococcal (ulcerative), or a combination of the two types. Symptoms are redness, burning, itching, and crusting of the lid margins. In the staphylococcal type, the scales are dry; small ulcerative lesions of the skin are observed; and the eyelashes may fall out. In the seborrheic type, the scales are oily; seborrhea of the scalp is usually present as well. Blepharitis is especially common in children with Down's syndrome and eczema.

Treatment of staphylococcal blepharitis consists of the instillation of antibiotic or sulfonamide ophthalmic ointment into the eye twice a day. Treatment should be continued for a week or so after all symptoms have disappeared. The crusts on the lids should be gently removed with a moist cotton applicator or warm compresses before the ointment is instilled. Occasionally, systemic antibiotics are required in severe cases of staphylococcal blepharitis.

The treatment of seborrheic blepharitis consists of controlling scalp seborrhea if it exists, removing the scales along the lid margins with a moist cotton applicator, and instilling sulfacetamide or an antistaphylococcal antibiotic ophthalmic ointment.

Seborrheic blepharitis can often be controlled by scrubbing the margin of the eyelids twice a day with a cotton applicator moistened in a bland, half-strength baby shampoo that does not irritate the eye.

Haesaert SP: *Clinical Manual of Ocular Microbiology and Cytology.* Mosby, 1993.
Tabbara KF, Hyndiuk RA (editors): *Infections of the Eye.* Little, Brown, 1986.

DISEASES OF THE CONJUNCTIVA

CONJUNCTIVITIS

Conjunctivitis is the most common of all pediatric ocular disorders. It is usually due to bacterial, viral, or fungal infections. Less commonly, it may result from an allergic reaction or physical or chemical irritation.

Symptoms consist of redness of the conjunctiva, foreign body sensation, a mucoid or purulent discharge, and sticking together of the eyelids in the morning. (See Table 17–4.) Vision is not affected. The cornea, anterior chamber, and intraocular pressure are normal.

Bacterial Conjunctivitis

The most common causes of bacterial conjunctivitis are the pneumococci, *Staphylococcus aureus, Haemophilus influenzae,* and β-hemolytic streptococci. There may be associated bacterial infections elsewhere in the body. Conjunctival membranes (diphtheritic conjunctivitis) or pseudomembranes (streptococcal conjunctivitis) may be present. Discharge, usually a prominent feature of bacterial conjunctivitis, is purulent or mucopurulent in character.

The causative organism should be identified, if possible, by obtaining smears and cultures. Empiric treatment with broad-spectrum antibiotics or sulfonamide ophthalmic drops or ointments instilled into the eye four to six times a day usually results in improvement within 48–72 hours. Treatment should be continued for 7–10 days. If improvement does not occur, it is important to make an etiologic diagnosis if this has not been done earlier. Bacterial conjunctivitis is usually a self-limited disease, but secondary corneal infection and ulceration occur rarely.

Inclusion Conjunctivitis

This disease is caused by the same chlamydial organism that produces inclusion conjunctivitis in the newborn. It is characterized by conjunctival redness, clear or mucoid discharge, and follicles in the lower palpebral conjunctiva. Treatment consists of the systemic administration of a tetracycline (but not to infants or young children) or erythromycin. Topical application of these drugs is not as effective as systemic treatment.

Chlamydial infection should be considered in any

Table 17–4. Clinical and laboratory features of conjunctivitis.[1]

	Viral	Bacterial	Chlamydial	Allergic
Itching	Minimal	Minimal	Minimal	Severe
Hyperemia	Generalized	Generalized	Generalized	Generalized
Tearing	Profuse	Moderate	Moderate	Moderate
Exudation	Minimal, mucoid	Profuse, purulent	Profuse, mucoid or mucopurulent	Minimal, slight mucus
Preauricular adenopathy	Common	Uncommon	Common only in inclusion conjunctivitis	None
Stained conjunctival smears and scrapings	Lymphocytes, plasma cells, multinucleated giant cells, eosinophilic intranuclear inclusions	Neutrophils, bacteria	Neutrophils, plasma cells, basophilic intracytoplasmic inclusions	Eosinophils
Associated sore throat and fever	Occasionally	Occassionally	Never	Never

[1]Modified from Vaughan D, Asbury T, Riordan-Eva P: *General Ophthalmology,* 13th ed. Appleton & Lange, 1992.

sexually active teenager with chronic conjunctivitis. Examination and treatment of the sexual partner should be undertaken.

Trachoma

Trachoma is infection of the conjunctiva with a bacterium of the genus *Chlamydia*. The disease is usually associated with poor hygiene and poor economic conditions. It is a major cause of blindness in the world but is rare in the USA except among Native Americans.

In the early stages, trachoma is characterized by a catarrhal type of reaction with diffuse redness, mild irritation, and a thin watery discharge. Subsequently, the conjunctiva becomes thickened, with papillary hypertrophy and formation of follicles, particularly in the tarsal region of the upper lids. Scarring of the conjunctiva develops later, and there is corneal vascularization and opacification.

Local therapy can probably control trachoma adequately, but systemic therapy is usually recommended also. Systemic sulfonamides, tetracyclines, and erythromycin are the agents most commonly used. For children over 9 years of age in whom dentition is complete, a 3- to 4-week course of oral tetracycline is given. Doxycycline is preferred, since administration is required only once a day. For children under age 9, the drug of choice is sulfisoxazole, 100 mg/kg/d orally in four divided doses for 1 week, followed by 60 mg/kg/d for an additional 2 weeks. It is sometimes necessary to repeat this treatment after 1 week without medication. Alternatively, a 3- to 4-week course of oral erythromycin may be given. The local treatment of choice is 1% tetracycline ointment applied twice a day, 6 days a week for 10 weeks. Since recurrences are common, follow-up evaluation is important.

Viral Conjunctivitis

Viral conjunctivitis is frequently due to infection with adenovirus type 3, 4, or 7 and may be associated with pharyngitis and preauricular adenopathy. The conjunctiva is quite hyperemic and shows follicular reaction. There is a thin watery discharge. The condition usually lasts 12–14 days. No treatment is of value. Sulfonamide preparations or broad-spectrum antibiotics are instilled locally to prevent secondary bacterial infection.

Epidemic keratoconjunctivitis is highly contagious, is usually due to infection with adenovirus type 8 or 19, and is often spread by the fingers of physicians during their examination of the eye or through contaminated instruments or eye drops. Conjunctivitis is followed in 5–14 days by photophobia and epithelial keratitis. Corneal subepithelial opacities may persist for months but will eventually fade without sequelae. While corticosteroids may relieve acute symptoms, their use should be avoided because of their many potential complications.

Measles conjunctivitis is characterized by a catarrhal reaction with mucopurulent discharge and, frequently, a swelling of the semilunar fold. Measles conjunctivitis may precede the skin eruption. If a secondary infection is present, it should be treated with antibiotics; otherwise, no specific treatment is indicated, because the disease is self-limited. Varicella-zoster conjunctivitis is characterized by vesicular lesions of the lids and lid margins and a hyperemia and infiltrative reaction of the conjunctiva. Preauricular lymph nodes are frequently present; secondary corneal involvement may occur.

Allergic Conjunctivitis

Allergic conjunctivitis produces symptoms of itching, lacrimation, mild redness, and a stringy mucoid discharge. Eosinophils may be seen on scrapings from the conjunctiva. For acute cases of conjunctivitis, use of topical weak ophthalmic corticosteroid drops (eg, 0.125% prednisolone) instilled five or six times a day or use of 1.5% hydrocortisone ophthalmic ointment or its equivalent instilled three or four times a day is quite effective. Topical corticosteroid therapy should not be continued beyond a few days unless supervised by an ophthalmologist. For chronic forms of allergic conjunctivitis, an attempt should be made to isolate the offending allergen and to eliminate contact with it. Desensitization to the allergen can be carried out if elimination of contact is not possible. Symptomatic relief may be obtained with the use of topical ophthalmic solutions containing vasoconstricting agents and antihistamines. Ophthalmic sodium cromolyn 4% and systemic antihistamines also are helpful.

Phlyctenular Keratoconjunctivitis

Phlyctenular keratoconjunctivitis appears as elevated clear nodules, situated near the limbus, with surrounding hyperemia. The disease has been associated with a hypersensitivity reaction to tuberculin; phlyctenules may also develop as a hypersensitivity reaction to other bacterial products or other antigens.

Treatment consists of the local application of corticosteroids. Systemic tuberculosis should be ruled out.

Vernal Conjunctivitis

This form of conjunctivitis is seen in patients ages 5–20. It tends to be seasonal and becomes less severe with age. Symptoms consist of lacrimation, itching, stringy discharge, and giant "cobblestone" papillary hypertrophy in the tarsal conjunctiva or grayish elevated areas at the limbus. (See Figure 17–7.) Many eosinophils are seen in the scraping of the lesions.

Treatment consists of the local application of corticosteroid ointment or drops several times a day. Topical solutions of 4% cromolyn sodium applied several times a day often provide relief from symptoms and may reduce the need for topical corticosteroids. Se-

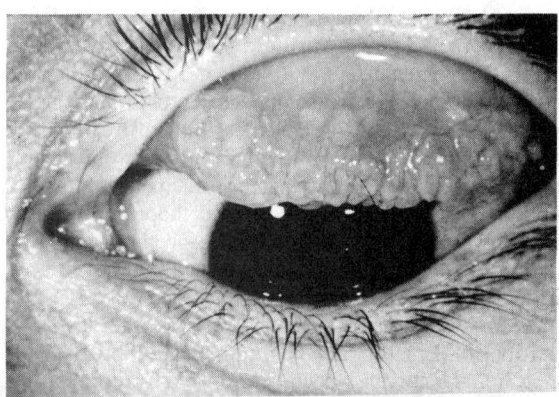

Figure 17–7. Vernal conjunctivitis. "Cobblestone" papillae in superior tarsal conjunctiva. (Courtesy of P Thygeson.) In: Vaughan D, Asbury T, Riordan-Eva P: *General Ophthalmology,* 13th ed. Appleton & Lange, 1992.)

vere cases may require more extensive therapy, but this should be conducted by an ophthalmologist.

Kawasaki Disease

Mucocutaneous lymph node syndrome (Kawasaki disease) is a disease of unknown cause that has conjunctivitis as one of its diagnostic features (see p 569). The conjunctivitis is usually not severe, and no other ocular findings have been described. Treatment is supportive only.

Ophthalmia Neonatorum

Ophthalmia neonatorum is inflammation of the conjunctiva of the newborn. It may be due to bacterial (gonococcal, staphylococcal, pneumococcal), chlamydial, or herpes simplex infections or to chemical irritation (silver nitrate). Bacterial conjunctivitis appears 2–5 days after birth; chlamydial conjunctivitis appears 5–10 days after birth. Herpes simplex conjunctivitis may be present within 2 weeks of birth. Conjunctivitis associated with silver nitrate usually is evident within the first 24–48 hours after birth. A definite diagnosis is established by smears and cultures of the material taken from the conjunctiva. Conjunctivitis due to silver nitrate is sterile, although secondary bacterial infections may occur.

Chlamydia is the most common cause of infectious neonatal conjunctivitis. Almost 50% of infants born to mothers with chlamydial cervicitis develop neonatal conjunctivitis. Because pneumonitis, otitis media, and vulvovaginitis often follow the conjunctivitis, systemic antibiotic treatment is necessary.

In most states in the USA, chemical (1% silver nitrate) or antibiotic prophylaxis of the newborn eye is required. These laws are highly variable in the different states. Various antibiotics such as erythromycin, tetracyclines, or bacitracin are currently used for prophylaxis of ophthalmia neonatorum.

It is most important to treat gonococcal conjunctivitis vigorously because corneal ulceration and perforation can occur in untreated or inadequately treated cases. Topical antibiotic therapy is unnecessary when systemic antibiotic therapy is given. However, normal saline may be used to irrigate the purulent discharge from the conjunctiva. The treatment of gonococcal conjunctivitis consists of administering penicillin 100,000 units/kg/d intravenously in two to four divided doses for 7 days. Penicillinase-producing strains should be treated with parenteral ceftriaxone, 25–50 mg/kg/d for 7 days, or cefotaxime, 25 mg/kg parenterally every 12 hours. Disseminated gonococcal infection should be excluded.

Other types of bacterial conjunctivitis of the newborn should be treated by the instillation of appropriate antibiotic ointments four times a day. Chlamydial conjunctivitis should be treated with erythromycin syrup, 50 mg/kg/d orally in four divided doses for 14 days. Herpes simplex infections should be treated with 1% trifluridine drops every 2 hours for 7 days in addition to intravenous acyclovir. Systemic herpes simplex must be ruled out.

In all cases of conjunctivitis, treatment should be continued for a few days after the symptoms have subsided; this will prevent early recurrences.

Abelson MB et al: Effects of Vasocon-A in the allergen challenge model of acute allergic conjunctivitis. Arch Ophthalmol 1990;108:520.

Foster CS: The Cromolyn Sodium Collaborative Study Group: Evaluation of topical cromolyn sodium in the treatment of vernal conjunctivitis. Ophthalmology 1988; 95:194.

Haesaert SP: *Clinical Manual of Ocular Microbiology and Cytology.* Mosby, 1993.

Hammerschlag MR et al: Efficacy of neonatal ocular prophylaxis for the prevention of chlamydial and gonococcal conjunctivitis. N Eng J Med 1989;320:769.

Isenberg SJ et al: Source of the conjunctival flora at birth and implications for ophthalmia neonatorum prophylaxis. Am J Ophthalmol 1988;106:458.

Leibowitz HM: Antibacterial effectiveness of ciprofloxacin 0.3% ophthalmic solution in the treatment of bacterial conjunctivitis. Am J Ophthalmol 1991;112:295.

Sandström I: Treatment of neonatal conjunctivitis. Arch Ophthalmol 1987;105:925.

MUCOCUTANEOUS DISEASES

Conjunctival lesions may be associated with mucocutaneous diseases, including erythema multiforme, Stevens-Johnson syndrome, Reiter's syndrome, Behçet's syndrome, and mucocutaneous lymph node syndrome (Kawasaki disease). The conjunctival involvement consists of erythema, vesicular lesions that frequently rupture, membrane formation, and the development of symblepharon (adhesion) between the raw edges of the bulbar and palpebral conjunctivae.

Goblet cells in the conjunctiva are destroyed in the cicatricial process. This decreases the mucus secretion that is essential for the spread of tears over the cornea. Keratitis sicca (corneal drying) may result.

Treatment of the conjunctival lesions associated with these conditions is symptomatic, ie, soothing eye drops and compresses. Topical corticosteroids are helpful in the acute stages in diminishing the intensity and complications of the acute inflammatory phase. Antibiotics are of no benefit except for prevention of secondary infection. Erythema multiforme and Stevens-Johnson disease may be precipitated by sulfonamide and antibiotic therapy. Topical antibiotic therapy may be used when secondary bacterial infection occurs; care must be taken to choose an antibiotic to which the patient is not sensitive. The use of topical lubricants and the application of soft contact lenses may prevent corneal drying and ulceration and the formation of conjunctival adhesions.

Friedlaender MH: *Allergy and Immunology of the Eye,* 2nd ed. Raven, 1993.
Gold DH, Weingeist TA (editors): *The Eye in Systemic Disease.* Lippincott, 1990.

DISEASES OF THE CORNEA

CORNEAL ULCERS

Corneal ulcers are serious ocular disorders, and ophthalmologic consultation always should be obtained. They may follow corneal injury or conjunctivitis or may be associated with systemic infections. Corneal ulcers are usually diagnosed by simple inspection. There is loss of anterior substance of the cornea, with surrounding opaque gray or white necrosis. Corneal ulcers may be peripheral or central. Several ulcers may be present in the same eye. The area of ulceration stains with fluorescein. A serious effort should be made to determine the etiology of any corneal ulcer. Cultures and scrapings should be taken, and sensitivity tests should be performed if bacterial organisms are found.

Bacterial Corneal Ulcers

Central bacterial corneal ulcers are due to infections with pneumococci, hemolytic streptococci, *P aeruginosa,* and, less commonly, gram-positive and other gram-negative rods. Marginal corneal ulcers may develop as a result of bacterial hypersensitivity reactions, most commonly to staphylococcal infections.

After material is obtained for cultures, treatment should be started immediately, before sensitivity tests

are completed. Subsequently, the antibiotic can be changed if necessary. For mild superficial bacterial ulcers, the topical use of antibiotic drops or ointment at frequent intervals is usually satisfactory. Until the susceptibility of the organism is known, treatment can be started with an ophthalmic antibiotic preparation that includes neomycin, bacitracin, and polymyxin B or a combination of trimethoprim sulfate and polymyxin B, or with a broad-spectrum antibiotic. Cycloplegic drops should be used to relieve the iridocyclitis that accompanies bacterial ulcers. In more severe corneal ulcers that involve the deeper portions of the stroma, more intensive antibiotic therapy should be given. Specially prepared fortified topical antibiotic solutions such as cefazolin or cefamandole (50 mg/mL) and gentamicin or tobramycin (10–20 mg/mL) are administered alternately every 30–60 minutes. Corticosteroids should not be given topically in these cases, since they interfere with the healing process and might exaggerate an infection that is not susceptible to the antibiotic treatment.

Marginal corneal ulcers respond to topical corticosteroids. If a staphylococcal infection of the conjunctiva or eyelid is present, it should be treated with appropriate antibiotics.

Viral Corneal Ulcers

A. Herpes Simplex Ulcer (Dendritic): Herpes simplex keratitis is becoming more common in children. Frequently it presents as a unilateral red eye with a preauricular lymph node. Lesions in the cornea may or may not be associated with herpes labialis. Corneal involvement is frequently precipitated by the topical application of corticosteroids and less commonly with the systemic use of corticosteroids. In the initial infection, the lesion has the appearance of a dendrite (Figure 17–8) that may be easily identified after the instillation of fluorescein. There are one or more branching vesicular lesions involving the anterior part of the cornea. These vesicles rupture. Subsequently, deeper involvement of the cornea may occur. Iritis may also develop as a complication.

Treatment of acute herpes infection of the cornea consists of topical application of antiviral medication: trifluridine, idoxuridine, or vidarabine. Trifluridine is applied in 1% solution (Viroptic) every 2 hours up to nine times a day. Idoxuridine is applied in 0.5% ointment (Stoxil) four times a day or in 0.1% solution (Herplex, Stoxil) hourly during the day and every 2 hours at night. Vidarabine in 3% ointment (Vira-A) is applied five times a day. Acyclovir in 3% ointment is effective, but no commercial preparation for ophthalmic use is available in the USA.

Mechanical denuding of the infected corneal epithelium is also an effective method of treating fresh cases of superficial herpes simplex keratitis. This procedure should be performed by an ophthalmologist. Deeper involvement of the cornea may represent a hypersensitivity reaction, and the use of topical cor-

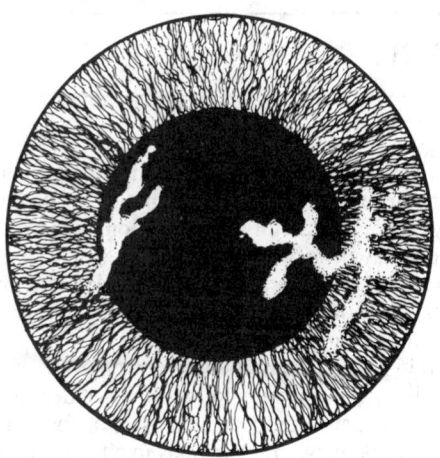

Figure 17–8. Dendritic type of lesion seen in herpes simplex keratitis. (Reproduced, with permission, from Vaughan D, Asbury T: *General Ophthalmology,* 8th ed. Lange, 1977.)

ticosteroids in conjunction with an antiviral medication sometimes improves the condition. Because the use of corticosteroids in an active herpes infection can lead to rapid deterioration of the cornea, this treatment should be conducted only by an ophthalmologist.

B. Herpes Zoster Infection: Herpes zoster keratitis is associated with zoster infection of the first branch of the trigeminal nerve. Corneal involvement may be superficial or deep and accompanied by uveitis. Topical and systemic acyclovir are often effective. Topical corticosteroids are used for the management of deep corneal involvement with uveitis. Relief is obtained with the use of topical corticosteroids. Cycloplegic drops should be used for relieving the iridocyclitis that accompanies herpes zoster infection. The physician must be certain of the diagnosis of herpes zoster before employing topical corticosteroids, since other viral diseases of the cornea are aggravated by these agents.

Cobo LM et al: Oral acyclovir in the treatment of acute herpes zoster ophthalmicus. Ophthalmology 1986;93: 763.

Cruz OA et al: Microbial keratitis in children. Ophthalmology 1993;100:192.

Kaufman HE: Update on antiviral agents. Ophthalmology 1985;92:533.

Leibowitz HM: *Corneal Disorders: Clinical Diagnosis and Management.* Saunders, 1984.

Leibowitz HM: Clinical evaluation of ciprofloxacin 0.3% ophthalmic solution for treatment of bacterial keratitis. Am J Ophthalmol 1991;112:34S.

Ostler HB, Ostler MW: *Disease of the External Eye and Adnexa: A text and Atlas.* Williams & Wilkins, 1993

Smolin G, Thoft RA (editors): The Cornea: Scientific Foundations and Clinical Practice, 2nd ed. Little Brown, 1987.

ALLERGIC REACTIONS

Allergic reactions in the cornea may involve either the superficial epithelial or deeper stromal layers. Most forms of deep keratitis probably represent hypersensitivity reactions. The allergen may be airborne, or it may enter the cornea by way of the circulation in the limbus. Treatment consists of determining the offending agent, if possible, and then eliminating its contact with the patient. Topical corticosteroids usually are required. They should be used only under the supervision of an ophthalmologist.

Interstitial Keratitis

Interstitial keratitis is an acute immune reaction in the cornea, usually associated with congenital syphilis. Symptoms consist of intense photophobia, tearing, pain, and decreased vision. On examination, the cornea has a diffuse opaque appearance. Fine vessels may be noted in the stroma. There may be aggregates of these vessels, which appear as orange-red areas (salmon patches). Other evidence of congenital syphilis may also be present. Serologic tests are often negative.

Interstitial keratitis may be associated with other diseases such as tuberculosis and the autoimmune disorders, and any such contributing condition should be ruled out.

Treatment consists of the use of topical corticosteroids and cycloplegics for relief of symptoms. If active syphilis is present, it should be appropriately treated.

Friedlaender MH: *Allergy and Immunology of the Eye,* 2nd ed. Raven, 1993.

Grayson M: *Diseases of the Cornea,* 2nd ed. Mosby, 1983.

Smolin G, O'Connor GR: *Ocular Immunology,* 2nd ed. Little, Brown, 1986.

CORNEAL DRYING & EXPOSURE

Keratoconjunctivitis Sicca

This condition is rare in children and results from a lacrimal gland insufficiency. The treatment of choice is tear replacement with artificial tear solutions as necessary to keep the cornea moist. Bland ophthalmic ointments (Duolube, Duratears, Lacri-Lube) may also be used, particularly at bedtime.

Exposure & Neuroparalytic Keratitis

Exposure keratitis may develop after facial nerve palsies or after a period of unconsciousness during which the eyes are exposed. Treatment is similar to that described above.

Familial Dysautonomia (Riley-Day Syndrome)

In this condition, there is a deficiency of tears and decreased corneal sensation. Corneal drying can occur. Tear replacement (see Keratoconjunctivitis Sicca, above) is indicated.

Xerophthalmia

Severe vitamin A deficiency reduces conjunctival secretion of mucus, and this leads to conjunctival and corneal drying and keratinization. The cornea may become soft and necrotic (keratomalacia), and corneal perforation may occur. The conjunctival changes are characterized by a foamy, triangular lesion that is usually on the temporal side and has its base at the limbus (Bitot's spot). The conjunctival and corneal changes together are known as xerophthalmia.

Patients are treated with systemic vitamin A. Topical antibiotic drops may be indicated to prevent secondary infection.

Levine MR: Medical and surgical treatment of the dry eye. Int Ophthalmol Clin (Fall) 1978;18:101.

Ostler HB, Ostler MW: *Disease of the External Eye and Adnexa: A text and Atlas.* Williams & Wilkins, 1993.

Smolin G, Thoft RA (editors): *The Cornea: Scientific Foundations and Clinical Practice.* Little, Brown, 1987.

Sommer A, Sugana T: Corneal xerophthalmia and keratomalacia. Arch Ophthalmol 1982;100:404.

CORNEAL INVOLVEMENT IN OTHER SYSTEMIC DISEASES

The cornea is involved in many systemic diseases. Small calcium deposits may be observed in the corneas of patients with hyperparathyroidism. Cystine crystals are observed in patients with cystinosis. Excessive intake of vitamin D may lead to calcification of the anterior part of the cornea in a band opacity of the exposed portion of the cornea. Deficiency of vitamin A may lead to drying (xerosis) and softening (keratomalacia) of the cornea. Corneal ulceration may occur in patients with severe debilitating diseases such as dysentery. Corneal opacities may occur in children with Hurler's disease (gargoylism) and other mucopolysaccharide disorders.

In all of these conditions, it is important to recognize the underlying disease and treat appropriately.

Grayson M: *Diseases of the Cornea,* 2nd ed. Mosby, 1983.

Smolin G, Thoft RA (editors): *The Cornea: Scientific Foundations and Clinical Practice.* Little, Brown, 1987.

Sugar J: Corneal manifestations of systemic mucopolysaccharidoses. Ann Ophthalmol 1979;11:531.

UVEITIS

Inflammation of the uveal tract may present anteriorly as iritis or cyclitis (inflammation of the ciliary body) or as posterior inflammations (choroiditis). Uveitis may be associated with other ocular diseases, such as corneal ulceration, keratitis, hypermature cataracts, necrotic intraocular tumors, or optic neuritis. It usually occurs with ocular trauma.

Uveitis may be classified as exogenous or endogenous. Exogenous uveitis follows the accidental introduction of pathogenic organisms or a foreign substance into the eye. Endogenous uveitis is a result of various systemic processes.

Endogenous uveitis, which is the more common form, may further be divided into granulomatous and nongranulomatous types. Nongranulomatous uveitis usually involves the iris and ciliary body and produces symptoms of photophobia, pain, redness, and blurred vision. The pupil is small and often irregular. There is circumcorneal injection. On examination with a slit lamp, cells in the anterior chamber and fine precipitates on the posterior surface of the cornea may be observed. Granulomatous uveitis may involve the iris, ciliary body, or choroid. Pain, redness, and photophobia are not so prominent as in the nongranulomatous form. Vision may be markedly disturbed, particularly if the involvement is in the macular area. On ophthalmoscopy, the vitreous may be quite hazy. Active lesions of choroiditis may be seen as swollen, white, indistinct irregular patches. As the choroiditis subsides, pigmentary changes may take place.

Uveitis presents a complex problem and may be associated with systemic disease. In children, the most common associated disease is juvenile rheumatoid arthritis, usually the pauciarticular form. Iritis may antedate joint symptoms. All patients with juvenile rheumatoid arthritis should have a slitlamp examination. Other common associated diseases are toxoplasmosis; histoplasmosis; tuberculosis; sarcoidosis, polyarteritis, and other collagen diseases; bacterial infections of the sinuses or teeth; food and pollen allergies; and viral diseases such as mumps, measles, chickenpox, influenza, herpes simplex, and herpes zoster. The relationship between systemic disease and uveitis may be incidental. There is pathologic evidence that the choroid and retina may be invaded with *Toxoplasma* and *Mycobacterium tuberculosis.* However, aside from these specific instances, causative organisms have not been found to enter the uveal tissue. There is accumulating evidence that most cases of uveitis are due to an immune reaction.

Treatment

If systemic disease is present, it should be appropriately treated. However, successful treatment of systemic disease does not always result in a cure of the uveitis. Nonspecific treatment of uveitis consists of the use of cycloplegics to dilate the pupil and to relieve the ciliary and iris spasm. Atropine, 1–2% solution, or scopolamine, 0.25% solution, should be used two or three times daily. In addition, the topical use of 10% phenylephrine hydrochloride to dilate the pupil widely is indicated. Corticosteroids should be used unless they are contraindicated by the presence of a specific bacterial or viral infection. For inflammations of the anterior uveal tract, topical and subconjunctival corticosteroids are useful in reducing the inflammation. For posterior uveitis, systemic corticosteroids should be used.

The management of uveitis is difficult. Many complications can occur, including glaucoma, cataract, and retinal detachment. Therefore, these cases should be managed by an ophthalmologist.

Giles CL: Pediatric intermediate uveitis. J Pediatr Ophthalmol Strabismus 1989;26:136.

Kanski JJ: Juvenile arthritis and uveitis. Surv Ophthalmol 1990;34:253.

Kanski JJ: Lensectomy for complicated cataract in juvenile chronic iridocyclitis. Br J Ophthalmol 1992;76:72.

Nussenblatt RB, Palestine AG: *Uveitis: Fundamentals and Clinical Practice.* Year Book, 1989.

Smith RE, Nozik A: *Uveitis: A Clinical Approach to Diagnosis and Management,* 2nd ed. Williams & Wilkins, 1988.

Wolf MD, Lichter PR, Ragsdale CG: Prognostic factors in the uveitis of juvenile rheumatoid arthritis. Ophthalmology 1987;94:1242.

SYMPATHETIC OPHTHALMIA

Sympathetic ophthalmia is a special form of bilateral granulomatous uveitis. It follows a penetrating ocular injury involving the uveal tract. It may occur at any time from 10 days after injury to many years later, but it usually presents within the first 2–4 months after initial injury. The etiology of sympathetic ophthalmia is not understood, but it probably represents a hypersensitivity response to uveal pigment. The diagnosis is based on a history of an injury to one (exciting) eye with the subsequent development of uveitis in the other (sympathizing) eye.

Treatment consists of the use of systemic and topical corticosteroids and topical cycloplegics. Immunosuppressive agents also are employed in resistant cases. Long-term therapy is usually necessary, and maintenance doses of corticosteroids are usually indicated to prevent a flare-up of this condition. The disease can be averted by early enucleation of the eye that has received a severe injury with no prospect of useful vision.

Nussenblatt RB, Palestine AG: *Uveitis: Fundamentals and Clinical Practice.* Year Book, 1989.

Smolin G, O'Connor GR: *Ocular Immunology,* 2nd ed. Little, Brown, 1986.

DISEASES OF THE RETINA

HEREDITARY RETINAL DISORDERS

Hereditary retinal disorders may be evident shortly after birth or not until the second decade of life. Many of these disorders involve primarily one layer of the retina (eg, the pigment epithelium, the rod and cone layer, or the ganglion cell layer), but other layers of the retina are usually secondarily involved.

Retinitis pigmentosa is a bilateral hereditary disease involving chiefly the retinal rods or the retinal pigment epithelium. Symptoms of night blindness usually begin early in the second decade. Restriction of visual fields subsequently occurs; this generally progresses, so that by middle age the visual fields are markedly contracted and the visual acuity severely depressed. However, certain forms of the disease are less severe, especially in the early stages. Ophthalmoscopic examination may reveal only some incipient pigmentary abnormalities in the midperiphery of the ocular fundus. The diagnosis may be confirmed by electroretinography, which shows markedly reduced or unrecordable activity. As the disease progresses, additional changes occur: narrowing of the retinal arteries and veins, waxy appearance of the optic disk, and "bone corpuscle" pigment deposits. Retinitis pigmentosa may be associated with many systemic diseases: renal abnormalities, deafness, convulsions and obesity, hypogenitalism, polydactyly, mental retardation (Laurence-Moon-Biedl syndrome), and abetalipoproteinemia. There is no satisfactory treatment for retinitis pigmentosa. The mode of inheritance varies. Genetic counseling is advisable for prospective parents with this disorder.

Rod-cone dystrophy is characterized by initial cone degeneration; rod function is affected later. Early symptoms and findings include poor visual acuity, color vision, and photophobia. A depigmented ring around the macula may be observed on ophthalmoscopy. Late changes are similar to those in retinitis pigmentosa.

Fundus flavimaculatus consists of multiple round and fishtail-like yellow-white lesions of the posterior and midperipheral fundus. The onset is in the first or second decade of life. Some patients with this disorder develop atrophic changes in the macula with severe visual loss (Stargardt's disease); others may retain good macular function and visual acuity.

Coats's disease is an exudative retinopathy characterized by hemorrhagic and exudative lesions and by telangiectatic vessels. The onset is usually within the first few years of life; males are affected more often than females. Usually only one eye is involved; vision is often severely impaired. The disorder may cause a white pupillary reflex (leukocoria) and must be differentiated from other causes of leukocoria, such as cataracts, persistent hyperplastic primary vitreous, and retinoblastoma.

Vitelliform degeneration (Best's disease) is a disorder of the retinal pigment epithelium that occurs in the macular region at or shortly after birth. Ophthalmoscopically, the macula has a yellow deposit resembling a "sunny side up" fried egg. During the first or second decade of life, the lesion changes; the sunny side up egg yolk becomes scrambled, and scarring and pigmentary changes may lead to loss of central vision.

Leber's congenital amaurosis is characterized by congenital blindness or reduced vision, nystagmus, and poor pupillary light responses. Other neurologic disorders may be present also. Initially, the ocular fundus appears normal or there may be some mild pigmentary changes. With time, the disk becomes atrophic, and pigmentary changes become more obvious. Electroretinographic testing shows changes similar to those seen in retinitis pigmentosa.

Color vision abnormalities are common, with approximately 7% of males and 0.5% of females affected. Many of the tests used clinically are not sensitive enough to detect small changes. Color vision is a retinal cone function; each cone has three distinct photosensitive pigments, with spectral sensitive patterns maximal at red, green, or blue. Hereditary color vision defects result from a deficiency or absence of one or more of the three cone photosensitive pigments.

Berson EL et al: Ocular findings in patients with autosomal dominant retinitis pigmentosa and a rhodopsin gene defect (Pro-23-His). Arch Ophthalmol 1991;109:92.

Breton ME, Nelson LB: What do color blind children really see? Guidelines for clinical prescreening based on recent findings. Surv Ophthalmol 1983;27:306.

Heckenlively JR et al: Clinical findings and common symptoms in retinitis pigmentosa. Am J Ophthalmol 1988;105:504.

Ryan SJ (editor): Retina. Vol I in: *Basic Science and Inherited Retinal Disease.* Ogden TE (editor). Mosby, 1989.

Schroeder R et al: Leber's congenital amaurosis. Retrospective review of 43 cases and a new fundus finding in two cases. Arch Ophthalmol 1987;105:356.

Silodor SW et al: Natural history and management of advanced Coats' disease. Ophthalmic Surg 1988;19:89.

RETINOPATHY OF PREMATURITY (Retrolental Fibroplasia)

Retinopathy of prematurity is a primary bilateral retinal vascular disorder of premature infants. The disease occurs most frequently in those with a birth weight under 1500 g who have received prolonged supplemental oxygen therapy for more than 50 days. Infants at highest risk are those born before 32 weeks of gestation and with a birth weight under 1250 g. For several years, after the role of oxygen in the development of retinopathy of prematurity was established, the disease became almost extinct with restricted oxygen therapy. However, prolonged supplemental oxygen therapy is again being employed in the management of increasing numbers of premature infants of very low birth weight. As a result, more cases of retinopathy of prematurity can be expected. The variability, severity and susceptibility to retinopathy in the extremely premature infant suggest that factors other than hyperoxia play a role in the etiology of this disease. Oxygen is probably only one factor among many and may not even be the major cause of retinopathy of prematurity.

In general, peripheral vascularization of the retina is not complete until about 2 weeks after full-term birth. However, this is variable; some eyes have complete vascularization at 8 months' gestational age. Until retinal vascularization is complete, the peripheral immature vessels, which are immediately posterior to the demarcation site of vascular to avascular retina, are extremely sensitive to hyperoxia and respond by vasoconstriction and obliteration. A vasoproliferative substance is released from the ischemic retina. When oxygen concentrations are subsequently reduced, the retinal vessels in the posterior pole often dilate as a result of peripheral vascular shunts formed near the site of vaso-obliteration. These shunts may take the form of neofibrovascular membranes on the surface of the retina or may extend into the vitreous cavity. Tractional retinal detachments may occur. In advanced stages, the retrolental space is filled with fibrovascular and retinal tissues, the anterior chambers are shallow, and the eyes are small and blind. In incomplete forms, myopia and strabismus are often observed; retinal detachment may occur as a late complication in the teenage years. Up to 85% of acute cases of retinopathy of prematurity regress as vascularization to the peripheral aspect of the retina is completed in a nearly normal manner.

Retinopathy of prematurity is related mainly to the degree of prematurity. Gestational age and birth weight are inversely correlated to the development of retinopathy of prematurity. The duration of supplemental oxygen rather than the level of arterial oxygenation correlates best with the disorder. Furthermore, retinopathy of prematurity usually develops in the smallest and the sickest premature infants. It is more common in infants with multiple complications of prematurity.

It is essential that pediatricians be aware of the relationship of oxygen therapy to the development of retinopathy of prematurity—not only the concentration of oxygen but also the duration of oxygen treatment and the degree of prematurity.

All premature infants receiving oxygen therapy should be followed as closely as possible to make certain that arterial blood oxygen levels do not remain excessively high for any period of time. Changes in the immature retinal vessels appear to be related not only to high arterial blood oxygen levels but also to the duration of hyperoxia. The value of the early administration of vitamin E (an antioxidant) in diminishing the severity of retinopathy of prematurity or in preventing its occurrence is under investigation.

All premature infants should have careful ophthalmoscopy performed by a skilled examiner by the sixth week of life, at which time severe forms of retinopathy of prematurity are first evident. The changes associated with retinopathy of prematurity are now staged from I to V, with V representing the most severe involvement (see Table 17–5). For stage III, cryotherapy—and, most recently, indirect laser photocoagulation—of the avascular retina have been shown to significantly reduce progression of the disease. If cryotherapy is unsuccessful in preventing progression of the disease and if retinal detachment occurs, surgical treatment of the detachment is sometimes indicted, but the prognosis for useful vision in such cases is poor.

Ophthalmologic examination for retinopathy of prematurity is necessary until the retina is completely vascularized or the condition has stabilized. Ongoing ophthalmologic assessment is crucial every 6–12 months because of the increased risk for development of strabismus, refractive errors, amblyopia, and visual loss.

Eichenbaum JW et al: *Treatment of Retinopathy of Prematurity.* Year Book, 1990.

Harnett ME et al: Anterior segment evaluation of infants with retinopathy of prematurity. Ophthalmology 1990;97:122.

Landers III MC et al: Treatment of retinopathy of prematurity with argon laser photocoagulation. Arch Ophthalmol 1992;110:44.

Multicenter trial of cryotherapy for retinopathy of prematu-

Table 17–5. Stages of retinopathy of prematurity.

Stage I	Demarcation line or border dividing the vascular from the avascular retina.
Stage II	Ridge. Line of previous stage acquires volume and rises above the surface retina to become a ridge.
Stage III	Ridge with extraretinal fibrovascular proliferation.
Stage IV	Subtotal retinal detachment.
Stage V	Total retinal detachment.

rity: 3½-year outcome—structure and function. Arch Ophthalmol 1993;111:339.

Palmer EA et al: Incidence and early course of retinopathy of prematurity. Ophthalmology 1991;98:1628.

Schaffer DB et al: Prognostic factors in the natural course of retinopathy of prematurity. Ophthalmology 1993; 100:230.

Sira IB, Nissenkorn I, Kremer I: Retinopathy of prematurity. Surv Ophthalmol 1988;33:1.

RETINAL DETACHMENT

Detachment of the retina in children is usually associated with severe ocular trauma or with high myopia. In the latter condition, there are degenerative changes in the periphery of the retina that lead to subsequent separation of the retina. Retinal detachments also occur in primary retinal vitreal diseases such as incontinentia pigmenti, persistent hyperplastic primary vitreous, familial exudative vitreoretinopathy, and retinopathy of prematurity. The visual disturbance may start with the sensation of flashing lights, or the patient may observe a dark cloud coming in from one section of the visual field. On ophthalmoscopy, the area of detachment appears elevated and gray. The retinal vessels appear darker, and the retina is seen with increased convex dioptric power in the ophthalmoscope.

The only treatment is surgical repair.

deJaun E Jr: The treatment of pediatric retinal detachment. Arch Ophthalmol 1993;111:599.

Michels RG, Wilkinson CP, Rice TA: *Retinal Detachment.* Mosby, 1990.

Rosner M, Treister G, Belkin M: Epidemiology of retinal detachment in childhood and adolescence. J Pediatr Ophthalmol Strabismus 1987;24:42.

RETINOBLASTOMA

Retinoblastoma is a comparatively rare malignant tumor of children; it affects approximately one infant in 20,000 live births. A family history of retinoblastoma is found in less than 10% of the cases. However, about 40% of all children with retinoblastoma may have a predisposition to tumor formation that can be inherited as an autosomal dominant trait. The remaining 60% of cases occur as a sporadic mutation and are not inherited. Mutations in a specific locus of chromosome 13 correlate with the development of retinoblastoma. Approximately 25% of cases are bilateral. Patients who survive bilateral retinoblastoma or who have a family history of retinoblastoma have about a 50% chance of transmitting the disease to their offspring. Genetic counseling is complex but advisable for survivors of retinoblastoma as well as for parents of children with retinoblastoma. Karyotype analysis is desirable.

The presenting symptom is usually an abnormal red reflex with a white spot in the pupil (see Figure 17–1). Strabismus may be present. If the tumor becomes very large, glaucoma may occur, with a steamy cornea and red eye. Occasionally, retinoblastoma ruptures through the globe and results in a painful red eye. The diagnosis is usually made by ophthalmoscopic examination. To accomplish ophthalmoscopy, wide pupillary dilatation is essential; general anesthesia is often necessary. The tumor appears as a solid yellow or white elevated mass. A small section of the eye may be involved, or the entire eye may be filled with tumor.

Retinoblastoma usually is confined to the eye for several months to years. It may spread outside the globe along the optic nerve into the subarachnoid space and then along the base of the brain. Hematogenous metastases to the bone marrow are frequent. The tumor also may extend outside the globe into the orbit and then to regional lymph nodes. Bone marrow aspiration, fluid cytology, CT scans of the orbits, and head and bone scans are recommended in all patients with retinoblastoma to determine the extent of the tumor.

Treatment is best provided in a medical center where there is an experienced team of ophthalmologists, pediatric oncologists and radiotherapists familiar with the disease. The goal of therapy is to maximize vision and patient survival. Enucleation is recommended in unilateral retinoblastoma involving more than half of the retina. Enucleation is also recommended (for the eye with the advanced lesion) in patients with bilateral tumors. It may also be necessary for advanced bilateral disease with no hope of useful vision and for eyes unresponsive to other forms of therapy. External beam radiotherapy is an option for patients with unilateral disease involving less than half of the retina, for therapy of the less advanced eye in bilateral cases, and in advanced bilateral cases as an alternative to bilateral enucleation. Laser photocoagulation may be used for small posterior primary tumors and cryotherapy for small anterior primary tumors. Chemotherapy is recommended for patients with tumor invasion of the optic nerve, with massive choroidal invasion, and with orbital involvement.

For parents who have an affected child but no previous family history of retinoblastoma, the risk of retinoblastoma in a second child is 1–6%. However, if two or more siblings are affected, the chances are approximately 50% that the next child will be affected. Approximately 16% of patients with bilateral retinoblastoma, almost all of which are hereditary, will develop a second primary neoplasm later in life, usually osteogenic sarcoma.

Ellsworth RM: Retinoblastoma. In: *Clinical Ophthalmology,* vol 3. Duane TD (editor). Harper & Row, 1992.

Kopelman JE, McLean IW, Rosenberg SH: Multivariate analysis of risk for metastasis in retinoblastoma treatment by enucleation. Ophthalmology 1987;94:371.

Musarella MA, Gallie BL: A simplified scheme for genetic counseling in retinoblastoma. J Pediatr Ophthalmol Strabismus 1987;24:124.

Sanders BM, Draper GJ, Kingston JE: Retinoblastoma in Great Britain 1969–80: Incidence, treatment and survival. Br J Ophthalmol 1988;72:576.

Seidman DJ et al: Early diagnosis of retinoblastoma based on dysmorphic features and karyotype analysis. Ophthalmology 1987;94:663.

Shields JA: *Diagnosis and Management of Intraocular Tumors.* Mosby, 1983.

Wiggs JL, Dryja TP: Predicting the risk of hereditary retinoblastoma. Am J Ophthalmol 1988;106:346.

RETINITIS

Cytomegalovirus

Cytomegalovirus infections of the retina occur in newborn infants and immunocompromised patients, often in HIV positive hosts. Ocular findings include disseminated retinal hemorrhages, perivascular infiltrates, and focal areas of white retinal necrosis. In the congenital form, other ocular findings include microphthalmia, cataract, and optic atrophy. Ganciclovir halts or slows the infection, but the disease often recurs after the drug is stopped.

Rubella

Maternal rubella infections occurring during the first trimester of pregnancy produce changes in the retinal pigment epithelial layer that appear as discrete areas of pigmentation and depigmentation on ophthalmoscopy. The retina has a mottled salt-and-pepper appearance. The optic disk and vessels are normal. The retinopathy does not progress.

Toxoplasmosis

Toxoplasmic retinitis is usually congenital, occurring as a result of infection in utero of mothers who have acquired the disease, particularly during the third trimester of pregnancy. The characteristic finding is a posterior central focal necrotizing retinitis. Inactive lesions are characterized by sharply demarcated pigment borders and atrophy of the retina and choroid with visible sclera. Satellite lesions may be present; active white lesions occur adjacent to the old, healed areas. Vitreous is usually clear, although there may be heavily cellular infiltration and exudation. The disease is usually self-limited. Treatment of the active, vision-threatening lesions consists of the combined administration of pyrimethamine and sulfadiazine. Clindamycin may be combined or used as an alternative single agent.

Herpes Simplex

Herpes simplex retinitis usually occurs in patients suffering from herpes encephalitis or in immunocompromised patients. A severe occlusive retinal vasculitis develops which is followed by retinal necrosis and sometimes retinal detachment. Treatment consists of intravenous acyclovir. Retinal detachment surgery may become necessary.

Duker JS, Blumenkranz MS: Diagnosis and management of the acute retinal necrosis (ARN) syndrome. Surv Ophthalmol 1991;35:327.

Hennis HL, Scott AA, Apple DJ: Cytomegalovirus retinitis. Surv Ophthalmol 1989;34:193.

Kuppermann BD et al: Correlation between CD4+ counts and prevalence of cytomegalovirus retinitis and human immunodeficiency virus-related retinal vasculopathy in patients with acquired immunodeficiency syndrome. Am J Ophthalmol 1993;115:575.

Lewis ML et al: Herpes simplex virus type 1: A cause of the acute retinal necrosis syndrome. Ophthalmology 1989; 96:875.

Rothova A et al: Therapy for ocular toxoplasmosis. Am J Ophthalmol 1993;115:517.

Tabbara KF: Ocular toxoplasmosis, In: *Clinical Ophthalmology,* vol 4. Duane TD (editor). Harper & Row, 1993.

OPTIC NEURITIS

Optic neuritis may involve only the head of the nerve (papillitis) or the orbital portion of the nerve (retrobulbar neuritis). Optic neuritis may occur in association with generalized infectious diseases, demyelinating diseases, blood dyscrasias, or metabolic diseases or may be due to exposure to toxins or drugs or extension of inflammatory disease such as sinusitis or meningitis. Clinically, there is an acute loss of vision. Involvement may be of one or both eyes; in children, the disease is frequently bilateral. Central visual defects are present. There may be some discomfort in the eyes on movement of the globes. On ophthalmoscopic examination, papilledema may be present or the disks may appear normal.

Optic neuritis in children often follows a viral illness and is usually a self-limited disease. The visual prognosis is generally favorable. Visual improvement commonly occurs in 1–4 weeks. If the cause can be determined, it should be treated. Systemic corticosteroid therapy has been advocated, but its effectiveness has not been established.

The presence of papilledema may be a sign of increased intracranial pressure. The differentiation between optic neuritis and papilledema secondary to increased intracranial pressure is not always easy. In general, papilledema due to increased intracranial pressure does not produce a severe loss of vision, and there often are associated neurologic signs. Radio-graphic imaging studies often are advisable to establish a diagnosis.

Beck RW et al: A randomized, controlled trial of corticosteroids in the treatment of acute optic neuritis. N Engl J Med 1992;326:581.

Burde RM, Savino PJ, Trobe JD: *Clinical Decisions in Neuro-Ophthalmology,* 2nd ed. Mosby, 1992.

Miller NR: *Walsh and Hoyt's Clinical Neuro-Ophthalmology,* 5th ed, vol 4. Williams & Wilkins, 1991.

Repka MX, Miller NR: Optic atrophy in children. Am J Ophthalmol 1988;106:191.

Walsh TJ: *Neuro-ophthalmology: Clinical Signs and Symptoms,* 3rd ed. Lea & Febiger, 1992

DISEASES OF THE ORBIT

ORBITAL CELLULITIS

Orbital cellulitis may exist in either a preseptal or a postseptal form. Periorbital edema, redness, congestion of the eyelids, pain, leukocytosis, and fever are present in both forms. However, proptosis, limited extraocular movement, and reduced visual acuity indicate deep orbital involvement. The depth of involvement may be determined accurately either by CT scan or MRI.

Orbital cellulitis is a serious illness. In children, orbital cellulitis is usually due to bacterial infection. The most common causative organisms are *S aureus* and gram-negative bacilli in neonates; *H influenzae* and *S pneumoniae* in children between ages 6 months and 5 years; *S aureus, H influenzae,* and *S pneumoniae* in older children; and gram-negative organisms in immunocompromised children. A distinct magenta discoloration of the skin of the eyelids is present in cases of *H influenzae* infection. There may be associated infections elsewhere in the body, particularly in the sinuses.

Treatment consists of hot packs and the vigorous use of systemic (primarily intravenous) antibiotics; a favorable response is usually obtained within 48–72 hours. If this does not occur, surgical drainage should be considered. Complications may include intracranial extension of the infection and cavernous sinus thrombosis.

Mauriello JA Jr, Flanagan JC (editors): *Management of Orbital and Ocular Adnexal Tumors and Inflammations.* Field & Wood, 1990.

Molarte AB, Isenberg SJ: Periorbital cellulitis in infancy. J Pediatr Ophthalmol Strabismus 1989;26:232.

Rootman J: *Diseases of the Orbit: A Multidisciplinary Approach.* Lippincott, 1988.

Weiss A et al: Bacterial periorbital and orbital cellulitis in childhood. Ophthalmology 1983;90:195.

ORBITAL TUMORS
& PSEUDOTUMORS

Orbital tumors are rare in children. The most common primary tumors are hemangiomas, lymphangiomas, neurofibromas, gliomas of the optic nerve, dermoids, rhabdomyosarcomas, and tumors of the lacrimal gland. Neuroblastoma, Wilms' tumor, leukemia, and lymphoma may spread into the orbit. The presenting symptoms are exophthalmos, congestion and ecchymosis of the globe and lids, extraocular muscle weakness, and displacement of the globe. Optic nerve gliomas may show enlargement of the optic foramen on x-ray examination.

Treatment includes surgical removal, x-ray therapy, or the use of chemotherapy in certain cases. For certain benign tumors, it is often better not to attempt total removal of the lesion.

Pseudotumor of the orbit is uncommon in children. It is an inflammation of the orbital tissues, sometimes granulomatous in character but usually unrelated to any specific granulomatous disease. As a rule, only one orbit is affected, but in about 25% of the cases the other orbit is involved. The symptoms may develop suddenly or over a period of months. Swelling of the eyelid and conjunctiva often precedes the proptosis and diplopia. The diagnosis is usually made by exclusion of other causes of swelling and proptosis. Spontaneous remission often occurs. However, dramatic improvement usually follows systemic corticosteroid therapy.

Casper DS Chi TL, Trokel SL: *Orbital Disease: Imaging and Analysis.* Thieme, 1993.

Rosenthal AR: Ocular Manifestations of leukemia: A review. Ophthalmology 1983;90:899.

Shields JA et al: *Diagnosis and Management of Orbital Tumors.* Saunders, 1989.

Weiss AH et al: Primary and secondary orbital teratomas. J Pediatr Ophthalmol Strabismus 1989;26:44.

DISEASES OF THE LACRIMAL APPARATUS

NASOLACRIMAL DUCT OBSTRUCTION

In a significant number of infants, the nasolacrimal duct fails to completely canalize at the time of birth; the obstruction is usually at the nasal end of the duct. Symptoms consist of persistent tearing and, often, mucoid discharge in the inner corner of the eye.

Most cases subside without treatment. The obstruction usually opens spontaneously, and relief of symptoms occurs. Massage over the lacrimal sac with

expression toward the nose may be helpful in establishing the patency. If a purulent discharge is evident, manual expression of the sac should be performed, followed by instillation of topical antibiotics. If a cure does not result within the first few months of life, probing of the nasolacrimal duct should be performed by an ophthalmologist.

El-Mansoury J et al: Results of late probing for congenital nasolacrimal duct obstruction. Ophthalmology 1986;93: 1052.

Kushner BJ: Congenital nasolacrimal system obstruction. Arch Ophthalmol 1982;100:597.

Migliori ME, Putterman AM: Silicone intubation for the treatment of congenital lacrimal duct obstruction: Successful results removing the tubes after six weeks. Ophthalmology 1988; 95:792.

Nucci P et al: Conservative management of congenital nasolacrimal duct obstruction. J Pediatr Ophthalmol Strabismus 1989;26:39.

CONGENITAL DACRYOCYSTOCELE

Congenital dacryocystocele of the lacrimal sac presents at birth as a bluish subcutaneous mass about 1 cm below the medial canthus. It occurs as a result of blockage of the nasolacrimal system with impairment of retrograde passage of the sac contents through the canaliculi. Without treatment, this condition often leads to infection and occasionally fistula formation. Probing of the nasolacrimal system may be required to drain the dacryocystocele and restore patency of the nasolacrimal system. Dacryocystocele must be differentiated from an encephalocele, which can be similar in appearance but generally presents above the medial canthus.

Birchansky LD et al: Management of congenital lacrimal sac fistula. Arch Ophthalmol 1990;108:388.

Grin TR, Mertz JS, Stass-Isern M: Congenital nasolacrimal duct cysts in dacrocystocele. Ophthalmology 1991;98: 1238.

Mansour AM et al: Congenital dacryocele: A collaborative review. Ophthalmology 1991;98:1744.

DACRYOCYSTITIS

Inflammation of the tear sac (dacryocystitis) is usually secondary to obstruction of the nasolacrimal duct. In newborns, the dacryocystitis almost always is observed in patients with a dacryocystocele. There is resultant stasis of the tears in the sac, with secondary bacterial infection. Symptoms consist of tearing and mucopurulent discharge. There is usually an acute inflammation in the region of the lacrimal sac. Fever and leukocytosis may be present. Occasionally, the sac may rupture to the skin surface.

If possible, cultures should be obtained and the organism identified. For mild cases, expression of the contents of the lacrimal sac followed by instillation of topical antibiotics in the region of the lacrimal puncta may be effective. More severe cases should also be treated with systemic antibiotics and warm compresses. Irrigation of the canaliculi and lacrimal sac with antibiotic solution is a more successful method of delivering adequate concentrations of antibiotics to the area of infection. Once the acute infection has subsided, an attempt should be made to establish the passage of tears. The nasolacrimal system should be probed under general anesthesia if the system does not permit passage of fluid irrigated through the canaliculi.

Hoyt CS, Good WV: The eyes. In: *Rudolph's Pediatrics.* Rudolph AM, Hoffman JI, Rudolph CD (editors). Appleton & Lange, 1991.
Isenberg SJ (editor): *The Eye in Infancy,* 2nd ed. Mosby, 1993.

DACRYOADENITIS

Acute inflammation of the lacrimal gland is usually nonbacterial and associated with systemic diseases such as mumps and infectious mononucleosis. The main symptoms are pain and tenderness in the upper outer portion of the orbit. An S-shaped curve of the eyelid is often present as a result of an outer mechanical ptosis produced by swelling of the lacrimal gland. There may be associated adenopathy and fever. Dacryoadenitis is usually self-limited. Treatment is largely symptomatic; hot or cold compresses over the lacrimal gland may give relief. If a specific bacterial infection is present, appropriate antibiotics are indicated.

Darrell RW: *Viral Diseases of the Eye.* Lea & Febiger, 1985.
Harris GJ, Snyder RW: Lacrimal gland abscess. Am J Ophthalmol 1987;104:193.
Linberg JV: *Oculoplastic and Orbital Emergencies.* Appleton & Lange, 1990.
Rootman J: *Diseases of the Orbit: A Multidisciplinary Approach.* Lippincott, 1988.

VISUAL FUNCTION IN LEARNING DISABILITIES

Learning disabilities are almost never associated with ocular disorders. However, a complete ophthalmologic examination is justified in children with learning disabilities with special attention to the visual function at near. The examination should include measurement of near and distant vision, near point of accommodation, convergence amplitudes and near points of convergence, and a cycloplegic refraction. Gross ocular problems may cause poor or double vision, which may be significant factors in learning disabilities. Weakness of accommodation or convergence or significant hyperopia (farsightedness) may be related to the comfort of reading, which rarely can be a factor in learning disabilities.

Lehmkuhle S et al: A defective visual pathway in children with reading disability. N Engl J Med 1993:328:989.
Menacker SJ, Breton ME, Breton ML et al: Do tinted lenses improve the reading performance of dyslexic children? A cohort study. Arch Ophthalmol 1993;111:213.

REFERENCES

Albert DM, Jakobiec FA (editors): *Principles and Practice of Ophthalmology,* 6 vols. Saunders, 1993.
Apt L, Urea PT: The eye. In: *Current Pediatric Therapy 13.* Gellis SS, Kagan BM (editors). Saunders, 1990.
Buckingham T (editor): *Visual Problems in Childhood.* Oxford Univ Press, 1993.
Cibis GW, Tongue AC, Stass-Isern ML (editors): *Decision Making in Pediatric Ophthalmology.* Decker, 1993.
Coles WH: *Ophthalmology, A Diagnostic Text.* Williams & Wilkins, 1989.
Dhillon B, Millar GT: *The Child's Eye.* Oxford Univ Press, 1993.
Duane TD (editor): *Clinical Ophthalmology,* 5 vols. Harper & Row, 1992.
Ellis PP: Diseases of the eye. In: *Pediatric Therapy,* 3rd ed. Eichenwald HF, Ströder J, Ginsburg CM (editors). Mosby, 1993.
Fraunfelder FT, Roy FH (editors): *Current Ocular Therapy,* 3rd ed. Saunders, 1990.

Hoyt CS, Good WV: The eyes. In: *Rudolph's Pediatrics,* 19th ed. Rudolph AM, Hoffman JI, Rudolph CD (editors). Appleton & Lange, 1991.
Isenberg SJ (editor): *The Eye in Infancy,* 2nd ed. Mosby, 1993.
Miller SJH: *Parson's Diseases of the Eye,* 18th ed. Churchill Livingstone, 1990.
Nelson LB, Calhoun JH, Harley RD (editors): *Pediatric Ophthalmology,* 3rd ed. Saunders, 1991.
Newell FW: *Ophthalmology: Principles and Concepts,* 7th ed. Mosby, 1992.
Newman NM: *Neuro-Ophthalmology. A Practical Text.* Appleton & Lange, 1992.
Pavan-Langston D (editor): *Manual of Ocular Diagnosis and Therapy,* 3rd ed. Little, Brown, 1991.
Vaughan D, Asbury T, Riordan-Eva P: *General Ophthalmology,* 13th ed. Appleton & Lange, 1992.

Oral Medicine & Dentistry

R.B. Abrams, DDS, & W.A. Mueller, DMD

Disease in the oral cavity can have a profound effect on systemic health, and the obverse is also true in that systemic disease can be reflected in the oral cavity. This chapter will discuss the interface between medicine and dentistry for the pediatric patient.

THE MOUTH OF THE NEWBORN & OF THE INFANT

The mouth of the newborn should be lined with an intact, smooth, moist and shiny mucosa. The alveolar ridges (Figure 18–1) should be continuous and relatively smooth. Within the alveolar bone are numerous tooth buds which at birth are mostly primary (baby) teeth with a few permanent teeth just starting.

Teeth

The primary teeth begin to form at approximately 6 weeks of gestation, and their calcification starts at some time in the second trimester. The permanent teeth are just beginning to develop at birth. There is enough development of permanent teeth to permit their damage by perinatal or antenatal trauma.

The primary teeth usually do not begin to erupt until approximately 6–7 months of age. However, on rare occasions (1:2000), teeth are present at birth (natal teeth) or erupt within the first month (neonatal teeth). These are most common in the anterior mandible and can be "real" primary teeth or supernumerary (extra) teeth. These can be differentiated radiographically. On occasion, these teeth will need to be removed to facilitate nursing, heal persistent ulceration of the ventral tongue, or eliminate the risk of aspiration. Consultation with a pediatric dentist is advisable.

Frena

There should be noticeable but small maxillary and mandibular labial frena (Figure 18–2). Sometimes these are slightly thick, but they are usually of no consequence. There may also be several small accessory frena farther posteriorly. The extreme is multiple thick tightly bound frena, as in oral-facial-digital syndrome.

Decisions about if and when a labial frenum should be surgically reduced are best left until adolescence. Many thick frena need not be corrected.

The tongue is connected to the floor of the mouth by the lingual frenum (Figures 18–1 and 18–3). This connection should not impede the free movement of the tongue. If the attachment is tight and high up on the alveolar ridge (Figure 18–4), it may restrict movement. This condition is called ankyloglossia (tongue-tie). If it needs to be surgically corrected, earlier (3–4 years) is better than later, but there is usually no urgency for surgery in the neonatal period.

The Palate

The palate of the newborn should be intact and continuous from the alveolar ridge anteriorly to the uvula (Figure 18–1). Cleft lip and palate are common defects (1:700). The cleft of the palate can be unilateral or bilateral (Figure 18–5). The cleft can involve just the alveolar ridge, as in Figure 18–5, or the ridge and entire palate. Clefts can be isolated soft palate defects also. This is common in the Robin anomalad. A final classification of cleft palate is submucous cleft, which is harder to detect. This is a muscular problem in the soft palate with no bony component. Sometimes these children will have a notched or bifid uvula.

Cleft lip and palate rehabilitation is an extensive program involving many specialties and can be lifelong. Owing to the complexity of the problem, children with cleft palate are best treated by a cleft palate team so that treatment can be coordinated between all the specialties.

Cleft lip and palate treatment begins immediately after birth with the fabrication of a palatal obturator to help the baby feed. This same appliance can be used to "mold" the alveolus closed once the initial lip repair has been accomplished. In the case of bilateral cleft lip and palate, the dentist will apply extraoral orthopedic traction to guide the protruding premaxilla back into the oral cavity to facilitate lip closure by the surgeon.

Dental involvement in children with cleft palate is extensive and may extend over a lifetime. A cleft palate team is a good place to find expertise to deal with this problem.

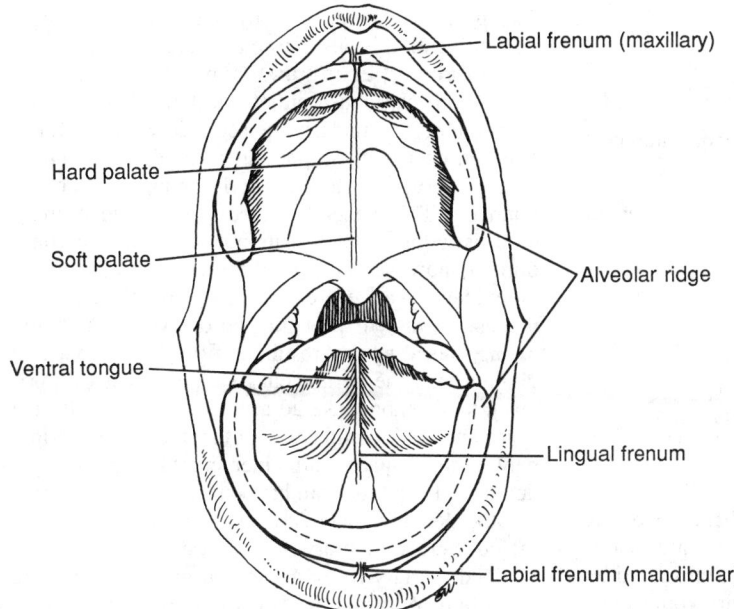

Figure 18–1. Normal anatomy of the newborn mouth.

Other Soft Tissue Variations

Other minor soft tissue variations can exist in the newborn mouth. Small (1–2 mm) round, smooth, whitish bumps can appear on the alveolar ridges or the palate. These are keratin cysts and are called Epstein's pearls or dental lamina cysts. They are benign and require no treatment as they usually disappear.

Some newborns may have small intraoral lymphangiomas on the alveolar ridge or the floor of the mouth. These and any other soft tissue variations that are more noticeable or larger than those just described should be evaluated by a dentist familiar with management of neonates.

Teething

A. Normal Eruption: As the child grows and begins to develop teeth, one encounters problems of teething. Primary teeth generally begin to erupt at around 6 months of age. They are usually mandibular

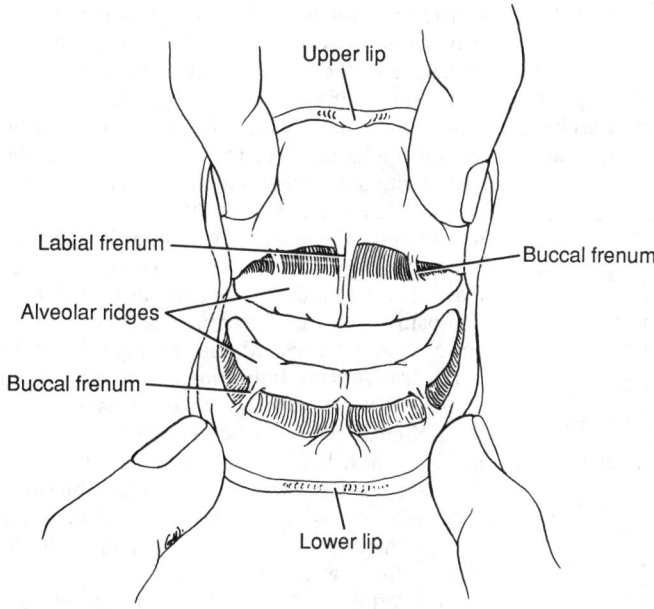

Figure 18–2. The frena.

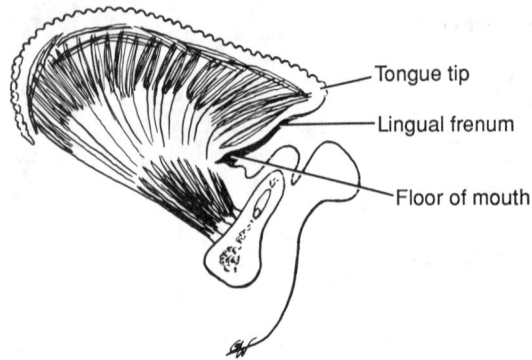

Figure 18–3. Normal position of lingual frenum.

incisors but can be maxillary first and can appear as early as 3–4 months or as late as 12–16 months. Concerns about sequence or timing of eruption should be discussed with a dentist comfortable with young children. There are many reported side effects from teething—diarrhea, drooling, fever, rash, etc—but any real correlation is questionable.

Common treatment for teething pain has been the application of a topical anesthetic or "teething gel." Most of these are benzocaine or, less commonly, lidocaine. They can cause profound numbness of the entire oral cavity and pharynx. Suppression of the gag reflex can be a serious sequela. Systemic analgesia (acetaminophen or ibuprofen) is more effective and safer. Solid rubber or chilled fluid-filled teething toys are beneficial if only for distraction purposes. Massaging the gums can be very soothing.

Occasionally, one encounters a noticeable swelling of the gingiva during teething. This condition can present as red to purple, round, raised, smooth lesions, which may be symptomatic but usually are not. They can appear in the anterior or posterior alveolar ridge and are always on the crest. These eruption cysts or eruption hematomas are fluid-filled areas immediately overlying an erupting tooth and generally

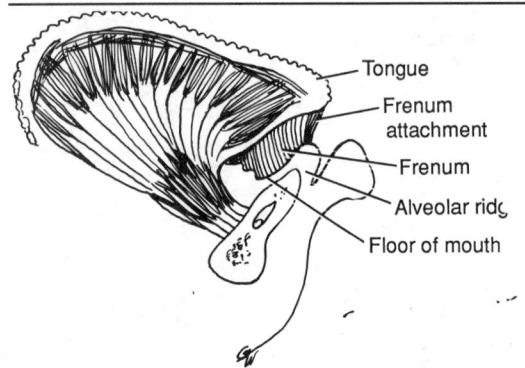

Figure 18–4. Ankyloglossia (tongue-tie).

disappear spontaneously. Any decision about surgical intervention is best left to a dental specialist.

B. Delayed Eruption: Premature loss of a primary tooth can cause either accelerated or delayed eruption of the underlying secondary tooth. Early eruption occurs if the permanent tooth is beginning its active eruption and the overlying primary tooth is removed. This generally occurs when the primary tooth is within 1 year of its normal time of exfoliation. If, however, loss of the primary tooth occurs more than a year before expected exfoliation, the permanent tooth will probably be delayed in eruption owing to healing that results in filling in of bone and gingiva over the permanent tooth. The loss of a primary tooth may cause adjacent teeth to tip into the space and lead to impaction of the underlying permanent tooth. A space maintainer should be placed by a dentist to keep this from happening.

Other local factors delaying or preventing eruption include supernumerary teeth, cysts, tumors, over-retained primary teeth, ankylosed primary teeth, and impaction. A generalized delay in eruption may be due to endocrinopathies (hypothyroidism, hypopituitarism) or other systemic conditions (cleidocranial dysplasia, rickets, trisomy 21).

C. Ectopic Eruption: Ectopic eruption occurs if the position of an erupting tooth is abnormal. In severe instances, the order in which teeth erupt is affected. If the dental arch provides insufficient room for permanent teeth, they may erupt abnormally. In the mandible, lower incisors may be lingually placed to such an extent that the primary incisors do not exfoliate. The parents' concern about a "double row of teeth" may be the reason for the child's first dental visit. If the primary teeth are not loose, they should be removed by the dentist. If they are loose, they should be allowed to exfoliate naturally. In the maxilla, inadequate room for eruption of the permanent first molar may cause abnormal resorption of the distal root structures of the second primary molar. If the problem is severe, the permanent molar may even become caught under the unresorbed enamel crown of the deciduous molar and thus require extraction of the primary tooth and orthodontic repositioning of the permanent first molar after it has erupted. If it is not repositioned, the second premolar is likely to become impacted. If problems are detected early, the dentist may be able to redirect the permanent molar's eruption pathway so that the permanent first molar erupts correctly and the second primary molar is not lost.

D. Impaction: Impaction occurs when a tooth is prevented from erupting for any reason. The teeth most often affected are the third molars and the maxillary canines. Because patients with impacted third molars are at risk for developing ameloblastomas or dentigerous cysts, if these teeth are not surgically removed, the impacted third molar (along with its opposing third molar) should be removed after it has been determined that eruption will not be possible,

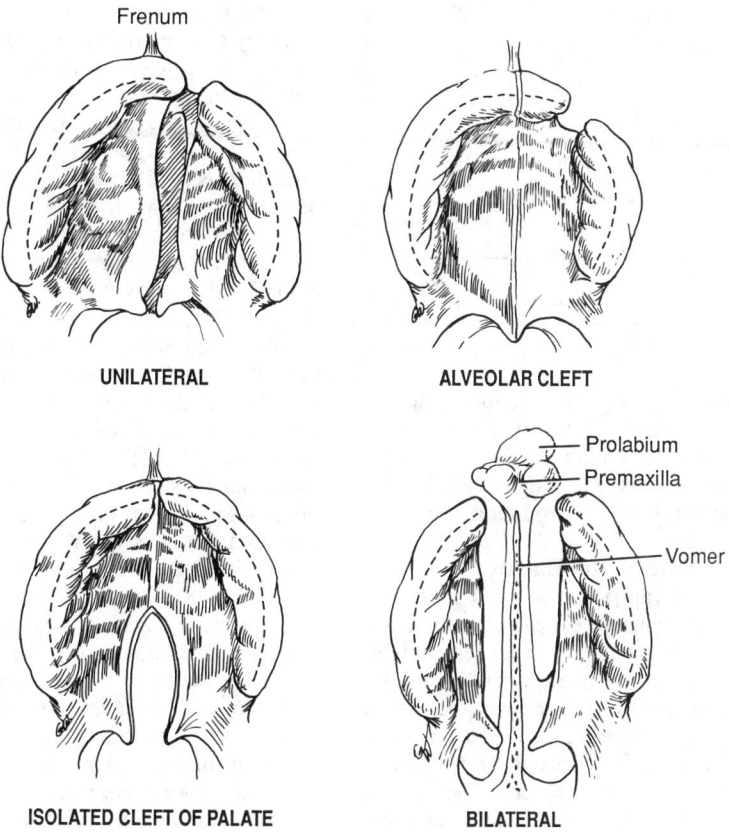

Figure 18–5. Types of clefts.

but this can sometimes not be assessed until the late teens. Maxillary canines, however, should not be extracted because of their aesthetic importance and key role in dental occlusion. They can often be brought into correct alignment through surgical exposure and orthodontic treatment.

E. Other Variations: Failure of teeth to develop– a condition sometimes called congenitally missing teeth—is quite rare in the primary dentition. How-

ever, it occurs in about 5% of permanent dentitions (exclusive of third molars), and one or more of the third molars is missing in about 25% of all individuals. The incidence of congenitally missing teeth varies among different genetic groups, but the most frequently missing are maxillary lateral incisors and mandibular second premolars.

Occasionally, there are extra teeth—most typically an extra (fourth) molar or extra (third) bicuspid.

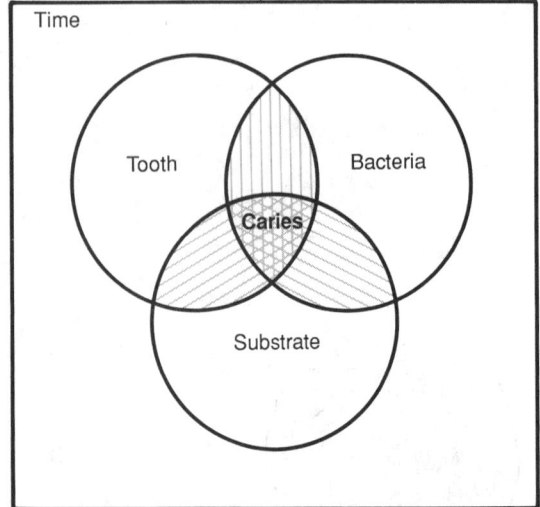

Figure 18–6. Conditions necessary for caries.

Mesiodentes, which are peg-shaped supernumerary teeth situated at the maxillary midline, are seen in about 5% of individuals and may interfere with eruption of permanent incisors. Mesiodentes should be considered for removal even if they do not erupt.

Dental Caries & Periodontal Disease

Once teeth begin to erupt, they are at risk for dental caries (decay). Parents must be educated about dental diseases and their causes and consequences. Almost all dental disease can be prevented, so the earlier the parents are indoctrinated, the better chance the child has to be disease-free. The best time to introduce the idea of oral hygiene is during prenatal care, followed by strong reinforcement after delivery. The current recommendation of the American Academy of Pediatric Dentistry is for children to have their first dental visit between 12 and 18 months of age.

Dental caries and periodontal disease are among the most common of all infectious diseases. They are also among the most easily preventable. Oral hygiene for the infant can start at birth. The gums can be gently cleaned with a moist soft cloth. Once the teeth begin to erupt, oral hygiene must be practiced in earnest. Again, a soft moist cloth can be used after feeding to gently rub the teeth. A very small, very soft toothbrush can be used as well. Toothpaste at the start is not necessary.

Figure 18–6 demonstrates the conditions that must be met for dental caries to start. Once teeth are present, they can be attacked by acidogenic bacteria, especially *Streptococcus mutans*. Dental plaque accumulates on the surface of the teeth as an adherent film. As plaque grows, bacteria accumulate within it in close proximity to the tooth. The third necessary ingredient is a substrate for the bacteria. In the case of dental caries, carbohydrate—especially refined carbohydrates such as sucrose—is the most active in that the bacteria metabolize sucrose and produce considerable acid as a by-product. This acid promptly reduces the oral pH. The acidic environment causes the enamel of the teeth to dissolve, which is the beginning of caries. Once the decay process has worked its way through the enamel, there is very little resistance to keep it from affecting the vital tissues (nerve) of the tooth. The tooth subsequently becomes necrotic, and an abscess occurs. Figure 18–7 demonstrates the progression of caries from the enamel through to the pulp and the subsequent formation of a dental abscess. This process is not always symptomatic, but it can lead to severe pain, fever, and swelling.

In the early stages of decay, the tooth may be sensitive to temperature changes or especially sweets. At this point, the tooth can be repaired by removing the caries and "filling" the defect. As the decay progresses, more pain may be involved, and generally one needs the equivalent of root canal therapy to save the tooth. Once there is an abscess, with or without swelling, a choice must be made between root canal therapy and removal of the tooth. In the presence of cellulitis or facial space abscess, extraction is usually the treatment of choice.

Many people will question the importance of the

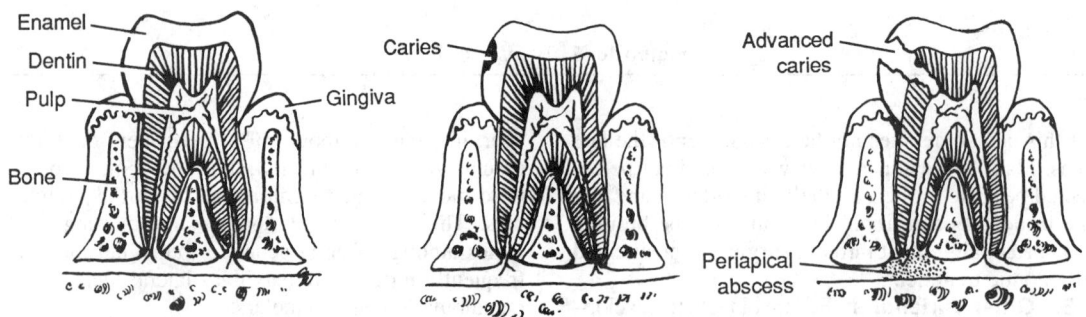

Figure 18–7. Tooth anatomy and progression of caries.

primary dentition. Baby teeth allow the child to eat properly, speak properly, have a good self-image, and preserve the space for the permanent dentition. Premature loss of primary teeth can cause major orthodontic and growth and development problems.

Preventing Dental Disease

To prevent dental caries, it is necessary to remove the bacteria on a regular basis. Brushing with a fluoride-containing toothpaste and flossing the teeth regularly (at least twice daily) will keep the oral flora to a minimum. A second step is to decrease the amount of substrate available to the bacteria. Limiting or eliminating refined carbohydrate is very effective (low sugar diets), as is limiting exposures to refined carbohydrates. The ideal schedule would be for a small "sugar" exposure at the end of each meal. The form of the substrate is important also. Caramels, licorice, raisins, gummy bears, etc, are concentrated sugar and because of their sticky texture will remain on the teeth for much longer than the same sugar in liquid form. The child's primary care physician can play an invaluable role in disseminating this information and reinforcing these ideas.

Fluoride

The final step in fighting the spread of dental caries is to strengthen the tooth. The addition of fluoride helps to create a more resistant tooth. Systemic fluoride, whether from water fluoridation or dietary supplementation, is incorporated into the crystalline structure of the enamel and creates a stronger, more acid-resistant covering. Topically applied fluoride is important in interfering with oral flora metabolism and in remineralizing early carious lesions. Table 18–1 demonstrates the current systemic fluoride dose recommended by the American Academy of Pediatrics and the American Academy of Pediatric Dentistry. It is important not to exceed these recommendations. To do so may lead to fluorosis, which is an unsightly staining of the permanent teeth.

Topical fluoride therapy is used in addition to all other oral hygiene measures in certain high-risk children. Children allowed to take their bottle to bed and those who nurse at will and fall asleep nursing are at risk for nursing bottle caries. This particular type of decay involves mostly the maxillary incisors. When a child is lying in bed sucking on a bottle, the contents of the bottle are "trapped" between the backs of the front teeth and the tongue. This allows for more concentrated damage to the teeth as the acid produced by bacteria fails to dissipate. In addition, as the child falls asleep, salivary function decreases dramatically. This further endangers the teeth by eliminating the buffering capacity of saliva and its remineralizing potential. Topical fluoride may slow the decay process. In combination with eliminating high-risk nursing practices and instituting good oral hygiene, these infants may avoid serious dental problems.

Patients with chronically low oral pH may benefit from topical fluoride. This includes those with gastroesophageal reflux, bulimia, or salivary dysfunction from radiation, graft-versus-host disease, or autoimmune disease. Saliva is the most effective oral cavity buffer there is. It also helps remineralize minor enamel dissolution. Xerostomia can lead to rampant caries. These children must have dental care more routinely than healthy children. Multiply handicapped children who cannot accomplish or receive proper oral hygiene can also benefit from additional topical fluoride.

Any child with a serious medical problem or handicapping condition should be referred to a pediatric dentist as early as possible.

Periodontal Disease

Periodontal disease is a problem with the supporting structures: bone, gums, and ligaments. It starts as an inflammation of the gum tissue adjacent to the tooth. Bacterial accumulation in the space between the tooth and gum (gingival sulcus) causes irritation that leads to inflamed tissue. This beginning phase is called gingivitis. As the inflammation spreads through the sulcus, there is more soft tissue involvement. Eventually, there is soft tissue destruction and loss of bone as disease spreads toward the apex of the tooth. This level of involvement is periodontitis and requires professional cleaning and often medication or surgery for correction. Figure 18–8 shows the different stages and progression of periodontal disease.

The prevention and initial management of periodontal disease in children involves the removal of bacteria from the teeth with proper oral hygiene.

Trauma

Managing orofacial trauma is a regular part of pediatric dentistry. Trauma often consists only of abrasions or lacerations of lips, gingiva, tongue, or mucosa, including frena, with no hard tissue damage. The lacerations should be cleansed and inspected for foreign bodies and sutured where appropriate. Occa-

Table 18–1. Fluoride dosages based on tap water fluoride supply.

Age (years)	Dose of Fluoride Administered (mg/d)	
	If <0.03 ppm F in Drinking Water	If 0.3–0.7 ppm F in Drinking Water[1]
Birth to age 2	0.25	Nil
2–3 years	0.5	0.25
3–13 years	1	0.5

[1]If there is >0.7 ppm F in drinking water, no supplement is needed.

Note: There is a reported risk of fluorosis associated with the above regimen; however, no consensus has been reached about revising it. Until that is done, practitioners can consider halving the fluoride dosage until age 6 for children who are considered at low risk for caries.

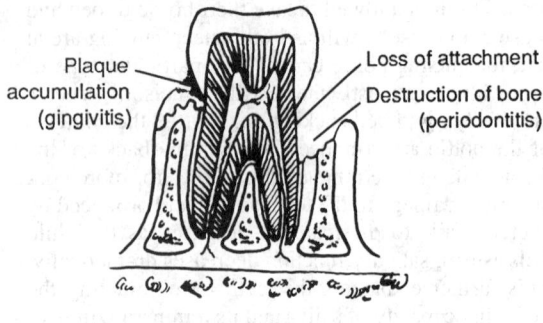

Figure 18–8. Periodontal disease.

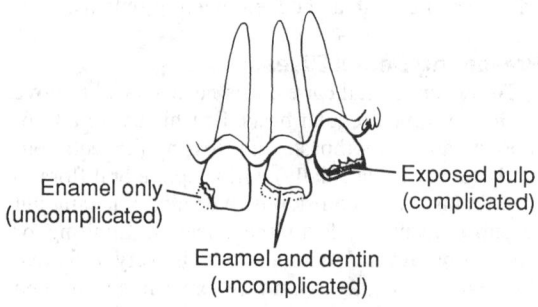

Figure 18–10. Patterns of crown fracture.

sionally, radiographs of the tongue, lips, or cheeks are used to look for tooth fragments or other foreign bodies.

Tooth-related trauma can consist of displacement (luxation), fracture, or loss of teeth (avulsion). Figure 18–9 demonstrates the different luxation injuries, and Figure 18–10 shows the different degrees of tooth fracture.

The most innocent luxation injury is mobility without displacement (subluxation). Unless mobility is extensive, this condition can be followed without active intervention. An intrusive luxation (Figure 18–9) in the primary dentition is usually observed for a period of time to discern whether the tooth or teeth in question will reerupt. If after several months this has not occurred or if the area becomes infected, the teeth are usually removed. There is a 30% chance of damage to the permanent teeth with any intrusive injury

of primary teeth. Permanent teeth intrusions are corrected with surgical or orthodontic repositioning of teeth and placement of a splint to stabilize the teeth. Stabilization is for 10–14 days. Root canal treatment may be necessary in the future. Lateral and extrusive luxations are generally repositioned and splinted also in permanent teeth. Severe luxations in any direction in primary teeth are treated with extraction.

Avulsed primary dentition is not replanted. The area is investigated for fractured roots or foreign bodies. Avulsed permanent teeth are gently cleansed and replanted with splinting. If replaced into the alveolar bone within an hour, these teeth have a good prognosis. The prognosis worsens rapidly with increased time outside of the mouth. Recent studies show that milk is the best storage and transport medium for avulsed teeth that will be replanted. Water, saline, and saliva can be used if milk is not accessible.

All luxated and replanted teeth need to be followed carefully and regularly by a dentist. These teeth can become abscessed or fused to the bone (ankylose) at any time during the healing process.

Fractured teeth should be seen promptly by a dentist. Many need to be protected quickly to avoid sensitivity, pain, or infection from exposed pulp. If the fractured tooth is severe enough, it may require immediate root canal surgery.

All facial trauma needs to be evaluated for jaw fracture. Blows to the chin are among the most common childhood oral-facial traumas. They are also a leading cause of condylar fracture in the pediatric population. One should be suspicious of pain or deviation when the jaw is opened.

Dental Emergencies

Dental emergencies other than trauma usually

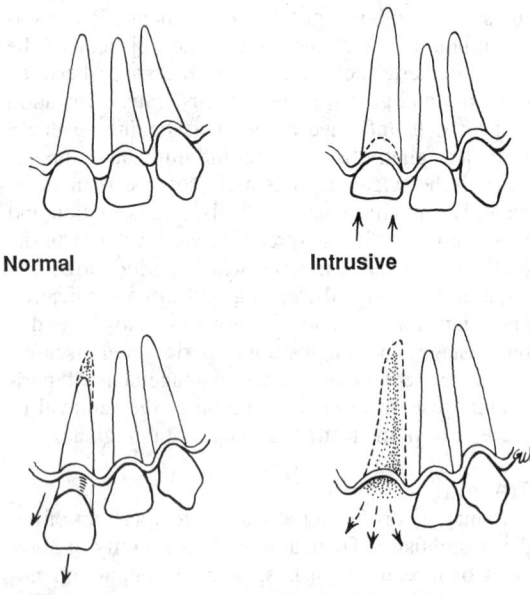

Figure 18–9. Patterns of luxation injuries.

present as pain or swelling due to advanced caries. Odontogenic pain usually responds to acetaminophen, ibuprofen, codeine, or, in severe cases, hydrocodone. As with teething, topical application of medicaments is of limited value.

Swelling confined to the gum tissue above or below the tooth is usually not an urgent situation. This "gumboil" or parulis represents infection that has spread outward from the root of the tooth through the bone and periosteum into the gum. Usually it will begin to drain and leave a fistulous tract. If the infection invades the facial spaces, cellulitis can occur. Swelling of the mid face, especially the bridge of the nose and the lower eyelid, is an urgent situation. All facial swelling needs to be evaluated by a dentist. Extraction of teeth or root canal therapy combined with antibiotics is the usual treatment. With extensive facial cellulitis, many young children will be admitted to hospital and managed with intravenous antibiotics.

Antibiotics in Pediatric Dentistry

Antibiotics of choice for odontogenic infection include penicillin G or V, or clindamycin for penicillin-allergic or refractory patients. When calculating the dose of oral antibiotics, one should keep in mind that penicillin and amoxicillin are only about 50% absorbed, so the dose should be chosen from the high end of the range. Intramuscular benzathine penicillin G is favored by many pediatric dentists because of the rapid rise in blood level that occurs with this preparation and the longer-acting feature.

Several patient groups require prophylactic antibiotic coverage prior to any invasive dental manipulation, including tooth cleaning. Cardiovascular patients at risk for subacute infective endocarditis are at the top of this list. The American Heart Association has made specific recommendations for premedication of cardiac patients. Immunosuppressed patients (oncology, HIV, posttransplant) also require coverage, as do children with indwelling central venous catheters. Patients with Broviac, Quinton, Hickman, etc, lines are routinely medicated prior to invasive dental treatment even though there are no reported dental-related catheter infections.

Children with a ventriculoperitoneal shunt may receive prophylaxis, though many practitioners refuse on the grounds that there is no circulatory connection to such a shunt and therefore no danger from bacteremia.

All of these children are premedicated using current American Heart Association guidelines. The most popular drug regimen is oral amoxicillin, 50 mg/kg 1 hour prior to appointment, followed by 25 mg/kg 6 hours later. Clindamycin is recommended for penicillin-allergic patients.

Selected orthopedic patients with prosthetic replacements will be "covered" with cephalosporins such as cephalexin, 1 g 1 hour before and 0.5 g 6 hours later. The dose is doubled at 60 lb.

The Pediatric Oncology Patient

The child with cancer needs to be evaluated by a dentist knowledgeable about pediatric oncology. The evaluation should be accomplished as soon after diagnosis and before chemotherapy as possible.

The aim of the consultation is to eliminate all existing and potential sources of infection before the child becomes neutropenic. Once chemotherapy begins, there is a brief interval before "counts" reach their nadir (7–10 days). Areas of concern to the dentist include abscessed teeth, teeth with extensive caries, soon to exfoliate teeth, ragged or broken teeth or fillings, and orthodontic appliances. Once the child becomes neutropenic, abscessed or infected or severely carious teeth can no longer be considered innocent, even if asymptomatic. Loose teeth that will soon exfoliate can also become a nidus for infection as well as a cause of bleeding if the patient becomes profoundly thrombocytopenic. Sharp, ragged teeth can be a source of irritation that can lead to infection. Chemotherapeutic drugs are cytotoxic to the oral mucosa. The oral mucosa becomes atrophic and ulcerates with ease (mucositis). This is painful and often leads to inadequate oral intake and nutrition. Once the mucosal barrier is breached by ulceration, the patient can become septic, especially with alpha-hemolytic streptococci and other mouth flora. Friction and damage to mucosa is the main concern with braces. Therefore, all orthodontic hardware is removed prior to chemotherapy.

The pediatric oncology patient should be monitored steadily during cancer therapy to screen for infection, manage oral bleeding, and control oral pain. These children can experience spontaneous oral hemorrhaging, especially when platelet counts are below 20,000/μL. Poor oral hygiene or areas of irritation can increase the chances of bleeding.

The child receiving radiation therapy to the head and neck is prone to develop extensive salivary dysfunction (xerostomia) if salivary tissue is in the path of the primary beam of radiation. This should be managed aggressively to avoid rapid extensive destruction of dentition. Customized fluoride applicators are used in this situation combined with close follow-up.

The child undergoing bone marrow transplantation must be similarly screened. These children may develop oral morbidity from an acute graft-versus-host reaction while they are in isolation before their marrow has become reconstituted. Long-term follow-up includes monitoring of growth, managing salivary dysfunction from total body radiation, and treatment of oral graft-versus-host disease.

The pediatric oncology patient also needs to be followed carefully after completion of therapy to manage oral and maxillofacial growth disturbances. Late effects of therapy are morphologic changes in tooth development (microdontia or extensive hypocalcification) and disturbances in eruption (no eruption, no root or delayed eruption). These side effects are seen in chemotherapy and radiation therapy patients, and must be managed by a dentist who is familiar with young children and their growth and development.

The Child With Hematologic Problems

The child with hemophilia needs to have "factor" levels managed before and after any invasive dental procedures (including the administration of local anesthesia, even for simple fillings). The rule of thumb is 50% of factor activity for factor VIII deficiency and 25% for factor IX. Some patients with very mild factor VIII or von Willebrand's disease may respond to desmopressin acetate. Antifibrinolytic medications such as aminocaproic acid or tranexamic acid are used successfully after dental treatment. Postoperative bleeding can also be treated with a wide variety of topical medicaments such as Gelfoam and thrombin.

Anticoagulant Therapy

The pediatric patient receiving anticoagulant therapy must undergo dosage adjustment before invasive dental treatment. This is a relatively simple matter when dealing with heparin, with its short half-life of 4–6 hours. It is a much more difficult problem with warfarin and its half-life of 40–70 hours.

Diabetic Patients

Children who are insulin-dependent are prone to problems with dental treatment. The diabetic child has a reduced capacity to heal, a higher incidence of periodontal disease, and a higher caries rate. These children need to be followed carefully managed on a routine basis. Care must be taken not to disturb the regular cycle of eating and insulin dosage. Anxiety associated with dental appointments can cause a major upset in the diabetic child's routine. Postoperative pain or pain from dental abscess can cause patients not to eat. Warning not to eat until the numbness wears off or until the filling gets hard can also create imbalances in the patients normal schedule of food intake and insulin dosage. Insulin levels must be adjusted to conform to treatment needs and vice versa. These children need to be monitored for hypoglycemic episodes as well as diabetic ketoacidosis.

HIV Infection

The child with HIV infection is especially prone to opportunistic infections, especially oral candidiasis. There may be recurrent bouts of major oral ulceration and extensive gingivitis, which could lead to problems with nutrition and infection.

Arthritis

The child with juvenile rheumatoid arthritis can have major disturbances in oral and maxillofacial growth. This is especially true if the temporomandibular joint is involved. These children may experience extensive growth retardation in the mandible and develop a decreased oral opening. Dental care can be very difficult to accomplish. The arthritic child's medication regimen must also be considered prior to invasive dental treatment. Methotrexate, because of its immune suppression, and aspirin and nonsteroidal anti-inflammatory agents, because they disturb platelet function, are of concern to the dental practitioner.

Renal Disease

The pediatric patient with chronic renal disease usually has a greatly decreased incidence of dental caries. This is presumably due to increased salivary urea concentration. There is, however, an increased incidence of enamel hypoplasia and xerostomia. Uremic stomatitis was once a prevalent finding in renal patients, but not now. Oral ecchymosis and petechiae are common. The renal transplant child must be managed in light of its immunosuppressed status and should be monitored for any signs of neoplasm secondary to his immunosuppression.

Reactive Airway Disease

The child with severe reactive airway disease can be a management problem for the dental practitioner. Managing behavior and medications are the two major concerns. The stress of an invasive dental procedure can trigger a reactive airway episode. The patient receiving multiple medications, including steroids, must be carefully managed through the stressful experience.

DENTAL REFERRAL

Referral to a dentist is appropriate whenever there is a question about a child's oral and maxillofacial health and development. Most pediatric dentists will want to see a child for a first visit between 12 and 18 months of age. The average child should be seen every 6 months for dental follow-up. This recommendation changes for any of the medically involved children whose problems are discussed in the text that precedes. They should be seen earlier and more frequently.

Close cooperation between physician and dentist can lead to improved outcomes for both the well child and the medically compromised child. Early intervention in the dental disease process will result in reduced morbidity and healthier children.

REFERENCES

Andreasen JO, Andreasen FM: *Essentials of Traumatic Injuries to the Teeth.* Munksgaard, 1990.

Bardach J, Morris, HL: *Multidisciplinary Management of Cleft Lip and Palate.* Saunders, 1990.

Brodsky L, Holt L, Ritter-Schmidt D: *Craniofacial Anomalies: An Interdisciplinary Approach.* Mosby Year Book, 1992.

Little JW, Falace D: *Dental Management of the Medically Compromised Patient,* 4th ed. Mosby Year Book, 1993.

Nelson JD: *Pocket Book of Pediatric Antimicrobial Therapy,* 9th ed. Williams & Wilkins, 1991.

Pinkham J: *Pediatric Dentistry.* Saunders, 1988.

Pizzo PA, Poplack DG: *Principles and Practice of Pediatric Oncology,* 2nd ed. Lippincott, 1993.

Proffit WR: *Contemporary Orthodontics,* 2nd ed. Mosby Year Book, 1993.

Redding SW, Montgomery M: *Dentistry in Systemic Disease.* JBK Publishing, 1990.

Rose LF, Kaye D: *Internal Medicine for Dentistry,* 2nd ed. Mosby, 1990.

Schluger S et al: *Periodontal Diseases.* Lea & Febiger, 1990.

Wei SHY: *Pediatric Dentistry.* Lea & Febiger, 1988.

19 Ear, Nose, & Throat

Stephen Berman, MD, & Barton D. Schmitt, MD

THE EAR: DISEASES & DISORDERS

OTITIS MEDIA

Otitis media, defined as an inflammation of the middle ear, is usually associated with an effusion or collection of fluid in the middle ear space. Otitis media is classified as acute, unresponsive, residual, persistent, or chronic according to its onset, response to therapy, duration, and complications. Each type of otitis media calls for a specific management plan. The term "acute otitis media" implies the onset of a new symptomatic infection. "Unresponsive otitis media" is characterized by continued tympanic membrane inflammation or acute symptoms despite initial antibiotic therapy. "Residual otitis media" is middle ear effusion without tympanic membrane inflammation or symptoms 3–6 weeks following initiation of antibiotic therapy for acute otitis media. "Persistent otitis media," sometimes referred to as otitis media with effusion, is the continued presence of a middle ear effusion 6 weeks or longer after initiation of antibiotic therapy. And the term "chronic otitis media" implies irreversible damage to middle ear structures. At the 3-week posttherapy visit for acute otitis media, resolution will be documented in approximately 50% of cases; 40% will have residual otitis media; and 10% with have unresponsive otitis media. Approximately 75% of cases of residual otitis media resolve spontaneously during the subsequent 4–6 weeks. The incidence and prevalence of asymptomatic middle ear effusions that are residual or persistent has been studied with tympanometry in Europe. During 1 year of observation, 42% of 3-year-olds develop an effusion. At any point in time, 20% of 2-year-olds have an effusion, of which half are persistent, lasting longer than 6 weeks. Classification based on the type of effusion (purulent, serous, or mucoid) has little clinical relevance, since it is often difficult to distinguish the type of effusion with otoscopy, and bacterial pathogens are frequently isolated from all three types of effusion.

In one clinical practice study, about one-third of the pediatrician's visits with sick children was spent in the diagnosis and management of otitis media. The National Center for Health Statistics reports that the percent of total (sick and preventive) office visits with a diagnosis of otitis media in 1990 for children 5 years and under was 18%. The annual visit rate for otitis media in children under 2 years of age was 102.1 per 100 children per year. In Boston, the incidence of otitis media in a cohort of children followed from birth was 1.3 episodes per child year during the first 2 years of life. By the time children reach 3 years of age, more than two-thirds of them have experienced one episode of otitis media and one-third have had three or more episodes. More children present with otitis media in the winter months, when respiratory syncytial virus and other viruses are present in the community. These upper respiratory tract infections adversely affect auditory tube (eustachian tube) function and predispose the child to middle ear inflammation. Since young children have shorter, more compliant, and more horizontally placed auditory tubes than older children and adults, colds in young patients will produce more severe auditory tube dysfunction. This dysfunction prevents middle ear secretions from draining and results in negative pressure in the middle ear space. Negative pressure predisposes the patient to periodic aspiration of contaminated nasopharyngeal secretions, which causes bacterial infection.

Specific conditions that cause auditory tube dysfunction and predispose children to recurrent or persistent otitis media include frequent viral upper respiratory tract infections, allergic and vasomotor rhinitis, trisomy 21, cystic fibrosis, hypothyroidism, and anatomic abnormalities such as cleft palate, obstructing adenoids, and nasopharyngeal tumors. Bottle feeding or propping, passive exposure to smoking, and day care outside the home also predispose children to recurrent or persistent otitis media. Infants who experience an initial episode of otitis media in the first 2 or 3 months of life are more likely to have recurrent or chronic otitis media during the first year. The main reason to treat children with recurrent acute otitis or persistent asymptomatic middle ear effusions is to restore normal hearing in order to promote language development and reduce the risk of behavior problems. Persistent effusions do not predispose to conditions such as retraction pockets, adhesive otitis, cholesteatoma, tympanic membrane atrophy, or tympanosclerosis. It is unclear whether fluctuating or long-term mild conductive hearing impairment during specific vulnerable age periods adversely impacts language development, behavior, and subsequent academic functioning. Lack of evidence establishing a causal relationship means that management guidelines should be flexible and take into account parental as well as physician preferences. Furthermore, the lack of conclusive evidence of a causal link because of insufficient data does not mean that such a link does not exist.

The diagnosis of otitis media with effusion is based on specific otoscopic findings, which include the appearance of the tympanic membrane and an assessment of its mobility. In recent years, tympanometry has also become a useful technique in documenting middle ear effusions in children and infants older than 7 months. Unfortunately, this procedure does not identify early acute otitis media prior to the development of an effusion and does not differentiate unresponsive from residual otitis media. In pediatric practice, tympanometry is useful for screening patients uncooperative to examination, clarifying questionable otoscopic findings, and providing an objective measurement that can be used to follow the course of persistent effusions. Otoscopy and tympanometry are discussed on p 445.

Dempster JH, MacKenzie K: Tympanometry in the detection of hearing impairments associated with otitis media with effusion. Clin Otolaryngol 1991;16:157.

Paradise JL: Does early-life otitis media result in lasting developmental impairment? Why the question persists, and a proposed plan for addressing it. Adv Pediatr 1992;39:157.

Schappert SM: Office visits for otitis media: United States, 1975–90. In: *Advance Data From Vital and Health Statistics.* Centers for Disease Control/National Center for Health Statistics, 1992.

Teele DW et al: Epidemiology of otitis media during the first seven years of life in children in Greater Boston: A prospective, cohort study. J Infect Dis 1989;160:83.

Teele DW et al: Otitis media in infancy and intellectual ability, school achievement, speech, and language at 7 years. J Infect Dis 1990;162:685.

Zielhuis GM et al: The prevalence of otitis media with effusion: A critical review of the literature. Clin Otolaryngol 1990;15:283.

1. ACUTE OTITIS MEDIA

Essentials of Diagnosis

- Recent onset
- Red or yellow, immobile tympanic membrane
- Ear discharge
- Earache

General Considerations

Bacteriologic findings in middle ear aspirates from Denver, Colorado, can be summarized as follows: *Streptococcus pneumoniae,* 42% of cases; *Haemophilus influenzae,* 41%; *Moraxella catarrhalis,* 9%; *Streptococcus pyogenes,* 2%; *Staphylococcus aureus,* 4%; and others (including enteric gram-negative organisms and anaerobic organisms), 2%. In 21% of cases, aspirates are sterile or grow presumed nonpathogens such as *Staphylococcus epidermidis* and diphtheroids. In about 10% of cases, multiple pathogens are isolated from a single middle ear aspirate. In children with bilateral acute otitis media, different pathogens can be recovered from each ear in 5–10% of cases. *S pneumoniae* is uniformly the most common pathogen throughout the country. *M catarrhalis* has become more frequently recognized as a causative agent of acute otitis media. *H influenzae* remains an important pathogen throughout childhood and into early adulthood. In Colorado, 25% of the pathogens are β-lactamase producers resistant to penicillins, while 6% are resistant to trimethoprim-sulfamethoxazole. In many areas, the prevalence of β-lactamase-producing isolates for *H influenzae* is greater than 30%; that for *M catarrhalis* and *S aureus* is 80% or higher. The problem of *S pneumoniae* resistance to trimethoprim-sulfamethoxazole and amoxicillin is also becoming more widespread.

The microbiologic causes of acute otitis media in early infancy differ from those in later life. The risk of gram-negative enteric infection is especially high in infants who are under 6 weeks of age and have been or are hospitalized in a neonatal intensive care nursery. In normal infants seen during the first 3 months of life, acute otitis media is caused by *S aureus* and *Chlamydia trachomatis* as well as *S pneumoniae, H influenzae,* and *M catarrhalis.*

Studies using antigen detection or culture of middle ear aspirates in cases of acute otitis media identify a virus in 16% of cases; 10% have mixed viral and bacterial isolates; and 6% have only viral isolates. It remains unclear whether viruses are the primary cause of acute otitis media or whether they promote bacterial superinfection by impairing auditory tube function and other host immune and nonimmune defenses. The presence of virus in the middle ear space may compromise eradication of bacterial pathogens by antibiotics and predispose to unresponsive otitis media.

Clinical Findings

A. Symptoms and Signs: Acute otitis media often presents with ear pain in association with symptoms of upper respiratory tract infection (eg, rhinorrhea, stuffy nose, and cough) or purulent conjunctivitis. While older children may complain of earache, young children demonstrate pain by crying, increased irritability, and difficulty in sleeping or feeding. Irritability may be related to hearing loss as well as pain.

Tugging at the ears is a nonspecific symptom that is not useful in identifying cases of acute otitis media. Fever is present in less than half the cases. Facial palsy or ataxia may occur on rare occasions.

The tympanic membrane appears either red or yellow, depending on the degree of inflammation and the amount of purulent material in the middle ear space. White exudate may be visible on the membrane. In early cases, bulging may be limited to the pars flaccida. Later, the entire eardrum bulges outward, giving a doughnut-like appearance. Tympanic membrane mobility is absent or markedly diminished. If the eardrum has spontaneously ruptured, cloudy to purulent discharge will be present in the ear canal, making examination of the tympanic membrane difficult. Cerumen that has melted with high fever or tears present in the ear canal can cause confusion with middle ear discharge. Occasionally, bullae form between the outer and middle layers of the tympanic membrane and produce acute bullous myringitis. This entity should be considered a form of acute otitis media caused by the same pathogens.

B. Laboratory findings: Nasopharyngeal and throat cultures are not useful because *S pneumoniae* and nontypable *H influenzae* are often present in well children and thus are of no significance. If perforation has occurred, it may be useful to culture the discharge, using a nasopharyngeal culture swab. If the discharge has been present for over 8 hours, the likelihood of demonstrating the pathogen is small because it frequently is overgrown with saprophytes.

Beyond the neonatal period, acute otitis media infrequently presents with signs of systemic toxicity; therefore, blood cultures, urine culture, and lumbar puncture are indicated in the child with acute otitis media who also appears toxic or shows signs of meningeal irritation. The likelihood of occult bacteremia in a febrile infant or young child is not altered by the presence or absence of acute otitis media.

Differential Diagnosis

Not all earaches are caused by acute otitis media. Mumps, toothache, otitis externa, a foreign body in the ear canal, an ear canal furuncle, ear canal trauma, hard cerumen, and temporomandibular joint dysfunction can all present with a chief complaint of earache. Injected vessels at the drum periphery and along the malleus are frequently overdiagnosed as "early otitis media." An infected-appearing tympanic membrane as well as a flushed face can occur with fever or crying. Cleaning wax from the ear canal can cause reactive hyperemia of the same vessels. Such an eardrum may be red, but it will be mobile and not require treatment. Because acute otitis media is the most common complication of a cold, an infant with a cold and fever should never be sent home without having submitted to examination of the eardrums. Cerumen removal (see below) will often be necessary for this purpose.

Complications

The most common complication associated with acute otitis media is a hearing loss of 20–35 dB, which may persist for several months. The tympanic membrane may rupture spontaneously because of pressure necrosis and produce a sizable perforation. Acute otitis media may also cause labyrinthitis with ataxia, facial paralysis, cholesteatoma, mastoiditis, ossicular necrosis, pseudotumor cerebri (otitic hydrocephalus), or cerebral thrombophlebitis.

Treatment

An algorithm for the management of acute otitis media is presented in Figure 19–1.

A. Specific Measures:

1. Systemic antibiotics–In areas where β-lactamase-producing pathogens are common, the initial treatment for otitis media should be 10 days of oral trimethoprim, 10 mg/kg/d, with sulfamethoxazole, 40 mg/kg/d, in two divided doses. The same holds true for children with associated purulent conjunctivitis, since in these children the organism is usually *H influenzae*. Otherwise, the drug of choice for acute otitis media in children of all ages is amoxicillin, 50 mg/kg/d orally in three divided doses, continued for 10 days. If symptoms persist beyond 48 hours of therapy, the patient should be reevaluated for an associated infection (eg, meningitis) versus and unresponsive otitis media.

Clinical trials comparing commonly prescribed antibiotics have documented similar cure rates in acute otitis media for amoxicillin, trimethoprim-sulfamethoxazole, erythromycin plus sulfisoxazole, amoxicillin plus clavulanate, and third-generation cephalosporins. While many cases of acute otitis media will clinically resolve without any therapy, recent work suggests that antibiotic treatment, especially in cases with high fever or earache, is more effective than placebo therapy. The use of amoxicillin or trimethoprim-sulfamethoxazole as first-line therapy is based primarily on cost and safety considerations. A 10-day course of antibiotic is current standard practice. However, it is possible that 5 days may be as effective as 10 days in the absence of a tympanic membrane perforation with drainage.

Tetracyclines are contraindicated for ear infections because about 50% of pneumococci and streptococci are resistant to these drugs and because they cause staining of the tooth enamel. Trimethoprim prescribed in combination with sulfamethoxazole is not effective against *S pyogenes* and should not be used if streptococcal pharyngitis is suspected.

Acute otitis media in infants less than 6 weeks of age with a complicated neonatal course requiring prolonged hospitalization is often caused by gram-negative enteric organisms. These infants require tympanocentesis, blood culture, and lumbar puncture and should receive intravenous ampicillin plus either gentamicin or cefotaxime in the hospital pending cul-

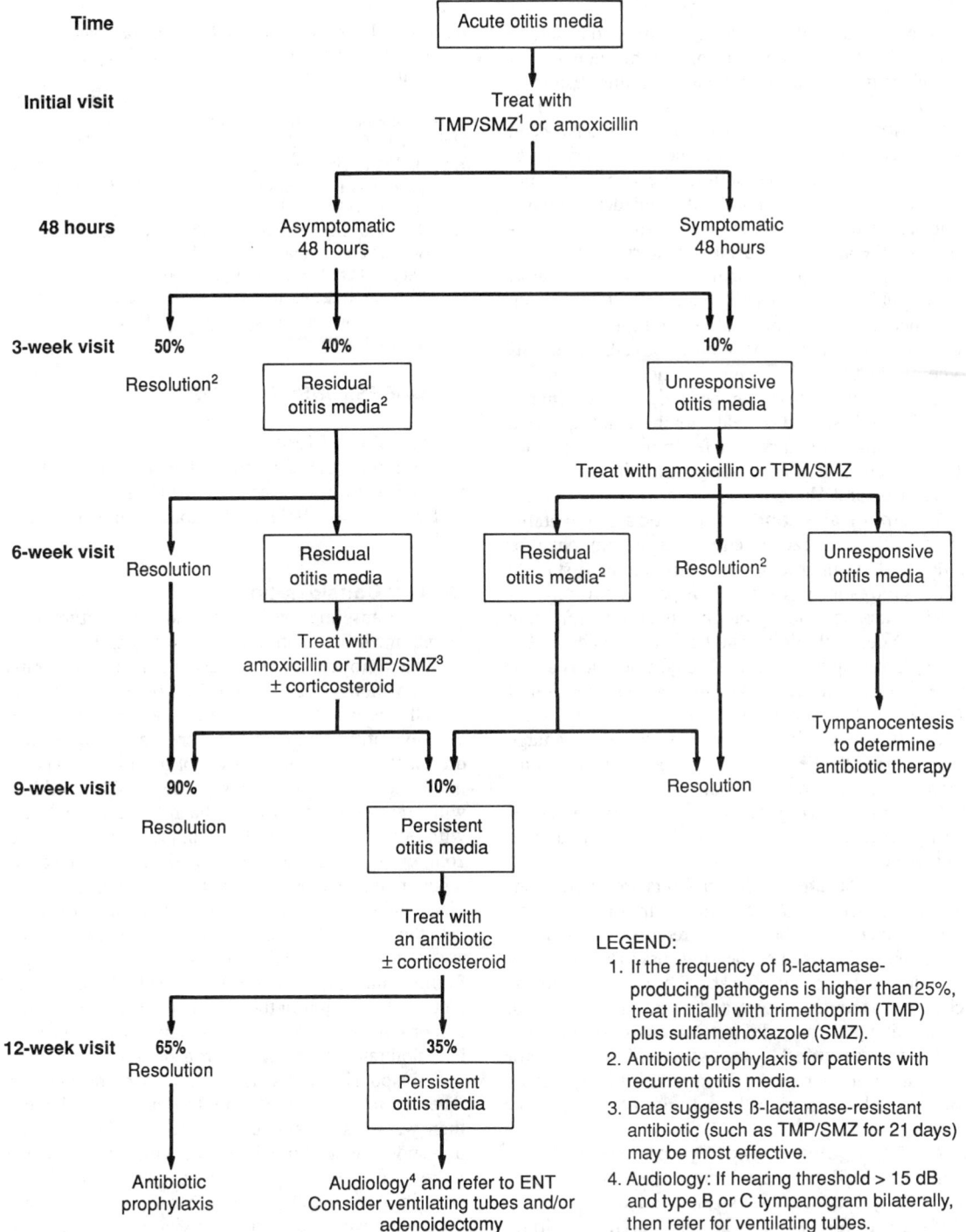

Figure 19–1. Algorithm for the management of otitis media. For prophylaxis in children with recurrent acute otitis media, see text.

ture results. Acute otitis media in infants under 3 months without additional risk factors or signs of serious illness can be treated on an outpatient basis. Because of a higher frequency of *S aureus* and perhaps *Chlamydia,* consider treatment with erythromycin plus sulfamethoxazole. Alternatives include third-generation cephalosporins or amoxicillin plus clavulanate (Augmentin). These children should be reexamined at 24 and 48 hours. If their condition worsens during this time period, they should be hospitalized. Infants who present with systemic symptoms or who fail to respond to outpatient management require tympanocentesis, blood culture, and usually a lumbar puncture. Ampicillin plus either gentamicin or cefotaxime should be initiated pending results of culture.

2. Antibiotic ear drops–If the eardrum has been perforated, there is usually a cloudy to watery material in the ear canal, and antibiotic ear drops are not required. However, the child with considerable purulent drainage from the ear may profit from this adjunctive therapy. The purulent material can be removed by gentle suction, using a syringe and a short plastic tubing such as can be made by cutting a scalp vein needle set. Normal saline solution can be instilled without force and then removed. After this type of cleansing has eliminated the pus, antibiotic-corticosteroid ear drops can be instilled three times a day. The child should be held with the head supported sideways and stationary for a few minutes after drops are instilled. Cotton plugs are contraindicated.

B. General Measures:

1. Analgesics and antipyretics–An irritable child with an earache requires acetaminophen or rarely codeine in order to sleep through the first night while on treatment. However, if pain is severe, consider tympanocentesis or myringotomy for pain relief. Young children can be given codeine, 0.5 mg/kg/dose, up to four times a day. Codeine is available in several cough medicines in a concentration of 10 mg/tsp. Antipyretics for fever control may be required for the relief of pain and have the disadvantage of obscuring the field of vision if the tympanic membrane needs to be reexamined.

2. Oral decongestants–Antihistamine-decongestant combinations are ineffective in the treatment of acute otitis media.

3. Reassurance–Some patients are overly concerned about ear infections and their complications. Reassurance should be given as required. There is little danger of permanent hearing loss. The child can be allowed to go outside, and the ears need not be covered. Mountain travel and flying are permitted. Swimming is permitted if perforation is not present.

4. Unwarranted measures–Vasoconstrictor nose drops are of no value because it is nearly impossible to deliver them to the entrance of the auditory tube.

C. Myringotomy and Tympanocentesis: A common pitfall in therapy is not performing myringotomy or tympanocentesis when it is indicated (see p 445). In a child with an acutely bulging eardrum, myringotomy is indicated if the patient has severe pain (as evidenced by inconsolable screaming) or if recurrent vomiting or ataxia is associated with the ear infection. In these circumstance, myringotomy is more effective than analgesics or antiemetics. Unfortunately, myringotomy does not appear to prevent the development of residual or persistent otitis media.

Berman S, Roark R: Factors influencing outcome in children treated with antibiotics for acute otitis media. Pediatr Infect Dis J 1993;12:20-4.

Hendricks WA et al: Five vs. ten days of therapy for acute otitis media. Pediatr Infect Dis 1988;7:14.

Howie VM: Otitis media. Pediatr Rev 1993;14:320.

Kaleida PH et al: Amoxicillin or myringotomy or both for acute otitis media: Results of a randomized clinical trial. Pediatrics 1991;87:466.

Le CT: Choosing an antibiotic: Efficacy, side effects and cost. Contemp Pediatr 1991;8:11.

Marchant CD et al: Measuring the comparative efficacy of antibacterial agents for acute otitis media: The "Pollyanna phenomenon." J Pediatr 1992;120:72.

2. UNRESPONSIVE OTITIS MEDIA

Essentials of Diagnosis

- Antibiotic treatment longer than 48 hours
- Persistent fever, earache, or irritability
- Red or yellow bulging, immobile tympanic membrane

General Considerations

Symptoms and otoscopic findings of tympanic membrane inflammation that persist after 48 hours of initial antibiotic therapy represent unresponsive otitis media, which occurs in about 10% of children treated initially with a 10-day course of antibiotics. Unresponsive otitis media occurs more frequently in children with a history of recurrent otitis or infection during the winter season. The majority (57%) of children with unresponsive otitis media following treatment with either amoxicillin, trimethoprim-sulfamethoxazole, or erythromycin plus sulfisoxazole have sterile repeat middle ear aspirates at the 3-week posttherapy visit. Therefore, failure of antibiotic therapy to eradicate the pathogen is not the usual cause of unresponsive otitis media. Persistent symptoms and otoscopic findings may be related to the effects of a concomitant viral infection in the middle ear space, since unresponsive otitis media is associated with high viral isolation rates from middle ear aspirates.

Unresponsive otitis media is also more common when antibiotic therapy fails to eradicate pathogens than when pathogens are eradicated. Children with unresponsive otitis media treated with amoxicillin are more likely to have β-lactamase-producing pathogens in a posttherapy middle ear aspirate than children who respond to initial amoxicillin treatment. Organisms sensitive to initial therapy are identified in 24% of posttherapy aspirates. Organisms resistant to initial therapy are identified in 19% of posttherapy aspirates. Eradication of a middle ear pathogen with antibiotic therapy is less likely after 2–4 days when a virus and bacteria are both isolated from a middle ear aspirate than when bacteria are isolated alone.

Treatment

A. Medical Treatment: Children who remain febrile and appear toxic despite 48 hours of antibiotic therapy for acute otitis media should be evaluated for associated occult infection and hospitalized for treatment with intravenous cefotaxime or ceftriaxone pending the results of cultures.

Unresponsive otitis media in the nontoxic child initially treated with trimethoprim-sulfamethoxazole should be treated with amoxicillin, and vice versa. The sequential administration of amoxicillin and trimethoprim-sulfamethoxazole provides excellent coverage for resistant pathogens. Trimethoprim-sulfamethoxazole covers β-lactamase-producing organisms resistant to amoxicillin such as *H influenzae, M catarrhalis,* and *S aureus,* while amoxicillin covers organisms resistant to trimethoprim-sulfamethoxazole such as *S pyogenes, group B streptococci,* enterococci, and resistant *S pneumoniae.* Third-generation cephalosporins, amoxicillin plus clavulanate, and erythromycin plus sulfamethoxazole offer minimal advantages in terms of coverage of resistant organisms. They are most useful as second-line antibiotics for children who are allergic to either amoxicillin or trimethoprim-sulfisoxazole. If the physician is concerned about compliance, the patient can be treated with an intramuscular injection of ceftriaxone or penicillin G benzathine and procaine combined (Bicillin C-R) and oral sulfisoxazole.

B. Surgical Treatment: If unresponsive otitis media still persists after a second course of antibiotics, myringotomy or tympanocentesis should be performed and the middle ear aspirate cultured to determine the most appropriate antibiotic therapy. Failure of unresponsive otitis media to resolve following a third course of antibiotic therapy based on culture results is an indication for referral to an otolaryngologist.

Arola M, Ziegler T, Ruushanen O: Respiratory virus infection as a cause of prolonged symptoms in acute otitis media. J Pediatr 1990;116:697.

Carlin SA et al: Host factors and early therapeutic response in acute otitis media. J Pediatr 1991;118:178.

Chonmaitree T et al: Effect of viral respiratory tract infection on outcome of acute otitis media. J Pediatr 1992;120:856.

Green SM, Rothrock SG: Single-dose intramuscular ceftriaxone for acute otitis media in children. Pediatrics 1993;91:23.

Ruuskanen O et al: Viruses in acute otitis media: Increasing evidence for clinical significance. Pediatr Infect Dis J 1991;10:425.

Teele DE et al: Bacteriology of acute otitis media unresponsive to initial antimicrobial therapy. J Pediatr 1981;98:537.

3. RESIDUAL OTITIS MEDIA

Essential of Diagnosis

- Middle ear effusion present 3–6 weeks after initial course of antibiotic therapy.
- Air-fluid levels or bubbles.
- Retracted tympanic membrane.
- Diminished or absent tympanic membrane mobility.
- Type B or C tympanogram (Figure 19–3).
- Hearing threshold 15 dB or higher.

General Considerations

Residual otitis media following appropriate antibiotic therapy for acute otitis media occurs in 40% of children. These middle ear effusions clear spontaneously within 6 weeks in 75–85% of cases. Residual otitis media results when the auditory tube fails to clear the effusion present in the middle ear space following antibiotic treatment of acute otitis media. The effusion is usually serous, resembling serum transudate, and histopathologic examination of the middle ear shows subepithelial edema. The effusion is usually associated with a low-grade (15- to 20-dB) conductive hearing loss.

Clinical Findings

Children with residual otitis media are usually asymptomatic and have a mild hearing loss. The patient may complain of fullness in the ear. An older patient may compare the feeling with "talking inside a barrel." In the preverbal child, hearing loss should be suspected if irritability, inattentiveness, or increased behavior problems are noted. Unlike acute otitis media, there is minimal pain.

The tympanic membrane may appear mildly injected and dull or may have a normal appearance. Mobility is diminished or absent. When fluid levels or air bubbles are visualized, the effusion is in a stage of resolution, with auditory tube function improving. When auditory tube dysfunction results in persistent negative pressure in the middle ear space, the tympanic membrane appears retracted, and the position of the short process of the *right* malleus changes from the 7 o'clock to the 9 o'clock position. Tympanic membrane mobility is altered, and the membrane may move only when negative pressure is applied.

The presence of auditory tube dysfunction and middle ear effusion predisposes the child to another episode of acute otitis media. In some children with recurrent otitis media, an effusion persists in the middle ear between episodes and a cycle of acute otitis media alternates with residual otitis media.

Treatment

Management of residual otitis media is outlined in Figure 19–1. When residual otitis media is present 3 weeks after initial antibiotic therapy, one should follow the patient without administering additional antibiotics. If the effusion is still present after another 3 weeks, the otitis can be considered persistent and requires further antibiotic treatment as outlined below.

Oral decongestants and antihistamines have not been shown to be effective in preventing or clearing residual otitis media.

Mandel EM et al: Efficacy of amoxicillin with and without decongestant antihistamine for otitis media with effusion in children. N Engl J Med 1987;316:432.

Teele DW, Klein JO, Rosner B: Epidemiology of otitis media during the first seven years of life in children in greater Boston: A prospective, cohort study. J Infect Dis 1989;160:83.

4. PERSISTENT OTITIS MEDIA OR OTITIS MEDIA WITH EFFUSION

Essentials of Diagnosis

- Middle ear effusion present 6 weeks or longer posttherapy.
- Dull, opaque tympanic membrane.
- Diminished or absent tympanic membrane mobility.
- Type B or C tympanogram (Figure 19–3).
- Hearing threshold 20 dB or higher.

General Considerations

Children with middle ear effusions that fail to resolve with antibiotics during a 6-week time period can be considered to have persistent otitis media. The rate of spontaneous resolution of middle ear effusions present at the 6-week follow-up visit is approximately 50% every 3 months during the subsequent year. In about 5% of ears the effusion will persist longer than one year.

The majority of effusions in persistent otitis media are mucoid; about 10% are serous and less than 10% purulent. However, middle ear aspirates of persistent otitis media often grow pathogenic organisms. The most common pathogens isolated from these effusions are H influenzae (15% of cases), M catarrhalis (9%), and S pyogenes (1%). Most strains of H influenzae and M catarrhalis are β-lactamase-positive. S epidermidis and diphtheroids are isolated in 33% of effusions. Evidence supporting the pathogenic role of these organisms includes the findings of type-specific antibody in middle ear fluid; studies in animals also suggest that the middle ear space should be sterile.

Antibiotic treatment of acute otitis media that results in a good clinical response may not correlate well with eradication of organisms. Ongoing low-grade bacterial infection of the middle ear space may persist and evoke local accumulation of lymphocytes and macrophages. Antibody production, complement activation, and release of chemical mediators may all occur. The mediators, together with bacterial products such as endotoxin and neuraminidase, cause tis-

sue edema, increased capillary leakage, and hemorrhage. In addition, the mediators stimulate the formation of goblet cells in the respiratory epithelium and these cells produce excessive secretions. The inflammatory response or bacterial toxins may destroy a surfactant-like substance present on the inner surface of the auditory tube, thereby reducing surface tension and predisposing the auditory tube to collapse.

Clinical Findings

Patients with persistent otitis media usually are asymptomatic or complain of a feeling of fullness in the ear. The tympanic membrane commonly appears dull and opaque; in severe cases, it may have a bluish tint. Tympanic membrane mobility is usually markedly diminished. Half of children with a persistent middle ear effusion have a hearing threshold of 25 dB or higher.

Complications

Children with persistent otitis media are at increased risk of developing retraction pockets, which predispose them to cholesteatoma and other complications such as erosion of the ossicles.

Treatment

The clinician can choose one of several management options to treat asymptomatic effusions that have persisted for 6–9 weeks: corticosteroid plus antibiotic, antibiotic alone, or observation without additional therapy. Available data suggest that the most cost-effective therapy is to administer corticosteroid (prednisone, 1 mg/kg/d in two divided doses) for 7 days combined with an antibiotic (trimethoprim-sulfamethoxazole, 1 mL/kg/d in two divided doses, or an alternative) for 21 days. Children without a history of varicella who have been exposed in the prior month should not receive prednisone because of the potential risk of disseminated disease if they are receiving corticosteroid therapy. Prednisone's side effects are similar to those noted in treating asthmatic episodes with short steroid courses: in rare cases, marked behavioral changes; occasionally, vomiting or increased appetite. If the patient clears the persistent middle ear effusion bilaterally, consider following the patient monthly and administering low-dose antibiotic prophylaxis with amoxicillin, 20 mg/kg/d in one or two doses, or sulfisoxazole, 75 mg/kg/d in one or two doses, for 3 months to prevent a recurrence of otitis media with effusion. If the patient is not clear bilaterally, consider treatment with another antibiotic. Consider low-dose prophylaxis for patients who, following this therapy, have cleared the persistent middle ear effusion bilaterally or still have a unilateral effusion with hearing intact on one side. When a bilateral effusion with hearing loss persists 12 weeks or longer despite this management, consider referral to an otolaryngologist for placement of ventilating tubes. However, prior to referral, obtain audiology testing to document a bilateral hearing loss (a hearing threshold > 15 dB) and assess the child for any behavioral difficulties such as easy distractibility or short attention span or developmental delays in language. The timing to place ventilating tubes in a child with a bilateral hearing loss should be individualized some time between 3 and 6 months depending on the child's developmental and behavioral status and the parents' preference.

The goal of surgical intervention in the management of persistent effusions is improvement in hearing. Appropriate interventions include myringotomy with ventilating tubes, adenoidectomy (only for children older than 4 years), or a combination of the two. Tonsillectomy alone or in combination with other surgical procedures offers no benefit and should not be performed.

The mean improvement in hearing by ventilation tubes or adenoidectomy compared with control therapy (observation) is about 12 dB 6 months post surgery and slightly less than 6 dB 12 months post surgery. The advantages of ventilating tubes over adenoidectomy are (1) the immediate clearing of fluid and improvement in hearing; (2) lower risks of complications particularly hemorrhage; and (3) lower cost. Disadvantages are (1) a spontaneous tube extrusion rate of 15–30% within 6 months, (2) tympanosclerosis, (3) bacterial infection at the site of the tube, and (4) higher risks of chronic perforation and subsequent cholesteatoma. The effect of tympanosclerosis, produced by a foreign body reaction to the tube, on hearing later in life is unclear. Fifteen years after surgery, 50% of patients have tympanosclerosis, but hearing remains normal. Data are not available on the hearing effects of tympanosclerosis after 15 years. In general, adenoidectomy should be considered in children older than 4 years who have required multiple tube reinsertions. Unfortunately, it is difficult to predict who will obtain the most benefit from adenoidectomy, as neither adenoidal size nor symptoms of obstruction are useful predictors. Therefore, guidelines for the surgical management of persistent otitis should be individualized, and one should solicit parental and, if appropriate, patient preferences.

Berman S, Roark R, Luckey D: Theoretical cost effectiveness of management options for children with persisting middle ear effusions. [Accepted for publication in Pediatrics, July, 1993.]

Dowell SF, Bresee JS: Severe varicella associated with steroid use. Pediatrics 1993;92:223.

Rosenfield RM et al: Systematic steroids for otitis media with effusion in children. Arch Otolaryngol Head Neck Surg 1991;117:984.

Rosenfield RM, Post JC: Meta-analysis of antibiotics for the treatment of otitis media with effusion. Arch Otolaryngol Head Neck Surg 1992;106:378.

Zielhuis GM et al: Analysis and presentation of data on the natural course of otitis media with effusion in children. Int J Epidemiol 1990;19:1037.

5. CHRONIC OTITIS MEDIA

Chronic otitis media is an appropriate diagnosis when irreversible damage to middle ear structures has occurred. Damage includes retraction pockets, adhesive otitis, atrophy or perforation of the tympanic membrane, cholesteatoma, cholesterol granuloma formation, and erosion of ossicles.

Clinical Findings

Otoscopic examination can identify damage to the middle ear structures. Tympanosclerosis is caused by chronic inflammation or trauma that produces granulation tissue, hyalinization, and calcification. The appearance of a small defect in the posterior superior area of the pars tensa or in the pars flaccida suggests a retraction pocket. Retraction pockets occur when chronic inflammation and negative pressure in the middle ear space produce atrophy and atelectasis of the tympanic membrane. Continued inflammation can cause adhesions between the retraction pocket and the ossicles. This condition, referred to as adhesive otitis, predisposes to formation of a cholesteatoma or fixation and erosion of the ossicles. Erosion of the ossicles results from osteitis and compromise of the blood supply. Ossicular discontinuity produces a severe hearing loss with a threshold of 25–50 dB. A tympanogram with very high compliance indicates ossicular discontinuity. The presence of a greasy-looking mass or debris seen in a retraction pocket or perforation suggests cholesteatoma regardless of the presence of discharge. The size of the perforation does not correlate with the extent of the cholesteatoma.

Treatment

Corrective surgery will be necessary for adhesive otitis media, cholesteatoma, or ossicular disarticulation. The aim of surgery is restoration of normal hearing thresholds and prevention of further damage to middle ear structures.

Bernard PAM et al: Randomized controlled trial comparing long term sulfonamide therapy to ventilation tubes for otitis media with effusion. Pediatrics 1991;88:215.

Gates GA et al: Effectiveness of adenoidectomy and tympanostomy tubes in the treatment of chronic otitis media with effusion. N Engl J Med 1987;317:1444.

Maw AR, Herod F: Otoscopic, impedance and audiometric findings in glue ear treated by adenoidectomy and tonsillectomy. Lancet 1986;1:1399.

Paradise JC et al: Efficacy of adenoidectomy for recurrent otitis media in children previously treated with tympanostomy tube placement. JAMA 1990;263:2066.

Pichichero ME, Bergjash LR, Hengever AS: Anatomic and audiologic sequelae after tympanostomy tube insertion or prolonged antibiotic therapy for otitis media. Pediatr Infect Dis J 1989;8:780.

Skinner DW, Lesser TH, Richards SH: A 15 year follow-up

of a controlled trial of the use of grommets in glue ear. Otolaryngology 1988;13:341.

6. CHRONIC PERFORATION OF THE TYMPANIC MEMBRANE

Essentials of Diagnosis

- Painless otorrhea, intermittent or persistent.
- Perforated tympanic membrane.
- Conductive hearing loss of 20–40 dB.

General Considerations

A perforation of the tympanic membrane can be considered chronic if it lasts for longer than 1 month. When the perforation is associated with a discharge, it is called chronic suppurative otitis media. Most perforations seen with acute otitis media heal within 2 weeks. Chronic perforations usually can be prevented by aggressive early treatment of acute otitis media. Reinfections of the exposed middle ear cavity are the most common complication of this disorder.

Clinical Findings

A. Symptoms and Signs: When a perforation is present, the condition is usually painless. If no infection is present, the middle ear cavity is seen to contain thickened, inflamed mucosa. If superimposed infection is present, serous or purulent drainage will be seen, and the middle ear cavity may contain granulation tissue or even polyps. A conductive hearing loss will usually be present depending on the size of the perforation.

The site of perforation is important. Central perforations are usually relatively safe from cholesteatoma formation. Peripheral perforations, especially in the pars flaccida, impose a risk for development of cholesteatoma because the ear canal epithelium adjacent to the perforation may invade it.

B. Laboratory Findings: Any discharge present should be cultured before treatment is initiated. Sensitivity tests are often necessary because the most common organisms are *Pseudomonas* and *S aureus*. The role of anaerobic organisms is unclear. A PPD test should be done to rule out tuberculosis.

C. Imaging: Mastoid CT films are helpful if a superimposed mastoiditis is suspected.

Complications

This disorder can have serious complications, but they are rare with proper therapy. They occur mainly in unattended cases of superinfected, chronically perforated eardrums. Cholesteatoma can be suspected if the discharge is foul-smelling and if a white, oily mass is seen within the perforation. The associated perforation may be pinpoint in size. If the discharge does not respond to 2 weeks of aggressive therapy, mastoiditis or cholesteatoma should be suspected. Serious central nervous system complications such as extradural abscess, subdural abscess, brain abscess, meningitis, labyrinthitis, or lateral sinus thrombophlebitis can occur with extension of this process. Therefore, patients with facial palsy, vertigo, or other central nervous system signs should be referred immediately to an otolaryngologist. Otogenous tetanus is another possible sequela.

Treatment

A. Specific Measures: If a serous or purulent discharge is present, antibiotic-corticosteroid ear drops (suspensions are less irritating than solutions) should be instilled three times daily for 1 week. Most products contain polymyxin, neomycin, and hydrocortisone. *Pseudomonas* is sensitive to the former. Gentamicin ear drops are also useful. The ear drops will not be effective unless the ear canals are aspirated free of discharge and debris before the drops are instilled. If the discharge is purulent or foul-smelling or if systemic signs are present, systemic antibiotics should also be prescribed. An antibiotic effective against β-lactamase-producing organisms can be given at the outset and another drug substituted depending on the culture results. This therapy can be continued for 2 weeks. If there is any recurrence of discharge, antibiotic ear drops should be instilled immediately.

Chronic suppurative otitis media with *Pseudomonas* is often resistant to outpatient therapy. If daily outpatient aspiration of discharge is unsuccessful, it may be necessary to hospitalize the patient for parenteral therapy with an antipseudomonal antibiotic. The role of oral quinolone antibiotics effective against *Pseudomonas for* outpatient management is unclear because of possible side effects on growing cartilage in children.

B. Surgical Treatment: Repair of the defect in the tympanic membrane is rarely successful during the time period when children have frequent colds and recurrent auditory tube dysfunction. Therefore, tympanoplasty is usually deferred until age 9–12. The perforated eardrum can be repaired earlier if the nonperforated one remains free of infection and effusion for a year. If drainage persists despite treatment, the patient must be referred to an otologist to rule out cholesteatoma, mastoiditis, or other complication.

C. Follow-Up Care: The patient should be seen once a week until the discharge has cleared and about once every 3 months until surgery has been done. This follow-up is imperative to prevent any serious complications.

D. Prevention of Recurrences:

1. Bathing–Before bathing and hair washing, cotton plugs should be put in the ear and the surface completely covered with petrolatum ointment.

2. Swimming–Swimming should be discouraged unless it is a matter of great importance to the patient, in which case it can be continued using custom-fitted ear molds plus a bathing cap for girls or a scuba cap for boys. Diving, jumping into the water, and underwater swimming must be absolutely forbidden.

3. Unwarranted measures–The constant use of a cotton plug in the ear canal will increase the risk of superinfection. Exposure to air is helpful.

Prognosis

With treatment, 80–90% of perforations heal spontaneously by 1 year. The remainder require careful follow-up.

Arguedas AG et al: Ceftazidime for therapy of children with chronic suppurative otitis media without cholesteatoma. Pediatr Infect Dis J 1993;12:246.

Fliss DM et al: Medical management of chronic suppurative otitis media without cholesteatoma in children. J Pediatr 1990;116:991.

Kenna MA, Bluestone CD: Microbiology of chronic suppurative otitis media. Pediatr Infect Dis J 1986;5:223.

Nelson JD: Chronic suppurative otitis media. Pediatr Infect Dis J 1988;7:446.

Schaad US: Role of the new quinolones in pediatric practice. Pediatr Infect Dis J 1992;11:1043.

7. RECURRENT OTITIS MEDIA

Recurrent otitis media is defined as three or more episodes of otitis media within a 6-month period. During the first 2 years of life, 15–20% of children experience recurrent otitis media. Because episodes of acute otitis media in infancy are frequently asymptomatic, high-risk infants with an initial episode during the first 3 months of life require close monitoring and monthly follow-up. Language development should be evaluated at 18, 24, and 36 months by use of the Early Language Milestone (ELM) scale. An appropriate home language stimulation program and guidelines for the management of behavior problems related to conductive hearing loss should be instituted for all infants and children with impaired hearing. (See Detection and Management of Hearing Deficits, below.)

Antibiotic Prophylaxis

Prophylaxis should be started following resolution of the third acute otitis media episode within a 6-month period. Effective antibiotic therapy can be provided with sulfisoxazole, 70 mg/kg/d in two divided doses, or amoxicillin, 20 mg/kg/d in two divided doses. One daily dose may also be effective.

Antibiotics should be administered daily for 3 months. During the next 3 months, it is often helpful to advise parents to restart the antibiotic at the first sign of a cold and give it for a minimum of 2 weeks or until cold symptoms resolve. However, during the winter respiratory infection season, it is more effective to provide continuous daily antibiotic prophylaxis rather than to start antibiotics only when respiratory symptoms occur. Antibiotics can reduce the frequency of recurrent acute otitis by 50%.

Otolaryngologic Referral

Failure to prevent a second new infection by giving continuous prophylaxis during 3 months and a third infection during a period of 4–6 months are indications for referral to an otolaryngologist for insertion of ventilating tubes. Reasons for surgical intervention include reducing the number of painful episodes for the child, physician and emergency room visits, days of lost work, and family anxiety level. It is possible (but has not been proved) that the fluctuating hearing loss associated with this condition delays language development or causes behavioral problems. Occasionally, patients with ventilating tubes continue to have recurrent acute otitis media and benefit from antibiotic prophylaxis. Children older than 2 years with recurrent otitis may benefit from receiving pneumococcal polysaccharide vaccine. The efficacy of new conjugate pneumococcal vaccines to prevent acute otitis media is being evaluated in field trials now under way.

Alho OP, Koivu M, Sorri M: What is an "otitis-prone" child? Int J Pediatr Otorhinolaryngol 1991;21:201.

Berman S et al: Effectiveness of continuous versus intermittent amoxicillin to prevent episodes of otitis media. Pediatr Infect Dis J 1992;11:63.

Casselbrant ML et al: Efficacy of antimicrobial prophylaxis and of tympanostomy tube insertion for prevention of recurrent acute otitis media: Results of a randomized clinical trial. Pediatr Infect Dis J 1992;11:278.

Gonzalez C et al: Prevention of recurrent acute otitis media chemoprophylaxis versus tympanostomy tubes. Laryngoscope 1986;96:1330.

Liston TE et al: The bacteriology of recurrent otitis media and the effect of sulfisoxazole chemoprophylaxis. Pediatr Infect Dis J 1984;3:20.

ACUTE BAROTITIS

Sudden changes in barometric pressure, as can occur with diving or flying, can lead to acute serous effusion into the middle ear cavity. The history itself is diagnostic. The patient presents with complaints of severe pain and loss of hearing in the affected ear. Otoscopic examination usually reveals a hemorrhagic tympanic membrane.

The process is self-limited, lasting for 2–3 days. The principal therapeutic agent is an analgesic, usually codeine. Decongestants are also prescribed, but antibiotics are not necessary.

The prognosis is excellent. The patient should be taught techniques for prevention, such as use of a nasal decongestant spray 30 minutes before descent and autoinflation maneuvers during descent.

ACUTE TRAUMA TO THE MIDDLE EAR

Head injuries, a blow to the ear canal, sudden impact with water, blast injuries, or the insertion of pointed instruments into the ear canal can lead to perforation of the tympanic membrane or hematoma of the middle ear. One study reported that 50% of serious penetrating wounds of the tympanic membrane were due to parental use of a cotton-tipped swab.

Treatment of middle ear hematomas consists mainly of watchful waiting. Prophylactic antibiotics are not necessary unless signs of superimposed infection appear. The prognosis for unimpaired hearing depends upon whether or not the ossicles are dislocated or fractured in the process. The patient needs to be followed with audiometrics until hearing has returned to normal.

Traumatic perforations of the tympanic membrane often do not heal spontaneously and should be referred to an otolaryngologist. Perforations caused by a foreign body must be attended to immediately, whereas those due to impact can be seen within 24 hours. Early debridement and placement of a graft virtually ensure closure.

Silverstein H et al: Penetration wounds of the tympanic membrane and ossicular chain. Trans Am Acad Ophthalmol Otolaryngol 1973;77:125.

MASTOIDITIS

Infection of the mastoid antrum and air cells may follow an episode of untreated or improperly treated acute otitis media. The most common etiologic agents are *Streptococcus pyogenes, Streptococcus pneumoniae,* and *Staphylococcus aureus. Haemophilus influenzae* causes mastoiditis much less frequently than might be expected. Other agents that can cause this disease include *Pseudomonas, Mycobacterium,* enteropathic gram-negative rods, and *Moraxella catarrhalis.* Anaerobic organisms appear to play a role in chronic mastoiditis; however, there are no data on how frequently they cause acute mastoiditis.

Mastoiditis is unusual before age 2, when air cells begin to develop.

Clinical Findings

The principal complaints are usually postauricular pain and fever. On examination, the mastoid area is often swollen and reddened. In the late stage, it may be fluctuant. The earliest finding is severe tenderness upon mastoid percussion. Acute otitis media is almost always present. Late findings are a pinna that is pushed forward by postauricular swelling and an ear canal that is narrowed in the posterior superior wall because of pressure from the mastoid abscess. In infants less than 1 year of age, the swelling occurs superior to the ear and pushes the pinna downward rather than outward.

Mastoiditis is a clinical diagnosis. It cannot be diagnosed on the basis of x-rays alone. In the acute phase, there is diffuse inflammatory clouding of the mastoid cells as in every case of acute otitis media. Only later is there evidence of bony destruction and resorption of the mastoid air cells. The best method to determine the extent of disease is by CT scanning.

Complications

Meningitis is a complication in up to 9% of cases of acute mastoiditis. This infection should be suspected when a child has high fever, stiff neck, severe headache, or other meningeal signs. A lumbar puncture should be performed to diagnose this condition. Brain abscess occurs in 2% of cases and may be associated with persistent headache, recurring fever, or changes in sensorium. A CT scan should be performed.

Treatment & Prognosis

The patient must be hospitalized, because this disorder represents osteitis. Before therapy is initiated, myringotomy (see below) should be performed in order to obtain material for culture and also to relieve the pressure in the middle ear-mastoid space.

The initial management of uncomplicated acute mastoiditis includes intravenous antibiotic therapy and perhaps surgery. Results of gram-stained smears taken during tympanocentesis may help in the choice of antibiotics. Ceftriaxone with nafcillin or with clindamycin would be a reasonable initial choice. Indications for immediate surgery include clear evidence of a major complication such as meningitis, brain abscess, cavernous sinus thrombosis, acute suppurative labyrinthitis, or facial palsy. Some otolaryngologists consider the destruction of septal bone (osteitis) and resorption of the mastoid air cells an indication for surgery as well.

Oral antibiotics should be continued for 4–6 weeks after the patient is discharged.

The prognosis is good if treatment is started early and continued until the process is inactive.

Myer CM: The diagnosis and management of mastoiditis. Pediatr Ann 1991;20:622.

Ogle JW, Lauer BA: Acute mastoiditis: Diagnosis and complications. Am J Dis Child 1986;140:1178.

Palva T, Virtanen H, Makinen J: Acute and latent mastoiditis in children. J Laryngol Otol 1985;99:127.

CONGENITAL EAR MALFORMATIONS

Agenesis of the external ear canal results in deafness that requires evaluation in the first month of life by hearing specialists and an otolaryngologist.

"Lop ears" (Dumbo ears) lead to much teasing and ridicule. To prevent secondary emotional problems, they can be corrected at age 5 or 6 by plastic surgery. The ear is of approximately adult size by then, and there is little risk of affecting growth of the tissues.

An ear is low-set if the upper pole is below eye level. This condition is often associated with renal malformations (eg, Potter's syndrome), and renal ultrasound examination is helpful.

Preauricular tags, ectopic cartilages, fistulas, sinuses, or cysts require surgical correction, mainly for cosmetic reasons. Most preauricular pits are asymptomatic. If one should become infected, the patient should receive antibiotic therapy and be referred to an otolaryngologist for eventual resection. Children with any of the above findings should have their hearing tested.

Brown FE et al: Correction of congenital auricular deformities by splinting in the neonatal period. Pediatrics 1986;78:406.
Jaffe BF: Pinna anomalies associated with congenital conductive hearing loss. Pediatrics 1976;57:332.

OTITIS EXTERNA

Otitis externa is inflammation of the skin lining the ear canals. The most common cause is accumulation of water in the ear, leading to maceration and desquamation of the lining and conversion of the pH from acid to alkaline (eg, from swimming or frequent showering). Swimming pools are worse than lakes because the chlorine kills the normal ear flora. Other causes are trauma to the ear canal from using cotton-tipped applicators to clean it or poorly fitted ear plugs for swimming; contact dermatitis due to hair sprays, perfumes, or self-administered ear drops; and chronic drainage from a perforated tympanic membrane. The superimposed infections are often due to *Staphylococcus aureus* or *Pseudomonas aeruginosa.*

Clinical Findings

There is pain and itching in the ear, especially with chewing or pressure on the tragus. Movement of the pinna or tragus causes considerable pain. Drainage is minimal. The ear canal is grossly swollen, and the patient resists any attempt to insert an ear speculum. Debris is noticeable in the canal. It is often impossible to visualize the tympanic membrane. Hearing is normal unless complete occlusion has occurred.

Treatment

Topical treatment usually suffices. The crucial initial step is removal of the desquamated epithelium and moist cerumen. This debris can be irrigated out or suctioned out using warm half-strength white vinegar, Burow's solution (one packet of Domeboro Pow-

der to 250 mL tap water), or normal saline. Once the ear canal is open, antibiotic-corticosteroid ear drops should be instilled three or four times daily. The corticosteroid is needed to reduce the inflammatory response. A follow-up visit in 1 week to document an intact tympanic membrane is imperative.

Oral antibiotics are indicated if any signs of invasiveness are present, such as fever, cellulitis of the auricles, or tender postauricular lymph nodes. An anti-staphylococcal antibiotic can be prescribed while awaiting the results of culture of the ear canal discharge. Systemic antibiotics alone without topical treatment will not clear up otitis externa. An analgesic such as codeine may be required temporarily. Children predisposed to this problem should instill 2 or 3 drops of a 1:1 solution of white vinegar and 70% ethyl alcohol into their ears before and after swimming. During the acute phase, swimming should be avoided. A cotton earplug is not helpful and may prolong the infection.

Marcy SM: Infections of the external ear. Pediatr Infect Dis J 1985;4:192.

EAR CANAL FOREIGN BODY

Numerous objects can be inserted into the ear canal by a child. An insect in the ear should be killed with alcohol solution (spirits will do for telephone advice). The patient should be immobilized on a papoose board with the head firmly grasped by an assistant.

An attempt should be made first to remove a foreign body by straightening the ear canal by pulling on the pinna and gently shaking the child's head. If a smooth object such as a bead is present, a cotton-tipped applicator with warmed dental wax or collodion should be inserted and placed against the object for 1–2 minutes, after which time it can be removed. An object with an irregular surface can perhaps be removed with a bayonet forceps. A steel object (eg, a ball bearing) can sometimes be removed with a magnetic probe. A right-angled hook or configured paper clip can sometimes be inserted past the object and then withdrawn, driving the object ahead of it.

If these methods fail, irrigation can be attempted. The tube should be inserted past the object so that the stream rebounds against the tympanic membrane and flushes the object out. Another approach for smooth objects is to use a suction machine. The end of the rubber tubing forms a better seal with the foreign body if it is first coated with petrolatum.

Irrigation with water is contraindicated with vegetable materials because they swell on contact with water. They can be irrigated with 70% alcohol solution. Wet tissue paper is also difficult to remove.

If the object is large or wedged in place, the patient should be referred to an otolaryngologist early rather than risk traumatizing the ear canal and causing edema that will require removing the foreign body under anesthesia.

Cunningham DG, Zanga JR: Myiasis of the external auditory meatus. J Pediatr 1974;84:857.

Stool SE, McConnell CS: Foreign bodies in pediatric otolaryngology: Some diagnostic and therapeutic pointers. Clin Pediatr (Phila) 1973;12:113.

EAR CANAL FURUNCLE

A furuncle in the outer cartilaginous portions of the ear canal is most often caused by *Staphylococcus aureus*. The patient usually complains of pain in the outer part of the ear opening and resists insertion of a speculum. A small red lump will be noticed by simply looking through the otoscope with a large speculum that is not inserted. Treatment consists of topical bacitracin ointment. When the furuncle has pointed, incision and drainage should be carried out, usually with a needle. Spread of this infection is rare; if it occurs, dicloxacillin, 25 mg/kg/d orally, should be added to the regimen. Recurrences point to manipulation of the ear canal (eg, with dirty fingernails, paper clips, hairpins, or cotton swabs).

EAR CANAL TRAUMA

Children may insert sticks or other objects into the ear canal. This normally results in abrasion of the ear canal, with more bleeding than might be suspected. Parents cause similar injuries by overzealous attempts to remove earwax. It is mandatory that the tympanic membrane be examined. If it is free of injury, no treatment is necessary because the abrasions heal readily.

HEMATOMA OF THE PINNA

Trauma to the earlobe can result in formation of a hematoma between the perichondrium and cartilage. The hematoma appears as a boggy purple swelling of the upper half of the earlobe. If this is unattended, it can cause pressure necrosis of the underlying cartilage and result in a boxer's "cauliflower ear." To prevent this cosmetic handicap, physicians should refer patients to a surgeon for aspiration and the application of a carefully molded pressure dressing.

PIERCED EAR PROBLEMS

The most common complication of ear piercing is superimposed infection, usually with *Staphylococcus aureus*. A small abscess develops at the site, and purulent material drains from both sides of the perfora-

tion. The infection usually stems from the use of contaminated needles or posts, touching the earlobes with dirty hands, or wearing earrings too tight. This localized infection can occasionally progress to life-threatening staphylococcal septicemia. Other potential complications are viral hepatitis, erysipelas, and keloid formation.

Treatment of a primary infection requires removal of the foreign body (the earring); administration of dicloxacillin, 25 mg/kg/d orally for 5 days while culture is being performed; and use of local bacitracin ointment. Infections acquired later can often be aborted with bacitracin ointment applied to the posts and reinserted three times a day.

Earrings, especially if they are made of nickel, can occasionally cause dermatitis of the earlobe. If this condition is suspected, the earrings should be removed and replaced with 14K gold or stainless steel earrings and topical corticosteroids applied to the posts several times a day.

A serious problem associated with pierced ears occurs when the earring post is grasped by a child in play and completely pulled through the earlobe, leaving a jagged laceration. The scar that develops can lead to deformity of the earlobe and may require plastic surgery. Another hazard is the possibility that an infant or young child may remove the earring and put it in its mouth, causing choking or aspiration. For this reason, the ears should not be pierced until the child is at least 4 years of age. The physician can train the office nurse to pierce ears under aseptic conditions with equipment purchased from a surgical supply house. This would prevent the majority of primary infections that occur.

Becker PG et al: Earring aspiration and other jewelry hazards. Pediatrics 1986;78:494.

Cortese TA, Dickey RA: Complications of ear piercing. Am Fam Physician (Aug) 1971;4:66.

Lovejoy FH: Life-threatening staphylococcal disease following ear piercing. Pediatrics 1970;46:301.

THE EAR: DIAGNOSTIC & THERAPEUTIC PROCEDURES

DETECTION & MANAGEMENT OF HEARING DEFICITS*

Hearing deficits are classified as conductive, sensorineural, or mixed. Conductive hearing loss results from a blockage of the transmission of sound waves

---

*Contributed by Dewey Walker, MD, Marion Downs, MA, and Jerry Northern, PhD.

from the external auditory canal to the inner ear and is characterized by normal bone conduction and reduced air conduction hearing. In children, conductive losses are most often caused by middle ear effusion. Sensorineural hearing loss occurs when the auditory nerve or cochlear hair cells are damaged. Mixed hearing loss is characterized by components of both conductive and sensorineural loss. The criteria for normal hearing levels in children are lower than those in adults, since children are in the process of learning language. In children, a hearing loss of 15–30 dB is considered mild, 31–50 dB moderate, 51–80 dB severe, and 81–100 dB profound.

Conductive Hearing Loss

By far the greatest number of conductive hearing losses during childhood are caused by otitis media and its sequelae. Other causes include atresia, stenosis, or collapse of the ear canal; furuncle, cerumen, or foreign body in the ear; aural discharge; bony growths; otitis externa; perichondritis; middle ear anomalies (eg, stapes fixation, ossicular malformation); and cleft palate.

The average hearing loss due to middle ear effusion (whether serous, purulent, or mucoid) is 27–31 dB, the equivalent of a mild hearing loss. This loss may be intermittent in nature and may occur in one or both ears.

The American Academy of Pediatrics recommends that hearing be assessed and language development skills be monitored in children who have frequently recurring acute otitis media or middle ear effusion persisting longer than 3 months. The effects of hearing loss may be insidious and may not be discernible until the explosive phase of expressive language development occurs between 16 and 24 months of age; therefore, the optimal times for screening very young children are 18 and 24 months. An acceptable tool for language screening at these ages is the Early Language Milestone (ELM) scale. Children 3, 4, and 5 years of age should also be screened for language delays.

To mitigate the likelihood of a communication disorder developing, the physician should inform the parents of a child with middle ear disease that the child's hearing may not be normal and should instruct the parents to (1) turn off sources of background noise (eg, televisions, radios, dishwashers) when speaking to the child; (2) focus on the child's face and gain his or her direct attention before speaking; (3) speak slightly louder than usual; and (4) have the teacher place the child in the front of the classroom.

Sensorineural Hearing Loss

Sensorineural hearing loss arises from a lesion in the cochlear structures of the inner ear or in the neural fibers of the auditory nerve (cranial nerve VIII). Most sensorineural losses in children are congenital, with an incidence of one in 750 live births. Causes of congenital deafness include perinatal infections, problems related to premature birth, and autosomal recessive and dominant inheritance of various deafness syndromes. In some hereditary diseases (eg, Alport's syndrome), hearing loss is progressive and becomes apparent later in childhood. The incidence of acquired sensorineural loss in children has decreased since the advent of effective immunization programs (eg, against rubella and mumps) and the control of erythroblastosis fetalis with $Rh_o(D)$ immune globulin. Meningitis remains the most common cause of acquired hearing loss, with deafness occurring in about 10% of children with bacterial meningitis.

In the past, the effect of unilateral deafness on school performance was thought to be insignificant. However, studies now show that more than one-third of affected children fail one or more grades in school. Therefore, merely recommending preferential classroom seating for these children is no longer sufficient; they should be referred for full evaluation of their hearing needs.

Acquisition of language skills is more severely affected by bilateral than unilateral sensorineural hearing loss. The earlier the deafness occurs, the graver the consequences for language development; the earlier a sensorineural loss is detected and treated (by sound amplification and language habilitation), the better the chances of a good outcome. For example, detection of deafness in a 3-month-old infant and treatment by 4 months of age will result in an optimal outcome. Unfortunately, an average of 2–3 years elapses between the time a hearing loss is recognized and treatment is instituted. The alert physician can eliminate this time lag by utilizing the screening techniques described below.

Screening for Hearing Deficits

Screening procedures are essential for early detection and diagnosis of hearing deficits. The procedures used will vary according to the child's age.

A. Screening of Newborns: During either the hospital stay or the infant's first office visit, records of the infant's neonatal course and family history should be reviewed to determine if the infant is at risk for hearing deficits. According to the Joint Committee on Infant Screening, the following factors place infants at high risk: (1) a family history of childhood hearing impairment; (2) perinatal infections (eg, cytomegalovirus, rubella, herpes simplex, toxoplasmosis, syphilis); (3) anatomic malformations involving the head or neck (eg, dysmorphic appearance, including syndromic and nonsyndromic abnormalities of the pinna); (4) birth weight less than 1500 g; (5) hyperbilirubinemia at levels exceeding indications for exchange transfusion; (6) bacterial meningitis; and (7) signs of severe asphyxia at birth (eg, Apgar scores of 0–3, failure to show spontaneous respiration by 10 minutes after birth, hypotonia persisting to 2 hours of age). If any of these risk factors are present, the infant should be screened by an audiologist, preferably prior to 3 months of age but not later than 6 months. The ideal screening test utilizes brain stem evoked response audiometry. If results of the screening test are positive for hearing deficit, the audiologist should do further diagnostic testing.

B. Screening of Infants: In the past, the parents' report of their infant's behavior was considered an adequate assessment of the infant's hearing. However, a deaf infant's behavior can appear normal and mislead the parents as well as the professional, especially if the infant has autosomal recessive deafness and is the firstborn child of carrier parents. The following office screening techniques should identify gross hearing losses, but they may or may not detect less severe hearing losses due to otitis media.

1. From birth to 4 months–In response to a sudden loud sound (70 dB or more) produced by a horn, clacker, or special electronic device, the infant should show a startle reflex or blink the eyes.

2. From 4 months to 2 years–While the infant is distracted with a toy or bright object, a noisemaker is sounded softly outside the field of vision at the child's waist level. Normal responses are as follows: at 4 months, there is widening of the eyes, interruption of other activity, and perhaps a slight turning of the head in the direction of the sound; at 6 months, the head turns toward the sound; at 9 months or older, the child should usually be able to locate a sound originating from below as well as turn to the appropriate side; after 1 year, the child should be able to locate sound whether it comes from below or above. After responses to these soft sounds are noted, a loud horn or clacker should be used to produce an eye blink or startle reflex. This last maneuver is necessary because deaf children are often visually alert and able scan the environment so actively that their scanning can be mistaken for an appropriate response to the softer noise test. A deaf child will not blink in response to the loud sound. Children who fail to respond appropriately should be referred for audiologic assessment.

C. Screening of Older Children: When children reach 3 years of age, their hearing can be tested by earphones and pure tone audiometry. The test frequencies for screening are 1000 Hz, 2000 Hz, and 4000 Hz, with the same tone presented at each frequency. Normally, the screening level is 20 dB. If a soundproof room is not available, the screening may be done at 25 dB. If the child does not respond at any one of the test frequencies in either ear, the test should be repeated within 1 week. Failures on rescreening should be referred for audiologic evaluation.

High-risk categories in older children include osteogenesis imperfecta and syndromes associated with deafness, such as Waardenburg's syndrome, Hurler's syndrome, Alport's syndrome, Treacher Collins' syndrome, Klippel-Feil syndrome, and fetal alcohol syndrome. Children with these disorders should receive audiologic evaluation as part of the complete workup. In addition, before any child is labeled as having mental retardation, autism, or severe behavior problems, the adequacy of his or her hearing must be determined. If a developmental speech delay is diagnosed, hearing should be tested as the first step in evaluating the language problem.

Referral

In addition to the referrals for audiologic testing mentioned above, a child with confirmed hearing loss should be referred to an otolaryngologist for evaluation and further management. Any child failing the language screen should be referred to a speech pathologist for language evaluation. Home language enrichment programs for children with mild language delays can be directed by the physician or by a speech pathologist. Programs for the deaf child vary from aural to total communication; the latter includes elements of aural programs plus signing. Each program should be thoroughly scrutinized for its relevance to the deaf child's age and hearing level.

Prevention

Appropriate pediatric care may help prevent many causes of hearing deficits. Erythroblastosis fetalis can be prevented by the use of $Rh_o(D)$ immune globulin, and hyperbilirubinemia can be controlled by phototherapy and exchange transfusions. Congenital rubella infections can be prevented by the use of rubella vaccine, and immunizations for other childhood diseases (eg, mumps) effectively prevent hearing losses from those conditions.

Aminoglycosides are potentially ototoxic and should be used judiciously and monitored carefully, especially in premature infants and in patients with renal insufficiency.

Reduction of exposure to loud noise in the child's environment will prevent high-frequency hearing losses. Repeated exposure to loud music, firecrackers, or shots from guns or cap pistols can impair hearing.

Bess FH, Tharpe AM: Unilateral hearing impairment in children. Pediatrics 1984;74:206.

Northern JL, Downs MP: *Hearing in Children,* 3rd ed. Williams & Wilkins, 1984.

Rowe LD: Hearing loss: The profound benefits of early diagnosis. Contemp Pediatr 1985;3(10):77.

Ruben RJ: Diagnosis of deafness in infancy. Pediatr Rev 1987;9:163.

Stewart JM, Downs MP: Congenital conducted hearing loss: The need for early identification and intervention. Pediatrics 1993;91:355.

CERUMEN REMOVAL

Cerumen removal is an essential skill for anyone who treats ear problems. Cerumen often prevents adequate visualization of the tympanic membrane. Impacted cerumen can also cause itching, pain, hearing loss, or otitis externa. If cerumen impinges on the eardrum, a chronic cough may be triggered and will persist until the cerumen is removed. The most common cause of impacted cerumen is the use of cotton-tipped swabs by parents in misguided attempts to clean the ear canal. Parents should be advised that earwax protects the ear (cerumen contains lysozymes and immunoglobulins that curtail infection) and will come out by itself; therefore, they should never put anything into the ear canal to accelerate the natural process.

The technique of removal depends on the consistency of the earwax. All the procedures described below require immobilization to prevent injury of the ear canal. The physician should remove cerumen under direct vision through the operating head of an otoscope. Frequently, cerumen that obstructs the view of the tympanic membrane can be pushed aside, the pneumatic seal reestablished, and mobility assessed without removing the speculum. Irrigation can also be used to remove cerumen.

(1) Very soft cerumen: Semiliquid earwax can be removed with cotton twisted on paper clips. Several passages with clean cotton are usually necessary. Nasopharyngeal culture swabs are an expensive substitute.

(2) Average cerumen: Sticky cerumen will adhere to an ear curette. If this technique fails, irrigation as described below should be instituted.

(3) Hard cerumen: Very hard cerumen may adhere to the wall of the ear canal and cause pain or bleeding if one attempts to remove it with a curette. This type of wax can be softened with Cerumenex or a few drops of detergent before irrigation is attempted. After 20 minutes, irrigation can be started with water warmed to 35–38 °C to prevent vertigo.

An easy-to-assemble ear syringe consists of a 12-mL plastic syringe plus a piece of small plastic tubing. The tubing can be made from any scalp vein needle set by cutting off the needle about 3 inches from the female connector. The front end of the tubing is placed in the canal, behind the cerumen if possible, and the water is ejected with maximal pressure on the syringe plunger. The advantage of this technique is that the very small tubing may be inserted into the ear canal itself, and the water stream is thus directed in the proper course without interfering with reflux.

A commercial jet tooth cleanser (eg, Water Pik) is also an excellent device for removing cerumen, but it is important to set it at low power (2 or less) to prevent damage to the intact tympanic membrane.

A perforated tympanic membrane is a contraindication to any form of irrigation.

Kravitz H et al: The cotton-tipped swab: A major cause of ear injury and hearing loss. Clin Pediatr (Phila) 1974; 13:965.

Schwartz RH et al: Cerumen removal. Am J Dis Child 1983;137:1064.

OTOSCOPY

Removal of cerumen (see above) may be necessary for adequate visualization of the ear and for assessment of the mobility of the tympanic membrane by pneumatic otoscopy.

The tympanic membrane is divided into four sections, based on the position of the long process of the malleus and the umbo, as shown in Figure 19–2. The anterosuperior quadrant contains the short process of the malleus; the posterosuperior quadrant, the incus and pars flaccida; the posteroinferior quadrant, the round window; and the anteroinferior quadrant, the pars tensa and light reflex. To assess mobility of the tympanic membrane, a pneumatic otoscope with a rubber suction bulb and tube is used. The speculum inserted into the patient's ear canal must be large enough to provide an airtight seal. When the rubber bulb is squeezed, the tympanic membrane will flap briskly if no fluid is present (normal finding); if fluid is present in the middle ear space, the mobility of the tympanic membrane will be diminished.

TYMPANOMETRY

Tympanometry utilizes an electroacoustic impedance bridge to measure tympanic membrane compliance and display it in graphic form. Compliance is determined at specific air pressures (from +200 to –400

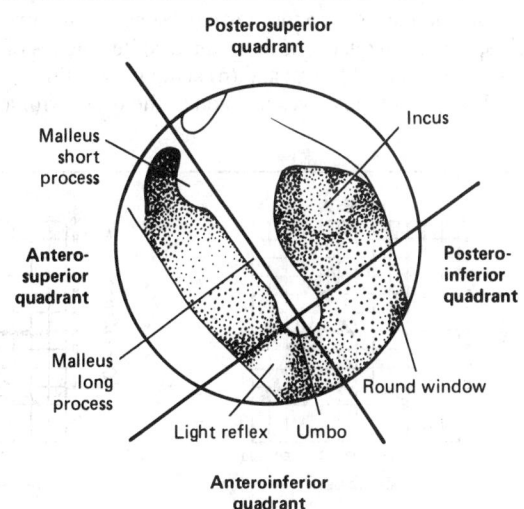

Figure 19–2. Schematic diagram of the left tympanic membrane. (Courtesy of the Department of Otolaryngology, University of Pittsburgh School of Medicine, and Eli Lilly and Co.)

mm H_2O air pressure) that are created in the hermetically sealed external ear canal. The existing middle ear pressure can be measured by determining the ear canal pressure at which the tympanic membrane is most compliant. Because total visualization of the tympanic membrane is not necessary, tympanometry does not require removal of cerumen unless the canal is completely blocked.

Tympanograms can be classified into three major patterns, as shown in Figure 19–3. The type A pattern, characterized by maximum compliance at normal atmospheric pressure (0 mm H_2O air pressure), indicates a normal tympanic membrane, good auditory tube function, and absence of effusion. The type B pattern identifies a nonmobile tympanic membrane, which may be associated with middle ear effusion, perforation, patent ventilation tubes, or excessive and hard-packed cerumen. The type C pattern indicates an intact mobile tympanic membrane with poor auditory tube function and excessive negative pressure (> –150 mm H_2O air pressure) in the middle ear. Middle ear effusion is present in about 20% of patients with a type C pattern.

MYRINGOTOMY & TYMPANOCENTESIS

Tympanocentesis (placement of a needle through the tympanic membrane) is mainly a diagnostic procedure, because the hole closes over quickly and provides little sustained drainage. Tympanocentesis is helpful in (1) acute otitis media in a hospitalized newborn, because the pathogens may be gram-negative; (2) acute otitis media in a patient with compromised host resistance, because the organism may be unusual; (3) painful bullae of the tympanic membrane; (4) a complete workup for presumed sepsis or meningitis; (5) unresponsive otitis media despite courses of two different antibiotics; and (6) acute mastoiditis.

Myringotomy involves incision of the drum with a myringotomy knife, leaving a flap through which drainage fluid may escape. This procedure is helpful for both diagnostic and therapeutic purposes. Myringotomy is indicated (1) when a patient on an initial visit with bulging acute purulent otitis media has severe pain or vomiting, because both symptoms are relieved by myringotomy; (2) when pain and fever fail to resolve after 48 hours of appropriate antibiotic treatment, because a middle ear abscess or resistant organism may exist; and (3) for acute mastoiditis, because it is important to permit drainage as well as to identify the particular organism.

Technique of Myringotomy

A. Premedication: In the conditions mentioned, the pain associated with myringotomy is only slightly greater than the pain that already exists from acute inflammation of the tympanic membrane. Therefore, no premedication is generally indicated. The patient who is extremely difficult to hold may be premedicated with meperidine, 1 mg/kg intramuscularly.

B. Restraint: The patient must be completely immobile while the incision is being made. A papoose board or a sheet can be used to immobilize the body. An extra attendant is required to hold the patient's head steady.

C. Site: With an open-headed operating otoscope, the operator carefully selects a target. This is generally in the posteroinferior quadrant. This site prevents disruption of the ossicles during the procedure.

D. Incision: The knife is lowered slowly until it touches the surface of the tympanic membrane at the chosen site. A quick 2- to 3-mm incision in the anterior direction is then made, leaving a curved flap in the area indicated (eg, from 8 o'clock to 4 o'clock on the right eardrum).

E. Culture: The myringotomy knife tip should be wiped on a cotton swab moistened with a few

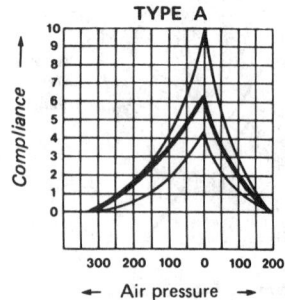
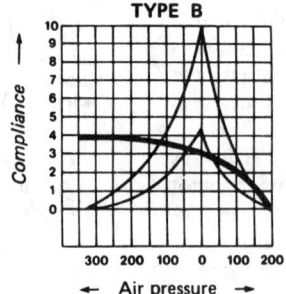
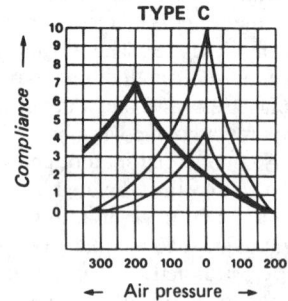

Figure 19–3. Type A tympanograms are characterized by maximum compliance at normal atmospheric pressure (0 mm H_2O air pressure). Type B tympanograms show little or no change in compliance of the tympanic membrane as air pressure in the external ear canal is varied. Type C tympanograms show near-normal compliance with significant negative middle ear pressures (typically more severe than –150 mm H_2O). (Reproduced, with permission, from Northern JL: Advanced techniques for measuring middle ear function. Pediatrics 1978;61:761.)

drops of normal saline solution. The material is then placed on a sheep blood agar plate, a chocolate agar plate, and a slide for Gram staining.

Technique of Tympanocentesis

Steps A, B, and C are as described in the preceding section.

In this procedure, the operator needs an assistant to hold the patient's head immobile. An 8.8-cm spinal needle (No. 18 or No. 20) with a short bevel is attached to a 1-mL syringe. The plunger is removed from the syringe, and a suction tube is placed over the syringe opening. The spinal needle is bent at a slight angle so that its end is out of the operator's line of vision. The operator moves the needle toward the posteroinferior quadrant, inserting it through the tympanic membrane, and aspirates the middle ear effusion into the syringe.

Kaplan SL, Feigen RD: Simplified technique for tympanocentesis. Pediatrics 1978;62:418.

THE NOSE & PARANASAL SINUSES

RHINITIS

1. ACUTE VIRAL RHINITIS (Common Cold)

The common cold is the most frequent infectious disease of humans, and the incidence is higher in early childhood than in any other period of life. Children under age 5 have 6–12 colds a year. Upper respiratory infections may be caused by over 200 different viruses, including rhinovirus, coronavirus, adenovirus, influenza virus, parainfluenza virus, respiratory syncytial virus, and coxsackievirus. Minor epidemics occur during the winter months and spread rapidly among susceptible people. The peak month (September) coincides with the opening of school.

Clinical Findings

The patient usually experiences a sudden onset of clear or mucoid rhinorrhea plus fever. The main symptoms are usually profound congestion of the nose and sinuses. Mild sore throat and cough also frequently develop. Although the fever is usually low-grade in older children, in the first 5 or 6 years of life it can be as high as 40.6 °C without superinfection. The nose and throat are usually inflamed. Several members of a family are often sick simultaneously.

Complications

Acute otitis media is the most common complication and is often heralded by return of fever or crying 4–7 days after onset of the of the cold symptoms. Other complications due to superinfection are purulent sinusitis, purulent conjunctivitis, pneumonia, and pyogenic adenitis.

The presence of a cold or upper respiratory tract infection in a child scheduled for surgery may require postponement of the operation. The primary physician can use the following guidelines when screening children for elective surgery: Surgery is usually postponed if fever or cough is present. Surgery can proceed if the child has only a runny nose, sore throat, or ear infection. If anesthesia will not require intubation (eg, as for placement of tympanoplasty tubes), surgery can be permitted even if the child has a cough (provided that findings on chest film are normal).

Treatment

Treatment is largely symptomatic. Acetaminophen is helpful for fever, sore throat, or muscle aches. A stuffy, congested nose can be treated with normal saline nose drops (mix ¼ tsp table salt with 6 oz of water), 3 drops in each nostril. After several minutes, a suction bulb can be used to remove the secretions of the infant unable to blow its nose. If this procedure fails after several attempts and the stuffy nose still interferes with feeding or sleep, phenylephrine, 0.125% nose drops, 1 drop every 4 hours as necessary, can be used in children 6 months to 2 years of age. Children over 2 years of age can use long-acting xylometazoline or oxymetazoline 0.05% nose drops. Drops should be used only when the nose is congested and discontinued by 5 days to prevent rebound chemical rhinitis. Antihistamines are probably not effective in relieving cold symptoms. In rhinoviral colds, increased levels of histamine are not observed. Antibiotics do not prevent superinfection and should not be used. Codeine and dextromethorphan should not be used since they do not alleviate the symptoms of acute cough.

Colds account for many unnecessary visits to the physician. Parents are often unduly worried about how many colds their children have or are overly concerned about noisy breathing, which they fear indicates pneumonia. Parents should be instructed that fast breathing or difficult breathing with retraction is a sign of a lower respiratory infection such as bronchiolitis or pneumonia. Most colds can be assessed and treated by telephone.

The prognosis is excellent. In the usual cold, the fever lasts for less than 3 days and the other symptoms persist for 1–2 weeks.

Doyle W et al: A double-blind, placebo-controlled clinical trial of the effect of chlorpheniramine on response of nasal airway, middle ear and eustachian tube to provocative rhinovirus challenge. Pediatr Infect Dis J 1988; 7:229.

Hutton N et al: Effectiveness of an antihistamine-decongestant combination for young children with the common cold: A randomized, controlled clinical trial. J Pediatr 1991;118:125.

Naclero RM et al: Is histamine responsible for symptoms of rhinovirus colds? A look at the inflammatory mediators following infection. Pediatr Infect Dis J 1988;7:215.

Szilagyi PG: What can we do about the common cold? Contemp Pediatr 1990;7(2):23.

Taylor JA et al: Efficacy of cough suppressants in children. J Pediatr 1993;122:799.

2. ACUTE PURULENT RHINITIS

Purulent yellow discharge that persists for more than 10 days usually represents purulent sinusitis, adenoiditis, or other bacterial superinfection of a common cold. The most likely organisms are *Streptococcus pneumoniae, Haemophilus influenzae,* group A β-hemolytic streptococci, and *Staphylococcus aureus.* Rare causes are diphtheria, pertussis, and syphilis. The common cold may also be associated with some mucopurulent discharge, but discharge is usually intermittent and worse upon awakening in the morning. The β-hemolytic streptococci are the most likely organisms if there is crusting around the nares that resembles impetigo, redness of the skin below the nares, or a blistering distal dactylitis.

Oral amoxicillin or trimethoprim-sulfamethoxazole, administered for 10 days will cure most of these patients. Occasionally, alternative antibiotics to cover resistant pathogens will be needed based on culture results. The purulent material should be removed as completely as possible with a suction bulb or cotton-tipped applicators and a washcloth and soap.

If the problem recurs after adequate treatment, the patient should be referred to an otolaryngologist to rule out the possibility of a foreign body. If the discharge is foul-smelling and unilateral, this possibility becomes especially likely. The response to treatment is usually excellent.

Wald ER: Purulent nasal discharge. Pediatr Infect Dis J 1991;10:329.

3. PERSISTENT RHINITIS IN NEWBORNS

Rhinorrhea or nasal congestion in a young infant may be due to various causes.

About half of newborns are obligate nasal breathers, and if the nose becomes congested, they have difficulty with air exchange and may become irritable and dyspneic. The problem is worse during feeding because sucking completely blocks the infant's oral airway. These infants gradually learn to become mouth breathers as well as nasal breathers by age 5 or 6 months.

Differential Diagnosis & Treatment

A. Transient Idiopathic Stuffy Nose of the Newborn: Many infants have unexplained, transient (about 3 weeks) stuffy noses with mucoid or clear discharge that bubbles during feeding. The cause is not known. The diagnosis is made by exclusion. Normal saline nose drops can be instilled and, after several minutes, removed with cotton-tipped applicators or gentle suction with a rubber bulb syringe.

B. Reserpine Side Effects: If the mother is taking reserpine and the drug is in her blood at an effective level during labor, the newborn may have a stuffy nose. Treatment is as above.

C. Chemical Rhinitis: Chemical rhinitis may be due to overtreatment of idiopathic stuffy nose with topical vasoconstrictors. The irritative nose drops should be discontinued. The patient can be helped with oral decongestants and a corticosteroid nasal spray for 1 week.

D. Pyogenic Rhinitis: Infants with pyogenic rhinitis can have a clear or mucoid discharge rather than the purulent discharge seen in older children. The diagnosis is based on cultures of nasal discharge. Treatment is as outlined above.

E. Congenital Syphilis: The onset is usually before 6 weeks of age. The diagnosis is established by checking the serology done on the mother during the prenatal period. If signs other than the nasal discharge exist, such as an unresponsive skin rash or hepatosplenomegaly, additional serologic testing should be performed on the infant. Treatment is discussed in Chapter 33.

F. Hypothyroidism: See Chapter 27.

G. Choanal Atresia: Choanal atresia occurs bilaterally in 25% of affected children and unilaterally in 75%. Bilateral cases can cause severe respiratory distresseven apnea at birth if the child is an absolute nasal breather. Both types eventually present with a chronic nasal discharge because the normal sinus and nasal secretions can escape only anteriorly. A No. 8 soft rubber catheter should be passed through the nose and visualized in the oropharynx. If this procedure cannot be accomplished, a diagnosis of choanal atresia should be confirmed by radiographic study.

An oral airway should be placed immediately if the infant has bilateral choanal atresia. A dentist can fashion a comfortable airway to tide the patient over until mouth breathing is established. Feeding by syringe or medicine dropper is preferred. An otolaryngologist should decide on the optimal timing for definitive surgery, but it is usually 1 year of age.

H. Nasal Fracture Secondary to Birth Trauma: Physical examination should reveal subluxation of the nasal septum occluding the nasal passages. The infant should be referred to an otolaryngologist for reduction.

I. Allergic Rhinitis Associated With Cow's Milk: An allergic reaction to cow's milk can cause noisy breathing and increased production of nasal and oral mucus in infants 1–2 months of age. The symptoms resolve 24–48 hours after eliminating cow's milk from the diet, and they return promptly if the infant is rechallenged with milk.

Myer CM, Cotton RT: Nasal obstruction in the pediatric patient. Pediatrics 1983;72:766.

4. RECURRENT RHINITIS IN THE OLDER CHILD

This problem is all too frequent in the office practice of pediatrics. A child is brought in with the chief complaint that he or she has "one cold after another," has "constant colds," or "is always sick." Such a patient may be in the office on almost a weekly basis. Although the problem is frustrating, the differential diagnosis is rather simple.* Approximately two-thirds of these children have recurrent colds, and another one-third have allergic rhinitis.

Differential Diagnosis & Treatment

A. Common Cold: The most common cause of recurrent runny nose is repeated viral upper respiratory infections. The onset is usually after 6 months of age. The bouts of rhinorrhea are usually accompanied by fever. Cultures are negative for bacteria. There is some evidence for contagion within the family or peer group in most of these cases. The nasal mucosa during attacks is often inflamed.

The most common reason for the office visit is that the parents are overly concerned because they do not understand that the average child has approximately 6–12 colds a year during the preschool years. Or the patient may be overly exposed to viruses as a result of close contact with a sibling at school who brings home many pathogens or by frequently being left with large numbers of children at a day care center or with a baby-sitter.

Treatment consists of reassurance and concerned follow-up. The parents can be told that their child's general health is good, as evidenced by adequate weight gain and a robust activity level; that the prognosis is good in that this number of colds will not persist for more than a few years; that the body's exposure and response to colds is building up an antibody supply; and that this problem is not their fault and that they are doing a good job as parents.

B. Allergic Rhinitis: The onset of "hay fever" is usually after 2 years of age after the child has had

---

*__Note:__ An excessively ordered test is serum immunoelectrophoresis. Children with immune defects do not have an increased number of colds. Therefore, immune globulin tests are worthless unless the patient suffers from recurrent pneumonia, recurrent sinusitis, recurrent adenitis, or other recurrent severe infections.

adequate exposure to allergens. There is no fever or contagion among close contacts. The attacks include frequent sneezing, rubbing of the nose, and a profuse clear discharge. The nasal turbinates are swollen. The nasal smear demonstrates over 20% of the cells to be eosinophils. (Nasal eosinophilia may be normal during the first 3 months of life.) Nasal secretions should be collected only when the patient is symptomatic. Between attacks or after receiving antihistamines, the eosinophil smear may be falsely negative.

Oral decongestants and antihistamines should be tried until the right drug and dosage are found to give the optimal effect. Avoidance of allergens (especially pets and tobacco smoke) should be encouraged and environmental controls initiated. If the symptoms persist, treatment with cromolyn nasal spray or corticosteroid nasal spray should be considered.

A full discussion of allergic rhinitis is presented in Chapter 30.

C. Chemical Rhinitis: Prolonged use of vasoconstrictor nose drops beyond 7 days results in a rebound reaction and secondary nasal congestion (rhinitis medicamentosa). The offending nose drops should be discontinued.

D. Vasomotor Rhinitis: Some children react to sudden changes in environmental temperature with prolonged congestion and rhinorrhea. Air pollution (especially tobacco smoke) may be a factor. Oral decongestants can be used periodically to give symptomatic relief.

E. Vasomotor Rhinitis: See p 452.

Complications

Because this problem is such a nuisance, iatrogenic overtreatment is the most common complication.

Giving immune globulin injections is the most common error made in treating this disorder. The injections may be initiated without determining the serum IgG level or as a consequence of misinterpreting the results of IgG testing by comparing them with adult levels rather than with norms for age. Many studies show that immune globulin injections do not benefit patients with frequent upper respiratory infections. In addition to being painful and expensive, they may cause anaphylaxis or isoimmunization.

Other worthless approaches to this problem include bacterial vaccines, prophylactic antibiotics, and tonsillectomy and adenoidectomy. High doses of vitamin C have been found to be ineffective in reducing the symptoms and duration of colds. Patients are not infrequently kept home from school, trips, sports activities, parties, etc, with little indication. As long as they do not have a fever or severe symptoms, they can attend these functions. They should be given suitable medications for symptomatic relief of mild symptoms so that they can participate normally in these important events of childhood. The risk to other children is almost irrelevant, because these infections are contagious even during the incubation period and because the best time to have them and develop immunity is during childhood.

Gentry S: Allergic rhinitis: Always in season. Contemp Pediatr 1991;8(4):88.

Shapiro G: Understanding allergic rhinitis. Pediatr Rev 1986;7:212.

MOUTH BREATHING SECONDARY TO NASAL OBSTRUCTION

A child is sometimes brought in with the complaint that "he always breathes through his mouth," "he snores," etc. With the mouth covered, each nostril should be tested individually for patency. One or both nostrils may be so severely occluded that adequate air exchange cannot occur. Even when the nasal passages are not completely occluded, the patient may prefer to breathe through the mouth because it is more comfortable. With complete obstruction, a constant nasal discharge ensues because the normal sinus and nasal secretions can escape only anteriorly. The sense of smell is also impaired.

Differential Diagnosis

A. Large Adenoids: Large adenoids can be suspected if the soft palate is depressed or has limited elevation, the patient has hyponasal speech, or perhaps if the tonsils are huge. They can be diagnosed more precisely by mirror examination or by lateral soft tissue films of the nasopharynx.

B. Nasal Polyps: Polyps appear as glistening, gray to pink, jelly-like masses that are prominent just inside the anterior nares and occur singly or in clusters. They occur in cystic fibrosis and severe allergic rhinitis. One must be careful not to mistake the turbinates for polyps.

C. Recurrent Sinusitis: See below.

D. Allergic Rhinitis: See above.

E. Chemical Rhinitis: See above.

F. Other Causes: Persistent mouth breathing may be due to obstruction by nasopharyngeal tumor or by meningocele or encephalocele herniated into the nasal cavity. If unilateral nasal obstruction and epistaxis are frequent, juvenile angiofibroma should be suspected.

Complications

Most children with prolonged mouth breathing eventually develop dental malocclusion and what has been termed an adenoidal facies. The face is pinched and the maxilla narrowed because the molding pressures of the orbicularis oris and buccinator muscles are unopposed by the tongue. If nasopharyngeal tumors, meningoceles, or encephaloceles are not diagnosed early, they can cause considerable destruction or may even become incurable. Children with severe snoring may also develop sleep apnea or pulmonary hypertension.

Treatment

Allergic rhinitis usually responds to antihistamines or to intranasal cromolyn or corticosteroids. Sinusitis usually resolves with antibiotics. All other patients with documented chronic mouth breathing should be referred to an otolaryngologist for definitive evaluation and treatment. Polyps should never be removed until a meningocele has been ruled out.

Bresolin D et al: Facial characteristics of children who breathe through the mouth. Pediatrics 1984;73:622.

Gentry S: Allergic rhinitis: Always in season. Contemp Pediatr 1991;8:88.

Myer CM et al: Nasal obstruction in the pediatric patient. Pediatrics 1983;72:766.

SINUSITIS

1. ACUTE SINUSITIS

Essentials of Diagnosis

- Purulent rhinorrhea or postnasal drip.
- Rhinorrhea and daytime cough persisting beyond 10 days.
- Bad breath.
- Facial pain or percussion tenderness.
- Periorbital swelling.
- Headache.

General Considerations

Acute inflammation of the paranasal sinuses, or sinusitis, may complicate up to 5% of upper respiratory infections. The maxillary and ethmoidal sinuses are most commonly involved because of poor drainage related to anatomic features. When mucociliary clearance and drainage are further compromised by an upper respiratory infection, the risk of secondary bacterial infection increases. Sinusitis is also commonly seen during pollen season in children with allergic rhinitis. In cases in which superinfection occurs, the organisms are usually *Streptococcus pneumoniae, Haemophilus influenzae* (nontypable), *Moraxella catarrhalis,* and β-hemolytic streptococci. Rarely, anaerobic bacterial infections can cause fulminant frontal sinusitis. Viruses can be isolated in 10% of sinus aspirates, but their pathogenic role is unclear.

The ethmoidal sinus is the only one that is significantly developed at birth. The maxillary sinus is rudimentary at birth and visible on x-ray film by 6 months. The frontal sinus is not visible until 3–9 years of age. Clinical ethmoiditis does not usually occur until 6 months of age. About half of cases occur between 1 and 5 years of age, during which time the most common presenting sign is periorbital cellulitis. Maxillary sinusitis is seen clinically after 1 year of age. Frontal sinusitis is unusual before 10 years of age.

Clinical Findings
(Figure 19–4)

A. Symptoms and Signs: The most common clinical presentation in children is persistence of nasal discharge or postnasal drip and daytime cough longer than 7–10 days. Persistent, low-grade fever is often present. Malodorous breath or intermittent, painless morning periorbital swelling is often noted.

Older patients may complain of acute onset of headache, a sense of fullness, or facial pain overlying the involved sinus. Ethmoiditis causes retro-orbital pain; maxillary sinusitis causes upper molar or zygomatic pain; and frontal sinusitis causes pain above the eyebrow. These signs are often associated with a high fever.

Physical examination reveals injected nasal mucosa, usually associated with nasal or postnasal mucopurulent discharge. Occasionally there is percussion tenderness overlying the sinusitis. In ethmoiditis,

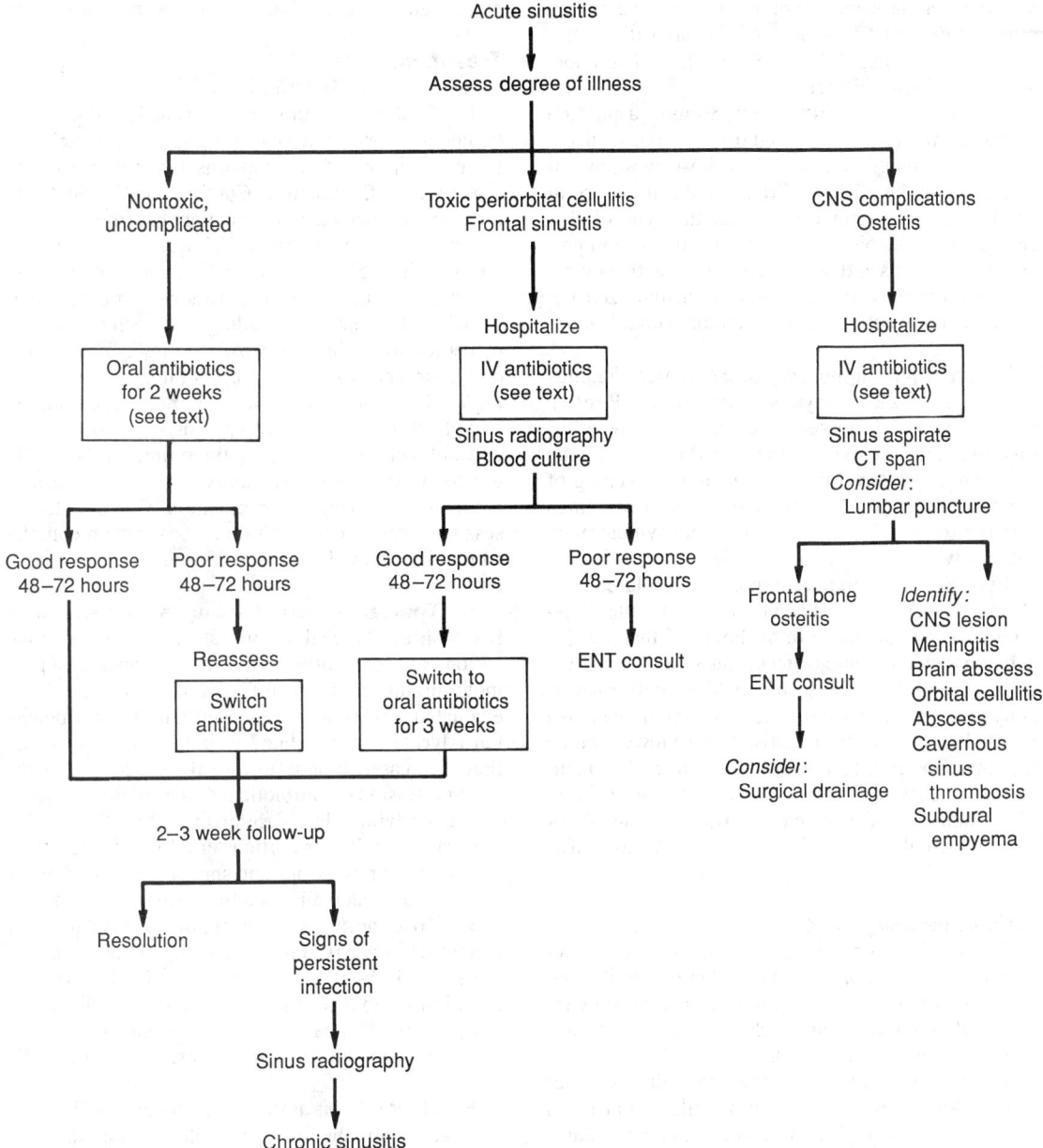

Figure 19–4. Algorithm for the management of acute sinusitis.

the tenderness is elicited by pressing medially on the inner canthus of the eye. Tenderness of the eyeball may also be present. Maxillary sinusitis reveals percussion tenderness on the maxillary bone. Frontal sinusitis reveals percussion tenderness when the physician presses upward on the floor of the supraorbital ridge. Periorbital swelling or mild discoloration may be present. The examination should identify exudative tonsillitis, a nasal foreign body, or dental caries and poor dental hygiene. Transillumination of the sinuses is difficult to perform and not very helpful unless it is grossly asymmetric. The chest should be auscultated for wheezing. Sinusitis precipitates intractable wheezing in some children with reactive airway disease. Vigorous treatment of the sinusitis eliminates the wheezing and the need for bronchodilators in many of these children.

B. Laboratory Findings: Sinus aspiration should be performed for diagnostic purposes in patients with complications and in those with an immunosuppressive disease. Gram's stain or culture of nasal discharge is unnecessary as the type of discharge (thin, mucoid, or purulent) is not a useful predictor of sinusitis and does not correlate with cultures of sinus aspirates. If the patient is hospitalized because of complications, a blood culture should be obtained.

C. Imaging: In most cases, the clinical findings are so classic that x-rays are not needed. Positive x-ray films in children over one year will show opacification of the involved sinuses, air-fluid levels if the obstruction is intermittent, or mucosal thickening of greater than 5 mm. It is notable that x-ray findings positive for sinusitis may be found in asymptomatic patients with colds or nasal allergies.

Sinus x-rays are indicated mainly in children with (1) facial swelling of unknown cause, (2) acute sinusitis that is unresponsive to 48 hours of therapy, (3) undocumented chronic or recurrent sinusitis, and (4) chronic asthma. A CT scan should be performed if bony erosions are present. Ultrasonography can also be used to document sinusitis. Sinus views include the anteroposterior (Caldwell) for the frontal and ethmoidal sinuses, occipitomental (Waters) for the maxillary sinuses, and submental-vertex and lateral for the sphenoidal sinus. A Waters view is usually sufficient.

Differential Diagnosis

Similar clinical presentations are associated with viral upper respiratory infection, allergic rhinitis and reactive airway disease, *Streptococcus pyogenes* infection during infancy and early childhood, and nasal foreign body. In older children, the main diagnostic problem is confusion with headaches due to other causes. An uncommon cause of maxillary sinusitis is extension of a periapical abscess of an upper molar.

Complications

The most frequent complication of paranasal sinusitis is preseptal periorbital cellulitis secondary to ethmoiditis. Less frequently, orbital cellulitis or abscess develops. These are associated with decreased extraocular movement, proptosis, edema, and altered visual acuity. The most common complication of frontal sinusitis is osteitis of the frontal bone, called Pott's puffy tumor. Additional serious intracranial complications include cavernous sinus thrombosis, subdural empyema, brain abscess, and meningitis. The most common maxillary complication is cellulitis of the cheek. Rarely, osteomyelitis of the maxilla can develop.

Treatment

A. Specific Measures:

1. Oral antibiotics–Acute sinusitis should be treated with oral antibiotics for 2–3 weeks to achieve more prompt relief of symptoms and more rapid resolution of inflammation. Continue antibiotic treatment for another week if the patient has improved but is not totally asymptomatic. The usual antibiotic is amoxicillin, 15 mg/kg, three times a day. In areas where β-lactamase-positive pathogens are common or when the patient is allergic to penicillin, use trimethoprim-sulfamethoxazole, 5 mg/kg/dose twice daily, or erythromycin plus sulfamethoxazole, 10 mg/kg/dose four times a day. Additional possibilities include third generation cephalosporins or amoxicillin-clavulanate, 15 mg/kg three times a day. Failure to improve after 48 hours suggests a resistant organism or potential complication. One should assess the patient for a central nervous system complication. If none is found, consider drainage or parenteral therapy.

2. Topical and oral decongestants and antihistamines–Topical decongestants and oral combinations are frequently used in acute sinusitis to promote drainage. Their effectiveness has not been evaluated, and concern has been raised about potential adverse effects related to impaired ciliary function, decreased blood flow to the mucosa, and reduced diffusion of antibiotic into the sinuses. Patients with underlying allergic rhinitis may benefit from intranasal cromolyn or corticosteroid nasal spray. Vasoconstrictor nose drops and sprays are all associated with rebound edema if used for more than 5–7 days.

3. Treatment of complications–Patients with evidence of invasive infection or any of the complications listed above should be immediately hospitalized. Intravenous therapy with nafcillin or clindamycin plus cefotaxime or with chloramphenicol alone should be initiated until culture results become available.

B. General Measures: A patient will often need acetaminophen or even codeine temporarily to permit sleep until drainage of the obstructed sinus is achieved. The application of ice over the sinus may help to relieve pain.

Dryness of the mucous membranesas occurs in many overheated homes in the winter if adequate humidification is not providedcan contribute to the obstruction. A humidifier in the patient's room and periodic warm showers may be of value. A child with sinusitis can be permitted to swim. Diving should be temporarily restricted unless nose plugs are used.

C. Surgical Treatment:

1. Lavage of the sinuses–If there is incapacitating initial pain or persistence of significant pain beyond several days, the patient should be referred to an otolaryngologist for lavage of the involved sinus.

2. External drainage–In complicated cases admitted to the hospital, an otolaryngologist should always be consulted. Sinus aspiration is helpful in many cases. For sinus intraorbital or intracranial complications, external drainage of the abscess is as important as antibiotic therapy.

D. Follow-Up Care: The patient should be seen in 48 hours if there is no improvement with antibiotic therapy and again at the end of the 2-week course. A confirmatory x-ray film should be obtained if symptoms persist at 2 weeks. Chronic or recurrent sinus infections suggest an underlying anatomic malformation, an allergy, cystic fibrosis, immotile cilia syndrome, or an immunodeficiency disorder.

Arruda LK et al: Abnormal maxillary sinus radiographs in children: Do they represent bacterial infection? Pediatrics 1990;85:553.

Brook I et al: Complications of sinusitis in children. Pediatrics 1980;66:568.

Feder HM Jr, Cates KL, Cementina AM: Pott puffy tumor: A serious occult infection. Pediatrics 1987;79:625.

Goldenhersh MJ et al: Sinusitis: Early recognition, aggressive treatment. Contemp Pediatr 1989;6(12):22.

Kovatch AL et al: Maxillary sinus radiographs in children with nonrespiratory complaints. Pediatrics 1984;73:306.

Wald ER: Management of sinusitis in infants and children. Pediatr Infect Dis J 1988;7:449.

Wald ER: Sinusitis in children. N Engl J Med 1992;326:319.

Wald ER et al: Subacute sinusitis in children. J Pediatr 1989;115:28.

2. RECURRENT OR CHRONIC SINUSITIS (Figure 19–5)

Chronic or frequent episodes of sinusitis occur in a small group of patients. The most common cause is allergic rhinitis. The second most common cause especially of frontal sinusitisis diving or jumping into water feet first. The remaining cases are caused by pressure against the ostia by a septal deviation, nasal malformation, polyp, or foreign body. In cases of chronic or recurrent pyogenic pansinusitis, poor host resistance (eg, an immune defect, Kartagener's syndrome, or cystic fibrosis) must be ruled out by immunoglobulin studies, cilia studies, and a sweat chloride test. Anaerobic and staphylococcal organisms are often responsible for chronic sinusitis. If allergies and diving do not offer a sufficient explanation for the problem, the patient should be referred to an otolaryngologist for complete evaluation. Functional endoscopic sinus surgery is being employed to manage patients with recurrent or persistent sinusitis. No data are available comparing the outcomes of surgical intervention with antibiotic management. There are large variations in use of this procedure by otolaryngologists.

Poole MD: Pediatric sinusitis is not a surgical disease. Ear Nose Throat J 1992;71:622.

Rachelefsky GS: Chronic sinusitis. Am J Dis Child 1989; 143:886.

RECURRENT EPISTAXIS

Most children have a few isolated nosebleeds, but recurrent nosebleed usually warrants a visit to the pediatrician. The nose is a very vascular structure. In most cases, epistaxis is due to mild trauma to the anterior portion of the nasal septum (Kiesselbach's area), sometimes as a result of falls or fistfights but usually due to vigorous nose rubbing, nose blowing, or nose picking. Less than 5% of children with recurrent epistaxis have a bleeding disorder.

Clinical Findings

A. Symptoms and Signs: The frequency of nosebleeds may be once a month to several times a day. If they are profuse, subsequent hematemesis or tarry stools may be reported. Examination of Kiesselbach's area reveals a red, raw surface with fresh clots or old crusts. There will often be blood under the fingernails.

B. Laboratory Findings: A baseline hematocrit is indicated in most patients. The true degree of anemia following a severe nosebleed may not be evident until 6–12 hours after bleeding has ceased.

Most patients do not need a hematologic workup, but bleeding tests are indicated if any of the following are present: a family history of a bleeding disorder, a past medical history of easy bleeding, spontaneous bleeding at other sites, bleeding that lasts for over 30 minutes or will not clot with direct pressure by the physician, onset before age 2, or a drop in the hematocrit due to epistaxis.

Differential Diagnosis

Although most cases of epistaxis occur following trauma to the normal nose, several contributing factors must be ruled out. If they are present, specific treatment will be needed.

A. Allergic Rhinitis: Boggy, inflamed mucosa

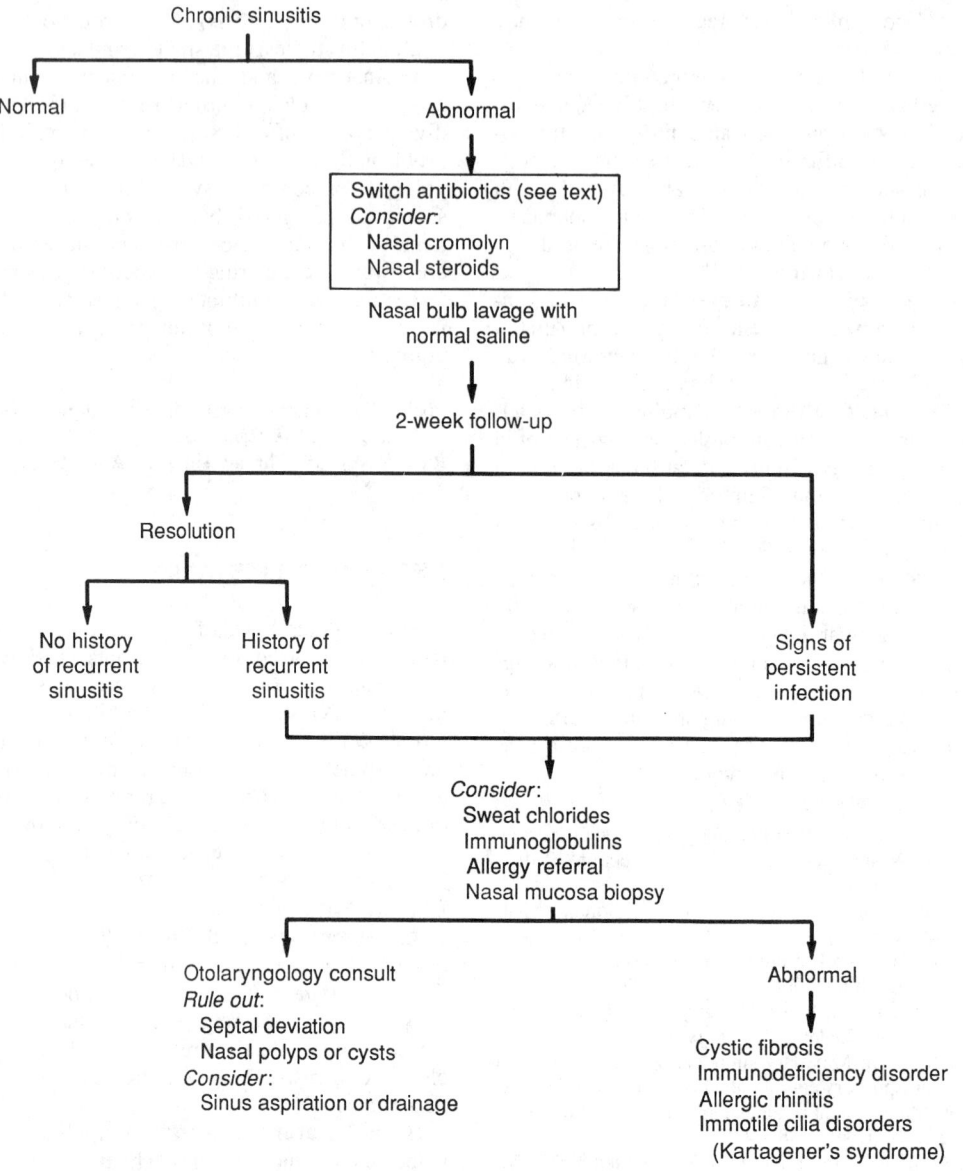

Figure 19–5. Algorithm for the management of chronic sinusitis.

is predisposed to epistaxis from itching and rubbing. This diagnosis is confirmed by a nasal smear for eosinophils. In such cases, antihistamines or cromolyn may help to decrease the amount of nasal pruritus and subsequent rubbing.

B. Chronic Bleeding Disorder: Numerous bleeding disorders (eg, von Willebrand's disease, thrombocytopenia) may present as recurrent epistaxis. A history of easy bleeding with circumcision, tonsillectomy, lacerations, venipuncture, or tooth eruption points to this type of disorder. A family history of hemophilia or other bleeding tendencies is suggestive. A history of spontaneous bleeding at other sites—gastrointestinal tract, hemarthrosis, menor-

rhagia, petechiae with crying, etc—or current physical findings of bleeding at other sites is suggestive. The presence of hepatomegaly or splenomegaly is also suggestive. These patients require bleeding screens.

C. Aspirin: Recent studies reveal that ingestion of normal doses of aspirin can interfere with platelet aggregation or adhesiveness and cause prolonged bleeding. The abnormal bleeding time is confirmatory.

D. Vascular Malformation: Kiesselbach's area must be carefully examined for telangiectasia, hemangiomas, or varicosities.

E. Hypertension: High blood pressure may predispose to prolonged nosebleeds.

F. Nasopharyngeal Angiofibroma: This tumor of adolescent males often presents with epistaxis. Bleeding confined to the back of the throat makes the elimination of this diagnosis mandatory. Lateral soft tissue films of the nasopharynx are diagnostic.

Complications

Unless an underlying bleeding disorder exists, the only complication of nosebleed is mild anemia. The latter is unusual and responds to iron therapy.

Treatment

A. Immediate Treatment: The following approach can be carried out in the office or given as phone advice: The patient should sit up and lean forward so as not to swallow the blood. The nose is pinched, with pressure over the bleeding site being maintained for 10 minutes by the clock. If bleeding continues, pressure is not being applied to the right spot, and it should be changed.

If this is not effective, clots should be removed by suction or blowing the nose. The bleeding site should be visualized. A pledget wet with 0.25% phenylephrine nose drops, 1% lidocaine with 1:1000 epinephrine or the most potent topical vasoconstrictor of all, 1% cocaineis inserted into the nose. Pressure is again applied for 10 minutes. Rarely does this technique fail.

Another approach involves the insertion of a small piece of gelatin sponge (Gelfoam) or topical thrombin over the bleeding site.

B. Preventive Treatment: The friability of the nasal vessels can be decreased with daily application of petrolatum or an antibiotic ointment by cotton-tipped applicator. The lubricant is applied daily until 5 days have passed without a nosebleed, then weekly for 1 month, and resumed only if the nosebleeds recur. In a very dry environment, humidification of the patient's room may be helpful. Aspirin should be avoided, as should vigorous blowing of the nose.

C. Reassurance: Parents mainly need education on how to stop nosebleeds. Parents also need reassurance regarding the amount of blood lostit always looks like more than it is. A normal hematocrit is usually comforting to the parents. The child should not be blamed regarding this problem. The parents should be told that simply rubbing a blocked nose or picking out dried mucus can cause nosebleeds.

D. Unwarranted Treatment: Electrocautery is contraindicated because it is painful and frightening to the child. Both electrocautery and chemical cautery can cause destruction of the septal tissue, resulting in scarring and an increased tendency for later bleeding.

Prognosis

Once home treatment and prophylaxis are mastered, nosebleeds become an insignificant problem for most families. In unusual cases where posterior bleeding occurs, the child must be referred to an otolaryngologist for a posterior nasal pack, evaluation for nasopharyngeal lesions, and perhaps a transfusion. If severe and repeated bleeding occurs, a skin graft over the scarred portion of the septum may be needed.

Mulbury PE: Recurrent epistaxis. Pediatr Rev 1991;12:213.

NASAL FURUNCLE

A nasal furuncle is an infection of a hair follicle in the anterior nares. Hair plucking or nose picking can provide a route of entry. The most common organism is *Staphylococcus aureus*. The diagnosis is made by finding an exquisitely tender, firm, red lump in the anterior naris. Treatment includes dicloxacillin or cephalexin orally for 5 days to prevent spread. The lesion should be gently incised and drained as soon as it points, usually with a needle. Topical bacitracin ointment may be of additional value. Since this lesion is in the drainage area of the cavernous sinus, the patient should be followed closely until healing is complete. Parents should be advised never to pick or squeeze a furuncle in this location, nor should the physician. Associated cellulitis or spread requires hospitalization for administration of intravenous antibiotics.

Some patients with recurrent skin abscesses as well as nasal furuncles are nasal carriers of *S aureus*. The skin problem will often not resolve until the nasal carrier state is eradicated by systemic antibiotics, topical antibiotics, and recolonization of the nasal mucosa with nonpathogenic staphylococci.

NASAL SEPTUM SUBLUXATION

Rarely, newborn infants have subluxation of the quadrangular cartilage of the septum. The tip of the nose deviates to one side, and the inferior septal border deviates to the other. There is also leaning of the columella and instability of the nasal tip. In the delivery room, reduction should be accomplished by lifting up the inferior border of the septum and replacing it in the septal groove of the floor of the nose. If any question about the procedure exists, an otolaryngologist should be consulted. This disorder must be distinguished from the more common transient flattening of the nose caused by the birth process.

Kent SE: Nasal septal deviation. J R Soc Med 1988;81:132.
Silverman SH et al: Dislocation of the triangular cartilage of the nasal septum. J Pediatr 1975;87:456.

NASAL FRACTURE

Most blows to the nose result in swelling and hematoma without fracture. A persistent nosebleed after trauma suggests nasal fracture. Crepitus or instability of the bones in the nasal bridge is diagnostic of fracture, as is marked deviation of the nose to one side. However, septal injury can only be ruled out by careful intranasal examination. If the parents feel that the appearance of the nose remains abnormal after the edema has resolved (usually 3–4 days), this should be taken as strong evidence for fracture. X-rays are not usually helpful because they are negative in half of cases of fracture. In general, they are warranted only in patients with symptoms and signs suggestive of fracture.

Patients with suspected nasal fractures should be referred to an ear, nose, and throat surgeon for definitive therapy. Resetting of the nasal fracture can be postponed up to 1 week without causing difficulty.

Olsen KD, Carpenter RJ, Kern EB: Nasal septal trauma in children. Pediatrics 1979;64:32.

NASAL SEPTUM HEMATOMA

After nasal trauma, it is essential to examine the inside of the nose with a nasal speculum. Hematoma of the nasal septum imposes a considerable risk of pressure necrosis and resorption of the cartilage, leading to septal perforation or a saddle-back nose in adulthood. This diagnosis is confirmed by the abrupt onset of nasal obstruction following trauma and the presence of a widened nasal septum. The normal nasal septum is 2–4 mm thick.

Treatment consists of prompt referral to an otolaryngologist for evacuation of the hematoma and packing of the nose.

East CA et al: Acute nasal trauma in children. J Pediatr Surg 1987;22:308.
Hematoma of the nasal septum. (Abstract.) Pediatr Rev 1992;13:225.

NASAL SEPTUM ABSCESS

A nasal septal abscess usually follows nasal trauma or a nasal furuncle. The symptoms include fever, nasal tenderness, and nasal occlusion. Physical findings reveal a fluctuant gray septal swelling, usually bilateral. The possible complications are the same as for nasal septal hematoma plus septicemia, meningitis, or cavernous sinus thrombosis.

Treatment consists of immediate hospitalization, incision and drainage by an otolaryngologist, and intravenous antibiotics.

Segal S et al: Bacterial meningitis secondary to abscess of the nasal septum. Pediatrics 1977;60:102.

FOREIGN BODIES IN THE NOSE

Most objects inserted into the nose are detected by the parent soon after insertion, and the child is brought in immediately. Occasionally, a nasal foreign body is detected only after unilateral purulent rhinitis occurs. Commonly inserted objects are pussy willow buds, beads, buttons, bullets, nuts, and marbles. In preparation for the object's removal, the nose should be suctioned and opened fully with a topical vasoconstrictor. The child's head should be held firmly to prevent movement and secondary injury during removal. The position of the head should be forward to prevent aspiration of the foreign body into a bronchus. A nasal speculum is sometimes helpful. Suction can be used to remove the layer of mucus that hides the object.

There are many ways to remove nasal foreign bodies. The obvious first maneuver is vigorous nose blowing if the child is old enough. If the object is round, such as a bead, collodion on a cotton-tipped applicator can be placed against it and left there for 1 or 2 minutes, after which it will usually be dry enough to remove the object. Irregular objects can sometimes be grasped with a bayonet forceps. If there is room to go past the object, a right-angled hook can be inserted and withdrawn, pushing the object ahead of it. If these techniques are not successful and there is some space between the object and the side of the nose, a lubricated No. 8 Bardex Foley catheter can be inserted. When the balloon is past the object, it can be inflated and then used to extract the object.

While the child's head remains tilted over a large basin, the noninvolved nostril can be flushed rapidly with normal saline from a nasal bulb syringe. The wave of fluid will wash around to the involved side and in most cases will force the object out. Closing the uninvolved nostril and placing one's mouth over the patient's mouth to administer a sudden blast of air will force the foreign body out if enough pressure is exerted. If the object seems inaccessible, is wedged in, or is quite large, the patient should be referred to an otolaryngologist without worsening its position through futile attempts.

Baker MD: Foreign bodies of the ears and nose in childhood. Pediatr Emerg Care 1987;3:67.
Stool SE, McConnell CS: Foreign bodies in pediatric otolaryngology. Clin Pediatr (Phila) 1973;12:113.

THE THROAT

ACUTE STOMATITIS

Recurrent Aphthous Stomatitis ("Canker Sore")

The main finding is single (two or three at most) small (3–10 mm) ulcers on the insides of the lips and throughout the remainder of the mouth. There is usually no associated fever or cervical adenopathy. The ulcers are very painful and last 1–2 weeks. They may recur numerous times throughout a patient's life span. The cause is not known, though an allergic or autoimmune basis is suspected. It is important to rule out offending agents that could be avoided (chocolate, nuts, tomatoes, etc). These lesions are commonly misdiagnosed as herpes simplex.

Treatment consists of topical antacids or sucralfate as a mouth coating four times daily. Topical corticosteroids, either in a dental pasteeg, triamcinolone acetonide 0.1% (Kenalog in Orabase)or in a mouthwash administered four times a day also have efficacy. Pain can be symptomatically improved by a bland diet, avoiding salty or acid foods, switching from a bottle to a cup in infants, 2% viscous lidocaine prior to meals, and acetaminophen or even codeine at bedtime. If the child is not old enough to expectorate the lidocaine, it must not be used. Measures that are unwarranted and sometimes harmful are smallpox vaccine, systemic antibiotics, chemical cautery, and *Lactobacillus*-containing agents.

Herpes Simplex Gingivostomatitis

Approximately 1% of children who have their first encounter with the herpes simplex virus develop multiple (ten or more) small (1–3 mm) ulcers of the buccal mucosa, anterior pillars, inner lips, tongue, and especially the gingiva, with associated fever, tender cervical nodes, and generalized inflammation of the mouth. The children are commonly under 3 years of age. This disorder lasts 7–10 days. Severe dysphagia interferes with eating and drinking. The primary disorder does not recur; herpes simplex recurs only in the form of cold sores that are found mainly at the labial mucocutaneous juncture.

Treatment is symptomatic as described for recurrent aphthous stomatitis (see above), with the exception that corticosteroids are contraindicated because they may result in spread of the infection. Oral acyclovir has not been approved for primary herpes gingivostomatitis. However, for severe cases, some physicians are prescribing acyclovir suspension (200 mg/5 mL), 10 mg/kg/dose three times daily for 7 days. The patient must be followed closely. Dehydration occasionally ensues despite liberal offerings of cold fluids, in which case the patient must be hospitalized so that intravenous fluids can be administered. Herpetic laryngotracheitis is a rare complication.

Stevens-Johnson Syndrome

The bullous form of erythema multiforme should be considered whenever there are vesicles and ulcers of the lips and oral mucosa with similar lesions on the conjunctiva and genitalia. In addition, most affected patients have a generalized erythema multiforme rash plus high fever and severe prostration. (For full discussion, see Chapter 13.)

Thrush

Oral candidiasis mainly affects bottle-fed infants and occasionally older children in a debilitated state. *Candida albicans* is a saprophyte that normally is not invasive unless the mouth is abraded. The use of broad-spectrum antibiotics may be a contributing factor. The symptoms include soreness of the mouth and refusal of feedings. Lesions consist of white curd-like plaques predominantly on the buccal mucosa. These plaques cannot be washed away after a water feeding.

Specific treatment consists of use of nystatin oral suspension, 1 mL four times a day for 1 week. This should be preceded by attempts to remove any large plaques with a moistened cotton-tipped applicator. The child should be fed temporarily with a spoon and cup to eliminate pain or continued abrasion. Pacifier use should be decreased.

Oral Syphilis

The primary chancre can occur on the lips or in the oral cavity. Secondary syphilis can present as mucous patches on any part of the oral cavity. These have a gray, slimy, concentric appearance and can occur in various sizes. Both of these lesions can be diagnosed by darkfield examination. By the time mucous patches are present, the serologic test for syphilis will be positive. Syphilis is discussed more fully in Chapter 33.

Traumatic Oral Ulcers

Ulcers are a nonspecific response of the oral mucosa to trauma. Mechanical trauma most commonly occurs on the buccal mucosa secondary to accidentally biting it with the molars. Thermal trauma, eg, from very hot foods, can also cause ulcerative lesions. Chemical ulcers can be produced by mucosal contact with aspirin, caustics, etc. Oral ulcers can also occur with leukemia or on a recurrent basis with cyclic neutropenia.

These lesions usually need no treatment. The pain subsides in 2 or 3 days.

Dunlap C, Parker BF, Lowe JW: Ten oral lesions you should know. Contemp Pediatr 1991;8:16.
Wright JM: A review of the oral manifestations of infections in pediatric patients. Pediatr Infect Dis J 1984;3:80.

ACUTE VIRAL PHARYNGITIS & TONSILLITIS

Over 90% of cases of sore throat and fever in children are due to viral infections. Most children develop associated rhinorrhea and mild cough and in fact are having a cold and nothing more. The findings seldom give any clue to the particular viral agent, but six types of viral pharyngitis are sufficiently distinctive to support an educated guess about the specific cause.

Clinical Findings

A. Infectious Mononucleosis: The findings are an exudative tonsillitis, generalized cervical adenitis, and fever, usually in a teenage patient. A palpable spleen or axillary adenopathy adds weight to the diagnosis. The presence of more than 20% atypical lymphocytes on a peripheral blood smear or a positive mononucleosis spot test (Monospot) confirms the diagnosis, although the Monospot is frequently negative in children under 5 years old. This diagnosis is often not considered until a patient with a presumptive diagnosis of streptococcal pharyngitis has failed to respond to 48 hours of treatment with penicillin.

B. Herpangina: Herpangina ulcers, 2–3 mm in size, are found on the anterior pillars and sometimes on the soft palate and uvula. There are no ulcers in the anterior mouth, as there are in herpes simplex. Fever is present. The disease lasts up to a week. Herpangina is caused by several members of the coxsackie A group of viruses, and a patient can have up to five bouts of herpangina in a lifetime.

C. Lymphonodular Pharyngitis: The classic finding is small, yellow-white nodules in the same distribution as the small ulcers in herpangina. In this condition, which is caused by coxsackievirus A10, the nodules do not ulcerate.

D. Hand, Foot, and Mouth Disease: This entity is caused by coxsackieviruses A5, A10, and A16. Ulcers occur on the tongue and oral mucosa. Vesicles, which usually do not ulcerate, are found on the palms, soles, and interdigital areas.

E. Pharyngoconjunctival Fever: This disorder is caused by an adenovirus. Exudative tonsillitis, conjunctivitis, and fever are the main findings.

F. Rubeola: The prodrome of measles looks like any nonspecific viral respiratory infection until one closely examines the buccal mucosa and the inner aspects of the lower lip. Small white specks the size of salt granules on an erythematous base (Koplik's spots) found at these sites are pathognomonic of early measles.

Treatment

The treatment of acute viral pharyngitis is strictly symptomatic. Older children can gargle with warm saline solution or antacid solution (eg, Mylanta). Younger children can suck on hard candy (especially butterscotch). Analgesics and antipyretics are sometimes helpful. Antibiotics are contraindicated.

McMillan JA et al: Pharyngitis associated with herpes simplex virus in college students. Pediatr Infect Dis J 1993;12:280.

Nakayama M et al: Pharyngoconjunctival fever caused by adenovirus type 11. Pediatr Infect Dis J 1992;11:6

ACUTE STREPTOCOCCAL PHARYNGITIS & TONSILLITIS

Approximately 10% of children with sore throat and fever have a streptococcal infection. Untreated streptococcal pharyngitis can result in acute rheumatic fever, glomerulonephritis, and suppurative complications (eg, cervical adenitis, peritonsillar abscess, otitis media, cellulitis, and septicemia). Vesicles and ulcers are suggestive of viral infection, whereas cervical adenitis, petechiae, a beefy-red uvula, and a tonsillar exudate are suggestive of streptococcal infection; the only way to make a definitive diagnosis is by obtaining a throat culture or a rapid identification test. Rapid identification tests are very specific but lack sensitivity. Therefore, a positive test indicates infection but a negative result requires confirmation with culture. A throat culture can be read 18 hours after being placed in an incubator. The bacteriology involved is simple, and an inexpensive office incubator is commercially available. Office throat cultures or rapid identification tests are essential for rational management of pharyngitis.

Treat cases of suspected or proved *S pyogenes* infection with a 10-day course of oral penicillin V potassium or or cephalosporin such as cephalexin or an intramuscular injection of penicillin G benzathine. Use erythromycin for patients with penicillin allergy. Treatment failure after 10 days of penicillin V administered three times daily varies from 6% to 23%. Approximately 5% of *S pyogenes* are resistant to erythromycin. Remember that trimethoprim-sulfamethoxazole is not an effective antibiotic for *S pyogenes*. Children should receive 24 hours of therapy prior to returning to school.

If the child has a history of recurrent streptococcal infection, one must document the presence of *S pyogenes* in an asymptomatic patient following a course of therapy. If compliance or the antibiotic dosage was questionable, treat with intramuscular penicillin; otherwise, treat with an antibiotic effective against β-lactamase-producing organisms (amoxicillin plus clavulanate, a cephalosporin, or erythromycin). If this therapy fails to eradicate the organism, consider a course of clindamycin for 10 days. In general, the carrier state is harmless, not contagious, and self-limited (2–6 months). An attempt to eradicate the carrier state is warranted only if the patient or another family member has frequent streptococcal infections or when a family member or patient has a history of rheumatic fever or glomerulonephritis. Consider also treatment for carriers who live in closed or semi-closed community settings. If the patient had three or more documented infections within 6 months, consider instituting daily penicillin prophylaxis during the winter season. Refer patients for tonsillectomy only if they continue to have frequent episodes despite antibiotic prophylaxis or when persistently enlarged tonsils cause chronic upper airway obstruction (see Figure 19–6).

Other rare causes of acute nonviral pharyngitis are *Corynebacterium diphtheriae, Neisseria gonorrhoeae,* group C streptococci, meningococci, *Chlamydia, Francisella tularensis,* and *Mycoplasma pneumoniae.*

Gerber MA, Markowitz M: Streptococcal pharyngitis: Clearing up the controversies. Contemp Pediat (October) 1992;9:118.

Pichichero ME et al: Comparative reliability of clinical, culture, and antigen detection methods for the diagnosis of group A beta-hemolytic streptococcal tonsillopharyngitis. Pediatr Ann 1992;21:798.

Pichichero ME: Cephalosporins are superior to penicillin for the treatment of streptococcal tonsillopharyngitis: Is the difference worth it? Pediatr Infect Dis J 1993;12:268.

Snellman L et al: Duration of positive throat cultures for group A streptococci after initiation of antibiotic therapy. Pediatrics 1993;91:1166.

Tanz RR et al: Clindamycin treatment of chronic pharyngeal carriage of group A streptococci. J Pediatr 1991;119:123.

RECURRENT PHARYNGITIS

School-age children are occasionally brought to a physician with a complaint of recurrent or persistent sore throat. Fever and other systemic manifestations are usually absent. There are three common causes of this problem: mouth breathing, postnasal drip, and school phobia.

Mouth breathing leads to dryness and irritation of the throat, especially in areas of low humidity. Occasionally, children will even complain upon awakening that their lips are stuck to their teeth. The causes of mouth breathing should be investigated. Symptomatic treatment consists of good hydration and environmental humidification.

Postnasal drip due to chronic sinusitis can lead to continuous irritation of the throat. Examination reveals mucopurulent secretions descending from the nasopharynx after the patient sniffs. The irritation is largely due to repeated clearing of the throat.

Children with **school avoidance problems** are brought in repeatedly for sore throats, but physical examination reveals a normal oropharynx and tonsillar area. The diagnosis is made by asking the parent if the problem has been interfering with the child's school attendance. The answer will be affirmative

and completely out of keeping with the degree of symptoms. Management is described in Chapter 6.

PERITONSILLAR CELLULITIS OR ABSCESS (Quinsy)

Tonsillar infection occasionally penetrates the tonsillar capsule, spreads to the surrounding tissues, and causes peritonsillar cellulitis. If untreated, necrosis occurs and a tonsillar abscess forms. This can occur at any age. The most common cause is β-hemolytic streptococci. Other pathogens are group D streptococci, α-hemolytic streptococci, *S pneumoniae,* and anaerobes.

The patient complains of a severe sore throat even before the physical findings become marked. A high fever is usually present. The process is almost always unilateral. The tonsil bulges medially, and the anterior pillar is prominent. The soft palate and uvula on the involved side are edematous and displaced medially toward the uninvolved side. In severe cases, there is trismus, dysphagia, and, finally, drooling. The quality of the voice is severely impaired by the fixation of the soft palate. On palpation, the tonsil is firm and exquisitely tender. A serious complication of inadequately treated peritonsillar abscess is a lateral pharyngeal abscess. This leads to fullness and tenderness of the lateral neck, as well as torticollis. Without intervention, the abscess eventually threatens life by airway obstruction or carotid artery erosion.

Aggressive treatment in early cases of peritonsillar cellulitis will usually abort the process and prevent suppuration. The treatment of choice is procaine penicillin by daily injection plus oral penicillin four times a day in high doses. Consider adding clindamycin for better coverage of β-lactamase-producing anaerobes if the rapid streptococcal test is negative. Daily follow-up is critical to detect possible abscess. If the initial swelling is marked, fluctuation develops, a neck mass develops, the patient appears toxic, or symptoms fail to respond to 48 hours of antibiotics, the patient should be hospitalized for intravenous penicillin or clindamycin. An otolaryngologist should be consulted. Incision and drainage under general anesthesia should be considered in children who fail to respond to intravenous antibiotics. Recurrent peritonsillar abscesses are so uncommon (7%) that routine tonsillectomy for a single bout is not indicated. Hospitalized patients can be discharged on oral antibiotics when fever is resolved for 24 hours and they can swallow easily.

Shoemaker M, Lampe R, Weir MR: Peritonsillitis: Abscess or cellulitis? Pediatr Infect Dis J 1986;5:43.

Stringer SP et al: Outpatient management of peritonsillar abscess. Arch Otolaryngol Head Neck Surg 1988;114:296.

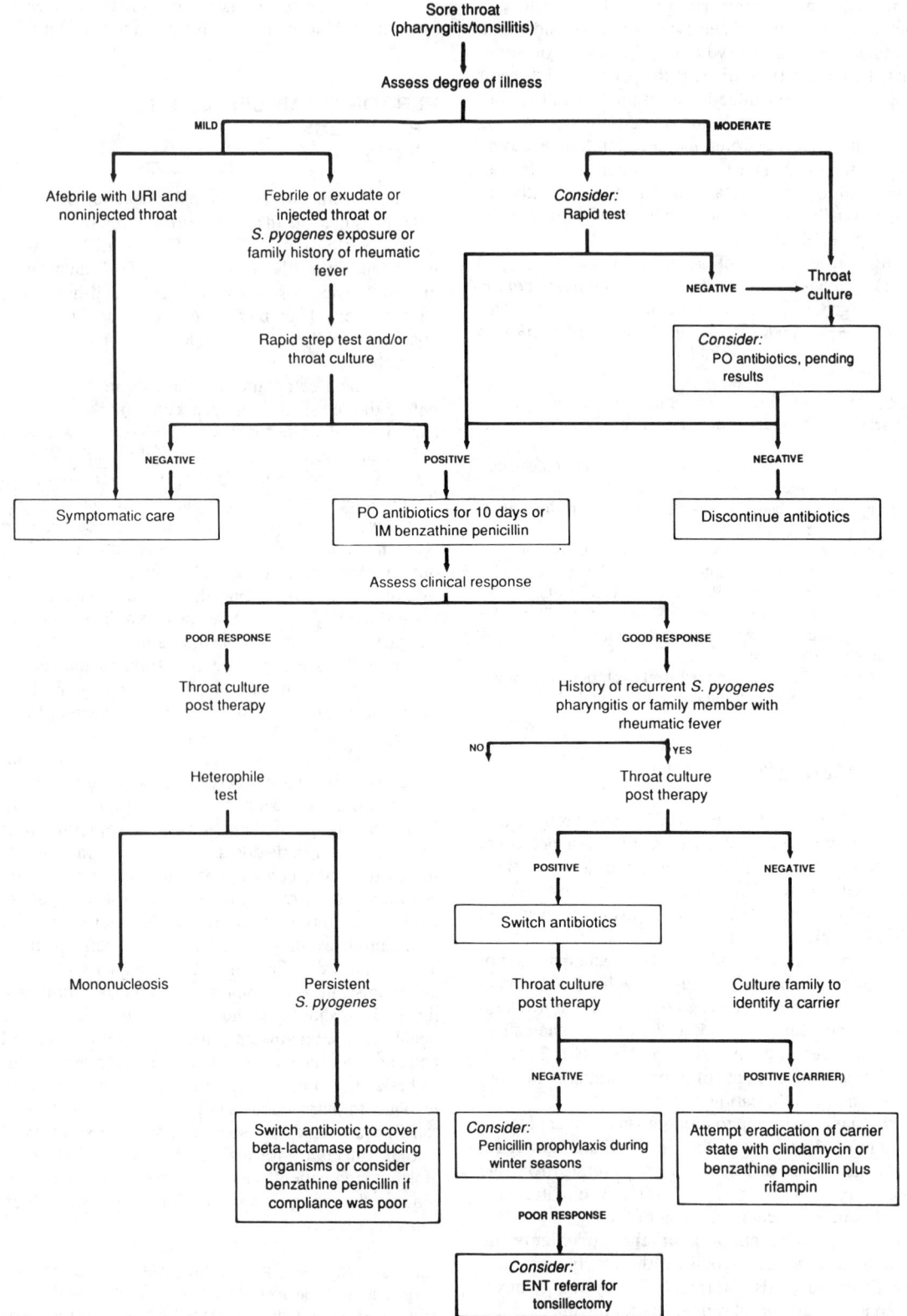

Figure 19–6. Algorithm for the management of streptococcal infection. (Modified and reproduced, with permission, from Berman S: *Pediatric Decision Making.* BC Decker, 1990.)

RETROPHARYNGEAL ABSCESS

Retropharyngeal nodes drain the adenoids, nasopharynx, and paranasal sinuses and can become infected. The most common causes are β-hemolytic streptococci and *S aureus*. If this pyogenic adenitis goes untreated, a retropharyngeal abscess forms. The process occurs most commonly during the first 2 years of life. Beyond this age, retropharyngeal abscess usually results from superinfection of a penetrating injury of the posterior wall of the oropharynx.

The diagnosis should be strongly suspected in an infant with fever, respiratory symptoms, and neck hyperextension. Dysphagia, drooling, dyspnea, and gurgling respirations are also found and are due to impingement by the abscess. Prominent swelling on one side of the posterior pharyngeal wall confirms the diagnosis. Swelling usually stops at the midline because a medial raphe divides the prevertebral space. Lateral neck soft tissue films show the retropharyngeal space to be wider than the C4 vertebral body.

Retropharyngeal abscess is a surgical emergency. Immediate hospitalization is required. A surgeon should incise and drain the abscess under general anesthesia to prevent its extension. The head should be kept down during incision to prevent aspiration of purulent material. Intravenous hydration and antibiotics should be instituted before surgery. A semisynthetic penicillin is the drug of choice pending the results of stained smear examination and culture.

Grosso J: Retropharyngeal abscess. Am J Dis Child 1990;144:1350.

LUDWIG'S ANGINA

Ludwig's angina is a rapidly progressive cellulitis of the submandibular space. The submandibular space extends from the mucous membrane of the tongue to the muscular and fascial attachments of the hyoid bone. The initiating factor in over half of cases is dental disease, including abscesses and extraction. Some patients have a history of lacerations and injuries to the floor of the mouth. Group A streptococci are the most common organisms identified, but other pathogens have been recovered.

The presenting symptoms are fever and tender swelling of the floor of the mouth. The tongue can become enlarged as well as tender and erythematous. Upward displacement of the tongue may cause dysphagia and drooling. Laboratory evaluation includes blood cultures and hypopharyngeal aspiration to attempt to identify the specific pathogen.

Treatment consists of giving high doses of intravenous clindamycin or ampicillin and nafcillin until the results of cultures and sensitivity tests are available. Since the most common cause of death in Ludwig's angina is sudden airway obstruction, the patient must be followed closely in the intensive care unit and intubation provided for any progressive respiratory distress. An otolaryngologist should be consulted to identify an abscess and consider the benefit of incision and drainage.

ACUTE UVULITIS

Infections involving the uvula are uncommon. In children under 5 years of age, the cause is usually *Haemophilus influenzae* type b. In children over 5 years of age, group A streptococcus is the usual pathogen. Associated bacteremia is common.

The main symptoms are fever, dysphagia, and drooling. The prominent physical finding is an erythematous, swollen uvula. Laboratory studies should include a complete blood count and blood culture. A lateral neck radiograph should be obtained to rule out associated epiglottitis. Patients with acute uvulitis should be admitted to the hospital and treated with intravenous antibiotics that cover β-lactamase-producing organisms.

Li KI et al: Isolated uvulitis due to *Haemophilus influenzae* type b. Pediatrics 1984;74:1054.

ACUTE CERVICAL ADENITIS

Essentials of Diagnosis

- Large, tender, unilateral cervical mass.
- Fever.
- Moderate to marked leukocytosis.

General Considerations

Local infections of the ear, nose, and throat can spread to the regional node and cause a secondary inflammation there. The most commonly involved node is the jugulodigastric node, which drains the tonsillar area. The problem is most prevalent among preschool children.

A classic case involves a large, unilateral, solitary, tender node. About 70% of these cases are due to β-hemolytic streptococci, 20% are due to staphylococci, and the remainder may be due to viruses. *Haemophilus influenzae* or anaerobes have rarely been reported as the cause. Surgeons report a higher incidence of staphylococcal infection, but they see a greater proportion of atypical cases that have failed to respond to penicillin therapy and thus require incision and drainage.

The most common site of invasion is from pharyngitis or tonsillitis. Other entry sites for pyogenic adenitis are periapical dental abscess (usually producing a submandibular adenitis), facial impetigo (infected cuts or bug bites), infected acne, and otitis externa (usually producing a preauricular adenitis).

Clinical Findings

A. Symptoms and Signs: The patient is brought in with a chief complaint of swollen neck or face. There is usually sustained high fever, especially in staphylococcal infections. The mass is often the size of a walnut or even an egg. It is taut, firm, and exquisitely tender. If left untreated, it may develop overlying erythema. The exact size of the node should be recorded for future follow-up. Each tooth should be examined for periapical abscess and percussed for tenderness. Protective torticollis is sometimes present.

B. Laboratory Findings: The white blood cell count is usually about 20,000/μL with a shift to the left. A throat culture and rapid streptococcal test are often helpful. A tuberculin skin test should be given. Aspirated material from fluctuant nodes should be Gram-stained and cultured for aerobes and anaerobes.

Differential Diagnosis

The causes of cervical adenopathy are numerous. Five general categories can be distinguished on the basis of the clinical findings.

A. Acute Unilateral Cervical Adenitis: See above.

B. Acute Bilateral Cervical Adenitis: Painful and tender nodes are present on both sides, and the patient usually has fever.

1. Infectious mononucleosis–This diagnosis can be aided by the findings of splenomegaly, over 20% atypical white blood cells on the Wright-stained smear, and a positive mononucleosis spot test (Monospot). Toxoplasmosis and cytomegalovirus infections can imitate this disorder.

2. Tularemia–There will be a history of wild rabbit or deerfly exposure.

3. Diphtheria–This occurs only in nonimmunized children.

C. Subacute or Chronic Adenitis: In this condition, an isolated node usually exists, but it is smaller and less tender than the acute pyogenic adenitis described previously.

1. Nonspecific viral pharyngitis–This accounts for about 80% of cases in this category.

2. β-Hemolytic streptococcal infection–Streptococci can occasionally cause a low-grade cervical adenitis; staphylococci never do.

3. Cat-scratch fever–Cat-scratch fever accounts for over 70% of cases of chronic cervical adenopathy. The diagnosis is aided by the finding of a primary papule in approximately 60% of cases. In over 90% of cases, cat scratches are present or there is a history of contact with cats. The node is usually mildly tender. The cat-scratch skin test is helpful and relatively safe.

4. Atypical mycobacterial infection–The node is generally nontender and submandibular (occasionally preauricular). The nodes become fluctuant after several months. Affected patients are usually 1–5 years of age. A history of drinking unpasteurized milk is helpful. A mildly positive PPD is suggestive. A PPD-standard test gives 5–10 mm of induration, whereas the PPD-Battey gives over 10 mm of induration. If skin tests for atypical mycobacteria are not available, the OT (old tuberculin) test can be substituted for screening.

D. Cervical Node Tumors: Malignant tumors usually are not suspected until the adenopathy persists despite treatment. Classically, the nodes are painless, nontender, and firm to hard in consistency. They may occur as a single node, as unilateral multiple nodes in a chain, as bilateral cervical nodes, or as generalized adenopathy. Cancers that may present in the neck are Hodgkin's disease, lymphosarcoma, fibrosarcoma, thyroid cancer, leukemia, and cancers with an occult primary in the nasopharynx (eg, rhabdomyosarcoma). A benign tumor that presents as enlarged cervical nodes is sinus histiocytosis.

E. Imitators of Adenitis: Several structures in the neck can become infected and resemble a node. The first three masses are of congenital origin and are listed in order of frequency.

1. Thyroglossal duct cyst–When superinfected, this congenital malformation can become acutely swollen. Helpful findings are the fact that it is in the midline, located between the hyoid bone and suprasternal notch, and moves upward upon sticking out the tongue or swallowing. Occasionally, the cyst develops a sinus tract and opening just lateral to the midline.

2. Branchial cleft cyst–When superinfected, this can become a tender mass 3–5 cm in diameter. Aids to diagnosis are the fact that the mass is located along the anterior border of the sternocleidomastoid muscle and is smooth and fluctuant, as a cyst should be. Occasionally, it is attached to the overlying skin by a small dimple or a draining sinus tract.

3. Cystic hygroma–Most of these lymphatic cysts are located in the posterior triangle just above the clavicle. The mass is soft and compressible and can be transilluminated. Over 60% are noted at birth, and the remainder usually present by 2 years of age. If cysts become large enough, they can compromise swallowing and breathing.

4. Mumps–The most common pitfall in differential diagnosis of cervical adenopathy is mistaking mumps for adenitis. However, a swollen parotid crosses the angle of the jaw, is associated with preauricular percussion tenderness, is bilateral in 70% of cases, and there is frequently a history of exposure to mumps and no mumps immunization. Submandibular mumps can present a diagnostic dilemma.

5. Ranula–This sublingual retention cyst can be mistaken for a submental node.

6. Sternocleidomastoid muscle hematoma– This cervical mass is noted at 2–4 weeks of age. On close examination, it is found to be part of the muscle body and not movable. An associated torticollis is usually confirmatory.

Complications

The most common complication in the untreated case is suppuration of the node, with eventual pointing and exterior drainage. In the preantibiotic era, extension sometimes occurred internally, resulting in jugular vein thrombosis, carotid artery rupture, septicemia, and compression of the esophagus or larynx. Poststreptococcal acute glomerulonephritis and bacteremia have also been reported.

Treatment

A. Specific Measures: Unless the rapid streptococcal test is positive or the patient has recently been exposed to β-hemolytic streptococci, dicloxacillin or cephalexin is usually started initially. An antistaphylococcal also must be started initially if the patient is under 6 months of age or the node is already fluctuant or erythematous. The patient should be referred to a dentist if periapical abscess is suspected. These dental patients should also be given prophylactic penicillin therapy prior to seeing the dentist to prevent progression to facial cellulitis or submandibular adenitis.

B. General Measures: Analgesics (even codeine) are necessary during the first few days. Patients may obtain significant relief from application of cold compresses or an ice cube to the inflamed node.

C. Surgical Treatment: Early treatment with antibiotics prevents many cases of pyogenic adenitis from progressing to suppuration. However, once fluctuation occurs, antibiotic therapy alone is not sufficient treatment. When fluctuation or pointing is present and the PPD skin test is negative, the primary physician or a surgeon should incise and drain the abscess. This can be done as an office procedure or in an ambulatory surgery unit. Hospitalization is required only if the patient is toxic, dehydrated, dysphagic, dyspneic, or less than 6 months of age.

D. Follow-Up Care: The patient must be seen daily. A good response includes resolution of the fever and improvement in the tenderness after 48 hours of treatment. Reduction in size of the nodes may take several more days. The antibiotic should be continued for 10 days. If there is no improvement in 48 hours and the PPD test is negative, the node should be aspirated with an 18-gauge needle and 0.5 mL of normal saline in the syringe to obtain material for Gram-stained smear, culture, and sensitivity tests. Aspirated material should be cultured aerobically and anaerobically.

E. Treatment of Nonpyogenic Adenitis:

1. Cat-scratch fever and atypical mycobacterial infection– Treatment is described in Chapter 33.

2. Persistent unexplained node–As previously mentioned, cancer of the cervical node is usually asymptomatic. The patient with a cervical node that continues to enlarge for more than 2 weeks despite treatment or is still large (> 3 cm) and unchanged in size for more than 2 months should be referred to a surgeon for possible biopsy.

3. Branchial cleft cyst and thyroglossal duct cyst–If superinfected, these lesions should be treated with antibiotics for 10 days. After the infection clears, the patient should be referred to a surgeon for definitive excision of the cyst.

Prognosis

With appropriate treatment, the prognosis is excellent. After the infection clears, the node may remain palpable for several months but will gradually decrease in size unless it is scarred. Recurrent pyogenic adenitis is rare. When it occurs, it is usually due to diseases such as chronic granulomatous disease of childhood or an immunologic disorder.

Caruthers HA: Cat scratch disease: An overview based on a study of 1200 patients. Am J Dis Child 1985;139:1124.

Knight PJ, Mulne AF, Vassy LE: When is lymph node biopsy indicated in children with enlarged peripheral nodes? Pediatrics 1982;69:391.

Marcy SM: Infections of lymph nodes of head and neck. Pediatr Infect Dis J 1983;2:397.

Margileth AM: Cervical adenitis. Pediatr Rev 1985;7:13.

Pounds LA: Neck masses of congenital origin. Pediatr Clin North Am 1981;28:841.

Zitelli BJ: Evaluating the child with a neck mass. Contemp Pediatr 1990;7(1):90.

TONSILLECTOMY & ADENOIDECTOMY (T&A)

Removal of the tonsils and adenoids has been described as a North American ritual. Although about 30% of children in the USA have their tonsils and adenoids removed, only 1–2% of children have adequate medical indications for this procedure.

Besides being usually unnecessary, the procedure is costly and carries considerable risk. The mortality rate under good conditions is still one death per 15,000 operations. Postoperative bleeding on the fifth to eighth day occurs in about 5% of cases and requires transfusion or suturing of the tonsillar bed. Some children with previously normal speech develop hypernasal speech. The emotional hazards of hospitalization and surgery in a child under 5 years of age have been well documented. There are still questions regarding the role of tonsils in immunologic response and disease prevention.

Invalid Reasons for T&A

The following conditions account for the removal of over 95% of tonsils and adenoids.

A. "Large Tonsils": Many parents feel that large tonsils mean bad tonsils. It is unfortunate that the peak incidence of infections correlates so well with tonsillar size. Normal lymphoid atrophy occurs spontaneously after age 8. The parent should be reassured that the patient's tonsils are within normal range. It is very important at well child checkups not to call a child's tonsils "big" or "bad."

B. Recurrent Colds and Sore Throats: T&A does not decrease the incidence of viral respiratory infections. Parents must be reassured that these infections are a natural event at this age and that contacts eventually give the patient increased immunity.

C. Recurrent Streptococcal Pharyngitis: At one time, repeated episodes of "strep throat" were considered an indication for tonsillectomy. However, it has been shown in several studies that the incidence of streptococcal infections does not decrease after the tonsils have been removed unless seven or more attacks occur per year. Moreover, the future diagnosis of streptococcal infections is made difficult by the lack of tonsillar exudates.

D. Recurrent Otitis Media: Most cases of recurrent purulent otitis media can be treated with prophylactic antibiotics. Most cases of chronic serous otitis media with hearing loss eventually resolve or require tympanoplasty tubes. An adenoidectomy may be helpful if the child also has symptoms of nasal obstruction.

E. Parental Pressure: Some parents place great demands on their doctor for a T&A and must be skillfully reeducated.

F. School Absence: For the child who misses school for vague symptoms, removing the tonsils will not relieve the problem.

G. "Chronic Tonsillitis": It is unclear whether this condition even exists. If it does, it is certainly very rare. The tonsil is allegedly so diseased that even antibiotics cannot eliminate the infections.

H. Miscellaneous Conditions: Poor appetite, allergic rhinitis, asthma, unexplained fevers, and halitosis are not indications for tonsillectomy.

Indications for Adenoidectomy

A. Persistent Nasal Obstruction and Mouth Breathing: Mouth breathing can have many causes. However, if this problem is due to large adenoids, they should be removed to prevent an adenoidal facies. Removal should be preceded by a 2-week trial of penicillin or clindamycin to rule out enlargement from subacute adenoiditis.

B. Snoring: The adenoids should be removed if they appear to be the cause of sleep apnea, uninterrupted nighttime snoring, or daytime snoring.

C. Hyponasal Speech: Large adenoids can cause hyponasal speech that leads to poor communi-

cation as well as teasing. On examination, large adenoids are found to be preventing the uvula from moving upward normally.

Indications for Tonsillectomy

A. Persistent Oral Obstruction and Dysphagia: Intermittent oral obstruction, dysphagia, and drooling can occur as a result of inflammation and swelling of the tonsils. If the problem is persistent and the tonsils are seen to almost touch in the midline, tonsillectomy should be considered. This is especially likely to happen in people who have small oral cavities.

B. Recurrent Peritonsillar Abscess: This problem implies that the tonsil is no longer inhibiting the spread of infection and needs to be removed. About 7% of peritonsillar abscesses recur.

C. Recurrent Pyogenic Cervical Adenitis: Again, the tonsil is no longer acting as an effective barrier to the spread of infection.

D. Suspected Tonsillar Tumor: The prominent unilateral tonsil, especially if it is rapidly enlarging, may be removed with the presumptive diagnosis of tonsillar neoplasm. On palpation, these tumors are usually firm and fixed. This is a grave diagnosis to miss.

Indications for Combined T&A

A. Cor Pulmonale: A patient with adenoidal hypertrophy can develop chronic hypoxia that leads to pulmonary hypertension and finally to cor pulmonale and right-sided heart failure. This is a rare but serious complication that is definitely helped by T&A, sometimes on an emergency basis.

B. Sleep Apnea Syndrome: Affected children all have loud snoring interrupted by apneic episodes. Many are referred because of excessive daytime sleepiness and worsening school performance. Acquired pectus excavatum and poor growth has also been reported in some of these children. Their symptoms are reversed by T&A.

Contraindications to T&A

A. Short Palate: Adenoids should not be removed in a child with a cleft palate, submucous cleft palate, or bifid uvula, because of the risk of aggravating the velopharyngeal incompetence and causing hypernasal speech and nasal regurgitation.

B. Bleeding Disorder: If a chronic bleeding disorder is present, it must be diagnosed and compensated for before a T&A.

C. Acute Tonsillitis: T&A should be postponed until an acute tonsillitis is resolved. This guideline may prevent superinfection of the wound.

Management of Parental Pressure

If parents are dissatisfied with the kind of treatment they are receiving, they can "doctor-shop" until they find someone who will remove their child's tonsils. This can be prevented by the following approach: The parents' complaint must be taken seriously. All of the reasonable indications for T&A must be competently investigated. The ear, nose, and throat examination must be performed carefully, and the parents must be assured that there are some valid reasons to take out the tonsils but only when the benefit outweighs the risk, discomfort, and inconvenience.

The parents can then be reassured that their child is basically healthy and does not have one of the valid indications. The prognosis for spontaneous involution of the tonsils and adenoids and a lower incidence of respiratory infections in years to come can be offered. In addition, it can be mentioned that the risk of taking the tonsils out is considerably greater than the risk of leaving them in.

If the parents are still unconvinced, a consultation is in order. Since it is in the child's best interest, an otolaryngologist should be chosen who shares the pediatrician's viewpoint on this subject.

Paradise JL et al: Efficacy of tonsillectomy for recurrent throat infection in severely affected children. N Engl J Med 1984;310:674.

Ridgway D et al: Unsuspected non-Hodgkin's lymphoma of the tonsils and adenoids in children. Pediatrics 1987; 79:399.

Stradling JR et al: Effect of adenotonsillectomy on nocturnal hypoxaemia, sleep disturbance, and symptoms in snoring children. Lancet 1990;335:249.

DISORDERS OF THE LIPS*

Labial Sucking Tubercle

A small baby may present with a small callus in the mid upper lip. It usually is asymptomatic and disappears after cup feeding is initiated.

Swollen Lip

Allergy can cause the sudden onset of angioedema of the lip. Possible causes include foods, contact dermatitis to lipstick, and insect bites. Treatment includes avoidance of the cause, cold compresses, and oral antihistamines.

Cheilitis

Dry, cracked, scaling lips are usually due to sun or wind exposure. Contact dermatitis from mouthpieces of various woodwind or brass instruments has also been reported. Licking the lips accentuates the process, and the patient should be warned of this. Liberal use of lip balms gives excellent results.

Perlèche

The angle of the mouth may become fissured and raw. This most commonly happens in children who

---

*Herpetic lesions are discussed in Chapter 35.

drool or lick the sides of the mouth, establishing a macerated area. The most common pathogen is *Candida albicans*. Sores at the corners of the mouth can also be due to use of wide teething rings with rough edges. Riboflavin deficiency is a rare cause. The lesions respond well to nystatin cream. Occasionally, a corticosteroid must be added.

Inclusion Cyst

Inclusion cysts, or retention cysts, are due to the obstruction of mucous glands or other mucous membrane structures. In the newborn, they occur on the hard palate or gums and are called Epstein's pearls. These small cysts resolve spontaneously in 1–2 months. In older children, inclusion cysts usually occur on the palate, uvula, or tonsillar pillars. They appear as taut, yellow sacs varying in size from 2 mm to 10 mm. They spontaneously resolve in several months to a year without requiring incision and drainage. They can be rechecked in 1 month to confirm that they are not enlarging rapidly and thereafter reevaluated only during regular visits. Occasionally, a mucous cyst on the lower lip (mucocele) will require drainage for cosmetic reasons. Minor salivary glands are present at this site, and biting the lip may sever their ducts and initiate the problem.

DISORDERS OF THE TONGUE

Geographic Tongue (Benign Migratory Glossitis)

This condition of unknown cause is marked by circular or elliptical smooth areas on the tongue devoid of papillae and surrounded by a narrow ring of hyperkeratosis. The pattern can change from day to day. The lesions are painless and may last months to years. This puzzling disorder is benign, uncommon after age 6, and requires no treatment.

Fissured Tongue (Scrotal Tongue)

This condition is marked by numerous irregular fissures on the dorsum of the tongue. It occurs in approximately 1% of people and is usually a dominant trait. It is also frequently seen in children with trisomy 21 and other retarded patients who have the habit of chewing on a protruded tongue.

Coated Tongue (Furry Tongue)

The tongue normally becomes coated if mastication is impaired and the patient is on a liquid or soft diet. Mouth breathing, fever, or dehydration can accentuate the process.

Macroglossia

Tongue hypertrophy and protrusion may be a clue

to Beckwith-Wiedemann syndrome, glycogen storage disease, cretinism, Hurler's syndrome, lymphangioma, or hemangioma. In trisomy 21, the normal-sized tongue protrudes because the oral cavity is small.

Acute Bacterial Glossitis

Reported causes of acute suppurative glossitis include *Haemophilus influenzae* type b, *Streptococcus pyogenes,* and *Pseudomonas.* This rare disease is characterized by fever and rapid swelling and tenderness of the tongue. Intravenous antibiotics are required.

Edwards MS, Reynolds GES: Acute glossitis due to *Hemophilus influenzae* type b. J Pediatr 1978;93:532.

ORAL TRAUMA

Puncture wounds of the floor of the mouth and soft palate are not uncommon in children. Most could be prevented if children were prevented from playing with sticks or pencils in their mouths. Treatment includes a tetanus booster if one has not been given in the previous 5 years. Prophylactic antibiotics are not helpful, but the patient should be seen after 48 hours to rule out the possibility of superinfection. Puncture wounds of the anterior pillar or posterior pharynx should be followed closely for carotid thrombosis or retropharyngeal abscess, respectively.

Lacerations of the lip require precise closure and alignment of the mucocutaneous juncture. Lacerations of the buccal mucosa usually heal without suturing. Most tongue lacerations heal without suturing; if they involve the edges of the tongue and are large enough to cause gaping of the wound, black silk sutures must be placed, sometimes under general anesthesia. Complicated wounds should be referred to an oral surgeon.

HALITOSIS

"Bad breath" is a puzzling and distressing complaint. In most cases, it is due to acute stomatitis, pharyngitis, or sinusitis. In children, there are two common causes of chronic halitosis: continual mouth breathing and thumb-sucking or blanket-sucking. Unusual causes of foul breath are a nasal foreign body, esophageal diverticulum, gastric bezoar, bronchiectasis, and lung abscess. In older children, the presence of orthodontic devices or dentures can cause halitosis if good dental hygiene is not maintained. Halitosis can also be caused by decaying food particles that are embedded in cryptic tonsils. In adolescents, tobacco use is a common cause. Also, offensive skin odors (eg, dirty feet) of long duration can become absorbed

and excreted through the lungs. Mouthwashes and chewable breath fresheners give limited improvement. The cause must be uncovered to help the patient with chronic halitosis.

SALIVARY GLAND DISORDERS*

Suppurative Parotitis

Pyogenic parotitis is an unusual clinical disorder found chiefly in newborns and debilitated older patients. The parotid gland is swollen, tender, and often reddened. The diagnosis is made by expression of purulent material from Stensen's duct. The material should be smeared and cultured. Fever and leukocytosis may be present.

Treatment includes hospitalization and intravenous nafcillin because the most common causative organism is *Staphylococcus aureus*. If fluctuation occurs and drainage through Stensen's duct is impaired, aspiration of the pus with an 18-gauge needle can avoid the necessity for incision and drainage. This procedure may have to be repeated three or four times.

Recurrent Idiopathic Parotitis

Some children experience repeated episodes of parotid swelling that lasts 1–2 weeks and then resolves spontaneously. There is usually mild pain and often no fever. The process is most often unilateral, a fact that argues against an autoimmune process as the underlying cause and suggests instead some sort of obstructive process. Serum amylase is normal, which speaks against a diagnosis of viral parotitis, as can occur with mumps, parainfluenza, and other viral infections. As many as ten episodes may occur from age 2 on. Antibiotic prophylaxis may reduce the number of episodes. The problem usually resolves spontaneously at puberty.

Treatment includes analgesics if pain is present. A 4-day course of corticosteroids can be recommended if it can be initiated early in an attack. A second attack of parotid swelling without fever should result in referral to an otolaryngologist for a sialogram to rule out calculus of Stensen's duct. The usual finding is sialectasis. The sialogram seems to improve as the recurrence rate diminishes.

Pneumoparotitis

Children with pneumoparotitis complain of a sudden onset of pain and swelling in the parotid area. A history of playing a musical wind instrument or blowing up balloons confirms the diagnosis. The cause of this transient condition is inflation of the parotid gland secondary to sudden increased intraoral pressure.

---

*Mumps is discussed in Chapter 35.

Tumors of the Parotid

Mixed tumors, hemangiomas, and leukemia can present in the parotid gland as a hard or persistent mass. The patient should be referred to a surgeon.

Ranula

A ranula is a retention cyst of a sublingual salivary gland. It is found on the floor of the mouth to one side of the lingual frenulum. Ranula has been described as resembling a frog's belly, because it is thin-walled and contains a clear bluish fluid. Referral to an otolaryngologist for excision of the cyst and associated sublingual gland is the treatment of choice.

Crysdale WS: Ranulas and their treatment. Laryngoscope 1988;98:296.

David RB et al: Suppurative parotitis in children. Am J Dis Child 1970;119:332.

Saunders HF: Wind parotitis. N Engl J Med 1973;289:689.

ORAL CONGENITAL MALFORMATIONS

Tongue-Tie

The tightness of the lingual frenulum varies greatly among normal people. A short frenulum prevents both protrusion and elevation of the tongue. A puckering of the midline of the tongue occurs with tongue movement. The condition in no way interferes with the ability to nurse. It is unlikely that it interferes with the ability to speak, because even children with ankyloglossia have normal speech.

Treatment consists of reassurance. Although there is no evidence to support it, clipping of the frenulum is sometimes recommended if the tongue does not protrude beyond the teeth or gums. If this degree of tongue-tie is associated with impairment of rapid articulation, the patient should be referred to an otolaryngologist for correction. Casual frenulum clipping can result in significant bleeding from a cut lingual artery or injury to the orifices of Wharton's duct.

Cleft Lip & Cleft Palate

Cleft lip, cleft palate, or both conditions are found in 1:800 live births. They are readily diagnosed in the newborn nursery. Treatment requires a multidisciplinary team approach—plastic surgeons, otolaryngologists, audiologists, speech therapists, orthodontists, and prosthodontists. Cleft lip repair is usually performed before 3 months of age. Cleft palate repair is usually performed at about 12 months of age. This is essential to permit normal speech development, which should begin at this time. Approximately 90% of children with cleft palate have chronic or persistent otitis media and must be carefully followed for this problem. Some otolaryngologists recommend prophylactic tympanoplasty tubes. See discussion in Chapter 29 for details of management.

Bifid Uvula & Submucous Cleft Palate

A bifid uvula is present in 3% of healthy children. However, there is a close association (as high as 75%) between this and submucous cleft palate. A submucous cleft can be diagnosed by noting a translucent zone in the middle of the soft palate. Palpation of the hard palate reveals absence of the posterior bony portion. Affected children have a 40% risk of developing persistent otitis media. They also are at risk of incomplete closure of the palate, resulting in hypernasal speech. During feeding, some of these infants experience nasal regurgitation of food. Children with a submucous cleft palate that causes abnormal speech or nasal regurgitation of food need referral to a plastic surgeon associated with a cleft palate clinic for repair.

Moss ALH et al: Submucous cleft palate. Arch Dis Child 1990;65:182.

Shprintzen JJ: Morphologic significance of bifid uvula. Pediatrics 1985;75:553.

High-Arched Palate

A high-arched palate is usually a genetic trait of no consequence. It is seen also in children who are chronic mouth breathers and in premature infants who undergo prolonged oral intubation. Some rare causes of high-arched palate are congenital disorders such as Marfan's syndrome, Treacher Collins' syndrome, and Ehlers-Danlos syndrome.

Pierre Robin Syndrome

This congenital malformation is characterized by the triad of micrognathia, cleft palate, and glossoptosis. Affected children present as emergencies in the newborn period because of infringement on the airway by the tongue. The main objective of treatment is to prevent asphyxia until the mandible becomes large enough to accommodate the tongue. In some cases, this objective can be achieved by leaving the child in a prone position while unattended. In severe cases, a custom-fitted oropharyngeal airway is often required. The child requires close observation and careful feeding until the problem is outgrown.

REFERENCES

Balkany TJ, Pashley NRT: *Clinical Pediatric Otolaryngology.* Mosby, 1986.

Bardach J, Morris HL: *Multidisciplinary Management of Cleft Palate.* Saunders, 1990.

Bluestone CD, Klein JO: *Otitis Media in Infants and Children.* Saunders, 1988.

Bluestone CD et al: *Pediatric Otolaryngology,* 2nd ed. 2 vols. Saunders, 1990.

Bordley JE: *Ear, Nose and Throat Disorders in Children.* Raven Press, 1986.

Healy GB: *Common Problems in Pediatric Otolaryngology.* Year Book, 1990.

Myer CM, Cotton RT: *A Practical Approach to Pediatric Otolaryngology.* Year Book, 1988.

Naspitz CK, Tinkelman DG: *Childhood Rhinitis and Sinusitis.* Marcel Dekker, 1990.

Northern JL, Downs MP: *Hearing in Children,* 4th ed. Williams & Wilkins, 1991.

Respiratory Tract & Mediastinum 20

Gary L. Larsen, MD, Steven H. Abman, MD, Leland L. Fan, MD,
Carl W. White, MD, & Frank J. Accurso, MD

Respiratory disorders are among the most common acute or chronic problems encountered by physicians who care for children. Pediatric pulmonary diseases account for slightly less than one-half of deaths in children under 1 year of age and about 20% of all hospitalizations of children under 15 years of age. It is estimated that approximately 7% of children suffer some sort of chronic disorder of the lower respiratory system.

Understanding the physiologic and pathologic consequences of these diseases in this age group requires an appreciation of the normal growth and development of the lung. In addition, the physician must be familiar with the common diagnostic aids and therapeutic options used in approaching these problems. These matters are dealt with here, followed by discussions of congenital and acquired diseases of the respiratory tract and mediastinum.

Mellins RB, Stripp B, Taussig LM: Pediatric pulmonology in North America: Coming of age. Am Rev Respir Dis 1987;134:849.

US Department of Health and Human Services, National Institutes of Health: *Pediatric Respiratory Disorders.* Department of Health and Human Services Publication No. (NIH) 86–2107, 1986.

GROWTH & DEVELOPMENT OF THE LUNG

Understanding the growth and development of the respiratory system requires understanding changes in its anatomy, mechanical properties, and metabolic and defense functions. In addition to traditional approaches, the techniques of molecular and cellular biology are now being used to investigate the normal growth and development of the respiratory system—as well as the response to injury—at different stages of development.

The lung derives from the foregut during the fourth week of gestation. Subsequent branching leads to the development of the conducting airways (bronchial tree) by about 16 weeks of gestation. The terminal respiratory units—the gas-exchanging portion of the lung—undergo development from the latter third of gestation through the first few months after birth, when alveoli morphologically similar to those in adults are formed. It is clear that alveoli increase in number throughout childhood, but the age at which this increase normally stops is a controversial topic, with estimates ranging from 2 years to adolescence. The development of the pulmonary arterial system in general occurs with the development of the airways, while capillary proliferation in the terminal respiratory units occurs with the development of the alveoli.

With birth, the lung assumes the gas-exchanging function served by the placenta in utero, placing immediate stress on all components of the respiratory system. Abnormalities in the lung, respiratory muscles, chest wall, airway, respiratory controller, or pulmonary circulation may therefore present at birth. Postnatal survival depends, for example, on the development of the surfactant system to maintain airway stability and allow gas exchange. Immaturity of the surfactant system, seen often in infants of less than 35 weeks' gestational age, can result in severe respiratory morbidity in the immediate neonatal period as well as subsequent chronic lung disease in infancy. Persistent pulmonary hypertension of the newborn—the failure of the normal transition to a low-resistance pulmonary circulation at birth—can complicate a number of neonatal respiratory diseases.

Several mechanical properties of the respiratory system in infants increase the risk of respiratory compromise in this age group. The upper airway in infants is smaller and less firm than the upper airway in adults; therefore, obstruction in response to infection, inflammation, or foreign body is more likely. The chest wall of the infant is more compliant than that of the adult. For this reason, respiratory efforts encountered in some disease states can result in collapse and more labored breathing. In addition, the infant has fewer fatigue-resistant diaphragmatic muscle fibers, a fact suggesting that respiratory muscle fatigue may occur earlier in response to an increased load.

The development of airway reactivity, ie, acute changes in airway resistance in response to a given stimulus, has been controversial. Earlier studies suggested that infants lack airway smooth muscle similar to that in adults; this finding would imply that bronchoconstriction cannot occur in infants. The evidence now suggests that infants can exhibit airway reactivity. The mechanisms of airway reactivity in infancy are not completely understood but probably include some contractile elements in the airway that respond to neural stimuli. Recent studies also suggest that genetic factors play a role in the development of airway reactivity.

Pulmonary defense mechanisms, including cough, mucociliary clearance, and local and circulating components of the immune system, are present at birth. However, specific defects in immunity may present over variable periods after birth. This time lapse perhaps reflects passive immunity from the mother and the timing of infectious challenges to the respiratory tract.

Bernfield M: Matrix regulation of cell proliferation: Implications for growth of the embryo. Semin Perinatol 1984;8:117.

Cagle PT, Thurlbeck WM: Postpneumonectomy compensatory lung growth. Am Rev Respir Dis 1988;138:1314.

Langston C et al: Human lung growth in late gestation and in the neonate. Am Rev Respir Dis 1984;129:607.

Laros CD, Westermann CJJ: Dilatation, compensatory growth, or both following pneumonectomy during childhood and adolescence. J Thorac Cardiovasc Surg 1987; 93:570.

Murray JF: The Normal Lung: *The Basis for Diagnosis and Treatment of Pulmonary Disease.* Saunders, 1986.

Reid LM: The pulmonary circulation: Remodeling in growth and disease. The 1978 J Burns Amberson Lecture. Am Rev Respir Dis 1978;119:531.

DIAGNOSTIC AIDS

PHYSICAL EXAMINATION OF THE RESPIRATORY TRACT

The physical examination is done to corroborate findings obtained from the history, to assess severity of illness and adequacy of gas exchange, and to localize disease processes. The traditional approach of inspection, palpation, percussion, and auscultation remain important, though these techniques have limitations in small infants. Assessing the rate, depth, ease, symmetry, and rhythm of respiration is critical to the detection of pulmonary disease. Attention should be given to tracheal position and thoracic configuration. Auscultation should be done to assess the quality of breath sounds and to detect the presence of abnormal sounds. Although there is confusion in the literature, the American Thoracic Society recommends classifying abnormal breath sounds as interrupted (fine or coarse crackles) or continuous (wheezing or rhonchi) sounds.

Extrapulmonary manifestations of pulmonary disease include growth failure, altered mental status (with hypoxemia or hypercapnia), cyanosis, clubbing, and osteoarthropathy. Evidence of cor pulmonale (loud pulmonic component of the second heart sound, hepatomegaly, elevated neck veins, and, rarely, peripheral edema) signifies advanced lung disease.

It is critical to establish whether respiratory derangements are (1) the primary abnormality, (2) secondary to some other disease process, or (3) part of a more generalized condition. Therefore, the physician should perform a complete physical examination to look for evidence of other conditions such as congenital heart disease (murmur, gallop), neuromuscular disease (muscle wasting, scoliosis), immunodeficiency (rash, diarrhea), and autoimmune disease or occult malignancy (arthritis, hepatosplenomegaly).

Pasterkamp H: The history and physical examination. In: *Disorders of the Respiratory Tract in Children,* 5th ed. Chernick V, Kendig EL Jr (editors). Saunders, 1990.

PULMONARY FUNCTION TESTS

An assessment of lung function in pediatric patients with either an acute or chronic respiratory disorder can aid in diagnosis, quantitate disease severity, define precipitants of symptoms, evaluate therapy, and chart the course of a disease. In addition, preoperative evaluation of pulmonary function in patients with lung disease can help define the risks of anesthesia and surgery and assist in the planning of respiratory care in the postoperative period. Balanced against these potential benefits of assessing lung function are several limitations, which must also be kept in mind. For example, the range of normal values for a test may be quite wide, and the predicted normal values change dramatically with growth. For this reason, serial determinations of lung function are often more informative than a single determination, especially when dealing with a disease in which values may vary as a reflection of disease severity (asthma) or progression (cystic fibrosis). In addition, patient cooperation is essential for almost all physiologic assessments. Most children are not able to perform the necessary maneuvers before 5–7 years of age. Therefore, tests for use in infants and small children are not widely available and are more of a research tool than a clinical adjunct to care. Despite these problems, tests of lung function may still contribute to the care of children.

The pulmonary function equipment most often available in an office or clinic is a spirometer on which forced vital capacity can be recorded either as a volume-time tracing (spirogram) or a flow-volume curve. The patient takes a slow, full inhalation of air to maximum inflation, holds in inhalation for a short period, and then performs a sudden, sustained maximal exhalation over at least 3 seconds. The tracing produced by the exhalation shows forced vital capacity (FVC), ie, the total amount of air that is exhaled from maximum inspiration, and the forced expiratory volume in the first second of the exhalation (FEV_1). The maximum midexpiratory flow rate (MMEF, or $FEF_{25-75\%}$), the mean flow rate during the middle portion of the FVC maneuver, is also commonly calculated. In addition to obtaining the absolute values for these three tests and comparing them with normal values, medical personnel may also determine the FEV_1/FVC ratio. A ratio greater than 0.8 in children and young adults is consistent with normal airflow without limitation.

An important use of these basic tests of lung function is differentiating an obstructive from a restrictive process. Examples of obstructive processes include asthma, chronic bronchitis, and cystic fibrosis, whereas restrictive problems include chest wall deformities that limit lung expansion and interstitial processes due to collagen-vascular diseases, hypersensitivity pneumonitis, and interstitial fibrosis. Classically, diseases that obstruct airflow decrease the FEV_1 more than the FVC, so that the FEV_1/FVC ratio is low. In restrictive problems, however, the decreases in the FEV_1 and FVC are proportionate; thus, the ratio of FEV_1 to FVC is either normal or high. Clinical suspicion of a restrictive disease is usually an indication for referral to a tertiary care center for more complete evaluation of lung function and the associated disease process.

A test of lung function that can be readily performed in the office or at home is the peak expiratory flow rate (PEFR), ie, the maximal flow recorded during an FVC maneuver. The test can be assessed by a number of hand-held devices specifically made for this one test of pulmonary function. Patients can measure the PEFR at home at regular intervals and record the results in a diary, a practice that may be helpful in following the course of various pulmonary disorders, especially those that are difficult to control and require multiple medications (eg, steroid-dependent asthma). These devices can also be used to give patients with poor perception of their disease an awareness of a decrease in lung function, thus facilitating earlier treatment.

Cross D, Nelson HS: The role of the peak flow meter in the diagnosis and management of asthma. J Allergy Clin Immunol 1991;87:120.

Lemen RJ: Pulmonary function testing in the office, clinic, and home. In: *Disorders of the Respiratory Tract in Chil-*
dren, 5th ed. Chernick V, Kendig EL Jr (editor). Saunders, 1990.

Wilson MC, Larsen GL: The assessment of lung function: Pulmonary function tests. In: *Allergic Disease of Infancy, Childhood and Adolescence,* 2nd ed. Bierman CW, Pearlman DS (editors). Saunders, 1988.

ARTERIAL BLOOD GASES & NONINVASIVE ASSESSMENT OF OXYGEN TENSION & SATURATION

Arterial blood gas determinations are the best indicators of how well the respiratory system is performing its gas-exchanging function and how well acid-base homeostasis is being maintained. Assessment of blood gases is essential in critically ill children and may be used also for determining the severity of lung involvement in chronic conditions. Abnormalities in blood gas tensions may occur with dysfunction of any part of the respiratory system, including the respiratory controller, the conducting airways, the gas-exchanging portions of the lung, the pulmonary circulation, the respiratory muscles, and the chest wall. In pediatrics, hypoxia (low PaO_2) most commonly results from mismatching of ventilation and perfusion. Hypercapnia (elevated $PaCO_2$) often results from increased work of breathing secondary to increased pulmonary resistance, decreased compliance, or an abnormal chest wall. Hypercapnia may also occur with normal lungs and a normal chest wall if there is a depressed respiratory controller or if respiratory muscles are weakened for any reason. Blood gases may be sampled by intermittent arterial puncture or through indwelling arterial lines. Table 20–1 gives normal values for arterial pH, PaO_2, and $PaCO_2$ at sea level and at an altitude of 5000 feet.

The noninvasive, transcutaneous techniques of measuring oxygen saturation and PO_2 allow on-line monitoring in many different settings. Monitoring oxygen saturation in the intensive care unit is vital to anticipating respiratory failure in critically ill patients. As another example, desaturation during sleep is an important finding in patients with upper airway obstruction. The importance of evaluating the gas-exchanging portions of the lung make arterial blood gas measurements or noninvasive measurements of oxygen saturation an important part of the evaluation of any pediatric patient with suspected lung disease.

Hay WW Jr, Thilo E, Curlander JB: Pulse oximetry in neonatal medicine. Clin Perinatol 1991;18:441.

Table 20–1. Normal arterial blood gas values on room air.

	pH	PaO_2 (mm Hg)	$PaCO_2$ (mm Hg)
Sea level	7.38–7.42	85–95	36–42
5000 feet	7.36–7.40	65–75	35–40

Levison H et al: Arterial blood gases, alveolar-arterial oxygen difference, and physiologic deadspace in children and young adults. Am Rev Respir Dis 1970;101:972.

Yahav J, Mindorff C, Levison H: The validity of transcutaneous oxygen tension method in children with cardiorespiratory problems. Am Rev Respir Dis 1981;124:586.

CULTURE OF MATERIAL FROM THE RESPIRATORY TRACT

Expectorated sputum is rarely available from patients under 5–6 years of age, but in older children a sputum Gram stain showing significant numbers of organisms within neutrophils may indicate the pathogen present. Stains and cultures for bacteria from nasopharyngeal secretions are frequently misleading.

Cultures from the lower respiratory tract can be obtained by (1) tracheal aspiration through an endotracheal tube or through a rigid or fiberoptic bronchoscope, (2) transtracheal percutaneous aspiration, (3) lung puncture, or (4) the double-brush technique through the fiberoptic bronchoscope. The latter technique can be used to obtain endobronchial secretions in older critically ill or debilitated children large enough to accommodate the large (4.9 mm) bronchoscope required for the procedure.

Complications are most likely to occur with transtracheal percutaneous aspiration or lung puncture. These complications are related to a lack of experience by most physicians in utilizing these techniques in children. The other methods, however, are more likely to produce samples contaminated with oropharyngeal flora and may not be the best guide to therapy. Lung puncture, directed to a consolidated area using physical examination, radiographic studies, or ultrasound, is the favored approach in the child who deteriorates after initial antibiotic treatment or in the critically ill or immunocompromised child. Pneumothoraces (1–10% of cases) that follow lung puncture are usually small. Open lung biopsy, though a major intervention, should be considered in the worsening or critically ill child when other approaches have not been successful. Thoracentesis should be performed when pleural fluid is present, and complete cultures should be obtained. Blood glucose and lactate dehydrogenase should be drawn simultaneously for comparison with pleural fluid chemistries. Blood cultures provide specific diagnoses and must be obtained in children with acute pneumonia.

If indeed a specimen is obtained through invasive means, it is critical that appropriate studies be obtained for the following: (1) viruses, (2) *Mycoplasma pneumoniae,* (3) *Chlamydia,* (4) *Legionella pneumophila,* (5) *Bordetella pertussis,* (6) fungi, (7) acid-fast bacteria, (8) anaerobes or other bacteria, and (9) *Pneumocystis carinii.* In addition, these specimens should be studied for potential pathogens using rapid diagnostic techniques such as immunofluorescent antibody and enzyme-linked immunosorbent assay (ELISA). Counterimmunoelectrophoresis performed on pleural fluid, serum, or concentrated urine may help identify disease due to *Streptococcus pneumoniae* or *Haemophilus influenzae.* Because these tests can be performed quickly, they may obviate further, more invasive studies.

Alpert BE, O'Sullivan BP, Panitch HB: Nonbronchoscopic approach to bronchoalveolar lavage in children with artificial airways. Pediatr Pulmonol 1992; 13:38.

Bromberg K, Hammerschlag MR: Rapid diagnosis of pneumonia in children. Semin Respir Infect 1987;2:159.

Koumbourlis AC, Kurland G: Nonbronchoscopic bronchoalveolar lavage in mechanically ventilated infants: Technique, efficacy, and applications. Pediatr Pulmon 1993; 15:257.

Peter G: The child with pneumonia: Diagnostic and therapeutic considerations. Pediatr Infect Dis J 1988;7:453.

IMAGING OF THE RESPIRATORY TRACT

The plain chest radiograph remains one of the most important techniques for investigating suspected lung disease. Both frontal and lateral views should be obtained in most instances. Hyperaeration, best demonstrated in the lateral projection as flattening of the diaphragm, is a common finding because of the propensity of young children to develop small airways obstruction and also because of the prevalence of asthma in all pediatric age groups. Parenchymal changes may be manifested by increased interstitial markings, consolidation, air bronchograms, or loss of diaphragm or heart contours. When pleural fluid is suspected, lateral decubitus films may be helpful in determining the extent and mobility of the fluid. When a foreign body is suspected, forced expiratory films may demonstrate focal air trapping and shift of the mediastinum to the contralateral side. Lateral neck films can be useful in assessing the size of adenoids and tonsils and also in differentiating croup from epiglottitis, the latter being associated with the "thumbprint" sign.

Barium swallow is indicated for patients with suspected aspiration so that the physician can look for swallowing dysfunction, tracheoesophageal fistula, gastroesophageal reflux, and achalasia. This technique is also very important in detecting vascular rings and slings, because most (not all) are also associated with esophageal compression. Airway fluoroscopy is another important tool for assessing both fixed airway obstruction (ie, subglottic stenosis) and dynamic airway obstruction (ie, tracheomalacia). Fluoroscopy of the diaphragm can detect paralysis by demonstrating paradoxic movement of the involved hemidiaphragm.

High-resolution computed tomography (CT scanning) enables the radiologist to better evaluate diffuse infiltrative lung disease, metastatic disease, mediastinal masses, and chest wall disease. Magnetic resonance imaging (MRI) is useful for defining subtle or complex abnormalities and vascular rings. Ventilation/perfusion scans can provide information about regional ventilation and perfusion and can help detect vascular malformations and pulmonary emboli (rare in children). Pulmonary angiography is occasionally necessary to define the pulmonary vascular bed more precisely. Bronchography is rarely done in the USA but can be useful in the specific circumstance when lobectomy is contemplated for suspected localized bronchiectasis.

Effmann EL, Kirks DR: Chest computed tomography in children. Pediatr Clin North Am 1985;32:1383.

Eggleston DE, Slovis TL, Watts FB: Update on pediatric chest imaging. Pediatr Pulmonol 1988;5:158.

Kirchner SG, Horev G: Diagnostic imaging in children with acute chest and abdominal disorders. Pediatr Clin North Am 1985;32:1363.

BRONCHOSCOPY

Pediatric patients with potential airway problems become candidates for laryngoscopy or bronchoscopy (or both) when less invasive modalities fail to define the lesion adequately. The diagnostic indications for laryngoscopy include hoarseness, stridor, and symptoms of obstructive sleep apnea; those for bronchoscopy include wheezing, suspected foreign body, pneumonia, atelectasis, chronic cough, hemoptysis, and placement of an endotracheal tube and assessment of patency. In general, the more specific the indication, the higher the diagnostic yield.

Currently, pediatric bronchoscopy can be done with either flexible fiberoptic instruments or with rigid open-tube instruments. Recent advances in fiberoptic technology and the development of ultrathin flexible bronchoscopes have greatly increased the physician's ability to explore the pediatric airway. The advantages of using a flexible bronchoscope include the following: (1) the procedure can be done at the bedside with sedation and topical anesthetics and requires no general anesthesia; (2) evaluation of the upper airway can be done with little risk in patients who are awake; (3) the distal airways of intubated patients can be examined without removing the endotracheal tube; (4) the instrument can be used as an obturator to intubate a patient with a difficult upper airway; (5) endotracheal tube placement and patency can be checked; (6) assessment of airway dynamics is generally better; and (7) it is possible to examine more distal airways. The advantages of using a rigid instrument are (1) easier removal of foreign bodies (for this reason, rigid bronchoscopy remains the procedure of choice for suspected foreign body aspiration); (2) better airway control, which allows the patient to be ventilated through the bronchoscope; and (3) superior optics. The choice of procedures depends largely on the expertise available, but in general, pediatric airway evaluation is optimal with a multidisciplinary approach involving pediatric anesthesia, surgery, otolaryngology, and pulmonology.

Fan LL, Sparks LM, Dulinski JP: Applications of an ultrathin flexible bronchoscope for neonatal and pediatric airway problems. Chest 1986;89:673.

Fan LL, Sparks LM, Fix EJ: Flexible fiberoptic endoscopy for airway problems in a pediatric intensive care unit. Chest 1988;93:556.

Godfrey S et al: Is there a place for rigid bronchoscopy in the management of pediatric lung disease? Pediatr Pulmonol 1987;3:179.

Green CG et al: Flexible endoscopy of the pediatric airway. Am Rev Respir Dis 1992; 145:233.

Whitehead B et al: Technique and use of transbronchial biopsy in children and adolescents. Pediatr Pulmonol 1992;12:240.

Wood RE: Endoscopy of the airway. J Pediatr 1988;112:1.

Wood RE: Spelunking in the pediatric airways: Explorations with the flexible fiberoptic bronchoscope. Pediatr Clin North Am 1984;31:785.

GENERAL THERAPY OF PEDIATRIC LUNG DISEASES

OXYGEN THERAPY

Oxygen therapy consists of administration of supplemental oxygen at concentrations greater than that of room air (21%) in order to increase arterial oxygen tension. Supplemental oxygen can be administered through an endotracheal tube during mechanical ventilation or through an inflatable anesthesia bag with a mask. In spontaneously breathing patients, delivery can be achieved by nasal cannula, head hood, or mask (including simple, rebreathing, nonrebreathing, or Venturi masks). The general goal of oxygen therapy is to correct for hypoxemia by attempting to achieve an arterial oxygen tension of 65–90 mm Hg or an oxygen saturation above 92%. The actual oxygen concentration achieved by nasal cannula or mask depends on the flow rate, the type of mask used, and the patient's age. For example, small changes in flow rate during oxygen administration by nasal cannula can lead to substantial changes in inspired oxygen concentration in young infants. In addition, the amount of oxygen required to correct hypoxemia may vary according to the child's activity. It is not unusual, for example, for an infant with chronic lung disease to require 0.75 L/min while awake but 1 L/min while asleep or feeding.

Although the head hood is an efficient device for maintaining oxygen delivery in young infants during hospitalization, the nasal cannula is used more often because it allows the infant greater activity. The cannula generally has nasal prongs that are inserted in the nares, but it can be modified by removing the prongs. This nasal catheter can then be taped under the nose or inserted in the nasopharynx. The flow through the nasal cannula should generally not exceed 3 L/min to avoid excessive drying of the nasal mucosa. In general, administration of supplemental oxygen by nasal cannula, even at high flow rates, can rarely achieve inspired oxygen concentrations greater than 40–45%. In contrast, partial rebreathing and nonrebreathing masks or head hoods can be used to achieve inspired oxygen concentrations as high as 90–100%.

Because the physical findings of cyanosis can be subtle, especially with milder degrees of hypoxemia, the adequacy of oxygenation must be assessed by measuring arterial oxygen tension via arterial blood gas or transcutaneous PO_2 monitoring. In addition, oxygen saturation can be determined by oximetry. The advantages of the noninvasive methods (transcutaneous PO_2 and oximetry) include the ability to obtain continuous measurements during various normal activities and to avoid artifacts caused by crying or breath holding during attempts at arterial puncture. For children with chronic cardiopulmonary disorders that may require supplemental oxygen therapy (such as bronchopulmonary dysplasia or cystic fibrosis), frequent noninvasive assessments are essential to ensure the safety and adequacy of treatment. In addition, long-term follow-up of children with chronic oxygen requirements should include serial electrocardiographic or echocardiographic assessments at regular intervals to observe for early signs of pulmonary hypertension and cor pulmonale, which may suggest that therapy has been inadequate.

Abman SH et al: Pulmonary vascular response to oxygen in infants with BPD. Pediatrics 1985;75:80.

Fan LL et al: Determination of inspired oxygen delivery by nasal cannula in infants with chronic lung disease. J Pediatr 1983;103:923.

National Conference on Oxygen Therapy. Chest 1984;86: 236.

INHALATION OF BRONCHODILATORS & OTHER MEDICATIONS

Various diseases in pediatric patients give rise to airway obstruction that may be reversed by an inhaled bronchodilator. Airway obstruction may be encountered in cystic fibrosis, bronchiolitis, and bronchopulmonary dysplasia as well as in acute and chronic asthma. Of the classes of inhaled drugs used in the treatment of these disorders, the β-adrenergic agonists and parasympatholytic agents may lead to the most prompt reversal of the obstruction. Other classes of inhaled drugs that may be beneficial, especially in the treatment of asthma, include corticosteroids and sodium cromoglycate. Inhalation therapy with these classes of drugs is discussed below. The cystic fibrosis section contains a discussion of the use of inhaled antibiotics.

The β-adrenergic agonists may be delivered by either a prepackaged, pressurized canister (metered-dose inhaler, or MDI) or a reusable nebulizer in which a solution of the medication is aerosolized by the flow of gas from a portable gas compressor or a source of compressed gas (such as 100% oxygen). The MDIs are convenient to use and carry and can be combined with spacing devices for younger children who lack the ability to coordinate actuation of the MDI with proper inhalation technique. On the other hand, the nebulizer is a more effective method of delivering medication to infants and young children. Several inhaled β_2-adrenergic agents that are more selective for the respiratory tract and have longer durations of action are now available (see Chapter 33 and discussion of asthma). In the treatment of acute episodes of airway obstruction, the inhaled adrenergic agents have been shown to be as effective as the injectable ones. In addition, delivery of the drug by the aerosol route has been associated with fewer side effects. Although concern has been raised about the safety of delivering this class of medication directly to the airways, most authorities believe that these drugs are safe when both physician and family realize that a poor response to the agents may signify the need for corticosteroids to help restore β-adrenergic responsiveness.

Anticholinergic agents may also acutely decrease airway obstruction. Furthermore, they may yield a longer duration of bronchodilation than do many adrenergic agents. Selected patients may benefit from receiving both β-adrenergic and anticholinergic agents. In general, this class of drugs is most effective in the treatment of chronic bronchitis.

Other classes of inhaled medications used primarily to treat asthma include corticosteroids, sodium cromoglycate, and nedocromil sodium. Currently in the United States, corticosteroids and nedocromil are available only in MDIs, whereas cromolyn may be prescribed as either an MDI or a solution for nebulization. Although these medications are not effective in acutely relieving airways obstruction, long-term use may lead to decreases in airway reactivity. In addition, corticosteroids may help maintain or restore responsiveness of the airways to adrenergic drugs.

Kerrebijn KF, van Essen-Zandvliet EEM, Neijens HJ: Effect of long-term treatment with inhaled corticosteroids and beta-agonists on the bronchial responsiveness in children with asthma. J Allergy Clin Immunol 1987; 79:653.

König P: Inhaled corticosteroids: Their present and future role in the management of asthma. J Allergy Clin Immunol 1988;82:297.

Levison H, Reilly PA, Worsley GH: Spacing devices and metered-dose inhalers in childhood asthma. J Pediatr 1985;107:662.

Nelson HS: Beta-adrenergic therapy. In: *Allergy: Principles and Practice,* 4th ed. Middleton E et al (editors). Mosby, 1993.

Ruddy RM et al: Aerosolized metaproterenol compared to subcutaneous epinephrine in the emergency treatment of acute childhood asthma. Pediatr Pulmonol 1986;2:230.

Shapiro GG et al: Double-blind evaluation of nebulized cromolyn, terbutaline, and the combination for childhood asthma. J Allergy Clin Immunol 1988;81:449.

Uchida DA, Brugman S, Larsen GL: New Insights into the mechanisms and treatment of childhood asthma. Semin Respir Med 1990;11:211.

PULMONARY PHYSIOTHERAPY

Chest physical therapy, including postural drainage with percussion and forced expiratory maneuvers, has been widely employed in an attempt to improve the clearance of secretions in patients with impaired clearance. However, there are few studies of the efficacy of techniques used. Studies have suggested that chest physical therapy is not helpful in adults with uncomplicated pneumonias. However, data indicating that postural drainage can be beneficial in children with cystic fibrosis are accumulating. A recent 3-year study indicates that there is less decline in pulmonary function of children treated with traditional postural drainage and percussion than with directed coughing alone. The experience of many pediatric pulmonary centers now suggests that chest physical therapy is an important adjunct to other therapies.

Postural drainage requires positioning of the patient to favor emptying each of the segmental bronchi. Percussion or vibration is used to loosen secretions and facilitate drainage. Physicians should carefully review the positions and the technique of percussion to perform this mode of therapy properly. In general, the patient spends 1–2 minutes in each of nine body positions (ie, 10–20 minutes for the duration of a treatment). Treatments may be given 1–4 times a day at home and sometimes more frequently in the hospital setting. Patients are encouraged to cough regularly during the procedure. Children who cannot be encouraged to cough may require pharyngeal suctioning by trained personnel.

"Blow bottles" that provide the patient feedback about respiratory efforts may also encourage deep breathing. This technique is particularly useful in patients recovering from surgery.

Desmond KJ et al: Immediate and long-term effects of chest physiotherapy in patients with cystic fibrosis. J Pediatr 1983;103:538.

Reisman JJ et al: Role of conventional physiotherapy in cystic fibrosis. J Pediatr 1988;113:632.

AVOIDANCE OF ENVIRONMENTAL HAZARDS

Parents of normal children as well as those of children with respiratory disorders should be counseled about environmental hazards to the lung. The list of potential hazards includes small objects that may be aspirated, allergens that can precipitate respiratory symptoms in atopic children, and cigarette smoke.

The harmful effects of smoking in the home deserve special emphasis. Children from families where the parents and others smoke have decreased lung growth as well as decreased pulmonary function in comparison with children raised in homes where there are no smokers. Exposure of children to tobacco smoke also leads to an increased frequency of lower respiratory tract infections and an increased incidence of respiratory symptoms, including recurrent wheezing. Health care providers must increase their efforts to educate patients and their families about the hazards of smoking. Resources within the community that will help smokers give up the habit should be utilized as part of the routine health maintenance for all children.

American Academy of Pediatrics Committee on Environmental Hazards: Involuntary smoking: A hazard to children. Pediatrics 1986;77:755.

Weitzman M et al: Maternal smoking and childhood asthma. Pediatrics 1990;85:505.

DISORDERS OF THE CONDUCTING AIRWAYS

The conducting airways consist of the nose, mouth, pharynx, larynx, trachea, bronchi, and bronchioles. These airways direct inspired air to the gas exchange units of the lung; they do not participate in gas exchange themselves. Airflow obstruction in the conducting airways occurs by any of three mechanisms: (1) external compression (eg, vascular ring, tumor), (2) abnormalities of the airway structure itself (eg, congenital defects, thickening of an airway wall due to inflammation), or (3) material in the airway lumen (eg, foreign body, mucus).

Airway obstruction can be fixed (airflow limited in both the inspiratory and expiratory phases of respiration) or variable (airflow limited more in one phase of respiration than the other). Variable obstruction is common in children because their airways are more compliant and susceptible to dynamic compression. With variable extrathoracic airway obstruction (eg, croup), airflow limitation is greater during inspiration, leading to inspiratory stridor. With variable intrathoracic obstruction, limitation is greater during expiration, producing expiratory wheezing. Thus, determining the phase of respiration in which obstruction is greatest may be helpful in localizing the site of obstruction.

CLINICAL FINDINGS IN EXTRATHORACIC AIRWAYS OBSTRUCTION

Patients with abnormalities of the extrathoracic airway may present with snoring and other symptoms of obstructive apnea, hoarseness, brassy cough, or stridor. When taking the history, the physician should obtain the following information: (1) the onset of symptoms; (2) the nature of the course of the illness, ie, acute (eg, infectious croup), recurrent (eg, spasmodic croup), chronic (eg, subglottic stenosis), or progressive (eg, laryngeal papillomatosis); and (3) risk factors (eg, difficult delivery, ductal ligation, intubation). A careful physical examination should determine if obstructive symptoms are present at rest or with agitation, if they are positional, or if they are related to sleep. The presence of agitation, air hunger, severe retractions, cyanosis, lethargy, or coma should alert the physician to a potentially life-threatening condition that may require immediate airway intervention. Helpful diagnostic studies in the evaluation of upper airway obstruction include chest and lateral neck films, airway fluoroscopy, and barium swallow. An ECG can provide evidence of pulmonary hypertension in patients with chronic obstruction. Patients with symptoms of obstructive sleep apnea may benefit from polysomnography (measurements during sleep of the motion of the chest wall, airflow at the nose and mouth, heart rate, oxygen saturation, and selected electroencephalographic leads to stage sleep), which can help define the severity of the illness. In older children, pulmonary function tests can differentiate fixed from variable airflow obstruction and determine the site of variable obstruction. Direct laryngoscopy and bronchoscopy remain the procedures of choice to establish the precise diagnosis. Treatment should be directed at relieving airway obstruction and correcting the underlying condition if possible.

CLINICAL FINDINGS IN INTRATHORACIC AIRWAY OBSTRUCTION

Patients with abnormalities of the intrathoracic airways usually present with wheezing that is most prominent during expiration. The history should in-

clude the following: (1) age at onset; (2) precipitating factors (exercise, upper respiratory illnesses, allergens, choking while eating, etc); (3) course, ie, acute (bronchiolitis, foreign body), chronic (tracheomalacia, vascular ring), recurrent (reactive airways disease), or progressive (cystic fibrosis, bronchiolitis obliterans); (4) presence and nature of cough; (5) production of sputum; (6) previous response to bronchodilators; (7) symptoms with positional changes (vascular rings); and (8) involvement of other organ systems (malabsorption in cystic fibrosis).

Physical examination should include growth measurements and vital signs. The examiner should look for cyanosis or pallor, barrel-shaped chest, retractions and use of accessory muscles, and clubbing. Auscultation should define the pattern and timing of respiration, detect the presence of crackles and wheezing, and determine whether findings are localized or generalized.

Routine tests include plain chest films, a sweat test, and pulmonary function tests in older children. Other diagnostic studies are dictated by the history and physical findings. Treatment should be directed toward the primary cause of the obstruction but generally includes a trial of bronchodilators.

CONGENITAL DISORDERS OF THE EXTRATHORACIC AIRWAY

LARYNGOMALACIA

Laryngomalacia is a benign congenital disorder in which the cartilaginous support for the supraglottic structures is underdeveloped. It is the most common cause of persistent stridor in infants and usually presents in the first 6 weeks of life. Stridor has been reported to be worse in the supine position, with increased activity, with upper respiratory infections, and during feeding; however, the clinical presentation can be variable. The condition usually improves with age and resolves by 2 years of age, but symptoms may persist for years. The diagnosis is established by direct laryngoscopy, in which inspiratory collapse of an "omega-shaped" epiglottis (with or without long, redundant arytenoids) is visualized. In mildly affected patients with a typical presentation (those without stridor at rest or retractions), this procedure may not be necessary. No treatment is needed except in the extremely rare circumstance of severe obstruction that requires airway intervention. A recent observation suggests that these patients may have slight desaturation during sleep, the clinical importance of which is unknown.

Belmont JR, Grundfast K: Congenital laryngeal stridor (laryngomalacia): Etiologic factors and associated disorders. Ann Otol Rhinol Laryngol 1984;93:430.

Macfarlane PI, Olinsky A, Phelan PD: Proximal airway function 8 to 16 years after laryngomalacia: Follow-up flow-volume loop studies. J Pediatr 1985;107:216.

McCray PB et al: Hypoxia and hypercapnia in infants with mild laryngomalacia. Am J Dis Child 1988;142:896.

Phelan PD et al: The clinical and physiological manifestations of the "infantile" larynx: Natural history and relationship to mental retardation. Aust Paediatr J 1971; 7:135.

OTHER CONGENITAL PROBLEMS

Other congenital lesions of the larynx are quite rare. These include laryngeal atresia, laryngeal web, laryngocele and cyst of the larynx, subglottic hemangioma, and laryngeal cleft. All these disorders are best diagnosed by direct laryngoscopy. Laryngeal atresia obviously presents immediately after birth with severe respiratory distress and is most often fatal, although a few survivors have been reported. Laryngeal web, representing fusion of the anterior portion of the true vocal cords, is associated with hoarseness, aphonia, and stridor. Surgical correction may be necessary, depending upon the degree of airway obstruction.

Congenital cysts and laryngoceles are believed to have similar origin. Cysts are more superficial, whereas laryngoceles communicate with the interior of the larynx. Cysts are generally fluid-filled, whereas laryngoceles may be air- or fluid-filled. Airway obstruction is usually prominent and requires surgical intervention. Laser therapy is commonly employed for this purpose.

Subglottic hemangiomas usually present in infancy with signs of upper airway obstruction and are often associated with similar lesions of the skin. Although these lesions tend to regress spontaneously over time, airway obstruction may require surgical treatment with laser or even tracheostomy.

Laryngeal cleft is a very rare condition resulting from failure of posterior cricoid fusion. Patients with this condition may have stridor but always aspirate severely, resulting in recurrent or chronic pneumonia and failure to thrive. Barium swallow is always positive for severe aspiration, but diagnosis can be very difficult even with direct laryngoscopy. Patients often require tracheostomy and gastrostomy, because surgical correction is not always successful.

Gatti WM, MacDonald E, Orfei E: Congenital laryngeal atresia. Laryngoscope 1987;97:966.

Richardson MA, Cotton RT: Anatomic abnormalities of the pediatric airway. Pediatr Clin North Am 1984;31:821.

Smith RJH, Catlin FI: Congenital anomalies of the larynx. Am J Dis Child 1984;138:35.

ACQUIRED DISORDERS OF THE EXTRATHORACIC AIRWAY

CROUP SYNDROME

Croup describes a series of acute inflammatory diseases of the larynx including viral croup (laryngotracheobronchitis), epiglottitis (supraglottitis), and bacterial tracheitis. In patients presenting with acute stridor, these entities form the main differential diagnosis, although spasmodic croup, angioneurotic edema, laryngeal or esophageal foreign body, and retropharyngeal abscess should be considered.

1. VIRAL CROUP

Viral croup generally affects younger children in the fall and early winter and is most often caused by parainfluenza virus type 1. Other organisms causing croup include parainfluenza virus types 2 and 3, respiratory syncytial virus, influenza virus, rubeola virus, adenovirus, and *Mycoplasma pneumoniae*. Although inflammation of the entire airway is usually present, edema formation in the subglottic space accounts for the predominant signs of upper airway obstruction.

Clinical Findings

A. Symptoms and Signs: There is usually a prodrome of upper respiratory tract symptoms followed by the development of a barking cough and stridor. Fever is usually absent or low-grade but may on occasion be as high as in patients with epiglottitis. Patients with mild disease may exhibit only stridor when agitated, but as obstruction worsens, symptoms may progress to stridor at rest, accompanied by retractions, air hunger, and cyanosis in severe cases. On examination, the presence of cough and the absence of drooling tend to favor the diagnosis of viral croup over epiglottitis.

B. Imaging: Lateral neck films can be diagnostically helpful by showing subglottic narrowing and a normal epiglottis. It is important to confirm that the epiglottis is normal by direct laryngoscopy, because the presentation of epiglottitis may be similar to that of croup. Although controversy exists regarding the safety of such a procedure, a recent study suggests that it is reasonably safe in patients with suspected viral croup. Direct inspection is necessary because some patients with suspected croup actually prove to have epiglottitis.

Treatment

Treatment of viral croup is supportive. Patients

without stridor at rest may be managed as outpatients with mist therapy, oral hydration, and minimal handling. Although mist is believed to be helpful in relieving symptoms, the only clinical study done to date failed to demonstrate its effectiveness. Patients with stridor at rest require hospitalization. Appropriate hospital management includes the same therapy given to outpatients. Additionally, oxygen should be administered with careful observation to patients demonstrating desaturation by pulse oximetry. Nebulized racemic epinephrine (0.5 mL of a 2.25% solution diluted with 1.5–3.5 mL of sterile water) has been shown to relieve airway obstruction for up to 2 hours, presumably by reducing edema. Nebulized L-epinephrine (5 mL of 1:1000 solution) is also effective. Other, more pure alpha-agonists are also effective but are shorter-acting. The use of corticosteroids remains controversial; all controlled studies to date have had methodologic shortcomings. Nonetheless, the efficacy demonstrated in some studies, coupled with the lack of identified side effects, seems to justify a short course in severe cases (those patients not responding to racemic epinephrine). Dexamethasone (0.5–1 mg/kg [up to 10 mg] given orally or parenterally as a single dose or repeated in 12 hours) is appropriate. Nebulized steroid may also be effective but is currently unavailable in the United States.

Patients with impending respiratory failure require an artificial airway. Although there is controversy regarding the choice between intubation and tracheostomy, recent studies suggest that intubation with an endotracheal tube of slightly smaller diameter than would ordinarily be used is reasonably safe. Extubation should be accomplished within 2–3 days to minimize the risk of laryngeal injury. If the patient fails extubation, tracheostomy should be performed.

Prognosis

Most children with viral croup have an uneventful course and improve within a few days. Recent studies suggest that patients with a history of croup may have airway hyperreactivity. However, it has not been determined if this was present prior to the croup episode or if the croup episode itself altered airway function. Recurrence of croup occurs in some instances, implying airway hyperreactivity.

Bourchier D, Dawson KP, Ferguson DM: Humidification in viral croup: A controlled trial. Aust Paediatr J 1984; 20:289.

Couriel JM: Management of croup. Arch Dis Child 1988; 63:1305.

Husby S et al: Treatment of croup with nebulized steroid (budesonide): A double blind, placebo controlled study. Arch Dis Child 1993;68:352.

Kairys SW, Olmstead EM, O'Connor GT: Steroid treatment of laryngotracheitis: A meta-analysis of the evidence from randomized trials. Pediatrics 1989;83:683.

Mauro RD, Poole SR, Lockhart CH: Differentiation of epiglottitis from laryngotracheitis in the child with stridor. Am J Dis Child 1988;142:679.

McEniery J et al: Review of intubation in severe laryngotracheobronchitis. Pediatrics 1991;87:847.

Waisman Y et al: Prospective randomized double-blind study comparing L-epinephrine and racemic epinephrine aerosols in the treatment of laryngotracheitis (croup). Pediatrics 1992;89:302.

2. EPIGLOTTITIS

Epiglottitis represents a true medical emergency. It is almost always caused by *Haemophilus influenzae* type B, although other organisms such as *Streptococcus pneumoniae* and groups A and C *Streptococcus pyogenes* have been implicated. Resulting inflammation and swelling of the supraglottic structures (epiglottis and arytenoids) can develop rapidly and lead to life-threatening upper airway obstruction.

Clinical Findings

A. Symptoms and Signs: Typically, patients present with a rather sudden onset of fever, dysphagia, drooling, muffled voice, inspiratory retractions, cyanosis, and soft stridor. They often sit in a "sniffing dog" position, which gives them the best airway possible under the circumstances. Progression to total airway obstruction may occur and result in respiratory arrest.

B. Imaging: Diagnostically, lateral neck films may be helpful in demonstrating a classic "thumbprint" sign. However, obtaining films may delay important airway intervention. The definitive diagnosis is made by direct inspection of the epiglottis, a procedure that should be done by an experienced airway specialist under controlled conditions (usually the operating room). The typical findings are a cherry-red and swollen epiglottis and arytenoids.

Treatment

Once the diagnosis is made, endotracheal intubation should be performed immediately. Most anesthesiologists favor the use of general anesthesia (but not muscle relaxants) to facilitate intubation. Once an airway is established, cultures of the blood and epiglottis should be obtained and the patient started on appropriate intravenous antibiotics to cover *Haemophilus influenzae* (ceftriaxone sodium, 150 mg/kg/d in two divided doses or equivalent cephalosporin; chloramphenicol, 100 mg/kg/d in four divided doses; or ampicillin, 200 mg/kg/d in four divided doses). Ampicillin should probably not be used alone unless cultures are positive and demonstrate a sensitive organism.

Careful attention should be given to respiratory care of the intubated patient to prevent accidental extubation and tube obstruction. This includes adequate restraint, humidification, and frequent suctioning.

Extubation can usually be accomplished in 24–48 hours, when direct inspection shows significant reduction in the size of the epiglottis. Some centers use the resolution of fever as a criterion for extubation. Intravenous antibiotics should be continued for 2–3 days, followed by oral antibiotics to complete a 10-day course.

If a physician who has little experience in treating airway disorders and is located far from a tertiary pediatric facility encounters a patient with epiglottitis, the following is recommended. Start the patient on oxygen, and assemble all the airway equipment available. Manipulate the patient as little as possible, and allow the child to remain sitting up. Enlist the help of the most experienced airway person available, or call a transport team. Carefully start an intravenous line, and give antibiotics. If the patient obstructs completely and suffers a respiratory arrest, attempt to establish an airway by any means possible: intubation, bag and mask ventilation, transtracheal ventilation with a large-bore angiocatheter attached to a 3-mm endotracheal tube adapter and resuscitation bag, or tracheostomy.

Complications

Complications related to *H influenzae* infection in other sites include pneumonia, cervical adenitis, and septic arthritis. Meningitis is extremely rare.

Prognosis

Prompt recognition and appropriate treatment usually results in rapid resolution of swelling and inflammation. Recurrence is unusual.

Butt W et al: Acute epiglottitis: A different approach to management. Crit Care Med 1988;16:43.
Crockett DM et al: Airway management of acute supraglottitis at the Children's Hospital, Boston: 1980–1985. Ann Otol Rhinol Laryngol 1988;97:114.

3. BACTERIAL TRACHEITIS

Bacterial tracheitis (pseudomembranous croup) represents a severe form of laryngotracheobronchitis that has received increased attention in the recent literature. It is not a new condition but one that has been "rediscovered." The organism most often isolated is *Staphylococcus aureus,* but organisms such as *Haemophilus influenzae,* group A *Streptococcus pyogenes, Neisseria* species, and others have been reported. The disease probably represents localized mucosal invasion of bacteria in patients with primary viral croup, resulting in inflammatory edema, purulent secretions, and pseudomembranes. Although cultures of the tracheal secretions are frequently positive, blood cultures are almost always negative.

Clinical Findings

A. Symptoms and Signs: The early clinical picture is similar to that of viral croup. However, instead of gradual improvement, patients develop high fever, toxicity, and progressive upper airway obstruction that is unresponsive to standard croup therapy. The incidence of sudden respiratory arrest or progressive respiratory failure is very high; in such instances, airway intervention is required.

B. Laboratory Findings: The white count is usually elevated, with left shift. Cultures of tracheal secretions usually demonstrate one of the causative organisms.

C. Imaging: Lateral neck films show a normal epiglottis but often severe subglottic and tracheal narrowing. Frequently, irregularity of the contour of the proximal tracheal mucosa and pseudomembrane formation in the airway are present.

Treatment

Patients with suspected bacterial tracheitis should be managed in a similar fashion to those with epiglottitis. Because of the high incidence of respiratory arrest or progressive respiratory failure, intubation is almost always necessary. Once intubated, patients often have thick, purulent, obstructive tracheal secretions. Therefore, extreme care (adequate humidification, frequent suctioning, intensive care monitoring) is required to prevent endotracheal tube obstruction. Appropriate intravenous antibiotics to cover *S aureus, H influenzae,* and the other organisms are indicated. Because thick secretions persist for several days, the period of intubation required is longer for bacterial tracheitis than for epiglottitis.

Prognosis

Despite the severity of this illness, the reported mortality rate is very low. Therefore, appropriate management is generally associated with a excellent outcome.

Hen J: Current management of upper airway obstruction. Pediatr Ann (April) 1986;15:274.
Liston SL et al: Bacterial tracheitis. Am J Dis Child 1983;137:764.
Nelson WE: Bacterial croup: A historical perspective. J Pediatr 1984;105:52.

VOCAL CORD PARALYSIS

Unilateral or bilateral vocal cord paralysis may be a congenital condition or, more commonly, a condition acquired from injury to the recurrent laryngeal nerves. Risk factors that predispose patients to acquired paralysis include difficult delivery (especially face presentation), neck and thoracic surgery (eg, ductal ligation, repair of tracheoesophageal fistula), trauma, mediastinal masses, pulmonary hypertension, and central nervous system disease (eg, Arnold-Chiari malformation). Patients usually present with varying degrees of hoarseness, aspiration, or high-pitched stridor. Unilateral cord paralysis is more likely to occur on the left because of the longer course of the left recurrent laryngeal nerve and its proximity to major thoracic structures. Patients with unilateral paralysis are usually hoarse but rarely have stridor. With bilateral cord paralysis, the closer to midline the cords are positioned, the greater the airway obstruction; the more lateral the cords are positioned, the greater the tendency to aspirate and experience hoarseness or aphonia. With partial function (paresis), the adductor muscles tend to operate better than the abductors, with a resultant high-pitched inspiratory stridor and normal voice. Airway intervention (intubation, tracheostomy) is rarely indicated in unilateral paralysis but is often necessary for bilateral paralysis. Recovery is related to the severity of nerve injury and the potential for healing.

Cohen SR et al: Laryngeal paralysis in children: A long-term retrospective study. Ann Otol Rhinol Laryngol 1982;91:417.

Emery PJ, Fearon B: Vocal cord palsy in pediatric practice: A review of 71 cases. Int J Pediatr Otorhinolaryngol 1984;8:147.

Fan LL et al: Paralyzed left vocal cord associated with patent ductus arteriosus ligation. J Thorac Cardiovasc Surg 1989;98:611.

SUBGLOTTIC STENOSIS

Subglottic stenosis can be a congenital condition or, more commonly, a lesion acquired from endotracheal intubation. Neonates and infants are particularly vulnerable to subglottic injury from intubation: the subglottis is the narrowest part of an infant's airway, and the cricoid cartilage, which supports the subglottis, is the only cartilage that completely encircles the airway. The clinical presentation may vary from patients who are totally asymptomatic to those who have typical evidence of severe upper airway obstruction. Patients with signs of stridor who fail extubation repeatedly are likely to have subglottic stenosis. As with other conditions, diagnosis is ultimately established by direct laryngoscopy and bronchoscopy. Tracheostomy is often required when airway compromise is severe. Although a number of surgical approaches to correct this problem have been tried, the failure rate is high. The most promising procedures are the "cricoid split," in which the cricoid cartilage is surgically opened (better for acquired than congenital lesions), and the laryngotracheoplasty, in which a cartilage graft from another source (eg, rib) is used to expand the framework.

Fan LL: Complications of intubation in children. Probl Anesth 1988;2:250.

Pashley NRT, Fan LL: Laryngeal injury from endotracheal intubation in the neonate. In: *Bronchopulmonary Dysplasia*. Bancalari E, Stocker JT (editors). Hemisphere Publishing, 1988.

LARYNGEAL TRAUMA

Injury to the larynx may result from external trauma, such as automobile accidents, snowmobile accidents (clothesline injury), and hanging, or internal trauma, such as noxious inhalation (burns and caustic substances) and intubation (already discussed). External trauma can cause laryngeal fracture, which requires an emergency tracheostomy to prevent death. After appropriate airway intervention, attention should be directed to debridement and closure of lacerations. Reduction of laryngeal fractures should be performed as soon as the patient is stabilized.

Myers EN: Assessing and repairing laryngeal injuries. J Respir Dis 1982;3:43.

LARYNGEAL PAPILLOMATOSIS

Papillomas of the larynx are benign, warty growths that are difficult to treat. The presumed cause is human papillomavirus infection. A substantial percentage of mothers of patients with laryngeal papillomas have a history of genital condylomas at the time of delivery, a fact suggesting that the virus is acquired at birth during passage through an infected birth canal.

The age at onset is usually 2–4 years, but the disease may present at any age. Patients usually develop hoarseness, croupy cough, or stridor that can lead to life-threatening airway obstruction. Diagnosis is established by direct laryngoscopy.

Treatment is directed at relieving airway obstruction, usually by surgical removal of the lesions. Occasionally, tracheostomy is necessary when life-threatening obstruction or respiratory arrest occurs. Although a number of surgical procedures (laser, cup forceps, cryosurgery) have been used to remove papillomas, none are satisfactory: recurrences are the rule, and repeated operations at frequent intervals to prevent airway compromise are required. Occasionally, the lesions will spread down the trachea and bronchi, making surgical removal more difficult. Fortunately, spontaneous remissions do occur, usually by puberty, so that the goal of therapy is to maintain an adequate airway until remission occurs.

McDonald GA, Strong MS: Respiratory papillomatosis: Keeping it under control. J Respir Dis 1984;5:36.

CONGENITAL DISORDERS OF THE INTRATHORACIC AIRWAYS

TRACHEOMALACIA

Tracheomalacia exists when the cartilaginous framework of the trachea is inadequate to maintain airway patency. Because cartilage of the infant airway is normally "soft," all infants may have some degree of dynamic collapse of the trachea during expiration, when pressure outside the trachea exceeds intraluminal pressure. In tracheomalacia, whether congenital or acquired, dynamic collapse leads to airway obstruction. The congenital variety may be isolated or associated with another developmental defect, such as tracheoesophageal fistula or vascular ring. It may be localized to part of the trachea or, more commonly, may involve the entire trachea as well as the remainder of the conducting airways. In severe cases, cartilage in the involved area may be missing or underdeveloped. The acquired variety has been associated with long-term ventilation of premature newborns that results in chronic tracheal injury.

Patients present with coarse wheezing, a prolonged expiratory phase, and a croupy cough, all of which increase with agitation and upper respiratory tract infections. Diagnosis can be made by cinefluoroscopy or bronchoscopy. Barium swallow may be indicated to rule out coexisting conditions. Usually, no treatment is indicated for the isolated condition, which generally improves over time. Coexisting lesions such as tracheoesophageal fistulas and vascular rings need primary repair. In severe cases of tracheomalacia, airway intervention by intubation or tracheostomy may be necessary; but this procedure alone is seldom satisfactory, because airway collapse continues to exist below the tip of the artificial airway. The application of continuous positive airway pressure through an artificial airway has occasionally been successful in stabilizing the collapsing airway.

Cogbill TH et al: Primary tracheomalacia. Ann Thorac Surg 1983;35:538.
Kanter et al: Treatment of severe tracheobronchomalacia with continuous positive airway pressure (CPAP). Anesthesiology 1982;57:54.
Sotomayor JL et al: Large-airway collapse due to acquired tracheobronchomalacia in infancy. Am J Dis Child 1986;140:367.

VASCULAR RINGS & SLINGS

Vascular anomalies of the aorta and its branches and the pulmonary arteries may compress the trachea or esophagus. The most common varieties include double aortic arch, right aortic arch with left ligamentum arteriosum or patent ductus arteriosus, pulmonary sling, anomalous innominate or left carotid artery, and aberrant right subclavian artery.

All but the aberrant right subclavian artery are associated with tracheal compression and, therefore, present in infancy with symptoms of chronic airway obstruction including stridor, course wheezing, and croupy cough. Symptoms are often worse in the supine position. Respiratory compromise is most severe with double aortic arch and may lead to apnea, respiratory arrest, or even death. Esophageal compression, present in all but anomalous innominate or carotid artery, may result in feeding difficulties, including dysphagia and vomiting. Therefore, barium swallow demonstrating this esophageal compression forms the mainstay of establishing the diagnosis. In the case of anomalous innominate or carotid artery, diagnosis is best established by cinefluoroscopy, MRI, or bronchoscopy.

Patients with significant symptoms require surgical correction, especially those with double aortic arch. Some controversy exists regarding whether angiography is necessary to define the anatomy prior to surgery. Patients usually improve following correction but may have persistent but milder symptoms of airway obstruction due to associated tracheomalacia.

Ashraf H, Subramanian S: Identifying the hallmarks of vascular rings in children. J Respir Dis 1985;6:31.
Keith HH: Vascular rings and tracheobronchial compression in infants. Pediatr Ann (Aug) 1977;6:91.

BRONCHOGENIC CYSTS

Bronchogenic cysts generally occur in the middle mediastinum (see Mediastinal Masses) near the carina and adjacent to the major bronchi but can be found elsewhere in the lung as well. Sizes are variable, ranging between 2 and 10 cm. Cyst walls are thick and may contain pus, mucus, or blood. These develop from abnormal lung budding of the primitive foregut. They do not contain distal lung parenchyma and generally do not communicate with the airway.

Clinically, respiratory distress can appear acutely in early childhood or present as chronic wheezing, chronic cough, tachypnea, recurrent pneumonia, or stridor, depending on location, size, and the degree of airway compression. On physical examination, tracheal deviation away from the midline may be noted, and the percussion note over involved lobes may be hyperresonant. Breath sounds over such areas will also be decreased. Air trapping and hyperinflation of the affected lobes is found on chest x-ray film. Smaller lesions or those detected early may not be appreciated on chest x-ray film or may appear spherical. Initial assessment of a suspected bronchogenic cyst usually includes a barium swallow to demonstrate the presence of a mass. This study also helps determine whether the lesion communicates with the gastrointestinal tract. CT scans or ultrasound can differentiate solid versus cystic mediastinal masses and define the cyst's relationship to the rest of the lung.

Treatment involves surgical resection of the bronchogenic cyst. Vigorous pulmonary physiotherapy is indicated in the postoperative period to prevent complications of the surgery (atelectasis, infection of lung distal to the site of resection of the cyst).

Stocker JT et al: Cystic and congenital lung disease in the newborn. In: *Perspectives in Pediatric Pathology.* Vol 4. Rosenberg H, Bolande T (editors). Year Book, 1978.

Turcios NL et al: When a neonate has cystic lung disease. J Respir Dis 1987;8:85.

ACQUIRED DISORDERS OF THE INTRATHORACIC AIRWAYS

FOREIGN BODY ASPIRATION

1. FOREIGN BODIES IN THE UPPER RESPIRATORY TRACT

Essentials of Diagnosis

- Acute onset of cyanosis and choking.
- Inability to vocalize or cough (complete obstruction) or with drooling and stridor (partial obstruction).

General Considerations

Foreign body aspiration contributes significantly to morbidity and mortality of early childhood, with many deaths resulting from upper airway obstruction each year. Most commonly, children between 6 months and 4 years of age are at particularly high risk for foreign body aspiration.

Clinical Findings

Foreign bodies lodged within the esophagus may compress the airway and cause respiratory distress. More typically, the foreign body lodges in the supraglottic airway, triggering protective reflexes that attempt to dislodge the object and causing laryngospasm. Onset is generally abrupt, with a history of the child running with food or other object in the mouth or playing with seeds, small coins, toys or other objects. Poor "child proofing" in the home and cases in which an older sibling feeds age-inappropriate foods (peanuts, hard candy, carrot slices, etc) to the younger child are typical. If the obstruction is only partial, coughing, stridor, and the ability to vocalize may persist. If complete, an inability to cough or vocalize (aphonia) and cyanosis with marked distress are observed. If untreated, progressive cyanosis, loss of consciousness, seizures, bradycardia, and cardiopulmonary arrest follow.

Treatment

The emergency treatment of upper airway obstruction due to foreign body aspiration is somewhat controversial. In general, it is recommended that if partial obstruction is present, children should be allowed to use their own cough reflex to extrude the foreign body. If after a brief observation period, the obstruction persists or the airway becomes completely obstructed, acute intervention is required. The AAP and AHA distinguish between children under or over 1 year of age. A choking infant under age 1 should be placed face-down position over the rescuer's arm, with the head positioned below the trunk. Four measured back blows are delivered rapidly between the infant's scapulas with the heel of the rescuer's hand. If obstruction persists, the infant should be rolled over and four rapid chest compressions performed (similar to CPR). This sequence is repeated until the obstruction is relieved. In children over age 1 year, abdominal thrusts (the "Heimlich maneuver") may be performed, with special care in younger children because of concern about possible intra-abdominal organ injury.

In both groups, blind probing of the airway to dislodge a foreign body is discouraged because of the risk of impaction. The airway may be opened by jaw thrust, and if the foreign body can be directly visualized, careful removal with the fingers or instruments (Magill forceps) can be attempted. Patients with persistent apnea and inability to achieve adequate ventilation may require emergency intubation, tracheostomy, or needle cricothyrotomy, depending on the setting and the rescuer's skills.

Abman SH et al: Emergency treatment of foreign body obstruction of the upper airway in children. J Emerg Med 1984;2:7.

American Heart Association: Standard guidelines for CPR and emergency cardiac care. JAMA 1986;255:2959.

Chameides L, (editor): *Textbook of Pediatric Advanced Life Support.* American Heart Association and American Academy of Pediatrics, 1990.

Committee on Accident and Poison Prevention, American Academy of Pediatrics: First aid for the choking child. Pediatrics 1981;67:744.

Greensher J, Mofenson HC: Emergency treatment of the choking child. Pediatrics 1982;70:110.

Heimlich JH: First aid for choking children: Back blows and chest thrusts cause complications and death. Pediatrics 1982;70:124.

2. FOREIGN BODIES IN THE LOWER RESPIRATORY TRACT

Essentials of Diagnosis

- Sudden onset of coughing, wheezing, or respiratory distress.
- Asymmetric physical findings of decreased breath sounds or localized wheezing.
- Asymmetric radiographic findings, especially with forced expiratory view.

General Considerations

The problem with diagnosing foreign body aspiration of the lower respiratory tract is the lack of parental observations documenting an acute aspiration. The abrupt onset of cough, choking or wheezing, especially in children between 6 months and 4 years who have access to high-risk objects such as peanuts, hard candy, small toys, and other objects, should heighten suspicion.

Clinical Findings

A. Symptoms and Signs: Clinically, the range of respiratory symptoms and signs varies, depending on the site of obstruction and the duration following the acute episode. For example, a large or central airway obstruction may cause marked distress and prompt early intervention. In contrast, if the foreign object remains in the lower respiratory tract, the acute cough or wheezing may diminish over time, only to recur later and present as chronic cough or persistent wheezing. Thus, foreign body aspiration should be suspected in children with chronic cough, persistent wheezing, or recurrent pneumonia. Long-standing foreign bodies may lead to bronchiectasis or lung abscess. On physical examination, asymmetric breath sounds or localized wheezing also suggest the presence of a foreign body.

B. Imaging: A physician who suspects foreign body aspiration should obtain inspiratory and forced expiratory chest x-rays. The latter study can be obtained in young children by manually compressing the abdomen during expiration. The initial inspiratory view may show localized hyperinflation due to the ball-valve effect of the foreign body, causing distal air trapping. A positive forced expiratory study shows a mediastinal shift away from the affected side. If airway obstruction is complete, atelectasis and related volume loss will be the major radiologic findings. Chest fluoroscopy is an alternative approach for detecting air trapping and mediastinal shift.

Treatment

If positive findings are absent but clinical suspicion persists, further evaluation with bronchoscopy is indicated. Rigid, not flexible, bronchoscopy is the recommended diagnostic and therapeutic approach to managing suspected or proved foreign body aspiration. Flexible bronchoscopy may be helpful for follow-up evaluations (after the foreign object has been removed).

Children with suspected acute foreign body aspiration should be admitted to the hospital for evaluation and treatment. Chest postural drainage was often performed in the past, prior to technologic improvements in bronchoscopy; however, postural drainage is no longer recommended because the foreign body may become dislodged and obstruct a major central airway. Rigid bronchoscopy under general anesthesia is the current treatment for foreign body aspiration. Bronchoscopy should not be delayed in children with respiratory distress but should be performed as soon as possible once the diagnosis is made, even in children with more chronic symptoms. Following the removal of the foreign body, β-adrenergic nebulization treatments followed by chest physiotherapy are recommended to help clear related mucus or bronchospasm. Current bronchoscopy skills facilitate foreign body removal with little risk. The relative dangers of missing a foreign body in the lower respiratory tract are much greater; these include the development of bronchiectasis and lung abscess over time. This risk justifies an aggressive approach to suspected foreign bodies in undocumented but suspicious cases.

Kosloske AM: Tracheobronchial foreign bodies in children: Back to the bronchoscope and a balloon. Pediatrics 1980;66:321.

Law D, Kosloske AM: Management of tracheobronchial foreign bodies in children: A reevaluation of postural drainage and bronchoscopy. Pediatrics 1976;58:362.

Wood RE, Gauderer MWL: Flexible fiberoptic bronchoscopy in the management of tracheobronchial foreign bodies in children: The value of a combined approach with open tube bronchoscopy. J Pediatr Surg 1984;19:693.

BRONCHITIS

Essentials of Diagnosis

- Cough that usually progresses from dry to productive.
- Rhonchi appearing predominantly during expiration.

General Considerations

Bronchitis refers to inflammation of the major conducting airways within the lung. As an isolated entity, this problem is probably unusual in children. However, inflammation within this section of the airways commonly occurs in association with disease processes involving other areas of the respiratory tract. From a temporal standpoint, bronchitis may be acute, chronic, or recurrent. In adults, the diagnosis of chronic bronchitis is based on a history of at least 3 months of productive cough occurring for 2 or more years, but no generally acceptable criteria for this diagnosis exist in children. However, if cough with sputum production persists in a child for a period of at least 3–4 weeks, the physician should consider the diagnoses discussed below (see Differential Diagnosis).

Clinical Findings

A. Symptoms and Signs: An acute bronchitis usually begins as a dry, nonproductive cough that may be associated with other features of an upper respiratory illness of viral origin. The longer the cough persists, the more likely the cough will become productive. In general, children with uncomplicated acute bronchitis appear nontoxic, and fever, if present, is low-grade. On examination of the chest, diffuse rhonchi appearing predominantly during expiration are noted. In uncomplicated acute bronchitis, mucus production decreases, and the cough disappears over a period of 7–10 days.

B. Laboratory Findings: The white blood count is usually normal and, if elevated, may suggest a viral infection. Pulmonary function tests may reveal variable degrees of airway obstruction.

C. Imaging: An x-ray examination of the chest may be normal or show a mild increase in bronchovascular markings.

Differential Diagnosis

Most attacks of acute bronchitis are caused by viral infections. Although episodes are usually self-limited, certain viral pathogens, such as the adenovirus, can produce a more severe clinical picture that resembles a pertussis-like illness. Bacteria that may produce disease in which bronchitis is a prominent symptom include *Bordetella pertussis, Mycobacterium tuberculosis, Corynebacterium diphtheriae,* and *Mycoplasma pneumoniae.*

Noninfectious diseases need to be considered in the evaluation of an acute bronchitis that differs from the clinical picture described above and in cases of chronic bronchitis or recurrent bronchitic episodes. Asthma may present as a persistent cough with little or no wheezing. Sinus infections may provide a source of persistent irritation to the respiratory tract and lead to a chronic cough. Cystic fibrosis, an immunodeficiency, or primary ciliary dyskinesia must also be considered if the bronchitic syndrome persists or recurs and if bronchiectasis is present or suspected. In the younger child, respiratory tract anomalies, foreign bodies, and recurrent aspiration must also be considered. Tobacco or marihuana smoking may contribute to this process in older children. In patients of all ages, the potential role of irritants within their environment must also be evaluated.

Complications

In otherwise healthy children, complications of an acute bronchitis secondary to a viral infection are few but include otitis media, sinusitis, and pneumonia. When the bronchitic syndrome is secondary to other underlying problems outlined in the differential diagnosis, the prognosis depends on the primary problem.

Treatment

When bronchitis is secondary to an uncomplicated acute viral infection, supportive therapy (stressing adequate hydration, rest, and patience) is all that is necessary. Expectorants and cough suppressants, though commonly used, are seldom indicated. Avoidance of irritants during the viral infection may also decrease symptoms and morbidity. When the bronchitic syndrome is due to other underlying problems, the treatment must address the primary process.

Florman AL, Cushing AH, Umland ET: Rapid noninvasive techniques for determining etiology of bronchitis and pneumonia in infants and children. Clin Chest Med 1987;8:669.

Loughlin GM: Bronchitis. In: *Disorders of the Respiratory Tract in Children,* 5th ed. Chernick V, Kendig EL Jr (editors). Saunders, 1990.

Morgan WJ, Taussig LM: The chronic bronchitis complex in children. Pediatr Clin North Am 1984;31:851.

Rossman CM, Newhouse MT: Primary ciliary dyskinesia: Evaluation and management. Pediatr Pulmonol 1988; 5:36.

BRONCHIOLITIS

Essentials of Diagnosis

- Young infant with acute onset of tachypnea, cough, rhinorrhea, and expiratory wheeze.
- Chest x-ray with streaky infiltrates and hyperaeration.

General Considerations

Bronchiolitis is a common cause of acute hospital admissions in young infants (under 2 years), especially during the winter months. Although respiratory syncytial virus is by far the most common pathogen, other viral agents include parainfluenza, influenza, and adenovirus. *Mycoplasma, Chlamydia, Ureaplasma,* and *Pneumocystis* are other potential causes of wheezing-associated respiratory illness during early infancy. Major concerns include not only the acute effects of bronchiolitis but also the possibility of long-term airway injury and the development of chronic airways hyperreactivity (asthma). In addition, bronchiolitis due to respiratory syncytial virus infection contributes substantially to morbidity and mortality in children with underlying cardiopulmonary disorders, including bronchopulmonary dysplasia, cystic fibrosis, and congenital heart disease, especially when pulmonary hypertension is present.

Clinical Findings

A. Symptoms and Signs: The usual course of respiratory syncytial virus bronchiolitis includes 1–2 days of fever, rhinorrhea, and cough, followed by wheezing, tachypnea, and respiratory distress. Typically, the breathing pattern is shallow, with rapid respirations. Nasal flaring, cyanosis, retractions, and rales may be present, along with prolongation of the expiratory phase and wheezing, depending on the severity of illness. Some young infants present with apnea and little auscultatory findings but may subsequently develop rales, rhonchi, and expiratory wheezing. Otitis media, superimposed bacterial pneumonia, and bacteremia may be observed.

B. Laboratory Findings: The peripheral white blood cell count may be normal or show a mild lymphocytosis.

C. Imaging: Chest x-ray findings typically include hyperinflation with mild interstitial infiltrates, but segmental atelectasis is not uncommon.

Treatment

Although most children infected with respiratory syncytial virus bronchiolitis are readily managed as outpatients with supportive therapy, hospitalization is required in children less than 2 months of age and in patients with hypoxemia in room air, a history of apnea, moderate tachypnea with feeding difficulties, marked respiratory distress with retractions, and underlying chronic cardiopulmonary disorders. Initial management includes an assessment of oxygenation and ventilation with an arterial blood gas and, if hypoxemia is present, the administration of supplemental oxygen. Noninvasive measurements of oxygenation by oximeter or transcutaneous PO_2 monitor should be used to assess the response to therapy and provide early warning of impending respiratory failure in infants. In one series, 7% of normal children admitted for viral bronchiolitis subsequently required mechanical ventilation; infants with bronchopulmonary dysplasia and cystic fibrosis hospitalized with respiratory syncytial virus bronchiolitis develop respiratory failure at higher rates. Progressive respiratory distress (including progressive hypoxemia and hypercapnia) and apnea are common indications for admission to the intensive care unit and mechanical ventilation.

Medical staff should also administer intravenous hydration to correct losses and poor intake, while carefully monitoring intake, output, and urinary specific gravity to avoid overhydration and the risk of fluid overload and pulmonary edema. Although β-adrenergic therapy, theophylline, and corticosteroids may attenuate airway obstruction, their use remains controversial and empiric, and patients should be assessed individually to determine the degree of responsiveness to drug therapy.

The availability of rapid diagnostic testing for respiratory syncytial virus infection may allow for early intervention with antiviral therapy (ribavirin), especially in children with marked respiratory distress or chronic cardiopulmonary disease. Although ribavirin's efficacy remains unclear, its use is currently recommended for hospitalized infants with severe disease or with coexistent congenital heart disease, bronchopulmonary dysplasia, cystic fibrosis, immunodeficiencies, and other chronic lung disorders, as well as recent transplant recipients and patients undergoing chemotherapy. In addition, children less than 6 weeks of age and those with underlying metabolic, neurologic, or congenital abnormalities should be considered for ribavirin therapy.

Prognosis

Although the outcome following bronchiolitis is good for the overall population, the mortality rate in patients with congenital heart disease has been reported to be near 50%. In addition, recurrent episodes of wheezing may follow acute infection in almost half of the hospitalized infants, a fact suggesting the possibility that early infection may contribute to the subsequent development of chronic reactive airways disease.

Abman SH et al: Role of RSV in early hospitalizations for respiratory distress of young infants with cystic fibrosis. J Pediatr 1988;113:826.

Groothius J et al: RSV in children with bronchopulmonary dysplasia. Pediatrics 1988;82:199.

MacDonald NE et al: RSV in infants with congenital heart disease. N Engl J Med 1982;307:397.

Outwater KM, Crone RK: Management of respiratory failure in infants with acute viral bronchiolitis. Am J Dis Child 1984;138:1071.

Volovitz B, Faden H, Ogra PL: Release of leukotriene C_4 in respiratory tract during acute viral infection. J Pediatr 1988;112:218.

Wohl MEB: Bronchiolitis. In: *Disorders of the Respiratory Tract in Children,* 5th ed. Chernick V, Kendig EL Jr (editors). Saunders, 1990.

BRONCHIECTASIS

Essentials of Diagnosis

- Chronic cough with sputum production.
- Persistent abnormalities on physical examination of the chest.
- Persistent abnormalities on chest x-ray.

General Considerations

The term "bronchiectasis" means dilatation of bronchi. The dilatation may be regular, with the airway continuing to have a smooth outline (cylindric bronchiectasis); irregular, with areas of dilatation and constriction (varicose bronchiectasis); or marked, with destruction of structural components of the airway wall (saccular bronchiectasis). Although the incidence of the disease in the general population is low (< 0.5%), the morbidity associated with the more severe forms of bronchiectasis is significant. For this reason, an appreciation of the pathogenesis of bronchiectasis is important. Medical treatment can halt the progression of a potentially reversible form (cylindric bronchiectasis) to an irreversible destructive airway disease (saccular bronchiectasis).

Two factors appear to be important in the development of bronchiectasis: obstruction of the airway resulting in poor drainage is a feature of many disease processes that lead to this disorder (cystic fibrosis, foreign bodies), and infection must be present to damage the airway. Thus, in the healthy airway, either self-limited infection without significant obstruction or obstruction without infection is unlikely to lead to the more severe forms of bronchiectasis. However, the combination of the two for a period of time favors the development of bronchiectatic areas of lung.

Clinical Findings

A. Symptoms and Signs: The clinical manifestations of bronchiectasis vary widely from the healthy-appearing child whose only symptom may be chronic cough with early morning sputum production to chronically ill children with recurrent pneumonia with or without hemoptysis. There may be a history of recurrent respiratory infections, dyspnea on exertion, and a productive cough precipitated by exercise. In addition, some children present with a history of recurrent fevers. Chronic cough, persistent atelectasis, and failure of a chest x-ray to clear after a respiratory infection should suggest the possibility of bronchiectasis. On physical examination, digital clubbing may be present, and there may be evidence of sinusitis suggested by sinus tenderness or postnasal drainage of purulent secretions. Persistent adventitious sounds (moist rales, rhonchi) and decreased air entry are often noted over the bronchiectatic area when saccular changes are present.

B. Laboratory Findings and Imaging: Cultures from the respiratory tract usually reveal mixed flora; *Haemophilus influenzae* is one of the more common isolates. Because of coexistent sinus disease in many patients, cultures of secretions from the upper airway may also assist in determining antimicrobial therapy.

Chest films may show mildly abnormal findings with slightly increased bronchovascular markings or areas of atelectasis, or they may demonstrate cystic changes in one or more areas of the lung. The anatomy of the airways is best defined by high-resolution CT scan of the lung, which often reveals far more extensive disease (in terms of involvement of other areas of lung) than expected from the plain chest film. Although bronchography has been used to determine whether disease is localized or diffuse and whether varicose or saccular bronchiectasis is present, this study may lead to significant morbidity and has been replaced by radiologic studies. However, bronchography may still be of assistance when surgery is being considered.

Pulmonary function testing often reveals an obstructive pattern even in the absence of asthma, cystic fibrosis, or other disease processes leading to airway obstruction. This obstruction may reflect difficulty in handling airway secretions or a more generalized pulmonary problem involving both large and small airways. Evaluation of lung function before and after inhalation of a bronchodilator is helpful in assessing the potential contribution of this class of medications to therapy. In addition, serial assessments of lung function help define the progression or resolution of the disease.

Differential Diagnosis

Infectious diseases have always been important factors predisposing to bronchiectasis. Both rubeola and pertussis were prominently associated with bronchiectasis in older reports of this disorder. In addition, tuberculosis still causes significant airway damage. More recently, adenoviral infections have been noted to lead to bronchiectasis. As a practical matter, however, any viral or bacterial infection of the lung that leads to significant obstruction and persistent inflammation has the potential to damage the airway wall.

Bronchiectasis also develops in patients with cystic fibrosis, immunodeficiencies involving humoral immunity, and abnormal mucociliary clearance (primary ciliary dyskinesia). Recurrent aspiration has also been associated with this disorder. Aspiration of a foreign body must also be considered, especially when bronchiectatic changes are confined to one area of the lung.

Although congenital causes of bronchiectasis are relatively uncommon compared to the predisposing factors listed above, they must still be considered in the differential diagnosis. Bronchiectasis may result from a developmental arrest of bronchial cartilage in which the involved areas give rise to cysts that are prone to infection. In addition, defective development of bronchial cartilage (Williams-Campbell syndrome) and developmental failure of elastic and muscular tissues of the trachea and bronchi (tracheobronchomegaly or Mounier-Kuhn syndrome) have been associated with bronchiectasis. Bronchial stenosis, either congenital or acquired, also predisposes to bronchiectasis.

Complications

Several complications may develop as a consequence of the more severe forms of bronchiectasis. The major concerns include severe pneumonia, hemoptysis, and cor pulmonale. More unusual complications include abscesses of the lung or central nervous system as well as empyema and bronchopleural fistula.

Treatment

The initial approach to almost all children with

bronchiectasis is medical and consists of identifying bacterial pathogens present in the bronchiectatic areas of lung. Based on the severity of airway damage, antibiotics can be delivered either systemically (for saccular changes) or orally. Coupled with use of antibiotics is optimal pulmonary physiotherapy, which consists of inhalation of bronchodilators followed by postural drainage and chest percussion to affected areas of lung. If present, sinusitis must also be vigorously treated.

Surgical removal of an area of lung that has severe saccular bronchiectasis is considered when the response to several months of optimal medical therapy has been poor. Other indications include extensive or repeated hemoptysis and recurrent pneumonia in one area of lung. In general, surgery is best performed when the bronchiectatic area is well localized and the rest of the lung appears to be normal. This clinical description is most likely to be found in a child who has saccular bronchiectasis due to foreign body aspiration or a congenital defect. In general, children with more serious underlying disorders (cystic fibrosis, hypogammaglobulinemia) are likely to have bronchiectatic changes in several areas of the lung and are not good candidates for surgery.

Prognosis

The outlook for patients with bronchiectasis depends on the underlying cause of the problem, the severity of the bronchiectatic changes, and the extent of lung involvement. As noted, good pulmonary hygiene and avoidance of infectious complications in the involved areas of lung may reverse cylindric bronchiectasis.

Barker AF, Bardana EJ Jr: Bronchiectasis: Update of an orphan disease. Am Rev Respir Dis 1988;137:969.

Brown MA, Lemen RJ: Bronchiectasis. In: *Disorders of the Respiratory Tract in Children,* 5th ed. Chernick V, Kendig EL Jr (editors). Saunders, 1990.

Lewiston NJ: Bronchiectasis in childhood. Pediatr Clin North Am 1984;31:865.

BRONCHIOLITIS OBLITERANS (Bronchiolitis Fibrosa Obliterans)

Bronchiolitis obliterans is a disease characterized by obstruction of bronchi and bronchioles by fibrous tissue after an insult to the lower respiratory tract. The disorder can be precipitated by inhalation of toxic gases, infections of the lower respiratory tract (adenovirus, influenza virus, rubeola virus, *Bordetella, Mycoplasma*), connective tissue diseases, transplantation, and aspiration. Many episodes of bronchiolitis obliterans are idiopathic (no cause can be identified). Studies of adenovirus-induced bronchiolitis obliterans indicate that the disease occurs more frequently in the Native American population in Canada and in

Polynesian children in New Zealand, suggesting that racial or socioeconomic factors predispose to this process.

Clinical Findings

A. Symptoms and Signs: Bronchiolitis obliterans should be considered when there is persistent cough or wheezing after an acute pneumonia. Prolonged rales or wheezing or persistent exercise intolerance following a pulmonary insult should also suggest this disease. Sputum production may accompany these complaints.

B. Laboratory Findings and Imaging: Chest x-ray abnormalities include evidence of localized or generalized air trapping as well as possibly nodular densities and alveolar opacification. Scattered areas of matched decreases in ventilation and perfusion are seen when the lung is scanned. Pulmonary angiograms reveal decreased vasculature in the area of lung involvement, whereas bronchograms demonstrate marked pruning of the bronchial tree. An assessment of lung function demonstrates an obstructive process that may be combined with evidence of restriction. Administration of an inhaled bronchodilator both before and after courses of corticosteroids leads to little improvement in lung function.

Differential Diagnosis

Poorly treated asthma, cystic fibrosis, and bronchopulmonary dysplasia must be considered in the pediatric patient with evidence of persistent airway obstruction and ruled out on the basis of the history and appropriate diagnostic tests. A trial of medications (including corticosteroids) employed in the treatment of asthma may help to define the reversibility of the process when the primary differential is between asthma and bronchiolitis obliterans. Although the results of imaging and pulmonary function testing are very suggestive, the best way to establish a definitive diagnosis is by open lung biopsy.

Complications

Sequelae of bronchiolitis obliterans include persistent airway obstruction, recurrent wheezing, bronchiectasis, chronic atelectasis, recurrent pneumonia, and unilateral hyperlucent lung syndrome.

Treatment

Supplemental oxygen should be given to patients with oxygen desaturation during normal activities or sleep. In addition, early treatment should be directed at preventing ongoing airway damage due to problems such as aspiration, which may be either the primary insult or an acquired problem secondary to marked hyperinflation. Other forms of treatment may be more difficult to evaluate in terms of effectiveness. Oral and inhaled bronchodilators may be helpful in reversing airway obstruction produced by a reactive component to the disease. Many children also receive at least one course of corticosteroid treatment in an attempt to reverse the obstruction or prevent ongoing damage. Antibiotics should be used as clinically indicated for pneumonia.

Prognosis

Prognosis may depend in part on the underlying cause as well as the age at which the insult occurred. The course varies from mild asthma-like symptoms to rapidly fatal deterioration despite therapy.

Hardy KA, Schidlow DV, Zaeri N: Obliterative bronchiolitis in children. Chest 1988;93:461.

Wohl MEB: Bronchiolitis. In: *Disorders of the Respiratory Tract in Children,* 5th ed. Chernick V, Kendig EL Jr (editors). Saunders, 1990.

BRONCHOPULMONARY DYSPLASIA

Essentials of Diagnosis

- Acute respiratory distress in first week of life.
- Required oxygen therapy or mechanical ventilation.
- Persistent respiratory abnormalities, including physical signs, radiographic findings, and increased O_2 requirement, after 1 month of age.

General Considerations

As mortality rates for premature newborns have fallen dramatically over the past 2 decades, bronchopulmonary dysplasia remains one of the most significant sequelae following the management of acute respiratory distress in the neonatal intensive care unit, with an estimated incidence ranging between 10% and 40% (depending on the criteria used for definition and the gestational age of the population base). This disease was first characterized in 1967 when Northway and coworkers reported the clinical, radiologic, and pathologic findings in a group of premature newborns who required prolonged mechanical ventilation and oxygen therapy to treat hyaline membrane disease. The progression from acute hyaline membrane disease to chronic lung disease was divided into four stages: acute respiratory distress shortly after birth, usually hyaline membrane disease (stage I); clinical and radiographic worsening of the acute lung disease, often due to increased pulmonary blood flow secondary to a patent ductus arteriosus (stage II); and progressive signs of chronic lung disease (stages III and IV). Although some of the clinical features of bronchopulmonary dysplasia have changed over the past 20 years along with changes in therapy, this seminal paper led to understanding of the evolution of the problem and the potential risk factors: immaturity, oxygen toxicity, barotrauma, and inflammation.

The precise definition of bronchopulmonary dysplasia remains controversial. For most purposes, however, the disorder can be defined clinically as a chronic respiratory disorder of infancy that follows treatment during the first week of life for acute respiratory distress and is subsequently associated with persistent signs of respiratory distress, a requirement for supplemental oxygen, and radiographic abnormalities beyond 30 days of age. This broad definition does not accommodate some key issues, including the following: (1) although most of these children were premature and had hyaline membrane disease, full-term newborns with such disorders as meconium aspiration or persistent pulmonary hypertension can also develop bronchopulmonary dysplasia; (2) some severely preterm newborns require minimal ventilator support yet subsequently develop a prolonged oxygen requirement despite the absence of severe acute manifestations of respiratory failure; (3) newborns dying within the first weeks of life can already have the aggressive, fibroproliferative pathologic lesions that resemble bronchopulmonary dysplasia; and (4) physiologic abnormalities (increased airway resistance) and biochemical markers of lung injury (altered protease and antiprotease ratios, increased inflammatory cells and mediators), which are predictive of bronchopulmonary dysplasia, are already present in the first week of life.

Although the exact mechanisms leading to chronic lung disease are not completely understood, bronchopulmonary dysplasia represents the consequences of lung injury caused by oxygen toxicity, barotrauma, and inflammation superimposed on a susceptible, generally immature lung. The premature lung often lacks the ability to make adequate amounts of functional surfactant; furthermore, the antioxidant defense mechanisms are not sufficiently mature to protect the lung from the toxic oxygen metabolites generated from hyperoxia, which cause further lung injury. Thus, abnormal lung mechanics due to structural immaturity, surfactant deficiency, atelectasis, and pulmonary edema—plus lung injury secondary to hyperoxia and mechanical ventilation—lead to further abnormalities of lung function, causing increases in ventilator and oxygen requirements and leading to a vicious circle that compounds the progression of lung injury. Other factors such as excessive fluid administration, patent ductus arteriosus, pulmonary interstitial emphysema, pneumothorax, infection, and inflammatory stimuli secondary to lung injury or infection also play important roles in the pathogenesis and pathophysiology of the disease.

Differential Diagnosis

The radiologic differential diagnosis includes meconium aspiration syndrome, congenital infection (such as cytomegalovirus or Ureaplasma), cystic adenomatoid malformation, recurrent aspiration, pulmonary lymphangiectasia, total anomalous pulmonary venous return, overhydration, or idiopathic pulmonary fibrosis.

Clinical Course & Treatment

The clinical course of infants with bronchopulmonary dysplasia is extremely variable, ranging from a mild increased oxygen requirement that gradually resolves over a few months to more severe disease requiring chronic tracheostomy and mechanical ventilation for the first 2 years of life. In general, patients show slow, steady improvements in oxygen or ventilator requirements but can have frequent respiratory exacerbations leading to frequent or prolonged hospitalizations. Clinical management generally includes careful attention to growth, nutrition, metabolic status, development, neurologic status, and related problems, along with the various cardiopulmonary abnormalities described below.

Because increased airways resistance and bronchial hyperreactivity are common in infants with the disorder, various combinations of β-adrenergic agonists, aminophylline, corticosteroids, and cromolyn are commonly part of the treatment plan. Part of the rationale for the use of corticosteroids is to decrease lung inflammation and enhance responsiveness to β-adrenergic drugs, as in the treatment of severe asthma. Because thick secretions are common and may contribute to airway obstruction or recurrent atelectasis, chest physiotherapy following the administration of β-adrenergic agonists is commonly part of the regimen.

Although bronchial hyperreactivity in affected infants is well recognized, structural lesions (such as subglottic stenosis, vocal cord paralysis, tracheal stenosis, tracheomalacia, bronchial stenosis, granulomatous bronchial polyps, and others) often contribute to airflow limitation. This possibility suggests the need for careful bronchoscopic evaluations in children with significant involvement.

Infants often have recurrent pulmonary edema, which may be due to increased permeability of the injured pulmonary circulation or to increases in hydrostatic pressure if left ventricular dysfunction is present. In addition, salt and water retention secondary to chronic hypoxemia, hypercapnia, or other stimuli may be present. Chronic or intermittent diuretic therapy with furosemide, hydrochlorothiazide, and spironolactone is commonly used if there are rales or signs of persistent pulmonary edema, with acute improvement in lung function demonstrated by clinical studies. Unfortunately, diuretics often cause major side effects, including severe volume contraction, hypokalemia, alkalosis, and hyponatremia. Potassium and arginine chloride supplements are commonly required.

Infants often have pulmonary hypertension, and in many children, even mild hypoxia can cause significant elevations of pulmonary artery pressure. To minimize the harmful effects of hypoxia, medical staff must constantly maintain PaO_2 above 55–60 mm Hg. Because even intermittent hypoxia contributes to the development or progression of pulmonary hypertension and cor pulmonale, noninvasive assessments of oxygenation must be made during all activities, including the infant's waking, sleeping, and feeding periods. Serial electrocardiographic and echocardiographic studies monitor the development of right ventricular hypertrophy. If hypertrophy persists or develops where it previously was not present, intermittent hypoxia should be considered and further assessments of oxygenation pursued, especially while the infant sleeps. In addition, barium swallow, esophageal pH probe studies, bronchoscopy, and cardiac catheterization may reveal previously unsuspected cardiac or pulmonary lesions—aspiration, tracheomalacia, obstructive sleep apnea, anatomic cardiac lesions, etc—that contribute to the underlying pathophysiology. In addition, long-term care should include monitoring systemic hypertension and the development of left ventricular hypertrophy.

Nutritional problems in infants may be due to increased O_2 consumption, feeding difficulties, gastroesophageal reflux, and chronic hypoxia. Hypercaloric formulas and gastrostomies are often required to ensure adequate intake while avoiding overhydration. In addition, influenza vaccine is recommended. With the onset of acute wheezing secondary to suspected viral infection, rapid diagnostic testing for respiratory syncytial virus infection may facilitate early treatment, which may diminish the late morbidity of bronchiolitis.

For children who remain ventilator-dependent, the authors believe that arterial CO_2 should be maintained below 60 mm Hg—even when pH is normal—because of the potential adverse effects of hypercapnia on salt and water retention, cardiac function, and perhaps pulmonary vascular tone. Changes in ventilator settings in children with severe lung disease should be slow, because the effects of many of the changes may not be manifested for days. These signs may include poor feeding, irritability, weight loss, vomiting, increased retractions, wheezing, and CO_2 retention. Medical staff should frequently meet with the parents to review progress and changes in treatment plans and thereby decrease some of the family stresses involved in caring for children with chronic severe disease. Patience, continued family support, attention to developmental issues, and speech and physical therapy help to improve the long-term outlook.

Prognosis

Although the mortality rate is high in infants with severe (stage IV) bronchopulmonary dysplasia, the long-term outlook is generally favorable. However, more time and further study is needed to assess the impact in adolescence and early adulthood of such sequelae as persistent airway hyperreactivity, exercise intolerance, and perhaps abnormal lung growth. New therapeutic approaches such as surfactant replacement and high-frequency ventilation have not yet been shown to reduce the severity or incidence of bronchopulmonary dysplasia. The possible role of antioxidant therapy or specific anti-inflammatory agents must be pursued.

Abman SH et al: Pulmonary vascular response to oxygen in infants with severe bronchopulmonary dysplasia. Pediatrics 1985;75:80.

Bancalari E, Stocker JT (editors): *Bronchopulmonary Dysplasia.* Hemisphere Publishing, 1988.

Gerhardt T et al: Serial determination of pulmonary function in infants with chronic lung disease. J Pediatr 1987;110:448.

Holtzman RB, Frank L (editors): *Bronchopulmonary Dysplasia.* Clinical Perinatology, vol 19. Saunders, 1992.

Kao LC et al: Effects of oral diuretics on pulmonary mechanics in infants with BPD: Results of a double-blind cross-over sequential trial. Pediatrics 1984;74:37.

Koops BL et al: Outpatient management and follow-up of BPD. Clin Perinatol 1984;11:101.

Northway WH, Rosan RC, Porter DY: Pulmonary disease following respiratory therapy of hyaline membrane disease: Bronchopulmonary dysplasia. N Engl J Med 1967;276:357.

Northway WH et al: Late pulmonary sequelae of bronchopulmonary dysplasia. N Engl J Med 1990;323:1793.

O'Brodovich HM, Mellins RM: Bronchopulmonary dysplasia. Unresolved neonatal acute lung injury. Am Rev Respir Dis 1985;132:694.

CYSTIC FIBROSIS

Essentials of Diagnosis

- Sweat chloride greater than 60 mmol/L.
- Pulmonary, gastrointestinal, or hepatic dysfunction or injury.

General Considerations

Cystic fibrosis is the most common lethal genetic disease in the United States, with an incidence of 1:2000 Caucasian births. It is a major cause of pulmonary and gastrointestinal morbidity in children and a leading cause of death in early adulthood. Although cystic fibrosis causes abnormalities in the hepatic, gastrointestinal, and male reproductive systems, the lung disease is the major cause of morbidity and mortality. Almost all patients develop obstructive lung disease associated with chronic infection that leads to progressive loss of pulmonary function. The prognosis has improved steadily over the past 20 years, so that the median survival is now 28 years—perhaps as a result of use of antibiotics, better treatment of malabsorption, and the development of a network of special cystic fibrosis care centers. The centers usually employ a multidisciplinary approach to patient care that involves contributions from physicians, nurses, social workers, nutritionists, and physical or respiratory therapists. This network of centers is funded and reviewed by the Cystic Fibrosis Foundation, which is also a major force in encouraging and funding basic and clinical research in cystic fibrosis.

The cystic fibrosis gene has recently been located. The area of interest on the long arm of human chromosome 7 spans approximately 250,000 base pairs of genomic DNA. Its messenger RNA codes for a 1480-amino-acid protein, the cystic fibrosis transmembrane conductance regulator (CFTR). The CFTR is involved in chloride channel activity, but its exact function is unknown. Approximately 75% of the mutations in cystic fibrosis patients correspond to a specific deletion of three base pairs that results in the loss of a phenylalanine residue at amino acid position 508 of the putative product of the cystic fibrosis gene. The remainder of the cystic fibrosis mutant gene pool consists of many different mutations. Part of the variability in clinical course in cystic fibrosis can be explained by differences in genotype.

Clinical Findings & Treatment

A. Clinical Presentations and Diagnosis: Fifteen percent of infants with cystic fibrosis present at birth with an intestinal obstruction known as meconium ileus. Abdominal distention and the presence of a thick, sticky meconium throughout the large colon on meglumine diatrizoate (Gastrografin) enema examination suggest the diagnosis. In the past, surgical removal of the meconium was common and often led to resection of bowel. However, improved techniques of enema administration under radiologic observation have reduced the need for surgery.

Roughly half of patients with cystic fibrosis present classically in infancy with failure to thrive, respiratory compromise, or both. However, the age at presentation can be quite variable; some patients are not diagnosed until adulthood. Neonatal screening based on elevations of immunoreactive trypsinogen in the blood has recently received attention as an alternative method of case identification. Newborn screening has facilitated studies of early abnormalities in cystic fibrosis, but the long-term benefits of early diagnosis are still uncertain.

Whether the clinical suspicion of cystic fibrosis is based on meconium ileus, failure to thrive, recurrent respiratory infections, or elevated immunoreactive trypsinogen in infancy, the diagnosis is made only after a positive sweat test. The sweat of individuals with cystic fibrosis contains elevated concentrations of chloride and sodium. Although elevated sweat electrolytes are associated with other conditions, a positive sweat test coupled with the clinical picture usually confirms the diagnosis. Laboratories routinely performing sweat tests give more reliable results than those that perform them only occasionally. The Gibson-Cooke quantitative technique is the only acceptable method. Measurements of electrical conductivity alone can be unreliable.

B. Gastrointestinal and Nutritional Findings and Treatment: Untreated patients with cystic fibrosis have abdominal distention and discomfort; bulky, greasy stools; and increased flatulence secondary to exocrine pancreatic insufficiency and malabsorption. Some infants present with hypoalbuminemia, anemia, edema, and hepatomegaly. Infants with severe protein-calorie malnutrition have particularly difficult courses, with high morbidity and mortality rates. Older patients are subject to intestinal blockage from inspissated stool. This "meconium ileus equivalent" is now most often treated with cathartics and enemas and only rarely requires surgery. Patients with cystic fibrosis are more prone to intussusception (especially of the appendix) than are normal individuals.

The cornerstone of gastrointestinal treatment is pancreatic enzyme supplementation. Patients are required to take the enzyme capsules with each meal and with snacks. Newer enzyme preparations contain more lipase per capsule than older preparations; therefore, patients take fewer capsules, making administration easier. Occasionally, enzyme supplementation alone does not control the malabsorption, and antacids are added to the regimen.

Individuals with cystic fibrosis may demonstrate abnormalities in nutritional status, including fat-soluble vitamin deficiency, hypoalbuminemia, and poor growth with decreased stores of body fat. In the past, fat-restricted diets were recommended. It is now recognized that patients with cystic fibrosis need all the calories they can take, and unrestricted diets are now the norm in most centers. Moreover, caloric supplements, such as high-calorie commercial supplements or formulas or food modules (including polycose and medium-chain triglycerides) are often added to the patient's diet. In patients who do not respond to oral supplementation, nighttime nasogastric feeding or feeding by means of gastrostomy or jejunostomy has been tried. Although there is general agreement that quality of life is enhanced by improved nutrition, it is not known whether aggressive nutritional treatment increases longevity.

C. Pulmonary Findings and Treatment: Infants with cystic fibrosis frequently have respiratory compromise. Cough, tachypnea, rales, and wheezing are common findings. Respiratory syncytial virus infection is associated with marked morbidity in early infancy. Some patients develop cough only later in childhood or adolescence, but by adulthood almost all patients with cystic fibrosis have productive coughs. In more advanced disease, hemoptysis due to bronchiectasis, exercise limitation, and cor pulmonale may be present. Rales may be heard on physical examination. Clubbing also develops as the lung disease progresses.

Pulmonary function abnormalities initially show obstructive patterns with diminished flow rates and increased lung volumes. As the disease progresses, vital capacity is also affected. The incidence of airway reactivity in cystic fibrosis has been estimated to be 25–50%, several times the incidence in the general population. Initially, the airway is colonized with *Staphylococcus aureus,* but in most patients, *Pseudomonas aeruginosa* becomes predominant at some point. The acquisition of the characteristic mucoid *Pseudomonas* is associated with a more rapid decline in pulmonary function. In addition, infection with *Pseudomonas cepacia* has been associated with rapid deterioration and death. Pathologically, the earliest lesions involve hyperplasia of the mucus glands of the bronchial epithelium and mucosal and submucosal cellular infiltrates. Bronchiolectasis and bronchiectasis usually follow throughout all lung fields.

Treatment of the pulmonary disease in cystic fibrosis includes chest physical therapy, antibiotics, bronchodilators, and (more recently) anti-inflammatory agents. Each of these treatments is controversial. A recent study of postural drainage and percussion has demonstrated benefit over a 3-year period in patients receiving the therapy. This study has put the use of postural drainage on firmer ground. Although controlled trials have yielded ambiguous results, there is general agreement that antibiotics play a major role in pulmonary treatment. Antibiotics are used liberally in outpatient treatment (eg, with a change in cough or respiratory symptoms) and are used extensively during inpatient admissions. Recent studies have suggested a benefit from inhaled antibiotics. The high incidence of airway reactivity suggests an important treatment role for bronchodilators, yet some studies have shown paradoxic responses to these medications. The paradoxic responses may be related in part to the fact that the increasing compliance of large airways leads to earlier airway closure.

Current speculation on the development of lung disease in cystic fibrosis includes not only the effects of the bacterial pathogens but also the host response to such pathogens. If activated neutrophils or immune complexes are important in the genesis of the airway injury, then anti-inflammatory agents may be helpful. Although corticosteroids may be beneficial in patients with increased airway reactivity, a multicenter trial has identified complications, including glucose intolerance and the development of diabetes, associated with alternate-day prednisone use.

A subgroup of patients with cystic fibrosis have frequent pulmonary exacerbations characterized by difficult breathing, increased sputum production, decreased exercise tolerance, and diminished pulmonary function. These patients often benefit from hospital treatment, including intensive physical therapy, intravenous antibiotics, bronchodilators, and concentrated efforts at nutritional rehabilitation. The length of hospitalization is determined by following the improvement in pulmonary function; discharge is planned once pulmonary function tests have plateaued. Increasingly, outpatient intravenous therapy is being used to shorten the hospital stay.

D. Hepatic Disease: Although most patients with cystic fibrosis demonstrate cirrhosis at autopsy, only a small percentage develop portal hypertension. In these individuals, however, the clinical manifestations of the liver disease may be severe, with esophageal varices leading to life-threatening gastrointestinal bleeding and hypersplenism requiring splenic embolization.

E. Reproductive Tract Involvement: More than 95% of males with cystic fibrosis are infertile, a condition secondary to failure of development of wolffian tract structures such as the vas deferens. Cystic fibrosis is occasionally diagnosed through infertility evaluations in men with relatively mild involvement of the respiratory and gastrointestinal tracts. In general, women with cystic fibrosis are fertile, but pregnancy may place considerable stress on patients with limited pulmonary function.

Prognosis

The rate of progression of lung involvement usually determines survival. Most patients now reach adulthood. Recent reports of successful lung transplantation have been encouraging. In addition, new treatments are being developed based on improved understanding of the disease at the cellular and molecular levels. Along these lines, inhaled recombinant human DNase therapy has been shown to improve pulmonary function in cystic fibrosis. Gene therapy trials are already under way.

Aitken ML et al: Recombinant human DNase inhalation in normal subjects and patients with cystic fibrosis: A phase 1 study. JAMA 1992:267:1947.

Kerem B-S et al: Identification of the cystic fibrosis gene: Genetic analysis. Science 1989;245:1073.

Kerem E et al: The relation between genotype and phenotype in cystic fibrosis: Analysis of the most common mutation (delta F$_{508}$). N Engl J Med 1990;323:1517.

Redding G et al: Serial changes in pulmonary function in children hospitalized with cystic fibrosis. Am Rev Respir Dis 1982;126:31.

Scott J et al: Heart-lung transplantation for cystic fibrosis. Lancet 1988;2:192.

Taussig LM: *Cystic Fibrosis*. Thieme-Stratton, 1984.

CONGENITAL DISEASES INVOLVING ALVEOLI

The clinical spectrum of congenital lung disorders can vary widely, ranging from severe, life-threatening respiratory distress in the neonate (which typically occurs with cystic adenomatoid malformation and most cases of congenital lobar emphysema) to chronic cough, wheezing, or stridor in the older child (with bronchogenic cyst, for example) to incidental radiologic findings in patients with very mild symptoms. The following is a limited discussion of selected congenital structural lesions that involve or compromise alveoli.

PULMONARY AGENESIS & HYPOPLASIA

Pulmonary agenesis or hypoplasia represents absent or incomplete lung development, which generally reflects an intrauterine interruption or alteration of the normal sequence of embryologic events and may be associated with other congenital abnormalities.

With unilateral **pulmonary agenesis** (the complete absence of one lung), the trachea continues into a main bronchus and often has complete tracheal rings. The left lung is affected more often than the right. With compensatory postnatal growth over time, the remaining lung often herniates into the contralateral chest. Chest x-ray study shows a mediastinal shift toward the affected side, and vertebral abnormalities may be present. The outcome is primarily related to the severity of associated congenital lesions. About 50% of patients survive; the mortality rate is higher with agenesis of the right lung than of the left lung. This difference is probably not related to the higher incidence of associated anomalies but rather to a greater shift in the mediastinum that leads to tracheal compression and distortion.

Pulmonary hypoplasia is incomplete development of one or both lungs, resulting in the reduction of the number of bronchial branchings or a decrease in expected lung weight, volume, or DNA content. It is part of a spectrum with a gradual transition. Pulmonary hypoplasia may be present in up to 10–15% of perinatal autopsies. The pathogenesis of hypoplasia is multifactorial and includes the presence of an intrathoracic mass, resulting in lack of space for the lungs to grow, decreased size of the thorax, decreased fetal breathing movements, decreased blood flow to the lungs, or possibly a primary mesodermal defect affecting multiple organ systems. Congenital diaphragmatic hernia is the most common cause of pulmonary hypoplasia, with an incidence of 1:2200 births. Other causes include extralobar sequestration, diaphragmatic eventration or hypoplasia, thoracic neuroblastoma, fetal hydrops, and fetal hydrochylothorax. Chest cage abnormalities, diaphragmatic elevation, oligohydramnios, chromosomal abnormalities, severe musculoskeletal disorders, and cardiac lesions also may lead to hypoplastic lungs. In addition, postnatal factors may play important roles; for example, infants with advanced bronchopulmonary dysplasia can have pulmonary hypoplasia.

Clinical Findings

A. Symptoms and Signs: The clinical presentation is highly variable and is related to the severity of hypoplasia as well as associated abnormalities. Frequently, lung hypoplasia is associated with pneumothorax. Some newborns present with perinatal stress, severe acute respiratory distress, and persistent pulmonary hypertension of the newborn secondary to primary pulmonary hypoplasia (without associated anomalies). Children with milder degrees of hypoplasia may present with chronic cough, tachypnea, wheezing, and recurrent pneumonia.

B. Laboratory Findings and Imaging: Chest x-ray findings include variable degrees of volume loss in a small hemithorax with mediastinal shift. Ventilation/perfusion scans, angiography, and bronchoscopy are often helpful in the clinical evaluation. The degree of respiratory impairment is defined by analysis of arterial blood gases.

Treatment & Prognosis

Treatment is primarily supportive and directed at the symptoms. The overall outcome is determined by the severity of underlying medical problems and the extent of the hypoplasia.

Askenazi SS, Perlman M: Pulmonary hypoplasia: Lung weight and radial alveolar count as criteria of diagnosis. Arch Dis Child 1979;54:614.

Langston C, Thurlbeck WM: Conditions altering normal lung growth and development. In: *Neonatal Pulmonary Care.* Thibeault DW, Gregory GA (editors). Appleton-Century-Crofts, 1986.

Stocker JT et al: Cystic and congenital lung disease in the newborn. In: Perspectives in Pediatric Pathology. Vol 4. Rosenberg H, Bolande T (editors). Year Book, 1978.

PULMONARY SEQUESTRATION

Pulmonary sequestration is a localized mass of disorganized growth that is classified as either extralobar or intralobar. **Extralobar sequestration** is a mass of pulmonary parenchyma anatomically separate from the normal lung, with a distinct pleural investment. Its blood supply derives from either the systemic circulation (more typical), pulmonary vessels, or both. Although it can rarely communicate with the esophagus or stomach, it does not communicate directly with the tracheobronchial tree. Pathologically, extralobar sequestration appears as a solitary thoracic lesion near the diaphragm. Abdominal sites are rare. Size varies between 0.5 cm and 12 cm. Histologic findings include uniformly dilated bronchioles, alveolar ducts, and alveoli. Occasionally, the bronchial structure appears normal; often, however, the cartilage in the wall is deficient, or no cartilage-containing structures can be found. On occasion, lymphangiectasia is found within the lesion. Extralobar sequestration can be associated with other anomalies, including bronchogenic cysts, heart defects, and diaphragmatic hernia.

Intralobar sequestration is an isolated segment of lung within the normal pleural investment but without connection to the tracheobronchial tree. The arterial supply is often provided by one or more arteries arising from the aorta or its branches. Intralobar sequestration is usually found within the lower lobes (98%) and is rarely associated with other congenital anomalies (less than 2% versus 50% with extralobar sequestration). It is rarely seen in the newborn period (unlike extralobar sequestration). Some have hypothesized that intralobar sequestration is an acquired lesion secondary to chronic infection. Clinical presentation includes chronic cough, wheezing or "recurrent pneumonias." Rarely, intralobar sequestration can present with hemoptysis. Diagnosis is often made by angiography, demonstrating large systemic arteries perfusing the lesion. Treatment is by surgical resection.

Alivizatos P et al: Pulmonary sequestration complicated by anomalies of pulmonary venous return. J Pediatr Surg 1985;20:76.

Savic B et al: Lung sequestrations: Report of 7 cases and review of 540 published cases. Thorax 1979;34:96.

CONGENITAL LOBAR EMPHYSEMA

Congenital lobar emphysema (also known as infantile lobar emphysema, congenital localized emphysema, unilobar obstructive emphysema, or congenital hypertrophic lobar emphysema) presents in most patients as severe neonatal respiratory distress or as progressive respiratory impairment during the first year of life. Rarely, the mild or intermittent nature of the symptoms in older children or young adults results in a delayed diagnosis. Most patients are white males. Although the cause of congenital lobar emphysema is not well understood, some lesions exhibit bronchial cartilaginous dysplasia due to abnormal orientation or distribution of the bronchial cartilage. This leads to expiratory collapse, producing obstruction and the symptoms outlined below.

Clinical Findings

A. Symptoms and Signs: Clinical features include tachypnea, cyanosis, wheezing, retractions, and cough. Physical examination reveals decreased breath sounds on the affected side, perhaps with hyperresonance to percussion, mediastinal displacement, and bulging of the chest wall on the affected side.

B. Imaging: Radiologic findings include overdistention of the affected lobe, with wide separation of bronchovascular markings, collapse of adjacent lung, shift of the mediastinum away from the affected side, and a depressed diaphragm on the affected side. Other diagnostic studies include chest x-ray with fluoroscopy, ventilation/perfusion study, and perhaps

CT scan followed by bronchoscopy with or without bronchography, angiography, and exploratory thoracotomy.

Differential Diagnosis

The differential diagnosis of congenital lobar emphysema includes pneumothorax, pneumatocele, atelectasis with compensatory hyperinflation, diaphragmatic hernia, and congenital cystic adenomatoid malformation. The most common site of involvement is the left upper lobe (42%) or right middle lobe (35%). Evaluation must differentiate regional obstructive emphysema from lobar hyperinflation secondary to an uncomplicated ball-valve mechanism due to extrinsic compression from a mass (bronchogenic cyst, tumor, lymphadenopathy, foreign body, "pseudotumor" or plasma cell granuloma, vascular compression, etc) or intrinsic obstruction from a mucus plug due to infection and inflammation from various causes.

Treatment

Management generally involves surgery, especially when respiratory distress is marked, with either segmental or complete lobectomy. Conservative management in less symptomatic older children may lead to an outcome not different from those treated surgically with lobectomy.

Eigen H et al: Congenital lobar emphysema: Long-term evaluation of surgically and conservatively treated children. Am Rev Respir Dis 1976;113:823.

Luck SR et al: Congenital bronchopulmonary malformations. Curr Probl Surg (April) 1986;23:245.

Man DWK et al: Congenital lobar emphysema: Problems in diagnosis and management. Arch Dis Child 1983;58:709.

McBride JT et al: Lung growth and airway function after lobectomy in infancy for congenital lobar emphysema. J Clin Invest 1980;66:962.

Michelson E: Clinical spectrum of infantile lobar emphysema. Ann Thorac Surg 1977;24:182.

CONGENITAL CYSTIC ADENOMATOID MALFORMATION

Congenital cystic adenomatoid malformations are unilateral hamartomatous lesions that generally present as marked respiratory distress within the first days of life. This disorder accounts for 95% of cases of congenital cystic lung disease. Right and left lungs are involved with equal frequency. These lesions appear as gland-like space-occupying masses or have an "adenomatoid" increase in terminal respiratory structures, forming intercommunicating cysts of various sizes, lined by cuboidal or ciliated pseudostratified columnar epithelium. They may have polypoid formations of mucosa, with focally increased elastic tissue in the cyst wall beneath the bronchial type of epithelium. Air passages appear malformed and tend to lack cartilage.

There are three types. Type 1 is most common (75%) and consists of single or multiple large cysts (1–5 cm in diameter) with features of mature lung tissue. Type 1 is amenable to surgical resection. A mediastinal shift is evident on examination or chest x-ray film in 80% of patients and can mimic infantile lobar emphysema. Approximately 75% of type 1 lesions are right-sided. A survival rate of 90% is generally reported.

Type 2 lesions (20% of cases) consist of multiple small cysts (0.5–1.5 cm) resembling dilated simple bronchioles and are often associated with other anomalies (60%), especially renal agenesis or dysgenesis, cardiac malformations, and intestinal atresia. Approximately 60% of type 2 lesions are on the left side. Mediastinal shift is evident less often than in type 1 (10%), and the survival rate is worse (40%).

Type 3 lesions consist of small cysts (< 0.5 cm). They appear as a bulky, firm mass. The reported survival rate is 50%.

Clinical Findings

A. Symptoms and Signs: Clinically, respiratory distress is noted soon after birth. Expansion of the cysts occurs with the onset of breathing and produces compression of normal lung areas with mediastinal herniation. Breath sounds are decreased. With type 3 lesions, dullness to percussion may be present. The disorder can present in older patients as a spontaneous pneumothorax or "pneumonia."

B. Imaging: In type 1, chest x-ray shows an intrapulmonary mass of soft tissue density with scattered radiolucent areas of varying sizes and shapes, usually with a mediastinal shift and pulmonary herniation. Placement of a radiopaque feeding tube into the stomach helps in the differentiation from diaphragmatic hernia. Type 2 lesions appear similar except that the cysts are smaller. Type 3 may appear as a solid homogeneous mass filling the hemithorax and causing a marked mediastinal shift.

Treatment

Treatment of types 1 and 3 is surgical removal of the affected lobe. Because type 2 is often associated with other severe anomalies, management may be more complex. Segmental resection is not feasible because smaller cysts may expand after removal of the more obviously affected area.

Adzick NS, Harrison MR, Glick PC: Fetal cystic adenomatoid malformation: Prenatal diagnosis and natural history. J Pediatr Surg 1985;20:483.

Stocker JT, Madewell JE, Drake RM: Congenital cystic adenomatoid malformation of the lungs: Classification and morphologic spectrum. Hum Pathol 1977;8:155.

ACQUIRED DISORDERS INVOLVING ALVEOLI

BACTERIAL PNEUMONIA

Essentials of Diagnosis

- Fever of acute onset.
- Respiratory signs: cough, dyspnea, tachypnea, grunting, or retractions.
- Abnormal chest examination (rales or decreased breath sounds) or abnormal chest radiograph.

General Considerations

Bacterial pneumonia is inflammation of the lung classified according to the infecting organism. It usually develops when one or more of the defense mechanisms normally protecting the lung is inadequate. Patients with the following problems are particularly predisposed to this disease: aspiration, immunodeficiency or immunosuppression, congenital anomalies (intrapulmonary sequestration, tracheoesophageal fistula, cleft palate), abnormalities in mucus clearance (cystic fibrosis, ciliary dysfunction, tracheomalacia, bronchiectasis), congestive heart failure, and perinatal contamination.

Clinical Findings

A. Symptoms and Signs: The bacterial pathogen, severity of disease, and age of the patient may cause substantial variations in the presenting manifestations of acute bacterial pneumonia. Infants may manifest few or nonspecific findings on history and physical examination. Immunocompetent older patients may not be extremely ill. Some patients may present with fever only or only with signs of generalized toxicity. Others may have additional symptoms or signs of (1) lower respiratory tract disease (respiratory distress, cough, sputum production), (2) pneumonia (rales, decreased breath sounds, dullness to percussion, abnormal tactile or vocal fremitus), or (3) pleural involvement (splinting, pain, friction rub, dullness to percussion). Some patients may manifest additional extrapulmonary findings, such as meningismus or abdominal pain, due to pneumonia itself. Others may have evidence of infection at other sites due to the same organism causing their pneumonia: meningitis, otitis media, sinusitis, pericarditis, epiglottitis, or abscesses.

B. Laboratory Findings: Elevated white blood cell counts (> 15,000/μL) frequently accompany bacterial pneumonia. However, a low white blood count (> 5000/μL) can be an ominous finding in this disease.

C. Imaging: Chest radiographic findings (lateral and frontal views) define bacterial pneumonia.

Patchy infiltrates, atelectasis, hilar adenopathy, or pleural effusion may be observed. Films should be taken in the lateral decubitus position to identify pleural fluid. Complete lobar consolidation is not a common finding in infants and children. Severity of disease may not correlate with radiographic findings. Clinical resolution precedes resolution by chest x-ray.

D. Special Examinations: Invasive diagnostic procedures (transtracheal aspiration, bronchial brushing or washing, lung puncture, or open biopsy) should be undertaken in critically ill patients when other means do not adequately define etiology (see Culture of Material From the Respiratory Tract, p 496).

Differential Diagnosis

The differential diagnosis of bacterial pneumonia also varies with the age and immunocompetence of the host. The full spectrum of potential pathogens must be considered in each host and includes aerobic and anaerobic bacteria; acid-fast bacteria, including *Mycobacterium tuberculosis; Chlamydia trachomatis* and *Chlamydia psittaci; Rickettsia quintana* (Q fever); *Pneumocystis carinii; Bordetella pertussis; Mycoplasma pneumoniae; Legionella pneumophila* and respiratory viruses.

Noninfectious pulmonary disease (including gastric aspiration, foreign body aspiration, atelectasis, congenital malformations, congestive heart failure, malignant growths, tumors such as plasma cell granuloma, chronic interstitial lung diseases, and pulmonary hemosiderosis) should be considered in the differential diagnosis of localized or diffuse infiltrates. When effusions are present, additional noninfectious disorders such as collagen diseases, neoplasm, and pulmonary infarction should also be considered.

Complications

Empyema may occur frequently with staphylococcal and group A β-hemolytic streptococcal disease. Pneumococcal effusions have a more benign course. Distal sites of infection—meningitis, otitis media, sinusitis (especially of the ethmoids) and septicemia—may be present, particularly with disease due to *Streptococcus pneumoniae* or *Haemophilus influenzae*. Certain immunocompromised patients, such as those who have undergone splenectomy or who have hemoglobin SS or SC disease or thalassemia, are especially prone to overwhelming sepsis with these organisms. Distal infection of the bones, joints, or other organs (eg, liver abscess) may occur in certain hosts with specific organisms.

Treatment

Appropriate antimicrobial therapy varies according to which organisms are the likely cause of the bacterial pneumonia. Treatment should be guided by (1) Gram stain of sputum, tracheobronchial secretions, or pleural fluid if available; (2) radiographic findings; and (3) age and known or suspected immunocompetence of the host. For initial coverage in a patient with an unknown pathogen, the physician should consider (1) appropriate penicillins or cephalosporins (or both) to cover gram-positive organisms, including *Staphylococcus aureus;* (2) an aminoglycoside to cover gram-negative enteric organisms (especially in the newborn or immunocompromised host); (3) suitable coverage for *Haemophilus influenzae* in patients at risk; and (4) erythromycin to cover *Mycoplasma pneumoniae, Legionella pneumophila, Chlamydia* species, and *Ureaplasma.* Therapy is also guided by results of studies for bacterial and viral pathogens (see Culture of Material From the Respiratory Tract, p 496) and is based on other diagnostic studies (see below).

Additional therapeutic considerations include (1) oxygen, (2) humidification of inspired gases, (3) hydration and electrolyte supplementation, (4) oral hygiene, and (5) nutrition. Removal of pleural fluid for diagnostic purposes is indicated initially to guide antimicrobial therapy. Many feel that early chest tube drainage of empyema fluid due to *S aureus* is indicated. Empyema due to group A β-hemolytic streptococci or *H influenzae* may also necessitate chest tube drainage, whereas pleural effusions due to *S pneumoniae* rarely do. Repeated pleural taps should be considered in the patient who has persistent high fever for more than 10 days in association with significant pleural effusions. The persistence of organisms in this fluid or the persistence of toxicity, malaise, anorexia, and wasting in the patient suggests the potential need for pleural decortication.

Endotracheal intubation or mechanical ventilation may be indicated in patients with respiratory failure or those too debilitated or overwhelmed to handle their secretions.

Prognosis

For the immunocompetent host in whom bacterial pneumonia is adequately recognized and treated, the survival rate is high. For example, the mortality rate from uncomplicated pneumococcal pneumonia is less than 1%. If the patient survives the initial illness, persistently abnormal pulmonary function following empyema is surprisingly uncommon, even when treatment has been delayed or inappropriate.

Bromberg K, Hammerschlag MR: Rapid diagnosis of pneumonia in children. Semin Respir Infect 1987;2:159.

Peter G: The child with pneumonia: Diagnostic and therapeutic considerations. Pediatr Infect Dis J 1988;7:453.

Scheld WM, Mandell GL: Nosocomial pneumonia: Pathogenesis and recent advances in diagnosis and therapy. Rev Infect Dis 1991;13(Suppl 9):S743.

Schutze GE, Jacobs RF: Management of community-acquired bacterial pneumonia in hospitalized children. Pediatr Infect Dis J 1992;11:160.

Timmons OD et al: Association of respiratory syncytial virus and Streptococcus pneumoniae infection in young infants. Pediatr Infect Dis J 1987;6:1134.

VIRAL PNEUMONIA

Essentials of Diagnosis
- Upper respiratory infection prodrome (fever, coryza, cough, hoarseness).
- Wheezing or rales.
- Myalgia, malaise, headache (older children).

General Considerations
Viral pneumonia constitutes the vast majority of pediatric pulmonary infections. Respiratory syncytial virus (RSV), parainfluenza (1, 2, and 3) viruses, and influenza (A and B) viruses are responsible for more than 75% of infections. Neither severity of the disease or height of fever, radiographic findings, nor characteristics of cough or lung sounds reliably differentiate viral from bacterial pneumonias. Substantial pleural effusions, pneumatoceles, abscesses, lobar consolidation with lobar volume expansion, and "round" pneumonias are generally inconsistent with viral disease.

Clinical Findings
A. Symptoms and Signs: An upper respiratory infection frequently precedes the onset of lower respiratory disease due to viruses. Although wheezing or stridor may be prominent in viral disease, cough, signs of respiratory difficulty (retractions, grunting, nasal flaring) and physical findings (rales, decreased breath sounds) may not be distinguishable from those in bacterial pneumonia.

B. Laboratory Findings: The peripheral white blood cell count may be normal or slightly elevated and is not useful in distinguishing viral from bacterial disease. A markedly elevated white count, however, indicates that viral disease is less likely.

Rapid viral diagnostic tests, such as fluorescent antibody tests or ELISA for RSV, are increasingly available and should be performed to confirm this diagnosis in high-risk patients and for purposes of epidemiology or infection control. Rapid diagnosis of RSV infection does not preclude the possibility of concomitant infection with other pathogens.

C. Imaging: Chest radiographs frequently show perihilar streaking, increased interstitial markings, peribronchial cuffing, or patchy bronchopneumonia. However, lobar consolidation, as in bacterial pneumonia, may occur. Patients with adenovirus disease may have severe necrotizing pneumonias, resulting in the development of pneumatoceles. Hyperinflation of the lungs may occur when involvement of the small airways is prominent.

Differential Diagnosis
Considerations for the differential diagnosis of viral pneumonia are the same as those for bacterial pneumonia. In patients in whom wheezing is a prominent feature, the physician should consider asthma, airway obstruction due to foreign body aspiration,

acute bacterial or viral tracheitis, and parasitic disease.

Complications

Bronchiolitis obliterans or severe chronic respiratory failure may follow adenovirus pneumonia. Bronchiolitis or viral pneumonia may contribute to persistent reactive airway disease in some patients. Bronchiectasis, persistent interstitial lung diseases (fibrosis and desquamative interstitial pneumonitis), and unilateral hyperlucent lung (Swyer-James syndrome) may follow measles, adenovirus, and influenzal pneumonias. Viral pneumonia or laryngotracheobronchitis may predispose the patient to subsequent bacterial tracheitis or pneumonia as immediate sequelae. Plasma cell granuloma may develop as a rare sequela of viral or bacterial pneumonia.

Treatment

General supportive care for viral pneumonia does not differ from that for bacterial pneumonia. Patients can be quite ill and should be hospitalized according to the level of their illness. Because bacterial disease often cannot be definitively excluded, appropriate concomitant antibiotic coverage may be indicated.

Patients at risk for life-threatening RSV infections, such as those with bronchopulmonary dysplasia or other severe pulmonary conditions, congenital heart disease, or significant immunocompromise, should be hospitalized and treated with ribavirin. Rapid viral diagnostic tests may be a useful guide for such therapy. These high-risk patients should be immunized annually against influenza A and B viruses. Despite immunization, however, influenza can still occur. When available epidemiologic data indicate an active influenza A infection in the community, amantadine hydrochloride should be considered early for high-risk infants and children who appear to be infected.

Children with suspected viral pneumonia should be placed in respiratory isolation, and careful attention should be given to good handwashing practices.

Prognosis

Although most children with viral pneumonia recover uneventfully, worsening reactive airway disease, abnormal pulmonary function or chest radiographs, persistent respiratory insufficiency, and even death may occur in high-risk patients such as newborns or those with underlying lung, cardiac, or immunodeficiency disease. Patients with adenovirus infection or those concomitantly infected with RSV and second pathogens such as influenza, adenovirus, cytomegalovirus or *Pneumocystis carinii* also have a poorer prognosis.

Hall CB: Hospital-acquired pneumonia in children: The role of respiratory viruses. Semin Respir Infect 1987;2:48.

Heidemann SM: Clinical characteristics of parainfluenza virus infection in hospitalized children. Pediatr Pulmonol 1992;13:86.

Khamapirad T, Glezen WP: Clinical and radiographic assessment of acute lower respiratory tract disease in infants and children. Semin Respir Infect 1987;2:130.

Stretton M et al: Intensive care course and outcome of patients infected with respiratory syncytial virus. Pediatr Pulmonol 1992;13:143.

Tristram DA et al: Simultaneous infection with respiratory syncytial virus and other respiratory pathogens. Am J Dis Child 1988;142:834.

CHLAMYDIAL PNEUMONIA

Essentials of Diagnosis

- Cough, tachypnea, rales, few wheezes, and no fever (most patients).
- Appropriate age: 2–12 weeks.
- With or without inclusion conjunctivitis.
- With or without peripheral eosinophilia.
- Elevated immunoglobulins: IgM > IgG > > IgA.

General Considerations

Pulmonary disease due to *Chlamydia trachomatis* usually evolves gradually as the infection descends the respiratory tract. Infants may appear quite well despite the presence of significant pulmonary illness. Infant infections are now at epidemic proportions in urban environments worldwide. Other sexually transmitted organisms such as *Ureaplasma urealyticum* may also be widespread and contribute to lung disease in infants. Unlike bacteria, the chlamydiae are unable to synthesize their own ATP and are sometimes called "energy parasites."

Clinical Findings

A. Symptoms and Signs: About half of patients with chlamydial pneumonia have active inclusion conjunctivitis or a history of it. Rhinopharyngitis with nasal discharge or otitis media may have occurred or be currently present. Female patients may have vulvovaginitis.

Cough is usually present. It can have a staccato character and resemble that accompanying pertussis. The infant is usually tachypneic. Scattered inspiratory rales are commonly heard, but wheezes are rarely present. Significant fever suggests another or additional diagnosis.

B. Laboratory Findings: Although patients may frequently be hypoxemic, CO_2 retention is not common. Absolute peripheral blood eosinophilia (> 400 cells/μL) has been observed in about 75% of patients. Serum immunoglobulins are usually abnormal. IgM is virtually always elevated, IgG is high in many, and IgA is less frequently abnormal. *C trachomatis* can usually be identified in nasopharyngeal washings employing a fluorescent antibody or culture techniques.

C. Imaging: Chest radiographs may reveal diffuse interstitial and patchy alveolar infiltrates, peribronchial thickening, or focal consolidation. A small pleural reaction can be present. Despite the usual absence of wheezes, hyperexpansion is commonly present.

Differential Diagnosis

Bacterial, viral, and parasitic *(P carinii)* pneumonias should be considered. Premature infants and those with bronchopulmonary dysplasia may also have chlamydial or associated pneumonias.

Treatment

Erythromycin or sulfisoxazole therapy should be administered for 14 days. Hospitalization may be required for infants with significant respiratory distress, coughing paroxysms, or posttussive apnea. Oxygen therapy may be required for prolonged periods in some patients.

Prognosis

An increased incidence of obstructive airway disease and abnormal pulmonary function tests may occur for at least 7–8 years following the initial infection.

Brayden RM et al: Apnea in infants with *Chlamydia trachomatis* pneumonia. Pediatr Infect Dis J 1987;6:423.
Grayston JT et al: A new respiratory pathogen: *Chlamydia pneumoniae,* strain TWAR. J Infect Dis 1990; 161:618.
Hammerschlag MR et al: Comparison of enzyme immunoassay and culture for diagnosis of chlamydial conjunctivitis and respiratory infections in infants. J Clin Microbiol 1987;25:2306.
Hammerschlag MR et al: Persistent infection with *Chlamydia pneumoniae* following acute respiratory infection. Clin Infect Dis 1992;14:178.
Katzman DK et al: The incidence of *Chlamydia pneumoniae* lower respiratory tract infections among university students in northern California. West J Med 1991: 155:136.
Paisley JW et al: Rapid diagnosis of *Chlamydia trachomatis* pneumonia in infants by direct immunofluorescence microscopy of nasopharyngeal secretions. J Pediatr 1986; 109:653.

MYCOPLASMAL PNEUMONIA

Essentials of Diagnosis

- Fever (usually > 39 °C).
- Cough.
- Appropriate age: over 5 years old.

General Considerations

Mycoplasma pneumoniae is a common cause of symptomatic pneumonia in older children. Endemic and epidemic infection can occur. The incubation period is long (2–3 weeks), and the onset of symptoms is slow. Although the lung is the primary infection site, a variety of extrapulmonary complications can arise.

Clinical Findings

A. Symptoms and Signs: Fever, cough, headache, and malaise are common symptoms as the illness evolves. Although cough is usually dry at the onset, sputum production may develop as the illness progresses. Sore throat, otitis media, otitis externa, and bullous myringitis may occur. Rales are frequently present on chest examination; decreased breath sounds or dullness to percussion over the involved area may be present. ·

B. Laboratory Findings: The peripheral blood leukocyte count and differential white blood cell count are usually normal. The cold hemagglutinin titer should be determined, because it may be elevated during the acute presentation. A titer of 1:64 or higher supports the diagnosis. Acute and convalescent titers for *M pneumoniae* demonstrating a fourfold or greater rise in specific antibodies confirm the diagnosis.

C. Imaging: Chest radiographs usually demonstrate interstitial or bronchopneumonic infiltrates, frequently in the middle or lower lobes. Pleural effusions are extremely uncommon.

Complications

Extrapulmonary involvement of the blood, central nervous system, skin, heart, or joints can occur. Direct Coombs-positive autoimmune hemolytic anemia, occasionally a life-threatening disorder, is the most common hematologic abnormality that can accompany *M pneumoniae* infection. Coagulation defects and thrombocytopenia can also occur. Cerebral infarction, meningoencephalitis, Guillain-Barré syndrome, cranial nerve involvement, and psychosis all have been described. A wide variety of skin rashes, including erythema multiforme and Stevens-Johnson syndrome, can occur. Myocarditis, pericarditis, and a rheumatic fever-like illness can also occur.

Treatment

Antibiotic therapy with erythromycin for 7–10 days usually shortens the course of illness. Supportive measures, including hydration, antipyretics, and bed rest, are helpful.

Prognosis

In the absence of the less common extrapulmonary complications, the outlook for recovery is excellent. However, the extent to which *M pneumoniae* can initiate or exacerbate chronic lung disease is not well understood.

Broughton RA: Infections due to *Mycoplasma pneumoniae* in childhood. Pediatr Infect Dis J 1986;5:71.
Leigh MW, Clyde WA Jr: Chlamydial and mycoplasmal pneumonias. Semin Respir Infect 1987;2:152.

McCracken GH Jr: Current status of antibiotic treatment for *Mycoplasma pneumoniae* infections. Pediatr Infect Dis J 1986;5:167.

Orlicek SL, Walker MS, Kuhls TL: Severe mycoplasma pneumonia in young children with Down syndrome. Clin Pediatr 1992;31:409.

TUBERCULOSIS

Essentials of Diagnosis

- Positive tuberculin skin test or anergic host.
- Positive culture for *Mycobacterium tuberculosis.*
- With or without history of contact.

General Considerations

Very recently, there has been a resurgence of tuberculosis in all age groups, including children. The clinical spectrum of pulmonary infection with tuberculosis includes a positive tuberculin skin test without evident disease, asymptomatic primary infection, the Ghon complex, bronchial obstruction with secondary collapse or obstructed airways, segmental lesions, calcified nodules, pleural effusions, progressive primary cavitating lesions, contiguous spread into adjacent thoracic structures, acute miliary tuberculosis, adult respiratory distress syndrome (ARDS), overwhelming reactivation infection in the immunocompromised host, occult lymphohematogenous spread, and metastatic extrapulmonary involvement at almost any site. Symptoms of airway obstruction, sometimes with secondary bacterial pneumonia resulting from hilar adenopathy, are common presenting features in children.

Clinical Findings

A. Symptoms and Signs: The most important aspect of the history is that of contact with an individual with tuberculosis. Frequently, this contact may be made through an elderly relative, a caretaker, or a person previously residing in a region with endemic tuberculosis or by travel of the patients themselves to such an area. Homeless and medically indigent children are at high risk, as are those in contact with high-risk adults (AIDS patients, residents of correctional institutions or nursing homes, intravenous or other drug users, and health care workers). Once exposed, pediatric patients at risk for developing active disease include infants and those with malnutrition, AIDS, diabetes mellitus, or immunosuppression (antitumor chemotherapy, corticosteroids). In suspected cases, the patient, immediate family, and suspected carriers of the disease should be tuberculin-tested. The route of contagion is through inhalation. Thus, isolated pulmonary parenchymal tuberculosis constitutes more than 95% of presenting cases. The primary focus, which is usually single, and the nodal involvement may or may not be radiographically visible. Because healing—rather than progression—is the usual course

in the uncompromised host, a positive tuberculin test may be the only manifestation of disease.

The tuberculous complications listed above most often occur during the first year of infection. Thereafter, infection remains quiescent until adolescence, when reactivation of pulmonary tuberculosis is common. At any stage, chronic cough, anorexia, weight loss or failure to gain weight, or fever are useful clinical signs if present. Except in cases with complications or advanced disease, physical findings are few. Most children with pulmonary tuberculosis are asymptomatic.

B. Laboratory Findings: A positive tuberculin skin test is defined as 10 mm or more of induration 48–72 hours after intradermal injection of 5 tuberculin units of PPD. Tine tests should not be used. Appropriate control skin tests, such as those for hypersensitivity to diphtheria/tetanus, mumps, *Candida albicans,* or dermatophyton/trichophyton, should be applied at the same time the PPD is applied. If the patient fails to respond to PPD and all of the controls, the possibility of tuberculosis is not excluded.

Chest radiographs, both anteroposterior and lateral views, should be obtained in all suspected cases. Culture for *M tuberculosis* is critical for proving the diagnosis and for defining drug susceptibility. Early morning gastric lavage following an overnight fast should be performed on three occasions in infants and children with suspected active pulmonary tuberculosis prior to the onset of drug therapy when the severity of illness allows. Although stains for acid-fast bacilli on this material are of little value, this is the ideal culture site. Despite the increasing importance of isolating organisms because of multiple drug resistance, only 40% of children will yield positive cultures.

Sputum cultures from older children and adolescents are similarly useful. Stains and cultures of bronchial secretions are useful if bronchoscopy is performed in the patient's evaluation. When pleural effusions are present, pleural biopsy for cultures and histopathologic examination for granulomas or organisms most consistently provide diagnostic information. Meningeal involvement is a real possibility in young children, and lumbar puncture should be considered in their initial evaluation.

Differential Diagnosis

Fungal diseases that primarily affect the lungs such as histoplasmosis, coccidioidomycosis, cryptococcosis, and North American blastomycosis may resemble tuberculosis and should be excluded by appropriate serologic studies if the diagnosis is uncertain. Atypical tuberculous organisms may involve the lungs, especially in the immunocompromised patient. Depending on the presentation, diagnoses such as lymphoreticular and other malignancies, collagen-vascular disorders, or other pulmonary infections may be considered.

Complications

In addition to those listed above, lymphadenitis, meningitis, osteomyelitis, arthritis, enteritis, peritonitis, and renal, ocular, middle ear, and cutaneous disease may occur. The infant born to tuberculous parents is at great risk for developing illness. The possibility of life-threatening airway compromise must always be considered in patients with large mediastinal or hilar lesions.

Treatment

Because the risk of hepatitis due to isoniazid is extremely low in children, this drug is indicated in children with a positive tuberculin skin test. This greatly reduces the risk of subsequent active disease and complications with minimal morbidity. Isoniazid plus rifampin treatment for 6 months, plus pyrazinamide during the first 2 months, is indicated when the chest radiograph is abnormal or when there is extrapulmonary disease. Without pyrazinamide, isoniazid plus rifampin must be given for 9 months. In general, the more severe tuberculous complications are treated with a larger number of drugs. Enforced, directly observed therapy (twice weekly or greater) is indicated when noncompliance is suspected. Recommendations for antituberculosis chemotherapy, based on disease stage, are continuously being updated. The most current edition of *The Red Book of the American Academy of Pediatrics* is a reliable source for these protocols.

Corticosteroids are used to control inflammation in selected patients with (1) potentially life-threatening airway compression by lymph nodes, (2) acute pericardial effusion, (3) massive pleural effusion with mediastinal shift, and, possibly, (4) miliary tuberculosis with respiratory failure.

Prognosis

In patients with an intact immune system, modern antituberculous therapy offers good potential for recovery. The outlook for patients with immunodeficiencies, organisms resistant to multiple drugs, poor drug compliance, or advanced complications is guarded. Organisms resistant to multiple drugs are increasingly common. Resistance emerges either because the physician prescribes an inadequate regimen or because the patient discontinues medications. When resistance to or intolerance of isoniazid and rifampin prevents their use, cure rates are 50% or less.

Anuntaseree W, Suntornlohanakul S, Mitarnun W: Disseminated tuberculosis in a 2-month-old infant. Pediatr Pulmonol 1992;13:255.

Snider D: Pregnancy and tuberculosis. Chest 1984;86(Suppl 3):10S.

Starke JR: Current chemotherapy for tuberculosis in children. Infect Dis Clin North Am 1992;6:215.

Starke JR: Modern approach to the diagnosis and management of tuberculosis in children. Pediatr Clin North Am 1988;35:464.

Starke JR, Jacobs RF, Jereb J: Resurgence of tuberculosis in children. J Pediatr 1992;120:839.

Steinhoff MC, Lionel J: Treatment of tuberculosis in newborn infants and their mothers. Indian J Pediatr 1988; 55:240.

ASPIRATION PNEUMONIA

Essentials of Diagnosis

- Patient at risk.
- Fever.
- Cough.

General Considerations

The risk of aspiration pneumonia occurs in patients when anatomic defense mechanisms are impaired. These include patients with (1) seizures; (2) depressed sensorium; (3) recurrent gastroesophageal reflux, emesis, or gastrointestinal obstruction; (4) neuromuscular disorders with suck/swallow dysfunction; (5) anatomic abnormalities (laryngeal cleft, tracheoesophageal fistula, vocal cord paralysis); (6) debilitating illnesses, (7) occult brain stem lesions; (8) near-drowning; (9) nasogastric, endotracheal, or tracheostomy tubes; and (10) severe periodontal disease. Acute disease is commonly caused by bacteria present in the mouth (especially gram-negative anaerobes), and multiple organisms may concomitantly cause infection in many patients. Chronic aspiration often causes recurrent bouts of acute febrile pneumonia. It may also lead to chronic focal infiltrates, atelectasis, or illness resembling asthma or interstitial lung disease.

Clinical Findings

A. Symptoms and Signs: Acute onset of fever, cough, respiratory distress, or hypoxemia in a patient at risk suggests aspiration pneumonia. Chest physical findings, such as rales, rhonchi, or decreased breath sounds, may initially be limited to the lung region into which aspiration occurred. Although any region may be affected, the right side, especially the right upper lobe in the supine patient, is commonly affected. In patients with chronic aspiration, diffuse wheezing may occur. Generalized rales may also be present. Such patients may not develop acute febrile pneumonias.

B. Laboratory Findings and Imaging: Chest radiographs may reveal lobar consolidation or atelectasis and focal or generalized alveolar or interstitial infiltrates. In some patients with chronic aspiration, perihilar infiltrates with or without bilateral air trapping may be seen.

In severely ill patients with acute febrile illnesses, a bacteriologic diagnosis should be made. In addition to blood cultures, cultures of tracheobronchial secretions and bronchoalveolar lavage or lung puncture specimens may be desirable (see Culture of Material From the Respiratory Tract, p 496).

In patients with chronic aspiration pneumonitis, solid documentation of aspiration as the cause of illness may be elusive. Barium contrast studies may provide evidence of suck-swallow dysfunction, laryngeal cleft, occult tracheoesophageal fistula, or gastroesophageal reflux. Overnight or 24-hour esophageal pH probe studies may also help establish the latter. Although radionuclide scans are commonly employed, the yield from such studies is disappointingly low. Rigid bronchoscopy in infants or flexible bronchoscopy in older children can be useful in (1) more definitively excluding tracheoesophageal fistula and (2) obtaining bronchoalveolar lavage specimens to search for lipid-laden macrophages as evidence of chronic aspiration.

Differential Diagnosis

In the acutely ill patient, routine bacterial, viral, or mycoplasmal pneumonias should be considered. In the chronically ill patient, the differential diagnoses may include disorders causing (1) recurrent pneumonia (immunodeficiencies, ciliary dysfunction, foreign body, etc); (2) chronic wheezing; or (3) interstitial lung disorders (see below), depending on the presentation.

Complications

Empyema or lung abscess may result from acute aspiration pneumonia. Chronic disease may result in bronchiectasis.

Treatment

Antimicrobial therapy for acute aspiration pneumonia includes appropriate coverage for gram-negative anaerobic organisms. This might include, for example, intravenous penicillin G, 12 million units/m²/d, *plus* metronidazole, imipenem, or a combination of a β-lactam drug and β-lactamase inhibitor. In hospital-acquired infections, additional coverage for methicillin-resistant *Staphylococcus aureus* and multiply resistant *Pseudomonas aeruginosa,* streptococci, and other organisms should be provided.

Treatment of recurrent and chronic aspiration pneumonia may include the following: (1) surgical correction of anatomic abnormalities; (2) improved oral hygiene; (3) improved hydration; and (4) inhaled bronchodilators, chest physical therapy, and suctioning. In patients with compromise of the central nervous system, exclusive feeding by gastrostomy and (in some) tracheostomy may be required to control airway secretions. Gastroesophageal reflux, often requiring surgical correction, is commonly present in such patients.

Prognosis

The outlook for patients with aspiration pneumonia is directly related to the disorder causing their aspiration.

Colombo JL, Hallberg TK, Sammut PH: Time course of lipid-laden macrophages with acute and recurrent milk aspiration in rabbits. Pediatr Pulmonol 1992;12:95.

Colombo JL, Hallberg TK: Recurrent aspiration in children: Lipid-laden alveolar macrophage quantitation. Pediatr Pulmonol 1987;3:86.

Finegold SM: Aspiration pneumonia. Rev Infect Dis 1991; 13(Suppl 9):S737.

Moran JR et al: Lipid-laden alveolar macrophage and lactose assay as markers of aspiration in neonates with lung disease. J Pediatr 1988;112:643.

PNEUMONIA IN THE IMMUNOCOMPROMISED HOST

Essentials of Diagnosis

- Immunodeficiency disease, HIV infection, leukemia, lymphoma, cancer chemotherapy, chronic corticosteroid or ACTH therapy, postsplenectomy, sickle hemoglobinopathies, or splenic dysfunction states.
- Fever.
- Cough.

General Considerations

The immunocompromised host with pneumonia may be infected with any common organism (streptococcus, staphylococcus, *M pneumoniae*) or with a less common organism of several classes. These include (1) parasites *(Pneumocystis carinii, Toxoplasma gondii),* (2) fungi *(Aspergillus* species, mucormycosis, *Candida* species, *Cryptococcus neoformans, Cryptosporidium),* (3) viruses (cytomegalovirus; varicella-zoster, herpes simplex, influenza, or respiratory syncytial virus; adenovirus), and (4) bacteria (gram-negative enteric and anaerobic bacteria, *Nocardia* and *Actinomyces* species, and *Legionella pneumophila.*) Multiple organisms and types of organisms are commonly present.

Clinical Findings

A. Symptoms and Signs: Patients often present with subtle signs such as mild cough, tachypnea, or low-grade fever. Unfortunately, these are commonly overlooked until a predictable, rapid progression manifested by worsening cough, fever, respiratory distress, and hypoxemia occurs. An obvious portal of infection, such as an intravascular catheter, may predispose a patient to bacterial or fungal infection and should be suspected as the cause.

B. Laboratory Findings and Imaging: Fungal, parasitic, or bacterial infection, especially with antibiotic-resistant bacteria, should be suspected in the neutropenic child. Cultures of peripheral blood, sputum, tracheobronchial secretions, urine, nasopharynx or sinuses, bone marrow, pleural fluid, biopsied lymph nodes, or skin lesions or cultures through intravascular catheters should be obtained as soon as infection is suspected.

Invasive methods are commonly required to make an adequately early diagnosis. The results of these procedures do appear, in the majority of cases, to lead to important changes in empiric preoperative therapy. Sputum is frequently unavailable. Transtracheal aspiration has a high complication rate in children. Percutaneous lung puncture has a very high false-negative rate in *P carinii* pneumonia, and this is a very common organism. Bronchoalveolar lavage frequently provides the diagnosis of one or more organisms and should be done early in evaluation. The combined use of a wash, brushing, and lavage has given a particularly high yield in such patients. In patients with very rapidly advancing or advanced disease, open lung biopsy becomes more urgent. Although the morbidity and mortality rates of this procedure in this setting are high, a thoracoscopic approach may improve this outcome. Because of the multiplicity of organisms that may cause disease, a comprehensive set of studies should be done on lavage or biopsy material. These consist of (1) rapid diagnostic studies, including fluorescent antibody studies for *Legionella;* ELISA for respiratory syncytial virus, etc; (2) Gram, acid-fast, fungal, and methenamine silver stains; (3) cytologic examination for viral inclusions; and (4) cultures for viruses, anaerobic and aerobic bacteria, fungi, mycobacteria, and *Legionella.* If available, newly developed rapid immunofluorescent studies for *P carinii* should be obtained.

Chest radiographs may be useful. However, dyspnea and hypoxemia may be marked despite minimal radiographic abnormalities in *P carinii* pneumonia.

Differential Diagnosis

The organisms causing disease vary with the type of immunocompromise present. For example, the splenectomized patient may be overwhelmed by infection with *S pneumoniae* or *H influenzae.* The infant receiving ACTH therapy may be more likely to have *P carinii* infection. The febrile, neutropenic child who has been receiving adequate doses of intravenous broad-spectrum antibiotics may have fungal disease or *Pneumocystis* pneumonia. However, the key to diagnosis is to remain open to all infectious possibilities and to neglect no diagnostic study.

Depending on the form of immunocompromise, perhaps only half to two-thirds of new pulmonary infiltrates in such patients represent infection. Such infiltrates may also represent the following: (1) pulmonary toxicity of radiation, oxygen, chemotherapy, or other drugs; (2) pulmonary disorders, including hemorrhage, embolism, atelectasis, aspiration, or adult respiratory distress syndrome; (3) recurrence or extension of primary malignant growths or immunologic disorders; (4) transfusion reactions, leukostasis, or tumor cell lysis; or (5) interstitial lung disease, such as lymphocytic interstitial pneumonitis with HIV infection or Epstein-Barr virus infection.

Complications

Respiratory failure, shock, multiple organ damage, disseminated infection, and death commonly occur in the infected, immunocompromised host.

Treatment

Broad-spectrum intravenous antibiotics are indicated early in febrile, neutropenic, or immunocompromised children. Trimethoprim-sulfamethoxazole and erythromycin are also indicated early in the treatment of immunocompromised children. Further therapy should be based on studies of specimens obtained from bronchoalveolar lavage or lung biopsy.

Prognosis

Prognosis is guarded and based upon the severity of the underlying immunocompromise, appropriate early diagnosis and treatment, and the infecting organisms.

Barbour SD: AIDS of childhood. Pediatr Clin North Am 1987;34:247.

Frankel LR et al: Bronchoalveolar lavage for diagnosis of pneumonia in the immunocompromised child. Pediatrics 1988;81:785.

Glaser JH et al: Cytomegalovirus and *Pneumocystis carinii* pneumonia in children with acquired immunodeficiency syndrome. J Pediatr 1992; 120:929.

Hughes WT et al: Successful intermittent chemoprophylaxis for *Pneumocystis carinii* pneumonitis. N Engl J Med 1987;316:1627.

Hughes WT: Pneumonia in the immunocompromised child. Semin Respir Infect 1987;2:177.

Martin WJ et al: Role of bronchoalveolar lavage in the assessment of opportunistic pulmonary infections: Utility and complications. Mayo Clin Proc 1987;62:549.

Shaw NJ, Elton R, Eden OB: Pneumonia and pneumonitis in childhood malignancy. Acta Paediatr 1992;81 :222.

Valteau D et al: Nonbacterial nonfungal interstitial pneumonitis following autologous bone marrow transplantation in children treated with high-dose chemotherapy without total-body irradiation. Transplantation 1988;45: 737.

Winters JL et al: *Bordetella bronchiseptica* pneumonia in a patient with Down syndrome: A case report and review. Pediatrics 1992;89:1262.

HYPERSENSITIVITY PNEUMONIA

Essentials of Diagnosis

- History of exposure (birds, organic dusts or molds, etc).
- Interstitial infiltrates on chest radiograph or diffuse rales.
- With or without recurrent cough, fever, wheezing, or weight loss.

General Considerations

Hypersensitivity pneumonitis is a disease involving peripheral airways, interstitium, and alveoli. Both acute and chronic forms may occur. In children, the most common forms are brought on by exposure to birds or bird droppings (pigeons, parakeets, parrots, doves, etc). However, inhalation of almost any organic dust (moldy hay, compost, logs or tree bark, sawdust, or aerosols from humidifiers) can cause disease. Although uncommon in children, many of the latter present as occupational lung diseases in adults.

Clinical Findings

A. Symptoms and Signs: Episodic cough and fever can occur with acute exposures. Chronic exposure results in weight loss, fatigue, dyspnea, cyanosis, and, ultimately, respiratory failure.

B. Laboratory Findings: Acute exposures may be followed by polymorphonuclear leukocytosis with eosinophilia and evidence of airway obstruction on pulmonary function testing. Chronic disease results in a restrictive picture on lung function tests. Arterial blood gases may reveal hypoxemia with a decreased $PaCO_2$ and normal pH (respiratory alkalosis, compensated).

The serologic key to diagnosis is the finding of precipitins (precipitating IgG antibodies) to the organic dusts that contain avian proteins or fungal or bacterial antigens. However, exposure without related disease may cause the presence of precipitins.

Differential Diagnosis

Patients with primarily acute symptoms must be differentiated from patients with atopic asthma. Those with chronic symptoms must be distinguished from those with collagen-vascular, immunologic, or primary interstitial pulmonary disorders.

Complications

Prolonged exposure to offending antigens may result in pulmonary hypertension due to chronic hypoxemia, cor pulmonale, irreversible restrictive lung disease due to pulmonary fibrosis, or respiratory failure.

Treatment

Complete elimination of exposure to the offending antigens is required. Corticosteroids may hasten recovery.

Prognosis

With appropriate diagnosis and avoidance of offending antigens, the prognosis is excellent. However, a good prognosis is dependent on early diagnosis before irreversible pulmonary damage has occurred.

Carlsen K-H et al: Allergic alveolitis in a 12-year-old boy: Treatment with budesonide nebulizing solution. Pediatr Pulmonol 1992;12:257.

Eisenberg JD, Montanero A, Lee RG: Hypersensitivity pneumonitis in an infant. Pediatr Pulmonol 1992;12:186.

Fink JN: Hypersensitivity pneumonitis. J Allergy Clin Immunol 1984;74:1.

Levy MG, Fink JN: Hypersensitivity pneumonitis. Ann Allergy 1985;54:167.

O'Connell EJ et al: Childhood hypersensitivity pneumonitis (farmer's lung): Four cases in siblings with long-term follow-up. J Pediatr 1989; 114:995.

INTERSTITIAL LUNG DISEASE

Essentials of Diagnosis

- Tachypnea, dyspnea, retractions, or hypoxemia.
- Cough or rales.
- Bilateral pulmonary infiltrates.

General Considerations

Interstitial lung disorders in children may have a wide variety of presentations, and these are often subtle and gradual in onset. Such disorders in the child—not so in the adult—are commonly caused by infection, immunodeficiency, aspiration, cardiac disease, or pulmonary vascular disease. Also unlike adults, children less commonly have primary pulmonary interstitial lung disorders (desquamative, usual, or lymphocytic interstitial pneumonitis, etc), hypersensitivity pneumonitis, or collagen-vascular diseases.

Clinical Findings

A. Symptoms and Signs: Children may present with a chronic dry cough or a history of dyspnea on exertion. The child with more advanced disease may have increased dyspnea, tachypnea, retractions, cyanosis, clubbing, failure to thrive, or weight loss. Physical examination may reveal these findings, and dry ("Velcro") rales may be present on chest auscultation, especially at the lung bases.

B. Laboratory Findings and Imaging: Chest radiographs may be normal in up to 10–15% of patients. More commonly, diffuse or perihilar bilateral reticular interstitial infiltrates are present. Nodular and reticulonodular diseases are uncommon in children except in cases of HIV infection. Although infiltrates may show a unilateral predominance, bilateral disease is the rule except in cases of infection and aspiration-related disorders.

On pulmonary function testing, interstitial disorders often show a restrictive pattern of decreased lung volumes, compliance, and diffusing capacity for carbon monoxide, whereas the FEV_1/FVC ratio may be normal or increased. However, exercise-induced hypoxemia is often the earliest detectable abnormality of lung function. Blood gas abnormalities, if present, are the same as those in chronic hypersensitivity pneumonitis.

Whereas acute fulminant illness requires immediate, definitive diagnosis, a methodical, staged approach can be used in many chronically ill patients. This consists of (1) "serologic," (2) bronchoscopic, and (3) biopsy stages. Although bronchoalveolar lavage may be useful in identifying patients with pulmonary hemosiderosis (hemosiderin-laden macrophages), aspiration (lipid-laden macrophages), and infectious disorders, lung biopsy is the most reliable method for definitive diagnosis.

During the initial phase, x-rays, barium swallow, tests of pulmonary function, skin tests (see Tuberculosis), complete blood count, erythrocyte sedimentation rate, sweat test for cystic fibrosis, ECG or echocardiogram, serum immunoglobulins, IgE, and other immunologic evaluations, sputum studies (see Pneumonia in the Immunocompromised Host, pp 525–526), and serologic studies for Epstein-Barr virus, cytomegalovirus, *Mycoplasma pneumoniae, Chlamydia, Pneumocystis,* and *Ureaplasma urealyticum* may appropriately be considered and performed.

During the second phase, rigid bronchoscopy should be performed to exclude anatomic abnormalities and obtain multiple specimens of the tracheobronchial wall for evaluation of cilia. At the same procedure, bronchoalveolar lavage, preferably through a flexible bronchoscope and an endotracheal tube if the patient is large enough, should be done. Material for stains and cultures for microorganisms and for cytologic studies should be processed. In patients with static or slowly progressing disease, one can await results of bronchoscopic studies before proceeding further. In patients with more rapidly progressive disease, this stage should be combined with open lung biopsy. Studies of lung tissue, including histopathology, cultures, stains, immunofluorescence for immune complexes, and electron microscopy, should be processed. Although transbronchial biopsy may be useful in diagnosing a few disorders (eg, sarcoid), its overall usefulness in pediatrics is limited.

Differential Diagnosis

Malignant disorders (histiocytosis X, disseminated carcinoma), congenital disorders (Gaucher's disease, neurofibromatosis, tuberous sclerosis, familial interstitial lung disease), pulmonary hemosiderosis, pulmonary telangiectasia or lymphangiectasia, bronchiolitis obliterans, sarcoidosis, and ciliary dyskinesia should be considered in addition to the groups of disorders mentioned above.

Complications

Respiratory failure or pulmonary hypertension with cor pulmonale may occur.

Treatment

Therapy of interstitial lung disease due to infection, aspiration, or cardiac disorders should be directed at the primary disorder. Most of the primary pulmonary interstitial disorders are treated initially with daily prednisone (2 mg/kg/d) therapy for a period of 6 weeks to 6 months, depending on the severity of disease and the response. Many patients require even more prolonged therapy with alternate-day prednisone. Chloroquine (5–10 mg/kg/d) may be useful in selected disorders such as desquamative interstitial pneumonitis. Use of additional cytotoxic drugs (azathioprine, cyclophosphamide) has not been shown in a controlled fashion to be more beneficial than prednisone alone.

Prognosis

The prognosis is guarded in children with interstitial lung disease due to collagen-vascular and primary pulmonary interstitial diseases, immunodeficiency diseases, and cancer.

Diaz RP, Bowman CM: Childhood interstitial lung disease. Semin Respir Med 1990;11:253.
Falloon J et al: Human immunodeficiency virus infection in children. J Pediatr 1989;114:1.
Fan LL et al: Clinical spectrum of chronic interstitial lung disease in children. J Pediatr 1992;121:867.
Fan LL, Langston C: Chronic interstitial lung disease in children. Pediatr Pulmonol 1993;16:184.
Fernald GW et al: Chronic lung disease in children referred to a teaching hospital. Pediatr Pulmonol 1986;2:27.
Stagno S et al: Infant pneumonitis associated with cytomegalovirus, *Chlamydia, Pneumocystis,* and *Ureaplasma:* A prospective study. Pediatrics 1981;68:322.

EOSINOPHILIC PNEUMONIA

Essentials of Diagnosis

- Pulmonary infiltrates, often migratory, on chest radiograph.
- Persistent cough; wheezes or rales on chest auscultation.
- Excessive eosinophils in peripheral blood or in lung biopsy specimens.

General Considerations

A spectrum of diseases should be considered under this heading: (1) transient pulmonary infiltrates with eosinophilia (Löffler's syndrome), (2) tropical eosinophilia, (3) pulmonary eosinophilia with asthma (allergic bronchopulmonary aspergillosis and related disorders), (4) hypereosinophilic mucoid impaction, (5) bronchocentric granulomatosis, and (6) collagen-vascular disorders. Many occur in children with personal or family histories of allergies or asthma. These disorders may be related to hypersensitivity to migratory parasitic nematodes *(Ascaris, Strongyloides, Ancylostoma, Toxocara, Trichuris),* larval forms of filariae *(Wuchereria bancrofti),* or fungi *(Aspergillus, Candida).* Eosinophilic pneumonias also can be associated with drug hypersensitivity, sarcoidosis, Hodgkin's disease or other lymphomas, and bacterial infections, including brucellosis and those caused by *M tuberculosis* and atypical mycobacteria.

Clinical Findings

A. Symptoms and Signs: Patients may present with a recent onset or exacerbation of asthma (Löffler's syndrome) or exacerbation of more severe, long-standing asthma or cystic fibrosis. In most cases, cough, wheezing, or dyspnea are presenting complaints. In Löffler's syndrome, fever, malaise, sputum production, and, rarely, hemoptysis may be present. In allergic bronchopulmonary aspergillosis, patients may present all of these findings and commonly produce brown mucus plugs. Anorexia, weight loss, night sweats, and clubbing can also occur.

B. Laboratory Findings and Imaging: Elevated absolute peripheral blood eosinophil counts (> 3000/μL and often exceeding 50% of leukocytes) are present in Löffler's syndrome, tropical eosinophilia, and allergic bronchopulmonary aspergillosis. Elevated serum IgE levels (often as high as 1000–10,000 IU/mL or more) are commonly present. In allergic bronchopulmonary aspergillosis, the serum IgE concentration appears to correlate with activity of the disease. Stools should be examined for ova and parasites, often several times, to clarify the diagnosis. Isohemagglutinin titers are often markedly elevated in Löffler's syndrome.

In allergic bronchopulmonary aspergillosis and related disorders, patients may have central bronchiectasis demonstrable by chest radiograph ("tramlines") or CT scan. Saccular proximal bronchiectasis of the upper lobes is pathognomonic. Although the chest radiograph may be normal, peribronchial haziness, focal or plate-like atelectasis, or patchy to massive consolidation can occur. Positive immediate skin tests, serum IgG precipitating antibodies, or IgE specific for the offending fungus are present.

Differential Diagnosis

These disorders must be differentiated from exacerbations of asthma, cystic fibrosis, or other underlying lung disorders that can be manifested by infiltrates on chest x-ray films.

Complications

Although Löffler's syndrome is usually self-limited, delayed recognition and treatment of allergic bronchopulmonary aspergillosis may cause progressive lung damage and bronchiectasis. Lesions of the conducting airways in bronchocentric granulomatosis can extend into adjacent lung parenchyma and pulmonary arteries, resulting in a secondary vasculitis.

Treatment

Therapy for parasites causing Löffler's syndrome should be given, and corticosteroids may be required when illness is severe. Treatment of disease due to microfilariae is both diagnostic and therapeutic. Al-

lergic bronchopulmonary aspergillosis and related disorders are treated with prolonged courses of oral corticosteroids, bronchodilators, and chest physical therapy. Antifungal agents are not useful in these latter disorders.

Ahmad M et al: Thoracic aspergillosis: 2. Primary pulmonary aspergillosis, allergic bronchopulmonary aspergillosis, and related conditions. Cleve Clin Q 1984;51:631.

Buchheit J et al: Acute eosinophilic pneumonia with respiratory failure: A new syndrome? Am Rev Respir Dis 1992;145:716.

Christensen WN, Hutchins GM: Hypereosinophilic mucoid impaction of bronchi in 2 children under 2 years of age. Pediatr Pulmonol 1985;1:278.

Howard WA: Pulmonary infiltrates with eosinophilia (Löffler syndrome). In: *Disorders of the Respiratory Tract in Children,* 5th ed. Chernick V, Kendig EL Jr (editors). Saunders, 1990.

Lee TM et al: Allergic bronchopulmonary candidiasis: Case report and suggested diagnostic criteria. J Allergy Clin Immunol 1987;80:816.

Vijayan V-K et al: Pulmonary eosinophilia in pulmonary tuberculosis. Chest 1992;101:1708.

LUNG ABSCESS

Essentials of Diagnosis

- Fever.
- Cavitary mass on chest radiograph.
- With or without cough, chest pain, dyspnea, sputum production, or hemoptysis.

General Considerations

Lung abscesses are most likely to occur in immunocompromised patients, in those with severe infections elsewhere (embolic spread), or in those with recurrent aspiration, malnutrition, or blunt chest trauma. Although organisms such as *Staphylococcus aureus, Haemophilus influenzae, Streptococcus viridans,* and *Streptococcus pneumoniae* more commonly affect the previously normal host, anaerobic and gram-negative organisms as well as *Nocardia, Legionella* species, and fungi *(Candida, Aspergillus)* should also be considered in the immunocompromised host.

Clinical Findings

A. Symptoms and Signs: High fever, malaise, and weight loss are often present. Symptoms and signs referable to the chest may or may not be present. In infants, evidence of respiratory distress can be present.

B. Laboratory Findings and Imaging: Elevated peripheral white blood cell count with a neutrophil predominance or an elevated erythrocyte sedimentation rate may be present. Blood cultures are rarely positive except in the overwhelmed host.

Chest radiographs usually reveal single or multiple

thick-walled lung cavities. Air-fluid levels can be present. Local compressive atelectasis, pleural thickening, or adenopathy may also occur. Chest CT scan may provide better localization of the lesions.

In patients producing sputum, stains and cultures may provide the diagnosis. Direct percutaneous aspiration of material for stains and cultures directed by fluoroscopy or ultrasound should be considered in the severely compromised or ill.

Differential Diagnosis

Loculated pyopneumothorax, *Echinococcus* cyst, neoplasms, plasma cell granuloma, and infected congenital cysts and sequestrations should be considered in the differential diagnosis.

Complications

Although complications due to abscesses are now rare, mediastinal shift, tension pneumothorax, and spontaneous rupture can occur. Diagnostic maneuvers such as lung puncture may also cause complications (pneumothorax).

Treatment

Because of the risks of lung puncture, uncomplicated abscesses are frequently treated in the uncompromised host with appropriate broad-spectrum antibiotics directed at *S aureus, H influenzae,* and streptococci. Additional coverage for anaerobic and gram-negative organisms should be provided for others. Prolonged therapy (3 weeks or more) may be required. Attempts to drain abscesses via bronchoscopy have caused life-threatening airway compromise. Surgical drainage or lobectomy is occasionally required, primarily in immunocompromised patients. However, such procedures may themselves cause life-threatening complications, and surgical intervention must be judicious and well planned.

Prognosis

Although radiographic resolution may be very slow, resolution occurs in most patients without propensity to lower respiratory tract infections or loss of pulmonary function. Nonetheless, in the immunocompromised host, the outlook is guarded and dependent on the underlying disorder.

Asher MI et al: Primary lung abscess in childhood: The long-term outcome of conservative management. Am J Dis Child 1982;136:491.

Bartlett JG: Antibiotics in lung abscess. Semin Respir Infect 1991;6:103.

DeBoeck K et al: Percutaneous drainage of lung abscess in a malnourished child. Pediatr Infect Dis J 1991;10:163.

Kosloske AM et al: Drainage of pediatric lung abscess by cough, catheter, or complete resection. J Pediatr Surg 1986;21:596.

Lee SK, Morris RF, Cramer B: Percutaneous needle aspiration of neonatal lung abscesses. Pediatr Radiol 1991;21:254.

Lewin S et al: Legionnaire's disease. A cause of severe abscess-forming pneumonia. Am J Med 1979;67:339.

Lui RC, Inculet RI: Job's syndrome: A rare cause of recurrent lung abscess in childhood. Ann Thoracic Surg 1990;50:992.

Shim C, Santos GH, Zelefsky M: Percutaneous drainage of lung abscess. Lung 1990;168:201.

Siegel JD, McCracken GH: Neonatal lung abscess. Am J Dis Child 1979;133:947.

PULMONARY TUMORS

Primary tumors of the airway and parenchyma of the lung are unusual in pediatrics. Most intrathoracic tumors occur in or close to the mediastinum (see Mediastinal Masses, p 539). Other pulmonary tumors may be classified as benign, malignant, or metastatic. Benign pulmonary tumors include plasma cell granulomas, hamartomas, adenomas, papillomas, angiomas, leiomyomas, lipomas, and neurogenic tumors. The most common malignant tumor in children is a bronchogenic carcinoma, but this is again very rare. Other malignant tumors include fibrosarcomas and leiomyosarcomas. Metastatic tumors in childhood include Wilms' tumor, hepatoblastoma, osteogenic sarcoma, chondrosarcoma, Ewing's tumor, reticulum cell sarcoma, and soft tissue sarcomas. Because metastatic pulmonary tumors are more common than primary malignant growths in the lungs of children, patients with symptoms and roentgenographic or other data suggesting a pulmonary cancer should be thoroughly evaluated for nonpulmonary malignant tumors.

Clinical Findings

A. Symptoms and Signs: When tumors produce symptoms, these may include pain, fever, cough, wheezing, weight loss, malaise, anemia, anorexia, and hemoptysis. On physical examination, signs of volume loss or consolidation may be present if the tumor has led to significant airway obstruction. Physical findings consistent with pleural effusions may also be present.

B. Laboratory Findings and Imaging: In addition to frontal and lateral chest x-rays, fluoroscopy, CT scans, and angiography may be helpful in defining and delineating the tumor. In approaching the differential diagnosis (below), sputum cultures and cytology, as well as tuberculin and fungal skin tests plus fungal serology, may be of benefit in ruling out conditions that may appear to be mass lesions.

Differential Diagnosis

The differential diagnosis includes acute, recurrent, or persistent viral and bacterial pneumonia, tuberculosis, and pulmonary infiltrates due to fungal infections. In infants, congenital malformations (pulmonary sequestration, cystic adenomatoid malformation) may also present as mass lesions.

Treatment & Prognosis

Both the appropriate therapy and the response to therapy depend on the type and location of the tumor. Benign lesions may be cured with surgical resection, but the prognosis is more guarded with both primary and metastatic malignant lesions.

Brooks JW: Tumors of the chest. In: *Disorders of the Respiratory Tract in Children,* 5th ed. Chernick V, Kendig EL Jr (editors). Saunders, 1990.

Hammer J et al: Plasma cell granuloma of the lung: Associated laboratory findings and ultrastructural evidence of inflammatory origin. Pediatr Pulmonol 1991;10:299.

Hartman GE, Shochat SJ: Primary pulmonary neoplasms in childhood: A review. Ann Thorac Surg 1983;36:108.

Monzon CM et al: Plasma cell granuloma of the lung in children. Pediatrics 1982;70:268.

DISEASES OF THE PULMONARY CIRCULATION

PULMONARY HEMORRHAGE

Acute pulmonary hemorrhage can be defined as bleeding within the lungs, with or without hemoptysis, and is usually accompanied by filling alveolar infiltrates on chest x-ray. Hemosiderin-laden macrophages are found in the sputum and tracheal or gastric aspirate. Many cases are secondary to infection (bacterial, mycobacterial, parasitic, viral, or fungal), lung abscess, bronchiectasis (cystic fibrosis or other causes), foreign body, coagulopathy (often with overwhelming sepsis), or elevated pulmonary venous pressure (secondary to congestive heart failure or anatomic heart lesions). Structural lesions including arteriovenous fistula, multiple telangiectasia, pulmonary sequestration, agenesis of a single pulmonary artery, and esophageal duplication or bronchogenic cyst are other related causes. Lung contusion from trauma and such tumors as bronchial adenoma or left atrial myxoma are other causes. Pulmonary infarction secondary to pulmonary embolus is another uncommon cause in pediatrics.

In addition, alveolar hemorrhage syndromes—alveolar bleeding that occurs as a primary manifestation—may be idiopathic or drug-related or may occur in association with several uncommon disorders or as uncommon manifestations of systemic disease: Goodpasture's syndrome, rapidly progressive glomerulonephritis, and systemic vasculitides (often associated with such collagen-vascular diseases as systemic lupus erythematosus, rheumatoid arthritis, Wegener's granulomatosis, polyarteritis nodosa, Schönlein-Henoch purpura, and Behçet's disease). Idiopathic pulmonary hemosiderosis refers to the accumulation of hemosiderin in the lung, especially the alveolar macrophage, as a result of chronic or recurrent hemorrhage (usually from pulmonary capillaries) that is not associated with the causes listed above. Children and young adults are primarily affected, with the age at onset ranging between 6 months and 20 years. This group of disorders includes young infants with milk allergy (Heiner's syndrome).

Clinical Findings

A. Symptoms and Signs: Idiopathic pulmonary hemosiderosis usually presents with nonspecific respiratory symptoms (cough, tachypnea, retractions), with or without hemoptysis, poor growth, and fatigue. Some children or young adults may present with massive hemoptysis, marked respiratory distress, stridor, or a pneumonia-like syndrome. Fever, abdominal pain, digital clubbing, and chest pain may be reported. Jaundice and hepatosplenomegaly may be present with chronic bleeding. Physical examination often reveals decreased breath sounds, rales, rhonchi, or wheezing.

B. Laboratory Findings and Imaging: Laboratory studies demonstrate iron deficiency anemia and heme-positive sputum. Nonspecific findings may include lymphocytosis and an elevated erythrocyte sedimentation rate. Peripheral eosinophilia is present in up to 25% of patients. Chest x-ray findings include a range of findings, from transient perihilar infiltrates to large, fluffy alveolar infiltrates with or without atelectasis and mediastinal adenopathy. Pulmonary function testing generally reveals a restrictive impairment, with low lung volumes and poor compliance. Hemosiderin-laden macrophages are found in bronchial or gastric aspirates. The usefulness of lung biopsy in reaching the diagnosis is controversial. Suspected cases of cow's milk-induced pulmonary hemosiderosis can be confirmed by laboratory findings that include high titers of serum precipitins to multiple constituents of cow's milk and positive intradermal skin tests to various cow's milk proteins. Improvement after an empiric trial of a diet free of cow's milk also supports the diagnosis.

Differential Diagnosis

In contrast to idiopathic pulmonary hemosiderosis, Goodpasture's syndrome presents in a slightly older age group (15–35 years), tends to have a more aggressive pulmonary course, and has renal involvement (crescentic proliferative glomerulonephritis and circulating anti-glomerular basement membrane antibody). Wegener's granulomatosis also has renal involvement (granulomatous glomerulitis with necrotizing vasculitis, but renal biopsy may be nonspecific) and other systemic manifestations, especially with upper and lower respiratory tract inflammation. Upper tract involvement includes sinusitis, rhinitis, recurrent epistaxis, otitis media, saddle nose deformity, and subglottic stenosis. Wegener's granulomatosis may present without renal involvement early in the course of the disease. The diagnosis can be made by biopsy or an elevated antineutrophil cytoplasmic antibody titer.

Treatment

Therapy should be aimed at direct treatment of the underlying disease. Supportive measures, including iron therapy, supplemental oxygen, and blood transfusions, are provided as clinically indicated. In selected cases, a trial of cow's milk-free diet should be tried. The usefulness of corticosteroids or cytotoxic agents is unproved in idiopathic pulmonary hemosiderosis but appears to be beneficial in Wegener's granulomatosis and perhaps Goodpasture's syndrome.

Prognosis

The outcome of idiopathic pulmonary hemosiderosis is markedly variable, typically characterized by a waxing and waning course of intermittent intrapulmonary bleeds and the gradual development of chronic lung disease over time. The severity of the underlying renal disease contributes to the mortality rates associated with Goodpasture's syndrome and Wegener's granulomatosis.

Bradley JD: Pulmonary hemorrhage syndromes. Clin Chest Med 1982;3:593.

Hall SL et al: Wegener granulomatosis in pediatric patients. J Pediatr 1985;106:739.

Kjellman B et al: Idiopathic pulmonary hemosiderosis in Swedish children. Acta Paediatr Scand 1984;73:584.

Leatherman JW et al: Alveolar hemorrhage syndromes. Medicine (Baltimore) 1984;63:343.

Miller RW et al: Pulmonary hemorrhage in pediatric patients with systemic lupus erythematosus. J Pediatr 1986;108:576.

PULMONARY EMBOLISM

Although apparently rare in children, the incidence of pulmonary embolism is probably underestimated in pediatrics because it is often not considered in the differential diagnosis of respiratory distress. It occurs most commonly in pediatrics in sickle cell anemia as part of the "acute chest syndrome" and in rheumatic fever, infective endocarditis, schistosomiasis, bone fracture, dehydration, polycythemia, nephrotic syndrome, atrial fibrillation, "complicated" pneumonia, and other settings. The emboli may be single or multiple, large or small, with the clinical signs and symptoms dependent on the severity of pulmonary vascular obstruction.

Clinical Findings

A. Symptoms and Signs: Most often, pulmonary embolism presents clinically as the acute onset of dyspnea and tachypnea. Heart palpitations or "a sense of impending doom" may be reported. Pleuritic chest pain and hemoptysis may be present (but are not common), along with splinting, cyanosis, and tachycardia. Massive emboli may present with syncope and cardiac dysrhythmias. Physical examination is usually normal (except for tachycardia and tachypnea) unless the embolism is associated with an underlying disorder. Mild hypoxemia, rales, focal wheezing, or a pleural friction rub may be noted.

B. Laboratory Findings and Imaging: Radiologic findings may be normal, but a peripheral infiltrate, small pleural effusion, or elevated hemidiaphragm can be present. If the emboli are massive, differential blood flow and pulmonary artery enlargement may be appreciated. The ECG is usually normal unless the pulmonary embolus is massive. Ventilation/perfusion scans show localized areas of ventilation without perfusion. If this study is normal, pulmonary embolus is virtually excluded. Further evaluation may include radiofibrinogen leg scanning and impedance plethysmography to search for findings of significant deep venous thrombosis. Coagulation studies, including assessments of antithrombin III and protein C or S deficiencies, or defective fibrinolysis may be indicated. However, 90% of adult patients with venous thromboembolism have no identified coagulopathy.

Treatment

Acute treatment includes supplemental oxygen, sedation, and anticoagulation. Although controversial, current recommendations include heparin administration to maintain an activated partial thromboplastin time that is 1½ or more times the control value. Thrombolytic therapy with streptokinase and urokinase may be necessary if the pulmonary embolus is massive. In patients with identifiable deep venous thrombosis of the lower extremities and significant pulmonary emboli (with hemodynamic compromise despite anticoagulation), inferior vena caval interruption may be necessary. However, long-term prospective data is lacking.

Malik AR, Johnson A: Role of humoral mediators in the pulmonary vascular response to pulmonary embolism. In: *Pulmonary Vascular Physiology and Pathophysiology.* Weir EK, Reeves JT (editors). Bryan Dekker, 1989.

Moser KM: Pulmonary embolism. In: *Textbook of Respiratory Medicine.* Murray JF, Nadel JA (editors). Saunders, 1988.

PULMONARY EDEMA

The morbidity of many cardiopulmonary disorders appears to be directly related to the severity of pulmonary edema, defined as the excessive accumulation of extravascular fluid in the lung. This occurs when fluid is filtered into the lungs faster than it can be removed, leading to detrimental changes in lung mechanics, eg, decreased lung compliance, worsening hypoxemia from ventilation/perfusion mismatch, bronchial compression, and, if advanced, decreased surfactant function. In the normal lung, the rate of fluid filtration is determined by the balance of hydrostatic and oncotic pressures in the microcirculation and interstitium, as well as vascular permeability, surface area, and lymphatic function. In general, there are two basic types of pulmonary edema: increased pressure (cardiogenic or hydrostatic) and increased permeability (noncardiogenic or "primary"). Hydrostatic pulmonary edema is usually due to excessive increases in pressure, which is most commonly due to congestive heart failure from multiple causes. In contrast, many lung diseases, especially adult respiratory distress syndrome (ARDS; see below) are characterized by the development of pulmonary edema secondary to changes in permeability due to injury to the alveolocapillary barrier. In these settings, pulmonary edema formation occurs primarily, independent of the elevations of pulmonary venous pressure.

Clinical Findings

A. Symptoms and Signs: Clinical findings depend on the underlying cause and clinical setting. In general, cyanosis, tachypnea, tachycardia, and respiratory distress are present. Physical findings include rales, diminished breath sounds, and (in young infants) expiratory wheezing. More severe disease is characterized by progressive respiratory distress with marked retractions, dyspnea, and severe hypoxemia.

B. Imaging: Chest x-ray findings are dependent on the cause of the edema. Typically, pulmonary vessels appear prominent, often with diffuse interstitial or alveolar infiltrates. Heart size is usually normal in permeability edema but enlarged when hydrostatic causes underlie the problem.

Treatment

Although specific therapy depends on the underlying cause of the pulmonary edema, supplemental oxygen therapy and, if needed, ventilator support for respiratory failure are instituted. Diuretics, digoxin, and vasodilators may be indicated for congestive heart failure, along with restriction of salt and water. Recommended interventions for permeability edema are reducing vascular volume and maintaining the lowest central venous or pulmonary arterial wedge pressure, without sacrificing cardiac output or causing hypotension (see below).

Malik AR: Mechanisms of neurogenic pulmonary edema. Circ Res 1985;57:1.

Staub NC: Pathogenesis of pulmonary edema. Prog Cardiovasc Dis 1980;23:53.

ADULT RESPIRATORY DISTRESS SYNDROME (Shock Lung Syndrome)

Essentials of Diagnosis

- Progressive respiratory distress following an acute catastrophic event such as shock.
- Low lung compliance, marked hypoxemia.
- Chest x-ray demonstrating bilateral fluffy infiltrates, usually with normal heart size.
- Normal pulmonary artery wedge pressure (as measured by pulmonary artery catheter).

General Considerations

Adult respiratory distress syndrome (ARDS) is a clinical syndrome characterized by the progressive development of respiratory failure associated with acute lung injury. The inciting insult may be indirect (septic or hemorrhagic shock, head trauma and other causes of neurogenic pulmonary edema, burns, drug overdose, pancreatitis, massive blood transfusion, and many others) or direct (smoke or chemical inhalation, aspiration, lung infection, emboli, contusion, radiation pneumonitis). First reported by Ashbaugh in 1967, the term "adult" respiratory distress syndrome was derived from histologic and physiologic similarities with the respiratory distress syndrome observed in premature newborns. Despite its name, ARDS can be observed at any age. Its pathophysiologic hallmark is the presence of nonhydrostatic pulmonary edema due to increased pulmonary capillary permeability secondary to acute lung injury, in contrast to pulmonary edema secondary to elevated pulmonary venous pressures more typical of congestive heart failure. The exact mechanisms contributing to lung injury are not completely understood and may vary according to the type of insult involved. Several studies, however, have implicated a central role for the accumulation of activated neutrophils within the pulmonary circulation, leading to the release of injurious mediators, including toxic oxygen metabolites, eicosanoids, and proteinases. These agents may directly damage the endothelium, causing the loss of its barrier function, leading to increased permeability and resultant pulmonary edema. The acute inflammatory response associated with adult respiratory distress syndrome and its experimental models may also include contributions from alveolar macrophages, platelets, lymphocytes, and fibroblasts. Along with cellular infiltration, early histologic findings include microthrombi within the pulmonary circulation, intra-alveolar proteinaceous material, alveolar septal edema, and type I epithelial cell damage. Later findings (a few days after the initial injury) include increased interstitial and alveolar inflammation, type II cell proliferation, interstitial thickening with early collagen accumulation, and increased fibroblasts.

Clinical Findings

The classic clinical course of adult respiratory distress syndrome consists of progressive cyanosis and respiratory distress associated with stiff lungs (low compliance) and diffuse pulmonary infiltrates after an acute catastrophic event. The rate of development of acute respiratory failure is variable, but often there may be little sign of respiratory distress in its earliest stages, with progressive hypoxemia appearing within the period of 6–48 hours following the acute event. Early chest x-ray films may appear normal, but serial studies subsequently reveal patchy alveolar infiltrates, air bronchograms, and loss of lung volume, with the progression of increasing tachypnea, dyspnea, and hypoxemia. Rales are common on auscultation. Although initially responsive to supplemental oxygen, hypoxemia often becomes refractory to treatment because of marked ventilation/perfusion mismatching (intrapulmonary shunting) and low lung compliance with loss of lung volume. At this stage, mechanical ventilation is required, often with high-peak positive end-expiratory pressure (PEEP) and mean airway pressure (MAP).

Treatment

Therapy is primarily supportive. The first step lies in recognizing patients at risk, thereby anticipating and monitoring for the earliest signs of acute respiratory failure. Along with treating the underlying disorder (antibiotics for sepsis, blood products for hemorrhagic shock, etc), appropriate monitoring should be established early. This includes placement of a systemic arterial line for frequent assessments of arterial pH and blood gas tensions and for continuous measurements of arterial blood pressure. Pulse oximetry or transcutaneous PO_2 measurements provide serial, continuous determinations of oxygenation. Assessments of fluid status require placement of a Foley catheter. Dependable peripheral and central venous lines provide access for the administration of medications, blood products, and fluids and for assessing volume status by central venous pressures. In some cases, placement of a pulmonary arterial catheter allows essential determinations of pulmonary capillary wedge pressure, cardiac output, and mixed venous oxygen tensions and saturations (see Chapter 15).

The overall goal of acute therapy is to maximize tissue oxygen delivery, which is determined by the oxygen content of arterial blood (reflecting hemoglobin concentration, percent saturation, and arterial oxygen tension) and the cardiac index. Therefore, treatment typically includes maintaining hematocrit above 40%, cardiac index over 4.5 L/min/m^2, and oxygen saturation over 90–92%. Because of the severity

and rapidity of the progression of lung disease, volume-limited ventilators are generally recommended to ensure the constant delivery of adequate tidal volume in the face of changing respiratory system compliance. With advanced disease, high levels of PEEP and MAP are needed to treat severe hypoxemia. In addition, this may allow the FIO_2 to be lowered below 1, thereby decreasing the potential risk of superimposed hyperoxic lung injury which, if prolonged, may paradoxically contribute to a worse outcome (see below). High PEEP appears to improve the clinical course by attenuating the alterations of lung mechanics caused by pulmonary edema (especially the loss of lung volumes, thereby decreasing the magnitude of intrapulmonary shunt), but does not appear to decrease the amount of edema fluid present within the lung itself. The amount of PEEP required to improve oxygenation will vary considerably, from 4–6 cm H_2O for mild distress to levels over 20 cm H_2O for more advanced disease. The potential harmful effects of high PEEP include barotrauma, increased pulmonary hypertension, and decreased cardiac output, potentially leading to worse O_2 delivery. Paralysis and sedation often facilitate more effective ventilation. Clinical studies have failed to demonstrate beneficial effects of corticosteroids. Inotropic support, careful fluid management, prophylaxis against gastrointestinal bleeding, early antibiotic therapy with suspected secondary sepsis, close attention to nutritional needs, and exact guidelines for the onset and duration of mechanical ventilation are important aspects of intensive care unit management (see Chapter 15).

Prognosis

Mortality rates of 50–60% are commonly reported. Death is often due to multiple organ system failure associated with secondary infection and progressive respiratory failure. As in the premature newborn who develops bronchopulmonary dysplasia, therapeutic efforts to support and treat underlying acute respiratory failure (with hyperoxia and high airway pressure) may paradoxically contribute to subsequent irreversibility or to the progression of the lung injury to chronic stages. Although tracheostomy and prolonged mechanical ventilation are required in some patients with chronic lung disease after the acute course of adult respiratory distress syndrome, most adults who survive have little respiratory sequelae at follow-up.

Ashbaugh et al: Acute respiratory distress in adults. Lancet 1967;2:319.

Demling RH: Role of mediators in human adult respiratory distress syndrome. J Crit Care 1988;3:56.

Royall JA, Levin DL: Adult respiratory distress syndrome in pediatric patients. 1. Clinical aspects, pathophysiology, pathology, and mechanisms of lung injury. 2. Management. J Pediatr 1988;112:169,335.

CONGENITAL PULMONARY LYMPHANGIECTASIA

Structurally, congenital pulmonary lymphangiectasia appears as dilated subpleural and interlobular lymphatic channels and may present as part of a generalized lymphangiectasis (in association with obstructive cardiovascular lesions, especially total anomalous pulmonary venous return) or as an isolated, idiopathic lesion. Pathologically, the lung appears firm, bulky, and noncompressible, with prominent cystic lymphatics visible beneath the pleura. On cut section, dilated lymphatics are present near the hilum, along interlobular septa, around bronchovascular bundles, and beneath the pleura. Histologically, dilated lymphatics have a thin endothelial cell lining overlying a delicate network of elastin and collagen.

Clinical Findings

Congenital pulmonary lymphangiectasia is a rare, usually fatal disease that generally presents as acute or persistent respiratory distress at birth. Although most patients do not survive the newborn period, some survive longer, and there are isolated case reports of its diagnosis later in childhood. It may be associated with features of Noonan's syndrome, asplenia, total anomalous pulmonary venous return, septal defects, atrioventricular canal, hypoplastic left heart, aortic arch malformations, and renal malformations. Chylothorax has been reported. Chest x-ray findings include a "ground glass" appearance, prominent interstitial markings suggesting lymphatic distention, diffuse hyperlucency of the pulmonary parenchyma, and hyperinflation with depression of the diaphragm.

Prognosis

The outcome is poor. Although the onset of symptoms may be delayed for as long as the first few months of life, prolonged survival is extremely rare. Most deaths occur within weeks after birth.

Gardner TW et al: Congenital pulmonary lymphangiectasis. Clin Pediatr 1983;22:75.

Noonan JA et al: Congenital pulmonary lymphangiectasis. Am J Dis Child 1970;120:314.

DISORDERS OF THE CHEST WALL

EVENTRATION OF THE DIAPHRAGM

Eventration of the diaphragm is characterized on x-ray film by elevation of part or all of the diaphragm. Degrees of clinical symptomatology vary. Pathologically, the layers of the diaphragm are incompletely formed, with fibrous or loose connective tissue found where striated muscle is normally located. This congenital disorder is thought to represent incomplete formation of the diaphragm in utero. When defects are small, there is no paradoxic movement of the diaphragm and little symptomatology. Small eventrations may be detected on a chest x-ray film taken for another reason. When defects are large, there may or may not be paradoxic movement of the diaphragm, depending upon the nature of the tissue replacing the normal diaphragm. The degree of respiratory distress depends in large part upon the amount of paradoxic motion of the diaphragm. When the diaphragm moves upward during inspiration, instability of the inferior border of the chest wall increases the work of breathing and can lead to respiratory muscle fatigue. Treatment for respiratory distress is surgical plication, which stabilizes the diaphragm.

The differential diagnosis of eventration includes phrenic nerve injury and partial diaphragmatic hernia. The former can result from birth or other trauma and may also be seen following cardiac surgery. Usually, only one phrenic nerve is involved. An elevated hemidiaphragm is noted on chest x-ray film, and paradoxic motion of the diaphragm may be seen by fluoroscopy or ultrasound. Often, patients cannot be extubated or have persistent respiratory compromise, particularly with feeding. If symptoms persist for 2–4 weeks, the diaphragm is surgically plicated as described above. Function returns to the diaphragm in about 50% of cases of phrenic nerve injury whether or not plication was performed. Recovery periods of up to 100 days have been reported in these cases.

Obara H et al: Eventration of the diaphragm in infants and children. Acta Paediatr Scand 1987;76:654.

SCOLIOSIS

Scoliosis—lateral curvature of the spine—can, if uncorrected, lead to severe restrictive lung disease and death from cor pulmonale. Most cases of idiopathic scoliosis occur in adolescent girls and are corrected before there is significant pulmonary impairment. Congenital scoliosis of a severe degree or with other major abnormalities carries a more guarded prognosis. Scoliosis may also occur in patients with progressive neuromuscular disease, such as Duchenne's muscular dystrophy, and can be a major contributor to respiratory failure.

DiRocco PJ, Vaccaro P: Cardiopulmonary functioning in adolescent patients with mild idiopathic scoliosis. Arch Phys Med Rehabil 1988;69:198.

Szeinberg A et al: Forced vital capacity and maximal respiratory pressures in patients with mild and moderate scoliosis. Pediatr Pulmonol 1988;4:8.

PECTUS EXCAVATUM

Pectus excavatum is an anterior depression of the chest wall that may be symmetric or asymmetric with respect to the midline. Reports of exercise testing and pulmonary function testing in patients with pectus excavatum have not clearly demonstrated any marked abnormalities. Therefore, the decision to repair the deformity is usually based on cosmetic considerations. Postoperative care of patients following pectus excavatum requires mechanical ventilation and careful respiratory monitoring because of the weak chest wall following surgery.

Peterson RJ et al: Noninvasive assessment of exercise cardiac function before and after pectus excavatum repair. J Thorac Cardiovasc Surg 1985;90:251.

PECTUS CARINATUM

Pectus carinatum is a bowing out of the sternum, usually apparent at birth. The abnormality may be associated with some systemic diseases such as the mucopolysaccharidoses. As with pectus excavatum, abnormalities of pulmonary function tests are unusual in the absence of other disorders. The decision to repair this deformity is based primarily on cosmetic grounds. Postoperative care similarly requires careful monitoring because of chest wall instability produced by the repair.

Cahill JL, Lees GM, Robertson HT: A summary of preoperative and postoperative cardiorespiratory performance in patients undergoing pectus excavatum and carinatum repair. J Pediatr Surg 1984;19:430.

NEUROMUSCULAR DISORDERS

Many neuromuscular diseases are associated with chronic or recurrent pulmonary problems secondary to weakness of the respiratory and pharyngeal muscles. These difficulties are manifested as chronic or recurrent pneumonia secondary to aspiration and infection, atelectasis, hypoventilation, and respiratory failure in severe cases. Scoliosis, which frequently accompanies long-standing neuromuscular disorders, may further compromise respiratory function. Typical physical findings include weak cough, decreased air exchange, rales, wheezing, and dullness to percussion. Signs of cor pulmonale (loud pulmonary component to the second heart sound, hepatomegaly, elevated neck veins) may be evident in advanced cases. Chest films generally show small lung volumes. If chronic aspiration is present, increased interstitial infiltrates and areas of atelectasis or consolidation may be present. Arterial blood gases demonstrate hypoxemia in the early stages and compensated respiratory

acidosis in the late stages. Typical pulmonary function abnormalities include low lung volumes and decreased inspiratory force generated against an occluded airway. Treatment is supportive and includes vigorous pulmonary toilet, antibiotics with infection, and oxygen to correct hypoxemia. Unfortunately, despite aggressive medical therapy, many neuromuscular conditions progress to respiratory failure and death. The decision to intubate and ventilate is a difficult one; it should be made only when there is real hope that deterioration, though acute, is potentially reversible or when chronic ventilation has been deemed a therapeutic option. Chronic mechanical ventilation utilizing either noninvasive or invasive techniques is being used more frequently in patients with chronic respiratory insufficiency.

Lantos JD, Kohrman AF: Ethical aspects of pediatric home care. Pediatrics 1992;89:920.
Kennedy AS et al: Decortication for childhood empyema: The primary provider's peccadillo. Arch Surg 1991; 126:1287.
Shaffner DH, Gioia FR: Neuromuscular disease and respiratory failure. In: Textbook of Pediatric Intensive Care, 2nd ed. Rogers MC (editor). Williams & Wilkins, 1992.

DISORDERS OF THE PLEURA & PLEURAL CAVITY

The pleural membranes cover the outer surface of the lungs (visceral pleura) and the inner surface of the chest wall (parietal pleura). Because they are normally in intimate contact, the "space" between them is more of a potential space. However, disease processes can lead to accumulation of air or fluid in the pleural space. Classically, pleural effusions have been classified as transudates or exudates. Transudates occur when there is imbalance between hydrostatic and oncotic pressure, so that fluid filtration exceeds reabsorption (eg, congestive heart failure). Exudates form as a result of inflammation of the pleural surface leading to increased capillary permeability (eg, parapneumonic effusions). Other forms of pleural effusions include chylothorax and hemothorax.

Thoracentesis is helpful in characterizing the fluid and providing definitive diagnosis. Recovered fluid is considered an exudate (as opposed to a transudate) if any of the following are found: a pleural fluid to serum protein ratio greater than 0.5, a pleural fluid to serum lactic dehydrogenase (LDH) ratio greater than 0.6, or a pleural fluid LDH greater than 200 IU/L. Important additional studies on pleural fluid include cell count; pH and glucose; Gram, acid-fast, and fungal stains; cultures; counterimmunoelectrophoresis for specific organisms; cytology; and, occasionally, amylase concentration.

Sahn SA: Pleural manifestations of pulmonary disease. Hosp Pract (March) 1981;16:73.

PARAPNEUMONIC EFFUSION & EMPYEMA

Bacterial pneumonia is often accompanied by pleural effusion. Some of these effusions harbor infection, and others represent inflammatory reactions to pneumonia. The nomenclature in this area is somewhat confusing. Some use the term empyema for grossly purulent fluid and parapneumonic effusion for nonpurulent fluid. However, it is clear that some nonpurulent effusions will also contain organisms and represent either partially treated or early empyema. Therefore, it is probably best to refer to all effusions associated with pneumonia as parapneumonic effusions, some of which are infected and some of which are not.

The organism most commonly associated with empyema is *Streptococcus pneumoniae.* Other common organisms include *Haemophilus influenzae* and *Staphylococcus aureus* (formerly the most common). Less common causes are group A streptococci, gram-negative organisms, and anaerobic organisms. Effusions associated with tuberculosis are almost always sterile and represent an inflammatory reaction.

Clinical Findings

A. Symptoms and Signs: Patients usually present with typical signs of pneumonia, including fever, tachypnea, and cough. In addition, they may have chest pain, decreased breath sounds, and dullness to percussion on the affected side. They may prefer to lie on the affected side. With large effusions, there may be tracheal deviation to the contralateral side.

B. Laboratory Findings: The white blood count is often elevated, with left shift. Blood cultures are sometimes positive. The tuberculin skin test is positive in most cases of tuberculosis except when anergy is present or when the disease process is in a very early stage. Thoracentesis reveals findings consistent with an exudate. Pleural fluid cell count usually reveals predominantly polymorphonuclear cells in bacterial disease and lymphocytes in tuberculous effusions. In bacterial disease, the pleural fluid pH and glucose is often low. Although in adults the presence of low pH and glucose necessitates aggressive and thorough drainage procedures, the prognostic significance of these findings in children is not known. Gram stain, cultures, or counterimmunoelectrophoresis is often positive for the offending organism.

C. Imaging: The presence of pleural fluid is suggested by a homogeneous density on chest x-ray that obscures the underlying lung. Large effusions may cause a shift of the mediastinum to the contralateral side. Small effusions may only blunt the costophrenic angle. Lateral decubitus films may help to detect freely movable fluid by demonstrating a "layering-out" effect. If the fluid is loculated, no such effect is perceived. Ultrasonography can be extremely valuable in localizing the fluid and detecting loculations, especially when thoracentesis is contemplated.

Treatment & Prognosis

Appropriate intravenous antibiotics for at least 14 days and adequate drainage of the fluid remain the mainstay of therapy. Although there is a trend toward conservative management (no chest tube) of smaller pneumococcal empyemas, most larger effusions require chest tube drainage. More aggressive procedures such as thoracotomy with open drainage or decortication are rarely indicated except for less common causes of this disorder such as infection with group A streptococci and gram-negative and anaerobic organisms.

The prognosis is related to the severity of disease but is generally excellent, with complete or nearly complete recovery expected in most instances.

Foglia RP, Randolph J: Current indications for decortication in the treatment of empyema in children. J Pediatr Surg 1987;22:28.

Kennedy AS et al: Decortication for childhood empyema: The primary provider's peccadillo. Arch Surg 1991;126: 1287.

McLaughlin FJ et al: Empyema in children: Clinical course and long-term follow-up. Pediatrics 1984;73:587.

Murphy D, Lockhart CH, Todd JK: Pneumococcal empyema: Outcome of medical management. Am J Dis Child 1980;134:659.

Solak H, Yuksek T, Solak N: Methods of treatment of childhood empyema in a Turkish university hospital. Chest 1987;92:517.

HEMOTHORAX

Accumulation of blood in the pleural space can be caused by surgical or accidental trauma, coagulation defects, and pleural or pulmonary tumors. With blunt trauma, hemopneumothorax may be present. Symptoms are related to blood loss and compression of underlying lung parenchyma. There is some risk of secondary infection resulting in empyema. Drainage of a hemothorax is required when significant compromise of pulmonary function is present, as with hemopneumothorax. In uncomplicated cases, observation is indicated, because blood is readily absorbed spontaneously from the pleural space.

Rowe MI, Marchildon MB: Pediatric trauma. In: *Critical Care: State of the Art,* vol 2. Shoemaker WC, Thompson WL (editors). Society of Critical Care Medicine, 1981.

CHYLOTHORAX

The accumulation of chyle in the pleural space usually results from accidental or surgical trauma to the thoracic duct. In the newborn, chylothorax can be congenital or secondary to birth trauma. This condition also occurs as a result of superior vena cava obstruction secondary to central venous lines and following Fontan procedures for tricuspid atresia. Symptoms of chylothorax are related to the amount of fluid accumulation and degree of compromise of underlying pulmonary parenchyma. Thoracentesis reveals typical milky fluid (unless the patient has been fasting) containing predominantly T lymphocytes.

Treatment should be conservative because many chylothoraces resolve spontaneously. This includes the use of oral feedings with medium-chain triglycerides to reduce lymphatic flow through the thoracic duct. Drainage of chylous effusions should be performed only in the event of respiratory compromise, because the fluid often rapidly reaccumulates. Repeated or continuous drainage may lead to protein malnutrition and T cell depression, rendering the patient relatively immunocompromised. If reaccumulation of fluid persists for a prolonged period, surgical ligation of the thoracic duct or sclerosis of the pleural space can be attempted, although the results may be less than satisfactory.

Dhande V, Kattwinkel JA, Alford B: Recurrent bilateral pleural effusions secondary to superior vena cava obstruction as a complication of central venous catheterization. Pediatrics 1983;72:109.

McWilliams BC, Fan LL, Murphy SA: Transient T-cell depression in post-operative chylothorax. J Pediatr 1981; 99:595.

Puntis JWL, Roberts KD, Handy D: How should chylothorax be managed? Arch Dis Child 1987;62:593.

PNEUMOTHORAX & RELATED AIR LEAK SYNDROMES

Pneumothorax can occur spontaneously in newborns and in older children or, more commonly, as a result of birth trauma, positive-pressure ventilation, underlying obstructive or restrictive lung disease, and rupture of a congenital or acquired lung cyst. Pneumothorax can also occur as an acute complication of tracheostomy. Usually, air dissects from the alveolar spaces into the interstitial spaces of the lung. Migration to the visceral pleura ultimately leads to rupture into the pleural space. Associated conditions include pneumomediastinum, pneumopericardium, pneumoperitoneum, and subcutaneous emphysema. These conditions are more commonly associated with dissection of air into the interstitial spaces of the lung with retrograde dissection along the bronchovascular bundles toward the hilum.

Clinical Findings

A. Symptoms and Signs: The clinical spectrum can vary from patients who are asymptomatic to those with severe respiratory distress. Associated symptoms include cyanosis, chest pain, and dyspnea. Physical examination may reveal decreased breath sounds and hyperresonance to percussion on the affected side with tracheal deviation to the opposite side. When the pneumothorax is under tension, cardiac function may be compromised, resulting in hypotension or narrowing of the pulse pressure. Pneumopericardium is a life-threatening condition that presents with muffled heart tones and shock. Pneumomomediastinum rarely causes symptoms by itself.

B. Imaging: Chest films usually demonstrate the presence of free air in the pleural space. If the pneumothorax is large and under tension, compressive atelectasis of the underlying lung and shift of the mediastinum to the opposite side may be demonstrated. Cross-table lateral and lateral decubitus films can aid in the diagnosis of free air. Pneumopericardium is identified by the presence of air completely surrounding the heart, whereas in patients with pneumomomediastinum, the heart and mediastinal structures may be outlined with air but the air does not involve the diaphragmatic cardiac border.

Differential Diagnosis

When a patient on a ventilator acutely deteriorates, one must consider not only tension pneumothorax but also obstruction or dislodgment of the endotracheal tube and failure of the mechanical ventilator. Radiographically, pneumothorax must be distinguished from diaphragmatic hernia, lung cysts, congenital lobar emphysema, and cystic adenomatoid malformation, but this task is usually not difficult.

Treatment

Small or asymptomatic pneumothoraces usually do not require treatment and can be managed with close observation. Larger or symptomatic ones usually require drainage, though inhalation of 100% oxygen to wash out blood nitrogen can be tried.

Needle aspiration should be used to relieve tension acutely, followed by chest tube placement. Pneumopericardium requires immediate identification and needle aspiration to prevent death, followed by pericardial tube placement.

In older patients with spontaneous pneumothorax, recurrences are common; sclerosing and surgical procedures are often required.

Fan LL et al: Giant pulmonary cyst simulating a pneumothorax. Am J Dis Child 1988;142:189.

Ogata ES et al: Pneumothorax in the respiratory distress syndrome: Incidence and effect on vital signs, blood gases, and pH. Pediatrics 1976;58:177.

Fackler JC, Yaster M: Multiple trauma in the pediatric patient. In: *Textbook of Pediatric Intensive Care,* 2nd ed. Rogers MC (editor). Williams & Wilkins, 1992.

DISORDERS OF THE MEDIASTINUM

MEDIASTINITIS

Acute infection involving the mediastinum in pediatric patients is usually due to perforation of the esophagus secondary to trauma. The trauma may be self-induced (foreign body, puncture injury to the pharynx with a sharp object) or iatrogenic (endoscopy, attempted endotracheal intubation). Spontaneous esophageal perforation leading to mediastinitis can accompany vomiting, but this is rare. In addition, acute suppurative mediastinitis without trauma does occur but is unusual.

Clinical Findings

A. Symptoms and Signs: The early symptoms and signs of acute mediastinitis may be vague and include the gradual onset of fever, chills, and dysphagia with substernal pain. Dyspnea and cough may also be present. Inspiration may be accompanied by discomfort due to stretching of inflamed mediastinal structures, leading to a pattern of spasmodic or "halting" inspiration. On physical examination, evidence of obstruction of venous return may be present, with substernal pain elicited on palpation of the structures of the thorax. In addition, subcutaneous emphysema may be appreciated in the thoracic and cervical areas.

B. Laboratory Findings and Imaging: The white blood count of the patient with mediastinitis is usually high, with neutrophils and band forms prominent on the differential. The frontal view of the chest x-ray may reveal widening of the upper mediastinum; the lateral view shows anterior displacement of the trachea and the esophagus. Mediastinal emphysema, pleural effusions, and pyopneumothorax may also be present.

Differential Diagnosis

The differential diagnosis includes diseases that lead to the toxic appearance of an infant or child. A primary bacterial pneumonia as well as septicemia must be considered. Retropharyngeal abscesses may also lead to the pattern of respiratory distress seen with a suppurative mediastinitis.

Complications

If not recognized and rapidly treated, this disease can progress rapidly and lead to death. Death may result from the infection or tracheal obstruction. The formation of a mediastinal abscess may also complicate the clinical course of the disease.

Treatment

As soon as the diagnosis is made, parenterally administered broad-spectrum antibiotics must be given. If significant tracheal obstruction is present, an airway must be provided. Drainage of abscesses in the mediastinum may also be indicated.

North J, Emanuel B: Mediastinitis in a child caused by perforation of pharynx. Am J Dis Child 1975;129:962.

Templeton JM: Thoracic emergencies. In: *Textbook of Pediatric Emergency Medicine,* 2nd ed. Fleisher GR, Ludwig S (editors). Williams & Wilkins, 1988.

MEDIASTINAL MASSES

Mediastinal masses may come to a physician's attention because of symptoms produced by pressure on the esophagus, airways, nerves, or vessels within the mediastinum or may be discovered unexpectedly on a routine chest x-ray. Once the mass is identified, localization to one of four mediastinal compartments aids in the differential diagnosis (Figure 20–1). The superior mediastinum is the area above the pericardium that is bordered inferiorly by an imaginary line from the manubrium to the fourth thoracic vertebra. The anterior mediastinum is bordered by the sternum anteriorly and the pericardium posteriorly, whereas the posterior mediastinum is defined by the pericardium and diaphragm anteriorly and the lower eight thoracic vertebrae posteriorly. The middle mediastinum is surrounded by these three compartments.

Clinical Findings

A. Symptoms and Signs: When present, respiratory symptoms are due to pressure on an airway and may include cough, wheezing, and complaints consistent with an infectious process caused by partial or complete obstruction of an airway (unresolving pneumonia in one area of lung, bronchitis). Hemoptysis can also occur but is an unusual presenting symptom. Dysphagia may occur secondary to compression of the esophagus. Encroachment of the mass on the recurrent laryngeal nerve can cause hoarseness due to paralysis of the left vocal cord. Superior vena caval obstruction can lead to dilatation of neck vessels as well as other signs and symptoms of obstruction of venous return from the upper part of the body (superior mediastinal syndrome).

B. Laboratory Findings and Imaging: The mass is initially defined by frontal and lateral chest x-rays together with thoracic CT scans and perhaps MRI. A barium swallow may also help define the extent of a mass. Other studies that may be required include angiography (to define the blood supply to large tumors), electrocardiography, echocardiography, ultrasound of the thorax, fungal and mycobacterial skin tests, and urinary catecholamine assays. A myelogram may be necessary in children suspected of having a neurogenic tumor in the posterior mediastinum.

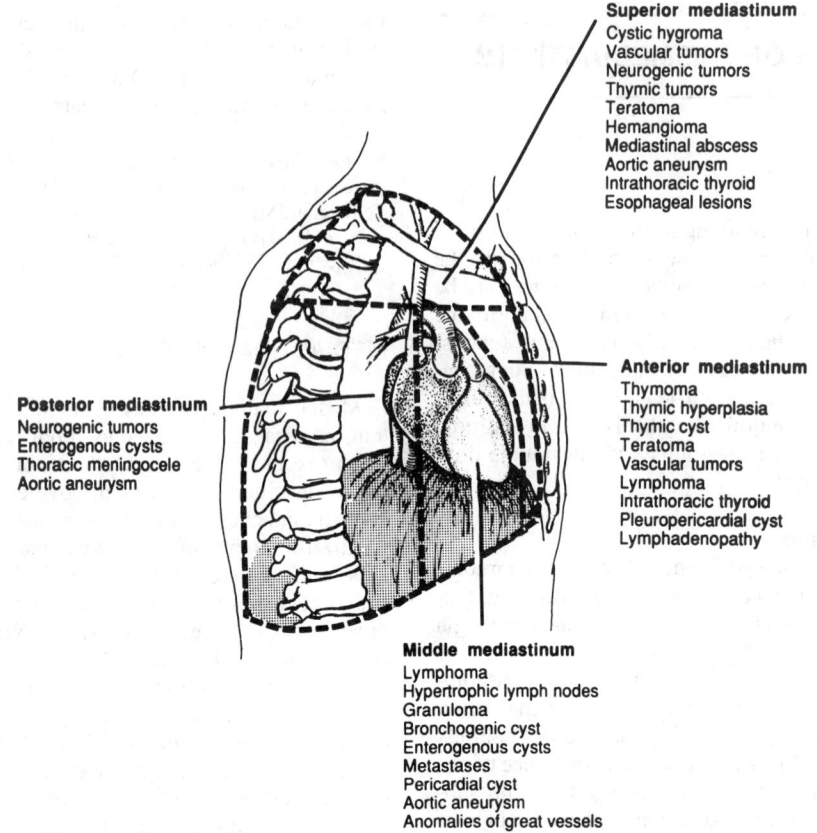

Superior mediastinum
Cystic hygroma
Vascular tumors
Neurogenic tumors
Thymic tumors
Teratoma
Hemangioma
Mediastinal abscess
Aortic aneurysm
Intrathoracic thyroid
Esophageal lesions

Anterior mediastinum
Thymoma
Thymic hyperplasia
Thymic cyst
Teratoma
Vascular tumors
Lymphoma
Intrathoracic thyroid
Pleuropericardial cyst
Lymphadenopathy

Posterior mediastinum
Neurogenic tumors
Enterogenous cysts
Thoracic meningocele
Aortic aneurysm

Middle mediastinum
Lymphoma
Hypertrophic lymph nodes
Granuloma
Bronchogenic cyst
Enterogenous cysts
Metastases
Pericardial cyst
Aortic aneurysm
Anomalies of great vessels

Figure 20–1. Anatomic compartments within the mediastinum. The differential diagnosis of mediastinal masses is based on location within these four compartments.

Differential Diagnosis

The differential diagnosis classified by the mediastinal compartment housing the mass is shown in Figure 20–1. Several general points should be kept in mind. In some series, more than 50% of mediastinal tumors occur in the posterior mediastinum and are mainly neurogenic tumors or enterogenous cysts. Most neurogenic tumors in children under 4 years of age are malignant (neuroblastoma, neuroganglioblastoma), whereas a benign ganglioneuroma is the most common histologic type in older children. In the mid and anterior mediastinum, tumors of lymphatic origin (lymphomas) are the primary concern. Bulky anterior mediastinal tumors that compress the trachea and the great vessels can lead to a superior mediastinal syndrome, and the children can present difficult diagnostic problems because of anesthesia hazards. Definitive diagnosis in most instances relies on surgery to obtain the mass or a part of the mass for a histologic assessment. In cases of lymphoma, the scalene nodes may also contain tumor and may be biopsied in an attempt to establish a diagnosis.

Treatment & Prognosis

Both the appropriate therapy and the response to therapy depend on the cause of the mediastinal mass.

Brooks JW: Tumors of the chest. In: *Disorders of the Respiratory Tract in Children,* 5th ed. Chernick V, Kendig EL Jr (editors). Saunders, 1990.

Filler RM, Simpson HS, Ein SH: Mediastinal masses in infants and children. Pediatr Clin North Am 1979;26:677.

Halpern S et al: Anterior mediastinal masses: Anesthesia hazards and other problems. J Pediatr 1983;102:407.

Templeton JM: Thoracic emergencies. In: *Textbook of Pediatric Emergency Medicine,* 2nd ed. Fleisher GR, Ludwig S (editors). Williams & Wilkins, 1988.

DISORDERS OF THE CONTROL OF BREATHING

ACUTE LIFE-THREATENING EPISODES IN INFANCY

A substantial number of infants are brought to medical attention following apparently acute life-threatening episodes of cardiorespiratory instability involving cyanosis, pallor, or apnea. In one-half of cases, a well-recognized medical entity that accounts for the episode can be found after a thorough and careful evaluation. The infants in whom no explanation for the episode can be found are said to have apnea of infancy. Initial interest in these infants was sparked in part by the observation that some died suddenly, leading some to speculate that such events may provide a clue to the identification of infants at risk for the sudden infant death syndrome (SIDS). After almost 2 decades of study, the picture emerging is that of a weak relationship between apnea of infancy and SIDS, with only a small percentage of patients with apnea of infancy at risk for sudden death. In addition, only a small percentage of infants succumbing to SIDS have identifiable episodes of apnea beforehand.

The following section describes an approach to the patient who has undergone an acute life-threatening episode, taking note of the very broad differential diagnosis in this syndrome and uncertainties in both evaluation and treatment. The clinical features of acute life-threatening episodes are discussed in relationship to the differential diagnosis.

Differential Diagnosis

Table 20–2 lists a classification of disorders associated with acute life-threatening events. A careful history is often the most helpful part of the evaluation. Attention must be focused on the details of episodes. It is useful to determine whether the infant has been chronically ill or essentially well. A report of several days of poor feeding, temperature instability, or respiratory or gastrointestinal symptoms suggests an infectious process. Reports of "struggling to breathe" or "trying to breathe" imply airway obstruction. Association of the episodes with feeding implies discoordinated swallowing, gastroesophageal reflux, or airway obstruction. Episodes that typically follow crying may be related to breath holding. Association of episodes with sleeping may also suggest gastroesophageal reflux or apnea of infancy. Attempts should be made to determine the duration of the episode, but this is often difficult. It is helpful to role-play the episode with the family. Details regarding the measures taken to resuscitate the infant and the

Table 20–2. Differential diagnosis of acute life-threatening episodes (ALTE).

Infectious	Viral: respiratory syncytial virus and other respiratory viruses Bacterial: sepsis, pertussis
Gastrointestinal	Gastroesophageal reflux with or without obstructive apnea
Respiratory	Airway abnormality; vascular rings, pulmonary slings, tracheomalacia Pneumonia
Neurologic	Seizure disorder CNS infection: meningitis, encephalitis Vasovagal response Leigh's encephalopathy Brain tumor
Cardiovascular	Congenital malformation Dysrhythmias Cardiomyopathy
Nonaccidental trauma	Battering Drug overdose Munchausen-by-proxy syndrome
No definable cause	Apnea of infancy

infant's recovery from the episode are often useful in determining the severity of the episode.

The physical examination provides further direction in pursuing the differential diagnosis. The presence of fever or hypothermia suggests infection. An altered state of consciousness implies a postictal state or drug overdose. Respiratory distress implies cardiac or pulmonary lesions.

Most patients are hospitalized for observation in order to reduce stress on the family and allow prompt completion of the evaluation. Laboratory evaluation includes a complete blood count for indications of infection. Serum electrolytes are usually obtained. Elevations in serum bicarbonate suggest chronic hypoventilation, whereas decreases suggest acute acidosis, perhaps due to hypoxia during the episode. Chronic acidosis is suggestive of an inherited metabolic disorder. The chest x-ray film is examined for infiltrates suggesting acute infection or chronic aspiration and for cardiac size as a clue to intrinsic cardiac disease. Arterial blood gas studies provide an initial assessment of oxygenation and acid-base status, and low PaO_2 or elevated $PaCO_2$ (or both) implies cardiorespiratory disease. A significant base deficit suggests that the episode was accompanied by hypoxia or circulatory impairment. On-line oxygen saturation measurements in the hospital assess the infant's oxygenation status during different activities and are more comprehensive than a single blood gas sample.

Because apnea has been associated with respiratory infections, diagnostic studies for infection with respiratory syncytial virus in particular but also other viruses and B pertussis may contribute to the diagnostic process. The apnea seen with infection often precedes other physical findings. If there is any possibility that the episode involved airway obstruction, a barium swallow and air laryngotracheogram should be done. Vascular rings, pulmonary slings, and other intrathoracic lesions impinging upon the trachea are often best demonstrated on barium swallow. The air laryngotracheogram also aids in identifying structural lesions or tracheomalacia. Fiberoptic bronchoscopy may also be used to evaluate the airway. The barium swallow is not done to identify gastroesophageal reflux, because it is presumed that the majority of normal infants demonstrate reflux. If reflux is suspected to be the cause of the apnea, it should be documented by esophageal pH monitoring coupled with respiratory pattern recording. In general, most infants with reflux and apnea can be treated with medical antireflux measures. Infants with reflux and repeated episodes of apnea may benefit from a surgical antireflux procedure.

There are several neurologic causes of acute life-threatening episodes. Apnea as the sole manifestation of a seizure disorder is unusual but may occur. In cases of repeated episodes, 24-hour electroencephalographic monitoring may be helpful in detecting a seizure disorder. Leigh's disease, a brain stem disorder characterized pathologically by neuronal dropout, may present with apneic episodes.

Apneic episodes have been linked to child abuse in several ways. Head injury following nonaccidental trauma may be first brought to medical attention because of apnea. Other signs of abuse are usually immediately apparent in these cases. Drug overdose, either accidental (eg, mistakes in application of anticolic medications containing barbiturates) or intentional, may also present with apnea. Several series document that apneic episodes may be falsely reported by parents seeking attention—one of the instances of Munchausen-by-proxy syndrome. In addition, parents may physically interfere with respiratory efforts. Pinch marks on the nares are sometimes found in these cases.

Treatment

Therapy is directed at the underlying cause if one is found. After blood cultures are taken, antibiotics should be administered to infants who appear toxic. Seizure disorders are treated with anticonvulsants. Vascular rings and pulmonary slings must be corrected surgically because of severe morbidity and high mortality rates in uncorrected cases.

The approach to care in apnea of infancy is controversial. These are infants presenting with acute life-threatening episodes where no definable cause can be ascertained. Treatment in this group of patients has centered around the use of electronic monitors for the detection of apnea or bradycardia in the home. Parents are then taught cardiopulmonary resuscitation so that they may intervene in the event of a serious episode. The rationale for the use of monitors implies that infants who are at risk for subsequent severe epi-

sodes can be identified. Medical personnel have made a number of attempts to predict which infants are at risk for subsequent severe episodes. These attempts have included hypoxic and hypercapnic challenges and determinations of the frequency of periodic breathing or apnea, usually through the use of pneumograms. None of these techniques are sufficiently specific or selective to be useful in prediction. In addition, the efficacy of home monitoring has never been demonstrated in controlled trials.

The decision to monitor these infants involves the participation of the family as well as the physician. Infants with severe initial episodes or repeated severe episodes are now thought to be at significant increased risk for sudden death and should probably be monitored in the home despite the uncertainty of the effectiveness of this step. Episodes in these children are so severe that the parents want to know the infant's condition at all times. Monitoring is not indicated in patients who have isolated episodes of lesser severity unless the parents clearly express a wish for it. Pneumograms can be used to determine whether apnea is occurring if there is uncertainty. However, pneumograms are not predictive and play no role in the decision to monitor or when to stop monitoring. Discontinuing the monitor is usually based on the infant's ability to go several months without triggering the alarm. Aminophylline has been suggested as treatment for apnea of infancy, but controlled trials are lacking; at this point, this drug is not recommended.

Brooks JG: Apparent life-threatening events and apnea of infancy. Clin Perinatol 1992;19:809.

National Institutes of Health Consensus Development Conference Statement: Infantile apnea and home monitoring. Sept 29 to Oct 1, 1986. Pediatrics 1987;79:292.

Southall DP: Role of apnea in the sudden infant death syndrome: A personal view. Pediatrics 1988;81:73.

SUDDEN INFANT DEATH SYNDROME

Essentials of Diagnosis

- Sudden and unexpected death in infancy.
- Adequate postmortem examination excluding known causes of death.

General Considerations

The sudden infant death syndrome (SIDS) is a poorly understood disorder encompassing cases of sudden and unexpected death of previously well or nearly well infants that remain unexplained after an adequate postmortem examination. The postmortem examination is an important feature of the definition because approximately 20% of cases of sudden death can be explained by autopsy findings. The incidence of SIDS in the United States (1–2:1000) makes it the leading cause of death in infancy after the neonatal period. The overall incidence of SIDS has steadily declined over the past few decades.

Epidemiologic and pathologic data constitute most of what is known about SIDS. The number of deaths peaks at age 2 months, and most deaths occur in infants a few weeks of age to 6 months of age. There is an increase in deaths during the peak respiratory virus season, and most deaths occur between midnight and 8:00 AM. The syndrome is more common among minorities and socioeconomically disadvantaged populations. There is a 3:2 male predominance in most series. Other risk factors include low birth weight, teenage or drug-addicted mothers, maternal smoking, and a family history of SIDS. Most of these risk factors are associated with a two- or threefold elevation of incidence but are not specific enough to be useful in predicting which infants will die unexpectedly. Recent immunization is not a risk factor.

The most consistent pathologic findings are intrathoracic petechiae and mild inflammation and congestion of the respiratory tract. Subtler pathologic findings include brain stem gliosis, extramedullary hematopoiesis, and increases in periadrenal brown fat. These latter findings suggest that infants who succumb to SIDS have had intermittent or chronic hypoxia before death.

The mechanism or mechanisms of death in SIDS are unknown. For example, it is not known whether the initiating event at the time of death is cessation of breathing or cardiac dysrhythmia or asystole. Suggested hypotheses have included upper airway obstruction, catecholamine excess, brain stem immaturity or injury, and increased fetal hemoglobin. It has been recognized that some infants who presented with apneic episodes subsequently died from SIDS; however, study of these infants and prospective studies of large numbers of newborns have indicated that most infants with apnea do not die from SIDS and that most infants with SIDS have no identifiable episodes of apnea (see discussion of acute life-threatening episodes, above).

A history of mild symptoms of upper respiratory infection before death is not uncommon, and SIDS victims are sometimes seen by physicians a day or so before death. When infants are discovered blue, cold, and motionless by parents or caretakers, they are most commonly taken to the emergency room, where resuscitative efforts are almost uniformly of no avail. Families must then be supported following the death. The National Sudden Infant Death Syndrome Foundation provides information about psychosocial support groups and counseling for families of SIDS victims. The postmortem examination can be of value to the family; when the diagnosis of SIDS is established, lingering questions about other possible causes of death are resolved. For this reason, as well as for ascertaining causes of death in infancy, postmortem examination should always be recommended. Some recent reports have suggested that a death scene investigation may also be important in determining the cause of sudden unexpected deaths in infancy.

Positioning & SIDS

A variety of recent studies from other countries have presented evidence that the incidence of SIDS is significantly higher when infants are placed in their beds for sleeping in the prone position. A Task Force on Infant Positioning and SIDS of the American Academy of Pediatrics has reviewed these studies and has made the following summary statement:

Based on careful evaluation of existing data indicating an association between Sudden Infant Death Syndrome (SIDS) and prone sleeping position for infants, the Academy recommends that healthy infants, when being put down for sleep, be positioned on their side or back.

This statement has been made with full knowledge of the limitations of many of the studies that were reviewed and with concern for the still valid reasons why certain infants—eg, preterm infants with respiratory distress, infants with gastroesophageal reflux, or certain airway anomalies—do better sleeping in the prone position. Nevertheless, the current evidence is compelling for recommending the side or back position for sleeping in healthy term infants.

AAP Task Force on Infant Positioning and SIDS: Positioning and SIDS. Pediatrics 1992;89:1120.

Bentele KH, Albani M: Are there tests predictive for prolonged apnoea in SIDS? A review of epidemiological and function studies. Acta Paediatr Scand [Suppl] 1988; 342:1.

Giulian GG, Gilbert EF, Moss RL: Elevated fetal hemoglobin levels in sudden infant death syndrome. N Engl J Med 1987;316:1122.

Hoffman HJ et al: Risk factors for SIDS: Results of the National Institute of Child Health and Human Development SIDS Cooperative Epidemiological Study. Ann N Y Acad Sci 1988;533:13.

Ponsonby A-L et al: Factors potentiating the risk of sudden infant death syndrome associated with the prone position. N Engl J Med 1993;329:377.

Southall DP, Talbert DG: Mechanisms for abnormal apnea of possible relevance to the sudden infant death syndrome. Ann N Y Acad Sci 1988;533:329.

Valdes-Dapena M: A pathologist's perspective on possible mechanisms in SIDS. Ann N Y Acad Sci 1988;533:31.

21 Cardiovascular Diseases

Robert R. Wolfe, MD, Mark M. Boucek, MD,
Michael S. Schaeffer, MD, & James W. Wiggins, MD

Cardiovascular disease is a significant cause of death and chronic illness in children. In North America, more than 1% of newborn infants have congenital heart disease, usually due to multifactorial causes. Preventive medicine is the most important aspect of pediatrics, and it is becoming obvious that the prevention of adult heart disease must begin in childhood (eg, prevention of atherosclerosis by diet modification). But prevention requires an understanding of the causes of disease, and in this there are wide discrepancies, ranging from significant accomplishments in the case of rheumatic fever to the very tentative steps being taken to understand the causes of congenital heart disease, atherosclerosis, and essential hypertension.

CLUES TO THE PRESENCE OF HEART DISEASE

Although there are traditional signs and symptoms that suggest heart disease in an infant or child, it is necessary to know how to determine which require immediate attention and which are insignificant. The presence of a heart murmur, for example, may suggest the possibility of heart disease in an infant, or the murmur may be a functional or innocent murmur (see p 519). Not all serious cardiovascular disorders are accompanied by an easily detectable murmur.

The most important clues to the presence of heart disease requiring prompt attention are congestive heart failure and cyanosis. These clinical conditions will be discussed in more detail in subsequent sections.

DIAGNOSTIC EVALUATION

Sequence of Evaluation
(1) History
(2) Physical examination
(3) Electrocardiogram
(4) Chest x-ray
(5) Echocardiogram
(6) Cardiac catheterization (with angiography)

HISTORY

In obtaining the history from the family or the patient, one must keep in perspective the age and relative activity of that patient. A history of increasing feeding difficulties and diaphoresis is the most common feature of early congestive heart failure.

Family History
Most cardiac diseases are familial, so the history of heart disease in a first-degree relative should be sought. These details might suggest the need to evaluate the child for hyperlipidemia.

Pregnancy
The history of pregnancy should elicit information regarding first-trimester exposure to illness or medications, which places infants at high risk for congenital heart disease. A history of significant problems related to labor and delivery, such as perinatal stress or asphyxia at birth, suggests causes of myocardial dysfunction in the neonate.

Growth & Development
Major cardiac problems frequently affect a child's ability to grow. There may be a history of poor feeding (early fatigue, vomiting, lethargy) or of failure to thrive despite adequate caloric intake. Gross motor development may also be delayed in children with significant congestive heart failure or cyanosis, although other aspects of development are less frequently affected.

Tachypnea
Parents frequently notice rapid or abnormal breathing in the child. Although infants at rest rarely breathe faster than 40 respirations per minute, infants in congestive heart failure usually have respiratory rates in excess of 60/min (and often as rapid as 80–

100/min). Tachypnea may be considered the cardinal sign of left-sided heart failure in the pediatric patient.

Cyanosis

Cyanosis is often missed by parents and physicians. The infant with a cyanotic heart lesion may be more gray than blue (and may have no heart murmur). Cyanotic heart disease may go unrecognized because of lack of appreciation of the subtleties of diagnosing cyanosis.

Hypoxemic Spells

It is important to determine if the patient with a cyanotic heart lesion such as tetralogy of Fallot is having hypoxemic spells, because prompt surgical intervention may be required. These spells usually occur on morning awakening or after a feeding or bowel movement; the infant begins breathing fast, becomes progressively more gray or blue, and cries as if having severe pain. Such a spell rarely may progress to unconsciousness, paresis, or even death.

Other Clinical Clues

Orthopnea, dyspnea, easy fatigability, growth failure, sweating, squatting, and pneumonia are frequent clues to the presence of heart disease.

PHYSICAL EXAMINATION

Careful examination of the patient frequently offers the best clues to significant cardiac problems and the probable diagnosis. The presence of other congenital abnormalities, particularly chromosomal disorders, increases the probability of congenital heart disease.

The examination should begin with a careful general inspection to note activity (agitation, lethargy) and skin perfusion and color. Vital signs, including temperature, pulse rate, respiratory rate, and particularly blood pressure (in all four extremities in symptomatic infants), can reflect the overall status of the patient. Auscultation of the heart and lungs should be performed early in the overall examination, because the infant's crying limits the physician's ability to hear even pronounced cardiac sounds. Abdominal examination for position and size of organs is also important.

1. CARDIOVASCULAR EXAMINATION

Inspection & Palpation

Conformation of the chest can give clues to past or present cardiomegaly. Prominence of the precordial chest wall is frequently seen in infants and children with cardiomegaly. Increased cardiac activity is often noted on inspection.

Palpation may reveal precordial activity, right ventricular lift, or left-sided heave; a diffuse point of maximal impulse; or the presence of a thrill due to a loud murmur. Thrills are typically located where the murmur is most intense and can sometimes be felt at the point of radiation, as in a suprasternal notch or carotid thrill with aortic stenosis. In patients with severe pulmonary hypertension, palpable pulmonary closure is frequently noted, usually at the mid to upper left sternal border.

Auscultation

To detect and differentiate abnormal heart sounds, one must be familiar with the pattern and timing of normal heart sounds.

A. Normal Heart Sounds: S_1 (the first heart sound) is the sound of atrioventricular valve closure. It is best heard at the lower left sternal border and is usually medium-pitched. Although four components of S_1 can be detected by phonocardiography, only one or two of these are usually heard with a stethoscope.

S_2 (the second heart sound) is the sound of semilunar valve closure. It has a higher pitch than S_1 and is best heard along the lower and upper left sternal border. S_2 has two component sounds, A_2 and P_2 (aortic and pulmonary valve closure). A_2 is best appreciated at the mid and lower left sternal border, whereas P_2 is best heard at the upper left sternal border and is normally softer than A_2. Splitting of S_2 varies with respirations, widening with inspiration and narrowing with expiration, and is best heard at the second left intercostal space at the sternal border.

S_3 (the third heart sound) is the sound of rapid filling of the left ventricle. It occurs in early diastole, after S_2, and is a medium- to low-pitched thud. When heard in normal children, the sound will diminish or disappear when there is a change from the supine to the sitting or standing position; it is usually also intermittent.

S_4 (the fourth heart sound) is associated with atrial contraction and increased atrial pressure and has a low pitch similar to that of S_3. It occurs just prior to S_1 and is not normally audible.

B. Abnormal Heart Sounds: Abnormalities in splitting or intensity of the component sounds of S_2 can be helpful in the diagnosis of major heart problems. With inspiration, there is a decrease in the intrathoracic pressure; this decrease causes increased filling of the right side of the heart, thereby prolonging the ejection time and delaying closure of the pulmonary valve. Normal intrathoracic pressure changes have little effect on the filling of the left side of the heart. Widening of splitting can be a clue to right-sided volume overload, whereas narrowing may indicate increased pulmonary artery pressure. A single S_2 is often heard in cases of malposition of the great vessels or severe pulmonary hypertension.

Ejection clicks are high-pitched and are usually related to dilated great vessels or valve abnormalities (or both). They can be heard throughout the ventricular systole and are classified as early, mid, or late. Early ejection clicks at the upper left sternal border are usually of pulmonary origin. Aortic clicks are heard in a wider distribution but best at the apex. Widespread clicks originating or loudest at the apex can be mitral or aortic in origin. The mid to late ejection click at the apex is most typically mitral valve prolapse. Early clicks may also be heard in spontaneous closure of ventricular septal defects.

S_3 can be a functional sound in childhood, although it often is associated with cardiac abnormalities.

S_4 is not normally audible; its finding on auscultation is almost always associated with cardiac abnormalities.

C. Murmurs: Murmurs are the most common cardiovascular finding. The presence of a murmur in a child almost always causes alarm in the parents, who associate murmurs with major heart disease. However, most children have functional or innocent murmurs.

1. Characteristics–Murmurs can be evaluated on the basis of the following characteristics:

a. Location and radiation–Where the murmur is best heard and where the sound extends.

b. Relationship to cardiac cycle and duration–Systolic (with the pulse), diastolic, continuous, or to-and-fro.

c. Intensity–Classified as grade I, soft and heard with difficulty; grade II, soft but easily heard; grade III, loud but without a thrill; grade IV, loud and associated with a precordial thrill; grade V, loud, with thrill, and audible with the edge of the stethoscope; or grade VI, very loud and audible with the stethoscope off the chest or with the naked ear.

d. Quality–Harsh, musical, or rough; high, medium, or low in pitch.

e. Variation with position–Audible when patient is supine, sitting, standing, or squatting.

2. Functional murmurs–The seven commonest functional murmurs heard in childhood are as follows:

a. Newborn murmur–As the name implies, this murmur is frequently heard within the first few days of life. Typically, it is located at the lower left sternal border, without significant radiation. Newborn murmur is a soft, short, vibratory grade I–II/VI early systolic murmur that often subsides when mild pressure is applied to the abdomen. Newborn murmur usually disappears by 2–3 weeks of age.

b. Functional murmur of peripheral arterial pulmonary stenosis– This murmur is frequently heard in the premature infant, often after closure of a patent ductus arteriosus. It is secondary to mild narrowing of the branches of the pulmonary artery. Typically, the murmur is heard with equal intensity at the upper left sternal border, back, and in both axillas. It is a soft, short, high-pitched, grade I–II/VI systolic ejection murmur and usually disappears by 6 months

of life. This murmur must be differentiated from true peripheral arterial pulmonary stenosis (rubella syndrome), coarctation of the thoracic aorta, valvular pulmonary stenosis, and atrial septal defect. These entities should, however, have other findings to suggest their organic nature.

c. Still's murmur–Probably the most common murmur of early childhood, this murmur can be heard in infancy, although it is most typically heard from the age of 2 years until adolescence. Classically, Still's murmur is loudest midway between the apex and the lower left sternal border, and often it may be transmitted (depending on loudness) to the remainder of the precordial area. Still's murmur is a musical or vibratory, short, high-pitched, grade I–III early systolic ejection murmur. It is loudest when the patient is in the supine position; it diminishes or disappears when the patient sits or stands or during Valsalva's maneuver. Still's murmur may be louder in patients with fever or tachycardia.

d. Pulmonary outflow ejection murmur–This murmur may be heard throughout childhood. It is usually a soft, short, systolic ejection murmur, grade I–II in intensity and well localized to the upper left sternal border. The murmur becomes louder when the patient is in the supine position or when cardiac output is increased and softens with standing or during Valsalva's maneuver. Pulmonary outflow ejection murmur must be differentiated from other murmurs, such as those associated with pulmonary stenosis, coarctation of the aorta, atrial septal defect, and peripheral pulmonary artery stenosis.

e. Venous hum–This very common murmur of childhood is usually heard after 3 years of age. The murmur is located at the upper right and left sternal borders and in the lower neck. It is described as a continuous musical hum of grade I–II intensity, and it may be accentuated in diastole and with inspiration. This murmur always disappears when the patient is placed in a supine position or when the jugular vein is compressed. Venous hum is thought to be produced by turbulence in the subclavian and jugular veins.

f. Innominate or carotid bruit–This murmur is more common in the older child and adolescent. It is heard in the right supraclavicular and neck areas. This is a long systolic ejection murmur, somewhat harsh and of grade II–III intensity. The bruit can be accentuated by light pressure on the carotid artery and must be differentiated from all types of aortic stenosis.

g. Hemic murmur–Hemic murmurs are heard whenever anemia, fever, stress, or any increase in cardiac output is present. Typically, they are heard best in the aortic and pulmonary areas. These systolic ejection murmurs are of grade I–II intensity and are high-pitched. They disappear with normalization of cardiac output.

Frequently, an experienced listener is able to ascertain that a murmur is functional without performing extensive and expensive laboratory evaluations.

When functional murmurs are found in a child, the physician should assure the parents that these are normal heart sounds of the developing child and that they represent no abnormality of the heart.

3. Organic murmurs–Organic murmurs are evaluated on the basis of the characteristics outlined above (location, intensity, etc). These murmurs will be discussed in relationship to specific lesions later in this chapter.

2. NONCARDIAC EXAMINATION

Arterial Pulse

A. Rate and Rhythm: Cardiac rate and rhythm are usually determined by palpation of the radial or brachial pulse. Throughout infancy and childhood, the rate is subject to great variation. Multiple determinations must be made under properly evaluated conditions before conclusions can be drawn about their significance. This cautious approach is particularly important in infants.

Marked variations in heart rate occur with activity; therefore, the resting heart rate may be most accurately determined during sleep. In older children, exercise and emotional factors have a marked effect upon the heart rate. All of these factors should be taken into account when examining the child, because many children are apprehensive and may react emotionally to the initial phases of the examination. It is possible for normal infants to have heart rates of 180 or 190 during the activity associated with a physical or electrocardiographic examination. Average resting heart rates range from 120/min in infants to 80/min in older children.

In the pediatric age group, the rhythm may be regular, or there may be a phasic variation in the heart rate (sinus arrhythmia), which is normal. Variations occasionally occur without relation to the respiratory cycle.

B. Quality and Amplitude of Pulse: Examination of the cardiovascular system should always include comparison of the pulses of the upper and lower extremities. A bounding pulse is characteristic of patent ductus arteriosus or aortic regurgitation. Narrow or thready pulses are found in patients with congestive heart failure or severe aortic stenosis.

The suprasternal notch should be examined, where visible pulsation is usually abnormal, although it may be seen in patients who are emotionally excited. A prominent pulsation is found in aortic insufficiency, patent ductus arteriosus, and coarctation of the aorta. A palpable thrill in the suprasternal notch is characteristic of aortic stenosis and is occasionally found with valvular pulmonary stenosis, coarctation of the aorta, and patent ductus arteriosus.

Assessment of the femoral pulse is an essential part of the physical examination of every infant and child. The femoral pulse should be readily palpable and equal in amplitude and time of appearance with the brachial pulse. A femoral pulse that is absent or weak or one that is delayed in comparison with the brachial pulse suggests coarctation of the aorta. An absent or diminished femoral pulse may be the only clue to the cause of a life-threatening problem.

Arterial Blood Pressure

Blood pressures should be obtained in the upper and lower extremities. Systolic pressure in the lower extremities determined by the auscultatory technique is usually higher than that found in the upper extremities in patients *over age 1 year*. In normal infants, the pressure in the arms may be higher. The cuff must cover the same relative area of the arm and leg; for this reason, a larger cuff usually must be used for the leg than for the arm.

A. Procedures: Because of variation of blood pressure with respiration and slower rhythmic variations (Mayer or Traube-Hering waves), pressure obtained by any method should be repeated several times.

1. Auscultatory method–Hearing Korotkoff sounds by stethoscope and sphygmomanometer is the commonest measure of blood pressure in children and correlates well with direct intra-arterial measurements. However, many factors affect its accuracy. Among these are the dimensions of the inflatable bag within the cuff. The length of the bag should be 100% and the width 50% of the circumference of the limb. A cuff that is too narrow or too short will produce a blood pressure reading that is higher than the true pressure.

2. Palpatory method–Palpation of the pulse characteristics distal to the occluding cuff provides an approximation of the systolic blood pressure in the infant.

3. Flush method–The flush method is also useful in small infants. The distal foot or hand is blanched by manual squeezing or application of an elastic bandage, and the cuff is inflated above the systolic pressure. The extremity is then observed as the cuff pressure is slowly reduced. The observed flush corresponds to a value approximating that of the systolic pressure. A useful technique for assessing coarctation of the aorta is to apply the cuffs to the upper and lower extremities simultaneously and observe flushing.

4. Doppler ultrasound or automated blood pressure method–The combination of a small ultrasound transducer and a sphygmomanometer has proved to be especially applicable to the small infant. Considerations of cuff dimensions are still critical, however.

B. Pulse Pressure: Pulse pressure is determined by subtracting the diastolic pressure from the systolic pressure. Normally, the pulse pressure is less than 50 mm Hg or less than half the systolic pressure. A widened pulse pressure (which is associated with a bounding pulse) is present in aorticopulmonary shunt (eg, patent ductus arteriosus), aortic insufficiency, fever, anemia, and complete heart block. A narrow pulse pressure is seen in congestive heart failure, severe aortic stenosis, and pericardial tamponade.

Venous Pressure & Pulse

The level of the distended jugular vein above the suprasternal notch when the patient is at a 45-degree angle is a measure of venous pressure in older children and adults. Normally, one may observe the level of the transition between collapse and distention of the jugular vein approximately 1–2 cm above the notch. In addition to the level of the pulse, the wave pattern should be observed. Two waves can frequently be seen: (1) The *a* wave, due to right atrial contraction, is a rather sharply rising wave and therefore occurs immediately before or with the first heart sound or point of maximum impulse. (2) The *v* wave, caused by filling of the right atrium during ventricular systole, is a more slowly rising wave and occurs toward the end of ventricular systole. The venous pulse is not too helpful in examining infants and young children, however, because their necks are short and fat.

Extremities

Cyanosis of the extremities usually indicates congenital heart disease, but severe pulmonary disease must be excluded. Cyanosis is characterized by a bluish discoloration of the nails, but the entire distal portion of the extremity may be involved.

A. Clubbing of Fingers and Toes: Clubbing implies fairly severe cyanotic congenital heart disease. It usually does not appear until approximately age 1, although occasionally, in patients with severe cyanosis, it may occur earlier. The first sign of clubbing is softening of the nail beds, followed by rounding of the fingernails and then by thickening and shininess of the terminal phalanx, with loss of creases.

Cyanosis is by far the most common cause, but clubbing occurs also in patients with infective endocarditis, severe liver disease, and lung abscess.

B. Edema: Edema of the lower extremities is characteristic of right ventricular heart failure in older children and adults. However, in infants and younger children, peripheral edema is more likely to affect first the face, then the presacral region, and eventually the extremities.

Abdomen

Hepatomegaly is the cardinal sign of right heart failure in the infant and child. Presystolic pulsation of the liver may occur with right atrial hypertension and systolic pulsation with tricuspid insufficiency. Congestive splenomegaly may be present in patients who have had long-standing congestive heart failure. Enlargement of the spleen is one of the characteristic features of subacute infective endocarditis. Ascites is occasionally present in right heart failure.

Ferencz C, Villasenor AC: Epidemiology of cardiovascular malformations: The state of the art. Cardiol Young 1991; 1:264.

Nelson WP, Egbert AM: How to measure blood pressure accurately. Primary Cardiol (Sept) 1984;10:14.

Smythe JF et al: Initial evaluation of heart murmurs: Are laboratory tests necessary? Pediatrics 1990;86:497.

ELECTROCARDIOGRAM & VECTORCARDIOGRAM

The electrocardiogram (ECG) is an essential part of the evaluation of the cardiovascular system. The ECG is the sine qua non for the diagnosis of dysrhythmias and may offer the best clue to the specific diagnosis of congenital lesions (eg, left axis deviation in a blue baby, suggesting tricuspid atresia). Conversely, the ECG may provide little or no help (as in assessing right ventricular hypertrophy in the newborn or left ventricular hypertrophy in the child with congenital aortic stenosis).

It is not possible, within the limitations of this presentation, to teach the interpretation of the ECG, but a few basic facts and definitions should help to orient the student.

A. Propagation of Electrical Force: As shown in Figure 21–1, a wave of electrical force traveling toward an electrode inscribes a positive (upward) deflection; away from an electrode, a negative deflection; and perpendicular to an electrode, a low-voltage, isodiphasic complex. These forces are inscribed as loops on the vectorcardiogram (VCG), and abnormalities are manifested as alterations in direction and duration of force or as increased or decreased electrical force (amplitude of QRS complex on ECG or loop on VCG).

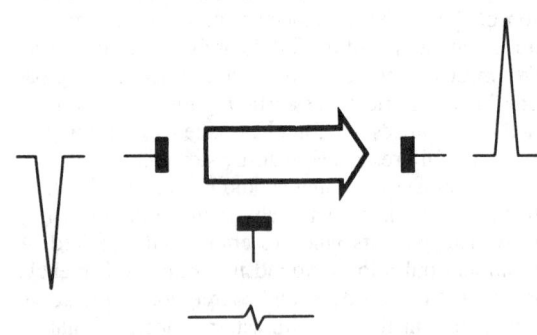

Figure 21–1. Depolarization of the myocardium. The arrow represents the wave of electrical force. As it travels toward the electrode, it inscribes a positive (upward) deflection; away from the electrode, a negative (downward) deflection; perpendicular to the electrode, a low-voltage, isodiphasic deflection.

B. Age-Related Variations: The ECG and VCG evolve with the age of the patient. The rate gradually decreases and intervals generally increase with age. There is also progressive change in dominance of ventricles from right ventricular dominance in the young infant to left ventricular dominance in the older infant, child, and adult. The normal ECG of the 1-week-old would be highly abnormal for a 1-year-old, and the ECG of a 5-year-old would not be normal for an adult.

C. Electrocardiographic Interpretation: Figure 21–2 defines the events recorded on the ECG. The sequence of recording the findings of the ECG is usually as follows: rate, rhythm, P wave, PR interval, QRS complex (including axis, amplitude, and duration), QT interval, ST segment, T wave, and impression.

1. Rate–The paper speed at which ECGs are usually taken is 25 mm/s. Each small square is 1 mm and each large square 5 mm. Therefore, five large squares represent 1 s, one large square 0.2 s, and one small square 0.04 s. A common method of estimating the ventricular rate is to count the number of large squares between two QRS complexes: If QRS complexes appear at a rate of one per large square (5/s), the ventricular rate is 300; if QRS complexes appear every two squares, the ventricular rate is 150, etc. The formula is to divide the number of large squares between QRS complexes into 300 and roughly interpolate for fractions of large squares.

2. Rhythm–Normal sinus rhythm consists of a normal P wave followed by a normal PR interval and a normal QRS complex.

3. P wave–The P wave represents atrial depolarization. In the pediatric patient, it is normally not taller than 2.5 mm or more than 0.08 s in duration.

4. PR interval–This interval is measured from the beginning of the P wave to the beginning of the QRS complex. It increases with age and with slower rates. The PR interval ranges from a minimum of 0.11 s in infants to a maximum of 0.18 s in older children with slow rates. The PR interval is commonly prolonged in rheumatic heart disease and by digitalis.

5. QRS complex–This represents ventricular depolarization, and its amplitude and direction of force (axis) reveal the relative size of (viable) ventricular mass in hypertrophy, hypoplasia, and infarction. Abnormal ventricular conduction (eg, right bundle branch block, anterior fascicular block) is also revealed. Interpretation of the QRS complex is one of the most important aspects of cardiologic diagnosis.

6. QT interval–This interval is measured from the beginning of the QRS complex to the end of the T wave. The QT duration is affected by drugs such as digitalis and electrolyte imbalances such as hypocalcemia and hypokalemia (really QU interval prolongation). The normal duration is rate-related, and must be corrected using the following formula:

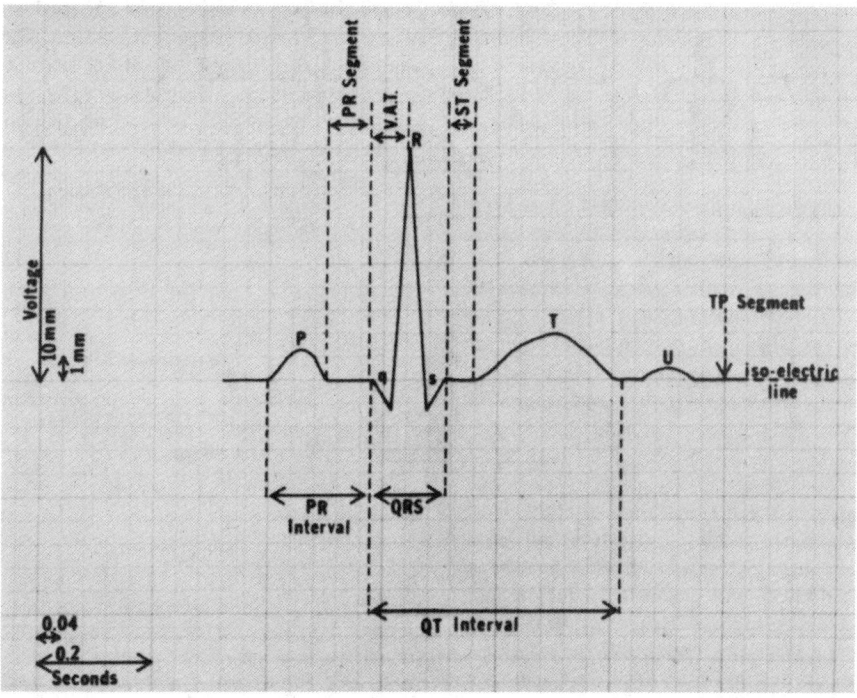

Figure 21–2. Complexes and intervals of the electrocardiogram.

$$QT_c = \frac{QT\ interval(s)}{\sqrt{R - R\ interval(s)}}$$

The normal QT_c is usually less than 0.44 s.

7. ST segment–This short segment lying between the end of the QRS complex and the beginning of the T wave is affected by drugs and electrolyte imbalances and reflects myocardial injury.

8. T wave–The T wave represents myocardial repolarization and is altered by electrolytes, myocardial hypertrophy, and ischemia.

9. Impression–The ultimate impression of the ECG is derived from a systematic analysis of features such as those described above as compared with expected normal values for the age of the child.

D. Vectorcardiographic Interpretation: The VCG reveals much of the same information as the ECG. In fact, it is possible to draw the QRS loop of the VCG with considerable accuracy from QRS complexes of the ECG. Figure 21–3 displays the ECG and VCG of the same patient. The vector interpretation of the ECG (eg, direction and shape of loop) derived by looking at the ECG is perhaps the major contribution of vectorcardiography. It is usually not necessary to obtain an actual VCG to know what the loops look like.

Gillette PC, Garson A Jr: *Pediatric Arrhythmias: Electrophysiology and Pacing.* Saunders, 1990.

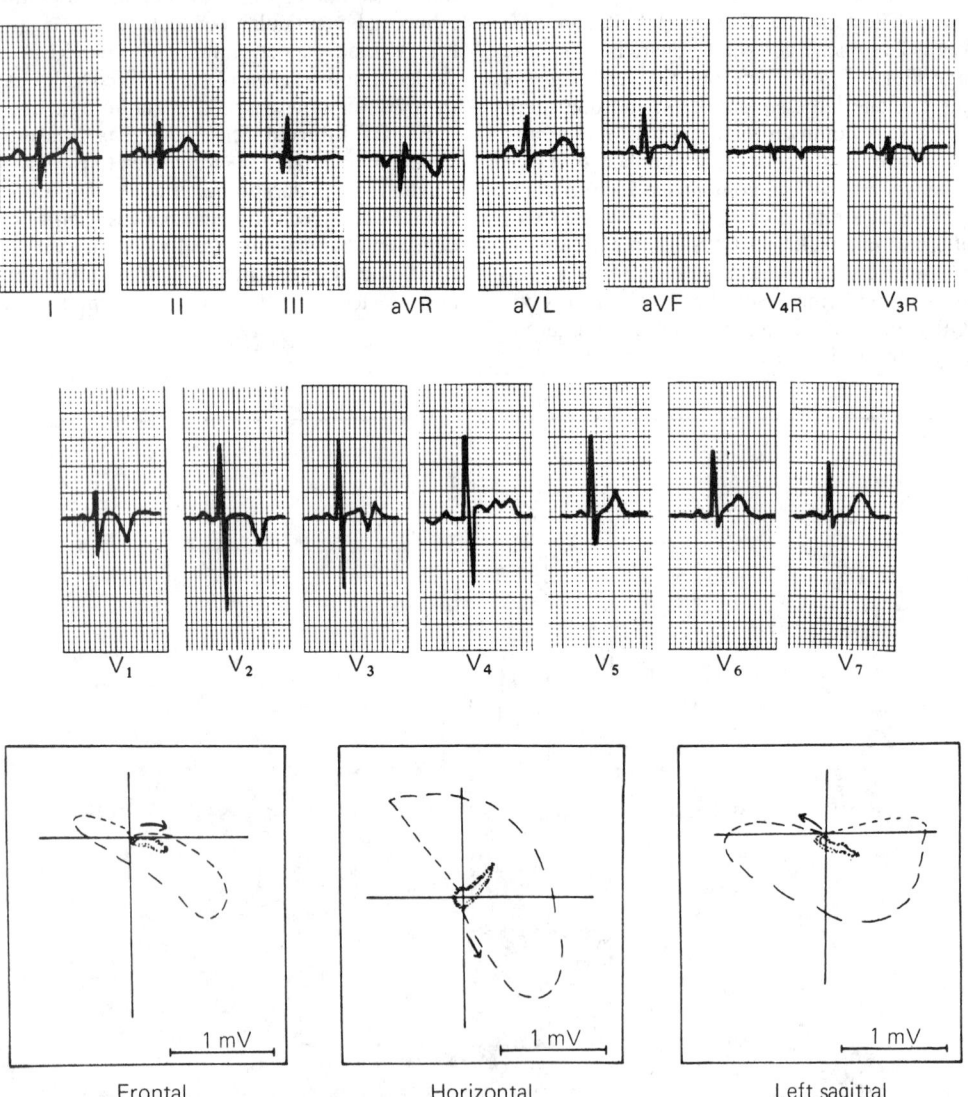

Figure 21–3. Electrocardiographic and vectorcardiographic findings in the same 10-month-old infant. The direction, duration, and magnitude of electrical force are comparable in each tracing.

Goldman MJ: *Principles of Clinical Electrocardiography,* 12th ed. Lange, 1986.

Liebman J, Plonsey R, Gillette PC: *Pediatric Electrocardiography.* Williams & Wilkins, 1982.

CHEST X-RAY

The chest x-ray requires systematic evaluation. Accurate conclusions about the presence or absence of congenital heart defects and bone abnormalities can only be drawn if the proper procedures were followed—eg, the penetration of x-ray was adequate, and the films were obtained on adequate inspiration (distortions due to inadequate inspiration may look like cardiomegaly and increased vascular markings). The size of the heart, as seen on the chest x-ray film, must be evaluated in relationship to the age and size of the patient. Chest films of the normal newborn will show a greater heart size and more pronounced vascular markings than those of the normal older child. These factors must all be taken into consideration in evaluating heart size and configuration and lung fields. The standard posteroanterior and left lateral chest films are usually adequate for this evaluation (Figure 21–4). If there is suspicion of vascular ring or mediastinal mass, multiple-view films with barium swallow are indicated.

Condon V: The heart and great vessels. In: *Caffey's Pediatric X-Ray Diagnosis: An Integrated Imaging Approach.* Silverman FN (editor). Year Book, 1985.

ECHOCARDIOGRAPHY & DOPPLER ULTRASONOGRAPHY

Echocardiography is now the major noninvasive method for diagnosis of congenital heart defects and is used to define anatomy, function, chamber and vessel size, and valve abnormalities. The use of M mode and two-dimensional echocardiography will in most instances allow accurate diagnosis. These methods, along with Doppler ultrasonography (color, pulsed, or continuous wave ultrasound measurements) can now be used to predict cardiac output, flow direction, valve gradients, and pulmonary artery pressure. Interpretation of the results of these studies requires the skill of the pediatric cardiologist. In cases of major heart disease, cardiac catheterization should also be performed.

Goldberg SJ et al: *Doppler Echocardiography,* 2nd ed. Lea & Febiger, 1988.

Seward JB et al: *Two Dimensional Echocardiographic Atlas: Congenital Heart Disease,* Springer-Verlag, 1987.

Snider AR, Serwer GA: *Echocardiography in Pediatric Heart Disease,* Year Book, 1990.

NUCLEAR CARDIOLOGY

Current use of radionuclide tracers in infants and children includes detection and quantification of left-to-right and right-to-left intracardiac shunting, quantification of cardiac output at rest and during exercise using gated blood pool scintigraphy, and myocardial imaging with thallium-201 for ischemia or infarction. In the older child, the latter method can be enhanced by exercise stress testing. These tests yield more objective data for evaluation of children with heart disease.

Schaffer MS, Gilday DL: Pediatric cardiovascular nuclear medicine. In: *Cardiovascular Nuclear Medicine,* Appleton & Lange, 1988.

Wiles HB: Nuclear cardiology. In: *The Science and Practice of Pediatric Cardiology.* Garson A Jr, Bricker JT, McNamara DG (editors). Lea & Febiger, 1990.

MAGNETIC RESONANCE IMAGING

Magnetic resonance imaging (MRI) is now a valuable tool in the evaluation and noninvasive follow-up of many congenital heart defects. Particularly in the

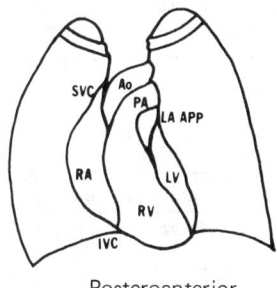

Posteroanterior

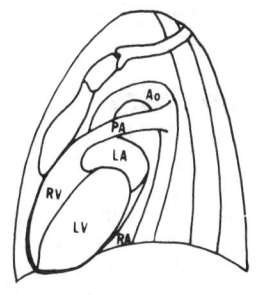

Left lateral

Figure 21–4. Position of cardiovascular structures in principal x-ray views. (RV, right ventricle; LA, left atrium; LA APP, left atrial appendage; LV, left ventricle; Ao, aorta; PA, pulmonary artery; SVC, superior vena cava; IVC, inferior vena cava.)

imaging of vascular structures of the thorax, MRI can only be matched by angiography. The addition of "gated" imaging or cine MRI now allows dynamic evaluation of the structure and blood flow patterns within the heart and great vessels. MRI is invaluable in the long-term follow up of coarctation of the aorta after angioplasty.

Boxer RA et al: Cardiac magnetic resonance imaging in children with congenital heart disease. J Pediatr 1986; 109:460.

Friedman BJ et al: Comparison of magnetic resonance imaging and echocardiography in determination of cardiac dimensions in normal subjects. J Am Coll Cardiol 1985; 5:1369.

Vick GW, Rohey R, Johnston DL: Nuclear magnetic resonance and positron emission tomography. In: *The Science and Practice of Pediatric Cardiology.* Garson A Jr, Bricker JT, McNamara DG (editors). Lea & Febiger, 1990.

ERGOMETRY

Pediatric ergometry is a newly evolving technique. It has long been hampered by lack of appreciation of its applications and availability of normal data. Most children with heart disease are capable of normal activity, and exercise data are essential to prevent overprotection. The response to exercise is valuable in determining the need for cardiovascular surgery and its timing. Bicycle ergometers or treadmills can often be employed to test children as young as 6 years. Important exercise parameters include stress ECGs, conditioning, and performance data. Significant stress ischemia or dysrhythmias warrant physical restrictions or appropriate therapy. Children demonstrating poor performance with suboptimal conditioning benefit from an exercise prescription. The pre- and postoperative child can then be objectively guided into appropriate recreational and competitive activities and given prevocational guidance.

Christianson JL, Strong WD: Exercise testing. In: *Heart Disease in Infants, Children and Adolescents,* 4th ed. Adams FH, Emmanouilides GC, Riemenschneider TA (editors). Williams & Wilkins, 1989.

ARTERIAL BLOOD GASES
(Arterial PO$_2$, Systemic O$_2$ Saturation)

Because cyanosis is difficult to measure (and sometimes to recognize) by inspection of the patient, objective laboratory determinations are required. The quantitative response of arterial PO$_2$ or O$_2$ saturation (eg, by pulse oximetry) to administration of 100% oxygen is one of the most useful methods of distinguishing cyanosis produced by heart disease from cyanosis

related to lung disease in sick infants. In cyanotic heart disease, PaO$_2$ increases very little from values obtained while breathing ambient room air as compared with values during 100% oxygen administration. However, there is usually a very significant increase in PaO$_2$ when oxygen is administered to a patient with lung disease. Continuous noninvasive methods for monitoring arterial PO$_2$ include the transcutaneous O$_2$ monitor and pulse oximetry. Inherent limitations have prevented the general substitution of these noninvasive methods for direct arterial sampling in this evaluation, but they are valuable in overall cardiopulmonary care of the sick infant. Table 21–1 illustrates the sort of response one might expect following at least 10 minutes of 100% oxygen administration to cyanotic infants with heart disease versus lung disease.

OTHER NONINVASIVE LABORATORY STUDIES

In children of all ages, but particularly in the infant and newborn, many metabolic abnormalities can have a major influence on the performance of the cardiovascular system. In evaluating the symptomatic infant, it is important to rule out infection, hypoglycemia, hypocalcemia, hypovolemia, hyperkalemia, inborn errors of metabolism, anemia, etc. Likewise, severe cardiovascular problems may be accompanied by some of these abnormalities.

CARDIAC CATHETERIZATION & ANGIOCARDIOGRAPHY

The definitive anatomic and physiologic study of infants and children with heart disease is cardiac catheterization. It is essential for the primary physician to distinguish those infants and children who require the specialized diagnostic and therapeutic facilities of the pediatric cardiac center from those who may be safely managed without such facilities and consultation. On the basis of the preceding steps of diagnostic evaluation—history, physical examination, ECG, chest x-ray, and other noninvasive laboratory studies—the consulting pediatric cardiologist has a rather precise assessment of the anatomic and

Table 21–1. Examples of responses to 10 minutes of 100% oxygen in lung disease and heart disease.

	Lung Disease		Heart Disease	
	Room Air	100% O$_2$	Room Air	100% O$_2$
Color	Blue →	Pink	Blue →	Blue
Oximetry	60% →	99%	60% →	62%
Pao$_2$ (mm Hg)	35 →	120	35 →	38

physiologic abnormalities in simple malformations and considerable useful information about complex malformations.

Indications & Objectives
A. Infants:
1. Indications–

a. Infants with cyanosis presumed to be cardiovascular in origin should be catheterized as soon as a reasonably stable clinical condition can be achieved. This should be performed for diagnosis of anatomic abnormalities not easily appreciated by echocardiography and for therapeutic interventions such as balloon atrial septostomy or valvuloplasty of a stenotic pulmonary or aortic valve.

b. Infants with severe congestive heart failure that does not respond promptly and satisfactorily to anticongestive measures.

c. Infants in whom early operation for congenital heart disease is contemplated.

d. Infants in whom the anatomic and physiologic abnormality is sufficiently vague that appropriate medical management is not possible.

e. Infants who have evidence of complicating or potentially progressive problems, such as pulmonary hypertension.

2. Objectives–(In descending order of importance.)

a. To perform the study with the lowest possible rate of death or serious complications. Pediatric cardiologists and pediatric cardiac catheterization laboratories with experience in studying infants are required so that these objectives can be met: to gain meaningful information promptly; to care for the critically ill infant with temperature and pH control, fluid management, and all essential pediatric treatment; and to anticipate and handle life-threatening crises.

b. To gain information which is not available by other methods and which will provide the basis for therapeutic decisions (medical or surgical).

c. To provide therapeutic intervention (eg, Rashkind septostomy, balloon valvuloplasty).

d. To obtain sufficient physiologic and anatomic data so that repeat catheterization to complete the study will not be necessary.

B. Children:
1. Indications–

a. All children for whom heart surgery is contemplated (with the exception of children with unequivocal patent ductus arteriosus or atrial septal defect [or both] or other uncomplicated anatomy or physiology).

b. All children in whom there is question about the anatomic or physiologic abnormality which would significantly influence management and which cannot be completely answered by noninvasive methods.

c. Children with progressive lesions that require careful physiologic monitoring (such as pulmonary hypertension).

d. Children who have had cardiovascular surgery and require assessment of the adequacy of the repair.

e. Children with mild to moderate cardiovascular lesions when important information about the natural history is required. This procedure should be done only in the setting of a well-designed protocol and fully informed consent.

2. Objectives–It goes without saying that conducting the study with the lowest possible risk is the most important objective of cardiac catheterization of the child as well as the infant; and the risk to the child ($< 0.2\%$) is certainly much less than to the sick infant (2%). Complete anatomic and physiologic data are important objectives of catheterization in children and infants. No physician or laboratory should undertake the catheterization of a child unless prepared to obtain a completely informative study and unless physicians and surgeons are available who are capable of proceeding with whatever medical or surgical therapy may be indicated.

Contraindications
Cardiac catheterization is contraindicated in infants and children who present with no clinical urgency and none of the indications listed above. It should not be done if personnel and facilities fail to meet high standards of patient safety and clinical diagnostic and therapeutic expertise.

Cardiac Catheterization Data
Figure 21–5 shows oxygen saturation (in percent) and pressure (in mm Hg) values obtained at cardiac catheterization from the chambers and great arteries of the heart. These values would be within the normal range for a child.

A. Oxygen Content and Saturation; Pulmonary and Systemic Blood Flow (Cardiac Output): In most laboratories, evidence of left-to-right shunt is determined by changes of blood oxygen content or saturation during passage of the catheter through the right side of the heart. A significant increase in oxygen content or oxygen saturation from one chamber to another indicates the presence of a left-to-right shunt at the site of the increase. The oxygen saturation of the peripheral arterial blood should always be determined during cardiac catheterization. Normal arterial oxygen saturation is 91–97%. A decrease (at sea level) below 91% suggests the presence of a right-to-left shunt, underventilation, or pulmonary disease.

The size of a left-to-right shunt is usually expressed as a ratio of the pulmonary to systemic blood flow or as liters per minute as determined by the Fick principle:

$$\frac{\text{Cardiac output}}{\text{(L/min)}} = \frac{\text{Oxygen consumption (mL/min)}}{\text{Arteriovenous difference (mL/L)}}$$

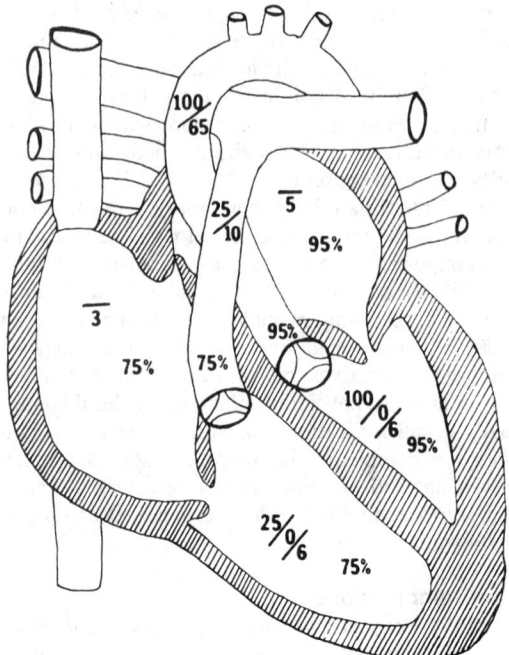

Figure 21–5. Pressures (in mm Hg) and oxygen saturation (in percent) obtained by cardiac catheterization in a normal child. (3 = mean pressure of 3 mm Hg in right atrium; 5 = mean pressure of 5 mm Hg in left atrium.)

B. Pressures: Pressures should be determined in all chambers and vessels entered. Pressures should always be recorded when a catheter is pulled back from a distal chamber or vessel into a more proximal chamber. It is not normal for systolic pressure in the ventricles to exceed systolic pressure in the great arteries or mean diastolic pressure in the atria to exceed end-diastolic pressure in the ventricles. If a "gradient" in pressure does exist, it means that there is obstruction, and the severity of the gradient is one criterion for the necessity of operative repair. A right ventricular systolic pressure of 100 mm Hg and a pulmonary artery systolic pressure of 20 mm Hg yield a gradient of 80 mm Hg. In this case, the patient would be classified as having severe pulmonary stenosis requiring repair.

C. Pulmonary and Systemic Vascular Resistance: The vascular resistance is calculated from the following formula and reported in units or in dynes-sec-cm^{-5}/m^2:

$$\text{Resistance} = \frac{\text{Pressure}}{\text{Flow}}$$

Pulmonary vascular resistance equals mean pulmonary artery pressure minus the mean pulmonary artery wedge or left atrial pressure divided by pulmonary blood flow per square meter of body surface area. (Pulmonary blood flow is determined from the Fick principle, as noted previously.) **Systemic vascular resistance** equals mean systemic arterial pressure minus the mean central nervous pressure divided by systemic blood flow.

Normally, the pulmonary vascular resistance ranges from 1 to 3 units, or 80 to 240 dynes-sec-cm^{-5}/m^2. If pulmonary resistance is above 10 units or the pulmonary/systemic resistance ratio is above 0.7, all other diagnostic findings should be reviewed carefully to confirm the presence of pulmonary hypertension that is so severe as to render the patient inoperable.

D. Special Techniques: Special techniques employed during cardiac catheterization include the following:

1. Hydrogen electrode catheter–Used to determine the presence of very small left-to-right shunts, this technique enables the operator to detect such shunts even in the absence of any increase in oxygen saturation.

2. Indicator dilution curves–This involves injection of an indicator, such as indocyanine green (Cardio-Green), at specific places in the heart and detection of the dye downstream, usually in a peripheral artery. This technique permits the detection of both right-to-left and left-to-right shunts at the specific points within the cardiovascular system. Cardiac output is frequently determined by this method.

3. Selective angiocardiography and cineangiocardiography–In this technique, contrast material is injected in a specific chamber or vessel and the course of the contrast material followed by serial large film x-rays (angiocardiography) or by motion pictures (cineangiocardiography).

4. Contrast echocardiography–Saline or indocyanine green is rapidly injected via the cardiac catheter, and downstream "clouding" is imaged with either M mode or two-dimensional echocardiography. Dynamic spatial or structural relationships of chambers, valves, and vessels are visualized; this procedure may be done repetitively without the risk of radiation.

5. Interventional catheterization–Specially designed catheters are now used for dilatation of stenotic valves and vascular structures. Balloon valvuloplasty/angioplasty is now the treatment of choice for valve pulmonary stenosis, coarctation of the thoracic aorta, aortic valve stenosis and pulmonary arterial stenoses. Other valve and vascular stenoses are being evaluated along with special occluding devices for closing patent ductus arteriosus and atrial septal defects. Many simple defects are now treated effectively through these and other procedures.

Nihil MR: Catheterization and angiography. In: *The Science and Practice of Pediatric Cardiology.* Garson A Jr, Bricker JT, McNamara DG (editors). Lea & Febiger, 1990.

Perry SB, Keane JF, Locke JE: Interventional catheterizations in pediatric congenital and acquired heart disease. Am J Cardiol 1988;61:109G.

PRENATAL & NEONATAL CIRCULATION

Fetal Circulation

In the fetus, the placenta is the organ of respiration and for exchange of waste products. Oxygenated blood (approximately 80% saturated) passes from the placenta through the umbilical vein to the heart. As it flows toward the heart, it mixes with blood from the inferior vena cava and from the portal vein, so that blood entering the right atrium is approximately 65% saturated. A considerable amount of this blood is shunted immediately across the foramen ovale into the left atrium. The venous blood derived from the upper part of the body is much less saturated (approximately 30%), and most of it enters the right ventricle through the tricuspid valve. Thus, the blood in the right ventricle is a mixture of both relatively highly saturated blood from the umbilical vein and desaturated blood from the venae cavae. This mixture results in a blood oxygen saturation of approximately 50% in the right ventricle.

The blood in the left atrium is derived from the blood shunting across the foramen ovale and the blood returning from the pulmonary veins. A great deal of the left ventricular output goes to the head, whereas the lower portion of the body is supplied by blood both from the right ventricle, through the patent ductus arteriosus, and from the left ventricle.

Physiologic Changes at Birth & in the Neonatal Period

At birth, two dramatic events that affect the cardiovascular and pulmonary system occur: (1) the umbilical cord is clamped, removing the placenta from the circulation; and (2) breathing commences. As a result, marked changes in the circulation occur. During fetal life, the placenta offers little resistance to the flow of blood, so that the systemic circuit is a low-resistance one. On the other hand, the pulmonary arterioles are markedly constricted and offer strong resistance to the flow of blood into the lung. Clamping the cord causes a sudden increase in resistance to flow in the systemic circuit. As the lung becomes the organ of respiration, the oxygen tension (PO_2) increases in the vicinity of the small pulmonary arterioles, resulting in a release of the constriction and thus a significant decrease in the pulmonary arteriolar resistance. Indeed, the pulmonary vascular resistance shortly after birth is less than that of the systemic circuit.

Because of the changes in resistance, the great majority of the right ventricular outflow now passes into the lung rather than through the ductus arteriosus into the descending aorta. In fact, functional closure of the ductus arteriosus begins to develop shortly after birth.

Recent studies have demonstrated that the ductus arteriosus remains patent for a variable period, usually 24–48 hours. During the first hour after birth, there is a small right-to-left shunt (as in the fetus). However, after 1 hour, bidirectional shunting occurs, with the left-to-right direction predominating. In most cases, right-to-left shunting completely disappears by 8 hours. However, in patients with severe hypoxia (eg, in respiratory distress syndrome), the pulmonary vascular resistance remains quite elevated, resulting in a continued right-to-left shunt. The cause of the functional closure of the ductus arteriosus is not completely known. However, evidence indicates that the increased PO_2 of the arterial blood causes spasm of the ductus. Anatomically, however, the ductus arteriosus does not close until approximately age 3 months.

In fetal life, the foramen ovale serves as a one-way valve, permitting shunting of blood from the inferior vena cava through the right atrium into the left atrium. At birth, because of the changes in the pulmonary and systemic vascular resistance and the increase in the quantity of blood returning from the pulmonary veins to the left atrium, the left atrial pressure rises above that of the right atrium. This functionally closes the flap of the one-way valve, essentially preventing flow of blood across the septum. It has been shown, however, that a small right-to-left shunt does continue for the first week of life. Although the foramen ovale remains functionally closed throughout life, it remains patent in about 25% of patients.

A clinical syndrome has been recognized that is characterized in term infants by onset of tachypnea, cyanosis, and clinical evidence of pulmonary hypertension during the first 8 hours after delivery. These infants have massive right-to-left ductal or foramen shunting or both for 3–7 days because of the high pulmonary vascular resistance. The clinical course is generally one of progressive cor pulmonale, hypoxia, and acidosis, terminating in early death unless the pulmonary resistance can be lowered. The resistance can usually be reversed by instituting appropriate means to increase alveolar PO_2: high-frequency, low tidal volume hyperventilation (to produce respiratory alkalosis) and intravenous administration of vasoactive drugs. Recently, extracorporeal membrane oxygenation (ECMO) and inhaled nitric oxide have shown promise in selected cases. At postmortem, the findings include increased thickness of the pulmonary arteriolar media, which is believed to represent persistence of the fetal circulation.

Changes in the First Year of Life

The most significant changes occur at birth and within the neonatal period. However, pulmonary vascular resistance and the pulmonary arterial pressure continue to fall during the first year of life. This phenomenon results from the involution of the pulmonary arteriole from a relatively thick-walled, small-lumen vessel to a thin-walled, large-lumen vessel.

Adult levels of resistance and pressure are usually achieved by age 6 months to 1 year.

Anderson HL et al: Extracorporeal membrane oxygenation for pediatric cardiopulmonary failure. J Thorac Cardiovasc Surg 1990;99:1011.

Heyman MA: Fetal and neonatal circulations. In: *Heart Disease in Infants, Children and Adolescents,* 4th ed. Adams FH, Emmanouilides GC, Riemenschneider TA (editors). Williams & Wilkins, 1989.

Kinsella JP et al: Clinical responses to prolonged treatment of persistent pulmonary hypertension of the newborn with low doses of inhaled nitric oxide. J Pediatr 1993;123:103.

MAJOR CLUES TO HEART DISEASE IN INFANTS & CHILDREN

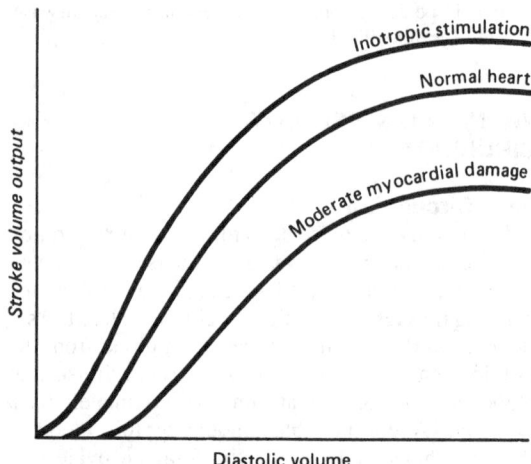

Figure 21–6. Ventricular performance curves.

CONGESTIVE HEART FAILURE

Congestive heart failure at the clinical level is the failure of the heart to meet the circulatory and metabolic needs of the body. Congestive heart failure is one of the two major clues to the presence of important heart disease. (The other is cyanosis; see below.) It has been estimated that congestive heart failure begins before age 1 year in over 90% of infants and children who ever develop the disorder in the pediatric age period—and most of these patients are less than 6 months of age.

Congestive heart failure beginning in infancy may persist throughout childhood until operation relieves the underlying malformation (unless surgery is not possible). Other infants with moderately severe heart failure in the first few months of life may gradually compensate (for a variety of reasons) and not require medical intervention after age 12 or 18 months even though their congenital heart lesions are still unrepaired.

Clinical Findings

The three cardinal signs of congestive heart failure in the pediatric patient are cardiomegaly (the sine qua non), tachypnea (left side), and hepatomegaly (right side).

Cardiomegaly represents a homeostatic (compensatory) mechanism that maintains adequate cardiac output by enlarging the capacity of the pump. This mechanism is frequently referred to as Starling's law of the heart. Up to a point, the enlarging heart can deliver a greater stroke volume output, but limits are soon reached (the descending limb of Starling's curve). Figure 21–6 shows a family of ventricular performance curves. The curve at the right depicts a damaged myocardium; the curve in the center, a normal myocardium; and the curve at the left, a myocardium under inotropic stimulation. One should be very cautious about the diagnosis of congestive heart failure in the absence of an enlarged heart (an exception being a condition such as total anomalous venous return below the diaphragm, which will for a short period of time be characterized by other signs of congestive heart failure without an enlarged heart). Cardiomegaly without other signs of congestive failure may well be taken as early or homeostatically compensated congestive heart failure.

Tachypnea may be considered the cardinal sign of left-sided heart failure. It may be present for a short time before hepatomegaly occurs, although pure left-sided or pure right-sided heart failure does not commonly exist independently for long.

Hepatomegaly is the cardinal sign of right-sided heart failure. The liver is capable of trapping relatively large amounts of edema fluid in the infant that would be more evident as peripheral edema in the older child and adult. It is therefore common rather than unusual for the infant in moderately severe heart failure to have an enlarged liver with no pretibial or even presacral or facial edema. Peripheral edema is found in infants only in the most severe cases of congestive heart failure.

Additional signs and symptoms of congestive heart failure are feeding difficulties, dyspnea, restlessness, easy fatigability, weak pulses, pallor, rales, peripheral edema, weight gain from fluid accumulation, tachycardia, sweating, pneumonia, orthopnea, and growth failure.

Underlying Causes of Heart Failure in the Pediatric Age Group

By far the most common cause of congestive heart failure in the pediatric patient is congenital heart disease. Causes in infancy and childhood appear in the outline below:

A. Heart Failure in Infancy:

1. Cardiovascular causes–Congenital heart disease (producing volume overload, outflow obstruction, myocardial impairment), congenital vascular disease (eg, coarctation of the aorta, an outflow-obstruction disorder, peripheral arteriovenous shunts, a volume overload disorder), acquired myocardial disease (eg, myocarditis), dysrhythmias, rheumatic fever (very rare in infants in the USA).

2. Noncardiovascular causes–Acidosis, respiratory disease, central nervous system disease, anemia, sepsis, hypoglycemia.

B. Heart Failure in Childhood: Cardiovascular causes are potentially the same as in infancy except that rheumatic fever plays a more important role in childhood. Noncardiovascular causes become less important with increasing age—especially such mechanisms as acidosis and hypoglycemia.

Treatment

The physician caring for children must have facility with routine measures and familiarity with some emergency measures for treating congestive heart failure.

A. Routine Measures:

1. Digitalis–Digitalis is the keystone of the treatment of congestive heart failure. The desired effect is improvement in myocardial performance (inotropic effect). shifting the patient to a more efficient ventricular performance in the family of curves shown in Figure 21–6. The preparation most widely used in pediatrics is digoxin, which may be administered (in order of rapidity of onset of effect) intravenously, intramuscularly, or orally. The clinical urgency of the individual case dictates how quickly digitalization should be accomplished. Although there are general guidelines, the ultimate dosage (on a milligram per kilogram basis) must be individualized for each patient.

a. Protocols for digitalization–

(1) In hospital–

Age	Parenteral	Oral
Premature	0.035 mg/kg	0.04 mg/kg
1 week to 2 years	0.05 mg/kg	0.07 mg/kg
< 2 weeks or > 2 years	0.04 mg/kg	0.06 mg/kg

Use of the elixir (0.05 mg/mL) is advisable even in older children because the bioavailability of the tablet preparations is unreliable.

The routine schedule consists of giving one-fourth the digitalizing dose intramuscularly or orally every 6 hours for four doses. For rapid digitalization, give half the digitalizing dose intravenously or intramuscularly and repeat in 4–6 hours. For very rapid digitalization, give the full digitalizing dose intravenously with very close monitoring. For maintenance, give one-fourth to one-third the oral digitalizing dose daily (divided into morning and evening doses).

(2) Digitalization of outpatients–Give the maintenance dose of digoxin (see above) divided in morning and evening doses. In less than a week, adequate digitalization is obtained without running the risk of a parent inadvertently failing to revert to a maintenance dosage schedule and continuing a high digitalizing dose to the point of toxicity (even death).

b. Digitalis toxicity–Slowing of the heart rate below 100 in infants, below 80 in young children, and below 60 in older children is often taken as a guide to reducing the dosage of digoxin. Any dysrhythmia that occurs during digitalis therapy should be attributed to the drug until proved otherwise, although ventricular bigeminy and various degrees of atrioventricular block are characteristic of digitalis toxicity. Age-specific serum levels suggestive of toxicity during maintenance therapy are as follows: newborn, over 4 ng/mL; 1 month to 1 year, over 3 ng/mL; after 1 year, over 2 ng/mL.

c. Digitalis poisoning–*This is an acute emergency that must be treated without delay.* The sooner the stomach is emptied, the better the prognosis, but even if many hours have passed, the stomach should still be emptied. Attention must then be paid to maintaining an adequate cardiac rate and output and to controlling the dysrhythmia. A useful basic intravenous solution is 10% glucose in water to which KCl (3 meq/kg/d) and regular insulin (20 units/1000 mL) have been added. KCl must be used with caution in patients with electrocardiographic high-grade block. It should be given in amounts not to exceed the maintenance requirement per 24 hours for the weight or surface area of the patient. To this solution may be added isoproterenol (in the calibrated administration set) titrated in quantities appropriate to maintain adequate heart rate and output in the face of complete heart block. Phenytoin may be administered through the intravenous tubing to treat dysrhythmias by beginning with a 1-mg/kg slow intravenous push followed every 5–10 minutes with doubling doses to a maximum total combined dose of 15 mg/kg. In severe cases, digoxin immune FAB (ovine) should be given intravenously. If this agent is not available, a temporary transvenous pacemaker may be required to control arrhythmias.

2. Diuretics–If digitalis alone is inadequate to achieve satisfactory compensation, diuretics may be required. For rapid inpatient diuresis, give furosemide intravenously or intramuscularly; for maintenance therapy, give thiazides or furosemide orally daily along with spironolactone.

The dosages are as follows:

a. Furosemide–

(1) Intravenously or intramuscularly, 1 mg/kg/dose, given two or three times daily while monitored in the hospital, monitor electrolytes.

(2) Orally, 2–5 mg/kg/d.

b. Thiazides–These drugs should be given daily with spironolactone (which helps to prevent excessive potassium loss). Do not give daily for prolonged periods unless spironolactone is being given also and serum electrolytes are being monitored periodically.

(1) Chlorothiazide suspension (250 mg/tsp), 20 mg/kg/d.

(2) Hydrochlorothiazide tablets, 2 mg/kg/d.

c. Spironolactone–Give 2–4 mg/kg/d in two divided doses.

3. Rest and sedation–The decompensated and mildly distressed patient requires rest; the severely distressed and anxious infant or child requires sedation. Parenteral morphine, 0.1 mg/kg, is useful for sedation as well as for control of acute pulmonary edema, but it should only be given with good airway control.

4. Oxygen–Oxygen will not make a patient with cyanotic heart disease pink, but it will raise the systemic PaO_2 in patients with severe congestive heart failure, overcoming the capillary-alveolar block of pulmonary edema and alleviating the hypoxemic contribution to congestive failure.

5. Salt restriction–Salt restriction must be approached with caution in infants and children. Treatment of the disease entity known as low-salt congestive heart failure is one of the more hazardous undertakings in medical management. Our feeling is that there is no place for salt-free formulas in the treatment of congestive failure in infants. Standard SMA or Similac 60/40 has about the same sodium content as human milk and about half the sodium content of cow's milk and other prepared formulas. Most cases of "low-salt failure" are largely due to overly vigorous salt restriction (sometimes combined with the other major factor, overly vigorous diuretic therapy). Clearly salty foods such as potato chips and bacon should be avoided, and no salt should be used beyond what is normally used in cooking. It is important that food be palatable enough to eat for a child, who may already be undernourished as a consequence of chronic, poorly compensated heart failure.

B. Emergency and Heroic Measures: The acute emergencies of congestive heart failure are usually related to fluid retention with pulmonary edema and low cardiac output. Some emergency therapeutic measures that may be lifesaving include the following:

1. Morphine–For acute pulmonary edema, give 0.1 mg/kg intravenously or subcutaneously.

2. Diuretics–Furosemide or ethacrynic acid may be given intravenously in an initial dosage of 1 mg/kg to produce a rapid diuresis.

3. Positive pressure breathing–Pulmonary edema may sometimes be managed by intubation or mask with bag-breathing or a respirator to raise the alveolar pressure above pulmonary capillary pressure.

4. Peritoneal dialysis–Although furosemide has largely met the need for the extremely rapid relief of fluid retention, there are three specific instances where peritoneal dialysis with a hypertonic solution may be indicated: (1) when fluid retention (especially pulmonary edema) is life-threatening and diuretics are unsuccessful; (2) in low-salt congestive heart failure when both the fluid retention and the electrolyte imbalance require correction; and (3) in the early postoperative care of an infant who may have transient renal failure with both fluid retention and hyperkalemia.

The advantages of hypertonic peritoneal dialysis are that the procedure promptly (within minutes) draws fluid into the peritoneal cavity, where it is subject to immediate removal, while simultaneously correcting the electrolyte imbalance, whether it is low-sodium, high-potassium, or both. For methods of dialysis, see Chapter 24. If the major problem is electrolyte imbalance, such as potassium retention, a hypertonic solution is not required and the usual "isotonic" dialyzing fluid is indicated.

5. Intravenous inotropic support–Use of agents such as dopamine (1–20 μg/kg/min), dobutamine (2–15 μg/kg/min), isoproterenol (0.1–1 μg/kg/min), and amrinone (0.75 mg/kg bolus then 5–10 μg/kg/min) may help in stabilizing patients with severe myocardial dysfunction, hypotension, or low cardiac output. These agents can be lifesaving in myocarditis and cardiogenic shock.

6. Afterload reduction–A relatively new form of therapy for "pump" failure is to effect afterload reduction by decreasing systemic vascular resistance with an intravenous infusion of vasodilators. Experience in children is limited. The procedure has been used largely in postoperative patients with reduced cardiac output and peripheral vasoconstriction. Agents such as nitroprusside have been lifesaving but must be used in a setting where central venous pressure, arterial pressure, cardiac output, etc, can be carefully monitored.

Beckman RH, Rocchini AP, Rosenthal A: Hemodynamic effects of nitroprusside in infants with a large ventricular septal defect. Circulation 1981;64:553.

Beckman RH et al: Vasodilator therapy in children. Pediatrics 1984;73:43.

Epstein SE (editor): Calcium channel blockers: Present and future directions. Am J Cardiol 1985;55:1.

Latson L: Captopril in children with cardiomyopathies. Circulation 1991;83:707.

Montigny M et al: Captopril in infants for congestive heart failure secondary to a large ventricular left to right shunt. Am J Cardiol 1989;63:631.

Padbury JF et al: Dopamine pharmacokinetics in newborn infants. J Pediatrics 1990;117:472.

Smith TW: Digitalis in the management of heart failure. Hosp Pract (March) 1984;19:67.

Zaritsky A, Chernow B: Use of catecholamines in pediatrics. J Pediatr 1984;105:341.

CYANOSIS

One of the two major clues to the presence of heart disease in the infant and child is cyanosis. (The other is congestive heart failure; see above.)

Cyanosis represents an increased concentration (4–5 g/dL) of reduced hemoglobin in the blood. Bluish discoloration is usually, but not always, a sign. Patients with anemia and cyanosis may not appear blue; patients with polycythemia may appear cyanotic, even though true cyanosis and inadequate blood oxygen content are not present. Visible cyanosis accompanies low cardiac output, hypothermia, and systemic venous congestion, even in the presence of adequate oxygenation.

In patients with true central cyanosis, the cause of cyanosis (cardiac, pulmonary, hematologic, or central nervous system disorder) must be determined. Most often, the physician is faced with differentiating between cardiac and pulmonary problems. Evaluation of arterial blood gases (see above) is one of the easiest ways to differentiate between lung and heart disease. Cyanosis in heart disease is also related to pulmonary blood flow. In some "cyanotic" congenital heart defects, the decrease in pulmonary blood flow is minimal and results in minimal cyanosis. Presence of pulmonary hypertension also influences pulmonary blood flow, and thus oxygen therapy may cause a partial increase in oxygen saturation; the increase is usually much less in patients with heart disease than in those with pulmonary disease.

Evaluation for methemoglobinemia may be necessary to rule out hematologic causes of cyanosis. If the cause of cyanosis is a disease of the central nervous system, the patient will usually respond to oxygen therapy.

Cyanotic heart disease is usually a medical emergency, most often requiring palliative or corrective surgery.

CONGENITAL HEART DISEASE

Congenital heart disease is present in about 1% of studied North American and British populations, making this the most common category of congenital structural malformation. Curative or palliative surgical correction is now available for over 90% of patients with congenital heart disease.

The customary division of congenital heart diseases into noncyanotic and cyanotic types is useful if one understands the basis for it. By convention, patients with right-to-left shunts fall into the cyanotic category whether they have readily recognizable cyanosis or not; patients who do not have right-to-left shunts—even if they are cyanotic for other reasons, such as low cardiac output—are placed in the noncyanotic category. The physiologic basis of cyanosis has been discussed above.

Etiologic Considerations

Only 8% of all congenital heart defects are known to be associated with single mutant gene or chromosome abnormalities, and the remainder are due to various other causes. Multiple environmental factors, including diabetes, alcohol consumption, progesterone use, certain viruses, and other teratogens, are now associated with an increased incidence of malformations. These factors probably represent environmental triggers in persons susceptible or predisposed to congenital heart defects. The effect of rubella virus is probably independent of hereditary factors and consequently predisposes to patent ductus arteriosus and pulmonary artery branch stenosis. Acquired heart diseases, such as rheumatic fever, appear to have much stronger environmental influence. Atherosclerosis clearly can have distinct familial patterns but in some circumstances can be influenced by diet, drugs, or life-style.

In dealing with families of children with congenital heart disease, the physician must often answer the question of risk to future pregnancies. Table 21–2 outlines the risk for certain lesions in patients with one affected first-degree relative. Studies indicate that the incidence in children of affected mothers may be as high as 10–15%. With more than one affected first-degree relative, recurrence is also much higher, and some families may have a hereditary predisposition to congenital heart disease.

Table 21–2. Observed and expected recurrence risks in siblings of 1478 probands with congenital heart lesion.[1]

Anomaly	Probands	Affected Siblings No.	Percent	Exp. ($\sqrt{p}$)
Ventricular septal defect	212	24/543	4.4	5.0
Patent ductus arteriosus	204	17/505	3.4	3.5
Tetralogy of Fallot	157	9/338	2.7	3.2
Atrial septal defect	152	11/342	3.2	3.2
Pulmonary stenosis	146	10/345	2.9	2.9
Aortic stenosis	135	7/317	2.2	2.1
Coarctation of aorta	128	5/272	1.8	2.4
Transpositions of great vessels	103	4/209	1.9	2.2
Atrioventricular canal	73	4/151	2.6	2.0
Tricuspid atresia	51	1/96	1.0	1.4
Ebstein's anomaly	42	1/96	1.1	0.7
Truncus arteriosus	41	1/86	1.2	0.7
Pulmonary atresia	34	1/77	1.3	1.0
Total	1478	95/3376		

[1]Reproduced, with permission, from Nora JJ: Etiologic factors in congenital heart disease. Pediatr Clin North Am 1971; 18:1059.

Ferencz C, Villasenor AC: Epidemiology of cardiovascular malformations: The state of the art. Cardiol Young 1991; 1:264.

Nora JJ, Nora AH: Maternal transmission of congenital heart disease: New recurrence risk figures and the questions of cytoplasmic inheritance and vulnerability to teratogens. Am J Cardiol 1987;59:459.

NONCYANOTIC HEART DISEASE

ATRIAL SEPTAL DEFECT OF THE OSTIUM SECUNDUM VARIETY

Essentials of Diagnosis

- S_2 widely split and usually fixed.
- Grade I–III/VI ejection systolic murmur at pulmonary area.
- Widely radiating systolic murmur mimicking peripheral pulmonary artery stenosis (common in infancy).
- Diastolic flow murmur at lower left sternal border (if shunt is significant in size).
- ECG with rsR' in lead V_1.

General Considerations

An atrial septal defect is an opening in the atrial septum permitting the shunting of blood between the two atria. There are three major types: (1) The ostium secundum type (discussed here) is the most common and is in an intermediate position. (2) The sinus venosus type is positioned high in the atrial septum, is the least common, and is frequently associated with partial anomalous venous return. (3) The ostium primum type is low in position and is a form of atrioventricular septal defect; it is discussed in that section.

Atrial septal defect of the ostium secundum variety occurs in approximately 10% of patients with congenital heart disease and is twice as common in females as in males. Diagnosis in infancy is becoming more common.

Pulmonary hypertension and growth failure are increasingly recognized in infancy and childhood. After the third decade, an increased pulmonary vascular resistance develops, the left-to-right shunting decreases, and right-to-left shunting begins.

Clinical Findings

A. Symptoms and Signs: Infants may present with congestive heart failure often unresponsive to medical management, necessitating early total corrective surgery. However, children with atrial septal defects often have no cardiovascular symptoms. Some patients remain asymptomatic throughout life; others develop easy fatigability as older children or adults. Cyanosis does not occur until pulmonary hypertension develops. This may never occur; if it does, it is not seen until after the third decade of life. Congestive heart failure is uncommon in infants and young children.

The arterial pulses are normal and equal throughout. In the usual case, the heart is hyperactive, with a heaving impulse felt best at the lower left sternal border and over the xiphoid process. There are usually no thrills. S_2 at the pulmonary area is widely split and sometimes fixed. The pulmonary component is normal in intensity. A grade I–III/VI ejection type systolic murmur is heard best at the left sternal border in the second intercostal space. An additional murmur of relative peripheral pulmonary artery stenosis may be heard, more commonly in infants. A middiastolic murmur can often be heard in the fourth intercostal space at the left sternal border. This murmur is due to increased blood flow across the tricuspid valve during diastole (tricuspid flow murmur). The presence of this murmur suggests a high flow (pulmonary to systemic blood flow ratio greater than 2:1).

B. Imaging: Chest x-ray films usually demonstrate cardiac enlargement. The main pulmonary artery may be dilated. The pulmonary vascular markings are increased as a result of increased pulmonary blood flow.

C. Electrocardiography and Vectorcardiography: The usual ECG shows right axis deviation with a clockwise loop in the frontal plane. In the right precordial leads, there is usually an rsR' pattern.

D. Echocardiography: M mode echocardiography shows (1) paradoxic motion of the ventricular septal wall (moving in the same direction rather than the direction opposite to that of the free left ventricular wall) and (2) dilated right ventricular cavity with increased tricuspid valve excursion. Direct visualization of the atrial septal defect by two-dimensional echocardiography, plus demonstration of a left-to-right shunt through the defect by color flow Doppler, confirms the diagnosis and may eliminate the need for cardiac catheterization.

E. Cardiac Catheterization: Oximetry reveals evidence of a significant increase in oxygen saturation at the atrial level. The pulmonary artery pressure is usually normal. The right ventricular pressure is occasionally greater than the pulmonary artery pressure, the increased right-sided "flow." Pulmonary vascular resistance is usually normal. The ratio of pulmonary to systemic blood flow may vary from 1.5:1 to 4:1. A catheter can easily be passed across the atrial septum into the left atrium.

Treatment

Surgical closure is generally recommended for ostium secundum type atrial septal defects in which the ratio of pulmonary to systemic blood flow is greater than 2:1. Operation is usually performed electively in patients between ages 2 and 4 years. The death rate for surgical closure is less than 1%. When surgical intervention is early, late complications of right ventricular dysfunction and significant dysrhythmias may be avoided or diminished. Early surgery is also indicated in infants presenting with congestive heart failure or significant pulmonary hypertension. Double-umbrella closure devices to close selected atrial septal defects by interventional cardiac catheterization are in clinical trials.

Course & Prognosis

Patients with atrial septal defects usually tolerate them very well in the first 2 decades of life, and an occasional patient may live a completely normal life without symptoms. Frequently, however, pulmonary hypertension and reversal of the shunt develop by the third or fourth decade. Heart failure may also occur at this time. Subacute infective endocarditis is a very rare complication. Spontaneous closure occurs and is sometimes associated with an aneurysm of the atrial septum. Exercise tolerance and oxygen consumption in surgically corrected children are generally normal, and physical limitations are unnecessary.

Ettedgui J et al: Diagnostic echocardiographic features of the sinus venosus defect. Br Heart J 1990;64:329.

Fukazawa M, Fukushige J, Ueda K: Atrial septal defects in neonates with reference to spontaneous closure. Am Heart J 1988;116:123.

Mahoney LT et al: Atrial septal defects that present in infancy. Am J Dis Child 1986;140:1115.

Pollick C et al: Doppler color flow imaging assessment of shunt size in atrial septal defect. Circulation 1987; 78:522.

Reybrouck T et al: Cardiorespiratory exercise capacity after surgical closure of atrial septal defect is influenced by the age at surgery. Am Heart J 1991;122 1073.

Rome JJ et al: Double umbrella closure of atrial defects. Circulation 1990;82:751.

VENTRICULAR SEPTAL DEFECTS

Essentials of Diagnosis

Small- to moderate-sized left-to-right shunt without pulmonary hypertension:
- Acyanotic, relatively asymptomatic.
- Grade II–IV/VI pansystolic murmur, maximal along the lower left sternal border.
- P_2 not accentuated.

Large left-to-right shunt:
- Acyanotic.
- Easy fatigability.
- Congestive heart failure in infancy (often).
- Hyperactive heart; biventricular enlargement.
- Grade II–V/VI pansystolic murmur, maximal at lower left sternal border.
- P_2 usually accentuated.
- Diastolic flow murmur at apex.

Insignificant left-to-right shunt or bidirectional shunt with pulmonary hypertension:
- Quiet precordium with right ventricular lift.
- Palpable P_2.
- Short ejection systolic murmur along left sternal border; single accentuated S_2.
- Systemic arterial oxygen desaturation may be present; pulmonary arterial pressure and systemic arterial pressures are equal; little or no oxygen saturation increase at right ventricular level by catheterization.

General Considerations

Simple ventricular septal defect (without other lesions) is the single most common congenital heart malformation, accounting for about 25% of all cases of congenital heart disease. Defects in the ventricular septum can occur both in the membranous portion of the septum (most common) and in the muscular portion.

There are five different courses that patients with ventricular septal defect may follow:

A. Spontaneous Closure: Thirty to 50 percent of all ventricular septal defects close spontaneously. The small defects close in 60–70% of cases. Larger defects may occasionally also close spontaneously, and there are many documented examples of spontaneous closure of ventricular septal defects in the second and third decades of life. Half of the defects that do not close become functionally or anatomically smaller.

B. Shunts Too Small to Justify Repair: Asymptomatic patients with hearts normal in size (as seen on x-ray film) and without pulmonary hypertension are generally not subjected to surgical repair. In those who have had cardiac catheterization, the ratio of pulmonary to systemic blood flow is usually found to be less than 2:1, and serial cardiac catheterizations demonstrate that the shunts get progressively smaller.

C. Disease Severe Enough to Require Surgery: The time of surgery depends upon the nature of the disease. Patients may require surgery in infancy because of intractable congestive heart failure; surgery before 2 years of age because of progression of pulmonary hypertension; or surgery between 2 and 5 years of age as an elective procedure.

D. Defect Inoperable Because of Pulmonary Hypertension: The vast majority of patients with inoperable pulmonary hypertension will develop this condition progressively. The combined data of the multicenter National History Study indicate that most cases of irreversible pulmonary hypertension can be prevented by surgical repair of the defect before 2 years of age.

E. Development of Infundibular Pulmonary Stenosis: Approximately 5% of infants with large left-to-right shunts will develop progressive infundibular obstruction effecting an outflow gradient and diminution of the shunt. A small proportion of these infants have precyanotic tetralogy of Fallot, as evidenced by coexistent right aortic arch or abnormal spatial orientation of the infundibulum.

Clinical Findings

A. Symptoms and Signs: Patients with small or moderate left-to-right shunts usually have no cardiovascular symptoms. There may be a history of frequent respiratory infections in infancy and early childhood. Patients with large left-to-right shunts frequently are sick early in infancy. Such patients have frequent respiratory infections, including bouts of pneumonitis. They grow slowly, with very poor weight gain. Dyspnea, exercise intolerance, and fatigue are quite common. Congestive heart failure may develop between 1 and 6 months of age. Patients who survive the first year usually improve, although easy fatigability may persist. With severe pulmonary hypertension (Eisenmenger's syndrome), cyanosis is present.

1. Small left-to-right shunt—There are usually no lifts, heaves, thrills, or shocks. The first sound at the apex is normal, and the second sound at the pulmonary area is split physiologically. The pulmonary component is normal. A grade II–IV/VI, medium- to high-pitched, blowing pansystolic murmur is heard best at the left sternal border in the third and fourth intercostal spaces. There is slight radiation over the entire precordium. No diastolic murmurs are heard.

2. Moderate left-to-right shunt—Slight prominence of the precordium is common. There is a moderate left ventricular thrust. A systolic thrill may be palpable at the lower left sternal border between the third and fourth intercostal spaces. The second sound at the pulmonary area is most often split but may be single. A grade IV/VI, harsh pansystolic murmur is heard best at the lower left sternal border in the fourth intercostal space. A diastolic flow murmur is heard and indicates that the pulmonary venous return across the mitral valve is large and that the pulmonary to systemic blood flow ratio is at least 2:1.

3. Very large ventricular septal defects with pulmonary hypertension—The precordium is prominent, and the sternum bulges. A left ventricular thrust and a right ventricular heave are palpable. A shock of the second sound can be felt at the pulmonary area. A thrill may or may not be present at the lower left sternal border. A second heart sound is usually single or narrowly split, with accentuation of the pulmonary component. The murmur ranges from grade II to grade V/VI and is usually harsh and pansystolic. Occasionally, when the defect is large, very little murmur can be heard. A diastolic flow murmur may or may not be heard, depending on the size of the shunt.

B. Imaging: X-ray findings of the chest vary, depending upon the size of the shunt. In patients with small shunts, x-ray findings may be normal. The heart is normal in size, and the pulmonary vascular markings may be just beyond the upper limits of normal. Patients with large shunts usually show significant cardiac enlargement involving both the left and right ventricles and the left atrium. The aorta is usually small to normal in size, and the main pulmonary artery segment is dilated. The pulmonary vascular markings are significantly increased in patients with large shunts.

C. Electrocardiography: There is some correlation between the electrocardiographic and the hemodynamic findings. The ECG is normal in patients with small left-to-right shunts and normal pulmonary arterial pressures. Left ventricular hypertrophy is usually found in patients with large left-to-right shunts and normal pulmonary vascular resistance. Combined ventricular hypertrophy (both right and left) is found in patients with pulmonary hypertension due to increased flow, increased resistance, or both. Pure right ventricular hypertrophy is found in patients with pulmonary hypertension due to pulmonary vascular obstruction.

D. Echocardiography: Two-dimensional echocardiography provides visualization of defects that are 4 mm or larger in about 65–75% of cases and often can pinpoint the anatomic location. Addition of color flow Doppler, however, allows detection of smaller defects.

E. Cardiac Catheterization and Angiocardiography: Oxygen saturation is increased at the right ventricular level. The pulmonary artery pressure may vary from normal to that in the systemic arteries. Left atrial pressure (pulmonary capillary pressure) may be normal to increased. Pulmonary vascular resistance varies from normal to markedly increased. The ratio of pulmonary to systemic blood flow may vary from 1.1:1 to 4:1. Hydrogen electrode curves and dye dilution curves may indicate a shunt at the ventricular level. Angiocardiographic examination defines the number, size, and location of the defects.

Treatment

A. Medical Management: Patients who develop congestive heart failure should be treated vigorously with anticongestive measures (see Congestive Heart Failure, above). If the patient does not respond to vigorous anticongestive measures or shows signs of progressive pulmonary hypertension, surgery is indicated without delay. Transcatheter closure of ventricular septal defects is being evaluated as an experimental procedure.

B. Surgical Treatment: The age for elective surgery is becoming progressively younger in most centers (range, < 2 years to 5 years). Patients with cardiomegaly, poor growth, poor exercise tolerance, or other clinical abnormalities who have cardiac catheterization findings of significant shunt (≥ 2:1) without significant pulmonary hypertension (> 10 units of resistance) are candidates for surgery. In general, patients with mean pulmonary artery pressures equal to systemic pressure who are unresponsive to oxygen administration, with little or no left-to-right shunt or bidirectional shunting, and pulmonary resistance calculated to be greater than 10 resistance units (or pulmonary/systemic resistance ratios > 0.7) are considered inoperable. There are patients who have pulmonary hypertension of lesser degree who remain operable, but there is a progressively greater risk with increasing pulmonary hypertension (from 1% risk for patients without pulmonary hypertension to 25% for those at the upper limits of operability).

In order to prevent pulmonary hypertension from reaching inoperable levels, early surgical intervention is recommended for patients who have increased pulmonary vascular resistance. In centers with the capability of doing total correction on infants with or without deep hypothermia, complete repair before 2 years of age is recommended. The presence of multiple muscular defects in a tiny symptomatic infant is still considered to be an indication for pulmonary artery banding as an initial palliative procedure. Transcatheter closure of selected defects is in clinical trials.

Course & Prognosis

Significant late dysrhythmias are uncommon. Functional exercise capacity and oxygen consumption are usually normal, and physical restrictions are unnecessary. Adults with corrected defects have a normal quality of life. Definite congenital heart disease occurred in approximately 3% of probands of male and female patients with ventricular septal defect.

Driscoll DJ et al: Occurrence risk for congenital heart disease in relative of patients with aortic stenosis, pulmonary stenosis, or ventricular septal defect. Circulation 1993;87(Suppl):I-121.

Hornberger LK et al: Elucidation of the natural history of ventricular septal defects by serial Doppler color flow mapping studies. J Am Coll Cardiol 1989;13:1111.

Lock JE et al: Transcatheter closure of ventricular septal defects. Circulation 1988;78:361.

Mehta AV et al: Ventricular septal defect in the first year of life. Am J Cardiol 1992;70:364.

Soto B, Ceballos R, Kirklen JW: Ventricular septal defects: A surgical viewpoint. J Am Coll Cardiol 1989;14:1291.

ATRIOVENTRICULAR SEPTAL DEFECT

Essentials of Diagnosis

- Murmur often inaudible in neonates.
- Loud pulmonary component of S_2.
- Common in infants with Down's syndrome.
- ECG with left axis deviation.

General Considerations

An atrioventricular septal defect is a congenital cardiac abnormality that results from incomplete fusion of the embryonic endocardial cushions. The endocardial cushions help to form the lower portion of the atrial septum, the membranous portion of the ventricular septum, and the septal leaflets of the tricuspid and mitral valves. These defects are not very common. They account for about 4% of all cases of congenital heart disease. The incidence of this abnormality is 20% in patients with Down's syndrome.

Atrioventricular septal defects may be divided into incomplete and complete forms. The complete form, also known as persistent common atrioventricular canal, consists of a high ventricular septal defect, a low atrial septal defect of the ostium primum variety that is continuous with the ventricular septal defect, and a cleft in both the septal leaflet of the tricuspid valve and the anterior leaflet of the mitral valve. In the incomplete form, any one of these components may be present. The most common partial form of atrioventricular septal defect is the ostium primum type of atrial septal defect with a cleft in the mitral valve.

The complete form (persistent common atrioventricular canal) results in large left-to-right shunts at both the ventricular and atrial levels, tricuspid and mitral regurgitation, and marked pulmonary hypertension, usually with some increase in pulmonary vascular resistance. When the latter is present, the shunts may be bidirectional. The hemodynamics in the incomplete form are dependent upon the lesions present.

Clinical Findings

A. Symptoms and Signs: The clinical picture varies depending upon the severity of the defect. In the incomplete form, these patients may be indistinguishable from patients with the ostium secundum type of atrial septal defect. They are often asymptomatic. On the other hand, patients with atrioventricular canal usually are severely affected. Congestive heart failure often develops in infancy, and recurrent bouts of pneumonitis are common.

In the complete form, the murmur may be inaudible in the neonate. After 4–6 weeks, a nonspecific systolic murmur develops; the murmur is usually not as harsh as that of an isolated ventricular septal defect. The heart is significantly enlarged (both right and left sides), and a systolic thrill may be palpated at the lower left sternal border. The second heart sound is split, with an accentuated pulmonary component. A pronounced diastolic flow murmur may be heard at the apex and lower left sternal border.

When severe pulmonary vascular obstruction is present, there is evidence of dominant right ventricular enlargement. A shock of the second sound can be palpated at the pulmonary area. No thrill is felt. The second sound is markedly accentuated and single. A nonspecific short systolic murmur is heard at the lower left sternal border. No diastolic flow murmurs are heard. Cyanosis is detectable in severe cases with predominant right-to-left shunts.

The physical findings in the incomplete form depend upon the lesions. In the most common variety (ostium primum atrial septal defect with mitral regurgitation), the findings are similar to those of the ostium secundum type of atrial septal defect with or without findings of mitral regurgitation.

B. Imaging: As indicated on x-ray film, cardiac enlargement is present depending on the degree of specific anatomic defect and the severity. In the complete (canal) form, there is enlargement of all four chambers. The pulmonary vascular markings are increased. In patients with pulmonary vascular obstruction, only the main pulmonary artery segment and its branches are prominent. The peripheral markings are usually decreased.

C. Electrocardiography: In all forms of atrioventricular septal defect, left axis deviation with a counterclockwise loop in the frontal plane is present. The mean axis varies from approximately –30 to –90 degrees. Since left axis deviation is present in all patients with this defect, the ECG is a very important diagnostic tool. First-degree heart block is present in over 50% of cases. Right, left, or combined ventricular hypertrophy is present depending upon the particular type of defect and the presence or absence of pulmonary vascular obstruction.

D. Echocardiography: On M mode echocardiography, excursion of the atrioventricular valve through the plane of the interventricular septal defect is characteristic. The anatomy can be directly visualized by two-dimensional echocardiography; the sensitivity of this method is equal to that of selective cineangiography.

E. Cardiac Catheterization and Angiocardiography: The results of cardiac catheterization vary depending upon the type of defect present. When catheterization is performed from the leg, the catheter is easily passed across the atrial septum in its lowest portion and frequently enters the left ventricle directly. This catheter course is a result of the very low atrial septal defect and the cleft in the mitral valve. Increased oxygen saturation in the right ventricle or right atrium identifies the level of the shunt. Angiocardiography reveals a characteristic "gooseneck" deformity in the complete canal form. Two-dimensional Doppler color flow echocardiography is extremely useful in identifying the subgroups of endocardial cushion defects.

Treatment

Treatment consists of anticongestive measures and eventual surgical correction. In the incomplete form, surgery is associated with a relatively low death rate (2–5%). The complete form is associated with a significantly higher death rate (about 15–25%), but complete correction in the first year of life, prior to the onset of irreversible pulmonary hypertension, is advisable.

Pulmonary artery banding procedures are contra-indicated in infants with shunts predominantly at the atrial level. They are less effective in patients with predominantly ventricular level shunts than in patients with simple ventricular septal defect. At corrective surgery, transesophageal echo is useful in assessing the adequacy of repair.

Hawort SG: Pulmonary vascular bed in children with complete atrioventricular septal defect: Relation between structure and hemodynamic abnormalities. Am J Cardiol 1986;57:833.

Marino B et al: Atrioventricular canal in Down syndrome. Am J Dis Child 1990;144:1120.

Moscoso G: Developmental morphology of atrioventricular cushions and atrioventricular septal structures: A clue to understanding atrioventricular septal defects. J Perinat Med 1991;19:215.

PATENT DUCTUS ARTERIOSUS

Essentials of Diagnosis

- Variable murmur, with active precordium and full pulses, in newborn premature infants.
- Continuous murmur and full pulses in older infants.

General Considerations

Patent ductus arteriosus is the persistence in extrauterine life of the normal fetal vessel that joins the pulmonary artery to the aorta. It closes spontaneously in normal term infants by 4 days of age. It is a common abnormality, accounting for about 12% of all cases of congenital heart disease. It is very common in children born to mothers who had rubella during the first trimester of pregnancy. There is a higher incidence of patent ductus arteriosus in infants born at high altitudes (over 10,000 feet). It is twice as common in females as in males. In intensive care premature nurseries in infants weighing less than 1500 g, the frequency of patent ductus arteriosus may be as high as 20–60%.

The defect occurs as an isolated abnormality, but associated lesions are not infrequent. Coarctation of the aorta, patent ductus arteriosus, and ventricular septal defect are commonly associated. Even more important to recognize are those patients with murmurs of patent ductus but without readily apparent findings of other associated lesions who are being kept alive by the patent ductus (eg, a patient with patent ductus with unsuspected pulmonary atresia).

Clinical Findings

A. Symptoms and Signs: The clinical findings and the clinical course depend on the size of the shunt and the degree of pulmonary hypertension.

1. Typical patent ductus arteriosus–The pulses are bounding, and pulse pressure is widened (pulse pressure is greater than half of the systolic pressure). The first heart sound is normal. The second heart sound is usually narrowly split and very rarely (when the shunt is maximal) paradoxically split (ie, the second sound closes on inspiration and splits on expiration). The paradoxic splitting is due to the maximal overload of the left ventricle and the prolonged ejection of blood from this chamber.

The murmur is quite characteristic. It is a very rough "machinery" murmur that is maximal at the second intercostal space at the left sternal border and inferior to the left clavicle. It begins shortly after the first heart sound, rises to a peak at the second heart sound, and passes through the second heart sound into diastole, where it becomes a decrescendo murmur and fades or disappears before the first heart sound. The murmur tends to radiate fairly well over the lung fields anteriorly but relatively poorly over the lung fields posteriorly. A diastolic flow murmur is often heard at the apex. Depending on the pulmonary artery pressure, the murmur may be only systolic in time. This characteristic should be fully appreciated when trying to reach a diagnosis of patent ductus arteriosus in infants.

2. Patent ductus arteriosus with pulmonary hypertension–The physical findings depend upon the cause of the pulmonary hypertension. If pulmonary hypertension is due primarily to a marked increase in blood flow and only a slight increase in pulmonary vascular resistance, the physical findings are similar to those listed above. The significant difference is the presence of an accentuated pulmonary component of S_2. Bounding pulses and a loud continuous heart murmur are present. In patients with pulmonary vascular resistance and predominant right-to-left shunt, the findings are quite different. There may be evidence of cyanosis. The second heart sound is single and quite accentuated, and there is no significant heart murmur. The pulses are normal rather than bounding.

3. Patent ductus arteriosus in the premature neonate with associated respiratory distress syndrome–A premature neonate during or after the clinical course of respiratory distress syndrome may have a significant associated patent ductus arteriosus that is paradoxically difficult to detect clinically but is often threatening in magnitude. A soft, nonspecific systolic murmur or no murmur is more common than the classic continuous murmur. The peripheral pulse and precordium are often bounding but typically are not characteristic for several days after the onset of a large left-to-right shunt. An early sign indicating the presence of a significant left-to-right shunt with concomitant congestive heart failure is increasing dependence on oxygen and respiratory support. In addition, increasing radiographic cardiomegaly and pulmonary edema plus increasing echocardiographic evidence of a left-to-right shunt differentiate this clinical and laboratory picture from bronchopulmonary dysplasia.

B. Imaging: In simple patent ductus arteriosus, the x-ray appearance depends upon the size of the shunt. If the shunt is relatively small or moderate in size, the heart is not enlarged. If the shunt is large, there is evidence of both left atrial and left ventricular enlargement. In both cases, the aorta is prominent, as is the main pulmonary artery segment.

C. Electrocardiography: The ECG may be normal or may show left ventricular hypertrophy, depending on the size of the shunt. In patients with pulmonary hypertension due to increased blood flow, there is usually biventricular hypertrophy. In those with pulmonary vascular obstruction, there is pure right ventricular hypertrophy. An anterior ST depression (V_1) of 2 mm suggests subendocardial ischemia due to a diastolic "steal" from the coronary arteries via the ductus; this finding indicates the need for closure.

D. Echocardiography: Enlargement of the left atrium as measured by M mode echocardiography is an important clue to the presence of congestive heart failure and is especially useful in diagnosing patent ductus arteriosus in the premature infant. A left atrial to ascending aorta ratio of less than 1.2 or 1.3 is considered evidence of a sizable left-to-right ductal shunt. Premature infants with patent ductus arteriosus who are undergoing medical or surgical therapy for closure should have a complete two-dimensional echocardiographic evaluation to rule out associated heart disease, especially ductus-dependent lesions. The use of color flow pulsed Doppler ultrasonography and two-dimensional echocardiography can provide visualization of the ductus and confirmation of the direction and degree of shunting and may eliminate the need for a diagnostic cardiac catheterization.

E. Cardiac Catheterization and Angiocardiography: Cardiac catheterization will reveal increased oxygen content or saturation at the level of the pulmonary artery. Hydrogen electrode curves are positive in the pulmonary artery and negative in the right ventricle. The catheter can often be passed through the ductus from the pulmonary artery into the descending thoracic aorta. Arteriograms taken following injection of contrast material into the aortic arch show a shunt at the level of the ductus. If catheterization is not performed, the cardiologist must be completely satisfied that there is neither an associated lesion nor pulmonary hypertension. Transcatheter closure of patent ductus arteriosus is once again being evaluated in selected centers staffed by personnel with expertise in interventional cardiology in older children.

Patients with patent ductus arteriosus and pulmonary hypertension due to large left-to-right shunts show a marked increase in oxygen saturation at the pulmonary artery level and normal systemic arterial saturation. Those with marked pulmonary vascular obstruction show little or no increase in oxygen content at the pulmonary artery and a decrease in systemic arterial saturation. In both cases, a catheter may be passed through the ductus into the descending thoracic aorta.

Cardiac catheterization is rarely indicated in the premature infant with symptomatic ductus.

Treatment

Treatment consists of surgical correction except in patients with pulmonary vascular obstruction. Patients with large left-to-right shunts and pulmonary hypertension should be operated on very early (even under the age of 1 year) to prevent the development of progressive pulmonary vascular obstruction. Simple patent ductus arteriosus should be corrected after the child reaches age 1, though the operation may be delayed until later without increasing the risk of death. Transcatheter closure with an occluder device is being evaluated as an experimental technique. Transcatheter closure of small defects with a coil is becoming standard therapy.

Patients with nonreactive pulmonary vascular obstruction who have resistance greater than 10 units and a pulmonary/systemic resistance ratio greater than 0.7 should not be operated upon. These patients are made worse by closure of the ductus, because the ductus serves as an escape route and limits the degree of pulmonary hypertension.

The premature infant with symptomatic ductus presents a special and controversial problem. At some institutions, it is customary to operate on virtually all premature infants weighing under 1200 g. At other institutions, surgery is rarely done, and most infants receive a maximum of three doses of either oral indomethacin (0.1–0.3 mg/kg every 8–24 hours) or parenteral indomethacin (0.1–0.3 mg/kg every 12 hours) if adequate renal, hematologic, and hepatic function are demonstrated. Contraindications to indomethacin treatment include hyperbilirubinemia of 12 mg/dL or greater, renal failure, shock, necrotizing enterocolitis, intracranial hemorrhage, hemorrhagic disease, and evidence of a spontaneously closing ductus. Efficacy and safety of indomethacin use are enhanced by the careful monitoring of serum levels of indomethacin. A serum level of less than 250 ng/mL is associated with treatment failure. Conventional conservative management includes fluid restriction with or without diuretics and ligation only if these fail. Factors to be considered in making a rational decision on modality of therapy include a high rate of spontaneous ductus closure without therapy and an extremely low surgical risk in experienced centers; the inability of a laboratory to monitor serum levels of indomethacin may influence the decision. Transcatheter occluder devices are in clinical trials.

Course & Prognosis

Patients with simple patent ductus arteriosus and small to moderate shunts usually do quite well even without surgery. However, in the third or fourth decade of life, symptoms of easy fatigability, dyspnea on exertion, and exercise intolerance appear, usually as a consequence of the development of pulmonary hypertension or congestive heart failure.

Spontaneous closure of a patent ductus arteriosus may occur within the first 2 years of life or beyond. This is especially true in infants who were born prematurely. After age 2, spontaneous closure is less common. Because subacute infective endocarditis is a potential complication, surgical ligation is recommended if the defect persists beyond age 2 years.

Patients with large shunts or pulmonary hypertension do much less well. Poor growth and development, frequent episodes of pneumonitis, and the development of congestive heart failure are not uncommon in patients with large left-to-right shunts. If these patients do not succumb to congestive heart failure in early infancy, they frequently go on to develop pulmonary vascular obstruction in later childhood or adolescence. Life expectancy is markedly reduced, and these patients often die in their second or third decade. Those rare patients with pulmonary vascular obstruction from very early infancy are actually less symptomatic than those with pulmonary hypertension without obstruction.

Cambier PA et al: Percutaneous closure of the small patent ductus arteriosus using coil embolization. Am J Cardiol 1992;69:815.

Goldberg SJ: Response of the patent ductus arteriosus to indomethacin treatment. Am J Dis Child 1987;141:250.

Rashkind WJ et al: Nonsurgical closure of patent ductus arteriosus. Circulation 1987;75:583.

Reller MD et al: Duration of ductal shunting in healthy preterm infants: An echocardiographic color flow Doppler study. J Pediatr 1988;112:441.

Reller MD et al: The timing of spontaneous closure of the Ductus arteriosus in infants with respiratory distress syndrome. Am J Cardiol 1990;66:75.

Valdez-Cruz M et al: Real-time Doppler color flow mapping for detection of patent ductus arteriosus. J Am Coll Cardiol 1986;8:1105.

MALFORMATIONS ASSOCIATED WITH OBSTRUCTION TO BLOOD FLOW ON THE RIGHT SIDE OF THE HEART

1. VALVULAR PULMONARY STENOSIS WITH INTACT VENTRICULAR SEPTUM

Essentials of Diagnosis

- No symptoms with mild and moderately severe cases.
- Cyanosis and a high incidence of right-sided congestive heart failure in very severe cases.
- Right ventricular lift; systolic ejection click at the pulmonary area in mild to moderately severe cases.
- S_2 widely split with soft to inaudible P_2; grade I–

VI/VI obstructive systolic murmur, maximal at the pulmonary area.

- Dilated pulmonary artery on posteroanterior chest x-ray film.

General Considerations

Obstruction of right ventricular outflow at the pulmonary valve level accounts for about 10% of all cases of congenital heart disease. In the usual case, the cusps of the pulmonary valve are fused to form a membrane or diaphragm with a hole in the middle that varies from 2 mm to 1 cm in diameter. Occasionally, there may be a fusion of only two cusps, producing a bicuspid pulmonary valve. Very frequently, especially in the more severe cases, there is secondary infundibular stenosis. The pulmonary valve ring is usually small. There is usually moderate to marked poststenotic dilatation of both the main and left pulmonary arteries. Patent foramen ovale is fairly common.

Obstruction to blood flow across the pulmonary valve results in an increase in pressure developed by the right ventricle to maintain an adequate output across that valve. Pressures greater than systemic are potentially life-threatening and are associated with "critical" obstruction. As a consequence of the increased work required of the right ventricle, severe right ventricular hypertrophy and eventual right ventricular failure can occur. In contrast to patients with right ventricular outflow obstruction, patients with this obstruction who also have a large ventricular septal defect (ie, tetralogy of Fallot) are not at great risk for heart failure; because of the septal defect, there is communication between the ventricles, which limits the amount of pressure developed in the right ventricle (pressure is equal to systemic pressure) and thereby makes heart failure extremely uncommon.

When the obstruction is severe and the ventricular septum is intact, a right-to-left shunt will often occur at the atrial level through a patent foramen ovale. Accordingly, patients with this condition may have a varying degree of cyanosis. The presence of cyanosis indicates a relatively severe degree of valvular obstruction.

Clinical Findings

A. Symptoms and Signs: The history depends upon the severity of the obstruction. Patients with a mild or even a moderate degree of valvular pulmonary stenosis are completely asymptomatic throughout infancy, childhood, and adolescence. Patients with a more severe type of valvular obstruction may develop cyanosis and congestive heart failure very early—even in the neonatal period. Hypoxemic spells characterized by a sudden onset of marked cyanosis and dyspnea are much less common than in tetralogy of Fallot.

Patients with mild to moderate obstruction are acyanotic. Patients with severe or critical stenosis usually show evidence of central cyanosis. These patients are usually well developed and well nourished. They often have a round face and widely spaced eyes. The pulses are normal and equal throughout. Clubbing may occur in severe cases in which cyanosis has persisted for a long time. On examination of the heart, there may be prominence of the precordium. A heaving impulse of the right ventricle can frequently be palpated. A systolic thrill is often palpated in the pulmonary area and occasionally in the suprasternal notch. The first heart sound is normal. In patients with mild to moderate stenosis, a prominent ejection click of pulmonary origin is heard best at the second left intercostal space. This click varies with respiration. It is much more prominent during expiration than inspiration. In patients with severe stenosis, the click tends to merge with the first heart sound. The second heart sound also varies with the degree of stenosis. In mild valvular stenosis, the second heart sound is normally split and the pulmonary component is normal in intensity. In moderate degrees of obstruction, the second heart sound is more widely split and the pulmonary component is softer. In severe pulmonary stenosis, the second heart sound is single, since the pulmonary component cannot be heard. An ejection type, rough, obstructive systolic murmur is best heard at the second interspace at the left sternal border. It radiates very well to the back. No diastolic murmurs are audible. In older children, a prominent "A" wave is seen in the jugular venous pulse. If there is congestive heart failure, the liver is enlarged.

B. Imaging: In the mild form of pulmonary stenosis, the heart may be normal in size. Poststenotic dilatation of the main pulmonary artery segment and the left pulmonary artery is often present. In moderate to severe cases, there may be a slight right ventricular enlargement, and there may or may not be poststenotic dilatation of the main pulmonary artery. In patients who are cyanotic, the pulmonary vascular markings are decreased; otherwise, they are normal.

C. Electrocardiography: Electrocardiographic findings are usually normal in patients with mild obstruction. Right ventricular hypertrophy is present in patients with moderate to severe valvular obstruction. In severe obstruction, right ventricular hypertrophy and the right ventricular strain pattern (deep inversion of the T wave) are seen in the right precordial leads. In the most severe form, right atrial hypertrophy is also present. Right axis deviation is also seen in the moderate to severe forms. Occasionally, the axis is greater than +180 degrees.

D. Echocardiography: M mode echocardiography reveals atrial contraction and elevated right ventricular diastolic pressure causing early opening of the pulmonary valve (ie, opening prior to the onset of ventricular systole). The pulmonary valve appears to be unusually echo-dense. The pulmonary valve image on two-dimensional echocardiography shows a thickened structure with less than normal excursion.

The transvalvular pressure gradient can be noninvasively and accurately estimated by echo Doppler technique.

E. Cardiac Catheterization and Angiocardiography: There is no increase in oxygen saturation or oxygen content in the right side of the heart. In the more severe cases, there is a right-to-left shunt at the atrial level. Pulmonary artery pressure is normal in milder cases and quite low in moderately severe to severe cases. Right ventricular pressure is always higher than pulmonary artery pressure. The gradient across the pulmonary valve varies from 10 to 200 mm Hg. In severe cases, the right atrial pressure is often elevated, with a predominant "A" wave. Cineangiocardiography with injection of contrast material into the right ventricle shows thickening of the pulmonary valve and the very narrow opening of the pulmonary valve. This produces a "jet" of contrast from the right ventricle into the pulmonary artery. Infundibular hypertrophy may be present.

Treatment

Elective valvotomy is recommended for children with right ventricular pressures of greater than 50 mm Hg or higher than two-thirds of systemic pressure. Immediate correction is indicated for patients with systemic or greater right ventricular pressure. Percutaneous balloon valvuloplasty has become the procedure of choice in most institutions. It appears to be as effective as surgery in relieving obstruction and causes less valve insufficiency.

The need for additional surgical resection of associated infundibular hypertrophy is controversial. Because additional surgery increases the risk and because the outflow obstruction usually regresses, many centers perform only the valvotomy.

Course & Prognosis

Patients with mild pulmonary stenosis live a normal life and have a normal life span. Those with stenosis of moderate severity rarely are symptomatic. Those with severe valvular obstruction may develop severe cyanosis and congestive heart failure in early life.

Postoperative follow-up suggests that most patients with right ventricular pressure equal to or less than systemic pressure who were treated surgically early in life have good voluntary maximum exercise capacity. If relief of valvular obstruction occurs prior to 20 years of age, longevity is essentially the same as that of the general population. Physical restriction is unwarranted in these patients. The quality of life of adults with pulmonary stenosis is comparable to that of the normal population . The risk of coronary heart disease is 1.7% in the offspring of males and approximately 4% in probands of females.

Driscoll DJ et al: Occurrence risk for congenital heart defects in relatives of patients with aortic stenosis, pulmonary stenosis, or ventricular septal defect. Circulation 1993;87(Suppl):I-121.

Kopecky SL et al: Long term outcome of patients undergoing surgical repair of isolated pulmonary valve stenosis. Circulation 1988;78:1150.

Lloyd T, Donnerstein R: Rapid T-wave normalization after balloon pulmonary valvuloplasty in children. Am J Cardiol 1989;64:399.

Marantz PM et al: Results of balloon valvuloplasty in typical and dysplastic pulmonary valve stenosis: Doppler echocardiographic follow up. J Am Coll Cardiol 1988; 12:476.

McCrindle B, Kan J: Long term results after balloon valvuloplasty. Circulation 1991;83:1915.

Rey C et al: Percutaneous transluminal balloon valvuloplasty of congenital pulmonary valve stenosis, with a special report on infants and neonates. J Am Coll Cardiol 1988;11:815.

2. INFUNDIBULAR PULMONARY STENOSIS WITHOUT VENTRICULAR SEPTAL DEFECT

Pure infundibular pulmonary stenosis is rare. One should suspect infundibular pulmonary stenosis where there is evidence of mild to moderate pulmonary stenosis and intact ventricular septum and (1) no pulmonary ejection click is audible and (2) the murmur is maximal in the third and fourth intercostal spaces rather than in the second intercostal space. Otherwise, the clinical picture may be identical.

3. DISTAL PULMONARY STENOSIS

Supravalvular Pulmonary Stenosis

Supravalvular pulmonary stenosis, a relatively rare condition, is due to coarctation of the body of the main pulmonary artery. The clinical picture may be identical with that of valvular pulmonary stenosis, although the murmur is maximal in the first intercostal space at the left sternal border and in the suprasternal notch. No ejection click is audible. A second heart sound is usually narrowly split, and the pulmonary component is quite loud as a result of closure of the pulmonary valve under high pressure. The murmur radiates extremely well into the neck and over the lung fields.

Peripheral Pulmonary Branch Stenosis

In peripheral pulmonary branch stenosis, there are multiple small coarctations of the branches of the pulmonary artery in the periphery of the lung. Systolic murmurs may be heard over both lung fields, both anteriorly and posteriorly. The transient pulmonary branch stenosis murmurs of infancy (previously described under heart murmurs) are innocent. Pulmonary artery branch stenosis murmurs may be the most audible murmurs in atrial septal defects in infancy and early childhood. The most common cause of significant pulmonary artery branch stenosis is maternal rubella. Several types of supravalvular aortic stenosis syndromes may be found in association with this condition.

Surgery is often unsuccessful. Transvenous angioplasty is currently being assessed but does not appear to be as efficacious in patients with peripheral pulmonary branch stenosis as in patients with pulmonary valvular stenosis.

Absence of a Pulmonary Artery

Absence of a pulmonary artery may be an isolated malformation or may occur in association with other congenital heart diseases. It is occasionally seen in patients with tetralogy of Fallot.

Dunkle LM, Rowe RD: Transient murmur simulating pulmonary artery stenosis in premature infants. Am J Dis Child 1972;124:666.

Rothma A et al: Early results and follow-up of balloon angioplasty for branch pulmonary artery stenosis. J Am Coll Cardiol 1990;15:1109.

MALFORMATIONS ASSOCIATED WITH OBSTRUCTION TO BLOOD FLOW ON THE LEFT SIDE OF THE HEART

1. COARCTATION OF THE AORTA

Essentials of Diagnosis

- Pulse lag in lower extremities.
- Blood pressure of 20 mm Hg or pressure greater in upper than in lower extremities.
- Blowing systolic murmur in left axilla.

General Considerations

Coarctation is a common cardiac abnormality accounting for about 6% of all cases of congenital heart disease. Three times as many males as females are affected. In the vast majority of cases, coarctation occurs in the thoracic portion of the descending aorta. The abdominal aorta is very rarely involved. Coarctations are usually in the juxtaductal position rather than the pre- or postductal position. The term **coarctation of aorta syndrome** is a useful concept, because most symptomatic infants will have associated patent ductus arteriosus, tubular hypoplasia of the aortic isthmus (frequently erroneously termed a coarctation), ventricular septal defect, and bicuspid aortic valve. The tubular hypoplasia of the aortic isthmus is probably related to paucity of blood flow in the fetus and often spontaneously enlarges with postnatal growth.

Clinical Findings

A. Symptoms and Signs: Patients with coarc-

tation may or may not have cardiovascular symptoms in infancy, childhood, and adolescence. Congestive heart failure may develop in early infancy, and symptoms of decreased exercise tolerance and fatigability may appear in childhood.

The important physical finding is diminution or absence of femoral pulses. However, a significant number of infants will initially have equal upper and lower extremity pulses until the coexistent patent ductus arteriosus closes. Normally, the blood pressure in the upper extremities is slightly higher than in the lower extremities during the first few months of life. After 1 year of age, blood pressure higher in the arms than in the legs is suggestive of coarctation of the aorta. The actual level of blood pressure in the arms may be only moderately elevated, even in severe coarctation, or it may be significantly elevated. In the presence of severe congestive heart failure, the differences in pulses in the upper and lower extremities may not be readily apparent, but with compensation, the pulses in the arms are palpably stronger than those of normal infants; the pulses in the legs remain diminished or absent in affected infants. The left subclavian artery is occasionally involved in the coarctation, in which case the left brachial pulse is weak. If the coarctation is uncomplicated, the heart sounds are normal. The aortic component of the second heart sound is occasionally increased in intensity. An ejection systolic murmur of grade II/VI intensity is often heard at the aortic area and the lower left sternal border. The pathognomonic murmur of coarctation is heard in the left axilla. This murmur is usually systolic in timing but may spill into diastole. If the coarctation is complicated by other malformations, murmurs associated with these other abnormalities will be audible.

B. Imaging: In the older child, x-ray findings may indicate a heart normal in size, although there is usually some evidence of left ventricular enlargement. The ascending aorta is usually normal in size. On barium swallow, the esophagus has a characteristic E shape. The first arc of the E is due to dilatation of the aorta just proximal to the coarctation. The second arc is due to poststenotic dilatation of the aorta. The middle bar of the E is due to the coarctation itself. In older children, notching or scalloping of the ribs caused by marked enlargement of the intercostal collaterals can be seen. Magnetic resonance imaging (MRI) has become extremely useful for determining noninvasively the anatomy of the coarctation.

In infants in congestive heart failure, there is evidence of marked cardiac enlargement and pulmonary venous congestion.

C. Electrocardiography: ECGs in children may be normal or may show evidence of slight left ventricular hypertrophy. In infants with or without congestive heart failure, the ECG usually demonstrates right ventricular hypertrophy.

D. Echocardiography: M mode echocardiography reveals only secondary evidence of the coarctation. In infants with congestive heart failure, dilated right and left ventricles are noted. A striking posterior displacement of the mitral valve in the left ventricular cavity with poor excursion is common. Real-time two-dimensional echocardiography may visualize the coarctation directly, and color flow Doppler may serve as a predictor of severity.

E. Cardiac Catheterization and Angiocardiography: These studies demonstrate the position, anatomy, and severity of the coarctation and will assess the adequacy of the collateral circulation.

Treatment

Infants with coarctation of the aorta and congestive heart failure require vigorous anticongestive measures. Dilation of the associated patent ductus arteriosus with a constant infusion of prostaglandin E_1 may stabilize the critically ill infant until operation can be performed. Many with isolated coarctation and no associated lesions respond well and do not require surgery in infancy. In infants with striking congestive heart failure and without associated cardiovascular abnormalities, severe systemic hypertension is often a contributing factor.

Infants with associated intracardiac defects sometimes need immediate surgery but frequently require revision of the recoarctation later in life. Modification of the surgical technique utilizing a subclavian flap anastomosis reduces the likelihood of this late complication. This technique has been used successfully in infants weighing as little as 1000 g. Patients repaired with patch aortoplasty must be followed frequently (every 1–2 years) because of the potential for rapid progression of aortic aneurysms.

Percutaneous balloon angioplasty has been used successfully as a palliative procedure to stabilize critically ill infants with coarctation of aorta syndrome. It is likely that surgical correction will be necessary after stabilization. Percutaneous balloon angioplasty is also being utilized to dilate recoarctations in postoperative patients.

Patients who do not require surgery early in life may be corrected electively at ages 3–5 years unless significant systemic hypertension develops.

Course & Prognosis

Children who survive the neonatal period without developing congestive heart failure do quite well throughout childhood and adolescence. Fatal complications (eg, hypertensive encephalopathy, intracranial bleeding) occur uncommonly. Subacute infective endocarditis is also rare before adolescence.

Children with coarctation corrected during school age are at significant risk for systemic hypertension and myocardial dysfunction. Careful exercise testing is mandatory prior to their participation in athletic activities.

Balderson S et al: Maximal voluntary exercise variables in children with postoperative coarctation of the aorta. J Am Coll Cardiol 1992;191:154.

Cohen M et al: Coarctation of the aorta: Long-term follow-up and prediction of outcome after surgical correction. Circulation 1989;80:840.

Mendelsohn AM et al: Rapid progression of aortic aneurysms after patch aortoplasty repair of coarctation of the aorta. J Am Coll Cardiol 1992;20:381.

Simpson IA et al: Color flow Doppler flow mapping in patients with coarctation of the aorta: New observations and improved evaluation with color flow diameter and proximal acceleration as predictors of severity. Circulation 1988;77:736.

Ward KE et al: Delayed detection of coarctation in infancy: Implications for timing newborn follow-up. Pediatrics 1990;86:972.

2. AORTIC STENOSIS

Essentials of Diagnosis

- Systolic ejection murmur at upper right sternal border.
- Thrill in carotid arteries.
- Systolic click at the apex.
- Dilatation of the ascending aorta on chest x-ray.

General Considerations

Aortic stenosis may be defined from the anatomic or physiologic point of view. Anatomically, it consists of an obstruction to the outflow from the left ventricle at or near the aortic valve. Physiologically, aortic stenosis may be defined as a condition in which a systolic pressure gradient of more than 10 mm Hg exists between the left ventricle and the aorta. Aortic stenosis accounts for approximately 5% of all cases of congenital heart disease. Anatomically, congenital aortic stenosis may be divided into four types:

A. Valvular Aortic Stenosis (75%): Critical aortic stenosis presenting in infancy usually consists of a unicuspid diaphragm-like structure without well-defined commissures. Preschool and school-age children more commonly present with a bicuspid valve. Teenagers and young adults characteristically present with tricuspid but partially fused leaflets. This lesion is more common in males than females.

B. Discrete Membranous Subvalvular Aortic Stenosis (20 %): This consists of a membranous or fibrous ring just below the aortic valve. The ring forms a diaphragm with a hole in the middle and results in obstruction to left ventricular outflow. The aortic valve itself and the anterior leaflet of the mitral valve are often deformed.

C. Supravalvular Aortic Stenosis: In this variety, there is a constriction of the ascending aorta just above the coronary arteries. This condition is often associated with a family history, abnormal facies, and mental retardation (Williams syndrome).

D. Idiopathic Hypertrophic Subaortic Stenosis (IHSS): In this case, there is a marked hypertrophy of the entire left ventricle and, predominantly, the ventricular septum. With contraction of the ventricle, the hypertrophic portion of the septum, together with the mitral valve, causes obstruction of left ventricular outflow. A family history is often present.

Obstruction to outflow from the left ventricle causes the left ventricle to work harder to maintain an adequate pressure and flow in the systemic arterial circuit, resulting in hypertrophy of the left ventricle and increased oxygen requirement. If the stenosis is severe, the oxygen requirements may exceed the capacity of the coronary arteries to supply oxygen, and relative coronary insufficiency may develop. In critical aortic stenosis, left ventricular failure may occur. The left ventricle is usually able to adapt to the increased pressure load for a considerable period of time before heart failure or coronary insufficiency develops.

Clinical Findings

A. Symptoms and Signs: Most patients with aortic stenosis have no cardiovascular symptoms. Except in the most severe cases, the patient may do well up until the third to fifth decades of life, although some patients have mild exercise intolerance and easy fatigability. A small percentage of patients have significant symptoms within the first decade, ie, dizziness and syncope. Sudden death, although uncommon, may occur in all forms of aortic stenosis, with the greatest risk being idiopathic hypertrophic subaortic stenosis.

Although isolated valvular aortic stenosis seldom causes symptoms in infancy, severe heart failure occasionally occurs when critical obstruction is present. The response to medical management is poor; therefore, an aggressive surgical approach is recommended.

The physical findings vary somewhat depending upon the anatomic type of lesion:

1. Valvular aortic stenosis–Affected patients are well developed and well nourished. The pulses are usually normal and equal throughout. If the stenosis is severe and there is a gradient of greater than 80 mm Hg, the pulses are small with a slow upstroke. Examination of the heart reveals a left ventricular thrust at the apex. A systolic thrill at the right base, the suprasternal notch, and both carotid arteries accompanies moderate disease. If only one carotid artery manifests a thrill, it is the right carotid (usually seen in milder disease).

The first heart sound is normal. A prominent aortic type ejection click or ejection sound is best heard at the apex. In infants, this click can be heard at the lower left sternal border and at the aortic area. It is separated from the first heart sound by a short but appreciable interval. It does not vary with respiration. The second heart sound at the pulmonary area is physiologically split. The aortic component of the second heart sound is of good intensity. There is a grade III–V/VI, rough, medium- to high-pitched ejection type systolic murmur, loudest at the first and second intercostal spaces, which radiates well into the suprasternal notch and along the carotids. The murmur also radiates fairly well down the lower left sternal border and can be heard at the apex. The murmur transmits to the neck, and its grade correlates roughly with the severity of the stenosis.

2. Discrete membranous subvalvular aortic stenosis–The findings are essentially the same as those of valvular aortic stenosis. Absence of an aortic ejection click is an important differentiating point, and the thrill and murmur are usually somewhat more intense at the left sternal border in the third and fourth intercostal spaces than at the aortic area. Frequently, however, the murmur is equally intense at both areas. A diastolic murmur of aortic insufficiency is commonly heard after 5 years of age.

3. Supravalvular aortic stenosis–Affected patients often have abnormal facies and are mentally retarded. The thrill and murmur are characteristically best heard in the suprasternal notch and along the carotids, although they are well transmitted over the aortic area and near the mid left sternal border. A difference in pulses and blood pressure between the right and left arms may be found, with the more prominent pulse and pressure in the right arm.

4. Idiopathic hypertrophic subaortic stenosis–The murmur in this case is ejection in quality, grade II–III/VI, and heard from the left sternal border toward the apex and sometimes associated with a murmur of mitral insufficiency. There is often an atrial fourth heart sound with a diastolic murmur. No ejection click is audible. The arterial pulse wave has a rapid upstroke and frequently a bisferiens quality.

B. Imaging: In most cases, x-ray findings indicate that the heart is not enlarged. The left ventricle, however, is slightly prominent. In valvular and discrete subvalvular aortic stenosis, dilatation of the ascending aorta is frequently seen (more commonly in the former). The ascending aorta is usually normal in idiopathic hypertrophic subaortic stenosis and in supravalvular aortic stenosis.

C. Electrocardiography: There is some correlation between the severity of the obstruction and the ECG. Patients with mild aortic stenosis have normal ECGs. Patients with severe obstruction frequently demonstrate evidence of left ventricular hypertrophy and left ventricular strain, but many do not. In about 25% of severe cases, the ECG is normal. Progressive increase in left ventricular hypertrophy on serial ECGs indicates a significant degree of obstruction. Left ventricular strain is taken as a potential indication for operation.

D. Echocardiography: This has become a reliable noninvasive technique for the initial diagnosis and follow-up evaluation of idiopathic hypertrophic subaortic stenosis. It also provides clues to the progression of other forms of aortic stenosis. Doppler echocardiographic techniques can now predict transvalvular gradients quite accurately.

E. Cardiac Catheterization and Angiocardiography: Left heart catheterization demonstrates the pressure differential between the left ventricle and the aorta and the level at which the gradient exists. Patients with severe aortic stenosis may be asymptomatic and have normal ECGs and chest x-rays. Serial cardiac catheterization is frequently the only reliable guide to the progression and the severity of the lesion. In the case of valvular aortic stenosis, an asymptomatic patient with a resting gradient of 60–80 mm Hg is considered to require surgery. In the face of symptoms, patients with lesser gradients are surgical candidates. Cineangiocardiography is helpful in demonstrating the level of the obstruction.

Treatment

Because the results of surgery are frequently unsatisfactory, surgical repair should only be considered in patients with symptoms or a large resting gradient (60–80 mm Hg). In many cases, the gradient can only be moderately to minimally relieved without producing aortic insufficiency (which is potentially more harmful than the lesion for which surgery was undertaken). Percutaneous balloon valvuloplasty is now accepted as standard treatment. Discrete subvalvular aortic stenosis requires a lesser gradient for surgical intervention, because continued trauma to the aortic valve by the subvalvular jet may destroy the valve. Unfortunately, simple resection is followed by recurrence in more than 25% of patients with subvalvular aortic stenosis. Asymmetric septal hypertrophy has even less satisfactory results than muscle resection; therefore, medical management with propranolol should be tried initially.

All patients should have close follow-up, and those over age 6 years should undergo yearly exercise testing. If exercise testing is normal, restriction of physical activity may not be necessary in patients with mild to moderate aortic stenosis; in many cases, these patients may participate in competitive sports.

Course & Prognosis

All forms of left ventricular outflow tract obstruction tend to be progressive diseases. However, regression of the obstruction has been documented in a few patients with supravalvular obstruction. Pediatric patients with left ventricular outflow tract obstruction—with the exception of those with critical aortic stenosis of infancy—are usually asymptomatic. Symptoms accompanying severe unoperated obstruction (angina, syncope, and congestive heart failure) are all rare currently because of detection and surgical intervention. The vast majority of children without asymmetric septal hypertrophy are not only asymptomatic but also tend to have the personality and capabilities

to compete in sports. There is increasing evidence that pre- or postoperative children whose obstruction is mild to moderate have above-average oxygen consumption and maximum voluntary working capacity. Children in this category with normal findings on resting and exercising ECG and normal heart size may safely participate in vigorous physical activity, including nonisometric competitive sports. Children with severe aortic stenosis tend to demonstrate ventricular dysrhythmias as adults.

Kasten-Sportas CH et al: Percutaneous balloon valvuloplasty in neonates with critical aortic stenosis. J Am Coll Cardiol 1991;13:1101.

Kennedy KD et al: Natural history of moderate aortic stenosis. J Am Coll Cardiol 1991;17:313.

Oh JK et al: Prediction of the severity of aortic stenosis by Doppler aortic valve area determination. J Am Coll Cardiol 1988;11:1227.

Sheddy RE et al: Gradient reduction aortic valve regurgitation and prolapse after balloon aortic valvuloplasty in 32 consecutive patients with congenital aortic stenosis. J Am Coll Cardiol 1990;16:451.

Witsenburg M et al: Short and midterm results of balloon valvuloplasty for valvar aortic stenosis in children. Am J Cardiol 1992;69:945.

Wolfe RR et al: Arrhythmias in patients with valvar aortic stenosis, valvar pulmonic stenosis, and ventricular septal defect. Circulation 1993;87(Suppl):I-89.

Zeevi B et al: Neonatal critical valvar aortic stenosis. Circulation 1989;80:831.

3. MITRAL VALVE PROLAPSE

Essentials of Diagnosis

- Midsystolic click best heard with patient in standing or squatting position.
- Occasional late systolic murmur.

General Considerations

Mitral valve prolapse is the most common entity to present with abnormal auscultatory findings in pediatric patients. It is secondary to redundant valve tissue or abnormal tissue comprising the mitral valve apparatus. The mitral valve prolapses, moving posteriorly or superiorly into the left atrium during ventricular systole. A systolic click occurs at the time of this movement and is the clinical hallmark of this entity. Mitral insufficiency may occur late in systole, causing an atypical, short, late systolic murmur with variable radiation. It is most commonly found in individuals with the following characteristics: over 6 years of age, female, slender habitus, and bony thoracic abnormalities. Its incidence is estimated to vary from 2% to 20%, with the higher part of the range representing incidence in slender teenage females.

Clinical Findings

A. Symptoms and Signs: The vast majority of

patients with mitral valve prolapse are asymptomatic. Chest pain, palpitations, and dizziness are reported, but it is not clear whether or not these symptoms are more common in affected patients than in the normal population. Significant dysrhythmias are uncommon, and true exercise intolerance is rare. The standard approach to auscultation must be modified to diagnose mitral valve prolapse; ie, auscultation should be performed with the patient placed in various positions. Clicks with or without systolic murmur are more commonly elicited in the standing and squatting positions than in the supine and sitting positions. The systolic click occurs earlier in children than in adults; ie, it tends to be midsystolic rather than late systolic. Although it is usually heard at the apex, it may be audible at the left sternal border or even occasionally may be panthoracic. A midsystolic or systolic murmur following the click implies mitral insufficiency and is much less common than isolated prolapse. The murmur tends to be atypical for mitral insufficiency in that it is not pansystolic and radiates to the sternum rather than to the left axilla. A coexistent diastolic murmur of relative or real mitral stenosis is rare. Occasionally, a systolic "honk" is heard.

B. Imaging: In the rare case of significant mitral insufficiency, the left atrium may be enlarged; this is visualized best on lateral film x-ray. Most chest x-rays show normal findings, and their use is therefore largely unwarranted.

C. Electrocardiography: Despite the fact that flat or inverted T waves in precordial lead V_6 have been reported, almost all electrocardiographic findings are normal. Disabling chest pain is rare and should be assessed with ergometric electrocardiography.

D. Echocardiography: Significant posterior systolic movement of the anterior mitral valve leaflet is considered diagnostic. Many false-positive results are due to multiple leaflet images (chevroning) or to the presence of insignificant (small duration and amplitude) posterior systolic valve movement. False-negative results are also common, partly owing to performance of the procedure when the patient is in the supine position. If the physical findings are typical for isolated prolapse, echocardiography is not warranted.

E. Cardiac Catheterization and Angiography: Invasive procedures are very rarely indicated.

Treatment & Prognosis

Use of oral propranolol may be effective in rare cases of disabling chest pain. Prophylaxis for subacute infectious endocarditis is indicated only in individuals with associated mitral insufficiency.

The natural course of disease is largely unknown. Twenty years of observation indicate, however, that mitral valve prolapse in childhood is a largely benign entity. It merges with a common variation from normal in slender children and is associated with an as-

thenic body build that presumably results from altered geometry of the left ventricle and mitral valve.

Alpert MA et al: Frequency of isolated panic attacks and panic disorder in patients with mitral valve prolapse syndrome. Am J Cardiol 1992;69(17):1489.

Arfken CL et al: Mitral valve prolapse: Associations with symptoms and anxiety. Pediatrics 1990;85:311.

Barlow JB, Pocock WA: Billowing, floppy, prolapsed or flail valves? Am J Cardiol 1985;55:501.

Kessler KM: Prolapse paranoia. J Am Coll Cardiol 1988; 11:48.

Levine RA: Reconsideration of echocardiographic standards for mitral valve prolapse: Lack of association between leaf displacement isolated to the apical 4-chamber view and independent echocardiographic evidence of abnormality. J Am Coll Cardiol 1988;11:1010.

4. OTHER CONGENITAL VALVULAR LESIONS

Congenital Mitral Stenosis

In this rare disorder, the valve leaflets are thickened and fused to produce a diaphragm-like or funnel-like structure with an opening in the center. Frequent associated malformations include subaortic and aortic stenosis and coarctation of the aorta. This lesion complex is known as Shone's syndrome. Most patients develop symptoms early in life. Early symptoms include tachypnea, dyspnea, and severe failure to thrive. Physical examination reveals a first heart sound that is accentuated, and the pulmonary closure sound is loud. No opening snap can be heard. In most cases, a presystolic crescendo murmur is heard at the apex. Occasionally, only a middiastolic murmur can be heard. Rarely, no murmur at all is heard. Electrocardiography shows right axis deviation, biatrial enlargement, and right ventricular hypertrophy. X-ray reveals evidence of left atrial enlargement and, fr11equently, pulmonary venous congestion. Echocardiography shows abnormal valve structures with reduced excursion and left atrial enlargement. Cardiac catheterization reveals an elevated pulmonary capillary pressure and wedge pressure and pulmonary hypertension.

Surgical treatment, including valve replacement with a prosthetic mitral valve, has become possible even in infants weighing 3–5 kg.

Cor Triatriatum

This is an extremely rare abnormality in which the pulmonary veins enter a separate chamber rather than pass directly into the left atrium. The chamber communicates with the left atrium through an opening of variable size. The physiologic consequences of this condition are very similar to those of mitral stenosis. The clinical findings depend upon the size of the opening. If the opening is extremely small, symptoms develop very early in life. If the opening is large, patients may be asymptomatic for a considerable period of time. Echocardiography may reveal a dense shadow in the left atrium. Two-dimensional color flow Doppler echocardiographic techniques have greatly enhanced the noninvasive accuracy of the diagnosis. Cardiac catheterization may be diagnostic. Finding a high pulmonary capillary pressure (high pulmonary venous pressure) and a low left atrial pressure (if the catheter can be passed through the foramen ovale into the true left atrial chamber) makes the diagnosis certain. Angiocardiographic studies may identify two "left atrial" chambers.

Surgical repair is usually successful.

Congenital Mitral Regurgitation

This is a relatively rare abnormality that is usually associated with other congenital heart lesions, including corrected transposition of the great vessels, endocardial cushion defect, and endocardial fibroelastosis. Uncomplicated congenital mitral regurgitation is very rare. It is sometimes present in patients with Marfan's syndrome. Occasionally, there is a congenital dilatation of the valve ring with an otherwise normal valve. In other cases, the chordae tendineae are malformed, resulting in mitral regurgitation.

Congenital Aortic Regurgitation

The most common causes of this disorder are bicuspid aortic valve, either uncomplicated or with coarctation of the aorta; ventricular septal defect and aortic insufficiency; and fenestration of the aortic valve cusp (one or more holes in the cusp).

Absence of the Pulmonary Valve

This rare abnormality is usually associated with ventricular septal defect. In about 50% of cases, pulmonary stenosis is present (tetralogy of Fallot).

Ebstein's Malformation of the Tricuspid Valve

This uncommon abnormality consists of downward displacement of the tricuspid valve such that the greater portion of the valve is attached to the ventricular wall rather than to the fibrous ring. As a result, the upper portion of the right ventricle is functionally within the right atrium. The portion of the ventricle below the apex of the tricuspid valve is very small and represents the true functioning right ventricle. Clinically, there is a wide spectrum of abnormalities ranging from relative absence of symptoms to death in early infancy. The severity depends upon the degree of malattachment of the valve and the associated abnormalities. Echocardiography is useful in diagnosis.

Surgical repair consists of an annuloplasty procedure to modify the level of tricuspid orifice and diminish mitral insufficiency. The procedure's rate of success is highly variable. Late dysrhythmias are common. Postoperative tolerance of exercise is significantly increased compared to preoperative status but decreased compared to normal individuals.

Driscoll DJ, Mottram CD, Danielson GK: Spectrum of exercise intolerance in 45 patients with Ebstein's anomaly and observations on exercise tolerance in 11 patients after surgical repair. J Am Coll Cardiol 1988;11:831.

Lang D et al: Pathologic spectrum of malformations of the tricuspid valve in prenatal and neonatal life. J Am Coll Cardiol 1991;17:1161.

Quaegebeur JN et al: Surgery for Ebstein's anomaly. J Am Coll Cardiol 1991;17:722.

Saxena A et al: The left ventricular function in patients 20 years of age with Ebstein's anomaly of the tricuspid valve. Am J Cardiol 1991;67:217.

Spevak PJ et al: Balloon angioplasty for congenital mitral stenosis. Am J Cardiol 1990;66:472.

MYOCARDIAL DISEASES

Myocardial diseases are characterized by significant cardiac enlargement. Murmurs may or may not be present. Electrocardiographic changes include left ventricular hypertrophy, ST depression, and T wave inversion.

1. GLYCOGEN STORAGE DISEASE OF THE HEART

At least ten types of glycogen storage disease are recognized. The type that primarily involves the heart is known as Pompe's disease. The deficient enzyme (acid maltase) is necessary for hydrolysis of the outer branches of glycogen, and its absence results in marked deposition of glycogen within the myocardium. Cardiac glycogenosis is a rare heritable (autosomal recessive) disorder.

Affected infants are usually normal at birth, but onset commonly begins by the sixth month of life. These children have a history of retardation of growth and development, feeding problems, poor weight gain, and then the findings of heart failure. Physical examination reveals generalized muscular weakness, a large tongue, cardiomegaly, no significant heart murmurs, and, occasionally, evidence of congestive heart failure. Chest x-rays reveal marked cardiomegaly with or without pulmonary venous congestion. The ECG shows a short PR interval with left ventricular hypertrophy and shows ST depression and T wave inversion over the left precordial leads. Echocardiography shows extremely thick ventricular wall structures.

Children with this disease usually die within the first year of life. Death may be sudden or due to progressive congestive heart failure.

2. ANOMALOUS ORIGIN OF THE LEFT CORONARY ARTERY

In this condition, the left coronary artery arises from the pulmonary artery rather than from the aorta. In the neonatal period, while the pulmonary arterial pressure is relatively high, blood is supplied to the left ventricle from the pulmonary artery. Accordingly, during this period the child is asymptomatic and does well. However, within the first 2 months of life, the pulmonary arterial pressure decreases to normal. This phenomenon results in a marked decrease of flow to the left coronary artery. Infarction of the heart usually occurs. If the patient survives, collateral channels appear that join the peripheral branches of the right with the branches of the left coronary artery. As a result, the direction of blood flow in the left coronary artery changes. Whereas previously there was some flow from the pulmonary artery into the myocardium through the left coronary, flow now occurs from the right coronary artery through the collateral into the left coronary artery and then into the pulmonary artery. In essence, then, an arteriovenous fistula is formed that further removes blood from the myocardium, resulting in further myocardial infarction and fibrosis. Death occurs eventually as a result of marked dilatation of the heart and congestive heart failure. At autopsy, the left ventricle is found to be markedly fibrosed and thin.

Clinical Findings

A. Symptoms and Signs: Patients appear to be normal at birth. Growth and development are relatively normal for a few months, although detailed questioning of the parents often discloses a history of intermittent episodes of severe abdominal pain, pallor, and sweating, especially during or after feeding. These episodes are thought to be secondary to "colic," and attacks are similar to anginal attacks in adults.

On physical examination, the patients are usually well developed and well nourished. The pulses are usually weak but equal throughout. The heart is enlarged but not very active. A murmur of mitral regurgitation is frequently present, although no murmur may be heard.

B. Imaging: Chest x-ray films show significant cardiac enlargement with or without pulmonary venous congestion.

C. Electrocardiography: The ECG is usually diagnostic. There are T wave inversions in leads I and aVL. The precordial leads show T wave inversions from V_{4-7}. Deep Q waves are often seen in leads I, aVL, and V_{4-6}. These findings of myocardial infarction are similar to those in adults.

D. Echocardiography: The diagnosis can be made with two-dimensional techniques by visualizing a single large right coronary artery arising from the aorta.

E. Cardiac Catheterization and Angiocardiography: A small left-to-right shunt (a result of the flow of blood from the right through the left coronary artery into the pulmonary artery) can often be detected at the pulmonary artery level. Frequently, however, the shunt is very small and can be detected only by the most sensitive techniques, eg, by the use of a hydrogen electrode catheter. Cineangiocardiography following injection of contrast material into the root of the aorta shows absence of origin of the left coronary artery from the aorta. A huge right coronary artery fills directly from the aorta, and the contrast material will flow through the right coronary system into the left coronary arteries and finally into the pulmonary artery.

Treatment & Prognosis

Treatment remains controversial. Medical management with anticongestives and afterload reduction is advocated by some. Lengthy operations requiring cardiopulmonary bypass to effect two functional coronary arteries from the aorta have a significant mortality rate in critically ill infants. Simple ligation of the left coronary artery or subclavian to coronary artery anastomosis (without cardiopulmonary bypass) should be considered for the most critically ill infants. More complex operations should only be considered for the more stable infants or older children.

The prognosis is guarded. No therapeutic modality has been shown to be superior in follow-up studies of survivors.

Midgley A et al: Repair of anomalous origin of the left coronary artery in the infant and small child. J Am Coll Cardiol 1984;4:1231.

Sauer U et al: Risk factors for perioperative mortality in children with anomalous origin of the left coronary artery from the pulmonary artery. J Thorac Cardiovasc Surg 1991;102:566.

3. ENDOCARDIAL FIBROELASTOSIS

The incidence of endocardial fibroelastosis has decreased dramatically over the past 2 decades, and this entity is now uncommon. The cause is not known, although intrauterine infection with mumps or coxsackievirus B has been suggested.

Pathologic examination discloses a marked milky white thickening of the endocardium, the subendocardial layers of the left ventricle, and, usually, the left atrium. The mitral valve is frequently involved also. The myocardial fibers themselves are fibrotic and disorganized, and associated hypervascularization is common. Serial sections often show coexistent evidence of myocarditis. Thus, endocardial fibroelastosis appears to be part of a continuum of primary endomyocardial diseases and may be a sequela to myocarditis.

Clinical Findings

A. Symptoms and Signs: Patients appear normal at birth, and growth and development during early infancy are normal. About half develop symptoms within the first 5 months of life, and most are symptomatic by age 1. An occasional patient may have no symptoms until age 5.

The symptoms and signs that do develop are associated with left ventricular heart failure. These include dyspnea, easy fatigability, feeding difficulties, and, eventually, findings of left and right heart failure.

On physical examination, these children are often small and undernourished. The heart is usually enlarged, and the heart tones are poor (when there is evidence of decompensation). A murmur of mitral regurgitation may be present.

B. Imaging: Chest x-ray films show generalized cardiac enlargement with or without pulmonary venous congestion.

C. Electrocardiography: The ECG almost always shows evidence of left ventricular hypertrophy and, quite frequently, ST depression and T wave inversion. If there has been pulmonary hypertension secondary to left heart failure, right ventricular hypertrophy may be present. Right atrial hypertrophy is sometimes present. Complete heart block is occasionally seen.

D. Echocardiography: M mode and two-dimensional techniques reveal dilatation of cardiac chambers and echo-dense endocardial images indicating decreased myocardial function.

E. Cardiac Catheterization and Angiocardiography: Catheterization reveals the absence of left-to-right shunts. Pulmonary hypertension may be present. Cineangiocardiography demonstrates diminished myocardial contractility. Transcatheter endomyocardial biopsy has become a more common technique in infants and children for primary myocardial disease but seldom reveals a cause.

Treatment & Prognosis

Treatment of endocardial fibroelastosis is medical and consists of adequate and prolonged use of digitalis and oral diuretics. If response to the usual dose is not satisfactory, the dosage of both digitalis and diuretics should be increased until a satisfactory response is noted or toxicity occurs. Afterload reduction would appear to be rational therapy for infants with this disease. Continue these agents for several years.

Some children appear to improve initially with treatment but then develop recurrent bouts of heart failure. Complete recovery in such patients is very infrequent, and unless transplanted most eventually die with intractable congestive heart failure. The prognosis is most favorable in patients who present between 6 months and 3 years of age and respond promptly to treatment.

Chan KY et al: Immunosuppressive therapy in the management of acute myocarditis in children: A clinical trial. J Am Coll Cardiol 1991;17:458.

CYANOTIC HEART DISEASE

TETRALOGY OF FALLOT

Essentials of Diagnosis

- Cyanosis after the neonatal period.
- Hypoxemic spells during infancy.
- Right-sided aortic arch in 25%.
- Systolic ejection murmur at upper left sternal border.

General Considerations

In Fallot's tetralogy, there is a ventricular septal defect and severe obstruction to right ventricular outflow such that the intracardiac shunt is predominantly from right to left. This is the most common type of cyanotic heart lesion, accounting for 10–15% of all cases of congenital heart disease. The ventricular defect is usually located in the membranous portion of the septum but may be totally surrounded by muscular tissue and is usually quite large. Obstruction to right ventricular outflow may be solely at the infundibular level (50–75%), at the valvular level alone (rarely), or at both levels (25% or more). The primary embryologic abnormality is in the septation of the conus and truncus arteriosus, resulting in an enlarged overriding aorta and hypoplasia of the pulmonary trunk. Experimental lesions in specific loci of ectodermal (neural crest) tissue which migrate to the conus can reproduce the defects seen in tetralogy of Fallot. The term tetralogy has been used to describe this combination of lesions, since there is always associated right ventricular hypertrophy and a varying degree of "overriding of the aorta." The overriding is present because of the position of the ventricular septal defect in relation to a dilated and often dextroposed aorta. These two factors (right ventricular hypertrophy and overriding aorta) plus the major lesions make up the tetralogy. A right-sided aortic arch is present in 25% of cases and an atrial septal defect in 15%.

Severe obstruction to right ventricular outflow plus a large ventricular septal defect results in a right-to-left shunt at the ventricular level and desaturation of the arterial blood. The degree of desaturation and the extent of cyanosis depend upon the size of the shunt. This in turn is dependent upon the resistance to outflow from the right ventricle, the size of the ventricular septal defect, and the systemic vascular resistance. The greater the obstruction, the larger the ventricular septal defect, and the lower the systemic vascular resistance, the greater the right-to-left shunt. Although the patient may be deeply cyanotic, the amount of pressure the right ventricle can develop is limited to that of the systemic (aortic) pressure. In other words, right ventricular pressure cannot exceed left ventricular pressure. The right ventricle is usually quite able to maintain this level of pressure without developing heart failure.

Clinical Findings

A. Symptoms and Signs: The clinical findings vary depending upon the degree of right ventricular outflow obstruction. Patients with a mild degree of obstruction are only minimally cyanotic or acyanotic and may even present initially with congestive heart failure. Those with maximal obstruction are deeply cyanotic from birth. However, few children are asymptomatic; most have cyanosis by 4 months of age; and the cyanosis usually is progressive. Growth and development are retarded, and easy fatigability and dyspnea on exertion are common. Squatting is seen when the children become old enough to walk.

Hypoxemic spells (cyanotic spells) are characterized by the following signs and symptoms: (1) sudden onset of cyanosis or deepening of cyanosis; (2) sudden onset of dyspnea; (3) alterations in consciousness, encompassing a spectrum from irritability to syncope; and (4) decrease in intensity or disappearance of the systolic murmur. These episodes may begin in the neonatal period and continue until nearly school age. It is unusual, however, for the initial episode to occur after 2 years of age. Acute treatment of cyanotic spells consists of giving oxygen and placing the patient in the knee-chest position. Acidosis, if present, should be corrected with intravenous sodium bicarbonate. Morphine sulfate should be administered cautiously by a parenteral route in a dosage of 0.1 mg/kg. Propranolol, 0.1–0.2 mg/kg intravenously, has been found to be useful. Chronic (daily) treatment of cyanotic spells with propranolol, 1 mg/kg orally every 4 hours while awake, remains controversial; however, in a significant number of patients, this regimen has prevented subsequent "spells" and made it possible to delay operation until total correction can be performed.

Patients with tetralogy are usually small and thin. The degree of cyanosis is variable. The fingers and toes show varying degrees of clubbing depending upon the age of the child and the severity of the cyanosis.

On examination of the heart, a right ventricular lift is palpable. No thrills are present. The first sound is normal; occasionally, there is an ejection click at the apex that is aortic in origin. The second sound is single and best heard at the lower left sternal border between the third and fourth intercostal spaces. The second heart sound at the pulmonary area is soft; however, aortic closure is loud and heard best in the third and fourth intercostal spaces at the left sternal border. There is a grade I–III/VI, rough, ejection type systolic murmur that is maximal at the left sternal border in the third intercostal space. This murmur radiates over the anterior and posterior lung fields. Diastolic murmurs are not present.

B. Laboratory Findings: The hemoglobin, hematocrit, and red blood count are usually mildly to markedly elevated, depending upon the degree of arterial oxygen desaturation.

C. Imaging: Chest x-rays reveal the overall heart size to be normal, and indeed the x-ray film may sometimes be interpreted as being entirely normal. However, the right ventricle is hypertrophied, and this is often shown in the posteroanterior projection by an upturning of the apex (boot-shaped heart). The main pulmonary artery segment is usually concave, and the aorta in 25% of cases arches to the right. The pulmonary vascular markings are usually decreased.

D. Electrocardiography: The cardiac axis is to the right, ranging from +90 to +180 degrees. The P waves are usually normal, although there may be evidence of slight right atrial hypertrophy. Right ventricular hypertrophy is always present, but right ventricular strain patterns are rare.

E. Echocardiography: Two-dimensional imaging reveals thickening of the free right ventricular wall, with overriding of the aorta and a membranous ventricular septal defect and can be diagnostic. Furthermore, obstruction at the level of the infundibulum and pulmonary valve can be identified, and the size of the proximal pulmonary arteries can be measured. The anatomy of the coronary arteries may be visualized.

F. Cardiac Catheterization and Angiocardiography: Cardiac catheterization reveals the presence of a right-to-left shunt in most cases. There is arterial blood desaturation of varying degree. The right-to-left shunt exists at the ventricular level. The right ventricular pressure is at systemic levels, and the pressure contour in the right ventricle is almost identical with that of the left ventricle. The pulmonary artery pressure is extremely low (mean ranges of 5–10 mm Hg). The gradients and pressure may be noted at the valvular level, the infundibular level, or both. The catheter frequently is passed from the right ventricle into the overriding ascending aorta but may cause a transient right bundle branch block.

Cineangiocardiography is diagnostic. Injection of contrast material into the right ventricle reveals the right ventricular outflow obstruction and the right-to-left shunt at the ventricular level. An aortic root injection or selective coronary angiography may be necessary to demonstrate anomalies of coronary artery distribution that can affect surgical technique.

Treatment

A. Palliative Treatment: Palliative treatment is recommended for very small infants who are markedly symptomatic (severely cyanotic, frequent severe anoxic spells) and in whom complete correction would be difficult or impossible. Medical (chronic oral beta-blocking agents) or, more often, surgical (creation of a systemic arterial to pulmonary arterial anastomosis) palliation can be used.

The earliest procedure employed for this disease (Blalock-Taussig) consists of an anastomosis between the subclavian artery and the pulmonary artery. It is usually done on the side opposite the aortic arch. A synthetic shunt anastomosis between the ascending aorta and the main pulmonary artery may be performed.

B. Total Correction: Total correction of tetralogy of Fallot is performed under the cardiopulmonary bypass. It involves opening the right ventricle, closing the ventricular septal defect, and removing the obstruction to right ventricular outflow. The surgical death rate varies from 2 to 15%. The major limiting anatomic feature of total correction is the size of the pulmonary artery and its branches. Children who survive the operation are markedly improved. There is complete disappearance of cyanosis, and clubbing disappears shortly thereafter. Growth and development improve markedly, and these patients often become asymptomatic within a short period of time. However, these patients may remain at risk for sudden death due to dysrhythmias. Currently, major cardiovascular centers are performing total correction for virtually all infants with this condition, including newborns.

Course & Prognosis

Infants with the most severe form of the disease are usually deeply cyanotic at birth. Hypoxemic spells may occur during the neonatal period. Death is extremely rare during a severe hypoxemic spell. Many patients who survive the first year of life seem to improve. This may be due to the development of systemic-to-pulmonary collateral vessels. Although hypoxemic spells may decrease in severity, these children remain deeply cyanotic and markedly limited in their activity. They seldom survive the second decade of life without surgical treatment.

Infants with moderate obstruction to right ventricular outflow do fairly well. Although cyanosis is present in very early life, it is usually not severe. The cyanosis may progress in severity, and anoxic spells may occur. These patients do fairly well in later childhood, but their condition progressively deteriorates during the second and third decades of life. Death occurs by the third decade as a result of cerebrovascular accidents, brain abscess, subacute infective endocarditis, anoxia, or pulmonary hemorrhage.

Patients with the mildest form of the disease are said to have the "acyanotic" variety. The degree of obstruction is very mild, and the right-to-left shunt is small. Very frequently, there is a predominant left-to-right shunt. However, the degree of obstruction often increases as the patient gets older. This, combined with the increased activity, results in progressively worsening cyanosis. Many of these patients live relatively normal lives without severe symptoms. Life expectancy, however, is definitely decreased, and death usually occurs by the third to fourth decade.

Complete repair prior to the school-age years usually results in fair to good function, although patients are occasionally subject to sudden death from dysrhythmias.

Friedli B, Bolens M, Taktak M: Conduction disturbances after correction of tetralogy of Fallot. J Am Coll Cardiol 1988;11:162.

Garson A Jr, Gillette PC, McNamara DG: Propranolol: The preferred palliation for tetralogy of Fallot. Am J Cardiol 1981;47:1098.

Murphy JG et al: Long-term outcome in patients undergoing surgical repair of tetralogy of Fallot. N Engl J Med 1993;9:593.

Vaksmann G et al: Frequency and prognosis of arrhythmias after operative "correction" of tetralogy of Fallot. Am J Cardiol. 1990;66:346.

Walsh EP: Late results in patients with tetralogy of Fallot repaired during infancy. Circulation 1988;77:1062.

Zahka KG et al: Long-term valvular function after total repair of tetralogy of Fallot: Relation to ventricular arrhythmias. Circulation 1988;78(Suppl 3):14.

PULMONARY ATRESIA WITH VENTRICULAR SEPTAL DEFECT

This condition consists of complete atresia of the pulmonary valve in association with ventricular septal defect. Essentially, it is an extreme form of tetralogy of Fallot. Since there is no flow outward from the right ventricle into the pulmonary artery, the pulmonary blood flow must be derived either from a patent ductus arteriosus or from collateral channels.

The clinical picture depends entirely upon the size of the ductus or the collateral channels (or both). If they are large, patients may do quite well and actually do better than those with severe tetralogy of Fallot. If effective pulmonary blood flow is small, death occurs secondary to severe anoxia early in life. This may occur suddenly with postnatal closure of a patent ductus arteriosus.

Echocardiography or cardiac catheterization and angiocardiography are diagnostic. If patent ductus arteriosus dependency is established, a prostaglandin E_1 infusion to dilate the patent ductus arteriosus may help stabilize the patient until surgery.

Infants who are severely hypoxemic require urgent systemic to pulmonary anastomosis in order to provide sufficient oxygenated blood to the body.

A corrective surgical procedure that has been successful in patients with adequate-sized pulmonary arteries consists of bypassing the obstructed right ventricular outflow and closing the ventricular septal defect. Success may depend on precise definition of pulmonary arterial and collateral blood supply to the lung and prior unifocalization of segments with dual arterial blood supply. More recently, an approach has been adopted to create initially a central connection between the right ventricle or aorta to the central pulmonary artery.

Hoffback KM et al: Analysis of survival in patients with pulmonic valve atresia and ventricular septal defect. Am J Cardiol 1991;67:737.

Sullivan ID et al: Surgical unifocalization in pulmonary atresia and ventricular septal defect: A realistic goal? Circulation 1988;78(Suppl 3):55.

PULMONARY ATRESIA WITH INTACT VENTRICULAR SEPTUM

Essentials of Diagnosis

- Cyanosis at birth.
- Chest x-ray film with concave pulmonary artery segment and apex tilted upward.

General Considerations

In this uncommon condition, the pulmonary valve is absent and is replaced by a small diaphragm consisting of the fused cusps. The ventricular septum is intact. The main pulmonary artery segment is somewhat hypoplastic but almost always patent. In the type 1 deformity (80%), the cavity volume of the right ventricle is extremely small and the wall is thickened and fibrotic. In type 2, the right ventricular cavity is frequently of normal size.

During intrauterine life, if the tricuspid valve is intact and normal, very little blood enters the right ventricle, since there is no outlet for this chamber. Almost all of the blood passes through the foramen ovale directly into the left side of the heart. In the type 2 deformity, there is usually an outlet for the right ventricle (tricuspid valve insufficiency), and the right ventricle receives a sufficient quantity of blood to permit it to develop in a relatively normal fashion.

Following birth, the pulmonary circulation is maintained primarily by a patent ductus arteriosus. Although a bronchial pulmonary collateral network is present, it is usually insufficient to maintain the pulmonary circulation. Accordingly, whether or not the patients live depends upon the patency of the ductus arteriosus. The ductus usually remains open for only a short period of time. As it closes, hypoxia becomes progressively more severe, and death eventually occurs.

Clinical Findings

A. Symptoms and Signs: Patients may be normal at birth, although they are usually cyanotic. Cyanosis becomes progressively more severe and is associated with severe dyspnea. A blowing systolic murmur due to the associated patent ductus arteriosus may be heard at the pulmonary area and under the left clavicle. In type 2 deformity, a loud pansystolic murmur due to the tricuspid insufficiency is heard at the lower left sternal border. Not infrequently, the liver is pulsating.

B. Imaging: Chest x-rays show a markedly enlarged heart with marked decrease in pulmonary vascular markings. With striking tricuspid insufficiency, right atrial enlargement may be massive and the cardiac silhouette may virtually fill the chest.

C. Electrocardiography: Electrocardiography reveals an axis that is usually normal in the frontal plane. Evidence for right atrial enlargement is usually striking. Voltage criteria for other chamber enlargement are variable.

D. Echocardiography: M mode and two-dimensional echocardiography shows absence of the pulmonary valve, with varying degrees of hypoplasia of the right ventricular cavity and tricuspid annulus. The severity of tricuspid regurgitation often correlates positively with right ventricular size.

E. Cardiac Catheterization and Angiocardiography: The diagnosis can be made on cardiac catheterization and cineangiocardiography. Right ventricular pressure is very high (greater than systemic). A cineangiocardiogram following injection of contrast material into the right ventricle reveals absence of filling of the pulmonary artery from the right ventricle. It also demonstrates the size of the right ventricular chamber, relative hypoplasia of the components of the tripartite right ventricle (inflow, trabecular, infundibulum), and the presence or absence of tricuspid regurgitation, and right ventricular sinusoids that anastomose with the coronary arteries may fill.

Treatment & Prognosis

As in pulmonary atresia with ventricular septal defect, a prostaglandin E_1 infusion is useful in stabilizing the patient and maintaining patency of the ductus until surgery can be performed. Surgery should be undertaken as soon as the diagnosis is made by cardiac catheterization. A Rashkind atrial septostomy is performed, depending on right ventricular size, to open up the communication across the atrial septum. Subsequent surgical approaches vary widely. In cases of type 1 deformity, it is necessary to immediately establish a surgical aorticopulmonary anastomosis (usually a Blalock-Taussig shunt). Later in infancy, a communication between the right ventricle and pulmonary artery should be created in an attempt to stimulate right ventricular cavity growth. In cases of type 2 deformity, a closed valvotomy may be all that is necessary initially, with a more definitive reconstruction of the right ventricular outflow tract accomplished at a later date.

The prognosis is unpredictable for patients with type 1 or type 2 deformity who survive the surgery. In type 1 patients, the dimensions of the right ventricle can increase significantly after the initial procedure. Overall, however, this disorder remains one of the least satisfactory forms of cyanotic congenital heart disease, because little progress has been made in surgical management.

Calder AL, Co EE, Sage MD: Coronary artery abnormalities in pulmonary atresia with intact ventricular septum. Am J Cardiol 1987;59:436.

Leung M et al: Echocardiographic assessment of neonates with pulmonary atresia and intact ventricular septum. J Am Coll Cardiol 1988;12:719.

Shaddy RE et al: Right ventricular growth after transventricular pulmonary valvotomy and central aortopulmonary shunt for pulmonary atresia and intact ventricular septum. Circulation 1990;82:IV–157.

TRICUSPID ATRESIA

Essential of Diagnosis

- Marked cyanosis present from birth.
- ECG with left axis deviation, right atrial enlargement, and left ventricular hypertrophy.

General Considerations

This relatively rare condition (< 1% of cases of congenital heart disease) is characterized by complete atresia of the tricuspid valve. As a result, no direct communication exists between the right atrium and right ventricle.

Tricuspid atresia may be divided into two types, depending upon the relationship of the great vessels:

Type 1. Without transposition of the great arteries: (a) No ventricular septal defect. Hypoplasia or atresia of the pulmonary artery. Patent ductus arteriosus. (b) Small ventricular septal defect. Pulmonary stenosis. Hypoplastic pulmonary artery. (c) Large ventricular septal defect and no pulmonary stenosis. Normal-sized pulmonary artery.

Type 2. With transposition of the great arteries: (a) With ventricular septal defect and pulmonary stenosis. (b) With ventricular septal defect but without pulmonary stenosis.

Because there is no direct communication between the right atrium and right ventricle, the entire systemic venous return must flow through the atrial septum (either an atrial septal defect or patent foramen ovale) into the left atrium. Accordingly, the left atrium receives both the systemic venous return and the pulmonary venous return. Complete mixing occurs in the left atrium, resulting in a greater or lesser degree of arterial desaturation.

As a result of this lack of direct communication, the development of the ventricle depends upon the presence of a left-to-right shunt at the ventricular level. Therefore, severe hypoplasia of the right ventricle occurs in those forms in which there is no ventricular septal defect or in which the ventricular septal defect is very small.

Clinical Findings

A. Symptoms and Signs: In the great majority of patients with tricuspid atresia, symptoms develop very early in infancy. Except in cases in which the pulmonary blood flow is great, cyanosis is present at birth. Growth and development are very poor, and there is usually easy fatigability on feeding, tachypnea, dyspnea, anoxic spells, and evidence of right heart failure. Patients with marked increase in pulmonary blood flow (types 1c and 2b) will develop evidence of left heart failure as well.

Clubbing is present if the child is old enough. On examination of the heart, a slight bulge on the right side of the sternum may occasionally be seen. The first heart sound is normal. The second heart sound is most often single (owing to aortic closure). A murmur is usually present, although it is variable. It ranges from grade I to grade III/VI in intensity and usually is a harsh blowing murmur heard best at the lower left sternal border.

B. Imaging: Chest x-ray findings are variable. The heart may be slightly to markedly enlarged. The main pulmonary artery segment is usually small or absent. The size of the right atrium varies from huge to only moderately enlarged, depending upon the size of the communication at the atrial level. The pulmonary vascular markings are usually decreased, although in types 1c and 2b they are increased.

C. Electrocardiography: The ECG is usually helpful. It often shows a left axis deviation with a counterclockwise loop in the frontal plane. The P waves are tall and peaked, indicative of right atrial hypertrophy. The size of the P wave depends upon the right atrial pressure, which in turn depends upon the size of the interatrial communication (the taller the P wave, the smaller the communication). Left ventricular hypertrophy or left ventricular preponderance is found in almost all cases. Voltage over the right precordium is usually low.

D. Echocardiography: M mode and two-dimensional methods are diagnostic and show absence of the tricuspid valve, the relationship of the great vessels, and the sources of pulmonary blood flow.

E. Cardiac Catheterization and Angiocardiography: This reveals the marked right-to-left shunt at the atrial level and desaturation of the left atrial blood. Because of the complete mixing in the left atrial chambers, oxygen saturation in the left ventricle, right ventricle, pulmonary artery, and aorta is identical to that in the left atrium. The right atrial pressure is increased. Left ventricular and systemic pressures are normal. The catheter cannot be passed through the tricuspid valve from the right atrium to the right ventricle. The course of the catheter is always from right atrium into left atrium and from there into left ventricle.

Treatment & Prognosis

In infants with high pulmonary artery flow, conventional anticongestive therapy should be given until the infant begins to outgrow the ventricular septal defect. At that point, a Fontan procedure (connection of right atrium to right ventricle or pulmonary artery) should be considered.

In infants with extremely low pulmonary artery flow, prostaglandin E₁ should be infused until an aorticopulmonary shunt can be performed. The Fontan procedure is rapidly gaining acceptance as the palliative procedure of choice. The optimal timing is controversial, but the procedure has been performed successfully in infants under 1 year of age.

The prognosis for all patients with tricuspid atresia depends on achieving a balance of pulmonary blood flow that permits adequate oxygenation of the tissues without producing intractable congestive heart failure. For children treated by the Fontan procedure, the prognosis is as yet undefined; initial results are moderately encouraging.

Gewillig MH et al: Impact on Fontan operation on left ventricular size and contractility in tricuspid atresia. Circulation 1990;81:118.

Ka Hung Tam C et al: Course of tricuspid atresia in the Fontan era. Am J Cardiol 1989;63:589.

Mair DD et al: Fontan operation on 176 patients with tricuspid atresia. Circulation Suppl 1990;82:IV–164.

HYPOPLASTIC LEFT HEART SYNDROME

Essentials of Diagnosis

- Mild cyanosis at birth. Minimal auscultatory findings.
- Rapid onset of shock with ductal closure.

General Considerations

Hypoplastic left heart syndrome includes a number of conditions in which there are either valvular or vascular lesions on the left side of the heart, resulting in hypoplasia of the left ventricle. The syndrome is found in 1.4–3.8% of infants with congenital heart disease.

The lesions that make up this syndrome are mitral atresia, aortic atresia, or both. In all of these conditions, there is severe obstruction to either filling or emptying of the left ventricle. As a result, during intrauterine life, the quantity of blood filling the left ventricle is extremely small, resulting in hypoplasia of this chamber. Following birth, survival depends upon a patent ductus arteriosus. there is marked impairment of the circulation because of the very small size of the left ventricle and the presence of obstructing lesions. Congestive heart failure develops rapidly, in most cases within several days to 3 months of life.

Patients with aortic atresia develop congestive heart failure very early, usually within the first week. Death occurs earliest in this group. Patients with mitral atresia who have large atrial and ventricular communications may live longer. Some patients have lived beyond the first decade. Patients with involvement of the aortic arch usually die within 1 month or less.

Clinical Findings

A. Symptoms and Signs: The clinical picture depends upon the type of obstructing lesion. Cyanosis is usually present early in life and is usually generalized. Patients with hypoplasia or atresia of the aortic arch may show differential cyanosis. Murmurs may or may not be present and are usually nondiagnostic. Congestive heart failure and shock accompany closure of the ductus arteriosus.

B. Imaging: Chest x-ray findings usually are relatively normal at birth. Rapid and progressive cardiac enlargement then occurs, frequently associated with pulmonary venous congestion. These changes occur earliest in patients with aortic atresia.

C. Electrocardiography: The ECG usually demonstrates right axis deviation, right atrial hypertrophy, and right ventricular hypertrophy with relative paucity of left ventricular forces and absence of a Q wave in V_6.

D. Echocardiography: Echocardiography is usually diagnostic and often eliminates the need for cardiac catheterization. A diminutive aorta and left ventricle with a poorly defined mitral valve in the presence of a normal and easily definable tricuspid valve are diagnostic. The systemic circulation is dependent on the patent ductus arteriosus. there is retrograde flow in the aortic arch with color Doppler.

Treatment & Prognosis

PGE₁ infusion is essential initial management, since systemic circulation depends on a patent ductus arteriosus. Further management depends on balancing pulmonary and systemic blood flow, because the right ventricle provides both. With increasing postnatal age, the pulmonary resistance falls, favoring pulmonary overcirculation and compromised systemic perfusion. Techniques to increase pulmonary vascular tone—such as hypoxia and hypercapnic ventilation, increased viscosity (hematocrit), and avoidance of pharmacologic pulmonary vasodilators—can improve systemic perfusion.

Definitive therapy at present is creation of single ventricle physiology operatively, as with the Norwood procedure and its variants. An increasing number of infants are receiving orthotopic cardiac transplantation in infancy to replace the defective cardiac anatomy.

The prognosis for this once uniformly lethal syndrome is improving. Palliative operations can now be performed with survival rates of 50–75%. Many palliated infants may ultimately require transplantation.

The 1-year survival rates with primary transplantation are over 80%. Further advances in surgery and immunology are likely to continue to improve the prognosis.

Boucek MM, Bernstein D: *Heart Transplantation in Infancy.* Progress in Pediatric Cardiology, 1993.

Boucek MM et al: Cardiac transplantation in infancy: Donors and recipients. J Pediatr 1990;116:171.

Morris CD, Outcalt J, Menashe VD: Hypoplastic left heart syndrome: Natural history in a geographically defined population. Pediatrics 1990;85:977.

Murdison KA et al: Hypoplastic left heart syndrome. Circulation Suppl 1990;82:IV–199.

COMPLETE TRANSPOSITION OF THE GREAT ARTERIES

Essentials of Diagnosis

- Cyanotic newborn without respiratory distress.
- More common in males.

General Considerations

Complete transposition of the great vessels is the second most common variety of cyanotic congenital heart disease, accounting for about 16% of all cases. The male/female ratio is 3:1. The disorder is due to an embryologic abnormality in the spiral division of the truncus arteriosus.

The aorta is located anterior to the pulmonary artery—either directly anterior or to the left or right. The pulmonary artery usually ascends parallel to the aorta rather than crosses it. In most cases, associated intracardiac abnormalities are present. These include ventricular septal defect, atrial septal defect, pulmonary stenosis, and patent ductus arteriosus. Obstructive changes within the pulmonary arteriolar bed are common in patients past infancy.

Transposition of the great vessels can be classified as follows:

Group 1. Transposition with intact ventricular septum: (a) Without pulmonary stenosis or (b) with pulmonary stenosis, subvalvular or valvular (or both).

Group 2. Transposition with ventricular septal defect: (a) With pulmonary stenosis, (b) with pulmonary vascular obstruction, or (c) without pulmonary vascular obstruction (normal pulmonary vascular resistance).

Since the aorta arises directly from the right ventricle, life would not be possible unless there were mixing between the systemic and pulmonary circulations; oxygenated blood from the pulmonary veins must in some way reach the systemic arterial circuit. In patients with intact ventricular septum (group 1), mixing occurs at the atrial and also at the ductal levels. However, in most patients, these communications are small, and the ductus arteriosus often closes shortly after birth. These patients are therefore severely cyanotic, and congestive heart failure occurs rapidly as a result of the marked increase in cardiac output. Patients with a ventricular septal defect show greater or lesser degrees of cyanosis, depending upon the ratio of the pulmonary to systemic blood flow. Patients with ventricular septal defect and pulmonary stenosis (groups 2a and 2b) are usually severely cyanotic because of the limited blood flow to the lungs. Patients with ventricular septal defect and pulmonary vascular obstruction (group 2b) show a moderate degree of cyanosis. Patients with ventricular septal defect and normal pulmonary vascular resistance (group 2c) show the least cyanosis but often develop heart failure very early because of the enormous pulmonary blood flow.

Congestive heart failure develops not only because of the high cardiac output but also because of the poor oxygenation of the myocardium and the presence of systemic pressure in both ventricles.

Clinical Findings

A. Symptoms and Signs: Many of the neonates are quite large, some weighing 4 kg (9 lb) at birth, and most are cyanotic at birth, although cyanosis occasionally does not develop until later. Patients in groups 1 and 2a are most cyanotic. Retardation of growth and development after the neonatal period is common. Congestive heart failure occurs in patients in groups 1 and 2c. Patients in group 2a show no evidence of congestive heart failure but often have severe anoxic spells in early life.

Although these infants are usually large at birth, growth and development are retarded before definitive surgery. The findings on cardiovascular examination depend somewhat upon the intracardiac defects. Group 1a patients have only soft murmurs or none at all. The first heart sound is usually normal. The second heart sound is single and accentuated and is best heard at the lower left sternal border. Patients in group 1b have loud obstructive systolic murmurs that are maximal at the second and third intercostal spaces and the left sternal border, radiating well to the first and second intercostal spaces. Group 2a patients have a murmur of pulmonary stenosis (obstructive systolic murmur at the base of the heart, best heard to the right of the sternum). Those in group 2c have a systolic murmur along the lower sternal border and a mitral diastolic flow murmur at the apex.

B. Imaging: In the sick, blue newborn, at a time when any diagnostic clues are greatly appreciated, the chest x-ray in transposition is often very nonspecific. In fact, at any age, the so-called characteristic findings may be lacking.

C. Electrocardiography: Early in infancy, the ECG is usually of little positive help. It reveals the usual amount of right ventricular hypertrophy expected for age. The absence of positive findings of other lesions, such as left axis deviation of tricuspid atresia, provides some deductive information.

D. Echocardiography: Two-dimensional imaging and Doppler evaluation can accurately describe the anatomy and physiology in infants with transposition. The abnormal relationship of the great vessels is the hallmark of transposition on echocardiography. Even the balloon septostomy may performed with echo guidance.

E. Cardiac Catheterization and Angiocardiography: Cardiac catheterization has a dual purpose in this malformation: diagnosis and therapy. As soon as the cardiologist has confidently demonstrated that complete transposition of the great arteries exists and that there are two well-developed ventricles, a Rashkind septostomy may be performed. The coronary anatomy can be delineated by ascending aortography.

Treatment

It has become increasingly apparent at many pediatric cardiology centers throughout the world that survival of patients with transposition of the great arteries depends on early, aggressive management. Cardiac catheterization is no longer routine for all types of transposition. Complex variations such as 2a, 2b, and 2c may still require invasive evaluation. PGE_1 infusion may improve mixing of oxygenated blood by opening the ductus arteriosus.

All patients with favorable anatomic and hemodynamic criteria (type 1) should be offered corrective surgery by 1 month of age. Surgery traditionally involved insertion of an intra-atrial baffle (by either a Mustard or a Senning operation) to redirect systemic and pulmonary venous blood to the appropriate pulmonary and aortic ventricles. Since 1975, surgical techniques to "switch" the great vessels to their anatomically appropriate locations have undergone a slow evolution. A key feature in the development of techniques has been careful patient selection. The left ventricular musculature in this entity rapidly loses its muscle mass and potential to meet systemic afterload unless a large ventricular septal defect or left ventricular outflow obstruction occurs; consequently, newborns with either of these conditions are appropriate candidates. The incidence of death from this type of surgery has fallen from 25% to approximately 10%. Although the death rate following an intra-atrial baffling procedure may be lower, there is growing concern about the long-term ability of an anatomic right ventricle to function as a systemic circulation pump. During the past several years, most institutions have begun using anatomic correction techniques in almost all patients. As the use of anatomic correction (vessel switch) techniques has spread to more centers, postoperative complications such as supravalvular pulmonary stenosis and stenoses or kinking of coronary arteries have been noted. The long-term exercise capacity of patients after interatrial rerouting operations has, in some studies, turned out to be better than that

projected by early studies. Long-term results for anatomic correction are yet to be determined. The intermediate-term results appear to be excellent for the arterial switch procedure.

Lupinetti FM et al: Intermediate-term survival and functional results after arterial repair for transposition of the great arteries. J Thorac Cardiovasc Surg 1992;103:421.

Muewe NN et al: Cardiopulmonary adaptation at rest and during exercise 10 years after Mustard atrial repair for transposition of the great arteries. Circulation 1988;77:1055.

Schmidt KG, Cloez JL, Silverman NH: Assessment of right ventricular performance by pulsed Doppler echocardiography in patients after intraatrial repair of aortopulmonary transposition in infancy and childhood. J Am Coll Cardiol 1989;13:1578.

Wernovsky G et al: Midtown results after the arterial switch operation for transposition of the great arteries with intact ventricular septum. Circulation 1988;77:1333.

ORIGIN OF BOTH GREAT VESSELS FROM THE RIGHT VENTRICLE

In this rare malformation, the aorta is completely transposed, but the pulmonary artery occupies a relatively normal position. Accordingly, both great vessels arise from the right ventricle. Ventricular septal defect is present in all cases and provides the only outlet for the left ventricle.

This malformation may be divided into five types on the basis of the relationship of the ventricular septal defect to the great arteries and the presence or absence of pulmonary stenosis: (1) ventricular septal defect related to the aorta, (2) ventricular septal defect related to the pulmonary artery (Taussig-Bing type), (3) ventricular septal defect committed to both great vessels, (4) ventricular septal defect uncommitted to the great vessels, and (5) ventricular septal defect related to the aorta, with pulmonary stenosis (tetralogy of Fallot type).

The clinical and laboratory features depend on which of the five anatomic types occurs. Two-dimensional echocardiography has proved to be extremely important in the diagnosis and classification of this entity.

Surgical correction is most satisfactory in patients with ventricular septal defect related to the aorta and is effected by closing the defect and creating a tunnel from the left ventricle to the aorta via the patch. Correction of uncommitted defects or defects related to the pulmonary artery requires patch closure and directing the blood to the pulmonary artery, thereby creating a transposition of the great vessels and an associated interatrial rerouting procedure. The use of a valued external conduit may be necessary in the complex varieties.

Roberson DA, Silverman NH: Malaligned outlet septum with subpulmonary ventricular septal defect and abnormal ventriculoarterial connection: A morphologic spectrum defined echocardiographically. J Am Coll Cardiol 1990;16:459.

Shen WK et al: Sudden death after repair of double outlet right ventricle. Circulation 1990;81:128.

TOTAL ANOMALOUS PULMONARY VENOUS RETURN WITH OR WITHOUT OBSTRUCTION

Essentials of Diagnosis

- Cyanosis.
- Systolic ejection murmur with left sternal border flow rumble and accentuated P_2.
- Right atrial and right ventricular hypertrophy.
- Pulmonary venous connection.

General Considerations

This malformation accounts for approximately 2% of all congenital heart lesions. The pulmonary venous blood does not drain into the left atrium but either directly or indirectly (via a systemic venous connection) into the right atrium. Thus, the entire venous drainage of the body drains into the right atrium.

This malformation may be classified according to the site of entry of the pulmonary veins into the right side of the heart.

> **Type 1 (55%):** Entry into the left superior vena cava (persistent anterior cardinal vein) or right superior vena cava.
> **Type 2:** Entry into the right atrium or into the coronary sinus.
> **Type 3:** Entry below the diaphragm (usually into the portal vein).
> **Type 4:** Multiple types of entry.

Since the entire venous drainage from the body drains into the right atrium, a right-to-left shunt is always present at the atrial level. This may take the form either of a large atrial septal defect or a patent foramen ovale. Relatively complete mixing of the systemic and pulmonary venous return occurs in the right atrium, so that the left atrial and hence the systemic arterial saturation levels approximately equal that of the right atrial saturation.

The degree of desaturation of the blood (and thus the degree of cyanosis present) is determined by the ratio of the quantity of pulmonary blood flow to that of the systemic blood flow. If pulmonary vascular resistance is normal, the flow of blood into the pulmonary artery is much greater than that into the left side of the heart. In this case, there is much greater return from the pulmonary than from the systemic venous system, and the saturation within the right atrium is high. Affected patients function very well, with relatively normal pulmonary artery pressures, and at least physiologically are very similar to patients with very large atrial septal defects and normal pulmonary venous return.

If pulmonary vascular resistance is elevated, the ratio of pulmonary to systemic blood flow is much lower. When the pulmonary vascular resistance equals that of the systemic vascular resistance, equal amounts of blood flow in both directions. When this occurs, marked desaturation of the mixed blood develops and the patient is markedly cyanotic. Such patients do much less well and eventually develop severe right heart failure.

Clinical Findings

A. With Normal Pulmonary Vascular Resistance: The great majority of patients in this group have some elevation of the pulmonary artery pressure owing to the marked increase in pulmonary blood flow. In most cases, the pressure does not reach systemic levels.

1. Symptoms and signs–These patients may have a history of mild cyanosis in the neonatal period and during early infancy. Thereafter, they do relatively well except for frequent respiratory infections. They are usually rather small and thin and resemble patients with very large atrial septal defects.

Careful examination discloses duskiness of the nail beds and mucous membranes, but definite cyanosis and clubbing are usually not present. The arterial pulses are normal. The jugular venous pulses usually show a significant V wave. Examination of the heart shows left chest prominence. A right ventricular heaving impulse is palpable.

The pulmonary component of the second sound is usually increased in intensity. A grade II–IV/VI ejection type systolic murmur is heard at the pulmonary area. It radiates very well over the lung fields anteriorly and posteriorly. An early to middiastolic flow murmur is often heard at the lower left sternal border in the third and fourth intercostal spaces (tricuspid flow murmur).

2. Imaging–Chest x-ray reveals evidence of cardiac enlargement primarily involving the right atrium, right ventricle, and pulmonary artery. There is a marked increase in pulmonary vascular markings. There is often a characteristic contour called a "snowman" or "figure of 8," which is seen where the anomalous veins drain into a persistent left superior vena cava.

3. Electrocardiography–Electrocardiography reveals right axis deviation and varying degrees of right atrial and right ventricular hypertrophy. There is often a QR pattern over the right precordial leads.

4. Echocardiography–Demonstration by echocardiography of a chamber posterior to the left atrium is strongly suggestive of the diagnosis. However, echocardiographic discrimination between anomalies of pulmonary venous return and persistence of pulmonary fetal circulation can still be challenging. The availability of two-dimensional echocardiography plus color flow Doppler has increased the diagnostic accuracy.

B. With Increased Pulmonary Vascular Resistance: This group includes patients in whom the pulmonary veins drain into a systemic venous structure below the diaphragm. It also includes a small number of patients in whom the venous drainage is into a systemic vein above the diaphragm.

1. Symptoms and signs–These infants are usually quite sick. Half die within the first 6 months; most are dead by age 1 year unless treated surgically. Cyanosis is common at birth and is quite evident by 1 week. Another common early symptom is severe tachypnea. Congestive heart failure develops later.

Cardiac examination discloses a striking right ventricular impulse. A shock of the second sound is palpable. The first heart sound is accentuated. The second heart sound is markedly accentuated and single. A grade I–II/VI ejection type systolic murmur is frequently heard over the pulmonary area with radiation over the lung fields. Diastolic murmurs are uncommon. In many cases, no murmur is heard at all.

2. Imaging–In the most severe and classic cases, the heart is small and pulmonary venous congestion is marked. In less severe cases, the heart may be slightly enlarged or normal in size, with only slight pulmonary venous congestion.

3. Electrocardiography–The ECG shows right axis deviation, right atrial hypertrophy, and right ventricular hypertrophy.

4. Echocardiography–Echocardiography may demonstrate the combination of a small left atrium and a vessel lying parallel and anterior to the descending aorta and to the left of the inferior vena cava. Color flow Doppler echocardiographic patterns are useful in establishing the diagnosis and are often diagnostic.

5. Cardiac catheterization and angiocardiography–These procedures are diagnostic. Cardiac catheterization demonstrates the presence of total anomalous pulmonary venous return and (usually) the site of entry of the anomalous veins. It also demonstrates the ratio of the pulmonary to systemic blood flow and the degree of pulmonary hypertension and pulmonary vascular resistance.

Cineangiocardiography following injection of contrast material into the right ventricle or pulmonary artery demonstrates the presence of anomalous pulmonary venous return and the site of entry of the anomalous veins.

Treatment

If immediate surgical intervention is not contemplated, atrial balloon septostomy should be performed during the initial diagnostic cardiac catheterization. This procedure coupled with vigorous medical management may sustain some infants for several months. Within the past few years, however, certain centers have reported excellent surgical results employing either cardiopulmonary bypass or deep hypothermia (cooling to 20 °C). A modification of the anastomosis allowing a larger communication has also greatly improved the surgical results. In such centers, the option of immediate surgical correction may be taken.

Course & Prognosis

Patients with normal pulmonary vascular resistance and only modest elevation of pulmonary artery pressures may do quite well through the first or second decade. Eventually, however, progressive increase in pulmonary vascular resistance and pulmonary hypertension does occur. Patients with increased pulmonary vascular resistance and pulmonary hypertension do poorly, and most die unless treated before age 1 year.

Smallhorn JF et al: Two-dimensional and pulsed Doppler echocardiography in the postoperative evaluation of total anomalous pulmonary venous connection. Circulation 1987;76:298.
VanMeter C et al: Partial anomalous pulmonary venous return. Circulation Suppl 1990;82:IV–195.

PERSISTENT TRUNCUS ARTERIOSUS

Essentials of Diagnosis

- Neonatal cyanosis.
- Systolic ejection click.

General Considerations

Persistent truncus arteriosus probably accounts for less than 1% of all congenital heart malformations. Only one (huge) great vessel arises from the heart and supplies both the systemic and pulmonary arterial beds. It develops embryologically as a result of complete lack of formation of the spiral ridges that divide the fetal truncus arteriosus into the aorta and pulmonary artery. A high ventricular septal defect is always present. The number of valve leaflets varies from two to 6, and the valve may be sufficient, insufficient, or stenotic.

The classification most commonly employed is divided into four types:

Type 1: One pulmonary artery that arises from the base of the trunk just above the semilunar valve and runs parallel with the ascending aorta (48%).

Type 2: Two pulmonary arteries that arise side by side from the posterior aspect of the truncus (29%).

Type 3: Two pulmonary arteries that arise independently from either side of the trunk (11%).

Type 4: No demonstrable pulmonary artery

(12%). Pulmonary circulation is derived from bronchials arising from the descending thoracic aorta. (The existence of this variety of truncus is controversial. Many authorities consider it an extreme form of tetralogy of Fallot with an atretic main pulmonary artery.)

In this condition, blood leaves the heart through a single common exit. Therefore, the saturation of the blood in the pulmonary artery is the same as that in the systemic arteries. The degree of systemic arterial oxygen saturation depends upon the ratio of the pulmonary to systemic blood flow. If pulmonary vascular resistance is normal, the pulmonary blood flow is much greater than the systemic blood flow and the saturation is relatively high. If pulmonary vascular resistance is great, owing either to pulmonary vascular obstruction or to very small pulmonary arteries, pulmonary blood flow is reduced and oxygen saturation is low. The systolic pressures in both ventricles are identical to that in the aorta.

Clinical Findings

A. Symptoms and Signs: The clinical picture varies depending upon the degree of pulmonary blood flow.

1. Large pulmonary blood flow–Patients with large pulmonary blood flow do well and are usually acyanotic, though the nail beds are commonly dusky. They function similarly to patients with large ventricular septal defects and pulmonary hypertension. Examination of the heart reveals a hyperactive impulse, felt both at the apex and over the xiphoid process. A systolic thrill is common at the lower left sternal border. The first heart sound is normal. A loud early systolic ejection click is commonly heard. The second sound is single and accentuated. A grade IV/VI, completely pansystolic murmur is audible at the lower left sternal border. A diastolic flow murmur can often be heard at the apex (mitral flow murmur).

2. Decreased pulmonary blood flow–Patients with decreased pulmonary blood flow have marked cyanosis early and do very poorly. The most common manifestations include retardation of growth and development, easy fatigability, dyspnea on exertion, and congestive heart failure. The heart is not unduly active. The first and second heart sounds are loud. A systolic grade II–IV/VI murmur is heard at the lower left sternal border. No diastolic flow murmur is heard. A continuous heart murmur is very uncommon except in type 4, in which the continuous murmur is due to the large bronchial collateral vessels. A very loud systolic ejection click is commonly heard.

B. Imaging: Most common x-ray findings are a boot-shaped heart, absence of the main pulmonary artery segment, and a large aorta that frequently arches to the right. The pulmonary vascular markings vary, depending upon the degree of pulmonary blood flow.

C. Electrocardiography: The axis is usually normal, though left axis deviation occurs rarely. Evidence of right ventricular hypertrophy or combined ventricular hypertrophy is commonly present. Left ventricular hypertrophy as an isolated finding is rare.

D. Echocardiography: A characteristic image would exhibit override of a single great artery (similar to tetralogy of Fallot) without a demonstrable right ventricular infundibulum. The origin or the pulmonary arteries and the degree of truncal valve abnormality can be seen. Color flow Doppler can aid in the description of pulmonary flow.

E. Angiocardiography: This procedure is usually diagnostic. Injection of contrast material into the right ventricle demonstrates the presence of a ventricular septal defect and the single vessel arising from the heart. The exact type of truncus, however, may be somewhat difficult to determine even from angiocardiograms.

Treatment

Anticongestive measures are indicated for patients with high pulmonary blood flow and congestive failure. Aortic homografting for "total correction" of the truncus has been performed in selected patients. During the past several years, the number of severely symptomatic infants undergoing successful "total correction" in the first 3 months of life has increased. Operative repair requires placement of a conduit from right ventricle to the pulmonary artery, and as the child grows replacement will be necessary.

Course & Prognosis

The outcome depends to a great extent upon the status of the pulmonary circulation. Patients with a low pulmonary blood flow usually do very poorly and die within 1 year. Those with increased pulmonary blood flow can survive for a variable period. A few cases of survival without surgery into the third decade have been reported. Death is usually due to congestive heart failure, hypoxia, subacute infective endocarditis, or brain abscess. Surgical repair has dramatically improved the prognosis.

Juanida E, Haworth SG: Pulmonary vascular disease in children with truncus arteriosus. Am J Cardiol 1984;54: 1315.

Pierpont MEM et al: Cardiac malformations in relatives of children with truncus arteriosus or interruption of the aortic arch. Am J Cardiol 1988;61:423.

Spicer B et al: Repair of truncus arteriosus in neonates with the use of a valveless conduit. Circulation 1984;70:26.

DEXTROCARDIA

This lesion consists of right-sided heart with or without reversal of position of other organs (situs inversus). If there is no reversal of other organs, the heart usually has other severe defects. With complete situs inversus, the heart is usually normal.

Apical pulse and sounds are heard on the right side of the chest. X-ray film shows the cardiac silhouette on the right side. On electrocardiography, the P waves are usually inverted in lead I; QRS is predominantly down in lead I; and lead II resembles normal lead III and vice versa. Two-dimensional echocardiography is extremely useful in defining the complex anatomy.

With situs inversus and no heart defects, the prognosis is excellent. If severe heart defects are present, definitive diagnosis is imperative, because corrective surgery is frequently beneficial.

Emmanouilides GC, Baylen BG: Dextrocardia and the cardiosplenic syndromes. In: *Neonatal Cardiopulmonary Distress.* Emmanouilides GC, Baylen BG (editors). Year Book, 1988.

Van Praagh R et al: Malposition of the heart. In: *Heart Disease in Infants, Children, and Adolescents,* 4th ed. Adams FH, Emmanouilides GC, Riemenschneider TA (editors). Williams and Wilkins, 1989.

ACQUIRED HEART DISEASE

RHEUMATIC FEVER

Rheumatic fever is a disease in transition. Although it is still an important disease in the USA, its frequency has diminished significantly over the past half century. Penicillin is largely responsible, but the decrease in frequency of rheumatic fever was already apparent before the antibiotic era. In the USA and other developed countries in the temperate zone, improvement in standards of living, general hygiene, and opportunities for medical care have greatly reduced the incidence of this disease. However, there has been a resurgence of acute rheumatic fever in several regions of the United States (the Midwest in 1984 and the intermountain West in 1987). In addition, the character of the illness is more malignant than that seen in the 1970s, with a high incidence of associated carditis and chorea. The reason for these regional epidemics is not as yet known, but it is clear that the disease is back.

Until the recent epidemic, the symptomatic presentation of the disease had also changed significantly in the USA within the past 2 decades. The frequency with which one encounters severe disabling carditis has greatly diminished, and the attack rate of acute rheumatic fever is considerably less than the original estimate of 0.3% in untreated children. Current manifestations of carditis are often mild and transient and require serial examinations by a skilled auscultator to confirm or rule out the diagnosis. One can only spec-

ulate on the reasons for these changes in the epidemiologic characteristics of the disease in different communities and on what role, if any, the liberal use of antibiotics may have played.

Group A β-hemolytic streptococcal infection of the upper respiratory tract is the essential environmental trigger that acts on predisposed individuals. The latest attempts to define host susceptibility implicate immune response (Ir) genes, which are present in approximately 15% of the population. The immune response triggered by colonization of the pharynx with group A streptococci consists of (1) sensitization of B lymphocytes by streptococcal antigens, (2) formation of antistreptococcal antibody, (3) formation of immune complexes that cross-react with cardiac sarcolemma antigens, and (4) myocardial and valvular inflammatory response.

The peak period of risk in the USA is age 5–15 years. The disease is slightly more common in girls and is now more common in blacks, perhaps reflecting socioeconomic factors. The average annual attack rate in the total North American population is less than one per 10,000, and the presence of rheumatic heart disease in the school-age population is less than one per 1000. The annual death rate from rheumatic heart disease in school-age children (whites and nonwhites) recorded a decade ago was less than one per 100,000.

Jones Criteria (Revised) for Diagnosis of Rheumatic Fever

Major manifestations
    Carditis
    Polyarthritis
    Sydenham's chorea
    Erythema marginatum
    Subcutaneous nodules
Minor manifestations
    Clinical
        Previous rheumatic fever or rheumatic heart disease
        Polyarthralgia
        Fever
    Laboratory
        Acute phase reaction: elevated erythrocyte sedimentation rate, C-reactive protein, leukocytosis
        Prolonged PR interval

Plus

Supporting evidence of preceding streptococcal infection, ie, increased titers of antistreptolysin O or other streptococcal antibodies, positive throat culture for group A *Streptococcus.*

Traditionally, two major or one major and two minor criteria (plus supporting evidence of streptococcal infection) justified the presumptive diagnosis of rheumatic fever. However, the major modern dilemma regarding diagnosis is that the physical findings may be so subtle and transient that the criteria are marginal. Since improper diagnosis has lifelong and serious consequences, it is justified to hospitalize patients with marginal findings so that serial clinical studies of the patient, including multiple examinations by a pediatric cardiologist, can be performed. If rheumatic fever appears likely on the basis of appropriate and careful evaluation but does not fully meet the Revised Jones Criteria, the diagnosis of suspect acute rheumatic fever is appropriate. This diagnosis mandates anti-infective prophylaxis but attempts to avoid the social and economic sequelae of the full diagnosis.

Major Manifestations of Rheumatic Fever

A. Active Carditis: Any one of the following–

1. A significant *new* murmur that is clearly mitral insufficiency (with or without a transient apical diastolic Carey-Coombs murmur) or aortic insufficiency. It should be remembered that mitral insufficiency, while commonly caused by rheumatic fever, has many other causes in childhood.

2. Pericarditis, manifested by a pericardial friction rub or evidence of pericardial effusion.

3. Evidence of congestive heart failure.

B. Polyarthritis: Two or more joints must be involved; involvement of one joint does not constitute a major manifestation. The joints may be involved simultaneously or (more diagnostically) in a migratory fashion. The most commonly involved joints are the ankles, knees, hips, wrists, elbows, and shoulders. Heat, redness, swelling, severe pain, and tenderness are usually all present. Arthralgia alone without the other signs of inflammation is not sufficient to meet the criterion of polyarthritis.

C. Subcutaneous Nodules: These are usually seen only in severe cases, and then most commonly over the joints, scalp, and spinal column. They vary from a few millimeters to 2 cm in diameter and are nontender and freely movable under the skin.

D. Erythema Marginatum: While this is a specific and major manifestation of acute rheumatic fever, many physicians fail to distinguish it from other skin lesions. It usually occurs only in severe cases and is rarely an essential diagnostic clue. It consists of a macular erythematous rash with a circinate border and appears primarily on the trunk and extremities. The face is usually not involved.

E. Sydenham's Chorea: Sydenham's chorea is characterized by emotional instability and involuntary movements. These findings become progressively more severe and are often followed by the development of ataxia and slurring of speech. Muscular weakness becomes apparent following the onset of the involuntary movements. The individual attack of chorea is self-limiting, although it may last up to 3 months. It is not uncommon to find involvement on only one side. Manifestations may not be apparent for months to years after the acute episode of rheumatic fever.

Minor Manifestations of Rheumatic Fever

A. Fever: The fever is usually low-grade, although occasionally it reaches 39.4–40 °C.

B. Polyarthralgia: Pain in two or more joints without heat, swelling, and tenderness is a minor rather than a major manifestation.

C. Electrocardiographic Changes: Prolongation of the PR interval represents only a minor manifestation and does not qualify as active carditis.

D. Acute Phase Reaction: The sedimentation rate is accelerated and, more specifically, the C-reactive protein is elevated. Congestive heart failure does not influence the C-reactive protein and usually does not affect the sedimentation rate. Leukocytosis is the rule.

E. History: There is a prior history of acute rheumatic fever or the presence of inactive rheumatic heart disease.

Essential Manifestation

Except in cases of rheumatic fever presenting solely as Sydenham's chorea or long-standing carditis, there should be clear supporting evidence of a streptococcal infection such as scarlet fever, a positive throat culture for group A β-hemolytic *Streptococcus,* and increased antistreptolysin O or other streptococcal antibody titers. The antistreptolysin O titer is significantly higher in rheumatic fever than in uncomplicated streptococcal infections.

Other Manifestations

Associated findings may include erythema multiforme; abdominal, back, and precordial pain; and nontraumatic epistaxis, vomiting, malaise, weight loss, and anemia. The abdominal pain may mimic a "surgical abdomen," and many negative laparotomies have been performed in patients with acute rheumatic fever.

Treatment & Prophylaxis

A. Treatment of the Acute Episode:

1. Anti-infective therapy–Eradication of the streptococcal infection is essential. Benzathine penicillin G is the drug of choice. Depending on the age and weight of the patient, give a single intramuscular injection of 0.6–1.2 million units, or give 125–250 mg orally four times a day for 10 days. Erythromycin, 250 mg orally four times a day, may be substituted if the patient is allergic to penicillin.

2. Anti-inflammatory agents–

a. Aspirin–Patients with the contemporary form of the disease need significantly less aspirin than in the past. Currently, 30–60 mg/kg/d is given in four divided doses; this dosage is often more than sufficient to effect dramatic relief of the arthritis and fever. In general, higher dosages carry a greater risk of side effects, and there are no proved short- or long-term benefits of giving high doses to effect salicylate blood levels of 20–30 mg/dL. The duration of therapy must be tailored to meet the needs of the patient, but use of aspirin for 2–6 weeks, with reduction in dosage toward the end of the course, is usually sufficient.

b. Corticosteroids–Corticosteroids are rarely indicated in current therapy. However, in the unusual patient with severe carditis and manifestations of congestive heart failure (as evidenced by radiographic findings of cardiomegaly or by cardiopulmonary symptoms or a gallop rhythm), therapy may not only be effective but lifesaving. Corticosteroid therapy may be given as follows: prednisone, 2 mg/kg/d orally for 2 weeks (or comparable doses of other corticosteroids); reduce prednisone to 1 mg/kg/d the third week, and begin aspirin, 50 mg/kg/d; stop prednisone at the end of 3 weeks, and continue aspirin for 8 weeks or until the C-reactive protein is negative and the sedimentation rate is falling.

3. Therapy of congestive heart failure–See Congestive Heart Failure, above.

4. Bed rest and ambulation–Strict bed rest is not required for patients with arthritis and mild carditis without congestive heart failure. It is preferable to maintain a regimen of bed-to-chair with bathroom privileges and meals at the table for patients who are relatively asymptomatic while on aspirin therapy. Asymptomatic patients can be kept in bed only under duress anyway. Patients with severe carditis (congestive heart failure) have no desire to get out of bed and should be at bed rest at least as long as corticosteroid therapy is required. *Gradual* indoor ambulation followed by modified outdoor activity may be ordered when symptoms have disappeared but there is still clinical and laboratory evidence of rheumatic activity. Modified bed rest for 2–6 weeks is generally adequate. Children should not return to school while there is clear evidence of rheumatic activity.

B. Treatment After the Acute Episode:

1. Prevention–The patient who has had rheumatic fever has a greatly increased risk of developing rheumatic fever following the next inadequately treated group A β-hemolytic streptococcal infection. *Prevention is thus the most important therapeutic course for the physician to emphasize.* The purpose of follow-up visits after the acute episode is not so much to evaluate the evolution of mitral insufficiency murmurs as to reinforce the physician's advice about the necessity for antibacterial prophylaxis with benzathine penicillin G. At such times, the physician should stress that greater protection is afforded by administration via the intramuscular route than via the oral route and that, in addition, failure to comply with regular oral medication programs increases the risk for recurrence of rheumatic fever. Thus, patients should be informed that the parenteral route will be favored

until they are adults, at which time their internists may elect oral medication.

If myocardial or valvular disease persists, antibacterial prophylaxis is a lifelong commitment. More commonly with transient cardiac involvement, 3–5 years of therapy or discontinuance at adolescence is a practical and effective approach.

The following regimens are in current use:

a. Benzathine penicillin G, 1.2 million units intramuscularly every 28 days, is the drug of choice.

b. Sulfadiazine, 500 mg daily as a single oral dose for patients weighing over 27 kg (60 lb), is the drug of second choice. Blood dyscrasias and a lesser effectiveness in reducing streptococcal infections make this drug less satisfactory than benzathine penicillin G.

c. Penicillin G (buffered), 250,000 units orally twice daily, offers approximately the same protection afforded by sulfadiazine but is much less effective than intramuscular benzathine penicillin G (5.5 versus 0.4 streptococcal infections per 100 patient years).

d. Erythromycin, 250 mg orally twice a day, may be given to those patients who may be allergic to both penicillin and sulfonamides.

2. Residual valvular damage–Chronic congestive heart failure may follow a single severe episode of acute rheumatic carditis or, more commonly, may follow repeated episodes. In children in the USA, the usual manifestations of residual valvular damage are heart murmurs of mitral and aortic insufficiency; murmurs are not accompanied by congestive heart failure during most of the pediatric age period *as long as repeated attacks are prevented.*

Methods of managing congestive heart failure have been previously discussed. Children with severe valvular damage who cannot be adequately managed on a medical regimen must be considered for valve replacement—and considered before the myocardium is irreversibly damaged.

Ayoub EM: Resurgence of rheumatic fever in the United States: The changing picture of a preventable illness. Postgrad Med 1992;92:139.

Kaplan EL, Hill HR: The return of rheumatic fever: Consequences, implications and needs. J Pediatr 1987;111:244.

Majeed H et al: Acute rheumatic polyarthritis. Am J Dis Child 1990;144:831.

Veasy LG et al: Resurgence of acute rheumatic fever in the intermountain west of the United States. N Engl J Med 1987;316:421.

RHEUMATIC HEART DISEASE

Mitral Insufficiency

Mitral insufficiency, the most common valvular residual of acute rheumatic carditis, is characterized by a pansystolic murmur that is localized at the apex. In patients with mitral involvement, the murmur appears early in the course of rheumatic carditis, and—depending on the severity of the damage—may disappear over a period of days or months or may persist for life.

Among the many other causes of mitral insufficiency, the most common is the mitral dysfunction syndrome, characterized by a mid to late apical systolic murmur introduced by a click.* Other causes are myocarditis, endocardial fibroelastosis, anomalous left coronary artery, and congenital anomalies of the mitral valve, which occur as isolated lesions or as part of a complex of anomalies (eg, endocardial cushion defects).

Mitral Stenosis

There are murmurs of mitral stenosis which are secondary to structural stenosis of the valve; those which are due to relative excess of flow (in large volumes of regurgitation); and those which are present during acute valvulitis (Carey-Coombs murmur). Mitral stenosis due to structural stenosis is rarely encountered in the USA before 5–10 years following the first episode of acute rheumatic carditis and is much more commonly discovered in adults than in children. Early structural mitral stenosis murmurs, flow murmurs, and Carey-Coombs murmurs are short and heard in mid diastole. Progressively more severe mitral stenosis murmurs become longer in duration until they attain the classic crescendo, presystolic configuration.

Aortic Insufficiency

This early decrescendo diastolic murmur is not commonly encountered as the sole valvular involvement of rheumatic carditis. It is the second most frequent valve affected in polyvalvular as well as in single valvular disease. It appears that the aortic valve is involved more often in males and in blacks. A short aortic systolic murmur due to excess flow may accompany the aortic insufficiency murmur.

Aortic Stenosis

Dominant aortic stenosis of rheumatic origin does not occur in pediatric patients. Aortic stenosis in children is congenital. In one large series, the shortest length of time observed for a patient to develop dominant aortic stenosis secondary to rheumatic heart disease was 20 years.

Horstkotte D et al: Pathomorphologic aspects, etiology, and natural history of acquired mitral stenosis. Eur Heart J 1991;12(Suppl B):55.

Lembo NJ et al: Mitral valve prolapse in patients with prior rheumatic fever. Circulation 1988;77:830.

---

*A word of caution about diagnosing the mitral dysfunction syndrome: The echocardiographic finding of prolapse (redundancy) of the mitral valve, which characterizes mitral dysfunction, may also be found in patients with acute rheumatic fever and recently acquired rheumatic heart disease.

MYOCARDITIS

In the great majority of cases, the cause of myocarditis is not determined. Coxsackievirus B is the commonest infectious agent isolated. Coxsackievirus A, rubella virus, cytomegalovirus, mumps virus, herpes virus, adenovirus, and many other viral agents have been implicated. Virtually every other infectious agent, including bacteria, fungi, rickettsiae, chlamydiae, spirochetes, parasites, and human immunodeficiency virus has been suggested as a cause of myocarditis, but laboratory confirmation is seldom possible. It is important to emphasize that myocarditis is part of a spectrum of primary endomyocardial diseases and may be one of the causes of endocardial fibroelastosis.

Clinical Findings

A. Symptoms and Signs: The clinical picture usually falls into two separate patterns: (1) Onset of congestive heart failure is sudden in a newborn who has been in relatively good health 12–24 hours previously. This is a malignant form of the disease and is thought to be solely secondary to overwhelming viremia and tissue invasion of multiple organ systems, including the heart. (2) In the older child, the onset of cardiac findings tends to be much more gradual. There is often a history of an upper respiratory tract infection or gastroenteritis within the month prior to the development of cardiac findings. This is a more insidious form of the disease and may have a late postinfectious or autoimmune component. Recovery from the initial infection is followed by gradual and progressive development of easy fatigability, dyspnea on exertion, and malaise.

In the newborn infant, the signs of congestive heart failure are usually quite apparent. The skin is pale and gray, and peripheral cyanosis may be present. The pulses are rapid, weak, and thready. Edema of the face and extremities may be present. Significant cardiomegaly is present, and the left and right ventricular impulses are weak. On auscultation, the heart sounds may be muffled and distant. Third and fourth heart sounds are common, resulting in a gallop rhythm. Murmurs are usually absent, though a murmur of tricuspid or mitral insufficiency can occasionally be heard. Moist rales are usually present at both lung bases. The liver is enlarged and frequently tender. The level of the jugular venous pulse is elevated.

B. Imaging: Generalized cardiomegaly can be seen on x-ray. There is evidence of moderate to marked pulmonary venous congestion. Pneumonitis is commonly present.

C. Electrocardiography: The ECG is variable. Classically, there is evidence of low voltage of the QRS throughout all frontal and precordial leads and depression of the ST segment and inversion of the T waves in leads I, III, and aVF and in the left precordial leads during the acute malignant stage. Dysrhythmias are common, and atrioventricular and intraventricular conduction disturbances may be present. With the more benign form—or during the recovery phase of the malignant form—high-voltage QRS complexes are commonly seen and are indicative of left ventricular hypertrophy.

D. Echocardiography: Echocardiography demonstrates four-chamber dilation with poor ventricular function and atrioventricular valve regurgitation.

Treatment

A. Digitalis: The use of digitalis in a rapidly deteriorating child with myocarditis is dangerous and should be undertaken with great caution. Because the inflamed myocardium is markedly sensitive to digitalis, only about two-thirds of the usual total digitalizing dose should be employed. During the initial phase of therapy, frequent ECGs should be taken. If serious dysrhythmias or other evidence of digitalis intoxication develops, the drug should be stopped and not reinstituted until all evidence of digitalis toxicity has disappeared. If toxicity is not evident and there is no clinical response, digitalis doses should be increased until one or the other is noted.

B. Diuretics: Diuretics should be administered with caution, since they may potentiate digitalis toxicity.

C. Corticosteroids: The administration of corticosteroids is controversial but seems more rational when used in the treatment of the more benign postinfectious autoimmune cases. If the patient's condition continues to deteriorate despite anticongestive measures, corticosteroids are commonly employed.

D. Systemic Vasodilators: The use of systemic vasodilators such as nitroprusside in a hypotensive deteriorating critically ill patient is risky but may be lifesaving.

Prognosis

The prognosis is related to the age at onset, the response to therapy, and the presence or absence of recurrences. If the patient is less than 6 months of age or older than 3 years, responds poorly to therapy, and manifests multiple recurrences of congestive heart failure, the prognosis is poor. Many patients recover clinically but have persistent cardiomegaly. It is possible that subclinical myocarditis in childhood is the pathophysiologic basis for some of the idiopathic myocardiopathies seen later in life.

Chan KY et al: Immunosuppressive therapy in the management of acute myocarditis in children. J Am Coll Cardiol 1991;17:458.

Rozkovec A et al: Natural history of left ventricular function in neonatal coxsackie myocarditis. Pediatr Care 1985; 6:151.

INFECTIVE ENDOCARDITIS

Essentials of Diagnosis

- Preexisting organic heart murmur.
- Persistent fever.
- Increasing symptoms of heart disease (ranging from easy fatigability to heart failure).
- Splenomegaly (70%).
- Embolic phenomena (50%).
- Leukocytosis, elevated erythrocyte sedimentation rate, hematuria, positive blood culture.

General Considerations

Bacterial infection of the endocardial surface of the heart or the intimal surface of certain arterial vessels (coarcted segment of aorta and ductus arteriosus) is a rare condition that usually occurs when an abnormality of the heart or great vessels exists. It may develop in a normal heart during the course of septicemia.

The incidence of infective endocarditis appears to be increasing owing to many factors, including (1) increased survival rates for children with congenital heart disease, (2) greater use of chronic central venous catheters, and (3) increased use of prosthetic material and valves. Pediatric patients without preexisting heart disease also are at increased risk for infective endocarditis owing to (1) increased survival rates for children with immune deficiencies, (2) greater use of chronic indwelling lines in critically ill newborns, and (3) increased incidence of intravenous drug abuse.

Patients at greatest risk include those with aorticopulmonary shunts, left-sided outflow obstruction, and ventricular septal defects. Predisposing factors can be identified approximately 30% of the time and include dental procedures, nonsterile surgical procedures, and cardiovascular surgery.

Organisms causing endocarditis include *Streptococcus viridans* (about 50% of cases), *Staphylococcus aureus* (about 30%), and fungal agents (about 10%).

Clinical Findings

A. History: Almost all patients have a history of heart disease. There may or may not be a history of infection or a surgical procedure (tooth extraction, tonsillectomy).

B. Symptoms, Signs, and Laboratory Findings: In one large study, the following symptoms, signs, and laboratory findings were reported (in order of decreasing frequency): changing murmurs, fever, positive blood culture, weight loss, cardiomegaly, elevated sedimentation rate, splenomegaly, petechiae, embolism, and leukocytosis. Other findings include hematuria, signs of congestive heart failure, clubbing, joint pains, and hepatomegaly. Echocardiography has become a valuable tool in diagnosing large vegetations.

Prevention

It is recommended that patients at risk for infective endocarditis be given appropriate antibiotics before any type of dental work (tooth extraction, cleaning) and before operations within the oropharynx, gastrointestinal tract, and genitourinary tract. Continuous antibiotic prophylaxis (as in the treatment of rheumatic fever) is *not* recommended in patients with congenital heart disease.

The following schedule is recommended: < 15 kg, 750 mg oral Amoxicillin; 15–30 kg, 1500 mg; > 30 kg, 3000 mg. This dose is to be given 1 hour prior to dental procedures and followed by one-half the initial dose 6 hours later.

Treatment

In a patient with known heart disease, the presence of an otherwise unexplained fever should alert the physician to the possibility of infective endocarditis. A positive blood culture or other major findings of infective endocarditis confirm the diagnosis. If a positive blood culture is obtained and the organism is identified, specific treatment should be begun immediately. Even if blood cultures are negative after 48 hours, it is advisable to begin penicillin therapy (if there is other evidence of infective endocarditis), because most positive cultures are obtained within the first 48 hours. Penicillin is the drug choice in most cases. Other antibiotics may be added (see Chapter 34). If congestive heart failure occurs and progresses unremittingly in the face of adequate antibiotic therapy, surgical excision of the infected area and prosthetic valve replacement should be considered.

Course & Prognosis

The prognosis depends upon how early in the course of the infectious process treatment is instituted. The prognosis is better in patients in whom blood culture is positive. If congestive heart failure develops, the prognosis is usually poor.

Even though bacteriologic cure of the infectious process is achieved, death may occur as a result of congestive heart failure secondary to severe valvular destruction. Intractable congestive heart failure may occur weeks or months following bacteriologic cure. Embolization may occur following bacteriologic cure when vegetations tear off from the involved area.

The death rate for infective endocarditis is still about 20%.

Awadallah SM et al: The changing pattern of infective endocarditis in childhood. Am J Cardiol 1991;68:90.

Biancaniello TM, Romero JR: Bacterial endocarditis after adjustment of orthodontic appliances. J Pediatr 1991; 118:248.

Dajani AS et al: Prevention of bacterial endocarditis: Recommendations by the American Heart Association. JAMA 1990;264:2919.

Jaffe WM et al: Infective endocarditis, 1983–1988: Echocardiographic findings and factors influencing morbidity and mortality. J Am Coll Cardiol 1990;15:1227.

PERICARDITIS

Essentials of Diagnosis

- Retrosternal pain made worse by deep inspiration and decreased by leaning forward.
- Fever.
- Shortness of breath and grunting respirations are common.
- Pericardial friction rub.
- Tachycardia.
- Hepatomegaly and distention of the jugular veins.
- ECG with elevated ST segment.

General Considerations

Involvement of the pericardium rarely occurs as an isolated event. In the great majority of cases, pericardial disease occurs in association with a more generalized process. Important causes include rheumatic fever, viral pericarditis, purulent pericarditis, rheumatoid arthritis, uremia, and tuberculosis.

In the pediatric age group, pericardial disease usually takes the form of acute pericarditis. In most cases, there is effusion of fluid into the pericardial cavity. The consequences of such effusion depend upon the amount, type, and speed of fluid accumulation. Under certain circumstances, serious compression of the heart occurs. The direct compression and the body's attempt to correct it result in cardiac tamponade. Unless the pericardial fluid is evacuated, death occurs very rapidly.

Clinical Findings

A. Symptoms and Signs: The symptoms depend to a great extent upon the cause of the pericarditis. Pain is common. It is usually sharp and stabbing, located in the mid chest and in the shoulder and neck, made worse by deep inspiration, and considerably decreased by sitting up and leaning forward. Shortness of breath and grunting respirations are common findings in all patients.

The physical findings depend upon whether or not a significant amount of effusion is present: (1) In the absence of significant accumulation of fluid, the pulses are normal and the level of the jugular venous pulse is normal. On examination of the heart, a characteristic scratchy, high-pitched friction rub may be heard. It is often systolic and diastolic and can be located at any point between the apex and the left sternal border. The location and timing vary considerably from time to time. The heart sounds are usually normal, and the heart is not enlarged to percussion. (2) If there is a considerable accumulation of pericardial fluid, the cardiovascular findings are different. The heart is enlarged to percussion, but on inspection of the precordium, it seems to be very quiet. Auscultation reveals distant and muffled heart tones. Friction rub is usually not present. In the absence of cardiac tamponade, the peripheral, venous, and arterial pulses are normal.

Cardiac tamponade is characterized by distention of the jugular veins, tachycardia, enlargement of the liver, peripheral edema, and "paradoxic pulse," in which the systolic pressure drops by more than 10 mm Hg during inspiration. The term paradoxic pulse is a misnomer, since the drop is only an accentuation of a normal event. (Normally, the systolic pressure drops by no more than 5 mm Hg.) This finding is best determined with the use of a blood pressure cuff. At this point, the patient is critically ill and has all the symptoms and signs suggestive of right-sided congestive heart failure.

Not all patients with marked cardiac compression demonstrate all the findings listed above. If the patient appears critically ill and has evidence of pericarditis and effusion, treatment should be instituted even though all the clinical signs of cardiac tamponade are not present.

B. Imaging: In pericarditis without effusion, chest x-ray findings are normal. With pericardial effusion, the cardiac silhouette is enlarged, often in the shape of a water bottle, with blunting of the cardiodiaphragmatic borders. When there is evidence of cardiac tamponade, the lung fields are clear. This is in contrast to patients with myocardial dilatation, who show evidence of pulmonary congestion.

C. Electrocardiography: A number of electrocardiographic abnormalities occur in patients with pericarditis. Low voltage is commonly seen in patients with significant pericardial effusion, although the voltage may be normal. The ST segment is commonly elevated during the first week of involvement. The T wave is usually upright during this time. Following this, the ST segment is normal and the T wave becomes flattened. After about 2 weeks, the T wave inverts and remains inverted for several weeks or months. In contrast to findings in patients with myocardial infarction, there is no reciprocal relationship between the findings in lead I and lead III in the frontal plane and the right and left precordial leads.

D. Echocardiography: Echocardiography has become a most reliable form of noninvasive diagnosis of pericardial effusion. The results must be considered in the light of the clinical picture in deciding whether or not to remove the fluid.

Treatment

Treatment depends upon the cause of the pericarditis. Cardiac tamponade due to any cause must be treated by evacuation of the fluid. It is usually desirable to perform a wide resection of the pericardium through a surgical incision. However, needle insertion into the pericardial sac may be lifesaving in an emergency situation.

Prognosis

The prognosis depends to a great extent upon the cause of the pericardial disease. Cardiac tamponade due to any cause will result in death unless the fluid is evacuated.

SPECIFIC DISEASES INVOLVING THE PERICARDIUM

Acute Rheumatic Fever

When pericarditis occurs during the course of acute rheumatic fever, it is almost always associated with involvement of the myocardium and endocardium (pancarditis). Thus, heart murmurs are almost always present. The pericarditis is usually of the serofibrinous variety and usually not associated with significant pericardial effusion.

Patients with acute rheumatic fever and pericarditis are usually very ill, with severe cardiac involvement. They respond extremely well to corticosteroid therapy. Pericarditis usually disappears rapidly (1 week) after corticosteroid therapy is started. Constrictive pericarditis almost never occurs secondary to this disease.

Viral Pericarditis

Viral pericarditis is uncommon in children and young adults. The most common cause is the coxsackievirus B4. Influenza virus has also been implicated. There is usually a history of a protracted upper respiratory tract infection.

The pericardial effusion usually lasts for several weeks. Cardiac tamponade is rare. Recurrences of pericardial effusion are quite common even months or years after the initial episode. Constrictive pericarditis has been reported in this disease.

Purulent Pericarditis

The most common causes of purulent pericarditis are pneumococci, streptococci, staphylococci, *Escherichia coli,* and *Haemophilus influenzae.* This disorder is always secondary to infection elsewhere, although occasionally the primary site is not obvious. In addition to demonstrating signs of cardiac compression, patients are quite septic and run extremely high fevers. The purulent fluid accumulating within the pericardial sac is usually quite thick and filled with polymorphonuclear leukocytes. Although antibiotics will sterilize the pericardial fluid, pericardial tamponade commonly develops, and evacuation of the pericardial sac is usually necessary. Wide resection of the pericardium through a surgical incision performed in the operating room is most desirable, but pericardiocentesis is often dramatically effective and lifesaving. Drainage of the purulent fluid is followed by marked improvement of symptoms.

Postpericardiotomy Syndrome

Postpericardiotomy syndrome is characterized by fever, chest pain, friction rub, and elevation of ST segment noted on ECG 1–2 weeks after open heart surgery. It appears to be an autoimmune disease with high titers of antiheart antibody and with detectable evidence of fresh or reactivated viral illness. The syndrome is often self-limited and responds well to short courses of aspirin or corticosteroid therapy. Occasionally, it lasts for months to years and may require pericardiocentesis or pericardiectomy.

Guindo J et al: Recurrent pericarditis: Relief with colchicine. Circulation 1990;82:1117.

Mason TG, Neal WA, DiBartolomeo AG: Elevated antinuclear antibody titers and the postpericardiotomy syndrome. J Pediatr 1990;116:403.

Sagrista-Sauleda J, Permanyer-Miralda G, Soler-Soler J: Tuberculous pericarditis: Ten-year experience with a prospective protocol for diagnosis and treatment. J Am Coll Cardiol 1988;11:724.

HYPERTENSION*

Blood pressure determinations are being more routinely obtained in the examination of infants and children; as a result, systemic hypertension has become more widely recognized as a pediatric problem. Pediatric standards for blood pressure have been published, but the studies from which these standards were derived suffered from three methodologic problems. The first and most important is that the widest cuff that would fit between the axilla and antecubital fossa was not routinely used. The use of a wide cuff either has no effect on blood pressure or decreases blood pressure by a maximum of 5 mm Hg. Use of a narrow cuff, however, routinely increases blood pressure by 10–50 mm Hg. The second methodologic problem was lack of an ethnic cross section. Third, the fact that systemic blood pressure decreases with increasing altitude of residence was not taken into consideration.

These three problems were addressed in a study of a triracial population at sea level and at an altitude of 10,000 feet. The widest cuff that would fit between the axilla and antecubital fossa was used in each case. Most children from 10–11 years of age needed a standard adult-size cuff (bladder width of 12 cm), and many high school students needed a large adult-size cuff (width of 16 cm) or leg cuff (width of 18 cm). Results of the study are shown in Table 21–3. The 95th percentile value for blood pressure was similar for both sexes and all three ethnic groups. Blood pressure varied more with altitude and body weight than

Table 21–3. The 95th percentile value for blood pressure (mm Hg) taken in the sitting position.[1]

Age (y)	Sea Level			10,000 Feet		
	S	Dm	Dd	S	Dm	Dd
5				92	72	62
6	106	64	60	96	74	66
7	108	72	66	98	76	70
8	110	76	70	104	80	70
9	114	80	76	106	80	70
10	118	82	76	108	80	70
11	124	82	78	108	80	72
12	128	84	78	108	80	72
13	132	84	80	116	84	76
14	136	86	80	120	84	76
15	140	88	80	120	84	80
16	140	90	80	120	84	80
17	140	92	80	122	84	80
18	140	92	80	130	84	80

[1]Blood pressures: S = systolic (Korotkoff's sound 1; onset of tapping); Dm = diastolic muffling (Korotkoff's sound 4); Dd = diastolic disappearance (Korotkoff's sound 5).

with sex or ethnic origin. If the blood pressure taken in a quiet atmosphere and sitting position exceeds the 95th percentile for systolic, diastolic muffle, or diastolic disappearance pressures, it should be repeated twice in 1- to 2-week intervals. If it is abnormal all three times, a pediatric hypertension diagnostic center should be consulted.

Essential hypertension is the most common form of pediatric hypertension. Coarctation of the thoracic or abdominal aorta, renal artery stenosis, renal disease, and pheochromocytoma should be ruled out.

Patients with essential hypertension often show improvement with reduction of obesity, reduction of excessive salt intake, institution of an exercise program, avoidance of cigarette smoking, and avoidance of use of oral contraceptives. The use of antihypertensive drugs in pediatric hypertension is controversial, but thiazide diuretics and propranolol are useful in selected cases.

Burke GL et al: Blood pressure and echocardiographic measures in children: The Bogalusa heart study. Circulation 1987;75:106.

Gifford RW et al: The fifth report of the Joint National Committee on detection, evaluation, and treatment of high blood pressure. Arch Intern Med 1993;153:154.

Gilman MW et al: Use of multiple visits to increase blood pressure tracking correlations in childhood. Pediatrics 1991;87:708.

Rocchini AP: Blood pressure in obese adolescents. Pediatrics 1988;82:16.

Steinfeld L et al: Sphygmomanometry in pediatric patients. J Pediatr 1978;92:934.

Task force on blood pressure control in children. Pediatrics 1987;79:1.

Weisman DN: Systolic or diastolic blood pressure. Pediatrics 1988;82:112.

*The diagnostic evaluation of renal hypertension and the treatment of hypertensive emergencies, as well as the ambulatory treatment of chronic hypertension, are discussed in Chapter 24.

ATHEROSCLEROSIS AS A PEDIATRIC PROBLEM

Awareness of the importance of coronary artery risk factors in general—and atherosclerosis in particular—has risen dramatically in the general population during the past 25 years. In adults, the incidence of death from ischemic heart disease has been decreasing over the last decade, presumably as a result of modifying the diet or life-style to avoid known risks for heart disease. During this same decade, a large number of serum samples from the pediatric population have been collected and analyzed for lipids, and epidemiologic studies have been performed to determine the relationship of lipid levels to coronary heart disease. The level of serum lipids in childhood usually remains the same through adolescence. Biochemical abnormalities in the lipid profile appear early in childhood and correlate with higher risk for coronary artery disease in adulthood. High-density lipoprotein has been identified as an antiatherogenic agent through these studies.

The concept of pediatric screening for hyperlipidemia has been evaluated carefully. Currently, only children at high risk—ie, children with a family history of early myocardial infarction (prior to 50–55 years) in parents or grandparents or with known familial hyperlipidemia—are screened routinely. In addition, some researchers consider adolescents with total cholesterol levels of greater than 180 mg/dL or low-density lipoprotein levels of greater than 110 mg/dL to be at risk for coronary artery disease in adulthood.

In the majority of cases, treatment consists of dietary restrictions, exercise, abstinence from smoking, and avoidance of other ischemic heart disease risk factors. In patients with life-threatening familial hyperlipidemia, pharmacologic and surgical intervention (ileal bypass or portacaval shunt) may be considered.

Jacobson MS, Lillienfeld DE: The pediatrician's role in atherosclerosis prevention. J Pediatr 1988;112:836.

Lauer RM, Clark WR: Use of cholesterol measurements in childhood for the prediction of adult hypercholesterolemia: The Muscatine Study. JAMA 1990;264:3034.

Lauer RM et al: National cholesterol education program (NCEP): Highlights of report. Pediatrics 1992;89:495.

Uauy R: Lovastatin therapy in receptor-negative homozygous familial hypercholesterolemia. J Pediatr 1988;113:387.

MUCOCUTANEOUS LYMPH NODE SYNDROME

Mucocutaneous lymph node syndrome, also known as Kawasaki disease, was first described in Japan in 1967. The acute illness is characterized by (1) prolonged fever (over 5 days) that is unresponsive to antibiotics; (2) conjunctivitis; (3) cracking and fissuring of the lips, with inflammation of mucous membranes; (4) cervical lymphadenopathy; (5) rash involving the trunk and extremities, with reddened palms and soles of the hands and feet and subsequent desquamation of tips of the toes and fingers; and (6) edema. Patients may also have associated arthritis. Thrombocytosis and increased sedimentation rate are seen on laboratory examination.

Cardiovascular complications during the acute illness include myocarditis, pericarditis, and arteritis that predisposes to aneurysm formation in the coronary arteries in approximately 20% of patients. Aneurysm formation may occur 7–45 days after the onset of illness. Acute myocardial infarction may occur during the acute illness secondary to thrombosis of these aneurysms. Death occurs in 1–2% of patients during this phase of the illness. Long-term follow-up of patients with aneurysms shows some resolution of aneurysms in half of those affected; the remainder may continue to have aneurysms, may develop stenosis, and, possibly later, may develop myocardial ischemia.

During the acute illness and for 2–3 months after, patients should be monitored closely by serial electrocardiography, chest x-ray, and M mode and two-dimensional echocardiography. Selective coronary angiography is recommended in those patients with coronary abnormalities detected by echocardiography.

The acute illness is now treated with high doses of intravenous immune globulin (IGIV), 2 g/kg as a single dose given over 10–12 hours. If fever recurs within 48–72 hours and no other source of the fever is detected, a repeat dose is recommended, and high doses of aspirin, 20 mg/kg/dose given four times a day until day 14 of illness, then 3–5 mg/kg/d for 2–3 months from the onset of illness if echocardiogram is normal or indefinitely if coronary abnormalities are present. Evidence of myocardial ischemia or infarction warrants early cardiac catheterization and bypass surgery if obstruction exists.

American Heart Association Committee on Rheumatic Fever, Endocarditis, Kawasaki Disease: Diagnostic guidelines for Kawasaki disease. Am J Dis Child 1990;144:1220.

Gersony WM: Diagnosis and management of Kawasaki disease. JAMA 1991;265:2699.

Management of Kawasaki syndrome: a consensus statement prepared by North American participants of the third international Kawasaki disease symposium, Tokyo, Japan, December 1988. Pediatr Infect Dis J 1989;8:663.

Newburger JW et al: A single intravenous infusion of gamma globulin as compared with four infusions in the treatment of acute Kawasaki syndrome. N Engl J Med 1991;324:1633.

Sundel RP et al: Gamma globulin re-treatment in Kawasaki disease. J Pediatr 1993;123:657.

DISORDERS OF RATE & RHYTHM & ELECTROLYTE IMBALANCE

The recognition and treatment of cardiac arrhythmias has markedly increased in the recent past for a number of reasons. Better monitoring (electrocardiography, bedside monitors, Holter monitors, etc) has increased the awareness and detection of rhythm disturbances. There is also a true rise in the incidence of arrhythmias. More children are now surviving cardiac surgery and acute carditis and live chronically with altered hemodynamics, physiology, and structural changes. These changes over time will create altered conduction and new arrhythmias.

The advent of invasive electrophysiology with recordings from the endocardium has greatly improved our understanding of the conduction system. And now, with cardiac ablation techniques, we can offer these children a "cure" rather than lifelong antiarrhythmia treatment.

In normal cardiac conduction, depolarization occurs in the following sequence: sinoatrial node (depolarization cannot be seen on ECG), atria (P wave), atrioventricular node (PR segment), and bundles and ventricles (QRS). Repolarization (T wave) then occurs. In evaluating cardiac dysrhythmias and abnormal findings on the ECG, it is important to keep in mind the normal sequence of cardiac conduction as well as the normal intervals of conduction (PR, QRS, QT, etc) and the normal rates in children. A systematic approach to electrocardiography is essential.

Sinus Arrhythmia

It is normal to have phasic variation in the heart rate (sinus arrhythmia). Typically, the sinus rate varies with the respiratory cycle, while P=QRS=T intervals remain normal. "Marked" sinus arrhythmia is defined as a greater than 100% variation in heart rate. It may be found in association with respiratory distress or increased intracranial pressure, or it may be present in normal children. It alone virtually never requires treatment. However, it may be associated with sinus node dysfunction (see below).

Sinus Bradycardia

Depending on the age of the patient, sinus bradycardia is defined as either (1) a heart rate below the normal limit for age (neonates to 6 years, 60 beats/min; 7–11 years, 45 beats/min; > 12 years, 40 beats/min) or (2) a heart rate inappropriately slow for the functional status of the patient (chronotropic incompetence). In critically ill patients, common causes of sinus bradycardia include hypoxia, central nervous system damage, and iatrogenic medication side effects. Only symptomatic bradycardia (syncope, low cardiac output, or exercise intolerance) requires treatment (atropine or artificial cardiac pacing).

Sinus Tachycardia

The heart rate normally accelerates in response to stress, (eg, fever, hypovolemia, anemia, or congestive heart failure). Tachycardia with decreased cardiac output is more ominous and warrants evaluation for shock or tachyarrhythmia. Treatment may be indicated for correction of the underlying cause of tachycardia (transfusion for anemia, correction of hypovolemia or fever, etc).

Gillette PC, Garson A Jr: *Pediatric Arrhythmias: Electrophysiology and Pacing.* Saunders, 1990.

PREMATURE ATRIAL CONTRACTIONS

Premature atrial contractions are triggered by an ectopic focus in the atrium. They are one of the most common premature beats seen in the pediatric population, particularly during the fetal and newborn period. They may be conducted (with associated QRS) or nonconducted (without associated QRS) (Figure 21–7). There is usually some delay until the next normal sinus beat. Depending on the ectopic focus of the premature contraction, the frontal plane vector of the P wave may be normal (+60 degrees) or abnormal. As an isolated finding, premature atrial contractions are benign and require no treatment. They may need to be suppressed with antiarrhythmic agents when they trigger tachyarrhythmias or produce bradycardia secondary to nonconduction.

PREMATURE JUNCTIONAL CONTRACTIONS

Premature junctional contractions arise within the AV node or the bundle of His. Most often they induce a normal QRS complex with no preceding P wave and may have retrograde atrial depolarization (P wave seen after QRS wave). When conducted aberrantly to the ventricles, premature junctional contractions look wide and bizarre and cannot be distinguished from premature ventricular contractions except by invasive electrophysiologic study. As an isolated finding, premature junctional contractions are usually benign and require no specific therapy.

PREMATURE VENTRICULAR CONTRACTIONS

Premature ventricular contractions may originate in either ventricle and are characterized by a bizarre QRS of > 80 ms duration in newborns and 120 ms in children, an abnormal T wave, not preceded by a P wave and a compensatory pause (interval between two beats including the premature contraction equal

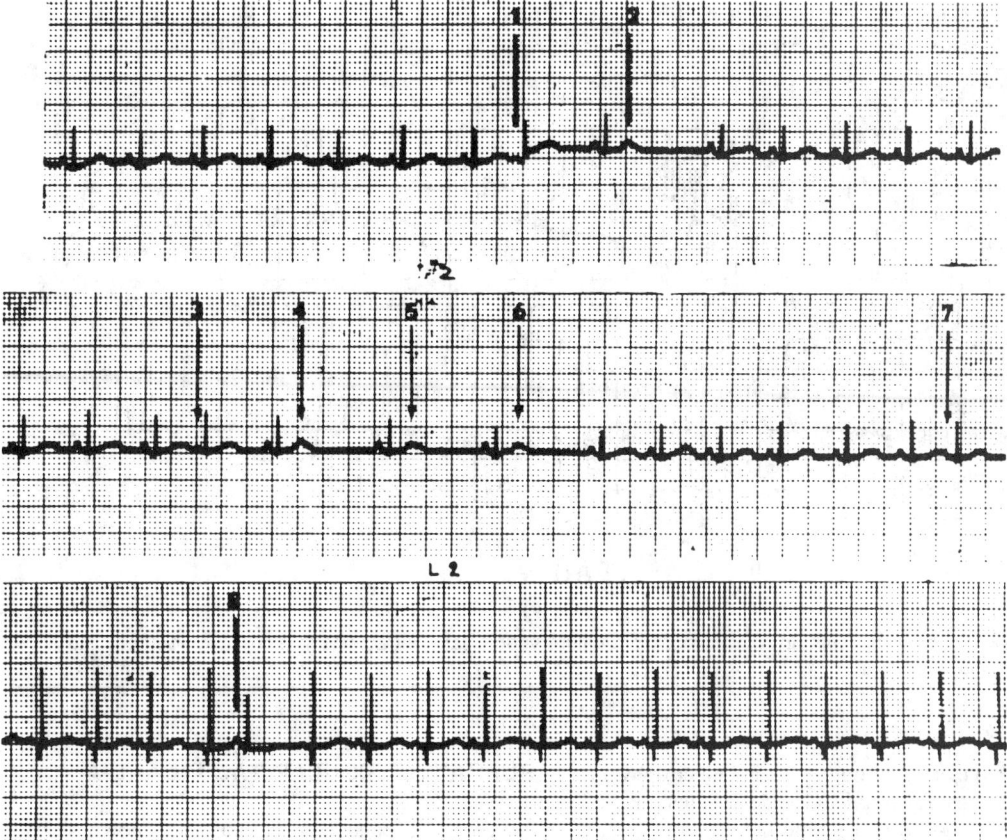

Figure 21–7. Lead II rhythm strip with premature atrial contractions. Beats 1, 3, 7, and 8 are conducted to the ventricles while beats 2, 4, 5, and 6 are not.

to two normal cardiac cycles (Figure 21–8). Premature ventricular contractions originating from a single ectopic focus all have the same configuration; those of multifocal origin show varying configurations. The consecutive occurrence of more than one beat can result in coupling (Figure 21–8) or ventricular tachycardia (three or more consecutive ventricular beats).

Most unifocal premature ventricular contractions in otherwise normal patients are benign. The nature of contractions can be confirmed by having the patient exercise. As the heart rate increases, benign premature contractions disappear. If exercise results in an increase or coupling of contractions, there may be underlying disease. Multifocal premature ventricular contractions are always abnormal and may be more dangerous. They may be associated with drug overdose (tricyclic antidepressants, digoxin toxicity, electrolyte imbalance, or hypoxia). Treatment is directed at correcting the underlying disorder.

SINUS NODE DYSFUNCTION

Sinus node dysfunction, or sick sinus syndrome, is a clinical syndrome of inappropriate sinus nodal function and rate. The abnormality may be a true anatomic defect of the sinus node or its surrounding tissue, or it may be an abnormality of the autonomic input. It is defined as one or more of the following: (1) sinus bradycardia, (2) "marked" sinus arrhythmia, (3) sinus pause or arrest, (4) sinoatrial exit block, (5) combined brady-and tachyarrhythmias, (6) sinus node reentry, and (7) atrial muscle reentry tachycardia. It is usually associated with postoperative repair of congenital heart disease (most commonly the Mustard or Senning repair for transposition of the great arteries), but it is also seen in unoperated congenital heart disease, acquired heart diseases and in normal hearts. Sometimes it is inherited. Symptoms usually present between 2 and 17 years and consist of syncope, presyncope, or disorientation. Some patients might experience palpitations, pallor, or exercise intolerance.

The evaluation of sinus node dysfunction involves

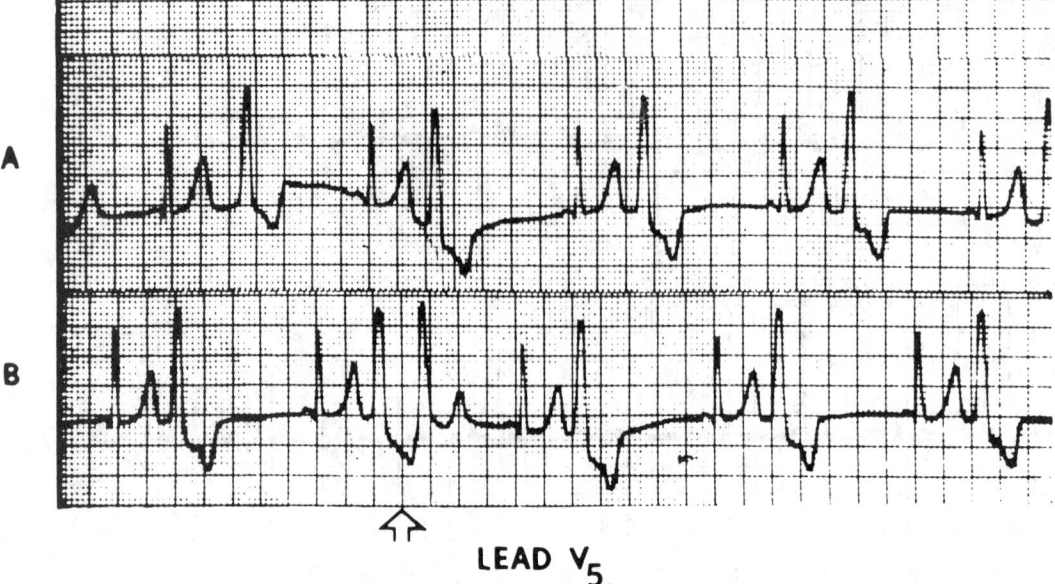

Figure 21–8. Lead V_5 rhythm strip with unifocal, premature ventricular contractions in a bigeminy pattern. The arrow shows a ventricular couplet.

both external electrocardiography and electrophysiologic recordings. Resting ECGs, exercise testing, and ambulatory monitoring help define the arrhythmia and correlate rhythm changes with symptoms. Invasive electrophysiologic recordings measure sinus node automaticity, sinoatrial conduction, and intrinsic heart rate with and without autonomic nervous system blockade. The correction of sinus node dysfunction during autonomic blockade with atropine and propranolol implies that the dysfunction is secondary to abnormal autonomic tone rather than an anatomic abnormality of the sinus node.

Treatment of sinus node dysfunction is usually reserved for symptomatic patients. Asymptomatic patients can just be observed since there is little chance of sudden death. Bradyarrhythmias are treated with vagolytic (scopolamine) or adrenergic (aminophylline) agents or permanent cardiac pacemakers. Antiarrhythmic treatment of tachyarrhythmias often produces or enhances bradycardia, thus requiring permanent pacing. In selected cases, permanent cardiac pacing is performed prophylactically prior to the initiation of antiarrhythmic medications. The prognosis for sinus node dysfunction is excellent when appropriate treatment is provided, with total morbidity and mortality rates nearly equal to those of the underlying heart disease. However, if left untreated, sinus node dysfunction may lead to chronic dysfunction and even sudden death.

SUPRAVENTRICULAR TACHYCARDIA

Supraventricular tachycardia, also known as paroxysmal supraventricular tachycardia or paroxysmal atrial tachycardia, is defined as an abnormal arrhythmia mechanism arising above or within the bundle of His (thus excluding sinus tachycardia). The mode of presentation is dependent upon the interaction of the rate of the tachycardia, the cardiovascular system, and the patient in general. A slow tachycardia may be poorly tolerated in a child with congestive heart failure or an underlying systemic disease such as anemia or sepsis or may go unnoticed in an otherwise normal child. Incessant tachycardia in an otherwise healthy individual, albeit slow (120–150 beats/min), may cause myocardial dysfunction and congestive heart failure if left untreated.

Tachycardia mechanisms can be divided into three groups: reentry, enhanced automaticity, and triggered dysrhythmias.

Reentry is conduction through two or more pathways, creating a sustained repetitive circular loop. The circuit can be confined to the atrium (intra-atrial reentry, a form of atrial flutter) (Figure 21–9). It may be confined within the atrioventricular node (atrioventricular nodal reentrant tachycardia) or it may encompass an atrioventricular accessory connection, producing orthodromic reciprocating tachycardia, where the electrical impulse travels anterograde down the atrioventricular node and then retrograde up the accessory connection and then back down the atrioventricular node to complete the reentrant loop

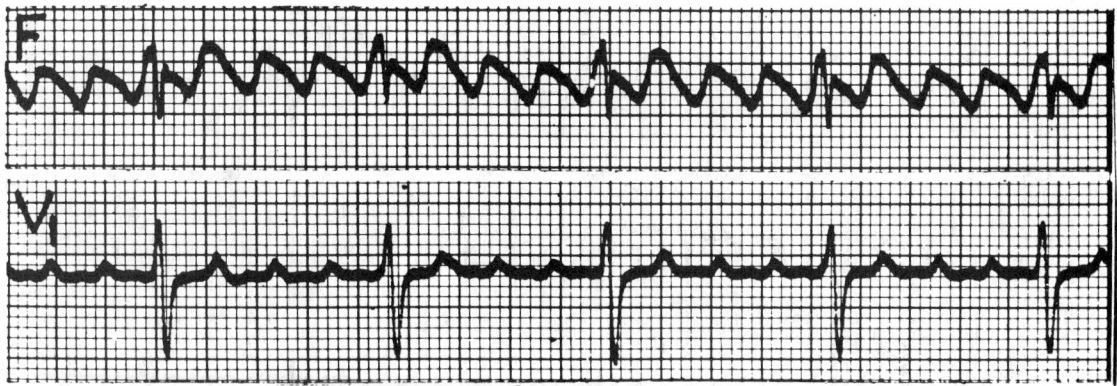

Figure 21–9. Leads aVF (F) and V$_1$, showing atrial flutter with "sawtooth" atrial flutter waves.

(Figure 21–10). Wolff-Parkinson-White syndrome is a subclass of these in which, during sinus rhythm, the impulse travels anterograde down the accessory connection, bypassing the atrioventricular node and creating ventricular preexcitation (early eccentric activation of the ventricle with a short PR interval and slurred upstroke of the QRS, a delta wave (Figure 21–11). Reentrant tachycardia represents approximately 80% of pediatric arrhythmias, have a wide range of rates, may or may not demonstrate P waves and initiate and terminate abruptly.

Enhanced automaticity (also known as automatic or ectopic tachycardia) is created when a focus of cardiac tissue develops an abnormally fast spontaneous rate of depolarization. These arrhythmias represent approximately 20% of childhood arrhythmias and are usually under autonomic influence. Electrocardiography demonstrates a normal QRS complex preceded by an abnormal P wave (Figure 21–12). Junctional ectopic tachycardia may show atrioventricular dissociation or 1:1 retrograde conduction (Figure 21–13). These tachycardias demonstrate a gradual onset and offset and may be paroxysmal or incessant. When they are incessant, they usually present with congestive heart failure and a clinical picture of dilated cardiomyopathy.

Triggered dysrhythmia is extremely rare. It is caused by enhanced afterdepolarizations of the action potential that reach the takeoff potential. It is one of the side effects of digitalis toxicity.

Clinical Findings

A. Symptoms and Signs: Clinical presentation varies with the age of the patient. Infants tend to turn pale and mottled with onset of tachycardia and may become irritable. With long duration of tachycardia, symptoms of congestive heart failure develop. Heart rates can be from 240 to 300 beats/min. Early diagnosis and prompt therapy are imperative in this group of patients. Older children may complain of dizziness, palpitations, fatigue, and chest pain. Heart rates usu-

ally range from 240/min in the younger child to 150–180/min in the teenager. Congestive heart failure is less common in children than in infants. Tachycardia may be associated with either congenital heart defects such as Ebstein's anomaly or acquired conditions such a cardiomyopathies and myocarditis. Complete noninvasive cardiovascular evaluation is indicated in all patients with a first episode of supraventricular tachycardia .

B. Imaging: Findings on chest x-ray are normal during the early course of tachycardia. If congestive heart failure is present, the heart is enlarged and there is evidence of pulmonary venous congestion.

C. Electrocardiography: Electrocardiography is the most important tool in the diagnosis of this condition.

1. The heart rate is rapid and out of proportion to the patient's physical status (ie, a rate of 140/min with an abnormal P wave while quiet and asleep) .

2. The rhythm is extremely regular. There is little variation in the rate throughout the entire tracing.

3. P waves may or may not be present. If they are present, there is no variation in the appearance or in the PR interval. P waves may be difficult to find because they are superimposed upon the preceding T wave. Furthermore, if the abnormal focus is located within the atrioventricular node, the P waves will not be seen (Figure 21–10).

4. The QRS complex is usually the same as during normal sinus rhythm. However, the QRS complex is occasionally widened, in which case the condition may be difficult to differentiate from ventricular tachycardia (supraventricular tachycardia with aberrant ventricular conduction).

Treatment

A. Acute Treatment: During initial episodes, patients require close monitoring. Correction of acidosis and electrolyte abnormalities is also indicated.

1. Vagal maneuvers–The "diving reflex," an icebag placed on the nasal bridge for 20 seconds (in-

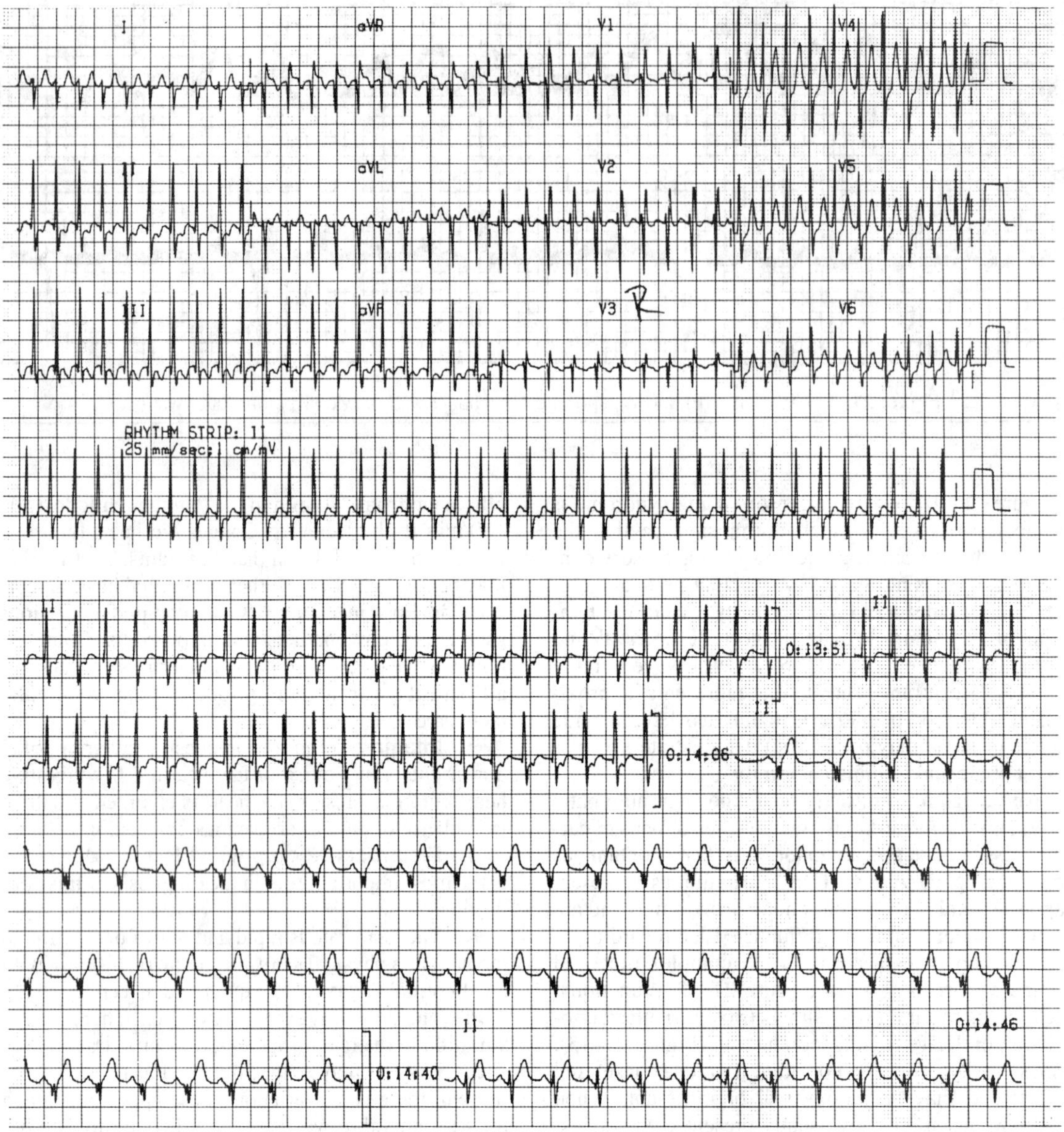

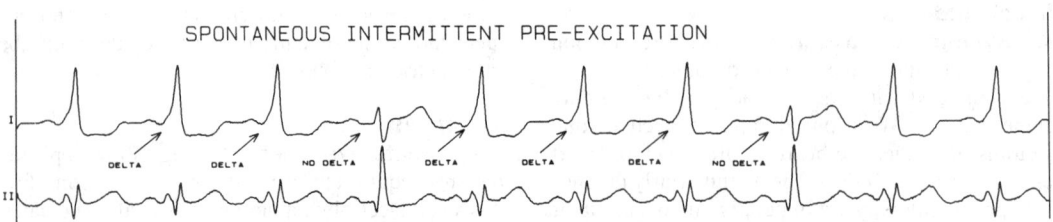

Figure 21–10. Supraventricular tachycardia. **A:** Twelve-lead ECG showing orthodromic reciprocating tachycardia (see text). **B:** Lead II rhythm strip showing spontaneous conversion to normal sinus rhythm with ventricular preexcitation (Wolff-Parkinson-White syndrome) and then spontaneous resolution with loss of the delta wave and a normal PR interval at the end of the tracing.

Figure 21–11. Leads I and II with spontaneous intermittent ventricular preexcitation (Wolff-Parkinson-White syndrome).

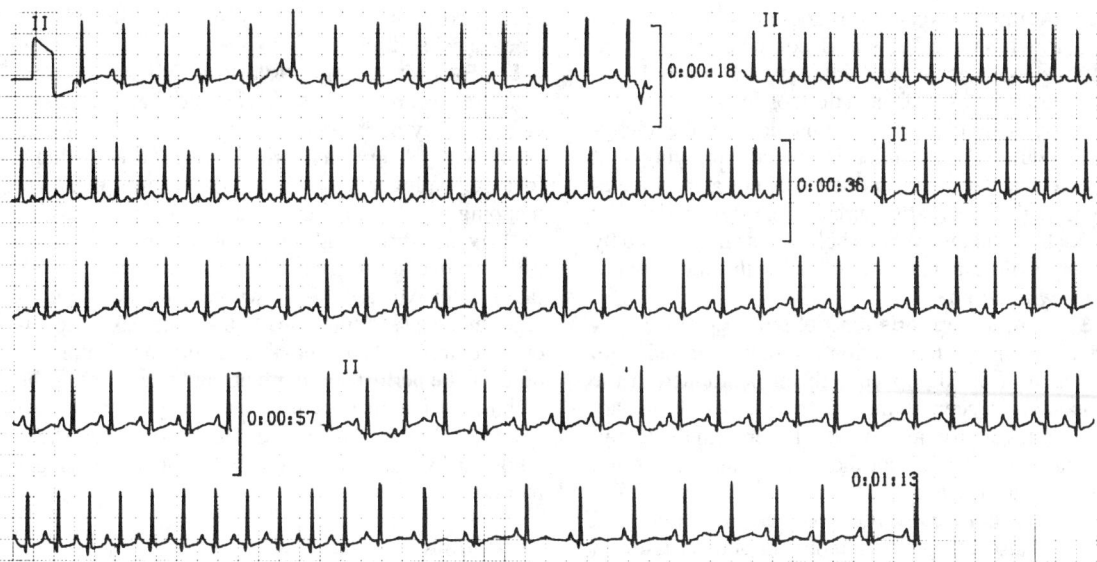

Figure 21–12. Lead II rhythm strip of ectopic atrial tachycardia. The tracing demonstrates a variable rate with a maximum of 260 beats/min, an abnormal P wave, and a gradual termination.

fants) or facial immersion in ice water (children or adolescents), will increase parasympathetic tone and terminate some tachycardias. The Valsalva maneuver, which can be performed by older compliant children, may also terminate supraventricular tachycardia.

2. Adenosine–Adenosine, an endogenous purine nucleoside, is a short-acting ($t_{1/2}$= 93 seconds) agent that transiently blocks conduction through the atrioventricular node and interrupts tachycardia circuits that utilize conduction through the node (atrioventricular nodal reentrant tachycardia, orthodromic

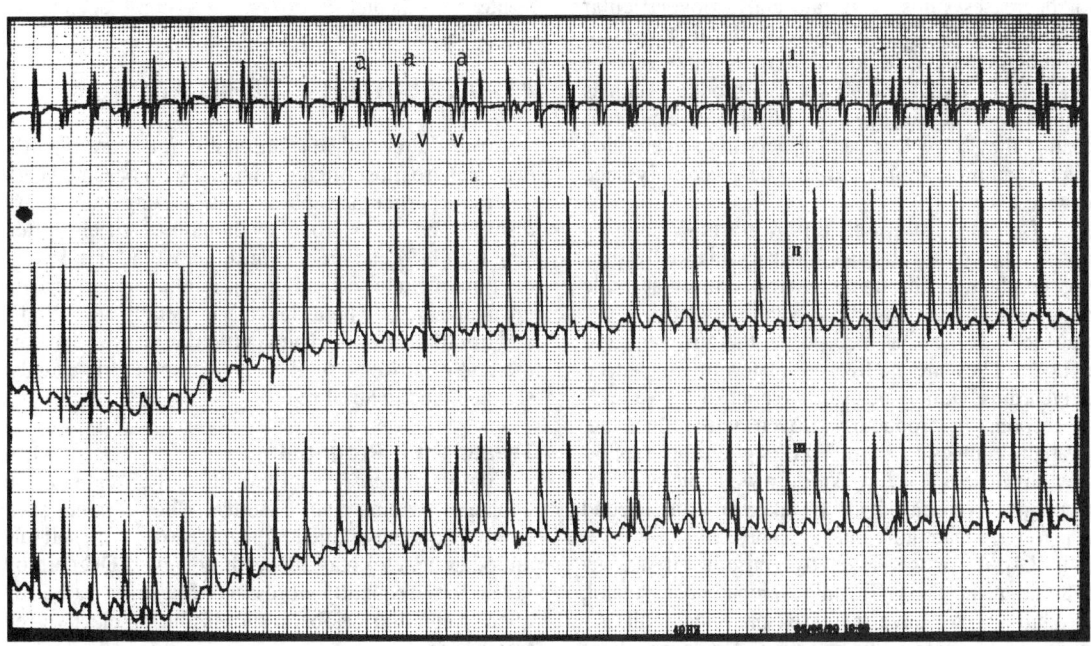

Figure 21–13. Three-lead rhythm strip of junctional ectopic tachycardia. Lead I is an atrial electrogram showing atrial (a)–ventricular (v) dissociation.

reciprocating tachycardia). It does not convert tachycardias whose mechanism is confined to the atria (atrial ectopic tachycardia, intra-atrial reentry). However, it serves as a diagnostic tool in these arrhythmias by demonstrating continuation of the tachycardia during atrioventricular block, implying that atrioventricular node conduction is not a crucial element of the tachycardia circuit. The dose is 50–250 μg/kg by rapid intravenous bolus. It is antagonized by aminophylline and should be used with caution in patients with asthma.

3. Transesophageal atrial pacing–Atrial overdrive pacing and termination can be performed from a bipolar electrode-tipped catheter positioned in the esophagus adjacent to the left atrium. Overdrive pacing at rates approximately 30% faster than the tachycardia rate will interrupt the tachycardia circuit and restore sinus rhythm.

4. DC cardioversion–DC cardioversion (1–2 J/kg) is also effective in more refractory cases of tachycardia and in critically ill infants. It should be used immediately when a patient presents in cardiovascular collapse and the above methods of cardioversion are not readily available. It will terminate virtually all reentrant arrhythmias but will only temporarily interrupt tachycardias caused by enhanced automaticity.

B. Chronic Treatment:

1. Digitalis–Digitalis is the drug of choice for long-term therapy. Conversion should be accomplished within 8–12 hours. Doses used are the same as those for congestive heart failure.

2. Beta-adrenergic blocking agents–Propranolol decreases sinus heart rate and atrioventricular nodal conduction. It is effective in the treatment of both reentrant and ectopic arrhythmias in doses ranging from 1 to 4 mg/kg/d. Newer beta-blockers such as atenolol and nadolol have recently become popular because they have less central nervous system side effects than propranolol and may be given only once or twice a day.

3. Calcium channel antagonists–Verapamil and other calcium channel blockers markedly prolong conduction through the atrioventricular node and are effective in interrupting and preventing reentrant tachycardias that incorporate the atrioventricular node. They are ineffective in terminating atrial tachycardias but may be useful to control the ventricular response by producing atrioventricular blockade. Verapamil comes in short- and long-acting preparations; the dose is 4–17 mg/kg/d. In well-tolerated, infrequent tachycardias, it can be taken on an as-needed basis to terminate individual episodes.

4. Other drugs–Recently introduced antiarrhythmic medications (flecainide, propafenone, sotalol, amiodarone, etc) have increased pharmacologic actions and are extremely effective. However, these drugs also have serious side effects, including proarrhythmia (production of arrhythmias) and sudden death, and should be used only under the direction of a pediatric cardiologist.

5. Radiofrequency ablation–This is a nonsurgical transvenous catheter technique that will desiccate an arrhythmia focus or accessory pathway and permanently "cure" an arrhythmia. The arrhythmia focus or pathway is localized by electrophysiologic mapping techniques, and a small 5 mm "burn" is created by delivering radiofrequency current from the catheter tip to a surface patch. The immediate success rate is approximately 85%, with a low rate of recurrence and a late failure rate of 10%. The risk of developing complete heart block is about 1%. The procedure can be performed in infants and adults and is the technique of choice in children over 3 years of age. In younger children, it should be reserved for those whose arrhythmias are refractory to medical management.

Prognosis

Supraventricular tachycardia has an excellent prognosis. When it presents in early infancy, 90% will respond to initial treatment. Approximately 30% will recur at an average age of 8 years.

Perry J, Garson A Jr: Supraventricular tachycardia due to Wolff-Parkinson-White syndrome in children: Early disappearance and late recurrence. J Am Coll Cardiol 1990;16:1215.

Van Hare GF et al: Percutaneous radiofrequency catheter ablation for supraventricular arrhythmias in children. J Am Coll Cardiol 1991;17:1613.

Van Hare GF, Stanger P: Ventricular tachycardia and accelerated ventricular rhythm presenting in the first month of life. Am J Cardiol 1991;67:42.

ATRIAL FLUTTER & FIBRILLATION

Atrial flutter and fibrillation are quite rare in children and are most often associated with organic heart disease—particularly postoperative congenital heart disease and sinus node dysfunction. Atrial flutter (Figure 21–9) can present in infancy, and if 1:1 conduction of flutter occurs, it can mimic supraventricular tachycardia. The atrial rate is usually > 240/min and often > 300/min. The ventricular rate depends on the rate of atrioventricular conduction and is usually slower than the atrial rate.

Treatment & Prognosis

Transesophageal atrial pacing is the treatment of choice to terminate atrial flutter. When it is not successful, antiarrhythmic medications (digoxin, sotalol, amiodarone, etc) may succeed; however, DC cardioversion is frequently necessary. Recently, radiofrequency ablation has been successful in selective refractory cases.

The prognosis in neonates without structural heart disease is excellent, and following conversion these patients may need no medications, while postoperative atrial flutter and fibrillation is often refractory to medical management. In extreme cases, creation of complete heart block and permanent pacing may be necessary.

VENTRICULAR TACHYCARDIA

Ventricular tachycardia (Figure 21–14) is uncommon in childhood. It is usually associated with underlying abnormalities of the myocardium (myocarditis, cardiomyopathy, myocardial tumors, or postoperative congenital heart disease) or toxicity (hypoxia, electrolyte imbalance, drug toxicity). Sustained tachycardia is generally an unstable situation and if left untreated will usually degenerate into ventricular fibrillation.

Acute termination of ventricular tachycardia involves restoration of the normal myocardium when possible (correct electrolyte imbalance, drug toxicity, etc) and DC cardioversion (1–4 J/kg), cardioversion with lidocaine (1 mg/kg), or both. Chronic suppression of ventricular arrhythmias with antiarrhythmic drugs has many side effects (including proarrhythmia and death), and it must be initiated in the hospital under the direction of a pediatric cardiologist.

LONG QT SYNDROME

The long QT syndrome in children is an arrhythmic disorder in which ventricular repolarization is irregular and prolonged ($QT_c > 0.44$ s). It presents as syncope or seizures in response to exercise or sudden death, and if untreated it has a very high mortality rate (5% per year). It is transmitted genetically in an autosomal dominant or recessive pattern (the latter associated with congenital deafness), or it may be sporadic.

Treatment is with beta blockade and exercise limitation and is only partially successful.

Garson A Jr et al: The long QT syndrome in children: An international study of 287 patients. Circulation 1993;87: 1866.

BENIGN VENTRICULAR ECTOPY

Single and couplet premature ventricular contractions—even nonsustained ventricular tachycardia—are benign arrhythmias in the setting of a normal heart. The investigation is directed at the evaluation of the heart and myocardium, and when findings are normal no treatment or exercise limitation is necessary. **Accelerated ventricular rhythm** is a sustained ventricular tachycardia seen in neonates with normal hearts. The rate is within 10% of the preceding sinus rate, and it is a self-limiting arrhythmia which requires no treatment.

HEART BLOCK

1. FIRST-DEGREE HEART BLOCK

First-degree heart block is an electrocardiographic diagnosis of prolongation of the PR interval. The block does not in itself cause problems, but it is frequently seen in association with such congenital heart defects as atrial septal defect and with diseases such as rheumatic carditis. The PR interval may also be prolonged as a result of digoxin therapy.

2. SECOND-DEGREE HEART BLOCK

Mobitz type I (Wenckebach) heart block is recognized by progressive prolongation of the PR interval

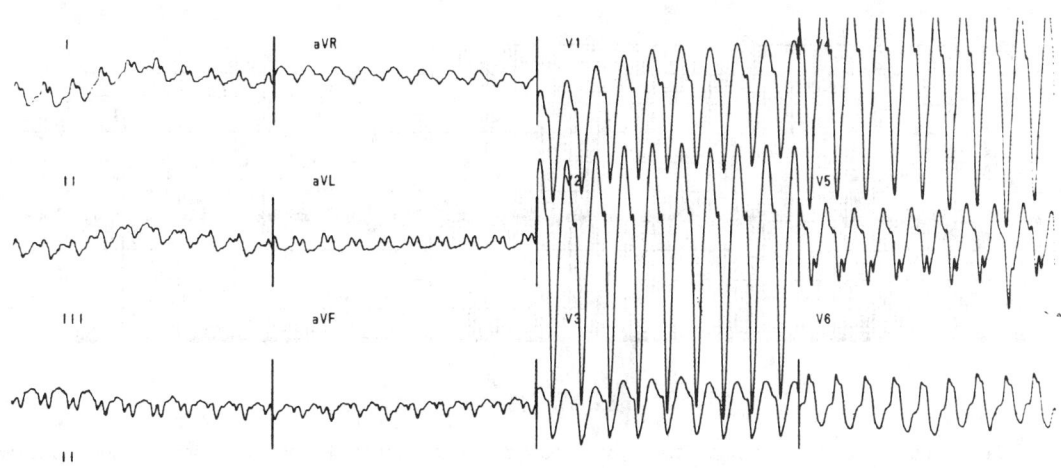

Figure 21–14. Twelve-lead ECG from a child with imipramine toxicity and ventricular tachycardia.

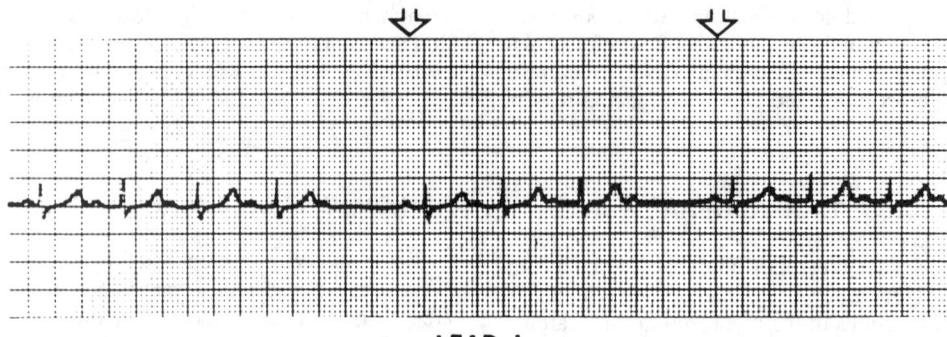

LEAD I

Figure 21–15. Lead I rhythm strip with Mobitz type I (Wenckebach) second-degree heart block. There is progressive lengthening of the PR interval prior to the nonconducted P wave.

until there is no QRS following a P wave (loss of atrioventricular conduction; Figure 21–15), whereupon the cycle may repeat itself. Mobitz type I heart block occurs in normal hearts and is usually benign. In **Mobitz type II** heart block, there is no progressive lengthening of the PR interval before the dropped beat (Figure 21–16). Mobitz type II heart block is frequently associated with organic heart disease, and a complete evaluation is necessary. In selected cases of Mobitz type II block, complete heart block may ensue, and prophylactic permanent pacemakers have been implanted.

3. COMPLETE HEART BLOCK

In complete heart block, the atria and ventricles beat independently. The atrial rate is usually more rapid than the ventricular rate (Figure 21–17). Ventricular rates can range from 40 to 80 beats/min, while atrial rates may be faster.

Congenital complete heart block, the most common form of complete heart block, has a very high association with maternal systemic lupus erythematosus (80% at our institution). Serologic screening should be performed in the mother of an infant with complete heart block even if she has no symptoms of collagen vascular disease. Congenital complete heart block is also associated with congenitally corrected transposition of the great vessels and endocardial cushion defect. Acquired complete heart block may be secondary to acute myocarditis, drug toxicity, electrolyte imbalance, hypoxia, and cardiac surgery.

Clinical Findings

Prenatal bradycardia is frequently noted in infants with congenital complete heart block. In the past, this finding occasionally indicated the need for emergency delivery of the infant; however, since the advent of fetal monitoring and fetal echocardiography, this is not often necessary. An overall assessment of postnatal adaptation to the heart block is important.

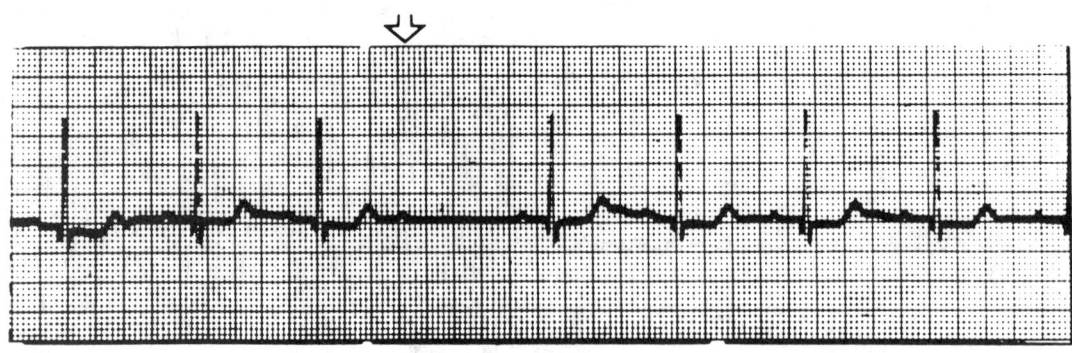

LEAD III

Figure 21–16. Lead III rhythm strip with Mobitz type II second-degree heart block. There is a consistent PR interval with occasional loss of atrioventricular conduction (arrow).

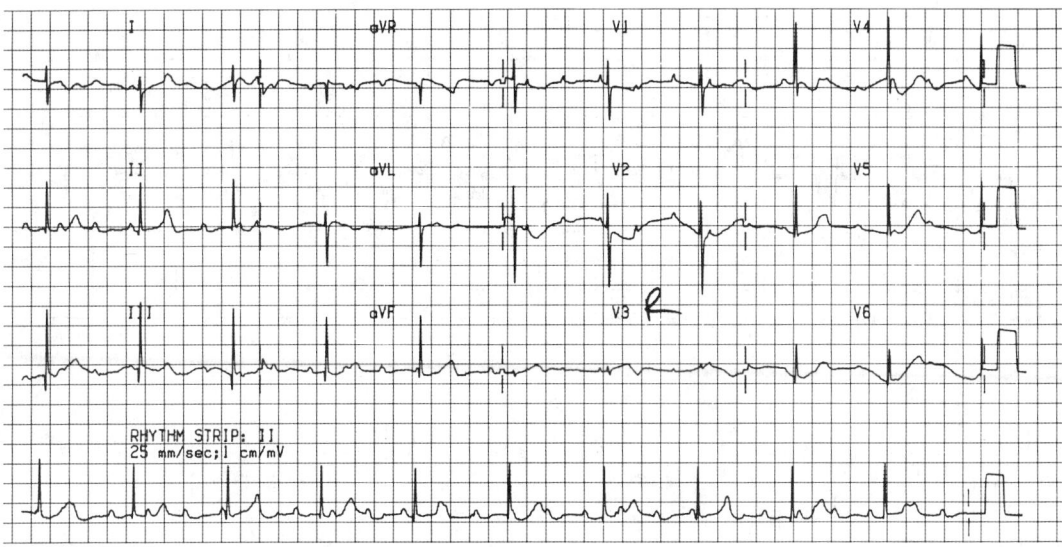

Figure 21–17. Twelve-lead ECG and lead II rhythm strip of complete heart block. The atrial rate is 150/min and the ventricular rate 60/min.

Adaptation is largely dependent on the heart rate; infants with heart rates < 55 beats/min are at significantly greater risk for low cardiac output, congestive heart failure, and death. Wide QRS complexes and a rapid atrial rate are also poor prognostic signs. Most patients have an innocent flow murmur from increased stroke volume. In symptomatic patients, the heart can be quite enlarged and pulmonary edema present. In older patients, Stokes-Adams syncope can be the presenting symptom, or heart block may be found unexpectedly on routine physical examination. Complete cardiac evaluation, including echocardiography and Holter monitoring, is necessary to assess the patient for ventricular dysfunction and to relate any symptoms to concurrent arrhythmias.

Treatment

In patients thought to be at risk for Stokes-Adams attacks or congestive heart failure, the treatment of choice for complete heart block is surgical insertion of a permanent pacemaker. Until permanent pacing can be instituted, patients can be temporarily assisted by infusions of isoproterenol or by temporary transcutaneous pacemakers.

Schmidt KG et al: Perinatal outcome of fetal complete atrioventricular block: A multicenter experience. J Am Coll Cardiol 1991;17:1360.

SYNCOPE
(Fainting)

Syncope is a sudden transient loss of consciousness that resolves spontaneously. The common form of syncope (simple fainting) occurs in 15% of children and is a disorder of control of heart rate and blood pressure by the autonomic nervous system which causes hypotension or bradycardia. It is often associated with rapid rising and postural hypotension, prolonged standing, or hypovolemia. Patients exhibit "vagal" symptoms such as pallor, nausea, or diaphoresis. Syncope, also known as autonomic dysfunction, can be evaluated with head-up tilt table testing. The patient is placed supine on a tilt table, and then—under constant heart rate and blood pressure monitoring—is tilted to the upright position. If symptoms develop, they can be classified as vasodepressor (hypotension), cardioinhibitory (bradycardia), or mixed. Treatment can then be directed accordingly. Syncope is usually self-limited and can be controlled with dietary salt and volume-loading to prevent hypovolemia. Syncope that occurs during exercise or stress or is associated with a positive family history is a warning sign that there may be a serious underlying dysrhythmia calling for further investigation.

Perry J, Garson A: The child with recurrent syncope: Autonomic function testing and beta-adrenergic hypersensitivity. J Am Coll Cardiol 1991;17:1168.

A.

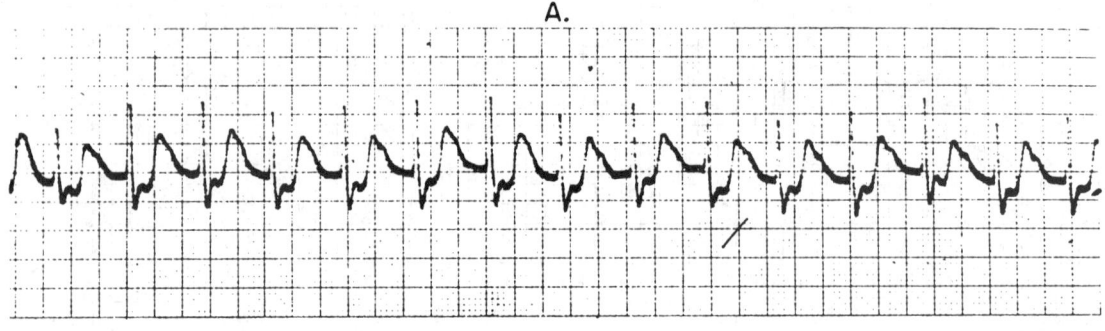

B.

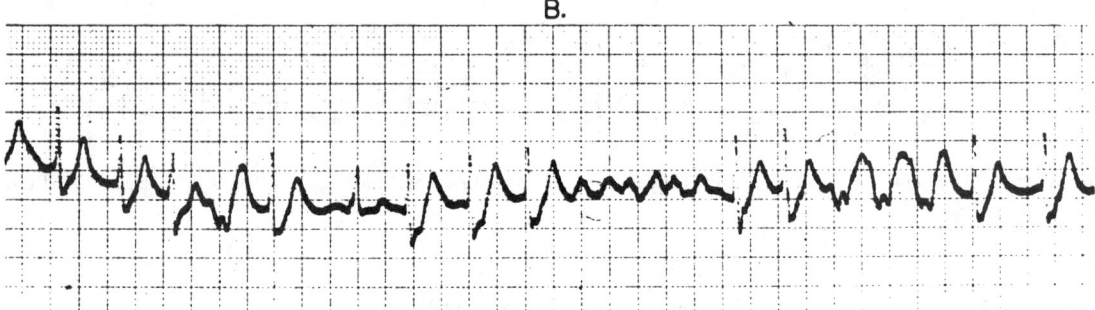

Figure 21–18. Rhythm strips of hyperkalemia beginning with tall peaked T waves and progressing to sinusoidal ventricular tachycardia.

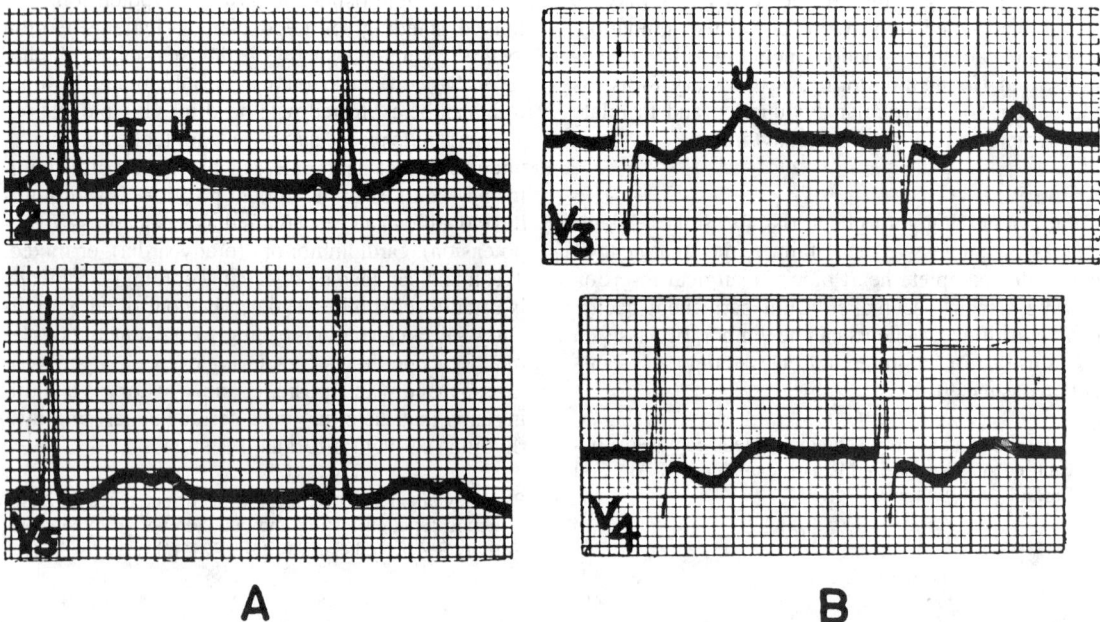

A   B

Figure 21–19. ECGs of hypokalemia showing ST segment depression and prominent U waves.

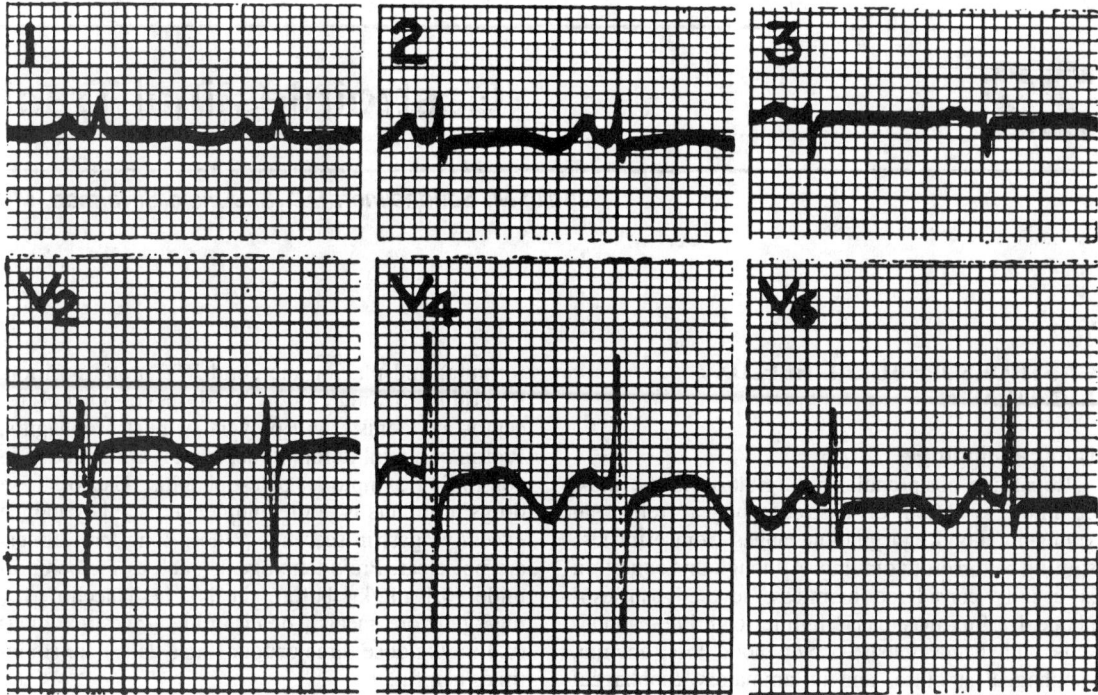

Figure 21–20. ECGs of hypocalcemia demonstrating QT interval prolongation and T wave inversion.

ELECTROLYTE IMBALANCE

Potassium, calcium, and to a lesser extent magnesium imbalances are reflected on the ECG. Electrolyte disturbances due to potassium and calcium excess or deficiency are of greatest concern to the pediatrician, and some familiarity with these abnormal tracings is essential. In hyperkalemia (Figure 21–18), there is gradual progression from tall peaked T waves (5–7 meq/L) through widening of the QRS complex (8–9 meq/L) to a broad, almost sinusoidal ventricular tachycardia configuration (> 10 meq/L). Hypokalemia (Figure 21–19) is characterized by progressive prominence of the U wave and prolongation of the QT interval with ST segment depression. In hypocalcemia (Figure 21–20), there is prolongation of the QT interval, and in extreme cases T wave inversion occurs.

Gastrointestinal Tract

Judith M. Sondheimer, MD & Arnold Silverman, MD

GASTROESOPHAGEAL REFLUX & CHALASIA

Clinical Findings

Repetitive postprandial regurgitation is the most common symptom of gastroesophageal reflux in young infants. Regurgitation ranges from effortless spitting to forceful vomiting. Although this condition is usually considered harmless, severe gastroesophageal reflux may cause failure to thrive, esophagitis with hematemesis, occult blood loss, anemia, esophageal stricture, and inflammatory esophageal polyps. Aspiration pneumonia, chronic cough, wheezing, and asthma-like attacks are reported. Dysphagia, discomfort or colic after feedings, and neck contortions (Sandifer's syndrome) may occur. Ruminative behavior is sometimes a symptom. Apneic spells in young infants, especially occurring with position change after feeding, may be caused by gastroesophageal reflux. Gastroesophageal reflux is common in neurologically impaired children. (See Table 22–1.) An associated sliding hiatal hernia is not rare.

Gastroesophageal reflux is usually diagnosed clinically in thriving infants under 6 months of age. It can be diagnosed on barium swallow by observing free regurgitation of barium from stomach to esophagus. However, both false-positive and false-negative tests are common. An upper GI series is important to rule out anatomic causes of vomiting. Prolonged monitoring of esophageal pH is a more sensitive test. Esophageal and gastric scintiscanning is sometimes helpful in identifying pulmonary aspiration. Esophageal manometry is not diagnostic but may identify hiatal hernia, hypotonic lower esophageal sphincter pressure, or motor disorders of the esophagus. Esophagoscopy is not diagnostic, but esophagitis can be identified visually or from biopsy material.

Treatment & Prognosis

In 85% of patients, gastroesophageal reflux is self-limited, disappearing between 6 and 12 months, often coincident with assumption of erect posture and initiation of solid feedings. Regurgitation is reduced by conservative measures such as small, frequent feedings thickened with rice cereal (2–3 tsp per ounce of formula) and placing the child in a prone position. Ranitidine (5.0 mg/kg/d in two doses) or other H_2 receptor antagonists will prevent or heal esophagitis. Proton pump inhibitors (omeprazole) are effective in controlling symptoms of esophagitis. Use of these drugs in infants is not recommended, as they induce excessive gastrin secretion, whose long-term effects are not clear. Prokinetic agents such as metoclopramide (0.1 mg/kg before meals), bethanechol (0.1 mg/kg before meals), or cisapride (investigational) (0.3 mg/kg/dose three or four times daily) are sometimes helpful.

Indications for surgery include (1) persistent vomiting with failure to thrive after 2–3 months of conservative treatment; (2) esophagitis refractory to medical treatment or persistent esophageal stricture; and (3) reflux causing apneic spells or chronic pulmonary disease. Children over 18 months, children with large hiatus hernias, and neurologically handicapped children respond less well to medical therapy for gastroesophageal reflux. Decreased vomiting is almost uniformly noted after a fundoplication. Dysphagia, gastric retention, decreased gastric capacity with early satiety, and retching are sometimes seen after surgery.

Boyle JT: Gastroesophageal reflux in the pediatric patient. Gastroenterol Clin North Am 1989;18:315.

Gunasekaran TS, Hassall EG: Efficacy and safety of omeprazole for severe gastrointestinal reflux in children. J Pediatr 1993;123:148.

Orenstein SR et al: Gastroesophageal reflux and respiratory disease in children. J Pediatr 1988;112:847.

Sondheimer JM: Gastroesophageal reflux: Update on pathogenesis and diagnosis. Pediatr Clin North Am 1988;35:103.

ACHALASIA OF THE ESOPHAGUS

Esophageal achalasia is characterized by failure of relaxation of the lower esophageal sphincter and lack of propulsive peristalsis in the esophageal body.

Clinical Findings

A. Symptoms and Signs: Achalasia is seen in all age groups but is uncommon under the age of 5

Table 22–1. Causes of vomiting and regurgitation.

GASTROINTESTINAL TRACT DISORDERS

Esophagus	**Intestine**
Achalasia	Atresia and stenosis
Gastroesophageal	Meconium ileus
reflux (chalasia)	Malrotation, volvulus
Hiatal hernia	Duplication
Peptic esophagitis	Intussusception
Atresia with or without	Foreign body, polyposis
fistula	Soy or cow's milk protein
Congenital vascular or	intolerance
mucosal rings, webs	Gluten enteropathy
Stenosis	Food allergy
Duplication and divertic-	Hirschsprung's disease
ulum	Chronic intestinal pseudo-
Foreign body	obstruction
Periesophageal mass	Appendicitis, perforations
Stomach	Crohn's disease
Hypertrophic pyloric	Gastroenteritis, infections
stenosis	**Other abdominal organs**
Pylorospasm	Hepatitis
Diaphragmatic hernia	Gallstones
Peptic disease and	Pancreatitis
gastritis	Peritonitis
Gastric volvulus, dia-	
phragm	
Duodenum	
Atresia, diaphragm	
Annular pancreas	
Duodenitis and ulcer	
Malrotation	
Mesenteric bands	
Superior mesenteric	
artery syndrome	

EXTRA-GASTROINTESTINAL TRACT DISORDERS

Sepsis	Adrenal insufficiency
Pneumonia	Renal tubular acidosis
Otitis media	Inborn errors
Urinary tract infection	Urea cycle disorders
Meningitis	Phenylketonuria
Subdural effusion	Maple syrup urine
Hydrocephalus	disease
Brain tumor	Organic acidemia
Reye's syndrome	Galactosemia
Rumination	Fructose intolerance
Intoxications	Tyrosinosis
Alcohol	Scleroderma
Aspirin	Epidermolysis bullosa
Acetaminophen	

years. The history of difficulty in swallowing solid food is intermittent at first and often goes back for many years. Typical symptoms include retrosternal pain and frequent episodes of food "sticking" in the throat or upper chest. Patients eat slowly and often drink large amounts of fluid with meals. Dysphagia is relieved by repeated forceful swallowing or by vomiting. Familial cases have been described. Chronic cough, wheezing, recurrent pneumonitis, anemia, and weight loss may occur.

B. Imaging and Manometric Studies: The barium swallow shows a grossly dilated esophagus (megaesophagus) with a short, tapered stricture at the distal end. In infants, dilation of the esophageal body may not be striking. Cinefluoroscopy may show ab-

sence of normal peristalsis. Esophageal manometry may demonstrate absence of peristalsis or non-peristaltic contractions after swallowing and failure of the lower esophageal sphincter to relax with swallowing.

Differential Diagnosis

Reflux esophagitis with peptic esophageal stricture must be ruled out by esophagoscopy, x-ray, pH probe, and manometric studies. Congenital esophageal stricture, esophageal webs, and esophageal masses may mimic esophageal achalasia.

Treatment & Prognosis

Pneumatic dilation of the lower esophageal sphincter is of value in most cases and can be repeated if symptoms recur. More definitive results can be achieved by surgically splitting the lower esophageal sphincter muscle (Heller myotomy). Because of the shorter duration of the illness in pediatric patients, the prognosis for return of the esophagus to normal caliber after surgical treatment is better than in adults.

Berquist WE et al: Achalasia: Diagnosis, management and clinical course in 16 children. Pediatrics 1983;71:798.

Nakayama DK et al: Pneumatic dilation and operative treatment of achalasia in children. J Pediatr Surg 1987;22: 619.

CAUSTIC BURNS OF THE ESOPHAGUS

Ingestion of caustic solids or liquids (pH > 12) may produce esophageal lesions ranging from superficial inflammation to coagulative necrosis with ulceration, perforation, and mediastinitis (or peritonitis if the stomach is involved). Children who have swallowed lye usually have painful, edematous lesions of the lips, oropharynx, and sometimes the larynx. The severity of oral lesions does not correlate well with the degree of esophageal injury. Esophageal or laryngeal obstruction secondary to edema and exudate occurs within 24 hours. Dysphagia caused by edema and tissue necrosis usually resolves over a few hours or days. The child may remain asymptomatic for a few months as an esophageal stricture develops. X-ray findings usually reveal esophageal stricture in the areas of anatomic narrowing, eg, the cervical region, at the point at which the left bronchus crosses the esophagus and at the gastroesophageal junction. Stricture of the esophagus occurs only if full-thickness necrosis of the deep muscle layers occurs. Single, dense, localized strictures may occur, or the entire esophagus may become twisted and narrowed. Shortening of the esophagus may lead to a hiatal hernia.

The child with a history of alkali ingestion should have a careful examination of the lips and mouth and evaluation of the airway. Drooling is common. Oral lesions are especially frequent if solid agents have been ingested. Stricture formation may occur slowly over months. Dysphagia is first manifest for solids and eventually for liquids.

Vomiting should not be induced following alkali ingestion. Hospitalization is recommended even if ingestion is only suspected. Intravenous corticosteroids (eg, methylprednisolone sodium succinate), 1–2 mg/kg/d, are started immediately if oral cavity swelling is severe and laryngeal edema is suspected. Intravenous fluids may be necessary if dysphagia is present. Esophagoscopy should be done within 24–48 hours after ingestion. Treatment is stopped if there is no visible lesion or if only a first-degree burn is seen. Corticosteroids may be beneficial if second-degree burns are noted but are not likely to prevent stricture formation from deep third-degree burns. Repeated esophageal dilations may be necessary as a stricture develops but are not performed acutely. When x-rays show erosion into the mediastinum or peritoneum, antibiotics are mandatory. Intraluminal esophageal stenting may be beneficial during early management.

Even with early treatment, stricture formation is inevitable in most cases with deep third-degree burns. Surgical replacement of the esophagus with a segment of colon may be necessary if dilation fails to control stricture.

Although other ingestants may cause esophageal irritation (eg, bleach, detergents, or acids), it is rare for any but the strongest acids and detergents to result in full-thickness necrosis and stricture.

Anderson KD, Rouse TM, Randolph JG: A controlled trial of corticosteroids in children with corrosive injury of the esophagus. N Engl J Med 1990;323:637.
Crain FC, Gershel JC, Mezey AP: Symptoms as predictors of esophageal injury. Am J Dis Child 1984;138:863.
Gaudreault P et al: Predictability of esophageal injury from signs and symptoms. A study of caustic ingestion in 378 children. Pediatrics 1983;71:767.
Goldman LP, Weigert JM: Corrosive substance ingestion: A review. Am J Gastroenterol 1984;79:85.

HIATAL HERNIA

Hiatal hernias are classified as (1) paraesophageal, in which the esophagus and gastroesophageal junction are normally placed with the gastric cardia herniated beside the esophagus through the esophageal hiatus; and (2) sliding, in which the gastroesophageal junction and a portion of the proximal stomach are herniated through the esophageal hiatus. Paraesophageal hernia is rare in childhood and presents with pain, or rarely esophageal obstruction or respiratory compromise. Sliding hernia is common in children. Gastroesophageal reflux may accompany sliding hiatal hernia, though many, even those of large size, cause no symptoms.

PYLORIC STENOSIS

Essentials of Diagnosis

- Vomiting, usually projectile.
- Constipation.
- Poor weight gain or weight loss.
- Dehydration and hypochlorhydric alkalosis.
- Palpable olive-sized mass in the right upper quadrant.
- Typical hypoechoic mass of 1.5 cm or greater in diameter on ultrasound.
- "String sign" and retained gastric contents on x-ray.

General Considerations

The cause of the increase in the size of the circular muscle of the pylorus is not known. There is a coincidence of the disease in twins or fathers and sons. The disease occurs in one out of 500 births, and males are affected 3–4 times more commonly than females. The reported increased incidence in firstborns and in the spring and fall months is controversial.

Clinical Findings

A. Symptoms and Signs: Vomiting usually begins between 2 and 4 weeks of age and rapidly becomes projectile after every feeding; it starts at birth in about 10% of cases. Presentation may be delayed in premature infants. The vomitus is rarely bilious but may be blood-streaked. The infant is hungry and nurses avidly, but constipation and failure to thrive occur. Dehydration, weight loss, fretfulness, and finally apathy occur. The upper abdomen may be distended after feeding, and prominent gastric peristaltic waves from left to right may be seen. An olive-sized tumor can almost always be felt in the subhepatic location to the right of the umbilicus, especially after the child has vomited.

B. Laboratory Findings: Elevated unconjugated bilirubin occurs in 2–3% of cases. There is hypochloremic alkalosis with potassium depletion. Hemoconcentration is reflected by elevated hemoglobin and hematocrit values.

C. Imaging: An upper gastrointestinal series reveals delay in gastric emptying and an elongated narrowed pyloric channel ("string sign"). The enlarged pyloric muscle causes characteristic semilunar impressions on the gastric antrum. Ultrasonography shows a hypoechoic ring in front of the right kidney and medial to the gallbladder.

Differential Diagnosis

Other causes of vomiting in young infants must be ruled out. (See Table 22–1.) In esophageal stenosis or achalasia, the emesis contains no gastric contents, and metabolic alkalosis is rare. With annular pancreas, malrotation, volvulus, and lesions causing small bowel obstruction, the emesis is bilious. The absence of virilization and hyperkalemia generally rules out congenital adrenal hyperplasia with adrenal insufficiency. Neurologic abnormalities and metabolic acidosis are often associated with other metabolic disorders. Sepsis and urinary tract infections should be checked by culture. Pylorospasm during barium x-ray may cause delay in gastric emptying, but the elongated narrow pyloric canal is not seen and no mass is palpable. Antral webs or diaphragms, duplications, cysts, and ulcers of the pyloric canal are rare causes of gastric outlet obstruction.

Treatment & Prognosis

Pyloromyotomy is the treatment of choice and consists of incision down to the mucosa and fully across the pyloric length. Prior to surgery, it is imperative to repair dehydration and electrolyte abnormalities even if it takes 24–48 hours.

The outlook is excellent following surgery. Sometimes there is continued vomiting postoperatively in cases with a long preoperative history. The postoperative barium x-ray remains abnormal despite relief of symptoms.

Khamapirad T, Athey PA: Ultrasound diagnosis of hypertrophic pyloric stenosis. J Pediatr 1983;102:23.

Moazam F, Kolts BE, Rodgers B: In pursuit of the etiology of congenital hypertrophic pyloric stenosis. J Pediatr Gastroenterol Nutr 1982;1:97.

EVALUATION OF THE CHILD WITH VOMITING

Assessment of the child with repetitive vomiting should start with a complete history, physical examination, and description of the vomitus. Emesis of gastric contents is characteristic of patients with gastric outlet obstruction, central nervous system infection or mass lesions, peptic disease, chronic urinary tract infection, chronic otitis or sinusitis, metabolic diseases (especially those causing acidosis), rumination, or psychogenic vomiting. Gastroesophageal reflux should be suspected in a healthy child with effortless postprandial spitting. A careful history will help to distinguish these entities. An upper gastrointestinal series is essential to rule out anatomic causes of vomiting. Further evaluations may include serum electrolytes, calcium, magnesium, urea nitrogen, urinalysis, and culture. The decision to obtain x-rays and scans of the central nervous system, chest, or sinuses requires a strong indication from historical information or from the physical examination.

The child who vomits bile-stained material may have small intestinal obstruction and should be investigated urgently. Bile staining may be gold or green in color. The history and physical examination are the essential starting points of the evaluation and should include duration of vomiting, the presence of blood in the vomitus, the presence of abdominal pain or distention, the character of the stools, and the presence of fever. Pain localized to the right lower quadrant suggests appendicitis. Midline or diffuse abdominal pain suggests pancreatitis or generalized peritonitis. Abdominal distention suggests intestinal obstruction. Viral and bacterial gastroenteritis may be associated with diarrhea and may produce a generalized ileus with bilious emesis. Gallbladder disease is uncommon in childhood but should be suspected in children with a positive family history or primary medical conditions promoting gallstones. The presence of mucus and blood in the stool should raise the suspicion of intestinal intussusception or bacterial or toxic colitis. Three-way radiographs of the abdomen are a first diagnostic step in localizing the site of intestinal obstruction. Historical and physical clues should direct further evaluation.

The evaluation of bloody vomitus should start with confirmation that the material vomited is indeed blood. Causes of bloody vomitus are listed in Table 22–11. Careful assessment of the cardiovascular stability of the child is essential before extensive evaluation is initiated. Passage of a nasogastric tube will help determine whether bleeding is ongoing. Hematocrit should be measured. The history and physical examination will provide specific clues to diagnosis which may make further testing unnecessary. If further diagnostic testing is desired, the most productive test will be upper intestinal endoscopy.

PEPTIC DISEASE

Peptic ulcers may occur at any age but are more frequent between 12 and 18 years. Boys are affected more commonly than girls. Up to age 6, most ulcers are secondary, associated with an underlying illness, toxin, or drug. A positive family history is present in about 30% of cases of primary duodenal ulcer.

Although the pathogenesis of peptic ulcer is multifactorial, the final common pathway appears to be a breakdown in the normal mucosal defense, which permits acid peptic digestion of the mucosa. Causes include (1) reduced mucous protective layer (aspirin, nonsteroidal anti-inflammatory drugs, hypoxia); (2) reduced metabolic activity of the gastric mucosal cell, which allows for the diffusion of hydrogen ions into the cell (hypoxia, hypotension); (3) increased gastric secretion of acid or pepsin (increased parietal cell mass, increased postprandial secretion of gastrin, increased vagal tone); (4) reflux of bile from duodenum to stomach; and (5) decreased neutralizing activity in duodenal secretions. The most common causes of secondary ulcer are toxins (alcohol, aspirin), sepsis, hypotension, burns, and injury of the central nervous system.

In adults there is a close association between gastric antral infection with *Helicobacter pylori*, antral gastritis and primary peptic ulcer of the duodenum and stomach. The incidence of *H pylori* infection is low in North American children but increases with age (50% of blood donors in the USA have *H pylori* antibodies). There is no evidence that *H pylori* infection causes recurrent abdominal pain of childhood or dyspepsia without gastritis.

Clinical Findings

A. Symptoms and Signs:

1. At 0–3 years of age–In infants past the neonatal period up to the age of 3, symptoms of primary ulcers include anorexia, vomiting, crying after meals, and melena or hematemesis. Secondary ulcers are more acute, and hemorrhage or perforation may be the first signs.

2. At 3–6 years of age–Vomiting related to eating is usually present. Gastric outlet obstruction may cause protracted vomiting. Periumbilical or generalized abdominal pain is common. The typical "ulcer pain" is rarely present. Melena, hematemesis, and perforation are common in cases of secondary ulcers.

3. At 6–18 years of age–Fewer than 50% of patients have "typical" ulcer symptoms. Melena or hematemesis (or both) is noted in over 50%; occult bleeding and anemia may occur without other symptoms. In addition to the acute illnesses responsible for secondary ulcers (central nervous system disease, burns, sepsis, multiple organ failure), chronic conditions such as pulmonary insufficiency, Crohn's disease, hepatic cirrhosis, and rheumatoid arthritis are associated with peptic disease.

B. Gastric Analysis: Gastric analysis is rarely performed. It may be useful in identifying extreme hypersecretion such as that associated with the Zollinger-Ellison syndrome, but a secretin stimulation test is much less cumbersome. Gastrin levels after a feeding tend to be higher in children with duodenal ulcers. They should be obtained in cases of recurrent ulcers if no other cause is found as a first step in identifying the rare child with hypergastrinemia syndrome.

C. Imaging: Radiologic signs of ulceration or a deformity should be present. The frequency with which the radiologic sign of duodenal irritability is found in normal infants makes this x-ray finding unreliable. In patients with severe degrees of duodenal irritability, a crater may not be demonstrated, because the barium is moved out of the bulb very rapidly.

D. Panendoscopy: Upper intestinal endoscopy should be performed if x-ray is negative or equivocal. If upper gastrointestinal bleeding (hematemesis or melena) is present, endoscopy should be the first diagnostic test if it can be done within 48 hours of the episode. Endoscopy also permits gastric biopsy necessary for the identification of *H pylori* by culture, histology and urease activity. The presence of serum anti-*H pylori* antibody appears to correlate well with infection; titers fall with eradication and rise with relapse.

Differential Diagnosis

Acute secondary ulcers should be suspected in any child with a severe underlying disease who suddenly presents with abdominal distention, hematemesis, or melena. The differential diagnosis of primary peptic ulcer includes recurrent abdominal pain, irritable colon syndrome, esophagitis, chronic pancreatitis, cholelithiasis, and recurrent midgut volvulus. Suspicion should increase when there is a family history of primary peptic ulcer disease, even if the gastrointestinal complaints are vague.

Treatment

Peptic ulcer disease may be treated with liquid antacids, 0.5–2.5 mL/kg given every 1–2 hours. For mild to moderate symptoms, antacids are given 1 and 3 hours after meals and before bed. Histamine H_2 receptor antagonists prevent histamine stimulation of gastric acid production. Cimetidine (5 mg/kg/dose given orally before meals and at bedtime) or ranitidine (2.5 mg/kg/dose given orally every 12 hours) produces effective healing of peptic ulceration in 4–8 weeks. Famotidine, another H_2 receptor antagonist, can be used, but the dose in children is not determined. None of the H_2 receptor antagonists are more effective than liquid antacids given appropriately. Proton pump inhibitors (omeprazole) are powerful inhibitors of gastric acid secretion. Appropriate dosage for children is not determined. The effects of prolonged hypergastrinemia seen with these agents are not known.

Recurrences may be prevented with a single nighttime dose of H_2 receptor antagonist. Anticholinergics should be given only in rare cases with significant hypersecretion.

Strict "ulcer diet" is not indicated. Foods that cause pain should be avoided. Caffeine should be avoided because it increases gastric secretion. Three regular meals are recommended; snacks are to be avoided, especially at bedtime. Aspirin and nonsteroidal antiinflammatory drugs should be avoided.

Surgical treatment is reserved for the complications, eg, perforation, hemorrhage, obstruction, or incapacitating, intractable pain.

Although symptoms may improve with antacids, cure of peptic disease associated with *H pylori* requires eradication of the organism. The optimal therapeutic regimen is still undetermined. In children, 2 weeks of an oral bismuth preparation (bismuth subsalicylate or subcitrate) plus antibiotics (amoxicillin and metronidazole) is most often prescribed in addition to the antisecretory agents listed above.

Prognosis

Long-term studies show that up to 80% of children with primary duodenal ulcers have recurrent symptoms on long-term follow-up. The prognosis for recurrence is much lower in the younger group (0–6 years). Surgery for duodenal ulcers (pyloroplasty and vagotomy) gives excellent results.

Graham DY et al: Factors influencing the eradication of *Helicobacter pylori* with triple therapy. Gastroenterology 1992;102:493.

Nord KS: Peptic ulcer disease in the pediatric population. Pediatr Clin North Am 1988;35:117.

Peterson WL: *Helicobacter pylori* and peptic ulcer disease. N Engl J Med 1991;324:1043.

CONGENITAL DIAPHRAGMATIC HERNIA

Diaphragmatic hernia may be secondary to a posterolateral defect in the diaphragm (foramen of Bochdalek) or, in about 5% of cases, to a retrosternal defect (foramen of Morgagni). It represents failure of division of the thoracic and abdominal cavities at the eighth to tenth weeks of fetal life. All degrees of protrusion of the abdominal viscera through the diaphragmatic opening into the thoracic cavity may occur. The extent of herniation determines the severity and the timing of the symptoms. Eighty percent of posterolateral defects involve the left diaphragm. In eventration of the diaphragm, a leaf of the diaphragm with hypoplastic muscular elements balloons into the chest and leads to identical but much milder symptoms.

Symptoms of mild to severe respiratory distress are usually present at birth. The abdomen may be scaphoid because of the displacement of the viscera. Breath sounds in the affected hemithorax are absent, with displacement of the point of maximal cardiac impulse. In asymptomatic patients, the diaphragmatic hernia may be found on incidental x-ray of the chest. Thirty percent of infants with diaphragmatic hernia die. The most common cause of death is pulmonary insufficiency. The lung on the affected side is hypoplastic, with decreased generations of airways and pulmonary arteries throughout with pulmonary hypertension. Other causes of morbidity and mortality include mediastinal shift with vascular kinking, pulmonary infection, prematurity, cardiac anomalies, and intestinal malrotation. Extracorporeal membrane oxygenation may decrease the early postoperative mortality rate in patients with poor lung compliance. There is growing enthusiasm for the use of nitric oxide for treatment of pulmonary vascular hypertension in these patients.

Adzick NS et al: Diaphragmatic hernia in the fetus: Prenatal diagnosis and outcome in 94 cases. J Pediatr Surg 1985; 20:357.

Kinsella JP et al: Clinical responses to prolonged treatment of persistent pulmonary hypertension of the newborn with low doses of inhaled nitric oxide. J Pediatr 1993; 123:103.

Van Meurs KP et al: Congenital diaphragmatic hernia: Long term outcome in neonates treated with extracorporeal membrane oxygenation. J Pediatr 1993;122:893.

CONGENITAL ATRESIAS & STENOSES OF THE GASTROINTESTINAL TRACT

The usual mode of presentation is neonatal intestinal obstruction or perforation. The presence of atresia or stenosis may produce polyhydramnios prenatally and can be diagnosed before birth by ultrasound. The triad of abdominal distention, bilious vomiting, and obstipation or failure to pass meconium constitutes the most important clue to diagnosis. Prematurity and other congenital anomalies may be present. The localization and relative incidence of atresias and stenoses are given in Table 22–2.

CONGENITAL DUODENAL OBSTRUCTION

Extrinsic duodenal obstruction is usually due to congenital peritoneal bands associated with intestinal malrotation (with or without volvulus); to annular pancreas; or, more rarely, to duplication of the duodenum. Intrinsic obstruction is due to stenosis, a mucosal diaphragm or "wind-sock" deformity, or duodenal atresia. The duodenal lumen may be obliterated by a membrane or completely interrupted with a fibrous cord between the two segments. Atresia may be proximal or distal to the ampulla of Vater.

Clinical Findings

A. Atresia: A history of polyhydramnios is common. Vomiting (usually bile-stained) begins within a few hours after birth, with epigastric distention. Meconium may be normally passed. Duodenal atresia is commonly associated with other congenital anoma-

Table 22–2. Localization and incidence of gastrointestinal atresias and stenoses.

	Area Involved	Type of Lesion	Relative Frequency
Pylorus		Atresia Web or diaphragm (66%)	1%
Duodenum	Distal to the ampulla of Vater (80%)	Atresia Web or diaphragm (40%)	45%
Jejunoileal	Proximal jejunum and distal ileum (66%)	Atresia (multiple in 6–29%) Stenosis (20%)	50%
Colon	Left colon and rectum (50%)	Atresia (may be associated with atresias of the small bowel)	5–9%

lies (30%), including esophageal atresia, other intestinal atresias, and cardiac and renal anomalies. Prematurity (25–50%) and Down's syndrome (20–30%) are associated conditions. Abdominal x-rays show gaseous distention of the stomach and proximal duodenum ("double bubble"). With protracted vomiting and dehydration, there may be little air in the stomach; it is then advisable to instill air into the stomach to elicit the typical pattern. Absence of gas in the intestinal tract distal to the obstruction suggests atresia or an extrinsic obstruction severe enough to completely occlude the lumen, whereas air scattered over the lower abdomen may indicate a partial duodenal obstruction of either the intrinsic or extrinsic variety. A barium enema may be helpful in determining the presence of a concomitant malrotation or atresia lower in the gastrointestinal tract.

B. Duodenal Stenosis: Obvious symptoms of duodenal obstruction may be delayed for weeks or years. Although the stenotic area is usually postampullary, the vomitus does not always contain bile.

Treatment & Prognosis

Thorough exploration is necessary at operation both to find the cause of the obstruction and to make sure no additional pathologic anomalies are present lower in the gastrointestinal tract.

The mortality rate (35–40%) is significantly affected by prematurity, Down's syndrome, and associated congenital anomalies. Postoperative duodenal dilation and hypomotility may cause continued symptoms.

CONGENITAL JEJUNAL & ILEAL OBSTRUCTION

Bile-stained vomiting with abdominal distention usually begins in the first 48 hours of life. Small amounts of meconium may be passed. Prematurity and severe congenital anomalies often coexist. Atresias, stenoses, and obstructing membranes may affect multiple sites. The small intestine may be significantly shortened. X-ray features include dilated loops of small bowel and absence of colonic gas. Barium enema will reveal a colon of restricted caliber (microcolon) if the atresia is in the lower small bowel. In over 10% of cases of jejunoileal atresia, there is absence of the mesentery, and the superior mesenteric artery cannot be identified beyond the origin of the right colic and ileocolic arteries. As a result, the ileum coils around one of these two arteries, giving rise to the "Christmas tree" deformity. The tenuous blood supply often leads to long areas of gangrenous bowel and compromises surgical anastomoses. Multiple intestinal atresias may be associated with immunodeficiency.

The differential diagnosis should include Hirschsprung's disease, paralytic ileus secondary to sepsis, gastroenteritis or pneumonia, midgut volvulus, and meconium ileus. Surgery is mandatory in newborn infants with small bowel atresia. Postoperative complications include short bowel syndrome and hypomotility.

Walker MW et al: Multiple areas of intestinal atresia associated with immunodeficiency and post transfusion graft versus host disease. J Pediatr 1993;123:93.

ANNULAR PANCREAS

Annular pancreas is a result of incomplete rotation and fusion of the dorsal and ventral pancreatic anlagen. The symptoms are those of partial or complete duodenal obstruction. Down's syndrome and congenital anomalies of the gastrointestinal tract occur frequently. As with other neonatal gastrointestinal obstructive lesions of the neonate, polyhydramnios is common. Clinical manifestations can develop late in childhood.

Treatment consists of duodenoduodenostomy or duodenojejunostomy without operative dissection or division of the pancreatic annulus.

Kiernan PD et al: Annular pancreas: Mayo Clinic experience from 1957 to 1976 with review of the literature. Arch Surg 1980;115:46.

Merrill JR, Raffensperger JG: Pediatric annular pancreas: Twenty years' experience. J Pediatr Surg 1976;11:921.

MIDGUT MALROTATION WITH OR WITHOUT VOLVULUS

Normally, the midgut (which extends from the duodenojejunal junction to the mid transverse colon and which is supplied by the superior mesenteric artery) returns to the intra-abdominal position during the tenth week of embryonic life. The root of the mesentery rotates in a counterclockwise direction during retraction. This causes the colon to cross ventrally; the cecum moves from the left to the right lower quadrant, and the duodenum crosses dorsally to become partly retroperitoneal. When this rotation is incomplete, the posterior fixation of the mesentery is defective, so that the bowel from the ligament of Treitz to the mid transverse colon may twist, causing a volvulus around the pedicle-like mesentery. Duodenal or ileal obstruction may later result through peritoneal bands from the mobile hepatic flexure or cecum. Most cases are asymptomatic.

Clinical Findings

A. Symptoms and Signs: Seventy-five percent of symptomatic cases show high intestinal obstruction within the first 3 weeks of life, with bile-stained vomitus, abdominal distention, and visible peristalsis. The first signs may occur later in life, with symptoms of intermittent intestinal obstruction (postprandial abdominal pain and vomiting) or, rarely, with malabsorption, a protein-losing enteropathy, or intermittent diarrhea. Diarrhea may be an early symptom in infants under the age of 6 months. Associated congenital anomalies, especially cardiac, occur in over 25% of symptomatic cases.

B. Imaging: An upper gastrointestinal series may show partial or complete small bowel obstruction. The duodenojejunal junction may lie to the right of the spine along with the jejunal loops. The diagnosis of malrotation can be further confirmed by barium enema, which may demonstrate a mobile cecum located in the midline.

Treatment & Prognosis

Midgut volvulus is a surgical emergency, Bowel ischemia results from occlusion of the superior mesenteric artery. When necrosis is extensive, it is recommended that a first operation include only reduction of the volvulus with lysis of mesenteric bands. Intestinal resection should be delayed if possible until a second-look operation 24–48 hours later can be undertaken in the hope that some bowel will recover and can be salvaged. The prognosis is guarded if there is associated perforation, peritonitis, or extensive intestinal necrosis.

Duke JH Jr, Yar MS: Primary small bowel volvulus. Arch Surg 1977;112:685.
Janik JS, Ein SH: Normal intestinal rotation with nonfixation: A cause of chronic abdominal pain. J Pediatr Surg 1979;14:670.
Millar AJW et al: The deadly vomit: Malrotation and midgut volvulus. Pediatr Surg Int 1987;2:172.
Stewart DR et al: Malrotation of the bowel in infants and children: A 15 year experience. Surgery 1976;79:716.

MECKEL'S DIVERTICULUM & OMPHALOMESENTERIC DUCT REMNANTS

Meckel's diverticulum is present in 1.5% of the population but rarely causes symptoms. Familial cases have been reported. Complications occur three times more frequently in males than in females, and in 50–60% of cases within the first 2 years of life. Heterotopic tissue (gastric mucosa mostly, but also pancreatic tissue and jejunal or colonic mucosa) is ten times as likely to be found in symptomatic diverticula. In adults, Meckel's diverticulum is usually located within 100 cm of the ileocecal valve on the antimesenteric side and has its own blood supply.

Clinical Findings

A. Symptoms and Signs: In 40–60% of symptomatic cases, painless rectal bleeding of dark maroon or even melanotic blood occurs. Acute blood loss may cause shock. Occult bleeding is less common but may cause anemia. Gastric mucosa and an ulcer of the adjacent ileal mucosa are found in the majority of diverticula that bleed.

Intestinal obstruction occurs in 25% of symptomatic cases. Ileocolic intussusception occurs with intestinal infarction. A mass is palpable.

Volvulus of the bowel around a fibrous remnant of the vitelline duct extending from the tip of the diverticulum to the abdominal wall may occur. In some cases, entrapment of a bowel loop under a band running between the diverticulum and the base of the mesentery has been associated with intestinal obstruction. The diverticulum may be trapped in an inguinal hernia (Littre's hernia).

Diverticulitis occurs in 10–20% of symptomatic cases and is clinically indistinguishable from acute appendicitis. Perforation and generalized peritonitis may occur. There may be chronic recurrent abdominal pain.

B. Imaging: Diagnosis of this condition is seldom made on barium x-ray. Radionuclide imaging with ^{99m}Tc pertechnetate may demonstrate the diverticulum lined with heterotopic gastric mucosa. Stimulation of ^{99m}Tc pertechnetate uptake by both pentagastrin and cimetidine can reduce the number of false-negative results. Angiography may be useful when bleeding is brisk.

Treatment

A. Diverticulum: Treatment is surgical. At operation, close inspection of the ileum proximal and distal to the diverticulum may reveal ulcerations and heterotopic tissue adjacent to the neck of the diverticulum.

B. Other Remnants of the Omphalomesenteric Duct: Fecal discharge from the umbilicus is evidence of a patent omphalomesenteric duct. The duct may be completely closed, leading to persistence of a fibrous cord joining ileum and umbilicus and potentially the origin of a volvulus. In other instances, a mucoid discharge may be indicative of a mucocele, which can protrude through the umbilicus and be mistaken for an umbilical granuloma, since it is firm and bright red. In all cases, surgical excision of the omphalomesenteric remnant is indicated.

Prognosis

The prognosis for Meckel's diverticulum is good. Marked hemorrhage may occur but is rarely exsanguinating.

Mackey WC, Dineen P: A fifty-year experience with Meckel's diverticulum. Surg Gynecol Obstet 1983;156:56.
Treves S, Grand RJ, Eraklis AJ: Pentagastrin stimulation of technetium-99m uptake by ectopic gastric mucosa in Meckel's diverticulum. Radiology 1978;128:711.

DUPLICATIONS OF THE GASTROINTESTINAL TRACT

Duplications of the gastrointestinal tract are congenital malformations most often discovered during infancy. Duplications are spherical or tubular structures of various size that may occur anywhere along the gastrointestinal tract. They usually contain fluid and sometimes blood if necrosis has taken place. Most duplications do not communicate with the intestinal lumen; they are attached to the mesenteric side of the gut and share a common muscular coat. The epithelial lining of the duplication is usually of the same type as that from which it originates; 20–30% contain ectopic gastric mucosa. Some duplications are attached to the spinal cord and are associated with hemivertebrae (neurenteric cysts). Esophageal duplications are rare.

Symptoms usually begin in infancy, with vomiting, abdominal distention, colicky pain, rectal bleeding, partial or total intestinal obstruction, or an abdominal mass. Physical examination reveals a rounded, smooth, freely movable mass, and x-ray films of the abdomen show a noncalcified mass displacing the intestines or compressing the stomach. Scanning with ^{99m}Tc pertechnetate is useful in duplications containing gastric mucosa. Involvement of the terminal small bowel can give rise to an intussusception.

Prompt surgical treatment is indicated.

Favara B, Franciosi RA, Akers DR: Enteric duplications. Thirty-seven cases: A vascular theory of pathogenesis. Am J Dis Child 1971;122:501.

Pruksapong C et al: Gastric duplication. J Pediatr Surg 1979;14:83.

PERITONITIS

Primary bacterial peritonitis is rare. The most common organisms responsible include *Escherichia coli* and other enteric organisms, hemolytic streptococci, and pneumococci. Primary peritonitis occurs in young patients with splenectomy, splenic dysfunction, or ascites (nephrotic syndrome, advanced liver disease, kwashiorkor). It also occurs in infants with pyelonephritis or pneumonia. Secondary peritonitis usually results from penetrating abdominal trauma or ruptured viscus. (Appendicitis, perforated peptic ulcer, cholecystitis, pancreatitis, inflammatory bowel disease, midgut volvulus, intussusception, and strangulated hernia are some primary events.) Intra-abdominal abscesses may form in pelvic, subhepatic, or subphrenic areas, but localization of infection is less common in young infants than it is in adults.

Symptoms include severe abdominal pain, fever, nausea, and vomiting. Respirations are shallow. The abdomen is tender, rigid, and distended, with involuntary guarding. Bowel sounds may be absent. Tenderness is present on rectal examination. In secondary peritonitis, these signs are accompanied by, and even overshadowed by, the signs and symptoms of the underlying cause of peritonitis. Diarrhea is fairly common in primary peritonitis and less so in secondary peritonitis.

The leukocyte count is initially high (greater than 20,000/μL) and later may fall to neutropenic levels, especially in primary peritonitis. Bacterial peritonitis should be suspected if paracentesis fluid contains more than 500 LEUKOCYTES/μL or more than 32 mg/dL of lactate, has a pH less than 7.34, or if the pH of ascites is more than 0.1 pH unit less than arterial pH. Etiologic diagnosis is made by Gram's stain and culture, preferably of 5–10 mL of fluid for optimal yield.

Antibiotic treatment and supportive therapy for dehydration, shock, and acidosis are indicated. Surgical treatment of the underlying cause of secondary peritonitis is critical. Drainage of localized abscess is often required.

Bell MJ: Peritonitis in the newborn: Current concepts. Pediatr Clin North Am 1985;32:1181.

Bell MJ et al: The microbiological flora and anti-microbial therapy of neonatal peritonitis. J Pediatr Surg 1980;15:569.

Clark JH et al: Spontaneous bacterial peritonitis. J Pediatr 1984;104:495.

Emanuel B et al: Perforation of gastrointestinal tract in infancy and childhood. Surg Gynecol Obstet 1978;146:926.

Garcia-Tsau G, Conn HO, Lerner E: The diagnosis of bacterial peritonitis: Comparison of pH, lactate concentration and leucocyte count. Hepatology 1985;5:91.

CONGENITAL AGANGLIONIC MEGACOLON (Hirschsprung's Disease)

Essentials of Diagnosis

- Partial or complete intestinal obstruction in the newborn period, with vomiting, diarrhea, abdominal distention, and shock.
- Obstinate constipation, abdominal enlargement, ribbon-like stools, and failure to thrive in infancy or childhood.
- Absence of fecal material on rectal examination.
- Absence of ganglion cells in the narrowed segment.
- Narrowed colonic segment proximal to the anus visible on barium enema examination.

General Considerations

Hirschsprung's disease is due to an absence of ganglion cells in the mucosal and muscular layers of the colon. During development of the fetus, there is a failure of neural crest cells to migrate to the mesodermal layers. The rectum alone (30%) or the rectosigmoid (44%) is usually affected. The entire colon is aganglionic in 8% of cases. Segmental aganglionosis is very rare and may be an acquired lesion secondary to ischemia. The denervated segment is narrowed, with dilation of the proximal uninvolved colon. In long-standing cases, the mucosa of the dilated colonic segment may become thin and inflamed (enterocolitis) with both blood and protein loss.

A familial pattern has been described, particularly in total colonic aganglionosis. The disease is four times more common in boys than in girls, and 10–15% of patients have Down's syndrome.

Clinical Findings

A. Symptoms and Signs: Failure of the newborn to pass meconium–followed by vomiting, abdominal distention, and reluctance to feed—suggests the diagnosis. The infant is irritable, and breathing may be rapid and grunting because of abdominal distention. The infant may pass meconium normally, and obvious symptoms may not develop until after discharge from the newborn nursery. In some cases, symptoms appear later and are those of partial intestinal obstruction, with abdominal distention and bilious vomiting. Bouts of enterocolitis manifested by fever, explosive diarrhea, and prostration are reported in about 50% of newborns with this disease. These episodes may lead to acute inflammatory and ischemic changes in the colon, with perforation (especially cecal) and sepsis. In later infancy, alternating obstipation and diarrhea predominate. The older child is more likely to present with constipation. The stools are offensive and ribbon-like, the abdomen enlarged, and the veins prominent; peristaltic patterns are readily visible, and fecal masses are palpable. Intermittent bouts of intestinal obstruction due to fecal impaction, hypochromic anemia, hypoproteinemia, and failure to thrive are common. Encopresis is rarely seen.

On digital examination, the anal canal and rectum are devoid of fecal material and may feel narrow despite fecal impaction obvious on abdominal examination or abdominal x-ray. If the involved segment is short, there may be a gush of flatus and of pale, liquid, offensive stool as the finger is withdrawn. The presence of fecal colonic impaction associated with an empty rectum is most suggestive of the disease.

B. Laboratory Findings: Ganglion cells are absent in both the submucosal and muscular layers of the involved bowel. Special stains may show nerve trunk hypertrophy and increased acetylcholinesterase activity. Rectal suction or grasp biopsies taken at 3, 4, and 5 cm from the anus readily establish the diagnosis, although some prefer a full-thickness rectal biopsy in order to have access to the ganglion cells between the muscular layers (plexus myentericus).

C. Imaging: X-ray examination of the abdomen may reveal dilated colonic loops and absence of gas

from the pelvic colon on an erect lateral film. A barium enema, introducing a small amount of radiopaque material through a catheter with the tip inserted barely beyond the anal sphincter, will usually demonstrate the narrowed segment distally with a sharp transition to proximal dilated colon. However, in neonates a "transition zone" may not be seen. Retention of barium for 24–48 hours is not diagnostic of Hirschsprung's disease but can be seen in retentive constipation as well.

D. Special Examinations: Manometric studies can be diagnostic, especially when a short, aganglionic segment is present. Failure of the internal sphincter muscle to relax after balloon distention of the rectum is seen in all patients with Hirschsprung's disease, regardless of the length of the aganglionic segment. Interpretation of acetylcholinesterase staining in newborns is sometimes difficult.

Differential Diagnosis

Hirschsprung's disease accounts for 15–20% of cases of neonatal intestinal obstruction. In childhood, this disease must be differentiated from retentive constipation with colon distention. It can also be confused with celiac disease because of the striking abdominal distention and failure to thrive.

Treatment

Diversion of the fecal stream is the first step in the surgical treatment. A colostomy (or ileostomy) is performed proximal to the aganglionic segment. If enterocolitis is present, saline irrigations should be repeatedly given through a rectal cannula. Plasma expanders and fluid and electrolyte homeostasis are essential before surgery.

Resection of the aganglionic segment is usually delayed until the infant is at least 6 months of age. During operation, it is essential to ascertain by biopsy the exact location of the transition between ganglionated and nonganglionated bowel. The endorectal pullthrough (Soave) procedure, in which the ganglionated proximal bowel is pulled through the seromuscular cuff of the remnant of distal rectum, is the surgical procedure most commonly performed in the United States for treatment of Hirschsprung's disease.

Prognosis

Enterocolitis before or after surgery is associated with a 30% mortality rate, especially in infants with a long aganglionic segment. Long-term complications following surgery include dysmotility of the remaining bowel and anastomotic breakdown or stricture with fecal incontinence or fecal impaction. Postoperative obstruction may result from inadvertent retention of a distal aganglionic segment or postoperative destruction of ganglion cells secondary to vascular impairment and chronic inflammatory changes at the time of surgery.

Dykes EH, Guiney EJ: Total colonic aganglionosis. J Pediatr Gastroenterol Nutr 1989;8:129.

Klein MD et al: Hirschsprung's disease in the newborn. J Pediatr Surg 1984;19:370.

Kleinhaus S et al: Hirschsprung's disease: A survey of the members of the Surgical Section of the American Academy of Pediatrics. J Pediatr Surg 1979;14:588.

CHYLOUS ASCITES

Chylous ascites due to congenital infection or developmental abnormality of the lymphatic system may be observed at birth. If the thoracic duct is involved, chylothorax may be present. Later in life, chylous ascites may result from congenital lymphatic abnormality, tumors, peritoneal bands, or trauma to major lymphatics.

Clinical Findings

A. Symptoms and Signs: In both congenital and acquired forms, diarrhea and failure to thrive are noted. The abdomen is distended, with a fluid wave and shifting dullness. Unilateral or generalized peripheral lymphedema may be present.

B. Laboratory Findings: Laboratory findings include hypoalbuminemia, hypogammaglobulinemia, and lymphopenia. Ascitic fluid will contain lymphocytes and have the biochemical composition of chyle if the patient has been fed; otherwise it is indistinguishable from ascites secondary to cirrhosis.

Differential Diagnosis

Chylous ascites must be differentiated from ascites due to liver failure and, in the older child, from constrictive pericarditis and neoplastic, infectious, or inflammatory diseases causing lymphatic obstruction.

Complications & Sequelae

Severe chylous ascites can be fatal. Chronic loss of albumin and gamma globulin through the gastrointestinal tract may lead to edema and increase the risk of infection. Rapidly accumulating chylous ascites may cause respiratory complications.

Treatment & Prognosis

If there is a congenital abnormality due to hypoplasia, aplasia, or ectasia of the lymphatics, little can be done for the patient. Shunting of peritoneal fluid into the venous system is sometimes effective. Attempts to relieve the ascites by bringing the saphenous vein into the peritoneal cavity have had partial success. A fat-free diet supplemented with medium-chain triglycerides decreases the formation of chylous ascitic fluid. Total parenteral nutrition may be necessary. The congenital form of chylous ascites may spontaneously disappear following paracentesis and a medium-chain triglyceride diet. The prognosis is guarded, although spontaneous cures have been reported.

Cochran WJ et al: Chylous ascites in infants and children: A case report and literature review. J Pediatr Gastroenterol Nutr 1985;4:668.

Guttman FM, Montupet P, Bloss RS: Experience with peritoneovenous shunting for congenital chylous ascites in infants and children. J Pediatr Surg 1982;17:368.

CONGENITAL ANORECTAL ANOMALIES

Anorectal anomalies occur once in every 3000–4000 births, and most types are more common in males. Inspection of the perianal area is essential in all newborns.

Classification

A. Anterior Displacement of the Anal Opening: This condition is more common in girls than in boys. It may be associated with a posterior rectal shelf and usually is characterized by constipation that responds poorly to medical management.

B. Anal Stenosis: The anal aperture is very small and filled with a dot of meconium. Defecation is difficult, and there may be ribbon-like stools, fecal impaction, and abdominal distention. This malformation accounts for perhaps 10% of cases of anorectal anomalies.

C. Imperforate Anal Membrane: The infant fails to pass meconium, and a greenish bulging membrane is seen. After excision, bowel and sphincter function are normal.

D. Anal Agenesis: This results from defective development of the anus. The anal dimple is present, and stimulation of the perianal area leads to puckering indicative of the presence of the external sphincter. If there is no associated fistula, intestinal obstruction occurs. Fistulas may be perineal or vulvar in the female and perineal or urethral in the male. A perineal fistula presents as a streak of meconium buried in thickened perineal skin.

E. Rectal and Anal Agenesis: Rectal and anal agenesis accounts for 75% of total anorectal anomalies. Fistulas are almost invariably present. In the female, they may be vestibular or vaginal or may enter a urogenital sinus, which is a common passageway for the urethra and vagina. In the male, fistulas are rectovesical or rectourethral. Associated major congenital malformations are common. Sacral defects, prematurity, and hypoplastic internal and external sphincters significantly influence the prognosis for life and function.

F. Rectal Atresia: The anal canal and lower rectum form a blind pouch that is separated for a variable distance from the blind upper rectal pouch.

Radiologic Findings

Careful radiologic evaluation is indicated immediately so that the anal anomaly and the extent of associated anomalies of the bowel and the urogenital tract can be fully appraised.

Treatment & Prognosis

Dilation of the anus should be undertaken in cases of anal stenosis. Treatment for imperforate anal membrane consists of excision of the membrane and dilation. Colostomy is advocated for all cases of rectal agenesis. In patients with anal agenesis and a visible fistula of sufficient size to pass meconium, treatment can be deferred. The male without a visible fistula may have a urethral fistula; therefore, colostomy is recommended.

Of the patients with "low" defects, 80–90% are continent after surgery; with "high" defects, only 30% achieve continence. Gracilis muscle transplants may improve continence. Levatorplasty may also be used as a secondary operation following surgery for anorectal agenesis.

The mortality rate is about 20%. The prognosis is worse in small premature infants and in infants with associated anomalies.

De Vries PA: The surgery of anorectal anomalies: Its evolution with evaluation of procedures. Curr Probl Surg 1984;21(5):1.

Ditesheim JA, Templeton JM: Short-term vs. long-term quality of life following repair of high imperforate anus. J Pediatr Surg 1987;22:581.

Reisner SH et al: Determination of anterior displacement of the anus in newborn infants and children. Pediatrics 1984;73:216.

Roy CC, Morin CL, Weber AM: Gastrointestinal emergency problems in paediatric practice. Clin Gastroenterol 1981;10:225.

Smith ED: The bathwater needs changing, but don't throw out the baby: An overview of anorectal anomalies. J Pediatr Surg 1987;22:335.

ACUTE ABDOMEN

Many disorders must be considered in the differential diagnosis of acute abdomen. Emergency surgery should not be considered until the differential diagnosis has been completed. The patient may be too young to describe symptoms, and the parent's description is a subjective interpretation of what he or she thinks is wrong. A partial etiologic classification of acute abdomen is shown in Table 22–3, with the most common causes noted. Some of the specific entities are discussed in subsequent sections. Reaching a speedy and accurate diagnosis in the patient with an acute abdomen is critical and requires skill in physical diagnosis, intimate acquaintance with the characteristic symptoms of a large number of conditions, and the judicious selection of laboratory and radiologic tests.

Hatch EI: The acute abdomen in children. Pediatr Clin North Am 1985;32:1151.

ACUTE APPENDICITIS

Essentials of Diagnosis

- Diffuse, crampy abdominal pain, followed by right lower quadrant pain.
- Anorexia, vomiting, and constipation.
- Low-grade fever (38–38.5 °C).
- Right lower quadrant tenderness with rebound tenderness and, eventually, guarding.
- White blood cell count < 15,000/μL, with raised neutrophil levels.

General Considerations

Acute appendicitis is the most common cause of abdominal surgery in childhood. The frequency increases with age and peaks between 15 and 30 years.

Table 22–3. Etiologic classification of acute abdomen.[1]

Mechanical Obstruction		Inflammatory Diseases and Infections			
Intraluminal Obstruction	Extraluminal Obstruction	Gastrointestinal Disease	Paralytic Ileus	Blunt Trauma	Miscellaneous
Foreign body	Hernia	Appendicitis	Sepsis	Accident	Lead poisoning
Bezoar	Intussusception	Crohn's disease	Pneumonia	Battered child	Sickle cell crisis
Fecalith	Volvulus	Ulcerative colitis	Pyelonephritis	syndrome	Familial Mediterranean fever
Gallstone	Duplication	Henoch-Schönlein	Peritonitis		
Parasites	Stenosis	purpura and other	Pancreatitis		Porphyria
Meconium ileus	Tumor	causes of vasculitis	Cholecystitis		Diabetic acidosis
equivalent	Mesenteric cyst	tis	Renal and gallbladder stones		Addisonian crisis
Tumor	Superior mesenteric	Peptic ulcer	Pelvic inflammation		Torsion of testis
Fecaloma	artery syndrome	Meckel's diverticulitis	Lymphadenitis due		Torsion of ovarian pedicle
	Pyloric stenosis	tis	to viral or bacterial		
		Acute gastroenteritis	infection		
		Pseudomembranous enterocolitis			

[1]Reproduced, with permission, from Roy CC, Morin CL, Weber AM: Gastrointestinal emergency problems in paediatric practice. Clin Gastroenterol 1981;10:225.

Luminal obstruction by fecaliths (25%) or parasites is a predisposing factor.

The incidence of perforation is high (40%) in infants and children. In order to avoid delay in diagnosis, it is important to maintain close communication with parents, perform a thorough physical examination and sequential examinations of the abdomen over a period of several hours, and interpret correctly the evolving symptoms and signs.

Clinical Findings

A. Symptoms and Signs: The triad of persistent localized right lower quadrant pain, localized abdominal tenderness, and slight fever strongly suggests appendicitis. Anorexia, vomiting, and constipation also occur. The clinical picture is often atypical, ie, generalized pain, tenderness around the umbilicus, and no leukocytosis. Diarrhea can substitute for constipation, and a subsiding upper respiratory tract infection may be found. Rectal examination should always be done and may reveal localized mass or tenderness. Examination of the stool may suggest other diagnoses, such as colitis or intussusception. Because many infections give rise to symptoms mimicking appendicitis and because physical findings are often inconclusive, it is important to repeat examinations of the abdomen. In children under 2 years old, the pain of appendicitis is poorly localized, and perforation before surgery is common.

B. Laboratory Findings: White blood cell counts are seldom higher than 15,000/μL. Fecal leukocytes and blood are rare.

C. Imaging: A radiopaque fecalith is reportedly present in two-thirds of cases of ruptured appendix. A barium enema examination showing a normal appendix and cecum usually rules out appendicitis. However, a positive diagnosis of nonperforated appendicitis cannot be made by barium enema. Ultrasonography of the acutely inflamed appendix shows a noncompressible tubular structure in 93% of cases. A localized fluid collection adjacent to or surrounding the appendix may also be seen. Enlarged mesenteric lymph nodes are a nondiagnostic finding.

Differential Diagnosis

The presence of intrathoracic infection (eg, pneumonia) or urinary tract infection should be kept in mind, along with other medical and surgical conditions leading to acute abdomen (see above).

Treatment & Prognosis

Appendectomy is indicated whenever the diagnosis of appendicitis cannot be ruled out after a period of close observation. Postoperative antibiotic therapy directed to the treatment of anaerobes and coliforms is reserved for cases with gangrenous or perforated appendix. A single intraoperative dose of cefoxitin or cefotetan is recommended for all cases in order to prevent postoperative complications. The mortality rate is less than 1% in patients during childhood, despite the high incidence of perforation. Laparoscopic removal of a nonruptured appendix is associated with a shortened hospital stay.

Antimicrobial prophylaxis in surgery. Med Lett Drugs Ther 1992;34:5.

Gilbert SR: Appendicitis in children. Surg Gynecol Obstet 1985;161:261.

Harrison MW et al: Acute appendicitis in children: Factors affecting morbidity. Am J Surg 1984;147:605.

INTUSSUSCEPTION

Essentials of Diagnosis

- Paroxysmal, episodic abdominal pain and vomiting.
- Sausage-shaped mass in upper abdomen.
- Rectal passage of bloody material (mucus and stool).
- Barium enema evidence of intussusception.

General Considerations

Intussusception is the most frequent cause of intestinal obstruction in the first 2 years of life. It is three times more common in males than in females. In most cases (85%) the cause is not apparent, although polyps, Meckel's diverticulum, Schönlein-Henoch purpura, lymphomas, lipomas, parasites, foreign bodies, or adenovirus or rotavirus infections with hypertrophy of Peyer's patches are predisposing factors. Intussusception of the small intestine occurs in patients with celiac disease and cystic fibrosis, usually related to the bulk of stool in the terminal ileum. In children older than 6 years of age, lymphoma is the most common lesion. Intermittent small bowel intussusception is a rare cause of recurrent abdominal pain.

The intussusception usually starts just proximal to the ileocecal valve, so that invagination is ileocolic. Other forms include ileoileal and colocolic. Swelling, hemorrhage, incarceration with necrosis of the intussuscepted bowel, and eventual perforation and peritonitis occur as a result of impairment of venous return.

Clinical Findings

Characteristically, a thriving infant 3–12 months of age suddenly develops periodic abdominal pain with screaming and drawing up of the knees. Vomiting occurs soon afterward (90% of cases), and bloody bowel movements with mucus appear within the next 12 hours (50%). Prostration and fever supervene. The abdomen is tender and becomes distended. On palpation, a sausage-shaped tumor may be found usually in the upper mid abdomen. In rare cases, the onset may be painless or with diarrhea. Some patients show signs of altered consciousness, particularly lethargy between spasms of pain, or may have seizures.

The intussusception can persist for several days when obstruction is not complete, and such cases may present as separate attacks of enterocolitis. In older children, sudden attacks of abdominal pain may be related to chronic recurrent intussusception with spontaneous reduction.

Treatment

A. Conservative Measures: A barium enema is both diagnostic and therapeutic. It is a safe procedure in experienced hands if the following recommendations are observed:

1. No attempt should be made at hydrostatic reduction if there are signs of strangulated bowel, perforation, or severe toxicity.

2. The barium solution should be allowed to drip by gravity through a Foley bag catheter inserted in the rectum from a height not more than 1 meter (3½ feet) above the fluoroscopy table.

3. There should be no manipulation of the abdomen during hydrostatic reduction under fluoroscopic examination, because this may increase intraluminal pressure and thus the risk of perforation.

4. Upon reduction, there should be free reflux of barium for a distance of 24–30 cm into the ileum; this is best demonstrated in a postevacuation film.

B. Surgical Measures: For patients not suitable for hydrostatic reduction or in whom it is unsuccessful (25%), surgery is required. This has the advantages of demonstrating any lead point (such as Meckel's diverticulum) and of a lower recurrence rate.

Prognosis

Intussusception is almost uniformly fatal if untreated. The prognosis relates to the duration of the intussusception before reduction. The mortality rate with treatment is 1–2%. The patient should be observed carefully in hospital after hydrostatic reduction because intussusception recurs in 3–4% of patients, usually within 24 hours after reduction.

Bruce J et al: Intussusception: Evolution of current management. J Pediatr Gastroenterol Nutr 1987;6:663.
Singer J: Altered consciousness as an early manifestation of intussusception. Pediatrics 1979;64:93.

FOREIGN BODIES
IN THE ALIMENTARY TRACT

Most foreign bodies pass through the esophagus and the rest of the gastrointestinal tract without difficulty, although anything longer than 3–5 cm may have difficulty passing the duodenal loop at the region of the ligament of Treitz. Ingested foreign bodies tend to lodge in areas of natural constriction—valleculae, thoracic inlet, gastroesophageal junction, pylorus, ligament of Treitz, and ileocecal junction. Foreign bodies lodged in the esophagus for more than 24 hours require removal. Smooth foreign bodies in the stomach, such as buttons or coins, may be watched without attempting removal for up to several months if the child is free of symptoms. Straight pins, screws, and nails generally pass without incident. Removal of open safety pins or wooden toothpicks is recommended. Camera batteries that contain 45% potassium hydroxide are hazardous and should be removed endoscopically if present in the esophagus or in the stomach after 24 hours. The use of balanced electrolyte lavage solutions containing polyethylene glycol (eg, Golytely) may help the passage of small, smooth foreign bodies lodged in the stomach or intestine. Lavage is especially useful in hastening the passage of button batteries or ingested tablets that may be toxic. Failure of a smooth foreign body to exit the stomach after several weeks suggests the possibility of gastric outlet obstruction.

Esophagogastroscopy will permit the removal of the majority of foreign bodies lodged in the esophagus and stomach. A Foley catheter may be used to dislodge smooth, round esophageal foreign bodies in healthy children with no previous esophageal disease. It is introduced into the esophagus, and the balloon at the distal end is inflated below the foreign body. Careful withdrawal of the catheter under fluoroscopic observation will bring the foreign body into the mouth where it can be extracted. Only an experienced radiologist should attempt this maneuver. If a foreign body remains in the bowel for longer than 5 days, surgical removal should be considered, especially if symptoms occur.

Bertoni G et al: A new protector device for safe endoscopic removal of sharp gastroesophageal foreign bodies in infants. J Pediatr Gastroenterol Nutr 1993;16:393.
Bloom RR et al: Foreign bodies of the gastrointestinal tract. Am Surg 1986;52:618.
Campbell JB, Foley LC: A safe alternative to endoscopic removal of blunt esophageal foreign bodies. Arch Otolaryngol 1983;109:323.
Litovitz TL: Battery ingestions: Product accessibility and clinical course. Pediatrics 1985;75:469.

ANAL FISSURE

Anal fissure consists of a slit-like tear in the anal canal, usually secondary to the passage of large, hard, dry fecal masses. Anal stenosis and trauma can be contributory factors, as can a crypt abscess following gastroenteritis. Sexual abuse must be considered in any child with large, irregular, or multiple anal fissures.

The infant or child cries with defecation and will try to hold back stools. Sparse, bright red bleeding is seen on the outside of the stool or on the toilet tissue following defecation. The fissure can often be seen if the patient is held in a knee-chest position and the buttocks spread apart.

When a fissure cannot be identified, it is essential to rule out other causes of rectal bleeding. If there is no history of constipation, the physician should consider juvenile polyp, perianal inflammation (due to group A streptococcal infection), or inflammatory bowel disease.

Anal fissures should be treated promptly, especially in infancy, to break the constipation-fissure-retention-constipation cycle. A stool softener should be given and is usually effective against constipation. The introduction of a gloved, lubricated finger twice daily lessens sphincter spasm. Warm sitz baths after defecation may be helpful. In rare cases, silver nitrate cauterization or surgery is indicated.

INGUINAL HERNIA

A peritoneal sac precedes the testicle as it descends from the genital ridge to the scrotum. The lower portion of this sac envelops the testis to form the tunica vaginalis, and the remainder normally atrophies by the time of birth. Persistence of the processus vaginalis presents as a mass in the inguinal region when an abdominal structure or peritoneal fluid is forced into it. The persistent sac may be very short or may extend into the scrotum. In some cases, peritoneal fluid may become trapped in the tunica vaginalis of the testis (noncommunicating hydrocele). If the processus vaginalis remains open, peritoneal fluid or an abdominal structure may be forced into it (indirect inguinal hernia).

Most inguinal hernias are of the indirect type and occur much more frequently in boys than in girls (9:1). Hernias may be present at birth or may appear at any age thereafter. The incidence in premature infants is close to 5%. In those weighing 1000 g or less, inguinal hernia is reported in 30%, and girls are more commonly affected.

Clinical Findings

There are no symptoms associated with an empty hernial sac. In most cases, the hernia is a painless inguinal swelling varying in size. There may be a history of inguinal fullness associated with coughing or long periods of standing; or there may be a firm, globular, and tender swelling, sometimes associated with vomiting and abdominal distention.

Spontaneous reduction frequently occurs while sleeping or with mild external pressure. In some instances, a herniated loop of intestine may become partially obstructed, leading to pain, irritability, and incomplete intestinal obstruction. Rarely, the loop of bowel becomes incarcerated, and signs of complete intestinal obstruction are present. Gangrene of the testis may occur; in the female, the ovary may prolapse into the hernial sac.

Inspection of the two inguinal areas may reveal a characteristic bulging or mass. Infants should be observed for evidence of swelling after crying and older children after bearing down.

A suggestive history is often the only criterion for diagnosis, along with the "silk glove" feel of the rubbing together of the two walls of the empty hernial sac.

Differential Diagnosis

An inguinal mass may represent lymph nodes. They are usually multiple and more discrete. Hydrocele of the cord transilluminates. An undescended testis may be moved along the canal and is associated with absence of the testicle in the scrotum.

Treatment

Surgery is indicated. There is still controversy about exploring the opposite side. Herniography is helpful in determining the patency of the processus vaginalis, but patency does not necessarily lead to a hernia.

Incarcerated inguinal hernias occur most often in the first 10 months of life and are more common in girls than in boys. Manipulative reduction can be attempted after placing the sedated infant in the Trendelenburg position with an ice bag on the affected side. This is contraindicated if the incarcerated hernia has been present for more than 12 hours or if bloody stools are noted.

McGregor DB et al: The unilateral pediatric inguinal hernia: Should the contralateral side be explored? J Pediatr Surg 1980;15:313.
Viidik T, Marshall DG: Direct inguinal hernias in infancy and early childhood. J Pediatr Surg 1980;15:646.

UMBILICAL HERNIA

Umbilical hernias are more common in premature than in full-term infants. This defect is also more common in black infants.

Excessive thinning of the skin distended by the hernia and progressive enlargement of the fascial defects are rarely reported unless there is increased intra-abdominal pressure due to organomegaly or ascites. Incarceration is the only dangerous problem and is limited to smaller hernias.

Most umbilical hernias regress spontaneously if the fascial defect has a diameter of less than 1 cm. Large defects may still disappear without treatment, but seldom before school age. Large defects and smaller hernias persisting up to school age should be treated surgically. Reducing the hernia and strapping the skin do not accelerate the healing process.

Hale DE et al: Umbilical hernia: What happens after age 5 years. J Pediatr 1981;98:415.

Erbe RW: Inherited gastrointestinal polyposis syndromes. N Engl J Med 1976;294:1101.

Haggitt RC, Reid BJ: Hereditary polyposis syndromes. Am J Surg Pathol 1986;10:871.

TUMORS OF THE GASTROINTESTINAL TRACT

1. JUVENILE POLYPS

Juvenile polyps are usually pedunculated and solitary, with a stalk covered in part by colonic mucosa. The head of the polyp is composed of hyperplastic glandular and vascular elements, often with cystic transformation. Juvenile polyps are benign, and 80% occur in the rectosigmoid. They are rare before age 1. Their incidence is highest between 3 and 5 years of age. They are rare after age 15 because of autoamputation. They are more frequent in boys. The painless passage of small amounts of bright red blood on a normal or constipated stool by an otherwise well child is the most frequent manifestation. Abdominal pain is infrequent, but a juvenile polyp can be the lead point for an intussusception. Low-lying polyps may prolapse during defecation.

Rarely, there are many juvenile polyps in the colon, causing anemia, diarrhea, and protein loss. A few cases have been reported of generalized juvenile polyposis involving the stomach and the small and large bowel. These cases are associated with a slightly increased risk of cancer.

Flexible fiberoptic colonoscopy is both diagnostic and therapeutic when polyps are suspected. After removal of the polyp by electrocautery, nothing further should be done if histologic findings confirm the diagnosis of juvenile polyp. There is a slight risk of developing further juvenile polyps.

Other polyposis syndromes are summarized in Table 22–4.

2. CANCER OF THE ESOPHAGUS & SMALL & LARGE INTESTINE

The most common small bowel cancer in children is lymphosarcoma. Intermittent abdominal pain, abdominal mass, intussusception, or a celiac-like picture may be present. Long-term survivals are reported in patients without lymph node involvement at surgery.

Carcinoid tumors of the appendix in children are not aggressive, regardless of the degree of invasion. However, carcinoid tumors of the ileum may metastasize.

Esophageal cancer is rare in childhood. Caustic injury of the esophagus increases the risk of squamous cell carcinoma, and chronic peptic esophagitis is associated with Barrett's esophagus, a precancerous lesion.

Adenocarcinoma of the colon is rare in the pediatric age group. The transverse colon and rectosigmoid are the two most commonly affected sites. The low 5-year survival relates to the nonspecificity of presenting complaints and the large percentage of undifferentiated types. Children with a family history of cancer and chronic ulcerative colitis or familial polyposis are at greater risk but seldom develop cancer before age 15.

Aiges HW et al: Adenocarcinoma of the colon in an adolescent with the family cancer syndrome. J Pediatr 1979; 94:632.

Collins RH et al: Colon cancer, dysplasia and surveillance in patients with ulcerative colitis: A critical review. N Engl J Med 1987;316:1654.

Table 22–4. Gastrointestinal polyposis syndromes.

	Location	Number	Histology	Extraintestinal Findings	Malignant Potential
Juvenile polyps	Colon	Usually single; rarely multiple	Hyperplastic, hamartomatous	None	None (single) Slight (multiple)
Familial polyposis	Colon; less commonly, stomach and small bowel	Multiple	Adenomatous	None	Very common
Peutz-Jeghers syndrome	Small bowel, stomach, colon	Multiple	Hamartomatous	Pigmented cutaneous and oral macules; ovarian cysts and tumors; bony exostoses	2–3%
Gardner's syndrome	Colon; less commonly, stomach and small bowel	Multiple	Adenomatous	Cysts, tumors, and desmoids of skin and bone; other tumors	Very common
Cronkhite-Canada syndrome	Stomach, colon; less commonly, esophagus and small bowel	Multiple	Hamartomatous	Alopecia; onychodystrophy; hyperpigmentation	Rare
Turcot syndrome	Colon	Multiple	Adenomatous	Thyroid and brain tumors	Possible

Gray GM et al: Lymphomas involving the gastrointestinal tract. Gastroenterology 1982;82:143.

Hassall E: Barrett's esophagus: New definitions and approaches in children. J Pediatr Gastroenterol Nutr 1993; 16:345.

3. MESENTERIC CYSTS

These rare tumors may be small or large, single or multiloculated. Invariably thin-walled, they contain either serous, chylous, or hemorrhagic fluid. They are commonly located in the mesentery of the small intestine but may also be seen in the mesocolon.

Most mesenteric cysts are asymptomatic. Traction on the mesentery eventually leads to colicky abdominal pain, which can be mild and recurrent but may present acutely with vomiting. Volvulus is reported, as is hemorrhage into the cyst. A rounded mass can occasionally be palpated or can be seen on x-ray film to displace adjacent intestine. Abdominal ultrasonography is usually diagnostic.

Surgical removal is indicated.

Christensen JA et al: Mesenteric cysts. Am Surg 1975;41: 352.

4. INTESTINAL HEMANGIOMA

Hemangiomas of the bowel may be a source of acute or chronic blood loss and anemia. They may also cause intestinal obstruction by triggering intussusception, by local stricture, or by intramural hematoma formation. Thrombocytopenia and consumptive coagulopathy are occasional systemic complications. Some lesions are telangiectasias (Rendu-Osler-Weber syndrome), and others are capillary hemangiomas. However, the largest group consists of cavernous hemangiomas, which are large, thin-walled vessels arising from the submucosal vascular plexus. They may protrude into the lumen as polypoid lesions or may invade the intestine from mucosa to serosa.

Abrahamson J, Shandling B: Intestinal hemangiomata in childhood and a syndrome for diagnosis: A collective review. J Pediatr Surg 1973;8:487.

Mestre JR, Andres JM: Hereditary hemorrhagic telangiectasia causing hematemesis in an infant. J Pediatr 1982; 101:577.

ACUTE INFECTIOUS DIARRHEA
(Gastroenteritis)

Acute gastroenteritis is one of the most common pediatric illnesses. Although bacteria (primarily *Shigella, Salmonella,* and *Campylobacter;* see Chapter 36) and parasites (*Entamoeba histolytica;* see Chapter 37) may be etiologic, rotavirus and other viruses (enteric adenovirus, Norwalk-like agents, calicivirus) cause most infections. They are generally hardy agents and are easily spread by fecal-oral transmission. Outbreaks are common; winter rotavirus epidemics and outbreaks in day-care centers and hospitals are well known. Toxin-secreting *E coli* are a common cause of acute enteritis in developing countries—nearly as important as viral causes. (See Table 22–5.)

Management of most cases of acute viral gastroenteritis consists of repair of fluid deficits either orally or intravenously. Specific etiologic agents may be diagnosed by culture (bacteria), antigen detection (rotavirus), and microscopic examination (parasites); electron microscopy is useful if specific viral agents are sought. (See Chapter 35.) In presumed acute viral gastroenteritis, specific etiologic diagnosis is usually unnecessary. Infants, especially those under 6 months of age, are at most risk of dehydration and secondary complications.

Clinical Findings

A. History: The incubation period for rotavirus infection is 2–4 days. There may be a history of exposure to others with similar illness.

B. Symptoms and Signs: Most symptoms of viral enteritis derive from dehydration (see Chapter 40). Fever is variable. Rash may be present in enteroviral infections. Vomiting in the first 24–48 hours of illness is present in 80–90%. Vomiting is usually nonbloody and nonbilious. Occasionally, there is abdominal distention due to ileus. Grossly bloody stools are rare in viral enteritis but common in bacterial enteritis involving the colon. In newborn infants, rotavirus may cause bloody diarrhea. In immunocompromised hosts, viral agents such as CMV, herpes simplex, varicella, and others may cause colitis with bloody stool.

C. Laboratory Findings: The leukocyte count is variable; marked elevation or left-shift is unusual for acute viral gastroenteritis. Electrolytes reflect the degree of dehydration and bicarbonate loss in the stools. Metabolic acidosis may be due to fecal bicarbonate loss, ketoacidosis from starvation, and lactic acidosis from hypovolemia. Measurement of stool electrolytes is usually unnecessary unless the diarrhea appears to be caused by a toxin or hormone stimulating intestinal water and electrolyte secretion. A stool sodium concentration of greater that 90 meq/L increases the likelihood of a secretory diarrhea.

Stool should be tested during the initial evaluation for blood and leukocytes. If positive for either, culture for enteric bacterial pathogens is indicated. Examination for ameba may also be done. If neither leukocytes nor blood is present, further testing is not usually needed as specific antibiotic treatment is not necessary. If an etiologic diagnosis is needed for patient isolation, public health requirements, or prolonged or unusual illness, the stool may be tested for

Table 22–5. Causes, characteristics, and treatment of acute enteritis.

Cause	Stool Exam	Symptoms	Treatment
Bacterial			
Salmonella	Liquid, foul, positive for white blood cells, positive for gross or occult blood	Fever, abdominal pain	None unless signs of extraintestinal infection or sepsis; ampicillin, amoxicillin, trimethoprim-sulfamethoxazole, third-generation cephalosporin.
Shigella	Small, grossly bloody, frequent	Fever, tenesmus, abdominal pain	Trimethoprim-sulfamethoxazole, ampicillin, if susceptible.
Campylobacter jejuni	Gross blood and mucus in streaks	Few systemic symptoms	None or erythromycin.
Yersinia enterocolitica	Similar to Salmonella	Similar to Salmonella	None effective for enteric disease.
Aeromonas hydrophilia	Watery; mild to moderate	Nausea, vomiting; probably enterotoxin-mediated	Usually self-limited; trimethoprim-sulfamethoxazole.
Plesiomonas shigelloides	Watery	Nausea, vomiting; possible enterotoxin	Usually self-limited; trimethoprim-sulfamethoxazole.
Escherichia coli invasive	Small, grossly bloody, positive for white blood cells	Abdominal pain, tenesmus	Trimethoprim-sulfamethoxazole; ampicillin; gentamicin.
Enterotoxigenic	Liquid, green, voluminous	Nausea, vomiting; heat labile toxin-mediated	Usually self-limited.
Enteropathogenic	Liquid, green, voluminous	Nausea, vomiting; adherence factors important	Usually self-limited.
Veratoxin-producing strains (0157:H7, others)	Small, grossly bloody, positive for white blood cells	Fever, tenesmus; organism produces Shigella-type toxin; may cause hemolytic-uremic syndrome	Antimicrobials may be detrimental.
Viral			
Rotavirus	Liquid, few white blood cells	Vomiting, nausea	None; fluid management.
Others: Caliciviruses, Norwalk, enteric adenovirus, enteroviruses	Same as above	As above	None; fluid management.
Parasitic			
Giardia lamblia	Very foul, liquid, negative for blood, negative for white blood cells, cysts present in 30–60%	Vomiting, nausea, abdominal distension, gas	Furazolidone (5 mg/kg/d for 7 days), metronidazole (15 mg/kg/d for 5 days).
Entamoeba histolytica	Blood and mucus, trophozoites on fresh stool exam	Abdominal pain, tenesmus	Metronidazole (35–50 mg/kg/d for 10 days).
Cryptosporidum	Watery or bloody, depending upon site of infestation	Incidence often in immunodeficient patients but also in healthy children; history of animal exposure	Clarithromycin may be tried.
Other toxic diarrheas E coli (see above)			
Clostridium difficile	Loose, positive for white blood cells, cytotoxin present in stool, hemocult positive	Abdominal pain, fever; history of prior antibiotic use is typical	Vancomycin (30–40 mg/kg/d for 7 days); metronidazole (25 mg/kg/d for 7 days); oral bacitracin (1500 units/kg/d for 7 days).
Staphylococcus aureus	Explosive, watery, positive for white blood cells	Nausea, vomiting, history of group outbreaks, onset after ingestion	Fluid management.
Clostridium perfringens	Explosive, watery, positive for white blood cells	Vomiting, abrupt onset; history of meat ingestion	Fluid management.

rotavirus antigen by a number of commercial methods or by electron microscopy, which can detect other enteric viruses.

D. Imaging: X-ray films are rarely needed. A nonspecific gas pattern including air-fluid levels in both large and small bowel is expected. Pneumatosis intestinalis may rarely be seen due to viral causes.

Differential Diagnosis

A high fever, febrile seizure, or change in mental status is typical of shigellosis. Significant abdominal tenderness or peritoneal signs suggest a more serious problem; a ruptured appendix in an infant is often misdiagnosed as acute gastroenteritis, as are intussusception, volvulus, pancreatitis, lower lobe pneumonia, meningitis, and urinary tract infection. Duration of vomiting longer than 24–48 hours or persistence of vomiting without diarrhea requires consideration of other causes. Elevated intracranial pressure, hepatitis, intestinal obstruction, metabolic disorders (adrenal insufficiency, acidosis), and poisoning are a few possibilities.

Complications & Sequelae

Dehydration and electrolyte abnormalities (eg, severe hypernatremia with cerebral damage) are the most important acute complications; improper attention to nutrition results in most secondary problems. Inappropriate continuation of a clear-liquid diet, often due to poor medical instruction, may result in persistent, loose "starvation" stools and weight loss. Secondary lactase deficiency is common but is not a contraindication to breast feeding in most infants. Persistent loose, acid stools (pH < 5.5) that are positive for reducing substances while drinking a milk-containing formula or breast milk suggests lactase deficiency; change to a sucrose- or glucose-based formula is curative. Occasionally, milk protein allergy follows acute gastroenteritis, and the persistent diarrhea responds only to an elemental formula. Small bowel colonization with enteric organisms may follow many intestinal insults, including acute gastroenteritis; this condition may produce a secretory diarrhea or malabsorption syndrome.

Systemic spread of enteric viruses that cause acute gastroenteritis never occurs except with enteroviruses; these, however, are not major causes of dehydrating enteritis (see Chapter 35).

Therapy & Prevention

For management of fluid and electrolyte balance, including oral rehydration regimens, see Chapter 40.

When stooling has markedly diminished, half-strength formula is offered as tolerated for 24–48 hours; full-strength formula must then be given so that secondary caloric deprivation can be avoided. Constipating solids (rice cereal, bananas, carrots, applesauce—not apple juice, which is hyperosmolar) may be given to older infants when feeding resumes.

Antidiarrheal agents (in particular, loperamide, which is now available over-the-counter) are usually unnecessary; those that block motility may be dangerous if used in inflammatory enteritis (such as shigellosis). Drugs with significant nonintestinal actions, such as diphenoxylate-atropine, may be fatal in young children.

Good hygiene reduces fecal-oral spread of these agents. Vaccines for rotavirus are being evaluated. There is no specific antiviral or oral therapy. Immunity is only partial, and repeated attacks may occur.

Guerrant RL, Lohr JA, Williams EK: Acute infectious diarrhea. 1. Epidemiology, etiology, and pathogenesis. Pediatr Infect Dis J 1986;5:353.
Williams EK, Lohr JA, Guerrant RL: Acute infectious diarrhea. 2. Diagnosis, treatment, and prevention. Pediatr Infect Dis J 1986;5:455.

CHRONIC DIARRHEA

What constitutes diarrhea is sometimes difficult to define because there are wide variations in normal bowel habit. Some infants pass one firm stool every second to third day, whereas others may have 5–8 soft small stools daily. A gradual or sudden increase in the number of stools, a reduction in their consistency coupled with an increase in their fluid content (> 15 g/kg/d), should raise a suspicion that an organic cause of chronic diarrhea is present.

Diarrhea may result from any of the following closely related pathogenetic mechanisms: (1) interruption of normal cell transport processes for water, electrolytes, or nutrients; (2) decrease in the surface area available for absorption, which may be due to shortening of the bowel or mucosal disease; (3) increase in intestinal motility; (4) increase in unabsorbable osmotically active molecules in the intestinal lumen; and (5) increase in intestinal permeability, leading to increased loss of water and electrolytes.

The differential diagnosis of chronic diarrhea is lengthy. Table 22–6 lists some disease categories and specific conditions in which diarrhea is a prominent feature.

Causes of Diarrhea Other Than Infectious

A. Antibiotic Therapy: Diarrhea accompanies antibiotic therapy in up to 30% of cases. Some antibiotics decrease carbohydrate transport and intestinal lactase levels. Eradication of normal gut flora and overgrowth of other organisms may cause diarrhea. Most antibiotic-associated diarrhea is watery in nature, is unassociated with systemic symptoms, and decreases when antibiotic therapy is stopped. Pseudomembranous colitis, caused by the toxins produced by *Clostridium difficile,* occurs in 0.2–10% of patients treated with antibiotics, especially clindamy-

Table 22–6. Guide to differential diagnosis of chronic diarrhea.

Disease	Age	Type of Diarrhea	Associated Features
Bacterial infections	Any age	Mucoid, bloody stool with polymorphonuclear leukocytes.	Rarely chronic except in immunocompromised hosts; *Salmonella* and *Yersinia* most likely.
Viral infections	Any age	Watery.	Rarely chronic except in immunocompromised hosts; cytomegalovirus, adenovirus, rotavirus.
Parasitic infections	Any age	Depends on organism.	*Entamoeba, Giardia, Cryptosporidium.*
Dietary factors Overfeeding (especially starches)	< 6 mo	Watery.	Colicky behavior without weight loss.
Protein allergy	< 2 mo	Watery with or without malabsorption of fat; at times, blood and mucus.	Colic, vomiting (anemia, hypoproteinemia).
Acrodermatitis enteropathica	< 12 mo	Voluminous with steatorrhea.	Malnutrition, skin rash; low serum zinc; usually genetic; sometimes secondary to severe dietary zinc deficiency.
Primary bile acid malabsorption	< 1 mo	Voluminous with steatorrhea.	Malnutrition; defective ileal transport of bile acids.
Irritable colon/chronic, nonspecific diarrhea	6–36 mo	Watery, frequent, with mucus, undigested food: no steatorrhea.	Healthy child; often starts with bout of gastroenteritis.
Toxic diarrhea (antibiotics, cancer chemotherapy, radiation)	Any age	Loose; sometimes steatorrhea, with occult blood or pus.	Vomiting; anorexia.
Functional tumors (neuroblastoma, carcinoid, pancreatic cholera, Zollinger-Ellison syndrome)	Any age	Secretory diarrhea, watery; persists when patient fasts.	Hypokalemia; other symptoms depend upon tumor.
Carbohydrate malabsorption Congenital deficiencies Sucrase-isomaltase	< 6 mo	Watery; low pH; reducing substance-positive after acid hydrolysis; volume varies with sucrose intake.	Abdominal distention; poor growth; deficiency present in 0.8% of North Americans, 10% of Alaskan natives.
Glucose-galactose malabsorption	< 1 mo	Intractable diarrhea with feeding; stool pH low; watery; reducing substances present.	Poor growth; defect in glucose transport.
Genetic deficiencies Lactase	> 4 y	Watery diarrhea with lactose; low pH; reducing substances present.	Deficiency develops in 100% of Asians, 80% of American blacks, 15% of American whites.
Acquired deficiencies Lactase and sucrase	Any age	Watery; low pH; reducing substances present.	Follows intestinal injury or infection.
Monosaccharide intolerance	< 6 mo	Watery; low pH; reducing substances present.	Rare; follows infection; made worse by malnutrition.
Pancreatic disorders Cystic fibrosis	< 6 mo	Steatorrhea; bulky, foul, pale.	Respiratory infection; poor weight gain.
Shwachman syndrome	< 2 y	Steatorrhea; bulky, foul, pale.	Neutropenia; short stature; bacterial infections; metaphyseal dysostosis.
Chronic pancreatitis	Any age	Steatorrhea; bulky, foul, pale.	Rare in children; usually associated with alcoholism.
Celiac disease	> 12 mo	Steatorrhea; bulky, foul, pale.	Vomiting, distention, irritability, anorexia.
Intestinal lymphangiectasia	3 mo	Voluminous; steatorrhea.	Lymphedema, lymphopenia, hypoalbuminemia.
Immune defects Hypogammaglobulinemia; IgA deficiency	Any age	Watery; sometimes steatorrhea.	Recurrent cutaneous and respiratory infection.
Combined immunodeficiency	< 1 mo	Severe; watery.	Stomatitis, skin rash, recurrent infection, opportunistic infection.

(continued)

Table 22–6. Guide to differential diagnosis of chronic diarrhea. (continued)

Disease	Age	Type of Diarrhea	Associated Features
HIV infection	Any age	Steatorrhea.	Other opportunistic infections.
Defective cellular immunity	< 2 y		
Genetic-metabolic disorders Chloride-losing diarrhea	< 1 mo	Watery.	Alkalosis; growth failure.
Abeta- and hypobetalipoproteinemia	< 3 mo	Profuse; steatorrhea.	Progressive neurologic symptoms; low serum cholesterol; acanthocytosis.
Wolman's disease	< 1 mo	Profuse; steatorrhea.	Vomiting; severe growth failure; adrenal calcification; hypercholesterolemia.
Folate malabsorption	< 1 mo	Watery.	Megaloblastic anemia, stomatitis, seizures, retardation.
Anatomic abnormalities Blind (stagnant) loop/bacterial overgrowth	Any age	Watery; fat and carbohydrate malabsorption.	Caused by surgical adhesions, intestinal duplication, abnormal gastrointestinal motility, partial obstruction.
Short bowel	Any age	Watery; malabsorption of all nutrients.	Rarely congenital; usually secondary to surgical resection.
Intestinal pseudo-obstruction	Any age	Watery; malabsorption of all nutrients.	Distention; May be acquired or congenital; diarrhea secondary to bacterial overgrowth.
Inflammatory bowel disease Crohn's disease	Usually > 10 y	Loose with or without steatorrhea.	Pain, fever, abdominal mass, growth failure; joint pain, perianal disease.
Ulcerative colitis	Usually > 10 y	Bloody stools with polymorphonuclear leukocytes.	Tenesmus, anemia, abdominal pain, fever, joint pain; less severe growth failure.
Eosinophilic gastroenteritis	Any age	Watery or bloody, depending upon site of disease.	Intestinal or gastric obstruction, eczema, asthma.
Hirschsprung's disease with enterocolitis	< 1 y	Foul, liquid with white and red blood cells.	Abdominal distention, fever, history of constipation.
Malnutrition	< 1 y	Loose, steatorrhea; sometimes with carbohydrate malabsorption.	Becomes temporarily worse with refeeding.
Endocrine disorders Hyperthyroidism	Any age	Frequent, loose stool without malabsorption.	Other signs of hyperthyroidism.

cin, cephalosporins, and amoxicillin. Patients develop fever, tenesmus, and abdominal pain with diarrhea which contains leukocytes and sometimes gross blood up to 8 weeks after antibiotic exposure. Treatment with oral vancomycin (30–50 mg/kg/d) or metronidazole (30 mg/kg/d) for 7 days is recommended. Relapse occurs after treatment in up to 10% of cases.

B. Parenteral Infections: Infections of the urinary tract and upper respiratory tract (especially otitis media) are at times associated with diarrhea. The mechanism remains obscure. Antibiotic treatment of the primary infection, toxins released by infective agents, and local irritation of the rectum (in patients with bladder infections) may play a role.

C. Malnutrition: Malnutrition is associated with an increased occurrence of enteral infections, decreased bile acid synthesis, decreased disaccharidase activity, altered motility, and changes in the intestinal flora, all of which may produce diarrhea.

D. Diet: Overfeeding may cause diarrhea, especially in young infants. Relative deficiency of pancreatic amylase in young infants may produce diarrhea after starchy foods. Fruit juices, especially those high in fructose or sorbitol, produce osmotic diarrhea. Intestinal irritants (spices and foods high in roughage) and histamine releasers (citrus and tomatoes) also cause diarrhea.

E. Allergic Diarrhea: Diarrhea caused by allergy to dietary proteins is a frequently entertained but rarely documented entity except in cases of milk and soy protein sensitivity. It is more common in infants under 12 months of age, who may experience mild to severe colitis. Older children may develop a celiac-like syndrome with a flat mucosal lesion, steatorrhea, hypoproteinemia, and occult blood loss. Skin testing is not reliable. Double-blind oral challenge with the suspected food under careful observation is necessary to confirm intestinal protein allergy. In infants, the condition usually disappears after 12 months. Allergies to fish, peanuts, and eggs are more likely to be lifelong.

F. Chronic, Nonspecific Diarrhea: Chronic, nonspecific diarrhea, sometimes called irritable colon syndrome, is the most common cause of loose stools in thriving children. The typical patient is a toddler 6–20 months of age who was a colicky baby and who has 3–6 loose, mucoid stools per day during the waking hours. The child is active, looks healthy, has a good appetite, and is growing normally. The diarrhea worsens with a low-residue, low-fat, or high-carbohydrate diet and during periods of stress and infection. It clears spontaneously at about 3½ years of age (usually coincident with toilet training). No organic disease is discoverable. The pathogenesis of the condition is obscure. Possible causes include abnormalities of bile acid absorption in the terminal ileum, incomplete carbohydrate absorption (excessive fruit juice ingestion seems to worsen the condition), and abnormal motor function. A high familial incidence of functional bowel disease is observed. Stool tests for blood, fat, parasites, and ova are negative.

The following measures are helpful: institution of a high-fat, low-carbohydrate, high-fiber diet; avoidance of between-meal snacks; and avoidance of chilled fluids, especially fruit juices. It may be helpful to give loperamide, 0.1–0.2 mg/kg/d in two or three divided doses; cholestyramine, 2–4 g in divided doses; or psyllium agents, 1–2 tsp twice daily.

Greene HL, Ghishan FK: Excessive fluid intake as a cause of chronic diarrhea in young children. J Pediatr 1983; 102:836.

Hoekstra JH et al: Apple juice malabsorption: Fructose or sorbitol? J Pediatr Gastroenterol Nutr 1993;16:39

Hyams JS et al: Carbohydrate malabsorption following fruit juice ingestion in young children. Pediatrics 1988;82:64.

Jonas A, Diver-Haber A: Stool output and composition in the chronic non-specific diarrhoea syndrome. Arch Dis Child 1982;57:35.

Kelly CP et al: *Clostridium difficile* colitis. N Engl J Med 1994;330:257.

Lloyd-Still JD: Chronic diarrhoea of childhood and the misuse of elimination diets. J Pediatr 1979;95:10.

THE MALABSORPTION SYNDROMES

Intestinal malabsorption is produced by shortening of the small bowel (short gut syndrome) or decreasing the amount of absorptive surface area (eg, celiac disease). Impaired motility of the small intestine may interfere with normal propulsive movements and mixing of food with pancreatic and biliary secretions. Anaerobic bacteria proliferate under these conditions and impair fat absorption by deconjugation of bile acids, (intestinal pseudo-obstruction, postoperative blind loop syndrome). Impaired intestinal lymphatic (congenital lymphangiectasis) or venous drainage and mucosal dysfunction secondary to hypoxia also cause malabsorption. Diseases reducing pancreatic exocrine function (cystic fibrosis, Shwachman syndrome) or the production and flow of biliary secretions cause nutrient malabsorption. Malabsorption of specific nutrients may be genetically determined—disaccharidase deficiency, glucose-galactose malabsorption, and abetalipoproteinemia.

Clinical Findings

Gastrointestinal symptoms such as diarrhea, vomiting, anorexia, abdominal pain, and bloating are not always present, and the presenting complaints may not refer to the gastrointestinal tract. Certain physical features such as potbelly and wasted buttocks may indicate celiac disease. Personal observation of the stools for abnormal color, consistency, bulkiness, odor, mucus, and blood is important. Microscopic examination of stools for neutral and split fat (fatty acids) is helpful because most malabsorption syndromes involve some fat malabsorption.

The following are the most helpful investigations:

A. Fat Absorption: Qualitative or quantitative (72-hour) fecal fat excretion, serum carotene, and prothrombin time.

B. Protein Absorption or Abnormal Protein Loss: Serum protein electrophoresis and fecal excretion of α_1-antitrypsin.

C. Carbohydrate Absorption: Stool pH and reducing substances, breath hydrogen analysis after carbohydrate ingestion, and disaccharidase levels in intestinal mucosa.

D. Absorption of Folic Acid and Vitamin B_{12}: Serum folic acid and vitamin B_{12}.

E. Bacteriology and Parasitology: Culture and microscopic examination of stool and duodenal juice.

F. Imaging: Upper gastrointestinal series with small bowel follow-through, barium enema, and bone age.

G. Sweat Test: Chloride determination.

H. Pancreatic Exocrine Function: Examination of duodenal aspirate (volume, viscosity, pH, and bicarbonate, trypsin, lipase, and amylase activity) and bentiromide excretion test.

I. Liver Function Tests: Bilirubin, aminotransferases, alkaline phosphatase, and prothrombin time.

J. Miscellaneous: Peroral small bowel biopsy, D-xylose absorption, rectosigmoidoscopy and rectal biopsy, immunoglobulin levels, lipoprotein electrophoresis, urine catecholamines, and endocrine function tests.

Differential Diagnosis

The pathophysiologic classification set forth in Table 22–7 may be helpful in view of the considerable variety of disorders giving rise to malabsorption.

Treatment & Prognosis

See specific syndromes (celiac disease, disaccharidase deficiency, etc).

Table 22–7. Malabsorption syndromes.

Intraluminal phase abnormalities
  Acid hypersecretion; Zollinger-Ellison syndrome
  Gastric resection
  Exocrine pancreatic insufficiency
    Cystic fibrosis
    Chronic pancreatitis
    Pancreatic pseudocysts
    Schwachman syndrome
    Enterokinase deficiency
    Lipase and colipase deficiency
    Malnutrition
  Decreased conjugated bile acids
    Liver production and excretion
      Neonatal hepatitis
      Biliary atresia: intrahepatic and extrahepatic
      Acute and chronic active hepatitis
      Disease of the biliary tract
      Cirrhosis
      Fat malabsorption in the premature infant
    Intestinal malabsorption of bile acids
    Short bowel syndrome
    Bacterial overgrowth
      Blind loop
      Fistula
      Strictures, regional enteritis
      Scleroderma, intestinal pseudo-obstruction
Intestinal phase abnormalities
  Mucosal diseases
    Infections, bacterial or viral
    Infections, parasitic
      Giardia lamblia
      Fish tapeworm
      Hookworm
    Malnutrition
      Marasmus
      Kwashiorkor
  Dermatitis herpetiformis
  Folic acid deficiency
  Drugs: methotrexate, antibiotics
  Crohn's disease
  Cow's milk and soy protein intolerance
  Secondary disaccharidase deficiency
  Secondary monosaccharide intolerance
  Hirschsprung's disease with enterocolitis
  Tropical sprue
  Celiac disease
  Radiation enteritis
  Lymphoma
	Intestinal phase abnormalities (cont'd)
	  Circulatory disturbances
	    Cirrhosis
	    Congestive heart failure
	  Abnormal structure of gastrointestinal tract
	    Dumping syndrome after gastrectomy
	    Malrotation
	    Stenosis of jejunum or ileum
	    Small bowel resection; short bowel syndrome
	    Polyposis
	  Selective inborn absorptive defects
	    Congenital malabsorption of folic acid
	    Selective malabsorption of vitamin B_{12}
	    Cystinuria, methionine malabsorption
	    Hartnup disease, blue diaper syndrome
	    Glucose-galactose malabsorption
	    Primary disaccharidase deficiency
	    Acrodermatitis enteropathica
	    Abetalipoproteinemia
	    Congenital chloridorrhea
	    Primary hypomagnesemia
	    Hereditary fructose intolerance
	    Familial hypophosphatemic rickets
	  Endocrine diseases
	    Diabetes
	    Addison's disease
	    Hyperthyroidism
	    Hypoparathyroidism, pseudohypoparathyroidism
	    Neuroblastoma, ganglioneuroma
	Delivery phase defects
	  Whipple's disease
	  Intestinal lymphangiectasis
	  Congestive heart failure
	  Regional enteritis with lymphangiectasis
	  Lymphoma
	  Abetalipoproteinemia
	Miscellaneous
	  Renal insufficiency
	  Carcinoid, mastocytosis
	  Immunity defects
	  Familial dysautonomia
	  Collagen disease
	  Wolman's disease
	  Histiocytosis X

Anderson CM: Malabsorption in children. Clin Gastroenterol 1977;6:355.

Friedman HI, Nylund B: Intestinal fat digestion, absorption, and transport: A review. Am J Clin Nutr 1980;33:1108.

CONSTIPATION

Constipation is the regular passage of firm or hard stools or the infrequent passage of stool. In the presence of fecal impaction, there may be encopresis (involuntary fecal soiling). Familial, cultural, and social factors influence the genesis, development, and course. Psychologic factors, toilet-training techniques, and diet (particularly excessive milk intake and low-residue diets) may also influence bowel habits. Neu-

rologic (spinal cord lesions) and anatomic (anorectal) disorders, hypothyroidism, and hypercalcemia, are all well-known causes of constipation.

Clinical Findings

Many symptoms, such as fever, convulsions, nervousness, school failure, bad breath, and the like have been improperly attributed to constipation. Normal infants often appear to have difficulty passing a stool. The child's face may turn red and the legs are drawn up on the abdomen even when the stool passed is soft. This pattern may be erroneously viewed as constipation. Similarly, the infant may become flushed, draw up the legs, and act as though struggling to pass stool, when in fact the infant is attempting to withhold stool. Failure to appreciate this normal developmental pattern may lead to the unwise use of laxatives or enemas. As children become ambulatory, many new and exciting activities interfere with the response to the "call to stool"; they may pass enough stool to relieve rectal distention while continuing to play, or they may gradually develop the ability to ignore the sensation of rectal fullness. In older children, school, games, social events, and the inadequate privacy and hygiene of school toilets may all interfere with regular defecation. Fecal retention may lead to impaction of the rectum, with involuntary fecal leakage. Leakage generally stops when impaction is relieved. Occasionally, fecal incontinence is a sign of primary emotional disturbance, especially if no impaction is present.

Differential Diagnosis

Constipation is prevalent among mentally retarded children with associated motor deficits and in those with hypothyroidism. Causes of constipation are listed in Table 22–8.

Features distinguishing retentive constipation from Hirschsprung's disease are summarized in Table 22–9.

Treatment

Reduced milk intake and increased intake of fluids and high-residue foods such as bran, whole wheat, fruits, and vegetables may be sufficient therapy in cases of mild constipation. The use of a barley malt extract such as Maltsupex, 1–2 tsp added to feedings two or three times daily, is helpful in small infants. Stool softeners such as dioctyl sodium sulfosuccinate, 5–10 mg/kg/d, prevent excessive drying of the stool and are effective unless there is voluntary stool retention. Cathartics such as standardized extract of senna

Table 22–9. Differentiation of retentive constipation and Hirschsprung's disease.

	Retentive Constipation	Hirschsprung's Disease
Onset	2–3 years	At birth
Abdominal distention	Rare	Present
Nutrition/growth	Normal	Poor
Soiling	Intermittent or constant	Never
Rectal examination	Ampulla full	Ampulla may be empty
Rectal biopsy	Ganglion cells present	Ganglion cells absent
Rectal manometry	Normal rectoanal reflex	Nonrelaxation of internal anal sphincter
Barium enema	Distended rectum	Narrow distal segment with proximal megacolon

fruit (eg, Senokot syrup), 1–2 tsp twice daily depending on age, can be used for short periods of time.

If encopresis is present, treatment should start with relieving fecal impaction. Following this step, an effective stool softener should be given in amounts sufficient to induce 3–4 loose stools per day (2–5 mL/kg/d of mineral oil in two doses). After several weeks to months of regular loose stools, the dosage of mineral oil can be tapered and stopped. Mineral oil should not be given to nonambulatory infants, retarded children, or those with gastroesophageal reflux. Aspiration of mineral oil may cause severe lipid pneumonia.

Table 22–8. Causes of constipation.[1]

Functional or retentive causes
Dietary causes
  Undernutrition, dehydration
  Excessive milk intake
  Lack of bulk
Drug and cathartic abuse
Structural defects of gastrointestinal tract
  Anus and rectum
    Fissure, hemorrhoids, abscess
    Anterior location of anus
    Anal and rectal stenosis
    Presacral teratoma
    Rectal prolapse
  Small bowel and colon
    Tumor, stricture
    Chronic volvulus
    Intussusception
    Internal hernia
Smooth muscle diseases of gastrointestinal tract
  Scleroderma and dermatomyositis
  Systemic lupus erythematosus
  Chronic intestinal pseudo-obstruction
	Abnormalities of myenteric ganglion cells
	  Hirschsprung's disease
	  Hypo- and hyperganglionosis
	  Recklinghausen's disease
	  Multiple endocrine neoplasia type IIB
	Absence of abdominal musculature
	Spinal cord defects
	Metabolic and endocrine disorders
	  Hypothyroidism
	  Hyperparathyroidism
	  Renal tubular acidosis
	  Diabetes insipidus (dehydration)
	  Vitamin D intoxication, hypercalcemia
	  Idiopathic hypercalcemia
	Neurologic and psychiatric conditions
	  Myotonic dystrophy
	  Amyotonia congenita
	  Brain tumors
	  Mental retardation
	  Psychosis

[1]Modified and reproduced, with permission, from Silverman A, Roy CC: *Pediatric Clinical Gastroenterology,* 3rd ed. Mosby, 1983.

The prevention of stool holding and the establishment of a regular bowel habit are accomplished by "toileting" the child at regular times each day and by the daily administration of mineral oil over a period of several months in a reduced dosage. Recurrence of encopresis should be treated promptly with a short course of laxatives or enemas. A multiple vitamin is recommended while mineral oil is administered.

Psychiatric consultation may be indicated for patients with recurrent symptoms or overt, severe emotional disturbances.

Hatch TF: Encopresis and constipation in children. Pediatr Clin North Am 1988;35:257.

Olness K, McParland FA, Piper J: Biofeedback: A new modality in the management of children with fecal soiling. J Pediatr 1980;96:505.

Schmitt BD: Encopresis. Prim Care 1984;11:497.

GASTROINTESTINAL BLEEDING

Vomiting or rectal evacuation of blood is an alarming symptom. The history should provide detailed answers to the following questions:

(1) *Is it really blood and is it coming from the gastrointestinal tract?* A number of substances may simulate hematochezia or melena; therefore, the presence of blood should be confirmed chemically. Information concerning genitourinary problems, coughing, or epistaxis may identify a source of bleeding elsewhere than in the gastrointestinal tract.

(2) *How much blood is there and what is its color and character?* Table 22–10 lists the sites of gastrointestinal bleeding in relationship to the amount and the appearance of the blood in the stools. Tables

Table 22–10. Identification of sites of gastrointestinal bleeding.

Symptom or Sign	Location of Bleeding Lesion
Effortless welling forth of bright red blood from the mouth	Nasopharyngeal or oral lesions; esophageal varices; lacerations of esophageal or gastric mucosa (Mallory-Weiss syndrome).
Vomiting of bright red blood or of "coffee grounds"	Lesion proximal to ligament of Treitz.
Melena	Lesion proximal to ligament of Treitz. Blood loss in excess of 50–100 mL/24 h.
Bright red or dark red blood in stools	Lesion in the ileum or colon. (Massive upper gastrointestinal bleeding may also be associated with bright red blood in stool.)
Streak of blood on outside of a stool	Lesion in the rectal ampulla or anal canal.

22–11 and 22–12 list clinical causes of hematemesis and rectal bleeding.

(3) *Is the child acutely or chronically ill?* The physical examination should be thorough no matter how ill the patient is. Alertness to signs of portal hypertension, intestinal obstruction, or blood dyscrasia is particularly important. The nasal passages should be inspected for signs of recent epistaxis; the vagina for menstrual blood; and the anus for fissures and hemorrhoids.

A systolic blood pressure below 100 mm Hg and a pulse rate above 100/min in an older child suggest at least a 20% reduction of blood volume. A pulse rate increase of 20/min or a drop in systolic blood pressure greater than 10 mm Hg when the patient sits up is also a sensitive index of significant volume depletion.

(4) *Is the child still bleeding?* A determination of vital signs every 15 minutes is essential to assess ongoing bleeding. Serial hematocrits are useful. An important maneuver for assessing the origin and severity of gastrointestinal bleeding is the introduction of a nasogastric tube in the stomach. Detection of blood in the gastric aspirate confirms a bleeding site proximal to the ligament of Treitz. However, its absence does not rule out the duodenum as the source.

Management

A hemorrhagic diathesis should be ruled out, and vitamin K should be given intravenously. In severe bleeding, needs for volume replacement are monitored by measurement of central venous pressure. In less severe cases, vital signs, serial hematocrits, and gastric aspirates are sufficient.

If blood is recovered from the gastric aspirate, gastric lavage with saline should be performed for 30–60 minutes, until only a blood-tinged return is obtained. Panendoscopy is then done to identify the bleeding site. Endoscopy is superior to barium contrast study for lesions such as esophageal varices, stress ulcers, and gastritis. Colonoscopy may identify the source of bright red rectal bleeding and should be performed if the extent of bleeding warrants immediate investigation and if plain x-ray films show no signs of intestinal obstruction.

Small or large bowel lesions that bleed briskly (> 0.5 mL/min) may be localized by angiography or radionuclide scanning following injection of labeled red cells.

Persistent vascular bleeding (varices, vascular anomalies) may be temporarily relieved using vasopressin (20 units/1.73 m^2 intravenously over a 20-minute period). Thereafter it may be necessary to sustain the infusion for 24 hours at a rate of 0.2–0.4 units/1.73 m^2/min. Bleeding from esophageal varices may be stopped by temporary compression with a pediatric Sengstaken-Blakemore tube. Sclerotherapy or banding of uncontrolled bleeding varices is the treatment of choice.

Table 22–11. Causes of hematemesis in infants and children.[1]

Entity	Age	Amount of Blood	Clinical Features	Cause
Swallowed maternal blood	Newborn	Variable	No other signs of illness; Apt test shows alkaline denaturation of blood.	Blood swallowed at delivery or during nursing.
Stress ulcer	Any age	Large	Sickliness; pallor; shock.	Central nervous system disease, sepsis, asphyxia, burns.
Hemorrhagic gastritis	Newborn	Large	Sickliness; pallor; shock.	Central nervous system disease, sepsis, asphyxia.
Hemorrhagic disease of newborn	Newborn to 2 months	Variable	Melena, bleeding elsewhere.	Vitamin K deficiency, liver disease, clotting defect.
Gastric volvulus	Newborn, infancy	Small	Intractable vomiting.	Congenital defect, eventration of diaphragm.
Peptic disease	Any age	Variable	Relatively good health, vomiting, pain.	Duodenal or antral ulcer.
Esophageal varices	Any age	Large	May have signs of liver disease.	Portal hypertension secondary to liver disease or portal obstruction.
Esophagitis	Any age	Small	Dysphagia, chronic vomiting.	Peptic; infection (in immunocompromised hosts).
Foreign body	Infancy to later childhood	Small	Dysphagia.	Trauma.
Gastric outlet obstruction	Any age	Small	Vomiting, failure to thrive.	Gastric or esophageal ulcer or mucosal tear.
Erosive gastritis or esophagitis	Any age	Small	Vomiting, pain, dysphagia.	Ingestion of acids, alkali, iron, aspirin.
Gastritis	Any age	Small	Protracted vomiting.	Infection, bile reflux, ingestion.
Mallory-Weiss syndrome	Preschool to adolescence	Moderate to large	Retching, vomiting.	Increased intraesophageal pressure and mucosal tear.
Swallowed blood	Any age	Moderate to large	Nausea, epistaxis.	Bleeding from mouth, gums, ears, nose, or throat.

[1]Modified and reproduced, with permission, from Silverman A, Roy CC: *Pediatric Clinical Gastroenterology,* 3rd ed. Mosby, 1983.

If gastric decompression, antacid therapy, and transfusion are ineffective in stopping ulcer bleeding, laser therapy, local injection of epinephrine, electrocautery, or emergency surgery may be necessary.

Hyams JS, Leichtner AM, Schwartz AN: Recent advances in diagnosis and treatment of gastrointestinal hemorrhage in infants and children. J Pediatr 1985;106:1.

McKusick KA et al: ^{99m}Tc red blood cells for detection of gastrointestinal bleeding. AJR 1981;137:1113.

Roy CC, Morin CL, Weber AM: Gastrointestinal emergency problems in paediatric practice. Clin Gastroenterol 1981;10:225.

RECURRENT ABDOMINAL PAIN

About 10% of healthy school children between 5 and 15 years of age will at some time experience recurrent episodes of abdominal pain severe enough to affect activity. An organic cause can be found in fewer than 10% of cases, and there is often evidence that the pain is a reaction to emotional stress.

Clinical Findings

A. Symptoms and Signs: Attacks of abdominal pain are characteristically of variable duration and intensity. Although the pain is usually located in the periumbilical area, location far from the umbilicus does not rule out recurrent abdominal pain. Pain may occur both day and night. Weight loss rarely occurs. Pain may be associated with dramatic reactions; patients may clutch the abdomen, double over, or even throw themselves to the ground. School attendance may suffer. Indeed, reluctance to attend school (school phobia) may be an important etiologic factor. The pain may be associated with pallor, nausea, vomiting, and slight temperature elevation.

The pain usually bears little relationship to bowel habits and activity, although constipation is present in some. At times, pain may occur during meals or before the child leaves for school. A definite precipitating or stressful situation in the child's life at the time the pains began can sometimes be elicited. A history of functional gastrointestinal complaints is often found in family members.

A thorough physical examination is essential and is usually negative in these children. Abdominal tender-

Table 22–12. Differential diagnosis of rectal bleeding in infants and children.

Cause	Usual Age Group	Additional Complaints	Amount of Blood	Color of Blood
Swallowed foreign body	Any age	Rarely, perforation and abscess	Usually small	Melena
Systemic bleeding	Any age	Other evidence of bleeding	Variable	Dark or bright
Hemorrhagic disease of the newborn	Newborn	Other evidence of bleeding	Variable	Dark or bright
Milk intolerance	Infants	Colicky abdominal pain, diarrhea	Moderate to large	Dark or bright; usually with diarrhea
Esophageal varices	> 4 years	Signs of portal hypertension	Variable	Usually dark; bright with massive bleed
Hemangioma or familial telangiectasia	Any age	Telangiectasia elsewhere	Variable	Dark or bright
Peptic ulcer, gastritis	Any age	Abdominal pain	Usually small; can be massive	Dark
Duplication of bowel	Any age	Pain, obstruction, mass	Usually small	Usually dark
Meckel's diverticulum	Any age; rare under 2 months	Anemia, painless bleeding	Small to large; usually large	Maroon
Volvulus	Infant or young child	Abdominal pain, intestinal obstruction	Small to large	Dark or bright
Intussusception	< 18 months	Abdominal pain, mass	Small to large	Dark or bright with "currant jelly" mucus
Ulcerative colitis	> 4 years	Diarrhea, cramps	Small to large	Usually bright, with diarrhea
Bacterial enteritis	Any age	Diarrhea, cramps, fever	Small to large	Usually bright, with diarrhea
Juvenile polyp	2–8 years	None	Small to large	Bright, with normal stool
Inserted foreign body	Child	Pain	Small	Bright with mucus
Anal fissure or proctitis	< 2 years	Pain with defecation	Small	Bright with mucus
Swallowed maternal blood	Newborn	None	Variable	Dark
Esophagitis	Any age	Dysphagia, hematemesis	Usually small	Dark
Schönlein-Henoch purpura	3–10 years	Purpuric rash, arthritis, abdominal pain, hematuria	Variable	Dark or bright
Lymphoid nodular hyperplasia	3–24 months	Loose stools	Small	Bright

ness, if present, is diffuse and mild, although discomfort over the descending colon is common.

B. Laboratory Findings: Complete blood count, sedimentation rate, urinalysis, and stool test for occult blood usually suffice. If the pain is atypical, further testing suggested by symptoms should be done.

Differential Diagnosis

Organic causes relating to the urinary and gastrointestinal tracts, as well as extra-abdominal causes (Table 22–3), should be ruled out by appropriate studies. Pinworms, "mesenteric lymphadenitis," and "chronic appendicitis" are improbable causes of recurrent abdominal pain. Milk intolerance due to lactose intolerance usually manifests itself by both pain and diarrhea. However, abdominal discomfort may at times be the only symptom. Abdominal migraine and abdominal epilepsy are rare conditions. The incidence of significant peptic gastritis, esophagitis, duodenitis, and ulcer disease is probably underappreciated. Upper intestinal endoscopy may be useful.

Treatment & Prognosis

Treatment consists of reassurance based on a thorough physical appraisal and a sympathetic explanation of the functional nature of the complaint. Therapy for emotional problems is sometimes required, but drugs should be avoided. The prognosis is good.

Appley J: *The Child With Abdominal Pain,* 2nd ed. Blackwell, 1975.

Liebman WM: Recurrent abdominal pain in children: A retrospective survey of 119 patients. Clin Pediatr 1978; 17:149.

Silverman A, Roy CC: Psychophysiologic recurrent abdominal pain. In: *Pediatric Clinical Gastroenterology,* 3rd ed. Mosby, 1983.

PROTEIN-LOSING ENTEROPATHIES

Excessive loss of plasma proteins into the gastrointestinal tract occurs in association with a number of disorders, some of which are listed below.

Disorders Associated With Protein-Losing Enteropathy

A. Vascular Obstruction: Congestive heart failure, constrictive pericarditis, atrial septal defect, primary myocardial disease, increased right atrial pressure.

B. Gastric: Giant hypertrophic gastritis, or Ménétrier's disease (may be a result of CMV infection); polyps.

C. Small Intestine: Celiac disease, intestinal lymphangiectasia, regional enteritis, Whipple's disease, lymphosarcoma, acute gastrointestinal infection, allergic gastroenteropathy, blind loop syndrome, abetalipoproteinemia, chronic mucosal ischemia (eg, from chronic volvulus or radiation enteritis).

D. Colon: Ulcerative colitis, Hirschsprung's disease, pseudomembranous colitis, polyposis syndromes, villous adenoma, solitary rectal ulcer.

E. Other: Immunologic deficiency states.

Clinical Findings

The signs and symptoms include edema, chylous ascites, poor weight gain, deficiencies of fat-soluble vitamins, and anemia. Serum albumin is usually less than 2.5 g/dL.

Differential Diagnosis

Hypoalbuminemia may be due to an increased catabolic rate or may be associated with poor protein intake, impaired hepatic protein synthesis, mechanical or functional obstruction of lymph flow, or congenital malformations of lymphatics outside the gastrointestinal tract. It is especially important to rule out malnutrition and to make certain that no significant proteinuria is present. Lymphangiography is useful after age 2 years.

Treatment

Temporary benefits can be derived from albumin infusions in conjunction with diuretics. Treatment must be directed toward the primary underlying cause.

Magazzu G et al: Reliability and usefulness of random fecal alpha-1-antitrypsin concentration: Further simplification of the method. J Pediatr Gastroenterol Nutr 1985;4:402.

Thomas DW et al: Random fecal alpha-1-antitrypsin concentration in children with gastrointestinal disease. Gastroenterology 1981;80:776.

CELIAC DISEASE
(Gluten Enteropathy)

Essentials of Diagnosis

- Diarrhea and steatorrhea.
- Failure to thrive; loss of weight involving mostly the limbs and buttocks.
- Abdominal distention.
- Depressed D-xylose absorption.
- Villous atrophy on small bowel biopsy.
- Improvement on gluten-free diet, and histologic relapse following reintroduction of gluten into the diet.
- Normal pancreatic and biliary secretions.

General Considerations

Celiac disease results from intestinal sensitivity to the gliadin fraction of gluten from wheat, rye, barley, and oats. Most cases present during the second year of life, but the age at onset and the severity are both variable. The disease is more common in Europe and in Canada than in the USA and is uncommon in blacks and Asians.

The underlying pathologic process is not yet clearly understood, but it is thought that the intestinal lesion is the result of a cell-mediated immune response susceptible to gliadin, the alcohol-soluble fraction of gluten. Ten percent of first-degree relatives may be affected. The inheritance is probably polygenic, but it might result from a single gene in combination with an environmental precipitant such as intestinal adenovirus infection. The adenovirus capsid protein shares some sequence homology with gliadin. The increased incidence of celiac disease in children with type I diabetes mellitus, IgA deficiency, and Down's syndrome suggests possible immunologic factors in etiology.

Clinical Findings

A. Symptoms and Signs:

1. Diarrhea–Affected children present with a history of digestive disturbances starting at 6–12 months of age—the age at which wheat, rye, or oat glutens are first fed. Initially, the diarrhea may be intermittent and related to upper respiratory tract infections. Subsequently, it is continuous, with bulky, pale, frothy, greasy, foul-smelling stools. During celiac crises, dehydration, shock, and acidosis are commonly seen. Diarrhea is absent in 10% of cases.

2. Constipation, vomiting, and abdominal pain–This triad of symptoms may in a small number of cases dominate the clinical picture and suggest a diagnosis of intestinal obstruction. Constipation generally results from a combination of anorexia, dehydration, muscle weakness, and very thick, fatty stools.

3. Failure to thrive–The onset of diarrhea is usually accompanied by loss of appetite, failure to gain weight, and increased irritability.

4. Wasting and retardation of growth–In established cases, there is a loss of weight, which is most marked in the limbs and buttocks. The face remains plump, and the abdomen becomes distended secondary to accumulation of gas and fluid in the intestinal tract. Growth failure may dominate the clinical picture.

5. Anemia and vitamin deficiencies–Anemia usually responds to iron and is rarely megaloblastic. Deficiencies in fat-soluble vitamins are common. Rickets can be seen when growth has not been completely halted by the disease. Osteomalacia is more common, however, and pathologic fractures may occur. Hypoprothrombinemia can be severe, and some patients present with severe bleeding diathesis.

B. Laboratory Findings:

1. Fat content of stools–A 3-day collection of stools usually reveals excessive fecal fat. A normal child will excrete 5–10% of ingested fats. The untreated celiac patient will excrete more than 15% of daily fat intake. Anorexia may be so severe that steatorrhea may not be present in 10–25% of cases until normal intake is established.

2. Impaired carbohydrate absorption–A low oral glucose tolerance curve is seen. Absorption of D-xylose is impaired, with blood levels lower than 20 mg/dL 60 minutes after ingestion.

3. Hypoproteinemia–Hypoalbuminemia can be severe enough to lead to edema. There is evidence of increased protein loss in the gut lumen and poor hepatic synthesis secondary to malnutrition.

C. Imaging: A small bowel series shows a malabsorptive pattern characterized by segmentation, clumping of the barium column, and hypersecretion. These changes are nonspecific, and x-ray films of the small bowel should therefore be taken to rule out structural defects that might cause malabsorption. (See Table 22–7.)

D. Biopsy Findings: Intestinal biopsy is the most reliable test for celiac disease. It is a safe and simple procedure even in infants. Under the dissecting microscope, the jejunal mucosa lacks the slender, finger-like projections that characterize normal villi. Under the light microscope, the celiac mucosa has shortened or absent villi, lengthened crypts of Lieberkühn, and intense plasma cell infiltration of the lamina propria. Normal to nearly normal appearance of the lamina propria can be expected after withdrawal of gluten from the diet.

E. Serologic Tests: Anti-gliadin antibody, anti-reticulin antibody, and anti-endomysial antibodies are useful screening tests. IgG antibodies to gliadin are present in 10% of normal children. IgA antibodies are more specific to celiac patients.

Differential Diagnosis

The differential diagnosis includes disorders that cause malabsorption. Strict adherence to two diagnostic criteria—ie, the characteristic small bowel microscopic changes and clinical improvement on a gluten-free diet—is essential. Whenever the mucosal lesion is not characteristic or the response to a gluten-free diet is not as good as expected, challenge with a gluten-containing diet is indicated. Repeat biopsy while on a gluten-free diet is not critical to the diagnosis.

Treatment

A. Diet: Treatment consists of dietary gluten restriction for life. All sources of wheat, rye, barley, and oat gluten must be eliminated during the initial treatment. Some patients may be able to tolerate oats in the diet, but this should be tested only after recovery has occurred. Dietary supervision is essential. Initially, the diet should provide 25% more calories than calculated for expected weight. Lactose is poorly tolerated in the acute stage because the extensive mucosal damage leads to acquired disaccharidase deficiency. Normal amounts of fat are advisable. Supplemental vitamins and minerals are indicated in the acute phase.

In treating a severely affected child, the diet should be tailored to the child's appetite and capacity to absorb. A full gluten-free diet can usually be given after 2–3 weeks. Clinical improvement is usually evident within a week, and histologic repair is complete after 3–12 months.

B. Corticosteroids: Corticosteroids can hasten clinical improvement but are indicated only in very ill patients with signs and symptoms of celiac crisis.

Prognosis

Improvement and clinical recovery are the rule but may be slow. Malignant lymphoma of the small bowel occurs with increased frequency in older adults with long-standing disease. Dietary treatment seems to decrease the risk of this serious complication.

Aurrichio S et al: Gluten-sensitive enteropathy in childhood. Pediatr Clin North Am 1988;35:157.

Burgin-Wolff A et al: A reliable screening test for childhood celiac disease: Fluorescent immunosorbent test for gliadin antibodies. J Pediatr 1983;102:655.

Cacciari E et al: Short stature and celiac disease: A relationship to consider even in patients with no gastrointestinal tract symptoms. J Pediatr 1983;103:708.

Cooper BT et al: Celiac disease and malignancy. Medicine 1980;59:249.

DISACCHARIDASE DEFICIENCY

Essentials of Diagnosis

- Watery diarrhea, explosive and frothy.
- Stool pH < 5.5.
- Reducing substances present in stools.
- Flat glucose tolerance test following disaccharide loading.
- A positive breath hydrogen test following an oral test dose of lactose or sucrose.

General Considerations

Carbohydrates account for a substantial proportion of the human diet. The polysaccharide starch and the disaccharides sucrose and lactose are quantitatively the most important and require hydrolysis by intestinal brush border disaccharidases before significant absorption can take place. Disaccharidase levels are higher in the jejunum and in the proximal ileum than in the distal ileum and duodenum. Some substrates can be hydrolyzed by more than one enzyme, and, conversely, some enzymes act on more than one substrate.

In primary disaccharidase deficiency, the enzyme deficit is isolated, the disaccharide intolerance is likely to persist, intestinal histologic findings are normal, and a family history is common.

Because disaccharidases are confined to the outer cell layer of the intestinal epithelium, they are susceptible to mucosal damage. A number of conditions are now known to give rise to secondary disaccharidase deficiency, which is transient and involves decrease in all mucosal enzymes with lactase usually most severely depressed. Histologic examination reveals changes compatible with the underlying disorder. A familial incidence is uncommon.

Clinical Findings

A. Primary (Congenital):

1. Lactase deficiency–Congenital lactase deficiency is a rare condition leading to diarrhea after lactose is ingested. The stools are frothy and acid; their pH may fall below 4.5 owing to the presence of organic acids. The osmotic action of unhydrolyzed lactose leads to catharsis. Vomiting is common. Severe malnutrition may occur. Reducing substances are usually present in the stools, and lactosuria may occur. Infants with lactosuria, aminoaciduria, proteinuria, acidosis, and elevated blood urea nitrogen have been described. An oral lactose tolerance test (2 g/kg) after dietary lactose has been withdrawn is likely to result in symptoms of intolerance within 8 hours; the blood glucose levels show no appreciable rise. A rise in breath hydrogen after oral administration of lactose is also diagnostic.

Patients respond to the exclusion of lactose from their diets.

2. Sucrase and isomaltase deficiency–This is a combined defect that is inherited as an autosomal recessive trait. Diarrhea usually occurs only when sucrose is fed. Abdominal distention, failure to thrive, and chronic diarrhea may be the presenting symptoms. Distaste for and avoidance of sucrose occurs even in young infants. Since sucrase-isomaltase deficiencies have been found in siblings who had few or no symptoms, it is likely that a number of persons with this trait—particularly adults—remain unrecognized.

Because sucrose is not a reducing sugar, the usual 5 drops of stool and 10 drops of water added to a Clinitest tablet will not give a positive reaction unless sucrose is hydrolyzed (1-N HCl is substituted for the water and the mixture allowed to boil for a few seconds before adding the tablet). A sucrose tolerance test (2 g/kg) is likely to be flat. Breath hydrogen will be elevated after ingestion of sucrose. Because many gastric and extraintestinal factors can account for very poor blood glucose rises, it is wise to check the stools for the presence of sucrose and to follow the sucrose tolerance test by the xylose absorption test. Shock may occur owing to osmotic water losses in some patients with lactase or sucrase-isomaltase deficiency with a standard dose of the disaccharide for the tolerance test. In sucrase-isomaltase deficiency, exclusion of sucrose is usually sufficient. Starch intolerance is rarely a problem, because the 1–6 linkages of starch hydrolyzed by isomaltase constitute only a small part of the molecule.

B. Secondary (Acquired):

1. Secondary lactase deficiency–Diarrhea may be produced in normal individuals if a large dose of lactose is ingested. The threshold for lactose tolerance is usually much lower than that for sucrose. There is a high prevalence of lactose intolerance in certain racial groups (70% in North American blacks and nearly 100% in Asian populations) after 3–5 years of age. Neomycin and kanamycin administration can reduce lactase activity in adults. Celiac disease, giardiasis, malnutrition, viral or bacterial gastroenteritis, abetalipoproteinemia, immunoglobulin deficiencies, and intestinal mucosal injury secondary to radiation and cancer chemotherapy all can decrease intestinal lactase activity.

2. Secondary sucrase deficiency–Intestinal mucosal damage tends to lower the levels of all disaccharidases. Signs of sucrose intolerance are usually masked by the more striking symptoms related to lactose. Infectious diarrhea is the most frequent cause of secondary sucrose intolerance.

Treatment

A. Lactose-Free Diet: Many commercially available infant formulas are lactose-free. Foods containing whey, dry milk solids, and curds should be excluded. It is important to see if labels indicate any lactose content, particularly in canned puréed baby foods. Cheeses (cottage, cheddar, cream), ice cream, sherbet, yogurt, and chocolate milk powders contain variable amounts of lactose, small amounts of which may be well tolerated.

B. Sucrose-Restricted Diet: Avoidance of sucrose prevents diarrhea. Glucose or dietetic sugar substitutes may be used as sweeteners in cooking and baking. A small amount of sucrose in grapes, cherries, strawberries, and blackberries may be tolerated. Other fruits contain significant sucrose and may cause diarrhea. Most green vegetables are sucrose-free, but peas, beans, and lentils should be avoided.

Prognosis

Primary disaccharidase deficiency is a lifelong defect. However, in both lactase and sucrase deficiencies, tolerance for the disaccharide may increase with age. The prognosis in the secondary or acquired forms of disaccharidase deficiency is that of the underlying illness. Normal tolerance for lactose may not be regained for many months after an acute mucosal injury.

Barilas-Mury C, Solomons NW: Test-retest reproducibility of hydrogen breath test for lactose maldigestion in preschool children. J Pediatr Gastroenterol Nutr 1987;6:281.

Heitlinger LA, Lebenthal E: Disorders of carbohydrate digestion and absorption. Pediatr Clin North Am 1988; 35:239.

Kilby A et al: Sucrase-isomaltase deficiency: A follow-up report. Arch Dis Child 1979;53:677.

Perman JA et al: Sucrose malabsorption in children: Noninvasive diagnosis by interval breath hydrogen determination. J Pediatr 1978;93:17.

GLUCOSE-GALACTOSE MALABSORPTION

Glucose malabsorption can also cause osmotic diarrhea. A decreased rate of tubular reabsorption of glucose is often associated with the intestinal cell transport defect.

In the congenital form of the disease, severe diarrhea begins within a few days after birth. Small bowel histologic findings are normal. Glycosuria and aminoaciduria may occur. The glucose tolerance test is flat. Fructose is well tolerated. The diarrhea promptly subsides on withdrawal of glucose and galactose from the diet. The stool pH is not as acid as that reported in disaccharidase deficiencies; fecal reducing substances are consistently found. The clinical features associated with acquired disease are the same as those seen with disaccharidase deficiency states. The acquired form is mainly seen in the perinatal period but is also described in older infants, usually following an acute viral or bacterial enteritis. Both disaccharides and monosaccharides, including fructose, are malabsorbed.

In the congenital form, total exclusion of glucose and galactose from the diet is mandatory. A satisfactory formula consists of fructose with a carbohydrate-free formula. The prognosis is good if the disease is diagnosed early, because tolerance for glucose and galactose improves with age. In the secondary form, prolonged parenteral nutrition may be required until intestinal transport mechanisms for monosaccharides return.

Fairclough PD et al: Absorption of glucose and maltose in congenital glucose-galactose malabsorption. Pediatr Res 1978;12:1112.

Klish WJ et al: Intestinal surface area in infants with acquired monosaccharide intolerance. J Pediatr 1978;92: 566.

Nichols VN et al: Acquired monosaccharide intolerance in infants. J Pediatr Gastroenterol Nutr 1989;8:51.

INTESTINAL LYMPHANGIECTASIA

This form of protein-losing enteropathy results from a congenital abnormality of the lymphatic system and is often associated with lymphatic aberrations in the extremities. Obstruction to lymphatic drainage of the intestine leads to rupture of the intestinal lacteals with leakage of lymph into the lumen of the bowel. Fat loss may be significant and lead to steatorrhea. Chronic loss of lymphocytes and of immunoglobulins is usual and increases the susceptibility to infections.

Clinical Findings

Peripheral edema, diarrhea, abdominal distention, lymphedematous extremities, chylous effusions, and repeated infections are common. Laboratory findings are low serum albumin, decreased immunoglobulin levels, lymphocytopenia, and anemia. Serum calcium is frequently depressed, and stool fat may be elevated. Lymphocytes may be seen in large numbers on a stool smear. Fecal α_1-antiprotease is elevated. X-ray studies reveal an edematous small bowel mucosal pattern, and biopsy reveals dilated lacteals in the villi and lamina propria. In certain cases where the disorder involves the submucosa, subserosa, mesentery, and omentum, the mucosal biopsy may be normal, and laparotomy is necessary to establish the diagnosis.

Differential Diagnosis

Other causes of protein-losing enteropathy must be considered, although an associated lymphedematous extremity strongly favors this diagnosis.

Treatment & Prognosis

Surgery is needed when the lesion is localized to a small area of the bowel or in cases of constrictive pericarditis or obstructing tumors. This may include placement of a LeVeen or Denver shunt or construction of a saphenous vein-peritoneal anastomosis in intractable cases.

A low-fat diet reduces lymph flow. Medium-chain triglycerides as a fat source are effective only in the mucosal type of lymphangiectasia. Water-soluble vitamin and calcium supplements should be given. Antibiotics are used for specific infections. Total parenteral nutrition is helpful on a temporary basis.

The prognosis at present is not favorable, although there may be remission with age.

Tift WL, Lloyd JK: Intestinal lymphangiectasia: Long-term results with MCT diet. Arch Dis Child 1975;50:269.

Vardy PA, Lebenthal E, Shwachman H: Intestinal lymphangiectasia: A reappraisal. Pediatrics 1975;55:842.

COW'S MILK PROTEIN INTOLERANCE

Milk intolerance is more common in males and in young infants with a family history of allergy and atopy. The estimated incidence is 0.5–1%. Colic, vomiting, and diarrhea are the major symptoms. Stools often contain blood and mucus. Sigmoidoscopic examination reveals a superficial colitis, often with an eosinophilic infiltrate. Pneumatosis intestinalis may be present on x-ray. Viral gastroenteritis sometimes precedes the onset of symptoms. Eosinophilic gastroenteritis with protein-losing enteropathy, hypoalbuminemia, and hypogammaglobulinemia is less common. A celiac-like syndrome with villous atrophy, malabsorption, hypoalbuminemia, occult blood in the stool, and anemia can occur in older children. Anaphylactic shock may occur in rare infants. Symptoms in these infants are IgE-mediated.

Breast-fed infants under 6 months of age can also develop blood-streaked stools and a sigmoidoscopic picture similar to that of infants with milk protein sensitivity. Tiny amounts of intact allergen passed in breast milk may be the cause. Elimination of whole cow's milk from the mother's diet sometimes causes resolution of bloody diarrhea. A switch to semielemental diet almost always results in improvement. Because the blood loss and diarrhea in these breast-fed infants are rarely severe, it is not essential that breast feeding be stopped. If symptoms are severe or prolonged, however, a trial of semielemental formula is recommended. The colitic pattern of milk protein sensitivity and colitis in breast-fed infants usually clears spontaneously by 6–12 months of age.

Patients with milk protein allergy have a 30% incidence of sensitivity to soy protein, with similar symptoms. It is best to use a casein hydrolysate formula as an elimination diet to prove the diagnosis. A normal 1-hour blood xylose level 4–12 weeks after clinical recovery, with a drop below 25 mg/dL 4 days after reintroduction of cow's milk protein, has also been shown to be a reliable means of diagnosis.

Estaban MM (editor): Adverse reactions to foods in infancy and childhood. J Pediatr 1992;121(Suppl):S1.

IMMUNOLOGIC DEFICIENCY STATES WITH DIARRHEA OR MALABSORPTION

Diarrhea is a frequent finding in immune deficiency states, but the cause is usually obscure. Standard pathogenic bacteria may not be found in the stools, but giardiasis is common. Fifty to 60 percent of patients with idiopathic acquired hypogammaglobulinemia have steatorrhea and intestinal villous atrophy. Lymphonodular hyperplasia is a common feature in this group of patients. Congenital or Bruton type agammaglobulinemics uniformly have diarrhea and abnormal intestinal morphology. Patients with isolated IgA deficiency may also present with chronic diarrhea, a celiac-like picture, lymphoid nodular hyperplasia, and giardiasis. Patients with isolated cellular immunity defects, combined cellular and humoral immune incompetence, and HIV infection may have severe chronic diarrhea leading to malnutrition. The cause of diarrhea may be recognized bacterial, viral, or parasitic pathogens, organisms usually considered nonpathogens (*Blastocystis hominis, Candida*), or unusual organisms (cytomegalovirus, *Cryptosporidium, Isospora belli, Mycobacterium* species, Microsporidia, and algal organisms such as Cyanobacteria). Often, the cause is not found. There is a high incidence of disaccharidase deficiency. Chronic granulomatous disease may be associated with intestinal symptoms suggestive of chronic inflammatory bowel disease. A rectal biopsy may reveal the presence of typical macrophages.

Treatment must be directed toward correction of the immunologic defect. Specific treatments are available or being developed for many of the unusual pathogens causing diarrhea in the immunocompromised host. Thus, a vigorous diagnostic search for specific pathogens is warranted in these individuals.

Ogra PL, Bienenstock J (editors): *The Mucosal Immune System in Health and Disease.* 81st Ross Conference on Pediatric Research, Columbus, Ohio. Ross Laboratories, 1981.

Smith PD et al: Gastrointestinal infections in AIDS. Ann Intern Med 1992;116:63.

INFLAMMATORY BOWEL DISEASE

Crohn's disease and ulcerative colitis are the two major idiopathic inflammatory bowel diseases of children. They share many features resulting from bowel inflammation, such as diarrhea, pain, fever, and blood loss, but they differ in important aspects, such as distribution of disease, histologic findings, incidence and type of extraintestinal symptoms, response to medications and surgery, and prognosis. A comparison of these two conditions is shown in Table 22–13. The cause is unknown but is probably a genetically determined immunologic response to an environmental antigenic trigger, possibly a virus or bacterium, which may cross-react with antigens in the gastrointestinal tract. There is no indication that diet or emotional factors are a primary cause of these diseases.

Differential Diagnosis

A. Crohn's Disease: When extraintestinal symptoms predominate, Crohn's disease can be mistaken for rheumatoid arthritis, systemic lupus erythematosus, or hypopituitarism. Frequently, the acute onset of ileocolitis is mistaken for acute appendicitis.

Symptoms sometimes suggest celiac disease, peptic ulcer, intestinal obstruction, or intestinal lymphoma.

B. Ulcerative Colitis: In the acute stage, bacterial pathogens and toxins causing colitis must be ruled out. These include *Shigella, Salmonella, Yersinia, Campylobacter, Entamoeba histolytica,* invasive *Escherichia coli, Aeromonas hydrophila,* and the toxin producers *E coli* serotype 0157:H7 and *Clostridium difficile.* Mild ulcerative colitis mimics irritable bowel symptoms. Connective tissue diseases must be considered. Crohn's disease of the colon is an important differential possibility.

Complications
(See Table 22–13.)

A. Crohn's Disease: Intestinal obstruction, fistula, and abscess formation are frequent. Perforation

Table 22–13. Features of Crohn's disease and ulcerative colitis.[1]

	Crohn's Disease	Ulcerative Colitis
Age at onset	10–20 years	10–20 years
Incidence	4–6 per 100,000	3–15 per 100,000
Relative incidence in children	2	1
Area of bowel affected	Oropharynx, esophagus, and stomach, rare; small bowel only, 25–30%; colon and anus only, 25%; ileocolitis, 40%; diffuse disease, 5%	Total colon, 90%; proctitis, 10%
Distribution	Segmental; disease-free skip areas common.	Continuous; distal to proximal.
Pathology	Full-thickness, acute, and chronic inflammation; noncaseating granulomas (50%), extraintestinal fistulas, abscesses, stricture, and fibrosis may be present.	Superficial, acute inflammation of mucosa with microscopic crypt abscess.
X-ray findings	Segmental lesions; thickened, circular folds, cobblestone appearance of bowel wall secondary to longitudinal ulcers and transverse fissures; fixation and separation of loops; narrowed lumen; "string sign"; fistulas.	Superficial colitis; loss of haustra; shortened colon and pseudopolyps (islands of nomal tissue surrounded by denuded mucosa) are late findings.
Intestinal symptoms	Abdominal pain, diarrhea (usually loose with blood if colon involved) perianal disease, enteroenteric/enterocutaneous fistula, abscess, anorexia.	Abdominal pain, bloody diarrhea, urgency, and tenesmus.
Extraintestinal symptoms Arthritis/arthralgia	15%	9%
Fever	40–50%	40–50%
Stomatitis	9%	2%
Weight loss	90% (mean 5.7 kg.)	68% (mean 4.1 kg.)
Delayed growth and sexual development	30%	5–10%
Uveitis/conjunctivitis	15% (in Crohn's colitis)	4%
Sclerosing cholangitis	—	4%
Renal stones	6% (oxalate)	6% (urate)
Pyoderma gangrenosum	1–3%	5%
Erythema nodosum	8–15%	4%
Laboratory findings	High erythrocyte sedimentation rate; microcytic anemia; low serum iron and total iron-binding capacity; increased fecal protein loss; low serum albumin.	High erythrocyte sedimentation rate; microcytic anemia, high white blood cell count with left shift.

[1]Source: Kirschner BS: Inflammatory bowel disease in children. Pediatr Clin North Am 1988;35:189.

and hemorrhage are rare. Malnutrition is caused by anorexia and compounded by malabsorption, protein-losing enteropathy, disaccharidase deficiency, and diarrhea induced by bile salts. Systemic complications include perianal disease, pyoderma gangrenosum, arthritis, amyloidosis, and growth retardation.

B. Ulcerative Colitis: Arthritis, uveitis, pyoderma gangrenosum, and malnutrition all occur. Growth failure and delayed puberty are less common than in Crohn's disease. Liver disease (chronic active hepatitis, sclerosing cholangitis) is more common. In patients with pancolitis, carcinoma of the colon occurs with an incidence of 1–2% per year after the first 10 years of disease. Cancer risk is a function of disease duration and not age of onset. Mortality with colon cancer is high, because the usual screening tests (occult blood in stool, pain, and abnormal x-ray findings) are not specific, may be ignored in a patient with colitis, and diagnosis may be delayed.

Treatment

Medical treatment for Crohn's disease and ulcerative colitis is similar and includes anti-inflammatory, antidiarrheal, and antibiotic medication. No medical therapy has proved uniformly effective.

A. Diet: A high-protein, high-carbohydrate diet with normal amounts of fat is recommended. Decreased amounts of roughage may help decrease symptoms in those with colitis or with partial intestinal obstruction. Lactose is poorly tolerated when disease is active. The main concern should be ensuring adequate caloric intake. Restrictive or "bland" diets are counterproductive because they usually result in poor intake. Vitamin and iron supplements are recommended. Zinc levels are often low in patients with Crohn's disease and should be repleted. Supplemental calories in the form of liquid diets are well tolerated. Total parenteral nutrition for periods of 4–6 weeks may induce remission of symptoms and stimulate linear growth and sexual development. Enteral administration of low-residue or elemental liquid diets may also be associated with rapid nutritional repletion and temporary remission of symptoms, perhaps because of reduced enteral antigen load. Home programs of both enteral and parenteral nutritional support have been used in many patients with intractable symptoms or growth failure.

B. Sulfasalazine: This drug is effective in mild cases of ulcerative colitis and possibly in cases of Crohn's disease of the colon. It prevents relapse of ulcerative colitis once remission is induced. The drug is not absorbed in the small intestine. It is hydrolyzed by colon flora into sulfapyridine and 5-aminosalicylate. The sulfa moiety is probably inactive but is responsible for the allergic side effects of the drug. The salicylate moiety probably has a local anti-inflammatory activity in the colon. Side effects are common, including skin rash, nausea, headache, and abdominal pain. More rarely, serum sickness, hemolytic anemia,

aplastic anemia, and pancreatitis occur. Response to therapy may be slow. Sulfasalazine inhibits folic acid absorption, and supplemental folic acid is recommended.

Two to 3 grams per day in three divided doses are recommended for children over 10, or 50 mg/kg/d for those under 10. Half of this dose is used as a maintenance medication for well-controlled ulcerative colitis. Salicylate polymers for both oral and rectal use (olsalazine, mesalamine) are available. They are no more effective than sulfasalazine but can be tolerated by sulfonamide-sensitive patients and have fewer side effects.

C. Corticosteroids: With more severe inflammatory bowel disease, corticosteroids are used.

1. Intravenous steroids–Methylprednisolone, 2 mg/kg/d, or hydrocortisone, 10 mg/kg/d, may be given when disease is severe. Adrenocorticotropic hormone (ACTH) has more side effects and is no more effective.

2. Prednisone–Prednisone, 1–2 mg/kg/d orally in two or three divided doses, is given for 6–8 weeks, followed by a gradual tapering. Alternate-day steroids are associated with fewer side effects as the dosage of drug is tapered. There is no evidence that corticosteroids prevent relapses. Prednisone is often given in conjunction with sulfasalazine. The patient or the parents should be warned about the risk of varicella infection and the other numerous side effects of high-dose steroids.

Hydrocortisone in the form of enema or foam can be instilled into the rectum in patients with severe tenesmus or ulcerative proctitis.

D. Azathioprine: Azathioprine, 1.5–2 mg/kg/d orally, is used only when a high maintenance dose of corticosteroids is necessary to keep the disease under control and there are serious risks of steroid-induced complications. The results of this therapy may be delayed weeks to months.

E. Metronidazole: This drug is now used routinely in Crohn's disease patients with perianal disease. Disease tends to recur when the drug is discontinued. It may also be effective in Crohn's disease of the colon. The dose of metronidazole is 15–30 mg/kg/d in three divided doses. Peripheral neuropathy may be a side effect with prolonged use.

F. Cyclosporine: This powerful immunosuppressant may be effective in severe inflammatory bowel disease but is usually used to "buy time" in severely affected patients who are at high risk for surgical complications.

G. Surgery:

1. Crohn's disease–Crohn's disease is not cured by surgery. However, 70% of patients will eventually require surgery to relieve obstruction, drain abscess, relieve intractable symptoms, or encourage growth and sexual maturation. The relapse rate 6 years after surgery is 60%. The recurrence usually occurs at the site of anastomosis. Recurrence of disease is most likely in the first 2 years after surgery. The rate of recurrence may be less in disease limited to the colon. Surgery performed for the alleviation of growth retardation must be performed before puberty.

2. Ulcerative colitis–Surgery is curative in this disease. It is reserved for those with uncontrolled hemorrhage, toxic megacolon, unrelenting pain and diarrhea, high-grade mucosal dysplasia, or malignant growths. There are now several surgical approaches (ileoanal anastomosis, Koch-type continent ileostomy) that allow a near normal life-style after colectomy. Liver disease may not be improved by the removal of the colon.

Prognosis

A. Crohn's Disease: Although the mortality rate is low (2% in the first 7 years), the morbidity is high. The disease is progressive in most cases, and its course is interspersed with both acute and chronic complications, leading to variable degrees of disability. Over 50% of patients experience symptoms that impose limits on the quality of their lives. About 20%

have severe disabling disease, and 20% have so few symptoms that they describe themselves as healthy.

B. Ulcerative Colitis: The overall prognosis for ulcerative colitis is good. About 5% of patients present with toxic megacolon and require immediate surgery. Seventy-five percent will have a relapsing remitting course. Twenty-five to 40% of patients will require surgery, especially those with pancolitis, anemia, and hypoalbuminemia at the time of presentation.

Chong SKF et al: Histologic diagnosis of chronic inflammatory bowel disease in childhood. Gut 1985;26:55.

Fonkalsrud EW, Loar N: Long term results after colectomy and endorectal ileal pullthrough procedure in children. Ann Surg 1991;215:57.

Greenstein AJ et al: The extraintestinal complications of Crohn's disease and chronic ulcerative colitis: A study of 700 patients. Medicine 1976;55:401.

Gryboski JD: Ulcerative colitis in children 10 years or younger. J Pediatr Gastroenterol Nutr 1993;17:24.

Kirschner BS: Inflammatory bowel disease in children. Pediatr Clin North Am 1988;35:189.

Noel RA, Ferry GD: Pediatric inflammatory bowel disease. Curr Opin Gastroenterol 1992;8:676.

REFERENCES

Balistreri WF, Stocker JT (editors): *Pediatric Hepatology.* Hemisphere, 1990.

Silverman A, Roy CC: *Pediatric Clinical Gastroenterology,* 3rd ed. Mosby, 1983.

Walker WA et al (editors): *Pediatric Gastrointestinal Disease.* BC Decker, 1991.

Wyllie R, Hyams JS (editors): *Pediatric Gastrointestinal Disease.* Saunders, 1993.

Liver & Pancreas

23

Ronald J. Sokol, MD, Michael R. Narkewicz, MD, & Arnold Silverman, MD

LIVER

PROLONGED NEONATAL CHOLESTATIC JAUNDICE

The main clinical features of the group of disorders causing prolonged neonatal cholestasis are (1) elevated direct-reacting bilirubin fraction (> 2 mg/dL or > 20% of total bilirubin), (2) elevated serum bile acids (> 10 μmol/L), (3) variably acholic stools, (4) dark urine, and (5) hepatomegaly.

Prolonged neonatal cholestasis (decreased bile flow) may be due to intrahepatic or extrahepatic causes. Though many specific causes of intrahepatic cholestasis have been identified, a specific cause is found only in about 25% of cases. With rare exceptions, extrahepatic cholestasis is due to anatomic defects that occur without specific known cause.

Attention to specific clinical clues distinguishes these two major categories of jaundice in 85% of cases. Histologic examination of tissue obtained by percutaneous liver biopsy increases the accuracy of differentiation to over 95% (Table 23–1).

INTRAHEPATIC CHOLESTASIS

Intrahepatic cholestasis is characterized by patency of the extrahepatic biliary system—despite cholestasis—and abnormalities on liver function tests. A specific cause can be identified in about 25% of cases. Patency of the extrahepatic biliary tract can least invasively be confirmed by hepatobiliary scintigraphy using ^{99m}Tc-diethyliminodiacetic acid (diethyl-IDA, DIDA). Radioactivity in the bowel within 4–14 hours is evidence of patency. Patency of the extrahepatic biliary system can also be determined by cholangiography carried out intraoperatively, percutaneously by transhepatic cholecystography, or by utilizing the newly designed pediatric-sized side-viewing endoscope.

1. PERINATAL OR NEONATAL HEPATITIS DUE TO INFECTION

This diagnosis is considered in infants with jaundice, hepatomegaly, vomiting, lethargy, and other systemic signs. A perinatally acquired viral, bacterial, or protozoal infection must be identified. Infection may occur by transplacental spread, via the ascending route from vaginal or cervical structures into amniotic fluid; from swallowed contaminated fluids (maternal blood, urine) during delivery; or from breast milk, contaminated hands, etc. The infectious agents most apt to be associated with neonatal intrahepatic cholestasis include herpesvirus, varicella virus, coxsackieviruses, cytomegalovirus, rubella virus, echoviruses, adenovirus, hepatitis B virus, human immunodeficiency virus, *Treponema pallidum*, and *Toxoplasma gondii*. The degree of liver cell injury caused by these agents is variable, ranging from massive hepatic necrosis (herpesvirus) to focal necrosis and mild inflammation (cytomegalovirus, hepatitis B virus). Serum bilirubin, bile acids, ALT, AST, and alkaline phosphatase are elevated. The infant is jaundiced and generally appears ill.

Clinical Findings

A. Symptoms and Signs: Clinical symptoms usually appear in the first 2 weeks of life but may appear as late as 2–3 months. Jaundice may be noted in the first 24 hours or may develop later. Loss of appetite, poor sucking reflex, lethargy, and vomiting are frequent. Stools may be normal to pale in color but are seldom acholic. Dark urine stains the diaper. Hepatomegaly is present, and the liver has a uniform firm consistency. Splenomegaly is variably present. Macular, papular, or petechial rashes may occur. In less severe cases, failure to thrive may be the major complaint. Unusual presentations include liver failure, hypoproteinemia, and anasarca (nonhemolytic hydrops) and hemorrhagic disease of the newborn.

B. Laboratory Findings: The blood count often shows neutropenia, thrombocytopenia, and signs of mild hemolysis. Mixed hyperbilirubinemia, elevated aminotransferases with near-normal alkaline phosphatase, prolongation of clotting studies, mild

Table 23–1. Differentiating clinical and pathologic features of intra- and extrahepatic neonatal cholestasis.

	Intrahepatic	Extrahepatic
Clinical features	Preterm, small for gestational age, appears ill; hepatosplenomegaly, other organ or system involvement; incomplete cholestasis (stools with some color); associated cause identified (infections, metabolic, familial, etc).	Full-term, seems well, hepatomegaly (firm to hard), complete cholestasis (acholic stools), polysplenia syndrome, equal right and left hepatic lobes.
Pathologic features	Cholestasis, lobular disarray, giant cells, portal inflammation, minimal fibrosis, rare neoductular formation, steatosis, extramedullary hematopoiesis.	Cholestasis, neoductular proliferation, portal fibrosis, bile lakes, normal lobular architecture, rare giant cells.

acidosis, and elevated cord serum IgM suggest congenital infection. Nasopharyngeal washings, urine, stool, and cerebrospinal fluid should be cultured for virus. Specific serologic tests may be useful (TORCH titers), as are long bone x-rays to determine the presence of "celery stalking" in the metaphysial regions of the humeri, femurs, and tibias. When indicated, CT and MRI can identify intracranial calcifications. Nuclear hepatobiliary imaging shows decreased hepatic clearance of the circulating isotope with excretion into the gut.

Histologic examination of liver biopsy tissue obtained by the percutaneous route is performed to distinguish intrahepatic from extrahepatic cholestasis rather than to identify a specific infectious agent within the liver tissue. Exceptions to this generalization include the finding of intracytoplasmic inclusions of cytomegalovirus in hepatocytes or bile duct epithelial cells and the finding of intranuclear acidophilic inclusions of herpesvirus. Variable degrees of lobular disarray characterized by focal necrosis, multinucleated giant cell transformation, and ballooned pale hepatocytes with loss of cord-like arrangement of liver cells are usual. Intrahepatocytic and canalicular cholestasis may be prominent. Portal changes are not striking, but modest neoductular proliferation and mild fibrosis may occur.

Differential Diagnosis

Great care must be taken to distinguish infectious causes of intrahepatic cholestasis from genetic or metabolic causes (inborn errors), because the clinical presentations are very similar. Galactosemia, congenital fructose intolerance, and tyrosinemia must be investigated promptly, because specific dietary therapy is available. Alpha$_1$-antitrypsin deficiency, cystic fibrosis, and neonatal iron storage disease must also be considered. Specific physical features may be helpful

when considering Alagille's or Zellweger's syndromes.

Unless the bile ducts have spontaneously perforated, infants with extrahepatic cholestasis do not appear ill; stools are usually completely acholic, and the liver is enlarged and firm. Histologic findings are shown in Table 23–1.

Treatment

Most forms of viral neonatal hepatitis are treated symptomatically. Infants with herpesvirus infections may be treated with acyclovir. Fluids and adequate calories are encouraged. Intravenous dextrose may be needed if feedings are not well tolerated. The consequences of cholestasis are treated as indicated (Table 23–2). Vitamin K orally or by injection and vitamins D and E orally should be provided. Choleretics (cholestyramine, phenobarbital, or ursodeoxycholic acid) are used if cholestasis persists. Corticosteroids are contraindicated. Penicillin for suspected syphilis or specific antibiotics for bacterial hepatitis need to be administered promptly. Infants born to women with hepatitis B should be given hepatitis B immune globulin immediately and subsequently immunized with hepatitis B virus vaccine, as outlined in Chapter 10.

Prognosis

Multiple organ involvement is commonly associated with neonatal infectious hepatitis and has a poor outcome. Death from hepatic or cardiac failure, intractable acidosis, or intracranial hemorrhage is seen, especially in herpesvirus or echovirus infection and occasionally in cytomegalovirus or rubella infection. Hepatitis B virus may rarely cause fulminant neonatal viral hepatitis; however, most infected infants become asymptomatic carriers of hepatitis B. On the other hand, infants with transplacental diseases may recover completely or suffer sequelae, especially neurologic ones. Persistent liver disease results in mild chronic hepatitis, portal fibrosis, or cirrhosis. Chronic cholestasis may lead to dental enamel hypoplasia, failure to thrive, biliary rickets, severe pruritus, and xanthoma.

Specific Infectious Agents

A. Neonatal Hepatitis Virus B Disease: Infection with hepatitis B virus (HBV) may occur at any time during perinatal life, but the risk is higher when acute maternal disease occurs during the last trimester of pregnancy. However, most cases of neonatal disease are acquired from mothers who are asymptomatic carriers of hepatitis B. Hepatitis B virus has been found in most body fluids besides blood, including breast milk, but it does not seem to be present in feces. In chronic HBsAg carrier mothers, fetal and infant acquisition risk is greatest if the mother (1) is also HBeAg-positive and HBeAb-negative, (2) has detectable levels of serum-specific hepa-

Table 23–2. Treatment of complications of chronic liver disease.

Indication	Treatment	Dose	Toxicity
Intrahepatic cholestasis	Phenobarbital	3–10 mg/kg/d	Drowsiness, irritability, interference with vitamin D metabolism
	Cholestyramine/colestipol hydro-chloride	250–500 mg/kg/d	Constipation, acidosis, binding of drugs, increased steatorrhea
Pruritus	Phenobarbital or cholestyramine/colestipol (or both)	Same as above	
	Antihistamines: Diphenhydramine hydrochloride Hydroxyzine	5–10 mg/kg/d 2–5 mg/kg/d	Drowsiness
	Ultraviolet light B	Exposure as needed	Skin burn
	Carbamazepine	20–40 mg/kg/d	Hepatotoxicity, marrow suppression, fluid retention
	Rifampin	10 mg/kg/d	Hepatotoxicity, marrow suppression
	Ursodeoxycholic acid	10–15 mg/kg/d	Transient increase in pruritus
Steatorrhea	Formula containing medium-chain triglycerides (eg, Pregestimil)	120–150 calories/kg/d for infants	Expensive
	Oil supplement containing medium-chain triglycerides	1–2 mL/kg/d	Diarrhea, aspiration
Malabsorption of fat-soluble vitamins	Vitamin A	10,000–25,000 units/d	Hepatitis, pseudotumor cerebri, bone lesions
	Vitamin D	800–5000 units/d	Hypercalcemia, hypercalciuria
	25-Hydroxycholecalciferol (vitamin D)	3–5 µg/kg/d	Hypercalcemia, hypercalciuria
	1,25-Dihydroxycholecalciferol (vitamin D)	0.05–0.2 µg/kg/d	Hypercalcemia, hypercalciuria
	Vitamin E (oral)	25–200 IU/kg/d TPGS,[1] 15–25 IU/kg/d	Potentiation of vitamin K deficiency
	Vitamin E (intramuscular)	1–2 mg/kg/d	Muscle calcifications
	Vitamin K (oral)	2.5 mg twice per week to 5.0 mg per day	
	Vitamin K (intramuscular)	2–5 mg each 4 weeks	
Malabsorption of other nutrients	Multiple vitamin	1–2 times the standard dose	
	Calcium	25–100 mg/kg/d	Hypercalcemia, hypercalciuria
	Phosphorus	25–50 mg/kg/d	Gastrointestinal intolerance
	Zinc	1 mg/kg/d	Interference with copper absorption
Ascites[2]	Sodium restriction	1–2 meq/kg/d	
	Spironolactone	3–5 mg/kg/d (up to 10 mg)	Gynecomastia, hyperkalemia
	Furosemide	1–2 mg/kg/d	Hyponatremia, hypokalemia
	Intravenous albumin	1 g/kg/dose	
	Paracentesis		Hypotension
	Peritoneovenous (Le Veen) shunt		
Hepatic encephalopathy[2]	Protein restriction	0.5–1 g/kg/d	
	Intravenous glucose (10% dextrose)	n8mg/kg/min	
	Oral neomycin	2–4 g/m^2 BSA in 4 doses	Renal toxicity
	Oral lactulose	1 mL/kg/dose each 4–6 hours	Diarrhea
	High branched-chain amino acid—enteral or parenteral supplements (unproved benefit)	0.5–1 g/kg/d	
	Plasmapheresis		
	Hemodialysis		

[1]Tocopheryl polyethylene glycol-1000 succinate (water-soluble vitamin E).
[2]In order of sequential management.

titis B DNA polymerase, or (3) has high serum levels of HBcAb. These findings are markers of high infectivity; however, hepatitis B can be transmitted even if HBsAg is the only marker present.

Neonatal liver disease due to HBV is extremely variable. The infant has a 70–90% chance of acquiring HBV at birth from HBsAg-positive mothers if nothing is done to prevent infection (ie, administration of HBIG or vaccine). Most infected infants become asymptomatic carriers of HBV, usually for life. Fulminant hepatic necrosis has rarely been reported, especially in association with intrapartum or postpartum transfusions of infected blood. However, it also can occur from maternally transmitted virus. In such cases, progressive jaundice, stupor, shrinking liver size, and coagulation abnormalities dominate the clinical picture. Respiratory, circulatory, and renal failure usually follow. Histologically, the liver shows massive hepatocyte necrosis, collapse of reticulum framework, minimal inflammation, and occasional pseudoacinar structures. Rare survivors are reported with reasonable restitution of liver architecture toward normal.

In less severe cases, focal hepatocyte necrosis is seen with a mild portal inflammatory response. Cholestasis is intracellular and canalicular. Chronic persistent and chronic active hepatitis may be present for many years, with serologic evidence of persisting antigenemia (HBsAg) and mildly elevated serum aminotransferases. Chronic active hepatitis may progress to cirrhosis within 1–2 years.

To prevent perinatal transmission, all infants of mothers who are HBsAg-positive (regardless of HBeAg status) should receive hepatitis B immune globulin and hepatitis B vaccine within the first 24 hours after birth and vaccine again at 1 and 6 months of age (see Chapter 10).

B. Neonatal Bacterial Hepatitis: Most bacterial liver infections in newborns are acquired by transplacental invasion from amnionitis with ascending spread from maternal vaginal or cervical infection. Onset is abrupt, usually within 48–72 hours after delivery, with signs of sepsis and often shock. Jaundice, seen in less than 25% of cases, appears early and is of the mixed type. The liver enlarges rapidly, and the histologic picture is that of diffuse hepatitis with or without micro- or macroabscess. The most common organisms are *Escherichia coli, Listeria monocytogenes,* and group B streptococci and rarely *Mycobacterium tuberculosis.* Isolated neonatal liver abscess due to *E coli* or *Staphylococcus aureus* is often associated with omphalitis or umbilical vein catheterization. Bacterial hepatitis and neonatal liver abscesses require specific antibiotics in large doses and, rarely, surgical drainage. Deaths are common, but survivors show no long-term consequences of liver disease.

C. Neonatal Jaundice With Urinary Tract Infection: Jaundice in affected infants–usually

males—typically appears between the second and fourth weeks of life. The manifestations of this disorder are lethargy, fever, poor appetite, jaundice, and hepatomegaly. Except for mixed hyperbilirubinemia, other liver function tests are not remarkable. Leukocytosis is present, and infection is confirmed by culture techniques. The mechanism for the liver impairment is unknown, though toxic action of bacterial products (endotoxins) and the inflammatory response have been incriminated.

Treatment of the infection leads to prompt resolution of the cholestasis without hepatic sequelae. Metabolic liver diseases may present with gram-negative bacterial urinary tract infection and should be considered.

Balistreri WF: Neonatal cholestasis. J Pediatr 1985;106:171.

Felber S, Sinatra F: Systemic disorders associated with neonatal cholestasis. Semin Liver Dis 1987;7:108.

Krugman S: Viral hepatitis: A, B, C, D, and E: Prevention. Pediatr Rev 1992;13:245.

Pickering LK: Management of the infant of a mother with viral hepatitis. Pediatr Rev 1988;9:315.

Spivak WF: Diagnostic utility of hepatobiliary scintigraphy with ^{99m}Tc-DISIDA in neonatal cholestasis. J Pediatr 1987;110:885.

Stevens CE et al: Perinatal hepatitis B virus transmission in the United States. JAMA 1985;253:1740.

2. INTRAHEPATIC CHOLESTASIS DUE TO INBORN ERRORS OF METABOLISM, FAMILIAL CAUSES, & "TOXIC" CAUSES

These cholestatic syndromes are caused by specific enzyme deficiencies or other inherited disorders; a positive history of certain precipitants associated with neonatal liver disease; and features of intrahepatic cholestasis—ie, jaundice, hepatomegaly, and normal to completely acholic stools. Some of the specific clinical conditions have characteristic clinical signs.

Enzyme Deficiencies & Other Inherited Disorders

Early specific diagnosis is important because dietary treatment may be available (Table 23–3). Reversal of liver disease and clinical symptoms is prompt and permanent in several disorders as long as the diet is maintained. As with other genetically inherited inborn errors of metabolism, genetic counseling for parents of the affected infant should be done as soon as possible.

Cholestasis due to metabolic diseases such as galactosemia, fructose intolerance, and tyrosinemia may be accompanied by vomiting, lethargy, poor feeding, and irritability. Hepatomegaly is a constant finding. The infants often appear septic; gram-nega-

Table 23–3. Metabolic and genetic causes of neonatal cholestasis.

Disease	Inborn Error	Hepatic Pathology	Diagnostic Studies
Galactosemia	Galactose-1-phosphate uridyltransferase	Cholestasis, steatosis, necrosis, pseudoacini, fibrosis	Galactose-1-phosphate uridyltransferase assay of red blood cells
Fructose intolerance	Fructose-1-phosphate aldolase	Steatosis, necrosis, pseudoacini, fibrosis	Liver fructose-1-phosphate aldolase assay or leukocyte DNA analysis
Tyrosinemia	Fumarylacetoacetase	Necrosis, steatosis, pseudoacini, portal fibrosis	Urinary succinylacetone, fumarylacetoacetase assay of red blood cells
Cystic fibrosis	Cystic fibrosis transmembrane regulator gene abnormality	Cholestasis, neoductular proliferation, excess bile duct mucus, portal fibrosis	Sweat test and leukocyte DNA analysis
Hypopituitarism	Deficient production of pituitary hormones	Cholestasis, giant cells	Thyroxine, TSH, cortisol levels
Alpha$_1$-antitrypsin deficiency	Abnormal α_1-antitrypsin molecule (Pi ZZ phenotype)	Giant cells, cholestasis, steatosis, neoductular proliferation, fibrosis, PAS-diastase resistant cytoplasmic granules	Serum α_1-antitrypsin phenotype
Gaucher's disease	β-Glucosidase	Cholestasis, cytoplasmic inclusions in Kupffer's cells (foam cells)	β-Glucosidase assay in leukocytes
Niemann-Pick disease	Lysosomal sphingomyelinase	Cholestasis, cytoplasmic inclusions in Kupffer's cells	Sphingomyelinase assay of leukocytes or liver
Glycogen storage disease type IV	Branching enzyme	Fibrosis, cirrhosis, PAS-diastase resistant cytoplasmic inclusions	Brancher enzyme analysis of leukocytes or liver
Neonatal hemochromatosis	Unknown	Giant cells, portal fibrosis, hemosiderosis, cirrhosis	Histology, iron stains
Peroxisomal disorders (eg, Zellweger's syndrome)	Deficient peroxisomal enzymes or assembly	Cholestasis, necrosis, fibrosis, cirrhosis, hemosiderosis	Plasma very long chain fatty acids, qualitative bile acids, plasmalogen, pipecolic acid, liver electron microscopy
Abnormalities in bile acid metabolism	Several enzyme deficiencies defined	Cholestasis, necrosis, giant cells	Urine, serum, duodenal fluid analyzed for bile acids by fast atom bombardment-mass spectroscopy
Byler's disease (familial progressive intrahepatic cholestasis)	Unknown	Cholestasis, necrosis, giant cells, fibrosis	Histology, family history, normal cholesterol, low or normal γ-glutamyltranspeptidase
Alagille's syndrome (syndromic paucity of interlobular bile ducts)	Unknown	Cholestasis, paucity of interlobular bile ducts, increased copper levels	Three or more clinical features, liver histology

tive bacteria can be cultured from blood in 25–50% of cases, especially in patients with galactosemia.

Other inherited conditions that present with neonatal intrahepatic cholestasis are outlined in Table 23–3. Treatment of these disorders is outlined in Chapter 34.

"Toxic" Causes of Neonatal Cholestasis

A. Neonatal Ischemic/Hypoxic Conditions: Perinatal events that result in hypoperfusion of the gastrointestinal system are sometimes followed in 1–2 weeks by cholestasis. This is seen in premature infants with respiratory distress, severe hypoxia, hypoglycemia, shock, and acidosis. When these perinatal conditions develop in association with gastrointestinal lesions such as ruptured omphalocele, gastroschisis, or later necrotizing enterocolitis, a subsequent cholestatic picture is common (25–50% of cases).

Liver function studies reveal mixed hyperbilirubinemia, elevated alkaline phosphatase and γ-glutamyl transpeptidase values, and variable elevation of the aminotransferases. Stools are seldom persistently acholic.

Choleretics (cholestyramine, phenobarbital, ursodeoxycholic acid), introduction of enteral feedings as soon as possible, and nutritional support are the mainstays of treatment until the cholestasis resolves (see Table 23–2). In some cases, this resolution may take 3–6 months. Complete resolution of the hepatic abnormalities is the rule, but portal fibrosis with perilobular scarring is occasionally seen on follow-up biopsy.

B. Prolonged Parenteral Nutrition: Cholestasis may develop after 1–2 weeks in premature newborns receiving total parenteral nutrition. The mechanism is multifactorial, including possible toxicity of intravenous amino acids, diminished stimulation of bile flow from prolonged absence of feedings, translocation of intestinal bacteria and their cell wall products, missing nutrients or antioxidants, photo-oxidation of amino acids, and the "physiologic cholestatic" propensity of the premature infant.

Early introduction of feedings has reduced the frequency of this disorder. The prognosis is generally good. Rare cases of portal fibrosis, cirrhosis, and hepatoma may develop, particularly in infants with intestinal resections or anomalies.

C. "Inspissated Bile Syndrome": This is the result of accumulation of bile in canaliculi and in the small and medium-sized bile ducts in hemolytic disease of the newborn (Rh, ABO) and in some infants receiving total parenteral nutrition. The same mechanisms may cause intrinsic obstruction of the common duct. An ischemia-reperfusion injury may also contribute to cholestasis in Rh incompatibility. In extreme hemolysis, the cholestasis may be seemingly complete, with acholic stools. Levels of bilirubin may reach 40 mg/dL, primarily direct-reacting. If inspissation of bile occurs within the extrahepatic biliary tree, differentiation from biliary atresia may be difficult. A trial of choleretics (cholestyramine, phenobarbital, or ursodeoxycholic acid) is indicated. Once stools show a return to normal color or ^{99m}Tc-DIDA scanning shows biliary excretion into the duodenum, patency of the extrahepatic biliary tree is ensured. Small bile-colored plugs in the stools are sometimes reported by parents at the time stool color becomes normal. Though most cases slowly improve over 2–6 months, persistence of complete cholestasis for more than 2 weeks requires further studies (ultrasonography, DIDA scanning, liver biopsy) with possible laparotomy for exploration of the extrahepatic biliary tree. Irrigation of the common bile duct is sometimes necessary to dislodge the obstructing inspissated biliary material.

Balistreri WF, Bove KE: Hepatobiliary consequences of parenteral alimentation. Prog Liver Dis 1990;9:567.

Bhatia J et al: Total parenteral nutrition-associated alterations in hepatobiliary function and histology in rats: Is light exposure a clue? Pediatr Res 1993;33:487.

Dunn L et al: Beneficial effects of early hypocaloric enteral feedings or neonatal gastrointestinal function: Preliminary report of a randomized trial. J Pediatr 1988;112:622.

Enzenauer RW et al: Total parenteral nutrition cholestasis: A cause of mechanical biliary obstruction. Pediatrics 1985;76:905.

Mock DM et al: Chronic fructose intoxication after infancy in children with hereditary fructose intolerance: A cause of growth retardation. N Engl J Med 1983;309:764.

Odievre M et al: Hereditary fructose intolerance in childhood. Am J Dis Child 1978;132:605.

Singh I et al: Peroxisomal disorders: Biochemical and clinical diagnostic considerations. Am J Dis Child 1988;142:1297.

3. NEONATAL HEPATITIS (Giant Cell Hepatitis)

This type of cholestatic jaundice of unknown cause presents with the usual features of cholestasis and a typical appearance on histologic examination of biopsied liver tissue; it accounts for up to 75% of cases of neonatal intrahepatic cholestasis. The degree of cholestasis is variable, and the disorder may be indistinguishable from extrahepatic causes in 10% of cases. Alpha$_1$-antitrypsin deficiency, Alagille's syndrome, and Byler's disease may present in a similar clinical and histologic manner.

Intrauterine growth retardation, prematurity, poor feeding, emesis, poor growth, and partially or intermittently acholic stools are typical clinical characteristics of intrahepatic cholestasis. Neonatal lupus erythematosus may present with giant cell hepatitis; however, thrombocytopenia, skin rash, or congenital heart block is usually present.

In cases of suspected idiopathic neonatal hepatitis (absence of infectious, metabolic, and toxic causes), patency of the biliary tree should be verified to exclude extrahepatic "surgical" disorders. DIDA scanning and ultrasonography may be helpful in this regard. Some have used the enteral string test during DIDA scanning to confirm bile duct patency. Liver biopsy findings are frequently diagnostic, especially after 6–8 weeks of age (see Table 23–1). Biopsy may be misleading before 4 weeks of age, however. Failure to detect patency of the biliary tree, nondiagnostic liver biopsy findings, or persisting complete cholestasis (acholic stools) are indications for minilaparotomy and intraoperative cholangiography by an experienced surgeon. Occasionally, a small but patent (hypoplastic) extrahepatic biliary tree is demonstrated and is probably the result rather than the cause of diminished bile flow; reconstruction of hypoplastic biliary trees should not be attempted.

Once a patent extrahepatic tree is confirmed, therapy should include choleretics (cholestyramine, phenobarbital, or ursodeoxycholic acid), a special formula with medium-chain triglycerides (Pregestimil or Alimentum), and supplemental fat-soluble vitamins in water-miscible form. (See Table 23–2.) These are continued as long as significant cholestasis remains (conjugated bilirubin > 1 mg/dL). Fat-soluble vitamin levels should be monitored while supplements are given.

Eighty percent of patients recover without significant hepatic fibrosis. However, if a relative previously had neonatal hepatitis, there is a 70–80%

probability of progression to cirrhosis ("Byler's disease").

Long-term consequences correlate best with the duration of the cholestasis. In general, failure to resolve the cholestatic picture is associated with progressive liver disease and evolving cirrhosis. This may occur either with normal numbers of interlobular bile ducts or when diminished numbers of ducts (paucity of interlobular ducts) result. Perilobular and intralobular fibrosis both progress, and portal hypertension eventually ensues, with splenomegaly and esophageal varices. Finally, ascites with rising bilirubin levels heralds the onset of hepatic failure. Liver transplantation has been successful when signs of hepatic decompensation are noted (rising bilirubin, intractable ascites).

Dick MC, Mowat AP: Hepatitis syndrome in infancy: An epidemiological survey with 10 year follow-up. Arch Dis Child 1985;60:512.

Laxer RM et al: Liver disease in neonatal lupus erythematosus. J Pediatr 1990;116:238.

Odievre M et al: Long-term prognosis for infants with intrahepatic cholestasis and patent extrahepatic biliary tract. Arch Dis Child 1981;56:373.

Rosenthal P et al: Hepatobiliary scintigraphy and the string test in the evaluation of neonatal cholestasis. J Pediatr Gastroenterol Nutr 1989;8:292.

Sokol RJ: Medical management of the infant or child with chronic liver disease. Semin Liver Dis 1987;7:155.

4. PAUCITY OF INTERLOBULAR BILE DUCTS

Forms of intrahepatic cholestasis caused by decreased numbers of interlobular bile ducts may be classified according to whether or not they are associated with other malformations. The syndromic form, Alagille's syndrome (arteriohepatic dysplasia), is sometimes recognized by identification of the characteristic facies, which becomes more obvious with age. The forehead is prominent, as is the nasal bridge. The eyes are set deep and sometimes widely apart (hypertelorism). Often the chin is small and slightly pointed and projects forward. Ears are prominent. The severity of cholestasis is variable; thus, stool color varies. Pruritus begins by 3–4 months of age. Firm, smooth hepatomegaly is present, and cardiac murmurs are frequent. Xanthomas develop later in the disease. Occasionally, early cholestasis is mild and not recognized.

Conjugated hyperbilirubinemia may be mild to severe (2–15 mg/dL). Serum alkaline phosphatase, γ-glutamyl transpeptidase, and cholesterol are markedly elevated, especially early in life. Serum bile acids are always elevated. Aminotransferases are slightly increased, but clotting factors and other liver proteins are usually normal.

The cardiovascular abnormalities include peripheral and valvular pulmonary stenoses (most common), atrial septal defect, coarctation of the aorta, and tetralogy of Fallot.

Vertebral arch defects are common, including incomplete fusion of the vertebral body or anterior arch (butterfly deformity) and diminished interpedicle distance in the thoracolumbar spine. Eye abnormalities (posterior embryotoxon) and renal abnormalities (dysplastic kidneys, renal tubular ectasia, single kidney, hematuria) are also associated with this disorder. Growth retardation with normal to increased levels of growth hormone is common. Although variable, the IQ is frequently low. Hypogonadism with micropenis may be present. A weak, high-pitched voice may develop. Neurologic disorders due to vitamin E deficiency (areflexia, ataxia, ophthalmoplegia) eventually develop in many children.

In the nonsyndromic form, paucity of interlobular bile ducts is seen in the absence of the extrahepatic malformations. Paucity may also be seen in α_1-antitrypsin deficiency, in Zellweger's syndrome and in association with lymphedema (Aagenaes' syndrome), in cystic fibrosis, in cytomegalovirus or rubella infection, and in inborn errors of bile acid metabolism.

High doses (4–8 g/d) of cholestyramine may control pruritus, lower cholesterol, and clear xanthomas. Phenobarbital may lower serum bilirubin. Ursodeoxycholic therapy (10–15 mg/kg/d) appears to be more effective and less toxic than cholestyramine or phenobarbital. Nutritional therapy to prevent wasting and deficiencies of fat-soluble vitamins is of particular importance because of the severity of cholestasis (see Table 23–2).

Prognosis is more favorable in the syndromic than in the nonsyndromic varieties. In the former, only 30–40% of patients have severe, progressive disease, whereas over 70% of patients suffering from the latter progress to cirrhosis. In Alagille's syndrome, cholestasis frequently improves by age 2–4 years, with minimal residual hepatic fibrosis. Survival into adulthood despite raised serum bile acids, aminotransferases, and alkaline phosphatase is common. Several patients have developed hepatocellular carcinoma. Hypogonadism has been noted; however, fertility is not obviously affected. Cardiovascular anomalies may shorten life expectancy. Some patients have persistent, severe cholestasis, rendering their quality of life poor; liver transplant has been performed under these circumstances.

The gene for Alagille's syndrome is located on chromosome 20p, though it has not yet been isolated and cloned.

Alagille D et al: Syndromic paucity of interlobular bile ducts (Alagille syndrome or arteriohepatic dysplasia): Review of 80 cases. J Pediatr 1987;110:195.

Balistreri WF et al: Biochemical and clinical response to ursodeoxycholic acid administration in pediatric patients with chronic cholestasis. In: *Bile Acids as Therapeutic*

Agents. Paumgartner G, Stiehl A, Gerok W (editors). Kluwer, 1991.

Riely CA: Familial intrahepatic cholestatic syndromes. Semin Liver Dis 1987;7:119.

Schnittger S: Molecular and cytogenic analysis of an interstitial 20p depletion associated with syndromic intrahepatic ductular hypoplasia (Alagille syndrome). Hum Genet 1989;83:239.

Schwarzenberg SJ et al: Long-term complications of arteriohepatic dysplasia. Am J Med 1992;93:171.

Sokol RJ et al: Multicenter trial of d-alpha tocopheryl polyethylene glycol-1000 succinate for treatment of vitamin E deficiency in children with chronic cholestasis. Gastroenterology 1993;104:1727.

EXTRAHEPATIC NEONATAL CHOLESTASIS

Extrahepatic neonatal cholestasis is characterized by complete and persistent cholestasis (acholic stools) in the first 1–4 weeks of life, surgically proved lack of patency of the extrahepatic biliary tree by intraoperative cholangiography, firm to hard hepatomegaly, and typical features on histologic examination of liver biopsy tissue. (See Table 23–1.) Causes include extrahepatic biliary atresia, choledochal cyst, intrinsic obstruction of the common duct, and spontaneous perforation of the extrahepatic ducts.

Extrahepatic Biliary Atresia

In Caucasians, extrahepatic biliary atresia occurs in 1:13,000–1:8000 births, and the incidence in both sexes is equal. In Asians, the incidence is higher, and the disorder is twice as common in girls. The abnormality found most commonly is complete atresia of all extrahepatic biliary structures, but there are variants. The specific cause is not known, though evidence supports an insult to the biliary structures in the perinatal period that progresses in postnatal life. Extrahepatic atresia has not been found in stillborn fetuses and is rarely seen in premature infants. Meconium and first-passed stools are usually normal in color, suggesting early patency of the ducts. Furthermore, the presence of patent intrahepatic bile ducts near the porta hepatis is not consistent with congenital absence of the primitive bile duct. Evidence obtained from surgically removed remnants of the extrahepatic biliary tree suggests an inflammatory or sclerosing cholangiopathy. Although an infectious cause seems reasonable, no agent has been consistently found in such cases. The role of reovirus type 3 in biliary atresia has been suggested but recently disputed. Preliminary studies suggest involvement of rotavirus group C. Although other congenital malformations, especially vascular ones, may occasionally be seen in extrahepatic biliary atresia, only polysplenia syndrome (situs inversus, levocardia, absence of the inferior vena cava, multiple spleens, midline liver) is consistently associated with extrahepatic biliary atresia.

Jaundice may be noted in the newborn period but is more often delayed until 2–3 weeks of age. The urine is dark and stains the diaper, and the stools are often pale yellow, buff-colored, gray, or acholic. Seepage of bilirubin products across the intestinal mucosa gives some yellow coloration to the stools. Hepatomegaly is common, and the liver may feel firm to hard; splenomegaly develops later. Pruritus, digital clubbing, xanthomas, and a rachitic rosary may be noted in slightly older patients. Murmurs reflecting increasing cardiovascular output or shunting through bronchial arteries may be heard over the entire precordium and back. By 2–6 months, the growth curves reveal poor weight gain, probably as a result of fat malabsorption and increased oxygen consumption. Late in the course, ascites and bleeding complications occur.

No single laboratory test will consistently differentiate this entity from other causes of "complete" obstructive jaundice. A DIDA excretion study performed early in the course of disease and after pretreatment with phenobarbital (3–5 mg/kg/d for 5–7 days) may distinguish intrahepatic from extrahepatic causes of cholestasis. Although biliary atresia is suggested by persistent elevation of serum γ-glutamyl transpeptidase or alkaline phosphatase levels, high cholesterol levels, and prolonged prothrombin times, these findings have also been reported in severe neonatal hepatitis, α_1-antitrypsin deficiency, and bile duct paucity. Furthermore, these tests will not differentiate the location of the obstruction within the extrahepatic system . Generally, the aminotransferases are only modestly elevated in biliary atresia. Serum proteins and blood clotting factors are not affected early in the disease. Routine chest x-ray may reveal abnormalities suggestive of polysplenia syndrome. Ultrasonography of the biliary system should be performed to ascertain the presence of choledochal cyst. Liver biopsy specimens can differentiate intrahepatic causes of cholestasis from biliary atresia in over 90% of cases.

The major diagnostic dilemma is between this entity and neonatal hepatitis, bile duct paucity, choledochal cyst, or intrinsic bile duct obstruction (stones, bile plugs). Though spontaneous perforation of extrahepatic bile ducts leads to jaundice and acholic stools, the infants are usually quite ill with chemical peritonitis from biliary ascites, and hepatomegaly is not found.

If the diagnosis of biliary atresia cannot be excluded by the diagnostic evaluation before 60 days of life, surgical exploration is necessary. Laparotomy must include liver biopsy and an operative cholangiogram if a gallbladder is present. The presence of yellow bile in the gallbladder implies patency of the proximal extrahepatic duct system. Radiographic visualization of dye in the duodenum excludes obstruction to the distal extrahepatic ducts.

In the absence of surgical correction, the following eventually develop: failure to thrive, marked pruritus, portal hypertension, hypersplenism, bleeding diathesis, rickets, ascites, and cyanosis. Bronchitis and pneumonia are common. Eventually, hepatic failure and death occur, almost always by age 18–24 months.

Except for the occasional example of "correctable" biliary atresia where choledocho- or cholecystojejunostomy is feasible, the standard procedure is hepatoportoenterostomy (Kasai procedure). Occasionally, portocholecystostomy (gallbladder Kasai procedure) may be performed if the gallbladder is present and the passage to the duodenum is patent. These procedures are best done in specialized centers where experienced surgical, pediatric, and nursing personnel are available. It is recommended that surgery be performed as early as possible (age 6–10 weeks); the Kasai procedure should generally not be undertaken in infants over 4 months of age, because the likelihood of bile drainage at this age is very low.

Orthotopic liver transplantation is now indicated for patients who fail to drain bile after the Kasai procedure or who progress to end-stage biliary cirrhosis despite surgical treatment. The 5-year survival rate following transplantation is 60–80%.

Whether or not the Kasai procedure is performed, supportive medical treatment measures consist of vitamin and caloric support (using water-miscible forms of vitamins A, D, K, and E and formulas containing medium-chain triglycerides [Pregestimil or Alimentum]). (See Table 23–2.) Bacterial infections (eg, ascending cholangitis) should be treated promptly with broad-spectrum antibiotics, and signs of bleeding tendency should be corrected with intramuscular vitamin K. Ascites can be managed with reduced sodium intake and spironolactone. Choleretics and bile acid-binding products (cholestyramine, aluminum hydroxide gel) are of little use. The value of ursodeoxycholic acid remains to be determined.

When bile flow is sustained, the 5-year survival rate is 35–50%. Complete surgical failures have the same outcome as nonoperated cases, but patients die sooner (age 8–15 months versus age 18–36 months). Death is usually due to liver failure, sepsis, acidosis, or respiratory failure secondary to intractable ascites. Surprisingly, terminal hemorrhage is unusual. Liver transplantation has dramatically changed the outlook for these patients.

Butler SN, Smith D: Living with chronic pediatric liver disease: The parent's experience. Pediatr Nurs 1992;18:453.

Karrer FM et al: Biliary atresia registry, 1976 to 1989. J Pediatr Surg 1990;25:1076.

Kaufman SS et al: Nutritional support for the infant with extrahepatic biliary atresia. J Pediatr 1987;100:679.

Laurent J: Long-term outcome after surgery for biliary atresia: Study of 40 patients surviving for more than 10 years. Gastroenterology 1990;99:1793.

Lilly JR et al: The surgery of biliary atresia. Ann Surg 1989;210:289.

Ohtomo Y et al: Glomerular alterations in children with biliary atresia. J Pediatr 1992;120:404.

Riepenhoff-Talty M et al: Group A rotaviruses produce extrahepatic biliary obstruction in orally inoculated newborn mice. Pediatr Res 1993;33:394.

Choledochal Cyst

Choledochal cysts cause 2–5% of cases of extrahepatic neonatal cholestasis; the incidence is higher in Asians. In most cases, the clinical manifestations, basic laboratory findings, and histopathologic features on liver biopsy are indistinguishable from those seen in biliary atresia. Neonatal symptomatic cysts are usually associated with atresia of the distal common duct—accounting for the diagnostic dilemma—and may simply be part of the spectrum of biliary atresia. However, a palpable subhepatic mass, positive ultrasound scan, or pressure deformity on the first and second portion of duodenum seen on upper gastrointestinal series promptly resolves the question. Immediate operation is indicated once abnormalities in clotting factors have been corrected and bacterial cholangitis, if present, has been treated with intravenous antibiotics. Discovery of such a mass eliminates the need for other studies. In older children, choledochal cyst presents as recurrent episodes of obstructive jaundice or abdominal pain or as a right abdominal mass.

Excision of the cyst and hepatojejunal anastomosis are recommended. In some cases, because of technical problems, only the mucosa of the cyst can be removed with jejunal anastomosis to the proximal bile duct. Anastomosis of cyst to jejunum is not recommended.

The prognosis depends upon the presence or absence of associated evidence of atresia and the appearance of the intrahepatic ducts. If atresia is found, the prognosis is similar to that described above. If an isolated cyst is encountered, the outcome is generally excellent, with resolution of the jaundice and return to normal liver cellular architecture the rule. However, bouts of ascending cholangitis, particularly if intrahepatic cysts are present, or obstruction of the anastomotic site may occur. The risk of biliary carcinoma developing within the cyst is about 5–15% at adulthood; therefore, cystectomy should be done whenever possible.

Cheney M et al: Choledochal cyst. World J Surg 1985;9:244.

Lilly JR et al: Forme fruste choledochal cyst. J Pediatr Surg 1985;20:449.

Saing H et al: Surgical management of choledochal cysts: A review of 60 cases. J Pediatr Surg 1985;20:443.

Voyles CR et al: Carcinoma in choledochal cysts: Age-related incidence. Arch Surg 1983;118:986.

Spontaneous Perforation of the Extrahepatic Ducts

The sudden appearance of obstructive jaundice, acholic stools, and abdominal enlargement with ascites in a sick newborn is suggestive of this condition. The liver is usually normal in size, and a yellow-green discoloration can often be discerned under the umbilicus or in the scrotum. In 24% of cases stones or sludge is found obstructing the common bile duct. DIDA scan shows leakage from the biliary tree, and ultrasound confirms ascites or fluid around the bile duct.

Treatment is surgical. Simple drainage, without attempt at oversewing the perforation is sufficient in primary perforations. A diversion anastomosis is constructed in cases associated with choledochal cyst or stenosis.

The prognosis is generally good.

Haller JO et al: Spontaneous perforation of the common bile duct in children. Radiology 1989;172:621.

Megison SM et al: Management of common bile duct obstruction associated with spontaneous perforation of the biliary tree. Surgery 1992;111:237.

OTHER NEONATAL HYPERBILIRUBINEMIC CONDITIONS (Noncholestatic Nonhemolytic)

This group of disorders associated with hyperbilirubinemia is of two types: (1) unconjugated hyperbilirubinemia, consisting of breast milk jaundice, Lucey-Driscoll syndrome, congenital hypothyroidism, upper intestinal obstruction, Gilbert's syndrome, Crigler-Najjar syndrome, and drug-induced hyperbilirubinemia; and (2) conjugated noncholestatic hyperbilirubinemia, consisting of Dubin-Johnson syndrome and Rotor's syndrome.

1. UNCONJUGATED HYPERBILIRUBINEMIA

Breast Milk Jaundice

Persistent elevation of the indirect bilirubin fraction may occur in up to 36% of breast-fed infants. Recent studies implicate an enhancer of intestinal absorption of unconjugated bilirubin in jaundice-causing human milk rather than an inhibitor of bilirubin conjugation acting upon hepatocytes. The increased enterohepatic shunting of unconjugated bilirubin exceeds the normal conjugating capacity in the liver of these infants.

Hyperbilirubinemia does not usually exceed 20 mg/dL, with most in the range of 10–15 mg/dL. In those whose bilirubin levels are above 4–5 mg/dL, the jaundice is noticeable by the fifth to seventh days of breast feeding. It may accentuate the underlying physiologic jaundice—especially early, when total fluid intake may be less than optimal. Except for jaundice, the physical examination is usually normal; urine does not stain the diaper, and the stools are golden-yellow.

The jaundice peaks by the third week and clears before 3 months in almost all infants, even when breast feedings are continued.

Kernicterus has never been reported in this condition. In special situations, breast feeding may be temporarily discontinued and replaced by formula feedings for 2–3 days until serum bilirubin decreases by 2–8 mg/dL. Cow's milk formulas inhibit the intestinal reabsorption of unconjugated bilirubin. When breast feeding is reinstituted, the serum bilirubin may increase slightly but not to the previous level. Phototherapy is not indicated in the healthy term infant with this condition.

Alonso EM et al: Enterohepatic circulation of nonconjugated bilirubin in rats fed with human milk. J Pediatr 1991;118:425.

Gourley GR, Aren RA: β-Glucuronidase and hyperbilirubinemia in breast-fed and formula-fed babies. Lancet 1986;1:644.

Hamosh M: Breast milk jaundice. (Editorial.) J Pediatr Gastroenterol Nutr 1990;11:145.

Newman TB, Maisels MJ: Evaluation and treatment of jaundice in the term newborn: A kinder, gentler approach. Pediatrics 1992;89:809.

Congenital Hypothyroidism

Though the differential diagnosis should always include consideration of congenital hypothyroidism as a cause of indirect hyperbilirubinemia, the diagnosis may be obvious from other clinical and physical clues or from the newborn screening results. The jaundice quickly clears with replacement thyroid hormone therapy, though the mechanism is unclear.

Labrune P et al: Bilirubin uridine diphosphate glucuronosyltransferase hepatic activity in jaundice associated with congenital hypothyroidism. J Pediatr Gastroenterol Nutr 1992;14:79.

Upper Intestinal Obstruction

The association of indirect hyperbilirubinemia with high intestinal obstruction—eg, duodenal atresia, annular pancreas, pyloric stenosis—in the newborn has been observed repeatedly; the mechanism is unknown. Diminished levels of hepatic glucuronyl transferase have been found on liver biopsy in pyloric stenosis.

Treatment is that of the underlying obstructive condition (usually surgical), and jaundice disappears once adequate nutrition is achieved.

Wolley MM et al: Jaundice, hypertrophic pyloric stenosis and hepatic glucuronyl transferase. J Pediatr Surg 1974; 9:359.

Gilbert's Syndrome

This is a common form (3–7% of the population) of familial hyperbilirubinemia associated with a partial reduction of hepatic bilirubin uridine diphosphate glucuronyl transferase activity and perhaps an abnormality in the function or amount of one or more hepatocyte membrane protein carriers. Mild fluctuating jaundice, especially with illness, and vague constitutional symptoms are common. Jaundice is first recognized after puberty. Shortened red cell survival time in some patients is thought to be due to reduced activity of enzymes involved in heme biosynthesis (protoporphyrinogen oxidase). Subsidence of hyperbilirubinemia has been achieved in patients by administration of phenobarbital (5–8 mg/kg/d), though this therapy is not justified.

The disease is inherited as an autosomal dominant with incomplete penetrance. Males are affected more often than females (4:1). Serum unconjugated bilirubin is less than 3–6 mg/dL. The findings on liver biopsy and most other liver function tests are normal except for prolonged indocyanine green and sulfobromophthalein (BSP) retention. An increase in the level of unconjugated bilirubin after a 2-day fast (300 kcal/d) of 1.4 mg/dL or more is consistent with the diagnosis of Gilbert's syndrome. The nicotinic acid provocation test is seldom used in pediatric patients.

Gentile S et al: Dose dependence of nicotinic acid-induced hyperbilirubinemia and its dissociation from hemolysis in Gilbert's syndrome. J Lab Clin Med 1986;107:166.

Gollan JL et al: Effect of dietary composition on the unconjugated hyperbilirubinemia of Gilbert's syndrome. Gut 1976;17:335.

Crigler-Najjar Syndrome

Patients with type I disease usually develop rapid severe elevation of unconjugated bilirubin, with neurologic consequences (kernicterus). Prompt recognition of this entity and treatment with exchange transfusions is required, followed by phototherapy. Some survive without neurologic signs until adolescence or early adulthood, at which time deterioration may suddenly occur. The bile is colorless and contains a predominance of unconjugated bilirubin, small amounts of monoconjugates, and only traces of conjugated bilirubin. Phenobarbital administration in these patients does not significantly alter these findings, nor does it lower serum bilirubin levels. The glucuronyl transferase deficiency is inherited in an autosomal recessive pattern. A combination of phototherapy and cholestyramine may keep bilirubin levels below 25 mg/dL. The use of tin protoporphyrin or tin mesoporphyrin remains experimental. Liver transplantation is curative and may prevent kernicterus if performed early. An auxiliary orthotopic transplantation also relieves the jaundice while the patient retains native liver.

A milder form (type II) with both autosomal dominant and recessive inheritance is rarely associated with neurologic complications. Hyperbilirubinemia is less severe, and the bile is pigmented and contains bilirubin mono- and diglucuronide. Patients with this form respond to phenobarbital with lowering of serum bilirubin levels. An increased proportion of mono- and diconjugated bilirubin in the bile follows phenobarbital treatment.

Liver biopsy findings and liver function tests are consistently normal in both types.

Galbraith RA et al: Suppression of bilirubin production in the Crigler-Najjar type I syndrome: Studies with the heme oxygenase inhibitor tin mesoporphyrin. Pediatrics 1992;89:175.

Shevell MI et al: Crigler-Najjar syndrome type 1: Treatment by home phototherapy followed by orthotopic liver transplantation. J Pediatr 1987;110:429.

Whitington PF et al: Orthotopic auxiliary liver transplantation for Crigler-Najjar syndrome type I. Lancet 1993; 342:779.

Drug-Induced Hyperbilirubinemia

Vitamin K_3 (menadiol) may elevate indirect bilirubin levels by causing hemolysis. Vitamin K_1 (phytonadione) can be safely used in neonates. Rifampin may cause unconjugated hyperbilirubinemia. Other drugs (eg, ceftriaxone, sulfonamides) may displace bilirubin from albumin, potentially increasing the risk of kernicterus—especially in the sick premature infant.

Fink S, Karp W, Robertson A: Ceftriaxone effect on bilirubin-albumin binding. Pediatrics 1987;80:873.

2. CONJUGATED NONCHOLESTATIC HYPERBILIRUBINEMIA (Dubin-Johnson Syndrome & Rotor's Syndrome)

The diagnosis is aided by a positive family history (autosomal recessive inheritance) and jaundice that persists or recurs.

The basic defect in Dubin-Johnson syndrome is impaired hepatocyte excretion of conjugated bilirubin into bile, with a variable degree of impairment in uptake and conjugation complicating the picture. In Rotor's syndrome, the defect lies in hepatic uptake and storage of bilirubin. Bile acids are normally handled so that cholestasis does not occur. Bilirubin values range from 2 to 5 mg/dL, and other liver function tests are normal. In Rotor's syndrome, the liver is normal; in Dubin-Johnson syndrome, it is darkly pigmented on gross inspection. Microscopic examination reveals numerous dark-brown pigment granules consisting of polymers of epinephrine metabolites, especially in the centrilobular regions. However, the amount of pigment varies within families, and some jaundiced members may have no demonstrable pigmentation in the liver. Otherwise, the liver is histologically normal. Oral cholecystography fails to visualize the gallbladder in Dubin-Johnson syndrome but is normal in Rotor's syndrome. Differences in the excretion patterns of sulfobromophthalein (BSP), in results of DIDA cholescintigraphy, in urinary coproporphyrin I and III levels, and in the serum pattern of mono- and diglucuronide conjugates of bilirubin can help distinguish between these two conditions.

The prognosis is excellent, and no treatment is needed.

Crawford JM, Gollan JL: Bilirubin metabolism and the pathophysiology of jaundice. In: *Diseases of the Liver*. Schiff L, Schiff ER (editors). Lippincott, 1993.

Rosenthal P et al: The distribution of serum bilirubin conjugates in pediatric hepatobiliary diseases. J Pediatr 1987; 110:201.

Shieh CC et al: Dubin-Johnson syndrome presenting with neonatal cholestasis. Arch Dis Child 1990;65:898.

Sotelo-Avila C et al: Cholecystitis in a 17-year-old boy with recurrent jaundice since childhood. J Pediatr 1988; 112:668.

HEPATITIS A

Essentials of Diagnosis

- Gastrointestinal upset (anorexia, vomiting, diarrhea).
- Jaundice.
- Liver tenderness.
- Abnormal liver function tests.
- Local epidemic of the disease.
- Specific antibody rise.

General Considerations
(See Table 23–4.)

Hepatitis A viral (HAV) disease is caused by a virus or strains of related viruses and tends to occur in both epidemic and sporadic fashion. Transmission by the fecal-oral route explains epidemic outbreaks from contaminated food or water supplies, particularly by food handlers. Particles 27 nm in diameter have been found in stools during the acute phase of type A hepatitis and are similar in appearance to the enterovirus group. Sporadic cases usually result from contact

HEPATITIS VIRUS ABBREVIATIONS	
HAV	**Hepatitis A virus**
Anti-HAV	Antibody to HAV
HBV	Hepatitis B virus
HBsAg	HBV surface antigen
HBcAg	HBV core antigen
HBeAg	HBV e antigen
Anti-HBs	Antibody to HBsAg
Anti-HBc	Antibody to HBcAg
Anti-HBc IgM	IgM antibody to HBcAg
Anti-HBe	Antibody to HBeAg
HCV	Hepatitis C virus
Anti-HCV	Antibody to HCV
HDV	Hepatitis D (delta) virus
Anti-HDV	Antibody to HDV
HEV	Hepatitis E virus
Anti-HEV	Antibody to HEV
NANBNC	Non-A, non-B, non-C hepatitis virus

with an affected individual. Transmission through blood products obtained during the viremic phase has occurred, though very rarely. The overt form of the disease is easily recognized by the clinical manifestations, but a large number of affected individuals have an anicteric and unrecognized form of the disease. This has been especially true in outbreaks of hepatitis A reported in day care centers accepting children younger than 3 years of age. Lifelong immunity to HAV is conferred following infection.

Antibody to HAV appears within 1–4 weeks of clinical symptoms. While the great majority of children with infectious hepatitis are asymptomatic or have mild disease and recover completely, some will develop fulminant hepatitis. Children who die during the initial attack of the disease do so from massive hepatic necrosis secondary to overwhelming viremia, an immunologic deficiency state, or perhaps exposure to a mutant strain of virus.

Clinical Findings

A. History: A history of direct exposure to a previously jaundiced individual or of eating seafood or drinking contaminated water in the recent past should be sought. Following an incubation period of

Table 23–4. Hepatitis viruses.

	HAV	HBV	HCV	HDV	HEV
Type of virus	Enterovirus (RNA)	Hepadnavirus (DNA)	Flavivirus (RNA)	Incomplete (RNA)	Calicivirus (RNA)
Transmission routes	Fecal-oral	Parenteral, sexual, vertical	Parenteral, sexual	Parenteral, sexual	Fecal-oral
Incubation period	15–40 days	50–150 days	1–5 months	20–90 days	2–9 weeks
Diagnostic test	Anti-HAV IgM	HBsAg, Anti-HBc IgM	Anti-HCV	Anto-HDV	Anti-HEV
Mortality rate	0.1–0.2%	0.5–2%	1–2%	2–20%	1–2% (in pregnant women, 20%)
Carrier state	No	Yes	Yes	Yes	No

15–40 days, the initial nonspecific symptoms usually precede the development of jaundice by 5–10 days.

B. Symptoms and Signs: Fever, anorexia, vomiting, headache, and abdominal pain are the usual symptoms. Darkening of the urine, suggesting the presence of bile, precedes jaundice. Jaundice reaches a peak in 1–2 weeks and then begins to subside. The stools may become light or clay-colored during this time. Clinical improvement can be noted as jaundice develops. Tender hepatomegaly and jaundice are typically present; splenomegaly is variable.

C. Laboratory Findings: Aminotransferases and conjugated and unconjugated bilirubin levels are elevated. The leukocyte count is normal to low; the sedimentation rate is elevated. Serum proteins are generally normal, but an elevation of the gamma globulin fraction (> 2.5 g/dL) can occur and indicates a worse prognosis. Hypoalbuminemia, hypoglycemia, and marked prolongation of prothrombin time are serious prognostic findings. Urine bile and urobilinogen are increased. Serologic tests are available for both the specific IgM and IgG antibodies to the type A hepatitis virus. A positive hepatitis A-IgM indicates acute disease, whereas the IgG remains elevated after recovery.

Percutaneous liver biopsy is rarely indicated but may be safely performed in most children—provided the partial thromboplastin time, platelet count, and bleeding time are normal and the prothrombin time is prolonged no more than 4 or 5 seconds. The presence of ascites may increase the risk of percutaneous liver biopsy. "Balloon cells" and acidophilic bodies are characteristic histologic findings. Liver cell necrosis may be diffuse or focal, with accompanying infiltration of inflammatory cells containing polymorphonuclear leukocytes, lymphocytes, macrophages, and plasma cells, particularly in portal areas. Some bile duct proliferation may be seen in the perilobular portal areas alongside areas of bile stasis. Regenerative liver cells and proliferation of reticuloendothelial cells are present. Occasionally, massive hepatocyte necrosis is seen, portending a bad prognosis.

Differential Diagnosis

Before jaundice appears, the symptoms are those of a nonspecific viral enteritis. Other diseases with somewhat similar onset include pancreatitis, infectious mononucleosis, leptospirosis, drug-induced hepatitis, Wilson's disease, and, most often, type B, type C, type E, or type non-A, non-B hepatitis. Acquired cytomegalovirus disease may also mimic HAV, though lymphadenopathy is usually present in the former.

Prevention

Some attempt at isolation of the patient is indicated, though most patients with type A hepatitis are noninfectious by the time the disease becomes overt. Stool, urine, and blood-contaminated objects should be handled with extreme care for 1 month after the appearance of jaundice.

Passive-active immunization of exposed susceptibles can be achieved by giving standard immune globulin, 0.02–0.04 mL/kg intramuscularly. Illness is prevented in 80–90% of individuals if immune globulin is given within 1–2 weeks of exposure. Individuals traveling to endemic disease areas should receive 0.02–0.06 mL/kg as prophylaxis, depending on length of stay. HAV vaccines are being developed and are promising.

Treatment

There are no specific measures. Sedatives and corticosteroids should be avoided.

At the start of the illness, a light diet is preferable. During the icteric phase, lower-fat foods may diminish gastrointestinal symptoms but do not affect overall outcome. Drugs and elective surgery should be avoided.

Prognosis

Ninety-five percent of children recover without sequelae. In rare cases of fulminant hepatitis, the patient may die in 5 days or may survive as long as 1–2 months. The prognosis is poor if the signs and symptoms of hepatic coma develop, with deepening of jaundice and development of ascites; orthotopic liver transplantation is indicated under these circumstances. Incomplete resolution leads to prolonged hepatitis or chronic cholestatic hepatitis but not to cirrhosis. Rare cases of aplastic anemia following acute infectious hepatitis have also been reported. A benign relapse of symptoms may occur in 10–15% of cases after 6–10 weeks of apparent resolution.

Feinstone SM, Purcell RH: New methods for the serodiagnosis of hepatitis A. Gastroenterology 1980;78:1092.

Hadler SC et al: Risk factors for hepatitis A in day care centers. J Infect Dis 1982;145:255.

Hoofnagle JH, DiBisceglie AM: Serologic diagnosis of acute and chronic viral hepatitis. Semin Liver Dis 1991; 11:73.

Krugman S: Viral hepatitis A, B, C, D, and E: Infection and prevention. Pediatr Rev 1992;13:203, 245.

Noble RC et al: Post transfusion hepatitis A in a neonatal intensive care unit. JAMA 1984;252:2711.

Tabor E et al: Asymptomatic viral hepatitis types A and B in an adolescent population. Pediatrics 1978;62:1026.

Werzberger A et al: A controlled trial of a formalin-inactivated hepatitis A vaccine in healthy children. N Engl J Med 1992;327:453.

HEPATITIS B

Essentials of Diagnosis

- Gastrointestinal upset, anorexia, vomiting, diarrhea.
- Jaundice, tender hepatomegaly, abnormal liver function tests.

- Serologic evidence of hepatitis B disease: HBsAg, HBeAg, Anti-HBc-IgM.
- History of parenteral, sexual, or household exposure or maternal HBsAg carriage.

General Considerations
(See Table 23–4.)

In contrast to hepatitis A, hepatitis B has a delayed onset with an incubation period of 21–135 days. The disease is due to a DNA virus (42-nm Dane particle) that is usually acquired perinatally from a carrier mother, blood products, shared needles, needle sticks, tattoos) or through sexual transmission. Breast milk, urine, and saliva have been shown to contain viral antigen. Transmission via blood products has been almost eliminated by HBsAg donor-screening protocols. Mutant viruses predispose to fulminant hepatitis.

The complete Dane particle is composed of a core (28-nm particle) that is found in the nucleus of infected liver cells and a double-shelled surface particle apparently formed in the cytoplasm where the completed virus particle is synthesized. The surface antigen in blood is termed HBsAg. This particle is found as a 22-nm spherical particle in the serum but occasionally occurs as a filamentous structure as well. The antibody to it is HBsAb. The core antigen is termed HBcAg and its antibody HBcAb. A specific HBcAb-IgM occurs during active viral replication.

Another important antigen-antibody system associated with hepatitis B virus disease is the "e" antigen system. HBeAg, a truncated soluble form of HBcAg, appears in the serum of infected patients early and correlates with active virus replication. Persistence of HBeAg is a marker of infectivity, whereas the appearance of HBeAb generally implies termination of viral replication. Other serologic markers indicating viral replication include the presence of DNA polymerase HBV DNA.

Clinical Findings

A. Symptoms and Signs: The symptoms are nonspecific, consisting only of slight fever (which may be absent) and mild gastrointestinal upset. Visible jaundice is usually the first significant finding. It is accompanied by darkening of the urine and pale or clay-colored stools. Hepatomegaly is present. Occasionally, a symptom complex of macular rash, urticarial lesions, and arthritis antedates the appearance of icterus. When acquired vertically at birth, chronic disease is frequently asymptomatic despite ongoing liver injury.

B. Laboratory Findings: To diagnose acute hepatitis B infection, the HBsAg and anti-HBc IgM are the only tests needed. To document recovery, immunity, or response to the HBV vaccine, the anti-HBs is useful. HBeAg is followed during chronic HBV infection and, if persisting after 8 weeks in acute infections, may signify a likelihood of chronic

infection. Vertical transmission to newborns is documented by positive HBsAg.

Liver function test results are similar to those discussed previously for hepatitis A. Liver biopsy seldom differentiates hepatitis A and B disease, though specific stains may detect HBcAg or HBsAg in liver.

Renal involvement may be suspected on the basis of urinary findings suggesting glomerulonephritis.

Differential Diagnosis

The differentiation between hepatitis A and hepatitis B disease is made easier by a history of parenteral exposure, a parent who is HBsAg-positive, and an unusually long period of incubation. Hepatitis B and hepatitis C infection are differentiated serologically. The history may suggest a drug-induced hepatitis, especially if a serum sickness prodrome is reported.

Non-A, non-B hepatitis is diagnosed in the absence of serologic markers of hepatitis types A, B, or C.

Prevention

Control of the incidence of hepatitis B in the population is based on screening of blood donors and pregnant women, use of properly sterilized needles and surgical equipment, avoidance of sexual contact with carriers, and vaccination of household contacts, sexual partners, medical personnel, and those at high risk. Universal immunization of all infants born in the USA is now recommended. When acquired vertically at birth, chronic disease is frequently asymptomatic despite ongoing liver injury. The vaccine is highly effective for preexposure prophylaxis (see Chapter 10). Postexposure administration of hepatitis B immune globulin (0.06 mL/kg intramuscularly, given as soon as possible after exposure, up to 7 days) and initiation of vaccination are also effective.

Treatment

Supportive measures such as bed rest and a nutritious diet are used during the active stage of disease. Corticosteroids are contraindicated. For patients with progressive disease (chronic active hepatitis), treatment with alpha-interferon (3–5 million units/1.73 m^2 body surface area three times a week for 4–6 months) inhibits viral replication in 40% of patients, though relapses may occur after completion of therapy. Asymptomatic HBsAg carriers do not respond. Liver transplantation is successful in acute fulminant hepatitis B; however, reinfection is common following liver transplantation performed as treatment for chronic hepatitis B.

Prognosis

The prognosis is good, though fulminant hepatitis, chronic persistent hepatitis, or chronic active hepatitis and cirrhosis may supervene in 10% of patients. The course of the disease is variable, but jaundice seldom persists for more than 2 weeks. HBsAg disappears in 95% of cases at the time of clinical recovery.

Persistent asymptomatic antigenemia may occur, particularly in children with Down's syndrome or leukemia and those undergoing chronic hemodialysis. Persistence of neonatally acquired HBsAg occurs in 70–90% of infants, and the presence of e antigen in the HBsAg carrier patient seems to imply a poorer prognosis. Chronic hepatitis B disease predisposes to development of hepatocellular carcinoma. After 8–10 years of HBV infection, surveillance for development of hepatocellular carcinoma with hepatic ultrasound and serum alpha-fetoprotein are performed annually.

Bortolotti F et al: Long-term outcome of chronic hepatitis type B in patients who acquired hepatitis B infection in childhood. Gastroenterology 1990;99:805.

Chang MH et al: Factors affecting clearance of hepatitis B e antigen in hepatitis B surface antigen carrier children. J Pediatr 1989; 115:385.

Hepatitis B virus: A comprehensive strategy for eliminating transmission in the United States through universal childhood vaccination. Recommendations of the Immunization Practices Advisory Committee. MMWR Morb Mortal Wkly Rep 1991;40:1.

Hoofnagle JH: Type A and type B hepatitis. Lab Med 1983; 14:705.

Ruiz-Moreno M et al: Prospective, randomized controlled trial of interferon-α in children with chronic hepatitis B. Hepatology 1991;13:1035.

Shapiro CN et al: Hepatitis B virus transmission between children in day care. Pediatr Infect Dis J 1989;8:870.

Xu Z-Y et al: Prevention of perinatal acquisition of hepatitis B virus carriage using vaccine: Preliminary report of a randomized, double-blind placebo-controlled and comparative trial. Pediatrics 1985;76:713.

HEPATITIS C

Hepatitis C virus (HCV) causes the chronic form of non-A, non-B hepatitis (90% of posttransfusion hepatitis cases). Risk factors include illicit use of intravenous drugs (40%), occupational or sexual exposure (10%), and transfusions (10%); 40% of cases have no known risk factors. Children with hemophilia or on chronic hemodialysis are particularly at risk. The risk from transfused blood products has greatly diminished (from 1–2:100 to 1:1000 units of blood) since the advent of blood testing for ALT and anti-HCV. Vertical transmission from HCV-infected mothers appears to occur only in mothers who are HIV-positive and is of unknown significance. HCV rarely, if ever, causes fulminant hepatitis in children or adults.

HCV is a single-stranded RNA virus in the flavivirus family. Several well-defined HCV antigens (C100-3, 5-1-1, C33c, C22) are the basis for serologic antibody tests. The second-generation ELISA test for anti-HCV is highly accurate, though anti-HCV may not develop until 6–12 months after infection. HCV RNA can be detected in serum by polymerase chain reaction and indicates active infection.

A history of intravenous drug use, previous transfusions, or chronic use of blood products is obtained in most pediatric cases.

Clinical Findings

A. Symptoms and Signs: The incubation period is 1–5 months, but the onset of symptoms is insidious. Many childhood cases are asymptomatic despite development of chronic hepatitis. More typical flu-like prodromal symptoms and jaundice occur in less than 25% of cases. Hepatosplenomegaly is evident in chronic hepatitis. Ascites, clubbing, palmar erythema, or spider angiomas indicate progression to cirrhosis.

B. Laboratory Findings: Fluctuating mild to moderate elevations of aminotransferases over long periods are characteristic of chronic HCV infection. Diagnosis is established by the presence of anti-HCV (second-generation ELISA) or HCV RNA by polymerase chain reaction, though anti-HCV may not appear for up to 6 months after infection.

Percutaneous liver biopsy is indicated in chronic cases. Histologic examination shows portal triaditis with chronic inflammatory cells, occasional lymphocyte nodules in portal tracts, mild macrovesicular steatosis, and variable bridging necrosis, fibrosis, and cirrhosis.

Differential Diagnosis

HCV should be distinguished from hepatitis A, B, and non-A, non-B, non-C cases by serologic testing. Other causes of childhood cirrhosis should be considered in chronic cases (eg, Wilson's disease, α_1-antitrypsin deficiency), or chronic hepatitis may be caused by drug or autoimmune reactions.

Treatment

Treatment of acute hepatitis is supportive. Chronic HCV infection responds to alpha interferon (3 million units/m^2 three time a week for 6 months) in 40–50% of cases. Relapses are common. Successful long term interferon regimens have not been reported. End-stage liver disease due to HCV responds well to liver transplantation. There appears to be no benefit (or harm) from using immune globulin in infants born to infected mothers.

Prognosis

In adults, 50% of HCV cases develop chronic hepatitis, and cirrhosis develops in 20% of those with chronic disease. A strong association exists between chronic HCV disease and the development of hepatocellular carcinoma as little as 15 years after infection. The outcome of infected children is less well defined, though cirrhosis may develop rapidly or after decades. Infants infected at birth have concomitant HIV infection; their outcome is unknown at present. In adults, chronic HCV infection has been associated with mixed cryoglobulinemia, polyarteritis nodosa, a sicca-like syndrome, and membranoproliferative glomerulonephritis.

Aach RD, et al: Hepatitis C infection in post-transfusion hepatitis: An analysis with first- and second-generation assays. N Engl J Med 1991;325:1325.

Choo Q-L et al: Isolation of a cDNA clone derived from a blood-borne non-A, non-B hepatitis genome. Science 1989;244:359.

Davis GL et al: Treatment of chronic hepatitis C with recombinant interferon alpha: A multicenter randomized, controlled trial. N Engl J Med 1989;321:1501.

Giovanninni M et al: Maternal-infant transmission of hepatitis C virus and HIV infection: A possible interaction. Lancet 1990;335:1166.

Tonas MM et al: Hepatitis C infection in a pediatric dialysis population. Pediatrics 1992; 89:707.

Lam JPH et al: Infrequent vertical transmission of hepatitis C virus. J Infect Dis 1993;167:527.

Ruis-Moreno et al. Treatment of children with chronic hepatitis C with recombinant interferon-α: A pilot study. Hepatology 1992;16:882.

HEPATITIS D
(Delta Agent)

The hepatitis D virus (HDV) is a 35-nm defective virus that requires a coat of HBsAg to be infectious. HDV infection thus can occur only in the presence of HBV infection. In developing countries, transmission is by intimate contact; in Western countries, by parenteral exposure. HDV is rare in the United states. HDV can coinfect simultaneously with HBV, causing acute hepatitis, or can superinfect a patient with chronic HBV infection, predisposing to chronic hepatitis or fulminant hepatitis. In children, there is a strong association between chronic HDV coinfection with HBV and chronic active hepatitis and cirrhosis. Vertical HDV transmission is rare. The diagnosis of HDV is made by anti-HDV IgM. Treatment is directed at therapy for HBV infection or for fulminant hepatic failure.

Bortolotti F et al: Long-term evaluation of chronic delta hepatitis in children. J Pediatr 1993;122:736.

Farci P et al: Infection with the delta agent in children. Gut 1985;26:4.

HEPATITIS E

Hepatitis E virus (HEV) is the cause of enterically transmitted, epidemic non-A, non-B hepatitis. It is rare in the United States. HEV is a calicivirus-like agent that is transmitted via the fecal-oral route. It occurs predominantly in developing countries, is associated with water-borne epidemics, and has only a 3% secondary attack rate in household contacts. Areas reporting epidemics include southeast Asia, China, the Indian subcontinent, the Middle East, northern and western Africa, Mexico, and Central America. Its clinical manifestations are similar to those of HAV except that it is rare in children but more common in adolescents and adults and is associated with a high mortality rate (10–20%) in pregnant women, particularly in the third trimester of pregnancy. Diagnosis is established by HEV antibody. The outcome in nonpregnant individuals is benign, with no chronic hepatitis or chronic carrier state reported to date. There is no effective treatment or vaccine.

Hyams KC et al: Acute sporadic hepatitis E in Sudanese children: Analysis based on a new Western blot assay. J Infect Dis 1992;165:1001.

Krawczynski K: Hepatitis E. Hepatology 1993;17:932.

FULMINANT HEPATITIS
(Acute Massive Hepatic Necrosis,
Acute Yellow Atrophy)

Fulminant hepatitis has a mortality rate of 80–90% in children. An unusual virulence of the infectious agent or peculiar host susceptibility is postulated in these cases. In the first few weeks of life, fulminant hepatic necrosis can be caused by herpesvirus, echovirus, or adenovirus. Metabolic disease that may be responsible include galactosemia, fructose intolerance, tyrosinemia, neonatal iron storage disease, and respiratory chain defects. Later, hepatitis B virus, non-A, non-B, non-C hepatitis virus, and hepatitis E virus are sometimes causative. Hepatitis A virus rarely is responsible for this dreaded disease. Patients with immunologic deficiency diseases and those receiving immunosuppressive drugs are especially vulnerable. In the older child, Wilson's disease, autoimmune chronic active hepatitis, and drugs (eg, acetaminophen, anesthetic agents) or toxins (eg, poisonous mushrooms) must also be considered.

Clinical Findings

In a number of patients, the disease proceeds in a rapidly fulminant course with deepening jaundice, coagulopathy, hyperammonemia, ascites, a rapidly shrinking liver, and progressive coma. Terminally, AST and ALT, which were exceptionally elevated (2000–10,000 IU/L) may improve at the time when the liver is getting smaller and undergoing massive necrosis and collapse. Another group of patients start with a course typical of "benign" hepatitis and then suddenly become ill once again during the second week of the disease. Fever, anorexia, vomiting, and abdominal pain may be noted, and worsening of liver function tests parallels changes in sensorium or impending coma. Hyperreflexia and a positive extensor plantar response are seen. A characteristic breath odor (fetor hepaticus) is present. A generalized bleeding tendency occurs at this time. Impairment of renal function, manifested by either oliguria or anuria, is an ominous sign. The striking laboratory findings include elevated serum bilirubin levels (usually > 20 mg/dL), high AST and ALT (> 5000 IU/L) that may decrease terminally, low serum albumin, hypoglycemia, and prolonged prothrombin time. Blood ammonia levels may be elevated, whereas blood urea nitrogen is often very low initially. Hyperpnea is frequent, and a mixed respiratory alkalosis and metabolic acidosis is present. A rise in the polymorphonuclear white cell count often presages acute liver failure.

Differential Diagnosis

Other known causes of fulminant hepatitis, such as drugs and other chemical poisons or naturally occurring plant toxins, may be difficult to exclude. Patients with Reye's syndrome are typically anicteric. A liver biopsy may be helpful. Wilson's disease, autoimmune chronic active hepatitis, acute leukemia, cardiomyopathy, and Budd-Chiari syndrome should be considered.

Complications

The development and depth of hepatic coma determine the prognosis. Patients in grade 3 or 4 coma (combativeness, unresponsive to verbal stimuli, or decorticate function) rarely survive without transplantation. Cerebral edema, which usually accompanies coma, is frequently the cause of death. Sepsis, hemorrhage, renal failure, or cardiorespiratory arrest is a common terminal event. Thus, when patients enter grade 3 coma, liver transplantation should be performed. The rare survivor without transplantation may have degrees of residual fibrosis or even cirrhosis.

Treatment

Many regimens have been tried, but controlled evaluation of therapy remains difficult. Exchange transfusion (with fresh heparinized blood) temporarily repairs both the chemical and hematologic abnormalities. Response may be delayed and repeated exchange transfusions necessary. Plasmapheresis with plasma exchange, total body washout, charcoal hemoperfusion, and hemodialysis using a special high-permeability membrane have been used in the treatment of fulminant hepatic failure. Removal of circulating toxins may be of greater benefit to extrahepatic organ function (brain) than to the liver itself. Reversal of hepatic encephalopathy may follow any of these therapeutic modalities but without improvement in the final prognosis. Survival in adults is not improved over the control group (about 20%). Orthotopic liver transplantation has met with success in approximately 50–60% of cases; however, patients in grade 4 coma may not always recover cerebral function. Therefore, patients in hepatic failure should be transferred to centers where liver transplantation can be performed. Criteria for deciding when to perform transplantation on these patients are not firmly established; however, serum bilirubin over 20 mg/dL, prothrombin time over 30 seconds, and factor V levels less than 20% are ominous signs.

Corticosteroids may actually be harmful. Sterilization of the colon with oral antibiotics such as metronidazole, neomycin, or gentamicin is recommended. An alternative is acidification of the colon with lactulose, 1–2 mL/kg three or four times daily, which reduces blood ammonia levels and traps ammonia in the colon. Preliminary studies suggest that intravenous infusions of prostaglandin E may be beneficial.

Close monitoring of fluid and electrolytes is mandatory and requires a central venous line. Ten percent dextrose solutions should be infused to maintain normal blood glucose. Diuretics, sedatives, and tranquilizers are to be used sparingly. Early signs of cerebral edema are treated with infusions of mannitol (0.5–1 g/kg). The experimental benzodiazepine antagonist flumazenil may improve encephalopathy.

Comatose patients are intubated, given mechanical ventilatory support, and monitored for signs of infection. Coagulopathy is treated with fresh-frozen plasma, other clotting factor concentrates, platelet infusions, or exchange transfusion. Plasmapheresis and hemodialysis may help maintain a patient while awaiting liver transplantation. Epidural monitoring for increased intracranial pressure in patients awaiting liver transplantation is advocated. Artificial hepatic support devices are being developed. Prophylactic immune globulin, 0.02 mL/kg intramuscularly, should be given to close contacts of the patient with hepatitis A and, perhaps, non-A, non-B, non-C hepatitis.

Prognosis

The overall prognosis remains grave. Exchange transfusions or other modes of heroic therapy do not improve survival figures. The presence of nests of liver cells seen on liver biopsy amounting to more than 25% of the total cells and rising levels of clotting factors V and VII coupled with rising levels of serum alpha-fetoprotein may signify a more favorable prognosis for early survival. Only the rare survivor escapes postnecrotic cirrhosis. Results of liver transplantation (60–85% survival) exceed survival in nontransplanted similar patients (20–25%).

Devictor D et al: Emergency liver transplantation for fulminant liver failure in infants and children. Hepatology 1992;16:1156.

Emond JC et al: Liver transplantation in the management of fulminant hepatic failure. Gastroenterology 1989;96:1583.

Fraser CL, Arieff AI: Hepatic encephalopathy. N Engl J Med 1985;313:865.

Grimm G et al: Improvement of hepatic encephalopathy treated with flumazenil. Lancet 1988;2:1392.

O'Grady JG et al: Early indicators of prognosis in fulminant hepatic failure. Gastroenterology 1989;97:439.

Psacharopoulos HT et al: Fulminant hepatic failure in childhood. Arch Dis Child 1980;55:252.

Russell GJ et al: Fulminant hepatic failure. J Pediatr 1987; 111:313.

Sokol RJ: Fulminant hepatic failure. In: *Pediatric Hepatology.* Balistreri WF, Stocker JT (editors). Hemisphere, 1990.

AUTOIMMUNE CHRONIC ACTIVE HEPATITIS
(Lupoid Hepatitis)

Autoimmune chronic active hepatitis is most common in teenage girls, though it does occur at all ages and in either sex. Chronic active hepatitis may also follow hepatitis B, hepatitis C, and delta hepatitis infections. Rarely, chronic active hepatitis evolves from drug-induced hepatitis (eg, pemoline) or may develop in conjunction with such diseases as ulcerative colitis, Sjögren's syndrome, or autoimmune hemolytic anemia. Wilson's disease and α_1-trypsin deficiency may also present as chronic active hepatitis. A positive HBsAg test indicates chronic active hepatitis caused by hepatitis type B, and anti-HCV and anti-HDV for types C and delta hepatitis, respectively. Positive antinuclear antibodies, smooth muscle antibodies or liver-kidney microsomal antibodies, and systemic manifestations (such as arthralgia, acne, and amenorrhea) are characteristic of autoimmune chronic active hepatitis.

A genetic susceptibility to development of this entity is suggested by the increased incidence of the histocompatibility antigens HLA-A1 and HLA-B8. These histocompatibility antigens may code for the defect in suppressor T cell function also noted in patients with chronic active hepatitis. Increased autoimmune disease in families of patients and a high prevalence of seroimmunologic abnormalities in relatives have been noted.

Clinical Findings

Fever, malaise, recurrent or persistent jaundice, skin rash, arthritis, amenorrhea, gynecomastia, acne, pleurisy, pericarditis, or ulcerative colitis may be found in the history of these patients, or asymptomatic hepatomegaly may be found on examination. Cutaneous signs of chronic liver disease may be noted (eg, spider angiomas, liver palms). Hepatosplenomegaly is frequently present. Digital clubbing may be found.

Liver function tests reveal moderate elevations of serum bilirubin, AST, ALT, and serum alkaline phosphatase. Serum albumin may be low. Serum IgG levels are strikingly elevated (in the range of 2–6 g/dL), with reports of values as high as 11 g/dL. Low levels of C3 complement have been seen. Three subtypes have been described based on autoantibodies present:

anti-smooth muscle (anti-actin), anti-liver-kidney microsome, and anti-soluble liver antigen.

Histologic examination of liver biopsy specimens shows loss of the lobular limiting plate, "piecemeal" necrosis, portal fibrosis, an inflammatory reaction of lymphocytes and plasma cells in the portal areas as well as perivascularly, and some bile duct and Kupffer cell proliferation and pseudolobule formation. Cirrhosis may be present at diagnosis in up to half of patients.

Differential Diagnosis

Laboratory and histologic findings differentiate other types of chronic hepatitis (eg, hepatitis types B, C, and D, Wilson's disease, chronic persistent hepatitis, α_1-antitrypsin disease, chronic pericholangitis, subacute hepatitis). Wilson's disease and α_1-antitrypsin deficiency must be excluded if hepatitis B and C studies are negative. Drug-induced (isoniazid, methyldopa) chronic active hepatitis should be ruled out. In acute, severe viral hepatitis, histologic examination may also show an "aggressive" lesion early in the disease (< 3 months).

Complications

Untreated disease that continues for months to years eventually results in postnecrotic cirrhosis. Persistent malaise, fatigue, and anorexia parallel disease activity. Bleeding from esophageal varices and development of ascites usually usher in hepatic failure.

Treatment

Corticosteroids (prednisone, 2 mg/kg/d) decrease the mortality rate during the early active phase of the disease. Azathioprine, 1 mg/kg/d, is of value in decreasing the side effects of long-term corticosteroid therapy but should not be used alone during the "induction" phase of treatment. Steroids are reduced over a 6- to 12-month period, and azathioprine is continued for 1–2 years. Relapses are treated similarly. Ursodeoxycholic acid or cyclosporine may be helpful in poorly responsive cases. Liver transplantation is indicated when disease progresses to cirrhosis despite therapy.

Prognosis

The overall prognosis for chronic active hepatitis has been significantly improved by early therapy. Some report cures (normal histologic findings) in 15–20% of cases. Relapses (seen clinically and histologically) occur in 40–50% of cases after cessation of therapy; remissions follow repeat treatment. Survival for 10 years is common despite residual cirrhosis. Progressive portal hypertension is seen, and complications (bleeding varices, ascites) require specific therapy. Liver transplantation is successful 70–80% of the time. Disease recurrence after transplantation is rare.

Davis GL, Czaja AJ, Ludwig J: Development and prognosis of histologic cirrhosis in corticosteroid-treated hepatitis B surface antigen-negative chronic active hepatitis. Gastroenterology 1984;87:1222.

Fitzgerald JF: Chronic hepatitis. J Pediatr 1984;104:893.

Maddrey WC: Subdivisions of idiopathic autoimmune chronic active hepatitis. Hepatology 1987;7:1372.

Maggiore G et al: Liver disease associated with anti-liver-kidney microsome antibody in children. J Pediatr 1986; 108:399.

Maggiore G et al: Treatment of autoimmune chronic active hepatitis in childhood. J Pediatr 1984;104:839.

Odievre M et al: Seroimmunologic classification of chronic hepatitis in 57 children. Hepatology 1983;3:407.

CIRRHOSIS

Cirrhosis is a pathologic condition of the liver characterized histologically by the presence of extensive fibrosis associated with regenerating liver nodules. It may be micro- or macronodular in appearance. Although the severity of this process may vary from one area of the liver to the next, the whole liver is typically involved. The architectural distortion is caused by the loss of hepatocytes, replacement by scar tissue (fibrosis), and the regrowth of liver cells, a combination of events that interferes with the flow of blood through this organ. The increased resistance to blood flow produces portal hypertension and its consequences. This also affects the microcirculation to regional hepatocytes, impairing their metabolic function, perpetuating the cirrhotic process by stimulating collagen deposition (fibrogenesis).

Many liver diseases may progress to cirrhosis. However, 30–50% of cases of cirrhosis have no discoverable cause at the time of diagnosis.

Two major forms of cirrhosis are described—postnecrotic and biliary—with different causes, symptomatology, and treatment requirements. Both forms can eventually lead to liver failure and death.

In the pediatric population, postnecrotic cirrhosis most often evolves as a result of acute liver disease (eg, idiopathic neonatal giant cell hepatitis, viral hepatitis type B or type C, non-A, non-B hepatitis, chronic active hepatitis, drug hepatitis) or certain inborn errors of metabolism (Table 23–3). Cirrhosis is an exceptional outcome of acute viral hepatitis A and usually follows massive hepatic necrosis. The course may be insidious, with no recognized icteric phase, as in some cases of hepatitis B, Wilson's disease, or α_1-antitrypsin deficiency. The underlying liver disease may be active, with abnormal liver function test results; or it may be quiescent, with only minimal derangement of liver tests. Most cases of biliary cirrhosis are due to congenital abnormalities of the bile ducts (biliary atresia, choledochal cyst, common duct stenosis), tumors of the bile duct, Caroli's disease, Byler's disease, sclerosing cholangitis, hypoplasia of the intrahepatic bile ducts, and cystic fibrosis.

Occasionally, the disease may follow a hypersensitivity reaction to certain drugs, such as phenytoin. Parasites (Clonorchis sinensis, Fasciola, Ascaris) may be causative in children living in endemic areas.

Clinical Findings

A. Symptoms and Signs: In postnecrotic causes of cirrhosis, general malaise, loss of appetite, failure to thrive, and nausea are frequent complaints, especially in the anicteric varieties. Easy bruising may be reported. Jaundice may or may not be present. The first indication of underlying liver disease may be ascites, gastrointestinal hemorrhage, or even signs of hepatic encephalopathy. There may be variable hepatosplenomegaly, spider angiomas, warm skin, and red "liver" palms. A small, shrunken liver may be detected by percussion over the right chest wall that reveals resonance rather than expected dullness. Most often, the liver is slightly enlarged, especially in the subxiphoid region, where it has a firm to hard quality and an irregular edge. Ascites may be detected as shifting dullness or a fluid wave. Gynecomastia may be noted in males. Digital clubbing is found in 10–15% of cases. Pretibial edema is often seen, reflecting underlying hypoproteinemia. In adolescent girls, irregularities of menstruation and amenorrhea may be early complaints.

In biliary cirrhosis, the patients usually have jaundice, dark urine, pruritus, and sometimes xanthoma in addition to the above clinical findings. Undernutrition and failure to thrive due to steatorrhea may be more apparent in this form of cirrhosis.

B. Laboratory Findings: In postnecrotic cirrhosis, mild abnormalities of aminotransferases (AST, ALT) are present, while serum protein determinations often reveal a decreased level of albumin and a variable increase in the level of gamma globulins. Prothrombin time is prolonged and usually unresponsive to vitamin K administration. Burr red cells may be noted on the peripheral blood smear. A mild anemia is present, and thrombocytopenia and leukopenia are present if hypersplenism exists.

In biliary cirrhosis, elevated conjugated bilirubin, bile acids, γ-glutamyl transpeptidase, alkaline phosphatase, and cholesterol are commonly found. The prolonged prothrombin time may respond to vitamin K administration (1–5 mg intramuscularly).

C. Imaging: As portal hypertension complicates cirrhosis, esophageal varices may be demonstrated by endoscopy or x-ray. Small amounts of ascitic fluid, esophageal or gastric varices, and portal venous flow can be seen by abdominal ultrasound examination. The evaluation process of biliary cirrhosis is often more involved and may require hepatobiliary scintigraphy, ultrasound scans of the biliary system, transhepatic cholangiography, or endoscopic or operative cholangiograms.

D. Pathologic Findings: Because sampling error by percutaneous needle biopsy in cirrhotic patients is high (50%), liver biopsy, preferably by laparoscopy or by surgical means, is advisable for confirmation of cirrhosis. Regenerating nodules and surrounding fibrosis are hallmarks of cirrhosis. Pathologic features of biliary cirrhosis also include canalicular and hepatocyte cholestasis, as well as plugging of bile ducts. The interlobular bile ducts may be increased or decreased, depending on the cause and the stage of the disease process.

Complications & Treatment

Major complications of cirrhosis in childhood include progressive nutritional disturbances, hormonal disturbances, the evolution of portal hypertension and its vagaries, and hepatic encephalopathy (see Table 23–2). Hepatocarcinoma occurs with increased frequency in the cirrhotic liver, especially in patients with the chronic form of hereditary tyrosinemia. At present, there is no proved treatment for cirrhosis, but wherever a treatable condition is identified (such as Wilson's disease, galactosemia, congenital fructose intolerance) or an offending agent eliminated (drugs, toxins), the disease's progression can be altered; in occasional cases, regression of fibrosis has been noted. Immunosuppressive treatment in autoimmune chronic liver disease also halts the progression of cirrhosis in most cases. Surgical correction of biliary tree abnormalities can stabilize the disease process or lead to a reversal in some situations.

Prognosis

Postnecrotic cirrhosis follows an unpredictable pattern. Prior to the development of liver transplantation, death occurred in the majority of patients within 10–15 years after diagnosis, usually from liver failure. A rising bilirubin coupled with diuretic refractory ascites in a cirrhotic patient portends demise from hepatic decompensation within 6–12 months or less. The terminal event in some patients may be generalized hemorrhage, sepsis, or cardiorespiratory arrest. For patients with biliary cirrhosis, the prognosis is good only for those with surgically corrected lesions that result in regression or stabilization of the underlying liver condition. For the remainder, without liver transplantation, this is a progressive, ultimately fatal disease. With liver transplantation, survival is 70–80%.

Conn HO, Atterbury CE: Cirrhosis. In: *Diseases of the Liver,* 7th ed. Schiff L, Schiff ER (editors). Lippincott, 1993.

Zironi G et al: Value of measurement of mean portal flow velocity by Doppler flowmetry in the diagnosis of portal hypertension. J Hepatol 1992;16:298.

ALPHA₁-ANTITRYPSIN DEFICIENCY LIVER DISEASE

Essentials of Diagnosis

- Serum α_1-antitrypsin level less than 80 mg/dL.
- Identification of specific phenotype (Pi ZZ, SZ).
- Detection of diastase-resistant glycoprotein deposits in periportal hepatocytes.
- Histologic evidence of liver disease.
- Family history of early-onset pulmonary disease or liver disease.

General Considerations

The disease is due to a deficiency in the protease inhibitor system (Pi), predisposing patients to chronic liver disease and an early onset of pulmonary emphysema. It is most often associated with the Pi phenotype ZZ. With the intermediate serum levels of α_1-antitrypsin present in the heterozygote phenotype (MZ), the incidence of liver disease in adults is only slightly greater than that in the general population despite the presence of glycoprotein deposits in hepatocytes. The exact relationship between low levels of serum α_1-antitrypsin and the development of liver disease is unclear. Emphysema develops because of a lack of inhibition of elastase, which destroys pulmonary connective tissue. Inclusion bodies in the liver contain a protein component immunologically cross-reactive with serum α_1-antitrypsin, containing excess mannose but lacking sialic acid. This structural abnormality leads to aggregation in the endoplasmic reticulum and is resistant to sialization by sialyltransferase. Although all patients with the ZZ genotype have antitrypsin inclusions in hepatocytes, that may be the only histologic evidence of liver disease. However, the likelihood of developing severe liver disease in response to hepatic injury is definitely increased in patients homozygous for this condition. From 30% to 50% of adults with α_1-antitrypsin deficiency have been found to have cirrhosis. A few children will have only pulmonary or pulmonary and hepatic involvement.

Clinical Findings

A. Symptoms and Signs: α_1-Antitrypsin deficiency should be suspected in all small-for-gestational-age newborns with neonatal cholestasis. Poor appetite, lethargy, slight irritability, and jaundice suggest neonatal hepatitis but are not pathognomonic of any one cause. Hepatosplenomegaly is present. Family history may be positive for emphysema or cirrhosis.

In the older child, hepatomegaly or physical findings suggestive of cirrhosis, especially in the face of a negative history of liver disease, should always lead one to suspect α_1-antitrypsin deficiency. Recurrent pulmonary disease (bronchitis, pneumonia) may be present in a few children.

B. Laboratory Findings: Low levels (< 0.2

mg/dL) of the α_1-globulin fraction may be noted on serum protein fractionation. Specific quantitation of α_1-antitrypsin reveals levels of less than 80 mg/dL in homozygotes (ZZ) deficient in this glycoprotein. Specific Pi genotyping should be done to confirm the diagnosis. Liver function tests often reflect underlying hepatic pathologic changes. Hyperbilirubinemia (mixed) and elevated aminotransferases, alkaline phosphatase, and γ-glutamyltranspeptidase are present early. Hyperbilirubinemia generally resolves, while aminotransferase elevation may persist. Signs of cirrhosis and portal hypertension may develop.

Liver biopsy shows diastase-resistant intracellular granules positive to periodic acid-Schiff staining, with hyaline masses, particularly in periportal zones.

Differential Diagnosis

In the newborn, other specific causes of neonatal cholestasis need to be considered. In the older child, other causes of insidious cirrhosis (eg, viral hepatitis A or B, autoimmune chronic active hepatitis, Wilson's disease, cystic fibrosis, glycogen storage disease) should be considered. If pulmonary symptoms predominate, then cystic fibrosis, immunodeficiency disease, tracheoesophageal anomalies, hiatal hernia, and hypoplastic pulmonary artery and lung disease should be considered.

Complications

Of all infants with Pi ZZ α_1-antitrypsin deficiency, only 20% develop liver disease in childhood. The complications of portal hypertension, cirrhosis, and chronic cholestasis predominate in affected children.

Early-onset pulmonary emphysema occurs in young adults (aged 30–40 years), particularly in smokers. An increased susceptibility to hepatocarcinoma has been noted in cirrhosis with α_1-antitrypsin deficiency.

Treatment

There is no specific treatment for the liver disease of this deficiency disorder. Affected infants who are breast-fed appear to have less severe liver disease. Replacement of the protein by transfusion therapy is successful in preventing pulmonary disease in affected adults. The neonatal cholestatic condition is treated with choleretics, medium-chain triglyceride-containing formula, and water-miscible vitamins (see Table 23–2). Portal hypertension, esophageal bleeding, ascites, and other complications are treated as described elsewhere. Genetic counseling is indicated whenever the diagnosis is made. Diagnosis by prenatal screening is possible. Liver transplantation has been shown to cure the deficiency.

Prognosis

Thirty to 50 percent of patients with liver injury either die from progressive liver disease or develop cirrhosis. A correlation between histologic patterns and clinical course has been documented in the infantile form of the disease. Liver failure can be expected 5–15 years after development of cirrhosis. Recurrence or persistence of hyperbilirubinemia along with worsening coagulation studies indicate the need for evaluation for possible liver transplantation. Decompensated cirrhosis caused by this disease is an excellent indication for liver transplantation; the survival rate is 70–90%.

Ibarguen E: Liver disease in alpha-1-antitrypsin deficiency: Prognostic indicators. J Pediatr 1990;117:864.

Schwarzenberg SJ, Sharp HL: Pathogenesis of alpha-1-antitrypsin deficiency-associated liver disease, 1990. J Pediatr Gastroenterol Nutr 1990;10:5.

Sharp HL: Alpha$_1$-antitrypsin: An ignored protein in understanding liver disease. Semin Liver Dis 1982;2:314.

Sveger T: Prospective study of children with alpha$_1$-antitrypsin deficiency: Eight-year old follow-up. J Pediatr 1984;104:91.

Wewers MD et al: Replacement therapy for alpha$_1$-antitrypsin deficiency associated with emphysema. N Engl J Med 1987;316:1055.

BILIARY TRACT DISEASE

1. CHOLELITHIASIS

Both calcium bilirubinate and cholesterol gallstones may develop at all ages in the pediatric population and in utero. Gallstone formation is a multifactorial process, the evolution of which is favored when the solubility of cholesterol (or calcium bilirubinate) in bile is exceeded. In the presence of poorly defined nucleation factors, cholesterol crystals begin to precipitate, incorporating proteins, mucus, and sometimes calcium bilirubinate as stone formation occurs. For some patients, gallbladder dysfunction is associated with biliary sludge formation, which may evolve into "sludge balls" or tumefaction bile and thence into gallstones. The process may be reversible in many patients.

Clinical Findings

A. History: Most symptomatic gallstones present with acute and recurrent episodes of moderate to severe, sharp epigastric or right upper quadrant pain. The pain may radiate substernally or to the right shoulder. On rare occasions, the presentation may include a history of jaundice, back pain, or generalized abdominal discomfort, where it is associated with pancreatitis, suggesting stone impaction in the common duct or ampulla hepatopancreatica. Nausea and vomiting may occur during attacks. Not infrequently, the pain episodes occur postprandially, and a relationship to the ingestion of fatty foods may be obtained but is not a consistent observation. The groups at risk for gallstones include the following: patients with known or suspected hemolytic disease (congenital spherocytosis, blacks with sickle cell disease); females; teenagers with prior pregnancy; obese individuals; certain racial or ethnic groups, particularly Native Americans (Pima Indians); Hispanics; and infants and children with ileal disease (Crohn's disease) or prior ileal resection. Fasting premature infants on prolonged parenteral hyperalimentation (with or without chronic furosemide therapy) are at particular risk for gallstone formation. Patients with cystic fibrosis or Wilson's disease also have an increased incidence of gallstones. Other, less certain risk factors include a positive family history, use of birth control pills, and diabetes mellitus.

B. Symptoms and Signs: During acute episodes of pain, tenderness in the upper abdomen, especially epigastric and right upper quadrant, can be elicited. Right flank pain may be noted. Referred pain is absent, as are peritoneal signs. The presence of scleral icterus should be sought. Evidence of underlying hemolytic disease in addition to icterus includes pallor (anemia), splenomegaly, tachycardia, and high-output cardiac murmur. Fever is unusual in uncomplicated cases.

C. Laboratory Findings: The white blood cell count is normal or slightly elevated. Liver function test results are not disturbed unless calculi have lodged in the extrahepatic biliary system, in which case elevated serum bilirubin and γ-glutamyl transpeptidase (or alkaline phosphatase) are noted. Serum pancreatic amylase may be increased if stone obstruction occurs at the ampulla hepatopancreatica.

D. Imaging: Plain abdominal x-rays are indicated in patients with acute, severe abdominal pain and may show calculi in the region of the gallbladder or bile ducts. Because most gallstones are radiolucent cholesterol stones, ultrasound evaluation is the diagnostic procedure of choice and reveals the presence of abnormal intraluminal contents (stones, sludge) as well as anatomic alterations of the gallbladder or dilation of the biliary ductal system. The presence of an anechoic acoustic shadow differentiates calculi from intraluminal sludge or sludge balls. Gallbladder function is best assessed by cholescintigraphy methods. Abdominal CT scanning may be helpful if tumor or other neighboring disease is suspected. Endoscopic retrograde cholangiopancreatography is particularly helpful in defining subtle abnormalities of the bile ducts and locating intraductal stones. In selected cases, therapeutic intervention such as sphincterotomy and stone removal can be done by endoscopic means.

Differential Diagnosis

Other abnormal conditions of the biliary system with similar presentation are summarized in Table 23–5. Liver disease (hepatitis, abscess, tumor, perihepatitis [Fitz-Hugh and Curtis syndrome]) can cause similar symptoms or signs. Peptic disease, reflux esophagitis, paraesophageal hiatal hernia, cardiac disease, and pneumomediastinum must be considered when the pain is epigastric or substernal in location. Renal or pancreatic disease is a possible explanation if the pain is located to the right flank or mid back. Subcapsular or supracapsular lesions of the liver (abscess, tumor, hematoma) or right lower lobe infiltrate may also be a cause of nontraumatic right shoulder pain.

Complications

Major problems are related to stone impaction in either the cystic or common duct and lead to stricture formation or perforation. Acute distention and subsequent perforation of the gallbladder may occur when gallstones cause obstruction of the cystic duct.

Exploration and surgical removal of calculi within the extrahepatic ducts requires T-tube drainage, and both procedures predispose the patient to bile duct stricture or ascending cholangitis. Stones impacted at the level of the ampulla hepatopancreatica often cause "gallstone pancreatitis."

Treatment

Symptomatic cholelithiasis is best treated by either open or laparoscopic cholecystectomy. Intraoperative cholangiography via the cystic duct is required so that the physician can be certain the ductal system is free of retained stones. Gallstones developing in premature infants being maintained on total parenteral nutrition can be followed by ultrasound examination. Most of the infants are asymptomatic, and the stones will resolve in 3–12 months. Gallstone dissolution using modalities such as cholelitholytics (ursodeoxycholic acid) or mechanical means (lithotripsy) has not been approved for use in children. Asymptomatic gallstones can be followed expectantly, because only 20% will eventually cause problems.

Prognosis

The prognosis is excellent in uncomplicated cases that come to surgery not requiring exploration and T-tube drainage of the common bile duct. Cystic duct "stump pain" is not reported to occur in the pediatric population.

Bowen JC et al: Gallstone disease: Pathophysiology, epidemiology, natural history, and treatment options. Med Clin North Am 1992;76:1143.

Debray D et al: Cholelithiasis in infancy: A study of 40 cases. J Pediatr 1993;122:385.

Sloven DG, Lebenthal E: Gallstones in children. Am J Dis Child 1991;145:105.

Ware RE et al: Laparoscopic cholecystectomy in young patients with sickle hemoglobinopathies. J Pediatr 1992; 120:58

Table 23-5. Biliary tract abnormalities.

	Acute Hydrops Transient Dilatation of Gallbladder[1,2]	Choledochal Cyst[3,4] (See Figure 23-1.)	Acalculous Cholecystitis[5]	Sclerosing Cholangitis[6,7,8]	Caroli's Disease[9] (Idiopathic Intrahepatic Bile Duct Dilatation)	Congenital Hepatic Fibrosis[10]
Predisposing or associated conditions	Premature infants with prolonged fasting or systemic illness. Hepatitis (giant cell, viral). Abnormalities of cystic duct. Kawasaki disease.	Congenital lesion. Female sex. Asians. Extrahepatic biliary atresia, idiopathic giant cell hepatitis. Rarely with Caroli's disease or congenital hepatic fibrosis.	Systemic illness, sepsis (*Streptococcus*, *Salmonella*, *Klebsiella*, etc). Gallbladder stasis, obstruction of cystic duct (stones, nodes, tumor).	Most have chronic ulcerative colitis (70%); 75% are males. Increased incidence of HLA-B8. Sicca syndrome, fibroinflammatory conditions, familial immunodeficiency syndrome.	Congenital lesion. Also found in congenital hepatic fibrosis or with choledochal cyst. Female sex. Autosomal recessive polycystic kidney disease.	Familial (autosomal recessive) 25% with autosomal recessive polycystic kidney disease. Choledochal cyst. Caroli's disease. Merkel-Gruber syndrome.
Symptoms	Absent in prematures. Vomiting, abdominal pain in older children.	Abdominal pain, vomiting, jaundice.	Acute severe abdominal pain, vomiting, fever.	Pruritus, jaundice, abdominal pain, fatigue.	Recurrent abdominal pain, vomiting. Fever, jaundice when cholangitis occurs.	Hematemesis, melena from bleeding esophageal varices.
Signs	Right upper quadrant abdominal mass. Tenderness in some.	Icterus, acholic stools, dark urine in neonatal period. Right upper quadrant abdominal mass or tenderness in older child.	Tenderness in midabdomen and right upper abdomen. Occasional palpable mass in right upper quadrant.	Icterus, hepatomegaly, splenomegaly.	Icterus, hepatomegaly.	Hepatosplenomegaly.
Laboratory abnormalities	Most are normal. Increased WBC count in sepsis (may be decreased in premature infants). Abnormal LFT's in hepatitis.	Conjugated hyperbilirubinemia, elevated GGTP, slightly increased AST. Elevated pancreatic serum amylase if ampulla hepatopancreatica is involved.	Elevated WBC, normal or slight abnormality of LFT's.	Elevated serum bile acids, bilirubin, GGTP. Slight elevation of AST.	Abnormal LFT's. Increased WBC with cholangitis. Urine abnormalities if associated with CHF.	Low platelet and WBC count (hypersplenism), slight elevation of AST, GGTP. Inability to concentrate urine.
Diagnostic studies most useful	Gallbladder ultrasound.	Gallbladder ultrasound hepatobiliary scintigraphy, and ERCP.	Scintigraphy to confirm nonfunction of gallbladder. Ultrasound or abdominal CT scan to rule out other neighboring disease.	Ultrasound of the biliary tree, ERCP, scintigraphy.	Transhepatic cholangiography, ERCP, scintigraphy, ultrasound, intravenous pyelography.	Liver biopsy (open is best). Ultrasound liver and kidneys. Upper endoscopy, splenoportogram.
Treatment	Treatment of associated condition. Needle or tube cystostomy may be required. Cholecystectomy seldom indicated.	Surgical resection rather than simple drainage.	Broad-spectrum antibiotic coverage, then cholecystectomy or cholecystostomy drainage and definitive surgery 3–4 weeks later.	Ursodeoxycholic acid, cholestyramine, immunosuppressive drugs, isomethotrexate. Liver transplant.	Antibiotics and surgical or endoscopic drainage for cholangitis. Liver transplant for some. Lobectomy for localized disease.	Endosclerosis or endoscopic ligation of varices, portacaval shunt. Liver transplantation.

(continued)

665

Table 23–5. Biliary tract abnormalities. (continued)

Complications	Perforation with bile peritonitis rare.	Progressive biliary cirrhosis. Increased incidence of cholangiocarcinoma. Cholangitis in some.	Perforation and bile peritonitis, sepsis, abscess or fistula formation. Pancreatitis.	Progressive biliary cirrhosis, portal hypertension, liver failure.	Sepsis with episodes of cholangitis, biliary cirrhosis, portal hypertension. Intraductal stones. Cholangiocarcinoma.	Bleeding from varices. Splenic rupture, severe thrombocytopenia. Progressive renal failure.
Prognosis	Excellent with resolution of underlying condition. Consider cystic duct obstruction if disorder fails to resolve.	Depends upon anatomic type of cyst, associated condition, and success of surgery. Liver transplant may be needed in some.	Good with early diagnosis and treatment.	Guarded; disease progression is expected even with medical treatment. Course not changed by colectomy.	Poor, with gradual deterioration of liver function. Multiple surgical drainage procedures expected. Liver transplant should alter long-term prognosis.	Good in absence of serious renal involvement and with control of portal hypertension. Slightly increased risk to cholangiocarcinoma. Liver/kidney transplant for some.

Ultrasound = refers to liver and biliary tract scanning; scintigraphy = refers to hepatobiliary scan using radiolabelled ^{99m}technetium; CHF = congenital hepatic fibrosis; ERCP = endoscopic retrograde cholangiopancreatography; LFT = liver function test; GGTP = gamma-glutamyl transpeptidase; AST = aspartate aminotransferase (SGOT); WBC = white blood count.

[1]Bowen A: Acute gallbladder dilatation in a neonate: Emphasis on ultrasonography. J Pediatr Gastroenterol Nutr 1984;3:304.
[2]Suddleson E et al: Hydrops of the gallbladder associated with Kawasaki syndrome. J. Pediatr Surg 1987;22:956.
[3]Kim S: Choledochal cyst: Survey by the Surgical Section of the American Academy of Pediatrics. J Pediatr Surg 1981;16:402.
[4]Sherman P et al: Choledochal cysts: Heterogeneity of clinical presentation. J Pediatr Gastroenterol Nutr 1986;5:867.
[5]Holcomb GW, O'Neill J Jr, Holcomb GW III: Cholecystitis, cholelithiasis and common duct stenosis in children and adolescents. Ann Surg 1980;191:626.
[6]El-Shabrawi M et al: Primary sclerosing cholangitis in childhood. Gastroenterology 1987;92:1226.
[7]LaRusso NF et al: Primary sclerosing cholangitis. N Engl J Med 1984;310:899.
[8]Sisto A et al: Primary sclerosing cholangitis in children: Study of 5 cases and review of the literature. Pediatrics 1987;80:918.
[9]Fagundes-Neto U et al: Caroli's disease in childhood: Report of 2 new cases. J Pediatr Gastroenterol Nutr 1983;2:708.
[10]Alvarez F et al: Congenital hepatic fibrosis in children. J Pediatr 1981;99:370.

2. ACUTE HYDROPS, CHOLEDOCHAL CYST, ACALCULOUS CHOLECYSTITIS, SCLEROSING CHOLANGITIS, CAROLI'S DISEASE, CONGENITAL HEPATIC FIBROSIS
(See Table 23–5.)

For a schematic representation of the various types of choledochal cysts, see Figure 23–1. See also the references associated with Table 23–5.

PYOGENIC & AMEBIC LIVER ABSCESS

Pyogenic liver abscesses are usually secondary to bacterial seeding via the portal vein from infected viscera and occasionally from ascending cholangitis or gangrenous cholecystitis. Solitary or mixed flora of intestinal origin (aerobes and anaerobes) are usually grown from aspirated material. Blood cultures are frequently positive in up to 60% of cases. The resulting lesion tends to be solitary and located in the right hepatic lobe. Bacterial seeding may also occur from infected burns, pyodermas, and osteomyelitis. Unusual causes include omphalitis, subacute infective endocarditis, pyelonephritis, and perinephric abscess. Multiple pyogenic liver abscesses are associated with severe sepsis. At particular risk are children receiving anti-inflammatory and immunosuppressive agents.

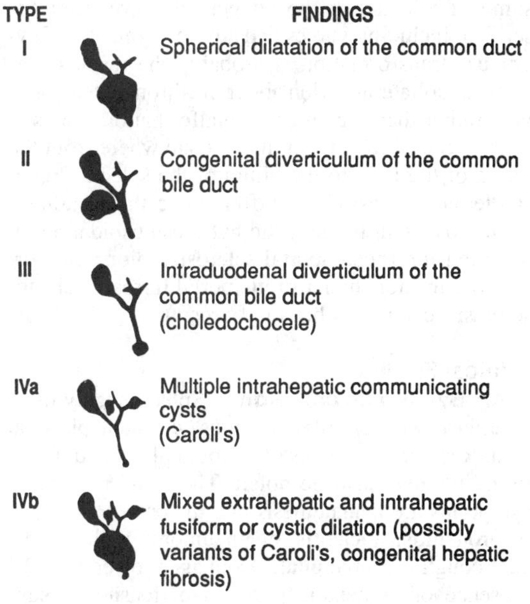

TYPE		FINDINGS
I		Spherical dilatation of the common duct
II		Congenital diverticulum of the common bile duct
III		Intraduodenal diverticulum of the common bile duct (choledochocele)
IVa		Multiple intrahepatic communicating cysts (Caroli's)
IVb		Mixed extrahepatic and intrahepatic fusiform or cystic dilation (possibly variants of Caroli's, congenital hepatic fibrosis)

Figure 23–1. Classification of cystic dilation of the bile ducts. Types I, II, and III are extrahepatic. Type IVa is solely intrahepatic, and type IVb is both intra- and extra-hepatic.

Likewise, children with defects in white blood cell function (chronic granulomatous disease) are more prone to pyogenic hepatic abscesses, especially those due to *Staphylococcus aureus*. In adults there is a male preponderance, and the abscesses are usually solitary.

Although amebic liver abscess is still rare in children, an increase in frequency has been noted, presumably as a result of increased travel through endemic areas (Mexico, Southeast Asia). *Entamoeba histolytica* invasion occurs via the large bowel, though a history of diarrhea (colitis-like picture) is not always obtained.

Clinical Findings

With pyogenic liver abscess, nonspecific complaints of low-grade to septic fever, chills, malaise, and abdominal pain are frequent. Weight loss is very common, especially in delayed diagnosis. A few patients have shaking chills and jaundice. The dominant complaint is a constant dull pain over an enlarged liver that is tender to palpation. An elevated hemidiaphragm with reduced or absent respiratory excursion may be demonstrated on physical examination and confirmed by fluoroscopy. Laboratory studies show leukocytosis and, at times, anemia. Liver function tests reveal low-grade bilirubin elevation and an elevated alkaline phosphatase. Elevated vitamin B_{12} levels are reported. Amebic liver abscesses are usually heralded by an acute illness with high fever, chills, and leukocytosis. Early in the course, liver tests may suggest mild hepatitis. An occasional prodrome may include cough, dyspnea, and shoulder pain as rupture of the abscess into the right chest occurs. Consolidation of the right lower lobe is common (30%).

Ultrasound liver scan is the most useful diagnostic aid in evaluating pyogenic and amebic abscesses, detecting lesions as small as 1–2 cm. Nuclear scanning with gallium or technetium sulfur colloid or CT imaging may be useful to differentiate tumor or hydatid cyst.

The distinction between pyogenic and amebic abscesses is best made by indirect hemagglutination test (which is positive in more than 95% of patients with amebic liver disease) and the prompt response of the latter to antiamebic therapy (metronidazole). Examination of material obtained by needle aspiration of the abscess using ultrasound guidance is often diagnostic.

Differential Diagnosis

Hepatitis, hepatoma, hydatid cyst, gallbladder disease, or biliary tract infections can mimic liver abscess. Subphrenic abscesses, empyema, and pneumonia may give a similar picture. Inflammatory disease of the intestines or of the biliary system may be complicated by liver abscess.

Complications

Spontaneous rupture of the abscess may occur with extension of infection into the subphrenic space, thorax, peritoneal cavity, and, occasionally, the pericardium. Bronchopleural fistula with large sputum production and hemoptysis can develop in severe cases. Simultaneously, the amebic liver abscess may be secondarily infected with bacteria (10–20% of cases). Metastatic hematogenous spread to the lungs and brain has been reported.

Treatment

When a solitary pyogenic liver abscess is suspected, needle aspiration using ultrasound guidance should be attempted. The decision regarding surgical drainage versus antibiotic treatment alone is best made on clinical grounds. Cultures (aerobic and anaerobic) are taken and specific antibiotic therapy started. Both solitary and multiple pyogenic liver abscesses can be treated by medical means.

Amebic abscesses should be treated promptly. Only those that are sufficiently large and threaten to rupture need to be aspirated. Uncomplicated cases can be treated with oral metronidazole, 30–50 mg/kg/d in three divided doses for 10 days. Intravenous metronidazole can be used in patients unable to take oral medication. In severe cases, give dehydroemetine, 1–1.5 mg/kg/d intramuscularly for 5 days, and chloroquine, 10–20 mg/kg/d in one or two divided doses for 21 days. Failure to improve after 72 hours of drug therapy indicates superimposed bacterial infection or an incorrect diagnosis. At this point, needle aspiration or surgical drainage is indicated. Once oral feedings can be tolerated, a 10-day course of diloxanide furoate (20 mg/kg/d in three doses) is started as a luminal amebicide. Resolution of the abscess cavity occurs over 3–6 months.

Prognosis

An unrecognized and untreated pyogenic liver abscess is universally fatal. The surgical cure rate is about 75%. Most amebic abscesses are cured with conservative medical management; the mortality rate is less than 3%. If extrahepatic complications occur (empyema, bronchopleural fistula, pericardial complications), 10–15% of patients will succumb.

Harrison HR, Crowe CP, Fulginiti VA: Amebic liver abscess in children: Clinical and epidemiologic features. Pediatrics 1979;64:923.

Knight R: Hepatic amebiasis. In: *Seminars in Liver Disease: Infectious Agents as Causes of Liver Diseases*, vol 4. Burke PD, Zuckerman AJ (editors). Thieme-Stratton, 1984.

Pineiro-Carrero VM, Andres AM: Morbidity and mortality in children with pyogenic liver disease: Am J Dis Child 1991;143:991.

Stain C et al: Pyogenic liver abscess: Modern treatment. Ann Surg 1991;126:991.

Thompson JE Jr, Forlenza S, Verma R: Amebic liver abscess: A therapeutic approach. Rev Infect Dis 1985; 7:171.

PREHEPATIC PORTAL HYPERTENSION

Essentials of Diagnosis

- Splenomegaly.
- Esophageal varices with hematemesis or melena.
- Elevated splenic pulp pressure.
- Normal wedge hepatic vein pressure.
- Normal liver histology.
- Impaired patency of splenic and portal veins shown by duplex Doppler ultrasound scanning, splenoportography, and venous phase of superior mesenteric or splenic angiography.

General Considerations

Prehepatic portal hypertension from acquired abnormalities of the portal and splenic veins accounts for 5–8% of cases of gastrointestinal bleeding in children. A history of neonatal omphalitis, sepsis, dehydration, and umbilical vein catheterization is present in 30–50% of cases. Less common known causes in older children include local trauma, peritonitis (pylephlebitis), and pancreatitis. Symptoms may occur before 1 year of age, but in most cases the diagnosis is not made until 3–5 years of age. Those with a positive neonatal history tend to become symptomatic earlier. Splenomegaly is often the first abnormal physical finding. Massive hematemesis or melena occurs within a few years.

A variety of portal or splenic vein malformations, some of which may be congenital, have been described, including valves and atretic segments. "Cavernous" transformation is probably the result of attempted collateralization about the thrombosed portal vein rather than a congenital malformation. The site of the venous obstruction may be anywhere from the hilum of the liver to the hilum of the spleen. Proper studies are necessary to differentiate this condition from those with intrahepatic but presinusoidal portal hypertension (hepatoportal sclerosis, idiopathic portal hypertension, noncirrhotic portal fibrosis, schistosomiasis, congenital hepatic fibrosis).

Clinical Findings

A. Symptoms and Signs: Splenomegaly in an otherwise well child is the most constant physical sign. Recurrent episodes of abdominal distention due to ascites may also be noted. The usual presenting symptoms are hematemesis and melena. An episode of bronchitis, tracheitis, or pneumonia with significant cough can precipitate esophageal bleeding. The presence of prehepatic portal hypertension is suggested by the following: (1) an episode of severe infection in the newborn period or early infancy—especially omphalitis, sepsis, gastroenteritis, severe dehydration, or prolonged or difficult umbilical vein catheterizations; (2) no previous evidence of liver disease; and (3) a history of well-being prior to onset or recognition of symptoms. In addition, transient ascites may occur following a bleeding episode.

B. Laboratory Findings and Imaging: Most other common causes of splenomegaly may be excluded by proper laboratory tests. Cultures, Epstein-Barr virus titers, blood smear examination, bone marrow studies, and liver function tests are necessary. Hypersplenism with mild leukopenia and thrombocytopenia are present in most cases. Fiberoptic esophagoscopy will reveal varices in symptomatic patients. In addition to normal liver function tests, confirmation of a normal liver is best obtained directly by liver biopsy or indirectly by measurement of wedge hepatic vein pressure (normal, 3–12 mm Hg). The finding of an elevated splenic pulp pressure (normal, 8–12 mm Hg) and demonstration of the block by simultaneous splenic portography confirm the diagnosis of prehepatic portal hypertension. Filling of collateral vessels to stomach and esophagus by the dye is frequently demonstrated. Selective arteriography using the superior mesenteric artery is recommended prior to definitive surgery to determine the patency of the superior mesenteric vein. Hypercoagulability due to antithrombin III, protein C, or protein S deficiency should be considered in the "idiopathic group."

Differential Diagnosis

All causes of splenomegaly must be included in the differential diagnosis, the most common ones being infections, blood dyscrasias, lipidosis, reticuloendotheliosis, cirrhosis of the liver, and cysts or hemangiomas of the spleen. When hematemesis or melena occurs, other causes of gastrointestinal bleeding are possible, ie, gastric or duodenal ulcers, tumors, Meckel's diverticulum, duplications, inflammatory bowel disease, and suprahepatic or hepatic venous obstructions.

Complications

The major manifestation and complication of this condition is bleeding esophageal varices. Fatal exsanguination appears to be uncommon, but hypovolemic shock or resulting anemia may require prompt treatment. Congestive splenomegaly with granulocytopenia and thrombocytopenia occurs but seldom causes major symptoms. Rupture of the enlarged spleen due to trauma is always a threat. Unexplained fluctuating episodes of ascites may develop, and retroperitoneal edema has been reported (Clatworthy's sign).

Treatment

A. Surgical Measures: Except in specialized centers, the surgical treatment of this disease has been disappointing. Portacaval anastomosis would be the most satisfactory procedure, but the portal vein is often involved in the basic disease process, making it unsuitable for anastomosis except in rare cases. Children have previously been treated by means of simultaneous splenectomy and splenorenal shunts. Sustained patency of the shunt is unlikely in children under the age of 8–10 years except when it is placed by an experienced surgeon. Thrombosis of the shunt is soon followed by recurrent and often more severe hemorrhage from esophageal varices. Splenectomy increases the risk of overwhelming sepsis. More importantly, however, it removes a "safe" group of collateral vessels running from the splenic capsule to the azygos veins, thereby bypassing the esophageal and gastric drainage system. Partial splenectomy or splenic embolization of one-third to one-half of the organ reduces concerns about traumatic rupture and improves the leukopenia and thrombocytopenia.

Other surgical decompression procedures include anastomosis of the superior mesenteric vein to the inferior vena cava (mesocaval shunt), distal splenorenal shunt (Warren procedure), and the interposition mesocaval shunt using knitted Dacron or Teflon for the graft. Esophageal and gastric resection of the varices and transthoracic ligation of the varices have been used as more desperate measures.

B. Medical Treatment: Because a few children with this disease will die as a result of esophageal bleeding, every effort should be made to control the disease medically. The chances for successful surgical shunting procedures improve as the child gets older. In addition, the patient may spontaneously develop a decompressive shunt adequate to prevent major bleeding from the esophageal varices.

Spontaneous cessation of hemorrhage from esophageal varices occurs frequently. Shock must be treated with crystalloid or colloid and then with blood transfusions. Platelet transfusions may be indicated if counts are below 10,000/μL. Gastric irrigation with iced 0.5% saline solution may help.

Early fiberoptic endoscopy is indicated to confirm the source of hemorrhage and, if possible, permit immediate treatment of ongoing bleeding. Intravariceal or paravariceal injection of a sclerosing agent or endoscopic variceal ligation is otherwise performed within 2–3 days after cessation of bleeding via the endoscope or via a rigid esophagoscope. Additional sessions may be needed to control the acute bleeding. Thereafter, elective sclerotherapy or ligation therapy is utilized to attempt obliteration of the varices.

A transient reduction of portal venous pressure may be achieved by the use of intravenous vasopressin. A dose of 0.1–0.3 unit/min given intravenously often stops the bleeding by constricting the splanchnic and hepatic arterioles and lowering portal venous pressure. Hypertension, bradycardia, diminished cardiac output, water retention, hyponatremia, and pulmonary edema may occur with this form of treatment. Transdermal nitroglycerin may reduce some of these side effects. Careful use of a pediatric Sengstaken-Blakemore tube can effectively stop the bleeding in over 90% of cases. In desperate cases, selective venous embolization can be life-saving but requires a minilaparotomy for access to the vessel in question.

An intravenous H_2 blocking agent is employed during the acute episode to reduce gastric acid output and its erosive effect on the varices by way of gastroesophageal reflux. Antitussive agents (eg, codeine) may be used when cough is excessive. Avoidance of contact sports in the presence of splenomegaly is advisable. Aspirin products should be avoided. Propranolol, a β-adrenergic antagonist, may reduce the risk of subsequent bleeding by lowering venous pressure in the portal drainage system.

Prognosis

The prognosis depends upon the site of the block, the effectiveness of sclerotherapy, the availability of suitable vessels for shunting procedures, and the experience of the surgeon. Each unsuccessful surgical procedure worsens the prognosis for life. In patients managed by medical means, bleeding episodes seem to diminish with adolescence.

The prognosis in patients managed by medical and supportive therapy may be better than in the surgically treated group, especially when surgery is performed at an early age. Portacaval encephalopathy is unusual in the postshunted child except when protein intake is excessive.

Alvarez F et al: Portal obstruction in children. (Two parts.) J Pediatr 1983;103:696, 703.

Bernard O et al: Portal hypertension in children. Clin Gastroenterol 1985;14:33.

Mowat AP: Prevention of variceal bleeding. J Pediatr Gastroenterol Nutr 1986;5:679.

Stiegmann GV et al: Endoscopic variceal ligation: An alternative of sclerotherapy. Gastrointest Endosc 1989;35:431.

SUPRAHEPATIC & INTRAHEPATIC (NONCIRRHOTIC) PORTAL HYPERTENSION

Etiologic Classification

In the absence of cirrhosis, suprahepatic or intrahepatic causes of portal hypertension are rare. The following entities should be considered.

A. Suprahepatic Vein Occlusion or Thrombosis (Budd-Chiari Syndrome): In most instances, no cause can be demonstrated. Endothelial injury to hepatic veins by bacterial endotoxins has been demonstrated experimentally. The occasional association of hepatic vein thrombosis in inflammatory bowel disease favors the presence of endogenous toxins traversing the liver. Allergic vasculitis leading to endophlebitis of the hepatic veins has been occasionally described. In addition, hepatic vein obstruction may be secondary to tumor, abdominal trauma,

hyperthermia, or sepsis, or it may occur following the repair of an omphalocele or gastroschisis. Congenital vena caval bands, webs, a membrane, or strictures above the hepatic veins are sometimes causative. Hepatic vein thrombosis may be a complication of oral contraceptive medications. Underlying thrombotic conditions (antithrombin III, protein C, or protein S deficiency) should be considered.

B. Intrahepatic Veno-occlusive Disease (Acute Stage): This entity is often the result of ingestion of pyrrolizidine alkaloids ("bush tea"), which causes widespread occlusion of the small- and medium-sized hepatic veins, with congestion and necrosis of the neighboring parenchymal cells. A familial form of the disease occurs in congenital immunodeficiency states. The disorder may develop after chemotherapy for acute leukemia. Veno-occlusive disease is being seen with increased frequency in patients who have undergone bone marrow transplantation.

The acute form of the disease generally follows a nonspecific respiratory illness. The disease may be rapidly fatal, though about 50% of patients recover. Subacute and chronic forms also exist. Increased use of herbal teas in the USA has been responsible for several reported cases.

C. Congenital Hepatic Fibrosis: This rare cause of intrahepatic presinusoidal portal hypertension is inherited as an autosomal recessive and usually requires open liver biopsy for diagnosis (Table 23–5). Splenoportography reveals patency of the portal venous system even though splenic pulp pressure is increased. The intrahepatic branches of the portal vein may be abnormal (duplicated). Renal abnormalities (microcystic disease) are often associated with the hepatic lesion; therefore, renal ultrasound and urography should be routinely performed.

D. Hepatoportal Sclerosis (Idiopathic Portal Hypertension, Noncirrhotic Portal Fibrosis), Noncirrhotic Nodular Transformation of the Liver, and Schistosomal Hepatic Fibrosis: These are also rare causes of intrahepatic presinusoidal portal hypertension.

Clinical, Laboratory, & Radiographic Findings

Most patients with suprahepatic portal hypertension present with abdominal enlargement due to ascites. Some have firm hepatomegaly. Abdominal pain and tender hepatosplenomegaly are frequently found. Jaundice is present in about 25% of cases. Vomiting, hematemesis, and diarrhea are less common. Cutaneous signs of chronic liver disease are lacking because the obstruction is usually acute. The presence of distended superficial veins on the back and anterior abdomen, along with dependent edema, is usually seen with inferior vena cava obstruction affecting hepatic vein outflow. Absence of hepatojugular reflux (jugular distention when pressure is applied to the liver) is a helpful clinical sign. Liver function tests are not usually helpful; liver function tends to be better preserved in other causes of this disorder than in the membranous obstruction of the Budd-Chiari syndrome. Localization is difficult. An inferior vena-cavogram using catheters from above or below the suspected obstruction may reveal an intrinsic filling defect, an infiltrating tumor, or extrinsic pressure and obstruction of the inferior vena cava by an adjacent lesion. A large caudate lobe of the liver suggests Budd-Chiari syndrome. Care must be taken in interpreting extrinsic pressure defects of the subdiaphragmatic inferior vena cava in the face of significant ascites.

Duplex Doppler-assisted ultrasound scanning of the suprahepatic inferior vena cava and the hepatic veins may be diagnostic of intrinsic disease. Simultaneous wedge hepatic vein pressure and hepatic venography are also useful procedures. Obstruction to major hepatic vein ostia and smaller vessels may be demonstrated by this procedure. In the absence of obstruction, reflux across the sinusoids into the portal vein branches can be accomplished. Pressures should also be taken from the right heart and supradiaphragmatic portion of the inferior vena cava. These should eliminate constrictive pericarditis and pulmonary hypertension from the differential diagnosis. Hepatic vein pressure is elevated to a greater degree than portal vein and splenic pulp pressure. In most instances, a liver biopsy should be done. Marked central venous congestion and necrosis without fibrosis are striking. Endothelial thickening of hepatic veins may also be found.

Differential Diagnosis

Because ascites is almost always present, cirrhosis due to any cause must be excluded. Suprahepatic (cardiac and pulmonary) or prehepatic causes of portal hypertension must also be excluded. Although ascites may occur in prehepatic portal hypertension, it is not common.

Complications

Without treatment, complete and persistent hepatic vein obstruction leads to liver failure, coma, and death. A nonportal type of cirrhosis may develop in the chronic form of hepatic veno-occlusive disease in which small- and medium-sized hepatic veins are affected. Hematemesis due to bleeding esophageal varices is frequent in the few survivors. Death from renal failure may occur in rare cases of congenital hepatic fibrosis.

Treatment

Efforts to correct underlying causes must be undertaken promptly. Surgical removal of the occluding tumor or of the hepatic vein thrombi is possible when the large ostia are involved. Transcardiac membranotomy can be attempted when the obstruction lies in the inferior vena cava. Mesocaval and portacaval

shunts and right atrial to inferior vena cava grafts have been attempted. Liver transplant should be seriously considered in refractory cases not amenable to other forms of surgical correction. Medical management with heparin, corticosteroids, and diuretics has had inconsistent results. Simple portacaval shunting is the treatment of choice in patients with congenital hepatic fibrosis and may be done prophylactically or after an esophageal bleed.

Prognosis

The mortality rate of hepatic vein obstruction is very high—95%. In veno-occlusive disease, the prognosis is better, with complete recovery possible in 50% of acute forms and 5–10% of subacute forms.

Etzioni A et al: Defective humoral and cellular immune functions associated with veno-occlusive disease of the liver. J Pediatr 1987;110:549.

Gentil-Kocher S et al: Budd-Chiari syndrome in children: Report of 22 cases. J Pediatr 1988;113:30.

Shulman HM et al: An analysis of hepatic venocclusive disease and centrilobular hepatic degeneration following bone marrow transplantation. Gastroenterology 1980;79:1178.

HEPATOMAS

Essentials of Diagnosis

- Abdominal enlargement and pain, weight loss, anemia.
- Hepatomegaly with or without a definable mass.
- Laparotomy and tissue biopsy.

General Considerations

Primary epithelial neoplasms of the liver represent 0.2–5.8% of all malignant conditions in the pediatric age group. After Wilms' tumor and neuroblastoma, it is the third most common intra-abdominal cancer. The incidence is higher in Southeast Asia, where childhood cirrhosis is more common. There are two basic morphologic types with certain clinical and prognostic differences. Hepatoblastoma predominates in male infants and children, with most cases appearing before age 3. Most lesions are found in the right lobe of the liver. Pathologic differentiation from hepatocarcinoma may be difficult.

Hepatocarcinoma, the other major malignant tumor of the liver, occurs more frequently after age 3. This type of neoplasm carries a poorer prognosis than hepatoblastoma and causes more abdominal discomfort. Hepatocarcinoma has been reported in chronic carriers of hepatitis B virus and in those with postnecrotic cirrhosis or biliary cirrhosis, but these are the exceptions rather than the rule. Patients with glycogen storage disease type I have an increased risk for hepatic adenoma and carcinoma. The association of hepatocarcinoma with tyrosinemia or α_1-antitrypsin deficiency cirrhosis has also been reported. The late development of hepatoma in patients treated with androgens for de Toni-Fanconi syndrome and aplastic anemia must also be kept in mind. The increased use of anabolic steroids by body-conscious adolescents poses a risk of hepatic neoplasia. An interesting aspect of primary epithelial neoplasms of the liver has been the increased incidence of associated anomalies and unusual conditions found in these children. Virilization has been reported as a consequence of gonadotropin activity of the tumor. Feminization with bilateral gynecomastia may occur in association with high estradiol levels in blood, the latter a consequence of increased aromatization of circulating androgens by the liver. Leydig cell hyperplasia without spermatogenesis is found on testicular biopsy. Hemihypertrophy, congenital absence of the kidney, macroglossia, and Meckel's diverticulum have been found in association with hepatocarcinoma.

Clinical Findings

A. History: Noticeable increase in abdominal girth with or without pain is the most constant feature of the history. A parent may note a "bulge" in the upper abdomen or report feeling a hard mass. Constitutional symptoms (anorexia, fatigue, fever, chills, etc) may be present. A teenage male may complain of gynecomastia.

B. Symptoms and Signs: Weight loss, pallor, and abdominal pain associated with a large abdomen are common. Physical examination reveals hepatomegaly with or without a definite tumor mass, usually to the right of the midline. Signs of chronic liver disease are usually absent. However, evidence of virilization or feminization in prepubertal children may be noted.

C. Laboratory Findings: Normal to slightly distorted liver function tests are the rule. Anemia is frequently seen, especially in cases of hepatoblastoma. Cystathioninuria has been reported. Alphafetoprotein levels may be elevated, especially in hepatoblastoma. Elevated estradiol levels are sometimes seen. Final tissue diagnosis is best obtained at laparotomy, though some physicians utilize fine needle aspiration of the liver mass guided either by ultrasound or CT.

D. Imaging: Plain abdominal x-ray is at times helpful in demonstrating the tumor shadow or calcified foci in the neoplasm. Ultrasound, CT, and MRI are useful for diagnosis and for following tumor response to therapy. A scintigraphic study of bone and lung and selective angiography are generally part of the preoperative workup to evaluate metastatic disease.

Differential Diagnosis

In the absence of a palpable mass, the differential diagnosis is that of hepatomegaly with or without anemia or jaundice. Hematologic and nutritional conditions should be ruled out, as well as α_1-antitrypsin deficiency disease, lipid storage diseases, histiocytosis X, glycogen storage disease, tyrosinemia, congenital hepatic fibrosis, hepatic abscess (pyogenic or amebic), cysts, adenoma, focal nodular hyperplasia, inflammatory pseudotumor, and hemangiomas. If fever is present, hepatic abscess (pyogenic or amebic) must be considered. Veno-occlusive disease and hepatic vein thrombosis are also rare possibilities. Tumors in the left lobe may be mistaken for pancreatic pseudocysts.

Complications

Progressive enlargement of the tumor, abdominal discomfort, ascites, respiratory difficulty, and widespread metastases (especially to lungs and abdominal lymph nodes) are the rule. Rupture of the neoplastic liver and intraperitoneal hemorrhage have been reported. Progressive anemia and emaciation predispose to an early septic death.

Treatment

An energetic surgical approach has resulted in the only long-term survivals. Complete resection of the lesion offers the only chance for cure. It appears that every isolated lung metastasis should also be surgically resected. Radiotherapy and chemotherapy have been disappointing in the treatment of primary liver neoplasms, though new combinations of drugs are continually being evaluated. These modalities are also used for initial cytoreduction of tumors found unresectable at the time of primary surgery. Second-look celiotomy has in some cases allowed resection of the tumor, resulting in a reduced mortality rate. Organ transplantation has been disappointing but continues to be performed in selected patients. The survival rate may be better for those patients in which the tumor is incidental to another disorder (tyrosinemia, biliary atresia, cirrhosis).

Prognosis

The survival rate if the tumor is completely removed is 60% for hepatoblastoma and 33% for hepatocellular carcinoma. Fibrolamellar oncocytic hepatocarcinoma has a more favorable prognosis. The overall survival and cure rate is less than 20%.

Ehren H, Mahour GH, Isaacs H: Benign liver tumors in infancy and childhood. Am J Surg 1983;145:325.

Haas JE et al: Histopathology and prognosis in childhood heptatoblastoma and hepatocellular cancer. Cancer 1989; 64:1082.

Mahour GH et al: Improved survival in infants and children with primary malignant liver tumors. Am J Surg 1983; 146:236.

Ni YH et al: Hepatocellular cancer in children: Clinical manifestations and prognosis. Cancer 1991;68:1737.

WILSON'S DISEASE
(Hepatolenticular Degeneration)

Essentials of Diagnosis

- Acute or chronic liver disease.
- Deteriorating neurologic status.
- Kayser-Fleischer rings.
- Elevated liver copper.
- Abnormalities in levels of ceruloplasmin and serum and urine copper.

General Considerations

In Wilson's disease, the increased hepatic copper may be due to an abnormal copper-binding protein or to a lysosomal defect that impairs the excretion of biliary copper. The disease should be considered in all children with evidence of liver disease or with suggestive neurologic signs. A family history is often present, and 25% of cases are identified by screening asymptomatic homozygous family members. The disease is autosomal recessive, occurs in 1:30,000 live births, and the gene defect is localized to chromosome 13.

Clinical Findings

A. Symptoms and Signs: Hepatic involvement may be fulminant, may masquerade as chronic active liver disease, or may progress insidiously to postnecrotic cirrhosis. Findings include jaundice, hepatomegaly early in childhood, splenomegaly, Kayser-Fleischer rings, and neurologic manifestations such as tremor, dysarthria, and drooling beginning after 10 years of age. Deterioration in school performance is often the earliest neurologic expression of disease. Psychiatric symptoms may also occur. The Kayser-Fleischer rings can sometimes be detected by unaided visual inspection as a brown band at the junction of the iris and cornea, but slitlamp examination is always necessary. Absence of Kayser-Fleischer rings does not exclude this diagnosis unless neurologic signs are present.

B. Laboratory Findings: The laboratory diagnosis is sometimes difficult. Serum ceruloplasmin levels are usually less than 20 mg/dL. (Normal values are 23–43 mg/dL.) Low values, however, are seen normally in infants under 3 months of age, and in 3–5% of homozygotes the levels may be low-normal. Serum copper levels are low, but the overlap with normal is too great for satisfactory discrimination. In acute fulminant Wilson's disease, serum copper levels are markedly elevated owing to hepatic necrosis and release of copper. The presence of anemia, hemolysis, very high serum bilirubin (> 20–30 mg/dL), and low alkaline phosphatase are characteristic of acute Wilson's disease. Urine copper excretion in children over 3 years of age is normally less than 30 µg/d; in Wilson's disease, it is greater than 190 µg/d. Finally, the tissue content of copper from a liver bi-

opsy, normally less than 20 µg/g wet tissue, is greater than 250 µg/g in Wilson's disease.

Glycosuria, aminoaciduria, and depressed serum uric acid levels have been reported. Hemolysis and gallstones may be present; bone lesions simulating those of osteochondritis dissecans have also been found.

The coarse nodular cirrhosis and glycogen nuclei seen on liver biopsy may distinguish Wilson's disease from other types of cirrhosis. Early in the disease, vacuolation of liver cells, steatosis, and lipofuscin granules can be seen, as well as Mallory bodies. The presence of the latter in a child is strongly suggestive of Wilson's disease. Stains for copper may sometimes be negative despite high copper content in the liver. Therefore, liver copper levels must be determined on biopsy specimens.

Differential Diagnosis

During the icteric phase, acute viral hepatitis, α_1-antitrypsin deficiency, chronic active hepatitis, Indian childhood cirrhosis, and drug-induced hepatitis are the usual diagnostic possibilities. Later, other causes of cirrhosis and portal hypertension need consideration. Laboratory testing for serum ceruloplasmin, urine copper excretion, and liver copper concentration will differentiate Wilson's disease from the others. The radiocopper ceruloplasmin incorporation test is sometimes needed to differentiate Wilson's disease with a normal ceruloplasmin level from other liver disease with increased liver and urine copper values. Urinary copper excretion during penicillamine challenge may help differentiate Wilson's disease from other causes.

Complications

Progressive liver disease, postnecrotic cirrhosis, hepatic coma, and death are not uncommon in the untreated patient. The complications of portal hypertension (variceal hemorrhage, ascites) are poorly tolerated by these patients. Progressive degenerating central nervous system disease and terminal aspiration pneumonia are common in untreated older people. Acute hemolytic disease may result in renal impairment and profound jaundice as part of the presentation of fulminant hepatitis.

Treatment

Penicillamine, 1000–2000 mg/d orally, is the drug of choice in all cases, whether symptomatic or not. It is best to begin with 250 mg/d and increase the dose weekly by 250-mg increments. The target dose is 20 mg/kg/d. Dietary restriction of copper intake is not practical. Supplementation with zinc sulfate may reduce copper absorption. Penicillamine is continued for life, though doses may be transiently reduced at the time of surgery or early in pregnancy. Vitamin B_6 (25 mg) is given daily while on penicillamine to prevent optic neuritis. For patients who cannot tolerate penicillamine, trientine hydrochloride is effective at a dose of 1–1.5 g/d.

General treatment measures for acute hepatitis are as outlined for infectious hepatitis. Liver transplantation is indicated for all cases of acute fulminant disease, progressive hepatic decompensation despite several months of penicillamine, and severe progressive hepatic insufficiency in patients who unadvisably discontinue penicillamine therapy.

Prognosis

The prognosis of untreated Wilson's disease is poor. Without transplantation, all patients with the fulminant presentation succumb. Copper chelation reduces hepatic copper content and reverses many of the liver lesions, but it does not have a profound effect on established cirrhosis. Neurologic symptoms generally respond to therapy. All siblings should be immediately screened and homozygotes treated with copper chelation even if asymptomatic.

DaCosta CM et al: Value of urinary copper excretion after penicillamine challenge in the diagnosis of Wilson's disease. Hepatology 1992;15:609.

Perman JA et al: Laboratory measures of copper metabolism in the differentiation of chronic active hepatitis and Wilson's disease in children. Pediatrics 1979;94:564.

Saito T: Presenting symptoms and natural history of Wilson's disease. Eur J Pediatr 1987;146:261.

Scheinberg IH, Sternlieb I: *Wilson's Disease.* Saunders, 1984.

Sokol RJ: Wilson's disease and Indian childhood cirrhosis. In: *Liver Disease in Children.* Suchy F (editor). Mosby, 1994.

Sternlieb I: Perspectives on Wilson's disease. Hepatology 1990;12:1234.

Werlin SL et al: Diagnostic dilemmas of Wilson's disease: Diagnosis and treatment. Pediatrics 1978;62:47.

REYE'S SYNDROME
(Encephalopathy With Fatty Degeneration of the Viscera)

Essentials of Diagnosis

- Prodromal upper respiratory tract infection, influenza A or B illness, or chickenpox.
- Vomiting.
- Lethargy, drowsiness progressing to semicoma.
- Elevated AST, hyperammonemia, normal or slightly elevated bilirubin, prolonged prothrombin time.
- Variable hypoglycemia.
- Microvesicular steatosis of liver, kidneys, brain, etc.

General Considerations

The number of reported cases of Reye's syndrome is decreasing, perhaps owing to a decline in the use of salicylates among younger children, who seem to be at greater risk. Varicella, influenza A and B, echovirus 2, coxsackie virus A, reovirus, and Epstein-Barr virus have been isolated from some patients. Epidemics of Reye's syndrome seem to cluster during influenza B epidemics. Salicylate use is associated with Reye's syndrome. Many cases in young children are actually caused by defects in fatty acid oxidation. The mode of onset may lead to confusion with other causes of coma, particularly toxic encephalopathy and hepatic coma.

The mechanism is thought to be damage to mitochondria caused by salicylate metabolites or some other toxin or chemical in the milieu of a viral infection. Mitochondrial dysfunction leads to elevated short-chain fatty acids and hyperammonemia as well as directly to cerebral edema.

Clinical Findings

A. Symptoms and Signs: Chickenpox or minor upper respiratory tract illness of short duration usually precedes the development of vomiting, irrational behavior, progressive stupor, and coma. Restlessness and convulsions may also occur. Striking physical findings are hyperpnea, irregular respirations, and dilated, sluggishly reacting pupils. Jaundice is minimal or absent. The liver may be normal or slightly enlarged. Splenomegaly is absent. A positive Babinski sign, hyperreflexia, and decorticate and decerebrate posturing are consistent with severe cerebral edema.

B. Laboratory Findings: Cerebrospinal fluid is acellular, and cerebrospinal fluid glucose may be low in younger patients. Cerebrospinal fluid pressure is variably elevated. The serum glucose is proportionately decreased. Moderate to severe elevations of AST, ALT, and lactate dehydrogenase are found. Serum bilirubin and alkaline phosphatase values are normal to slightly elevated. The prothrombin time is usually prolonged, and the blood ammonia is usually elevated. A mixed respiratory alkalosis and metabolic acidosis is seen. In a few cases, the blood urea nitrogen has been elevated. Hyperaminoacidemia (glutamine, alanine, lysine) and hypocitrullinemia are present.

Histopathologic changes in Reye's syndrome are most striking in the brain, liver, and kidneys, less so in the heart and pancreas. The brain shows gross cerebral edema, occasionally with evidence of herniation. Histologically, loss of neurons and fatty vacuolation around small vessels has been noted. The liver shows diffuse microvesicular steatosis with minimal inflammatory changes. Glycogen is virtually absent from the hepatocytes in biopsy specimens taken before administration of hypertonic glucose. Ultrastructural changes are mitochondrial.

The kidney changes include swelling and fatty degeneration of the proximal lobules.

C. Electroencephalography: The EEG shows diffuse slow wave activity.

Differential Diagnosis

Differentiation of Reye's syndrome from acute toxic encephalopathy, hepatic coma, or fulminant hepatitis can be made on clinical and laboratory grounds. A negative history and urine screen for ingestion of poisons and drugs, absence of cells in the cerebrospinal fluid, and absence of jaundice favor a diagnosis of Reye's syndrome. The fatty acid oxidation defects (eg, medium-chain acyl-CoA dehydrogenase deficiency) and other metabolic disorders may resemble Reye's syndrome; urine gas chromatographic analysis will help differentiate them. Liver biopsy and electron microscopy can be diagnostic, and the procedure is indicated in atypical cases.

Complications

Aspiration pneumonitis and respiratory failure are common, as with any comatose patient. Most patients die of cerebral edema rather than hepatic or renal failure. Cardiac dysrhythmias may develop, as may inappropriate vasopressin excretion, diabetes insipidus, and acute pancreatitis.

Treatment

Treatment is supportive. A nasogastric tube, Foley catheter, and arterial and central venous pressure lines should be inserted immediately. Mechanical ventilation may become necessary if the patient reaches grade 3 (Lovejoy). Intracranial pressure should be monitored directly and kept below 15–20 mm Hg, and systemic blood pressure should be kept sufficiently high to maintain cerebral perfusion pressure above 45–50 mm Hg. Hyperventilation, mannitol infusions (0.5–1 g/kg every 4 hours), barbiturates, or ventricular drainage is used to lower intracranial pressure. Maintenance fluids using 10% glucose should be given at a rate sufficient to produce a urine flow of 1–1.5 mL/kg/h. Careful attention to central venous pressure is needed when using hyperosmolar agents. Vitamin K_1, 3–5 mg intramuscularly, should be administered. Hypothermia (30–33 °C) and pharmacologic doses of pentobarbital (10–50 mg/kg/d) have been employed to decrease body (brain) metabolic needs during the period of uncontrolled intracranial pressure.

Prognosis

At least 70% of these patients survive. The prognosis is related to the depth of coma and the peak ammonia level on admission. Because Reye's syndrome is less common than before, many patients are diagnosed only when comatose. Severe neurologic residuals are not uncommon in younger children (< 2 years) who recover from prolonged grade 3–4 coma (Lovejoy). If relapse occurs, the patient should be screened for other metabolic defects.

Arrowsmith JB et al: National patterns of aspirin use and Reye's syndrome reporting, United States, 1980 to 1985. Pediatrics 1987;79:858.

Heubi JE et al: Grade I Reye's syndrome: Outcome and predictors of progression to deeper coma grades. N Engl J Med 1984;311:1539.

Heubi JE et al: Reye's syndrome: Current concepts. Hepatology 1987;7:155.

Hurwitz ES et al: Public Health Service study on Reye's syndrome and medications. N Engl J Med 1985;313:849.

Orlowski JP et al: A catch in the Reye. Pediatrics 1987;80:638.

Shaywitz BA, Rothstein P, Venes JL: Monitoring and management of increased intracranial pressure in Reye's syndrome: Results in 29 patients. Pediatrics 1980;66:198.

LIVER TRANSPLANTATION

Orthotopic liver transplantation is no longer considered experimental. Children with end-stage liver disease, acute fulminant hepatic failure, or complications from metabolic liver disorders should be considered for liver transplantation. Recent advances in immunosuppression (eg, introduction of cyclosporine and use of monoclonal antibodies against T cells), better candidate selection, improvements in surgical techniques, and experience in postoperative management have contributed to improved results.

The major indications for childhood transplantation are (1) a failed Kasai operation or decompensated cirrhosis caused by extrahepatic biliary atresia, (2) α_1-antitrypsin deficiency, (3) posthepatitic (autoimmune chronic active hepatitis, hepatitis B or C disease) cirrhosis, (4) tyrosinemia, (5) Crigler-Najjar syndrome type I, (6) Wilson's disease, (7) acute fulminant hepatic failure when recovery is unlikely, and (8) cases in which the consequences of chronic cholestasis severely impair the patient's quality of life. Children should be referred early for evaluation as transplantation candidates, because the limiting factor for success is the small donor pool. Pared-down adult livers are being used in children in many centers, and living related donors in several centers. In general, 75–85% of children survive at least 2–5 years after transplantation, with long-term survival expected to be comparable. Lifetime immunosuppression therapy using combinations of cyclosporine, prednisone, or azathioprine, with its incumbent risks, appears necessary to prevent rejection. Newer, more effective immunosuppressive agents (eg, FK 506) are being tested. The overall quality of life for children with transplanted livers appears to be excellent.

Broelsch CE et al: Application of reduced-size liver transplants as split grafts, auxiliary orthotopic grafts, and living related segmental transplants. Ann Surg 1990;212:368.

Emond JC et al: Improved results of living-related liver transplantation with routine application in a pediatric program. Transplantation 1993;55:835.

Lloyd-Still JD: Impact of orthotopic liver transplantation on mortality from pediatric liver disease. J Pediatr Gastroenterol Nutr 1991;12:305.

Rand EB et al: Measles vaccination after orthotopic liver transplantation. J Pediatr 1993;123:87.

Shaw BW et al: Liver transplantation therapy for children. (Two parts.) J Pediatr Gastroenterol Nutr 1988;7:157, 797.

Whitington PF, Balistreri WF: Liver transplantation in pediatrics: Indications, contraindications, and pretransplant management. J Pediatr 1991;118:169.

Zitelli BJ et al: Changes in life-style after liver transplantation. Pediatrics 1988;82:173.

PANCREAS

ACUTE PANCREATITIS

Most cases of acute pancreatitis are due to drugs, viral infections, systemic diseases, or accidental or nonaccidental abdominal trauma, though more than 20% are idiopathic. Other cases resulting in obstruction to pancreatic flow include stones in the ampulla hepatopancreatica, choledochal cysts, tumors of the duodenum, pancreas divisum, and ascariasis. The exact mechanisms by which intra-acinar or intraductal activation of pancreatic zymogens occurs are controversial. Acute pancreatitis has been seen with high-dosage corticosteroid therapy and administration of sulfasalazine, thiazides, valproic acid, azathioprine, mercaptopurine, asparaginase, and other drugs. It may also occur in cystic fibrosis, systemic lupus erythematosus, α_1-antitrypsin deficiency, diabetes, Crohn's disease, glycogen storage disease type I, hyperlipidemia types I and V, hyperparathyroidism, Schönlein-Henoch purpura, Reye's syndrome, Kawasaki disease, chronic renal failure, during rapid refeeding in cases of malnutrition, and in familial cases. Alcohol-induced pancreatitis should be considered in the teenage patient.

Clinical Findings

A. Symptoms and Signs: An acute onset of persistent (hours to days), severe upper abdominal and midabdominal pain occasionally referred to the back, with vomiting and fever, is the common presenting picture. The abdomen is tender but not rigid, and bowel sounds are diminished, suggesting peritoneal irritation. Abdominal distention is common in infants and younger children. In cases due to trauma, an abdominal mass that is suggestive of pseudocyst may be felt. Jaundice is unusual. Ascites may be noted, and a left-sided pleural effusion is present in some. Cullen's and Grey Turner's signs indicate hemorrhagic pancreatitis.

B. Laboratory Findings: Leukocytosis and an elevated serum ($> 1\frac{1}{2}–2$ times normal) and urine amylase should be expected early, except in infants under 6 months of age who may have hypoamylasemia. Serum lipase is elevated and persists longer than serum amylase. The immunoreactive trypsinogen test may also be of value. Pancreatic amylase isoenzyme determination can help differentiate nonpancreatic causes (salivary, intestinal, tubo-ovarian, etc) of serum amylase elevation. Hyperglycemia (serum glucose > 300 mg/dL), hypocalcemia, falling hematocrit, rising blood urea nitrogen, hypoxemia, and acidosis may all occur in severe cases and impart a poor prognosis.

C. Imaging: Plain x-ray films of the abdomen may show a localized ileus (sentinel loop). Ultrasonography shows decreased echodensity of the gland in comparison to the left lobe of the liver. Pseudocyst formation can also be seen early in the course. CT scanning is better for detecting pancreatic phlegmon or abscess formation. Endoscopic retrograde pancreatography may be useful in confirming patency of the main pancreatic duct in cases of abdominal trauma, in recurrent acute pancreatitis, or in revealing stones, strictures, pancreas divisum, etc.

Differential Diagnosis

Other causes of acute upper abdominal pain include lesions of the stomach, duodenum, liver, and biliary system; acute gastroenteritis or atypical appendicitis; pneumonia; volvulus; intussusception; and nonaccidental trauma.

Complications

Complications early in the disease include shock due to fluid and electrolyte disturbances, ileus, and hypocalcemic tetany. Impairment of oxygenation and respiratory distress (pancreatic lung) may require assisted ventilation in some patients. Hypervolemia is seen between the third and fifth days, at which time renal tubular necrosis may occur. The gastrointestinal, neurologic, musculoskeletal, hepatobiliary, dermatologic, and hematologic systems may also be involved.

Later, 5–10% of patients develop a pseudocyst heralded by recurrence of abdominal pain and rise in the serum amylase. From 15% to 25% of these will resolve spontaneously. Infection, hemorrhage, rupture, fistulization, or obstruction may occur. Phlegmon formation is frequently seen (30–50%) and may extend from the gland into the retroperitoneum or into the lesser sac. Most regress, but some require drainage. Infection in this inflammatory mass is a constant threat. Pancreatic abscess formation is fortunately rare (3–5%) and develops 2–3 weeks after the initial insult. Fever, leukocytosis, and pain occur; diagnosis is by ultrasound or CT scanning.

Chronic pancreatitis, pancreatic insufficiency, and

pancreatic lithiasis are rare sequelae of acute pancreatitis.

Treatment

Medical management includes rest, gastric suction, fluids, electrolyte replacement, and blood or colloid as needed. Peritoneal lavage is still being evaluated in severe cases. Pain should be controlled with meperidine. Oxygen may be required if desaturation occurs. An H_2 blocker helps to maintain gastric neutrality at a pH greater than 4.5. Nutrition is provided by the parenteral route. Broad-spectrum antibiotic coverage is employed only in severe hemorrhagic pancreatitis. Recurrence of pain after oral feedings may be prevented by giving pancreatic enzymes with the meal.

Surgical treatment is reserved for traumatic disruption of the gland, intraductal stone, unresolved or infected pseudocysts or abscesses, and other anatomic obstructive lesions. Early endoscopic decompression of the biliary system reduces the morbidity associated with biliary pancreatitis. Drugs known to produce acute pancreatitis should be discontinued.

Prognosis

In the pediatric age group, the prognosis is surprisingly good with conservative management. The mortality rate is 5–10% in patients treated by operation and 1% in those treated medically. The morbidity rate is high in the surgical group as a result of fistula formation.

Fan ST et al: Early treatment of acute biliary pancreatitis by endoscopic papillotomy. N Engl J Med 1993;328:228.

Siegel MJ, Martin KW, Worthington JL: Normal and abnormal pancreas in children: US studies. Radiology 1987; 165:15.

Weizman Z, Durie PR: Acute pancreatitis in childhood. J Pediatr 1988;113:24.

Ziegler DW et al: Pancreatitis in childhood. Ann Surg 1988;207:256.

CHRONIC PANCREATITIS

Two forms of chronic pancreatitis have been reported: chronic fibrosing pancreatitis and the more common familial autosomal dominant chronic relapsing pancreatitis.

The causes include stenotic lesions of the ampulla hepatopancreatica, strictures of the pancreatic ducts, intraductal stones, or persisting pseudocyst following acute pancreatitis. The role of pancreas divisum in chronic pancreatitis remains controversial. Chronic disease rarely follows acute nontraumatic pancreatitis. Choledochal and duplication cysts may give rise to episodes of pancreatitis before they are recognized as the cause of the pancreatitis. Hyperlipidemias (types I and V), hyperparathyroidism, and cystic fibrosis should be considered.

In hereditary pancreatitis, the morphologic findings are not specific. The ductus pancreaticus is dilated but not obstructed.

Clinical Findings

The diagnosis of the hereditary form is usually not made in childhood unless there is a similar history in other family members. The diagnosis of chronic fibrosing pancreatitis is made by surgical exploration demonstrating a normal duct system and typical histologic findings in the pancreatic biopsy.

A. Symptoms and Signs: There is usually a history of recurrent upper abdominal pain of variable severity but prolonged (1–6 days) duration. Radiation of the pain into the back is a frequent complaint. Fever and vomiting are not common in the chronic form. Abnormal stools and symptoms of diabetes may develop later in the course of this disease, and malnutrition due to failure of pancreatic exocrine secretions may also occur.

B. Laboratory Findings: The serum or urine amylase is usually elevated during early acute attacks. Pancreatic insufficiency and reduced volume and bicarbonate response may be found at duodenal intubation after intravenous administration of synthetic cholecystokinin (0.2 µg/kg) and secretin (2 units/kg). A threefold increase of normal serum amylase values is considered a positive test for obstruction. An indirect screening test for pancreatic insufficiency with bentiromide, a synthetic peptide, measures urine excretion of the chymotrypsin cleaved marker *p*-aminobenzoic acid (PABA). Normal subjects excrete over 50% of the ingested dose, with some overlap occurring in normal and diseased patients who have mild pancreatic insufficiency.

Blood lipids and urinary amino acids are elevated in familial forms of the disease associated with hyperlipoproteinemia and should be studied in all cases. Elevated blood glucose and glycohemoglobin levels and glycosuria are frequently found in protracted disease. Sweat chloride should be checked for cystic fibrosis and serum calcium for hyperparathyroidism.

C. Imaging: X-rays of the abdomen may show pancreatic or gallbladder calcifications. Contrast studies may demonstrate other obstructive lesions in the region of the duodenum. Endoscopic retrograde cholangiopancreatography is a helpful tool in nonsurgical diagnosis. Pancreatograms show ductal dilation, stones, strictures, or stenotic segments.

Differential Diagnosis

Other causes of recurrent abdominal pain must be considered. Specific causes such as hyperparathyroidism, systemic lupus erythematosus, infectious disease, and ductal obstruction by tumors, stones, or helminths must be excluded by appropriate tests.

Complications

Disabling abdominal pain, steatorrhea, nutritional deprivation, and diabetes are the most frequent long-term complications. Pancreatic carcinoma occurs more frequently in hereditary pancreatitis, especially in patients with calcifications within the gland.

Treatment

When the hereditary form of chronic pancreatitis is suspected or proved, medical management of acute attacks is indicated (see Acute Pancreatitis, above). If ductal obstruction is strongly suspected, surgical exploration should be undertaken if endoscopic means of therapy fail (balloon dilation, stenting, stone removal, sphincterotomy). Pancreatography and cholangiography can also be performed at laparotomy. Sphincterotomy and biopsy are recommended even when obvious obstruction is not found. Relapses seem to occur in most patients. Orally ingested pancreatic enzymes at mealtime may reduce pain episodes in some patients. The daily injection of a somatostatin analogue (octreotide acetate) has shown promise in relieving pain episodes and decreasing the serum amylase of some patients. Pseudocysts may be marsupialized to the surface or drained into the stomach or into a loop of jejunum in those failing to regress spontaneously. Recent experience in pediatric patients indicates that lateral pancreaticojejunostomy can reduce pain in appropriately selected patients. Prophylactic total or subtotal pancreatic resection is advocated by some workers.

Prognosis

In the absence of a correctable lesion, the prognosis is not good. Disabling episodes of pain, pancreatic insufficiency, and diabetes may ensue. Narcotic addiction and suicide are risks in teenagers with disabling disease.

Crombleholme TM et al: The modified Puestow procedure for chronic relapsing pancreatitis in childhood. J Pediatr Surg 1990;25:749.

Ghishan FK et al: Chronic relapsing pancreatitis in childhood. J Pediatr 1983;102:514.

Little JM et al: Chronic pancreatitis beginning in childhood and adolescence. Arch Surg 1992;127:90.

Niederau C, Glendell JH: Diagnosis of chronic pancreatitis. Gastroenterology 1985;88:1973.

GASTROINTESTINAL & HEPATOBILIARY MANIFESTATIONS OF CYSTIC FIBROSIS

Cystic fibrosis is a disease with protean manifestations. Although pulmonary and pancreatic involvement dominates the clinical picture for most patients (see Chapter 20), a variety of other organs can be involved. Table 23–6 lists the important gastrointestinal, pancreatic, and hepatobiliary conditions that may affect cystic fibrosis patients along with their clinical findings, incidence, most useful diagnostic studies, and preferred treatment.

Park RW, Grand RJ: Gastrointestinal manifestations of cystic fibrosis: A review. Gastroenterology 1981;81:1143.

Roy CC et al: Hepatobiliary disease in cystic fibrosis: A survey of current issues and concepts. J Pediatr Gastroenterol Nutr 1982;1:469.

Rubenstein S, Moss R, Lewiston N: Constipation and meconium ileus equivalent in patients with cystic fibrosis. Pediatrics 1986;78:473.

Scott RB, O'Loughlin EV, Gall DG: Gastroesophageal reflux in patients with cystic fibrosis. J Pediatr 1985;106:223.

Stern RC, Rothstein FC, Doershuk CF: Treatment and prognosis of symptomatic gallbladder disease in patients with cystic fibrosis. J Pediatr Gastroenterol Nutr 1986;5:35.

PANCREATIC EXOCRINE HYPOPLASIA & CHRONIC NEUTROPENIA (Shwachman's Syndrome)

This uncommon disease, characterized by diarrhea and failure to thrive, is due to pancreatic exocrine insufficiency. Pathologically, there is widespread fatty replacement of the glandular acinar tissue. This is easily recognized on abdominal CT scan. There is no fibrosis or inflammation, and the pancreatic ducts appear to be normal. The islet cells are spared. There is evidence that the disease is genetically determined.

The history of failure to thrive, diarrhea, fatty stools, and, in most cases, freedom from respiratory infections should make one suspect this entity. Important laboratory findings include normal sweat electrolytes but absent or reduced pancreatic lipase, amylase, and trypsin on duodenal intubation. Leukopenia is often present, and the platelet count is sometimes depressed. Small bowel is normal on histologic examination, and studies of absorption not dependent upon pancreatic enzymes yield normal results. The bone marrow is typically hypocellular, showing a "maturation arrest" of the granulocyte series. Metaphysial dysostosis and an elevated fetal hemoglobin may occur. Immunoglobulin deficiencies and hepatic dysfunction are also reported in some cases.

Normal sweat electrolytes and a negative history of repeated pulmonary infections differentiate this disease from cystic fibrosis. Small bowel biopsy supported by absorption tests, particularly with D-xylose, distinguishes the disorder from celiac disease. Cases of isolated lipase or enterokinase deficiency may be more difficult to distinguish by functional tests alone. Cyclic neutropenia, transient neutropenia, and pancreatic exocrine hypofunction due to viral causes must be considered.

Other causes of exocrine pancreatic insufficiency

Table 23–6. Gastrointestinal and hepatobiliary manifestations of cystic fibrosis.

Organ	Condition	Symptoms	Age of Presentation	Incidence	Diagnostic Evaluation	Management
Esophagus	Gastroesophageal reflux, esophagitis	Pyrosis, dysphagia, epigastric pain, hematemesis.	School age and older.	10–20%	Endoscopy and biopsy, overnight pH study.	H_2 blocker, antacids, surgical antireflux procedure.
	Varices	Hematemesis, melena.	Childhood and adolescents.	3–10%	Endoscopy, barium swallow.	Endosclerosis, drugs (see p 669), portacaval shunt, liver transplant.
Stomach	Gastritis	Upper abdominal pain, vomiting, hematemesis.	School age and older.	10–25%	Endoscopy and biopsy.	H_2 blockers, antacids, carafate, omeprazole.
	Hiatal hernia	Reflux symptoms (see above), epigastric pain.	School age and older.	3–5%	Endoscopy, barium swallow.	As above. Surgery in some.
Intestine	Meconium ileus	Abdominal distention, bilious emesis.	Neonate.	10–15%	X-ray studies, plain abdominal films; contrast enema shows microcolon. Neonatal CF screening test (immunoreactive trypsinogen [IRT]), then sweat chloride test.	Dislodgement of obstruction with gastrografin enema. Surgery if unsuccessful or if case complicated by atresia, perforation, or volvulus.
	Meconium ileus equivalent syndrome	Abdominal pain, acute and recurrent; distention; occasional vomiting.	Any age, usually school age through adolescence.	10–15%	Palpable mass in right lower quadrant, x-ray studies.	Gastrografin enema, intestinal lavage solution, diet, bulk laxatives, adjustment of pancreatic enzyme intake.
	Intussusception	Acute, intermittent abdominal pain; distention; emesis.	Infants through adolescence.	1–3%	X-ray studies, barium enema.	Reduction by barium enema or surgery if needed, diet, bulk laxatives. Adjustment of pancreatic enzyme intake.
	Rectal prolapse	Anal discomfort, rectal bleeding.	Infants and children to age 4–5 years.	15–25%	Visual mass protruding from anus.	Manual reduction, adjustment of pancreatic enzyme dosage, reassurance as problem resolves by age 3–5 years.
	Carbohydrate intolerance	Abdominal pain, flatulence, continued diarrhea with adequate replacement therapy.	Any age.	10–25%	Intestinal mucosal biopsy and disaccharidase analysis. Breath hydrogen after lactose load.	Reduce lactose intake; reduction of gastric hyperacidity if mucosa shows partial villous atrophy. Beware concurrent celiac disease or *Giardia* infection.
Pancreas	Total exocrine insufficiency	Diarrhea, steatorrhea, malnutrition, failure to thrive. Specific fat-soluble vitamin deficiency states.	Neonate through infancy.	80–90%	Quantitative sweat chloride iontophoresis test.	Pancreatic enzyme replacement, may need elemental formula, fat-soluble vitamin supplements.
	Partial exocrine insufficiency (pancreatic sufficiency)	Occasional diarrhea, mild growth delay.	Any age.	10–15%	Sweat test, 72-hour fecal fat evaluation, direct pancreatic function tests.	Pancreatic enzyme replacement in selected patients. Fat-soluble vitamin supplements as indicated by biochemical evaluation.

(continued)

Table 23–6. Gastrointestinal and hepatobiliary manifestations of cystic fibrosis. (continued)

Organ	Condition	Symptoms	Age of Presentation	Incidence	Diagnostic Evaluation	Management
Pancreas	Pancreatitis	Recurrent abdominal pain, vomiting.	Older children through adolescence.	0.1%	Increase serum lipase and amylase, pancreatic provocative test, endoscopic pancreatogram.	Addition of pancreatic enzymes to feeds, endoscopic removal of sludge or stone(s) if present, endoscopic papillotomy.
	Diabetes	Weight loss, polyuria, polydipsia.	Older children through adolescence.	5–7%	Glucose tolerance test and insulin levels.	Diet, insulin.
Liver	Steatosis	Hepatomegaly.	Neonates and infants, but some cases are seen at all ages.	15–30%	Liver biopsy.	Improved nutrition, replacement of pancreatic enzymes and vitamins.
	Focal biliary cirrhosis	Hepatomegaly.	Infants and older patients.	20–25%	Liver biopsy.	As above. Taurine supplements (still experimental), ursodeoxycholic acid (unproved benefit).
	Multilobular biliary cirrhosis	Hepatosplenomegaly, hematemesis from esophageal varices; hypersplenism, jaundice, ascites late in course.	School age through adolescence.	1–3%	Liver biopsy, endoscopy.	Improved nutrition, ursodeoxycholic acid (unproved benefit) endosclerosis of varices, splenic embolization, liver transplantation.
	Neonatal jaundice	Cholestatic jaundice hepatomegaly; often seen with meconium ileus.	Neonates.	0.1–1%	Neonatal CF screening (IRT), sweat chloride test, liver biopsy.	Nutritional support, special formula with medium-chain triglyceride-containing oil, pancreatic enzyme replacement.
Gallbladder	Microgallbladder	None.	Congenital–present at any age.	15–20%	Ultrasound or by hepatobiliary scintigraphy.	None needed.
	Cholelithiasis	Recurrent abdominal pain, rarely jaundice.	School age through adolescence.	3–5%	Ultrasound, CT scan.	Surgery (laparoscopic or open) if symptomatic and low risk, trial of cholelitholytics in others.
Extrahepatic bile ducts	Obstruction Intraluminal (sludge, stones, tumor)	Jaundice, hepatomegaly, abdominal pain.	Neonates, then older children through adolescence.	Rare in neonates (< 0.1%)	Ultrasound and hepatobiliary scintigraphy, endoscopic cholangiography, surgery.	Surgery in neonates, endoscopic intervention in older patients or surgery.
	Extraluminal (intrapancreatic compression, tumor)	As above.	As above.	Rare (< 1%)	As above.	Surgical biliary drainage procedure or biliary stent placement endoscopically.
	Stenosis	As above.	As above	1–40%	As above.	Endoscopic balloon dilatation, surgical drainage procedure.

must also be considered in the evaluation of a child with suspected pancreatic insufficiency. Such causes include (1) exocrine pancreatic insufficiency with aplastic alae, aplasia cutis, deafness (Johanson-Blizzard syndrome); (2) exocrine pancreatic insufficiency with aplastic anemia, developmental delay, seizures (Pearson bone marrow pancreas syndrome); (3) exocrine pancreatic insufficiency associated with duodenal atresia or stenosis; (4) exocrine pancreatic insufficiency associated with malnutrition; and (5) exocrine pancreatic insufficiency associated with pancreatic hypoplasia or agenesis.

The complications and sequelae of deficient pancreatic enzyme secretion are malnutrition, diarrhea, and growth failure. The degree of steatorrhea may lessen with age. Intragastric lipolysis mainly due to lingual lipase may be the compensatory mechanism in patients with low or absent pancreatic function. The major sequela seems to be short stature, though long-term follow-up studies are not available. Increased numbers of infections may be the results of chronic neutropenia. Neutrophil mobility is also impaired in many patients and perhaps contributes to their susceptibility to infections.

Pancreatic enzyme replacement therapy and fat-soluble vitamin replacement have been fairly successful, though some patients get along without it. The prognosis appears to be good for those able to survive the increased number of bacterial infections early in life. However, an increased incidence of leukemia has been noted in these patients.

Aggett PJ: Shwachman's syndrome. Arch Dis Child 1980; 55:331.

Cleghorn GJ et al: Exocrine pancreatic dysfunction in malnourished Australian aboriginal children. Med J Aust 1991;154:45.

Dosseter JF et al: Immunoreactive trypsin in Schwachman's syndrome. Arch Dis Child 1989;64:395.

Dupont C et al: Pancreatic lipomatosis and duodenal stenosis or atresia in children. J Pediatr 1990;115:603.

Hill RE et al: Steatorrhea and pancreatic insufficiency in Shwachman's syndrome. Gastroenterology 1982;83:22.

McShane MA et al: Pearson syndrome and mitochondrial encephalomyopathy in a patient with a deletion of mtDNA. Am J Hum Genet 1991;48:39.

Sarles J, Guys JM, Sauniere JF: Pancreatic function and congenital duodenal abnormalities. J Pediatr Gastroenterol Nutr 1993;16:284.

Winter WE et al: Congenital pancreatic hypoplasia: A syndrome of exocrine and endocrine pancreatic insufficiency. J Pediatr 1986;109:465.

Wright NM et al: Permanent neonatal diabetes mellitus and pancreatic exocrine insufficiency resulting from congenital pancreatic agenesis. Am J Dis Child 1993;47:607.

ISOLATED EXOCRINE PANCREATIC ENZYME DEFECT

Normal premature infants and most newborns produce little if any pancreatic amylase following meals or exogenous hormonal stimulation. This temporary physiologic insufficiency may persist for the first 3–6 months of life and be responsible for diarrhea when complex carbohydrates (cereals) are introduced into their diet.

Congenital pancreatic lipase deficiency and congenital colipase deficiency are extremely rare disorders, causing diarrhea and variable malnutrition with malabsorption of dietary fat and fat-soluble vitamins. The sweat chloride iontophoresis test is normal, and neutropenia is absent. Treatment involves use of oral replacement of pancreatic enzymes and a low-fat diet or formula containing medium-chain triglycerides.

Exocrine pancreatic insufficiency of proteolytic enzymes (trypsinogen, trypsin, chymotrypsin, etc) is in fact due to enterokinase deficiency, a duodenal mucosal enzyme required for activation of the pancreatic proenzymes. These patients present with malnutrition associated with hypoproteinemia and edema but are free of respiratory symptoms and have a normal sweat test. They respond to pancreatic enzyme replacement therapy and feeding formulas that contain a casein hydrolysate (eg, Nutramigen or Pregestimil).

Gaskin KJ et al: Colipase and lipase secretion in childhood-onset pancreatic insufficiency. Gastroenterology 1984; 86:1.

Ghishan FK et al: Isolated congenital enterokinase deficiency. Gastroenterology 1983;85:727.

Lebenthal E: The development of pancreatic function in premature infants after milk-based and soy-based formulas. Pediatr Res 1981;15:1240.

PANCREATIC TUMORS

Pancreatic tumors, whether benign or malignant, are rare lesions. They most often arise from ductal or acinar epithelium (malignant adenocarcinoma) or from islet (endocrine) components within the gland, such as the benign insulinoma (adenoma) derived from B cells. Other pancreatic tumors also originate from these pluripotential endocrine cells (gastrinoma, VIPoma, glucagonoma). These malignant lesions produce diverse symptoms, because they release biologically active polypeptides from this ectopic location. The clinical features of these tumors are summarized in Table 23–7. The differential diagnosis of these abdominal tumors includes Wilms' tumor, neuroblastoma, and malignant lymphoma. The development of endoscopic ultrasound shows promise in localizing these tumors.

Table 23–7. Pancreatic tumors.

	Age	Major Findings	Diagnosis	Treatment	Associated Conditions
Insulinoma	After age 3–4	Hypoglycemia, seizures; high serum insulin; abdominal pain and mass infrequent	Ultrasound, CT scan, MRI	Surgery	
Adenocarcinoma	Any age	Epigastric pain, mass, weight loss, anemia, biliary obstruction	Ultrasound, CT scan, MRI	Surgery	Hereditary (calcific) pancreatitis
Gastrinoma	Over age 5–8	Male sex, gastric hypersecretion, peptic symptoms, multiple ulcers, gastrointestinal bleeding, anemia, diarrhea	Elevated fasting gastrin and postsecretin suppression test (> 300 pg/mL), CT scan, MRI, laparotomy	Histamine H_2 blockers, omeprazole, surgical resection, total gastrectomy	Zollinger-Ellison syndrome, multiple endocrine neoplasia syndrome type I, neurofibromatosis
VIP	Any age	Secretory diarrhea, hypokalemia, weight loss	Elevated vasoactive intestinal polypeptide (VIP) levels; sometimes, elevated serum gastrin and pancreatic polypeptide	Surgery, octreotide therapy	
Glucagonoma	Older patients	Necrolytic rash, diarrhea, anemia, thrombotic events	Elevated glucagon, gastrin, VIP	Surgery	

Tersigni R et al: Pancreatic carcinoma in childhood: Case report of long survival and review of the literature. Surgery 1984;96:560.

Wolfe MM, Jensen RT: Zollinger-Ellison syndrome. N Engl J Med 1987;317:1200.

Wynick D, Williams SJ, Bloom SR: Symptomatic secondary hormone syndromes in patients with established malignant pancreatic endocrine tumors. N Engl J Med 1988;319:605.

REFERENCES

Alagille D, Odievre M: *Liver and Biliary Tract Disease in Children.* Wiley, 1978.

Lebenthal E (editor): Pediatric gastroenterology. (Two parts.) Pediatr Clin North Am 1988;35:1, 215.

Mowat A: *Liver Disorders in Childhood.* Butterworths, 1979.

Schiff L, Schiff ER: *Diseases of the Liver,* 7th ed. Lippincott, 1993.

Silverman A, Roy CC: *Pediatric Clinical Gastroenterology,* 3rd ed. Mosby, 1983.

Suchy F (editor): *Liver Disease in Children.* Mosby Year Book, 1994.

Walker WA et al: *Pediatric Gastrointestinal Disease: Pathophysiology, Diagnosis, Management.* BC Decker, 1991.

Kidney & Urinary Tract

24

Gary M. Lum, MD

EVALUATION OF THE KIDNEY & URINARY TRACT

HISTORY

When renal disease is suspected, a history should elicit the following: (1) family history of cystic disease, hereditary nephritis, deafness, dialysis, or renal transplantation; (2) preceding acute or chronic illnesses (eg, urinary tract infection, pharyngitis, impetigo, or endocarditis); (3) rashes or joint pains; (4) growth delay or failure to thrive; (5) polyuria, polydipsia, enuresis, frequency, or dysuria; (6) hematuria or discolored urine; (7) pain (abdominal, costovertebral angle, or flank) or trauma; (8) sudden weight gain or edema; and (9) drug or toxin exposure. In the newborn or small infant, additional information should be obtained regarding birth history, eg, prenatal ultrasonographic studies, birth asphyxia, Apgar scores, oligohydramnios, dysmorphic features, abdominal masses, voiding patterns, anomalous development, and umbilical artery catheterization.

PHYSICAL EXAMINATION

Important aspects of the physical examination include the height, weight, skin lesions (café au lait or ash leaf spots), pallor, edema, or skeletal deformities. Anomalies of the ears, eyes or external genitalia may be associated with renal disease. The blood pressure should be measured in a quiet setting. The cuff should cover two-thirds of the child's upper arm, and peripheral pulses should be noted. An ultrasonic device is useful for measurements in infants. The abdomen should be palpated, with attention to the kidneys, abdominal masses, musculature, and the presence of ascites.

LABORATORY EVALUATION OF RENAL FUNCTION

Urinalysis

A carefully performed urinalysis is the keystone in the evaluation of possible renal disease. Commercially available dipsticks can be used to screen for the presence of red blood cells, hemoglobin, leukocytes, nitrites, and protein and to approximate pH. The urinary sediment must be examined by microscope. The use of low illumination and a urine stain facilitates the examination. Casts should be sought at the periphery of the coverslip. Bacteria and cells are studied with the high-power objective. Crystals should be carefully described. The urine, collected properly, can be sent for culture when indicated.

Serum Analysis

The standard indicators of renal function are serum levels of creatinine and urea nitrogen. The ratio of serum urea nitrogen to creatinine is normally about 10:1. The ratio may increase in cases where renal perfusion or urine flow is decreased, because serum urea nitrogen levels are more affected by these and other factors (eg, nitrogen intake, catabolism, use of tetracyclines) than are creatinine levels. Therefore, the most reliable, easily assessed blood indicator of glomerular function is the serum level of creatinine.

Most laboratories report a "normal" range of serum creatinine. However, small children should have serum creatinine levels well under 0.8 mg/dL, and only the larger adolescents should have levels exceeding 1 mg/dL. Thus, one must interpret with caution the "normal" creatinine levels reported. For example, serum creatinine increasing from 0.5 mg/dL to 1 mg/dL represents a 50% decrease in GFR.

Less precise but nonetheless important indicators of the presence of renal disease are abnormalities of serum electrolytes, pH, calcium, phosphorus, magnesium, albumin, or complement.

Measurement of Glomerular Filtration Rate (GFR)

The determination of GFR is of paramount importance in the evaluation of suspected renal disease or in the serial follow-up of the child with established renal insufficiency.

An estimate of GFR may be made by measurements of the endogenous creatinine clearance (C_{Cr}) in milliliters per minute. A 24-hour urine collection is usually obtained; however, in small children from whom collection is difficult, a 12-hour daytime specimen, collected when urine flow rate is greatest, is acceptable. The procedure for collecting a quantitative urine specimen should be carefully explained so that the parent or patient understands fully the rationale of (1) first emptying the bladder (discarding that urine) and noting the time; and (2) putting all urine subsequently voided into the collection receptacle, including the last void, 12 or 24 hours later. Reliability of the 24-hour collection can be approximated by measurement of the total 24-hour creatinine excretion in the specimen. Total daily creatinine excretion (creatinine index) should be in the range of 14–20 mg/kg. If the creatinine index does not fall within this range, collections may be either inadequate or excessive. Calculation by the following formula requires measurements of plasma creatinine (P_{Cr}) in mg/mL, urine creatinine (U_{Cr}) in mg/mL, and urine volume (V) expressed as mL/min.

$$C_{Cr} = \frac{U_{Cr}\,V}{P_{Cr}}$$

Creatinine is a reflection of body muscle mass. Because accepted ranges of normal creatinine clearance are based on adult parameters, "correction" for size is needed to determine normal ranges in children. Clearance is "corrected" to a standard body surface area of 1.73 m^2, as shown in the following formula:

$$\text{"Corrected" } C_{Cr} = \frac{\text{Patient's } C_{Cr} \times 1.73 \text{ m}^2}{\text{Patient's body surface area}}$$

Although 80–125 mL/min/1.73 m^2 is considered a normal range for creatinine clearance, estimates at the lower end of this range may nonetheless suggest problems.

A simple and tested formula for quick approximation of creatinine clearance incorporates use of the plasma creatinine level and the child's length in centimeters:

$$C_{Cr} \text{ (mL/min/1.73 m}^2) = \frac{0.55 \times \text{Height in cm}}{P_{Cr} \text{ in mg/dL}}$$

Note: This formula takes into consideration an expression of body surface area; thus, further correction is not necessary. Use 0.45 × length in centimeters in newborns less than 1 year old. This method of calculation is not meant to detract from the importance of clearance determinations but is of great help to the clinician who desires a quick estimate of the appropriateness of a suspect level of plasma creatinine.

Urine Concentrating Ability

Inability to concentrate urine is associated with polyuria, polydipsia, or enuresis and is often the first sign of chronic renal failure. Except under unusual circumstances, a first morning void is expected to be concentrated. Evaluation of other abnormalities of urinary concentration or dilution is discussed under specific disease entities, eg, diabetes insipidus.

Microhematuria or Isolated Proteinuria

Hematuria and proteinuria occur with glomerular lesions. In children with *asymptomatic* hematuria or proteinuria, the search for *renal* origins will yield the most results. Dipstick detection of microhematuria should be followed by microscopic analysis. The presence of red cell casts supports the diagnosis of glomerulonephritis, but the absence of casts does not rule out the disease.

The diagnosis of benign hematuria, including benign familial hematuria, is by exclusion. In this group are children who are found to have asymptomatic hypercalciuria as an explanation for their hematuria. Figure 24–1 depicts a suggested approach to the renal workup of hematuria. Further discussion of glomerulonephritis follows.

The association of proteinuria with hematuria is characteristic of more significant glomerular disease. Proteinuria alone, however, may indicate the presence of some benign as well as some more serious entities.

The dipstick test for proteinuria should be followed by quantitation of urinary protein excretion. Significant proteinuria exceeds 150 mg/d. A spot urine sample which reveals a protein:creatinine ratio of > 0.1 is considered abnormal.

A timed (usually 24-hour) urine collection can still be useful, especially to demonstrate orthostatic or "postural" proteinuria. Urine voided during the night or upon awakening in the morning is collected in one container and urine formed in the upright position is collected in a separate container which is completed with a void just before going to bed. The two quantities can then be used to calculate total protein excretion, and the amount of protein can be compared in upright versus recumbent specimens to determine an orthostatic component. If the upright collection contains 80–100% of the measured protein and does not exceed a total of 1.5 g, the diagnosis of orthostatic (benign) proteinuria is acceptable. Even when a creatinine clearance is not required from a specimen, measuring the creatinine in the specimen and calculating the creatinine index can confirm specimen reliability.

An approach to the workup of isolated proteinuria is shown in Figure 24–2. Note that corticosteroid therapy is indicated in the algorithm. Since therapy may be initiated prior to referral and since it also may support a presumed diagnosis of "minimal change"

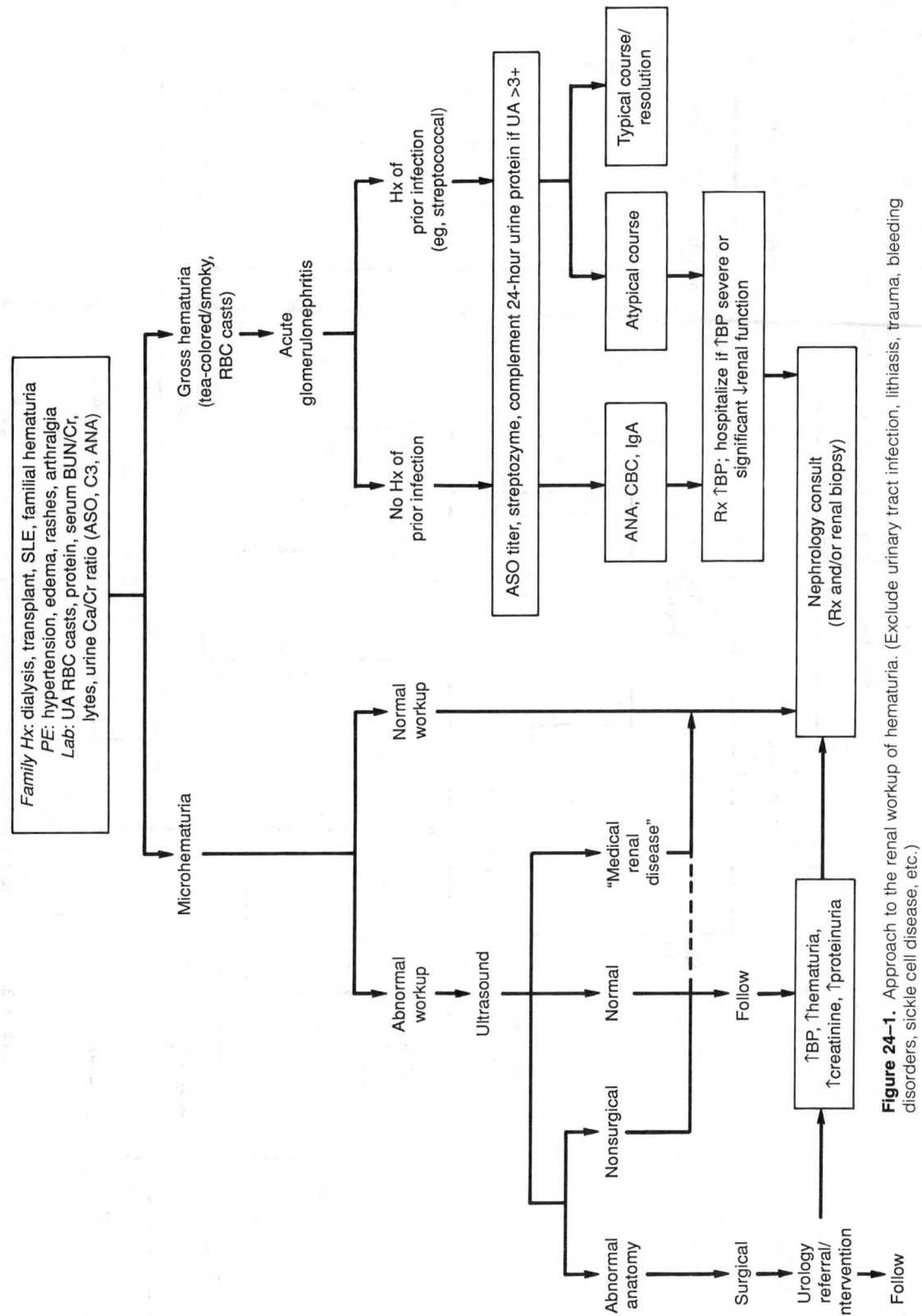

Figure 24–1. Approach to the renal workup of hematuria. (Exclude urinary tract infection, lithiasis, trauma, bleeding disorders, sickle cell disease, etc.)

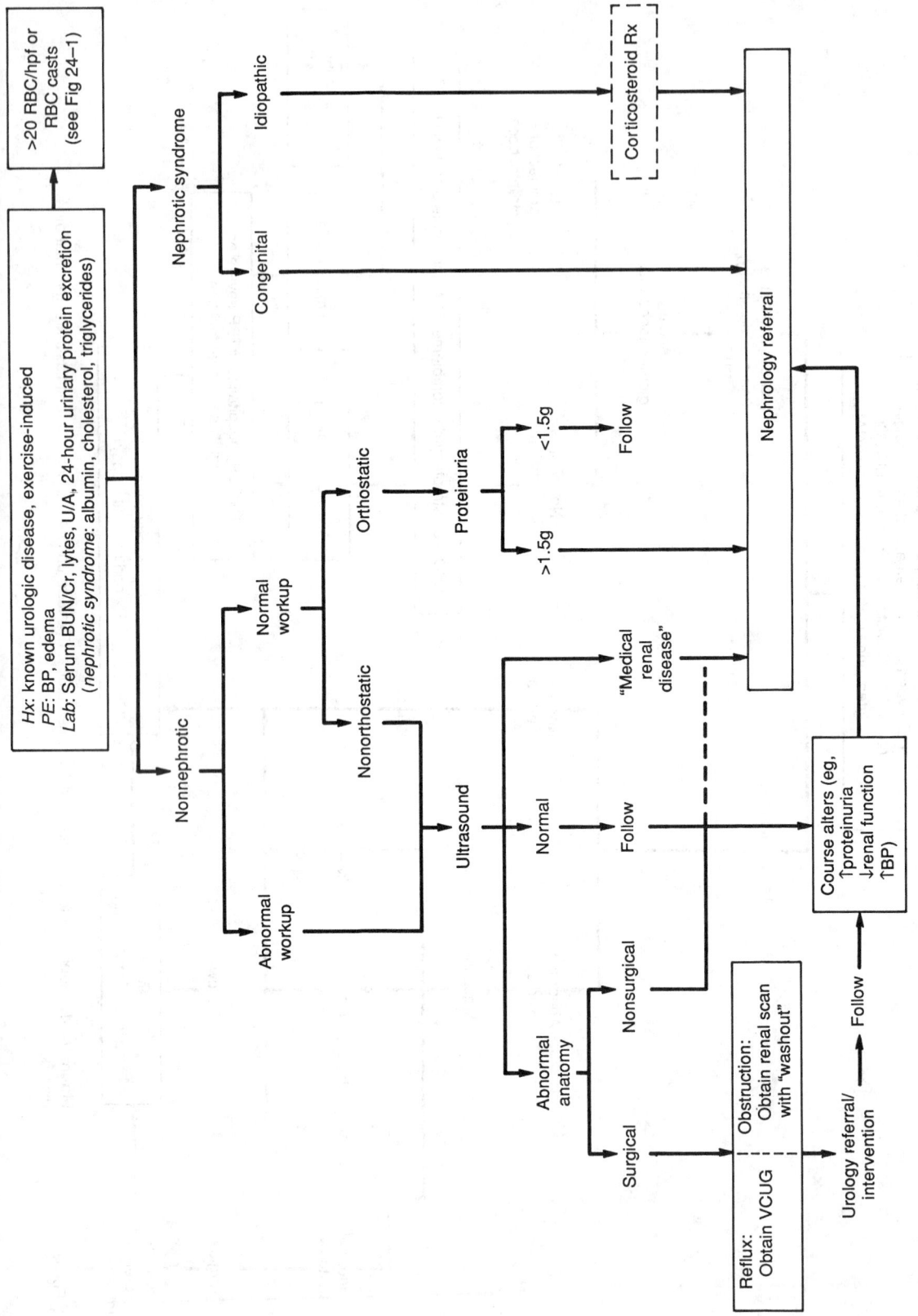

Figure 24–2. Approach to the workup of isolated proteinuria. Approach to the workup of isolated proteinuria.

disease, it may be considered a step in the workup. Discussion of other renal lesions with proteinuric presentations follows.

Special Tests of Renal Function

Measurements of urinary sodium, creatinine, and osmolality are useful in differentiating prerenal causes of renal insufficiency from renal causes when the possibility of acute tubular necrosis is raised.

The physiologic response to decreased renal perfusion is an increase in urine concentration (osmolality usually > 800 mosm/L), a rise in urinary solutes, and a decrease in urinary sodium (usually < 20 meq/L). Therefore, when an increase in serum creatinine or blood urea nitrogen concentration or a decrease in urinary output suggests the possibility of renal failure, appropriate steps can be taken to assess the status of renal function by qualitative and quantitative urinalysis. (See Acute Renal Failure.)

The presence of some substances in urine suggests tubular dysfunction. For example, glucose should not be present in concentrations greater than 5 mg/dL. Hyperphosphaturia is usual where there are significant tubular abnormalities (eg, Fanconi's syndrome). Measurement of the phosphate concentration of a 24-hour urine specimen and evaluation of tubular reabsorption of phosphorus (TRP) will help document renal tubular diseases as well as hyperparathyroid states. TRP (expressed as percentage of reabsorption) is calculated as follows:

$$TRP = 100 \left[1 - \frac{S_{Cr} \times U_{PO_4}}{S_{PO_4} \times U_{Cr}} \right]$$

where S_{Cr} = serum creatinine; U_{Cr} = urine creatinine; S_{PO4} = serum phosphate; and U_{PO4} = urine phosphate. All values for creatinine and phosphate are expressed in milligrams per deciliter for purposes of calculation. A TRP value of 80% or more is considered normal, though it depends somewhat on the S_{PO4}.

The urinary excretion of amino acids in generalized tubular disease reflects a quantitative increase rather than a qualitative change.

The ability of the proximal tubule to reabsorb bicarbonate is affected in several disease states—including isolated renal tubular acidosis, Fanconi's syndrome (which is present in diseases such as cystinosis), and chronic renal failure—and is discussed later under specific entities.

LABORATORY EVALUATION OF IMMUNOLOGIC FUNCTION

Much of parenchymal renal disease is mediated by immune mechanisms, many of which are not well defined or known. Examples of mechanisms in the kidney include (1) deposition of circulating antigen-antibody complexes that are themselves injurious or incite injurious responses and (2) formation of antibody directed against the glomerular basement membrane itself (rare in children).

Total serum complement, the C3 and C4 complement components and serum immunoglobulins should be measured when immune-mediated renal injury or chronic glomerulonephritis is suspected. Abnormal serum protein levels are often associated with immune complex deposition; in such cases, tests should be performed to detect antinuclear antibodies, hepatitis-associated antigen, rheumatoid factor, and cold-precipitable proteins (cryoglobulins). Where indicated, special studies to measure circulating immune complexes, C3 "nephritic" factor, and anti-glomerular basement membrane (anti-GBM) antibody may be performed. Very often, the diagnosis rests on the description of renal histology.

RADIOGRAPHIC EVALUATION

Renal ultrasonography is often the initial procedure in evaluation of a child's urinary tract. It is noninvasive and helpful in evaluating small infants with renal insufficiency; abdominal masses (eg, Wilms' tumor, neuroblastoma); or renal enlargement due to obstructive uropathy, renal vein thrombosis, or cystic disease. The integrity of the fetal urinary tract can also be evaluated by ultrasonography. Excretory urography is useful in assessing the anatomy and function of the kidney, collecting system, and bladder.

Radioisotope studies provide valuable information concerning renal anatomy, blood flow, and glomerular, tubular, and collecting system function.

Evaluation of the lower urinary tract (voiding cystourethrography or cystoscopy) is indicated when vesicoureteral reflux or bladder outlet obstruction is suspected. Cystoscopy is rarely indicated in the evaluation of asymptomatic hematuria or proteinuria in children because the yield is minimal.

When clinically indicated, computed tomography or magnetic resonance imaging may be helpful if less costly studies have failed to produce desired results.

Renal arteriography or venography is rarely indicated in children, except when necessary for defining vascular abnormalities (eg, renal artery stenosis) prior to surgical intervention. Less invasive measures such as ultrasonography and Doppler studies can be employed to demonstrate renal blood flow or thromboses.

Although excretory urogram and voiding cystourethrogram are used in the diagnosis of ureteral reflux, bladder dysfunction, and various levels of urinary tract obstruction, the aforementioned less invasive diagnostic tools are helpful in many of these cases as well.

Gusmano R et al: Natural history of reflux nephropathy in children. Contrib Nephrol 1988;61:200.

RENAL BIOPSY

The ultimate diagnostic procedure in children with suspected renal parenchymal disease is renal biopsy. Histologic information valuable for diagnosis, treatment, and prognosis can be obtained from a well-performed renal biopsy followed by proper tissue preparation, examination, and interpretation of findings. Satisfactory evaluation of renal tissue requires examination by light microscopy, immunofluorescence microscopy, and electron microscopy.

When a biopsy is anticipated, a pediatric nephrologist should be consulted. In children, percutaneous renal biopsy is an acceptable low-risk procedure when performed by an experienced physician; it avoids the risks of general anesthesia. An experienced surgeon should perform the biopsy if operative exposure of the kidney is necessary, if an increased risk factor (eg, bleeding disorder) is present, or if a wedge biopsy is preferred.

CONGENITAL ANOMALIES OF THE URINARY TRACT

RENAL PARENCHYMAL ANOMALIES

Congenital anomalies of the genitourinary tract are present in about 10% of children. Severity ranges from abnormalities which remain asymptomatic through adult life to malformations incompatible with intrauterine or extrauterine life.

Some asymptomatic abnormalities have significant complications. For example, in patients with horseshoe kidney (ie, kidneys fused in their lower poles), there is a reported higher incidence of renal calculi. Unilateral agenesis can occur and is usually accompanied by compensatory hypertrophy of the contralateral kidney and thus should be compatible with normal renal function. Supernumerary and ectopic kidneys can also occur and are usually of no significance. Abnormal genitourinary development can result in varying degrees of renal maldevelopment and function, of which complete renal agenesis is the most severe. When the agenesis is bilateral it causes early death. Oligohydramnios is present and probably is the cause of the pulmonary hypoplasia and peculiar (Potter) facies of infants with this anomaly.

Renal Hypoplasia & Dysplasia

Renal hypoplasia and dysplasia represent a spectrum of anomalies. In simple hypoplasia, which may be unilateral or bilateral, histologic findings on renal biopsy are normal, but the affected organs are smaller than normal. In the various forms of dysplasia, immature, undifferentiated renal tissue persists. In some of the dysplasias, the number of normal nephrons is insufficient to sustain life once the child reaches a critical body size. Such lack of renal tissue may not be readily discernible in the newborn period because the infant's urine production, although poor in concentration, may be adequate in volume. Often, the search for renal insufficiency is initiated only when growth failure or (unfortunately) even later manifestations of chronic renal failure are noted.

Other forms of renal dysplasia include oligomeganephronia (characterized by the presence of only a few large glomeruli) and the cystic dysplasias (characterized by the presence of renal cysts). This group includes microcystic disease (congenital nephrosis). A simple cyst within a kidney may be clinically unimportant because it does not predispose to progressive polycystic development. An entire kidney lost to multicystic development with concomitant hypertrophy and normal function of the contralateral side may also be of little clinical consequence. Nonetheless, even a simple cyst could pose problems if it becomes a site for lithiasis, infection or even symptomatic hematuria.

Polycystic Kidney Disease

The autosomal recessive form of polycystic kidney disease ("infantile" polycystic kidney disease) is characterized by large cystic kidneys, often associated with multiple organ systems affected by cystic malformations. Some children with this type die in the newborn period, but many will develop progressive deterioration toward end-stage renal failure. When autosomal recessive polycystic kidney disease is diagnosed at a later age, it may be predominantly manifested by liver rather than renal involvement. Autosomal dominant disease ("adult" form), though rarely of clinical significance (if at all) before the fourth decade, may also be detected in the newborn period and, depending on degree of severity, could be fatal. Although renal insufficiency and hypertension usually occur late in this type, there are exceptions. Detailed discussion of this entity is beyond the scope of this text. Careful documentation (usually by ultrasonography), close monitoring and management of the complications of renal insufficiency, and strict attention to hypertension control—as well as genetic counseling—are suggested. Management of end stage renal failure is by dialysis or renal transplantation.

Medullary Cystic Disease (Juvenile Nephronophthisis)

Medullary cystic disease is characterized by varying sizes of cysts in the medulla and is associated with tubular and interstitial nephritis. Children present with renal failure and signs of tubular dysfunction (decreased concentrating ability, Fanconi's syndrome). This lesion should not be confused with medullary sponge kidney (renal tubular ectasia), a frequently asymptomatic cystic disease usually found in adults.

Gabow PA: Autosomal dominant polycystic kidney disease. N Eng J Med 1993;329:332.

Kissane JM: Renal cysts in pediatric patients. Pediatr Nephrol 1990;4:69.

Pretorius DH et al: Diagnosis of autosomal dominant polycystic kidney disease in utero and in the young infant. J Ultrasound Med 1987;6:249.

DISTAL URINARY TRACT ANOMALIES

Obstruction of urine flow, infection, and stone formation, alone or in combination, are the hallmarks of distal urinary tract anomalies. Many of these abnormalities may be noted upon abdominal palpation and subsequently demonstrated by ultrasonography, excretory urography, or cystourethography. Some may be managed surgically; in others, therapy is limited to supportive treatment and prompt recognition and management of infection and chronic renal failure. Early recognition of reversible lesions is of the greatest importance. However, immediate postnatal detection and intervention may not be able to reverse damage sustained in utero.

Obstruction at the ureteropelvic junction may be the result of intrinsic muscle abnormalities, aberrant vessels, or fibrous bands. The lesion can cause hydronephrosis and usually presents as an abdominal mass in the newborn. Obstruction can occur in other parts of the ureter, especially at its entrance into the bladder, with resulting proximal hydroureter and hydronephrosis. Whether impediments to normal flow of urine are intrinsic or extrinsic, steps should immediately be taken to rectify the problem and minimize damage to the renal parenchyma.

Severe bladder malformations such as exstrophy are clinically obvious and provide a surgical challenge. More subtle—but urgent in terms of diagnosis—is obstruction of urine flow from aberrant posterior urethral valves. This anomaly, almost invariably confined to males, usually presents as anuria or a poor voiding stream in the newborn period; with severe obstruction of urine flow. Ascites may occur and the kidneys and bladder may be easily palpable. Provided that severe, irreversible damage to renal development has not occurred in utero, prompt intervention must be taken to avert further renal damage. The same can be said of many such complex genitourinary anomalies, including those of the external genitalia.

Complex Anomalies

The prune-belly syndrome is an association of urinary tract anomalies with cryptorchidism and absent abdominal musculature. Although complex anomalies, especially renal dysplasia, usually cause early death or the need for dialysis or transplantation, some patients have lived into the third decade with varying degrees of renal insufficiency. Early urinary diversion is essential to sustain renal function. At the time of this surgery, a renal biopsy can be obtained and may suggest the likelihood of adequate function in the future.

Discussion of other complex malformations, as well as such external genitalia anomalies as hypospadias, is beyond the scope of this text. Overall, urologic abnormalities resulting in severe compromise and destruction of renal tissue provide therapeutic and management challenges aimed at preserving all remaining function and treating the complications of progressive chronic renal failure.

Aliabadi H et al: Management of ureteropelvic junction obstruction in infants and neonates. Eur Urol 1988;15:103.

Lennert T et al: Multicystic renal dysplasia: Nephrectomy versus conservative treatment. Contrib Nephrol 1988; 67:183.

Rittenberg MH et al: Protective factors in posterior urethral valves. J Urol 1988;140:993.

HEMATURIA & GLOMERULAR DISEASE

Children with symptomatic (ie, painful) hematuria should be investigated for causes of direct injury to the urinary tract whether the pain is dysuria, associated with cystitis or urethritis; back pain secondary to pyelonephritis; or colicky flank pain accompanying the passage of a stone. "Bright red" blood or clots in the urine occur with bleeding disorders, trauma, and arteriovenous malformations. Abdominal masses suggest the presence of urinary tract obstruction, cystic disease, or tumors involving the renal or perirenal structures.

Asymptomatic hematuria is a challenge because clinical and diagnostic data must be obtained to determine whether the problem is transient or whether the child should be referred to a nephrologist for further diagnostic steps (such as renal biopsy) or management. Figure 24–1 suggests the outpatient approach to renal hematuria. The concern regarding the differential diagnosis is the possible presence of glomerular disease.

Acute poststreptococcal glomerulonephritis is the commonest form of postinfectious glomerulonephritis and the most frequently encountered in childhood. The epidemiologic relationship between certain strains of streptococci and glomerulonephritis is well recognized. Antigen-antibody complexes induced by the infection are formed in the bloodstream and deposited in the glomeruli. These deposited complexes may cause glomerular damage through activation of the complement system.

The diagnosis of poststreptococcal disease may be supported by a recent history (7–14 days previously) of group A β-hemolytic streptococcal infection. Recent streptococcal infection is demonstrated by an elevated antistreptolysin titer or by elevation of one or more antibody titers in the streptozyme panel. Other infections have been shown to cause similar glomerular injury; thus, postinfection glomerulonephritis is the better term for this type of acute glomerulonephritis.

The clinical presentation of glomerulonephritis is usually with gross hematuria ("coffee- or tea-colored" urine), with or without some (eg, periorbital) edema. Any symptoms reported are usually nonspecific, eg, malaise; in cases of severe hypertension, there may be headache. Fever is not expected. Severe glomerular injury (which usually occurs in severe, acute presentations of the more chronic or destructive forms of glomerulonephritis) may be accompanied by massive proteinuria (nephrotic syndrome), anasarca or ascites, and severe compromise in renal function.

There is no specific treatment for the nephritis. Appropriate antibiotic therapy is indicated for infection, if still present. The disturbances in renal function and resulting hypertension may require dietary management, diuretics, or antihypertensive drugs. In severe cases with rapidly deteriorating renal function, renal

Table 24–1. Glomerular diseases encountered in childhood.

Entity	Clinical Course	Prognosis
Postinfection glomerulonephritis (GN). Onset occurs 10–14 days after acute illness, commonly streptococcal. Characteristics include acute onset, tea-colored urine, mild to severe renal insufficiency (severe insufficiency is rare), edema.	Acute phase is usually over in 2 wks. There is complete resolution in 95% of cases. Severity of renal failure and hypertension varies. Microhematuria may persist to 18 months. Hypocomplementemia resolves in 1–30 days.	Excellent. Chronic disease is rare. Severe proteinuria, atypical presentation/course, or persistent hypocomplementemia suggest another entity is likely.
Membranoproliferative glomerulonephritis. Presentation ranges from mild microhematuria to acute GN syndrome. Diagnosis is made by renal biopsy. Etiologic origin is unknown. Type I and Type II are most common. Lesion is chronic.	Course can be mild to severe (rapid deterioration in renal function). May mimic postinfection GN. Proteinuria can be severe. Complement depression is intermittent to persistent. Hypertension is usually significant.	Type I may be responsive to medication (e.g. corticosteroids). Type II (dense deposit disease) is less treatable; functions decrease immediately to as long as 15 years later in 30–50% of untreated cases.
IgA Nephropathy. Classic presentation consists of asymptomatic gross hematuria during acute unrelated illness, with microhematuria between episodes. There are occasional instances of acute GN syndrome. Etiologic origin is unknown. Diagnosis is made by biopsy.	90% of cases resolve in 1–5 years. Gross hematuric episodes resolve with recovery from acute illness. Severity of renal insufficiency and hypertension varies. Proteinuria occurs in more severe, atypical cases.	Generally good. Small percentage develops chronic renal failure. Proteinuria in the nephrotic range is a poor sign. There is no universally accepted medication. (Corticosteroids may be useful in severe cases.)
Schönlein-Henoch purpura glomerulonephritis. Degree of renal involvement varies. Asymptomatic microhematuria is most common, but GN syndrome can occur. Renal biopsy is recommended in severe cases; it can provide prognostic information.	Presentation varies with severity of renal lesion. In rare cases, course may progress rapidly to serious renal failure. Hypertension varies. Proteinuria in the nephrotic range and severe decline in function can occur.	Overall, prognosis is good. Cases presenting with greater than 50% reduction in function or proteinuria exceeding 1 g/24 h may develop chronic renal failure. Severity of renal biopsy picture can best guide approach in such cases. There is no universally accepted medication.
Glomerulonephritis of systemic lupus erythematosus (SLE). Microhematuria and proteinuria on rare occasions are first signs of this systemic disease. Renal involvement varies. GN often causes the most concern. Histologic picture is variable.	Renal involvement is mild to severe. Clinical complexity depends on degree of renal insufficiency and other systems involved. Hypertension is significant. Manifestations of the severity of the renal lesion guide therapeutic intervention.	Renal involvement accounts for most of significant morbidity in SLE. Control of hypertension affects renal prognosis. Medication is guided by symptoms, serology, and renal lesion. End-stage renal failure can occur.
Hereditary glomerulonephritis (eg, Alport's syndrome). Transmission is autosomal dominant/x-linked, with family history marked by end-stage renal failure, especially in young males. Deafness and eye abnormalities are associated.	There is no acute syndrome. Females are generally less affected but are carriers. Hypertension and increasing proteinuria occur with advancing renal failure. There is no known medication. Management of manifestations of renal failure is appropriate.	Progressive proteinuria and hypertension occur early, with gradual decline in renal function in those most severely affected. Disease progresses to end-stage renal failure in most males.

biopsy and hemodialysis or peritoneal dialysis may be necessary; corticosteroids may also be administered in an attempt to influence the course.

The acute abnormalities generally resolve in 2–3 weeks and serum complement may be normal as early as 3 days or as late as 30 days. Although microscopic hematuria may persist for 1–2 years, most children recover completely. Persistent deterioration in renal function, urinary abnormalities beyond 18 months, persistent hypocomplementemia, and associated presence of nephrotic syndrome are ominous signs and are indications for renal biopsy.

Although the clinical presentations of the variety of glomerulonephritides are similar, the severity of presentation and clinical course influence differential diagnostic pursuits. The most commonly encountered entities in childhood and their clinical and histopathologic descriptions are listed in Table 24–1. Severe glomerular histopathologic and clinical entities, such as anti-glomerular basement membrane (anti-GBM) antibody disease (Goodpasture's syndrome) and idiopathic, rapidly progressive glomerulonephritis, may be considered in the differential diagnosis of acute glomerulonephritis, but these disorders are exceedingly rare in children.

Cameron JS: The treatment of lupus nephritis. Pediatr Nephrol 1989;3:350.

Couser WG: Pathogenesis of glomerulonephritis. Kidney Int 1991;44:5.

Ford DM et al: Childhood membranoproliferative glomerulonephritis type I: Limited steroid therapy. Kidney Int 1992;41:1606.

Jennetti JC, Falk RJ: Diagnosis and management of glomerulonephritis and vasculitis presenting as acute renal failure. Med Clin North Am 1990;74:893.

Oliviera DBG, Peters DK: Autoimmunity and the pathogenesis of glomerulonephritis. Pediatr Nephrol 1990;4:185.

Williams DG: Pathogenesis of idiopathic IgA nephropathy. Pediatr Nephrol 1993;7:303.

ACUTE INTERSTITIAL NEPHRITIS

Acute interstitial nephritis is characterized by diffuse or focal inflammation and edema of the renal interstitium and secondary involvement of the tubules but little or no secondary glomerular damage unless a combined or chronic picture is encountered. It seems to be related most often to drugs (eg, antibiotics, especially methicillin).

Fever, rigor, abdominal or flank pain, and rashes may occur in drug-associated cases. Urinalysis should reveal leukocyturia and hematuria. Hansel's staining of the urinary sediment is helpful in demonstrating the presence of eosinophils. The inflamma-

tion can be severe enough to cause rapid deterioration of renal function. Histologic demonstration of tubular and interstitial inflammation of the kidneys is helpful for diagnosis. Immediate identification and removal of the causative agent is imperative. A relentless course with progressive renal insufficiency or nephrotic syndrome may require supportive dialysis and treatment with corticosteroids.

PROTEINURIA & RENAL DISEASE

Urine is not normally completely protein-free, but the average excretion is well below 150 mg/24 h. Although isolated asymptomatic proteinuria may be secondary to renal disease or genitourinary tract abnormalities, proteinuria is not always associated with renal disease. Small increases in urinary protein can accompany febrile illnesses or exertion and can be noted in some cases only in urine produced while in the upright posture.

An approach to the workup of isolated proteinuria is shown in Figure 24–2. In idiopathic nephrotic syndrome without associated features of glomerulonephritis, treatment with corticosteroids may be initiated as described below. Nephrologic advice or follow-up should be pursued, especially in difficult or frequently relapsing cases.

CONGENITAL NEPHROSIS

Congenital nephrosis is a rare, uniformly fatal renal disorder that is often observed in more than one sibling in a family. Autosomal recessive inheritance is suggested. The kidneys are pale and large and may show microcystic dilations (microcystic disease) of the proximal tubules and glomerular changes. The latter consist of proliferation, crescent formation, and thickening of capillary walls. The pathogenesis is not well understood.

Infants with congenital nephrosis commonly have low birth weight (with an obstetric history of a large placenta), wide cranial sutures, delayed ossification, and mild edema. The edema may become apparent after the first few weeks or months of life. Anasarca follows, and the abdomen can become greatly distended by ascites. Massive proteinuria associated with typically appearing nephrotic syndrome and hyperlipidemia is the rule. Hematuria is common. If the patient lives long enough, progressive renal failure occurs. Most affected infants succumb to infections at the age of a few months.

Treatment has little to offer other than nutrition support and management of the chronic renal failure (qv).

IDIOPATHIC NEPHROTIC SYNDROME OF CHILDHOOD
("Nil" Disease, Lipoid Nephrosis, Minimal Change Disease)

Nephrotic syndrome is characterized by proteinuria, hypoproteinemia, edema, and hyperlipidemia. It may occur as a result of any form of glomerular disease and may be associated with a variety of extrarenal conditions. In children under 5 years of age, the disease usually takes the form of idiopathic nephrotic syndrome of childhood ("nil" disease, lipoid nephrosis), which has characteristic clinical and laboratory findings.

Clinical Findings

Affected patients are generally under 5 years of age at the time of their first episode. Often following an influenza-like syndrome, the child is noted to have periorbital swelling and perhaps oliguria. Within a few days, increasing edema—even anasarca—becomes evident. Other than vague malaise and, occasionally, abdominal pain, complaints are few. However, with significant "third spacing" of plasma volume, some children may even present with shock. With marked edema, there may also be dyspnea due to pleural effusions.

Despite heavy proteinuria, the urine sediment is usually normal. Microscopic hematuria (>20 rbc/hpf) should raise the suspicion of a glomerular lesion (such as focal glomerular sclerosis). Serum chemistries reveal hypoalbuminemia and hyperlipidemia. Abnormal immunoglobulin levels such as high IgM and low IgG have also been reported. However, no other evidence of immunologic disorder is present (eg, complement is normal, and there is no cryoglobulinemia). Some azotemia may occur but is related to intravascular volume depletion rather than to impairment of function.

Glomerular morphology is unremarkable except for fusion of foot processes of the visceral epithelium of the glomerular basement membrane. This finding, however, is nonspecific and is seen in many proteinuric states. There may be "minimal changes" in the glomerular mesangium, with unremarkable findings on immunofluorescence and electron microscopic examination.

Complications

Infectious complications (eg, peritonitis) are occasionally encountered, and pneumococci are frequently responsible. Immunization with pneumococcal vaccine is helpful. Hypercoagulability may be present, and thromboembolic phenomena are commonly reported.

Treatment & Prognosis

As soon as the diagnosis of idiopathic nephrotic syndrome is made, therapy with corticosteroids should be initiated. Prednisone, 2 mg/kg/d (maximum of 60 mg), is given daily for a maximum of 8 weeks until the dipstick test reveals trace to negative protein in the urine. The same dose is then administered on an alternate-day schedule for 1–2 months; thereafter, the dose is very gradually tapered and discontinued over an ensuing month. Lack of response—either total or partial—to treatment raises the suspicion of a true glomerular histopathologic lesion. If remission is achieved only to be followed by another relapse, the treatment course may be repeated. If at any time the nephrosis becomes refractory to treatment or if there are three relapses within a year's time, renal biopsy should be considered. If the histologic findings are consistent with "minimal change disease," other cytotoxic agents can be considered; however, these agents are generally most helpful when there is steroid dependence and not resistance.

Other therapeutic measures may be directed to the complications of the nephrotic syndrome itself. Unless the edema is of symptomatic proportions (eg, respiratory compromise due to ascites), diuretics should be used with extreme care; the patients are expected to have a decreased circulating volume and are also at risk for intravascular thrombosis. However, careful restoration of compromised circulating volume with intravenous albumin infusion and administration of diuretics is helpful in mobilizing edema. Immediate attention to infections (eg, acute peritonitis) is important to reduce morbidity.

Prognosis is often suggested by the initial response to corticosteroids. A prompt remission lasting for 3 years is almost always permanent. Failure to respond or early relapse usually heralds a prolonged series of relapses, which may indicate the presence of more serious nephropathy. Chlorambucil or other cytotoxic drug therapy is predictably successful only in children who respond to corticosteroids. As mentioned above, renal biopsy is recommended in atypical cases. Referral to a pediatric nephrologist should be made if steroid resistance or dependence is encountered.

Kher KK, Sweet M, Makker SP: Nephrotic syndrome in children. Curr Probl Pediatr (April) 1988;18:197.

Mendosa SA, Tune BM: Treatment of childhood nephrotic syndrome. J Am Soc Nephrol 1992;3:889.

Shulman SL et al: Predicting the response to cytotoxic therapy for childhood nephrotic syndrome: Superiority of response to corticosteroid therapy over histopathologic patterns. J Pediatr 1988;113:996.

FOCAL GLOMERULAR SCLEROSIS

Presentations of nephrotic syndrome that are resistant to corticosteroids or which relapse frequently may have as their histologic basis one of three most frequently encountered renal lesions. Therefore, referral to a pediatric nephrologist is necessary.

Focal glomerular sclerosis is characterized by the presence in renal biopsy specimens of normal-appearing glomeruli as well as some partially or completely sclerosed glomeruli. At presentation, the disease is often quite similar to idiopathic nephrotic syndrome; however, in most cases the response to corticosteroid therapy is poor. The lesion has serious prognostic implications; as many as 15–20% of cases can progress to end-stage renal failure. The clinical response to treatment is variable; experience with cyclosporine shows some promise.

Niaudet P et al: Treatment of severe childhood nephrosis. Adv Nephrol 1988;17:151.
Ponticelli C et al: A randomized trial of cyclosporine in steroid-resistant idiopathic nephrotic syndrome. Kidney Int 1993;43:1377.
Wyszynska T et al: Evaluation of prednisolone pulse therapy in steroid-resistant nephrotic syndrome: A multicenter collaborative study. Contrib Nephrol 1988;67:183.

MESANGIAL NEPHROPATHY
(Mesangial Glomerulonephritis)

Another lesion seen in cases of nephrosis poorly responsive to steroids is mesangial nephropathy, in which there is noted a distinct increase in the mesangial matrix of the glomeruli. Very often the expanded mesangium contains deposits of IgM demonstrated on immunofluorescent staining. Again, nephrologic consultation is helpful, as in a case where histologic diagnosis and therapy are needed.

MEMBRANOUS NEPHROPATHY
(Membranous Glomerulonephritis)

Membranous nephropathy is occasionally seen in children. The usual presenting feature is proteinuria of variable degree. This lesion has been reported to occur in children of all ages, but the diagnosis is more frequently made in older children.

Although largely idiopathic in nature, this renal lesion can be found in association with diseases such as hepatitis B antigenemia, systemic lupus erythematosus, congenital and secondary syphilis, and renal vein thrombosis; with immunologic disorders such as autoimmune thyroiditis; and with administration of drugs such as penicillamine. The pathogenesis is unknown, but it is thought that the glomerular lesion is the result of prolonged deposition of circulating antigen-antibody complexes.

The onset of membranous nephropathy is often insidious, but onset may be similar to that of idiopathic nephrotic syndrome of childhood (see above). Unlike that entity, membranous nephropathy is not expected to respond dramatically (ie, exhibit decreased proteinuria or complete remission of the nephrotic state) to corticosteroid therapy. However, low-dose exposure to steroid therapy has been shown to result in long-term favorable prognosis regarding the development of chronic renal insufficiency. The diagnosis is made by renal biopsy.

Cameron JS: Membranous nephropathy in childhood and its treatment. Pediatr Nephrol 1990;4:193.

DISEASES OF THE RENAL VESSELS

RENAL VEIN THROMBOSIS

In the newborn period, renal vein thrombosis may suddenly complicate the course of sepsis or dehydration. It may be observed in an infant of a diabetic mother, or it may be the result of umbilical vein catheterization. In older children and adolescents, renal vein thrombosis may develop following trauma or without any apparent predisposing factors; in these cases, nephrotic syndrome may be associated with renal vein thrombosis. There may also be an underlying membranous glomerulonephropathy.

Clinical Findings

In the newborn, renal vein thrombosis generally presents with the sudden development of an abdominal mass. If the thrombosis is bilateral, oliguria may be present; urine output may be normal with a unilateral thrombus. In older children, flank pain, sometimes with a palpable mass, is a common presentation. In some children with proteinuria, however, the nephrotic syndrome may be the first sign of renal vein thrombosis.

No single laboratory test is diagnostic of renal vein thrombosis. Hematuria usually is present and occasionally is gross. Proteinuria is less constant. In the newborn, thrombocytopenia may be found; this is rare in older children. Thrombosis may be demonstrated by ultrasonography and Doppler-flow studies.

Treatment

Anticoagulation with heparin is the treatment of choice both in newborns and in older children. In the newborn, a course of heparin combined with treatment of the underlying problem is usually all that is required. Management in other cases is less straightforward. The tendency for recurrence and embolization has led some workers in this field to recommend long-term anticoagulation. If an underlying membranous glomerulonephritis is suspected, biopsy should be performed.

Course & Prognosis

The rate of deaths due to renal vein thrombosis in the newborn is usually related to the underlying cause. If the child survives the acute phase, the prognosis for adequate renal function is good. The entity is much less common in older children, but they may be expected to follow the course known to occur in adults. Renal vein thrombosis may recur in the same kidney or occur in the other kidney years after the original episode of thrombus formation. Extension into the vena cava, with fatal pulmonary emboli, is a known complication.

The nephrotic syndrome, often with membranous glomerulonephritis, is associated with renal vein thrombosis. In some cases, thrombosis may be a complication of nephrotic syndrome. There is also evidence that the thrombus itself may result in glomerulonephritis, possibly through the release of renal tubular antigens.

RENAL ARTERIAL DISEASE

Children are susceptible to renovascular hypertension due to fibromuscular hyperplasia, congenital stenosis, or other renal arterial lesions. The proportion of hypertensive children with such demonstrable abnormalities, however, is quite small. Unfortunately, there are few clinical clues to underlying arterial lesions. Nonetheless, arterial lesions should be suspected in children whose hypertension is severe, beginning at 10 years of age or under, or associated with delayed visualization on excretory urogram. The diagnosis is established by renal arteriography with selective renal vein renin measurements. Some of these lesions may be repaired surgically (see Hypertension, below), but repair may be technically impossible in many small children. Although thrombosis of renal arteries is rare, it should be considered in a patient with acute onset of hypertension and hematuria in an appropriate setting (eg, in association with hyperviscosity or umbilical artery catheterization). Early diagnosis and treatment (eg, heparin) provides the best chance of reestablishing renal blood flow.

HEMOLYTIC-UREMIC SYNDROME

Although the glomerulonephritides as a group account for the majority of renal parenchymal causes of renal failure, the hemolytic-uremic syndrome is the most common single cause of renal failure due to glomerular vascular injury in childhood. Because of the usual gastrointestinal prodrome, severe fluid imbalances contribute to the degree of renal insufficiency; however, direct renal glomerular injury is primarily responsible.

The cause of the hemolytic-uremic syndrome is not well established, but epidemiologic studies have suggested both a genetic and an infectious or immunologic component. The primary lesion seems to be one of the endothelium of arterioles, especially in the kidney, with formation of platelet thrombi and resulting microangiopathic hemolysis. Recent data suggest that hemolytic-uremic syndrome involves a disorder of immunoregulation and that a unique class of anti-endothelial cell antibodies which may take part in the pathogenesis of the vascular injury is produced. However, the epidemic form of the disease in most cases is precipitated by *E coli* O157 verotoxin.

Clinical Findings

Hemolytic-uremic syndrome is found most often in children under 2 years of age. Older children may be expected to have a more severe course and thus a more guarded prognosis. It usually begins with a prodromal phase characterized by gastrointestinal symptoms, including abdominal pain, diarrhea, and vomiting. Oliguria, pallor, and bleeding manifestations, principally cutaneous and gastrointestinal, occur next. Hypertension and seizures develop in some infants, especially those who develop severe renal failure and fluid overload.

The triad of anemia, thrombocytopenia, and renal failure characterizes the syndrome. Anemia is profound and is associated with findings of red blood cell fragments on smear. A high reticulocyte count confirms the hemolytic nature of the anemia. The platelet count is almost invariably below $100,000/\mu L$. Other coagulation abnormalities are less consistent. Serum fibrin split products are often present, but fulminant disseminated intravascular coagulation is rare. Hematuria is often present. The serum complement level is normal.

Complications

The complications of hemolytic-uremic syndrome are usually those associated with the degree of renal failure. Neurologic problems, particularly seizures, may result from electrolyte abnormalities such as hyponatremia, hypertension, or central nervous system vascular disease. Severe bleeding, transfusion requirements, and complicating infections must be anticipated.

Treatment

As with any case of acute renal failure, meticulous attention to fluid and electrolyte status is crucial. There is evidence that early dialysis improves the prognosis; the size of the patient and the bleeding tendency will usually dictate peritoneal dialysis as the technique of choice. Seizures usually respond to control of hypertension and electrolyte abnormalities. It has been suggested that the plasma in some cases lacks a prostacyclin-stimulating factor, which is a potent inhibitor of platelet aggregation. Therefore, plasma infusion or plasmapheresis has been advocated in severe cases. Platelet inhibitors have also been tried, but the results have not been impressive, especially late in the disease. Nonetheless, it appears beneficial to use a platelet inhibitor early in the disease, which may obviate the need for platelet transfusion and has been observed to reduce, in some cases, the progression of renal failure. Red cell and platelet transfusions may be necessary; although the risk of volume overload is significant, it can be minimized by use of dialysis. The use of human recombinant erythropoietin (epoetin alfa) may be of benefit in minimizing red cell transfusion. While there is no universally accepted therapy for patients with this syndrome, the strict control of hypertension and nutrition and the use of dialysis appear to affect the long-term outcome. Renal failure may mandate dialysis.

Course & Prognosis

Geographic factors may determine the severity of hemolytic-uremic syndrome. Most commonly, children recover from the acute episode within 2–3 weeks, and follow-up examination reveals no residual renal insufficiency. However, some patients who recover from the acute episode have severe and occasionally progressive renal dysfunction or hypertension. Thus, follow-up of children recovering from hemolytic-uremic syndrome should include serial determinations of renal function for 1–2 years and meticulous attention to blood pressure for 5 years. Although a very small group of patients die in the early phase from the complications of central nervous system disease or acute renal failure, most children— even those with renal failure requiring dialysis—recover completely.

Kaplan BS et al: Recent advances in understanding the pathogenesis of the hemolytic uremic syndromes. Pediatr Nephrol 1990;4:276.

Rizzoni G et al: Plasma infusion for hemolytic-uremic syndrome in children: Results of a multicenter controlled trial. J Pediatr 1988;112:284.

Southwest Pediatric Nephrology Study Group: A clinicopathologic study of 24 children with hemolytic uremic syndrome. Pediatr Nephrol 1990;4:52.

Van Damme-Lombaerts J et al: Heparin plus dipyridamole in childhood hemolytic-uremic syndrome: A prospective, randomized study. J Pediatr 1988;113:913.

RENAL FAILURE

ACUTE RENAL FAILURE

Acute renal failure can be defined as the sudden inability to excrete urine of sufficient quantity or adequate composition to maintain normal body fluid homeostasis. It has many causes, including impaired renal perfusion, acute renal disease, renal ischemia, renal vascular compromise, or obstructive uropathy. Pre-renal, renal, and postrenal causes are shown in Table 24–2.

Clinical Findings

The hallmark of early renal failure is oliguria. The initial approach to an oliguric child should be aimed at classifying the problem in one of the categories outlined in Table 24–2. While an exact etiologic diagnosis is not necessary, accurate classification is helpful before initiating appropriate therapy.

If the cause of renal failure or oliguria is not clear, entities that can be treated (eg, volume depletion) should be considered first. After treatable problems or glomerular diseases are ruled out, a diagnosis of

Table 24–2. Classifications of causes of renal failure.

Prerenal
Dehydration due to gastroenteritis, malnutrition, or diarrhea
Hemorrhage, blood loss, aortic or renal vessel injury, trauma, surgery, cardiac surgery, renal arterial thrombosis
Diabetic acidosis
Pooling of interstitial fluid into local area of injury–burns, operative site, peritonitis
Hypovolemia associated with nephrotic syndrome
Shock
Heart failure
Renal
Hemolytic-uremic syndrome
Acute glomerulonephritis
Extension of prerenal hypoperfusion
Nephrotoxins
Acute tubular necrosis or vascular nephropathy
Renal (cortical) necrosis
Intravascular coagulation—septic shock, hemorrhage
Diseases of the kidney and vessels
Iatrogenic disorders
Severe infections
Drowning, especially fresh water
Treatment of neoplasms—hyperuricacidemia, hyperuricaciduria
Postrenal
Obstruction due to tumor, hematoma, or the presence of posterior urethral valves or ureteropelvic junction stricture, uretovesicle junction stricture, ureterocele
Sulfonamide crystals
Uric acid crystals
Stones
Trauma to a solitary kidney or collecting system
Renal vein thrombosis

acute tubular necrosis (eg, vasomotor nephropathy, ischemic injury) may be entertained.

A. Postrenal Causes: Postrenal failure, which is quite rare in children, is found in newborns with anatomic abnormalities. Obstruction of the bladder outlet should be relieved by insertion of a urethral catheter, followed by surgical correction. Timely intervention may prevent irreversible renal injury and chronic renal failure. Delayed voiding in the newborn period, anuria, or poor urinary stream usually suggests obstruction. Ureteropelvic junctional obstruction usually presents as an abdominal mass. Obstructive uropathy is accompanied by variable degrees of renal insufficiency.

B. Prerenal Causes: The commonest cause of decreased renal function in children is compromised renal perfusion. It is usually secondary to dehydration, although abnormalities of renal vasculature and poor cardiac performance may also be considered. Possible secondary causes should be addressed and, if possible, eliminated in order to determine if true renal functional disturbances are present.

C. Renal Causes: The various acute glomerulonephritides, the hemolytic-uremic syndrome, acute interstitial nephritis, and nephrotoxic injury are examples of "renal" entities that would be expected to produce varying degrees of acute renal failure. The diagnosis of acute tubular necrosis or vasomotor nephropathy is considered in clinical situations where—with no evidence of specific renal parenchymal diseases—the elimination of any prerenal or postrenal factors produces no improvement in renal performance.

Table 24–3 lists the urinary indices that are helpful in distinguishing prerenal conditions from acute tubular necrosis.

Complications

The clinical severity of the complications depends on the degree of renal functional impairment and oliguria. Common complications include (1) fluid overload (hypertension, congestive heart failure, pulmonary edema), (2) electrolyte disturbances (hyperkalemia), (3) metabolic acidosis, (4) hyperphosphatemia, and (5) uremia.

Table 24–3. Urine studies.

Prerenal Failure	Acute Tubular Necrosis
Urine osmolality 50 mosm/kg greater than plasma osmolality	Urine osmolality equal to or less than plasma osmolality
Urine sodium < 10 meq/L	Urinary sodium > 20 meq/L
Ratio of urine creatinine to plasma creatinine > 14:1	Ratio of urine creatinine to plasma creatinine < 14:1
Specific gravity > 1.020	Specific gravity 1.012–1.018

Treatment

An indwelling catheter is inserted and urine output monitored hourly. If insignificant quantities of urine are produced and renal failure is established, the catheter should be removed, as it will be more of a hazard than an aid. Prerenal or postrenal factors should be excluded or rectified and the circulating volume maintained with appropriate fluids. The patient's response is assessed by physical examination and observed urinary output. Measurement of central venous pressure may be indicated. If diuresis does not occur in response to the above measures, give furosemide, 1–5 mg/kg intravenously, the dose being higher with higher serum creatinine levels. Allow 1 hour for a response to occur. If the urine output remains low (< 200–250 mL/m^2/24 h), repeat the furosemide (up to 5 mg/kg). If no diuresis occurs, the further administration of diuretics will not be helpful.

If these maneuvers produce return of urine flow but biochemical evidence of acute renal failure persists, the resulting "nonoliguric" acute renal failure or acute tubular necrosis should, at the very least, be more manageable. Fluid overload and its attendant problems may then be avoided, and dialysis may be averted. However, if clinically necessary indicated medications and nutrients threatens to exceed the urinary output, or if reduction in such medications and nutrients would result in less than optimal care, dialysis is indicated. Institution of dialysis before the early complications of acute renal failure develop is likely to improve clinical management and outcome.

A. Indications for Dialysis: The need for dialysis is determined on the basis of individuals' clinical findings. However, there are some immediate, clinical indications for dialysis: (1) severe hyperkalemia; (2) unrelenting metabolic acidosis (usually in a situation where fluid overload prevents sodium bicarbonate administration); (3) fluid overload with or without severe hypertension or congestive heart failure (a situation that would seriously compromise caloric or drug administration); and (4) symptoms of uremia, usually manifested in children by central nervous system depression. The rate of rise of both blood urea nitrogen and serum creatinine levels may indicate the need for dialysis; it is generally accepted that the blood urea nitrogen level should not be allowed to exceed 100 mg/dL in small children.

Early dialysis, when properly performed, can simplify management and reduce morbidity and mortality of acute renal failure.

B. Methods of Dialysis: The choice between peritoneal dialysis and hemodialysis depends largely on the availability of either technique and the relative indications or contraindications of each procedure in a given patient. Peritoneal dialysis is generally preferred in children because of the ease of performance and patient tolerance. Although peritoneal dialysis is technically less efficient than hemodialysis, hemodynamic stability and metabolic control can be better sustained because this technique can be applied on a relatively continuous basis. However, hemodialysis should be considered in the following situations: (1) if rapid removal of toxins is desired; (2) if the size of the patient makes hemodialysis less technically cumbersome and hemodynamically well-tolerated; or (3) if impediments to efficient peritoneal dialysis are present (eg, ileus).

C. Complications of Dialysis: Complications of peritoneal dialysis include peritonitis, volume depletion, and technical complications such as dialysate leakage or respiratory compromise from intra-abdominal dialysate fluid. Peritonitis can be avoided by strict adherence to aseptic technique. Experienced personnel are largely responsible for minimizing the incidence of this complication. Peritoneal fluid cultures are obtained as clinically indicated. Dialysate can leak around the dialysis catheter or through tissue planes, causing dissection. However, leakage can be reduced by good catheter placement technique and appropriate intra-abdominal dialysate volumes. Any technical problems that result in abnormal flow of dialysate in and out of the peritoneal cavity require the attention of the nephrology consultant. Dialysis is useful in maintaining electrolyte balance; because potassium is absent from standard dialysate solutions, potassium may be added to the dialysate as clinically indicated. Phosphate is also absent because hyperphosphatemia is an expected problem in renal failure. Nonetheless, in situations where nutritional impairments result in inadequate phosphate intake, care must be taken to avert hypophosphatemia when implementing dialysis. Because dextrose is used in the dialysate to produce osmotic removal of water, hyperglycemia may result, especially when the higher dextrose concentrations are used (maximum 4.25%). Using the higher concentrations of dextrose can achieve relatively rapid correction of fluid overload. Fluid removal may also be increased with more frequent exchanges of the dialysate. However, rapid osmotic transfer of water may result in hypernatremia. Careful monitoring of all these parameters must accompany the process.

Hemodialysis can rapidly correct major metabolic and electrolyte disturbances, as well as volume overload. Technology that permits hemodialysis of even the small infant is available. The process is highly efficient, but there can be significant symptomatology and pathophysiologic responses to the rapidity of the induced physiologic and metabolic changes. Problems arising from these changes are minimized or avoided when experienced personnel under the direction of a nephrology consultant administer hemodialysis. Hemodynamic instability during the procedure is a common problem but can be controlled. Anticoagulation is usually required for the procedure, but under appropriate conditions it may be performed with minimal exposure to the risks associated with heparin administration. Careful monitoring of all

these factors, as well as appropriate biochemical parameters, must be performed. Note, however, that during or immediately following the procedure, blood sampling will produce misleading results because equilibration between extravascular compartments and the blood will not yet have been completed.

Access devices (eg, subclavian catheters) must be inspected for thrombotic or infectious complications. Such problems are greatly reduced when only experienced personnel are permitted to manipulate the various cannulas or catheters employed in the procedure.

The chronic applications of these forms of dialysis are also available for children. Continuous ambulatory peritoneal dialysis (CAPD) and continuous cycling peritoneal dialysis (CCPD) are both extremely useful for children and adults alike. These methods carry the advantages of simple application in the home setting and avoidance of the vascular access problems inherent with chronic hemodialysis. Although eventual renal transplantation is the ultimate goal for most children with end stage renal failure, the improvement in the techniques of dialysis has greatly enhanced the long-term management of these children.

Course & Prognosis

The period of severe oliguria, if it occurs, usually lasts about 10 days. If oliguria lasts longer than 3 weeks or if there is complete anuria, a diagnosis of acute tubular necrosis is very unlikely; vascular injury, severe ischemia (cortical necrosis), glomerulonephritis, or obstruction is more probable. The diuretic phase begins with progressive increases in urinary output, followed by the passage of large volumes of isosthenuric urine containing sodium levels of 80–150 meq/L. During the recovery phase, signs and symptoms subside rapidly, although polyuria may persist for several days or weeks. Urinary abnormalities usually disappear completely within a few months.

CHRONIC RENAL FAILURE

Chronic renal failure in children most commonly results from developmental abnormalities of the kidneys or urinary tract. The kidneys may develop poorly (hypoplasia, dysplasia) or not at all (aplasia). Cystic development may result in immediate or progressive insufficiency. Abnormal development of the urinary tract may not permit normal renal development. However, depending on the degree of interference with normal renal parenchymal development, timely surgery may minimize parenchymal injury and perhaps even achieve totally normal function. In older children, the chronic glomerulonephritides and nephropathies, irreversible nephrotoxic injury, or the hemolytic-uremic syndrome may also result in chronic renal failure.

In early life, when chronic renal failure is the result of an inadequate amount of normally functioning renal tissue, the clinical presentation is marked by inability to produce a concentrated urine (polyuria, polydipsia, enuresis). Depending on the degree of renal insufficiency, failure to thrive may be the chief concern. If abnormalities of the collecting system are responsible, there may be a history of urinary tract infection that had somehow missed medical attention and intervention. However, progressive deterioration of renal function may occur in the absence of infection. Usually, it is only in situations where appropriate health maintenance has not been available that such children present with overt complications of long-standing chronic renal failure, such as rickets or growth delay.

Chronic renal failure resulting from glomerulonephritis does not characteristically present with polyuria. Growth failure depends on age at presentation and the rapidity of functional decline. Given the usually acute initial presentation, it is likely that such a child would have early intervention and follow-up by a nephrologist. However, some of the chronic glomerulonephritides (eg, membranoproliferative glomerulonephritis) can progress unnoticed if subtle abnormalities of the urinary sediment are undetected or ignored. Any child with a history of chronic glomerulonephritis or significant renal injury (eg, hemolytic-uremic syndrome with residual renal insufficiency) needs close follow-up and monitoring of renal function, as well as careful attention directed at controlling associated abnormalities that contribute to the rate of functional decline (eg, hypertension, urinary tract infection).

Complications

Despite the kidney's ability to compensate for gradual loss of functioning nephrons in chronic renal failure progression, there are resulting complications that are expected early as well as those that occur toward end-stage renal disease (GFR < 15 mL/min/$1.73 m^2$); at this point, the compensatory capability is exhausted. In children who have developmentally reduced function but who are unable to concentrate the urine, polyuria and thus dehydration is more likely to be a problem than fluid overload. As renal homeostatic capability approaches end-stage, there may be a reduction in output; however, many such children can continue to produce generous quantities of urine (but not "good quality" urine), even when renal replacement therapies are initiated. Moreover, a "salt-wasting" state can occur. On the other hand, those children who develop chronic renal failure due to the glomerular disease will characteristically have difficulty with sodium and water retention and hypertension relatively early in the course of chronic renal failure.

Other rather early manifestations of chronic renal failure include metabolic acidosis and growth retardation. Disturbances in calcium, phosphorus, and vitamin D metabolism leading to renal osteodystrophy require prompt attention. Although renal compensation and increased parathyroid hormone can maintain a normal serum phosphate early in the course, there is a price to be paid: tertiary hyperparathyroidism with resulting skeletal abnormalities. This can be reflected early by an increase in serum alkaline phosphatase.

Overt uremic symptoms are late manifestations of chronic renal failure, (eg, severe hyperkalemia, and pericarditis). These complications are best averted by timely renal replacement therapy, ie, dialysis or transplant. Keep in mind that if left unchecked, chronic renal failure eventually will adversely affect every organ system. The subjective symptoms of uremia (eg, anorexia, nausea, lethargy) may be somewhat ameliorated by dietary protein restriction. However, compromise in adequate caloric intake can result from the protein restriction. Considerable interference with growth occurs in the uremic state anyway. The most difficult aspect of any dietary restriction is patient compliance. A diet restricted in sodium, potassium, and phosphorus that at the same time provides adequate caloric intake is often rejected. Dietary supplementation with essential amino or keto acids is helpful if the child will accept it. Therefore, utilization of dialysis may be indicated for successful dietary and nutritional control. Nasogastric feeding may be necessary, especially for the infant or small child, even while the child is maintained on chronic dialysis.

Anemia is usual in chronic renal failure. It is usually normochromic and normocytic and results from decreased renal erythropoietin synthesis as renal parenchyma atrophies. The anemia responds to erythropoitin treatment. Platelet dysfunction and other abnormalities of the coagulation system may be present. Bleeding phenomena, especially gastrointestinal bleeding, may be a problem.

Central nervous system manifestations of the condition range from subtle to confusion, apathy, and lethargy. These symptoms usually occur late in the course of disease and may be unsuspected clinically until the patient is carefully evaluated. With advancing uremia, stupor and coma may be present. Associated electrolyte abnormalities (eg, hyponatremia) may precipitate seizures (more commonly, a result of untreated hypertension).

Cardiovascular manifestations may be life-threatening. Uremic pericarditis may develop. Congestive heart failure or hypertension may be seen with volume overload, excessive renin excretion, or both.

Patients with chronic renal failure tend to be more susceptible to infections. Because of their generally debilitated state, they often handle infections poorly.

Treatment

The aim of treatment in chronic renal failure prior to dialysis is to minimize the occurrence of the aforementioned complications. However, presuming nothing more can be done for the underlying renal disease, efforts are still aimed at preserving as much renal function for as long as possible, provided that the patient tolerates the withholding of renal replacement therapies.

Controlling hypertension (see Treatment of Hypertension), hyperphosphatemia, and urinary tract infection can contribute greatly toward this endeavor. Acidosis may be treated with sodium citrate solutions, provided that the added sodium will not aggravate hypertension. Hyperphosphatemia is controlled by attempts at dietary restriction and the use of dietary phosphate binders (eg, calcium carbonate). Vitamin D should be administered to maintain normal serum calcium. When the blood urea nitrogen exceeds approximately 50 mg/dL, or if the child is lethargic or anorexic, dietary protein restriction should be initiated. Sodium restriction is advisable when hypertension is present. Potassium restriction will be necessary as the GFR falls to a level where urinary output decreases sharply. Meanwhile, the diet must continue to meet the child's specific daily requirements.

Renal function must be regularly monitored (creatinine and blood urea nitrogen), as well as serum electrolytes, calcium, phosphorus, and alkaline phosphatase. Results will guide changes in dietary management as well as adjustment in phosphate binder, citrate buffer, vitamin D, fluid intake, and blood pressure medications. Anemia may be effectively treated with recombinant human erythropoietin (epoetin alfa). All of these areas require careful monitoring in order to minimize symptomatology while continuing to assess the success or failure of the chronic renal failure treatment regimen and the need for the institution of chronic dialysis and transplantation.

Caution must also be taken to avoid medications that (1) aggravate the uremic condition (eg, tetracyclines, which increase blood urea); (2) depend upon renal excretion (eg, compounds containing magnesium); (3) raise blood pressure (eg, over-the-counter cold preparations containing vasoconstrictive agents); or (4) contain high amounts of substances of particular concern in the management of chronic renal failure (eg, sodium, potassium, and phosphate). Successful management relies greatly upon the education of patient and family.

Attention must also be directed to the psychosocial needs of the patient and family during their adjustment to severe chronic illness. The strategy for patient management, and the need for family education and adjustment, changes once a plan for chronic dialysis and possible renal transplantation is initiated. These changes may include a reduction in medications or dietary limitations, with the potential for improving growth.

Dialysis & Transplantation

The method of treatment of end-stage renal disease best tolerated by the child is a successful and uncomplicated renal transplant. Transplantation at first seems ideal; however, despite the advances that have been made in organ transplantation procedures, there are some problems. Adequate growth and well-being are directly related to acceptance of the graft, the degree of normal function, and the side effects of medications employed.

Great advances have also been made in peritoneal dialysis and hemodialysis, both in technique and in our understanding of the specialized approach required by the treatments. Hemodialysis is now performed in major centers that devote their entire effort in dialysis toward the management of pediatric patients, and it is now regarded as a reasonable long-range method of treating the child with end-stage renal disease. Treatment of terminal renal failure in children may thus consist of transplantation or dialysis, as the situation warrants. The demonstrated feasibility of chronic peritoneal dialysis in children has made this treatment most often the initial choice of dialysis therapy for children. Peritoneal dialysis via an indwelling chronic catheter is well accepted by children and can be performed in the home.

The best measure of the success of chronic dialysis in children is the level of physical and psychosocial rehabilitation achieved. Patients continue to participate in day-to-day activities and attend school; they have even recorded reasonable growth. Although catch-up growth rarely occurs, patients can grow at an acceptable rate even though they remain in the 3rd percentile. Associated problems such as chronic anemia and bone disease are being better controlled, and contribute to improved outcomes.

Beckman et al: Measurement of erythropoietin in anephric children: A report of the Southwest Pediatric Nephrology Study Group. Pediatr Nephrol 1989;3:75.

Lum GM: Peritonitis in infants and children on CAPD/CCPD. In: *Chronic Ambulatory Peritoneal Dialysis (CAPD) and Chronic Cycling Peritoneal Dialysis (CCPD) in Children.* Fine RN (editor). Martinus Nijhoff, 1987.

McEnery PT et al: Renal transplantation in children: A report of the North American Pediatric Renal Transplant Cooperative study. N Eng J Med 1992;326:1721.

Nakano M et al: Protein intake and renal function in children. Am J Dis Child 1989;143:160.

Tejani A et al: Strategies for optimizing growth in children with kidney transplants. Transplantation 1989;47:229.

RENAL HYPERTENSION

Hypertension in children is commonly of renal origin. It is usually encountered as an anticipated complication of known renal parenchymal disease, but it may be found on routine physical examination in an otherwise normal child. Increased understanding of the roles of water and salt retention on the one hand and overactivity of the renin-angiotensin system on the other has done much to guide therapy; it is nevertheless clear that not all forms of hypertension can be explained by these two mechanisms.

Hypertension in the newborn period is frequently encountered in the ill infant, usually in an intensive care setting. Etiologic origins include (1) congenital anomalies of the kidneys or renal vasculature, (2) obstruction of the urinary tract, (3) thrombosis of renal vasculature or kidneys, and (4) volume overload. There are also reported instances of apparent paradoxical elevations of blood pressure in clinical situations where chronic diuretic therapy is employed, eg, bronchopulmonary dysplasia. Asymptomatic hypertension in the newborn also elicits a search for renal, vascular, or aortic abnormalities (eg, polycystic kidneys, obstruction, renal vascular stenosis, thrombosis, neurofibromatosis, coarctation, etc), as well as some endocrine disorders.

Diagnosis

A child is felt to be normotensive if the average recorded systolic and diastolic blood pressures are less than the 90th percentile for age and sex. The 90th percentile in the newborn period is approximately 85–90/55–65 mm Hg for both sexes. In the first year of life, the acceptable levels are 90–100/60–67 mm Hg. Incremental increases with growth occur, gradually approaching young adult ranges of 100–120/65–75 mm Hg in the late teens. Careful measurement of the blood pressure includes ensuring that the size of the cuff is correct and that the equipment is reliable. The cuff should be wide enough to cover two-thirds of the upper arm and should encircle the arm completely without causing an overlap in the inflatable bladder. Although an anxious child may have an elevation in blood pressure, abnormal readings must not be too hastily attributed to this cause. Repeat measurement is helpful, especially after the child has been consoled.

Evaluation of renal hypertension in children is particularly directed toward the possibility of a unilateral lesion or other abnormality that might be susceptible to remedy by surgery. The evaluation of nonrenal possibilities suggested by the history or physical signs is detailed under these respective conditions.

Routine laboratory studies include a complete blood count, urinalysis, and urine culture and radiographic delineation of the urinary tract. A renal biopsy (which rarely reveals the cause of hypertension unless there is clinical evidence of renal disease) should always be undertaken with special care in the hypertensive patient and preferably after pressures have been controlled by therapy. Ureteric catheterization is not used now in lateralizing lesions; instead, the appropriate information is obtained from renal size, a rapid-sequence intravenous urogram, the renal scan, aortography with renal arteriography, and differential renal vein renin levels. A suggested approach to the outpatient work-up is shown in Figure 24–3.

Treatment

A. Treatment of Acute Emergent Hypertension: A hypertensive emergency may be said to exist when central nervous system signs of hypertension appear, eg, papilledema or seizures. Retinal hemorrhages or exudates also indicate a need for prompt and effective control. However, it is quite common in children to see no end organ abnormalities secondary to hypertension. Treatment varies with the clinical presentation. The primary classes of useful antihypertensive drugs are (1) diuretics, (2) alpha- and beta-adrenergic blockers, (3) angiotensin-converting enzyme (ACE) inhibitors, (4) calcium channel blockers, and (5) vasodilators.

1. One of the most effective drugs for use in a true hypertensive emergency is diazoxide, 5 mg/kg by a single, rapid intravenous injection.

2. Intravenous hydralazine can be effective in some cases. Dosage varies according to the severity of the hypertension and should begin at around 0.15 mg/kg.

3. Sodium nitroprusside is also effective in an intensive care setting for reducing severely elevated blood pressure. Intravenous administration of 0.5–10 µg/kg/min will reduce blood pressure in seconds, but the dose must be carefully monitored.

4. Furosemide, 1–5 mg/kg intravenously, will reduce blood volume and enhance the effectiveness of other drugs.

5. Sublingual nifedipine, a calcium channel blocker, is rapid-acting and in appropriate doses should not result in hypotensive blood pressure levels. The liquid from a 10 mg capsule can be withdrawn with a syringe, and dosage can be approximated. The exact dosage for children who weigh less than 10–30 kg is difficult to ascertain by this method, but 5 mg is a safe starting point. Because the treatment is directed at emergent levels of blood pressure, it is unlikely that the effects will be greater than desired. Larger children with malignant hypertension require 10 mg. In such cases, the capsule may simply be pierced and the medication squeezed under the patient's tongue. Whatever method is used to control emergent hypertension safely and rapidly, concomitant administration of oral medications for sustained control should also be initiated so that the effect will be maintained and the emergent measures reduced and discontinued. (See Table 24–4.)

Acute elevations of blood pressure not exceeding the 95th percentile for age may be approached with oral medication, and measures should be aimed at progressive improvement and control within 48 hours.

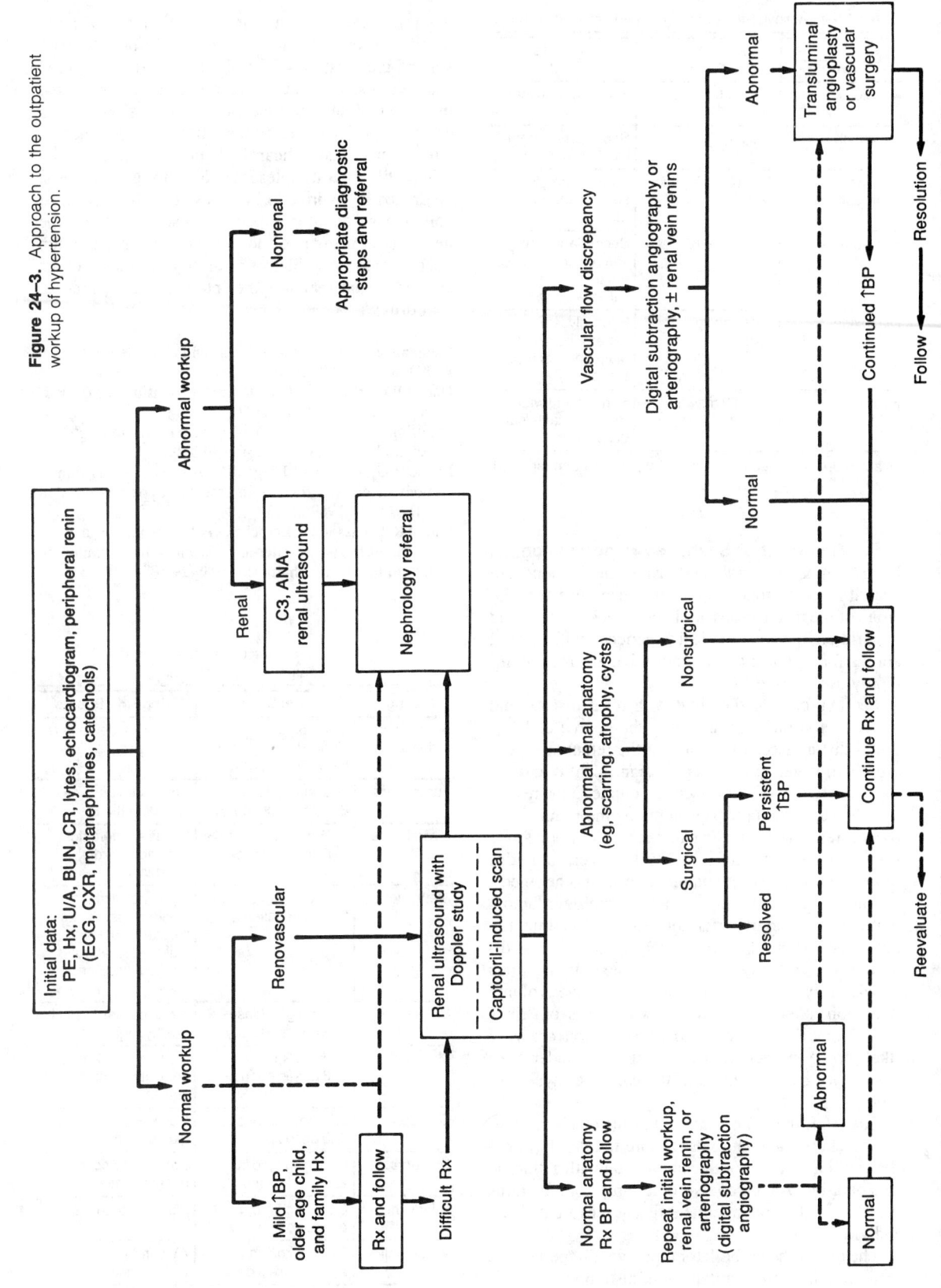

Figure 24-3. Approach to the outpatient workup of hypertension.

Table 24–4. Antihypertensive drugs for emergent treatment.

Drug	Dose	Major Side Effects[1]
Nifedipine	0.25–0.5 mg/kg SL	Flushing, tachycardia
Labetalol	1–3 mg/kg/h IV	Secondary to beta-blocking activity
Sodium nitroprusside	0.5–10 mg/kg/min IV drip	Cyanide toxicity, sodium and water retention
Furosemide	1–5 mg/kg IV	Secondary to severe volume contraction, hypokalemia
Diazoxide	2–10 mg/kg IV bolus	Hyperglycemia, hyperuricemia, sodium and water retention
Hydralazine	0.1–0.2 mg/kg IV	Sodium and water retention, tachycardia, flushing

[1]Many more side effects than those listed have been reported.

B. Treatment of Sustained Hypertension:

A large number of antihypertensive medications are available for the treatment of sustained hypertension. None of the medications has been extensively studied in children, but wide clinical experience with several allows for a choice among those that are more commonly used (Table 24–5).

The approach to the child with renal disease and hypertension includes assessing the degree of functional disturbances that result in the retention of sodium and water. When there is significant retention, the contribution of intravascular volume to the resulting elevated blood pressure supports the rational use of a diuretic. Thus, in some instances a diuretic alone may offer therapeutic benefit; however, diuretics more often are used in combination with other medications aimed at the other pathophysiologic factors that contribute to hypertension. As a single drug, the beta-blockers may be more widely applicable than diuretics and certainly lack the possible complications of electrolyte disturbances and excessive volume depletion. Nonetheless, these two classes of "first-order" medications for mild hypertension are very likely to be inadequate in the control of moderate to severe (ie, greater than the 95th percentile) hypertension.

The ACE inhibitors—as well as the calcium channel blockers—are being used more frequently in pediatrics, either alone or in combination with a diuretic or a beta-blocker. Of course, other drug combinations are used as their therapeutic efficacy is evaluated and individualized.

The use of the vasodilator type of antihypertensive drug requires concomitant administration of a diuretic to counter the effect of vasodilation on increas-ing renal sodium and water retention and a beta-blocker to counter reflex tachycardia. Minoxidil, considered the most powerful of the orally administered vasodilators, can be extremely efficacious in the treatment of severe, sustained hypertension, but its effect is greatly offset by the other effects described. Hirsutism is a significant side effect; consequently, minoxidil is a troublesome drug to use in girls. Hydralazine hydrochloride may still be the most common vasodilator in pediatric use, but, again, the necessity of using two additional drugs for maximum benefit keeps vasodilators in reserve for those severe situations that mandate the intervention of three or four drugs.

Flamanbaum W: Beta-blockers and hypertension. Am J Hypertens 1989;2:865.

Hanna JD, Chan JCM, Gill JR Jr: Hypertension and the kidney. J Pediatr 1991;118:327.

Ingelfinger JR: Investigating hypertension in children. Nephrol News Issues (Feb) 1989;3:29.

Leonetti G, Terzoli L, Bragato R: Advantages and limitations of diuretic therapy in essential hypertension. Am J Hypertens 1989;2:825.

Parent R, Chiasson JL, Larochelle P: Hemodynamic and endocrine effects of acute and chronic administration of nifedipine. J Clin Pharmacol 1989;29:107.

Table 24–5. Antihypertensive drugs for ambulatory treatment.

Drug	Oral Dose	Major Side Effects[1]
Hydrochlorothiazide	2–4 mg/kg/24 h as single dose or in 2 individual doses	Potassium depletion, hyperuricemia.
Furosemide	1–5 mg/kg/dose, 2–3 doses per day	Potassium and volume depletion.
Hydralazine	0.75 mg/kg/24 h in 4–6 divided doses	Lupus erythematosus, tachycardia, headache.
Methyldopa	10–40 mg/kg/24 h in 3 divided doses	False-positive Coombs test, hemolytic anemia, fever, leukopenia, abnormal liver function tests.
Propranolol	0.2–5 mg/kg/dose, 2–3 doses per day	Syncope, cardiac failure, hypoglycemia.
Minoxidil	0.15 mg/kg/dose, 2–3 doses per day	Tachycardia, angina, fluid retention, hirsutism.
Captopril	0.3–2 mg/kg/dose, 2–3 doses per day	Rash, hyperkalemia, glomerulopathy.
Enalapril	0.2–5 mg/kg/d in 2 divided doses	Proteinuria, cough, hyperkalemia.
Nifedipine	0.5–1 mg/kg/d, 3 doses per day	Flushing, tachycardia.
Verapamil	3–7 mg/kg/d in 2 or 3 divided doses	AV conduction disturbance.

[1]Many more side effects than those listed have been reported.

INHERITED OR DEVELOPMENTAL DEFECTS OF THE URINARY TRACT

Numerous entities and syndromes involve developmental, hereditary, or metabolic abnormalities of the kidneys and collecting system. The clinical problems encountered include concerns with overall metabolic consequences, failure to thrive, nephrolithiasis, renal glomerular or tubular dysfunction, and chronic renal failure. Specific discussion of all such entities is beyond the scope of this text. However, Table 24–6 lists some of the major entities and groups them into clinically, metabolically, or anatomically related problems.

DISORDERS OF THE RENAL TUBULES

Three subtypes of renal tubular acidosis are well recognized: (1) the "classic" form, called type I or distal renal tubular acidosis; (2) the bicarbonate "wasting" form, designated as type II or proximal renal tubular acidosis; and (3) type IV, or hyperkalemic renal tubular acidosis (rare in children), which is associated with hyporeninemic hypoaldosteronism. Type I and type II and their variants are encountered most frequently in children. Thus, discussion will focus on these two most commonly seen problems of urinary acidification.

Primary tubular disorders in childhood, such as glycinuria, hypouricemia, or renal glycosuria, may result from a defect in a single tubular transport pathway (see Table 24–6).

DISTAL RENAL TUBULAR ACIDOSIS (TYPE I)

The most common form of distal renal tubular acidosis in childhood is the hereditary form. The clinical presentation is one of failure to thrive, anorexia, vomiting, and dehydration. Hyperchloremic metabolic acidosis occurs, with hypokalemia and a urinary pH exceeding 6.5. The severity of the acidosis depends usually on the presence of a bicarbonate "leak." (This variant of distal renal tubular acidosis with bicarbonate wasting has been called type III but for clinical purposes need not be considered as a distinct entity.) Concomitant hypercalciuria may lead to rickets, nephrocalcinosis, nephrolithiasis, and renal failure.

Table 24–6. Inherited or developmental defects of the urinary tract.

Cystic diseases of genetic origin
  Polycystic disease
    Autosomal recessive form (infantile)
    Autosomal dominant form (adult)
    Other syndromes that include either form
  Cortical cysts
    Several syndromes are known to have various renal cystic manifestations, including "simple" cysts; may not have significant effect on renal functional status nor be associated with progressive disease
  Medullary cysts
    Medullary sponge kidney
    Medullary cystic disease (nephronophthisis)
  Hereditary and familial cystic dysplasia
    Congenital nephrosis
    "Finnish" disease

Dysplastic renal diseases
  Renal aplasia (unilateral, bilateral)
  Renal hypoplasia (unilateral, bilateral, total, segmental)
  Multicystic renal dysplasia (unilateral, bilateral, multilocular, postobstructive, etc)
  Familial and hereditary renal dysplasias
  Oligomeganephronia

Hereditary diseases associated with nephritis
  Hereditary nephritis with deafness and ocular defects (Alport's syndrome)
  Nail-patella syndrome
  Familial hyperprolinemia
  Hereditary nephrotic syndrome
  Hereditary osteolysis with nephropathy
  Hereditary nephritis with thoracic asphyxiant dystrophy syndrome

Hereditary diseases associated with intrarenal deposition of metabolites
  Angiokeratoma corporis diffusum (Fabry's disease)
  Heredopathia atactica polyneuritiformis (Refsum's disease)
  Various storage diseases (eg, G_{M1} monosialogangliosidosis, Hurler syndrome, Niemann-Pick disease, familial metachromatic leukodystrophy, glycogenosis type I [von Gierke's disease], glycogenosis type II [Pompe's disease])
  Hereditary amyloidosis (familial Mediterranean fever; heredofamilial urticaria with deafness and neuropathy; primary familial amyloidosis with polyneuropathy)

Hereditary renal diseases associated with tubular transport defects
  Hartnup disease
  Immunoglycinuria
  Fanconi's syndrome
  Oculocerebrorenal syndrome of Lowe
  Cystinosis (infantile, adolescent, adult types)
  Wilson's disease
  Galactosemia
  Hereditary fructose intolerance
  Renal tubular acidosis (many types)
  Hereditary tyrosinemia
  Renal glycosuria
  Vitamin D-resistant rickets
  Pseudohypoparathyroidism
  Vasopressin-resistant diabetes insipidus
  Hypouricemia

Hereditary diseases associated with lithiasis
  Hyperoxaluria
  L-Glyceric aciduria
  Xanthinuria
  Lesch-Nyhan syndrome and variants, gout
  Nephropathy due to familial hyperparathyroidism
  Cystinuria (types I, II, III)
  Glycinuria

Miscellaneous
  Hereditary intestinal vitamin B_{12} malabsorption
  Total and partial lipodystrophy
  Sickle cell anemia
  Bartter's syndrome

Other situations that may be responsible for distal renal tubular acidosis are listed in Table 24–6.

The pathogenesis of distal renal tubular acidosis has not yet been clearly defined. Basically, there appears to be a defect in the distal nephron, in the tubular transport of hydrogen ion, or in the maintenance of a steep enough gradient for proper excretion of hydrogen ion. This defect can be accompanied by degrees of bicarbonate wasting, or the defect may not be severe enough to lead to frank acidosis. More studies are needed to clarify the role of a variety of abnormalities that may be associated with the distal defect.

The classic method for determining the ability to handle an acid load in suspected distal renal tubular acidosis is the administration of NH_4Cl. However, this approach has been challenged. Recent evidence has shown that during sodium bicarbonate loading, the CO_2 tension of the urine does not increase in patients with distal renal tubular acidosis as it does in normal controls; this reflects a problem with the dehydration of H_2CO_3 in these patients.

Because acid load testing can be somewhat cumbersome to perform and could produce severe acidosis, it is best to use a simplified method of bicarbonate titration (described in the next section) and alkali administration to rule out proximal (type II) renal tubular acidosis. The dose of alkali required to achieve a normal plasma HCO_3^- concentration in patients with distal renal tubular acidosis is low (seldom exceeds 2–3 meq/kg/24 h) in contrast to that required in proximal renal tubular acidosis (> 10 meq/kg/24 h). Higher doses are, however, needed if distal renal tubular acidosis is accompanied by bicarbonate wasting. Alkali therapy can result in reduced complications and improved growth.

Distal renal tubular acidosis is usually a permanent disorder, although it sometimes occurs as a secondary complication. If irreversible renal damage is prevented, the prognosis is good.

PROXIMAL RENAL TUBULAR ACIDOSIS (TYPE II)

In the proximal tubule, the dominant process in the control of acid-base balance is the exchange of tubule cell hydrogen ion for intraluminal sodium. Proximal renal tubular acidosis is characterized by an alkaline urine pH, loss of bicarbonate in the urine, and mildly reduced serum bicarbonate concentrations. About 85–90% of bicarbonate reabsorption occurs in the proximal tubules. The lesion in proximal renal tubular acidosis is a lowering of the renal bicarbonate threshold, ie, the concentration of serum bicarbonate above which bicarbonate appears in the urine. With more severe acidosis, the concentration of serum bicarbonate drops and bicarbonate disappears from the urine; this reflects normal distal tubular acidification.

The proximal type is the most common type of renal tubular acidosis encountered in children. It is often an isolated defect, and in the small or preterm infant, it can be considered to be a factor of renal immaturity. The onset in infants is accompanied by failure to thrive, hyperchloremic acidosis, hypokalemia, and, rarely, nephrocalcinosis. Secondary forms are the result of reflux or obstructive uropathy and are seen in association with other tubular disorders (see Table 24–6).

Bicarbonate titration can be used to demonstrate the lowered renal threshold for bicarbonate reabsorption in proximal renal tubular acidosis, thereby distinguishing the proximal defect from the distal defect. This procedure is rather cumbersome and requires strict adherence to a protocol of bicarbonate infusion and measurement of urine pH and bicarbonate levels. A practical differentiation can be made by oral administration of citrate or bicarbonate, gradually increasing the dose until the serum level of bicarbonate reaches 22 meq/L. Larger doses, usually exceeding 5 meq/kg/24 h, are generally required to achieve the described level of serum bicarbonate in proximal renal tubular acidosis.

The available forms of bicarbonate therapy that are somewhat more easily tolerated than sodium bicarbonate are the citrate solutions (eg, Bicitra, Polycitra). Bicitra contains 1 meq of Na^+ and citrate per milliliter. Polycitra contains 2 meq per milliliter of citrate and 1 each of Na^+ and K^+. The required daily dosage is given in three divided doses. Potassium supplementation may be required, because the added sodium load presenting to the distal tubule may exaggerate potassium losses.

In cases of isolated defects, especially where the problem is related to renal immaturity, the prognosis is excellent. Alkali therapy can usually be discontinued after several months to 2 years. Growth should be normal, and the gradual increase in the serum bicarbonate level to above 22 meq/L heralds the presence of a raised bicarbonate threshold in the tubules. If the defect is part of a more complex tubular abnormality, the prognosis depends on the underlying disorder or syndrome.

OCULOCEREBRORENAL SYNDROME (Lowe's Syndrome)

Lowe's syndrome has been described in males only and is therefore thought to be transmitted as an X-linked recessive gene leading to anomalies involving the eyes, brain, and kidneys. The physical stigmas and the degree of mental retardation are variable. In addition to congenital cataracts and buphthalmos, the typical facies includes prominent epicanthal folds, frontal prominence, and a tendency to scaphocephaly. Muscle hypotonia is a prominent finding. The incidence of hypophosphatemic rickets is variable; it is characterized by low serum phosphorus levels, low to normal serum calcium levels, and elevated serum alkaline phosphatase levels. Some degree of renal tubular acidosis is usually present, characterized by hyperchloremic acidosis, an alkaline urine, and a diminution in both titratable acidity and urinary ammonia in response to an ammonium chloride challenge. The aminoaciduria is usually generalized. Mothers of affected males have punctate lens opacities.

Alkaline therapy should be given to those presenting with tubular acidosis. Vitamin D requirements range from 10,000 to 20,000 IU daily.

CONGENITAL HYPOKALEMIC ALKALOSIS
(Bartter's Syndrome)

Bartter's syndrome is characterized by severe hypokalemic, hypochloremic metabolic alkalosis; extremely high levels of circulating renin and aldosterone; and a paradoxic absence of hypertension. On renal biopsy, there is a striking juxtaglomerular hyperplasia. Most patients present in early infancy with severe failure to thrive.

The cause and pathogenesis are not known. The pathogenesis is thought to be related to sodium reabsorption defects in the proximal or distal tubule. Studies have associated elevated levels of prostaglandins with the syndrome, and treatment with inhibitors of prostaglandin (eg, indomethacin) has been advocated. A prostaglandin-independent chloride-reabsorptive defect has been proposed.

Treatment with prostaglandin inhibitors and potassium-conserving diuretics (eg, amiloride combined with magnesium supplements) may be beneficial. Although the prognosis is guarded, a few patients seem to have less severe forms of the disease that are compatible with long survival.

CYSTINOSIS

Three types of cystinosis have been identified: adult, adolescent, and infantile. The adult type is a relatively benign condition characterized by cystine deposition in the corneas, granulocytes, and fibroblasts but no renal disease. The adolescent type is also characterized by cystine deposition but is accompanied by the development of mild renal failure with Fanconi's syndrome during adolescence; growth is normal. The infantile type is both the most common and the most severe. Characteristically, children present in the first or second year of life with polyuria and on investigation are found to have renal rickets, generalized aminoaciduria, glycosuria, and a variable degree of renal tubular acidosis.

Cystinosis is an autosomal recessive condition that may be diagnosed in utero by obtaining fetal cells by amniocentesis, growing them in tissue culture, and measuring the avidity with which they incorporate ^{35}S-cystine.

The exact biochemical nature of the disease remains obscure. Cystine is stored in cellular lysosomes in virtually all tissues—the consequence of a now-recognized lysosomal cystine afflux transport system. Eventually, cystine accumulation results in cell damage and cell death, particularly in the renal tubules. Renal failure between ages 6 and 12 is common.

Whenever the diagnosis of cystinosis is suspected, slitlamp examination of the corneas should be performed, as cystine crystal deposition causes an almost pathognomonic ground-glass "dazzle" appearance. Cystine crystals may also be readily observed in bone marrow aspirates (especially with phase microscopy) and in the thyroid. Thyroxine or thyroid-stimulating hormone levels should be obtained in order to check for hypothyroidism.

Phosphocysteamine therapy is giving good results in the treatment of cystinosis. Depending on the progression of chronic renal failure, management is directed toward all side effects of renal failure with particular attention being paid to the control of renal osteodystrophy. Dialysis and renal homotransplantation are available for renal replacement therapy.

Markello TC, Bernadini IM, Gahl WA: Improved renal function in children with cystinosis treated with cysteamine. N Eng J Med 1993;328:1157.

PHOSPHATE-LOSING RENAL TUBULAR SYNDROMES & OTHER FORMS OF RICKETS

Recent investigation of the metabolic products of vitamin D_3 has done much to clarify the causes of various forms of rickets. Those forms due primarily to a lack of available calcium are described in Chapter 11. They include idiopathic hypercalciuria, in which there is low calcium intake or excessive urinary calcium loss; lack of vitamin D_3 because of low dietary intake or from steatorrhea; and vitamin D dependency and azotemic rickets. In vitamin D_3 dependency, there is an inborn or acquired inability to synthesize 1,25-dihydroxycholecalciferol (the calcium transport stimulating factor, type I), or there may be end-organ insensitivity to this factor (type II). Treatment consists of giving supplementary calcium or vitamin D in appropriate doses.

Diseases associated with decreased availability of phosphorus also cause rickets. Excessive use of antacids may be responsible. Most commonly, the defect is an inherited or acquired one in which a defect of phosphorus reabsorption is variably associated with other transport defects (eg, defects in transporting amino acids, glucose, bicarbonate, hydrogen ion, or potassium). Certain generalized metabolic diseases—notably Wilson's disease, galactosemia, fructose intolerance, and cystinosis—may cause similar tubular damage. Treatment of the primary type is to give extra phosphorus. Treatment of the acquired forms is that of the basic disease.

Familial hypophosphatemic vitamin D-resistant rickets is an example of a tubular nephropathy in which only phosphorus transport is affected. The majority of cases present during the second year of life, but some have been reported to occur in the first 6 months.

Clinical features vary. Changes may be only biochemical, with a strikingly low serum phosphorus level and an elevated alkaline phosphatase level. Muscle hypotonia may be severe; growth failure, bowing of the legs, and enlargement of the wrists, knees, and costochondral junctions are often associated with spinal deformities. Craniosynostosis has been described in infants with this disease. Pathologic fractures may be seen on x-ray, as well as certain unique findings consisting of an irregular mosaic formation of the haversian system and trabecular "halos" of low-density bone.

In most cases, the serum phosphorus level is less than 2 mg/dL. The urinary calcium level is low, and the serum calcium level may be normal or slightly low. Serum levels of 1,25-dihydroxycholecalciferol are low, probably because high levels of phosphate in the tubule cell shut off the 1α-hydroxylase activity. Aminoaciduria is rare.

Treatment consists of giving 1–3 g of phosphorus daily either as a buffered monosodium and disodium hydrogen phosphate solution at pH 7.4 or as Fleet's Phospho-Soda. Magnesium oxide, 10–15 mg/kg/d by mouth, may be of value. Supplementary calcitriol, up to 40 ng/kg/d, should be given if the serum calcium levels remain below normal.

Normal growth is never achieved unless every effort is made to keep the serum phosphorus level over 3 mg/dL.

NEPHROLITHIASIS

Renal calculi in children may occur as a consequence of certain inborn errors of metabolism, eg, cystine in cystinosis, glycine in hyperglycinuria, urates in Lesch-Nyhan syndrome, and oxalates in oxalosis. Stones may occur secondary to hypercalciuria in distal tubular acidosis, and large stones are quite often seen in children with spina bifida who have paralyzed lower limbs. Treatment is limited to that of the primary condition, if possible. Surgical removal of stones should be considered only for obstruction, intractable severe pain, and chronic infection.

Cystinuria

Cystinuria, like Hartnup disease and a number of other disorders, is primarily an abnormality of amino acid transport across both the enteric and proximal renal tubular epithelium. There appear to be at least three biochemical types. In the first type, the bowel transport of basic amino acids and cystine is impaired, but transport of cysteine is not impaired. In the renal tubule, basic amino acids are again rejected by the tubule, but cystine absorption into kidney slices in vitro seems to be normal. The reasons for the cystinuria are, therefore, still obscure. Heterozygotes have no aminoaciduria. The second type is similar to the first, except that the heterozygotes excrete excess cystine and lysine in the urine, and cystine transport in the bowel is normal. In the third type, only the nephron is involved.

The only clinical manifestations relate to stone formation. These include ureteral colic, dysuria, hematuria, proteinuria, and secondary urinary tract infection. The urinary excretion of cystine, lysine, arginine, and ornithine is increased.

The most reliable way to prevent stone formation is to maintain a constantly high free water clearance. This involves a water intake of about 400 mL/m^2 every 4 hours night and day. If this is not effective, treatment with sodium bicarbonate, 6 g/m^2/d, should also be given. Such measures will certainly prevent increases in stone formation and very often lead to dissolution.

Operative removal of the stone may occasionally be required. Penicillamine in doses of 1000–1500 mg/m^2/d will also decrease cystine excretion and bring about partial or complete dissolution of stones. This drug is expensive, however, and may give rise to rashes that are just as objectionable as the problem of maintaining a high water intake.

Primary Hyperoxaluria

Oxalate production in humans is derived from the oxidative deamination of glycine to glyoxalate (about 40%), from the serine-glycolate pathway (about 50%), and from ascorbic acid. At least two enzymatic blocks have been described. Type 1 is a 2-oxo-glutarate; glyoxalate carboligase deficiency that inhibits the diversion of glyoxalate to γ-hydroxy-α-ketoglutarate. Type 2 is glyoxalate reductase deficiency.

Excess oxalate combines with calcium to form insoluble deposits in the kidneys, lungs, and other tissues. The onset is during childhood. The joints are occasionally involved, but the main impact is on the kidneys, where progressive oxalate deposition leads to fibrosis and eventual renal failure.

Pyridoxine supplementation and a low-oxalate diet have been tried as therapy, but the overall prognosis is poor, and most patients succumb to uremia by early adulthood. Renal transplantation is not very successful, due to the destruction of the transplant kidney. However, there are encouraging results with concomitant liver transplants correcting the metabolic defect. Calcium carbimide, 1 mg/kg/24 h, has been tried as an inhibitor of the serine-glycolate pathway of oxalate production and was shown to substantially diminish oxalate excretion in type 1 oxalosis. The use of methylene blue has also been reported.

Hyperoxaluria may also occur secondary to ileal disease or after ileal resection.

Coe FL, Parks JH, Asplin JR: The pathogenesis and treatment of kidney stones. N Engl J Med 1992;327:1721.

Leumann E, Hoppe B, Neuhaus T: Management of primary hyperoxaluria: Efficacy of oral citrate administration. Pediatr Nephrol 1993;7:207.

NEPHROGENIC DIABETES INSIPIDUS

In the normal kidney, the interstitial fluid of the papilla is hyperosmolar to the fluid in the collecting duct. The luminal cells have a specific receptor for antidiuretic hormone (ADH), which, acting via cAMP, permits water to move across the cell membrane in response to the osmotic gradient. In the common X-linked recessive form (type I) of nephrogenic diabetes insipidus, there is a disorder of the ADH:adenylyl cyclase receptor, and urinary adenylyl cyclase is not increased after administration of vasopressin. In the type II variety, cAMP is formed by ADH action but has no effect on water transport. There are probably many variants of this complex mechanism, which is also influenced by prostaglandin E_1 and by its inhibitor, indomethacin.

The symptoms are limited to polyuria, polydipsia, and failure to thrive. In some children, particularly if the solute intake is unrestricted, some acclimatization to an elevated serum osmolality may develop. However, these children are particularly liable to episodes of dehydration, fever, vomiting, and convulsions.

Clinically, the diagnosis can be made on the basis of a history of polydipsia and polyuria that are not sensitive to the administration of vasopressin, desmopressin acetate (DDAVP), or lypressin. It is wise to confirm this in all cases by performing a vasopressin test. Maximal water restriction, overnight if possible, does not increase the tubular reabsorption of water (T^cH_2O) to above 3 mL/min/m². If 5% dextrose is administered at the rate of 275 mL/m² for 2 hours and vasopressin is given after 1 hour as an intravenous bolus of 0.005 unit/kg, the urine osmolality will not change during the period of infusion. The intravenous infusion of 2.5% saline at the rate of 0.25 mL/kg/min for not more than 45 minutes will result in only a small rise in urine osmolality in comparison to control infusion periods of normal saline. Theoretically, in psychogenic diabetes insipidus, vasopressin and hypertonic saline increase urine osmolality, but constant water loading seems to diminish renal response to ADH. Urine concentrating ability is impaired in a number of conditions—sickle cell anemia, pyelonephritis, potassium depletion, hypercalcemia, cystino-

sis and other renal tubular disorders, and obstructive uropathy—and as a result of nephrotoxic drugs.

In infants, it is usually best to allow water as demanded and to restrict salt. Serum sodium levels should be evaluated at intervals to ensure against hyperosmolality from inadvertent water restriction. In later childhood, sodium intake should continue to be restricted to 2–2.5 meq/kg/24 h. Studies have suggested that levels of C_{H2O} are significantly decreased by use of chlorothiazide, 60 mg/m²/24 h orally; ethacrynic acid, 120 mg/m²/24 h orally; and indomethacin, 3 mg/kg/24 h. When ethacrynic acid is given, potassium chloride, 2–3 meq/kg/24 h orally, should also be given to prevent alkalosis due to excessive potassium loss.

Roth KS, Diagnosis of renal tubular disorders: A guide for the clinician. Clin Pediatr (Phila) 1988;27:463.

URINARY TRACT INFECTIONS

Predisposing Factors

Urinary tract infections occur in approximately 1% of premature infants and newborns. Many of these infections are hematogenously spread; however, outside the clinical setting of perinatal acute illness and prematurity, urinary tract infections raise the possibility of urinary tract abnormalities. Within the first year of life, males are more likely to have an anatomic basis for developing urinary tract infection; nevertheless, the initial infection in a small child should alert the physician to the possibility of abnormal anatomy regardless of the patient's sex.

Older boys with a first infection should be examined for urinary tract abnormalities, whereas a more conservative, watchful approach may be taken with older girls, especially if sexual activity or poor personal hygiene is a possible cause. Such an approach, of course, assumes there are no other clinical abnormalities present that raise the suspicion of significant urinary tract disease (eg, enuresis or short stature).

Bacteria are by far the most common cause of urinary tract infections. The most predominant organisms are *Escherichia coli, Klebsiella, Staphylococcus,* and the enteric streptococci (all present in normal rectal and perineal flora). Unless there is reason to suspect that bacteremia is responsible for the development of the urinary tract infection, bacteria usually are presumed to gain access to the urinary tract via the urethra. The problem is greatly aggravated by poor hygiene, perineal infection (eg, pinworms), sexual activity, and instrumentation. Despite the fact that voiding provides some safeguard against such contamination developing into infection, abnormalities of the collecting system contribute to clinical infection and may lead to upper tract disease and renal parenchymal damage.

Clinical Findings

A. Symptoms and Signs: Newborns may present with fever, hypothermia, poor feeding, jaundice, failure to thrive, or sepsis. Infants may have fever of unknown origin, poor feeding, failure to thrive, strong-smelling urine, and irritability. Preschool children may have abdominal pain, vomiting, strong-smelling urine, fever, enuresis, increased frequency of urination, dysuria, or urgency. School-age children may develop the "classic" signs of urinary tract infection, including enuresis, increased frequency of urination, dysuria, urgency, fever, and costovertebral angle tenderness (flank pain). Occasionally, children with bacterial urinary tract infection will present with hemorrhagic cystitis.

Not all symptoms suggestive of urinary tract infection will actually prove to be related to bacterial infection. Anatomic abnormalities producing voiding discomfort, irritation of the external genitalia, or viral hemorrhagic cystitis are examples of such problems. On the other hand, some infections may actually be relatively asymptomatic. In either case, the presence of a urinary tract infection should be documented through the performance of a urinalysis and urine culture.

B. Laboratory Tests: A properly obtained clean-catch, midstream specimen is useful for urine culture, but poor technique can result in specimen contamination and subsequent false-positive test results. The clean-catch, midstream method may be satisfactory for children who can void upon request and who can be assisted in obtaining a proper specimen or be relied upon to obtain one unassisted. A bladder catheterization or suprapubic bladder tap may be performed when necessary (eg, highly suspicious clinical picture with the inability to obtain a satisfactory clean-catch specimen). Any procedure, however, carries the risk of contamination; for this reason, the more invasive procedures demand appropriate indication as well as the proper technique.

After the specimen is obtained care must be taken to decant an aliquot for urinalysis prior to sending the specimen for culture and sensitivity. The aliquot is then spun and prepared for microscopic analysis. The presence of bacteria in the specimen is highly suggestive of a urinary tract infection, provided that the aforementioned conditions of specimen collection have been met. The presence of pyuria (more than five white blood cells per high-power field) is also consistent with infection, but, again, specimen reliability is important because the perineal region, vagina, or external genitalia may be responsible for the presence of white or red cells in urine specimens. Nonetheless, such findings in the face of highly suspicious clinical symptoms should prompt

the initiation of antibiotic treatment until the culture results are obtained.

The mainstay in the diagnosis of urinary tract infection is a reliably obtained culture of the urine. The presence of multiple organisms suggests specimen contamination; however, this possibility must be evaluated in light of the method used in obtaining the specimen, as well as the level of confidence in the technical performance of the procedure employed. If the child is not already receiving the appropriate antibiotic as indicated by the sensitivities, a change should be made accordingly.

Nonculture methods, such as the nitrite sticks, for early detection of the possible presence of a urinary tract infection may be useful in following the child who is being watched for recurrent infection or being treated prophylactically with antibiotic suppression therapy.

Treatment

A. Initial Treatment: Once urinary tract infection is confirmed, initial therapy should be based on the patient's history of antibiotic use, the location of the infection, and the cost of alternative antibiotics. Many drugs are available for treating urinary tract infection, but all of them will occasionally be ineffective because of inherent resistance of the organism.

For uncomplicated cases of urethritis or cystitis, a single oral antibiotic (eg, ampicillin, a sulfonamide, nitrofurantoin) that the patient has not used recently can be administered for 10 days. The choice of antibiotic therapy must be verified by prior culture and sensitivity. A patient with suspected pyelonephritis need not always be admitted to the hospital but antibiotic coverage should be broad (ampicillin, a sulfonamide, or a cephalosporin plus gentamicin). This regimen ensures adequate coverage until the patient improves and the results of antibiotic sensitivity tests are available, allowing selection of a single effective oral antibiotic. Antibiotic dosages (depending on choice of drug) are appropriately modified in patients with acute or chronic renal failure.

Most urinary tract infections can be successfully treated with inexpensive drugs given orally. Followup urinalysis or use of nitrite sticks within 2–3 days can confirm therapeutic success. If symptoms persist, reexamination and repeat urine culture are necessary.

B. Treatment of Refractory Infection: Persistent bacteriuria indicates superinfection with a different organism or with the same organism due to obstruction, the presence of a foreign body, or conversion of the organism to a variant form.

Voiding cystourethrography should be considered with proved infection. Renal ultrasonography is a helpful, noninvasive tool for evaluating the anatomy of the urinary tract.

Obvious structural or obstructive anomalies require referral to a urologist experienced in dealing with children. Vesicoureteral reflux is common in younger children. If not severe, it will not result in renal damage and will disappear in time if repeated infections can be prevented. The presence of mild reflux does not ordinarily necessitate urologic consultation.

In patients without structural or functional urinary tract abnormalities, possible causes of recurrent infection include infrequent or incomplete voiding, poor perineal hygiene, pinworms, constipation, and the use of bubble bath. If attempts to deal with these problems are unsuccessful, single-dose prophylaxis at bedtime with agents such as nitrofurantoin or trimethoprim-sulfamethoxazole may be useful in combination with a program of frequent voiding.

C. Follow-Up of Patients With Urinary Tract Infection: All patients with urinary tract infection should be checked for recurrence every 1–2 months until they have remained free of infection for 1 year. Use of the nitrite test for home testing of first morning concentrated urine specimens may significantly reduce the cost of follow-up without compromising accuracy.

Prognosis

As long as urinary tract infections can be confined to the lower urinary tract (bladder and below), the prognosis is excellent. Once an infectious process has entered the kidney, the prognosis becomes more guarded. Hence, every diagnostic and therapeutic effort should be made to prevent recurrences.

Bailey RR: Vesico-ureteric reflux and reflux nephropathy. Kidney Int 1991;44:5.

REFERENCES

Edelmann CM Jr et al (editors): Pediatric Kidney Disease, 2nd ed. Little, Brown, 1992.

Holliday MA, Barratt TM, Avner ED: *Pediatric Nephrology, 4th ed.* Williams & Wilkins, 1994.

25

Neurologic & Muscular Disorders

Paul G. Moe, MD, & Alan R. Seay, MD

NEUROLOGIC ASSESSMENT & NEURODIAGNOSTIC PROCEDURES

NEUROLOGIC HISTORY & EXAMINATION

The history is usually taken with the child and parents together. Questions can be addressed directly to the older child with further details supplemented by the parent. If time permits, a teenager should be interviewed alone. If strong psychosocial factors become evident by the end of the joint interview, the parent may be asked to leave. Sensitive issues (eg, drug use, sexual activity) can then be reexplored with the older child.

A patient data form filled out by the parent in advance of the visit or in the physician's waiting room is helpful. The form should include the chief complaint, the patient's strengths and talents, birth and family history, medical history, and school and behavioral history. A checklist of behavioral issues such as hyperactivity, depression, short attention span, etc, can bring attention to areas that need to be more carefully explored during the interview. Developmental delays suspected in the infant or older child can also be addressed in a checklist. A physician interviewing a child aged 5–7 can begin with neutral questions regarding age and birthday. It is often informative to see whether these children know their birthday or even year of birth.

The core of the history is the present illness. What the parent or child sees as important should be the initial focus. In recurrent conditions (eg, seizures or headaches), it is important to find out what happened during the first as well as the most recent episode. Details of recurrent episodes should be thoroughly discussed, including frequency, duration, change in character over time, and precipitating and alleviating factors. The effect of emotions, medications, and environmental manipulations such as diet change should be reviewed. The physician should ascertain, if possible, whether the disease is congenital or age-acquired and whether it is progressive.

As the interview progresses, the clinician begins to form ideas about a possible diagnosis; these can be explored with searching questions. Occasionally, the patient and parent see things from different viewpoints. The child, for instance, may consider the headaches a trivial matter that does not interfere with activity; the mother may feel quite differently. It may be helpful to observe the emotional interchange between parent and child and to note each one's opinions regarding the severity of disease, the degree of interference with peer group and school activities, side effects and efficacy of medications, etc.

Depending on the nature of the complaint, the past medical history may or may not be extremely detailed. For example, in the case of a teenager with headaches, the history of pregnancy and birth is of little importance. In the case of a 2-month-old child with hypotonia, detailed information about those events is essential. The family and genetic history are often important. A strong family history of migraine or a history of myotonic dystrophy in an uncle might be the key to diagnosis in the examples cited. The parents may have to do some searching with inquiries to relatives or hospitals to assemble family history details.

Available health records, roentgenograms, electroencephalograms, and school records may complement the interview. Developmental history is essential in the assessment of any infant. The Denver Developmental Screening Test (DDST) is one helpful tool for reviewing each major area of behavior in infancy, ie, gross motor, fine motor, personal/social, and language. Some developmental expectations and landmarks are listed in Table 25–1.

In the older child, the developmental history can be explored with questions concerning school progress. The clinician should ask how the patient is getting along with the peer group, in physical activities, and in the family setting. Open-ended questions (eg, "What is she like? What is an average day in her life? What does she do?") can help the clinician assess the child's social functioning.

During examination, the infant or toddler is often held in the mother's lap. Much information can be obtained by *observing* a child and noting spontaneous movements, curiosity, ability to understand direc-

Table 25–1. Neurologic developmental landmarks.

	Birth	3 Months	6 Months	9 Months	12–15 Months	24 Months
Motor	Flexor posture, lifts head prone, hands grasped	Sits: head forward, bobbing, lifts head supine, hands open, retains briefly	Rolls both ways, begins to sit alone, supports (erect), bounces	Creeps, pulls up standing, pincer grasp, sits well	Walks with 1 or 2 hands held, stands alone briefly, releases on command	Walks and runs well, walks downstairs, turns pages singly
Special senses	Regards (vision), may follow 45 degrees	Looks at hands, follows 90–180 degrees	Discriminates voices, localizes sounds	Picks up raisin, "bye-bye"	Localizes noises, localizes pain	Towers 6–7 cubes, imitates scribble
Adaptive	Startles to sound, delayed nociceptive response	Smiles socially, vocalizes socially, follows vertically	Holds cube, palmar grasp, retrieves toy, transfers and rakes raisin	Bangs toys together, pat-a-cake	Assists in dressing, attempts spoon feeding, tries 2-cube tower	Asks for toilet, pulls on garments, spoon-feeds well, parallel play
Language	Throaty noises	Coos, chuckles, vocal social response	Babbles (polysyllables), "mmm-mmm"	"Ma-ma, Da-da," one other "word"	Understands simple command, speaks 1–3 words	Speaks in phrases, names 3–5 pictures, pronouns: "I, me, you"
Reflex	Tonic neck, palmar grasp	Disappearing tonic neck, Moro reflex	Begins voluntary stepping	Parachute response		
Automatisms	Moro reflex, sucks, roots, stepping, supporting, traction: head lag	Landau response, traction: no head lag	Neck righting, blinks to threat			

tions, and alertness to visual and auditory cues (eg, a tinkling bell).

Part of the neurologic examination includes a brief **general physical examination** with emphasis on the skin (birth marks), spine, neck, and skull (including palpation of the fontanelle and measurement of head circumference). Simple explanations to parent and child during the exam can reassure both the patient and the parent: "I'm checking the soft spot to be sure the headache isn't causing high pressure in the head; it feels soft. That is normal. The pressure is fine." At some point in the examination, the baby should be inspected virtually unclothed. In an older child, asking about birthmarks and inspecting the spine with the shirt pulled up and the child bent over for evaluation of scoliosis may be sufficient. Again, an explanation may be useful: "It is very important that I look at your spine to be sure there isn't any curvature. It looks straight. That's fine."

Developmental assessment should be included in the neurologic examination of the infant. At an appropriate age (eg, 6–18 months), the physician may start with handing blocks to the baby, offering a raisin, and evaluating reach and type of grasp. A younger baby often enjoys a bell, the older child a reflex hammer. Using the block and the raisin, the clinician can assess the items on the DDST that have not been elucidated by the history.

Running around the room and retrieving a ball is a test of the child's **station and gait.** Children usually enjoy having their **reflexes** tested. Be sure reflexes

are present proximally and distally, eg, knee jerk/ankle jerk, triceps/brachial radialis. Sometimes, a subtle case of hemiparesis can be suggested by a unilateral absence of abdominal or cremasteric cutaneous reflexes. Occasionally, tapping one's finger over a hamstring or biceps reflex can show an absent reflex or asymmetry in a lumbosacral plexus or brachial plexus injury.

Infantile automatisms—their presence, absence, or asymmetry—are important in examination of the newborn and very young infant (see Table 25–1).

Running around the room, squatting, jumping, etc, are tests of the child's **motor function.** In infants, tone—the subjective feeling that results while manipulating the limb—is important. (See the section on hypotonic infant.) Occasionally, formal muscle testing is necessary, eg, abduction at the shoulder and hand grasp, rising from a squat, and dorsiflexion of the foot to test proximal and distal strength. **Sensory testing** is rarely contributory, but touch, tickle, and pinprick testing can be used in small children.

By this time, the infant's **cranial nerves** have usually been satisfactorily assessed by observation (eg, extraocular movements, vision, and hearing). If there is concern about swallowing or tongue size or function, these areas can be examined with a flashlight and tongue blade. Lastly, the fundi should be assessed by having the infant look at a distant object or by having the parent attract the child's attention with a pinwheel or bell. The physician can approach from the side to observe the disk before light on the macula causes miosis. Sometimes, mydriatics to dilate the pupil are necessary.

In the older child, formal examination of **mental status** is rarely necessary. Simple assessment of cognition can be achieved by having the child obey right-and-left commands (eg, "Put your right hand on your left ear"), do simple math problems, and read paragraphs appropriate for grade level (see Table 25–2).

In the older child, the Romberg test (standing with eyes closed, feet together, and hands straight out), tandem walking, and standing and hopping on each foot are tests for **station and gait. Limb coordination** can be tested by finger pursuit, ie, having children touch the clinician's moving finger with their own. Finger-nose alternating movements and patting the palm and the back of the hand alternately on the lap are other tests of lateral coordination. In the older child, tests for sense of position, vibration, and even cortical sensory status (eg, position of the limb in space and finger writing) are occasionally important.

Because children can be uncooperative and findings uncertain, serial examinations are sometimes necessary. The reasons for the follow-up examination should be explained in detail to the parent. No neurologic examination is a complete failure. The clinician has the opportunity to observe the child during the interview and during play; these observations may give a reasonable assessment of neurologic function.

Finally, it must be emphasized that a complete examination should be performed and results told to the parents in plain language, even when the complaint seems trivial.

LUMBAR PUNCTURE

The principal purpose of lumbar puncture is to obtain an aliquot of cerebrospinal fluid for the diagnosis of infectious and inflammatory conditions of the central nervous system (Table 25–3). The uses of specimens of cerebrospinal fluid in cytologic studies, bioassays of enzymes and neurotransmitters, and specific rapid tests for viruses are widening the clinical (and research) applicability of lumbar puncture. However, performing lumbar puncture for manometric determinations, cellular content, and protein levels in many conditions—including head injuries, brain and spinal cord tumors, and seizure disorders—has been superseded by the use of brain imaging and biochemical techniques that are far more specific.

Therapeutically, lumbar puncture may be employed for drainage of cerebrospinal fluid to reduce its hematotoxic effects in hemorrhagic conditions (eg, intraventricular hemorrhage in newborns, ruptured berry aneurysm) and to lower intracranial pressure in pseudotumor cerebri. Symptoms may be improved in viral meningitis.

Lumbar puncture is usually performed with the patient in the lateral recumbent or decubitus position. Entry is at the level of the iliac crest or the L3–4 interspace, with the patient's head initially flexed and then extended. In small infants—especially premature infants and neonates in the first months of life—lumbar puncture is more safely and satisfactorily performed with the infant in the sitting position and the head only slightly flexed or supported with a pillow propped between the outstretched arms and legs resting against the infant's chest and abdomen. The wrists and ankles should be held by an assisting nurse, and the needle should be pointed slightly cephalad.

Note: Before lumbar puncture is performed, the fundi should always be checked for papilledema. Lumbar puncture is contraindicated in the presence of elevated intracranial pressure, especially when there are focal neurologic deficits, because of the risk of tentorial or tonsillar herniation. This risk is less likely when there is diffuse cerebral swelling than when elevated pressure is due to a mass lesion. Therefore, if equipment for CT brain scanning is readily available, lumbar puncture should usually be delayed until a scan can be done; it should not be delayed, however, if examination of cerebrospinal fluids is indispensable for diagnosis and vital therapeutic intervention.

Lumbar puncture must be performed promptly when a diffuse central nervous system infection (meningitis, meningoencephalitis, encephalitis, cerebritis) is suspected. Only a small-gauge needle should be used, and only enough fluid should be withdrawn to permit cell count, protein and glucose determination, and such stains and cultures (bacterial, fungal, and viral) and other studies as may be helpful. A specimen of 2–3 mL is usually adequate for microchemical determinations.

It is occasionally important to obtain opening and closing cerebrospinal fluid pressures. To obtain valid pressure readings, the head, neck, and legs should be gently brought into a straight line. Pressure in the sitting position should be measured with the level of the foramen magnum as "zero"; the length of the fluid column above that level is the pressure in millimeters of water.

Table 25–2. Mental status examination.

Orientation: Time, place, situation, name, date, year.

Memory: Recent and remote, eg, "What did you have for lunch?" "What did you do on your birthday?" Remember (for 10 minutes): "Red flag, Washington's birthday, Christmas presents."

Calculation: Depends on educational background. Example: Subtract serial sevens.

Proverbs: Interpret: "Too many cooks spoil the broth." "A rolling stone gathers no moss."

Situation: "What would you do if you saw a fire?"

Aphasia: "What 's this?" (chalk). "Stick out your tongue." "Put your right finger on your left ear." Sample speech, reading, and writing.

Table 25–3. Characteristics of cerebrospinal fluid (CSF) in the normal child and in central nervous system infections and inflammatory conditions.

Condition	Initial Pressure (mm H₂O)	Appearance	Cells/μL	Protein (mg/dL)	glucose (mg/dl)	Other Tests	Comments
Normal¹	< 180	Clear	0–5 lymphocytes. First 3 months, 1–3 PMNs. Neonates, up to 30 lymphocytes, 20–50 RBCs.	15–35 (lumbar). 5–15 (ventricular). Up to 150 (lumbar) for short time after birth; to 6 months, up to 65.	50–80 (two-thirds of blood glucose). May be increased after seizure.	CSF IgG index; < 0.7 units = CSF IgG/Serum IgG. CSF albumin/Serum albumin Lactate dehydrogenase (LDH), 2–27 IU/L.	CSF protein in first month may be up to 170 mg/dL in small-for-dates or premature infants. No increase in WBCs due to seizure.
Bloody tap	Normal or low	Bloody (sometimes with clot)	One additional WBC/700 RBCs.¹ RBCs not crenated.	One additional mg/800 RBCs.¹	Normal.	RBC number should fall between first and third tube; wait 5 minutes between tubes.	Spin down fluid; supernatant will be clear and colorless.
Bacterial meningitis, acute	200–750 +	Opalescent to purulent	Up to 1000s, mostly PMNs. Early, few cells	Up to 100s.	Decreased; may be none.	Smear and culture mandatory. LDH > 24 IU/L. Bacterial antigen tests.	Very early, glucose may be normal. Immunofluorescence tests.
Bacterial meningitis, partially treated	Usually increased	Clear or opalescent	Usually increased. PMNs usually predominate.	Elevated.	Normal or decreased.	LDH usually > 24 IU/L. Bacterial antigen tests.	Smear and culture often negative.
Tuberculous meningitis	150–750 +	Opalescent; fibrin web or pellicle	250–500, mostly lymphocytes. Early, more PMNs.	45–500; parallels cell count.	Decreased; may be none.	Smear for acid-fast organism; CSF culture and inoculation.	*Note:* Bacterial meningitis may be superimposed.
Fungal meningitis	Increased	Variable; often clear	10–500. Early, more PMNs; then mostly lymphocytes.	Elevated and increasing.	Decreased.	India ink preparations, cryptococcal antigen, culture, inoculations, immunofluorescence tests.	Often superimposed in patients who are debilitated or on immunosuppressive therapy.
Aseptic meningoencephalitides (poliomyelitis)	Normal or slightly increased	Clear unless cell count > 300	0 to few hundred, mostly lymphocytes; PMNs predominate early.	20–125.	Normal; may be low in mumps.	CSF, stool, throat wash for viral cultures. LDH < 28 IU/L (90% < 24 IU/L).	Acute and convalescent antibody titers. In mumps, up to 1000 lymphocytes; serum amylase often elevated. Rarely, several thousand cells present in enteroviral infection.
Neurosyphilis	Normal to 400	Clear unless protein is very high	10–100, mostly lymphocytes.	25–150; higher in meningitis.	Normal.	Positive CSF serology. CSF IgG index increased.	Blood serology positive in untreated cases; *Treponema pallidum* immobilization test positive.
Parainfectious encephalomyelitis	80–450, usually increased	Usually clear	0–50, mostly lymphocytes.	15–75.	Normal.	CSF IgG index may be increased. Oligoclonal bands variable.	No organisms. Fulminant cases resemble bacterial meningitis.
Polyneuritis Early	Normal and occasionally increased	Normal	Normal; occasionally slight increase.	Normal.	Normal.	Bacterial cultures negative; gamma globulin may be elevated.	Try to find cause (viral infections, toxins, lupus, infectious mononucleosis, diabetes, etc).
Late		Xanthochromic if protein high		45–1500.			
Meningeal carcinomatosis	Often elevated	Clear to opalescent	Cytologic identification of tumor cells.	Often mildly to moderately elevated.	Often depressed.	Cytology.	Seen with leukemia, medulloblastoma, meningeal melanosis, histiocytosis X. *Note:* May mimic meningitis.
Brain abscess	Normal or increased	Usually clear	5–500 in 80%; mostly PMNs.	Usually slightly increased.	Normal; occasionally decreased.		Cell count related to proximity to meninges; findings as in purulent meningitis if abscess perforates.

¹Many studies document pitfalls in using these ratios due to WBC lysis. Clinical judgment and repeat taps may be necessary to rule out meningitis in this situation. (See references.)

Table 25–4. Cerebrospinal fluid: Other useful constituents.

Cytology	Leukemia, brain tumor cells, lipomacrophages (CNS damage), iron-laden macrophages (subarachnoid hemorrhage)
Immunoglobulins: IgA, IgM, IgA, IgD, IgE, oligoclonal bands	Demyelinating disease, infections, neoplasms
Polyamines (eg, putrescine)	Some childhood brain tumors (diagnosis, monitoring); neural tube defects
Neurotransmitters (metabolites, eg, homovanillic acid)	Epilepsy, febrile seizures, Lesch-Nyhan syndrome, attention deficit hyperactivity disorder
Lactate/pyruvate; pH	Anoxia, hemorrhage, meningitis, metabolic disease
Enzymes: LDH, CK	Newborn anoxia, infection (bacterial versus viral), cerebrovascular accident

Multiple other components of cerebrospinal fluid have useful clinical applications. See Table 25–4.

Anbar R: Pitfalls in interpretation of traumatic lumbar puncture formula. (Letter.) Am J Dis Child 1986;140:638.

Anderson G: Neurotransmitter precursors and metabolites in CSF of human neonates. Dev Med Child Neurol 1985; 27:207.

Chow G, Schmidley JW: Lysis of erythrocytes and leukocytes in traumatic lumbar puncture. Arch Neurol 1984; 41:1984.

Jaffe M et al: The ameliorating effect of lumbar puncture in viral meningitis. Am J Dis Child 1989;143:682.

Markowitz H, Kokmen E: Neurologic diseases and the cerebrospinal fluid immunoglobin profile. Mayo Clin Proc 1983;58:273.

Novak RW: Lack of validity of standard corrections for white blood cell counts of blood-contaminated cerebrospinal fluid in infants. Am J Clin Pathol 1984;82:95.

Phillips P et al: Cerebrospinal fluid polyamines: Biochemical markers of malignant childhood brain tumors. Ann Neurol 1986;19:360.

Portnoy J, Olson L: Normal cerebrospinal fluid values in children: Another look. Pediatrics 1985;75:484.

Ricevuti G: Meningeal leukemia diagnosed by cytocentrifuge study of cerebrospinal fluid. Arch Neurol 1986; 43:466.

Rubenstein S, Yager R: What represents pleocytosis in blood-contaminated ("traumatic tap") CSF in childhood? J Pediatr 1985;107:249.

Shaywitz S, Shaywitz B: Attention deficit disorder: Current perspectives. Pediatr Neurol 1987;3:129.

Ward EM, Gushurst D: Uses and techniques of pediatric lumbar puncture. Am J Dis Child 1992;196:1160.

Wood J (editor): Neurology of CSF. Plenum Press, 1982.

ELECTROENCEPHALOGRAPHY

This widely used, noninvasive electrophysiologic method for recording cerebral activity has its greatest clinical applicability in the study of seizure disorders. "Activation" techniques to accentuate abnormalities or disclose latent abnormalities include photic stimulation, well-sustained hyperventilation for 3 minutes, and depriving the patient of sleep from about midnight until after breakfast, at which time the EEG is recorded. The latter is an excellent though less widely employed "activation" method.

Electroencephalography is also used in the evaluation of tumors, cerebrovascular accidents, neurodegenerative diseases, and other neurologic disorders causing brain dysfunction; but with some notable exceptions, it is nonspecific. Recordings over a 24-hour period or all-night recordings are invaluable in the diagnosis of sleep disturbances and narcolepsy. Electroencephalography with telemetry or simultaneous monitoring of behavior on videotape, has great usefulness in selected cases. The EEG can be helpful in determining a possible cause or mechanism of coma and is frequently used to aid in determining whether coma is irreversible and brain death has occurred.

The limitations of electroencephalography are considerable: In most cases, the duration of the actual tracing is about 45 minutes and reflects only surface cortical function. Many drugs—especially barbiturates and benzodiazepines, have considerable effects on the EEG and may obfuscate interpretation. About 15% of nonepileptic individuals, especially children, may have an abnormal EEG. Electroencephalographic findings such as those seen in migraine, learning disabilities, or behavior disorders do not reflect permanent "brain damage." A major usefulness of EEG is to show epileptiform activity in children with seizure disorders; sometimes the findings are virtually diagnostic, as in the hypsarrhythmia EEG of infantile spasms or the prolonged 3/second spike-wave of absence seizures.

At present, use of CT scans, evoked potentials, positron emission tomography, regional cerebral blood flow studies, and MRI supplements the use of electroencephalography as a diagnostic and prognostic tool.

EVOKED POTENTIALS

Cortical auditory, visual, or somatosensory evoked potentials (evoked responses) may be recorded from the scalp surface over the temporal, occipital, or frontoparietal cortex after repetitive stimulation of the retina by light flashes, of the cochlea by sounds, or of a never by galvanic stimuli of varying frequency and intensity, respectively. Computer averaging is used to recognize and enhance these responses while subtracting or suppressing the asynchronous background electroencephalographic activity. The presence or absence of evoked potential waves and their latencies (time from stimulus to wave peak or time between peaks) figure in the clinical interpretation.

The reproducible and quantifiable results obtained from brain stem auditory, pattern-shift visual, and short-latency somatosensory evoked potentials (see below) indicate the level of function of the relevant sensory pathway or system and identify the site of anatomic disruption. While results of these tests alone are usually not diagnostic, the tests are noninvasive, sensitive, objective, and relatively inexpensive extensions of the clinical neurologic examination. Because the auditory and somatosensory tests and one type of visual test are totally passive, requiring only that the patient remain still, they are particularly useful in the evaluation of functions in neonates and small children as well as in patients unable to cooperate (eg, as a result of mental retardation, degenerative disorder, anesthesia, or coma). Knowledge of normal values and experience in testing of the applicable patient group are mandatory.

Brain Stem Auditory Evoked Potentials

A brief auditory stimulus (click) of varying intensity and frequency is delivered to the ear to activate the auditory nerve (nerve VIII) and sequentially activate the cochlear nucleus, tracts and nuclei of the lateral lemniscus, and inferior colliculus. Thus, this technique assesses hearing and function of the brain stem auditory tracts.

Hearing in the neonate or uncooperative (but sedated) patient can be objectively assessed, making the technique particularly useful in high-risk infants—especially those in intensive care nurseries—and in retarded and autistic patients. Brain stem auditory evoked potentials are used to judge brain stem dysfunction in sleep apnea and in Arnold-Chiari malformation, and achondroplasia. Because high doses of anesthetic agents or barbiturates do not seriously affect results, the test is used to assess and monitor brain stem function of patients during surgery (in the operating room) and those in hypoxic-ischemic coma or coma following head injury. Absence of evoked potential waves beyond the first wave from the auditory nerve usually signifies brain death. Brain stem auditory evoked potentials are also useful in the early evaluation of diseases affecting myelin—ie, the various leukodystrophies and multiple sclerosis (although auditory evoked potentials are less valuable than visual evoked potentials in the latter)—and in intrinsic brain stem gliomas. They are sometimes useful in evaluation of hereditary ataxias, Wilson's disease (hepatolenticular degeneration), and other degenerative disorders affecting the brain stem.

Pattern-Shift Visual Evoked Potentials

The preferred stimulus is a shift (reversal) of a checkerboard pattern, and the response is a single wave (called P100) generated in the striate and parastriate visual cortex. The absolute latency of P100 (time from stimulus to wave peak) and the difference in latency between the two eyes are sensitive indicators of disease. The amplitude of response is affected by any process resulting in poor fixation on the stimulus screen or affecting visual acuity. Ability to focus on a checkerboard pattern is necessary. (An LED—light emitting diode—goggles or bright flash stimulus can be used in younger and uncooperative children, but the norms are less standardized.) Evoked potentials suggest that visual acuity may be 20/20 in infants by 6–7 months of age.

Clinical application of the test includes detection and monitoring of strabismus (ie, in amblyopia ex anopsia), optic neuritis, and lesions near the optic nerve and chiasm such as optic gliomas and craniopharyngiomas. Degenerative and immunologic diseases that affect visual transmission and may be detected early and followed by serial evaluations by this technique include adrenoleukodystrophy, Pelizaeus-Merzbacher disease, some spinocerebellar degenerations, sarcoidosis, and even multiple sclerosis. Flash visual evoked potentials are used to monitor function during surgery involving the eyes and optic nerve; to assess cortical or hysterical blindness; and to evaluate patients with photosensitive epilepsy, who may have exaggerated responses.

Short-Latency Somatosensory Evoked Potentials

Responses are commonly produced by electrical stimulation of peripheral sensory nerves, as this evokes potentials of greatest amplitude and clarity; finger tapping and muscle stretching may also be used. The function of this test is similar to that of the auditory test in closely correlating wave forms with function of the sensory pathways and permitting localization of conduction defects.

Short-latency somatosensory evoked potentials are used in the assessment of a wide variety of lesions of the peripheral nerve, root, spinal cord, and central nervous system following trauma, neuropathies (eg, in diabetes mellitus or Guillain-Barré syndrome), myelodysplasias, cerebral palsy, and many other disorders. The test procedure is often performed on an outpatient basis. One method is to stimulate the median nerve at the wrist with small (nonpainful) electrical shocks and record responses from the brachial plexus above the clavicle, the neck (cervical cord), and the opposite scalp area overlying the sensorimotor cortex. After stimulation from the knee (peroneal nerve) or ankle (tibial nerve), impulses are recorded from the lower lumbar spinal cord, cervical cord, and sensorimotor cortex. Such potentials are used to monitor spinal cord sensory functioning during surgery for disorders including scoliosis, myelodysplasias, and tumors and other lesions of the spinal cord or blood vessels supplying the cord. The technique is also used in leukodystrophies involving peripheral nerves, in multiple sclerosis, and in hysteria and malingering (anesthetic limbs). In the diagnosis of coma and brain death, somatosensory evoked potentials supplement the results of auditory evoked potentials.

Aldrich MS, Jahnke B: Diagnostic value of video EEG polysomnography. Neurology 1991;41:1060.

Chiappa KH, Ropper AH: Evoked potentials in clinical medicine. (Two parts.) N Engl J Med 1982;306:1140, 1205.

Cohen BA, Schenk VA, Sweeney DB: Meningitis-related hearing loss evaluated with evoked potentials. Pediatr Neurol 1988;4:18.

DeMeirleir LJ, Taylor MJ: Prognostic utility of SEPs in comatose children. Pediatr Neurol 1987;3:78.

Eyre JA (editor): The neurophysiologic examination of the newborn infant. *Clinics in Developmental Medicine,* No. 120. MacKeith Press, 1992.

Fagan ER, Taylor MJ, Logan WJ: Somatosensory evoked potentials. P2. A review of the clinical applications in pediatric neurology. Pediatr Neurol 1987;3:189.

Goldie WD et al: Brain stem auditory evoked potentials as a tool in the clinical assessment of children with posterior fossa tumors. J Child Neurol 1987;2:272.

Hecox KE, Cone B, Blaw ME: Brain stem auditory evoked response in the diagnosis of pediatric neurologic disease. Neurology 1981;31:832.

Kamimura N et al: Spinal somatosensory evoked potentials in infants and children with spinal cord lesions. Brain Dev 1988;10:355.

Mutoh K et al: Maturation of somatosensory evoked potentials upon posterior tibial nerve stimulation. Pediatr Neurol 1988;4:342.

Rotteveel JJ et al: The applications of evoked potentials in the diagnosis and follow-up of children with intracranial tumors. Childs Nerv Syst 1985;1:172.

Roy M et al: Evaluation of children and young adults with tethered spinal cord syndrome. Surg Neurol 1986;26:241.

Stockard J: Brain stem auditory evoked potentials in adult and infant sleep apnea syndrome, including sudden infant death syndrome, and near-miss for sudden infant death. Ann N Y Acad Sci 1982;388:443.

Stockard J et al: Prognostic value of brain stem auditory evoked potentials in neonates. Arch Neurol 1983;40:360.

Whyte HE et al: Prognostic utility of visual evoked potentials in term asphyxiated neonates. Pediatr Neurol 1986;2:220.

BRAIN ELECTRICAL ACTIVITY MAPPING (BEAM)

Brain electrical activity mapping is a relatively new technique in which electroencephalographic and evoked potential data recorded from multiple scalp electrodes are graphically displayed in color on a computer-driven video screen. Values between electrodes are obtained by interpolation. Learning-disabled, dyslexic, and epileptic children are being studied in research protocols. Expense, lack of normative data, and lack of numbers of homogeneous clinical patients preclude current use of this modality in pediatric practice.

Duffy FH: The BEAM method for neurophysiological diagnosis. Ann N Y Acad Sci 1985;457:19.

Nuwer M: Quantitative EEG. 1. Techniques and problems of frequency, analysis, and topographic mapping. Neurol Clin 1988;5:1.

Nuwer M, Sharbrough F: American EEG Society statement on clinical use of quantitative EEG. Neurology 1987; 37:28A.

PEDIATRIC NEURORADIOLOGIC PROCEDURES

Sedation for Procedures

Radiologic procedures in infants and children are usually performed by pediatric radiologists, but sedation for these procedures remains largely the responsibility of the physician caring for the child. The choice of sedation must take into account the patient's age and physical condition, the type of neurologic disorder, the effect and duration of the procedure, and whether immediate neurosurgery is anticipated. The prescribing physician should be familiar with the agent used.

Oral or rectal chloral hydrate, 30–60 mg/kg/dose, is safest. However, many radiology departments use only nonoral administration because of the risks of vomiting and aspiration. One favorite is pentobarbital, 6 mg/kg for children weighing less than 15 kg and 5 mg/kg for larger children (up to a maximum of 200 mg) given intramuscularly or rectally (at least 20 minutes before a procedure) or 2–4 mg/kg given intravenously. Equipment to support blood pressure and respiration must be available. This dosage usually achieves sedation for up to 2 hours. However, if sedation is inadequate 30 minutes after injection— and if the condition of the child permits—a second dose of pentobarbital, 2 mg/kg, is given. A "cardiac cocktail," usually of intramuscularly administered meperidine hydrochloride, secobarbital, and promethazine hydrochloride or chlorpromazine, may be employed by pediatricians who are familiar with it. General anesthesia may be indicated, especially if the child is to undergo surgery immediately on completion of a radiologic examination.

Computed Tomography (CT Scanning)

CT scanning consists of a series of cross-sectional ("axial") roentgenograms and can be performed on an outpatient basis. Radiation exposure is approximately the same as that from a skull roentgenogram series. The images can be viewed on an oscilloscope as the scan is being done and later examined on printed-out films; both oscilloscope views and films record variations in tissue densities. CT scanning is of high sensitivity (88–96% of lesions larger than 1–2 cm can be seen) but low specificity (a tumor, focus of infection, or infarct may have the same appearance).

The CT scan is often repeated after intravenous injection of iodized contrast for "enhancement," which reflects the vascularity of a lesion or its surrounding tissues. Precautions should be taken to ensure that the patient is not hypersensitive to iodinated dyes and that allergic reactions can be managed promptly. Sufficient information is often obtained from a non-enhanced scan; in these cases, cost and risk are minimized.

Sedation may be required for CT scanning. For positioning the head of children up to 8 years of age, a specially shaped headrest may be needed. The indications for CT scanning and the findings in specific conditions are discussed below in the sections on specific disorders.

There have been rapid advances in the application of CT techniques to further refine brain imaging, eg, with MRI and positron emission tomography, which are discussed below. Coupling regional cerebral blood flow techniques with CT procedures in exploring physiologic processes is also under investigation.

Magnetic Resonance Imaging (MRI)

Magnetic resonance imaging is a noninvasive technique that uses the magnetic properties of certain nuclei to produce signals known as the proton spin-lattice relaxation time and the spin-spin relaxation time—signals that are based on the density of nuclei at a given point and on their immediate environment (lattice). Currently, the technique is based on detecting the response (resonance) of hydrogen proton nuclei to applied radiofrequency electromagnetic radiation; these nuclei are abundant in the body and more sensitive to magnetic resonance imaging than other nuclei. The strength of relaxation signals varies with the relationship of water to protein and the amount of lipids present. The image displayed, which is made up of a mixture of signals and is similar to the CT film, provides high-resolution contrast of soft tissues. Magnetic resonance imaging can, in fact, provide information about the histologic, physiologic, and biochemical status of tissues in addition to gross anatomic data.

Clinically, MRI has been applied chiefly to the study of lesions in the head, but it can be used in examinations of the spine, body organs, and tissues such as muscles and nerves. It has been used to delineate brain tumors, edema, ischemic and hemorrhagic lesions, hydrocephalus, vascular disorders, inflammatory and infectious lesions, and degenerative processes. MRI can be used to study myelination and demyelination and, through the demonstration of changes in relaxation time, metabolic disorders of the brain, muscles, and glands. Because bone causes no artifact in the images, the posterior fossa and its contents can be studied far better using MRI than with CT scans; even blood vessels and the cranial nerves can be imaged. On the other hand, the inability of MRI to detect calcification limits its usefulness in the investigation of calcified lesions such as craniopharyngioma or leptomeningeal angiomatosis.

It is believed that the strong magnetic fields used in this procedure do not cause molecular or cellular damage. Work is progressing on imaging from nuclei other than hydrogen, such as phosphorus and sodium.

The cost of MRI is two or three times that of a contrast-enhanced CT scan. The procedure can be frightening and requires sedated sleep or light anesthesia for the child to ensure complete immobility. Magnetic resonance angiography (MRA) is a noninvasive (no arterial or venous puncture or dye injection) technique to show large extra- and intracranial blood vessels; it often now replaces the more hazardous intra-arterial injection angiogram.

Positron Emission Tomography (PET)

Positron emission tomography is an imaging technique that measures the metabolic rate at a given site by CT scanning to detect positron (proton) emission. For measurement of local cerebral metabolism, the radiolabeled substrate most frequently used has been fluorodeoxyglucose ^{18}F by injection. Gray matter and white matter are clearly distinguishable; the skull and air- or fluid-filled cavities are least active metabolically.

PET has been used to study the cerebral metabolism of neonates and brain activation by visual or auditory stimuli. Pathologic states that have been studied include epilepsy (during and between seizures), brain infarcts and tumors, and dementias. This functional test of brain metabolism is clinically useful in preoperative evaluation for epilepsy surgery. The "epileptogenic zone" will often be hypermetabolic during ictal events and hypoactive during the time between seizures. The information complements electrical (EEG) and imaging (MRI) findings to aid in the decision about what tissue to remove.

With this technique, infants with infantile spasms have occasionally been found to have a focal lesion, sometimes leading to successful surgical removal.

Clinical application is limited by the cost of the procedure and the clinician's need for access to a nearby cyclotron where the radiopharmaceuticals can be prepared.

Ultrasonography

Ultrasonography offers a pictorial display (eg, echoencephalogram, echocardiogram) of the varying densities of tissues in a given anatomic region or structure by recording the echoes of ultrasonic waves reflected from it. These waves, modulated by pulsations, are introduced into the tissue by means of a piezoelectric transducer. The many advantages of ultrasonography include the ability to make quick assessment of a structure and its positioning by means of portable equipment, without ionizing radiation and at about one-fourth the cost of CT scanning. Sedation is usually not necessary, and ultrasonography can be repeated as often as indicated. In brain imaging, B mode and real-time sector scanners are usually employed, permitting excellent detail in the coronal and sagittal planes. Contiguous structures can be studied by a continuous sweep and reviewed on videotape.

Ultrasonography has been used for in utero diagnosis of hydrocephalus and other anomalies. In neonates, the thin skull and the open anterior fontanelle have facilitated imaging of the brain, and ultrasonography is now used in many nurseries to screen and follow all infants of less than 32 weeks' gestation or under 1500 g for intracranial hemorrhage. Other uses in neonates include detection of hydrocephalus, major brain and spine malformations, and even calcifications from intrauterine infection with cytomegalovirus or *Toxoplasma*.

Cerebral Angiography

Arteriography remains a useful procedure in the diagnosis of many cerebrovascular disorders, particularly vascular malformations, and is sometimes used when a potentially operable lesion is suspected. In some instances of brain tumor, arteriography may be necessary to define the precise location or vascular bed, to differentiate among tumors, or to distinguish tumor from abscess or infarction. Noninvasive CT, MRI, and MRA are often satisfactory in cases of static or flowing blood disorders (eg, sinus thromboses). Thus, invasive arteriography is being used less often.

Myelography

X-ray examination of the spine following injection of a dye, water-soluble contrast medium, or air into the subarachnoid space via the lumbar or, rarely, the cervical route may be indicated in cases of spinal cord tumors or various forms of spinal dysraphism and in rare instances of herniated disks in children. However, in most institutions, MRI or CT metrizamide myelography is employed instead.

Adams C et al: Comparison of SPECT, EEG, CT, MRI, and pathology in partial epilepsy. Pediatr Neurol 1992;8:97.

Altman NR, Purser RK, Post MJ: Tuberous sclerosis: Characteristics at CT and MR imaging. Radiology 1988; 167:527.

Barkovich AJ: *Pediatric Neuroimaging.* Raven Press, 1989.

Brody AS, Gooding CA: Magnetic resonance imaging: Review article. Pediatr Rev 1986;8:87.

Chugani K: The role of positron emission tomography in childhood epilepsy. Int Pediatr 1992;7:260.

Doyle LW et al: Regional cerebral glucose metabolism of newborn infants measured by positron emission tomography. Dev Med Child Neurol 1983;25:143.

Edelman RR, Warach S: Magnetic resonance imaging. (Two parts.) N Engl J Med 1993;11:708, 785.

Nowell MA et al: Magnetic resonance imaging of white matter disease in children. AJR 1988;151:359.

Powers TA et al: Central nervous system lesions in pediatric patients. Radiology 1988;169:723.

Roach E et al: Magnetic resonance imaging in pediatric neurologic disorders. J Child Neurol 1987;2:110.

Taylor MJ, McCulloch D: Prognostic value of VEP's in young children with acute onset cortical blindness. Pediatr Neurol 1992;7:111.

DISORDERS AFFECTING THE NERVOUS SYSTEM IN INFANTS & CHILDREN

ALTERED STATES OF CONSCIOUSNESS

Essentials of Diagnosis

- Reduction or alteration in cognitive and affective mental functioning and in arousability or attentiveness.
- Acute onset.

General Considerations

Coma and other states of unconsciousness are imprecisely defined. Many terms are used to describe the continuum from full alertness and attentiveness or consciousness to complete unresponsiveness and deep coma. This continuum might include clouding, obtundation, somnolence or stupor, semicoma or light coma, and deep coma. Several scales have been used to grade the depth of unconsciousness. Tables 25–5 and 25–6 delineate some of these. Physicians should use one of these tables and further describe in their narratives what they mean. These descriptions help subsequent observers quantify unconsciousness and decide whether the patient is improving or deteriorating.

The neurologic substrate for consciousness is the reticular activating system in the brain stem, up to and including the thalamus and paraventricular hypothalamus. Large lesions of the cortex, especially of the left hemisphere, can also cause coma. "Locked-in syndrome" is a term used for patients who are conscious but have no access to motor or verbal expression because of massive loss of motor function of the brain stem. "Coma vigil" is the term used for patients who seem to be comatose but have some spontaneous motor behavior, such as eye opening or eye tracking, almost always at a reflex level. "Persistent vegetative state" denotes a chronic condition in which there is preservation of the sleep-wake cycle but no awareness and no recovery of mental function; this has been documented in infants.

Table 25–5. Gradation of coma.

	"Deep Coma"		"Light coma"		
	Grade 4	Grade 3	Grade 2	Grade 1	Stupor
Response to pain	0	+	Avoidance	Avoidance	Arousal unsustained
Tone/posture	Flaccid	Decerebrate	Variable	Variable	Normal
Tendon reflexes	0	+/−	+	+	+
Pupil response	0	+	+	+	+
Response to verbal stimuli	0	0	0	0	+
Other corneal reflex	0	+	+	+	+
Gag reflex	0	+	+	+	+

Emergency Measures

The clinician's first response is to ensure that the patient will survive the initial examination. The "ABCs" of resuscitation are pertinent: *A*irway must be kept open with positioning or even endotracheal intubation. *B*reathing and adequate air exchange can be assessed by auscultation; hand bag respiratory assistance with oxygen might be needed. *C*irculation must be assured by assessing pulse and blood pressure. An intravenous line will always be necessary. Fluids, plasma, blood, or even a dopamine drip (5–20 µg/kg/min) might be necessary in cases of hypotension. An extremely hypothermic or febrile child may require vigorous cooling or warming to save life. The assessment of vital signs may signal the diagnosis. Slow, insufficient respirations suggest poisoning by hypnotic drugs; apnea might indicate diphenoxylate hydrochloride poisoning. Rapid, deep respirations suggest acidosis, possibly metabolic, as with diabetic coma; toxic, eg, that due to aspirin; or neurogenic, as in Reye's syndrome. Hyperthermia might indicate infection or heat stroke; hypothermia might indicate cold exposure, ethanol poisoning, or hypoglycemia (especially in infancy).

The signs of impending brain herniation are another priority of the initial assessment. Bradycardia, high blood pressure, irregular breathing, increased extensor tone, and third nerve palsy with the eye deviated outward and the pupil dilated are possible signs of impending temporal lobe or brain stem herniation. These signs suggest a need for hyperventilation, reducing cerebral edema, prompt neurosurgical

Table 25–6. "Glasgow Coma Scale" for recording assessment of consciousness.[1,2]

		Date				
		Time	Time	Time	Time	etc
Best motor response	6 Obeys commands 5 Localizes pain 4 Withdraws 3 Abnormal flexing 2 Extensor response 1 None					
Best verbal response	5 Oriented 4 Confused conversation (words) 3 Inappropriate words (vocal sounds) 2 Incomprehensible sounds (cries) 1 None					
Eye opening	4 Spontaneous 3 To speech 2 To pain 1 None					
	Total Score					

[1]Modified and reproduced, with permission, from Jennett B, Teasdale G: Aspects of coma after severe head injury. Lancet 1977;1:878.

[2]The scale can also be modified for infants. The sections regarding motor response and eye opening remain unchanged; items in parentheses in verbal response section are to be applied to infants. Under 6 months of age, the best verbal response is a cry (score 2) and the best motor response is usually flexion (score 3), for a total maximal score of 9. Adjusted maximal scores are as follows:

Birth–6 months:	9	2–5 years:	13
6–12 months:	11	Over 5 years:	14–15
1–2 years:	12		

consultation, and possibly, in an infant with a bulging fontanelle, subdural or ventricular tap (or both).

Initial intravenous fluids should contain glucose until further assessment disproves hypoglycemia as a cause.

A history obtained from parents or witnesses is desirable. Sometimes the only history will be obtained from ambulance attendants. An important point is whether the child is known to have a chronic illness, eg, diabetes, hemophilia, epilepsy, or cystic fibrosis. Recent acute illness raises the possibility of coma caused by Reye's syndrome, viral or bacterial meningitis, or the much rarer hemolytic-uremic syndrome. A combination of viral illness with 1–3 days of sudden and intractable vomiting invariably precedes the coma of Reye's syndrome. (The illness is usually respiratory, sometimes varicella.)

Trauma is a common cause of coma. Lack of a history of trauma, especially in infants, does not rule it out; nonaccidental trauma or a fall unwitnessed by caretakers may have occurred.

In coma of unknown cause, poisoning is always a possibility. Absence of a history of ingestion of a toxic substance or of medication in the home does not rule out poisoning as a cause.

Often the history is obtained concurrently with a brief pediatric and neurologic screening examination. After the assessment of vital signs and their meaning, the general examination proceeds with an assessment for trauma. Palpation of the head and fontanelle, inspection of the ears for infection or hemorrhage, and a careful examination for neck stiffness are indicated. If circumstances suggest head or neck trauma, the head and neck must be immobilized so that any fracture or dislocation will not be aggravated. The skin must be inspected for petechiae or purpura that might suggest bacteremia, infection, bleeding disorder, or traumatic bruising. Examination of the chest, abdomen, and limbs is important to exclude enclosed hemorrhage, traumatic fractures, etc.

Neurologic examination quantifies the stimulus response and depth of coma, eg, responsiveness to verbal or painful stimuli. Examination of the eyes in reference to pupils, fundi, and eye movements is important. Are the eye movements spontaneous, or is it necessary to do the doll's-eye maneuver, ie, rotating the head rapidly to see whether the eyes follow? Motor and sensory examinations assess reflex asymmetries, Babinski sign, and evidence for spontaneous posturing or posturing induced by noxious stimuli (eg, decorticate or decerebrate posturing).

If the cause of the coma is not obvious, emergency laboratory tests must be obtained. Tables 25–7 and 25–8, respectively, list some of the causes of coma in children and mnemonics for its investigation. An immediate blood glucose (or Dextrostix), complete blood count, urine obtained by catheterization if necessary, pH and electrolytes (including bicarbonate), serum urea nitrogen, and AST are initial screens.

Urine, blood, and even gastric contents must be saved for toxin screen if the underlying cause is not obvious. Spinal tap is often necessary to rule out central nervous system infection. Papilledema is a relative contraindication to lumbar puncture. Occasionally, blood culture is obtained, antibiotics started, and imaging study of the brain done prior to a diagnostic spinal tap. If meningitis is suspected and a tap is believed to be hazardous, antibiotics should be started and the diagnostic spinal puncture done later. Tests that are less readily available but helpful in obscure cases of coma include PO_2, PCO_2, ammonia levels, serum and urine osmolality, porphyrins, lead levels, and, in the newborn, urine and serum amino acids and urine organic acids.

If there is any suspicion of head trauma or increased pressure, an emergency CT scan or MRI is necessary. Bone windows on the former study or skull x-rays can be done at the same sitting. The absence of skull fracture, of course, does not rule out coma caused by life-threatening closed head trauma; injury that results from shaking a child is one example. In a child with an open fontanelle, a real-time ultrasound may be substituted for the other, more definitive imaging studies if there is good local expertise.

Rarely, an emergency EEG aids in diagnosing the cause of coma. A nonconvulsive status epilepticus or focal finding seen with herpes encephalitis (periodic lateralized epileptiform discharges) or focal slowing as seen with stroke or cerebritis are cases in which the EEG might be helpful. The EEG also may correlate with the stage of coma (eg, in Reye's syndrome) and add prognostic information. (See Table 25–9.) An improving (or deteriorating) EEG may herald clinical improvement, aid in predicting outcome, and suggest the need for more (or less) heroic therapy.

Treatment

Treatment, of course, depends on the underlying cause. Emergency measures were outlined at the beginning of this section.

A. General Measures: Vital signs must be monitored and maintained. Most emergency rooms and intensive care units have flow sheets to monitor vital signs. The flow sheets provide space for repeated monitoring of the coma; one of the coma scales can be a useful tool for this purpose. The patient's response to vocal or painful stimuli and orientation to time, place, and situation when coming out of the coma are monitored. Posture and movements of the limbs, either spontaneously or in response to pain, are serially noted. Pupillary size, equality, and reaction to light and movement of the eyes to the doll's-eye maneuver or ice-water calorics should be recorded. Intravenous fluids can be tailored to the situation, eg, for treatment of acidosis, shock, or hypovolemia. Nasogastric suction is initially important; when the coma is prolonged, nasogastric feedings are sometimes part of treatment. The patient

Table 25–7. Some causes of coma in childhood.[1]

Mechanism of Coma	Likely Cause	
	Newborn, Infant	**Older Child**

Anoxia
  Asphyxia
  Respiratory
    obstruction
  Severe anemia
	Birth asphyxia
	Meconium aspiration, infection (especially respiratory syncytial virus)
	Hydrops fetalis
		CO poisoning
		Croup, epiglottitis
		
		Hemolysis, blood loss

Ischemia
  Cardiac
  Shock
	Shunting lesions, hypoplastic left heart
	Asphyxia (cardiac), sepsis
		Shunting lesions, aortic stenosis
		Blood loss, infection

Trauma	Birth contusion, hemorrhage, nonaccidental trauma	Falls, auto accidents
Infection	Gram-negative meningitis, herpes encephalitis, postimmunization encephalitis	Bacterial meningitis, viral encephalitis, postinfectious encephalitis
Vascular	Intraventricular hemorrhage (premature), sinus thrombosis	Arterial, venous occlusion with congenital heart disease
Neoplasm	Rare; variety, medulloblastoma	Brain stem glioma, increased pressure with posterior fossa tumors
Drugs	Maternal sedatives, injected analgesics	"Any" drugs
Epilepsy	Constant minor motor seizures	Constant minor motor seizures, petit mal status, postictal state
Toxins	Lead	Arsenic, alcohol, drugs, pesticides
Hypoglycemia	Birth injury, diabetic progeny, toxemic progeny	Diabetes, "prediabetes," "idiopathic," hypoglycemic agents
Increased intracranial pressure	Anoxic brain damage, hydrocephalus, unusual metabolic disorders (urea cycle; amino, or organic acidurias)	Toxic encephalopathy, Reye's syndrome, head trauma, tumor of posterior fossa
Hepatic causes	Hepatitis, fulminant (rare), bile duct atresia, inborn metabolic errors in bilirubin conjugation	Acute hepatitis, chronic aggressive hepatitis
Renal causes	Hypoplastic kidneys	Nephritis, acute and chronic
Hypertensive encephalopathy		Acute nephritis, vasculitis
Hypercapnia	Congenital lung anomalies, bronchopulmonary dysplasia	Cystic fibrosis

Electrolyte abnormalities
  Hypernatremia
  Hyponatremia
 	
  Severe acidosis
  Hyperkalemia
	Iatrogenic ($NaHCO_3$ use), salt poisoning
	Inappropriate antidiuretic hormone, adrenogenital syndrome, dialysis (iatrogenic)
	Septicemia, cold injury, metabolic errors
	Renal failure, adrenogenital syndrome
		Diarrhea, dehydration
		Diarrhea, dehydration, gastroenteritis
		
		Infection, diabetic coma, poisoning (aspirin, etc)
		Poisoning (aspirin, etc)

Purpuric	Disseminated intravascular coagulation (many causes), hemolytic-uremic syndrome	Disseminated intravascular coagulation (many causes), leukemia, thrombotic purpura (rare)

[1]Modified and reproduced, with permission, from Lewis J, Moe PG: The unconscious child. In: *Current Diagnosis,* 5th ed. Conn H, Conn R (editors). Saunders, 1977.

Table 25–8. Mnemonics for investigating coma in children.[1]

Seven H's	Five I's
Hypoglycemia	Ictal (or postictal)
Hyperosmotic	Ingestion
Hyponatremia	Infection
Hypertensive	Injury
Hypoxia	Illness
Hemorrhage	(extracranial, intracranial)
Hepatic (Reye's syndrome)	

[1]Modified and reproduced, with permission, from Lewis J, Moe PG: The unconscious child. In: *Current Diagnosis,* 5th ed. Conn H, Conn R (editors). Saunders, 1977.

Table 25–9. Electroencephalogram-coma correlates.[1]

Rhythmic 4–7/sec (1–3/sec)	I Lethargy
Dysrhythmic 1–3/sec (4–7/sec)	II Disorientation, delirium
Disorganized 1–3/sec, low amplitude	III Coma-decorticate
Low amplitude (< 50 microvolt), burst suppression	IV Coma-decerebrate
Almost isoelectric	V "Coma dépassé"

[1]Modified and reproduced, with permission, from Aoki Y, Lombroso CT: Prognostic value of electroencephalography in Reye's syndrome. Neurology 1973;23:333.

needs to be catheterized for monitoring urine output and for urinalysis. The child should be protected from decubiti with frequent turning and, if necessary, by providing a foam mattress. The eyes should be protected with pads and artificial tears.

B. Seizures: An EEG should be ordered if there is a question of ongoing seizures. If there are obvious motor seizures, treatment for status epilepticus is given with intravenous drugs (see below). If there is suggestion of brain stem herniation or increased pressure, an intracranial monitor may be necessary. (This procedure is described in more detail in Chapter 15.) Initial treatment of this possible complication includes keeping the patient's head up (15–30 degrees) and hyperventilation. Mannitol, diuretics, corticosteroids, and drainage of the spinal fluid are more heroic measures covered in detail elsewhere.

Prognosis

About half of children with nontraumatic causes of coma have a good outcome. In studies of adults assessed on admission or within the first days after the onset of coma, an analysis of multiple variables was most helpful in assessing prognosis. Abnormal neuro-ophthalmologic signs (eg, the absence of pupillary movement or of movement in response to the doll's-eye maneuver or ice-water calorics and the absence of corneal responses) were unfavorable. Delay in the return of motor responses, tone, or eye opening was also unfavorable. In children, the assessment done on admission is about as predictive as one done in succeeding days. Approximately two-thirds of outcomes can be successfully predicted at an early stage on the basis of coma severity, extraocular movements, pupillary reactions, motor patterns, blood pressure, temperature, and seizure type. Other characteristics, eg, the need for assisted respiration, the presence of increased intracranial pressure, and the duration of coma, were not significantly predictive.

Published reports suggest that an anoxic (as compared to traumatic, metabolic, toxic, etc) cause of coma, eg, that caused by near drowning, has a much grimmer outlook.

BRAIN DEATH

Many medical and law associations have endorsed the following definition of death: "An individual who has sustained either (1) irreversible cessation of circulatory and respiratory functions, or (2) irreversible cessation of all functions of the entire brain, including the brain stem, is dead. A determination of death must be made in accordance with accepted medical standards." Representatives from several pediatric and neurologic associations have endorsed the Guidelines for the Determination of Brain Death in Children (see reference below). The criteria in term infants (> 38 weeks) were applicable 1 week after the neurologic insult. Difficulties in assessing premature infants and term infants shortly after birth were acknowledged.

Prerequisites

The history is important. The physician must determine proximate causes to make sure there are no remediable or reversible conditions. Examples of such causes are metabolic conditions, toxic agents, sedative-hypnotic drugs, surgically remediable conditions, hypothermia, and paralytic agents.

Physical Examination Criteria
(See Chapter 15.)

The following criteria are those established by the Task Force on Brain Death in Children (see reference, below).

(1) Coexistence of coma and apnea. The patient must exhibit complete loss of consciousness, vocalization, and volitional activity.

(2) Absence of brain stem function as defined by the following: (a) Midposition or fully dilated pupils that do not respond to light. Drugs may influence and invalidate pupillary assessment. (b) Absence of spontaneous eye movements and those induced by oculocephalic and caloric (oculovestibular) testing. (c) Absence of movement of bulbar musculature, including facial and oropharyngeal muscles. The corneal, gag, cough, sucking, and rooting reflexes are absent. (d) Absence of respiratory movements when the patient is off the respirator. Apnea testing using standardized methods can be performed but is done after other criteria are met.

(3) The patient must not be significantly hypothermic or hypotensive for age.

(4) Tone is flaccid, and spontaneous or induced movements, excluding spinal cord events such as reflex withdrawal or spinal myoclonus, are absent.

(5) The examination should remain consistent with brain death throughout the observation and testing period.

Confirmation

Details of apnea testing suggest documentation of a PCO_2 level reaching > 60 mm Hg, with oxygenation maintained throughout; this level may be reached 3–15 minutes after taking the patient off the respirator. The recommended observation period to confirm brain death (repeated examinations) is 12–24 hours (longer in infancy); reversible causes *must* be ruled out.

If an irreversible cause is documented, laboratory testing is not essential. Helpful tests to support the clinical contention of brain death include the following:

(1) Electroencephalography: Electrocerebral silence should persist for 30 minutes. Drug concentrations must be insufficient to suppress EEG activity.

(2) Angiography: Failure of arterial intracerebral blood flow confirms brain death. Carotid arteriography and cerebral radionuclide angiography are two methods. Dural sinus flow may persist and not invalidate the diagnosis of brain death.

Other laboratory studies have not been sufficiently documented to be considered definitive; cerebral evoked potentials and ultrasound blood pulsations are two common examples. Xenon-enhanced computer tomography is a more elaborate method.

In rare cases, preserved intracranial perfusion in the presence of electroencephalographic silence has been documented, and the converse has also been reported. Controversy attends the definition and criteria of brain death in the newborn. This debate inevitably acknowledges the issue of withdrawing support from the infant with a hopeless prognosis who is not brain dead.

Ashwal S, Schneider S, Thompson J: Xenon computed tomography measuring cerebral blood flow in the determination of brain death in children. Ann Neurol 1989; 25:539.

Ashwal S, Schneider S: Brain death in the newborn. Pediatrics 1989;84:427.

Ashwal S: Brain death in the newborn. Clin Perinatol 1989; 16:501.

Celesia GG: Persistent vegetative state. Neurology 1993;43: 1457.

Childs NL, Mercer WN, Childs HW: Accuracy of diagnosis of persistent vegetative state. Neurology 1993;43:1465.

Freeman JM, Ferry PC: New brain death guidelines in children: Further confusion. Pediatrics 1988;81:301.

Goldie WD: Physiologic parameters for evaluating severe brain injury in infants and young children. Am J EEG Technol 1988;28:153.

Jones KM, Barnes PD: MR diagnosis of brain death. AJNR Am J Neuroradiol 199 2;13:65.

Levin HS et al: Vegetative state after closed head injury: Traumatic coma data bank report. Arch Neurol 1991;48: 580.

Lewis J, Moe PG: The unconscious child. In: *Current Diagnosis,* 5th ed. Conn H, Conn R (editors). Saunders, 1977.

Mizrahi EM, Pollack MA, Kellaway P: Neocortical death in infants: Behavioral, neurologic, and electroencephalographic characteristics. Pediatr Neurol 1985;1:302.

Shewmon DA: Commentary on guidelines for the determination of brain death in children. Ann Neurol 1988; 24:789.

Task Force on Brain Death in Children: Guidelines for the determination of brain death in children. Ann Neurol 1987;21:616. [Also Arch Neurol 1987;44:587. Neurology 1987;37:1077. Pediatr Neurol 1987;3:242. Pediatrics 1987;80:298.]

Teasdale G, Jennett B: Assessment of coma and impaired consciousness: A practical scale. Lancet 1974;2:81.

Toffol GJ et al: Pitfalls in diagnosing brain death in infancy. J Child Neurol 1987;2:134.

Vegetative state: Report of the American Neurological Association Committee on Ethical Affairs. Ann Neurol 1993;33:386.

Yager JY, Johnston B, Seshia SS: Coma scales in pediatric practice. Am J Dis Child 1990;144:1088.

SEIZURE DISORDERS (Epilepsies)

Essentials of Diagnosis

- Recurrent nonfebrile seizures.
- Often, interictal electroencephalographic changes.

General Considerations

A seizure is a sudden, transient disturbance of brain function, manifested by involuntary motor, sensory, autonomic, or psychic phenomena, alone or in any combination, often accompanied by alteration or loss of consciousness. A seizure may occur after a transient metabolic, traumatic, anoxic, or infectious insult to the brain.

Repeated seizures without evident time-limited cause justify the label of epilepsy. Seizures and epilepsy occur most commonly at the extremes of life. The incidence is highest in the newborn and higher in childhood than in later life. Epilepsy in childhood often remits. Prevalence (the number of people with epilepsy in the population at any given time) flattens out after age 10–15. The chance of having a second seizure after an initial unprovoked episode is 30%. The chance of remission from epilepsy in childhood is 50%. The recurrence rate after the withdrawal of drugs is about 30%. Factors adversely influencing recurrence include (1) difficulty in getting the seizures under control (ie, the number of seizures occurring before control is achieved), (2) neurologic dysfunction or mental retardation, (3) age at onset under 2 years, and (4) abnormal EEG at the time of discontinuing medication. The type of seizures also often determines prognosis.

Seizures are caused by any factor that can disturb brain function. Seizures and epilepsy are often classified as symptomatic (the cause is strongly identified or presumed) or idiopathic (the cause is unknown, or genetic influences are strongly etiologic). The younger the infant or child, the more likely that the cause can be identified. Idiopathic or genetic epilepsy most often appears between ages 4 and 16. A seizure disorder or epilepsy should not be considered idiopathic unless a searching history, examination, and appropriate laboratory tests have turned up no apparent cause.

Clinical Findings

A. Symptoms and Signs: The key to the diagnosis of epilepsy is, of course, the history. The initial symptom often identifies the aura to the seizure itself. A feeling of fear, numbness or tingling in the fingers, or bright lights in one visual field might be examples of an aura (really the onset of the seizure). Sometimes the patient recalls nothing because there has been no aura or warning. The parent might report that the patient's eyes went off to one side or that extreme pallor, trismus, or overall body stiffening occurred first. Occasionally there is a prodrome, eg, a feeling of "unwellness," of something about to happen, or a recurrent thought over minutes or hours prior to the aura and seizure itself.

Minute details of the seizure can help determine the site of onset and aid in classification of the seizure. Did the patient become extremely pale before falling? Was the patient able to respond to queries during the episode? Did the patient become completely unconscious? Did the patient fall stiffly or gradually slump to the floor? Was there an injury? How long did the stiffening or jerking last? Where were the sites of jerking?

Events after the seizure can be helpful in diagnosis. Was there loss of speech? Was the patient able to respond accurately before going to sleep?

All these events prior to, during, and after the seizure can help to classify the seizure and, indeed, may help to determine if the event actually was a probable epileptic seizure or a pseudoseizure, ie, a nonepileptic phenomenon mimicking a seizure. Classifying the seizure type may aid in diagnosis and prognosis and suggest desirable or necessary laboratory tests and medication choices. (See Tables 25–10 and 25–11.)

B. Status Epilepticus: Status epilepticus is a clinical or electrical seizure lasting at least 30 minutes or a series of seizures without complete recovery over the same period of time. After 30 minutes, the brain begins to suffer from hypoxia and acidosis, with depletion of local energy stores, cerebral edema, and structural damage. Eventually, high fever, hypotension, respiratory depression, and even death may occur. Thus, status epilepticus is a relative medical emergency.

Status epilepticus is classified as (1) convulsive, ie, the common tonic-clonic, or "grand mal" status epilepticus; or (2) nonconvulsive, eg, simple motor status without loss of consciousness. Other nonconvulsive types include absence status, or "spike-wave stupor," and (very rare) partial complex status epilepticus.

An EEG may be necessary to aid in diagnosing the less common variants, such as a patient with known absence who now is in a partially-in-contact, stuporous state.

A child with status epilepticus often has a high fever with or without intracranial infection, eg, viral encephalitis or bacterial meningitis. Status epilepticus may be the initial seizure; various studies show that one-fourth to three-fourths of children experience status epilepticus as the initial seizure. Often, it is a reflection of a remote insult (eg, anoxic or traumatic). Tumor, vascular disease (strokes), or head trauma, which are common causes of status epilepticus in adults, are uncommon causes in childhood. One-half of cases are symptomatic of acute (25%) or chronic (25%) central nervous system disorders. Infection or metabolic disorders are the most common symptomatic causes in children. The cause is unknown in half of cases, but many of these will be febrile.

Table 25–10. Clinical seizure correlation with electroencephalographic patterns.[1]

Clinical Seizure Type	EEG ictal	EEG Interictal
Focal Simple partial ("focal") Motor Sensory	Local contralateral discharge (spike, slow wave, etc)	Same
Complex partial ("psychomotor")	Focal or bilateral frontal, temporal discharge	Temporofrontal local or asynchronous discharge
Partial seizures with generalization	Above discharges become lateralized	
Generalized Absence ("petit mal") Simple (impairment of consciousness only) Complex (with tonic, clonic, autonomic component)	3/sec spike-wave	Normal
Atypical absence	Irregular 1–4/sec spike-wave	Abnormal, often slow spike-wave, asymmetric
Myoclonic seizures	Multiple spike-wave	Same
Tonic-clonic ("grand mal")	10/sec spike/ slowing, then spike/slow wave	Multiple spikes, spike-wave sharp, slow
Atonic (astatic, akinetic)	Multiple spike-wave	Same

[1]According to the International Classification of Epileptic Seizures. Some subtypes are not listed. Some age-limited syndromes occurring in childhood are not easily incorporated into this scheme.

Status epilepticus is more common in children under 1 year of age, with 37% of cases occurring under that age and 85% under age 5. Thus, the pediatrician sees status epilepticus most commonly in infants and preschoolers. For treatment, see Table 25–12.

C. Febrile Seizures: Criteria for febrile seizures are (1) age of 3 months to 5 years (most occur between the ages of 6 months and 3 years), (2) fever of 38.8 °C, and (3) non-central nervous system infection. Most (greater than 90%) are generalized and brief (less than 5 minutes) and occur early in an OMPA (otitis media, pharyngitis, adenitis) illness. Febrile seizures occur in 2–3% of children. Gastroenteritis, especially due to *Shigella* or *Campylobacter,* and urinary tract infections are less common causes. Roseola infantum is a rare but classic cause. One study implicated viral causes in 86% of cases. Immunizations may be a cause.

Rarely, status epilepticus may occur; fever is a common cause of status epilepticus in early child-

Table 25–11. Seizures by age at onset, pattern, and preferred treatment.

Age Group and Seizure Type	Age at Onset	Clinical Manifestations	Causative Factors	Electroencephalographic Pattern	Other Diagnostic Studies	Treatment and Comments (Anticonvulsants by Order of Choice)
Neonatal seizures	Birth to 2 weeks	Often "atypical": sudden limpness or tonic posturing, brief apnea, and cyanosis; odd cry; eyes "rolling up"; blinking or mouthing or chewing movements; nystagmus, twitchiness or clonic movements—focal, multifocal, or generalized.	Neurologic insults (hypoxia/ischemia; intracranial hemorrhage) present more in first 3 days or after eighth day; metabolic disturbances alone between third and eighth days; hypoglycemia, hypocalcemia, hyper- and hyponatremia. Drug withdrawal. Pyridoxine deficiency and other metabolic causes. CNS infections and structural abnormalities.	May correlate poorly with clinical seizures. Focal spikes or slow rhythms; multifocal discharges.	Lumbar puncture: serum Ca^{2+}, PO_4^{3-}, glucose, Mg^{2+}; BUN, amino acid screen, blood ammonia, organic acid screen, TORCHES[1] screen. Ultrasound or CT scan for suspected intracranial hemorrhage and structural abnormalities.	Phenobarbital, IV or IM; if seizures not controlled, add phenytoin IV (loading dose 20 mg/kg each). Diazepam, approximately 0.2 mg/kg. Treat underlying disorder. Seizures due to brain damage often resistant to anticonvulsants. When cause in doubt, stop protein feedings until enzyme deficiencies of urea cycle or amino acid metabolism ruled out.
West's syndrome "infantile spasms." (See also Lennox-Gastaut syndrome, below.)	3–18 months; occasionally up to 4 years	Sudden, usually symmetric adduction and flexion of limbs with concomitant flexion of head and trunk; also abduction and extensor movements like Moro reflex. Tendency for spasms to occur in clusters, on waking or falling asleep, or when fatigued, or may be noted particularly when the infant is being handled, is ill, or is otherwise irritable. Tendency for each patient to have own stereotyped pattern.	Pre- or perinatal brain damage or malformation in approximately one-third; biochemical, infectious, degenerative causes in approximately one-third; unknown in approximately one-third. With early onset, pyridoxine deficiency, amino- or organic aciduria. Tuberous sclerosis in 5–10%. Chronic inflammatory disease and toxoplasmosis. Aicardi syndrome (females with mental retardation, agenesis of corpus callosum, ocular and vertebral anomalies).	Hypsarrhythmia; chaotic high-voltage slow waves, random spikes, all leads (90%); other abnormalities in rest. Rarely "normal" EEG normalization usually correlates with reduction of seizures; not helpful prognostically regarding mental development.	Funduscopic and skin examination, trial of pyridoxine. Amino- and organic acid screen. Chronic inflammatory disease. TORCHES[1] screen, CT or MRI scan shall be done to (1) establish definite diagnosis, (2) aid in genetic counseling.	Corticotropin preferred (2–4 units/kg/d IM Acthar gel 1/d, then slow withdrawal). Some prefer oral corticosteroids. Clonazepam, valproic acid. In resistant cases, ketogenic or medium-chain triglyceride (MCT) diet (see text). Retardation of varying degree in approximately 90% of cases.
Febrile convulsions	3 months to 5 years	Usually generalized seizures, less than 15 minutes; rarely focal in onset. May lead to status epilepticus.	Nonneurologic febrile illness (temperature rises to 102.5 °F or higher); family history frequently positive for febrile convulsions.	Normal interictal EEG, especially when obtained 8–10 days after seizure. In older infants, 3/s spikes often seen.	In infants or whenever suspicion of meningitis exists, perform lumbar puncture.	Treat underlying illness, fever. Diazepam orally or rectally as needed 0.3–0.5 mg/kg 3 times daily during illness. Prophylaxis with phenobarbital (valproic acid if phenobarbital not tolerated), with neurologic deficits, prolonged seizure, family history of epilepsy.
Myoclonic-astatic (akinetic, atonic) seizures; formerly atypical absence. With mental retardation, Lennox-Gastaut syndrome.	Any time in childhood; normally 2–7 years	Shocklike violent contractions of one or more muscle groups, singly or irregularly repetitive; may fling patient suddenly to side, forward, or backward. Usually no or only brief loss of consciousness. Half of patients or more also have generalized grand mal seizures.	Multiple causes, usually resulting in diffuse neuronal damage. History of West's syndrome; prenatal or perinatal brain damage; viral meningoencephalitides; subacute sclerosing panencephalitis; CNS degenerative disorders; lead or other encephalopathies; structural cerebral abnormalities, eg, porencephaly.	Atypical slow (1–2.5 Hz) spike-wave complexes ("petit mal variant") and bursts of high-voltage generalized spikes, often with diffusely slow background frequencies. See text.	As dictated by index of suspicion. Lumbar puncture with measles antibody titer and CSF IgG index. Nerve conduction studies. Urine for lead, arylsulfatase A, etc. Skin biopsy for electron microscopy and enzyme studies. CT scan and brain biopsy may be justified.	Difficult to treat. Valproic acid, clonazepam, or ethosuximide. Felbamate. Imipramine as adjunct. Diazepam. Ketogenic or medium-chain triglyceride (MCT) diet. ACTH or corticosteroids as in West's syndrome. Protect head with helmet and chin padding.
Absence ("petit mal"). Also juvenile and myoclonic absence.	3–15 years	Lapses of consciousness or vacant stares, lasting about 10 seconds, often in "clusters." Automatisms of face and hands; clonic activity in 30–45%. Often confused with complex partial seizures but no aura or postictal confusion.	Unknown. Genetic component: probably an autosomal dominant gene.	Three-second bilaterally synchronous, symmetric, high-voltage spikes and waves. EEG "normalization" correlates closely with control of seizures.	Hyperventilation when patient on inadequate or no medication often provokes attacks. CT scan is rarely of value.	Valproic acid or ethosuximide: with latter, add phenobarbital if EEG suggests other abnormalities (grand mal). In resistant cases, ketogenic or MCT diet. Also, in resistant cases, valproic acid and ethosuximide together.

(continued)

Table 25–11. Seizures by age at onset (continued)

Age Group and Seizure Type	Age at Onset	Clinical Manifestations	Causative Factors	Electroencephalographic Pattern	Other Diagnostic Studies	Treatment and Comments (Anticonvulsants by Order of Choice)
Simple partial or focal seizures (motor/sensory/jacksonian). (Complex partial or psychomotor seizures, below.)	Any age	Seizure may involve any part of body; may spread in fixed pattern (jacksonian march), becoming generalized. In children, epileptogenic focus often "shifts," and epileptic manifestations may change concomitantly.	Often secondary to birth trauma, inflammatory process, vascular accidents, meningoencephalitis, etc. If seizures are coupled with new or progressive neurologic deficits, a structural lesion (eg, brain tumor) is likely.	Focal spikes or slow waves in appropriate cortical region; sometimes diffusely abnormal or even normal.	If seizures are difficult to control or progressive deficits occur, neuroradiodiagnostic studies, particularly CT brain scan, imperative (see text).	Carbamazepine, phenytoin, phenobarbital or primidone. Valproic acid useful adjunct.
Complex partial seizures (psychomotor, temporal lobe, or limbic seizures).	Any age	Aura may be a sensation of fear, epigastric discomfort, odd smell or taste (usually unpleasant), visual or auditory hallucination (either vague and "unformed" or well-formed image, words, music). Aura and seizure stereotyped for each patient. Seizure may consist of vague stare; facial, tongue, or swallowing movements and throaty sounds; or various complex automatisms. Unlike absences, complex partial seizures tend not to occur in clusters but singly and to last longer (1 minute or more), followed by confusion. History of aura (or child running to adult from "vague fear") and of automatisms involving more than face and hands establishes diagnosis. About 60% also develop generalized grand mal seizures.	As above. Temporal lobes especially sensitive to hypoxia; thus, this seizure type may be sequela of birth trauma, febrile convulsions, etc. Also especially vulnerable to certain viral infections, especially herpes simplex. Remediable other causes are small cryptic tumors or vascular malformations.	As above, but occurring in temporal lobe and its connections, eg, frontotemporal, temporoparietal, temporo-occipital regions.	CT scan when structural lesions suspected. Temporal lobe biopsy when herpes simplex encephalitis suspected. Carotid amobarbital injection when lateralization of speech dominance in question.	Carbamazepine, phenytoin, phenobarbital, or primidone. More than one drug may be necessary. Valproic acid may be useful. Phenacemide in seizures difficult to control. In cases uncontrolled by drugs and where a primary epileptogenic focus is identifiable, excision of anterior third of temporal lobe. Adjunctive psychotherapy required frequently. Felbamate and gabapentin.
"Benign epilepsy of childhood" (with "centrotemporal" or "rotandic" foci).	5–16 years	Partial motor or generalized seizures. Similar seizure patterns may be observed in patients with focal cortical lesions.	Seizure history of abnormal EEG findings in relatives of 40% of affected probands and 18–20% of parents and siblings, suggesting transmission by a single autosomal dominant gene, possibly with age-dependent penetrance.	Centrotemporal spikes or sharp waves ("rolandic discharges") appearing paroxysmally against a normal EEG background.	Serum Ca^{2+} and glucose, BUN, urinalysis. Seldom need CT scan.	Carbamazepine or phenytoin. Primidone or phenobarbital.
Juvenile myoclonic epilepsy (of Janz).	Late childhood and adolescence, peaking at 13 years	Mild myoclonic jerks of neck and shoulder flexor muscles after waking up ("awakening" grand mal seizures). Intelligence usually normal.	40% of relatives have myoclonias, especially in females; 15% have the abnormal EEG pattern with clinical attacks.	Interictal EEG shows fast variety of spike-and-wave sequences or 4- to 6-Hz multispike and wave complexes.	Differentiate from progressive myoclonic encephalopathy of Unverricht-Latora and other degenerative disorders by appropriate biopsies (muscle, liver, etc).	Valproic acid. Phenobarbital. Primidone.
Generalized tonic-clonic seizures (grand mal).	Any age	Loss of consciousness; tonic-clonic movements, often preceded by vague aura or cry. Bladder and bowel incontinence in approximately 15%. Postictal confusion; sleep. Often mixed with or masking other seizure patterns.	Often unknown. Genetic component. May be seen with metabolic disturbances, trauma, infection, intoxication, degenerative disorders, brain tumors, etc.	Bilaterally synchronous, symmetric multiple high-voltage spikes, spikes and waves, mixed patterns. Often normal under age 4.	As above.	Phenobarbital in first 12 months; carbamazepine or valproic acid; phenytoin; primidone. Combinations may be necessary.

[1]TORCHES is a mnemonic formula for toxoplasmosis, rubella, cytomegalovirus, herpes simplex, and syphilis.

Table 25–12. Status epilepticus treatment.

1. ABCs
   a. Airway: Maintain oral airway; intubation may be necessary.
   b. Breathing: Oxygen by mouth (if available).
   c. Circulation: Assess pulse, blood pressure; support with IV fluids, drugs. Monitor vital signs.
2. Start glucose-containing IV; draw Dextrostix/blood glucose; evaluate electrolytes, HCO_3^-, CBC, BUN , anticonvulsant levels.
3. Arterial blood gases, pH.
4. Give 50% glucose if dextrose low (1–2 mL/kg).
5. Begin IV drug therapy; goal is to control status in 20–60 minutes.
   a. Diazepam 0.1–0.3 mg/kg over 1–5 minutes (20 mg maximum); may repeat in 5–20 minutes (short action: 20 minutes; watch for respiratory depression). *or,* lorazepam 0.05–0.2 mg/kg, less effective with repeated doses, longer-acting than diazepam. Midazolam hydrochloride; ICU use only. IM, IV; intubation desirable.
   b. Phenytoin 10–20 mg/kg over 5–20 minutes (*not* IM) 1000 mg maximum); monitor with blood pressure and ECG if available.
   c. Phenobarbital 5–20 mg/kg (sometimes higher for newborns, refractory status in intubated patients in hospital and with monitored blood levels.
6. Correct metabolic perturbations (eg, low-sodium, acidosis).
7. Other drug approaches in refractory status:
   a. Repeat phenytoin, phenobarbital (5–10 mg/kg); monitor blood levels. Support respiration, BP as necessary.
   b. IV paraldehyde 4% solution or rectal paraldehyde 0.1–0.3 mL/kg diluted 1:1 in olive oil.
   c. Valproic acid suspension 50 mg/mL diluted 1:1, 30–60 mg/kg orally or rectally.
8. General anesthetic.
9. Consider underlying causes:
   a. Structural disorders or trauma (even nonaccidental trauma). Consider CT scan.
   b. Infection: Spinal tap, blood culture, antibiotics.
   c. Metabolic disorders: Lactic acidosis, toxins, uremia. May need HCO_3^-, medication, toxin screen, judicious fluid administration.
10. Give maintenance drug (if diazepam only was sufficient to halt status epilepticus): phenytoin 10 mg/kg, phenobarbital 5–10 mg/kg, etc.

hood. Febrile seizures rarely (2–4%) lead to epilepsy or recurrent nonfebrile seizures in later childhood and adult life. The chance of later epilepsy is higher if the febrile seizures have complex features, eg, a duration of over 15 minutes, more than one seizure in the same day, or focal features. Other adverse factors are an abnormal neurologic status preceding the seizures (eg, cerebral palsy or mental retardation), early onset of febrile seizure (before 1 year of age), and a family history of epilepsy. Even with adverse factors, the risk of epilepsy in later life is low, in the range of 15–20%.

Recurrent febrile seizures occur in 20–40% of cases but, in general, do not worsen the long-term outlook.

The child with a febrile seizure must be examined. Routine studies such as serum electrolytes, glucose, calcium, skull x-rays, or brain imaging studies are seldom helpful. A white count above 20,000/μL or

with an extreme left shift may correlate with bacteremia; a complete blood count and blood cultures may be appropriate studies. Serum sodium is often slightly low but not low enough to require treatment or to cause the seizure. *Meningitis must be ruled out.* Bacterial meningitis can present with a fever and seizure. Signs of meningitis (eg, bulging fontanelle, stiff neck, stupor, and irritability) may all be absent, especially in a child under 18 months of age.

After controlling the fever and stopping an ongoing seizure, the physician must decide whether to do a spinal tap. The fact that the child has had a previous febrile seizure does not rule out meningitis as the cause of the current episode. The younger the child, the more important the tap, because physical findings are less reliable in diagnosing meningitis. Although the yield is low, a tap should probably be done if the child is under age 2, if recovery is slow, if no other cause for the fever is found, or if close follow-up will not be possible. Occasionally, observation in the emergency room for several hours obviates the need for a tap. A negative tap does not rule out the emergence of meningitis during the same febrile illness; sometimes a second tap needs to be done.

Treatment after the seizure is problematic. Many clinicians choose to treat the child with maintenance dosage of anticonvulsant medication during the course of that febrile illness. Diazepam, 0.5 mg/kg two or three times a day orally or rectally, has been used in Europe and Japan with success both for prophylaxis and for prevention of subsequent seizures. (Suppositories are not currently available in the United States.) Phenobarbital and valproate sodium are other possible choices; however, the somnolence due to the phenobarbital load (about 5–10 mg/kg) is often discomforting to both the doctor and parent and sometimes confuses follow-up assessments. Valproic acid imposes greater risks and should not be given if there is vomiting or acidosis.

Most clinicians choose to follow the patient without administering anticonvulsant medication. Measures to control fever (sponging, antipyretics, and appropriate antibiotics if a bacterial illness is suspected or found) are the mainstays of treatment. The family can be reassured that simple febrile seizures are not thought to have any long-term adverse consequences. An EEG should be ordered if the febrile seizure is complicated or unusual; in the uncomplicated febrile seizure, the EEG is most often normal. About 10% will have slowing or other occipital abnormalities. Ideally, the study should be done at least a week after the illness to avoid transient findings due to the fever or seizure itself. In older children, 3 per second spike-wave discharge, suggestive of a genetic propensity to epilepsy, may occur. In the young infant, electroencephalographic findings seldom aid in assessing the chance of recurrence of febrile or nonfebrile seizures.

Prophylactic anticonvulsants are not indicated in the uncomplicated febrile seizure patient. If febrile seizures are complicated or prolonged or if medical reassurance fails to relieve family anxiety, anticonvulsant prophylaxis may be indicated and can reduce the incidence of recurrent febrile or nonfebrile seizures. One remedy is to use diazepam at the first onset of fever for the duration of the febrile illness as noted above. Phenobarbital, 3–5 mg/kg/d as a single bedtime dose, is an inexpensive and safe alternative. Often, increasing the dose gradually (eg, starting with 2 mg/kg/d the first week and increasing to 3 mg/kg/d the second week, etc) decreases side effects and noncompliance. A plasma phenobarbital level in the range of 15–40 μg/mL is desirable.

Valproate sodium is more hazardous. In infants, the liquid suspension must often be used but has a short half-life and causes more gastrointestinal upset than the coated capsules used in older children. The dose is 15–60 mg/kg/d in three or four divided doses. Precautionary laboratory studies are necessary.

Phenytoin and carbamazepine have not shown effectiveness in the prophylaxis of febrile seizures.

D. Laboratory Findings and Imaging: Ordering of laboratory tests depends on the age of the child, the severity and type of the seizure, whether the child is ill or injured, and the clinician's suspicion about the underlying cause. Every case of suspected seizure disorder warrants an EEG. Other studies are used selectively. Seizures in early infancy are often symptomatic. Therefore, the younger the child, the more careful must be the laboratory assessment (see Table 25–13).

Metabolic abnormalities are seldom found in the well child with seizures; unless there is a high clinical suspicion of uremia, hyponatremia, etc, laboratory tests are not necessary. Special studies may be necessary in unusual circumstances, eg, if hemolytic ure-

Table 25–13. Laboratory studies in first seizure of epilepsy (nonneonatal).

Well infant: EEG. Calcium, BUN, or urinalysis, and perhaps CT or MRI (abnormal examination or focally abnormal EEG may prompt an imaging study).
Well older child: EEG. Consider CT or MRI.
Ill infant: Calcium, magnesium, CBC, BUN, electrolytes, blood culture, lumbar puncture (LP), EEG, possibly CT or MRI.
Ill older child: CBC, BUN, LP, EEG, CT, or MRI.
Generalized tonic-clonic seizure: As above.
Generalized absence: EEG only.
Atypical absence: EEG, CT, MRI: Consider studies for mental retardation: serum and urine amino and organic acids, and chromosomes, including fragile X. If there is progressive worsening, consider lysosomal enzymes, LP (protein, enzymes, IgG), perhaps long-chain fatty acids, skin/conjunctival biopsies.
Infantile spasms: See atypical absence.
Myoclonic, progressive seizure with mental retardation: See Atypical absence.
Focal: EEG. In cases of mental retardation, positive neurologic examination, EEG focal slow wave, or poorly controlled seizures, do CT or MRI. In refractory cases, consider surgical evaluation.

mic syndrome or lead poisoning is a suspected cause. CT scans are overused in patients with seizures. The youngster with a routine febrile seizure, a nonfebrile generalized seizure with normal examination and normal EEG, or an absence seizure does not need a CT scan or MRI scan. The yield in a child with normal neurologic examination and EEG is less than 5%. Conversely, in children with symptomatic epileptic syndromes, the yield of positive results is as high as 60–80%. Examples include infantile spasms, Lennox-Gastaut syndrome, and progressive myoclonic epilepsy.

In focal seizures, children with benign rolandic epilepsy do not need a CT scan; it will invariably be normal. The yield with other focal seizures is 15–30%, with most of the findings unimportant in relation to diagnosis and prognosis (eg, a mildly dilated single ventricle, superficial atrophy). Nonetheless, an imaging study eases anxiety and rules out the remote possibility of tumor or vascular malformation. Other indications for CT scan or MRI include difficulty in controlling seizures, progressive neurologic findings on serial examinations, worsening focal findings on the EEG, suspicion of increased pressure, and, of course, any case in which surgery is being considered. A previous normal scan does not rule out an emerging tumor; if the course is unsatisfactory, repeating the scan may be necessary. A neoplasm or other unexpected treatable lesion is found in a small number, perhaps 2–3%, of CT scans.

E. Electroencephalography: The limitations of electroencephalography–even in epilepsy, where it is most useful—are considerable. *A seizure is a clinical phenomenon;* an EEG showing epileptiform activity may confirm and even extend the clinical diagnosis, but it cannot make the diagnosis.

The EEG need not be abnormal in the presence of a definite seizure disorder. Normal EEGs are seen following a first generalized seizure in one-third of children under 4 years of age; the initial EEG is normal in about 20% of older epileptic children and in about 10% of adults with epilepsy. These percentages are reduced when serial tracings are obtained. On the other hand, various grades of "dysrhythmias" are frequently observed in children; focal spikes and generalized spike-wave discharges are seen in 30% of close nonepileptic relatives of patients with centrencephalic epilepsy.

1. Diagnostic value–The greatest value of the EEG in convulsive disorders is in helping to classify seizure types and thus to select appropriate therapy (Table 25–10). Petit mal absences and partial complex or psychomotor seizures are sometimes difficult to distinguish, especially when the physician must rely on the history and cannot observe one; their differing electroencephalographic patterns will then prove most helpful. Another rather frequent illustration of the role of the EEG in guiding therapy is the finding of mixed seizure patterns in a child who clinically has only grand mal or only petit mal absences, since some anticonvulsants efficacious for one seizure type may provoke the other. The EEG may often help in diagnosing neonatal seizures with minimal and "atypical" clinical manifestations; it may show "hypsarrhythmia" in infantile spasms or the pattern associated with the Lennox-Gastaut syndrome, both expressions of diffuse brain dysfunctioning of multiple causes and generally of grave significance. The EEG may help differentiate "convulsive equivalents" from somatic complaints of psychogenic origin.

The EEG may show focal slowing that, if constant—particularly when there are corresponding focal seizure manifestations and abnormal neurologic findings—will alert the physician to the presence of a structural lesion, in which case brain imaging may establish the cause and help determine further investigation and treatment.

2. Prognostic value–A normal EEG following a first convulsion suggests (but does not guarantee) a favorable prognosis. Markedly abnormal EEGs may become normal with treatment (1) immediately following intravenous injection of 50 mg of vitamin B_6 in pyridoxine dependency or deficiency; (2) in infantile spasms and sometimes the Lennox-Gastaut syndrome (corticotropin or corticosteroids); (3) in petit mal absences (anticonvulsants); and (4) in petit mal and other minor motor seizures, including the Lennox-Gastaut syndrome (ketogenic diet). If so, it is likely that seizure control will be achieved (though this offers no clues to the mental status of the patient).

Electroencephalography should be repeated when there is an increase in the severity and frequency of seizures despite exhaustive and adequate anticonvulsant therapy; when there is a significant change in the clinical seizure pattern; or when there are progressive neurologic deficits. Focal or diffuse slowing may indicate a progressive lesion.

The EEG may be quite helpful in determining when to discontinue anticonvulsant therapy. The presence or absence of epileptiform activity on the EEG prior to withdrawal of anticonvulsants after a seizure-free period of several years on the medications has been shown to be correlated with the degree of risk of recurrence of seizures.

Differential Diagnosis

It is extremely important that a nonepileptic condition be accurately labeled. To the lay person, epilepsy often has connotations of brain damage and limitation of activity; a person so diagnosed may be precluded from certain occupations in later life. It is often very difficult to change an inaccurate diagnosis of many years' standing.

Some of the common nonepileptic events that mimic seizure disorder are listed in Table 25–14.

Complications

Emotional disturbances—notably anxiety, depression, anger, feelings of guilt and inadequacy—often occur as a reaction to the seizures in the parents of the affected child as well as in the child old enough to understand. The seizures—and particularly the hallucinatory auras and psychomotor attacks—frequently set off in the prepubescent and adolescent patient fantasies (and sometimes obsessive ruminations) about dying and death that may become so strong that they lead to suicidal behavior and attempts. The limitations many school systems place on epileptic children add to the problem. Commonly, the child expresses feelings by "acting out."

Pseudoretardation may occur in poorly controlled epileptic children because their seizures—or the subclinical paroxysms sustained—may interfere with their learning ability. Anticonvulsants are less likely to "slow the child down" but may do so when given in toxic amounts; phenobarbital is particularly implicated.

True mental retardation is most commonly part of the same pathologic process that causes the seizures but may occasionally occur when seizures are frequent, prolonged, and accompanied by hypoxia.

Physical injuries, especially lacerations of the forehead and chin, are frequent in astatic or akinetic seizures (drop attacks). In all other seizure disorders in childhood, injuries as a direct result of an attack are impressively rare.

Treatment

The ideal treatment of seizures is the correction of specific causes. However, even when a biochemical disorder (eg, leucine hypoglycemia), a tumor, or septic meningitis is being treated, anticonvulsant drugs are often still required.

A. Precautionary Management of Individual Brief Seizures: Protect the patient against self-injury and aspiration of vomitus. Beyond that, no specific therapy is necessary. The less done to the patient during a relatively brief seizure (up to 10 or 15 minutes), the better. Thrusting a spoon handle or tongue depressor into the clenched mouth of a convulsing patient or trying to restrain tonic-clonic movements may cause worse injuries than a bitten tongue or bruised limb. Mouth-to-mouth resuscitation is rarely (if ever) necessary.

B. General Management of the Young Epileptic:

1. Education–The patient and the parents must be helped to understand the problem of seizures and their management. Many children—some even as young as 3 years of age—are capable of cooperating with the physician in problems of seizure control.

All bottles containing antiepileptic drugs should bear a contents label. The parents should know the names and dosage of the anticonvulsants being administered.

Materials on epilepsy—including pamphlets (some in Spanish), monographs, films, and videotapes suit-

Table 25–14. Nonepileptic peroxysmal events.

Breath-holding attacks: Age 6 months to 3 years. Always precipitated by trauma and fright. Cyanosis; sometimes stiffening, tonic (or jerking-clonic), convulsion (anoxic seizure). Patient may sleep following attack. Family history positive in 30%. EEG is normal. Treatment is interpretation and reassurance.

Infantile syncope (pallid breath holding): No external precipitant (perhaps internal pain, cramp, or fear?). Pallor may be followed by seizure (anoxic/ischemic). Vagally (heart-slowing) mediated, like adult syncope. EEG normal; may get cardiac slowing with vagal stimulation (eyeball pressure, cold cloth on face) during EEG.

Tics or Tourette's syndrome: Simple or complex stereotyped (the same time after time) jerks or movements, coughs, grunts, sniffs. Worse at repose or with stress. May be suppressed during physician visit. Family history often positive. EEG negative. Nonanticonvulsant drugs may benefit.

Night terrors, sleep talking, walking, "sit-ups": Age 3–10. Usually occur in first sleep cycle (30–90 minutes after going to sleep), with crying, screaming, and "autonomic discharge" (pupils dilatated, perspiring, etc). Lasts minutes. Child goes back to sleep and has no recall of event the next day. Sleep studies (polysomnogram and EEG) are normal. Disappears with maturation. Sleep talking and walking and short "sit-ups" in bed are fragmentary arousals. If a spell is recorded, EEG shows arousal from deep sleep, but the behavior seems wakeful. The youngster needs to be protected from injury and gradually settled down and taken back to bed.

Nightmares: Nightmares or vivid dreams occur in subsequent cycles of sleep, often in the early morning hours, and generally are partially recalled the next day. The bizarre and frightening behavior may sometimes be confused with complex partial seizures. These occur during REM (rapid eye movement) sleep; epilepsy usually does not occur during that phase of sleep. In extreme or difficult cases, an all-night sleep EEG may help to differentiate seizures from nightmares.

Migraine: One variant of migraine can be associated with an acute confusional state. There may be the usual migraine prodrome with spots before the eyes, dizziness, visual field defects, and then agitated confusion. A history of other, more typical migraine with severe headache and vomiting but without confusion may aid in the diagnosis. The severe headache with vomiting as the youngster comes out of the migraine may aid in distinguishing the attack from epilepsy. Other seizure manifestations are practically never seen, eg, tonic-clonic movements, falling, and complete loss of consciousness. The EEG in migraine is usually normal and seldom has epileptiform abnormalities often seen in patients with epilepsy. Lastly, migraine and epilepsy are sometimes linked: migraine-caused ischemia on the brain surface sometimes leads to later epilepsy.

Syncope: Syncope often has a precipitant. The patient may remember feeling dizzy, lightheaded, and nauseated or ill, and sensing the room going dark. Observers will often notice extreme pallor at the onset. The fall is often but not necessarily gradual; injury may occur. Heart rate is often very slow. Patient may often have memory of beginning to fall. Occasionally, a tonic or tonic-clonic seizure due to anoxia may occur, especially if the patient is held upright and circulation to the head not restored. An EEG is invariably normal. The family history is often positive for syncope.

Shuddering: Shuddering or shivering attacks can occur in infancy and be a forerunner of essential tremor in later life. Often, the family history is positive for tremor. The shivering may be very frequent. EEG is normal. There is no clouding or loss of consciousness.

Gastroesophageal reflux: Seen more commonly in children with cerebral palsy or brain damage, reflux of acid gastric contents may cause pain that cannot be described by the child. At times, there may be unusual posturings (dystonic or other) of the head and neck or trunk, an apparent attempt to stretch the esophagus or close the opening. There is no loss of consciousness, but there may be eye rolling, apnea, occasional vomiting that may simulate a seizure. An upper GI series, cine of swallowing, sometimes even in EEG (which is always normal) may be necessary to distinguish this from seizures.

Masturbation: Rarely in infants, repetitive rocking or rubbing motions may simulate seizures. The youngster may look out of contact, be poorly responsive to the environment, and have autonomic expressions (eg, perspiration, dilatated pupils) that may be confused with seizures. Observation by a skilled individual, sometimes even in a hospital situation, may be necessary to distinguish this from seizures. EEG is of course normal between or during attacks. Interpretation and reassurance are the only necessary treatment.

Conversion reaction/pseudoseizures: As many as 50% of patients with pseudoseizures are epileptic. The episodes may be writhing, intercourselike movements, tonic episodes, bizarre jerking and thrashing around, or even apparently sudden unresponsiveness. Often, there is ongoing psychological trauma. Often, but not invariably, the patients are developmentally delayed. The spells must often be seen or recorded on videotape in a controlled situation to distinguish them from epilepsy. A normal EEG during a spell is a key diagnostic feature. Often the spells are so bizarre that they are easily distinguished. Sometimes, pseudoseizures can be precipitated by suggestion with injection of normal saline in a controlled situation. Combativeness is common, self-injury and incontinence rare.

Temper tantrums and rage attacks: These are sometimes confused with epilepsy. The youngster is often amnesic or at least claims amnesia for events during the spell. The attacks are usually precipitated by frustration or anger and are often directed either verbally of physically and subside with behavior modification and isolation. EEGs are generally normal but unfortunately seldom obtained during an attack. Anterior temporal leads may be helpful in ruling out temporal or lateral frontal abnormalities, the latter sometimes seen in partial complex seizures. Improvement of the attacks with psychotherapy, milieu therapy, or behavioral modification helps rule out epilepsy.

Benign paroxysmal vertigo: These are brief attacks of vertigo in which the youngster often appears frightened and pale and clutches the parent. The attacks last 5–30 seconds. Sometimes, nystagmus is identified. There is no loss of consciousness. Usually, the child is well and returns to play immediately afterward. The attacks may occur in clusters, then disappear for months. Attacks are usually seen in infants and preschoolers aged 2–5. EEG is normal. If caloric tests can be obtained (often very difficult in this age group), abnormalities with hypofunction of one side are sometimes seen. Medications are usually not desirable or necessary.

Staring spells: Teachers often make referral for absence or petit mal seizures in youngsters who stare or seem preoccupied at school. Helpful in the history is the lack of these spells at home, eg, in the early morning hours prior to breakfast, as might be seen with absence seizures. A lack of other epilepsy in the child or family history often is helpful. Sometimes, these children have difficulties with school and a cognitive or learning disability. The child can generally be brought out of this spell by a firm command. An EEG is sometimes necessary to confirm that absence seizures are not occurring. A 24-hour ambulatory EEG to record attacks during the child's everyday school activities is occasionally necessary.

able for children and teenagers, parents, teachers, and medical professionals—may be purchased through the Epilepsy Foundation of America, Materials Service Center, 4351 Garden City Drive, Landover, MD 20785. The Foundation's local chapter and other community organizations are eager to provide guidance and other services. In many cities, there are support groups for older children and adolescents and for their parents and others concerned.

2. Privileges and precautions in daily life– Encourage normal living within reasonable bounds. Children should engage in physical activities appropriate to their age and social group. After seizure control is established, swimming is generally permissible with a "buddy system" or adequate lifeguard coverage. High diving and high climbing should not be permitted. Physical training and sports (other than "contact" sports) are usually to be welcomed rather than restricted. Driving is discussed below.

Loss of sleep should be avoided. Emotional disturbances may need to be treated. Alcoholic intake—a serious problem usually beginning in adolescence—should be avoided, as it may precipitate seizures. Prompt attention should be given to infections. Further neurologic disturbances should be brought to the physician's attention promptly.

Although every effort should be made to control seizures, this must not interfere with a child's ability to function. Sometimes a child is better off having an occasional mild seizure than being so heavily sedated that function at home, in school, or at play is impaired. This often requires much art and fortitude on the part of the physician. Indeed, some pediatricians and pediatric neurologists, after discussion with the parents, are now not instituting anticonvulsant therapy after up to three nonfebrile convulsions in an otherwise neurologically intact child.

3. Driving–Driving becomes important to most young people at age 15 or 16. Restrictions vary from state to state; in most, a learner's permit or driver's license will be issued if the patient has been under a physician's care and free of seizures for at least 2 years, provided that the treatment or basic neurologic problem does not interfere with the ability to drive. A guide to this and other legal matters pertaining to persons with epilepsy is published by the Epilepsy Foundation of America, whose legal department may be able to provide additional information (see reference below).

4. Pregnancy–In the pregnant teenager with epilepsy, the possibility of teratogenic effects of anticonvulsants, such as facial clefts (about 5%), must be weighed against the risks from seizures. Such malformations occur in the infants of about 2.5% of untreated epileptic mothers.

C. Principles of Anticonvulsant Therapy:

1. Treat with the drug appropriate to the clinical situation, as outlined in Table 25–15.

2. Start with one drug in conventional dosage, and increase the dosage until seizures are controlled. If seizures are not controlled on the tolerated maximal dosage of one major anticonvulsant, gradually switch over to another before adding a second anticonvulsant. The dosages and usually effective blood levels listed in Table 25–14 are guides. Individual variations must be expected. The "therapeutic range" may also vary somewhat with the method used to determine levels. *Note:* Blood levels of antiepileptic drugs are discussed below.

3. Advise the parents and the patient that the prolonged use of anticonvulsant drugs will not produce significant or permanent "mental slowing" (although the underlying cause of the seizures might) and that prevention of seizures for 3–4 years or so substantially reduces the chances of recurrence. Advise them also that anticonvulsants are given to prevent further seizures and that they should be taken as prescribed. Changes in medications or dosages should not be made without the physician's knowledge. Unsupervised sudden withdrawal of anticonvulsant drugs may precipitate severe seizures or even status epilepticus.

Anticonvulsants must be kept where they cannot be ingested by small children or suicidal patients.

4. Check the patient at intervals, depending on the underlying cause of the seizures, the degree of control, and the toxic properties of the anticonvulsant drug or drugs used. Blood counts, urinalyses, and liver function or other biologic tests must be obtained periodically in the case of some anticonvulsants, as indicated in Table 25–15.

Periodic neurologic reevaluation is important. CT scanning may be indicated. Repeat EEGs are not needed to achieve seizure control. Indications for repeat EEGs are discussed above.

5. Continue anticonvulsant treatment until the patient is free of seizures for 2 or more years or, in some cases, through adolescence. In about 75% of cases, seizures may not recur. Such variables as younger age at onset, normal EEG, and ease of controlling seizures carry a favorable prognosis, whereas later onset, slowing or spikes on EEG, a history of atypical febrile convulsions, and possibly an abnormal neurologic examination carry a higher risk of recurrence.

6. In general, there is no need to withdraw anticonvulsants before taking an EEG.

7. Discontinue anticonvulsants gradually. If it becomes necessary to withdraw anticonvulsants abruptly, the patient should be under close medical surveillance. If seizures recur during or after withdrawal, anticonvulsant therapy should be reinstituted and again maintained for at least 2 or more years.

D. Blood Levels of Antiepileptic Drugs:

1. General comments–Most anticonvulsants take two or three times the length of their half-life to reach the "steady states" indicated in Table 25–15. This must be considered when blood levels are assessed after anticonvulsants are started or dosages are changed.

Table 25–15. Guide to pediatric anticonvulsant drug therapy.

Drug	Average Total (mg/Kg/d)	In	Divided Doses	Steady State: Days	Effective Blood Levels (µg/mL)[1]	Side Effects and Precautions[2]	Usage and Remarks
Primary anticonvulsant							
Carbamazepine (Tegretol)	15–25	:	2–4	3–6	4–12 (> 15)	Dizziness, ataxia, diplopia. Thrombocytopenia, leukopenia, rash. Rare: hepatotoxicity; bone marrow depression; dystonia; inappropriate ADH secretion; bizarre behaviors; tics.	Monitor CBC, platelet count, liver functions first 6 months closely; then periodically. Blood effects usually early and transient.
Valproic acid (Depakene, Depakote)	15–60[2]	:	2–4	2–4	50–120 (>140)	Few side effects. Occasional gastric discomfort, constipation. Rare: hepatotoxicity; hyperammonemia, leukopenia. Tremor, hair loss in 5%.	For prophylaxis in febrile convulsion, see text. Monitor CBC, platelets, liver functions first 6 months then periodically. Can be given rectally (suspension: 250 mg/5 mL).
Phenytoin (Dilantin)	5–10	:	1–2	5–10	5–20 (> 25)	Gum hypertrophy, hirsutism, ataxia, nystagmus, diplopia, rash, anorexia, nausea, osteomalacia. Severe toxicity may cause pseudodementia and liver damage. Rare: macrocytic anemia, lymph node involvement, exfoliative dermatitis, peripheral neuropathy.	Generally very effective and safe effect on behavior. Good dental hygiene reduces gum hyperplasia. May aggravate absence and myoclonic seizures. Consider supplemental vitamin D. Poorly absorbed by neonatal gut. Absorption after intramuscular injection erratic. Useful (IV) in neonatal seizures and status epilepticus. *Note:* Suspension not recommended.
Phenobarbital	3–8	:	1	10–21	15–40 (> 45)	Irritability and overactivity in many children; sedative effects in others. Mild ataxia, nystagmus, skin rash. May interfere with learning.	Safest overall drug. Bitter taste. Higher blood levels sometimes required and tolerated in severe chronic epileptics. Check linear growth periodically; obtain Ca^{2+} and bone films as indicated; consider supplemental vitamin D. Useful in neonatal seizures and status epilepticus.
Primidone (Mysoline)	10–25	:	3–4	1–5	4–12 (> 15)	Drowsiness, ataxia, vertigo, anorexia, nausea, vomiting, rash.	Start slowly with 25–35% of expected maintenance dose; increase every 2 days until full dose reached. Most useful when phenobarbital not tolerated. Suspension not pleasant.
Ethosuximide (Zarontin)	10–40	:	1–2	5–6	40–100 (> 150)	Nausea, gastric discomfort. Rare: Bone marrow depression; hepatotoxicity, lupus.	May aggravate generalized seizures. Combine with valproic acid in refractory absence seizures.
Clonazepam (Clonopin)	0.1–0.2	:	2–3	5–10	15–80 ng/mL (> 80)	Drowsiness (> 50%); soporific effects greatest drawback. Behavior problems (25%). Slurred speech, ataxia, salivation.	Start slowly with 25% of expected maintenance dose; increase every 2–3 days. Useful with difficult to treat minor motor seizures (astatic, myoclonic, infantile spasms; absences). Tolerance often occurs after a few months, but drug may be restarted after period of withdrawal.
Adjunctive or secondary drug							
Acetazolamide (Diamox)	5–20	:	2–3	(Not known)	…	Anorexia; numbness and tingling. Increase in urinary frequency; hence, do not give in evening. Renal stones.	Supplement to other medications, especially in absence and complex partial seizures. Also in females 4 days prior to and in the first 2–3 days of menstrual periods.
Methsuximide (Celontin)	15–30	:	3–4	(Not known)	10–40 (Normethsuximide)	Drowsiness, ataxia, headache, diplopia. Skin rash (15%).	Useful in complex partial and myoclonic-astatic seizures.
Clorazepate (Tranxene)	0.3–1	:	2–3	(Not known)	0.2–1.5 (> 2)	Lethargy.	May be useful adjunct in generalized tonic-clonic, partial, and astatic seizures.

Drug	Dosage		Frequency	Blood level	Adverse effects	Comments
Felbamate (Felbatol)	15–45	:	3–4	(Not known)	Anorexia, vomiting, insomnia, headache, somnolence, rash (1%).	New. Safe. In children with Lennox-Gastaut syndrome. (Adults: complex partial seizures.) May interact with other anticonvulsants.
Phenacemide (Phenurone)	25–50	:	2–4	(Not known)	Rash, anorexia, nausea. *Warning:* Hepatitis, psychosis, blood dyscrasias.	Especially effective in complex partial seizures when all other drugs fail. Frequent CBC, liver function tests initial 3–4 months, then 2–4/yr.
Diazepam (Valium)	0.20 ± 0.05	:	3	(Not known)	Somnolence.	Useful in myoclonic-astatic and absence seizures and infantile spasms. Often ineffective after a few months. First choice in status epilepticus, below.
Dextroamphetamine (Dexedrine)	0.25–0.75	:	Breakfast and noon	(Not known)	Nervousness, palpitations, anorexia, insomnia.	To counteract sedative effect of other drugs. Narcolepsy. ADHD (attention deficit hyperactivity disorder).
Trimethadione (Tridione)	20–50	:	3–4	470–1200 (dimethadione)	Rash, photophobia, irritability. *Warning:* Leukopenia, agranulocytosis, nephrosis. LE phenomenon.	Useful primary in absences if ethosuximide and valproic acid fail. May aggravate generalized seizures; if so, add phenobarbital. Monthly CBC, urinalysis.
Mephobarbital (Mebaral)	4–10	:	1–2	15–40 (phenobarbital)	As with phenobarbital.	Twice the quantity of phenobarbital required for comparable effect.

Treatment of status epilepticus

Drug	Dosage	Administration	Comments
Diazepam (Valium)	0.3 mg/kg IV initially. Repeat dose 0.1–0.3.	Administer slowly IV. Monitor pulse and blood pressure. May cause respiratory depression in presence of phenobarbital.	May need to be repeated every 3–4 hours. Follow with phenytoin or phenobarbital for long-range control. *Note:* Administration IM for status epilepticus ineffective.
Lorazepam	0.05–0.2 mg/kg IV. May repeat.	Mild respiratory depression.	May be more effective than diazepam. Longer-acting.
Phenobarbital	5–20 mg/kg IV initially. Repeat dose 5–10 mg/kg IV.	See above.	Rule out pyridoxine deficiency. In neonatal seizures, load with 15–30 mg/kg IV (IM if IV impossible).
Phenytoin (Dilantin)	10–20 mg/kg IV initially. Repeat dose 5–10 mg/kg IV.	Administer IV over a 5-minute period. IM absorption uncertain. Monitor blood levels.	Adjunct in neonatal seizures (20 mg/kg IV) if phenobarbital alone fails.
Paraldehyde	0.1–0.15 mL/kg IV; 0.2–0.3 mL/kg rectally.	Administer slowly IV mixed in saline; rectal dose in vegetable oil 1:1. Avoid in patient with pulmonary disease or in croupette.	Avoid IM administration if possible: may cause fat necrosis. Do not use plastic syringes. (No longer manufactured in USA.)
Lidocaine (Xylocaine)	2 mg/kg IV.	Administer slowly.	Useful especially when reluctant to give more diazepam, barbiturates, or paraldehyde. Effect brief (about 30 min).

General anesthesia if other measures fail.

Treatment of infantile spasms

See text regarding use of corticotropin or corticosteroids. Also, clonazepam, or valproic acid, especially with recurrences.

[1] In monotherapy, level at which clinical toxicity becomes manifest.

[2] The interaction of antiepileptic drugs is outlined in Table 25–16.

Individuals vary in their metabolism and their particular pharmacokinetic characteristics. These and external factors, including, for example, food intake or illness, also affect the blood level. Thus, the level reached on a milligram per kilogram or surface area basis varies among patients.

Experience and clinical research in the determination of antiepileptic blood levels have shown that there is some correlation between (1) drug dose and blood level, (2) blood level and therapeutic effect, and (3) blood level and some toxic effects.

2. Effective levels–The ranges given in Table 25–14 are those within which seizure control without toxicity will be achieved in most patients. The level for any given individual will vary not only with metabolic makeup (including biochemical defects) but also with the nature and severity of the seizures and their underlying cause, with other medications being taken, and other factors. Seizure control may be achieved at lower levels in some, and higher levels may be reached without toxicity in others. When control is achieved at a lower level, the dose should not be increased merely to get the level into the "therapeutic range." Likewise, toxic side effects will be experienced at different levels even within the "therapeutic range"; lowering the dose will usually resolve the problem, but sometimes the drug must be withdrawn or another added (or both). Some serious toxic effects, including allergic reactions, LE phenomenon, and bone marrow or liver toxicity, are independent of dosage; liver toxicity especially may be the effect not just of a particular drug but also of its use in a patient who is or has been on several—and often a whole gamut—of other drugs.

3. Interaction of antiepileptic drugs–Blood levels of anticonvulsants may be affected by other drugs used. Examples are shown in Table 25–16. In-

dividual variations occur; adjustment of doses may be required.

4. Indications for determination of blood levels–Drug blood levels should be measured in a new patient or after a new drug is introduced and seizure control without toxicity is achieved to determine the "effective level" for that patient. Blood level monitoring is useful also when expected control on a "usual" dosage has not been achieved, either with a single drug or after adding another; when seizures recur in a previously well-controlled patient; or when control is poor in a patient taking anticonvulsants being seen for the first time. A low level may indicate inadequate dosage, drug interaction, or—quite frequently—noncompliance with the prescribed regimen. A high level may indicate refractoriness, drug interaction, or a worsening neurologic process. *Note:* Brief and limited "breakthroughs" are common in children (particularly younger ones) with intercurrent infections or significant excitement or other stresses, and they do not necessitate blood levels.

Blood levels are mandatory when there are signs and symptoms of toxicity—particularly where there is polydrug therapy, the dosage of a drug has been raised, or another drug has been added. Blood levels may be the only means of detecting intoxication in a comatose patient or very young child. Toxic levels also occur with drug abuse or liver disease.

Finally, when the patient is well controlled (or is controlled as well as one may hope for in a patient refractory to antiepileptics or one with difficult-to-control seizures) and free of toxic signs, blood levels are desirable once or twice a year.

E. Side Effects of Antiepileptic Drugs: (See also Table 25–15.)

1. Serious allergic reactions usually necessitate discontinuance of a drug. However, not every rash in

Table 25–16. Interaction of epileptic drugs.

Level of–	Increased by –	Decreased by–	Variable or Unchanged by–
Carbamazepine	Felbamate, erythromycin[1]	Phenobarbital,[2] phenytoin,[2] primidone,[2] felbamate[3]	Valproic acid[2,4]
Felbamate		Phenytoin, carbamazepine	
Ethosuximide	Valproic acid[1]	Carbamazepine[2]	
Phenobarbital (primidone similar)	Valproic acid[4]		Phenytoin
Phenytoin	High level of phenobarbital,[1] felbamate	Aspirin,[4] low level of phenobarbital, valproic acid,[4] carbamazepine[2]	
Valproic acid[5]	Felbamate	Phenobarbital, carbamazepine,[5] phenytoin	

[1]Impairs metabolism.
[2]Increases (hepatic) metabolism.
[3]Carbamazepine-epoxide increased?
[4]May unbind from protein, causing overall lower blood level but increased free drug; the latter may cause toxicity despite overall normal or low total blood level.
[5]Carbamazepine and valproic acid may decrease each other.

a child receiving an anticonvulsant is due to the drug. If a useful antiepileptic drug is discontinued for this reason and the rash disappears, restarting the drug in a smaller dosage is often warranted to see if the reaction recurs.

2. Signs of drug toxicity will often disappear when the daily dosage is reduced by 25–30%.

3. The sedative effect of many of the anticonvulsants is often easily counteracted by the judicious use of coffee or dextroamphetamine sulfate, 2.5–5 mg at breakfast and 2.5 mg at noon.

4. Gingival hyperplasia secondary to phenytoin is best minimized through good dental hygiene but occasionally requires gingivectomy. This condition (but not hypertrichosis) usually disappears within about 6 months after the drug is discontinued.

F. Corticotropin and Corticosteroids:

1. Indications–These drugs are indicated for infantile spasms not due to causes amenable to specific therapy and in the Lennox-Gastaut syndrome which cannot be controlled by anticonvulsant drugs.

The duration of the therapy is guided by cessation of clinical seizures and normalization of the EEG. Corticotropin or the oral corticosteroids are usually continued in full doses for 2 weeks and then, if seizures have ceased, tapered over 1 week. Others use a total treatment period of about 2 months. If seizures recur, the dosage is increased to the last effective level and repeated for 2–4 weeks, or switching to or from prednisone is tried. Some clinicians maintain the patient for up to 6 months on this dosage before attempting withdrawal. There is no strong evidence, however, that longer courses of treatment are more beneficial.

2. Dosages–

a. Corticotropin gel, starting with 2–4 units/kg/d intramuscularly in a single morning dose. Parents can be taught to give injections.

b. Prednisone, starting with 2–4 mg/kg/d orally in two or three divided doses.

3. Precautions–Give additional potassium, guard against infections, and discuss the cushingoid appearance and its disappearance. Do not withdraw oral corticosteroids suddenly. Side effects in some series occur in up to 40% of cases, especially with higher doses than those listed here (used by some authorities).

G. Ketogenic or Medium-Chain Triglyceride Diet in Treatment of Epilepsy: A ketogenic diet should be recommended in astatic and myoclonic seizures and absence seizures not responsive to drug therapy; it is occasionally recommended for infantile spasms that do not respond to corticotropin or the corticosteroids. Ketosis is induced by a diet high in fats and very limited in carbohydrates with sufficient protein for body maintenance and growth; by the feeding of medium-chain triglycerides (MCT); or by a combination of these methods. The MCT diet induces ketosis more readily than does a high level of dietary fats

and thus requires less carbohydrate restriction. The mechanism for the anticonvulsant action of the ketogenic diet is not understood, though various hypotheses have been put forth. However, it is the ketosis, not the acidosis, that raises the seizure threshold.

The diet is usually most effective in young children (ie, those under the age of 8 years), but when all other measures fail, it should be tried even in adolescents.

As ketosis is achieved, a repeat EEG may be helpful; seizure control by the diet is more likely to occur if the EEG shows improvement.

The ketogenic diet is difficult and expensive, tends to be monotonous, and depends upon the ability of the caregiver to weigh out the foods as well as upon absolute adherence to the diet prescribed. Whether the ketosis is achieved by high-fat meals or an MCT diet is often a matter of the physician's, the dietitian's, or the patient's preference. The result may also depend on which form of the diet is better tolerated. Full cooperation of all family members is required, including the patient if old enough. However, when seizure control is achieved by this method, the child is alert, often needs no anticonvulsants or only small amounts, and parental and patient satisfaction is most gratifying.

H. Surgery: In seizure disorders intractable to anticonvulsant therapy and primarily of focal origin, neurosurgery should be considered. Useful procedures, depending on the lesion, include corticectomy, hemispherectomy, anterior temporal lobectomy (for complex partial seizures), callosotomy (or commissurotomy), and stereotactic ablation.

Annegars J: Factors prognostic of unprovoked seizures after febrile convulsions. N Engl J Med 1987;316:493.

Bobele GB, Bodensteiner JB: Infantile spasms. Neurol Clin 1990;8:633.

Camfield CS, Camfield PR: Febrile seizures: An Rx for parent fears and anxieties. Contemp Pediatr 1993;10:26.

Camfield P et al: A randomized study of carbamazepine versus no medication after a first unprovoked seizure in childhood. Neurology 1989;39:851.

Camfield PR et al: Epilepsy after a first unprovoked seizure in childhood. Neurology 1985;35:1657.

Chugani HT et al: Infantile spasms: I. PET identifies focal cortical dysgenesis in cryptogenic cases for surgical treatment. Ann Neurol 1990;27:406.

Committee on Drugs, American Academy of Pediatrics: Behavioral and cognitive effects of anticonvulsant therapy. Pediatrics 1985;76:644.

Crawford TO et al: Lorazepam in childhood status epilepticus and serial seizures. Neurology 1987;37:190.

Duchowny MS: Surgery for intractable epilepsy, issues and outcomes. Pediatrics 1989;84:886.

Dulac O, Plouin P, Jambaqué I: Predicting favorable outcome in idiopathic West syndrome. Epilepsia 1993;34:747.

Farwell JR et al: Phenobarbital for febrile seizures: Effects on intelligence and on seizure recurrence. N Engl J Med 1990;322:364.

First Seizure Trial Group: Randomized clinical trial on the efficacy of antiepileptic drugs in reducing the risk of relapse after a first unprovoked tonic-clonic seizure. Neurology 1993;43:478.

Freeman J: The best medicine for febrile seizures. N Engl J Med 1992;327:1161.

Gates JR: Epilepsy and sports participation. Physician Sports Med 1991;19:3.

Holmes G: Use of EEG in management of childhood epilepsy. Int Pediatr 1992;7:223.

Hrachovy R, Glaze DG, Frost JD: A retrospective study of spontaneous remission and long term outcome in patients with infantile spasms. Epilepsia 1991;32:212.

Ito M, Okuno T, Fujii T: ACTH therapy in infantile spasms: Relationship between dose of ACTH and initial effect on long-term prognosis. Pediatr Neurol 1990;6:240.

Jayakar P: The role of EEG in management of childhood epilepsy. Int Pediatr 1993;8:253.

Kotagal P, Rothner AD: Complex partial seizures in children: Diagnosis and management. Int Pediatr 1987;2:182.

Krumholz A et al: Driving and epilepsy. JAMA 1991;265:622.

Maytal J, Moshe S, Shinnar S: Status epilepticus. Pediatrics 1990;84:939.

Maytal J, Shinnar S: Febrile status epilepticus. Pediatrics 1990;86:611.

Maytal, J: Low Morbidity and Mortality of Status Epilepticus in Children. Pediatrics 1989;83:323.

McAbee GN, Barasch ES, Kurfist LA: Results of computed tomography in "neurologically normal" children after initial onset of seizures. Pediatr Neurol 1989;5:102.

Meador KJ et al: Comparative cognitive effects of anticonvulsants. Neurology 1990;40:391.

Painter MJ, Gaines L: Neonatal seizures: Diagnosis and treatment. J Child Neurol 1991;6:101.

Pellock JM: The classification of childhood seizures and epilepsy syndromes. Neurol Clin 1990;8:619.

Phillips S, Shanohan R: Etiology and morbidity of status epilepticus in children. Ann Neurol 1989;46:74.

Prats JM et al: Infantile spasms treated with high doses of sodium valproate: Initial response and follow-up. Dev Med Child Neurol 1991;33:617.

Reitter B, Walther B (editors): Proceedings of the symposium on infantile spasms, Mainz, Germany. Brain Dev 1987;9:345.

Rosman NP et al: A controlled trial of diazepam administered during febrile illnesses to prevent recurrence of febrile seizures. N Engl J Med 1993;328:79.

Shields WD: Status epilepticus. Pediatr Clin North Am 1989;36:383.

Shinnar S et al: Discontinuing antiepileptic medication in children with epilepsy after two years without seizures: A prospective study. N Engl J Med 1985;313:976.

Shinnar S et al: Risk of seizure recurrence following a first unprovoked seizure in childhood: a prospective study. Pediatrics 1990;85:1076.

Shinnar S et al: Sleep state and the risk of seizure recurrence following a first unprovoked seizure in childhood. Neurology 1993;43:701.

Snead OC: Treatment of infantile spasms. Pediatr Neurol 1990;6:147.

Taylor DC, McKinlay I: When not to treat epilepsy with drugs: Annotations. Dev Med Child Neurol 1984;26:822.

Trimble MR: Neurobehavioral effects of anticonvulsants. (Editorial.) JAMA 1991;265:1307.

Wallace SJ: Anti-epileptic drug monitoring: An overview. Dev Med Child Neurol 1990;32:923.

Working Group on Status Epilepticus: Treatment of convulsive status epilepticus. Bone RC (editor). JAMA 1992;270:854.

Wyllie E: Temporal lobe epilepsy in children. Int Pediatr 1993;8:267.

HEADACHES

Headache is not usually a psychosomatic symptom in very young children, whereas it is more apt to be so in older children and adolescents. Headaches occur in 37% and migraine in 2.7% of children by 7 years of age; by 14 years, the rates are 69% and 10.9%, respectively. A careful description of the headaches, associated circumstances, and other neurologic and systemic symptoms should be obtained. The family history and emotional problems should be discussed in detail. Systemic and neurologic examination, including blood pressure, ophthalmoscopic examination, and station and gait, will usually distinguish organic from psychogenic headaches. Differential features are given in Table 25–17.

If there is evidence of a specific intracranial cause or systemic disorder (eg, renal disease), diagnosis and treatment should be directed at the primary disorder.

Table 25–17. Differential features of headaches in children.

	Muscle Contraction (Tension/Psychogenic)	Vascular (Migraine)	Traction and Inflammatory (Increased Intracranial Pressure)
Time course	Chronic, recurrent.	Acute, paroxysmal, recurrent.	Chronic or intermittent but increasingly frequent; *progressive severity*.
Prodromes	No.	Yes.	No.
Description	Diffuse, bandlike, tight.	Intense, pulsatile, unilateral in older child (70%).	Diffuse; more occipital with infratentorial mass, more frontal with supratentorial mass.
Characteristic findings	Feelings of inadequacy, depression, or anxiety.	Neurologic symptoms and signs usually transient.	Positive neurologic signs, especially papilledema.
Predisposing factors	Problems at home or school or socially (sexually).	Positive family history (75%); trivial head trauma may precipitate.	No.

The most frequent headache with onset in adolescence is tension headache. Unlike vascular headache of migraine, the typical tension headache is variable in location, frontal, generalized ("hatband-like"), or occipital, not accomplished by visual, gastrointestinal, neurologic (eg, dizziness) symptoms. Unless accompanied by depression (a linkage quite common in adults, less common in children), noteworthy decreased school attendance or diminished athletic prowess seldom occurs. Adolescents with tension headaches usually, in spite of head pain, continue to function well. If there is fall-off in peer group or family relationships or schoolwork, more extensive interviewing in reference to adverse events or stress in those areas is needed.

Physical and neurologic examination in tension headaches is normal. Underlying depression must be ruled out. Laboratory studies are unnecessary. Treatment includes searching out and avoiding precipitants (stress, noise, etc) and use of minor analgesics, relaxation techniques, even biofeedback. Prophylactic medication (eg, amitriptyline) may be helpful.

The prognosis is guarded. Minor morbidity and decreased school and work efficiency may persist. Psychogenic etiology or enmeshment may be sought out in the especially difficult headache patient; psychiatric consultation may be needed.

A chronic progressive headache may represent brain tumor causing headache because of its midline location, obstructing spinal fluid flow, resulting in a painful, progressive hydrocephalus. Or, the tumor mass may distort pain-sensitive structures, eg, blood vessels, meninges, or dura.

While brain tumor headache may initially mimic migraine, tension, or sinus headaches, certain history and physical findings alert the clinician.

Headache of recent onset in a child in the age group from 3 to 10, the peak age for brain tumors, is worrisome. A progressive headache with worsening frequency (eg, from weekly to daily) and severity (eg, from mild to prostrating) suggests tumor.

Headache in the morning, perhaps due to change of position and change in intracranial dynamics, with vomiting (often without nausea) is ominous.

A child with headache who is deteriorating in social, school and athletic (coordination) prowess causes concern.

Even more important are positive neurologic findings. *The usual headache patient has a normal physical and neurological examination.* Strabismus, weakness of extraocular muscles, visual loss, poor pupillary response, and papilledema or optic atrophy must be ruled out. Coordination and gait must be assessed with finger-nose-finger pursuit, balancing on each leg, hopping, and tandem walking forward and backward on a straight line.

If suspicion remains high in spite of a normal neurologic examination, a follow-up examination is essential. An imaging study should be strongly considered.

The preferred if expensive ($1000) study is MRI. This modality is superior to CT scan for posterior fossa tumors and for visualization around bony structures such as the sella and foramen magnum. However, if suspicion for tumor is low, the more available and less expensive ($400–500) CT scan is a sensible alternative.

To summarize, a reasonable history with the key points listed above and a good physical and neurological examination will usually pick up the rare headache with brain tumor. A recent study of 104 children with onset of headaches prior to 7 years of age, seen by age 9, found mostly (75%) migraine. A pertinent quote from that article: "No child who presented for evaluation of headaches with a normal neurologic exam was found to have a brain tumor."

Migraine attacks are usually paroxysmal, throbbing, pulsating, or pounding in character (initial vasoconstriction of intracranial vessels followed by vasodilation of extracranial vessels). The pain in children is as often bilateral as unilateral, frontal or retro-orbital as hemicranial. Between attacks, the child is asymptomatic. Migraine in children is associated (in order of frequency) with nausea, gastric discomfort, or vomiting; dizziness or vertigo; photophobia, visual auras, and, less frequently, visual loss; sensory and motor disturbances, especially involving the face and arms; speech disturbances; and, occasionally, hemiplegia (sometimes alternating), acute confusional states, or impairment of space, time, and body image perceptions (termed the "Alice-in-Wonderland syndrome"). The child frequently seeks rest in a dark, quiet room.

Migraine of varying severity may occur in up to 6.6% of children between 7 and 14 years of age. Onset by age 4 is not uncommon. After 10 years of age, it is twice as common in girls as in boys. The family history is positive for migraine in up to 75% of patients and not infrequently also for epilepsy. School stresses (headache often occurs after school) and foods occasionally precipitate migraine. Head trauma may precipitate onset. In most instances, the migraine attack is brief (hours, not days), and sleep gives relief. Motion sickness is an associated feature in 45% of cases.

EEG may be abnormally slow to mildly or moderately dysrhythmic in up to 80% of patients soon after an attack of complicated migraine (emphasizing the relationship between migraine and epilepsy). Neuroradiologic studies, such as CT scanning, are usually not warranted unless there are definite neurologic or progressive abnormalities.

Acetaminophen or ibuprofen is often effective in children. The patient should be allowed to remain quiet in a darkened room. In children over 12 years of age, severe migraine may often be controlled by Fiorinal, Fioricet, or Midrin, one or two capsules every 4 hours. If these measures are ineffective, especially in the older child, and when anxiety and nausea are prominent symptoms, Cafergot is often useful.*

In the prevention of severe, frequent, and disabling migraine—especially in children too young to alert an adult to their symptoms or to follow the above regimen—prophylaxis is recommended as follows: propranolol, 10–40 mg three times daily depending on weight (contraindications are respiratory and cardiac disorders); cyproheptadine, 2–4 mg every 8–12 hours; or calcium channel blockers (in varying forms and dosages; they may have anticonvulsant action as well). Antidepressants such as imipramine or amitriptyline may be useful (25–50 mg at bedtime). In children, methysergide maleate is not recommended.

Operant conditioning and biofeedback are lengthy and expensive options, studied almost exclusively in children in conjunction with vascular, not tension, headaches. Biofeedback was studied and reported in a position paper of the American College of Physicians in 1985 and was thought unproved. A recent pediatric study suggested utility of these therapies in vascular headaches in children.

Barlow CF: Headaches and brain tumors. Am J Dis Child 1982;136:99.

Cady RK et al: Treatment of acute migraine with subcutaneous sumatriptan. JAMA 1991;265:2831.

Cho C, Pruitt AW: Therapeutic uses of calcium channel blocking drugs in the young. Am J Dis Child 1986;140: 360.

Chu ML, Shinnar S: Headaches in children younger than 7 years of age. Arch Neurol 1992;49:79.

Elser JM: Easing the pain of childhood headaches. Contemp Pediatr 1991;8:108.

Fenichel GM: Migraine in children. Neurol Clin 1985;3:77.

Honig PJ, Charney EB: Children with brain tumor headaches: Distinguishing features. Am J Dis Child 1982; 136:121.

Igarashi M et al: Pharmacologic treatment of childhood migraine. J Pediatr 1992;120:653.

Larson B et al: Therapist-assisted self-help relaxation treatment of chronic headaches in adolescents: A school-based intervention. J Child Psychol Psychiatry 1987;28: 127.

Linet MS et al: An epidemiologic study of headache among adolescents and young adults. JAMA 1989;261:2211.

Rothner AD: Classification, pathogenesis, evaluation, and management of headaches in children and adolescents. Curr Opin Pediatr 1992;4:949.

Singer HS et al: Chronic recurrent headaches in children. Pediatr Ann 1992;21:369.

*One capsule of Fiorinal contains butalbital, 50 mg; aspirin, 325 mg; and caffeine, 40 mg. One capsule of Fioricet contains butalbital, 50 mg; acetaminophen, 325 mg; and caffeine, 40 mg. Midrin contains isometheptene mucate, 65 mg; dichloralphenazone, 100 mg; and acetaminophen, 325 mg. Cafergot contains ergotamine tartrate, 1 mg, and caffeine, 100 mg. One capsule of Fiorinal or Lanorinal contains butalbital, 50 mg; aspirin, 325 mg; and caffeine, 40 mg.

The Childhood Brain Tumor Consortium: The epidemiology of headache among children with brain tumor: Headache in children with brain tumors. J Neurooncol 1991; 10:31.

SLEEP DISORDERS

Sleep Apnea Syndrome in Older Children

Sleep apnea syndrome should be considered if there is a history of restless sleep with snoring or respiratory noise during sleep and frequent awakenings from sleep in an older child who shows poor school performance associated with excessive daytime sleepiness or irritability and hyperactivity. Children with these problems frequently have hypertrophied tonsils or adenoids, causing partial airway obstruction; occasionally, they have facial dysmorphism, neuromuscular disorders with muscle hypotonia and poor pharyngeal muscle control, and hyperplastic tissues, as seen in myxedema, Hodgkin's disease, or pickwickian syndrome. Evaluation includes soft tissue x-rays of the lateral neck; chest x-ray; electrocardiography to rule out cardiomegaly, sinus dysrhythmias, and incipient or actual right-sided heart failure; arterial blood gas determinations while awake and during sleep; and polysomnography. Therapy is generally surgical, ranging from tonsillectomy and adenoidectomy when appropriate to tracheostomy when medical measures fail.

Narcolepsy

Narcolepsy, a primary disorder of sleep and wakefulness, is characterized by chronic, excessive daytime sleeping that occurs regardless of activity or surroundings and is not relieved by increased sleep at night. Onset occurs as early as 3 years of age and has been reported before 10 years of age in about 18% of patients and between puberty and the late teens in 60%. Narcolepsy usually interferes severely with normal living. Often months to years after onset, there may also be cataplexy (transient partial or total loss of muscle tone, often triggered by laughter, anger, or other emotional upsurge), hypnagogic hallucinations (visual or auditory), and the sensation of paralysis on falling asleep. Studies have shown that rapid eye movement (REM) sleep, with loss of muscle tone and an electroencephalographic low-amplitude mixed frequency pattern, occurs soon after sleep onset in patients with cataplexy, whereas normal subjects experience 80–100 minutes or longer of non-REM (NREM) sleep before the initial REM period.

Narcolepsy is treated with a central nervous system stimulant (dextroamphetamine or long-acting methylphenidate is preferred); occasionally, a tricyclic antidepressant, in low doses titrated to the need of the patient, is added to the treatment regimen. The condition persists throughout life.

Somnambulism

Somnambulism has been assigned to a group of sleep disturbances known as disorders of arousal. It is characterized by abrupt onset early in the night of an episode of veiled consciousness and coordinated activity (eg, walking, sometimes moving objects without seeming purpose). The episode is of relatively brief duration and ceases spontaneously. There is poor recall of the event on waking in the morning. Somnambulism may be related to mental activities occurring in stages 3 and 4 of NREM sleep. The incidence has been estimated at only 2–3%, but up to 15% of cases are reported in children 6–16 years of age, with boys affected more often than girls and many having recurrent episodes. No psychopathologic features can usually be demonstrated, but a strong association (30%) between childhood migraine and somnambulism has been noted, and episodes of somnambulism may be triggered in predisposed children by stresses, including febrile illnesses.

No treatment of somnambulism is required, and it is not necessary to seek psychiatric consultation.

Night Terrors

Night terrors (pavor nocturnus) are a disorder of arousal from NREM sleep. Most cases occur in children 3–8 years of age, and the disorder rarely occurs after adolescence. It is characterized by sudden (but only partial) waking, with the severely frightened child unable to be fully roused or comforted. Concomitant autonomic symptoms include rapid breathing, tachycardia, and perspiring. The next morning, the child has no recall of any nightmare. Psychopathologic mechanisms are unclear, but falling asleep after watching scenes of violence on television or hearing frightening stories may play a role. Elimination of such causes and administration of a mild antianxiety agent such as chlordiazepoxide may be helpful. It is important to differentiate these episodes from complex partial (psychomotor) seizures.

Aldrich MS: Narcolepsy. Neurology 1992;42(Suppl 6):34.

Barabas G, Ferrari M, Matthews WS: Childhood migraine and somnambulism. Neurology 1983;33:948.

Guilleminault C: Obstructive sleep apnea syndrome and its treatment in children. Pediatr Pulmonol 1987;3:429.

Klackenberg G: Somnambulism in childhood: Prevalence, course and behavioral correlations. Acta Paediatr Scand 1982;71:495.

Kotagal S, Hartse KM, Walsh JK: Characteristics of narcolepsy in preteenaged children. Pediatrics 1990;85:205.

Sheldon S, Spire JP, Levy H: *Pediatric Sleep Medicine.* Saunders, 1992.

HEAD & SPINAL INJURIES

Serious accidental injury constitutes one of the most common causes of childhood hospitalization and death in the United States.

Injury of the brain can result from sudden acceleration-deceleration movements or from sudden rotational or torsional movements of the head. Direct impact of the brain against the inner table of the skull, together with blood vessel rupture and dural tears, leads to parenchymal damage.

"Closed head injury" includes those injuries in which the skull remains intact or in which there is only a small linear fracture. "Open head injury" consists of those injuries involving major scalp lacerations and compound or depressed skull fractures. Brain parenchymal injury can occur in either closed or open head injuries but is more frequent and often more severe with open head injury.

The clinical severity of head injury is classified as mild, moderate, or severe, depending on the type and extent of brain damage, the presence of brain edema, and the presence or absence of intracranial hemorrhage. Intracranial hemorrhages can occupy a variety of potential spaces within the cranial vault, including epidural, subdural, and subarachnoid spaces. Cerebral contusions consist of a localized region of petechial hemorrhage and edema. Intraparenchymal hemorrhages can be small, or they can be massive, rapidly expanding to produce markedly elevated intracranial pressure and cerebral herniation.

Clinical Findings

A. Symptoms and Signs: In mild head injuries, loss of consciousness may not occur or may be only momentary. Frequently, patients experience mild to moderate headache, nausea, vomiting, vertigo, and light-headedness. Although tachycardia may be present, blood pressure and other vital signs are normal. There is rapid resolution of all symptoms. Occasionally, a brief, generalized clonic seizure may occur shortly after the head injury, but posttraumatic epilepsy is rare.

Moderately severe head injuries are associated with loss of consciousness for several minutes to 1 hour. Headache may be severe, and the patient may experience severe irritability, drowsiness, emotional lability, and signs of mild to moderate delirium. Nausea and vomiting can be prominent. Vertigo, tinnitus, and light-headedness can be moderately severe for a short period. Symptoms resolve in 1–2 days, though vertigo and some alteration in behavior, mood, and concentration persist for several days. Some children also experience relatively protracted problems regarding attention, concentration, and school performance after seemingly mild or moderate head injury.

Severe head injury is associated with prolonged loss of consciousness, usually longer than 1 hour. Headache, nausea, vomiting, and tinnitus are severe and at times incapacitating. Marked behavioral changes and seizures can develop immediately after the head injury, and posttraumatic epilepsy occurs in approximately 10% of children. Symptoms usually persist for several days or weeks, in some patients for months.

When intracranial hemorrhages occur, symptoms of progressively increasing intracranial pressure may develop. Patients have progressive loss of consciousness and severe nausea and vomiting. Seizures occur in about 50–70% of children with subdural hematomas. Fever and nuchal rigidity are often present with subdural hematomas, and meningitis may be suspected. Epidural and acute subdural hematomas may be acute and require emergency surgical drainage. These forms of intracranial hemorrhage can rapidly lead to death, particularly if they occur in the posterior fossa. Subarachnoid hemorrhages are unusual in childhood unless they are associated with an underlying cerebrovascular malformation. Intracerebral hematomas, particularly in the frontal and temporal regions, can occur after either a closed or open head injury. When intracerebral hemorrhages occur, an underlying bleeding diathesis should be excluded by appropriate laboratory testing.

B. Physical Examination: Initial assessment of patients who have suffered head injury includes frequent monitoring of heart rate, blood pressure, and temperature. Sudden changes in blood pressure, particularly hypotension, may be an indication of intrathoracic, intra-abdominal, or other systemic injury associated with bleeding.

Head circumference should be measured in infants after head injury, and the fontanelle size and tension should be carefully documented. Evaluation of the head and neck region is important in the search for signs of cerebrospinal fluid leakage from the ear and nose. Care should be taken to move the head as little as possible because injury to the spinal cord and cervical vertebrae may not be initially apparent. The patient should be examined thoroughly for signs of injury to extremities, abdomen, back, and chest. The skin should also be carefully examined for evidence of recent or remote injury. The possibility of nonaccidental trauma should be suspected when multiple sites of injury or injuries of different ages are present.

Neurologic examination includes assessment of pupillary size, symmetry, and light reflexes. Evidence of ocular and orbital injury may be associated with basilar skull fracture. Funduscopic examination may disclose retinal flame-shaped hemorrhages that can be indicative of subdural or subarachnoid hemorrhages. Increased intracranial pressure related to intracranial hemorrhages or cerebral edema may result in dilated, nonpulsating retinal veins and swelling of the optic disk. Assessment of muscle tone, strength, and reflexes may provide evidence of focal or lateralized neurologic dysfunction.

C. Laboratory Studies and Imaging: A sudden or progressive decrease in hematocrit may suggest rapidly evolving acute subdural hematoma. Injury may result in fluid and electrolyte abnormalities

as a consequence of inappropriate secretion of antidiuretic hormone or diabetes insipidus.

Radiographic studies, particularly CT scanning, should be conducted to search for skull fracture, intracranial hemorrhage, and intracranial foreign bodies. Skull films in general are not as helpful as CT scanning; however, in certain situations when CT scanning is not available, skull films may demonstrate clinically significant depressed or comminuted skull fractures. In addition, plain radiographs of the neck, chest, abdomen, and extremities are important in searching for more generalized evidence of injury. X-ray films of the neck should be obtained on all patients with head injury because unsuspected spinal injury can be present and require immediate stabilization. MRI can also demonstrate intracranial hemorrhage and some types of foreign bodies. However, MRI is not as helpful as CT scanning at defining bony abnormalities. Cerebral angiography may be required at times when major vascular damage is suspected or when the patient develops clinical signs suggesting arterial dissection.

Lumbar puncture is rarely needed in the evaluation of patients with head injury and in most instances is contraindicated. Infants with tense fontanelles and fever may be suspected initially of having bacterial meningitis, and in this situation lumbar puncture may be necessary.

Subdural tap is an important immediate diagnostic as well as therapeutic maneuver in acute and rapidly progressing subdural or epidural hematomas. When an acute subdural hematoma is clinically suspected and the patient is deteriorating rapidly, a subdural tap should be performed as an emergency procedure. The tap should not be delayed in order to obtain a CT scan. With posterior fossa subdural and epidural hematomas, a cisternal tap can also be life-saving.

EEGs after acute head injury are frequently abnormal but nonspecific, and their role is quite limited in the initial evaluation and management of head injury. EEGs may be useful in monitoring seizure activity and can complement serial neurologic examinations and assessments of a patient's progress after head injury.

Differential Diagnosis

Whenever the cause for the head injury is not readily apparent, nonaccidental trauma should be suspected. Intracranial hemorrhage may occur with relatively minor injuries in patients with bleeding diatheses. Some metabolic disorders, such as scurvy, rickets, and Menkes' disease, may predispose the patient to pathologic fractures and intracranial hemorrhage.

Complications

Seizures, either focal or generalized, have been reported in 5–15% of children with head injury. Usually the seizures are brief, but a few patients experience status epilepticus. Chronic posttraumatic epilepsy develops in 10% of children who have suffered brain lacerations or who have experienced prolonged loss of consciousness immediately after head injury. When posttraumatic seizures develop, approximately 50% will occur in the first 6 months after the injury, and 80% will have developed within 2 years. Antiepileptic medications may be started when patients have one or more immediate posttraumatic seizures and continued for up to 6 months. If seizures develop later, chronic antiepileptic medication is continued for 2–4 years.

Massive cerebral swelling, cerebral edema, and intracranial hematomas may lead to herniation of the temporal lobe through the tentorial notch with subsequent brain stem compression and rapid deterioration of the patient's mental status and neurologic function. Cerebellar tonsillar herniation results from posterior fossa hematomas and leads to clinical evidence of lower brain stem dysfunction, progressive loss of consciousness, and impaired cardiorespiratory functions.

Cerebrospinal fluid leakage through basilar skull fractures predisposes the patient to chronic, recurrent bacterial meningitis with organisms that normally inhabit the upper airway, such as *Streptococcus pneumoniae* and *Haemophilus influenzae*. Most cerebrospinal fluid leaks stop spontaneously, but chronic leaks require surgical closure. If the patient develops signs of fever, nuchal rigidity, or other evidence of possible meningitis, antibiotics are necessary.

Hydrocephalus can develop after head injury, particularly when subarachnoid hemorrhage leads to basilar arachnoiditis or impairment of the cerebrospinal fluid absorption through the arachnoid villi.

Some patients develop pseudotumor cerebri shortly after head injury, but the mechanism is not clear.

Patients with diastatic linear fractures develop leptomeningeal cysts. This cyst develops when a tear in the dura and arachnoid is followed by entrapment of the arachnoid between the margins of the diastatic fracture. Spinal fluid accumulates within the cyst and produces a progressively enlarging, fluid-filled mass over the fracture line. Removal of the cyst and closure of the dural tear requires surgical repair.

Postconcussion syndrome is seen in children, adolescents, and adults, but its pathogenesis is not clear. Principal manifestations are changes in behavior, personality, and sleep pattern, headache, vertigo, tinnitus, and various head and neck pains. School or job performance deteriorates, and the ability to concentrate is impaired. Hyperactivity can impair the child's normal daily function. Treatment is symptomatic, and postconcussion syndrome usually abates gradually over a period of days to weeks.

Treatment

Immediate treatment of a patient with serious head injury consists of securing the airway and supporting the cardiovascular system. Seizures, particularly status epilepticus, may require acute anticonvulsant medication. As described above, subdural or cisternal taps are required if the patient is rapidly deteriorating because of an acute subdural or epidural hematoma.

After the initial assessment, the patient must be observed carefully for several hours after head injury, whether in the emergency room, in an ambulatory clinic setting, or at home. The patient's arousability, pupillary light reflexes, extraocular movements, and extremity movements must be serially documented. Hospitalization of patients after head injury is necessary when the patient has focal or asymmetric neurologic deficits that do not rapidly resolve or when loss of consciousness is prolonged. It is important to admit and monitor carefully patients who show signs of deterioration and to initiate rapid treatment to relieve intracranial pressure.

Severe headache, nausea, vomiting, and restlessness can usually be treated symptomatically. Tetanus prophylaxis (0.5 mL tetanus toxoid) should be given to patients with scalp lacerations or open head injuries. Most patients do not require prophylactic antibiotics. However, patients with cerebrospinal fluid leakage from the nose or ears should be monitored carefully and antibiotics started if meningitis is suspected. Cerebral edema may be treated with diuretics, osmotic agents, or glucocorticoids or by lowering the patient's PCO_2. If acute obstructive hydrocephalus occurs, a ventricular drain aids in controlling increased intracranial pressure.

Patients with depressed or displaced fractures, epidural hematomas, progressive acute subdural hematomas, and some chronic subdural hematomas require operation. Evacuation of intracerebral hematomas is usually not indicated, though superficial intracerebral hematomas occasionally may be evacuated in an attempt to relieve severe and rapidly increasing mass effect.

Prognosis

Ninety percent or more of children who suffer from mild to moderate head injuries become free of symptoms and do not develop serious, long-term complications. Severe head injury is associated with a mortality rate of 5–10%. From 3% to 5% of children with severe head injury have severe, long-term neurologic deficits, and another 5–6% have moderate long-term deficits. Over 80% of children with severe head injury, however, enjoy good functional recovery.

SPINAL CORD INJURY

Spinal cord injury can occur at any age and often coexists with head injury. A high degree of suspicion is required to promptly diagnose and treat spinal injuries in infants and children. In neonates, spinal cord injury results from traction and hyperextension during difficult delivery. Generalized flaccidity and respiratory failure are frequently the predominant acute clinical manifestations, with spasticity and hyperreflexia developing later. In older children, the clinical signs of spinal cord injury depend on the level at which the injury occurs. Cervical cord injury results in respiratory weakness, flaccid weakness, and areflexia in the upper extremities; loss of bowel and bladder control; and spasticity and hyperreflexia in the lower extremities. A sensory level may be detectable in older children with low cervical, thoracic, and lumbosacral cord injury.

Diagnosis is based upon the clinical history, pattern of neurologic deficits, and MRI. Plain films can be useful in the initial evaluation if fractures and bone displacements are present, but a normal plain x-ray of the spinal column does not exclude spinal cord injury or replace the need for MRI if a spinal cord injury is clinically suspected. Initial management of suspected spinal cord injury involves stabilizing the neck, minimizing movement of the patient, and supporting respiratory and cardiovascular functions. Additional treatment measures include use of osmotic agents and corticosteroids to reduce edema, surgery to remove epidural or subdural hematoma, and surgery to stabilize bone fractures and displacements. Long-term management of residual neurologic dysfunction requires intensive rehabilitation; bowel and bladder care; treatment of spasticity with baclofen, diazepam, or dantrolene sodium; and psychologic counseling.

The prognosis varies with the severity of the injury. Children with complete cord transections have a poor prognosis for recovery. Late complications include progressive spinal deformity, contractures, dysesthetic pain syndromes, recurrent infections, and decubitus ulcers.

Davis PC et al: Spinal injuries in children: Role of MR. AJNR Am J Neuroradiol 199 1993;14:607.

Edwards MSB, Cogen PH: Craniospinal trauma in children. In: *Neurologic Aspects of Pediatrics.* Berg BO (editor). Butterworth-Heinemann, 1992.

Sneed RC, Stover SL: Undiagnosed spinal cord injuries in brain-injured children. Am J Dis Child 1988;142:965.

PERINATAL HEAD INJURY

Injury to the scalp and skull occurs during the perinatal period in association with prolonged pressure on the infant's skull, breech presentation, shoulder dystocia, or malpositioned forceps. Several types of head and scalp injury may be visibly apparent at the time of birth. Caput succedaneum is characterized by hemorrhagic edema of the scalp skin and muscles. Cephalhematoma is a localized subperiosteal hemorrhage; this type of hemorrhage is limited in extent by the periosteum that attaches at suture margins. Caput

and cephalhematomas resolve spontaneously and require no specific treatment. Cephalhematomas occasionally prolong neonatal jaundice, and approximately 25% of them overlie linear skull fractures. Subgaleal hemorrhage represents the most dangerous extracranial hemorrhage in the neonate. The blood of this hemorrhage dissects underneath the fascia of muscles of the head and neck. Blood may dissect and extend into the face, down the neck, and over the chest and back. Massive blood loss can take place, and subgaleal hemorrhage can result in exsanguination. Subgaleal hemorrhage usually occurs in association with an underlying bleeding disorder or after severe head trauma that results in tears of the dura that form the dural sinuses.

Skull fractures in the perinatal period involving the skull base and occipital region can be associated with dural tears and massive intracranial hemorrhage. Hemorrhage secondary to dural tear often results in catastrophic, rapid clinical deterioration and death.

Intracranial hemorrhage is the most serious consequence of head injury during the perinatal period. Epidural hematomas are usually associated with depressed skull fractures. Emergency surgical removal is mandatory. Subarachnoid hemorrhage is relatively frequent in the perinatal period and is often asymptomatic. However, hydrocephalus may develop after subarachnoid hemorrhage and may require ventriculoperitoneal shunting. Subdural hematomas are occasionally seen in the perinatal period and are often associated with cerebral laceration or contusion. Acute subdural hematomas may progress rapidly, and the patient may require emergency surgery for evacuation of the hematoma. Chronic subdural hematomas are manifested by increasing head circumference and the gradual appearance of neurologic deficits, anemia, poor weight gain, irritability, and somnolence.

Intracerebral hematomas usually indicate severe head trauma in the perinatal period and are frequently associated with dural lacerations or with bleeding disorders.

Intracranial Hemorrhage in the Premature

Approximately 25–40% of all newborns weighing less than 2000 g develop periventricular-interventricular hemorrhage. This type of hemorrhage originates in the germinal matrix and is related to immature blood vessel structure, poor blood vessel support by the germinal matrix, and the unusual tortuous course of veins in the region of the germinal matrix in the premature brain. Germinal matrix hemorrhages are classified as grade I, II, or III. Grade I indicates a hemorrhage limited to the subependymal, germinal matrix region with little or no intraventricular extension. Grade II represents the germinal matrix hemorrhage with moderate extension into the ventricular system. Grade III represents germinal matrix hemorrhage with massive intraventricular extension and usually ventriculomegaly. Furthermore, intraventricular hemorrhage may be associated with hemorrhagic infarction of the white matter dorsal and lateral to the anterior lateral ventricle.

Clinical symptoms of intraventricular-periventricular hemorrhage are related to the size of the hemorrhage and its degree of extension into the ventricular system. In addition, clinical symptoms are modified by the degree of the infant's systemic illness. Small grade I hemorrhages limited to the germinal matrix can be asymptomatic and are often diagnosed by ultrasound but not suspected clinically. Some patients develop a waxing and waning course with a gradual, stuttering evolution of neurologic deficits. The most dramatic presentation of intraventricular-periventricular hemorrhage, however, is the sudden catastrophic onset of seizures, anemia, and cardiovascular instability. Acute grade III hemorrhages combined with periventricular hemorrhagic infarction are associated with a mortality rate of more than 60% (see Table 25–18).

Laboratory evaluation of infants with periventricular-intraventricular hemorrhage includes assessment of the hematocrit, electrolytes, calcium, magnesium, blood glucose concentration, coagulation system, and acid-base status. Examination of spinal fluid after intraventricular hemorrhage is usually not necessary but reveals grossly bloody spinal fluid with elevated protein and decreased glucose concentration.

The primary diagnostic test in neonates suspected of having periventricular-intraventricular hemorrhage is cranial ultrasonography. This test is excellent for displaying germinal matrix hemorrhage with or without intraventricular extension and can be used for serial monitoring of ventricular size. However, ultrasonography is not an adequate method for evaluating cerebral hemispheres or structures of the posterior fossa. CT or MRI scanning is necessary for full evaluation of the cerebral parenchyma, the posterior fossa, and the subarachnoid, subdural, and epidural spaces.

Table 25–18. Prognosis of periventricular-intraventricular hemorrhage (IVH) in premature infants.

	Acute		Long-Term
	Mortality (%)	Hydrocephalus (%)	Neurologic Impairment (%)
Grade I	15	5	15
Grade II	20	25	30
Grade III	40	55	40
IVH and periventricular hemorrhagic infarction (grade IV)	> 60	80	90

Treatment

Treatment of infants with periventricular-intraventricular hemorrhage is directed at stabilizing and supporting the cardiovascular system. Abnormalities of the cardiovascular, renal, gastrointestinal, and other organ systems require specific monitoring and management. Fluid, electrolyte, and acid-base disturbances should be identified and corrected. Secondary infections and seizures should be treated with antibiotics and anticonvulsant medications. Any underlying bleeding diathesis should be corrected, and vitamin K_1 should be given to infants to ensure that a bleeding diathesis secondary to vitamin K deficiency does not contribute to the patient's problems.

For patients with progressive ventriculomegaly and hydrocephalus, ventricular drains and subsequent ventriculoperitoneal shunting are often required. The value of serial lumbar punctures is controversial, but this procedure can be useful in some patients if ventriculostomy is not readily available to relieve acute posthemorrhagic ventriculomegaly.

Prognosis

The outcome of intracranial hemorrhage is related to the extent of underlying brain injury. Brain lacerations and contusions predispose to the development of posttraumatic epilepsy and focal or multifocal areas of cerebral atrophy.

The outcome of neonatal intraventricular-periventricular hemorrhage is related to the size and extent of the hemorrhage and associated factors such as the presence of hemorrhagic infarction and systemic complications secondary to cardiovascular, renal, gastrointestinal, and other systemic abnormalities. Table 25–18 displays the overall mortality rates and morbidity rates with regard to neurologic deficits and hydrocephalus.

Jenkins A et al: Brain lesions detected by magnetic resonance imaging in mild and severe head injuries. Lancet 1986;2:445.

Kraus JF et al: Incidence, severity, and external causes of pediatric brain injury. Am J Dis Child 1986;140:687.

Kraus JF et al: Pediatric brain injuries: The nature, clinical course, and early outcomes in a defined United States population. Pediatrics 1987;79:501.

NEOPLASMS OF THE CENTRAL NERVOUS SYSTEM

1. INTRACRANIAL TUMORS

Neoplasms of the central nervous system account for approximately 20% of all malignant neoplasms of childhood and are second only to leukemia in frequency. The incidence of primary central nervous system tumors in people under 20 years of age is 20–25 per million per year, or about one-third to one-half of the incidence of childhood leukemia. The incidence of central nervous system tumors in children under age 2 is approximately one-tenth of that in older children, or approximately 2–2.5 per million per year. Approximately 1500 new cases of brain tumor occur each year in the United States, including 150–200 cases in children under 2 years old. The peak incidence of brain tumors occurs between the ages of 5 and 10 years, and the male:female ratio is approximately 1.2:1. Primary brain tumors can be classified generally by their cell of origin (see Table 25–19). In children over the age of 2, approximately 65% of brain tumors are infratentorial and 35% supratentorial. Secondary involvement of the nervous system is common in the early stages of acute leukemia, and the brain may be invaded directly by tumors that involve extraneural tissue in the head and neck region. Hematogenous metastatic spread from solid malignant tumors outside the nervous system is rare in childhood, but the true incidence of this phenomenon is unknown. Some highly aggressive and malignant intracranial tumors in childhood, such as medulloblastoma, commonly spread throughout the subarachnoid spaces within the central nervous system. Rarely, primary central nervous system tumors may metastasize to extraneural sites such as bone marrow, lung, and viscera. The cause and pathogenesis of brain tumors is unknown.

Clinical Manifestations

Manifestations of intracranial tumors consist of nonspecific signs due to increased intracranial pressure (see Table 25–20). Infratentorial tumors, regardless of histologic type, frequently present with gait disturbance, incoordination, multiple and often asymmetric cranial nerve deficits, and nystagmus. The patient may tilt the head in an attempt to relieve discomfort at the base of the skull due to cerebellar tonsillar

Table 25–19. Classification of primary brain tumors of childhood.

Tumor Type	Incidence (%)	Common Examples
Glial cell tumors	50–60	Astrocytoma Optic nerve glioma Brain stem glioma Ependymoma
Neuroectodermal tumors	25–35	Medulloblastoma Pinealoblastoma
Craniopharyngioma	5–10	
Germ cell tumors	< 10	Teratoma Dermoid Germinoma
Meningeal tumors	< 5	Meningioma Meningeal sarcoma
Lymphoma (non-Hodgkin's)	< 1	

Table 25–20. Signs of increased intracranial pressure.

Acute
Macrocephaly
Excessive rate of head growth
Altered behavior
Decreased level of consciousness
Vomiting
Blurred vision
Double vision
Optic disk swelling
Abducens nerve paresis
Chronic
Macrocephaly
Growth impairment
Developmental delay
Optic atrophy
Visual field loss

herniation, or head tilt may be a compensatory adjustment to correct double vision.

Specific neurologic manifestations of supratentorial tumors are dictated by the location of the tumor. Focal motor and sensory abnormalities and focal seizures occur frequently in the more common types of hemispheric tumors. Abnormalities of eye movements and vision are also common. Endocrine and autonomic disturbances may indicate the presence of a hypothalamic or thalamic tumor.

Diagnosis

When the clinical history and the findings of physical examination suggest the presence of an intracranial mass, a CT scan or MRI scan of the head should be obtained to define the precise anatomic site and extent of the tumor. Skull x-rays may show scalloping of the inner table of the skull, truncation of the sella turcica, or widening of the suture lines as evidence of increased intracranial pressure. Electroencephalographic findings in brain tumors are nonspecific, and EEGs are rarely necessary in the initial diagnostic evaluation of brain tumor. However, EEGs done on patients who have focal or generalized seizures as a manifestation of their tumor may show localized epileptiform discharges. An EEG done before initiation of treatment for the brain tumor may provide a useful baseline assessment of electrocerebral activity for future reference. Examination of cerebrospinal fluid is usually not necessary in the diagnosis of localized mass lesions within the nervous system. However, examination of spinal fluid—particularly cytopathologic examination—may be helpful when tumors are disseminated throughout the subarachnoid space.

Treatment

Some tumors, such as cerebellar astrocytomas, may be completely removed by surgery and require no additional treatment. However, most primary central nervous system tumors are currently treated by a combination of surgery, radiation, and chemotherapy. Surgery is frequently used to reduce the mass of tumor and is followed by localized radiation to the tumor bed. Some tumors with a propensity for subarachnoid seeding and spread (eg, medulloblastoma) are also treated with prophylactic total craniocerebral radiation. Chemotherapeutic agents currently being used for treatment of childhood brain tumors include prednisone, vincristine sulfate, etoposide, methotrexate, carmustine, cisplatin, and thiotepa. These drugs are often used in combinations over a period of several weeks. Current recommendations are that children with brain tumors be enrolled in multicenter protocols that use combinations of surgery, radiation, and chemotherapy.

2. PSEUDOTUMOR CEREBRI

Pseudotumor cerebri is a condition characterized by increased intracranial pressure in the absence of an identifiable intracranial mass or hydrocephalus. Clinical manifestations of pseudotumor cerebri are those of increased intracranial pressure as outlined in Table 25–20. The precise cause is usually not known, but pseudotumor cerebri has been described in association with a variety of inflammatory, metabolic, toxic, and connective tissue disorders (Table 25–21). The diagnosis of pseudotumor cerebri is one of exclusion. CT scans or MRI scans of the head are needed to exclude hydrocephalus and intracranial masses; these studies demonstrate ventricles of small or normal size but no other structural abnormalities. Lumbar puncture should be performed to document elevated cerebrospinal fluid pressure. Examination of cerebrospinal fluid reveals a normal cell count, a normal glucose concentration, and a normal or low protein concentration. In some inflammatory and connective tissue diseases, however, the cerebrospinal fluid protein may be increased.

Table 25–21. Conditions associated
with pseudotumor cerebri.

Metabolic-toxic disorders
  Hypervitaminosis A
  Hypovitaminosis A
  Prolonged steroid therapy
  Steroid withdrawal
  Tetracycline therapy
  Nalidixic acid therapy
  Iron deficiency
  Plumbism
  Hypocalcemia
  Hyperparathyroidism
  Adrenal insufficiency
  Lupus erythematosus
  Chronic CO_2 retention
Infectious and parainfectious disorders
  Chronic otitis media
  Poliomyelitis
  Guillain-Barré syndrome
Dural sinus thrombosis
Minor head injury

Specific treatment of pseudotumor cerebri is aimed at correcting any identifiable underlying predisposing condition. In addition, some patients may benefit from the use of furosemide or acetazolamide to decrease the volume and pressure of cerebrospinal fluid within the central nervous system. These drugs may be used in combination with repeated lumbar punctures to remove cerebrospinal fluid. If a program of repeated spinal fluid removal and medical management is not successful or if visual field loss is detected despite these measures, lumboperitoneal shunt or another surgical decompression procedure may be necessary to prevent irreparable visual loss and damage to the optic nerves.

3. SPINAL CORD TUMORS

The incidence of tumors within the spinal canal is one-sixth to one-fifth that of tumors within the intracranial compartment. The peak age at occurrence is approximately 4 years. Spinal tumors can be classified as intradural or extradural. Intradural tumors within the substance of the spinal cord are referred to as intramedullary and those outside as extramedullary. Recent reports suggest that approximately one-third of intraspinal tumors are intramedullary, approximately one-third are intradural extramedullary, and approximately one-third are extradural. About 10% of intraspinal tumors arise in the sacral region, and the remainder are distributed equally in the cervical, thoracic, and lumbar regions. Neurofibromas, meningiomas, dermoid cysts, teratomas, and metastatic tumors constitute the most frequent tumors that are extradural or intradural extramedullary. Astrocytomas and ependymomas are the most common intramedullary tumors.

Clinical manifestations of spinal cord tumors result from direct invasion of the tumor into neural tissue as well as from compression of neural tissue. Symptoms of gait disturbance, pain, and bowel and bladder dysfunction occur in association with abnormal muscle stretch reflexes, weakness, and sensory loss. The specific patterns of neurologic deficits are determined by the location and size of tumor mass.

When the clinical course and physical examination suggest the presence of an intraspinal mass, neuroimaging procedures are required. Spinal CT scan, metrizamide myelography, and spinal MRI scans are currently the methods by which a tumor can be defined. The use of gadolinium with MRI scanning enhances the definition of tumors within the spinal cord and within the spinal subarachnoid and extradural spaces. Although examination of cerebrospinal fluid may demonstrate the presence of neoplastic cells and markedly elevated protein concentrations, this test is not required for the diagnosis of intraspinal tumors and is contraindicated when significant cord compression is suspected clinically.

Primary intraspinal tumors may be totally removed by surgery, but many intramedullary tumors require a combination of surgery, radiation, and chemotherapy similar to the treatment of intracranial tumors discussed in the preceding section.

In addition to primary intraspinal tumors, the spinal cord and intraspinal compartment may be the site of direct invasion or hematogenous metastatic spread of tumors that arise outside the nervous system. Important examples include spinal neuroblastoma that may be an extension of paraspinous retroperitoneal neuroblastoma. Lymphoma, sarcoma, and leukemia may involve paraspinous tissue and spread to the intraspinal compartment through neural foramina. Treatment of these secondary neoplasms usually requires some combination of surgical excision, radiation, and chemotherapy.

Allen JC: Childhood brain tumors: Current status of clinical trials in newly diagnosed and recurrent disease. Pediatr Clin North Am 1985;32:633.

Baker RS, Baumann RJ, Buncic JR: Idiopathic intracranial hypertension (pseudotumor cerebri) in pediatric patients. Pediatr Neurol 1989;5:5.

Cohen ME, Duffner PK: *Brain Tumors in Children: Principles of Diagnosis and Treatment.* Raven Press, 1984.

Haft H, Ransohoff J, Carter S: Spinal cord tumors in children. Pediatrics 1959;23:1152.

Kadota RP et al: Brain tumors in children. J Pediatr 1989; 114:511.

Maria BL et al: Brainstem glioma: I. Pathology, clinical features, and therapy. J Child Neurol 1993;8:112.

Simpson DA, Carter RF, Ducrou W: Intracranial tumors in infancy. Dev Med Child Neurol 1968;10:190.

Weisberg LA, Chutorian AM: Pseudotumor cerebri of childhood. Am J Dis Child 1977;131:1243.

CEREBROVASCULAR DISEASE

Cerebrovascular disease, or stroke, occurs with an incidence in the pediatric population of approximately 1.2–2.5:100,000 per year. Although stroke occurs most frequently between the ages of 1 and 5 years, it may occur at any age during infancy and childhood. Congenital cyanotic heart disease is the most common underlying systemic disorder predisposing to stroke.

The initial approach to the patient should take into account the patient's age and any underlying systemic or neurologic illness. A systematic search for evidence of cardiac, vascular, or hematologic disease and intracranial disorders should be undertaken (Table 25–22).

Clinical Findings

A. Symptoms and Signs: The clinical manifestations of stroke in childhood vary according to the vascular distribution to the brain that is involved. Because many conditions leading to childhood stroke

Table 25–22. Etiologic risk factors for stroke in children.

Cardiac disorders
  Cyanotic heart disease
  Valvular disease
    Rheumatic
    Endocarditis
  Cardiomyopathy
  Cardiac dysrhythmia
Vascular occlusive disorders
  Arterial trauma (carotid dissections)
  Homocystinuria
  Mitochondrial encephalomyopathy
  Vasculitis
    Meningitis
    Polyarteritis nodosa
    Systemic lupus erythematosus
    Drug abuse (amphetamines)
  Fibromuscular dysplasia
  Moya-Moya syndrome
  Diabetes
  Nephrotic syndrome
  Systemic hypertension
  Dural sinus and cerebral venous thrombosis
    Meningitis
    Hyperviscosity
    Hypovolemia
  Cortical venous thrombosis
  Carotid-cavernous fistula
Hematologic disorders
  Polycythemia
  Thrombotic thrombocytopenia (TTP)
  Thrombocytopenic purpura (ITP)
  Thrombocythemia
  Hemoglobinopathies
    Sickle cell disease
    S-C disease
  Coagulation defects
    Hemophilia
    Vitamin K deficiency
  Hypercoagulable states
    Pregnancy
    Use of oral contraceptives
    Antithrombin III deficiency
    Protein C and S deficiencies
  Leukemia
Intracranial vascular anomalies
  Arteriovenous malformation
  Arterial aneurysm
  Carotid-cavernous fistula

result in emboli, multifocal neurologic involvement is common. Children may present with acute hemiplegia similar to stroke in adults. Symptoms of unilateral weakness, sensory disturbance, dysarthria, and dysphasia may develop over a period of minutes, but at times progressive worsening of symptoms may evolve over several hours. Bilateral hemispheric involvement may lead to a depressed level of consciousness. The patient may also demonstrate disturbances of mood and behavior and experience focal or multifocal seizures. Physical examination of the patient is aimed not only at identifying the specific deficits related to impaired cerebral blood flow but also at seeking evidence for any predisposing disorder. Retinal hemorrhages, splinter hemorrhages in the nail beds, cardiac murmurs, and signs of trauma are especially important findings.

When stroke is ushered in by a focal hemiconvulsion followed by hemiplegia, a chronic epilepsy syndrome may persist for years in association with hemiplegia. This combination of hemiconvulsion, hemiplegia, and chronic epilepsy has been referred to as the "HHE syndrome."

B. Laboratory Findings: Laboratory investigation can be carried out systemically, with particular attention to disorders involving the heart, blood vessels, platelets, red cells, hemoglobin, and coagulation proteins. Additional laboratory tests for systemic disorders such as systemic lupus erythematosus and polyarteritis nodosa are usually indicated.

Examination of spinal fluid is indicated in patients with fever, nuchal rigidity, or marked obtundation when the diagnosis of intracranial infection requires exclusion. The lumbar puncture, however, may be deferred until a neuroimage excluding brain abscess or a space-occupying lesion that might contraindicate lumbar puncture has been obtained. In the absence of infection and frank intracranial subarachnoid hemorrhage, the spinal fluid examination is rarely helpful in defining the cause of the cerebrovascular disorder.

C. Imaging: CT scans and MRI of the brain are often helpful in defining the extent of cerebral involvement with ischemia or hemorrhage. CT scans, however, may be normal within the first few hours of an ischemic stroke and, therefore, may need to be repeated several hours later. A CT scan early after the onset of neurologic deficits is valuable in excluding significant intracranial hemorrhage. This information may be helpful in the early stages of management and in the decision to treat with anticoagulants.

Cerebral angiography is usually not urgently needed but may be needed to confirm such disorders as fibromuscular dysplasia and cerebral arteritis. If angiography is done, all major vessels should be studied. If evidence of fibromuscular dysplasia is present in the intracranial or extracranial vessels, renal arteriography is indicated. With additional technical advances, MRA will soon replace conventional contrast angiography for most cases of childhood stroke.

When seizures are prominent, an EEG may be used as an adjunct in the patient's evaluation. An EEG and sequential electroencephalographic monitoring may help in the evaluation of patients with severely depressed levels of consciousness.

Electrocardiography and echocardiography are useful both in the diagnostic approach to the patient and in ongoing monitoring and management, particularly when hypotension or cardiac irregularities complicate the clinical course.

Differential Diagnosis

Patients with an acute onset of neurologic deficits must be evaluated not only for cerebrovascular disease but also for other disorders that can cause focal neurologic deficits. Hypoglycemia, prolonged focal seizures, a prolonged postictal paresis (Todd's paralysis), meningitis, encephalitis, and brain abscess should all be considered. Migraine with focal neurologic deficits may be difficult to differentiate initially from ischemic stroke. Occasionally, the onset of a neurodegenerative disorder (eg, adrenoleukodystrophy) may begin with the abrupt onset of seizures and focal neurologic deficits. The possibility of drug abuse—particularly cocaine—and other toxic exposures must be investigated diligently.

Treatment

The initial management of children with stroke is aimed at providing support for pulmonary, cardiovascular, and renal function. Appropriate fluid and electrolyte infusions should be started, and careful monitoring of heart rate and rhythm and blood pressure are required. Specific treatment of stroke depends in part upon the underlying pathogenesis and the specific predisposing disorder. In some situations, heparinization for emboli and consumption coagulopathies is indicated. In other disorders, such as fibromuscular dysplasia, treatment aimed at decreasing platelet adhesiveness may be an acceptable alternative to anticoagulation.

Long-term management requires intensive rehabilitation efforts, anticonvulsant treatment, and therapy aimed at improving the child's language, educational, and psychologic performance.

Prognosis

The outcome of stroke in infants and children is variable. Underlying predisposing conditions and the vascular territory involved all play a role in dictating the outcome for an individual patient. When the stroke involves extremely large portions of one hemisphere or large portions of both hemispheres and cerebral edema develops, the patient's level of consciousness may deteriorate rapidly, and death may occur within the first few days. Some patients may achieve almost complete recovery of neurologic function within several days if the cerebral territory is small. Seizures, either focal or generalized, may occur in 30–50% of patients at some point in the course of their cerebrovascular disorder. Chronic problems with learning, behavior, and activity are seen in many patients.

Broderick J et al: Stroke in children within a major metropolitan area: The surprising importance of intracerebral hemorrhage. J Child Neurol 1993;8:250.

Edwards MSB, Hoffman B: *Cerebral Vascular Disease in Children and Adolescents.* Williams & Wilkins, 1989.

Kerr LM et al: Ischemic stroke in the young: Evaluation and age comparison of patients six months to thirty-nine years. J Child Neurol 1993;8:266.

Reila AR, Roach ES: Etiology of stroke in children. J Child Neurol 1993;8:201.

Young RSK: Neurologic aspects of cardiovascular disease. In: *Neurologic Aspects of Pediatrics.* Berg BO (editor). Butterworth-Heinemann, 1992.

CONGENITAL MALFORMATIONS OF THE NERVOUS SYSTEM

Malformations of the nervous system occur in 1–3% of living neonates and are present in 40% of infants who die. Developmental anomalies of the central nervous system may result from a variety of causes, including infectious, toxic, metabolic, and vascular insults that affect the fetus. The specific type of malformation that results from such insults, however, may depend more upon the gestational period during which the insult occurs than on the specific cause. The period of induction, 0–28 days of gestation, is the period during which the neural plate appears and the neural tube forms and closes. Insults during this phase can result in a major absence of neural structures, such as anencephaly, or in a defect of neural tube closure, such as spina bifida, meningomyelocele, or encephalocele. Cellular proliferation and migration characterize neural development that occurs after 28 days of gestation. Lissencephaly, pachygyria, agyria, and agenesis of the corpus callosum represent disorders caused by insults that occur during the period of cellular proliferation and migration.

1. ABNORMALITIES OF NEURAL TUBE CLOSURE

Defects of neural tube closure constitute some of the most common forms of congenital malformations affecting the nervous system. Spina bifida with associated meningomyelocele or meningocele is commonly found in the lumbosacral region. Depending on the extent and severity of the involvement of the spinal cord and peripheral nerves, clinical findings include lower extremity weakness, bowel and bladder dysfunction, and hip dislocation. Operation to close meningoceles and meningomyeloceles is usually indicated. Additional treatment is necessary to manage chronic abnormalities of the urinary tract, orthopedic abnormalities such as kyphosis and scoliosis, and paresis of the lower extremities. Hydrocephalus commonly associated with meningomyelocele usually requires ventriculoperitoneal shunting.

Arnold-Chiari Malformations

Arnold-Chiari malformation type I consists of elongation and displacement of the caudal end of the brain stem into the spinal canal with protrusion of the cerebellar tonsils through the foramen magnum. In association with this hindbrain malformation, there are often minor to moderate abnormalities of the base of the skull, including basilar impression (platybasia) and small foramen magnum. Arnold-Chiari malformation type I may remain asymptomatic for years, but in older children and young adults it may cause progressive ataxia, paresis of the lower cranial nerves, and progressive vertigo. Posterior cervical laminectomy may be necessary to provide relief from cervical cord compression. Ventriculoperitoneal shunting is required for hydrocephalus.

Arnold-Chiari malformation type II consists of the malformations found in Arnold-Chiari type I plus an associated lumbosacral meningomyelocele. Hydrocephalus is present in approximately 90% of children with Arnold-Chiari type II. These patients may also have aqueductal stenosis, hydromyelia, or syringomyelia. The clinical manifestations of Arnold-Chiari type II are most commonly caused by the associated hydrocephalus and meningomyelocele. In addition, dysfunction of the lower cranial nerves may be present.

Arnold-Chiari malformation type III is characterized by occipital encephalocele, a closure defect of the rostral end of the neural tube. Hydrocephalus is extremely common with this malformation.

In general, the diagnosis of neural tube defects is obvious at the time of birth. Diagnosis may be strongly suspected prenatally on the basis of ultrasonographic findings and the presence of elevated alpha-fetoprotein in the amniotic fluid.

2. DISORDERS OF CELLULAR PROLIFERATION AND MIGRATION

Lissencephaly

Lissencephaly is a severe malformation of brain characterized by an extremely smooth cortical surface with minimal sulcal and gyral development. Such a smooth surface is characteristic of fetal brain at the end of the first trimester. In addition, many brains with lissencephaly have a primitive cytoarchitectural construction with a four-layered cerebral mantle instead of the mature six-layered cerebral mantle. Pachygyria and agyria are closely associated with lissencephaly but represent more restricted forms of migrational abnormalities. Patients with lissencephaly usually suffer from severe neurodevelopmental delay, microcephaly, and seizures (including infantile spasms) and frequently have additional associated malformations and dysmorphic features. Walker-Warburg syndrome or Miller-Dieker syndrome can often be identified in some of these patients. It is particularly important to identify these syndromes because of their genetic importance; Walker-Warburg syndrome is an autosomal recessive disorder, and Miller-Dieker syndrome is associated with defects of chromosome 17. In addition to these two syndromes, lissencephaly may be a component of Zellweger's syndrome, a metabolic peroxisomal abnormality. Zellweger's syndrome is diagnosed by the presence of elevated concentrations of very long chain fatty acids in plasma. A peroxisomal defect in fatty acid degradation in cultured skin fibroblasts confirms the diagnosis. No specific treatment for lissencephaly is available. Seizures may be controlled by the use of phenobarbital, phenytoin, or clonazepam.

MRI studies have helped to define a number of presumed migrational defects that are similar to but anatomically more restricted than lissencephaly. A distinctive example is bilateral persylvian cortical dysplasia. Patients have pseudobulbar palsy, variable cognitive deficits, facial diplegia, dysarthria, developmental delay, and epilepsy. Seizures are often difficult to control with antiepileptic drugs, and some patients have benefited from corpus callosotomy. The cause of this syndrome is as yet unknown, though intrauterine cerebral ischemic injury has been postulated. Therapy is aimed at improving speech and oromotor functions and controlling seizures.

Agenesis of the Corpus Callosum

Agenesis of the corpus callosum, once thought to be a relatively rare cerebral malformation, has been seen frequently with modern neuroimaging techniques such as CT and MRI. The cause of this malformation is unknown. Occasionally, it appears to be inherited in an autosomal dominant or autosomal recessive pattern. X-linked recessive patterns have also been described. Agenesis of the corpus callosum has been found in some patients with pyruvate dehydrogenase deficiency and in others with nonketotic hyperglycinemia. Most cases, however, are sporadic. Maldevelopment of the corpus callosum may be partial or complete. No specific clinical syndrome is typical of agenesis of the corpus callosum, although many patients have seizures, developmental delay, microcephaly, or mental retardation. Neurologic abnormalities may be related to microscopic cytoarchitectural abnormalities of the brain that occur in association with the agenesis of the corpus callosum. The malformation may be found coincidentally by neuroimaging studies in otherwise normal patients and has been described as a coincidental finding at autopsy in neurologically normal individuals. A special form of agenesis of the corpus callosum occurs in Aicardi's syndrome. In this X-linked disorder, agenesis of the corpus callosum is associated with infantile spasms, mental retardation, lacunar chorioretinopathy, and vertebral body abnormalities.

Dandy-Walker Malformation

Dandy-Walker malformation is characterized by aplasia of the vermis, cystic enlargement of the fourth ventricle, rostral displacement of the tentorium, and absence or atresia of the foramina of Magendie and Luschka. Although hydrocephalus is usually not present congenitally, it develops within the first few months of life, and 90% of patients who develop hydrocephalus do so by the age of 1 year. On physical examination, there is often a rounded protuberance or exaggeration of the occiput of the cranium. In the absence of hydrocephalus and increased intracranial pressure, there may be few physical findings to suggest neurologic dysfunction. An ataxic syndrome occurs in fewer than 20% of patients and is usually late in appearing. Many long-term neurologic deficits result directly from hydrocephalus. Diagnosis of Dandy-Walker malformation is confirmed by CT or MRI scanning of the head. Treatment is directed at the management of hydrocephalus.

3. CRANIOSYNOSTOSIS

Craniosynostosis, or premature closure of cranial sutures, is usually sporadic and idiopathic. However, some patients have hereditary disorders, such as Apert's syndrome and Crouzon's disease, that are associated with abnormalities of the digits, extremities, and heart. Occasionally, craniosynostosis may be associated with an underlying metabolic disturbance such as hyperthyroidism and hypophosphatasia. The most common form of craniosynostosis involves the sagittal suture and results in scaphocephaly, an elongation of the head in the anterior to posterior direction. Premature closure of the coronal sutures causes brachycephaly, an increase in cranial diameter from left to right. Unless many or all cranial sutures close prematurely, intracranial volume will not be compromised, and the brain's growth will not be impaired. Closure of only one or a few sutures will not cause impaired brain growth or neurologic dysfunction. Management of craniosynostosis is directed at preserving normal skull shape and consists of excising the fused suture and applying material to the edge of the craniectomy to prevent reossification of the bone edges. The best cosmetic effect on the skull is achieved when surgery is done during the first 6 months of life.

4. HYDROCEPHALUS

Hydrocephalus is characterized by an increased volume of cerebrospinal fluid in association with progressive ventricular dilation. In communicating hydrocephalus, cerebrospinal fluid can circulate through the ventricular system and into the subarachnoid space without obstruction. In noncommunicating hydrocephalus, an obstruction blocks the flow of spinal fluid within the ventricular system or blocks the egress of spinal fluid from the ventricular system into the subarachnoid space. A wide variety of disorders, such as hemorrhage, infection, tumors, and congenital malformations, may play an etiologic role in development of hydrocephalus.

Clinical features of hydrocephalus include macrocephaly, an excessive rate of head growth, irritability, vomiting, loss of appetite, impaired upgaze, impaired extraocular movements, hypertonia of the lower extremities, and generalized hyperreflexia. Without treatment, optic atrophy may occur. In infants, papilledema may not be present, whereas older children with closed cranial sutures can eventually develop swelling of the optic disk.

Hydrocephalus can be diagnosed on the basis of the clinical course, findings on physical examination, and CT scan or MRI findings. Radionuclide scans also demonstrate impaired cerebrospinal fluid circulation through the ventricular and subarachnoid systems but are rarely needed for clinical diagnosis or management.

Treatment of hydrocephalus is directed at providing an alternative outlet for cerebrospinal fluid from the intracranial compartment. The most common method is ventriculoperitoneal shunting. Other treatment should be directed, if possible, at the underlying cause of the hydrocephalus.

Barth PG: Disorders of neuronal migration. Can J Neurol Sci 1987;14:1.
Dobyns WB: Agenesis of the corpus callosum and gyral malformations are frequent manifestations of nonketotic hyperglycinemia. Neurology 1989;39:817.
Dobyns WB: The neurogenetics of lissencephaly. Neurol Clin 1989;7:89.
Hirsch JF et al: The Dandy-Walker malformation. J Neurosurg 1984;61:515.
Hoffman HJ, Epstein F (editors): *Disorders of the Developing Nervous System: Diagnosis and Treatment.* Blackwell, 1986.
Kuzniecky R et al: Congenital bilateral persylvian syndrome: Study of 31 patients. Lancet 1993;341:608.

ABNORMAL HEAD SIZE

Bone plates of the skull have almost no intrinsic capacity to enlarge or grow—unlike long bones—and are dependent upon extrinsic forces to stimulate new bone formation at the suture lines. Although gravity and traction on bone by muscle and scalp probably stimulate some growth, the single most important stimulus for head growth during infancy and childhood is brain growth. Therefore, the accurate assessment of head growth is one of the most important aspects of the neurologic examination of young children. A head circumference that is 2 SD above or below the mean for age requires investigation and explanation.

1. MICROCEPHALY

A head circumference more than 2 SD below the mean for age and sex is by definition microcephaly. More important, however, than a single head circumference measurement is the rate or pattern of head growth through time. Head circumference measurements that progressively drop to lower percentiles with increasing age are indicative of a process or condition that has impaired the brain's capacity to grow. The causes of microcephaly are numerous. Some examples are listed in Table 25–23.

Clinical Findings

A. Symptoms and Signs: Microcephaly may be suspected in the full-term newborn and in infants up to 6 months of age whose chest circumference exceeds the head circumference (unless the child is very obese). Microcephaly may be discovered when the child is examined because of delayed developmental milestones or neurologic problems, such as seizures or spasticity. There may be a marked backward slope of the forehead (as in familial microcephaly) with narrowing of the bitemporal diameter. The fontanelle may close earlier than expected, and sutures may be prominent.

B. Laboratory Findings: These vary with the cause. Abnormal dermatoglyphics may be present when the injury occurred before the 19th week of gestation. If clinical factors warrant, antibody titers for toxoplasmosis, rubella, cytomegalovirus, herpes simplex virus, and syphilis must be assessed. Elevated specific IgM titer, if obtained at birth, is indicative of congenital infection. Serum and urine amino and organic acid determination on the baby are occasionally diagnostic. The mother may need to be screened for phenylketonuria. Karyotyping, including fragile X, should be considered.

Table 25–23. Microcephaly.

Causes	Examples
Prenatal chromosomal	Trisomy 13, 18, 21
Malformation	Lissenencephaly, schizencephaly
Syndromes	Rubenstein-Taybi, Cornelia de Lange
Toxins	Alcohol, anticonvulsants (?), maternal phenylketonuria
Infections (intrauterine)	TORCHES[1]
Radiation	Maternal pelvis, 1st and 2nd trimester
Placental insufficiency	Toxemia, infection
Familial	Autosomal dominant, autosomal recessive
Perinatal hypoxia, trauma	Birth asphyxia, injury
Infections (perinatal)	Bacterial meningitis (especially group B streptococci) Viral encephalitis (coxsackie B, herpes simplex)
Metabolic	Hypoglycemia, phenylketonuria, maple syrup urine disease
Postnatal sequela from earlier insult	As above
Degenerative disease	Tay-Sachs, Krabbe's

[1]A mnemonic formula for *to*xoplasmosis, *r*ubella, *c*ytomegalovirus, *her*pes simplex and *s*yphilis.

C. Imaging: CT or MRI may aid in diagnosis (eg, of intracranial calcification, malformations, atrophy) and prognosis. These studies may demonstrate calcifications, malformations, or atrophic patterns that suggest specific congenital infections or genetic syndromes. Plain skull x-rays may show closed sutures, but these studies are of limited value in diagnosis and have been replaced by more sensitive and more informative scanning procedures. Genetic counseling should be done in any infant with significant microcephaly.

Differential Diagnosis

Congenital craniosynostosis involving multiple sutures is easily differentiated by inspection (head shape), history, identification of syndromes, hereditary pattern, and sometimes signs and symptoms of increased intracranial pressure. Common forms of craniosynostosis involving sagittal, coronal, and lambdoidal sutures are associated with abnormally shaped heads but do not cause microcephaly. Treatable undergrowth of the brain due to hypopituitarism or severe protein-calorie undernutrition is recognized by the history and clinical findings.

Treatment & Prognosis

Except for the treatable disorders noted above, treatment is usually supportive and directed at the multiple neurologic and sensory deficits, endocrine disturbances (eg, diabetes insipidus) and seizures. Many children with head circumferences more than 2 SD below the mean show variable degrees of mental retardation. The notable exceptions are found in cases of hypopituitarism (rare) or familial autosomal dominant microcephaly.

Ahlfors K et al: Microcephaly and congenital cytomegalovirus infection: Prospective and retrospective study. Pediatrics 1986;78:1058.

Ishihara T et al: Growth and achievement of large and small headed children in a normal population. Brain Dev 1988;10:295.

Jaffe M et al: The dilemma in prenatal diagnosis of idiopathic microcephaly. Dev Med Child Neurol 1987;29:187.

Jawarski M et al: Computed tomography of the head in evaluation of microcephaly. Pediatrics 1986;78:1064.

2. MACROCEPHALY

A head circumference more than 2 SD above the mean for age and sex denotes macrocephaly. Excessive head growth rate through time suggests increased intracranial pressure most likely caused by hydrocephalus, extra-axial fluid collections, or neoplasms. Macrocephaly with normal head growth rate suggests familial macrocephaly or true megalencephaly, as might occur in neurofibromatosis. Other example of causes of macrocephaly are listed in Table 25–24.

Table 25–24. Macrocephaly.

Causes	Examples
"Pseudomacrocephaly," "pseudohydrocephalus," "catch-up growth" crossing percentiles	Premature "grower," cystic fibrosis treatment, congenital heart disease recovery, parenteral alimentation.
Increased intracranial pressure	
With dilated ventricles	Progressive hydrocephalus, subdural effusion.
With other mass	Arachnoid cyst, porencephalic cyst, brain tumor.
Benign familial macrocephaly (idiopathic external hydrocephalus)	"External hydrocephalus," "benign enlargement of the subarachnoid spaces," "congenital communicating hydrocephalus," "benign subdural collections of infancy."
Megalencephaly (large brain)	Benign familial (see above).
With neurocutaneous disorder	Neurofibromatosis, tuberous sclerosis, etc.
With gigantism	Sotos syndrome.
With dwarfism	Achondroplasia.
Metabolic	Mucopolysaccharidoses.
Lysosomal	Metachromatic leukodytrophy.
Other leukodysrtrophy	Canavan's spongy degeneration.
Thickened skull	Fibrous dysplasia (bone), hemolytic anemia (marrow), sicklemia, thalassemia.

Clinical Findings

Clinical and laboratory findings vary with the underlying process. In infants, transillumination of the skull with an intensely bright light in a completely darkened room may disclose chronic subdural effusions, hydrocephalus, hydranencephaly, and large cystic defects.

A surgically or medically treatable condition must be ruled out. Thus, the first decision is whether and when to perform an imaging study.

A. Imaging Study Deferred:

1. "Catch-up growth," as in the thriving, neurologically intact premature infant whose rapid head enlargement is most marked in the first weeks of life, or the infant in the early phase of recovery from deprivation dwarfism. As the expected "normal" is reached, head growth slows down, then resumes a normal growth pattern. If the fontanelle is open, cranial ultrasonography can assess ventricular size and diagnose or exclude hydrocephalus.

2. Familial macrocephaly, where another family member may have an unusually large head and there are no signs or symptoms referable to such disorders as neurocutaneous dysplasias (especially neurofibromatosis) or cerebral gigantism (Sotos syndrome) nor significant mental or neurologic abnormalities in the child.

B. Brain Scan Indicated: CT or MRI–or ultrasonography, if the anterior fontanelle is open—is used to define any structural cause of macrocephaly and to determine an operable disorder. Even when the condition is not treatable (or is benign), the information gained may permit more accurate diagnosis and prognosis, guide management and genetic counseling, and serve as a basis for comparison should future abnormal cranial growth or neurologic changes necessitate a repeat study. An imaging study is necessary if there are any signs or symptoms of increased intracranial pressure (see Table 25–20).

Gooskens RHJM et al: Megalencephaly: Definition and classification. Brain Dev 1988;10:1.

Lorber J, Priestley BL: Children with large heads: A practical approach to diagnosis in 557 children with special reference to 109 children with megalencephaly. Dev Med Child Neurol 1981;23:494.

Wilms G et al: CT and MR in infants with pericerebral collections and macrocephaly: Benign enlargement of the subarachnoid spaces versus subdural collections. AJNR Am J Neuroradiol 1993;14:855.

NEUROCUTANEOUS DYSPLASIAS

Neurocutaneous dysplasias are diseases of the neuroectoderm and sometimes involve endoderm and mesoderm. Birth marks and skin growths appearing later often suggest a need to look for brain, spinal cord, and eye disease. Hamartomas (histologically normal tissue growing abnormally rapidly or in aberrant sites) are common. The most common dysplasias are dominantly inherited. Benign and even malignant tumors may develop.

1. NEUROFIBROMATOSIS (Recklinghausen's Disease)

Essentials of Diagnosis

- More than six café au lait spots 5 mm in greatest diameter in prepubertal individuals and over 15 mm of greatest diameter in postpubertal individuals.
- Two or more neurofibromas of any type or one plexiform neurofibroma.
- Freckling in the axillary or inguinal regions.
- Optic glioma.
- Two or more Lisch nodules (iris hamartomas).
- Distinctive osseous lesions, such as sphenoid dysplasia or thinning of long bone with or without pseudarthroses.
- First-degree relative (parent, sibling, offspring) with neurofibromatosis type 1 by above criteria.

Clinical Findings

A. Symptoms and Signs: The most common presenting symptoms are cognitive or psychomotor problems, eg, school difficulties; 40% of patients have learning disabilities, and mental retardation is seen in 8%. The family history is important in identifying dominant gene manifestations in parents; they should be examined in detail. The history should focus on lumps or masses causing disfigurement, functional problems, or pain. The clinician should ask about visual problems; strabismus or amblyopia dictates a search for optic glioma, a common tumor in this disease. Any progressive neurologic deficit might call for studies to rule out tumor of the spinal cord or central nervous system. Tumors of the eighth nerve are virtually never seen in the common neurofibromatosis type 1.

The physician should check blood pressure and examine the spine for scoliosis and the limbs for pseudarthroses. Head measurement often shows macrocephaly. Hearing and vision need to be assessed. The eye examination should include a check for proptosis and iris Lisch nodules; the optic disk should be examined for atrophy or papilledema. Short stature and precocious puberty are occasional findings. An examination for neurologic manifestations of tumors (eg, asymmetric reflexes, spasticity) is important.

B. Laboratory Findings: Laboratory tests are not likely to be of any value in asymptomatic patients. Selected patients require brain MRI or CT with special cuts through the optic nerves to rule out optic glioma. Hypertension necessitates a look at renal arteries for dysplasia and stenosis as a cause. Cognitive and school achievement testing may be indicated. Scoliosis or limb abnormalities should be studied by appropriate roentgenograms—even an MRI scan of the spinal cord and roots.

Differential Diagnosis

Patients with Albright's syndrome often have larger café au lait spots with precocious puberty. Many normal individuals have one or two café au lait spots.

Treatment

Genetic counseling is important. The risk to siblings is up to 50%. The disease may be progressive, with serious complications rarely seen. Patients sometimes worsen during puberty or pregnancy. Family members need to be evaluated for the presence of the gene. Annual or semiannual visits are important in the early detection of school problems or bony or neurologic abnormalities.

Multidisciplinary clinics are being established at medical centers around the United States and are often an excellent resource. Prenatal diagnosis is probably on the horizon, but the variability of manifestations (trivial to severe) will make therapeutic abortion an unlikely option. Chromosomal linkage studies are under way (chromosome 17).

Information for lay people and physicians is available from the National Neurofibromatosis Foundation, Inc., 70 West 40th Street, New York, NY 10018.

Aoki S et al: Neurofibromatosis types 1 and 2: Cranial MR findings. Radiology 1989;172:527.

Gomez MR (editor): *Neurocutaneous Diseases.* Butterworths, 1987.

Hoffman KJ, Boehm CD: Familial neurofibromatosis type 1: Clinical experience with DNA testing. J Pediatr 1992; 120:394.

Korf BR, Carranza E, Holmes GL: Patterns of seizures observed in association with neurofibromatosis I. Epilepsia 1993;34:616.

Listernick R, Charrow J, Greenwald M: Emergence of optic pathway gliomas in children with neurofibromatosis is type I after neuroimaging results. J Pediatr 1992;121: 584.

Neurofibromatosis: National Institutes of Health Consensus Statement Vol 6, No. 12, 1987.

Riccardi VM: Neurofibromatosis: Past, present, and future. N Engl J Med 1991;324:1283.

Sevick RJ et al: Evolution of white matter lesions in neurofibromatosis type I: MR findings. AJR Am J Roentgenol 1992;159:171.

2. TUBEROUS SCLEROSIS (Bourneville's Disease)

Essentials of Diagnosis

- Facial angiofibromas or subungual fibromas.
- Often hypomelanotic macules, gingival fibromas.
- Retinal hamartomas.
- Cortical tubers or subependymal glial nodules often calcified.
- Renal angiomyolipomas.

General Considerations

Tuberous sclerosis, a disease of unknown cause, is of autosomal dominant inheritance. The classic triad of seizures, mental retardation, and adenoma sebaceum is seen in only one-third of patients. The disease was earlier thought to have a high rate of mutation. As a result of more sophisticated techniques such as MRI, parents formerly thought not to harbor the gene are now being diagnosed as asymptomatic carriers.

Like neurofibromatosis, tuberous sclerosis may present with a wide variety of symptoms. The patient may be asymptomatic but for skin findings or may be devastated by severe infantile spasms in early infancy, continuing epilepsy, and mental retardation. Seizures in early infancy correlate with later mental retardation.

Clinical Findings

A. Symptoms and Signs:

1. Dermatologic features–Skin findings bring most cases to the physician's attention. Ninety-six percent have one or more hypomelanotic macules, facial angiofibromas, ungual fibromas, or shagreen patches. Adenoma sebaceum or the facial skin hamartomas may first appear in early childhood, often on the cheek, chin, and dry sites of the skin where acne is not usually seen. They often have a reddish hue. The off-white hypomelanotic macules are more easily seen in tanned or dark-skinned individuals. They often are oval or "ash leaf" in shape and follow dermatomes. A Wood lamp (ultraviolet light) shows the macules more clearly—a great help in the light-skinned patient. In the scalp, poliosis, or whitened hair, is the equivalent. In infancy, the presence of these macules accompanied by seizures is virtually diagnostic of the disease. Subungual or periungual fibromas are more common in the toes. Leathery, orange peel-like shagreen patches support the diagnosis. Café au lait spots are occasionally seen. Fibrous or raised plaques may resemble coalescent angiofibromas.

2. Neurologic features–Seizures are the most common presenting symptom. Five percent of cases of infantile spasm (a serious epileptic syndrome) occur in patients with tuberous sclerosis. Thus, any patient presenting with infantile spasms (and the parents as well) should be carefully examined for this disorder. An imaging study of the central nervous system, such as a CT scan, may show calcified subependymal nodules; MRI may show dysmyelinating white matter lesions or cortical tubers. Virtually any kind of symptomatic seizure—eg, atypical absence, partial complex, and generalized tonic-clonic seizures—may occur.

3. Mental retardation–Mental retardation is seen in up to 50% of patients referred to centers; the incidence is probably much lower in randomly selected patients. Patients with seizures are more prone to retardation or learning disabilities.

4. Renal lesions–Renal cysts or angiomyolipomas may be asymptomatic. Hematuria or obstruction of urine flow sometimes occurs; the latter requires operation. Ultrasound examination of the kidneys should be done in any patient suspected of having tuberous sclerosis, both to aid in diagnosis if lesions are found and to rule out renal obstructive disease.

5. Cardiopulmonary involvement–Rarely, cystic lung disease may occur. Rhabdomyomas of the heart may be asymptomatic but can lead to outflow obstruction, conduction difficulties, and death. Chest x-rays and echocardiograms can detect these rare manifestations.

6. Eye involvement–Retinal hamartomas are often near the disk; if distant from the disk, they are more "diagnostic" for this syndrome.

7. Skeletal involvement–Findings sometimes helpful in diagnosis are cystic rarefactions of the bones of the fingers or toes.

B. Diagnostic Studies: Plain radiographs may detect areas of thickening within the skull, spine, and pelvis and cystic lesions in the hands and feet. Chest x-rays may show lung honeycombing. More helpful is CT scanning, which can show the virtually pathognomonic subependymal nodular calcifications and sometimes widened gyri or tubers and brain tumors. Contrast material may show the often classically located tumors near the foramen interventriculare. Hypomyelinated lesions may be seen with magnetic resonance imaging.

The EEG is helpful in delineating the presence of seizure discharges.

Treatment

Therapy is as indicated by underlying disease, eg, seizures and tumors of the brain, kidney, and heart. Skin lesions on the face may need dermabrasion or other removal. Genetic counseling emphasizes identification of the carrier. There is a 50% risk for appearance in offspring if either parent is a carrier. The patient should be seen annually for counseling and re-examination in childhood. Identification of the chromosome and gene marker may in the future make intrauterine diagnosis possible.

Aicardi J: Tuberous sclerosis. Int Pediatr 1993;8:171.
Martin N et al: Gadolinium-DTPA enhanced MR imaging in tuberous sclerosis. Neuroradiology 1990;31:492.
Oppenheimer EY et al: Late appearance of hypopigmented maculae in tuberous sclerosis. Am J Dis Child 1985; 139:408.
Stefanson K: Tuberous sclerosis. Mayo Clin Proc 1991;66: 868.
Sugita K et al: Tuberous sclerosis: Report of two cases studied by computer assisted cranial tomography within one week after birth. Brain Dev 1985;7:438.

3. ENCEPHALOFACIAL ANGIOMATOSIS (Sturge-Weber Disease)

Sturge-Weber disease consists of a facial port wine nevus involving the upper part of the face (in the first division of the fifth nerve), a venous angioma of the meninges in the occipitoparietal regions, and choroidal angioma. The syndrome has been described without the facial nevus.

Clinical Findings

In infancy, the eye may show congenital glaucoma, or buphthalmos, with a cloudy, enlarged cornea. In early stages, the facial nevus may be the only indication, with no findings in the brain even on radiologic studies. The characteristic atrophy and calcifications of the cortex and meningoangiomatosis may appear with time, solidifying the diagnosis.

Physical examination may show focal seizures or hemiparesis on the side opposite the cerebral lesion. The facial nevus may be much more extensive than just the first division of the fifth nerve; eg, it can involve the lower face, mouth, lip, neck, and even torso. Hemiatrophy of the opposite limbs may occur. Mental handicap may result from poorly controlled seizures. Late-appearing glaucoma and, rarely, central nervous system hemorrhage occur.

Radiologic studies may show calcification of the cortex; CT scanning may show this much earlier than plain film studies. MRI scans often show underlying brain involvement.

The EEG often shows depression of voltage over the involved area in early stages; later, epileptiform abnormalities may be present focally.

Treatment

The disease is sporadic. Early control of seizures is important to avoid consequent developmental setback. If seizures do not occur, normal development can be anticipated. Careful examination of the newborn, with ophthalmologic assessment to detect early glaucoma, is indicated. Rarely, surgical removal of the involved meninges and the involved portion of the brain may be indicated, even hemispherectomy.

Strauss RP, Resnick SD: Pulsed dye laser therapy for port-wine stains in children: Psychosocial and ethical issues. J Pediatr 1993;122:505.
Tallman B et al: Location of port-wine stains and the likelihood of ophthalmic and/or central nervous system complications. Pediatrics 1991;87:323.
Taly AB et al: Sturge-Weber-Dimitri disease without facial nevus. Neurology 1987;37:1063.

4. VON HIPPEL-LINDAU DISEASE (Retinocerebellar Angiomatosis)

Von Hippel-Lindau disease is a rare, dominantly inherited condition with retinal and cerebellar hemangioblastomas, cysts of the kidneys, pancreas, and epididymis, and sometimes renal cancers. The patient may present with ataxia, slurred speech, and nystagmus due to a hemangioblastoma of the cerebellum or with a medullary spinal cord cystic hemangioblastoma. Retinal detachment may occur from hemorrhage or exudate in the retinal vascular malformation. Rarely, a pancreatic cyst or renal tumor may be the presenting symptom.

The diagnostic criteria for the disease are a retinal or cerebellar hemangioblastoma with or without a positive family history, intra-abdominal cyst, or renal cancer.

Coulam CM et al: Hippel-Lindau syndrome. Semin Roentgenol 1976;11:61.

CENTRAL NERVOUS SYSTEM DEGENERATIVE DISORDERS OF INFANCY & CHILDHOOD

Essentials of Diagnosis

- Arrest of psychomotor development.
- Loss, usually progressive but at variable rates, of mental and motor functioning and often vision.

- Seizures are common in some disorders.
- Symptoms and signs vary with age at onset and primary sites of involvement of specific types.

General Considerations

The central nervous system degenerative disorders of infancy and childhood are fortunately rare. An early clinical pattern of decline often follows normal early development. Referral for sophisticated biochemical testing is usually necessary before definitive diagnosis can be made. (See Tables 25–25 and 25–26.)

Aubourg P et al: Brain MRI and electrophysiologic abnormalities in preclinical and clinical adrenomyeloneuropathy. Neurology 1992;42:85.

Brown FR et al: Paroxysmal disorders: Neurodevelopmental and biochemical aspects. Am J Dis Child 1993;147:617.

Dyken PR: The neuronal ceroid lipofuscinoses. J Child Neurol 1989;4:165.

Goebel HH: Neuronal ceroid-lipofuscinoses: The current status. Brain Dev 1992;14:203.

Jaeken J, Carchon H: The carbohydrate-deficient glycoprotein syndromes: Recent developments. Int Pediatr 1993;8:60.

Jaeken J, Stibler H, Hagberg B: The carbohydrate-deficient glycoprotein syndrome. Acta Paediatr Scand Suppl 1991;375:1.

Mehler M, Rabinowich L: Inflammatory myeloclastic diffuse sclerosis. Ann Neurol 1988;23:413.

Menkes J: Huntington disease: Finding the gene and after. Pediatr Neurol 1988;4:73.

ATAXIAS OF CHILDHOOD

1. ACUTE CEREBELLAR ATAXIA

Acute cerebellar ataxia occurs most commonly in children 2–6 years of age. The onset is abrupt, and the evolution of symptoms is rapid. In about half of cases, there is a prodromal illness with fever, respiratory or gastrointestinal symptoms, or an exanthem within 3 weeks of onset. Associated viral infections include varicella, rubeola, mumps, rubella, echovirus infections, poliomyelitis, infectious mononucleosis, and influenza. Bacterial infections such as scarlet fever and salmonellosis have also been incriminated.

Clinical Findings

A. Symptoms and Signs: Ataxia of the trunk and extremities may be severe, so that the child exhibits a staggering, reeling gait and inability to sit without support or to reach for objects; or there may be only mild unsteadiness. Hypotonia, tremor of the extremities, and horizontal nystagmus may be present. Speech may be slurred. The child frequently is irritable, and vomiting may occur.

There are no clinical signs of increased intracranial pressure. Sensory and reflex testing usually shows no abnormalities.

B. Laboratory Findings: Cerebrospinal fluid pressure and protein and glucose levels are normal; slight lymphocytosis (up to about 30/µL) may be present. Attempts should be made to identify the etiologic viral agent.

C. Imaging: CT scans and x-rays of long bones are normal. The EEG may be normal or may show nonspecific slowing.

Differential Diagnosis

Acute cerebellar ataxia must be differentiated from acute cerebellar syndromes due to phenytoin, phenobarbital, primidone, or lead intoxication. For phenytoin, the toxic level in serum is usually above 25 µg/mL; for phenobarbital, above 50 µg/mL; for primidone, above 14 µg/mL. (See Seizure Disorders.) With lead intoxication, papilledema, anemia, basophilic stippling of erythrocytes, proteinuria, typical x-rays, and elevated cerebrospinal fluid protein are clinical clues, confirmed by serum, urine, or hair lead levels. An occult neuroblastoma, usually seen with the polymyoclonus-opsoclonus syndrome (see below) that once was included in acute cerebellar ataxia, must also be ruled out.

In rare cases, acute cerebellar ataxia may be the presenting sign of acute bacterial meningitis or may be mimicked by corticosteroid withdrawal, vasculitides such as in polyarteritis nodosa, trauma, the first attack of ataxia in a metabolic disorder such as Hartnup disease, or the onset of acute disseminated encephalomyelitis or of multiple sclerosis. The history and physical findings may differentiate these disturbances, but appropriate laboratory studies are often necessary. For ataxias with more chronic onset and course, see the sections on spinocerebellar degeneration (below) and the other degenerative disorders.

Treatment & Prognosis

Treatment is supportive. The use of corticosteroids has no rational justification.

Between 80% and 90% of children with acute cerebellar ataxia not secondary to drug toxicity recover without sequelae within 6–8 weeks. In the remainder, neurologic disturbances, including disorders of behavior and of learning, ataxia, abnormal eye movements, and speech impairment, may persist for months or years, and recovery may remain incomplete.

Cohen HA et al: Mumps-associated acute cerebellar ataxia. Am J Dis Child 1992;146:930.

Dunn DW, Patel H: Ataxia: From the benign to the ominous. Contemp Pediatr 1991;88:82.

Swaimen K: Ataxia in childhood. Int Pediatr 1990;5:153.

Table 25–25. Central nervous system degenerative disorders of infancy.

Disease	Enzyme Defect and Genetics	Onset	Early Manifestations	Vision and Hearing	Somatic Findings	Motor System	Seizures	Laboratory and Tissue Studies	Course
WHITE MATTER									
Globoid (Krabbe's) leukodystrophy	Recessive. Galactocerebrosidase and lactosylceramidase 1 deficiency.	First 6 months; "late-onset forms."	Feeding difficulties. Shrill cry. Irritability. Arching of back.	Optic atrophy, mid-course to late. Hyperacusis occasionally.	Head often small. Often underweight.	Early spasticity, occasionally preceded by hypotonia. Prolonged nerve conduction.	Early. Myoclonic and generalized.	CSF protein elevated; usually normal in late-onset forms. Sural nerve: nonspecific myelin breakdown. Enzyme deficiency in leukocytes, cultured skin fibroblasts.	Rapid. Death usually by 1½–2 years. Late-onset cases may live 5–10 years.
Metachromatic leukodystrophy	Recessive. Arylsulfatase A deficiency.	Second year. Less often, later in childhood.	Incoordination, especially gait disturbance; then general regression. Reverse in juveniles.	Optic atrophy, usually late. Hearing normal.	Head enlarged late. None in juvenile form.	Combined upper and lower motor neuron signs. Ataxia. Prolonged nerve conduction.	Infrequent, usually late and generalized.	Metachromatic cells in urine; negative sulfatase A test. CSF protein elevated; occasionally normal early. Sural nerve biopsy: metachromasia. Enzyme deficiency in leukocytes, cultured skin fibroblasts.	Moderately slow. Death in infantile form by 3–8 years, in "juvenile" form by 10–15 years.
Adrenoleukodystrophy and variants	X-linked recessive. Neonatal form recessive.	5–10 years. Newborn.	Impaired intellect, behavioral problems.	"Cortical blindness and deafness."		Ataxia, spasticity. Motor deficits may be asymmetric, or one-sided initially.	Occasionally.	Hyperpigmentation and adrenocortical insufficiency.¹ ACTH elevated. Accumulation of very long chain fatty acids. Plasma test available.	Fairly rapid, death usually within 2–3 years after onset.
Pelizaeus-Merzbacher disease	X-linked recessive; rare female.	(?) Birth to 2 years.	"Eye rolling" often shortly after birth. Head bobbing. Slow loss of intellect.	Slowly developing optic atrophy. Hearing normal.	Head and body normal.	Cerebellar signs early, hyperactive deep reflexes. Spasticity usually only very late.	Usually only late.	None specific. Brain biopsy: extensive dymyelination with small perivascular islands of intact myelin.	Exceedingly slow, often seemingly stationary. Many survive well into adult life.
DIFFUSE, BUT PRIMARILY GRAY MATTER									
Poliodystrophy (Alpers' disease)	Occasionally familial, recessive. Possibly viral. Metabolic forms.	Infancy to adolescence.	Variable: loss of intellect, seizures, incoordination.	"Cortical blindness and deafness."	Head normal initially; may fail to grow.	Variable: incoordination, spasticity.	Often initial manifestation: myoclonic, akinetic, and generalized.	Nonspecific. CSF protein normal or slightly elevated. Extensive neuronal loss in cortex; may occur very late. Citric acid cycle defects. Increased serum pyruvate, lactate.	Usually rapid, with death within 1–3 years after onset.
Tay-Sachs disease and G$_{M2}$ gangliosidosis variants: Sandhoff disease; juvenile; chronic-adult.	Recessive. Hexosaminidase deficiencies. Tay-Sachs 93% East European Jewish; hexosaminidase A and S. Others panethnic. Sandhoff hexosaminidase A and B.	Tay-Sachs, Sandhoff similar: 3–6 months. Others 2–6 years or later. Juvenile: partial hexosaminidase A.	Variable: shrill cry, loss of vision, infantile spasms, arrest of development. In juvenile and chronic forms; motor difficulties; later, mental difficulties.	Cherry-red macula, early blindness. Hyperacusis early. Strabismus in juvenile form, blindness late.	Head enlarged late. Liver occasionally enlarged. None in juvenile or chronic forms.	Initially floppy. Eventual decerebrate rigidity. In juvenile and chronic forms; dysarthria, ataxia, spasticity.	Frequent, in mid-course and late. Infantile spasms and generalized.	Blood smears: vacuolated lymphocytes; basophilic hypergranulation. Enzyme deficiencies in serum, leukocytes, culture skin fibroblasts.	Moderately rapid. Death usually by 2–5 years. In juvenile form, 5–15 years.
Niemann-Pick disease and variants	50% Jewish. Recessive. Sphingomyelinase deficiency. In variants, enzyme defects unknown.	First 6 months. In variants, later onset: often non-Jewish.	Slow development. Protruding belly.	Cherry-red macula in 35–50%. Blindness late. Deafness occasionally.	Head usually normal. Spleen enlarged more than liver. Occasional xanthomas of skin.	Initially floppy. Eventually spastic. Occasionally extrapyramidal signs.	Rare and late.	Blood: vacuolated lymphocytes; increased lipids. X-rays: "mottled" lungs, decalcified bones. "Foam cells" in bone marrow, spleen, lymph nodes; lipid analysis of nodes.	Moderately slow. Death usually by 3–5 years.

756

Disease	Genetics/Enzyme defect	Age of onset	Early signs	Eye findings	Head/organ findings	Motor/tone	Seizures	Laboratory/diagnostic findings	Course
Infantile Gaucher's disease (glucosyl ceramide lipidosis)	Recessive. Glucocerebrosidase deficiency.	First 6 months; rarely, late infancy.	Stridor or hoarse cry. Retraction. Feeding difficulties.	Occasional cherry-red macula. Convergent squint. Deafness occasionally.	Head usually normal. Liver and spleen equally enlarged.	Opisthotonos early, followed rapidly by decerebrate rigidity.	Rare and late.	Anemia. Increased acid phosphatase. X-rays: thinned cortex, trabeculation of bones. "Gaucher cells" in bone marrow, spleen. Enzyme deficiency in leukocytes or cultured skin fibroblasts.	Very rapid.
Lipogranulomatosis (Farber's disease)	Ceramidase deficiency.	Early in infancy.	Hoarseness, irritability, restricted joint movements.	Usually normal.	Painful nodular swelling of joints; subcutaneous nodules.	Psychomotor retardation and progressive paralysis.	Usually none.	Chest x-rays may show pulmonary infiltrates. Nodules: granulomatous lesions, resembling those in reticuloendotheliosis.	Rapid: death usually in 1–2 years.
Generalized gangliosidosis and juvenile type (G$_{M1}$ gangliosidoses)	Recessive. Beta-galactosidase deficiency.	First year; less often, second year.	Arrest of development. Protruding belly. Coarse facies in infantile (generalized) form.	50% "cherry-red spot." Hearing usually normal. In juvenile type, occasionally retinitis pigmentosa.	Head enlarged early. Liver enlarged more than spleen.	Initially floppy, eventually spastic.	Usually late.	Blood: vacuolated lymphocytes. X-rays: dorsolumbar kyphosis, "beaking" of vertebrae. "Foam cells" similar to those in Niemann-Pick disease.	Very rapid. Death within a few years. Slower in juvenile type.
Subacute necrotizing encephalomyelopathy (Leigh's disease)	Recessive Variable: thiamine triphosphate "inhibitor." Also deficiency of pyruvate carboxylase, pyruvate dehydrogenase.	Infancy to late childhood.	Difficulties in feeding. Feeble or absent cry. Floppiness.	Optic atrophy, often early. Roving eye movements.	Head usually normal, occasionally small. Cardiac and renal tubular dysfunction occasionally	Flaccid and immobile; may become spastic. Spinocerebellar forms.	Rare and late.	Increased blood lactate and pyruvate. CSF, urine for "inhibitor." "Inhibitor" in brain, liver, heart, skeletal muscle.	Usually rapid in infants, but may be slow with death after several years. Central hypoventilation a frequent cause of death.
"Steel wool," or "kinky hair," disease (Menkes')	X-linked recessive. Defect in copper absorption.	Infancy.	Peculiar facies. Secondary hair white, twisted, split. Hypothermia.	May show optic disk pallor and microcysts of pigment epithelium.	Normal to small.	Variable: floppy to spastic.	Myoclonic infantile spasms, status epilepticus.	Defective adsorption of copper. Cerebralangiography shows elongated arteries. Hair shows pili torti, split shafts. CT scan may show diffuse multifocal areas of low density.	Moderately rapid. Death usually by 3–4 years.
Huntington's disease	Dominant. Genetic marker on chromosome 4.	10% childhood onset.	Rigidity, dementia.	Ophthalmoplegia late.	None.	Rigidity, Chorea frequently absent in children.	50% with major motor seizures.	CT Scan may show "butterfly" atrophy of caudate and putamen.	Moderately rapid with death in 5–15 years.
Bassen-Kornzweig disease	Recessive. Primary defect unknown.	Early childhood.	Diarrhea in infancy.	Retinitis pigmentosa; late ophthalmoplegia.	None.	Ataxia, late extrapyramidal movement disorder.	None.	Abetalipoproteinemia: acanthocytosis, low serum vitamin E.	Progression arrested with vitamin E.

[1] CSF gamma globulin (IgG) is considered elevated in children when above 9% of total protein (possibly even > 8.3%); definitely elevated when > 14%.

Table 25–26. Central nervous system degenerative disorders of childhood.[1]

Disease	Enzyme Defect and Genetics	Onset	Early Manifestations	Vision and Hearing	Motor System	Seizures	Laboratory and Tissue Studies	Course
Neuroaxonal degeneration (Seitelberger's disease). Same as, or resembling, Hallervorden-Spatz disease	Familial. (?) recessive. Girls more frequent than boys. Defect unknown.	1–3 years.	Arrest of development and dementia. Loss of motor functions. Occasionally hypesthesia over trunk and legs.	Nystagmus frequent; optic atrophy, hearing impairment.	Combined upper and lower motor neuron lesions. Early, may lie in "frog" position.	Variable, but usually not a prominent feature.	Denervation on EMG; elevated serum LDH and transaminase. Increased iron uptake in region of basal ganglia by scintillation counter probes over the temples. Brain and sural nerve: axonal swellings or "spheroids." Iron deposition in globus pallidus.	Very slowly progressive, with death early in second decade or earlier.
Neuronal ceroid lipofuscinosis (cerebromacular degeneration); Late infantile cerebral sphingolipidosis (Bielschowsky-Jansky disease)	Recessive. Defect unknown.	2–4 years.	Ataxia. Visual difficulties. Arrested intellectual development.	Pigmentary degeneration of macula. Optic atrophy. Hearing may be impaired.	Ataxia, spasticity progressing to decerebrate rigidity.	Often early; myoclonic and later generalized; difficult to control.	Blood: vacuolated lymphocytes, azurophilic dispersed hypergranulation of polymorphonuclear cells. Electroretinography helpful. Bone marrow: sea-blue histiocytes. In skin, skeletal muscle, peripheral nerves, brain: "curvilinear bodies" and "fingerprint profiles"; autofluorescent lipopigments.	Moderately slow. Death in 3–8 years.
Subacute sclerosing panencephalitis (Dawson's disease, SSPE)	None. Relatively common. Measles "slow virus" infection. Also reported as result of rubella.	3–22 years. Rarely earlier or later.	Impaired intellect, emotional lability, incoordination.	Occasionally chorioretinitis or optic atrophy. Hearing normal.	Ataxia, slurred speech, occasionally involuntary movements, spasticity progressing to decerebrate rigidity.	Myoclonic and akinetic seizures relatively early; later, focal and generalized.	CSF protein normal to moderately elevated. High CSF gamma globulin,[2] oligoclonal bands. Elevated CSF and serum measles (or rubella) antibody titers. Characteristic EEG. Brain biopsy: inclusion body encephalitis; culturing of measles virus, possibly rubella virus.	Variable, from death in months to years. Remissions of variable duration may occur. Isoprinosine produces long-term remissions.
Multiple sclerosis (See also Chapter 30.)	None. Diagnosis difficult in childhood. Defect unknown. ?Slow virus infection.	2 years on.	Highly variable: may strike one or more sites of CNS. Paresthesias common.	Optic neuritis; diplopia, nystagmus at some time. Vestibulocochlear nerves occasionally affected.	Motor weakness, spasticity, ataxia, sphincter disturbances, slurred speech, mental difficulties.	Rare: focal or generalized.	CSF may show slight pleocytosis, elevation of protein and gamma globulin;[2] oligoclonal bands present. CT scan may show areas of demyelination. Auditory, visual, and somatosensory evoked responses often show lesions in respective pathways. Changes in T cell subsets.	Variable: complete remission possible. Recurrent attacks and involvement of multiple sites are prerequisites for diagnosis.
Cerebrotendinous xanthomatosis	?Recessive. Abnormal accumulation of cholesterol.	Late childhood to adolescence.	Xanthomas in tendons. Mental deterioration.	Cataracts; xanthelasma.	Cerebellar deficits. Late: bulbar paralysis.	Myoclonus.	Xanthomas may appear in lungs. Xanthomas in tendons (especially Achilles).	Very slowly progressive into middle life. Replace deficient bile acid.
Carbohydrate-deficient glycoprotein syndrome	Recessive glycoprotein abnormality.	Infancy.	Failure to thrive, retardation.	Strabismus.	Variable.	Rare.	Transferrin decreased. Liver steatosis. Cerebellar hypoplasia.	Cardiomyopathy, thrombosis
Refsum's disease	Recessive. Phytanic acid oxidase deficiency.	5–10 years.	Ataxia, ichthyosis, cardiomyopathy.	Retinitis pigmentosa.	Ataxia.	None.	Serum phytanic acid elevated; slow nerve conduction velocity, elevated CSF protein. Peroxisomal disease.	Treat with low phytanic acid diet.

[1] For late infantile metachromatic leukodystrophy, Pelizaeus-Merzbacher disease, poliodystrophy, Gaucher's disease of later onset, and subacute necrotizing encephalomyelopathy, see Table 25–25.

[2] CSF gamma globulin (IgG) is considered elevated in children when > 9% of total protein (possibly even > 8.3%); definitively elevated when > 14%.

2. POLYMYOCLONIA-OPSOCLONUS SYNDROME OF CHILDHOOD (Infantile Myoclonic Encephalopathy, "Dancing Eyes-Dancing Feet" Syndrome)

The symptoms and signs of this syndrome are at first similar to those of "acute cerebellar ataxia." Often of sudden onset, the disorder is characterized by severe incoordination of the trunk and extremities with lightning-like jerking or flinging movements of a group of muscles, causing the child to be in constant motion while awake. Extraocular muscle involvement results in sudden irregular eye movements (opsoclonus). Irritability and vomiting are often present, but there is no depression of level of consciousness. This syndrome occurs in association with viral infections, tumors of neural crest origin, and many other disorders. Immunologic mechanisms have been postulated. There are usually no signs of increased intracranial pressure. Cerebrospinal fluid may show normal or mildly increased protein levels. Special techniques show increased cerebrospinal fluid levels of plasmacytes and abnormal immunoglobulins. The EEG may be slightly slow, but when performed together with electromyography, it shows no evidence of association between cortical discharges and the muscle movements. An assiduous search must be made to rule out tumor of neural crest origin by x-rays of the chest and CT scan or ultrasound (or both) of the adrenal area as well as by assays of urinary catecholamine metabolites (vanilmandelic acid, etc) and cystathionine.

The symptoms respond (often dramatically) to large doses of corticotropin. Otherwise, treatment is as for specific entities. When a neural crest (or possibly other) tumor is found, surgical excision should be followed by irradiation and chemotherapy. Life span is determined by the biologic behavior of the tumor.

The syndrome is usually self-limited but may be characterized by exacerbations and remissions. However, even after removal of a neural crest tumor and without other evidence of its recurrence, symptoms may reappear. A high incidence of mild mental retardation has also been recorded.

Boltshauser E, Deonna TH, Hirt HR: Myoclonic encephalopathy of infants or "dancing eyes syndrome": Report of seven cases with long-term follow-up and review of the literature (cases with and without neuroblastoma). Helv Paediatr Acta 1979;34:119.

Mitchell WG, Snodgrass SR: Opsoclonus-ataxia due to childhood neural crest tumors: A chronic neurologic syndrome. J Child Neurol 1990;5:153.

Pranzatelli MR: The neurobiology of the opsoclonus-myoclonus syndrome. Clin Neuropharmacol 1992;15:186.

3. SPINOCEREBELLAR DEGENERATION DISORDERS

Spinocerebellar degeneration disorders may be hereditary or may occur in sporadic distribution. Hereditary disorders include Friedreich's ataxia, dominant hereditary ataxia, and a group of miscellaneous diseases.

Friedreich's Ataxia

This is a recessive disorder characterized by onset of gait ataxia or scoliosis before puberty, becoming progressively worse in the first 2 years and later. Reflexes, light touch, and position sensation are reduced. Dysarthria becomes progressively more severe. Cardiomyopathy usually develops, and diabetes mellitus is found in 40% of patients, with half of these requiring insulin. Pes cavus typically is found.

Treatment includes surgery for scoliosis and intervention as needed for cardiac disease and diabetes. Patients are usually confined to a wheelchair after age 20 years. Death occurs, usually from heart failure or dysrhythmias, in the third or fourth decade; some patients survive longer.

Dominant Ataxia

This disease (also known as olivopontocerebellar atrophy, Holmes's ataxia, Marie's ataxia, etc) occurs with varying manifestations, even among members of the same family. Ataxia occurs at onset, and progression continues with ophthalmoplegias, extrapyramidal tract and motor neuron degeneration, and later dementia. Levodopa may ameliorate rigidity and bradykinesia, but no other therapy is available. Only 10% have onset in childhood, and their course is often more rapid.

Miscellaneous Hereditary Ataxias

Associated findings permit identification of these recessive disorders. These include ataxia-telangiectasia (telangiectasia, immune defects; see below), Wilson's disease (Kayser-Fleischer rings), Refsum's disease (ichthyosis, cardiomyopathy, retinitis pigmentosa, large nerves), Rett's syndrome (regression to autism at 7–18 months in girls, loss of use of hands, progressive failure of brain growth), and abetalipoproteinemia (infantile diarrhea, acanthocytosis, retinitis pigmentosa). Patients with juvenile and chronic gangliosidoses and some hemolytic anemias and long-term survivors of Chédiak-Higashi disease may develop spinocerebellar degeneration. Idiopathic familial ataxia is called Behr's syndrome. Neuropathies such as Charcot-Marie-Tooth disease produce ataxia.

Haas R, Rapin I, Moser H: Rett syndrome and autism. J Child Neurol 1988;3(Suppl):52.

Sheu KFR et al: Mitochondrial enzymes in hereditary ataxias. Metab Brain Dis 1988;3:151.

Stumpf DA: The inherited ataxias. Neurol Clin 1985;3:47.

ATAXIA-TELANGIECTASIA
(Louis-Bar Syndrome)

Ataxia-telangiectasia is a multisystem disorder inherited as an autosomal recessive trait. It is characterized by progressive ataxia; telangiectasia of the bulbar conjunctiva, external ears, nares, and (later) other body surfaces, appearing in the third to sixth year; and recurrent respiratory, sinus, and ear infections. Ocular dyspraxia, slurred speech, choreoathetosis, hypotonia and areflexia, and psychomotor and growth retardation may be present. Endocrinopathies are common. Nerve conduction velocities may be reduced. The entire nervous system may be affected in late stages of the disease. A spectrum of involvement may be seen in the same family. Immunodeficiencies of IgA and IgE are common (see Chapter 29), and the incidence of certain cancers is high.

Ataxia-telangiectasia: A multisystem hereditary disease with immunodeficiency, impaired organ maturation, x-ray hypersensitivity, and a high incidence of neoplasia. (NIH Conference.) Ann Intern Med 1983;99:367.
Swift M et al: Incidence of cancer in 161 families affected by ataxia-telangiectasia. N Engl J Med 1991;325:1831.

EXTRAPYRAMIDAL DISORDERS

Extrapyramidal disorders are characterized by the presence in the waking state of one or more of the following features: dyskinesias, athetosis, ballismus, tremors, rigidity, and dystonias.

For the most part, precise pathologic and anatomic localization is not completely understood. Motor pathways synapsing in the striatum (putamen and caudate nucleus), globus pallidus, red nucleus, substantia nigra, and the body of Luys are involved; this "system" is modulated by pathways originating in the thalamus, cerebellum, and reticular formation.

1. SYDENHAM'S POSTRHEUMATIC CHOREA

Sydenham's chorea is characterized by an acute onset of choreiform movements and variable degrees of psychologic disturbance. It is frequently associated with endocarditis and arthritis. Although the disorder follows infections with β-hemolytic streptococci, the interval between infection and chorea may be greatly prolonged; throat cultures and antistreptolysin O (ASO) titers may therefore be negative. Psychic predisposition may also play a role. Chorea has also been associated with hypocalcemia, with vascular lupus erythematosus, and with toxic, viral, infectious and parainfectious, and degenerative encephalopathies.

Clinical Findings

A. Symptoms and Signs: Chorea, or rapid involuntary movements of the limbs and face, is the hallmark physical finding. In addition to the jerky incoordinate movements, the following are noted: emotional lability, waxing and waning ("milkmaid's") grip, darting tongue, "spooning" of the extended hands and their tendency to pronate, and knee jerks slow to return from the extended to their prestimulus position ("hung up"). Seizures, while uncommon, may be masked by choreic jerks.

B. Laboratory Findings: Anemia, leukocytosis, and an increased erythrocyte sedimentation rate may be present. The ASO titer may be elevated and C-reactive protein present. Throat culture is sometimes positive for β-hemolytic streptococci.

Electrocardiography and echocardiography are often essential to detect cardiac involvement. Antineuronal antibodies are present in most patients but are not specific. Electroencephalography may show nonspecific slowing or seizure activity.

Differential Diagnosis

The diagnosis is usually not difficult. Tics, drug-induced extrapyramidal syndromes, Huntington's chorea, and hepatolenticular degeneration (Wilson's disease), as well as other rare movement disorders, can usually be ruled out on historical and clinical grounds.

Other causes of chorea can be ruled out by laboratory tests, eg, ANA (antinuclear antibody) for lupus, TSH, T_4 for thyroid disease, serum calcium for hypocalcemia, Monospot for mononucleosis.

Treatment

There is no specific treatment. Dopaminergic blockers such as haloperidol, 0.5 mg to 3–6 mg/d, or pimozide, 4–12 mg /d, have been utilized. Parkinsonian side effects such as rigidity and masked facies and, with high doses, tardive dyskinesia rarely occur in childhood. Phenothiazines such as chlorpromazine, 25–50 mg three times a day, involve similar risks. A variety of other drugs have been utilized with success in individual cases, eg, the anticonvulsant sodium valproate, 50–60 mg/kg/d in divided doses, or prednisone, 0.5–2 mg/kg in divided doses. Emotional lability and depression sometimes warrant antidepressants such as amitriptyline, 25 or 50 mg/d.

All patients should be given antistreptococcal prophylaxis with benzathine penicillin, 0.6–1.2 million units/25 days intramuscularly, or oral penicillin or sulfonamides.

Prognosis

Sydenham's chorea is a self-limiting disease that may last from a few weeks to months. Two-thirds of patients relapse one or more times, but the ultimate outcome does not appear to be worse in those with recurrences. Valvular heart disease occurs in about one-third of patients, particularly if other rheumatic manifestations appear. Psychoneurotic disturbances, if not already present at the onset of illness, occur in a significant percentage of patients.

Dhanaraj M et al: Sodium valproate in Sydenham's chorea. Neurology 1985;35:114.

Kiessling LS, Marcotte AC, Culpepper L: Antineuronal antibodies in movement disorders. Pediatrics 1993;92:39.

Nausieda PA et al: Sydenham chorea: An update. Neurology 1980;30:331.

Peters ACB et al: ECHO 25 focal encephalitis and subacute hemichorea. Neurology 1979;29:676.

Pranzetelli MR: An approach to movement disorders in childhood. Pediatr Ann 1993;22:13.

Swedo SE et al: Sydenham's chorea: Physical and psychological symptoms of St Vitus dance. Pediatrics 1993;91:706.

2. TICS
(Habit Spasms)

Tics, or habit spasms, are quick repetitive but irregular movements, often stereotyped, and briefly suppressible. Coordination and muscle tone are not affected. A psychogenic basis is seldom discernible.

Transient tics of childhood (12–24% incidence in school-age children) last from 1 month to 1 year and seldom need treatment. Many children with tics have a history of encephalopathic past events, "soft signs" on neurologic examination, and school problems.

Facial tics such as grimaces, twitches, and blinking predominate, but the trunk and extremities are often involved and there are twisting or flinging movements. Vocal tics are less common.

Gilles de la Tourette's syndrome is a chronic disorder of multiple fluctuating motor and vocal tics, with onset in childhood, lasting more than a year, with absence of other recognizable causes for tics. Tics evolve slowly, new ones being added to or replacing old ones. Coprolalia and echolalia are relatively infrequent. Partial forms are common. The usual age at onset is 2–15 years, and the familial incidence is 35–50%; the disorder is now reported in almost all ethnic groups. Gilles de la Tourette's syndrome may be triggered by stimulants such as methylphenidate and dextroamphetamine. An imbalance of neurotransmitters, especially dopamine and serotonin, has been hypothesized.

In relatively mild cases, tics are self-limited and, when disregarded, disappear. When attention is paid to one tic, it may disappear only to be replaced by another that is often worse. If the tic and its underlying anxiety or compulsive neurosis are severe, psychiatric evaluation and treatment are needed.

Important comorbidities are attention deficit hyperactivity disorder and obsessive-compulsive disorder. Medications such as methylphenidate and dextroamphetamine may have to be carefully titrated to treat ADHD and avoid worsening tics. Fluoxetine and clomipramine may be useful for obsessive-compulsive disorder in patients with tics.

When medication is required to treat Tourette's syndrome, the most effective agents are dopamine blockers. However, many pediatric patients can manage without drug treatment. Generally, medications are reserved for patients with disabling symptoms; treatment may be relaxed or discontinued when the symptoms abate.

Nonpharmacologic treatment of Tourette's syndrome includes education of patients, family members, and school personnel. In some cases, restructuring the school environment to prevent tension and teasing may be necessary; supportive counseling, either at or outside school, should be provided.

Usually, medications will not eradicate the tics. Accordingly, the goal of treatment should be to reduce the tics to tolerable levels without inducing undesirable side effects. Dosage should be increased at weekly intervals until a satisfactory response is obtained. Often, a single dose at bedtime is sufficient. The two neuroleptic agents used most often are haloperidol and fluphenazine; side effects to be avoided include akathisia and tardive dyskinesia. The newest neuroleptic agent in use is pimozide; motor side effects of this drug are the same as those encountered with the use of other dopamine blockers.

Clonidine, clonazepam, and calcium channel blockers have been used in individual patients with some success; sometimes these agents are used for combined therapy (eg, haloperidol with nifedipine).

Barbas G (editor): [Many articles on Tourette's syndrome.] Psychiatr Ann (July) 1988;18:393.

Caine ED: Gilles de la Tourette's syndrome: A review of clinical and research studies and consideration of future directions for investigation. Arch Neurol 1985;42:393.

Calderone-Gonzales R, Calderone-Sepulveda R: Tourette syndrome: Current concepts. Int Pediatr 1993;8:176.

Como PG, Kurlan R: An open-label trial of fluoxetine for obsessive-compulsive disorder in Gilles de la Tourette's syndrome. Neurology 1991;41:872.

Harlan R et al: Sensory tics in Tourette's syndrome. Neurology 1989;39:731.

Harlan R et al: Transient tic disorder and the spectrum of Tourette syndrome. Arch Neurol 1988;45:1200.

Singer H: Tic disorders. Pediatr Ann 1993;33:33.

Stokes A et al: Peer problems in Tourette's disorder. Pediatrics 1991;87:936.

INFECTIONS & INFLAMMATORY DISORDERS OF THE CENTRAL NERVOUS SYSTEM

Infections of the central nervous system are among the most common neurologic disorders encountered by the pediatrician. While infections are among the central nervous system disorders most amenable to treatment, they are also among the disorders that have the highest potential for causing catastrophic destruction of the nervous system. It is imperative for the clinician to recognize such infections early. Appropriate therapy must be started as early as possible in order to prevent massive tissue destruction.

Clinical Manifestations

Patients with central nervous system infections, whether caused by bacteria, viruses, or other microorganisms, present with similar manifestations. Systemic signs of infection include fever, generalized malaise, or impaired heart, lung, liver, or kidney function. General features suggesting central nervous system infection consist of headache, stiff neck, fever or hypothermia, changes in mental status (including hyperirritability evolving into lethargy and coma), seizures, and focal sensory and motor deficits. On examination, meningeal irritation is manifested by the presence of Kernig's and Brudzinski's signs. In very young infants, signs of meningeal irritation may be absent, and temperature instability and hypothermia are often more prominent than fever. In young infants, a bulging fontanelle and an increased head circumference are common. Papilledema may eventually develop, particularly in older children and adolescents. Cranial nerve palsies may develop acutely or gradually during the course of neurologic infections. No specific clinical sign or symptom is reliable in distinguishing bacterial infections from infections caused by other microbes.

During the initial clinical assessment, conditions that predispose the patient to infection of the central nervous system should be sought. Infections involving the sinuses or other structures in the head and neck region can result in direct extension of infection into the intracranial compartment. Open head injuries, recent neurosurgical procedures, immunodeficiencies, and the presence of a mechanical shunt may provide strong evidence regarding the nature of the underlying illness.

Laboratory Investigation

When central nervous system infections are suspected, blood should be obtained for a complete blood count, general chemistry panel, and culture. Most important, however, is obtaining cerebrospinal fluid. In the absence of focal neurologic deficits or signs of increased intracranial pressure, spinal fluid should be obtained immediately from any patient in whom serious central nervous system infection is suspected. When papilledema or focal motor signs are present, a lumbar puncture may be delayed until a neuroimaging procedure has been done to exclude brain abscess or other space-occupying lesion. It is generally safe to obtain spinal fluid from infants with nonfocal neurologic examination even if the fontanelle is bulging. Once spinal fluid is obtained, it should be examined for the presence of red and white blood cells, protein concentration, glucose concentration, bacteria and other microorganisms, and a sample should be cultured. In addition, serologic and immunologic tests may be performed on the spinal fluid in an attempt to identify the specific organism. As a general rule, spinal fluid that contains a high proportion of polymorphonuclear leukocytes, a high protein concentration, and a low glucose concentration strongly suggests bacterial infection. Spinal fluid containing predominantly lymphocytes, a high protein concentration, and a low glucose concentration suggests infection with mycobacteria, fungi, uncommon bacteria, and some viruses such as lymphocytic choriomeningitis virus, herpes simplex virus, mumps virus, and arboviruses. Cerebrospinal fluid that contains a high proportion of lymphocytes, normal or only slightly elevated protein concentration, and a normal glucose concentration is most suggestive of viral infections, though partially treated bacterial meningitis and parameningeal infections may also result in this type of cerebrospinal fluid formula. Typical spinal fluid findings in a variety of infectious and inflammatory disorders are shown in Table 25–3.

Neuroimaging procedures such as CT and MRI may be helpful in demonstrating the presence of brain abscess, meningeal inflammation, or secondary problems such as venous and arterial infarctions, hemorrhages, and subdural effusions when these are expected. In addition, these neuroimaging procedures may identify sinus infections or other focal infections in the head or neck region that are related to the central nervous system infection. CT scanning may demonstrate bony abnormalities, such as basilar fractures, that are etiologically important to the central nervous system infection.

EEGs may be helpful in the assessment of patients who have had seizures at the time of presentation. The changes are often nonspecific and characterized by generalized slowing. In some instances, such as herpes simplex virus infection, focal electronegative activity may be seen early in the course and may be one of the earliest laboratory abnormalities to suggest the diagnosis. EEGs may also show focal slowing over regions of abscesses. Unusual, characteristic electroencephalographic patterns are seen in some patients with subacute sclerosing panencephalitis.

In some cases, brain biopsy may be needed to identify the presence of specific organisms and clarify the diagnosis. Herpes simplex virus infections are confirmed by histologic examination or culture of brain tissue. Brain biopsy is often needed to distinguish herpes simplex encephalitis from parasitic infections, brain tumors, and other structural abnormalities.

BACTERIAL MENINGITIS

Bacterial infections of the central nervous system may present acutely (symptoms evolving rapidly over 1–24 hours), subacutely (symptoms evolving over 1–7 days), or chronically (symptoms evolving over more than 1 week). Diffuse bacterial infections involve the leptomeninges, superficial cortical structures, and blood vessels. Although the term "meningitis" is used to describe these infections, it should not be forgotten that the brain parenchyma is also inflamed and that blood vessel walls may also be infiltrated by inflammatory cells that result in endothelial cell injury, vessel stenosis, and secondary ischemia and infarction.

Symptoms and findings of bacterial meningitis are described above. No specific features reliably distinguish infections caused by bacteria from infections caused by viruses, fungi, parasites, or other microbes.

Pathologically, the inflammatory process involves all intracranial structures to some degree. Acutely, this inflammatory process may result in cerebral edema or impaired cerebrospinal fluid flow through and out of the ventricular system resulting in hydrocephalus. Many bacterial infections are characterized by early and extensive involvement of blood vessels, both arteries and veins, resulting in ischemia, ischemic infarction, or hemorrhagic infarction.

Treatment

A. Specific Measures: (See also Chapter 36, *Haemophilus influenzae* type B infections, and Chapter 34.) Children under 3 months of age are treated initially with cefotaxime (or ceftriaxone if over 1 month of age) and ampicillin; the latter agent is used to treat *Listeria* and enterococci, agents that rarely affect older children. Children older than 3 months are treated with ceftriaxone, cefotaxime, or ampicillin plus chloramphenicol. If *S pneumoniae* cannot be ruled out by the initial Gram stain, the vancomycin is added until cultures are reported, since penicillin-resistant pneumococci are becoming more common in this country. Therapy may be narrowed if organism sensitivity allows. Duration of therapy is 7 days for meningococcal infections 10 days for *H influenzae* or pneumococcal infection, and 14–21 days for other organisms. Slow clinical response or the occurrence of complications may prolong the need for therapy. Although therapy for 7 days has proved successful in many children with *Haemophilus* infection, it cannot be recommended if steroids are also used (see below) without further study.

B. General and Supportive Measures: Children with bacterial meningitis are often systemically ill. The following complications should be looked for and treated aggressively: hypovolemia, hypoglycemia, hyponatremia, acidosis, septic shock, increased intracranial pressure, seizures, disseminated intravascular coagulation, and metastatic infection (eg, pericarditis, arthritis, and pneumonia). Children should initially be monitored closely (cardiorespiratory monitor, strict fluid balance and frequent urine specific gravity assessment, daily weights, neurologic assessment every few hours), not fed until neurologically very stable, isolated until the organism is known, rehydrated with isotonic solutions until euvolemic, and then given intravenous fluids containing dextrose and sodium at no more than maintenance rate (assuming no unusual losses occur).

Complications

Abnormalities of water and electrolyte balance result from either excessive or insufficient production of antidiuretic hormone and require careful monitoring and appropriate adjustments in fluid administration. Monitoring serum sodium every 8–12 hours during the first 1 or 2 days—and urine sodium if the inappropriate secretion of antidiuretic hormone is suspected—usually uncovers significant problems.

Seizures occur in up to 30% of children with bacterial meningitis. Seizures tend to be most frequent in neonates and less common in older children. Persistent focal seizures or focal seizures associated with focal neurologic deficits strongly suggest subdural effusion, abscess, or vascular lesions such as arterial infarct, cortical venous infarcts, or dural sinus thrombosis. Because generalized seizures in a metabolically compromised child may have severe sequelae, early recognition and therapy are critical; some practitioners prefer phenytoin for acute management because it is less sedating than phenobarbital.

Subdural effusions occur in as many as 50% of young children with *H influenzae* meningitis. Subdural effusions are often seen on CT scans of the head during the course of meningitis. They do not require treatment unless they are producing increased intracranial pressure or progressive mass effect. Although subdural effusions may be detected in children with persistent fever, such effusions do not usually have to be sampled or drained if the infecting organism is *Haemophilus*, meningococcus, or pneumococcus. These are usually sterilized with the standard treatment duration, and slowly waning fever during an otherwise uncomplicated recovery may be followed clinically. Under any other circumstance, however, aspiration of the fluid for documentation of sterilization or relief of pressure should be considered.

Cerebral edema can participate in the production of increased intracranial pressure, requiring treatment with dexamethasone, osmotic agents, diuretics, or hyperventilation; continuous pressure monitoring may be needed.

Long-term sequelae of meningitis result from direct inflammatory destruction of brain cells, vascular injuries, or secondary gliosis. Focal motor and sensory deficits, visual impairment, hearing loss, seizures, hydrocephalus, and a variety of cranial nerve deficits can result from meningitis. Sensorineural hearing loss in *H influenzae* meningitis occurs in approximately 5–10% of cases during long-term follow-up. Recent studies have suggested that the early addition of dexamethasone to the antibiotic regimen may modestly decrease the risk of hearing loss in some children with *H influenzae* meningitis (see Chapter 36).

In addition to the variety of disorders mentioned above, some patients with meningitis suffer from mental retardation and severe behavioral disorders that limit their function at school and later performance in life. Table 25–27 lists the overall mortality and morbidity figures for the most common organisms associated with acute bacterial meningitis in childhood.

BRAIN ABSCESS

Patients with brain abscess often appear to have systemic illness similar to patients with bacterial meningitis, but in addition they show signs of focal neurologic deficits, papilledema, and other evidence of increased intracranial pressure or evidence of a mass lesion. Symptoms may be present for a week or more; children with bacterial meningitis usually present within a few days. Conditions predisposing to development of brain abscess include penetrating head trauma; chronic infection of the middle ear, mastoid, or sinuses (especially the frontal sinus); chronic infection; cardiovascular lesions allowing right-to-left shunting of blood (including arteriovenous malformations); endocarditis; and meningeal infection, especially with necrotizing organisms such as enterics or staphylococci.

When brain abscess is strongly suspected, a neu-roimaging procedure such as CT or MRI should be done prior to lumbar puncture. If a brain abscess is identified, lumbar puncture may be dangerous and rarely alters the choice of antibiotic or clinical management since the spinal fluid abnormalities usually reflect only parameningeal inflammation. Table 25–28 lists organisms most often recovered from brain abscesses in children. Unfortunately, cultures from a large number of brain abscesses remain negative and the organisms responsible unknown.

The diagnosis of brain abscess is based primarily on a strong clinical suspicion and confirmed by a neuroimaging procedure. As mentioned earlier, electroencephalographic changes are nonspecific but frequently demonstrate focal slowing in the region of brain abscess. Treatment includes antibiotic management (as outlined in Table 25–28), neurologic consultation, and anticonvulsant and edema therapy if necessary. In their early stages, brain abscesses are areas of focal cerebritis and can be "cured" with antibiotic treatment alone, without surgical intervention. Well-developed abscesses require surgical drainage.

Differential diagnosis of brain abscess includes any condition that produces focal neurologic deficits and increased intracranial pressure, such as neoplasms, subdural effusions, cerebral infarctions, and cerebral edema.

The surgical mortality rate in the treatment of brain abscess is less than 5%. Untreated cerebral abscesses lead to irreversible tissue destruction and may rupture into the ventricle, producing catastrophic deterioration in neurologic function and death. Because brain abscesses are often associated with systemic illness and systemic infections, the death rate is frequently high in these patients.

VIRAL INFECTIONS

Viral infections of the central nervous system can involve primarily meninges (meningitis) (see Chapter 35) or cerebral parenchyma (encephalitis). All patients, however, have some degree of involvement of both the meninges and cerebral parenchyma (menin-

Table 25–27. Outcome of acute bacterial meningitis by organism.

Organism	Mortality (%)	Motor Handicap (%)		Intellect (%)	
		None	Severe	Normal	Severe Mental Retardation
Escherichia coli gram-negative organisms	20–50	62	25	75	25
Haemophilus influenzae	5–10	87	3	82	5
Streptococcus pneumoniae	10–30	96	0	83	0
Neisseria meningitidis	5–10	100	0	93	0
Group B streptococci	20	85	10–15	100	0
Overall total	10–25	85	5	82	6

Table 25–28. Initial antibiotic coverage for organisms commonly found in brain abscesses.

Suspected Organism	Drug
Staphylococcus aureus	Nafcillin or methicillin
β-Hemolytic streptococcus	Penicillin G
Viridans streptococci	Penicillin G
Gram-negative bacteria	Cefotaxime, ceftriaxone, or chloramphenicol
Anaerobic bacteria or unknown (cultures pending)	Penicillin G and chloramphenicol or metronidazole (unless *Staphylococcus* is suspected)

goencephalitis). Many viral infections are generalized and diffuse, but some viruses, notably herpes simplex and some arboviruses, characteristically cause prominent focal disease. Focal cerebral involvement is clearly evident on neuroimaging procedures. Some viruses have an affinity for specific central nervous system cell populations. Poliovirus and other enteroviruses can selectively infect anterior horn cells (poliomyelitis) and some intracranial motor neurons.

Although most viral infections of the nervous system present with an acute or subacute course in childhood, chronic infections can occur. Subacute sclerosing panencephalitis, for example, represents a chronic indolent infection caused by measles virus and is characterized clinically by progressive neurodegeneration and seizures.

Inflammatory reactions within the nervous system may occur during the convalescent stage of systemic viral infections. Parainfectious or postinfectious inflammation of the central nervous system results in several well-recognized disorders: acute disseminated encephalomyelitis, transverse myelitis, optic neuritis, polyneuritis, and Guillain-Barré syndrome.

Congenital viral infections can also affect the central nervous system. Cytomegalovirus, herpes simplex virus, and rubella virus are the most notable causes of viral brain injury in utero.

Treatment of viral infections of the nervous system is usually limited to symptomatic and supportive measures, except for herpes simplex virus. Acyclovir is the treatment of choice in suspected or proved cases of herpes simplex virus encephalitis. Acyclovir is also useful in some patients with varicella-zoster virus infections of the central nervous system.

Encephalopathy of HIV Infection

Neurologic syndromes associated directly with HIV infection (Table 25–29) include subacute encephalitis, meningitis, myelopathy, polyneuropathy, and myositis. In addition, secondary opportunistic infections of the central nervous system occur in patients with HIV-induced immunosuppression; toxoplasmal and cytomegaloviral infections have been

particularly common. Progressive multifocal leukoencephalopathy, a secondary papovavirus infection, and herpes simplex virus and herpes zoster virus infections also occur frequently in patients with HIV infection. A variety of fungal, mycobacterial, and bacterial infections have been described also.

Neurologic abnormalities in these patients can also be the result of noninfectious neoplastic disorders. Primary central nervous system lymphoma and metastatic lymphoma to the nervous system are the most frequent neoplasms involving the nervous system in these patients. See Chapters 29 and 35 for the diagnosis and management of HIV infection.

OTHER INFECTIONS

A wide variety of other microorganisms, including *Toxoplasma*, mycobacteria, spirochetes, rickettsiae, amebas, and mycoplasmas, can cause central nervous system infections. Central nervous system involvement in these infections is usually secondary to systemic infection or other predisposing factors. Appropriate cultures and serologic testing are required to confirm infections by these organisms. Parenteral antimicrobial treatment for these infections is discussed elsewhere in this text.

NONINFECTIOUS INFLAMMATORY DISORDERS OF THE CENTRAL NERVOUS SYSTEM

In the differential diagnosis of bacterial, viral, and other microbial infections of the central nervous system are disorders that cause inflammation but for which no specific etiologic organism has been identified. Sarcoidosis, Behçet's syndrome, systemic lupus erythematosus, other collagen-vascular disorders, and Kawasaki disease are examples. In these disorders, central nervous system inflammation usually occurs

Table 25–29. Neurologic aspects of HIV infection.

Direct HIV effects
  Encephalopathy
  Meningitis
  Myelopathy
  Neuropathy-neuritis
  Myositis
Secondary infections
  Toxoplasma meningoencephalitis
  Cytomegalovirus infections
  Herpes simplex virus infections
  Papovavirus infection (progressive multifocal leukoencephalopathy)
  Fungal infections
  Mycobacterial infections
Neoplasms
  Primary CNS lymphoma
  Metastatic lymphoma

in association with characteristic systemic manifestations that allow proper diagnosis. Management of central nervous system involvement in these disorders is the same as the treatment of the systemic illness.

OTHER PARAINFECTIOUS ENCEPHALOPATHIES

In association with systemic infections or other illnesses, central nervous system dysfunction may occur in the absence of direct central nervous system inflammation or infection. Reye's syndrome is a prominent example of this type of encephalopathy that often occurs in association with varicella virus or other respiratory or systemic viral infections. In Reye's syndrome, cerebral edema and cerebral dysfunction occur, but there is no evidence of any direct involvement of the nervous system by the associated microorganism or inflammation. Cerebral edema in Reye's syndrome is accompanied by liver dysfunction and fatty infiltration of the liver. Perhaps as a result of recent efforts to discourage use of aspirin in childhood febrile illnesses, there has been a marked decrease in the number of patients with Reye's syndrome. The precise relationship, however, between aspirin and Reye's syndrome is not clear.

Ashwal S et al: Bacterial meningitis in children. Neurology 1992;42:739.
Burns D: The neuropathology of pediatric acquired immunodeficiency syndrome. J Child Neurol 1992;7:332.
DeCarli C et al: The prevalence of computed tomographic abnormalities of the cerebrum in 100 consecutive children symptomatic with the human immune deficiency virus. Ann Neurol 1993;34:198.
Epstein LG, Gendelman HE: Human immunodeficiency virus type 1 infection of the nervous system: Pathogenetic mechanisms. Ann Neurol 1993;33:429.
Kohl S: Herpes simplex virus encephalitis in children. Pediatr Clin North Am 1988;35:465.
McCracken GH: Current management of bacterial meningitis in infants and children. Pediatr Infect Dis 1992;11:169.
Patrick CC, Kaplan SL: Current concepts in the pathogenesis and management of brain abscesses in children. Pediatr Clin North Am 1988;35:625.
Pomeroy SL et al: Seizures and other neurologic sequelae of bacterial meningitis in children. N Engl J Med 1990;323:1651.
Quagliarello V, Scheld WM: Bacterial meningitis: Pathogenesis, pathophysiology, and progress. N Engl J Med 1992;327:864.
Saez-Llorens X, McCracken GH: Bacterial meningitis in neonates and children. Infect Dis Clin North Am 1990;4:623.
Saez-Llorens X et al: Molecular pathophysiology of bacterial meningitis: Current concepts and therapeutic implications. J Pediatr 1990;116:671
Whitley RJ: Viral encephalitis. N Engl J Med 1990;323:242.

SYNDROMES PRESENTING AS ACUTE FLACCID PARALYSIS

Flaccid paralysis evolving over hours or a few days suggests involvement of the lower motor neuron complex (see Floppy Infant Syndrome). **Anterior horn cells** (spinal cord) may be involved by viral infection (paralytic poliomyelitis) or paraviral or postviral immunologically mediated disease (acute transverse myelitis). The **nerve trunks** (polyneuritis) may be diseased as in Guillain-Barré syndrome or affected by toxins (diphtheria, porphyria). The **neuromuscular junction** may be blocked by tick toxin or botulinum toxin. The paralysis rarely will be due to metabolic (periodic paralysis) or inflammatory muscle disease (myositis). *A lesion compressing the spinal cord must be ruled out.*

Clinical Findings

A. Symptoms and Signs: (Table 25–30.) The features that aid in diagnosis are age, a history of preceding or waning illness, the presence (at time of paralysis) of fever, rapidity of progression, cranial nerve findings, and sensory findings. The examination may show "long tract" findings (pyramidal tract), causing increased reflexes and positive Babinski sign. The spinothalamic tract may be interrupted, causing loss of pain and temperature. Back pain—even tenderness to percussion—may occur, as well as bowel and bladder dysfunction (incontinence). Often, the paralysis is ascending, symmetric, and painful (muscle tenderness or myalgia). Laboratory findings occasionally are diagnostic.

B. Laboratory Findings: (Table 25–30.) The examination of spinal fluid is most helpful. Imaging studies of the spinal column (plain films) and spinal cord (MRI, myelogram) are occasionally essential. Viral cultures (spinal fluid, throat, stool) and titers aid in diagnosing poliomyelitis. A high sedimentation rate may suggest tumor or abscess; antinuclear antibody (ANA) may suggest lupus arteritis.

Electromyography and nerve conduction velocity can be helpful in diagnosing polyneuropathy. Nerve conduction is usually slowed after 7–10 days. Findings in botulism and tick-bite paralysis can be specific and diagnostic. Rarely, elevation of muscle enzymes—or even myoglobinuria—may aid in diagnosis of myopathic paralysis. Porphyrin urine studies and heavy metal assays (arsenic, thallium, lead) can reveal those rare toxic causes of polyneuropathic paralysis.

Differential Diagnosis

The child who is "well" and becomes paralyzed often has polyneuritis. Acute transverse myelitis sometimes occurs in an afebrile child. The child who is ill and febrile at the time of paralysis often has acute transverse myelitis (or poliomyelitis); *acute epidural spinal cord abscess* (or other compressive le-

Table 25–30. Acute flaccid paralysis in children.

	Poliomyelitis (Paralytic, Spinal, and Bulbar), With or Without Encephalitis	Landry-Guillain-Barré Syndrome ("Acute Idiopathic Polyneuritis")	Botulism	Tick-Bite Paralysis	Transverse Myelitis and Neuromyelitis Optica
Etiology	Poliovirus types I, II, and III; Other enteroviruses; Immunization virus (rare).	Likely delayed hypersensitivity-immunologic. Mycoplasmal and viral infections (including infectious mononucleosis) and various systemic or toxic disorders may be underlying cause. *Campylobacter* enteritis. Hepatitis B.	*Clostridium botulinum* toxin. Block at neuromusclar junction. Under age one, toxin forms in bowel from ingested dust or honey in formula. At older ages, contaminated food (preformed toxin). Rarely from wound infection.	Probable interference with transmission of nerve impulse caused by toxin in tick saliva.	Usually unknown; immunodeficiency state (?)
History	None, or inadequate polio immunization. Upper respiratory or gastrointestinal symptoms followed by brief respite. Bulbar paralysis more frequent after tonsillectomy. Often in epidemics, in summer and early fall.	Nonspecific respiratory or gastrointestinal symptoms in preceding 5–14 days common. Any season, though slightly lower incidence in summer.	Infancy: dusty environment (eg, construction area), suburbs; honey. Older: "food poisoning." Multiple cases hours to days after ingesting contaminated food.	Exposure to ticks (dog tick in eastern USA; wood ticks). Irritability 12–24 hours before onset of a rapidly progressive ascending paralysis.	Occasionally, symptoms compatible with multiple sclerosis or optic neuritis. Progression from onset to paraplegia very rapid, usually without a history of bacterial infection.
Presenting complaints	Febrile at time of paralysis. Meningeal signs, muscle tenderness, and spasm. Asymmetric weakness widespread or segmental (cervical, thoracic, lumbar). Bulbar symptoms early or before extremity weakness. Anxiety. Delirium.	Symmetric weakness of lower extremities, which may ascend rapidly to arms, trunk, and face. Verbal child may complain of paresthesias. Fever uncommon. Facial weakness early. Miller-Fisher variant presents as ataxia and ophthalmoplegia.	Infancy: constipation, poor suck and cry. "Floppy." Apnea. Lethargy. Choking (cause of SIDS?). Older: blurred vision, diplopia, ptosis, choking, weakness.	Rapid onset and progression of ascending flaccid paralysis; often accompanied by pain and paresthesias. Paralysis of upper extremities usually occurs on second day after onset.	Root and back pain in about one-third of cases. Sensory loss below level of lesion accompanying rapidly developing paralysis. Sphincter difficulties common.
Findings	Flaccid weakness, usually asymmetric. Lumbar: legs, lower abdomen. Cervical: shoulder, arm, neck, diaphragm. Thoracic: intercostals, spine, upper abdomen. Bulbar: respiratory, lower cranial nerves. Fever in first days.	Flaccid weakness, symmetric, usually greater proximally, but may be more distal or equal in distribution. Facial diplegia in about 85%, then IX–X, XI, III–VI. Bulbar involvement may occur. Slight distal impairment of position, vibration, touch; difficult to assess in young children.	Infants: flaccid weakness. Alert. Eye, pupil, facial weakness. Deep tendon reflexes (DTR) decreased to 0? Absent suck, gag. Constipation. Older: paralysis accommodation, eye movements. Weak swallow. Respiratory paralysis.	Flaccid, symmetric paralysis. Cranial nerve and bulbar (respiratory) paralysis, ataxia, sphincter disturbances, and sensory deficits may occur. Some fever. Diagnosis rests on finding tick, which is especially likely to be on occipital scalp.	Paraplegia with areflexia below level of lesion early; later, may have hyperreflexia. Sensory loss below and hyperesthesia or normal sensation above level of lesion. Paralysis of bladder and rectum. Optic atrophy or neuritis may be present.
CSF	Pleocytosis (20–500 + cells) with PMN predominance in first few days, followed by rapid decrease and monocytic preponderance. Glucose normal. Protein frequently elevated (50–150 mg/dL).	Cytoalbuminologic dissociation; 10 or fewer mononuclear cells with high protein after first week. Normal glucose. Gamma globulin may be elevated.	Normal.	Normal.	Usually no manometric block; CSF may show increased protein, pleocytosis with predominantly mononuclear cells, increased gamma globulin.

(*continued*)

Table 25–30. Acute flaccid paralysis in children. (continued)

	Poliomyelitis (Paralytic, Spinal, and Bulbar), With or Without Encephalitis	Landry-Guillain-Barré Syndrome ("Acute Idiopathic Polyneuritis")	Botulism	Tick-Bite Paralysis	Transverse Myelitis and Neuromyelitis Optica
EMG	Denervation after 10–21 days. Nerve conduction normal.	Nerve conduction velocities markedly decreased, may be normal early.	EMG distinctive: BSAP ("brief small abundant potentials").	Nerve conduction slowed; returns rapidly to normal after removal of tick.	Normal early. Denervation at level of lesion after 10–21 days.
Other studies	Initially, leukocytosis. Virus in stool and throat. Serologic titers.	Search for specific cause such as infection, intoxication, metabolic or endocrine disease, allergic phenomena, neoplasm. Lymphocyte transformation demonstrated. *Mycoplasma pneumoniae* implicated.	Infancy: stool culture, toxin. Rare serum toxin +. Older: serum (or wound) toxin.	Leukocytosis, often with moderate eosinophilia.	Normal spine x-rays do not exclude spinal epidural abscess. MRI has largely replaced myelography to rule out cord-compressive lesions. Cord may be swelled in myelitis.
Course and prognosis	Paralysis usually maximal 3–5 days after onset. Transient bladder paralysis may occur. Outlook varies with extent and severity of involvement. *Note:* Threat greatest from respiratory failure and superinfection. Early muscle atrophy common.	Course progressive over a few days to about 2 weeks. Transient bladder paralysis may occur. *Note:* Threat greatest from respiratory failure, autonomic crises (eg, BP arrhythmia) and superinfection. Majority recover completely. Plasmapheresis may have a role. Intravenous IgG (IGIV) a new therapy.	Infancy: supportive. Penicillin ? Purge stool ? Antitoxin unnecessary. Respiratory support (prolonged often), gavage feeding. Avoid aminoglycosides. Older: penicillin, antitoxin, prolonged respiratory support. Prognosis: excellent with good quality intensive care. Fatality 3%.	Total removal of tick is followed by rapid improvement and recovery. Otherwise, mortality rate due to respiratory paralysis is very high.	Large degree of functional recovery possible. Corticosteroids are of controversial benefit in shortening duration of acute attack but not in preventing recurrences or altering the overall course.

sion) must be ruled out. Poliomyelitis is very rare in our immunized population. Paralysis due to tick bites occurs seasonally (spring and summer). The tick is usually found in the occipital hair. Removal is curative.

Paralysis due to botulism occurs most commonly under age 1; food-borne and wound botulism are very rare. An investigative history and laboratory studies are diagnostic. Intravenous drug abuse can lead to myelitis and paralysis. Furthermore, *chronic* myelopathy is emerging as a result of two human immunodeficiency viruses, HTLV-I and HTLV-III (now called HIV-1).

Complications

A. Respiratory Paralysis: Early and careful attention to oxygenation is essential; administration of oxygen, intubation, mechanical respiratory assistance, and careful suctioning of secretions may be required. Increasing anxiety and a rise in diastolic and systolic blood pressures are early signs of hypoxia. Cyanosis is a late sign. Deteriorating spirometric findings (forced expiratory volume in 1 second [FEV_1] and total vital capacity) may indicate the need for controlled intubation and respiratory support.

B. Infections: Pneumonia is common, especially in cases of respiratory paralysis. Prophylactic antibiotic administration is generally contraindicated. Antibiotic therapy is best guided by results of cultures. Bladder infections occur most commonly when an indwelling catheter is required because of bladder paralysis. Recovery from myelitis may be delayed by urinary tract infection.

C. Autonomic Crisis: This may be a cause of death in Guillain-Barré syndrome; strict attention to vital signs to detect and treat hypotension or hypertension and cardiac arrhythmias in an intensive care setting is advisable, at least early in the course in severely ill patients.

Treatment

There is no specific treatment in most of these syndromes; however, ticks causing paralysis must be removed. Other therapies include the use of erythromycin in *Mycoplasma* infections and botulism equine antitoxin in wound botulism. Recognized associated disorders (eg, endocrine, neoplastic, toxic) should be treated by appropriate means. Supportive care also involves "pulmonary toilet," adequate fluids and nutrition, bladder and bowel care, prevention of decubiti, and, in many cases, psychiatric support.

A. Corticosteroids: These agents are believed by most to be of no benefit in Guillain-Barré syndrome. Autonomic symptoms (eg, hypertension) in polyneuritis may require treatment.

B. Plasmapheresis: Plasma exchange has been beneficial in severe cases of Guillain-Barré syndrome.

C. Physical Therapy: Rehabilitative measures are best instituted when acute symptoms have subsided and the patient is stable.

D. Antibiotics: Appropriate antibiotics and drainage are required for epidermal abscess.

Prognosis

The prognosis varies greatly with the extent of involvement, duration of the inflammatory process, complications, and other factors.

Bleck TP: IVIg for GBS: Potential problems in the alphabet soup. Neurology 1993;43:857.

Briscoe DM et al: Prognosis in Guillain-Barré syndrome. Arch Dis Child 1987;62:733.

D'Cruz OF et al: Acute inflammatory demyelinating polyradiculoneuropathy (Guillain-Barré syndrome) after immunization with *Haemophilus influenzae* type b conjugate vaccine. J Pediatr 1989;115:743.

Dunne K et al: Acute transverse myelopathy in childhood. Dev Med Child Neurol 1986;28:198.

Freeman JM: Diagnosis and evaluation of acute paraplegia. Pediatr Rev 1983;4:328.

Griffen JW, Ho T: The Guillain-Barré syndrome at 75. Ann Neurol 1993;34:125.

Irani DN et al: Relapse in Guillain-Barré syndrome after treatment with human immune globulin. Neurology 1993;43:872.

Johnson RT, McArthur J: Myelopathic and retrovirus infections. Ann Neurol 1987;21:113.

Khatri BO et al: Plasmapheresis with acute inflammatory polyneuropathy. Pediatr Neurol 1990;6:17.

Kleyweg RP et al: Treatment of Guillain-Barré syndrome with high dose gammaglobulin. Neurology 1988;38:1639.

McKhahn G, Griffin JW: Plasmapheresis and GB syndrome. (Editorial.) Ann Neurol 1987;22:762.

Novak RW, Jones G, Chi'ien LT: Acute transverse myelopathy in childhood: A study of four cases. Clin Pediatr 1978;17:894.

Packer RJ et al: Magnetic resonance imaging of spinal cord disease in childhood. Pediatrics 1986;78:251.

Parry GJ: *Guillain-Barré Syndrome.* Thieme, 1993.

Ropper AH, Wijdicks EFM, Truax BT: *Guillain-Barré Syndrome.* Davis, 1993.

Shahar E, Murphy EG, Roifman DM: Benefit of intravenously administered immune serum globulin in patients with Guillain-Barré syndrome. J Pediatr 1990;116:141.

Vriesendorp FJ et al: Serum antibodies to GM1, GD1b, peripheral nerve myelin, and *Campylobacter jejuni* in patients with Guillain-Barré syndrome and controls: Correlation and prognosis. Ann Neurol 1993;34:130.

DISORDERS OF CHILDHOOD AFFECTING MUSCLES

This section is concerned with specific muscle and neuromuscular disorders, including the muscular dystrophies, myasthenia gravis, and miscellaneous congenital neuromuscular disorders. (See Table 25–31.)

Certain studies that are commonly used in the diagnosis of muscle diseases merit special consideration.

Serum Enzymes

Among muscle enzymes—creatine kinase (CK), aspartate aminotransferase (AST), and lactic dehydrogenase—helpful in diagnosing and following the course of some muscle disorders, usually only CK is now followed. CK (or CPK) reflects muscle damage or "leak" from muscle into plasma; the other enzymes are less available (aldolase) or also have liver origin. Normal CK values may vary in different laboratories. Blood should be drawn before electromyography or muscle biopsy, which may lead to release of the enzyme. Corticosteroids may suppress levels despite very active muscle disease.

Muscle Imaging

Ultrasonography, CT scanning, and MRI are employed in research studies to aid in the diagnosis and assessment of muscular dystrophies, congenital myopathies and myotonias, spinal muscular atrophies, and some neuropathies.

Electromyography (EMG)

Electromyography is often helpful in grossly differentiating "myopathic" from "neurogenic" processes. Fibrillations occur in both. In the myopathies, very low spikes are more typical, and the motor unit action potentials seen during contraction characteristically are of short duration, polyphasic, and increased in number for the strength of the contraction (increased interference pattern). "Neurogenic" findings include decreased numbers of motor units, which may be polyphasic, larger than normal, or both. The interference pattern is decreased.

In myotonic dystrophy, the EMG is characterized by prolonged discharge of electrical activity on movement of the probing needle ("dive bomber" sound), though these discharges may be found to a lesser degree in other conditions. During attempted relaxation after a contraction, electrical activity persists in parallel with the protracted relaxation of muscle.

Muscle Biopsy

Properly executed (by "open" biopsy or by using the Bergstrom muscle biopsy needle), this procedure

Table 25–31. Muscular dystrophies and myotonias of childhood.

Disease	Genetic Pattern	Age at Onset	Early Manifestations	Involved Muscles	Reflexes
Muscular dystrophies Duchenne's muscular dystrophy (pseudohypertrophic infantile)	X-linked recessive; autosomal recessive unusual Thirty to 50% have no family history.	2–6 years; rarer in infancy.	Clumsiness, easy fatigability on walking, running, and climbing stairs. Walking on toes; waddling gait. Lordosis. (Climbing up on legs rising from supine possition—Gower's maneuver.)	Axial and proximal before distal. Pelvic girdle; pseudophypertrophy of gastrocnemius (90%), triceps brachii, and vastus lateralis. Shoulder girdle usually later, also articulation difficulties. Eventually cardiomyopathy (50%).	Knee jerks ± or 0; ankle jerks + to ++.
Becker's muscular dystrophy (late onset)	X-linked recessive. (Allele at xp21)	Childhood (usually later than in Duchenne's).	Similar to Duchenne's.	Similar to Duchenne's.	Similar to Duchenne's.
Limb-girdle muscular dystrophy A. Pelvifemoral (Leyden-Möbius) B. Scapulohumeral (Erb's juvenile) (Chromosome 15)	Autosomal recessive in 60%; high sporadic incidence. A. Relatively common. B. Rare.	Variable; early childhood to adulthood.	Weakness, with distribution according to type. Waddling gait, difficulty climbing stairs. Lordosis.	A. Pelvic girdle usually involved first and to greater extent. B. Shoulder girdle often asymmetric. Quadriceps and hamstrings may be weakest. Pseudohypertrophy of calves uncommon.	Usually present.
Facioscapulohumeral muscular dystrophy (Landouzy-Déjérine) Scapuloperoneal variant (Chromosome 4)	Autosomal dominant; sporadic cases not uncommon.	Usually late in childhood and adolescence; rare in infancy; not uncommon in twenties.	Diminished facial movements with inability to close eyes, smile, or whistle. Face may be flat, unlined. Difficulty in raising arms over head. Lordosis. Tripping in scapuloperoneal type.	Facial muscles followed by shoulder girdle, with occasional spread to hips or distal legs (scapuloperoneal variant).	Present.
Spinal muscular atrophy (SMA) Infantile SMA (Werdnig-Hoffman disease)	Autosomal recessive.	0–2 years.	Floppy infant.	Big muscles: shoulder, hip. Tongue. Intercostals. Fingerstoes spared.	0 or nearly so.
Juvenile SMA (Kugelburg-Welander disease)	Autosomal recessive.	Onset after age 2 usually (age 5–15 typical).	Weakness. "Fasciculations" 50%. Rarely a cause of "floppy infant."	Same.	Same.
Metabolic myopathies Carnitine deficiency (lipid storage myopathy) Primary (rare) Secondary: multiple forms	Genetics variable.	Infancy to adolescence.	Fasting hypoglycemia and coma; less ketosis than expected. Myopathy. Cardiomyopathy. Fatty liver. Don't confuse with Reye's, SIDS.	Weakness variable; may be precipitated by exercise (with resultant myoglobulinuria) or fasting.	Normal to decreased.
"Oculocraniosomatic syndrome" (ophthalmoplegia and "ragged reds"; progressive external ophthalmoplegia) Kearns-Sayer	(?) Acquired; 80% female; other hereditary neurologic disorders may be found in patient or family.	Variable; from infancy to adult life; most at about 10 years of age.	Ptosis and limitation of eye movements; hearing and visual loss (retinitis pigmentosa); intellectual loss; cerebellular disturbance (ataxia).	Extraocular muscles, often asymmetric. Variable involvement of axial muscles; cardiac muscles, with conduction defect.	Depressed to ± or 0.
Myasthenia gravis Transient neonatal	Variable.	At birth.	Difficulty sucking, swallowing; trouble with secretions.	Somatic and cranial muscles.	Normal to decreased.
Persistent neonatal	Variable.	Variable: birth, neonatal, infancy.	Same.	Same.	Same.

(*continued*)

Table 25–31. Muscular dystrophies and myotonias of childhood. (continued)

Muscle Biopsy Findings	Other Diagnostic Tests	Treatment	Prognosis
Degeneration and variation in fiber size; proliferation of connective tissue. Basophilia, phagocytosis. Poor differentiation of fiber types on ATPase reaction; deficiency of type 2B fibers. Dystrophin absent.	EMG myopathic. CK (4000–5000 IU) very high with decrease toward normal over the years. ECG. Chest x-ray. Cloned dystrophin cDNA probes to detect deletions on xp21 chromosome from blood, amniotic fluid, chorionic villi.	Physical therapy, braces, wheelchair eventually, weight control.	Ten percent show nonprogressive mental retardation. Death from pneumonia 10–15 years after diagnosis with 75% of patients dead by age 20.
Similar to above, except type 2B fibers present. Reduced dystrophin.	Similar to above, although muscle enzymes may not be as elevated.	As above. Wheelchair in late childhood or early adult life.	Slower progression than Duchenne's, with death usually in adulthood.
Variation in muscle fiber size with many very large fibers. Fiber splitting and internal nuclei common. Many "moth-eaten" whorled fibers. Dystrophin normal.	EMG myopathic. CK variable; often normal but may be elevated ECG.	Physical therapy, weight control.	Mildly progressive: spread from lower to upper limbs may take 15–20 years. Life expectancy mid to late adulthood.
Predominantly large fibers with scattered tiny atrophic fibers, "moth-eaten" and whorled fibers. Inflammatory response. Little or no fiber splitting, fibrosis, or type 1 fiber predominance.	EMG myopathic. Muscle enzymes usually normal.	Physical therapy where indicated. Wheelchair in old age. ? steroids in inflammatory infant variant.	Very slowly progressive, often with plateaus, except in infantile form where there may be difficulties in walking by adolescence. Usually normal life span.
Small, group atrophy. Twin peak fiber size. Fiber type grouping. Minimal fibrosis. Same.	EMG "neuropathic." Nerve conduction, CSF, muscle enzymes normal. Chromosome 5; linkage studies for prenatal diagnosis. Same CK ("enzymes") may be mildly elevated.	Supportive: respiratory care, positioning, secretion management. Genetic counseling. Physical therapy, wheelchair positioning to avoid scoliosis. May walk, usually later lose this.	80–95% of patients 0–4 years die of pneumonia and respiratory failure. Fairly normal life expectancy. 4–40+ years.
Normal or lipid droplets ("Ragged red" fibers with lipid stain, eg, oil red O).	Muscle biochemistry (carnitine, CPT enzyme) Urine organic acids (at time of illness). Plasma carnitine. WBC, fibroblast enzyme studies.	Avoid fasting and mitochondrial toxins, eg, ASA, valproic acid. Carbohydrate. Treat acidosis. Carnitine orally.	Variable: occasionally fatal in infants. Progressive weakness, developmental delay, cardiomyopathy may occur.
Mitochondrial abnormalities. "Ragged red" fibers. Changes in fiber size, usually due to type 2 fiber atrophy.	CK usually normal. ECG with conduction block. CSF protein elevated. Nerve conduction slowed. CT, brain scan, and brain stem auditory evoked response may be abnormal. Mitochondrial deletions.	Plastic retraction of eyelids. Cardiac support. Anticipate diabetes mellitus. Coenzyme Q?	Dysphagia may develop (50%) as well as generalized muscle weakness. Prognosis fair if disease is confined to ocular muscles. In severe cases, spongy vacuolization of brain and brain stem.
Unnecessary.	Edrophonium or neostigmine tests. Acetylcholine receptor (AChR) antibodies. Repetitive nerve stimulation, EMG.	Supportive. Anticholinergic drugs.	Usually transient (< 2 months).
Sophisticated end plate, nerve terminal ultrastructural studies may be necessary.	May be similar to above. AChR antibodies negative.	May not respond to ACh-ase drugs, steroids, or immunosuppressants.	Variable, may have long-term severe course.

(continued)

Table 25–31. Muscular dystrophies and myotonias of childhood. (continued)

Disease	Genetic Pattern	Age at Onset	Early Manifestations	Involved Muscles	Reflexes
Congenital myopa-thies Myotonic dystrophy	Autosomal dominant.	At birth.	Same as myasthe-nia. Ptosis. Facial di-plegia. Arthrogyposis, club feet, thin ribs.	Cranial and somatic, pharyngeal.	Decreased to 0.
"Other" Central core Nemaline (rod body) Myotubular (cen-tronuclear) Congenital fiber type dispropor-tion	Variable, often auto-somal recessive.	Severe variants present at birth; milder variants (more common) infancy, child-hood.	Severe variant, as in myasthenia, myo-tonic dystrophy. Later presentation—facial weakness, mild to moderate weak-ness, even "toe walk-ing" only.	Similar to myotonic dystrophy.	Decreased to 0.
Congenital muscu-lar dystrophy (Fukayama)	? Genetic. ?Infectious.	Birth.	Hypotonia. Facial weakness, joint con-tractures, mental re-tardation.	Heterogenous. Fa-cial (cranial) and so-matic. Contracture common.	Variable.
Congenital muscu-lar dystrophy ("oc-cidental")	Unknown. Usually not familial.	Birth (or early in-fancy).	As above. Normal IQ.	Same.	Same.
Benign congenital hypotonia (Op-penheim)	Variable.	Variable.	Hypotonia only. Deep tendon reflexes +. Laboratory tests, biopsy normal.	Somatic muscles (respiratory muscles spared).	Normal to decreased.
Myotonias Myotonia congenita (Thomsen)	Autosomal dominant (autosomal recessive cases reported).	Early infancy to late childhood.	Difficulty in relaxing muscles after con-tracting them, espe-cially after sleep; aggravated by cold, excitement.	Hands especially; muscles may be dif-fusely enlarged, giv-ing patient Herculean appearance.	Normal.
Myotonic dystrophy (Steinert) (child-hood and adult form)	Autosomal dominant.	Late childhood to adolescence; neonatal and in-fantile forms in-creasingly recognized (see above).	Myotonia of grasp, tongue; worsened by cold, emotions. "Hatchet-face." Nasal voice. Weakness and easy fatigability. Mild to moderate mental retardation noted.	Wasting and weak-ness of facial mus-cles, including muscles of mastica-tion; sternocleido-mastoids, hands. Myotonic phenom-ena: "bunching up" of muscles of tongue, thenar eminance, fin-ger extensors after tapping with percus-sion hammer.	In infantile form, marked hyporeflexia.

(continued)

is usually most helpful. Histochemical techniques, histogram analysis of muscle fiber types, and electron microscopy are offering new classifications of the myopathies. Findings common to the myopathies in-clude variation in the size and shape of muscle fibers, increase in connective tissue, interstitial infiltration of fatty tissue, degenerative changes in muscle fibers, and central location of nuclei.

Staining the muscle for dystrophin amount aids in differentiating Duchenne's from Becker's dystrophy. Electrophoresis can confirm whether the dystrophin is absent or present in small amounts and whether there is a qualitative difference from normal dys-trophin, the latter two patterns being characteristic of Becker's dystrophy.

Dystrophin is a normal intracellular plasma mem-brane protein in muscle, the "gene product" missing in Duchenne's (and Becker's) dystrophy. Assays in muscle biopsies have shown very low levels or absent dystrophin in severe Duchenne's dystrophy, low con-centrations in "intermediate" forms (eg, manifesting

Table 25–31. Muscular dystrophies and myotonias of childhood. (continued)

Muscle Biopsy Findings	Other Diagnostic Tests	Treatment	Prognosis
Generalized fiber hypertrophy, delay in maturation. Type I atrophy. Internal nuclei.	EMG "myotonic" in some (waning amplitude and pitch). Test mother. CK often normal. DNA testing (chromosome 19) for GCT repeat.	Supportive, even respiratory support. Genetic counseling.	Severely involved infant may improve dramatically over months; expect mental retardation.
Distinctive diagnostic histochemistry, eg, "central cores," "nemaline rods."	Myopathic EMG.	Supportive. Genetic counseling.	Variable. May shorten life. Death in infancy or severe handicap. Scoliosis prominent.
"Dystrophic" changes. Fibrosis. Necrotic fibers. Internal nuclei. ? regenerative fibers.	Myopathic EMG. CK increased or normal. Positive CT, MRI scans: white matter low density, polymicrogyria, lissencephaly, etc.	Supportive.	Physical and mental handicap lifelong.
Same.	As above, CT, MRI variably low density.		May improve, walk. Scoliosis.
Normal with sophisticated studies (histochemistry, electron microscopy, even metabolic studies.)	Use of this diagnosis is shrinking with increasingly sophisticated biochemical (eg, cytochrome oxidase) studies.	Supportive.	Good (by definition). (Few documented long-term studies.)
Nonspecific and minor changes; type 2B fibers may be absent.	EMG "myotonic."	Usually none. Phenytoin, especially in cold weather, may improve muscle functioning.	Normal life expectancy, with only mild disability.
Type I fiber atrophy, type 2 hypertrophy, sarcoplasmic masses, internal nuclei, phagocytosis, fibrosis, and cellular reaction.	EMG markedly "myotonic." Glucose tolerance test, thyroid tests. ECG. Chest x-ray and pulmonary function tests. Immunoglobulins. PCR amplification of GCT repeat on chromosome 19q13 to distinguish normal from mutant alleles.	Procainamide, 250 mg 3 times daily orally, increased to tolerance; phenytoin 5–7 mg/kg/d orally. (Drugs usually little role.)	Frontal baldness, cataracts (85%), gonadal atrophy (85% of males), thyroid dysfunction, diabetes mellitus (20%). Cardiac conduction defects; impaired pulmonary function. Low IgG. Life expectancy decreased.

female carrier), and qualitatively abnormal dystrophin at intermediate levels in Becker's dystrophy.

Genetic Testing & Carrier Detection

To date, detection of carriers for Duchenne's dystrophy (mothers and sisters of involved boys) has rested on CK enzyme elevations (two-thirds will have this), physical findings of mild dystrophy (large calves, muscle weakness), abnormal muscle EMGs, or biopsy results. All are unreliable for diagnostic purposes.

DNA probes are now available for carrier detection and prenatal diagnosis of Duchenne's and Becker's dystrophy. Deletions are often found on the short arm of the X chromosome; it is postulated that all patients and most mothers will show deletions when sufficient probes are developed to search the whole Duchenne genome (perhaps 4000 kb in length).

Amplification of DNA is possible by the polymerase chain reactions (PCR) and can pin down the site of the deletion. Moreover, this technique plus Southern blot analysis can pick up DNA base repeats. For example, in myotonic dystrophy, a GCT triplet excess is currently the most sensitive test for that disease. The tests can be used for intrauterine diagnosis and prediction of whether the triplet is within the normal or mutant range. Thus, in many cases, the greater the number of repeats, the more severely involved the fetus or patient.

The DNA linkage analysis is utilized to predict current risk for infantile spinal muscular atrophy on chromosome 5.

Lastly, Kearns-Sayer progressive external ophthalmoplegia with retinopathy is inherited via maternal cytoplasmic mitochondria. Assay of mutations and deletions from blood or muscle samples are now commercially available to aid in diagnosis of that entity.

Therapy for Duchenne's muscular dystrophy continues to be frustrating. Prednisone in low doses has increased muscle strength and prolonged ambulation. Myoblast transfer—injecting muscle cells at multiple sites—has had poor therapeutic efficacy. Research emphasis is on gene therapy, but there is great difficulty in finding viral vectors able to carry the very large dystrophin gene into muscle cells.

Arahata K: Mosaic expression of dystrophin in symptomatic carriers of Duchenne's muscular dystrophy. N Engl J Med 1989;320:138.

Bartlett RJ: Duchenne muscular dystrophy: High frequency of deletions. Neurology 1989;38:1.

Darras BT: Molecular genetics of Duchenne and Becker muscular dystrophy. J Pediatr 1990;117:1.

Engel A: Gene therapy for Duchenne dystrophy. Ann Neurol 1993;34:3.

Fenichel GM et al: Long-term benefit from prednisone therapy in Duchenne muscular dystrophy. Neurology 1991; 14:1874.

Hilton T et al: End of life care in Duchenne muscular dystrophy. Pediatr Neurol 1993;9:165.

Karpati G et al: Myoblast transfer in muscular dystrophy. Ann Neurol 1993;34:8.

Hoffman EP: Characterization of dystrophin in muscle biopsy specimens from patients with Duchenne's or Becker's muscular dystrophy. N Engl J Med 1988;318:1363.

Holt IF et al: Mitochondrial myopathies: Clinical and biochemical features of 30 patients with major deletions of muscle mitochondrial DNA. Ann Neurol 1989;26:699.

Lanzi G et al: Myotonic dystrophy in childhood. Acta Neurol Belg 1982;82:150.

Martinez BA: Childhood nemaline myopathy: A review. Dev Med Child Neurol 1987;29:815.

McMenamin JB, Becker LE, Murphy EG: Congenital muscular dystrophy: A clinicopathologic report of 24 cases. J Pediatr 1982;100:692.

Milu JM, Gilbert-Barnes E: Type I spinal muscular atrophy (Werdnig-Hoffman disease). Am J Dis Child 1993;147:908.

Redman JB et al: Relationship between parental trinucleo-

tide GTC repeat length and severity of myotonic dystrophy in offspring. JAMA 1993;269:1960.

Russman BS: Rehabilitation of the pediatric patient with a neuromuscular disease. Neurol Clin 1990;8:727.

Stanley CA: New genetic defects in mitochondrial fatty acid oxidation and carnitine deficiency. Adv Pediatr 1987; 34:59.

Tritschler HJ, Medori R: Mitochondrial DNA alterations as a source of human disorders. Neurology 1993;43:280.

Wessel HB: Dystropin: A clinical perspective. Pediatric Neurology 1990;6:3.

Wolff JA: Gene therapy for neuromuscular disorders. Int Pediatr 1993;8:14.

BENIGN ACUTE CHILDHOOD MYOSITIS

Benign acute childhood myositis (myalgia cruris epidemica) is characterized by transient severe muscle pain and weakness affecting mainly the calves and occurring 1–2 days following an upper respiratory tract infection. Though symptoms involve mainly the gastrocnemius muscles, all skeletal muscles appear to be invaded directly by virus; recurrent episodes are due to different viral types. By demonstration of seroconversion or by isolation of the virus, acute myositis has been shown to be largely due to influenza types B and A and occasionally due to parainfluenza and adenovirus.

Ruff RL, Secrist D: Viral studies in benign acute childhood myositis. Arch Neurol 1982;39:261.

THE PERIODIC PARALYSES

Hypokalemic Periodic Paralysis

This rare condition is inherited as a dominant trait, with decreased occurrence in females, but it may appear sporadically. Onset occurs during childhood. The proximal muscles are affected first. Cranial and respiratory muscles are spared. Attacks of weakness may be precipitated by rest after exercise, exposure to cold, emotional stress, and high dietary intake of carbohydrate and sodium.

Attacks usually last for hours but may last for days and may be shortened by rest. The disease may progress to permanent weakness and atrophy.

The serum potassium level is low during an attack. Provocative tests that induce weakness and thus confirm the diagnosis include (1) exercise and (2) giving insulin, 0.25 unit/kg subcutaneously, simultaneously with glucose, 0.8 g/kg orally.

Hyperthyroidism, particularly in Japanese patients, may produce similar periodic weakness.

Acetazolamide, 5–30 mg/kg/d orally, is usually effective in preventing attacks. Alternative treatment consists of giving potassium chloride, 2–10 g orally to terminate an attack and 2–10 g at bedtime between attacks. The patient should be encouraged to eat a low-carbohydrate, low-sodium diet. Thiamine may abort the effects of carbohydrates. Unnecessary exposure to cold should be avoided.

The disorder is consistent with a normal life span. There are rare hyperkalemic and normokalemic variants.

Hyperkalemic Periodic Paralysis

This form of periodic paralysis has its onset in the first decade of life and is usually detected in infancy because of "staring" eyes (myotonic form of lid lag) or a very feeble cry (especially on waking). It is inherited as an autosomal dominant. Pseudohypertrophy of the calves is often present. There is an increased incidence of diabetes mellitus. The attacks are relatively short, lasting 30 minutes to 2 hours, and may be precipitated by rest after exercise, cold, and fatigue. Attacks usually occur in children of school age and then abate, although permanent muscle weakness may develop.

The serum potassium level rises during attacks. The EMG may show myotonia of the external ocular and facial muscles.

Treatment is with hydrochlorothiazide, 50 mg/d orally, or acetazolamide, 250 mg/d orally. Dichlorphenamide, 50 mg/d orally, has also been recommended. The dose must be adjusted for each case. The disorder is consistent with a normal life span.

Normokalemic Periodic Paralysis

The onset of this disorder occurs in the first decade of life. It is inherited as an autosomal dominant. Attacks come on during rest after exercise, with exposure to cold, following ingestion of foods high in potassium (eg, many fruit juices), and following ingestion of alcohol. The attacks may last for days.

In normokalemic paralysis, serum electrolyte levels do not change during attacks. Muscle biopsy may show vacuolar myopathy.

Treatment consists of increasing salt intake and giving acetazolamide, 250 mg/d orally, with dosage adjusted for each case; and fludrocortisone, 0.1 mg/d orally. The prognosis is good.

Bendheim P et al: Beta adrenergic treatment of hyperkalemic periodic paralysis. Neurology 1985;35:746.

Pearson CM: The periodic paralyses: Differential features and pathological observations in permanent myopathic weakness. Brain 1964;87:341.

MYASTHENIA GRAVIS

Essentials of Diagnosis

- Weakness, chiefly of muscles innervated by the brain stem, usually coming on or increasing with use (fatigue).
- Positive response to neostigmine and edrophonium.
- Acetylcholine receptor antibodies in serum (except in congenital form).

General Considerations

Myasthenia gravis is characterized by easy fatigability of muscles, particularly the extraocular muscles and those of mastication, swallowing, and respiration. However, in the neonatal period or in early infancy, the weakness may be so constant and general that an affected infant may present nonspecifically as a "floppy infant." Girls are affected more frequently than boys. The age at onset is over 10 years in 75% of cases, often shortly after menarche. If diagnosed before age 10, congenital myasthenia should be considered in retrospect. Thyrotoxicosis is found in almost 10% of affected female patients. The essential abnormality is a circulating antibody that binds to the acetylcholine receptor protein and thus reduces the number of motor end plates for binding by acetylcholine.

Clinical Findings

A. Symptoms and Signs:

1. Neonatal (transient) myasthenia gravis– This disorder occurs in 12% of infants born to myasthenic mothers. The condition is due to maternal acetylcholine receptor antibody transferred across the placenta; a thymic factor in the infant may also be involved. A sibling may have died in the neonatal period with similar symptoms and nondiagnostic autopsy.

2. Congenital (persistent) myasthenia gravis–In this form of the disease, the mothers of the affected infants rarely have myasthenia gravis, but other relatives may. Sex distribution is equal. Symptoms are often subtle and not recognized initially. Differential diagnosis includes many other causes of the "floppy infant" syndrome, such as infant botulism, ocular myopathy, congenital ptosis, and Möbius' syndrome (facial nuclear aplasia and other anomalies). This condition is not caused by receptor antibodies and often responds poorly to therapy. It may result from a genetic abnormality of the acetylcholine receptor protein or other neurotransmitter vagaries.

3. Juvenile myasthenia gravis–In this autoimmune form, the symptoms and signs are similar to those in adults. Receptor antibodies are usually present. The patient may be first seen by an otolaryngologist or psychiatrist. The more prominent signs are difficulty in chewing, dysphagia, a nasal voice, ptosis, and ophthalmoplegia. Pathologic fatigability of limbs, chiefly involving the proximal limb and neck muscles, may be more prominent than the bulbar signs and may lead to an initial diagnosis of conversion hysteria, muscular dystrophy, or polymyositis. Weakness may be limited to ocular muscles only. Associated disorders include autoimmune conditions, especially thyroid disease.

An acute fulminant form of myasthenia gravis has been reported in children of age 2–10 years and presents with rapidly progressive respiratory difficulties. Bulbar paralysis may evolve within 24 hours. There is no history of myasthenia. The differential diagnosis includes Guillain-Barré syndrome and bulbar poliomyelitis. Administration of anticholinesterase agents establishes the diagnosis and is lifesaving.

B. Laboratory Findings:

1. Neostigmine test–In newborns and very young infants, the neostigmine test may be preferable to the edrophonium (Tensilon) test because the longer duration of its response permits better observation, especially of sucking and swallowing movements. The test dose of neostigmine is 0.02 mg/kg subcutaneously, usually given with atropine, 0.01 mg/kg subcutaneously. There is a delay of about 10 minutes before the effect may be manifest. The physician should be prepared to suction secretions.

2. Edrophonium test–Testing with edrophonium is used in older children who are capable of cooperating in certain tasks, such as raising and lowering their eyelids and squeezing a sphygmomanometer bulb or the examiner's hands. The test dose is 0.1–1 mL intravenously, depending on the size of the child. Maximum improvement occurs within 2 minutes.

3. Other laboratory tests–Serum acetylcholine receptor antibodies are often found in the neonatal and juvenile forms. Ophthalmologic tests of ocular motility with edrophonium are often positive in patients able to cooperate. In juveniles, thyroid studies are appropriate.

C. Electrical Studies of Muscle: Repetitive stimulation of a motor nerve at slow rates (3/s) with recording over the appropriate muscle reveals a progressive fall in amplitude of the muscle potential in myasthenic patients. A maximal stimulus must be given. At higher rates of stimulation (50/s), there may be a transient repair of this defect before the progressive decline is seen.

If this study is negative, single fiber electromyography is now employed to determine if "mean jitter" exceeds normal.

D. Imaging: Chest x-ray and CT scanning in older children may disclose benign thymus enlargement. Thymus tumors are rare in children.

Treatment

A. General and Supportive Care: In the newborn or in a child in myasthenic or cholinergic crisis (see below), suctioning of secretions is essential. Respiratory assistance may be required.

Treatment should be conducted by physicians with experience in this disorder.

B. Anticholinesterase Drug Therapy:

1. Pyridostigmine bromide–The dose must be adjusted for each patient. A frequent starting dose is 15–30 mg orally every 6 hours.

2. Neostigmine–Fifteen milligrams of neostigmine are roughly equivalent to 60 mg of pyridostigmine bromide. Neostigmine often causes gastric hypermobility with diarrhea, but it is the drug of choice in newborns, in whom prompt treatment may be lifesaving. It may be given parenterally.

3. Atropine–Atropine may be added on a maintenance basis to control mild cholinergic side effects such as hypersecretion, abdominal cramps, and nausea and vomiting.

4. Immunologic intervention–This is primarily by use of prednisone. Plasmapheresis is effective in removing acetylcholine receptor antibody in severely affected patients.

5. Myasthenic crisis–Relatively sudden difficulties in swallowing and respiration may be observed in myasthenic patients. Edrophonium results in dramatic but brief improvement; this may make evaluation of the condition of the small child difficult. Suctioning, tracheostomy, respiratory assistance, and fluid and electrolyte maintenance may be required.

6. Cholinergic crisis–Cholinergic crisis may result from overdosage of anticholinesterase drugs. The resulting weakness may be similar to that of myasthenia, and the muscarinic effects (diarrhea, sweating, lacrimation, miosis, bradycardia, hypotension) are often absent or difficult to evaluate. The edrophonium test may help to determine whether the patient is receiving too little of the drug or is manifesting toxic symptoms due to overdosage. Improvement after the drugs are withdrawn suggests cholinergic crisis. Respirator facilities should be available. The patient may require atropine and tracheostomy.

C. Surgical Measures: Early thymectomy is beneficial in many patients whose disease is not confined to ocular symptoms; the effects may be delayed. Experienced surgical and postsurgical care are prerequisites.

Prognosis

Neonatal (transient) myasthenia presents a great threat to life, primarily due to aspiration of secretions. With proper treatment, the symptoms usually begin to disappear within a few days to 2–3 weeks, after which the child usually requires no further treatment.

In the congenital (persistent) form, the symptoms may initially be as acute as in the transient variety; more commonly, however, they are relatively benign and constant, with gradual worsening as the child grows older. Fatal cases occur.

In the juvenile form, patients may become resistant or unresponsive to anticholinesterase compounds and require corticosteroids or treatment in a hospital, where respiratory assistance can be given as needed. The overall prognosis for survival, for remission, and for improvement after therapy with prednisone and thymectomy is favorable.

Death in myasthenic or cholinergic crisis may occur unless prompt treatment is given.

Engel AG: Myasthenia gravis and myasthenic syndromes: Neurologic progress. Ann Neurol 1984;16:519.

Gordon N: Congenital myasthenia. Dev Med Child Neurol 1986;28:810.

Lefvert AK, Osterman PO: Newborn infants to myasthenic mothers: A clinical study and investigation of acetylcholine receptor antibodies in 17 children. Neurology 1983;33:133.

Morel E et al: Neonatal myasthenia gravis: A new clinical and immunologic appraisal in 30 cases. Neurology 1988;38:138.

Pascuzzi RM, Coslett HB, Johns TR: Long-term corticosteroid treatment of myasthenia gravis: Report of 116 patients. Ann Neurol 1984;15:291.

Rodriguez M et al: Myasthenia gravis in children: Long-term follow-up. Ann Neurol 1983;13:504.

Snead OC et al: Juvenile myasthenia gravis. Neurology 1980;30:732.

CONGENITAL ABSENCE OF MUSCLES*

Congenital absence (sometimes only partial) of one or more muscles, usually unilateral, and particularly of the pectoralis (sternal portion), trapezius, serratus anterior, quadratus femoris, or omohyoid, is not unusual. Heredofamilial cases have been reported. Other deformities—eg, syndactyly, microdactyly, and muscular dystrophy—may be present. Absence of muscles of the abdominal wall (prune belly) may be associated with anomalies of the gastrointestinal tract, urinary tract (Eagle's syndrome), or extremities or with cryptorchidism. Treatment is determined by the specific abnormalities present.

PERIPHERAL NERVE PALSIES

1. FACIAL WEAKNESS

Facial asymmetry may be present at birth or may develop later, either suddenly or gradually, unilaterally or bilaterally. Nuclear or peripheral involvement of the facial nerves results in sagging or drooping of the mouth and inability to close one or both eyes, particularly when newborns and infants cry. Inability to wrinkle the forehead may be demonstrated in infants and young children by getting them to follow an object (light) moved vertically above the forehead. Loss of taste of the anterior two-thirds of the tongue on the involved side may be demonstrated in intelligent, cooperative children by age 4 or 5; playing with a younger child and the judicious use of a tongue blade

may enable the physician to note whether the child's face puckers up when something sour (eg, lemon juice) is applied with a swab to the anterior tongue. Ability to wrinkle the forehead is preserved, owing to bilateral innervation, in supranuclear or central facial paralysis.

Injuries to the facial nerve at birth occur in 0.25–6.5% of consecutive live births. Forceps delivery is the cause in some cases; in others, the side of the face affected may have abutted in utero against the sacral prominence. Often, no cause can be established.

Facial asymmetry due to hypoplasia of one side of the cranium associated with contralateral hemiatrophy and spastic hemiparesis (due, in most instances, to an intrauterine cerebrovascular accident affecting one hemisphere) is usually differentiated easily, as is the hemiatrophy of one side of the body seen in Silver's syndrome.

Acquired peripheral facial weakness (Bell's palsy) of sudden onset and unknown cause is common in children. It often follows a viral illness (postinfectious) or physical trauma (eg, cold). It may be a presenting sign of a disorder such as tumor, hypertension, infectious mononucleosis, or Guillain-Barré syndrome, usually diagnosable by the history, physical examination, and appropriate laboratory tests.

Bilateral facial weakness in early life may be due to agenesis of the affected muscles or to nuclear causes (part of Möbius' syndrome) or may even be familial. Myasthenia gravis, polyneuritis, and myotonic dystrophy must be considered.

"Asymmetric crying facies," in which one side of the lower lip depresses with crying (this is the normal side) and the other does not, is a common innocent congenital malformation inherited as an autosomal dominant. The defect in the parent (the asymmetry often improves with age) may be almost inapparent. Electromyography suggests congenital absence of the depressor anguli oris muscle of the lower lip. Forceps pressure is often incriminated as a cause of this innocent congenital anomaly. Occasionally, other major (eg, cardiac septal) congenital defects accompany the palsy.

In the vast majority of cases of isolated peripheral facial palsy—both those present at birth and those acquired later—improvement begins within 1–2 weeks, and near or total recovery of function is observed within 2 months. Methylcellulose drops, 1%, should be instilled into the eyes to protect the cornea during the day; at night, the lid should be taped down with cellophane tape. Upward massage of the face for 5–10 minutes three or four times a day may help maintain muscle tone. Prednisone therapy reduces the pain of Bell's palsy and promotes recovery of facial strength and reduction of motor synkinesis ("crocodile tears").

Faradic or galvanic stimulation of facial muscles is not advised.

In the few children with permanent and cosmeti-

---

*Arthrogryposis multiplex, or contractures and fixation about multiple joints, is discussed briefly in a later section on the floppy infant. Clubfoot, Sprengel's deformity, and torticollis are discussed in Chapter 26.

cally disfiguring facial weakness, plastic surgical intervention at 6 years of age or older may be of benefit. New procedures, such as attachment of facial muscles to the temporal muscle or transplantation of cranial nerve XI, are being developed.

2. BRACHIAL PLEXUS INJURIES (Erb's Palsy, Klumpke's Paralysis)

Traction injuries of the brachial plexus are most common in newborns, occurring in 0.1% of spontaneous, 1.2% of breech, 1.3% of forceps, and 0.25% of all deliveries. The complexity of the brachial plexus precludes any absolute classification, but injuries are usually divided into those affecting the upper plexus (Erb's palsy) and those affecting the lower plexus (Klumpke's paralysis).

Erb's palsy, involving chiefly the fifth and sixth cervical roots, is seen in 99% of cases. It is usually associated with difficult breech delivery, forceps delivery (especially in brow and face presentations), or misapplication of the vacuum extractor. The arm is maintained in adduction and internal rotation at the shoulder, with the lower arm pronated, assuming the "waiter's tip" position. Loss of sensation may be difficult to assess in newborns.

In Klumpke's paralysis, involving chiefly the lower brachial plexus (eighth cervical and first thoracic roots), the small muscles of the hand and wrist flexors are affected, causing a "claw hand." Horner's syndrome may also be present. The injury, usually caused by manipulation during delivery, results from hyperabduction of the arm at the shoulder.

Swinging a child by one arm or jerking the arm may also cause lower plexus injuries ("nursemaid's palsy").

The palsies observed are usually due to avulsion of the plexus, with contusion, edema, and some hemorrhage. X-ray studies of the shoulder will rule out fractures of the clavicle or cervical spine as well as dislocations.

In most instances, recovery occurs spontaneously within a few days or weeks. However, contractures of the shoulder and especially the elbow joints and atrophy of the affected muscles may occur; positioning in the so-called Statue of Liberty or airplane wing position, formerly advised, has been said to contribute to these problems. Passive range-of-motion exercises, which can be taught to the parents, are most helpful in preventing contractures. Electromyography and MRI can delineate the extent of injury and aid in prognosis as well as identify those patients for whom surgical exploration and reparative procedures may be justified.

Adour KK: Current concepts in neurology: Diagnosis and management of facial paralysis. N Engl J Med 1982; 307:348.

Greenwald AG, Schute PC, Shiveley JL: Brachial plexus at birth palsy: A 10-year report on the incidence and prognosis. J Pediatr Orthop 1984;4:689.

Hunt D: Surgical management of brachial plexus injuries at birth. Dev Med Child Neurol 1988;30:824.

Miller M, Hall J: Familial asymmetric crying facies. Am J Dis Child 1979;133:743.

Painter ML, Bergman I: Obstetrical trauma to the neonatal central and peripheral nervous system. Semin Perinatol 1982;6:89.

Reroque H et al: Möbius' syndrome and transposition of the great vessels. Neurology 1988;38:1894.

Sudarshan A, Goldie WD: The spectrum of congenital facial diplegia (Moebius syndrome). Pediatr Neurol 1985; 1:180.

Urabe F et al: MR imaging of birth brachial palsy in a two-month old infant. Brain Dev 1991;13:130.

CHRONIC POLYNEUROPATHY

Polyneuropathy, usually insidious in onset and slowly progressive, occurs in children of any age. The presenting complaints are chiefly disturbances of gait and easy fatigability in walking or running and, slightly less often, weakness or clumsiness of the hands. Pain, tenderness, or paresthesias are less frequently mentioned. Neurologic examination discloses muscular weakness, greatest in the distal portions of the extremities, with steppage gait and depressed or absent deep tendon reflexes. Cranial nerves are sometimes affected. Sensory deficits (difficult to demonstrate in fearful children or those under 5 years of age) occur in a stocking and glove distribution. The muscles may be tender, and trophic changes such as glassy or "parchment" skin and absent sweating may occur. Thickening of the ulnar and peroneal nerves may be felt. Pure sensory neuropathies show up as chronic trauma, ie, the patient does not feel minor trauma and burns to the fingers and toes.

Known causes include (1) toxins, eg, lead, arsenic, mercurials, vincristine, and benzene; (2) systemic disorders, eg, diabetes mellitus, chronic uremia, recurrent hypoglycemia, porphyria, polyarteritis nodosa, and lupus erythematosus; (3) "inflammatory" states, eg, chronic or recurrent Guillain-Barré syndrome and neuritis associated with mumps or diphtheria; (4) hereditary, often degenerative conditions, which in some classifications include certain storage diseases, leukodystrophies, spinocerebellar degenerations with neurogenic components, and Bassen-Kornzweig syndrome (Table 25–32); and (5) the hereditary sensory or combined motor and sensory neuropathies. Polyneuropathies associated with carcinomas, beriberi or other vitamin deficiencies, or excessive vitamin B_6 intake are not reported or are exceedingly rare in children.

The most common chronic neuropathy of insidious onset often has no identifiable cause. This "chronic

Table 25–32. Hereditary neuropathies with known metabolic error.[1]

Disorder	Characteristics
Amyloidosis	Rarely seen in children.
Acute intermittent porphyria (AD)	Abdominal pain, emotional disease.
Krabbe's disease and metachromatic leukodystrophy (AR)	Onset usually in infancy. Dementia. WBC enzyme to diagnose.
Adrenoleukodystrophy (XLR) and myeloneuropathy (AR)	Peroxisomal disease. Long-chain fatty acid to diagnose either one.
Abetalipoproteinemia (AR), Fabry's disease (XLR), Tangier disease (AR), Refsum's disease (AR)	Disordered lipid metabolism in these 4 diseases.

[1]AD = autosomal dominant; AR = autosomal recessive; XLR = sex-linked recessive.

idiopathic neuropathy" is assumed to be immunologically mediated and may have a relapsing course. Sometimes there is facial weakness. Spinal fluid protein is elevated. Nerve conduction is slowed, and nerve biopsies are abnormal. Immunologic abnormalities are seldom demonstrated, though nerve biopsies may show round cell infiltration. Steroids and other immunosuppressants may give long-term benefit.

Of the four defined hereditary sensory neuropathies, the prototype is familial dysautonomia, also called Riley-Day syndrome and hereditary sensory neuropathy type III. Transmitted as an autosomal recessive trait and seen mostly in Jewish children, this disorder has its onset in infancy. It is characterized by vomiting and difficulties in feeding that are due to abnormal esophageal motility, pulmonary infections, decreased or absent tearing, indifference to pain, diminished or absent tendon reflexes, absence of fungiform papillae of the tongue, emotional lability, abnormal temperature control with excessive sweating, labile blood pressure, abnormal intradermal histamine responses, and other evidences of autonomic dysfunction. Mental retardation may be present. Neurologic findings include a marked decrease in unmyelinated fibers of cutaneous nerves and decreased myelinization in dorsal root fibers and the posterior columns of the spinal cord.

A careful genetic history (pedigree) and examination and electrical testing (motor and sensory nerve conduction, electromyography) of relatives are keys to diagnosis of hereditary neuropathy.

Other hereditary neuropathies may have ataxia as a prominent finding often overshadowing the neuropathy. Examples are Friedreich's ataxia, dominant cerebellar ataxia, and Marinesco-Sjögren's syndrome. Finally, some hereditary neuropathies are associated with identifiable and occasionally treatable metabolic errors (see Table 25–33). These disorders are described in more detail in other sections.

Laboratory diagnosis of chronic polyneuropathy is made by measurement of motor and sensory nerve conduction velocities; electromyography may show a neurogenic polyphasic pattern. Cerebrospinal fluid protein levels are often elevated, sometimes with an increased IgG index as well. Nerve biopsy, with teasing of the fibers as well as staining for metachromasia, is advised to demonstrate loss of myelin and (to a lesser degree) loss of axons and increased connective tissue or concentric lamellas ("onion skin appearance") around the nerve fiber. Muscle biopsy may show the pattern associated with denervation. Other laboratory studies—directed toward specific causes mentioned above—include screening for heavy metals and for metabolic, renal, or vascular disorders. Chronic lead intoxication, which rarely causes neuropathy in childhood, may escape detection until the child is given edetate calcium disodium (EDTA) and lead levels are determined in timed urines. Three- and fourfold rises are then diagnostic.

Therapy is directed at specific disorders whenever possible. Occasionally, the weakness is profound and involves bulbar nerves, in which case tracheostomy and respiratory assistance are required. Corticosteroid therapy may be of considerable benefit in cases where the cause is unknown or neuropathy is considered to be due to "chronic inflammation" (this is not the case in acute Guillain-Barré syndrome). Prednisone, 1–2.5 mg/kg/d orally, with tapering to the lowest effective dose—discontinued if the process seems to be arresting and reinstituted when symptoms recur—is recommended. Prednisone should probably not be used for treatment of peroneal muscular atrophy. In all cases considered for corticosteroid therapy, the risks and benefits should be carefully weighed. When treatment is available, symptoms regress and may disappear altogether over a period of months.

The long-term prognosis varies with the cause and the ability to offer specific therapy. In the "corticosteroid-dependent" group, residual deficits and deaths within a few years are more frequent.

Axelrod FB, Pearson J: Congenital sensory neuropathies: Diagnostic distinction from familial dysautonomia. Am J Dis Child 1984;138:947.

Bird SJ, Slodky JT: Corticosteroid responsive dominant neuropathy in childhood. Neurology 1991;41:437.

Chance PF et al: Trisomy 17p associated with Charcot-Marie-Tooth neuropathy type 1A phenotype. Neurology 1992;42:2295.

Chatorian, AM: Chronic polyneuropathy in childhood. Int Pediatr 1988;3:125.

Dyck PJ et al: The 10 P's: A mnemonic helpful in characterization and differential diagnosis of peripheral neuropathy. Neurology 1992;42:14.

Evans OB: Polyneuropathy in childhood. Pediatrics 1979; 64:96.

Hagberg B: Polyneuropathies in paediatrics. Eur J Pediatr 1990;149:296.

Table 25–33. Hereditary motor and sensory neuropathies; metabolic error unknown.

Name	Prototype Unknown	Inheritance	Clinical Features	Nerve Biopsy
Sensory and auto-nomic neuropathy	(1) Familial dysau-tonomia (2) Other	Autosomal recessive (AR) AR, ? autosomal dom-inant (AD)	See text Rare (see references)	(1) Decreased unmyelin fi-bers posterior column and cord (2) Variable (see references)
HMSN I (if tremor is present, Roussy-Lévy syndrome)	"Classic" Charcot-Marie-Tooth dis-ease	AD Chromosome 1, 17 pp 11.2 (segmental trisomy)	Onset 0–15 y. Weakness, atrophy of feet, calves (pes cavus, "stork legs"), hands. Sensory loss 0 or variable. Deep tendon reflexes (DTR) 0. MNCV slowed. Often hypertrophic (palpa-ble) nerves. Linked to Duffy blood group.	Segmental demyelination.
HMSN II	Neuronal/axonal Charcot-Marie-Tooth disease	AD	Less severe; onset 10–20. Leg cramps, numbness, MNCV normal or slightly slow. CSF protein often nor-mal.	Axonal loss, secondary demyelinization
HMSN III	Hypertrophic Char-cot-Marie-Tooth disease; Déjérine-Sottas disease	AR	Onset in infancy. Severe. CSF protein increased. Very slow MNCV. Slowly progressive.	Hypertrophic ("onion bulb") interstitial changes
HMSN IV	Refsum disease		Severe sensory, mild motor. Thick nerves. CSF protein elevated. Ichthyosis, retini-tis pigmentosa, ataxia, deaf-ness. Urine phytanic acid.	See HMSN III
HSMN V	Charcot-Marie-Tooth disease with spastic paraparesis		Abnormal pyramidal tract findings. Rule out adreno-myelopathy.	Defined in pedigrees
HMSN VI, VII	Optic atrophy, reti-nitis pigmentosa, etc.		Poorly defined. Multiple-sys-tems involved.	See HMSN V

MNCV = motor nerve conduction velocities.
HMSN = hereditary motor and sensory neuropathy.

Prensky AL, Dodson WE: The steroid treatment of heredi-tary motor and sensory neuropathy. Neuropediatrics 1984;15:203.

MISCELLANEOUS NEUROMUSCULAR DISORDERS

FLOPPY INFANT SYNDROME

Essentials of Diagnosis

- In early infancy, decreased muscular activity, both spontaneous and in response to postural reflex test-ing and to passive motion.
- In young infants, "frog posture" or other unusual positions at rest.
- In older infants, delay in motor milestones.

General Considerations

In the young infant, ventral suspension, ie, sup-porting the infant with a hand under the chest, nor-mally results in the infant's holding its head slightly up (45 degrees or less), the back straight or nearly so, the arms flexed at the elbows and slightly abducted, and the knees partly flexed. The floppy infant droops over the hand like an inverted U. Even the normal newborn attempts to keep the head in the same plane as the body when pulled up from supine to sitting by the hands ("traction response"). Marked head lag is characteristic of the floppy infant. Hyperextensibility of the joints is not a dependable criterion.

The usual reasons for seeking medical evaluation in older infants are delays in walking, running, or climbing stairs or motor difficulties and lack of en-durance.

Hypotonia or decreased motor activity is a frequent presenting complaint in neuromuscular disorders but may also accompany a variety of systemic conditions or may be due to certain disorders of connective tissue.

Clinical Types

A. Paralytic Group: There is significant lack of movement against gravity (eg, failure to kick the legs, hold up the arms, or attempt to stand when held) or in response to stimuli such as tickling or slight pain.

B. Nonparalytic Group: There is floppiness without significant paralysis.

Note: Deep tendon reflexes may be depressed or absent in the nonparalytic group also. Brisk reflexes with hypotonia point to suprasegmental or general cerebral dysfunction.

1. PARALYTIC GROUP

The hypotonic infant who is weak ("paralyzed") usually has a lesion of the lower motor neuron complex. (See Table 25–34.) Infantile progressive spinal muscular atrophy (Werdnig-Hoffman disease) is the most common cause. Neuropathy is rare. Botulism and myasthenia gravis (rare) are neuromuscular junction causes. Myotonic dystrophy and rare myopathies (eg, central core myopathy) are muscle disease entities.

In anterior horn cell or muscle disease, weakness is proximal, eg, shoulder and hips; finger movement is preserved. Tendon reflexes are absent or depressed; strength (to noxious stimuli) is decreased ("paralytic"). Intelligence is preserved. Fine motor, personal/social, and language milestones are normal, eg, on a Denver Developmental Screening Test (DDST).

Myopathies

The congenital, relatively nonprogressive myopathies, muscular dystrophy, myotonic dystrophy, polymyositis, and periodic paralysis are discussed elsewhere. Most cases of congenital or early infantile muscular dystrophy reported in the past probably represented congenital myopathies (Table 25–31). Congenital muscular dystrophy, diagnosed by muscle biopsy, occurs in two forms: (1) a benign form, with gradual improvement in strength; and (2) a severe form, in which there is either rapid progression of weakness and death in the first months or year of life or severe disability with little or no progression but lifelong marked limitation of activity.

Glycogenosis With Muscle Involvement

Glycogen storage diseases are described in Chapter 31. Patients with type II (Pompe's disease, due to a deficiency of acid maltase) are most likely to present as floppy infants. The weakness in type III (limit dextrinosis) is less marked than in type II, while the rare instances of type IV (amylopectinosis) are severely hypotonic. Muscle cramps on exertion or easy fatigability, rather than floppiness in infancy, is the presenting complaint in type V (McArdle's phosphorylase

Table 25–34. Floppy infant: paralytic causes.

Disease	Genetic	Early Manifestations
IPSMA (Infantile Progressive Spinal Muscular Atrophy) "Malignant" form	Autosomal recessive (AR)	In utero movements decreased by one-third. Gradual weakness, delay in gross motor milestones. Weak cry. Abdominal breathing. Poor limb motion ("no kicking"). Deep tendon reflexes (DTR)—0. Fasciculations of tongue. Normal personal-social behavior.
"Intermediate" form	AR	Onset under age 1 usual. *Progression slower:* may be impossible to predict early course of IPSMA. Hand tremors common.
Infantile botulism	Acquired under age 1 (mostly under 6 months); botulism spore in stool makes toxin	Poor feeding. Constipation. Weak cry. Failure to thrive. Lethargy. Facial weakness, ptosis, ocular muscle palsy. Inability to suck, swallow. Apnea. Source: soil dust (outdoor construction workers may bring it home on clothes), honey.
Myasthenia gravis Neonatal transient	12% of infants born from a myasthenia mother	Floppiness. Poor sucking and feeding; choking. Respiratory distress. Weak cry.
Congenital persistent	Mother normal. Rare AR (AD)	As above; may improve and later exacerbate.
Myotonic dystrophy	Autosomal dominant (AD) (almost always *mother* transmits gene in neonatal/infant severe form)	Polyhydramnios; failure of suck, respirations. Facial diplegia. Ptosis. Arthrogryposis. Thin ribs. Later, developmental delay.
Neonatal "rare myopathy," severe variant Nemaline central core "minimal change" myotubular (centronuclear) reducing body	AR, AD	Virtually all of the rare myopathies may have a severe (even fatal) neonatal or early infant form. Clinical features similar in infancy to infantile myotonic dystrophy.
Congenital muscular dystrophy Fukayama	? Genetic ? Infectious	Early onset. Facial weakness. Joint contractures. Severe mental retardation. Ill-defined.
Other		Severe or benign (improve). No mental retardation.
Essential hypotonia ("benign congenital hypotonia")	Unknown cause	Diagnosis of exclusion. Family history variable. Mild to moderate hypotonia with weakness.

deficiency) or the glycogenosis due to phosphofruc-tokinase deficiency or phosphohexose isomerase in-hibition.

Myasthenia Gravis

Neonatal transient and congenital persistent myas-thenia gravis, with patients presenting as "paralytic" floppy infants, is described elsewhere in this chapter.

Arthrogryposis Multiplex (Congenital Deformities About Multiple Joints)

This symptom complex, sometimes associated with hypotonia, may be of "neurogenic" or "myo-pathic" origin (or both) and may be associated with a wide variety of other anomalies. Orthopedic aspects are discussed in Chapter 26.

Spinal Cord Lesions

Severe limpness in newborns following breech ex-traction with stretching or actual tearing of the lower cervical to upper thoracic spinal cord is rarely seen today, owing to improved obstetric delivery. Klumpke's lower brachial plexus paralysis may be present; the abdomen is usually exceedingly soft, and the lower extremities are flaccid. Urinary retention is present initially; later, the bladder may function au-tonomously. Myelography or MRI scanning may de-fine the lesion. After a few weeks, spasticity of the lower limbs becomes obvious. Treatment is symp-tomatic and consists of bladder and skin care and eventual mobilization on crutches or in a wheelchair.

2. NONPARALYTIC GROUP

The nonparalytic group often has "brain damage." (See Table 25–35.) Intrauterine or perinatal insults to brain or spinal cord, while sometimes difficult to doc-ument, are major causes. (Occasionally, severe con-genital myopathies presenting in the newborn period cause confusion.) Persisting severe hypotonia is omi-nous. Tone will often vary. Spasticity and other forms of cerebral palsy may emerge; hypertonia and hypo-tonia may occur at varying times in the same infant. Choreoathetoid or ataxic movements and develop-mental delay can clarify the diagnosis. Reflexes are often increased; pathologic reflexes (Babinski, tonic neck) may persist or worsen.

The creatine kinase level and the EMG are usually normal. Prolonged nerve conduction velocities point to polyneuritis or leukodystrophy. Muscle biopsies, utilizing special stains and histographic analysis, often show a remarkable reduction in size of type II fibers associated with decreased voluntary motor ac-tivity.

Limpness in the neonatal period and early infancy and subsequent delay in achieving motor milestones

Table 25–35. Floppy infant: nonparalytic causes.

	Causes	Manifestations
Central ner-vous system disorders		
Atonic diple-gia ("pre-spastic di-plegia")	Intrauterine, perinatal as-phyxia, cord in-jury	Limpness, stupor; poor suck, cry, Moro reflex, grasp; later, irritability, increased tone and re-flexes
Choreoatheto-sis	As above; kernicterus	Hypotonic early; move-ment disorder emerges later (6–18 months)
Ataxic cere-bral palsy	Same	Same
Syndromes with hypoto-nia (CNS origin)		
Trisomy 21	Genetic	100% have hypotonia early
Prader-Willi syndrome	Genetic dele-tion 15q11	Hypotonia, hypomentia, hypogonadism, obesity
Marfan syn-drome	AD[1]	Arachnodactyly
Dysautonomia	AR[1]	Respiratory, corneal anesthesia
Turners syn-drome	45 X, or mosaic	Somatic stigmata (Chapter 32)
Degenerative disorders Tay-Sachs	AR	Macular cherry-red spot
Metachromatic leukodystro-phy	AR	Deep tendon reflexes increased early, poly-neuropathy late; men-tal retardation
Systemic dis-eases Malnutrition	Deprivation, cystic fibrosis, celiac disease	See underlying dis-ease elsewhere in text
Chronic illness	Congenital heart disease; chronic pulmo-nary disease (eg, broncho-pulmonary dys-plasia); uremic, renal acidosis	
Metabolic	Hypercalcemia, Lowe's disease	
Endocrine	Hypothyroid	

[1]AD = autosomal dominant
AR = autosomal recessive

are the presenting features in a large number of chil-dren with a variety of central nervous system disor-ders, including mental retardation, as in trisomy 21. In many such cases, no specific diagnosis can be made. Close observation and scoring of motor pat-terns and adaptive behavior, as by the Denver Devel-opmental Screening Test, are most helpful.

Crawford TO: Clinical evaluation of the floppy infant. Pediatr Ann 1992;21:348.

Dobyns WB: Classification of the cerebro-oculo-muscular syndrome(s). Brain Dev 1993;15:242.

Dubowitz V: *The Floppy Infant,* 2nd ed. No. 76 of: *Clinics in Developmental Medicine.* Heinemann, 1980.

Gamstorp I, Sarnat HG (editors): *Progressive Spinal Muscular Atrophies.* Raven Press, 1984.

Gay CT, Bodensteiner JB: The floppy infant: Recent advances in the understanding of disorders affecting the neuromuscular junction. Neurol Clin 1990;8:715.

Long SS: Botulism in infancy. Pediatr Infect Dis J 1984; 3:266.

Milu JM, Gilbert-Barnes E: Myotubular myopathy. Am J Dis Child 1993;147:905.

Thilo EK, Townsend SF, Deacon J: Infant botulism at 1 week of age: Report of two cases. Pediatrics 1993;92: 151.

CEREBRAL PALSY

Essentials of Diagnosis

- Impairment of movement and posture since birth or early infancy.
- Nonprogressive and nonhereditary.

General Considerations

Cerebral palsy is a term of clinical convenience for disorders of impaired motor functioning and posture with onset before or at birth or during the first year of life, basically nonprogressive, and varying widely in their causes, manifestations, and prognosis. The most obvious manifestation is impaired function of voluntary muscles. In the USA, cerebral palsy affects about 0.2% of neonatal survivors.

Classification

Classification is commonly based on the predominant motor deficit.

A. Spastic Forms: About 75% of cases. Often associated with other forms.

1. Quadriplegia (tetraplegia)–The four extremities may be involved about equally, or upper limbs may show more severe involvement. The main lesion is in the cerebral white matter. Quadriplegia due to perinatal damage often shows symptoms earlier than that due to fetal undernutrition or prematurity. Nearly 90% of patients are profoundly retarded.

2. Diplegia–Legs involved more than arms.

3. Hemiplegia–One side involved primarily.

4. Paraplegia–Legs only involved.

5. Monoplegia–One extremity only involved.

6. Triplegia–Three extremities involved.

B. Ataxia: About 15% of cases. Pure and in combination with other forms.

C. Dyskinesia (Choreoathetosis): About 5% of cases. Often associated with rigidity or spastic quadriplegia or diplegia.

D. Hypotonic Form: Fewer than 1% of cases. Persistent hypotonia with variable degrees of weakness.

Etiology

The cause is often obscure or multifactorial. No definite etiologic diagnosis is possible in over one-third of cases. The incidence is high among infants small for gestational age. Intrauterine hypoxia is a frequent cause. Other known causes are intrauterine bleeding, infections, toxins, congenital malformations, obstetric complications (including birth hypoxia), neonatal infections, kernicterus, neonatal hypoglycemia, acidosis, and a small number of genetic syndromes (about 2%).

Associated Deficits

A. Seizures: Seizures afflict about 50% of all children with cerebral palsy and are more prevalent in those with severe involvement.

B. Mental Retardation: Mild to moderate retardation is seen in 26% of patients and profound retardation in 27%. The incidence is correlated with the severity of cerebral palsy.

C. Sensory and Speech Deficits: Impairment of speech, vision, hearing, and perceptual functions is found often in varying degrees and combinations.

Clinical Findings

A. Symptoms and Signs: The typical spastic child exhibits muscular hypertonicity of the clasp-knife type that may eventually end in contractures. In the limb or limbs involved, tendon reflexes, if sufficient muscle relaxation can be achieved, are hyperactive; clonus may be present, and the plantar responses are often extensor. While voluntary control, especially of fine movements, is decreased, there is spread or overflow of associated movements. In extreme cases, the child may lie with elbows flexed and fists clenched (straphanger's posture) and legs crossed or scissored. In early infancy, the child may appear floppy, although tendon jerks are abnormally increased (hypotonic, atonic, or prespastic diplegia). Rigidity often accompanies cerebral palsy.

Ataxia may be difficult to delineate in the presence of spasticity or hyperkinetic movements.

Microcephaly (head circumference < 2 SD below the mean for age and sex and decreasing) is present in about 25% of spastic quadriplegics and diplegics.

Partial atrophy of the cranium on the involved side or of involved extremities is observed frequently, but dependable statistics are not available.

A smaller hand or foot, when coupled with mild weakness on muscle testing or hyperreflexia, often justifies a diagnosis of mild cerebral palsy of which the patient or the family may not even have been aware. Occasionally, multiple minor malformations will suggest an intrauterine origin.

B. Laboratory and Other Findings: No routine workup can be outlined. The clinical findings, the presence or absence of seizures, and the overall outlook for the child—particularly with respect to intelligence and the ability to carry on activities of daily living—determine what studies, if any, should be performed. Hip films in abduction are indicated to rule out dislocations secondary to spasticity. Electroencephalography is indicated when seizures are present or suspected. MRI scans may be helpful in determining timing of insult or malformation, eg, prenatal-intrauterine or perinatal.

Urine screening tests for amino and organic acidurias are indicated. In choreoathetosis with self-injury, serum uric acid determinations should be considered to rule out Lesch-Nyhan syndrome. Macrocephaly and dystonia suggest glutaricaciduria (organic acid).

Differential Diagnosis

The diagnosis is usually not difficult. Progressive deterioration in the first 3 months is more likely to denote a metabolic disorder; subsequently, it denotes one of the central nervous system degenerative disorders (Tables 25–25 and 25–26). In the ataxic form, cerebellar dysgenesis (sometimes familial) or a spinocerebellar degeneration may have to be ruled out.

Prevention

Obstetric advances involving late third-trimester management and delivery have resulted in significant gains. Much more needs to be done in prenatal care, especially during the second and early third trimester. Examples are maternal counseling to avoid cocaine and alcohol abuse and earlier detection of hypertensive disorders of pregnancy. The number of cases in which cerebral palsy is associated with aggressive efforts to salvage premature infants has decreased as a result of advances in neonatal care.

Treatment

Realistically, a child with cerebral palsy should be helped to achieve maximum potential rather than "normality." Special educational programming depends on the physical and mental potential of the child. The degree of improvement with physical therapy correlates positively with better intelligence. Treat seizures in the same way as those occurring in other children. The orthopedic aspects of cerebral palsy are discussed in Chapter 26.

Spasticity occasionally is reduced by diazepam or baclofen. Optimal doses vary according to the degree of spasticity, the size and age of the child, and other medications taken. Surgical amelioration of moderate to severe spasticity in cerebral palsy has been attempted by various procedures over many years; dorsal rhizotomy is the newest procedure.

Management of "hyperactivity" is dealt with in Chapter 6 in connection with attention deficit hyperactivity disorder.

Psychologic counseling and support of the child and family are of paramount importance.

Prognosis

In patients with severe cerebral palsy, especially spastics with profound retardation and seizures that are difficult to control, death due to intercurrent infections is not uncommon; nearly half die by 10 years of age. In nearly 30% of patients, chiefly in those with mild involvement, motor deficits resolve by the seventh birthday. Many children with cerebral palsy and average or near-average intelligence lead fairly normal, satisfying, and productive lives.

Abbott R, Forem SL, Johann M: Selective posterior rhizotomy for the treatment of spasticity: A review. Child Nerv Syst 1989;5:337.

Bergman I et al: Acute profound dystonia in infants with glutaric acidemia. Pediatrics 1989;83:228.

Cooke RWI: Cerebral palsy in very low birthweight infants. Arch Dis Child 1990;65:201.

Coorssen EA, Msall ME, Duffy LC: Multiple minor malformations as a marker for prenatal etiology of cerebral palsy. Dev Med Child Neurol 1991;33:730.

Freeman JM, Nelson BL: Intrapartum asphyxia and cerebral palsy. Pediatrics 1988;82:240.

Hughes I, Newton R: Genetic aspects of cerebral palsy. Dev Med Child Neurol 1992;34:80.

Molnar GE: Rehabilitation medicine, adding life to years: Rehabilitation in cerebral palsy. West J Med 1991;154:569.

Nelson KB: What proportion of cerebral palsy is related to birth asphyxia? (Editorial.) J Pediatr 1988;112:572.

Palmer FB et al: The effects of physical therapy on cerebral palsy: A controlled trial in infants with spastic diplegia. N Engl J Med 1988;318:803.

Scheuerle AE et al: Arginase deficiency presenting as cerebral palsy. Pediatrics 1993;91:995.

Torfs CP et al: Prenatal and perinatal factors in cerebral palsy. J Pediatr 1990;116:615.

Truwit CL: Cerebral palsy: MR findings in 40 patients. AJNR Am J Neuroradiol 199 1992;13:67.

Volpe JJ: Value of MR in definition of the neuropathology of cerebral palsy in vivo. AJNR Am J Neuroradiol 199 1992;13:79.

REFERENCES

Aicardi J: *Diseases of the Nervous System in Childhood.* MacKeith Press, 1992.

Illingworth RS: *The Development of the Infant and Young Child: Normal and Abnormal,* 8th ed. Churchill Livingstone, 1984.

Guilleminault C: *Sleep and Its Disorders in Children.* Raven Press, 1987.

Holmes GL: *Diagnosis and Management of Seizures in Childhood.* Saunders, 1987.

Menkes JH: *Textbook of Child Neurology,* 4th ed. Lea & Febiger, 1990.

Plum F, Posner J: *The Diagnosis of Stupor and Coma,* 3rd ed. Davis, 1980.

Swaiman KF: *Pediatric Neurology: Principles and Practice,* vols 1 and 2. Mosby, 1990.

Volpe JJ: *Neurology of the Newborn.* Saunders, 1987.

Orthopedics

Robert E. Eilert, MD, & Gaia Georgopoulos, MD

Orthopedics is the medical discipline that deals with disorders of neuromuscular and skeletal systems. Patients with orthopedic problems usually present with pain, loss of function, or deformity. Their symptoms must be considered not only in terms of the bones and joints but also in a more general sense relating to the anatomy, particularly of the extremities, and the blood vessels, skin, nerves, tendons, and muscles. As is true of most medical and surgical disorders, the diagnosis of orthopedic disorders can often be made on the basis of a carefully taken history. However, the physical examination is the most important feature of orthopedic diagnosis and depends upon an intimate knowledge of human anatomy.

DISTURBANCES OF PRENATAL ORIGIN

CONGENITAL AMPUTATIONS

Congenital amputations may be due to teratogens (eg, drugs or viruses), amniotic bands, or metabolic diseases (eg, diabetes in the mother) or, in rare cases, may be hereditary defects. Most are spontaneous and not genetically determined. The history of the pregnancy must be carefully reviewed in a search for possible teratogenic factors. There is a 30% incidence of multiple limb involvement, and children with congenital limb deficiencies also have a high incidence of associated congenital anomalies, including genitourinary and cardiac defects and cleft palates. According to the currently accepted international classification, amputations are either terminal or longitudinal. In terminal amputation, all parts are missing distal to the level of involvement—eg, absence of the forearm, wrist, and hand in the case of a terminal below-the-elbow amputation. A longitudinal amputation consists of partial absence of structures in the extremity along one side or the other. In radial clubhand, the entire radius is absent, but the thumb may be either hypoplastic or completely absent—ie, the effect on

structures distal to the amputation may vary. Complex tissue defects are nearly always associated with longitudinal amputations in that the associated nerves and muscles are usually not completely represented when a bone is absent. Bones within the axial skeleton likewise may be absent. Congenital absence of the sacrum is often associated with diabetes in the mother.

Terminal amputations are treated by means of a prosthesis, eg, to compensate for shortness of one leg. With longitudinal deficiencies, reconstructive surgery may be feasible with the objective of reducing deformity and stabilizing joints. In certain types of severe anomalies, operative treatment is indicated to remove a portion of the malformed foot so that a prosthesis can be fitted early. This applies to such anomalies as congenital absence of the fibula, which is the lower extremity bone most commonly congenitally absent. Fortunately, there is rarely a problem with tenting of the skin by relative overgrowth of bone within the stump in congenital amputations.

Lower extremity prostheses are best fitted at about the time of normal walking (12–15 months of age). Lower extremity prostheses are consistently well accepted, as they are necessary for balancing and walking. Upper extremity prostheses are not as well accepted. Fitting the child with a dummy type prosthesis as early as 6 months of age has the advantage of instilling an accustomed pattern of proper length and bimanual manipulation. Children fitted later than age 2 years nearly always reject upper extremity prostheses.

Children quickly learn how to function with their prostheses and can lead active lives, participating in sports with peers.

Choi DH, Kumar SJ, Bowen JR: Amputation or limb lengthening for partial or total absence of the fibula. J Bone Joint Surg [Am] 1990;72:1391.

Rosenfelder R: Infant amputees: Early growth and care. Clin Orthop 1980;148:41.

Scotland TR, Gallway HR: A long-term view of children with congenital and acquired upper limb deficiency. J Bone Joint Surg [Br] 1983;65:346.

Swanson AB, Swanson GD, Tada K: A classification of congenital limb malformation. J Hand Surg [Am] 1983; 8:693.

DEFORMITIES OF THE EXTREMITIES

1. METATARSUS VARUS

Metatarsus varus is a common congenital foot deformity characterized by inward deviation of the forepart of the foot. The longitudinal arch is often creased vertically when the deformity is more rigid. The lateral border of the foot demonstrates sharp angulation at the level of the base of the fifth metatarsal, and this bone will be especially prominent. The deformity varies from flexible to rigid. Most flexible deformities are secondary to intrauterine posture and usually resolve spontaneously. Several investigators have noticed a relationship between metatarsus varus and hip dysplasia, an incidence of 10–15%. The hips in these children should be very carefully checked.

If the deformity is rigid and cannot be manipulated past the midline, it is worthwhile to use a plaster cast changed at intervals of 2 weeks to correct the deformity. "Corrective" shoes do not live up to their name, though they can be used to maintain correction obtained by casting.

The prognosis for this common deformity of the foot is excellent, and few long-term problems are reported. If the deformity persists, the child will exhibit an in-toed gait and may have some problems with shoe wear secondary to the prominence of the base of the fifth metatarsal.

Bleck EE: Metatarsus adductus: Classification and relationship to outcomes of treatment. J Pediatr Orthop 1983;3:2.

Rushforth GF: The natural history of the hooked forefoot. J Bone Joint Surg [Br] 1978;60:530.

2. CLUBFOOT
(Talipes Equinovarus)

When foot deformity consists of the following three elements, the diagnosis of classic talipes equinovarus, or clubfoot, is made: (1) equinus or plantar flexion of the foot at the ankle joint, (2) varus or inversion deformity of the heel, and (3) forefoot varus. The incidence of talipes equinovarus is approximately 1:1000 live births. There are three major categories of clubfoot: (1) idiopathic; (2) neurogenic; and (3) those associated with syndromes, such as arthrogryposis and Larsen's syndrome. Any infant with a clubfoot should be examined carefully for associated anomalies, especially of the spine. Idiopathic clubfeet tend to follow a hereditary pattern in some families.

Treatment consists of manipulation of the foot to stretch the contracted tissues on the medial and posterior aspects, followed by splinting to hold the correction. When this treatment is instituted in the nursery shortly after birth, correction is achieved much more rapidly. When treatment is delayed, the foot tends to become more rigid within a matter of days. Treatment in the nursery by strapping and splinting is often effective. As the child gets older, casting following manipulation and stretching is necessary. The casts are applied sequentially, correcting first the forefoot adduction, then the inversion of the heel, and finally the equinus of the ankle. Treatment by means of casting requires patience and experience; if it is not done properly in sequence, iatrogenic deformities of the foot may result, such as rocker-bottom foot.

After full correction is obtained, a night brace is often prescribed for long-term maintenance of correction.

About half of children with clubfoot eventually need an operative procedure to lengthen the tightened structures about the foot.

A supple foot that is easily corrected by strapping and casting has a more favorable prognosis. If the foot is rigid and requires prolonged treatment to obtain correction, perhaps combined with surgery, the prognosis must be guarded.

Carroll NC: Congenital clubfoot: Pathoanatomy and treatment. Instr Course Lect 1987;36:117.

Cummings RJ, Lovell WW: Operative treatment of congenital idiopathic club foot. J Bone Joint Surg [Am] 1988; 70:1108.

Howard CB: Clubfoot: Its pathological anatomy. J Pediatr Orthop 1993;13:654.

3. CONGENITAL DYSPLASIA
OF THE HIP JOINT
(Developmental Dislocation of the Hip)

Developmental dysplasia of the hip encompasses a spectrum of conditions in which there is an abnormal relationship between the proximal femur and the acetabulum. In the most severe condition, the femoral head is located completely outside of the acetabulum; the hip may be either reducible or irreducible. This most severe condition is termed a dislocated hip. A dislocatable hip is one in which the hip is within the socket but can be dislocated with a provocative (Barley) maneuver. A subluxatable hip is one in which the femoral head comes partially out of the joint with a provocative maneuver. In acetabular dysplasia, the acetabulum is shallower than normal.

Developmental dysplasia of the hip occurs in approximately 1:1000 live births. At birth, there is lack of the development of both the acetabulum and the femur in cases of congenital hip dysplasia. The dysplasia becomes progressive with growth unless the dislocation is corrected. If the dislocation is corrected in the first few days or weeks of life, the dysplasia is completely reversible and a normal hip will develop. As the child becomes older and the dislocation or subluxation persists, the deformity will worsen to the point where it will not be completely reversible, especially after the walking age. For this reason, it is important to diagnose the deformity in the nursery or, at the latest, the 6-week checkup.

Clinical Findings

The diagnosis of developmental hip dislocation in the newborn depends upon demonstrating instability of the joint by placing the infant on its back and obtaining complete relaxation by feeding with a bottle if necessary. The examiner's long finger is then placed over the greater trochanter and the thumb over the inner side of the thigh. Both hips are flexed 90 degrees and then slowly abducted from the midline, one hip at a time. With gentle pressure, an attempt is made to lift the greater trochanter forward. A feeling of slipping as the head relocates is a sign of instability (as first described by Ortolani). In other infants, the joint is more stable, and the deformity must be provoked by applying slight pressure with the thumb on the medial side of the thigh as the thigh is adducted, thus slipping the hip posteriorly and eliciting a jerk as the hip dislocates. This sign was first described by Barlow. The signs of instability are the most reliable criteria for diagnosing congenital dislocation of the hip in the newborn. X-rays of the pelvis are notoriously unreliable until about 6 weeks of age; however, ultrasound has recently been used in both screening for and confirmation of developmental dysplasia. Asymmetric skin folds are present in about 40% of newborns and therefore are not particularly helpful.

After the first month of life, the signs of instability as demonstrated by Ortolani's test or Barlow's test become less evident. Contractures begin to develop about the hip joint, causing limitation of abduction. Normally, the hip should abduct fully to 90 degrees on either side during the first few months of life. It is important that the pelvis be held level to detect asymmetry of abduction. When the hips and knees are flexed, the knees are at unequal heights, with the dislocated side lower (Allis's sign). After the first few weeks of life, x-ray examination becomes more valuable, with lateral displacement of the femoral head being the most reliable sign. In mild cases, the only abnormality may be increased steepness of acetabular alignment, so that the acetabular angle is greater than 35 degrees.

If congenital dislocation of the hip has not been diagnosed during the first year of life and the child begins to walk, there will be a painless limp and a lurch to the affected side, as first described by Trendelenburg. When the child stands on the affected leg, there is a dip of the pelvis on the opposite side owing to weakness of the gluteus medius muscle. This has been termed Trendelenburg's sign and accounts for the unusual swaying gait. In children with bilateral dislocations, the loss of abduction is almost symmetric and may be deceiving. Abduction, however, is never complete, and x-ray of the pelvis is indicated in children with incomplete abduction in the first few months of life. As a child with bilateral dislocation of the hips begins to walk, the gait is waddling. The perineum is widened as a result of lateral displacement of the hips, and there is flexion contracture as a result of posterior displacement of the hips. This flexion contracture contributes to marked lordosis, and the greater trochanters are easily palpable in their elevated position. Treatment is still possible in the first 2 years of life, but the results are not nearly as effective as in children treated in the nursery.

Treatment

Dislocation or dysplasia diagnosed in the first few weeks or months of life can easily be treated by splinting, with the hip maintained in flexion and abduction. Full abduction is contraindicated, as this often leads to avascular necrosis of the femoral head. The use of double or triple diapers is never indicated for medical reasons, because diapers are not adequate to obtain proper positioning of the hip. In cases of joint laxity without true dislocation, improvement will be spontaneous; diapers are excessive treatment.

Various splints to maintain flexion and abduction of the hip, such as the ones designed by Pavlik, Ilfeld, or von Rosen, are available. Treatment of children requiring splints is best supervised by an orthopedic surgeon with a special interest in the problem.

In the first 4 months of life, reduction can be obtained by simply flexing and abducting the hip; no other manipulation is usually necessary. If force is used to reduce the hip, the excessive pressure may cause avascular necrosis. In such cases, preoperative traction for 2–3 weeks is important to relax soft tissues about the hip. Following traction in which the femur is brought down opposite the acetabulum, reduction can be easily achieved without force under general anesthesia. It is then necessary to place the child in a plaster cast, which is used for approximately 6 months. The position in the cast should be carefully adjusted in order to avoid stretching of the delicate blood supply to the femoral head. The hip is flexed slightly more than 90 degrees and abducted only 45–60 degrees. Internal rotation is avoided, because this tends to "wring out" the blood vessels in the capsule of the joint. If the reduction is not stable within a reasonable range following closed reduction, open reduction, combined with tightening of the lax capsule in order to maintain reduction, may be necessary.

If reduction is done at an older age, operations to correct the deformities of the acetabulum and femur may be necessary during growth.

Ando A, Gotoh E: Significance of inguinal folds for diagnosis of congenital dislocation of the hip in infants aged three to four months. J Pediatr Orthop 1990;10:331.

Boal DK, Schwenkter EP: The infant hip: Assessment with real-time US. Radiology 1985;157:667.

Forlin E et al: Prognostic factors in congenital dislocation of the hip treated with closed reduction: The importance of arthrographic evaluation. J Bone Joint Surg [Am] 1992; 74:1140.

Hensinger RN: Congenital dislocation of the hip: Treatment in infancy to walking age. Orthop Clin North Am 1987; 18:597.

Morrissy RT, Cowie GH: Congenital dislocation of the hip: Early detection and prevention of late complications. Clin Orthop (Sept) 1987;222:79.

Treadwell SJ: Economic evaluation of neonatal screening for congenital dislocation of the hip. J Pediatr Orthop 1990;10:327.

Viere RG, Birch JG, Herring JA: Use of the Pavlik harness in congenital dislocation of the hip: An analysis of failure of treatment. J Bone Joint Surg [Am] 1990;72:238.

Yngve D, Gross R: Late diagnosis of hip dislocation in infants. J Pediatr Orthop 1990;10:777.

4. TORTICOLLIS

Wryneck deformities in infancy may be due either to injury to the sternocleidomastoid muscle during delivery or to disease affecting the cervical spine. In the case of muscular deformity, the chin is rotated to the side opposite to the affected sternocleidomastoid muscle contracture, and the head is tilted toward the side of the contracture. A mass felt in the midportion of the sternocleidomastoid muscle does not represent a true tumor but fibrous transformation within the muscle.

In mild cases, passive stretching is usually effective. If the deformity has not been corrected by passive stretching within the first year of life, surgical division of the muscle will correct it. It is not necessary to excise the "tumor" of the sternocleidomastoid muscle, because this tends to resolve spontaneously. If the deformity is left untreated, an unsightly facial asymmetry will result.

Torticollis is occasionally associated with congenital deformities of the cervical spine, and x-rays of the spine are indicated in all cases. In addition, there is a 20% incidence of hip dysplasia.

Acute torticollis may follow upper respiratory infection or mild trauma in children. Rotatory subluxation of the upper cervical spine should be sought by appropriate x-ray views. Traction or a cervical collar usually results in resolution of the symptoms within 1 or 2 days. Other causes of torticollis include spinal cord or cerebellar tumors, syringomyelia, and rheumatoid arthritis.

Binder H, Eng GE, Gaiser JF: Congenital muscular torticollis: Results of conservative management with long-term follow-up in 85 cases. Arch Phys Med Rehabil 1987; 68:222.

Dawson EG, Smith L: Atlantoaxial subluxation in children due to vertebral anomalies. J Bone Joint Surg [Am] 1979; 61:582.

Phillips WA, Hensiger RN: The management of rotary atlanto-axial subluxation in children. J Bone Joint Surg [Am] 1989;71:664.

GENERALIZED AFFECTIONS OF SKELETON OR MESODERMAL TISSUES

1. ARTHROGRYPOSIS MULTIPLEX CONGENITA (Amyoplasia Congenita)

Arthrogryposis multiplex congenita consists of incomplete fibrous ankylosis (usually symmetric) of many or all of the joints of the body. There may be contractures either in flexion or extension. Upper extremity deformities usually consist of adduction of the shoulders, extension of the elbows, flexion of the wrists, and stiff, straight fingers with poor muscle control of the thumbs. In the lower extremities, common deformities are dislocation of the hips, extension of the knees, and severe clubfoot. The joints are fusiform and the joint capsules decreased in volume, producing contractures. Various investigations have attributed the basic defect to an abnormality of muscle or of the lower motor neuron. Muscular development is poor, and muscles may be represented only by fibrous bands. The joint deformities appear to be secondary to a lack of active motion during intrauterine development.

Passive mobilization of joints should be done early. Because of poor muscle control, however, joint mobility cannot be maintained by active motion. Prolonged casting for correction of deformities is contraindicated in these children because further stiffness is often produced. Use of removable splints combined with vigorous therapy is the most effective conservative treatment. Surgical release of the affected joints is often necessary. The clubfoot associated with arthrogryposis is very stiff and nearly always requires an operation. Surgery about the knees, including capsulotomy, osteotomy, and tendon lengthening, is used to correct deformity. Dynamic correction by two-pin skeletal traction may be effective in some knee contractures when combined with therapy to maintain motion while in traction. In the young child, a single vigorous attempt at reduction of the dislocated hip is worthwhile. Multiple operative procedures about the hip are contraindicated because further stiffness may be produced with consequent impairment of motion. The dislocation of the hip that occurs in arthrogryposis is associated with severe dysplasia of the bones and does not respond to treatment as ordinary congenital hip dislocation does. Affected children are often able to walk with bilateral dislocation of the hips, and in cases of severe rigidity it is better to leave the hips out of joint. With lesser demands, the long-term disability is not as severe as it would be in a person with normal mobility and strength.

The long-term prognosis for physical and vocational independence is poor. Patients usually have normal intelligence, but they have such severe physical restrictions that gainful employment is hard to find.

Hahn G: Arthrogryposis: Pediatric review and habilitative aspects. Clin Orthop (April) 1985;194:104.

Sarwark JF et al: Amyoplasia: A common form of arthrogryposis. J Bone Joint Surg [Am] 1990;72:465.

Segal LS et al: Equinovarus deformity in arthrogryposis and myelomeningocele: Evaluation of primary talectomy. Foot Ankle 1989;10:12.

2. MARFAN'S SYNDROME

Marfan's syndrome is a connective tissue disorder characterized by unusually long fingers and toes (arachnodactyly); hypermobility of the joints; subluxation of the ocular lenses; other eye abnormalities including cataract, coloboma, megalocornea, strabismus, and nystagmus; a high-arched palate; a strong tendency to scoliosis; pectus carinatum; and thoracic aortic aneurysms due to weakness of the media of the vessels. Serum mucoproteins may be decreased and urinary excretion of hydroxyproline increased. The condition is easily confused with homocystinuria, as the phenotypic presentation is identical. The two diseases may be differentiated by the presence of homocystine in the urine in homocystinuria.

Treatment is usually supportive for associated problems such as flatfeet. Scoliosis may involve more vigorous treatment by bracing or spine fusion. The long-term prognosis has improved for patients as better treatment for their aortic aneurysms has been devised.

Bornstein D, Byers DH: Collagen metabolism. In: *Current Concepts.* Upjohn, 1980.

Cohn DH, Byers RH: Clinical screening for collagen defects in connective tissue disease. Clin Perinatol 1990; 17:793.

3. CLEIDOCRANIAL DYSOSTOSIS

Cleidocranial dysostosis is an autosomal dominant disorder consisting of absence of part or all of the clavicle and delay in ossification of the skull. The facial bones are often underdeveloped, with absence of the sinuses, a high-arched palate, and defective teeth. The skull is enlarged, especially in the parietal and frontal regions. Coxa vara deformity of the proximal femur is sometimes present but usually is not of sufficient magnitude to require surgery. Deficiency of ossification of the symphysis pubica may persist into adult life. The clavicular deformity allows affected patients to touch their shoulders in the midline but otherwise presents no difficulty. The pelvic deformities do not prevent normal pregnancy and childbirth.

4. CRANIOFACIAL DYSOSTOSIS (Crouzon's Disease)

Craniofacial dysostosis is a syndrome consisting of acrocephaly, hypoplastic maxilla, beaked nose, protrusion of the lower lip, exophthalmos, exotropia, and hypertelorism. It is usually familial. No orthopedic treatment is necessary. Heroic efforts have been made by neurosurgeons and plastic surgeons to correct the grotesque deformity of patients, who generally have normal intelligence. These operative procedures are complicated and hazardous, involving multiple osteotomies of the skull and facial bones.

5. KLIPPEL-FEIL SYNDROME

Klippel-Feil syndrome is characterized by fusion of some or all of the cervical vertebrae. Multiple spinal anomalies may be present, with hemivertebrae and scoliosis. The neck is short and stiff, the hairline is low, and the ears are often low-set. Common associated defects include congenital scoliosis, cervical rib, spina bifida, torticollis, web neck, high scapula, renal anomalies, and deafness. Examination of the urinary tract by urinalysis, and renal ultrasound is indicated as well as a hearing test.

Scoliotic deformities, if progressive, may require treatment. Occasionally, it is necessary to correct the high scapula, also called **Sprengel's deformity** (see below).

Hensinger RN et al: Klippel-Feil syndrome. J Bone Joint Surg [Am] 1974;56:1246.

6. SPRENGEL'S DEFORMITY

Sprengel's deformity is a congenital condition in which one or both scapulas are elevated and small. The child cannot raise the arm completely on the affected side, and there may be torticollis. The deformity occurs alone or may be associated with Klippel-Feil syndrome.

If the deformity is functionally limiting, the scapula may be surgically relocated lower in the thorax. Excision of the upper portion of the scapula improves cosmetic appearance but has little effect on function.

Leibovic SJ et al: Sprengel deformity. J Bone Joint Surg [Am] 1990;72:192.

Samilson RL: Congenital and development anomalies of the shoulder girdle. Orthop Clin North Am 1980;11:219.

7. OSTEOGENESIS IMPERFECTA

Osteogenesis imperfecta is a rare, mainly dominantly inherited connective tissue disease characterized by multiple and recurrent fractures, The severe fetal type (osteogenesis imperfecta congenita) is characterized by multiple intrauterine or perinatal fractures. Affected children continue to have fractures and are dwarfed as a result of bony deformities and growth retardation. Intelligence is not affected. The shafts of the long bones are reduced in cortical thickness, and wormian bones are present in the skull. Other features include blue scleras, thin skin, hyperextensibility of ligaments, "otosclerosis" with significant hearing loss, and hypoplastic and deformed teeth. Recurrent epistaxis, easy bruisability, mild hyperpyrexia (which may increase significantly during anesthesia), and excessive diaphoresis are common. In the tarda type, fractures begin to occur at variable times after the perinatal period, resulting in relatively fewer fractures and deformities in these cases. The patients are sometimes suspected of having suffered induced fractures, and the condition should be ruled out in any case of nonaccidental trauma.

Metabolic defects include elevated serum pyrophosphate, decreased platelet aggregation, and decreased incorporation of sulfate into acid mucopolysaccharides by skin fibroblasts. Normal parents can be counseled that the likelihood of a second affected child is negligible.

There is no effective treatment by medication. Surgical treatment involves correction of deformity of the long bones. Multiple intramedullary rods have been used to prevent deformity from poor healing of fractures.

The overall prognosis is poor, and patients are often confined to wheelchairs during adulthood.

Albright JA, Miller EA: Osteogenesis imperfecta. (Editorial.) Clin Orthop (Sept) 1981;159:2.

Dent JA, Patterson CR: Fractures in early childhood: Osteogenesis imperfecta or child abuse. J Pediatr Orthop 1991;11:184.

Hanscom DA et al: Osteogenesis imperfecta. J Bone Joint Surg [Am] 1992;74:598.

8. IDIOPATHIC JUVENILE OSTEOPOROSIS

Idiopathic juvenile osteoporosis is an acute bone disease characterized by unexplained pathologic fractures of the spine and long bones. It affects boys and girls equally in the prepubertal years, and the degree of severity is variable. There is evidence of gross enteric malabsorption of calcium, which may reflect an abnormality of 1,25-dihydroxyergocalciferol synthesis.

9. OSTEOPETROSIS
(Osteitis Condensans Generalisata; Marble Bone Disease; Albers-Schönberg Disease)

Osteopetrosis is an unusual disorder of osteoclastic resorption of bone resulting in abnormally dense bones. The marrow spaces are smaller, resulting in anemia. There are two types—a milder autosomal dominant type and a more malignant type inherited as an autosomal recessive trait. The findings may appear at any age. On x-ray examination, the bones show increased density, transverse bands in the shafts, clubbing of ends, and vertical striations of long bones. There is thickening about the cranial foramina, and there may be heterotopic calcification of soft tissues. Treatment with corticosteroids to ameliorate the hematologic abnormalities should be tried.

The autosomal recessive form of osteopetrosis has recently been successfully treated by allogeneic bone marrow transplantation.

Kaplan FS, August CS, Fallon MD: Successful treatment of infantile malignant osteopetrosis by bone marrow transplantation: A case report. J Bone Joint Surg [Am] 1988;70:617.

10. ACHONDROPLASIA
(Classic Chondrodystrophy)

Achondroplasia is the most common form of short-limbed dwarfism. The upper arms and thighs are proportionately shorter than the forearms and legs. Findings frequently include bowing of the extremities, a waddling gait, limitation of motion of major joints, relaxation of the ligaments, short stubby fingers of almost equal length, frontal bossing, moderate hydrocephalus, depressed nasal bridge, and lumbar lordosis. Mentality and sexual function are normal. The disorder is transmitted as an autosomal dominant trait, but 80% of cases result from a random mutation. X-rays demonstrate short, thick tubular bones and irregular epiphysial plates. The ends of the bones are thick, with broadening and cupping. Epiphysial ossification may be delayed.

Osteotomies of the long bones are occasionally necessary if deformities are severe.

The spinal canal is narrowed, so that herniated disk in adulthood may lead to acute paraplegia.

Vilarrubias JM, Ginabreda I, Jimeno E: Lengthening of the lower limbs and correction of lumbar hyperlordosis in achondroplasia. Clin Orthop 1990;250:143.

11. OSTEOCHONDRODYSTROPHY
(Morquio's Disease)

Morquio's disease is an autosomal recessive disorder of mucopolysaccharide storage. Skeletal abnormalities include shortening of the spine, kyphosis, scoliosis, shortened extremities, pectus carinatum, genu valgum, and a hypoplastic odontoid with atlantoaxial instability. The child may appear normal at birth but begins to develop deformities between 1 and 4 years of age as a result of abnormal deposition of mucopolysaccharides.

X-rays demonstrate wedge-shaped flattened vertebrae and irregular, malformed epiphyses. The ribs are broad and have been likened to canoe paddles. The lower extremities are more severely involved than the upper ones.

There is no treatment, and the prognosis is poor, although many individuals survive into adulthood. Progressive clouding of the cornea leads to increasing visual impairment.

Stanescu V, Stanescu R, Maroteaux P: Pathogenic mechanisms in osteochondrodysplasias. J Bone Joint Surg [Am] 1984;66:817.

GROWTH DISTURBANCES OF THE MUSCULOSKELETAL SYSTEM

SCOLIOSIS

The term scoliosis denotes lateral curvature of the spine, which is always associated with some rotation of the involved vertebrae. Scoliosis is classified by its anatomic location, in either the thoracic or lumbar spine, with rare involvement of the cervical spine. The convexity of the curve is designated right or left. Thus, a right thoracic scoliosis would denote a thoracic curve in which the convexity is to the right, and this is the most common type of idiopathic curve. Posterior curvature of the spine (kyphosis) is normal in the thoracic area, though excessive curvature may become pathologic. Anterior curvature is called lordosis and is normal in the lumbar and cervical spines. Idiopathic scoliosis generally begins at about 8 or 10 years of age and progresses during growth. In rare instances, infantile scoliosis may be seen in children 2 years of age or less.

Idiopathic scoliosis is about four or five times more common in girls than in boys. The disorder is usually asymptomatic in the adolescent years, but severe curvature may lead to impairment of pulmonary function or low back pain in later years. It is important to examine the back of any adolescent coming in for a routine physical examination in order to identify scoliosis early. The examination is performed by having the patient bend forward 90 degrees with the hands joined in the midline. An abnormal finding consists of asymmetry of the height of the ribs or paravertebral muscles on one side, indicating rotation of the trunk associated with lateral curvature.

Diseases that may be associated with scoliosis include neurofibromatosis, Marfan's syndrome, cerebral palsy, muscular dystrophy, poliomyelitis, and myelodysplasia. Neurologic examination should be performed in all children with scoliosis to determine whether these disorders are present.

Five to 7% of cases of scoliosis are due to congenital vertebral anomalies such as a hemivertebral or unilateral vertebral bridge. These curves are more rigid than the more common idiopathic curve (see below) and will often increase with growth, especially during the rapid growth spurt during adolescence.

The most common type of scoliosis is so-called idiopathic scoliosis and constitutes 80% of all cases. In 30% of cases, other family members are affected also; thus, a family survey is valuable for detecting the problem in siblings if one child has been found to have scoliosis.

Idiopathic infantile scoliosis, occurring in children 2–4 years of age, is quite uncommon in the USA; it is more common in Great Britain. If the curvature is less than 30 degrees, the prognosis is excellent, as 70% resolve spontaneously. If the curvature is more than 30 degrees, there may be progression, and the prognosis is therefore guarded.

Postural compensation of the spine may lead to lateral curvature from such causes as unequal length of the lower extremities. Antalgic scoliosis may result from pressure on the spinal cord or roots by infectious processes or herniation of the nucleus pulposus; the underlying cause must be sought. The curvature will resolve as the primary problem is treated.

Clinical Findings

A. Symptoms and Signs: Scoliosis in adolescents is classically asymptomatic. It is imperative to seek the underlying cause in any case where there is pain, since in these instances the scoliosis is almost always secondary to some other disorder such as a bone or spinal cord tumor. Deformity of the rib cage and asymmetry of the waistline are evident with curvatures of 30 degrees or more. A lesser curvature may be detected by the forward bending test as described above, which is designed to detect early abnormalities of rotation that are not apparent when the patient is standing erect.

B. Imaging: The most valuable x-rays are those taken of the entire spine in the standing position in both the anteroposterior and lateral planes. Usually, there is one primary curvature with a compensatory curvature that develops to balance the body. At times there may be two primary curvatures, usually in the right thoracic and left lumbar regions. Any left thoracic curvature should be suspected of being secondary to neurologic or muscular disease, prompting a more meticulous neurologic examination. If the curvatures of the spine are balanced (compensated), the head is centered over the center of the pelvis and the patient is "in balance." If the spinal alignment is uncompensated, the head will be displaced to one side, which produces an unsightly deformity. Rotation of the spine may be measured by use of spirit level as described by Bunnell (1984). This rotation is associated with a marked rib hump as the lateral curvature increases in severity. Deformity of the rib cage produces a decrease in the space available for the lung and is the cause of long-term problems.

Treatment

Treatment of scoliosis depends on curve magnitude, skeletal maturity, and risk of progression. Curvatures of less than 20 degrees usually do not require treatment unless they show progression. Bracing is indicated for curvature of 20–40 degrees in a skeletally immature child. Treatment is indicated for any curvature that demonstrates progression on serial x-ray examination. Curvatures greater than 40 degrees are resistant to treatment by bracing. Thoracic curvatures greater than 60 degrees have been correlated with poor pulmonary function in adult life. Curvatures of such severity are an indication for surgical correction of the deformity and posterior spinal fusion to maintain the correction. Curvatures between 40 and 60 degrees may also require spinal fusion if they appear to be progressive or are causing decompensation of the spine or are cosmetically unacceptable.

Surgical fusion involves decortication of the bone over the laminas and spinous processes, with the addition of autogenous bone graft from the iliac crest. Postoperative correction is usually maintained by a Harrington or Luque rod, with activity restriction for several months until the fusion is solid.

Treatment is prolonged and difficult and is best done in centers where full support facilities are available.

Prognosis

Compensated small curvatures that do not progress may be well tolerated throughout life, with very little cosmetic concern. The patients should be counseled regarding the genetic transmission of scoliosis and cautioned that their children should be examined at regular intervals during growth. Large thoracic curvatures greater than 60 degrees are associated with shortened life span and may progress even during adult life. Large lumbar curvatures may lead to subluxation of the vertebrae and premature arthritic degeneration of the spine, producing disabling pain in

adulthood. Early detection allows for simple brace treatment. In patients so treated, the long-term prognosis is excellent, and surgery is not necessary. For this reason, school screening programs for scoliosis have gained popular support in many sections of the country.

Bunnell WP: An objective criterion for scoliosis screening. J Bone Joint Surg [Am] 1984;66:1381.

Byrd JA: Current theories on the etiology of idiopathic scoliosis. Clin Orthop (April) 1988;229:114.

Clayson D et al: Long-term psychological sequelae of surgically versus nonsurgically treated scoliosis. Spine 1987; 12:983.

Montgomery F, Willner S, Applegren G: Long term follow up of patients with adolescent idiopathic scoliosis treated conservatively: An analysis of the clinical value of progression. J Pediatr Orthop 1990;10:48.

Piazza MR, Bassett GS: Curve progression after treatment with the Wilmington brace for idiopathic scoliosis. J Pediatr Orthop 1990;10:39.

Raso VJ et al: Thoracic lordosis in idiopathic scoliosis. J Pediatr Orthop 1991;11:599.

Weinstein SL: Idiopathic scoliosis: Natural history. Spine 1986;11:780.

SLIPPED CAPITAL FEMORAL EPIPHYSIS

Slipped capital femoral epiphysis is separation of the proximal femoral epiphysis through the growth plate. The head of the femur is usually displaced medially and posteriorly relative to the neck of the femur. The condition occurs in adolescence and is most common in obese males. The cause is not clear, although some authorities have shown experimentally that the decreased strength of the perichondrial ring stabilizing the epiphysial area is sufficiently weakened by hormonal changes during the adolescent years that the simple overload of excessive body weight can produce a pathologic fracture through the growth plate. Hormonal studies in these children have not demonstrated any abnormality. Anatomic study of the area of separation demonstrates a histologic picture identical to that seen with traumatic separation, and the condition occasionally occurs as an acute episode resulting from a fall or direct trauma to the hip.

More commonly, however, there are vague symptoms over a protracted period of time in an otherwise healthy child who presents with pain and limp. The pain is often referred into the thigh or the medial side of the knee. It is important to examine the hip joint in any child complaining of knee pain, particularly in adolescents. The consistent finding on physical examination is limitation of internal rotation and abduction of the hip. There usually is also an associated hip flexion contracture as well as local tenderness about the hip. X-rays should be taken in both the anteroposterior and lateral planes and should include both hips.

Treatment is based on the same principles that govern treatment of fracture of the femoral neck in adults in that the head of the femur is fixed to the neck of the femur and the fracture line allowed to heal. Unfortunately, the severe complication of avascular necrosis occurs in 30% of these patients. There has been a positive correlation between forceful reduction of the slip and avascular necrosis. In cases of acute slip, as evidenced by the absence of any callus formation about the growth plate, it may be possible to reduce the hip by gentle traction. In more chronic cases, a more expeditious procedure is to pin the slip as it lies. Remodeling of the fracture site often improves the position of the hip without further surgery.

The long-term prognosis is guarded because most of these patients continue to be overweight and overstress their hip joints. Follow-up studies have shown a high incidence of premature degenerative arthritis in this group of patients—even those who do not develop avascular necrosis. The development of avascular necrosis almost guarantees a poor prognosis, because new bone does not replace the femoral head at this late stage of skeletal growth.

About 30% of patients have bilateral involvement, and patients should be followed for slipping of the opposite side, which may occur as long as 1 or 2 years after the primary episode.

Aronson DD, Carlson WE: Slipped capital femoral epiphysis: A prospective study of fixation with a single screw. J Bone Joint Surg [Am] 1992;74:810.

Carney BT et al: Long term follow up of slipped capital femoral epiphysis. J Bone Joint Surg [Am] 1991;73:667.

Crawford AH: Slipped capital femoral epiphysis: Current concepts review. J Bone Joint Surg [Am] 1988;70:1422.

Spero CR et al: Slipped capital femoral epiphysis in black children: Incidence of chondrolysis. J Pediatr Orthop 1992;12:444.

Wells D et al: Review of slipped capital femoral epiphysis associated with endocrine disease. J Pediatr Orthop 1992;610.

GENU VARUM & GENU VALGUM

Genu varum (bowleg) is normal from infancy through 2 years of life. The alignment then changes to genu valgum (knock-knee) until about 8 years of age, at which time adult alignment is attained. Criteria for referral to an orthopedist include persistent bowing beyond age 2, bowing that is increasing rather than decreasing, bowing of one leg only, and knock-knee associated with short stature.

Bracing may be appropriate, or, rarely, an osteotomy is necessary for a severe problem such as Blount's disease (proximal tibial epiphysial dysplasia).

Brighton CT: Structure and function of the growth plate. Clin Orthop (Oct) 1978;136:22.

Staheli LT: Torsional deformity. Pediatr Clin North Am 1977;24:799.

Vankka E, Salenius P: Spontaneous correction of severe tibiofemoral deformity in growing children. Acta Orthop Scand 1982;53:567.

TIBIAL TORSION

The physician is often asked about "toeing in" in small children. The disorder is routinely asymptomatic. Tibial torsion is rotation of the leg between the knee and the ankle. Internal rotation amounts to about 20 degrees at birth but decreases to neutral rotation by 16 months of age. The deformity is sometimes accentuated by laxity of the knee ligaments, allowing excessive internal rotation of the leg in small children. In children who have a persistent internal rotation of the tibia beyond 16–18 months of age, the condition is often due to sleeping with feet turned in and can be reversed with an external rotation splint worn only at night.

FEMORAL ANTEVERSION

"Toeing in" beyond 2 or 3 years of age is usually secondary to femoral anteversion, which produces excessive internal rotation of the femur as compared to external rotation. This femoral alignment follows a natural history of progressive decrease toward neutral up to 8 years of age, with slower change to 16 years of age. Studies comparing the results of treatment with shoes or braces to the natural history have shown that little is gained by active treatment. Active external rotation exercises such as ballet, skating, or bicycle riding may be worthwhile. Osteotomy for rotational correction is rarely required. Refer those who have no external rotation of hip in extension.

Fabry G, MacEwen GD, Shands AR Jr: Torsion of the femur. J Bone Joint Surg [Am] 1973;55:1726.

Wedge JH, Munkacsi I, Loback D: Anteversion of the femur and idiopathic osteoarthritis of the hip. J Bone Joint Surg [Am] 1989;71:1040.

COMMON FOOT PROBLEMS

When a child begins to stand and walk, the long arch of the foot is flat with a medial bulge over the inner border of the foot. The forefeet are mildly pronated or rotated inward, with a slight valgus alignment of the knees. As the child grows and muscle power improves, the long arch is better supported and more normal relationships occur in the lower extremities. (See also Metatarsus Varus and Talipes Equinovarus.)

1. FLATFOOT

Flatfoot is a normal condition in infants. Children presenting for examination should be checked to determine that the heel cord is of normal length when the heel is aligned in the neutral position, allowing complete dorsiflexion and plantar flexion. As long as the foot is supple and the presence of a longitudinal arch is noted when the child is sitting in a non-weight-bearing position, the parents can be assured that a normal arch will probably develop. There is usually a familial incidence of relaxed flatfeet in children who have prolonged malalignment of the foot. In any child with a shortened heel cord or stiffness of the foot, other causes of flatfoot such as tarsal coalition or vertical talus should be ruled out by a complete orthopedic examination and x-ray.

In the child with an ordinary relaxed flatfoot, no active treatment is indicated unless there is calf or leg pain. In children who have leg pains attributable to flatfeet, an orthopedic shoe with Thomas heel or an orthotic that holds the heel in neutral and supports the arch may relieve discomfort. An arch insert should not be prescribed unless passive correction of the arch is easily accomplished; otherwise, there will be irritation of the skin over the medial side of the foot.

Gonzalez PK, Kumar SJ: Calcaneonavicular coalition treated by resection and interposition of the extensor digitorum brevis muscle. J Bone Joint Surg [Am] 1990; 72:71.
Mosier KM, Asher M: Tarsal coalitions and peroneal spastic flatfoot: A review. J Bone Joint Surg [Am] 1984;66:976.
Wenger DR et al: Corrective shoes and inserts as treatment for a flexible flatfoot in infants and children. J Bone Joint Surg [Am] 1989;71A:800.

2. TALIPES CALCANEOVALGUS

Talipes calcaneovalgus is characterized by excessive dorsiflexion at the ankle and eversion of the foot. It is often present at birth and almost always corrects spontaneously. The deformity is due to intrauterine position.

Treatment consists of passive exercises by the mother, stretching the foot into plantar flexion. In rare instances, it may be necessary to use plaster casts to help with manipulation and positioning.

Complete correction is the rule.

3. CAVUS FOOT

In cavus foot, the deformity consists of an unusually high longitudinal arch of the foot. It may be hereditary or associated with neurologic conditions such as poliomyelitis, Charcot-Marie-Tooth disease, Friedreich's ataxia, or diastematomyelia. There is usually an associated contracture of the toe extensor, producing a claw toe deformity in which the metatarsal phalangeal joints are hyperextended and the interphalangeal joints acutely flexed. Any child presenting with cavus feet should have a careful neurologic examination including x-rays of the spine.

Stretching exercises for the heel cord and arch of the foot are indicated for conservative therapy. In resistant cases that do not respond to shoe adjustments (metatarsal bars and supports), operation may be necessary to lengthen the contracted extensor and flexor tendons and to release the plantar fascia and other tight plantar structures. Arthrodesis of the foot may be necessary later. If these feet are left untreated, they are often painful and limit walking.

The overall prognosis is much poorer than with low arch or pes planus.

4. CLAW TOES

In patients with claw toes, there is a flexion deformity of either or both interphalangeal joints, which results in the "claw." The condition is usually congenital or may be seen in association with disorders of motor weakness, such as Charcot-Marie-Tooth disease or pes cavus. Surgical correction can alleviate symptoms if the toes are painful.

5. BUNIONS
(Hallux Valgus)

Girls may present in adolescence with lateral deviation of the great toe associated with a prominence over the head of the first metatarsal. This deformity is painful only with shoe wear and almost always can be relieved by fitting shoes that are wide enough. Surgery should be avoided in the adolescent age group, because the results are much less successful than in adult patients with the same condition.

Coleman SS: *Complex Foot Deformities in Children*. Lea & Febiger, 1983.
Geissle AE, Stanton RP: Surgical treatment of adolescent hallux valgus. J Pediatr Orthop 1990;10:642.
Groiso J: Juvenile hallux: A conservative approach to treatment. J Bone Joint Surg [Am] 1992;74:1375.

EPIPHYSIAL GROWTH DISTURBANCES SECONDARY TO INFECTION OR TRAUMA

In the child under 1 year of age, there is direct vascular communication from the metaphysis to the epiphysis across the growth plate. For this reason, osteomyelitis occurring in the infant may produce permanent damage to the growth cartilage of the epiphysis with resulting angular deformity or decreased growth potential for the bone. Likewise, trauma, particularly of a compression variety, may damage part or all of the epiphysis. Once such damage occurs, deformity is progressive and may be severe, requiring osteotomy for angular deformity or epiphysiodesis for correction of leg length discrepancy.

DEGENERATIVE PROBLEMS
(Arthritis, Bursitis, & Tenosynovitis)

Degenerative arthritis may follow childhood skeletal problems such as infection, slipped capital femoral epiphysis, avascular necrosis, trauma, or may occur in association with hemophilia. Early effective treatment of these disorders will prevent arthritis. Late treatment is often unsatisfactory.

Degenerative changes in the soft tissues around joints may occur as a result of overuse syndrome in adolescent athletes. Young boys throwing excessive numbers of pitches, especially curve balls, may develop "little leaguer's elbow," consisting of degenerative changes around the humeral condyles associated with pain, swelling, and limitation of motion. In order to enforce the rest necessary for healing, a plaster cast may be necessary. A more reasonable preventive measure is to limit the number of pitches thrown by children.

Acute bursitis is quite uncommon in childhood, and other causes should be ruled out before this diagnosis is accepted.

Tenosynovitis is most common in the region of the knees and feet. Children taking dancing lessons, particularly toe dancing, may have pain around the flexor tendon sheaths in the toes or ankles. Rest is effective treatment. At the knee level, there may be irritation of the patellar ligament, with associated swelling in the infrapatellar fat pad. Synovitis in this area is usually due to overuse and is also treated by rest. Corticosteroid injections are contraindicated.

Kunnamo I et al: Clinical signs and laboratory tests in the differential diagnosis of arthritis in children. Am J Dis Child 1987;141:34.

TRAUMA

SOFT TISSUE TRAUMA
(Sprains, Strains, & Contusions)

A sprain is the stretching of a ligament, and a strain is a stretch of a muscle or tendon. In either of these injuries, there may be some degree of tissue tearing. Contusions are generally due to tissue compression, with damage to blood vessels within the tissue and the formation of hematoma.

A severe sprain is one in which the ligament is completely divided, resulting in instability of the joint. A mild or moderate sprain is one in which incomplete tearing of the ligament occurs, but in which there is associated local pain and swelling.

Mild or moderate sprains are treated by rest of the affected joint, with ice and elevation to prevent prolonged symptoms. By definition, mild or moderate sprain is not associated with instability of the joint.

If there is more severe trauma resulting in tearing of a ligament, instability of the joint may be demonstrated by gross examination or by stress testing with x-ray documentation. Such deformity of the joint may cause persistent instability resulting from inaccurate apposition of the ligament ends during healing. If instability is evident, surgical repair of the torn ligament may be indicated. If a muscle is torn at its tendinous insertion, it should be repaired.

The initial treatment of any sprain consists of ice, compression, and elevation. The purpose of the treatment is to decrease local edema and residual stiffness resulting from gelling of blood proteins in the interstitial space. Splinting of the affected joint protects against further injury and relieves swelling and pain.

1. ANKLE SPRAINS

The history will indicate that the injury was by either forceful inversion or eversion. The more common inversion injury results in tearing or injury to the lateral ligaments, whereas an eversion injury will injure the medial ligaments of the ankle. The injured ligaments may be identified by means of careful palpation for point tenderness around the ankle. The joint should be supported or immobilized at a right angle, which is the functional position. Adhesive taping may be effective to maintain this position but should be applied by one skilled in the use of tape and changed frequently in order to prevent the formation of blisters and skin damage. A posterior plaster splint is more easily applied and gives good joint rest if the extremity is protected by using crutches for weight bearing. Prolonged use of a plaster cast is usually not necessary, but the sprained ankle should be rested sufficiently to allow complete healing. This may take 3–6 weeks. Because fractures usually receive more attention and adequate follow-up, the results are often better. A properly treated ankle sprain should not be the source of prolonged and repeated disability.

2. KNEE SPRAINS

Sprains of the collateral and cruciate ligaments are uncommon in children. These ligaments are so strong that it is more common to injure the epiphysial growth plates, which are the weakest structures in the region of the knees of children. In adolescence, however, the physes have started to close, and the knee joint is more like that of an adult, so that rupture of the anterior cruciate ligament can result from a twisting injury. If the injury produces avulsion of the tibial spine, open anatomic reduction is often required.

Effusion of the knee after trauma deserves referral to an orthopedic specialist. The differential diagnosis includes torn ligament, torn meniscus, and osteochondral fracture. Nontraumatic effusion should be evaluated for inflammatory conditions (such as juvenile rheumatoid arthritis) or patellar malalignment.

3. INTERNAL DERANGEMENTS OF THE KNEE

Meniscal injuries are uncommon under age 12. Clicking or locking of the knee may occur in young children as a result of a discoid lateral meniscus, which is a rare type of congenital anomaly. As the child approaches adolescence, internal damage to the knee from a torsion weight-bearing injury may result in locking of the knee if tearing and displacement of the meniscus occur. Osteochondral fractures secondary to osteochondritis dissecans may also present as internal derangements of the knee in adolescence. Posttraumatic synovitis may mimic a meniscal lesion as well. In any severe injury to the knee, epiphysial injury should be suspected; stress films will sometimes demonstrate separation of the distal femoral epiphysis in such cases. Epiphysial injury should be suspected whenever there is tenderness on both sides of the metaphysis of the femur after injury.

Twyman RS, Desai K, Aichroth PM: Osteochondritis dissecans of the knee: A long term study. J Bone Joint Surg [Br] 1991;73:461.
Zaman M, Leonard MA: Meniscectomy in children: Results in 59 knees. Injury 1981;12:425.

4. BACK SPRAINS

Sprains of the ligaments and muscles of the back are unusual in children but may occur as a result of violent trauma from automobile accidents or athletic injuries. A child with back pain should not be presumed to have had trauma to the spine unless the history warrants that conclusion. The reason for back pain should be carefully sought by x-ray and physical examination. Inflammation, infection, and tumors are more common causes of back pain in children than sprains.

5. CONTUSIONS

Contusion of muscle with hematoma formation produces the familiar "charley horse" injury. Treatment of such injuries is by application of ice, compression, and rest. Exercise should be avoided for 5–7 days. Local heat may hasten healing once the acute phase of tenderness and swelling is past.

6. MYOSITIS OSSIFICANS

Ossification within muscle occurs when there is sufficient trauma to cause a hematoma that later heals in the manner of a fracture. The injury is usually a contusion and occurs most commonly in the quadriceps of the thigh or the triceps of the arm. When such a severe injury with hematoma is recognized, it is important to splint the extremity and avoid activity. If further activity is allowed, ossification may reach spectacular proportions and resemble an osteosarcoma.

Disability is great, with local swelling and heat and extreme pain upon the slightest motion of the adjacent joint. The limb should be rested, with the knee in extension or the elbow in 90 degrees of flexion, until the local reaction has subsided. Once local heat and tenderness have decreased, gentle active exercises may be initiated. Passive stretching exercises are not indicated, because they may stimulate the ossification reaction. It is occasionally necessary to excise excessive bony tissue if it interferes with muscle function once the reaction is mature. Surgery should not be attempted before 9 months to a year after injury, because it may restart the process and lead to an even more severe reaction.

Micheli LJ (editor): Injuries in the young athlete. Clin Sports Med 1988;7:459.

TRAUMATIC SUBLUXATIONS & DISLOCATIONS

Dislocation of a joint is always associated with severe damage to the ligaments and joint capsule. In contrast to fracture treatment, which may be safely postponed, dislocations must be reduced immediately. Dislocations can usually be reduced by gentle sustained traction. It often happens that no anesthetic is necessary for several hours after the injury, because of the protective anesthesia produced by the injury. Following reduction, the joint should be splinted for transportation of the patient.

The dislocated joint should be treated by immobilization for at least 3 weeks, followed by graduated active exercises through a full range of motion. Physical therapy is usually not indicated for children with injuries. As a matter of fact, vigorous manipulation of the joint by a therapist may be harmful. The child should be permitted to perform therapy alone. No stretching should be permitted.

1. SUBLUXATION OF THE RADIAL HEAD (Nursemaid's Elbow)

Infants frequently sustain subluxation of the radial head as a result of being lifted or pulled by the hand. The child appears with the elbow fully pronated and painful. The usual complaint is that the child's elbow will not bend. X-ray findings are normal, but there is point tenderness over the radial head. When the elbow is placed in full supination and slowly moved from full flexion to full extension, a click may be palpated at the level of the radial head. The relief of pain is remarkable, as the child usually stops crying immediately. The elbow may be immobilized in a sling for comfort for a day. Occasionally, symptoms will last for several days, requiring more prolonged immobilization.

Pulled elbow may be a clue to battering. This should be remembered during examination, especially if the problem is recurrent.

2. RECURRENT DISLOCATION OF THE PATELLA

Recurrent dislocation of the patella is more common in loose-jointed individuals, especially adolescent girls. If the patella completely dislocates, it nearly always goes laterally. Pain is severe, and the patient is brought to the doctor with the knee slightly flexed and an obvious bony mass lateral to the knee joint and a flat area over the usual location of the patella anteriorly. X-ray findings confirm the diagnosis. The patella may be reduced by extending the knee and placing slight pressure on the patella while gentle traction is exerted on the leg. In subluxation of the patella, the symptoms may be more subtle, and the patient may say that the knee "gives out" or "jumps out of place."

In the case of complete dislocation, the knee should be immobilized for 3–4 weeks, followed by a physical therapy program for strengthening the quadriceps muscle. Operation may be necessary to tighten the knee joint capsule if dislocation or subluxation is recurrent. In such instances, if the patella is not stabilized, repeated dislocation produces damage to the articular cartilage of the patellofemoral joint and premature degenerative arthritis.

Gao GX, Lee EH, Bose K: Surgical management of congenital and habitual dislocation of the patella. J Pediatr Orthop 1990;10:255.

EPIPHYSIAL SEPARATIONS

In children, epiphysial separations and fractures are more common than ligamentous injuries. This finding is based on the fact that the ligaments of the joints are generally stronger than the associated growth plates. In instances where dislocation is suspected, an x-ray should be taken in order to rule out epiphysial fracture. Films of the opposite extremity, especially around the elbow, may be valuable for comparison. Reduction of a fractured epiphysis should be done under anesthesia in order to align the growth plate with the least amount of force necessary. Fractures across the growth plate may produce bony bridges that will cause premature cessation of growth or angular deformities in the growth plate. Epiphysial fractures around the shoulder, wrist, and fingers can usually be treated by closed reduction, but fractures of the epiphyses around the elbow often require open reduction. In the lower extremity, accurate reduction of the epiphysial plate is necessary to prevent joint deformity if a joint surface is involved. Unfortunately, some of the most severe injuries to the epiphysial plate occur from compression injuries, where the amount of force is not immediately apparent. If angular deformities result, corrective osteotomy may be necessary.

Mizuta T et al: Statistical analysis of the incidence of physical injuries. J Pediatr Orthop 1987;7:518.

TORUS FRACTURES

Torus fractures consist of "buckling" of the cortex as a result of minimal angular trauma. They usually occur in the distal radius or ulna. Alignment is satisfactory, and simple immobilization for 3–5 weeks is sufficient.

GREENSTICK FRACTURES

With greenstick fractures there is frank disruption of the cortex on one side of the bone but no discernible cleavage plane on the opposite side. These fractures are angulated but not displaced, as the bone ends are not separated. Reduction is achieved by straightening the arm into normal alignment, and reduction is maintained by a snugly fitting plaster cast. It is necessary to x-ray children with greenstick fractures again in a week to 10 days to make certain that the reduction has been maintained in plaster. A slight angular deformity will be corrected by remodeling of the bone. The farther the fracture is from the growing end of the bone, the longer the time required for healing. The fracture can be considered healed when there are no findings of tenderness and local swelling or heat and when adequate bony callus is seen on x-ray.

FRACTURE OF THE CLAVICLE

Clavicular fractures are very common injuries in infants and children. They can be immobilized by a figure-of-eight dressing that retracts the shoulders and brings the clavicle to normal length. The healing callus will be apparent when the fracture has consolidated, but this unsightly lump will generally resolve over a period of months to a year.

SUPRACONDYLAR FRACTURES OF THE HUMERUS

Supracondylar fractures tend to occur in the age group from 3 to 6 years and are potentially dangerous because of the proximity to the brachial artery in the distal arm. They are usually associated with a significant amount of trauma, so that swelling may be severe. **Volkmann's ischemic contracture** of the forearm may occur as a result of vascular embarrassment. When severe swelling is present, the safest course is to place the arm in traction and carefully observe nerve function and the vascular supply to the hand. In these cases, the children should be hospitalized and followed carefully by experienced nurses. If the blood supply is compromised, exposure of the brachial artery may be necessary, although this is rarely needed when satisfactory reduction and traction are employed. Most often, these fractures are treated by closed reduction and percutaneous pinning. Complications associated with supracondylar fractures also include a resultant cubitus varus secondary to poor reduction. It is often difficult to ascertain adequacy of the reduction because a flexed position is necessary to maintain normal alignment. Such a "gunstock" deformity of the elbow may be somewhat unsightly but does not usually interfere with joint function.

Kurer MH, Regan MW: Completely displaced supracondylar fracture of the humerus in children: A review of 1708 comparable cases. Clin Orthop 1990;256:205.

Millis MB, Singer U, Hall JE: Supracondylar fracture of the humerus in children: Further experience with a study in orthopaedic decision-making. Clin Orthop (Sept) 1984; 188:90.

Royce RO et al: Neurologic complications after K-wire fixation of supracondylar humerus fractures in children. J Pediatr Orthop 1991;11:191.

GENERAL COMMENTS ON OTHER FRACTURES IN CHILDREN

Reduction of fractures in children is usually accomplished by simple traction and manipulation; open reduction is rarely indicated. Remodeling of the fracture callus will usually produce an almost normal appearance of the bone over a matter of months. The younger the child, the more remodeling is possible. Angular deformities remodel with ease. Rotatory deformities do not remodel, and this produces the cubitus varus deformity sometimes seen after supracondylar fractures.

The physician should be suspicious of child abuse whenever the age of a fracture does not match the history given or when the severity of the injury is more than the alleged accident would have produced. In suspected cases of battering where no fracture is present on the initial x-ray film, a repeat film 10 days later is in order. Bleeding beneath the periosteum will be calcified by 7–10 days, and the x-ray appearance is almost diagnostic of severe closed trauma characteristic of a battered child.

Cumming WA: Neonatal skeletal fractures: Birth trauma or child abuse? J Can Assoc Radiol 1979;30:30.

Dent JA, Patterson CR: Fractures in early childhood: Osteogenesis imperfecta or child abuse? J Pediatr Orthop 1991;11:184.

Ogden JA: *Skeletal Injury in the Child.* Lea & Febiger, 1982.

Rang M: *Children's Fractures,* 2nd ed. Lippincott, 1983.

Weber BG, Brunner C, Freuler F (editors): *Treatment of Fractures in Children and Adolescents.* Springer-Verlag, 1980.

INFECTIONS OF THE BONES & JOINTS

OSTEOMYELITIS

Osteomyelitis is an infectious process that usually starts in the spongy or medullary bone and then extends to involve compact or cortical bone. It is more common in boys than in girls. The lower extremities are most often affected, and there is commonly a history of trauma. Osteomyelitis may occur as a result of direct invasion from the outside through a penetrating wound (nail) or open fracture, but hematogenous spread of infection (eg, pyoderma or upper respiratory tract infection) from other infected areas is more common. The most common infecting organism is *Staphylococcus aureus,* which seems to have a special tendency to infect the metaphyses of growing bones. Anatomically, circulation in the long bones is such that the arterial supply to the metaphysis just below the growth plate is by end arteries, which turn sharply to end in venous sinusoids, causing a relative stasis. In the infant under 1 year of age, there is direct vascular communication with the epiphysis across the growth plate, so that direct spread may occur from the metaphysis to the epiphysis and subsequently into the joint. In the older child, the growth plate provides an effective barrier and the epiphysis is usually not involved, although the infection spreads retrograde from the metaphysis into the diaphysis and, by rupture through the cortical bone, down along the diaphysis beneath the periosteum.

1. EXOGENOUS OSTEOMYELITIS

In order to avoid osteomyelitis by direct extension, all wounds must be carefully examined and cleansed. Puncture wounds are especially liable to lead to osteomyelitis if not carefully debrided. Cultures of the wound made at the time of exploration and debridement may be useful if signs of inflammation and infection develop subsequently. Copious irrigation is necessary, and all nonviable skin, subcutaneous tissue, fascia, and muscle must be excised. In extensive or contaminated wounds, antibiotic coverage is indicated. Contaminated wounds should be left open and secondary closure performed 3–5 days later. If at the time of delayed closure further necrotic tissue is present, it should be excised. Leaving the wound open allows the infection to stay at the surface rather than extend inward to the bone.

Initially, broad-spectrum antibiotics should be used; after cultures have been read, an appropriate alternative antibiotic can be chosen if there is lingering inflammation. A tetanus toxoid booster is indicated for any questionable wound, but gas gangrene is better prevented by adequate debridement than by antitoxin.

Once exogenous osteomyelitis has become established, treatment becomes more complicated, requiring extensive surgical debridement and drainage followed by careful antibiotic management. These cases require hospitalization and the use of intravenous antibiotics.

2. HEMATOGENOUS OSTEOMYELITIS

Hematogenous osteomyelitis is usually caused by pyogenic bacteria; 85% of cases are due to staphylococci. Streptococci are rare causes of osteomyelitis today, but *Pseudomonas* organisms have often been documented in cases of nail puncture wounds. Children with sickle cell anemia are especially prone to osteomyelitis caused by salmonellae.

Clinical Findings

A. Symptoms and Signs: In infants, the manifestations of osteomyelitis may be quite subtle, presenting as irritability, diarrhea, or failure to feed properly; the temperature may be normal or slightly low; and the white blood count may be normal or only slightly elevated. There may be pseudoparalysis of the involved limb. In older children, the manifestations are more striking, with severe local tenderness and pain, high fever, rapid pulse, and elevated white blood count and sedimentation rate. Osteomyelitis of a lower extremity often presents around the knee in a child 7–10 years of age. Tenderness is most marked over the metaphysis of the bone where the process has its origin. The child may limp or refuse to bear weight.

B. Laboratory Findings: Blood cultures are often positive early. The most significant test in infancy is the aspiration of pus when suspicion arises because of lack of movement in a painful extremity. It is useful to insert a needle to the bone in the area of suspected infection and aspirate any fluid present. This fluid can be smeared and stained for organisms as well as cultured. Even edema fluid may be useful for determining the causative organism. The white blood cell count is usually elevated, as is the sedimentation rate.

C. Imaging: The first manifestation to appear on x-ray film is nonspecific local swelling. This is followed by elevation of the periosteum, with formation of new bone from the cambium layer of the periosteum occurring after 3–6 days. As the infection becomes chronic, areas of cortical bone are isolated by pus spreading down the medullary canal, causing rarefaction and demineralization of the bone. Such isolated pieces of cortex become ischemic and form sequestra (dead bone fragments). These x-ray findings are late, and osteomyelitis should be diagnosed clinically before significant x-ray findings are present. Bone scan is valuable in suspected cases before x-ray findings become positive.

Treatment

A. Specific Measures: Antibiotics should be started intravenously as soon as the diagnosis of osteomyelitis is made. Agents that cover *Staphylococcus aureus* and *Streptococcus pyogenes* (eg, oxacillin, nafcillin, or cefazolin, all at 150 mg/kg/d) are appropriate for most cases. For possible *Pseudomonas* infection, add ceftazidime (150 mg/kg/d) or an aminoglycoside. Parenteral antibiotic therapy should be continued until all clinical signs, the white blood count, and the sedimentation rate are improved, usually for 5–10 days. For a reliable family an oral antibiotic may then be begun; the dosage of most antistaphylococcal drugs (dicloxacillin, cephalexin, cephradine) must be 100–150 mg/kg/d in four divided doses to achieve adequate serum killing powers. At least 4 weeks of therapy (with normalization of the sedimentation rate and resolution of all local signs) should be completed. Chronic infections are treated for months. Following surgical debridement, *Pseudomonas* foot infections usually respond to 1–2 weeks of treatment.

B. General Measures: Splitting of the limb minimizes pain and decreases spread of the infection by lymphatic channels through the soft tissue. The splint should be removed periodically to allow active use of adjacent joints and prevent stiffening and muscle atrophy. In chronic osteomyelitis, splinting may be necessary to guard against fracture of the weakened bone.

C. Surgical Measures: Aspiration of the metaphysis is a useful diagnostic measure in any case of suspected osteomyelitis. Osteomyelitis represents a collection of pus under pressure within the body. In the first 24–72 hours, it may be possible to abort osteomyelitis by the use of antibiotics alone. However, if frank pus is aspirated from the bone, surgical drainage is indicated. If the infection has not shown a dramatic response within 24 hours in questionable cases, surgical drainage is also indicated. It is important that all devitalized soft tissue be removed and adequate exposure of the bone obtained in order to permit free drainage. Excessive amounts of bone should not be removed when draining acute osteomyelitis, because they may not be completely replaced by the normal healing process.

In questionable cases, little damage has been done by surgical drainage, but failure to drain the pus in acute cases may lead to more severe damage.

Prognosis

When osteomyelitis is diagnosed in the early clinical stages and prompt antibiotic therapy is begun, the prognosis is excellent. If the process has been unattended for a week to 10 days, there is almost always some permanent loss of bone structure, as well as the possibility of growth abnormality.

Faden H, Grossi M: Acute osteomyelitis in children: Reassessment of etiologic agents and their clinical characteristics. Am J Dis Child 1991;145:65.

Jacobs RF et al: Management of Pseudomonas osteochondritis complicating puncture wounds of the foot. Pediatrics 1982;69:432.

LaMont RL et al: Acute hematogenous osteomyelitis in children. J Pediatr Orthop 1987;7:579.

Scott RJ et al: Acute osteomyelitis in children: A review of 116 cases. J Pediatr Orthop 1990;10:649.

Tudisco C et al: Influence of chronic osteomyelitis on skeletal growth: Analysis at maturity of 26 cases affected during childhood. J Pediatr Orthop 1991;11:353.

PYOGENIC ARTHRITIS

The source of pyogenic arthritis varies according to the age of the child. In the infant, pyogenic arthritis often develops by spread from adjacent osteomyelitis. In the older child, it presents as an isolated infection, usually without bony involvement. In teenagers with pyogenic arthritis, an underlying systemic disease is usually the cause, eg, an obvious generalized infection or an organism that has an affinity for joints, such as the gonococcus.

The infecting organism varies with age: group B streptococcus and *Staphylococcus aureus* in those under 4 months; *Haemophilus influenzae* and *Staphylococcus* in those 4 months to 4 years old; and *Staphylococcus* and *Streptococcus pyogenes* in older children.

The initial effusion of the joint rapidly becomes purulent. An effusion of the joint may accompany osteomyelitis in the adjacent bone. A white blood cell count exceeding $100,000/\mu L$ in the joint fluid indicates a definite purulent infection. Generally, spread of infection is from the bone into the joint, but unattended pyogenic arthritis may also affect adjacent bone. The sedimentation rate is elevated.

Clinical Findings

A. Symptoms and Signs: In older children, the signs are striking, with fever, malaise, vomiting, and restriction of motion. In infants, paralysis of the limb due to inflammatory neuritis may be evident. Infection of the hip joint in infants can be diagnosed if suspicion is aroused by decreased abduction of the hip in an infant who is irritable or feeding poorly. A history of umbilical catheter treatment in the newborn nursery should alert the physician to the possibility of pyogenic arthritis of the hip.

B. Imaging: Early distention of the joint capsule is nonspecific and difficult to measure by x-ray. In the infant with unrecognized pyogenic arthritis, dislocation of the joint may follow within a few days as a result of distention of the capsule by pus. Later changes include destruction of the joint space, resorption of epiphysial cartilage, and erosion of the adjacent bone of the metaphysis. The bone scan shows increased flow and symmetrical increased uptake about the joint, unless there is a concomitant osteomyelitis.

Treatment

Diagnosis may be made by aspiration of the joint. In the hip joint, pyogenic arthritis is most easily treated by surgical drainage because the joint is deep and difficult to aspirate as well as being inaccessible to thorough cleaning through needle aspiration. In more superficial joints, such as the knee, aspiration of the joint at least twice daily may maintain adequate drainage. More recently, arthroscopic irrigation and debridement has been successful in treating pyogenic arthritis of the knee. If fever and clinical symptoms do not subside within 24 hours after treatment is begun, open surgical drainage is indicated. Antibiotics can be selected based on age and smears and cultures of the aspirated pus. Reasonable empiric therapy in infants includes cefuroxime (200 mg/kg/d in four divided doses) or oxacillin (150 mg/kg/d) plus a third-generation cephalosporin. An antistaphylococcal alone is usually adequate for children over 5 years. For staphylococcal infections, 3 weeks of therapy is recommended; for other organisms, 2 weeks is usually sufficient. Oral therapy may be begun when clinical signs have markedly improved. It is not necessary to give intra-articular antibiotics, since good levels are achieved in the synovial fluid.

Prognosis

The prognosis is excellent if the joint is drained early, before damage to the articular cartilage has occurred. If infection is present for more than 24 hours, there is dissolution of the proteoglycans in the articular cartilage, with subsequent arthrosis and fibrosis of the joint. Damage to the growth plate may also occur, especially within the hip joint, where the epiphysial plate is intracapsular.

Barton LL, Dunkle LM, Habib FH: Septic arthritis in childhood. A thirteen-year review. Am J Dis Child 1987; 141:898.
Betz RR et al: Late sequelae of septic arthritis of the hip in infancy and childhood. J Pediatr Orthop 1990;10:365.
Shaw BA, Kasser JR: Acute septic arthritis in infancy and childhood. Clin Orthop 1990;257:212.

TUBERCULOUS ARTHRITIS

Tuberculous arthritis is now a rare disease in the USA. It must be considered, however, in children with resistant infections of the joints, especially if there is a history of tuberculosis in family members. Generally, the infection may be ruled out by skin testing. The joints most commonly affected in children are the intervertebral disks, resulting in gibbus or dorsal angular deformity at the site of the involvement.

Treatment is by local drainage of the "cold abscess," followed by antituberculosis therapy with isoniazid, rifampin, and ethambutol. Prolonged immobilization in a plaster cast or prolonged bed rest is necessary in order to promote healing. Spinal fusion may be required to preserve stability of the vertebral column.

TRANSIENT SYNOVITIS OF THE HIP

The most common cause of limping and pain in the hip of children in the USA is transitory synovitis, an acute inflammatory reaction that often follows an upper respiratory infection and is generally self-lim-

ited. In questionable cases, aspiration of the hip yields only yellowish fluid, ruling out pyogenic arthritis. Generally, however, toxic synovitis of the hip is not associated with elevation of the erythrocyte sedimentation rate, the white blood count or a temperature above 38.3 °C. It classically affects children 3–10 years of age and is more common in boys. There is limitation of motion of the hip joint, particularly internal rotation, and x-ray changes are nonspecific, with some swelling apparent in the soft tissues around the joint.

Treatment consists of bed rest and the use of traction with slight flexion of the hip. Nonsteroidal antiinflammatory medications may shorten the course of the disease, although even with no treatment the disease usually is self-limited to a matter of days. It is important to maintain x-ray follow-up because toxic synovitis may be the precursor of avascular necrosis of the femoral head (see next section) in a small percentage of patients. X-ray films can be obtained at 1 month and 3 months, or earlier if there is persistent limp or pain.

Hodges DL, McGuire TJ: Hip pain in children: An anatomic approach. Orthop Rev 1988;17:251.
Kallio P, Tyoppy S, Kunnamo I: Transient synovitis and Perthes disease. Is there an aetiological connection? J Bone Joint Surg [Br] 1986;68:808.
Landin LA, Danielsson LG, Wattsgard C: Transient synovitis of the hip: Its incidence, epidemiology and relation to Perthes disease. J Bone Joint Surg [Br] 1987;69:238.
Terjesen T, Osthus P: Ultrasound in the diagnosis and follow-up of transient synovitis of the hip. J Pediatr Orthop 1991;11:608.

VASCULAR LESIONS & AVASCULAR NECROSIS (Osteochondroses)

AVASCULAR NECROSIS OF THE PROXIMAL FEMUR (Legg-Calvé-Perthes Disease)

The vascular supply of bone is generally precarious, and when it is interrupted, necrosis results. In contrast to other body tissues that undergo infarction, bone removes necrotic tissue and replaces it with living bone in a process called "creeping substitution." This replacement of necrotic bone may be so complete and so perfect that a completely normal bone results. Adequacy of replacement depends upon the age of the patient, the presence or absence of associated infection, congruity of the involved joint, and other physiologic and mechanical factors.

Because of their rapid growth in relation to their

blood supply, the secondary ossification centers in the epiphyses are subject to avascular necrosis. Despite the number of different names referring to avascular necrosis of the epiphyses, the process is identical, ie, necrosis of bone followed by replacement (see Table 26–1).

Even though the pathologic and radiologic features of avascular necrosis of the epiphyses are well known, the cause is not generally agreed upon. Necrosis may follow known causes such as trauma or infection, but idiopathic lesions usually develop during periods of rapid growth of the epiphyses. Thus, the highest incidence of Legg-Calvé-Perthes disease is between 4 and 8 years of age.

Clinical Findings

A. Symptoms and Signs: Persistent pain is the most common symptom, and the patient may present with limp or limitation of motion.

B. Laboratory Findings: Laboratory findings, including studies of joint aspirates, are normal.

C. Imaging: X-ray findings correlate with the progression of the process and the extent of necrosis. The early finding is effusion of the joint associated with slight widening of the joint space and periarticular swelling. Decreased bone density in and around the joint is apparent after a few weeks. The necrotic ossification center appears more dense than the surrounding viable structures, and there is collapse or narrowing of the femoral head.

As replacement of the necrotic ossification center occurs, there is rarefaction of the bone in a patchwork fashion, producing alternating areas of rarefaction and relative density or "fragmentation" of the epiphysis.

In the hip, there may be widening of the femoral head associated with flattening, giving rise to the term **coxa plana.** If infarction has extended across the growth plate, there will be a radiolucent lesion within the metaphysis. If the growth center of the femoral head has been damaged so that normal growth does not occur, varus deformity of the femoral neck will occur as a result of overgrowth of the greater trochanteric apophysis.

Table 26–1. The osteochondroses.

Ossification Center	Eponym	Typical Age
Capital femoral	Legg-Calvé-Perthes disease	3–5
Tarsal navicular	Köhler's bone disease	6
Second metatarsal head	Freiberg's disease	12–14
Vertebral ring	Scheuermann's disease	13–16
Capitellum	Panner's disease	9–11
Tibial tubercle	Osgood-Schlatter disease	11–13
Calcaneus	Sever's disease	8–9

Eventually, complete replacement of the epiphysis will become apparent as new bone replaces necrotic bone. The final shape of the head will depend upon the extent of the necrosis and collapse that has been allowed to occur.

Differential Diagnosis

Differential diagnosis must include inflammatory and infectious lesions of the joints or apophyses. Transient synovitis of the hip may be distinguished from Legg-Calvé-Perthes disease by serial x-rays.

Treatment

Treatment consists simply of protection of the joint. If the joint is deeply seated within the acetabulum and normal joint motion is maintained, a reasonably good result can be expected. The hip is held in abduction and internal rotation in order to fulfill this purpose. Braces are generally used. Surgery may be necessary for an uncooperative patient or one whose social or geographic circumstances do not allow use of a brace (living in a house trailer, in an unpaved rural area, etc).

Prognosis

The prognosis for complete replacement of the necrotic femoral head in a child is excellent, but the functional result will depend upon the amount of deformity that develops during the time the softened structure exists. In Legg-Calvé-Perthes disease, the prognosis depends upon the completeness of involvement of the epiphysial center. In general, patients with metaphysial defects, those in whom the disease develops late in childhood, and those who have more complete involvement of the femoral head have a poorer prognosis.

Osteochondrosis due to vascular lesion may affect various growth centers. Table 26–1 indicates the common sites and the typical ages at presentation.

Martinez AG, Weinstein SL, Dietz FR: Weight bearing abduction brace treatment of Legg-Calvé-Perthes disease. J Bone Joint Surg [Am] 1992;74:12.

McAndrew MP, Weinstein SL: A long-term follow-up of Legg-Calvé-Perthes disease. J Bone Joint Surg [Am] 1984;66:860.

Thompson GH, Salter RB: Legg-Calvé-Perthes disease: Current concepts and controversies. Orthop Clin North Am 1987;18:617.

Wenger DR, Ward WT, Herring JA: Legg-Calvé-Perthes disease. J Bone Joint Surg [Am] 1991;73:778.

OSTEOCHONDRITIS DISSECANS

In osteochondritis dissecans, there is a pie-shaped necrotic area of bone and cartilage adjacent to the articular surface. The fragment of bone may be broken off from the host bone and displaced into the joint as a loose body. If it remains attached, the necrotic fragment may be completely replaced by creeping substitution.

The pathologic process is precisely the same as that described above for avascular necrosing lesions of ossification centers. However, because these lesions are adjacent to articular cartilage, there may be joint damage.

The most common sites of these lesions are the knee (medial femoral condyle), the elbow joint (capitellum), and the talus (superior lateral dome).

Joint pain is the usual presenting complaint. However, local swelling or locking may be present, particularly if there is a fragment free in the joint. Laboratory studies are normal.

Treatment consists of protection of the involved area from mechanical damage. If there is a fragment free within the joint as a loose body, it must be surgically removed. For some marginal lesions, it may be worthwhile to drill the necrotic fragment in order to encourage more rapid vascular ingrowth and replacement. If large areas of a weight-bearing joint are involved, secondary degenerative arthritis may result.

Hughston JC, Hergenroeder PT, Courtenay BG: Osteochondritis dissecans of the femoral condyles. J Bone Joint Surg [Am] 1984;66:1340.

NEUROLOGIC DISORDERS INVOLVING THE MUSCULOSKELETAL SYSTEM

ORTHOPEDIC ASPECTS OF CEREBRAL PALSY

Early physical therapy to encourage completion of the normal developmental patterns may be of benefit in patients with cerebral palsy. The greatest gains from this type of therapy are obtained during the first few years of life, and therapy should not be continued with unrealistic goals when no improvement is apparent.

Bracing and splinting are of questionable benefit, although night splints may be useful in preventing equinus deformity of the feet or adduction contractures of the hips. Orthopedic surgery can offer procedures to weaken hyperactive spastic muscles, to transfer function of deforming spastic muscles, or to stabilize joints. In general, muscle transfers are unpredictable in cerebral palsy, and most orthopedic procedures are directed at weakening deforming forces or bony stabilization by osteotomy or arthrodesis. Recently, selective dorsal rhizotomy has been used in select cases.

Flexion and adduction of the hip due to hyperactivity of the adductors and flexors may produce a progressive paralytic dislocation of the hip. Congenital dislocation of the hip is unusual in cerebral palsy, but in more severely involved children, paralytic dislocation can lead to pain and dysfunction. Treatment of the dislocation once it has occurred is difficult and unsatisfactory. The principal preventive measure is abduction bracing, but this must often be supplemented by release of the adductors or hip flexors in order to prevent dislocation. In severe cases, osteotomy of the femur may also be necessary to correct the bony deformities of femoral anteversion and coxa valga that are invariably present.

Patients with a predominantly athetotic pattern are poor candidates for any surgical procedure or bracing. Neurosurgical procedures may be of some help.

Because it is difficult to predict the outcome of surgical procedures in cerebral palsy, the surgeon must examine patients on several occasions before any operative procedure is undertaken. Follow-up care by a physical therapist to maximize the anticipated long-term gains should be arranged before the operation.

Bleck EE: *Orthopaedic Management of Cerebral Palsy.* MacKeith, 1987.

Harris SR: Early neuromotor predictors of cerebral palsy in low birthweight infants. Dev Med Child Neurol 1987; 29:508.

Palmer FB et al: The effects of physical therapy on cerebral palsy: A controlled trial in infants with spastic diplegia. N Engl J Med 1988;318:803.

ORTHOPEDIC ASPECTS OF MYELODYSPLASIA

Patients born with spina bifida cystica (aperta) should be examined early by an orthopedic surgeon. The level of neurologic involvement determines the muscle imbalance that will be present and apt to produce deformity with growth. The involvement is often asymmetric and tends to change during the first 12–18 months of life. Early closure of the sac is the rule, although there has been some hesitancy to treat all of these patients because of the extremely poor prognosis associated with congenital hydrocephalus, high levels of paralysis, and associated congenital anomalies. Associated musculoskeletal problems may include clubfoot, congenital dislocation of the hip, arthrogryposis type changes of the lower extremities, and congenital scoliosis, among others. The most common lesions are at the level of L3–4 and tend to affect the hip joint, with progressive dislocation occurring during growth. Foot deformities may be in any direction and are complicated by the fact that sensation is generally absent. Spinal deformities develop in a high percentage of these children, with scoliosis being present in approximately 40%. Ambulation is impossible without braces or splints, and careful urologic follow-up must be obtained to prevent complications from incontinence. A high percentage of these children have hydrocephalus, which may be evident at birth or shortly thereafter, requiring shunting. The shunts are sources of infection and may require frequent replacement.

In children who have a reasonable likelihood of walking, operative treatment consists of reduction of the hip and alignment of the feet in the weight-bearing position as well as stabilization of the scoliosis. In children who do not have extension power of the knee, ie, those who lack active quadriceps function, the likelihood of ambulation is greatly decreased. In such patients, aggressive surgery in the hip region may result in stiffening of the joints, thus preventing sitting. Multiple foot operations are also contraindicated in these children.

The overall management of the child with spina bifida should be coordinated in a multidiscipline clinic where all doctors working in cooperation with each other can work also with therapists, social workers, and teachers to provide the best possible care.

Charney EB, Melchianni JB, Smith DR: Community ambulation by children with myelomeningocele and high level paralysis. J Pediatr Orthop 1991;11:579.

Findley TW et al: Ambulation in the adolescent with myelomeningocele. 1. Early childhood predictors. Arch Phys Med Rehabil 1987;68:518.

Menelaus MB: *The Orthopaedic Management of Spina Bifida Cystica,* 2nd ed. Churchill Livingstone, 1980.

MISCELLANEOUS DISEASES OF BONE

FIBROUS DYSPLASIA

Dysplastic fibrous tissue replacement of the medullary canal is accompanied by the formation of metaplastic bone in fibrous dysplasia. Three forms of the disease are recognized: monostotic, polyostotic, and polyostotic with endocrine disturbances (precocious puberty in females, hyperthyroidism, and hyperadrenalism, ie, Albright's syndrome).

Clinical Findings

A. Symptoms and Signs: The lesion or lesions may be asymptomatic. Pain, if present, is probably due to pathologic fractures. In females, endocrine disturbances may be present in the polyostotic variety and associated with café au lait spots.

B. Laboratory Findings: Laboratory findings are normal unless endocrine disturbances are present, in which case there may be increased secretion of gonadotropic, thyroid, or adrenal hormones.

C. Imaging: The lesion begins centrally within the medullary canal, usually of a long bone, and expands slowly. Pathologic fracture may occur. If metaplastic bone predominates, the contents of the lesion will be of the density of bone. Marked deformity of the bone may result, and a shepherd's crook deformity of the upper femur is a classic feature of the disease. The disease is often asymmetric, and limb length disturbances may occur as a result of stimulation of epiphysial cartilage growth.

Differential Diagnosis

The differential diagnosis may include other fibrous lesions of bone as well as destructive lesions such as bone cyst, eosinophilic granuloma, aneurysmal bone cyst, nonossifying fibroma, enchondroma, and chondromyxoid fibroma.

Treatment

If the lesion is small and asymptomatic, no treatment is needed. If the lesion is large and produces or threatens pathologic fracture, curettage and bone grafting are indicated.

Prognosis

Unless the lesions impair epiphysial growth, the prognosis is good. Lesions tend to enlarge during the growth period but are stable during adult life. Malignant transformation has not been recorded.

UNICAMERAL BONE CYST

Unicameral bone cyst appears in the metaphysis of a long bone, usually in the femur or humerus. It begins within the medullary canal adjacent to the epiphysial cartilage. It probably results from some fault in enchondral ossification. The cyst is "active" as long as it abuts onto the metaphysial side of the epiphysial cartilage and "inactive" when a border of normal bone exists between the cyst and the epiphysial cartilage. The lesion is usually identified when a pathologic fracture occurs, producing pain. Laboratory findings are normal. On x-ray films, the cyst is identified centrally within the medullary canal, producing expansion of the cortex and thinning over the widest portion of the cyst.

Treatment consists of injection with corticosteroid. Several injections may be required. If injection fails, then curettage and bone grafting may be required. The cyst may heal after a fracture and not require treatment.

The prognosis is excellent. Many cysts will heal following pathologic fracture.

dePalma L, Santuccil A: [Treatment of bone cysts with methylprednisolone acetate.] Int Orthop 1987;11:23. [French.]

ANEURYSMAL BONE CYST

Aneurysmal bone cyst is similar to unicameral bone cyst, but it contains blood rather than clear fluid. It usually occurs in a slightly eccentric position in the long bone, expanding the cortex of the bone but not breaking the cortex, although some extraosseous mass may be produced. On x-ray films, the lesion appears somewhat larger than the width of the epiphysial cartilage, and this feature distinguishes it from unicameral bone cyst.

The aneurysmal bone cyst is filled by large vascular lakes, and the stoma of the cyst contains fibrous tissue and areas of metaplastic ossification.

The lesion may appear quite aggressive histologically, and it is important to differentiate it from osteosarcoma or hemangioma. Treatment is by curettage and bone grafting, and the prognosis is excellent.

INFANTILE CORTICAL HYPEROSTOSIS (Caffey's Syndrome)

Infantile cortical hyperostosis is a benign disease of unknown cause that has its onset before 6 months of age and is characterized by irritability, fever, and nonsuppurating, tender, painful swellings. Swellings may involve almost any bone of the body and are frequently widespread. Classically, there are swellings of the mandible and clavicle in 50% of cases as well as of the ulna, humerus, and ribs. The disease is limited to the shafts of bones and does not involve subcutaneous tissues or joints. It is self-limited but may persist for weeks or months. Anemia, leukocytosis, an increased sedimentation rate, and elevation of the serum alkaline phosphatase are usually present. Cortical hyperostosis is demonstrable by a typical x-ray appearance and may be diagnosed on physical examination by an experienced pediatrician.

Fortunately, the disease appears to be decreasing in frequency. Corticosteroids are effective in severe cases.

The prognosis is good, and the disease usually terminates without deformity.

GANGLION

A ganglion is a smooth, small cystic mass connected by a pedicle to the joint capsule, usually on the dorsum of the wrist. It may also be seen in the tendon sheath over the flexor surfaces of the fingers. These ganglions can be excised if they interfere with function or cause persistent pain.

BAKER'S CYST

Baker's cyst is a herniation of the synovium in the knee joint into the popliteal region. In children, the diagnosis may be made by aspiration of mucinous fluid, but the cyst nearly always disappears with time. Whereas Baker's cysts may be indicative of intraarticular disease in the adult, they usually are of no clinical significance in children and rarely require excision.

Dinham JM: Popliteal cysts in children: The case against surgery. J Bone Joint Surg [Br] 1975;57:69.

Rheumatic Diseases

27

J. Roger Hollister, MD

JUVENILE RHEUMATOID ARTHRITIS
(Juvenile Chronic Arthritis)

Essentials of Diagnosis

- Nonmigratory monarticular or polyarticular arthropathy, with a tendency to involve large joints or proximal interphalangeal joints and lasting more than 3 months.
- Systemic manifestations with fever, erythematous rashes, nodules, leukocytosis, and, occasionally, iridocyclitis, pleuritis, pericarditis, anemia, fatigue, and growth failure.

General Considerations

Juvenile rheumatoid arthritis patients exhibit different immunogenetic traits from adult rheumatoid arthritis patients. In juvenile rheumatoid arthritis, HLA-DR5 is associated with iritis and the production of antinuclear antibodies, whereas HLA-DR4 is found in seropositive, polyarticular disease. These traits may be important in the formation of anti-suppressor cell antibodies, immune complex generation, and consequent chronic inflammatory disease.

Clinical Findings

A. Symptoms and Signs: There are four patterns of presentation in juvenile rheumatoid arthritis that provide clues to the prognosis and possible sequelae of the disease. In the acute febrile form, an evanescent salmon-pink macular rash, arthritis, hepatosplenomegaly, leukocytosis, and polyserositis characterize the constellation described by George Still. These patients have episodic illness, and remission of the systemic features can be expected within 1 year. They do not develop iridocyclitis.

The polyarticular pattern resembles the adult disease, with chronic pain and swelling of many joints in a symmetric fashion. Both large and small joints are usually involved. Systemic features are less prominent, though low-grade fever, fatigue, rheumatoid nodules, and anemia may be present. These patients tend to have long-standing arthritis, though the disease may wax and wane. Iridocyclitis is occasionally seen in this group. Older children may have a positive latex fixation test.

The third pattern consists of pauciarticular disease characterized by chronic arthritis of a few joints—often the large weight-bearing joints—in asymmetric distribution. The synovitis is usually mild and may be painless. Systemic features are uncommon, but there is severe extra-articular involvement with inflammation in the eye. Up to 30% of children with pauciarticular juvenile rheumatoid arthritis develop insidious, asymptomatic iridocyclitis, which may cause blindness if untreated. The activity of the eye disease does not correlate with that of the arthritis. Therefore, routine ophthalmologic screening with slitlamp examination must be performed every 6 months for 4 years, after which the risk is much lower.

The fourth pattern occurs in late childhood, mainly in boys, of whom 75% have HLA-B27. The early clinical pattern is of pauciarticular disease involving the lower limbs; later, the sacroiliac joints may be involved, and ultimately the lumbar and thoracic spine.

B. Laboratory Findings: There is no diagnostic test for juvenile rheumatoid arthritis. Rheumatoid factor is positive by the latex fixation test in about 15% of cases, usually when onset of polyarticular disease occurs after age 8 years. Antinuclear antibodies are most often present in pauciarticular disease with iridocyclitis and may serve as an indication of this complication; they are also fairly common in the late-onset rheumatoid factor-positive group. A normal erythrocyte sedimentation rate does not exclude the diagnosis.

In Table 27–1 are listed the general characteristics of joint fluid in various conditions. A positive Gram stain or culture is the only definitive test. A leukocyte count over 2000/μL suggests inflammation; this may be due to infection, any of the collagen-vascular diseases, leukemia, or reactive arthritis. A very low glucose concentration (< 40 mg/dL) or very high polymorphonuclear leukocyte count (> 60,000/μL) is highly suggestive of bacterial arthritis in a child. Chemical analysis of synovial fluid is otherwise of little diagnostic benefit.

C. Imaging: In the early stages of the disease, only soft tissue swelling and regional osteoporosis are seen. Cervical subluxation should be monitored by radiographs in patients with neck pain. MRI of involved joints may show joint damage earlier in the

Table 27–1. Joint fluid analysis.

Disorder	Cells/μL	Glucose[1]
Trauma	More red cells than white cells; usually < 2000 white cells	Normal
Reactive arthritis	3000–10,000 white cells, mostly mono-nuclears	Normal
Juvenile rheumatoid arthritis and other inflammatory arthritides	5000–60,000 white cells, mostly neutrophils	Usually normal or slightly low
Septic arthritis	> 60,000 white cells, > 90% neutrophils	Low to normal

[1] Normal value is 75% or more of serum glucose value.

course of the disease than with other imaging modalities.

Differential Diagnosis

Table 27–2 lists the most common causes of limb pain in childhood. A few points of information may indicate the most likely diagnosis. For instance, orthopedic causes are due to increased physical activity, not major trauma. Reactive arthritides are suggested by a preceding viral infection, strep throat, or purpuric rash, and their course is waxing and waning over several days. The characteristics of collagen-vascular and psycho-organic pain are covered in this chapter.

Monarticular arthritis is the most important differential disorder to establish. Pain in the hip or lower extremity is a frequent symptom with childhood cancer, especially leukemia, neuroblastoma, and rhabdomyosarcoma. Infiltration of bone by tumor and actual joint effusion may be seen. X-rays of the affected site and a careful examination of the blood smear for unusual cells and thrombocytopenia are necessary. In doubtful cases, bone marrow examination is indicated.

Bacterial arthritis is usually acute and monarticular except for arthritis associated with *Haemophilus influenzae* infection and gonorrhea, both of which may be associated with a migratory pattern. Fever, leukocytosis, and increased sedimentation rate with an acute process in a single joint demand synovial fluid examination and culture to identify the pathogen. An elevated synovial fluid white count and low glucose (relative to plasma glucose) suggest sepsis.

The arthritis of rheumatic fever is migratory, transient, and often more painful than that of juvenile rheumatoid arthritis. Rheumatic fever is very rare under the age of 5 years. Evidence of rheumatic carditis should be carefully sought. Evidence of recent streptococcal infection is essential to the diagnosis. The fever pattern in rheumatic fever is low-grade and persistent in comparison to the intermittent fever in the systemic form of juvenile rheumatoid arthritis.

Table 27–2. Differential diagnosis of limb pain in children.

Orthopedic
  Stress fracture
  Overuse syndrome
  Chondromalacia patellae
  Osgood-Schlatter disease
  Slipped capital femoral epiphysis
  Legg-Calvé-Perthes disease
  Hypermobility syndrome
Reactive arthritis
  Schönlein-Henoch purpura
  Reactive arthritis following diarrhea
  Toxic synovitis of the hip
  Transient synovitis following viral infection
  Rheumatic fever
Infections
  Bacterial
    Lyme arthritis
    Osteomyelitis
    Septic arthritis
    Discitis
  Viral
    Parvovirus (in adolescents)
    Rubella
    Hepatitis B arthritis
Collagen-vascular
  Juvenile rheumatoid arthritis
  Spondyloarthropathy
  Systemic lupus erythematosus
  Dermatomyositis
Neoplastic
  Leukemia
  Lymphoma
  Neuroblastoma
  Reticuloendotheliosis
  Osteoid osteoma
  Bone tumors (benign or malignant)
Syndromes of psycho-organic origin
  Growing pains
  Fibromyalgia
  Reflex neurovascular dystrophy

Lyme arthritis resembles pauciarticular juvenile rheumatoid arthritis, but it occurs as discrete, recurrent episodes of arthritis lasting 2–6 weeks. A negative test for antibodies to *Borrelia burgdorferi* argues strongly against this diagnosis.

Treatment

The objective of therapy is to restore function, relieve pain, and maintain joint motion. In recent years, other nonsteroidal anti-inflammatory drugs (NSAIDs) have replaced salicylates in the medical treatment of juvenile rheumatoid arthritis. Although their anti-inflammatory potency is not different from that of aspirin, their liquid form, decreased frequency of dosing, and diminished side effects appear to enhance compliance, cause fewer side effects, and justify their increased cost. Naproxen, 7.5 mg/kg twice daily; ibuprofen, 10 mg/kg four times daily; and tolmetin sodium, 10 mg/kg three times daily, may be used. If benefit occurs in the first 2 days, there will be continued improvement, with the maximum effect at 6 weeks. Aspirin, 75–100 mg/kg/d in three divided doses, is equally effective. Salicylates are withheld if the patient is exposed to chickenpox or Asian flu. Range-of-motion and muscle strengthening should be taught and supervised by a therapist, and a home program should be instituted. Bed rest is to be avoided except in the most acute stages. Joint casting is almost never indicated.

In patients who fail to respond to aspirin, there are a number of alternatives. Methotrexate has replaced injectable gold salt therapy as a second-line medication. Symptomatic response usually occurs within 3–4 weeks. The low doses used (5–10 mg/m^2/wk as a single dose) have been associated with few side effects. Stomatitis usually resolves with continued administration. Nausea may be prevented by splitting the dose. Hepatotoxicity, including fibrosis, is a concern. A CBC and liver function test should be obtained at 1- to 2-month intervals. Liver biopsy may be performed if there are recurrent elevations of aminotransferases. Injectable gold salts are an alternative in refractory cases.

Iridocyclitis should be treated by an ophthalmologist, and methotrexate may be used in difficult cases. Local steroid injections into joints, synovectomy, or joint replacement may be indicated in selected patients.

Prognosis

In the primarily articular forms, disease activity progressively diminishes with age and ceases in about 95% of cases by puberty. In a few instances, this will persist into adult life. Problems after puberty therefore relate primarily to residual joint damage. Cases presenting in the teen years usually presage adult disease. The children most liable to be permanently handicapped are those with unremitting synovitis, hip involvement, or positive rheumatoid factor tests.

Foster CS, Barrett F: Cataract development and cataract surgery in patients with juvenile rheumatoid arthritis-associated iridocyclitis. Ophthalmology 1993;100:810.

Graham LD et al: Morbidity associated with long-term methotrexate therapy in juvenile rheumatoid arthritis. Pediatr Pharm Ther 1992;120:468.

Giannini EH et al: Methotrexate in resistant juvenile rheumatoid arthritis: Results of the U.S.A.-U.S.S.R. double-blind, placebo-controlled trial. New Engl J Med 1992; 326:1043.

Lang BA, Shore A: A review of current concepts on the pathogenesis of juvenile rheumatoid arthritis. J Rheumatol 1990;21(Suppl, March):1.

Ostrov BE et al: Differentiation of systemic juvenile rheumatoid arthritis from acute leukemia near the onset of disease. J Pediatr 1993;122:595.

Rosenberg AM: Advanced drug therapy for juvenile rheumatoid arthritis. J Pediatr 1989;114:171.

Schneider R et al: Prognostic indicators of joint destruction in systemic onset juvenile rheumatoid arthritis. J Pediatr 1992;120:200.

Steele RW et al: Usefulness of scanning procedures for diagnosis of fever of unknown origin in children. J Pediatr 1991;119:526.

Szer IS et al: Long term course of Lyme arthritis in children. N Engl J Med 1991;325:159.

SPONDYLOARTHROPATHY

Lower extremity arthritis, particularly in males over 10 years of age, suggests a form of spondyloarthropathy. Inflammation of tendinous insertions (enthesopathy) such as the tibial tubercle or the heel occurs in these diseases and not in juvenile rheumatoid arthritis. Low back pain and sacroiliitis are quite specific for this form of arthritis. Carriage of HLA-B27 antigen occurs in 80% of these individuals. Specific syndromes of Reiter's disease, inflammatory bowel disease, psoriasis, or postdiarrheal reactive arthritis are suggested by the associated clinical findings and epidemiology. No autoantibodies are found, but inflammatory indicators such as an elevated erythrocyte sedimentation rate or C-reactive protein are usually present. The episodes are usually intermittent, in contrast to the more chronic symptoms of juvenile rheumatoid arthritis. Acute, not chronic, uveitis may occur.

The nonsteroidal medications, particularly indomethacin (2–4 mg/kg/d) and naproxen (15 mg/kg/d), are more effective than salicylates in the spondyloarthropathies. Refractory cases may respond to sulfasalazine. Local corticosteroid injections are contraindicated in Achilles tendinitis.

The arthritis is usually episodic. Unlike adults, children do not frequently progress to joint destruction or ankylosis.

Buxbaum J: Therapy for seronegative spondyloarthropathies. Curr Opin Rheumatol 1992;4:500.

SYSTEMIC LUPUS ERYTHEMATOSUS

Essentials of Diagnosis

- Multisystem inflammatory disease of joints, serous linings, skin, kidneys, and central nervous system.
- Antinuclear antibodies must be present in active, untreated disease.

General Considerations

Systemic lupus erythematosus is the prototype of immune complex diseases; its pathogenesis is related to deposition in the tissue of soluble immune complexes existing in the circulation. The spectrum of symptoms appears to be due not to tissue-specific autoantibodies but rather to damage to the tissue by lymphocytes, neutrophils, and complement evoked by the deposition of antigen-antibody complexes. Many such antigen-antibody systems are present in this disorder, but the best correlation exists between DNA-anti-DNA complexes and the activity of the disease. Laboratory tests of these antibodies and complement components give an objective assessment of disease pathogenesis and response to therapy. The trigger for the formation of immune complexes in systemic lupus erythematosus has not been identified. Autoreactive T lymphocytes that have escaped clonal deletion and unregulated B lymphocyte production of autoantibodies may initiate the disease.

A drug-related syndrome resembling systemic lupus erythematosus may be produced by procainamide, phenytoin, and isoniazid, among others. Affected patients recover on stopping the drug and do not manifest renal disease.

Clinical Findings

A. Symptoms and Signs: The onset is most common in girls (8:1) between the ages of 9 and 15 years. The symptoms depend on what organ is involved with immune complex deposition.

1. Joint symptoms are the commonest presenting feature. Nondeforming arthritis may involve any joint, often in a symmetric manner. Myositis may also occur and is more painful than the inflammation in dermatomyositis.

2. Systemic manifestations include weakness, anorexia, fever, fatigue, and loss of weight.

3. Skin lesions include butterfly erythema and induration, small ulcerations in skin and mucous membranes, purpura, alopecia, and Raynaud's phenomenon. The sun sensitivity of the dermal lesions may be striking.

4. Polyserositis may include pleurisy with effusions, peritonitis, and pericarditis. Libman-Sacks endocarditis may be seen in patients with antiphospholipid antibodies.

5. Hepatosplenomegaly and lymphadenopathy may occur.

6. Renal systemic lupus erythematosus produces few symptoms at onset but is often progressive and is the leading cause of death. Renal biopsy is indicated in patients who do not respond to steroids or who cannot have steroids tapered to a less toxic alternate-day regimen. The histologic pattern of diffuse proliferative nephritis requires the most aggressive treatment. Late complications are nephrosis and uremia.

7. Central nervous system involvement produces a variety of symptoms such as seizures, coma, hemiplegia, focal neuropathies, and behavior disturbances, including psychosis. The psychosis may be impossible to distinguish from corticosteroid-induced psychosis.

B. Laboratory Findings: Leukopenia and anemia are frequently found with a low incidence of Coombs positivity. Thrombocytopenia and purpura may be early manifestations even in the absence of other organ involvement. The erythrocyte sedimentation rate is elevated, and hypergammaglobulinemia is often present. Renal involvement is indicated by the presence in the urine of red cells, white cells, red cell casts, and proteinuria.

The antinuclear antibody test is the most sensitive diagnostic test and has supplanted the LE preparation. The antinuclear antibody test is invariably positive in patients with active untreated systemic lupus erythematosus, and a negative antinuclear antibody test effectively excludes the diagnosis. For patients with a positive antinuclear antibody test, a profile identifying individual disease-specific antibodies should be ordered. Anticardiolipin antibody and the lupus anticoagulant are two recently described autoantibodies that identify lupus patients at risk for thrombotic events.

In managing the disease, elevated titers of anti-DNA antibody and depressed levels of serum complement (hemolytic, C3, or C4) accurately reflect active disease, especially renal, central nervous system, and skin disease. A CT or MRI scan may identify pathologic conditions of the brain in lupus cerebritis, such as infarction, vasculitis, or atrophy.

Differential Diagnosis

Systemic lupus erythematosus may simulate many inflammatory diseases such as rheumatic fever, rheumatoid arthritis, and viral infections. It is essential to review all organ systems carefully to establish a clinical pattern. Renal and central nervous system involvement is unique to systemic lupus erythematosus. A negative antinuclear antibody test excludes the diagnosis of systemic lupus erythematosus. Tests yielding false-positive results are usually of low titer (< 1:320).

An overlap syndrome known as mixed connective tissue disease, with features of several collagen-vascular diseases, has recently been described in adults and children. The symptom complex is diverse and does not readily fit previous classifications. Arthritis, fever, skin tightening, Raynaud's phenomenon, muscle weakness, and rashes are most commonly present. Important factors in recognition of this disease entity are the relative infrequency of renal disease, which implies a better prognosis than systemic lupus erythematosus, and the corticosteroid responsiveness of symptoms, which distinguishes mixed connective tissue disease from scleroderma. The definition of the disease includes the presence of serum antibody to an extractable nuclear antigen. Patients are initially identified by a speckled pattern of immunofluorescence in the antinuclear antibody test. The specialized extractable nuclear antigen test demonstrates very high titers of up to 1:1,000,000 of the antibody. Pulmonary disease in childhood produces major morbidity.

Treatment

The treatment of systemic lupus erythematosus should be tailored to the organ system involved so that toxicities may be minimized. Prednisone, 0.5–1 mg/kg/d orally, has significantly lowered the mortality rate in systemic lupus erythematosus and should be used in all cases with renal, cardiac, or central nervous system involvement. The dose should be varied using clinical and laboratory parameters of disease activity, and the minimum amount of corticosteroid to control the disease should be used. Alternate-day regimens of corticosteroid are frequently possible. Skin manifestations may frequently be treated with antimalarials, eg, hydroxychloroquine, 5–7 mg/kg/d orally. Pleuritic pain or arthritis can often be managed with salicylates alone.

If disease control is inadequate with prednisone or if the dose required produces intolerable side effects, an immunosuppressant should be added. Either azathioprine, 2–3 mg/kg/d orally, or cyclophosphamide, 0.5–1 g/m², administered intravenously once a month, has been most widely used. These drugs are ineffective during acute crises such as seizures.

The toxicities of the regimens must be carefully considered. In life-threatening disease, the choices are easier. Growth failure, osteoporosis, Cushing's syndrome, adrenal suppression, and aseptic necrosis are serious side effects of chronic use of prednisone. When high doses of corticosteroids are used (> 2 mg/kg/d), the risk of sepsis is very real. Cyclophosphamide causes bladder epithelial dysplasia, hemorrhagic cystitis, and sterility. Azathioprine has been associated with liver damage and bone marrow suppression. Immunosuppressant treatment should be withheld if the total white count falls below 3000/μL or the neutrophil count below 1000/μL. Retinal damage from chloroquine derivatives has not been observed with recommended dosages. Intravenous pulse steroid therapy and plasmapheresis are treatments that may be useful in selected cases.

Amenorrhea may result from uncontrolled systemic lupus erythematosus but may also be a consequence of prednisone, cyclophosphamide, or azathioprine administration.

Course & Prognosis

The prognosis in systemic lupus erythematosus relates to the presence of renal involvement or infectious complications of treatment. With improved diagnosis, milder cases are now identified. Nonetheless, the survival rate improved from 51% at 5 years in 1954 to 90% today. The disease has a natural waxing and waning cycle, and periods of complete remission are not unusual.

Cervera R et al: Systemic lupus erythematosus: Clinical and immunologic patterns of disease expression in a cohort of 1,000 patients. Medicine 1993;72:113.
Friedman DM et al: Acute myocardial infarction in pediatric systemic lupus erythematosus. J Pediatr 1990;117:263.
Lehman TJA et al: Intermittent intravenous cyclophosphamide therapy for lupus nephritis. J Pediatr 1989;114:1055.
Lindsley CB: Lupus: A brighter outlook, a continuing challenge. Contemporary Pediatr 1992;9:19.

Lockshin MD: Therapy for systemic lupus erythematosus. N Engl J Med 1991;324:189.
Singsen BH: Mixed connective tissue disease in childhood. Pediatr Rev 1989;7:309.

DERMATOMYOSITIS
(Polymyositis)

Essentials of Diagnosis

- Pathognomonic skin rash.
- Weakness of proximal muscles and occasionally of pharyngeal and laryngeal groups.
- Pathogenesis related to vasculitis.

General Considerations

Dermatomyositis, a rare inflammatory disease of muscle and skin in childhood, is uniquely responsive to corticosteroid treatment. The vasculitis observed in childhood dermatomyositis differs pathologically from the adult disease. Small arteries and veins are involved, with an exudate of neutrophils, lymphocytes, plasma cells, and histiocytes. The lesion progresses to intimal proliferation and thrombus formation. These vascular changes are found in the skin, muscle, kidney, retina, and gastrointestinal tract. Postinflammatory calcinosis is frequent.

The autoimmune pathogenesis of dermatomyositis has been difficult to prove. Recent studies have shown that both cellular and humoral mechanisms may be involved. Lymphocytes from patients are stimulated to undergo blastogenesis in the presence of muscle tissue and will release lymphotoxin, which destroys cultured fetal muscle cells. Biopsies studied with immunofluorescence techniques demonstrate immunoglobulin and complement in perivascular distribution. The putative antigen has not been identified. Suggestive data relating adult myositis to toxoplasmosis have not been found in children, and results of viral studies have been negative.

Clinical Findings

A. Symptoms and Signs: The predominant symptom is muscular weakness in proximal distribution affecting pelvic and shoulder girdles. Tenderness, stiffness, and swelling may be found but are not striking. Neurologic findings such as absence of tendon reflexes are not seen until late in the disease. Pharyngeal and respiratory involvement can be life-threatening. Flexion contractures and muscle atrophy produce significant residual deformities. Calcinosis may follow the inflammation in muscle and skin. Vasculitis of the intestine causing hemorrhage or perforation is less frequently seen in recent years, perhaps owing to corticosteroid treatment.

The rash of dermatomyositis is very helpful in the diagnosis of unknown muscle disease. Characteristically, the rash involves the upper eyelids and extensor surfaces of the knuckles, elbows, and knees with a distinctive heliotrope color that progresses to a scaling and atrophic appearance. Periorbital edema is not uncommon. Nail fold capillary abnormalities may identify patients with a poorer prognosis. None of the rashes associated with other childhood rheumatic diseases have these features of distribution. The activity of the rash frequently does not parallel the muscle disease.

B. Laboratory Findings: Determination of muscle enzyme levels is the most helpful tool in diagnosis and treatment. All enzymes, including serum aldolase, should be screened to detect an abnormality that reflects activity of the disease. The blood count, erythrocyte sedimentation rate, and acute phase reactants are frequently normal. No autoantibodies are found. Electromyography is useful to distinguish myopathic from neuropathic causes of muscle weakness. Muscle biopsy is indicated in doubtful cases of myositis without the pathognomonic rash.

Treatment

Prednisone in high doses (1–2 mg/kg/d orally) has been shown to speed recovery. The dose should be maintained or increased until muscle enzymes have returned to normal. Functional recovery will lag somewhat behind laboratory improvement. With improvement, the dose may be cut to that level which maintains disease control and normal muscle enzymes. Treatment must be continued for an average of 2 years. Immunosuppressant agents are occasionally required in childhood dermatomyositis. Intravenous immune globulin or cyclosporine therapy may be tried in refractory cases. Physical therapy is critical to prevent or allay contractures.

Course & Prognosis

Most children will recover and discontinue medications in 1–3 years. Relapses may occur. Functional ability is very good in most patients. Myositis in childhood is not associated with an increased risk of cancer.

Hattori H et al: Benign acute myositis associated with rotavirus gastroenteritis. J Pediatr 1992;121:748.

Hechmatt J et al: Cyclosporin in juvenile dermatomyositis. Lancet 1989;1:1063.

Lang BA et al: Treatment of dermatomyositis with intravenous gammaglobulin. Am J Med 1991;91:169.

Martin A et al: Recurrent juvenile dermatomyositis and cutaneous necrotizing arteritis with molecular mimicry between streptococcal type 5 M protein and human skeletal myosin. J Pediatr 1992;121:739.

Sigurgeirsson B et al: Risk of cancer in patients with dermatomyositis or polymyositis. N Engl J Med 1992; 326:363.

POLYARTERITIS NODOSA

Polyarteritis nodosa is a rare disease, but a significant number of cases have been reported in childhood and infancy. No single cause has been found, but evidence of a streptococcal trigger and poorly controlled parvovirus infection have been found in some series.

Pathologically, the disease is a vasculitis of medium-sized arteries with fibrinoid degeneration in the media extending to the intima and adventitia. Neutrophils and eosinophils comprise the inflammatory reaction. Aneurysms may be palpated or seen radiographically. Thrombosis of diseased arteries may cause infarction in many organs. Fibrosis of vessels and surrounding tissues accompanies the healing stages.

Symptomatology involves many tissues, and diagnosis is difficult. In childhood, unexplained fever, conjunctivitis, central nervous system involvement, and cardiac disease are more prominent than is the case in adult disease. Many cases appear as acute myocarditis, and the peripheral neuropathy so common in the adult is unusual. Diagnosis depends on biopsy-proved vasculitis or characteristic aneurysms on angiography.

The mortality rate is high, especially with cardiac involvement. Treatment consists of prednisone, 1–1.5 mg/kg/d orally, and azathioprine, 1–2 mg/kg/d orally, but controlled studies of the efficacy of therapy of this rare disease are not yet available.

Corman LC, Dolson DJ: Polyarteritis nodosa and parvovirus B19 infection. Lancet 1992;339:491.

Magilavy DB et al: A syndrome of childhood polyarteritis. J Pediatr 1977;91:25.

Ozen S et al: Diagnostic criteria for polyarteritis nodosa in childhood. J Pediatr 1992;120:206.

Park JM et al: Right atrial myxoma with a nonembolic intestinal manifestation. Pediatr Cardiol 1990;11:164.

DIFFUSE SCLERODERMA
(Progressive Systemic Sclerosis)

Scleroderma is a rare disease in childhood. Both the generalized systemic type and the more localized benign form (morphea) have been described. The diagnosis is made on a clinical basis with the finding of a skin disease that progresses from an edematous phase to an atrophic, taut, immobile dermis involving some or all of the skin. Systemic involvement may include Raynaud's phenomenon, arthralgias, pulmonary fibrosis, and renal disease. Involvement of the lungs and kidneys leads to rapid demise. Histologically, the diagnosis may not be specific but includes dermal atrophy with increased fibrosis and collagen content. The pathogenesis remains obscure, but studies indicate an increased synthesis of immature collagen by cultured scleroderma fibroblasts.

Penicillamine and newer antihypertensive agents may provide effective treatment in the future. Physical therapy is sometimes helpful in reducing debilitation from contractures and muscle wasting.

Birdi N et al: Localized scleroderma progressing to systemic disease. Arthritis Rheum 1993;36:410.
Miller JJ: The fasciitis-morphea complex in children. Am J Dis Child 1992;146:733.

NONRHEUMATIC PAIN SYNDROMES

Reflex Sympathetic Dystrophy

Reflex sympathetic dystrophy is a painful condition that is frequently confused with arthritis. There appears to be both an increased prevalence and increased recognition of the condition. Severe extremity pain leading to nearly complete loss of function is the hallmark of the condition. Evidence of autonomic dysfunction is demonstrated by color changes, temperature differences, and dyshidrosis in the affected extremity. Foot involvement is more common than hand involvement. A puffy swelling of the entire hand or foot is common. On examination, there is marked cutaneous hyperesthesia to even the slightest touch. Results of laboratory tests are negative. X-ray findings are normal except for late development of osteoporosis. Bone scans are very helpful and demonstrate either increased or decreased blood supply to the painful extremity.

The cause of this condition remains elusive. Unlike adults, children only occasionally have a history of significant physical trauma at onset. How the autonomic dysfunction causes severe somatic pain is not known, but the feedback cycle does provide the basis for treatment. In mild cases, a program of rehabilitative physical therapy in combination with desensitization techniques will restore function and relieve pain. Refractory cases need family counseling and may respond to steroids or ganglionic blocks by local anesthesia. Long-term prognosis is good if recovery is rapid; recurrent episodes imply a less favorable prognosis.

Wilder RT et al: Reflex sympathetic dystrophy in children. J Bone Joint Surg [Am] 1992;74:910.

Fibromyalgia

Fibromyalgia is a diffuse pain syndrome in which patients experience pain all over their bodies without objective swelling. Weather changes and fatigue exacerbate symptoms. A sleep disturbance, such as insomnia or prolonged waking periods in the night, is an almost universal symptom; therefore, patients should be carefully questioned in this regard. On examination, patients are normal except for characteristic trigger points at the insertion of muscles, especially along the neck, spine, and pelvis.

Treatment consists of physical therapy and relieving the sleep disorder. Low-dose antidepressant medication (amitriptyline, 25 mg) taken before sleep may produce remarkable benefit in reduction of pain. Physical therapy should emphasize a graded rehabilitative approach to stretching and exercise. Analgesic medications provide poor pain relief and should be avoided because their use leads to escalation of medication, including narcotics.

The prognosis for young patients is not clear, and long-term strategies may be necessary to enable them to cope with the condition.

Sherry D et al: Psychosomatic musculoskeletal pain in childhood: Clinical and psychological analyses of 100 children. Pediatrics 1991;88:1093.
Sigal LH, Patella SJ: Lyme arthritis as the incorrect diagnosis in pediatric and adolescent fibromyalgia. Pediatrics 1992;90:523.

Chronic Fatigue Syndrome

Since 1985, chronic fatigue syndrome has become an increasingly common diagnosis. The distinction between this apparent organic fatigue and emotional causes of fatigue is not easily made. Criteria have been developed by NIH to assist in classification. The fatigue should have a defined date of onset, and there is a long list of excludable diagnoses. Other clinical manifestations include low-grade fevers, sore throat, painful lymph nodes, and neuropsychiatric problems. Epstein-Barr virus infection does not account for all of the patients described. Treatment is symptomatic and somewhat unsatisfactory.

Gold D et al: Chronic fatigue: A prospective clinical and virologic study. JAMA 1990;164:48.
Holmes GP et al: Chronic fatigue syndrome: A working case definition. Ann Intern Med 1988;108:387.
Marshall GS et al: Chronic fatigue in children: Clinical features, Epstein-Barr virus and human herpesvirus 6 serology and long term follow-up. Pediatr Infect Dis J 1991; 10:287.

HYPERMOBILITY SYNDROME

Ligamentous laxity, which previously was thought to occur only in Ehlers-Danlos syndrome or Down's syndrome, is now recognized as a frequent cause of joint pain in our physically competitive society.

Children are now participating in a wide range of physically demanding sports and activities. Patients with hypermobility present with episodic joint pain and occasionally with swelling that lasts a few days after increased physical activity. Depending on the activity, almost any joint may be affected.

Physical examination may reveal joint swelling and tenderness, but the key to diagnosis is the demonstration of ligamentous laxity. Five criteria have been established: (1) passive opposition of the thumb to the flexor surface of the forearm, (2) passive hyperextension of the fingers so that they are parallel to the extensor surface of the forearm, (3) hyperextension of the elbow, (4) hyperextension of the knee (genu recurvatum), and (5) palms on floor with knees extended. Results of laboratory tests are normal. The pain associated with the syndrome is produced by improper joint alignment, due to the laxity, during exercise.

Treatment consists of a graded conditioning program designed to provide muscular support of the joints to compensate for the loose ligaments. The prognosis is good provided conditioning before activities is adequate.

Gedalia A, Press J: Articular symptoms in hypermobile schoolchildren: A prospective study. J Pediatr 1991; 119:944.

REFERENCES

Ansell B: *Rheumatic Disorders in Childhood.* Butterworth, 1980.

Cassidy JT, Petty RE: *Textbook of Pediatric Rheumatology,* 2nd ed. Churchill Livingstone, 1990.

Hematologic Disorders

28

Peter A. Lane, MD, Rachelle Nuss, MD, & Daniel R. Ambruso, MD

NORMAL VALUES

Knowledge of the normal ranges for peripheral blood counts is essential to the diagnosis of hematologic disorders in infancy and childhood. These values vary significantly with age and are shown in Table 28–1.

Normal neonates show a relative polycythemia with a hematocrit of 45–65%. The normal reticulocyte count at birth is also relatively high at 2–8%. Within the first few days of life, erythrocyte production decreases and the levels of hemoglobin and hematocrit fall to a nadir at about 2–3 months. During this period, known as physiologic anemia of infancy, normal infants have hemoglobins as low as 10 g/dL and hematocrits as low as 30%. (In premature infants, a nadir of 7–8 g/dL may be noted at 8–10 weeks.) Thereafter, the normal values for hemoglobin gradually increase until adult values are reached after puberty.

The red cells of normal neonates are also larger than in later life. The normal MCV at birth is greater than 94 fL. The MCV subsequently falls to a nadir at about 6 months of age, when the normal is 70–84 fL. Thereafter, the MCV gradually increases until it reaches adult normal values after puberty.

The normal number of white blood cells is higher in infancy and early childhood than later in life. The differential white count shows a predominance of neutrophils at birth and in the older child, while a predominance of lymphocytes (up to 80%) is noted in later infancy through the first 6 years of life.

Normal values for the platelet count are 150,000–400,000/μL and vary little with age.

BONE MARROW FAILURE

Failure of the marrow to produce adequate numbers of circulating blood cells may be congenital or acquired and may cause pancytopenia (aplastic anemia) or involve only one cell line (single cytopenia).

Constitutional and acquired aplastic anemia will be discussed in detail here, while the more common single cytopenias (Table 28–2) will be dealt with in subsequent sections. Bone marrow failure caused by malignancy or other infiltrative disease is discussed elsewhere in the text. It is also important to remember that many drugs and toxins may affect the marrow and cause single or multiple cytopenias.

Suspicion of bone marrow failure should be high in children with pancytopenia and in children with single cytopenias and without evidence of peripheral red cell, white cell, or platelet destruction. Macrocytosis often accompanies bone marrow failure, and many of the constitutional bone marrow disorders are associated with a variety of congenital anomalies.

Alter DP, Young NS: The bone marrow failure syndromes. In: *Hematology of Infancy and Childhood,* 4th ed. Nathan DG, Oski FA (editors). Saunders, 1993.

CONSTITUTIONAL APLASTIC ANEMIA (Fanconi's Anemia)

Essentials of Diagnosis

- Thrombocytopenia progressing to pancytopenia.
- Macrocytosis.
- Multiple congenital anomalies.
- Increased chromosome breakage in peripheral blood lymphocytes.

General Considerations

Fanconi's anemia is a familial disorder thought to be inherited in an autosomal recessive manner. Hematologic manifestations typically begin with thrombocytopenia or neutropenia and subsequently progress over the course of months to years to pancytopenia. Typically, the diagnosis is made between the ages of 2 and 15 years.

Clinical Findings

A. Symptoms and Signs: Symptoms are due principally to the degree of hematologic abnormality: thrombocytopenia may cause purpura, petechiae, and bleeding; neutropenia may cause severe or recurrent infections; and anemia may cause weakness, fatigue,

Table 28-1. Normal peripheral blood values at various ages.[1]

	1st Day	2nd Day	6th Day	2 weeks	1 Month	2 Months	3 Months	6 Months	1 Year	2 Years	5 Years	8–12 Years	Adults	
													Males	Females
Red blood cells (millions/μL)	5.9 (4.1–7.5)	6 (4.0–7.3)	5.4 (3.9–6.8)	5 (4.5–5.5)	4.7 (4.2–5.2)	4.1 (3.6–4.6)	4 (3.5–4.5)	4.5 (4–5)	4.6 (4.1–5.1)	4.7 (4.2–5.2)	4.7 (4.2–5.2)	5 (4.5–5.4)	5.4 (4.6–6.2)	4.8 (4.2–5.4)
Hemoglobin (g/dL)	19 (14–24)	19 (15–23)	18 (13–23)	16.5 (15–20)	14 (11–17)	12 (11–14)	11 (10–13)	11.5 (10.5–14.5)	12 (11–15)	13 (12–15)	13.5 (12.5–15)	14 (13–15.5)	16 (13–18)	14 (11–16)
White blood cells (per μL)	17,000 (8–38)		13,500 (6–17)	12,000 (5–16)	11,500 (5–15)	11,000 (5–15)	10,500 (5–15)	10,500 (5–15)	10,000 (5–15)	9,500 (5–14)	8,000 (5–13)	8,000 (5–12)	7,000 (5–10)	7,000 (5–10)
PMNs[2] (%)	57	55	50	34	34	33	33	36	39	42	55	60	57–68	57–68
Eosinophils (total) (per μL)	20–1000				150–1150		70–550	70–550					100–400	100–400
Lymphocytes[2] (%)	20	20	37	55	56	56	57	55	53	49	36	31	25–33	25–33
Monocytes[2] (%)	10	15	9	8	7	7	7	6	6	7	7	7	3–7	3–7
Immature white cells (%)	10	5	0–1	0	0	0	0	0	0	0	0	0	0	0
Platelets[2] (per μL)	350,000		325,000	300,000			260,000			260,000		260,000	260,000	260,000
Nucleated red cells/100 white cells[3]	0–10		0–0.3	0	0	0	0	0	0	0	0	0	0	0
Reticulocytes (%)	3 (2–8)	3 (2–10)	1 (0.5–5)	0.4 (0–2)	0.2 (0–0.5)	0.5 (0.2–2)	2 (0.5–4)	0.8 (0.2–1.5)	1 (0.4–1.8)	1 (0.4–1.8)	1 (0.4–1.8)	1 (0.4–1.8)	1 (0.5–2)	1 (0.5–2)
Mean diameter of red cells (μm)	8.6				8.1		5–7		7.4		7.4		7.5	
MCV[4] (fL)	85–125		89–101	94–102	90		80	78	78	80	80	82	82–92	82–92
MCHC[4] (%)	36		35	34				33		32	34	34	34	34
MCH[4] (pg)	35–40		36	31	30		27	26	25	26	27	28	27–31	27–31
Hematocrit (%)	54 ± 10		51	50	40		35	35	36	37	38	40	40–54	37–47

[1]Modified and reproduced, with permission, from Merenstein GB, Kaplan DW, Rosenberg AA: *Silver, Kempe, Bruyn & Fulginiti's Handbook of Pediatrics*, 16th ed. Appleton & Lange, 1991.
[2]Usual or average values; considerable individual variation may occur.
[3]Total nucleated red cells: first day, <1000/μL.
[4]MCV = mean corpuscular volume. MCHC = mean corpuscular hemoglobin concentration. MCH = mean corpuscular hemoglobin.

Table 28–2. Important single cytopenias.

Red cell aplasia
 Congenital hypoplastic anemia (Diamond-Blackfan anemia)
 Transient erythroblastopenia of childhood
 Transient aplasia with chronic hemolysis
Neutropenia
 Kostmann's syndrome
 Schwachman-Diamond syndrome
 Cyclic neutropenia
Thrombocytopenia
 Thrombocytopenia with absent radii
 Amegakaryocytic thrombocytopenia

and pallor. Congenital anomalies are present in at least 50% of patients. The most common defects are skeletal and include hypoplasia, anomalies, or absence of the thumb and radius. The thenar eminence may be hypoplastic. Associated renal anomalies include aplasia, horseshoe kidney, and duplication of the collecting system. Other anomalies include microcephaly, short stature, microphthalmia, strabismus, ear anomalies, hypogenitalism, and patchy brown pigmentation of the skin.

B. Laboratory Findings: Laboratory findings depend upon the extent of the progression of bone marrow failure. Thrombocytopenia typically occurs first, followed over the course of months to years by neutropenia, anemia, and progression to severe aplastic anemia. Macrocytosis is virtually always present, usually associated with an elevation in fetal hemoglobin, and is an important diagnostic clue. The bone marrow usually reveals hypoplasia or aplasia consistent with the degree of peripheral cytopenias. The diagnosis is confirmed by the demonstration of an increased number of chromosome breaks and rearrangements in peripheral blood lymphocytes. The use of diepoxybutane to stimulate these breaks and rearrangements provides for a sensitive assay that is virtually always positive in children with Fanconi's anemia, even before the onset of hematologic abnormalities. Such testing is often capable of identifying heterozygous carriers and can be used for prenatal diagnosis as well.

Differential Diagnosis

Because Fanconi's anemia frequently presents with thrombocytopenia, the disorder must be differentiated from idiopathic thrombocytopenic purpura (ITP) and other more common causes of decreased platelets. In contrast to ITP, the thrombocytopenia of Fanconi's anemia usually presents with a gradual fall in the platelet count, and counts less than 20,000/μL are often accompanied by neutropenia or anemia. Furthermore, children with ITP do not have macrocytosis and would not typically have short stature, microcephaly, or other congenital anomalies. Fanconi's anemia may also present initially with pancytopenia and must be differentiated from acquired aplastic anemia and from diseases associated with

bone marrow infiltration such as acute leukemia. Examination of the bone marrow in conjunction with chromosome studies of lymphocytes are usually sufficient to differentiate these disorders.

Complications

The most important complications of Fanconi's anemia are those related to thrombocytopenia and neutropenia. In addition, individuals with Fanconi's anemia have a significantly increased risk of developing malignancies, especially acute nonlymphocytic leukemia. Death is usually the result of thrombocytopenic hemorrhage, overwhelming infection, or malignancy.

Treatment

Attentive supportive care is a critical feature of management. Patients with neutropenia who develop fever require prompt evaluation and parenteral broad-spectrum antibiotics. Transfusions are important but should be used judiciously, especially in the management of thrombocytopenic patients, who frequently become refractory to platelet transfusions as a consequence of alloimmunization. Transfusions from family members should be discouraged because of the negative impact on the outcome of bone marrow transplantation. Peripheral blood counts improve in many patients with androgen treatments; however, such treatments are associated with significant side effects, and masculinization is particularly troublesome in females.

Bone marrow transplantation has recently become the treatment of choice for children with Fanconi's anemia who are fortunate enough to have an HLA-identical sibling donor. First, it is important to exclude the possibility of Fanconi's anemia in the donor by testing lymphocytes for chromosome breakage.

Prognosis

Many patients succumb to bleeding, infection, or malignancy in adolescence or early adulthood. The long-term outlook for those undergoing successful bone marrow transplantation is uncertain.

Alter BP. Fanconi's anemia: Current concepts. Am J Pediatr Hematol/Oncol 1992;14:170.
Giampietro PF, et al: The need for more accurate and timely diagnosis in Fanconi anemia: A report from the International Fanconi Anemia Registry. Pediatrics 1993;91:1116.
Strathdee CA, Buchwald M: Molecular and cellular biology of Fanconi anemia. Am J Pediatr Hematol/Oncol 1992;14:177.

ACQUIRED APLASTIC ANEMIA

Essentials of Diagnosis

- Weakness and pallor.
- Petechiae, purpura, and bleeding.

- Frequent or severe infections.
- Pancytopenia with empty bone marrow.

General Considerations

Acquired aplastic anemia is characterized by peripheral pancytopenia with a hypocellular bone marrow. Approximately half of the cases in childhood are idiopathic, without evidence of any etiologic agent or associated abnormality. Other cases appear to be secondary to idiosyncratic reactions to drugs such as chloramphenicol, oxyphenbutazone, and quinacrine. Toxic causes include exposure to benzene, insecticides, and heavy metals. Infectious causes include viral hepatitis and infectious mononucleosis. In immunocompromised children, aplastic anemia has been associated with human parvovirus.

Clinical Findings

A. Symptoms and Signs: Symptoms and signs are usually those caused by pancytopenia. Weakness, fatigue, and pallor are the result of anemia; petechiae, purpura, and bleeding occur because of thrombocytopenia; and fevers due to generalized or localized infections are the result of neutropenia. Hepatosplenomegaly and significant lymphadenopathy are unusual.

Anemia is usually normocytic, with a low reticulocyte count. The white blood cell count is low, with a marked neutropenia. The platelet count is typically below 50,000/μL and frequently below 20,000/μL. Bone marrow aspiration and biopsy are essential to the diagnosis and show hypocellularity, often marked, with the marrow space replaced with fat.

Differential Diagnosis

Examination of the bone marrow usually excludes pancytopenia caused by infiltrative processes such as acute leukemia, storage diseases, and myelofibrosis. Many of these other conditions are associated with hepatosplenomegaly. Occasionally, children with pancytopenia and hypocellular bone marrows ultimately prove to have preleukemic conditions. In this regard, cytogenetic analysis of the marrow is helpful, since the finding of a clonal abnormality may predict the subsequent development of frank malignancy. Some children with Fanconi's anemia do not have congenital anomalies, and for that reason all children with newly diagnosed aplastic anemia should be studied for the presence of chromosome breaks and rearrangements in peripheral blood lymphocytes.

Complications

The disease is characteristically complicated by overwhelming infection and severe hemorrhage, and these two complications are the leading causes of death. Other complications are those associated with therapy.

Treatment

Comprehensive supportive care is most important in the management of children with acute acquired aplastic anemia. All febrile illnesses require prompt evaluation and usually parenteral antibiotics. Transfusions are important in the management of these patients. Packed red blood cells should be administered to alleviate symptoms of anemia when they develop. Platelet transfusions are important in the management of severe thrombocytopenia and may be lifesaving, but they should be used sparingly as most patients eventually develop platelet alloantibodies.

Bone marrow transplantation is the treatment of choice for patients with severe aplastic anemia when an HLA-compatible sibling donor is available. Because the likelihood of success with transplantation is adversely influenced by multiple transfusions, HLA typing of family members should be undertaken as soon as the diagnosis of aplastic anemia is made. The development of the National Bone Marrow Registry has made bone marrow transplantation from HLA-matched unrelated donors a viable therapeutic option for some patients.

Currently, the best alternative to bone marrow transplantation in the treatment of acquired aplastic anemia is immunotherapy with antithymocyte globulin (ATG), cyclosporine, or corticosteroids, singly or in combination. Hematologic improvement has occurred in over 50% of children treated with ATG, but remissions are often incomplete or not sustained. Recent studies suggest that a combination of ATG and cyclosporine may prove more effective than either therapy alone.

Prognosis

The prognosis for patients with severe aplastic anemia is extremely poor if bone marrow transplantation is not available and if immunotherapy is not effective. In such cases, patients usually die of infection or hemorrhage within 6–12 months after diagnosis. Children treated early with bone marrow transplantation from an HLA-identical sibling are now expected to have a long-term survival rate of greater than 80%.

Casper JT et al: Bone marrow transplantation for severe aplastic anemia in children. Am J Pediatr Hematol Oncol 1990;12:434.

Frickhofen N et al: Treatment of aplastic anemia with antilymphocyte globulin and methylprednisolone with or without cyclosporin. N Engl J Med 1991;324:1297.

Gluckman E et al: Bone marrow transplantation for severe aplastic anemia: Influence of conditioning and graft-versus-host disease prophylaxis regimens on outcome. Blood 1992;79:269.

Gluckman E et al: Multicenter randomized study comparing cyclosporin-A alone and antithymocyte globulin with prednisone for treatment of severe aplastic anemia. Blood 1992;79:2540.

Werner EJ et al: Immunosuppressive therapy versus bone

marrow transplantation for children with aplastic anemia. Pediatrics 1989;83:61.

ANEMIAS

APPROACH TO THE CHILD WITH ANEMIA

Anemia is a relatively common finding in pediatrics, and ascertainment of the cause is always important. The causes of anemia in childhood are myriad, but the correct diagnosis can usually be established with relatively little laboratory cost.

Frequently, the cause is suggested by a careful history. The possibility of nutritional causes should be addressed by inquiry about dietary intake, growth and development, and symptoms of chronic disease, malabsorption, or blood loss. Hemolytic disease may be suggested by a history of jaundice (including neonatal jaundice) or by a family history of anemia, jaundice, gallbladder disease, splenomegaly, or splenectomy. The child's ethnic background may suggest the possibility of certain hemoglobinopathies or of deficiencies of red cell enzymes such as glucose-6-phosphate dehydrogenase (G6PD). The review of systems may reveal clues to a previously unsuspected systemic disease with which anemia may be associated. Finally, the age of the patient should be considered, since some causes of anemia occur most commonly at certain ages. For example, iron deficiency anemia and β globin disorders present more commonly between 6 and 24 months of age than at other times in life.

The physical examination may also reveal clues to the cause of anemia. Poor growth may suggest chronic disease or hypothyroidism. Congenital anomalies may be associated with constitutional aplastic anemia (Fanconi's anemia) or with constitutional hypoplastic anemia (Diamond-Blackfan anemia). Other disorders may be suggested by the findings of petechiae or purpura (leukemia, aplastic anemia, hemolytic uremic syndrome), jaundice (hemolysis or liver disease), generalized lymphadenopathy (leukemia, juvenile rheumatoid arthritis, HIV infection), splenomegaly (leukemia, sickle syndromes, hereditary spherocytosis, liver disease, hypersplenism), or evidence of chronic or recurrent infections.

The initial laboratory evaluation of the anemic child generally consists of a complete blood count with differential and platelet count, review of the peripheral blood smear, and usually a reticulocyte count. The algorithm in Figure 28–1 shows the extent to which this limited amount of laboratory information, in conjunction with the history and physical examination, may lead to a specific diagnosis or focus additional laboratory investigations to a limited diagnostic category (eg, microcytic anemia, bone marrow failure, pure red cell aplasia, or hemolytic disease). This diagnostic scheme depends principally on the MCV to determine whether the anemia is microcytic, normocytic, or macrocytic, and the percentile curves of Dallman and Siimes (Figure 28–2) should be used to make this determination.

With regard to microcytic anemias, the incidence of iron deficiency in the United States has decreased significantly with improvements in infant nutrition. Still, iron deficiency is an important cause of microcytic anemia, especially between 6 and 24 months of age. A trial of therapeutic iron is appropriate in such children, provided the dietary history is compatible with the development of iron deficiency and the physical examination does not suggest an alternative cause for the anemia. If this is not the case—or if a trial of therapeutic iron fails to correct the anemia and microcytosis—then further laboratory evaluation is warranted.

Another key element of Figure 28–1 is the use of both the reticulocyte count and the peripheral blood smear to determine whether a normocytic or macrocytic anemia is due to hemolysis. Typically, hemolytic disease is associated with an elevated reticulocyte count, but many children with chronic hemolysis initially present during a period of virus-induced aplasia when the reticulocyte count is not elevated. Thus, review of the peripheral smear for evidence of hemolysis (eg, spherocytes, red cell fragmentation, sickle forms) is important in the evaluation of children with normocytic anemias and low reticulocyte counts. When hemolysis is suggested, the correct diagnosis may be suspected by specific abnormalities of red cell morphology or by clues from the history or physical examination. Autoimmune hemolysis can be excluded by Coombs testing, and review of blood counts and the peripheral smears of the mother and father may suggest congenital disorders such as hereditary spherocytosis. Children with normocytic or macrocytic anemias, with relatively low reticulocyte counts and no evidence of hemolysis on the blood smear, usually have anemias caused by inadequate erythropoiesis in the bone marrow. The presence of neutropenia or thrombocytopenia in such children suggests bone marrow failure and the possibility of aplastic anemia or malignancy and dictates examination of the bone marrow. Pure red cell aplasia may be constitutional (Diamond-Blackfan anemia), acquired and transient (transient erythroblastopenia of childhood), a manifestation of a systemic disease such as renal disease or hypothyroidism, or due to malnutrition or deficiencies of folate or cobalamin.

Dallman PR et al: Percentile curves for hemoglobin and red cell volume in infancy and childhood. J Pediatr 1979; 94:26.

Lane PA, Nuss R: Hematologic disorders. In: *Pediatric De-*

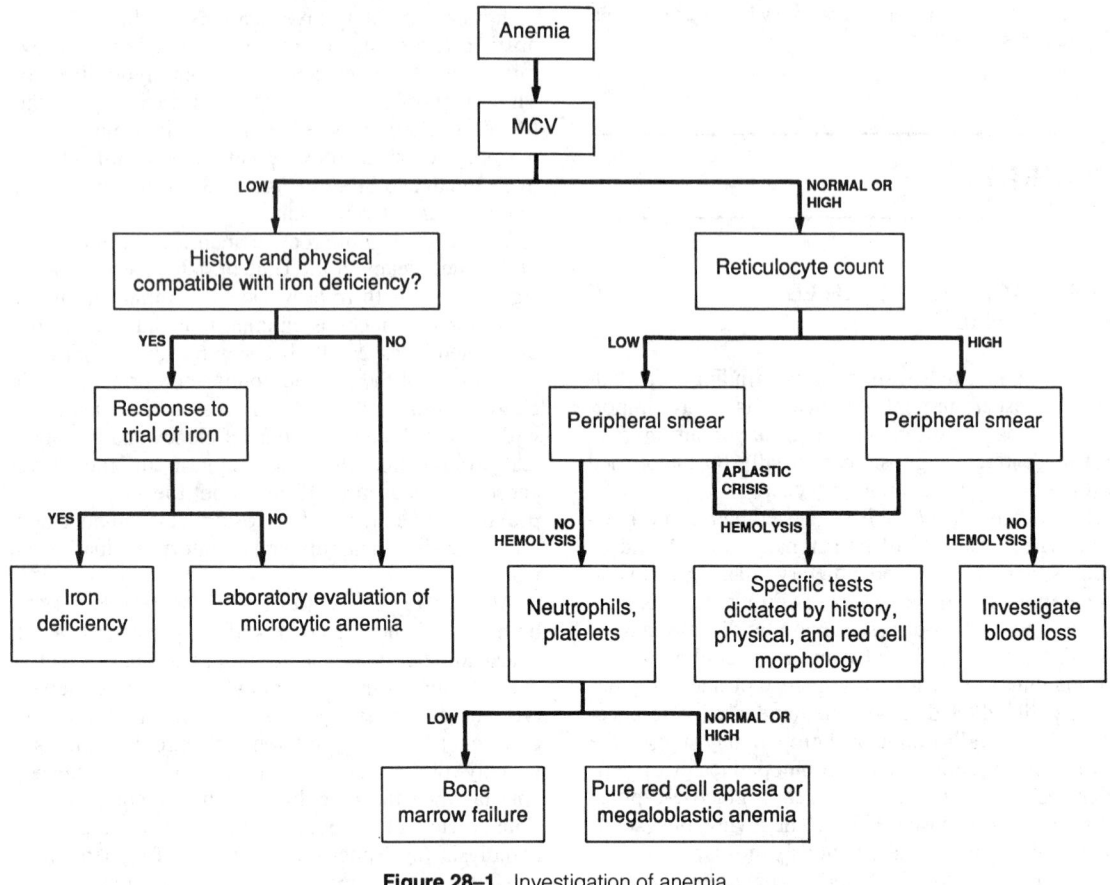

Figure 28–1. Investigation of anemia.

cision Making, 2nd ed. Berman S (editor). BC Decker, 1991.

Novak RW: Red blood cell distribution width in pediatric microcytic anemias. Pediatrics 1987;80:251.

Oski FA: Differential diagnosis of anemia. In: *Hematology of Infancy and Childhood,* 4th ed. Nathan DG, Oski FA (editors). Saunders, 1993.

PURE RED CELL APLASIA

Infants and children with normocytic or macrocytic anemia, a low reticulocyte count, and normal or elevated numbers of neutrophils and platelets should be suspected of having pure red cell aplasia. Examination of the peripheral smear in such cases is important because signs of hemolytic disease suggest the possibility of chronic hemolysis complicated by an aplastic crisis due to parvovirus infection. Appreciation of this phenomenon is important because children with chronic hemolytic disease may not be diagnosed until the anemia is exacerbated by an episode of red cell aplasia that results in a rapidly falling hemoglobin. In such cases, cardiovascular compromise and congestive heart failure are imminent threats.

1. CONGENITAL HYPOPLASTIC ANEMIA (Diamond-Blackfan Anemia)

Essentials of Diagnosis

- Age: birth to 1 year.
- Macrocytic anemia with reticulocytopenia.
- Bone marrow with erythroid hypoplasia.
- Short stature or congenital anomalies in one-third.

General Considerations

Diamond-Blackfan anemia is a relatively rare cause of anemia that usually presents in infancy or early childhood. Early diagnosis is important because the prompt initiation of therapy with corticosteroids results in increased erythropoiesis in about two-thirds of patients, thus avoiding the difficulties and complications of long-term chronic transfusion therapy. The cause of the disorder is unclear, and both autosomal dominant and autosomal recessive modes of inheritance have been suggested.

Clinical Findings

A. Symptoms and Signs: Signs and symptoms of the disorder are generally those of chronic anemia,

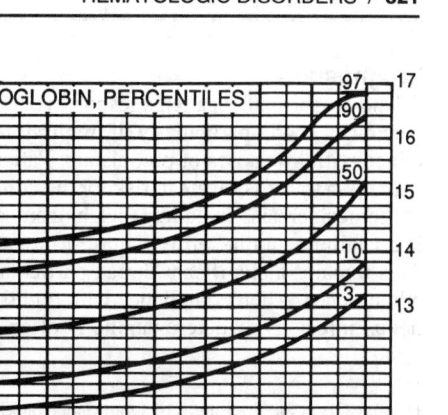

Figure 28–2. Hemoglobin and red cell volume in infancy and childhood. (From Dallman PR, Siimes MA: Percentile curves for hemoglobin and red cell volume in infancy and childhood. J Pediatr 1979;94:26.)

such as pallor, and in some cases cardiovascular compromise and congestive heart failure. Jaundice, splenomegaly, or other evidence of hemolysis is absent. Short stature or other congenital anomalies are present in one-third of patients. A wide variety of anomalies have been described, and abnormalities of the thumbs are probably the most common.

B. Laboratory Findings: The disorder is characterized by severe anemia and marked reticulocytopenia. The neutrophil count is usually normal or slightly decreased, and the platelet count is normal or elevated. The bone marrow shows a marked decrease in erythroid precursors but is otherwise normal. In older children, levels of fetal hemoglobin are usually increased and there is evidence of persistent fetal erythropoiesis such as the presence of the i antigen on erythrocytes. In addition, the level of adenosine deaminase in erythrocytes is elevated.

Differential Diagnosis

The principal disorder from which Diamond-Blackfan anemia must be differentiated is transient erythroblastopenia of childhood. In contrast to that condition, patients with Diamond-Blackfan anemia generally present at an earlier age, often have macrocytosis, and have evidence of fetal erythropoiesis and

an elevated level of red cell adenosine deaminase. In addition, short stature and congenital anomalies, which occur in one-third of patients with Diamond-Blackfan anemia, are not associated with transient erythroblastopenia. Lastly, transient erythroblastopenia of childhood usually resolves within 6–8 weeks after diagnosis, while Diamond-Blackfan anemia is generally a lifelong affliction. Other disorders associated with decreased red cell production such as renal failure, hypothyroidism, and the anemia of chronic disease need to be considered.

Treatment

Oral corticosteroids should be initiated as soon as the diagnosis is made. Two-thirds of patients will respond to prednisone, 2 mg/kg/d, and many of those who respond subsequently tolerate significant tapering of the dose. Patients who are unresponsive to prednisone generally require chronic red cell transfusion therapy, which inevitably causes transfusion-induced hemosiderosis and the need for chelation with parenteral deferoxamine. Bone marrow transplantation is an alternative therapy that should be considered for transfusion-dependent patients who have HLA-matched siblings. Hematopoietic growth factors have been used in some cases with limited success.

Prognosis

The prognosis for patients responsive to steroids is generally good, particularly if remission is maintained with low doses of prednisone. Patients dependent upon transfusion are at risk for the complications of hemosiderosis, including death from congestive heart failure, cardiac arrhythmias, or hepatic failure. This remains a significant threat, particularly during adolescence, when compliance with nightly subcutaneous infusions of deferoxamine is often a difficult issue.

Dunbar CE et al: Treatment of Diamond-Blackfan anaemia with haematopoietic growth factors, granulocyte-macrophage colony stimulating factor and interleukin 3: Sustained remissions following IL-3. Br J Haematol 1991; 79:316.
Glader BE et al: Elevated erythrocyte adenosine deaminase activity in congenital hypoplastic anemia. N Engl J Med 1983;309:1486.
Greinix HT et al: Long-term survival and cure after marrow transplantation for congenital hypoplastic anaemia (Diamond-Blackfan syndrome). Br J Haematol 1993;84:515.
Halperin DS et al: Diamond-Blackfan anemia: Etiology, pathophysiology and treatment. Am J Pediatr Hematol Oncol 1989;11:380.

2. TRANSIENT ERYTHROBLASTOPENIA OF CHILDHOOD

Essentials of Diagnosis

- Age 6 months to 4 years.
- Normocytic anemia with reticulocytopenia.
- Absence of hepatosplenomegaly or lymphadenopathy.
- Bone marrow with marked absence of erythroid precursors initially, followed by erythroid hyperplasia during recovery.

General Considerations

Transient erythroblastopenia of childhood is a relatively common cause of acquired anemia in early childhood. The disorder is generally suspected when a normocytic anemia is discovered during evaluation of pallor or when a complete blood count is obtained for another reason. Because the anemia is due to decreased red cell production and thus develops slowly, the cardiovascular system has time to compensate, and children with hemoglobins as low as 3 or 4 g/dL may look remarkably well. The disorder is thought to be autoimmune in most cases, since IgG from some patients has been shown to suppress erythropoiesis in vitro.

Clinical Findings

Pallor is the most frequent sign, and hepatosplenomegaly and lymphadenopathy are absent. The anemia is normocytic, and the smear shows no evidence of hemolysis. The platelet count is normal or elevated, and the neutrophil count is normal or, in some cases, somewhat decreased. The Coombs test is negative, and there is no evidence of chronic renal disease, hypothyroidism, or other systemic disorder. Bone marrow examination shows severe erythroid hypoplasia initially; subsequently, erythroid hyperplasia develops along with reticulocytosis and the anemia resolves.

Differential Diagnosis

Transient erythroblastopenia of childhood must be differentiated from Diamond-Blackfan anemia, particularly in infants less than 1 year of age. In contrast to Diamond-Blackfan anemia, transient erythroblastopenia is not associated with macrocytosis, short stature, or congenital anomalies, or evidence of fetal erythropoiesis prior to the phase of recovery. Also in contrast to Diamond-Blackfan anemia, levels of red cell adenosine deaminase are normal. Transient erythroblastopenia of childhood must also be differentiated from chronic disorders associated with decreased red cell production, such as renal failure, hypothyroidism, and other chronic states of infection or inflammation. As with other single cytopenias, the possibility of malignancy (ie, leukemia) should always be considered in children with red cell aplasia, especially if features not typical of transient erythroblastopenia of childhood are present, such as fever, bone pain, hepatosplenomegaly, or lymphadenopathy. In such cases, examination of the bone marrow is generally diagnostic. Confusion may sometimes arise when the anemia of transient erythroblastopenia is first identified during the early phase of recovery when the reticulocyte count is high. In such cases, the disorder may be confused with the anemia of acute blood loss or with hemolytic disease. In contrast to hemolytic disorders, however, there is no jaundice and no morphologic evidence of hemolysis on the blood smear.

Treatment & Prognosis

By definition, this is a transient disorder. Some children require red cell transfusions if signs of cardiovascular compromise are present. Resolution of the anemia is heralded by an increase in the reticulocyte count, which generally occurs within 4–8 weeks of diagnosis. In contrast to other autoimmune disorders of childhood (eg, ITP, autoimmune hemolytic anemia), the use of corticosteroids is of no proved benefit and is not indicated.

Bhambhani K et al: Seasonal clustering of transient erythroblastopenia of childhood. Am J Dis Child 1988;142:175.
Dickerman JD: Transient erythroblastopenia of childhood presenting with reticulocytosis and erythroid hyperplasia in the bone marrow. Pediatrics 1981;67:562.
Hays T et al: Transient erythroblastopenia of childhood: A review of 26 cases and reassessment of indications for bone marrow aspiration. Am J Dis Child 1989;143:605.

Rogers ZR et al: Reduced neutrophil counts in children with transient erythroblastopenia of childhood. J Pediatr 1989; 115:746.

Ware RE, Kinney TR: Transient erythroblastopenia in the first year of life. Am J Hematol 1991;37:156.

NUTRITIONAL ANEMIAS

1. IRON DEFICIENCY ANEMIA

Essentials of Diagnosis

- Pallor and fatigue.
- Poor dietary intake of iron (age 6–24 months).
- Chronic blood loss (age > 2 years).
- Microcytic, hypochromic anemia.

General Considerations

Long the most common cause of anemia in pediatric practice, iron deficiency has seen a dramatic decrease in incidence during the past 2 decades. This is the direct result of improved nutrition and the increased availability of iron-fortified infant formulas and cereals. Thus, the current approach to anemia in childhood must take into consideration a relatively greater chance of other causes than was formerly the case.

Normal term infants are born with sufficient iron stores to prevent the development of iron deficiency during the first 4 months of life. Thereafter, maintenance of iron sufficiency requires that absorption of dietary iron keep pace with the needs of rapid growth. For this reason, nutritional iron deficiency occurs with greatest frequency between 6 and 24 months of life. A deficiency prior to 6 months of age may occur if iron stores at birth are less than normal (prematurity, small birth weight, neonatal anemia, or perinatal blood loss) or if there is subsequent iron loss due to hemorrhage. The diagnosis of iron deficiency in children older than 24 months of age should trigger investigation for blood loss.

A significant body of evidence indicates that iron deficiency, in addition to causing anemia, has adverse effects on behavior and upon the development of cognitive function. Thus, the importance of the identification of iron deficiency and of its treatment extends past the resolution of any symptoms directly attributable to a lowered hemoglobin concentration.

Clinical Findings

A. Symptoms and Signs: Symptoms and signs vary with the severity of the deficiency. In infants with significant iron deficiency, pallor, fatigue, irritability, and delayed motor development are common. Children whose iron deficiency is due in part to ingestion of unfortified cow's milk may be fat and flabby, with poor muscle tone. A history of pica is common.

B. Laboratory Findings: The severity of anemia depends on the degree of iron deficiency, and hemoglobin values may be as low as 3–4 g/dL in severe cases. Red cells are microcytic and hypochromic, with a low MCV and low MCH. The red blood cell distribution width (RDW) is typically elevated, even with mild iron deficiency. The reticulocyte count is usually normal but may be slightly elevated in severe cases. Iron studies show a decreased serum ferritin as well as a low serum iron, elevated total iron-binding capacity, and decreased transferrin saturation. Free erythrocyte protoporphyrin is elevated. All of these laboratory abnormalities are usually present with moderate to severe iron deficiency, but mild cases may show variable laboratory results.

The bone marrow examination is not helpful in the diagnosis of iron deficiency in infants and small children because normal children deposit little or no iron in the form of hemosiderin in the marrow.

Differential Diagnosis

The differential diagnosis is that of microcytic, hypochromic anemia. The possibility of thalassemia should be considered, especially in infants of African, Mediterranean, or Asian ethnic background. In contrast to iron deficiency, infants with thalassemia generally have an elevated number of erythrocytes (the index of the MCV divided by the red cell number is usually < 13) and are less likely to have an elevated RDW. Thalassemias are associated with normal or increased levels of serum iron and ferritin and with normal iron-binding capacity and free erythrocyte protoporphyrin levels. The hemoglobin electrophoresis in β thalassemia trait typically shows an elevation of hemoglobin A_2, but coexistent iron deficiency may result in a falsely normal hemoglobin A_2 level. Iron deficiency anemia must also be differentiated from the anemia associated with lead poisoning and from hemoglobin E disorders. Thus, laboratory evaluation of microcytic anemias should include determination of serum lead levels in children thought to be at risk and hemoglobin electrophoresis to identify hemoglobin E in infants of Southeast Asian ancestry.

The anemia of chronic inflammation or infection may also be microcytic. This anemia is usually suspected because of the presence of a chronic systemic disorder. The level of serum iron is low, but serum ferritin is elevated. Finally, it should be appreciated that relatively mild infections, particularly during infancy, may cause transient anemia. For this reason, caution should be exercised when the diagnosis of mild iron deficiency is entertained in infants and young children who have had recent viral or bacterial infections. Ideally, screening tests for anemia should not be obtained within 3–4 weeks of such infections.

Treatment

The recommended oral dose of elemental iron is 4–6 mg/kg/d in three divided daily doses. Mild cases may be treated with 3 mg/kg/d given once daily before breakfast. Parenteral administration of iron is rarely necessary. Iron therapy results in an increased reticulocyte count within 3–5 days which is maximal between 5 and 7 days. The hemoglobin level begins to increase thereafter. The rate of hemoglobin rise is inversely related to the hemoglobin level at diagnosis. In moderate to severe cases, an elevated reticulocyte count 1 week after initiation of therapy confirms the diagnosis and documents compliance and response to therapy. When iron deficiency is the only cause of anemia, adequate treatment usually results in a resolution of the anemia within 4–6 weeks. Treatment is generally continued for an additional month or so to make certain that iron stores are replenished.

Calvo EB et al: Iron status in exclusively breast-fed infants. Pediatrics 1992;90:375.
Lozoff B et al: Long-term developmental outcome of infants with iron deficiency. N Engl J Med 1991;325:687.
Oski FA: Iron deficiency in infancy and childhood. N Engl J Med 1993;329:190.
Wasserman G et al: Independent effects of lead exposure and iron deficiency anemia on developmental outcome at age 2 years. J Pediatr 1992;121:695.

2. MEGALOBLASTIC ANEMIAS

Essentials of Diagnosis

- Pallor and fatigue.
- Nutritional deficiency or intestinal malabsorption.
- Macrocytic anemia.
- Megaloblastic bone marrow changes.

General Considerations

Megaloblastic anemia is a macrocytic anemia caused by deficiency of cobalamin (vitamin B_{12}), folic acid, or both. Cobalamin deficiency due to dietary insufficiency may occur in infants who are breast-fed by mothers who are strict vegetarians or who have pernicious anemia. Intestinal malabsorption is the usual cause of cobalamin deficiency in pediatrics and occurs with Crohn's disease, chronic pancreatitis, bacterial overgrowth of the small bowel, infection with the fish tapeworm (*Diphyllobothrium latum*), or after surgical resection of the terminal ileum. Deficiencies due to inborn errors of metabolism (transcobalamin II deficiency, methylmalonic aciduria) have also been described. Malabsorption of cobalamin due to deficiency of intrinsic factor (pernicious anemia) is rare in childhood.

Folic acid deficiency may be caused by inadequate dietary intake, malabsorption, increased folate requirements, or some combination of the three. Folate deficiency due to dietary deficiency alone is rare but occurs in severely malnourished infants and has been reported in infants fed goat's milk not fortified with folic acid. Folic acid is absorbed in the proximal small bowel, and deficiencies are encountered in malabsorptive syndromes such as celiac disease. Anticonvulsant medications (eg, phenytoin and phenobarbital) and cytotoxic drugs (eg, methotrexate) have also been associated with folate deficiency, caused by interference with folate absorption or metabolism. Finally, folic acid deficiency is more likely to develop in infants and children with increased requirements. This occurs during infancy because of rapid growth and also in children with chronic hemolytic anemia. Premature infants are particularly susceptible to the development of the deficiency because of low body stores of folate.

Clinical Findings

A. Symptoms and Signs: Infants with megaloblastic anemia may show pallor and mild jaundice due to ineffective erythropoiesis. Classically, the tongue is smooth and beefy red. Infants with cobalamin deficiency may be irritable and may be poor feeders. Older children with cobalamin deficiency may complain of paresthesias, weakness, or an unsteady gait and may show decreased vibratory sensation and proprioception on neurologic examination.

B. Laboratory Findings: The laboratory findings of megaloblastic anemia include an elevated MCV and MCH. The blood smear shows numerous macro-ovalocytes with anisocytosis and poikilocytosis. Neutrophils are large and have hypersegmented nuclei. The white cell count and the platelet count are normal with mild deficiencies but may be decreased in more severe cases. Examination of the bone marrow typically shows erythroid hyperplasia with large erythroid and myeloid precursors. There is nuclear-cytoplasmic dissociation and ineffective erythropoiesis. The serum indirect bilirubin concentration may be slightly elevated.

Children with cobalamin deficiency have a low serum vitamin B_{12} level. In addition, the urinary concentration of methylmalonic acid is significantly elevated. This latter test is useful in the diagnosis because decreased levels of serum vitamin B_{12} may also be seen in about 30% of patients with folic acid deficiency. Assessment of folate stores is best done by measuring the level of red cell folate rather than the serum folic acid.

Differential Diagnosis

It is important to recognize that most macrocytic anemias in pediatrics are not megaloblastic. Other causes of an increased MCV include an elevated reticulocyte count (hemolytic anemias), bone marrow failure syndromes (Fanconi's anemia, Diamond-Blackfan anemia), liver disease, and hypothyroidism.

Treatment

Treatment of cobalamin deficiency due to inadequate dietary intake is readily accomplished with oral supplementation. Most cases, however, are due to intestinal malabsorption and require parenteral treatment. In severe cases, parenteral therapy may induce life-threatening hypokalemia and require supplemental potassium. Folic acid deficiency is effectively treated with oral folic acid in most cases. Children at risk for the development of folic acid deficiencies such as premature infants and those with chronic hemolysis are usually given supplementary folic acid prophylactically.

Graham SM, et al: Long-term neurologic consequences of nutritional vitamin B_{12} deficiency in infants. J Pediatr 1992;121:710.

Meyers PA: Megaloblastic anemias. In: *Blood Diseases of Infancy and Childhood,* 6th ed. Miller DR, Baehner RL (editors). Mosby, 1989.

Skidmore MD et al: Biochemical evidence of asymptomatic vitamin B_{12} deficiency in children after ileal resection for necrotizing enterocolitis. J Pediatr 1989;115:102.

ANEMIA OF CHRONIC DISORDERS

Anemia is a frequent manifestation of many chronic illnesses in children. In some instances, causes may be mixed. For example, children with chronic disorders involving intestinal malabsorption or blood loss may have anemia of chronic inflammation in combination with nutritional deficiencies of iron, folate, or cobalamin. In other settings, the anemia is due to dysfunction of a single organ (eg, renal failure, hypothyroidism), and correction of the underlying abnormality causes resolution of the anemia.

1. ANEMIA OF CHRONIC INFLAMMATION

Anemia is frequently associated with chronic illness, particularly those with a significant inflammatory component. The anemia is usually mild to moderate in severity, with a hemoglobin of 8–12 g/dL. In general, the severity of the anemia corresponds to the severity of the underlying disorder. The reticulocyte count is low, and the anemia is thought to be due to inflammatory cytokines that inhibit erythropoiesis and impair iron release by reticuloendothelial cells. The serum iron concentration is low, but in contrast to iron deficiency, the iron-binding capacity is not elevated and the serum ferritin is high. Treatment consists of correction of the underlying disorder, which, if controlled, generally results in improvement in hemoglobin level.

Means RT Jr, Krantz SB: Progress in understanding the pathogenesis of the anemia of chronic disease. Blood 1992;80:1639.

2. ANEMIA OF CHRONIC RENAL FAILURE

Severe normocytic anemia occurs in most forms of renal disease that have progressed to renal insufficiency. Although white cell and platelet production remain normal, the bone marrow shows significant hypoplasia of the erythroid series and the reticulocyte count is low. The principal mechanism responsible for this anemia is deficiency of erythropoietin, a hormone normally produced in the kidney. In the presence of significant uremia, there may also be a component of hemolysis. In the past, treatment of the anemia of chronic renal failure depended on transfusions of packed red blood cells. However, recombinant human erythropoietin (epoetin alfa) has been shown to correct the anemia, and its use has largely eliminated the need for transfusions.

Boineau FG et al: The prevalence of anemia and correlations with mild and chronic renal insufficiency. J Pediatrics 1990;116:S60.

Montini G et al: Benefits and risks of anemia correction with recombinant human erythropoietin in children maintained by hemodialysis. J Pediatr 1990;117:556.

Montini G , et al: Pharmacokinetics and hematologic response to subcutaneous administration of recombinant human erythropoietin in children undergoing long-term peritoneal dialysis: A multicenter study. J Pediatr 1993; 122:297.

Siimes MA et al: Factors limiting the erythropoietin response in rapidly growing infants with congenital nephrosis on a peritoneal dialysis regimen after nephrectomy. J Pediatr 1992;120:44.

3. ANEMIA OF HYPOTHYROIDISM

Some patients with hypothyroidism develop significant anemia. Occasionally, anemia may be detected prior to the diagnosis of the underlying disorder. The anemia is usually normocytic or macrocytic, but it is not megaloblastic and hence not due to deficiencies of cobalamin or folate. This disorder emphasizes the importance of assessing growth and development during the evaluation of any anemic child, since the cause of the anemia of hypothyroidism is typically suggested by decreased growth velocity.

Replacement therapy with thyroid hormone is usually effective in correcting the anemia.

Cheu J-Y et al: Anemia in children and adolescents with hypothyroidism. Clin Pediatr 1981;20:696.

CONGENITAL HEMOLYTIC ANEMIAS: RED CELL MEMBRANE DEFECTS

The congenital hemolytic anemias are usually divided into three categories: defects of the red cell membrane, hemoglobinopathies, and disorders of red cell metabolism. This section will address the first of these groups of disorders and focus primarily on hereditary spherocytosis and hereditary elliptocytosis.

In most cases, the diagnosis of a red cell membrane disorder is suggested by the peripheral blood smear, which shows characteristic red cell morphology (eg, spherocytes, elliptocytes). These disorders are usually inherited in an autosomal dominant fashion, and the diagnosis thus may also be suggested by a family history of hemolytic disease. The hemolysis is usually due to the deleterious effect of the membrane abnormality on red cell deformability. Decreased cell deformability leads to entrapment of the abnormally shaped red cells in the spleen. Thus, many patients with red cell membrane defects have splenomegaly, and the hemolysis is often alleviated by splenectomy.

Becker PS, Lux SE: Disorders of the red cell membrane. In: *Hematology of Infancy and Childhood*, 4th ed. Nathan DG, Oski FA (editors). Saunders, 1993.
Clark MR, Wagner GM: Disorders of the erythrocyte membrane. In: *The Hereditary Hemolytic Anemias*. Mentzer WC, Wagner GM (editors). Churchill Livingstone, 1989.

1. HEREDITARY SPHEROCYTOSIS

Essentials of Diagnosis

- Anemia and jaundice.
- Splenomegaly.
- Positive family history of anemia, jaundice, or gallbladder disease.
- Spherocytosis with increased reticulocytes.
- Increased osmotic fragility.
- Negative Coombs test.

General Considerations

Hereditary spherocytosis is a relatively common inherited hemolytic anemia that occurs in all ethnic groups but is most common in persons of Northern European ancestry, in whom the incidence is 1:5000. The disorder is a heterogeneous one, marked by variable degrees of anemia, jaundice, and splenomegaly. In some persons, the disorder is mild and there is no anemia because erythroid hyperplasia fully compensates for hemolysis. At the other extreme, severe cases are transfusion-dependent prior to splenectomy. The hallmark of hereditary spherocytosis is the presence of microspherocytes in the peripheral blood. The disease is inherited in an autosomal dominant fashion in about 80% of cases; the remainder are thought to be autosomal recessive or to be caused by new mutations.

Hereditary spherocytosis is the result of a partial deficiency of spectrin, an important structural protein of the red cell membrane. Spectrin deficiency weakens the attachment of the cell membrane to the underlying membrane skeleton and causes the red cell to lose membrane surface area. This process creates spherocytes that are poorly deformable and have a shortened life span because they are trapped in the microcirculation of the spleen and engulfed by splenic macrophages. The extreme heterogeneity of hereditary spherocytosis is directly related to variable degrees of spectrin deficiency. In general, children who inherit hereditary spherocytosis in an autosomal dominant fashion have lesser degrees of spectrin deficiency and mild or moderate hemolysis. In contrast, those with nondominant forms of spherocytosis tend to have greater deficiencies of spectrin and a more severe anemia.

Clinical Findings

A. Symptoms and Signs: Symptoms and signs are those related to hemolytic anemia. Fifty percent of affected children have significant hyperbilirubinemia in the newborn period. Splenomegaly subsequently develops in the majority and is usually present by the age of 5 years. Jaundice is variably present and in many patients may only be noted during infection. Patients with significant chronic anemia may complain of pallor, fatigue, or malaise. Intermittent exacerbations of the anemia are caused by increased hemolysis or by aplastic crises and may be associated with severe weakness, fatigue, fever, abdominal pain, or even congestive heart failure.

B. Laboratory Findings: Most patients have mild chronic hemolysis with hemoglobin values between 9 and 12 g/dL. In some cases, the hemolysis is fully compensated and the hemoglobin is in the low-normal range. Rare cases of severe disease require frequent transfusions. The anemia is usually normocytic and hyperchromic. An elevation of the MCHC is noted in many patients. The blood smear shows numerous microspherocytes and polychromasia. The reticulocyte count is elevated and is often higher than one might expect for the degree of anemia. White blood cells and platelets are usually normal.

Osmotic fragility is increased, particularly after incubation at 37 °C for 24 hours. Serum bilirubin usually shows an elevation in the unconjugated fraction. Coombs testing is negative.

Differential Diagnosis

Spherocytes are frequently present in persons with immune hemolysis. Thus, in the newborn, hereditary spherocytosis must be distinguished from hemolytic disease caused by ABO or Rh incompatibilities. In older patients, autoimmune hemolytic anemia frequently presents with jaundice and splenomegaly and with spherocytes on the blood smear. The direct Coombs test is positive in most cases of immune hemolysis and readily distinguishes these disorders from hereditary spherocytosis, which is not caused by antibody. Occasionally, diagnostic confusion may arise in other patients with splenomegaly from other causes, especially when hypersplenism increases red cell destruction and when some spherocytes are noted on the blood smear. In such cases, the true cause of the splenomegaly is frequently suggested by signs or symptoms of portal hypertension or by laboratory evidence of chronic liver disease. In contrast to children with hereditary spherocytosis, those with hypersplenism typically have some degree of thrombocytopenia or neutropenia.

Complications

Severe jaundice may occur in the neonatal period and may occasionally require exchange transfusion if not controlled by phototherapy. Surgical splenectomy is associated with an increased risk of overwhelming bacterial infections, particularly with pneumococci. Pigmented gallstones occur in 60–70% of adults who have not undergone splenectomy and may form as early as 8–10 years of age.

Treatment

General supportive measures include the administration of folic acid to prevent the development of red cell hypoplasia due to folate deficiency. Acute exacerbations of anemia due to increased rates of hemolysis or to aplastic crises due to infection with human parvovirus may be severe enough to require red cell transfusions. Surgical splenectomy is the treatment of choice for most cases and always results in significant improvement. The procedure increases the survival of the spherocytic red cells and leads to complete correction of the anemia in most cases. Patients with more severe disease may show some degree of hemolysis after splenectomy. Except in unusually severe cases, the procedure should be postponed until the child is at least 5 or 6 years of age because of the great risk of postsplenectomy sepsis prior to this age. Alternatively, partial splenectomy may be considered for young children with severe hemolysis. All patients scheduled for splenectomy should be immunized with pneumococcal vaccine prior to the procedure, and some recommend prophylactic penicillin afterward. The need for splenectomy in mild cases is somewhat controversial. Splenectomy in the middle childhood years prevents the subsequent development of cholelithiasis and eliminates the need for the activity restrictions recommended for children with splenomegaly. However, these benefits must be weighed against the risks of the surgical procedure and the subsequent lifelong risk of postsplenectomy sepsis.

Prognosis

Splenectomy eliminates all signs and symptoms in all but the most severe cases and prevents the development of cholelithiasis. The abnormal red cell morphology and increased osmotic fragility persist without clinical consequence.

Agre P et al: Inheritance pattern in clinical response to splenectomy as a reflection of erythrocyte spectrin deficiency in hereditary spherocytosis. N Engl J Med 1986;315: 1579.

Eber SW et al: Variable clinical severity of hereditary spherocytosis: Relation to erythrocytic spectrin concentration, osmotic fragility, and autohemolysis. J Pediatr 1990;117:409.

Manno CS et al: Splenectomy in mild hereditary spherocytosis: Is it worth the risk? Am J Ped Hematol Oncol 1989;11:300.

Tchernia G et al: Initial assessment of the beneficial effect of partial splenectomy in hereditary spherocytosis. Blood 1993;81:2014.

2. HEREDITARY ELLIPTOCYTOSIS

Hereditary elliptocytosis is a heterogeneous disorder characterized by the presence in the peripheral blood of variable numbers of elliptocytes. The severity of the disorder ranges from an asymptomatic carrier state with normal red cell morphology to severe hemolytic anemia. Most affected individuals have numerous elliptocytes on the blood smear but mild or no hemolysis. Those with hemolysis have an elevated reticulocyte count and may have jaundice and splenomegaly. These disorders are caused by mutations of red cell membrane skeletal proteins, and most are inherited in an autosomal dominant fashion. Because most cases are asymptomatic, no treatment is indicated. Patients with significant degrees of hemolytic anemia may benefit from folate supplementation or from splenectomy.

Some infants with hereditary elliptocytosis present in the neonatal period with moderate to marked hemolysis and significant hyperbilirubinemia. This disorder has been termed transient infantile poikilocytosis because such infants exhibit bizarre erythrocyte morphology with elliptocytes, budding red cells, and small misshapen cells that defy description. The MCV is low, and the anemia may be severe enough to require red cell transfusions. Typically, one parent has hereditary elliptocytosis, usually mild or asymptomatic. The infant's hemolysis gradually abates during the first year of life, and the erythrocyte morphology subsequently becomes more typical of hereditary elliptocytosis.

Mentzer WC et al: Modulation of erythrocyte membrane mechanical stability by 2,3-diphosphoglycerate in the neonatal poikilocytosis/elliptocytosis syndrome. J Clin Invest 1987;79:943.

Palek J: Hereditary elliptocytosis and related disorders. Clin of Haematol 1985;14:45.

CONGENITAL HEMOLYTIC ANEMIAS: HEMOGLOBINOPATHIES

The hemoglobinopathies are an extremely heterogeneous group of congenital disorders that occur in many different ethnic groups. The relatively high frequency of these genetic variants is thought to be related to the protection afforded heterozygotes from malaria. The hemoglobinopathies are generally classified in two major groups. The first, the thalassemias, constitute a group of disorders caused by quantitative deficiencies in the production of globin chains. These quantitative defects in globin synthesis result in anemia which is microcytic and hypochromic. The second group of hemoglobinopathies are those caused by structural abnormalities of globin chains. The most important of these, hemoglobins S, C, and E, are all the result of point mutations and a single amino acid substitution in the β globin.

Figure 28–3 shows the normal developmental changes that occur in globin chain production during gestation and the first year of life. At birth, the predominant hemoglobin is fetal hemoglobin, which is composed of two α globin chains and two gamma globin chains. Subsequently, the production of gamma globin decreases and the production of β globin increases so that adult hemoglobin (two α chains and two β chains) is the predominant hemoglobin after 4–6 months. Because α globin chains are present in both fetal and adult hemoglobin, disorders of α globin synthesis (α thalassemia) are clinically manifest in the newborn as well as later in life. In contrast, β globin disorders such as β thalassemia and sickle cell disease are generally asymptomatic during the first 3–4 months of age and present clinically after gamma chain production—and hence fetal hemoglobin levels—have decreased substantially.

1. ALPHA THALASSEMIA

Essentials of Diagnosis
- African, Mediterranean, Middle Eastern, Chinese, or Southeast Asian ancestry.

- Microcytic, hypochromic anemia of variable severity.

General Considerations
Most of the α thalassemia syndromes are the result of deletions of one or more of the α globin genes on chromosome 16. Normal diploid cells have four α globin genes, and thus the variable severity of the α thalassemia syndromes is related to the number of gene deletions. Persons with one α globin gene deletion (silent carrier) are asymptomatic and have normal blood findings. Persons with two α globin gene deletions (α thalassemia trait) have a normal or slightly decreased hemoglobin level and some hypochromia and microcytosis. Persons with three α globin gene deletions (hemoglobin H disease) have a moderately severe anemia. The deletion of all four α globin genes results in fetal demise due to hydrops fetalis.

The severity of the α thalassemia syndromes varies among affected ethnic groups depending upon the genetic abnormalities prevalent in the population. In persons of African descent, α thalassemia is usually caused by the deletion of only one of the two α globin genes on one chromosome. Thus, heterozygotes in the African population are silent carriers, and homozygotes have α thalassemia trait. In Asians, however, deletions of one or of both α globin genes on the same chromosome are common. Thus, heterozygotes are either silent carriers or have α thalassemia trait and homozygotes or compound heterozygotes have α thalassemia trait, hemoglobin H disease, or hydrops fetalis. Thus, the presence of α thalassemia in a child of Asian ancestry has important implications for genetic counseling, whereas this is not usually the case in families of African ancestry.

Clinical Findings
The clinical findings depend upon the number of α

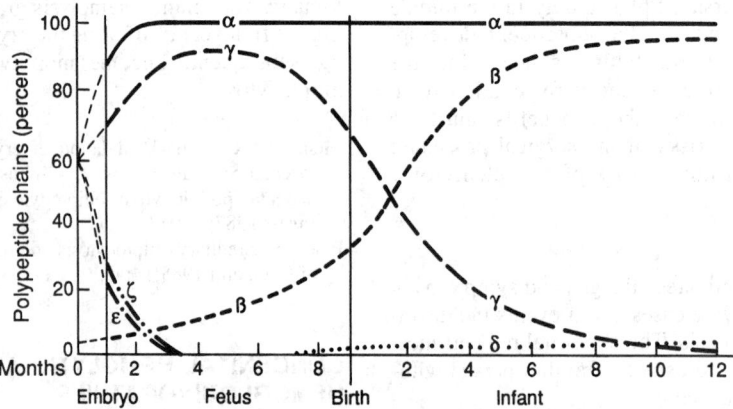

Figure 28–3. Changes in hemoglobin polypeptide chains during human development. (From Miller DR, Baehner RL: *Blood Diseases of Infancy and Childhood*, 6th ed. Mosby, 1989.)

globin genes deleted. The thalassemia syndromes and associated laboratory findings in newborns are shown in Table 28–3.

Persons with three α globin genes (one-gene deletion) are asymptomatic and have no hematologic abnormalities. Hemoglobin levels and MCV are normal. Hemoglobin electrophoresis in the neonatal period shows 1–2% hemoglobin Barts, a variant hemoglobin composed of four gamma globin chains. Hemoglobin electrophoresis after the first few months of life is normal. Thus, this condition is usually suspected only in the context of family studies.

Persons with two α globin genes (two-gene deletion) are typically asymptomatic. The MCV is usually < 100 fL at birth. Hematologic studies in older infants and children show a normal or slightly decreased hemoglobin level with a low MCV and a slightly hypochromic blood smear with some target cells. The hemoglobin electrophoresis typically showed 7–8% hemoglobin Barts in the neonatal period but is normal in older children and adults.

Persons with one α globin gene (three-gene deletion) have a moderately severe microcytic hemolytic anemia (Hb 7–9 g/dL), which is often accompanied by hepatosplenomegaly and some bony abnormalities due to the expanded medullary space. The reticulocyte count is elevated, and the red cells show marked hypochromia and microcytosis with significant poikilocytosis and some basophilic stippling. Hemoglobin electrophoresis in the neonatal period typically shows 15–25% hemoglobin Barts. Later in life, hemoglobin H (composed of four β globin chains) is detected and may comprise as much as 20–30% of the hemoglobin. Incubation of red cells with brilliant cresyl blue (hemoglobin H preparation) shows inclusion bodies formed by denatured hemoglobin H.

The deletion of all four α globin genes causes severe intrauterine anemia and asphyxia and results in hydrops fetalis and fetal demise or neonatal death shortly following delivery. There is extreme pallor and massive hepatosplenomegaly. Hemoglobin electrophoresis reveals a predominance of hemoglobin Barts with a complete absence of normal fetal or adult hemoglobin.

Differential Diagnosis

Alpha thalassemia trait (two-gene deletion) must be differentiated from other mild microcytic anemias including iron deficiency, β thalassemia trait, and the anemia of chronic disease. In contrast to children with iron deficiency, those with α thalassemia trait show normal or increased levels of ferritin and serum iron, and the free erythrocyte protoporphyrin is not elevated. In contrast to children with β thalassemia trait, those with α thalassemia trait have a normal hemoglobin electrophoresis after 4–6 months of age. Because α thalassemia trait is a mild disorder that is usually asymptomatic, signs of chronic disease and inflammation are usually absent. Finally, the history of a low MCV (< 96 fL) at birth or of a "fast" migrating hemoglobin band on the neonatal hemoglobinopathy screening test suggests α thalassemia.

Children with hemoglobin H disease may have jaundice and splenomegaly, and the disorder must be differentiated from other hemolytic anemias. The key to the diagnosis is the decreased MCV and the marked hypochromia on the blood smear. With the exception of β thalassemia, most other significant hemolytic disorders have a normal or elevated MCV and are not hypochromic.

Infants with hydrops fetalis due to severe α thalassemia must be distinguished from those with hydrops due to other causes of anemia such as isoimmunization.

Complications

The principal complication of α thalassemia trait is the needless administration of a therapeutic iron, which is frequently administered in the belief that a mild microcytic anemia is due to iron deficiency. Persons with hemoglobin H disease may have intermittent exacerbations of their anemia which require blood transfusions. Splenomegaly may become a significant problem, may exacerbate the anemia, and

Table 28–3. Clinical and laboratory findings in newborns with alpha thalassemia.[1]

Syndrome (Clinical Features)	Usual Genotype	α Gene Number	Hb (g/dL)	MCV (fL)	Hb Barts (%)
Normal	αα/αα	4	14–22	> 100	None
Silent carrier (no clinical abnormalities)	–α/αα	3	13.6–21	87–116	0–5.8
Alpha thalassemia trait (mild anemia)	– –αα or – α/ – α	2	14.3–19.3	84–101	2–10
Hemoglobin H disease (hemolytic anemia)	– –/ – α	1	12.4–14.2	80–93	19–27
Homozygous alpha thalassemia (stillborn—hydrops fetalis)	– –/– –	0	3–10	110–119	> 75

[1]From Embury SH, Mentzer WC: The thalassemia syndromes. In: *The Hereditary Hemolytic Anemias.* Mentzer WC, Wagner GM (editors). Churchill Livingstone, 1989.

may require splenectomy. Women pregnant with hydropic α thalassemia infants are subject to increased complications of pregnancy, particularly toxemia.

Treatment

Persons with α thalassemia trait require no treatment. Those with hemoglobin H disease should receive supplemental folic acid and avoid the same oxidant drugs that cause hemolysis in persons with G6PD deficiency, because exposure to these drugs may exacerbate their anemia. The anemia may also be exacerbated during periods of infection, and transfusions may be required. Occasionally, infants with hemoglobin H disease may show failure-to-thrive without red cell transfusions. Hypersplenism may develop later in childhood and require surgical splenectomy. Genetic counseling and prenatal diagnosis should be offered to families at risk for children with hemoglobin H disease or fetal hydrops.

Embury SH et al: The thalassemia syndromes. In: *The Hereditary Hemolytic Anemias.* Mentzer WC, Wagner GM (editors). Churchill Livingstone, 1989.

Giardina P, Hilgartner MW: Update on thalassemia. Pediatr Rev 1992;13:55.

2. BETA THALASSEMIA

Essentials of Diagnosis

Beta thalassemia minor:
- African, Mediterranean, Middle Eastern, or Asian ancestry.
- Mild microcytic, hypochromic anemia.
- No response to iron therapy.
- Elevated A$_2$ hemoglobin.

Beta thalassemia major:
- African, Mediterranean, Middle Eastern, or Asian ancestry.
- Moderate to very severe microcytic, hypochromic anemia with marked hepatosplenomegaly.
- Elevated fetal and A$_2$ hemoglobin.

General Considerations

In contrast to the four α globin genes, only two β globin genes are present in diploid cells, one on each chromosome 11. Some β thalassemia genes produce no β globin chains and are termed β^0 thalassemia. Other β globin genes produce some β globin but in diminished quantities and are termed β$^+$ thalassemia. Persons affected by β thalassemia may be heterozygous or homozygous. Heterozygotes for most β thalassemia genes have β thalassemia minor. Most homozygotes have β thalassemia major (Cooley's anemia), which is a severe transfusion-dependent anemia. Other homozygotes have a condition known as thalassemia intermedia that is more severe than thalassemia minor but not generally transfusion-dependent.

The worldwide importance of β thalassemia cannot be overstated. Beta thalassemia major is the most common cause of transfusion-dependent anemia in childhood. In addition, β thalassemia interacts with structural β globin variants such as hemoglobin S and hemoglobin E to cause serious disease in compound heterozygotes. These disorders are discussed further in the sections dealing with sickle hemoglobinopathies and hemoglobin E disorders.

Clinical Findings

A. Symptoms and Signs: Persons with β thalassemia minor are usually asymptomatic, and the only physical sign may be slight enlargement of the spleen. Persons with β thalassemia major are normal at birth but develop a significant anemia during the first year of life as fetal hemoglobin production decreases. If the disorder is not identified and treated with blood transfusions, such children develop massive hepatosplenomegaly and enlargement of the medullary space with thinning of the bony cortex. The skeletal changes cause characteristic facial deformities (prominent forehead and maxilla) and predispose the child to pathologic fractures. Poor growth and development also occur in inadequately treated children.

B. Laboratory Findings: Laboratory findings in β thalassemia minor include a normal or modestly decreased hemoglobin level. The MCV is almost always decreased. The blood smear typically shows hypochromia, target cells, and sometimes basophilic stippling. Hemoglobin electrophoresis is usually diagnostic when hemoglobin A$_2$ or hemoglobin F is elevated. Infants with β thalassemia major are hematologically normal at birth but develop severe anemia after the first few months of life. The blood smear typically shows a severe hypochromic, microcytic anemia with marked anisocytosis and poikilocytosis. Target cells are prominent, and nucleated red blood cells often exceed the number of circulating white blood cells. The hemoglobin usually falls to 5–6 g/dL or less, and the reticulocyte count is significantly elevated. Platelet and white blood cell counts may be increased, and the serum bilirubin is elevated. The bone marrow shows marked erythroid hyperplasia but is rarely needed for diagnosis. Hemoglobin electrophoresis shows only fetal and A$_2$ hemoglobin in children with homozygous β^0 thalassemia. Those with β$^+$ thalassemia genes make some hemoglobin A$_1$ but have a marked increase in fetal and in A$_2$ hemoglobin. The diagnosis of homozygous β thalassemia may also be suggested by the finding of β thalassemia minor in both parents.

Differential Diagnosis

Beta thalassemia minor must be differentiated from other causes of mild microcytic, hypochromic anemias, principally iron deficiency and α thalassemia. In contrast to those with iron deficiency anemia, individuals with β thalassemia minor typically have an elevated number of red blood cells, and the index of the MCV divided by the red cell count is under 13. Generally, the finding of an elevated hemoglobin A_2 is diagnostic; however, the A_2 level is lowered by coexistent iron deficiency, and this may lead to some confusion. Thus, in children thought to be iron deficient, hemoglobin electrophoresis testing is best performed after a course of iron therapy.

Beta thalassemia major is rarely confused with other disorders. Hemoglobin electrophoresis and family studies readily distinguish it from hemoglobin E-β thalassemia, which is another important cause of transfusion-dependent anemia. Generally, infants with hemoglobin E-β thalassemia develop anemia more slowly than those with homozygous β thalassemia.

Complications

The principal complication of β thalassemia minor is the unnecessary use of iron therapy in a futile attempt to correct the microcytic anemia. Children with β thalassemia major who do not receive blood transfusions or who are inadequately transfused suffer from poor growth and recurrent infections and have massive hepatosplenomegaly, thinning of the cortical bone, and pathologic fractures. Without treatment, most children die within the first decade of life. The principal complications of β thalassemia major in transfused children are hemosiderosis, splenomegaly and hypersplenism, viral infections, and alloimmunization. Transfusional hemosiderosis requires chelation therapy with deferoxamine to prevent cardiac, hepatic, and endocrine dysfunction. Noncompliance with chelation in adolescents and young adults may lead to death from congestive heart failure, cardiac arrhythmias, or hepatic failure. Even with adequate transfusions, most patients develop splenomegaly and some degree of hypersplenism which necessitates splenectomy because of the increasing transfusion requirements, usually between ages 5 and 10 years. This procedure subsequently places the child at risk for overwhelming septicemia. Children with β thalassemia major treated with bone marrow transplantation are subject to the many complications associated with that procedure.

Treatment

Beta thalassemia minor requires no specific therapy but has important implications for genetic counseling. For those with β thalassemia major, two approaches to treatment are now available: hypertransfusion with iron chelation or bone marrow transplantation. Programs of blood transfusion are generally targeted to maintain a nadir hemoglobin level above 11 g/dL. Such therapy has been associated with increased vigor and well-being, improved growth, and fewer overall complications. However, maintenance of good health currently requires iron chelation with nightly subcutaneous infusion of deferoxamine. Small doses of supplemental ascorbic acid may enhance the iron chelation in some children. Newly developed oral iron chelators are under study. Patients on chronic transfusion programs generally develop hypersplenism and require splenectomy when their yearly transfusion requirement of packed red cells exceeds 200–250 mL/kg. Splenectomy results in a decrease in the transfusion requirement and hence a lesser rate of iron loading but is associated with a high risk of postsplenectomy sepsis. For this reason, thalassemic patients should receive pneumococcal vaccine prior to the procedure and prophylactic penicillin afterward.

During the past decade, it has become clear that bone marrow transplantation is an important therapeutic option for children with β thalassemia major who have an HLA-identical sibling donor. Reports from numerous centers show excellent results. In a large study from Italy, the probability of 3-year event-free survival was 94% when transplantation was performed prior to the development of hepatomegaly or portal fibrosis.

Ehlers KH: Prolonged survival in patients with beta-thalassemia major treated with deferoxamine. J Pediatr 1991;118:540.

Embury SH, Mentzer WC: The thalassemia syndromes. In: *The Hereditary Hemolytic Anemias.* Mentzer WC, Wagner GM (editors). Churchill Livingstone, 1989.

Fosburg MT, Nathan DJ: Treatment of Cooley's anemia. Blood 1990;76:435.

Lucarelli G et al: Bone marrow transplantation in patients with thalassemia. N Engl J Med 1990;322:417.

Lucarelli G et al: Marrow transplantation in patients with thalassemia responsive to iron chelation therapy. N Engl J Med 1993;329:840.

Piomelli S, Loew T: Management of thalassemia major (Cooley's anemia). Hematol Oncol Clin North Am 1991; 5:557.

Weatherall DJ: The treatment of thalassemia: Slow progress and new dilemmas. N Engl J Med 1993;329:877.

3. SICKLE CELL DISEASE

Essentials of Diagnosis

- Black African, Mediterranean, Middle Eastern, or Indian ancestry.
- Anemia, elevated reticulocyte count, jaundice.
- Recurrent episodes of musculoskeletal or abdominal pain.
- Hemoglobin electrophoresis with hemoglobins S and F, hemoglobins S and C, or hemoglobins S, F, and A with S > A.
- Splenomegaly in early childhood with later disappearance.
- High risk of overwhelming sepsis.

General Considerations

Sickle hemoglobin is found with high frequency in persons of central African origin. It also occurs in other racial groups in Sicily, Italy, Greece, Turkey, Saudi Arabia, and India. Sickle cell anemia is caused by homozygosity for the sickle gene and is the most common form of sickle cell disease. Other clinically important sickling disorders are caused by compound heterozygous conditions in which the sickle gene interacts with genes for hemoglobin C, D, O_{Arab}, C_{Harlem}, or β thalassemia.

Overall, sickle cell disease occurs in about one of every 500 African-American infants. Eight percent of African-Americans are heterozygous carriers of the sickle gene and are said to have sickle cell trait.

The protean clinical manifestations of sickle hemoglobinopathies all can be linked directly or indirectly to the propensity of deoxygenated hemoglobin S to polymerize. Polymerization of sickle hemoglobin distorts erythrocyte morphology, decreases red cell deformability, causes a marked reduction in red cell life span, increases blood viscosity, and predisposes to episodes of vaso-occlusion.

During the past decade, neonatal screening for sickle hemoglobinopathies has been established in many regions of the United States. The identification of affected infants during the first few months of life, when coupled with follow-up programs of parental education, comprehensive medical care, and prophylactic penicillin, has been demonstrated to markedly reduce the mortality rate in early childhood.

Clinical Findings

A. Symptoms and Signs: The symptoms and signs of sickle cell disease are related to the hemolytic anemia and to tissue ischemia caused by vaso-occlusion. Children are normal at birth, and onset of symptoms is unusual before 3–4 months of age because high levels of fetal hemoglobin inhibit sickling. A moderately severe hemolytic anemia is generally present by 1 year of age, causes pallor, fatigue, and jaundice, and predisposes to the development of pigmented gallstones during adolescence and early adulthood. Intense congestion of the spleen with sickled cells causes splenomegaly in early childhood and results in functional asplenia as early as 3 months of age. This places children at great risk for overwhelming infection with encapsulated bacteria, particularly pneumococci. About one-third of patients experience one or more episodes of acute splenic sequestration, characterized by sudden enlargement of the spleen with pooling of red cells, acute exacerbation of anemia, and, in severe cases, shock and death.

Recurrent episodes of vaso-occlusion and tissue ischemia cause a myriad of acute and chronic problems. Dactylitis, or hand-and-foot syndrome, is the most common initial symptom of the disease and occurs in about 50% of children before the age of 3 years. Recurrent episodes of ischemic pain—particularly abdominal and musculoskeletal pain—occur throughout life. Strokes occur in about 10% of children and tend to be recurrent. The acute chest syndrome, characterized by fever, pleuritic chest pain, and acute pulmonary infiltrates with hypoxemia, is caused by pulmonary infection, infarction, or fat embolism from ischemic bone marrow. All tissues are susceptible to damage from vaso-occlusion, and multiple organ dysfunction is common by adulthood. Table 28–4 lists the common manifestations of sickle cell disease in children and adults.

B. Laboratory Findings: Children with sickle cell anemia (Hb SS) generally show a baseline hemoglobin level between 7 and 10 g/dL. This value may fall to life-threatening levels at the time of a sequestration or hypoplastic episode. The baseline reticulocyte count is markedly elevated. The anemia is normocytic or macrocytic, and the blood smear typically shows the characteristic sickle cells as well as numerous target cells. Patients with sickle β thalassemia generally have a low MCV and hypochromia as well. Those with sickle β⁺ thalassemia tend to have lesser degrees of hemolysis and anemia. Persons with sickle hemoglobin C (Hb SC) disease have fewer sickle forms and more target cells, and the hemoglobin level may be normal or only slightly decreased as the rate of hemolysis is much less than in sickle cell anemia.

The diagnosis of sickle hemoglobinopathy may be suspected by the finding of a positive sickle preparation. However, such sickling or solubility testing does not distinguish between sickle cell diseases and sickle cell trait, and false negatives are common during the first year of life, when elevated levels of fetal

Table 28–4. Common clinical manifestations of sickle cell disease.

	Acute	**Chronic**

Children	Bacterial sepsis or meningitis[1]
	 Splenic sequestration[1]
	 Aplastic crisis
	 Vaso-occlusive events
	   Dactylitis
	   Bone infarction
	   Acute chest syndrome[1]
	   Stroke[1]
	   Priapism
		Functional asplenia
		 Delayed growth and development
		 Aseptic necrosis of the hip
		 Hyposthenuria
		 Choletithiasis

Adults	Bacterial sepsis[1]
	 Aplastic crisis
	 Vaso-occlusive events
	   Bone infarction
	   Acute chest syndrome[1]
	   Stroke[1]
	   Priapism
	   Acute multi-organ failure syndrome[1]
		Malleolar ulcers
		 Proliferative retinopathy
		 Aseptic necrosis of the hip
		 Cholecystitis
		 Chronic organ failure[1]
		   Liver
		   Lung
		   Kidney
		   Decreased fertility

[1]Associated with significant mortality rate.

hemoglobin interfere with the detection of sickle hemoglobin. Thus, hemoglobin electrophoresis is always necessary to establish the diagnosis. Children with sickle cell anemia and with sickle β^0 thalassemia have only hemoglobins S and F. Persons with sickle β^+ thalassemia have a preponderance of hemoglobin S with 10–20% hemoglobin A_1. Persons with sickle hemoglobin C disease have equal amounts of hemoglobin S and hemoglobin C.

Serum chemistries are often abnormal depending on the severity of the hemolysis and on the presence of hepatic or renal dysfunction. X-rays of the skull and spine reveal cortical thinning, enlargement of the marrow spaces, and increased trabecular markings.

Differential Diagnosis

Hemoglobin electrophoresis and hematologic studies of the parents are usually sufficient to confirm the correct diagnosis of a sickle cell disorder. Infants whose electrophoresis shows only hemoglobin S and F occasionally have disorders other than sickle cell anemia or sickle β^0 thalassemia. The most important of these is a compound heterozygous condition of sickle hemoglobin and pancellular high persistence of fetal hemoglobin. Such children typically have 30% fetal hemoglobin and 70% hemoglobin S, but they do not have significant anemia nor are they subject to vaso-occlusive episodes.

Complications

Repeated tissue ischemia and infarction causes damage to virtually every organ system. The most important complications are listed in Table 28–4. Patients who require multiple transfusions are at risk for transfusional hemosiderosis and the development of red cell alloantibodies as well as transmission of infectious agents.

Treatment

The cornerstone of treatment is enrollment in a program that provides for patient and family education, comprehensive outpatient care, and appropriate treatment of acute complications. Important to the success of such a program are psychosocial services, blood bank services, and the ready availability of baseline patient information in the setting where acute problems are handled. Treatment of children with sickle cell anemia and sickle β^0 thalassemia includes prophylactic penicillin, which should be initiated by 3 months of age and continued at least until 5 years of age. Many recommend the continuation of prophylactic penicillin past this age, but conclusive evidence of benefit in older patients has not yet been obtained. The routine use of penicillin prophylaxis in hemoglobin SC disease and sickle β_+ thalassemia is controversial. Pneumococcal vaccine should be administered to all children with sickle cell disease at 2 years of age and again 3–5 years later. Other routine immunizations, including yearly vaccination against influenza, should be provided. All illnesses associated with fever greater than 38.5 °C should be evaluated promptly with bacterial cultures, administration of parenteral broad-spectrum antibiotics, and careful inpatient or outpatient observation.

Treatment of painful vaso-occlusive episodes includes the maintenance of good hydration, correction of acidosis if present, administration of adequate analgesia, maintenance of normal oxygen saturation, and the treatment of any associated infections.

Red cell transfusions play an important role in management. Transfusions are indicated to improve oxygen-carrying capacity during acute exacerbations of anemia, as occurs during episodes of splenic sequestration or marrow hypoplasia. Red cell transfusions are not indicated for the treatment of chronic steady-state anemia, which is usually well tolerated, or for uncomplicated episodes of vaso-occlusive pain. Partial exchange transfusion to reduce the percentage of circulating sickle cells is indicated for a number of severe acute vaso-occlusive events and may be life-saving. These include stroke or transient ischemic attack, severe acute chest syndrome, or acute life-threatening failure of other organs. Transfusions may also be used prior to high-risk procedures such as surgery with general anesthesia or arteriograms with ionic contrast materials. A subset of patients are treated with chronic hypertransfusion programs. The most important indication for this type of transfusion is stroke. Without transfusions, children with stroke have a 70% chance of recurrent stroke within a 2-year period. This risk of recurrent neurologic events is markedly reduced by the transfusion therapy.

Successful bone marrow transplantation cures sickle cell disease, but to date its use has been limited because of the risks associated with the procedure as well as the current inability to predict in young children the severity of future complications. Experimental therapy using chemotherapeutic agents such as hydroxyurea and butyrate to ameliorate the disease by increasing levels of fetal hemoglobin is under study.

Prognosis

Early identification by neonatal screening of infants with sickle cell disease, combined with comprehensive care that includes prophylactic penicillin, has markedly reduced the mortality rate in childhood. Most patients are now expected to live well into adulthood, but they eventually succumb to complications. Life expectancy is shortened, though occasional patients survive past 60 years of age.

Gaston MH et al: Prophylaxis with oral penicillin in children with sickle cell anemia: A randomized trial. N Engl J Med 1986;314:1593.

Miller ST et al: Role of *Chlamydia pneumoniae* in acute chest syndrome of sickle cell disease. J Pediatr 1991; 118:30.

Milner PF et al: Sickle cell disease as a cause of osteonecrosis of the femoral head. N Engl J Med 1991;325:1476.

National Institutes of Health Consensus Development Panel: Newborn screening for sickle cell disease and other hemoglobinopathies. JAMA 1987;258:1205.

Ohene-Frempong K: Stroke in sickle cell disease: Demographic, clinical, and therapeutic considerations. Semin Hematol 1991;28:213.

Serjeant JR: *Sickle Cell Disease.*, 2nd ed. Oxford Univ Press, 1992.

Wang WC et al: High risk of recurrent stroke after discontinuance of five to twelve years of transfusion therapy in patients with sickle cell disease. J Pediatr 1991;118:377.

Wilimas JA et al: A randomized study of outpatient treatment with ceftriaxone for selected febrile children with sickle cell disease. N Engl J Med 1993;329:472.

4. SICKLE CELL TRAIT

Individuals who are heterozygous for the sickle gene are said to have sickle cell trait. This genetic carrier state occurs in 8% of African-Americans and is even more common in some areas of Africa and the Middle East. Accurate identification of persons with sickle cell trait depends upon hemoglobin electrophoresis, which typically shows about 60% hemoglobin A_1 and about 40% hemoglobin S with normal levels of hemoglobin A_2 and F. There is no anemia or hemolysis, and the physical examination is normal. Individuals with sickle cell trait are generally healthy, and the overwhelming majority experience no illness attributable to the presence of sickle hemoglobin in their red cells. Life expectancy is normal.

Sickle trait erythrocytes are capable of sickling, particularly under conditions of significant hypoxemia, and a number of clinical abnormalities have been linked to this genetic carrier state. Exposure to environmental hypoxia (altitude > 10,000 feet above sea level) may precipitate splenic infarction or splenic sequestration. However, the vast majority of persons with sickle cell trait who choose to visit such altitudes for skiing, hiking, or climbing do so without difficulty. Many individuals with sickle trait develop some degree of hyposthenuria, and about 4% experience painless hematuria, usually microscopic but occasionally macroscopic. For the most part, these renal abnormalities are subclinical, and they do not progress to significant renal dysfunction. The incidence of bacteriuria and pyelonephritis may be increased during pregnancy, but overall rates of maternal and infant morbidity and mortality are not affected by the presence of sickle cell trait in the pregnant woman.

An epidemiologic study of army recruits in military basic training found a higher risk of sudden unexplained death following strenuous exertion in recruits with sickle cell trait than in those with normal hemoglobin. This study has raised concerns about exercise and exertion for persons with the trait. However, considerable evidence suggests that exercise is generally safe and that athletic performance is not adversely affected by sickle cell trait. Exercise tolerance is normal, and the incidence of sickle cell trait in African-American professional football players is similar to that of the general African-American population, suggesting no barrier to achievement in such a physically demanding profession. Thus, restrictions on athletic competition for children with sickle cell trait are not warranted. Sickle cell trait continues to be most significant for its implications regarding genetic counseling, not for any associated health risks.

Committee on Sports Medicine, American Academy of Pediatrics: Recommendations for participation in competitive sports. Pediatrics 1988;81:737.

Kark JA et al: Sickle cell trait as a risk factor for sudden death in physical training. N Engl J Med 1987;317:781.

Lane PA, Githens JH. Splenic syndrome at mountain altitudes in sickle cell trait: Its occurrence in nonblack persons. JAMA 1985;253:2251.

Pearson HA: Sickle cell trait in competitive athletics: Is there a risk? Pediatrics 1989;83:613.

5. HEMOGLOBIN C DISORDERS

Two percent of African-Americans are heterozygous for hemoglobin C and are said to have hemoglobin C trait. Such individuals have no symptoms, anemia, or hemolysis, but the blood smear shows some target cells. The principal importance of the identification of persons with hemoglobin C trait relates to genetic counseling, particularly with regard to the possibility of hemoglobin SC disease in offspring.

Persons with homozygous hemoglobin C have a mild to moderate hemolytic anemia and may have associated splenomegaly. The blood smear shows polychromasia and prominent target cells. As with other hemolytic anemias, complications of homozygous hemoglobin C include gallstones and aplastic crises.

6. HEMOGLOBIN E DISORDERS

Hemoglobin E is the second most common hemoglobin variant worldwide, with a gene frequency greater than 10% in some areas of Thailand and Cambodia. In Southeast Asia, an estimated 30 million people have hemoglobin E trait. Persons heterozygous for hemoglobin E are asymptomatic, but the hemoglobin level is normal or slightly decreased, and there may be mild microcytosis. Persons homozygous for hemoglobin E are also asymptomatic but usually have a mild anemia with microcytosis and some target cells on the blood smear. Splenomegaly may be present.

Hemoglobin E is most important because of its interaction with β thalassemia. Compound heterozygotes for hemoglobin E and β thalassemia are normal at birth but subsequently develop a moderate to severe hemolytic anemia that resembles homozygous β thalassemia. Such children may show jaundice, hepatosplenomegaly, and poor growth if the disorder is not recognized and treated appropriately. In about half of cases, the anemia becomes severe enough to require lifelong transfusion therapy. In some areas of the United States, hemoglobin E-β thalassemia has become a more common cause of transfusion-dependent anemia than homozygous β thalassemia.

Hurst D et al: Anemia and hemoglobinopathies in Southeast Asian refugee children. J Pediatr 1983;102:692.
Johnson JP et al: Differentiation of homozygous hemoglobin E from compound heterozygous hemoglobin E-β°-thalassemia by hemoglobin E mutation analysis. J Pediatr 1992;120:775.

7. UNSTABLE HEMOGLOBIN DISORDERS (Congenital Heinz Body Anemias)

Unstable hemoglobin disorders differ from most other structural hemoglobin variants because heterozygotes are affected by hemolytic anemia and often have jaundice. The anemia may be exacerbated during hemolytic crises precipitated by fever or by the ingestion of oxidant drugs. Splenomegaly is variably present, and patients are susceptible to the development of gallstones later in life. Patients with more severe hemolysis may report a dark brown urine.

Laboratory findings include a variable hemolytic anemia with a significant elevation in the reticulocyte count. The blood smear may show basophilic stippling. Inclusion bodies of precipitated denatured hemoglobin called Heinz bodies are demonstrated by special stains. Some of the unstable hemoglobins may be detected by hemoglobin electrophoresis, but many are electrophoretically silent. Thus, the diagnosis depends upon the demonstration of hemoglobin instability, usually with the isopropanol precipitation test.

The differential diagnosis includes most other causes of congenital hemolytic anemias. The autosomal dominant genetic transmission may arouse suspicion of a red cell membrane defect, but abnormalities on the peripheral smear are not typical of either spherocytosis or elliptocytosis. The exacerbation of hemolysis during infection or with ingestion of oxidant drugs and the presence of Heinz bodies may suggest a G6PD deficiency, but normal or elevated levels of G6PD and the increased hemoglobin precipitation with isopropanol are usually sufficient to differentiate unstable hemoglobin disorders from G6PD deficiency.

Treatment of children with unstable hemoglobin disorders generally depends on the severity of the hemolysis. Some prescribe supplemental folic acid to prevent the development of a folate deficiency. The avoidance of oxidant drugs is important for some of these disorders, as their use may precipitate hemolytic crises. The role of splenectomy is unclear.

Vichinsky EP, Lubin PH: Unstable hemoglobins, hemoglobins with altered oxygen affinity, and M-hemoglobins. Pediatr Clin North Am 1980;27:421.
Wagner GM et al: Sickling syndromes and unstable hemoglobin disease. In: *The Hereditary Hemolytic Anemias.* Mentzer WC, Wagner GM (editors). Churchill Livingstone, 1989.

8. OTHER HEMOGLOBINOPATHIES

Hundreds of other human globin chain variants have been identified and described. Some, such as hemoglobins D and G, are relatively common. Heterozygotes, who are frequently detected during the course of screening programs for hemoglobinopathies, are generally asymptomatic and usually have no anemia or hemolysis. The principal significance of most hemoglobin variants is the potential for disease in compound heterozygotes who also inherit a gene for β thalassemia or sickle hemoglobin. For example, children compound heterozygous for hemoglobins S and D_{Punjab} ($D_{Los\ Angeles}$) have a severe hemolytic anemia with a peripheral blood smear and clinical problems virtually identical to those of children with sickle cell anemia.

CONGENITAL HEMOLYTIC ANEMIAS: DISORDERS OF RED CELL METABOLISM

Erythrocytes are dependent upon the anaerobic metabolism of glucose for the maintenance of ATP levels sufficient for normal homeostasis. Glycolysis also produces the 2,3-DPG levels needed to modulate the oxygen affinity of adult hemoglobin. In addition, glucose metabolism via the hexosemonophosphate shunt is necessary to generate levels of NADPH sufficient to maintain adequate levels of reduced glutathione to protect the red cell against oxidant damage. Congenital deficiencies of many (not all) of the enzymes of the Embden-Meyerhof and hexosemonophosphate shunt pathways have been associated with hemolytic anemias. In general, the morphologic abnormalities present on the blood smear are nonspecific, and the inheritance of these disorders is autosomal recessive or X-linked. Thus, the possibility of a red cell enzyme defect should be considered during the evaluation of a congenital hemolytic anemia when the blood smear does not show red cell morphology typical of membrane or hemoglobin defects (eg, spherocytes, sickle forms, target cells), when hemoglobin disorders are excluded by hemoglobin electrophoresis and by isopropanol precipitation tests, and when family studies do not suggest an autosomal dominant disorder. The diagnosis is confirmed by finding a low level of the deficient enzyme.

This section will focus on the two most common disorders of erythrocyte metabolism: G6PD deficiency and pyruvate kinase deficiency.

1. GLUCOSE-6-PHOSPHATE DEHYDROGENASE (G6PD) DEFICIENCY

Essentials of Diagnosis
- African, Mediterranean, or Asian ancestry.
- Neonatal hyperbilirubinemia.
- Sporadic hemolysis associated with infection or with ingestion of oxidant drugs or fava beans.
- X-linked inheritance.

General Considerations
Deficiency of G6PD is easily the most common red cell enzyme defect that causes hemolytic anemia. The disorder has X-linked recessive inheritance and occurs with high frequency among persons of African, Mediterranean, and Asian ancestry. Hundreds of different G6PD variants have now been identified and characterized. In most instances, enzyme deficiency is due to the instability of the abnormal enzyme, and older red cells are thus more deficient than younger ones. The consequence of the deficiency is the inability of erythrocytes to generate the sufficient amounts of NADPH to maintain the levels of reduced glutathione necessary to protect the red cell against oxidant stress. Thus, most persons with G6PD deficiency do not have a chronic hemolytic anemia, but they do have episodic hemolysis at times of exposure to the oxidant stress of infection of certain drugs or food substances. The severity of the disorder varies among ethnic groups; G6PD deficiency in persons of African ancestry is less severe than in other ethnic groups.

Clinical Findings
A. Symptoms and Signs: Infants with G6PD deficiency may exhibit evidence of neonatal hemolysis in the absence of exogenous oxidant stress. Such hemolysis may result in significant hyperbilirubinemia and may require the use of phototherapy or exchange transfusion to prevent kernicterus. The deficiency is an important cause of neonatal hyperbilirubinemia in Mediterranean and Chinese infants but not in black infants. Older children with G6PD deficiency are asymptomatic and appear normal between episodes of hemolysis. Hemolytic episodes are often triggered by infection or by the ingestion of oxidant drugs, most importantly antimalarial compounds and sulfonamide antibiotics (Table 28–5). Ingestion of fava beans may trigger hemolysis in Mediterranean and Asian children but not in African children. Episodes of hemolysis are associated with pallor, jaundice, hemoglobinuria, and sometimes cardiovascular compromise.
B. Laboratory Findings: The hemoglobin, re-

Table 28–5. Some common drugs and chemicals that can induce hemolytic anemia in persons with G6PD deficiency.[1]

Acetanilid	Niridazole
Doxorubicin	Nitrofurantoin
Furazolidone	Phenazopyridine
Methylene blue	Primaquine
Nalidixic acid	Sulfamethoxazole

[1]From Beutler E: Glucose-6-phosphate dehydrogenase deficiency. N Engl J Med 1991;324:171.

ticulocyte count, and blood smear are usually normal in the absence of oxidant-induced hemolysis. Episodes of hemolysis are associated with a variable fall in hemoglobin. "Bite" cells or blister cells may be seen, along with a few spherocytes. Hemoglobinuria is common, and the reticulocyte count increases within a few days. Heinz bodies may be demonstrated with appropriate stains. The diagnosis is confirmed by the finding of reduced levels of G6PD in erythrocytes. Because this enzyme is present in increased quantities in reticulocytes, the test is best performed at a time when the reticulocyte count is normal or near normal.

Complications
Kernicterus is a risk for infants with significant neonatal hemolysis. Episodes of acute hemolysis in older children may be life-threatening if severe enough to cause cardiovascular compromise. Rare G6PD variants that are associated with chronic hemolytic anemia may be complicated by splenomegaly and by the formation of pigmented gallstones.

Treatment
The most important issue is avoidance of drugs known to be associated with hemolysis. These are listed in Table 28–5. For Mediterranean and Asian patients, the consumption of fava beans must also be avoided. Infections should be treated promptly and antibiotics given when appropriate. Most episodes of hemolysis are self-limiting, but red cell transfusions may be lifesaving when signs and symptoms suggest cardiovascular compromise.

Beutler E: Glucose-6-phosphate dehydrogenase deficiency. N Engl J Med 1991;324:169.

Kaplan M, Abramov A: Neonatal hyperbilirubinemia associated with glucose-6-phosphate dehydrogenase deficiency in Sephardic-Jewish neonates: Incidence, severity, and effect of phototherapy. Pediatrics 1992;90:401.

Mentzer WC, Glader BE: Disorders of erythrocyte metabolism. In: *The Hereditary Hemolytic Anemias.* Mentzer WC, Wagner GM (editors). Churchill Livingstone, 1989.

2. PYRUVATE KINASE DEFICIENCY

Pyruvate kinase deficiency is an autosomal recessive disorder that has been described in all ethnic groups but is most common in northern Europeans. The deficiency is associated with a chronic hemolytic anemia of varying severity. Approximately one-third of cases present in the neonatal period with jaundice and hemolysis that require phototherapy or occasionally exchange transfusion. In older children, the hemolysis may require intermittent support with red cell transfusions or may be mild enough to go unnoticed for many years. Jaundice and splenomegaly are frequently present in the more severe cases. The diagnosis may occasionally be suggested by the presence of echinocytes on the blood smear, but these are often absent prior to splenectomy. Measurement of 2,3-DPG and ATP levels in red cells may suggest the diagnosis if 2,3-DPG levels are elevated and ATP levels are reduced. The diagnosis depends upon the demonstration of low levels of pyruvate kinase activity in red cells.

Treatment depends upon the severity of the hemolysis. Blood transfusions may be required for significant anemia, and splenectomy may be beneficial. The procedure does not cure the disorder but does ameliorate the anemia and its symptoms. Characteristically, the reticulocyte count *increases* after splenectomy, despite the decreased hemolysis and increased hemoglobin level. In addition, echinocytes frequently become more prevalent.

Mentzer WC, Glader BE: Disorders of erythrocyte metabolism. In: *The Hereditary Hemolytic Anemias.* Mentzer WC, Wagner GM (editors). Churchill Livingstone, 1989.
Mentzer WC Jr: Pyruvate kinase deficiency and disorders of glycolysis. In: *Hematology of Infancy and Childhood,* 4th ed. Nathan DG, Oski FA (editors). Saunders, 1993.

ACQUIRED HEMOLYTIC ANEMIA

1. AUTOIMMUNE HEMOLYTIC ANEMIA

Essentials of Diagnosis

- Pallor, fatigue, and jaundice.
- Splenomegaly common.
- Positive Coombs test.
- Reticulocytosis and spherocytosis.

General Considerations

Acquired autoimmune hemolytic anemia is rare during the first 4 months of life but is one of the more common causes of acute anemia after the first year. Its appearance may be associated with other diseases such as infections (hepatitis, upper respiratory tract infections, mononucleosis, cytomegalovirus infection), systemic lupus erythematosus and other autoimmune syndromes, immunodeficiency states, and malignancies. Often, however, it is not associated with any other disease entity.

Clinical Findings

A. Symptoms and Signs: The disease usually has an acute onset, presenting with weakness, pallor, and fatigue. Jaundice is a prominent finding, and splenomegaly is often present. Some cases are chronic and insidious in onset. Clinical evidence of the underlying disease may be present.

B. Laboratory Findings: The anemia is normochromic and normocytic and may vary from mild to severe (hemoglobin concentration < 5 g/dL). The reticulocyte count is usually increased but occasionally may be normal or low. Spherocytes are usually present, and nucleated red cells may be seen on the peripheral smear. Although leukocytosis and elevated platelet counts are a common finding, thrombocytopenia is occasionally seen. Other laboratory data consistent with hemolysis are present such as increased indirect and total bilirubin, LDH, AST, and urinary urobilinogen. Hemoglobinemia or hemoglobinuria defines intravascular hemolysis. Examination of bone marrow shows a marked erythroid hyperplasia.

Serologic studies provide important information about the disease which is helpful in defining the pathophysiology, planning therapeutic strategies, and assessing prognosis (Table 28–6). In almost all cases, the direct and indirect antiglobulin (Coombs) tests are positive. Further evaluation allows distinction of three syndromes. The presence of IgG, maximal in vitro activity at 37 °C, and either no antigen specificity or an Rh-like specificity constitute warm autoimmune hemolytic anemia with extravascular destruction by the reticuloendothelial system. In contrast, the detection of complement alone and optimal reactivity in vitro at 4 °C with I or i antigen specificity are diagnostic of cold autoimmune hemolytic anemia with intravascular hemolysis. Paroxysmal cold hemoglobinuria appears identical to cold autoimmune hemolytic anemia but has a different antigen specificity and exhibits hemolysis as well as agglutination in vitro.

Differential Diagnosis

The principal condition to be differentiated in childhood is hereditary spherocytosis in crisis, because both diseases present with acute hemolysis and spherocytosis. The direct antiglobulin test is negative in hereditary spherocytosis. This test likewise differentiates autoimmune hemolytic anemia from essentially all other hemolytic anemias except neonatal alloimmune hemolysis.

Complications

The anemia may be very severe and result in cardiovascular collapse requiring emergency management. The complications of the underlying disease such as disseminated lupus erythematosus or lymphoma may be present.

Treatment

Medical management of the underlying disease is

Table 28–6. Classification of autoimmune hemolytic anemia (AIHA) in children.

Syndrome	Warm AIHA	Cold AIHA	Paroxysmal Cold Hematuria
Specific antiglobulin test IgG Complement	Strongly positive Negative or mildly positive	Negative Strongly positive	Negative Strongly positive
Temperature at maximal reactivity	37 °C	4 °C	4 °C
Antigen specificity	May be panagglutinin or may have an Rh-like specificity	I or i	P
Other	. . .	. . .	Positive biphasic hemolysin test
Pathophysiology	Extravascular hemolysis, destruction by the RES (eg, spleen)	Intravascular hemolysis	Intravascular hemolysis
Prognosis	May be more chronic (>3 months) with significant morbidity and mortality. May be associated with a primary disorder (lupus, immunodeficiency, etc)	Generally acute (<3 months). Good outlook. Often associated with infection.	Acute, self-limited. Associated with infection.
Therapy	Should respond to strategies which cause RES blockade, including steroids (prednisone, 2 mg/kg/d), IGIV (1 g/kg/d for 3 days), or splenectomy	May not respond to RES blockade. Severe cases may benefit from plasmapheresis.	Usually self-limited. Symptomatic management.

RES = reticuloendothelial system.

important in symptomatic cases. Defining the clinical syndrome provides a useful guide to treatment. Prednisone, intravenous immune globulin (IGIV), and splenectomy have all been effective approaches to warm autoimmune hemolytic anemia with its extravascular hemolysis in the spleen. Most cases will respond to steroids. After the initial treatment, the dose of steroids may be decreased slowly. Patients may respond to a high dose of IGIV, but fewer patients respond to IGIV than to prednisone. Although the rate of remission with splenectomy may be as high as 50%, particularly in warm autoimmune hemolytic anemia, this approach should be withheld until other treatments have been tried. In severe cases unresponsive to more conventional therapy, immunosuppressive agents such as cyclophosphamide, azathioprine, or busulfan may be tried alone or in combination with steroids.

Patients with cold autoimmune hemolytic anemia and paroxysmal cold hemoglobinuria are less likely to respond to the treatments described above. Since both of these syndromes are most apt to be associated with infections and have an acute, self-limited course, supportive care may be all that is required. Plasma exchange is effective in cold autoimmune (IgM) hemolytic anemia (and may be helpful in severe cases) because the offending antibody has only an intravascular distribution.

Supportive therapy is crucial to treatment. Patients with cold-reacting antibodies, particularly paroxysmal cold hemoglobinuria, should be kept in a warm environment. Transfusion may be necessary because of the complications of severe anemia but should be used only when there is no alternative. In most patients, crossmatch-compatible blood will not be found, and the least incompatible unit should be identified. Transfusion must be conducted carefully, beginning with a test dose (see Transfusion Medicine, p 821). Identification of the patient's phenotype for major red cell alloantigens may be helpful in avoiding alloimmunization or providing appropriate transfusions should alloantibodies arise after initial transfusions during the period of supportive care. Patients with severe intravascular hemolysis may have associated disseminated intravascular coagulation, and heparin therapy should be considered in such cases.

Prognosis

The outlook for autoimmune hemolytic anemia in childhood is positive. The presence of other associated diseases (congenital immunodeficiency, AIDS, lupus erythematosus, malignancy) portends a more chronic course (> 3 months). In general, children with warm autoimmune hemolytic anemia are at greater risk for more severe and chronic disease and higher morbidity and mortality rates. Hemolysis and positive antiglobulin tests may continue for months or years. Patients with cold autoimmune hemolytic anemia or paroxysmal cold hemoglobinuria are more likely to have acute, self-limited disease (< 3 months). Paroxysmal cold hemoglobinuria is almost always associated with infection (with *Mycoplasma*, cytomegalovirus, Epstein-Barr virus, etc).

Bussel JB et al: Intravenous treatment of autoimmune hemolytic anemia with gammaglobulin. Pediatr Res 1984; 12:237.

Heidemann SM et al: Exchange transfusion for autoimmune

hemolytic anemia. Am J Pediatr Hematol Oncol 1988; 9:302.

Petz LD, Garratty G: Unusual problems regarding autoimmune hemolytic anemias. In: *Acquired Immune Hemolytic Anemias.* Churchill Livingstone, 1980.

Salama A, Mueller-Eckhardt C: Autoimmune haemolytic anaemia in childhood associated with noncomplement binding IgM autoantibodies. Br J Haematol 1987;65:67.

2. NONIMMUNE ACQUIRED HEMOLYTIC ANEMIA

Hepatic disease may alter the lipid composition of the red cell membrane. This usually results in the formation of target cells and is not associated with significant hemolysis. Occasionally, however, severe hepatocellular damage is associated with the formation of "spur" cells and brisk hemolytic anemia. Renal disease may also be associated with significant hemolysis; hemolytic uremic syndrome is the best-known example. In this disorder, hemolysis is associated with the presence on the blood smear of echinocytes, fragmented red cells, and spherocytes.

A microangiopathic hemolytic anemia with fragmented red cells and some spherocytes may be observed in a number of conditions associated with intravascular coagulation and fibrin deposition within vessels. This occurs with disseminated intravascular coagulation such as may complicate overwhelming infection, but it may also occur when the intravascular coagulation is localized, as with giant cavernous hemangiomas (Kasabach-Merritt syndrome).

POLYCYTHEMIA & METHEMOGLOBINEMIA

CONGENITAL ERYTHROCYTOSIS (Familial Polycythemia)

In pediatrics, polycythemia is usually secondary to some hypoxemic disorder. However, a number of families with congenital erythrocytosis have been described. The disorder differs from polycythemia vera in that it affects only the erythroid series; the white cell count and platelet count are normal. It frequently occurs as an autosomal dominant, though it may also occur as an autosomal recessive. There are usually no physical findings except for plethora and splenomegaly. The hemoglobin may be as high as 27 g/dL, with a hematocrit of 80% and a red cell count of 10 million/μL. There are usually no symptoms other than headache and lethargy. Recent studies in a number of families have revealed (1) an abnormal hemoglobin

with increased oxygen affinity, (2) reduced red cell diphosphoglycerate, (3) autonomous increase in erythropoietin production, or (4) hypersensitivity of erythroid precursors to erythropoietin.

Treatment is not indicated unless symptoms are marked. Phlebotomy is the treatment of choice.

Buchanan GR: Congenital erythrocytosis in the absence of detectable erythropoietin. J Pediatr 1982;100:593.

Juvonen E et al: Autosomal dominant erythrocytosis caused by increased sensitivity to erythropoietin. Blood 1991; 78:3066.

Prchal JT: Autosomal dominant polycythemia. Blood 1985; 66:1208.

Walterspiel JN et al: Erythropoietin-induced congenital erythrocytosis: Treatment with myelosuppressive agents and hookworm infestation. J Pediatr 1985;107:575.

SECONDARY POLYCYTHEMIA

Secondary polycythemia occurs in response to hypoxemia in any condition that results in a lowered oxygen saturation of the blood. The most common cause of secondary polycythemia in pediatrics is cyanotic congenital heart disease. It also occurs in chronic pulmonary disease such as cystic fibrosis and in pulmonary arteriovenous shunts. Persons living at extremely high altitudes, as well as those with methemoglobinemia and sulfhemoglobinemia, develop polycythemia. It has on rare occasions been described without hypoxemia in association with renal tumors, brain tumors, Cushing's disease, or hydronephrosis.

Polycythemia occurs normally in the neonatal period; it is particularly exaggerated in infants who are preterm or small for gestational age. In these infants, polycythemia is frequently associated with other symptoms. It may occur in infants of diabetic mothers, and it has been described as a manifestation of Down's syndrome in the newborn and as a complication of congenital adrenal hyperplasia.

Iron deficiency may complicate polycythemia and aggravate the hyperviscosity. This complication should always be suspected when the MCV falls below the normal range. Multiple coagulation and bleeding abnormalities have also been described in severely polycythemic cardiac patients. These abnormalities include thrombocytopenia, mild consumption coagulopathy, and elevated fibrinolytic activity. Bleeding at surgery may be severe.

The ideal treatment of secondary polycythemia is correction of the underlying disorder. When this cannot be done, phlebotomy is often necessary to control the symptoms. Iron sufficiency should be maintained. Adequate hydration of the patient and phlebotomy with plasma replacement are indicated prior to major surgical procedures; these measures prevent the complications of thrombosis and hemorrhage. Isovolumetric exchange transfusion is the treatment of choice in severe cases.

Balcerzak SP, Bromberg PA: Secondary polycythemia. Semin Hematol 1975;12:353.

METHEMOGLOBINEMIA

Methemoglobin is formed when hemoglobin in a deoxygenated state is oxidized to the ferric form. Methemoglobin is being formed continuously in the red cells and is simultaneously reduced to hemoglobin by enzymes in the erythrocyte. Methemoglobin becomes unavailable for transport of oxygen and causes a shift in the dissociation curve of the residual oxyhemoglobin. Cyanosis is produced with methemoglobin levels of approximately 15% or greater. There are several mechanisms for the production of methemoglobinemia, which occurs as a congenital or acquired disorder.

1. HEMOGLOBIN M

The designation M is given to several abnormal hemoglobins associated with methemoglobinemia. Affected individuals are heterozygous for the gene, and it is transmitted as an autosomal dominant. A number of different types have been described in which various amino acid substitutions produce an abnormal hemoglobin molecule that cannot bind oxygen normally because iron remains in the ferric instead of the ferrous state. The defect may be on either the α globin or β globin chain. Hemoglobin electrophoresis at the usual pH will not always demonstrate the abnormal hemoglobin, and special techniques are necessary to detect it by electrophoresis as well as spectroscopically. The patient has marked and persistent cyanosis but is otherwise usually asymptomatic. Exercise tolerance may be normal, and life expectancy is not affected. This type of methemoglobinemia does not respond to any form of therapy.

Vichinsky EP, Lubin BH: Unstable hemoglobins, hemoglobins with altered oxygen affinity, and M-hemoglobins. Pediatr Clin North Am 1980;27:421.

2. CONGENITAL METHEMOGLOBINEMIA DUE TO ENZYME DEFICIENCIES

Congenital methemoglobinemia is most frequently caused by congenital absence of a reducing factor in the erythrocyte that is responsible for conversion of methemoglobin to hemoglobin in normal red cells. Most patients with this disease suffer from a deficiency of the reducing enzyme diaphorase I (coenzyme factor I). It is transmitted as an autosomal recessive trait. These patients may have as high as 40% methemoglobin but usually have no symptoms,

though a mild compensatory polycythemia may be present. Patients with methemoglobinemia associated with a deficiency of diaphorase I respond readily to treatment with ascorbic acid and with methylene blue (see below). However, treatment is not usually indicated.

3. ACQUIRED METHEMOGLOBINEMIA

A number of compounds activate the oxidation of hemoglobin from the ferrous to the ferric state, forming methemoglobin. These include the nitrites and nitrates (contaminated water), chlorates, and quinones. Drugs in this group are the aniline dyes, sulfonamides, acetanilid, phenacetin, bismuth subnitrate, and potassium chlorate. Poisoning with a drug or chemical containing one of these substances should be suspected in any infant or child who presents with sudden cyanosis. Methemoglobin levels in cases of poisoning may be extremely high and can produce severe anoxia and dyspnea with unconsciousness, circulatory failure, and death. Young infants and newborns are more susceptible to poisoning because their red cells have difficulty reducing hemoglobin, probably on the basis of a transient deficiency of NADH methemoglobin reductase. Infants with diarrhea and dehydration (acidosis) may show elevated levels of methemoglobin.

Patients with the acquired form of methemoglobinemia respond dramatically to methylene blue in a dosage of 1–2 mg/kg given intravenously. For infants and young children, a smaller dose (1–1.5 mg/kg) is recommended. Ascorbic acid administered orally or intravenously also reduces methemoglobin, but it acts more slowly.

Avner JR et al: Acquired methemoglobinemia: The relationship of cause to course of illness. Am J Dis Child 1990;144:1229.

Mansouri A, Lurie AA: Concise review: Methemoglobinemia. Am J Hematol 1993;42:7.

Murray KF, Christie DL: Dietary protein intolerance in infants with transient methemoglobinemia and diarrhea. J Pediatr 1993;122:90.

DISORDERS OF LEUKOCYTES

NEUTROPENIA

Essentials of Diagnosis

- Increased frequency of infections.
- Ulceration of oral mucosa and gingivitis.
- Normal numbers of red cells and platelets.

General Considerations

Neutropenia in infancy and childhood is usually defined as an absolute neutrophil (granulocyte) count of less than 1500/μL. However, in the first 2 years of life, normal infants may have absolute counts as low as 1000/μL. During the first few days of the newborn period, the absolute neutrophil count is higher than at later ages, and an absolute neutrophil count less than 3500 cells/μL may be considered neutropenia.

Neutropenias may result from absent or defective granulocyte stem cells, ineffective or suppressed myeloid maturation, decreased production of hematopoietic cytokines (G-CSF, GM-CSF, etc), decreased marrow release, increased neutrophil destruction, or an increased neutrophil "marginating pool" (pseudoneutropenia). A classification of neutropenic disorders is presented in Table 28–7.

The most severe types of congenital neutropenias include reticular dysgenesis (congenital aleukocytosis), Kostmann's syndrome (severe neutropenia with maturation defect in the marrow progenitor cells), Schwachman's syndrome (neutropenia with pancreatic insufficiency), neutropenia with immune deficiency states, cyclic neutropenia, and myelocathexis or dysgranulopoiesis. Neutropenia may also be associated with storage and metabolic diseases and immunodeficiency states. The most common causes of neutropenia are viral infection or drugs resulting either in decreased production in the marrow or increased destruction. Severe bacterial infections may be associated with neutropenia. Although rare, neonatal alloimmune neutropenia can be severe and associated with increased risk for infection. Autoimmune neutropenia in the mother can result in passive transfer of antibody and neutropenia in the neonate. Malignancies, osteopetrosis, marrow failure syndromes, and hypersplenism are not usually associated with isolated neutropenia.

Clinical Findings

A. Symptoms and Signs: Acute severe bacterial or fungal infection is the most significant complication of neutropenia. Although the risk is increased when the absolute neutrophil count is less than 500/μL, the actual susceptibility is quite variable and depends on the cause of neutropenia, marrow reserves, and other factors. The most frequent types of infection include septicemia, cellulitis, abscesses, pneumonia, and perirectal abscesses. Aphthous ulcers, gingivitis, and periodontal disease also cause significant problems for these patients. In addition to local signs and symptoms, patients may have chills, fever, and malaise. In most cases, the spleen and liver are not enlarged. *Staphylococcus aureus* and gram-negative bacteria are the most significant causes of infections.

B. Laboratory Findings: Neutrophils are absent or markedly reduced in the peripheral blood. In most forms of neutropenia or agranulocytosis, the monocytes and lymphocytes will be normal and the red cells and platelets not affected. The bone marrow usually shows a normal erythroid series, with adequate megakaryocytes but a marked reduction in the myeloid cells or a significant delay in maturation of this series.

In the evaluation of neutropenia, careful attention should be paid to the duration and pattern of neutropenia, the types of infections and their frequency, and phenotypic abnormalities on physical examination. A careful family history as well as blood counts

Table 28–7. Classification of neutropenia of childhood.

Congenital neutropenia with stem cell abnormalities
  Reticular dysgenesis
  Cyclic neutropenia
Congenital neutropenia with abnormalities of committed myeloid progenitor cells
  Neutropenia with immunodeficiency disorders (T cells and B cells)
  Severe congenital neutropenia (Kostmann)
  Chronic benign neutropenia of childhood
  Myelokathexis of dysmyelopoiesis
  Schwachman's syndrome
  Cartilage-hair hypoplasia
  Dyskeratosis congenita
  Fanconi's syndrome
  Hyperglycinemia and isovaleric, propionic, and methylmalonic acidemia
  Glycogenosis Ib
  Osteopetrosis
Acquired neutropenias affecting stem cells
  Malignancies (leukemia, lymphoma) and preleukemic disorders
  Drugs or toxic substances
  Ionizing radiation
  Aplastic anemia
Acquired neutropenias affecting committed myeloid progenitors or survival of mature neutrophils
  Ineffective granulopoiesis (vitamin B_{12}, folate, and copper deficiency)
  Infection
  Immune (neonatal alloimmune or autoimmune; autoimmune neutropenia of childhood)
  Hypersplenism

from the parents will be useful. If there is no obvious acquired cause such as viral infection or drug ingestion and no other primary disease, white blood cell counts should be done once or twice weekly for 2 months to evaluate the possibility of cyclic neutropenia. Bone marrow aspiration and biopsy are most important to characterize the morphologic features of myelopoiesis. Measuring the neutrophil counts in response to steroid infusion will document the marrow reserves. Elevated urinary muramidase levels and elevated serum lactoferrin may be found if increased neutrophil destruction is the cause of neutropenia. Other more specific tests to identify the mechanism of neutropenia include measurement of neutrophil antibodies or other tests for specific associated disease states such as serologic studies for lupus, immunoglobulin levels, and qualitative and quantitative assessment of lymphocytes. Cultures of bone marrow are important to define the numbers of stem cells and progenitors committed to the myeloid series or the presence of cytotoxic lymphocytes or humoral inhibitory factors. Direct measurement of cytokines is now available.

Treatment

If one can be identified, removal of the toxic agent or treatment of the associated disease is essential. As with neutrophil dysfunction syndromes, the hallmark of management includes diagnosis of infections and administration of appropriate antibiotics. Prophylactic antimicrobial therapy is not indicated.

Recent studies have shown administration of recombinant G-CSF and GM-CSF to be efficacious in management of neutropenia and its complications in patients with malignancies, marrow failure diseases, and congenital syndromes. Initially, patients may be started on 5 μg/kg/d of G-CSF (filgrastim) given subcutaneously or intravenously once a day. Depending on the response, the dose may be escalated to 10 μg/kg. For patients with congenital neutropenia, the dose should be regulated to keep the absolute neutrophil count less than 10,000/μL.

Prognosis

The prognosis varies greatly with the cause and severity of the neutropenia. In severe cases with persistent agranulocytosis, the prognosis is very poor in spite of antibiotic therapy; in mild or cyclic forms of neutropenia, symptoms may be minimal and the prognosis for normal life expectancy excellent. Recombinant hematopoietic hormones hold hope in the future for treatment of the more severe syndromes.

Ambruso DR et al: Infectious and bleeding complications in patients with glycogenosis Ib. Am J Dis Child 1985; 139:691.

Bussel J, Lalezari P, Fikrig S: Intravenous treatment with γ-globulin of autoimmune neutropenia of infancy. J Pediatr 1988;112:298.

Dale DC et al: A randomized controlled phase III trial of recombinant human granulocyte colony-stimulating factor (filgrastim) for treatment of severe chronic neutropenia. Blood 1993;81:2496.

Lange RD, Jones JB: Cyclic neutropenia: Review of clinical manifestations and management. Am J Pediatr Hematol Oncol 1981;3:363.

Stork LC et al: Pancytopenia in propionic acidemia: Hematologic evaluation and studies of hematopoiesis in vitro. Pediatr Res 1986;20:783.

Weetman RM, Boxer LA: Childhood neutropenia. Pediatr Clin North Am 1980;27:361.

NEUTROPHILIA

Neutrophilia is an increase in the peripheral blood absolute neutrophil count greater than 7500–8500 cells/μL for infants, children, and adults. To support the increased peripheral count, neutrophils may be mobilized from bone marrow storage or peripheral marginating pools. Acutely, neutrophilia is seen with bacterial or viral infections, inflammatory diseases (juvenile rheumatoid arthritis, inflammatory bowel disease, Kawasaki disease, etc), surgical or functional asplenia, liver failure, diabetic ketoacidosis, azotemia, and patients with congenital disorders of neutrophil function (eg, chronic granulomatous disease and leukocyte adherence deficiency) and hemolysis. Drugs such as steroids, lithium, and epinephrine are associated with an increase in the peripheral blood neutrophil count. Steroids cause release of neutrophils from the marrow pool and inhibit egress from capillary beds. Epinephrine causes release of the marginating pool. Acute neutrophilia has been reported after stress such as electric shock, trauma, burns, surgery, and emotional upset. Tumors involving the bone marrow such as lymphomas, neuroblastomas, and rhabdomyosarcoma may be associated with leukocytosis and the presence of immature myeloid cells in the peripheral blood.

Infants with Down's syndrome exhibit defective regulation of proliferation and maturation of the myeloid series and may develop neutrophilia. At times this process may affect other cell lines and mimics myeloproliferative disorder or acute myelogenous leukemia.

The neutrophilias must be distinguished from myeloproliferative disorders such as chronic myelogenous leukemia and juvenile chronic myelogenous leukemia. In general, abnormalities involving other cell lines, the presence of immature cells on the blood smear, and the presence of hepatosplenomegaly are important differentiating characteristics.

DISORDERS OF NEUTROPHIL FUNCTION

Neutrophils play a key role in host defenses. Circulating in capillary beds, they adhere to the vascular endothelium adjacent to sites of infection and inflammation. Moving between endothelial cells, the neutrophil migrates toward the offending agent. Contact with a microbe which is properly opsonized with complement or antibodies triggers ingestion, a process in which cytoplasmic streaming results in the formation of pseudopods that fuse around the invader, encasing it in a phagosome. During the ingestion phase, there is assembly and activation of the oxidase enzyme system, which takes oxygen from the surrounding medium and reduces it to form toxic oxygen metabolites critical to microbicidal activity. Concurrently, granules from the two main classes (azurophil and specific) fuse and release their contents into the phagolysosome. The concentration of toxic oxygen metabolites (hydrogen peroxide, hypochlorous acid, hydroxyl radical, and others) as well as other compounds (proteases, cationic proteins, cathepsins, defensins, and others) increases dramatically, resulting in the death and dissolution of the microbe. Complex physiologic and biochemical processes subserve and control these functions. Defects in any of these may lead to inadequate cell function and an increased risk of infection.

Neutrophil dysfunction may be organized according to the various phases of cell function: adherence, chemotaxis, ingestion, and killing. In addition, defective phagocytic activity may also arise in clinical disease states where there are abnormalities in the complement system or antibody production. Complement and antibodies are important in mediating cell motility and ingestion and are discussed in other chapters.

Classification

A summary of the major well-defined congenital defects in neutrophil function is presented in Table 28–8. In addition, there are a number of other congenital or acquired disorders associated with mild to moderate dysfunction of phagocytes. These include direct effects of drugs, metabolic defects (glycogenosis Ib, diabetes mellitus, renal disease, hypophosphatemia), and viral infections. Neutrophils from newborn infants exhibit multiple abnormalities, including deficiencies of adherence, chemotaxis, and bactericidal activity. Underlying these defects are problems with up-regulation of adhesion glycoproteins, altered oxidative metabolism, and deficiency of specific granules and their contents. Cells from patients with thermal injury, trauma, and overwhelming infection have defects in cell motility and bactericidal activity and exhibit similar biochemical abnormalities with neutrophils from newborn infants.

Clinical Findings

Recurrent bacterial or fungal infections are the hallmark of neutrophil dysfunction. Although many will have infection-free periods, episodes of pneumonia, sinusitis, cellulitis, cutaneous infections (including perianal or peritonsillar abscesses), and lymphadenitis are frequent. As with neutropenia, aphthous ulcers of mucous membranes, severe gingivitis, and periodontal disease are also major complications. In general, *Staphylococcus aureus,* along with gram-negative organisms, are commonly isolated from infected sites; other organisms may be specifically associated with a defined neutrophil function defect. In some disorders, fungi account for an increasing number of infections. Deep or generalized infections such as osteomyelitis, liver abscesses, sepsis, meningitis, and necrotic or even gangrenous soft tissue lesions occur in specific syndromes (eg, leukocyte adherence deficiency or chronic granulomatous disease). Patients with severe neutrophil dysfunction may die in childhood from severe infections or associated complications. Pertinent laboratory findings are summarized in Table 28–8.

Treatment

The mainstays of management of these patients remain the anticipation of infections and aggressive attempts to identify the foci and the causative agents. Surgical procedures to achieve these goals may be both diagnostic and therapeutic. Broad-spectrum antibiotics covering the range of possible organisms should be initiated without delay, switching to specific antimicrobial agents when the appropriate microbiologic diagnosis is made. When infections are unresponsive or when they recur, granulocyte transfusions may be helpful.

Chronic management includes prophylactic antibiotics. Trimethoprim-sulfamethoxazole and other antibiotic compounds enhance the bactericidal activity of neutrophils from patients with chronic granulomatous disease. Some patients with Chédiak-Higashi syndrome improve clinically when given ascorbic acid. Recently, recombinant gamma interferon has been shown to decrease the number and severity of infections in patients with chronic granulomatous disease. Demonstration of this activity with one patient group raises the possibility that cytokines, growth factors, and other biologic response modifiers may be helpful in other conditions in preventing recurrent infections. Bone marrow transplantation has been attempted in most major congenital neutrophil dysfunction syndromes, and reconstitution with normal cells and cell function has been documented. Combining genetic engineering with autologous bone marrow transplant may provide a future strategy for curing these disorders.

Prognosis

For mild to moderate defects, anticipation and conservative medical management will ensure a reasonable outlook. For severe defects, excessive morbidity and significant mortality still exist. In some diseases, the development of noninfectious complications, such as the lymphoproliferative phase of Chédiak-

Table 28–8. Classification of congenital neutrophil function deficits.

Disorder	Clinical Manifestations	Functional Defect	Biochemical Defect	Inheritance
Chédiak-Higashi syndrome	Oculocutaneous albinism, photophobia, nystagmus, ataxia. Recurrent infections of skin, respiratory tract, and mucous membranes caused by gram-positive and gram-negative organisms. Many die from lymphoproliferative phase with hepatomegaly, fever. This may be a viral associated hemophagocytic syndrome secondary to Epstein-Barr virus infection.	Neutropenia. Neutrophils, monocytes, lymphocytes, platelets, and all granule-containing cells have giant granules. Most significant defect is in chemotaxis. Also milder defects in microbicidal activity and degranulation.	Unknown. Alterations in membrane fusion with formation of giant granules. Other biochemical abnormalities in cAMP and cGMP, microtubule assembly.	Autosomal recessive.
Leukocyte adherence deficiency I	Recurrent soft tissue infections, including gingivitis, otitis, mucositis, periodontitis, skin infections. Delayed separation of the cord in newborn and problems with wound healing.	Neutrophilia. Diminished adherence to surfaces, leading to decreased chemotaxis.	Absence or partial deficiency of CD11/CD18 cell surface adhesive glycoproteins.	Autosomal recessive.
Leukocyte adherence deficiency II	Recurrent infections, mental retardation, craniofacial abnormalities, short stature. Red cells have Bombay phenotype.	Neutrophilia. Deficient "rolling" interaction with endothelial cells.	Deficient fucosyl transferase results in deficient sialyl Lewis X antigen, which interacts with P selection on endothelial cell to establish neutrophil rolling, a prerequisite for adherence and diapedesis.	Autosomal recessive.
Chronic granulomatous disease	Recurrent purulent infections with catalase-positive bacteria and fungi. May involve skin, mucous membranes. Also develop deep infections (lymph nodes, liver, bones).	Neutrophilia. Neutrophils demonstrate deficient bactericidal activity in the presence of normal chemotaxis and ingestion. Defect in the oxidase, resulting in absence or diminished production of toxic oxygen metabolites.	A number of molecular defects in oxidase components. Absent cytochrome b558 with decreased mRNA for either (1) or (2): (1) gp91 phox (2) gp22 phox Absent p47 phox or p67 phox (cytosolic components).	(1) X-linked (60–65% of cases). (2) Autosomal recessive (<5% of cases). Autosomal recessive (30% of cases)
Myeloperoxidase deficiency	Generally healthy.	Diminished capacity to enhance hydrogen peroxide-mediated microbicidal activity.	Diminished or absent myeloperoxidase; posttranslational defect in processing protein.	Autosomal recessive.
Specific granule deficiency	Recurrent skin and deep tissue infections.	Decreased chemotaxis and bactericidal activity.	Failure to produce specific granules or their contents during myelopoiesis.	Autosomal recessive.

Higashi syndrome, may be of significant prognostic importance.

Ambruso DR, Johnston RB Jr: Chronic granulomatous disease. In: *Pediatric Respiratory Disease: Diagnosis and Treatment.* Hilman BC (editor). Saunders,1993.

Etzioni A et al: Brief report: Recurrent severe infections caused by a novel leukocyte adhesion deficiency. N Engl J Med 1992;327:1789.

The International Chronic Granulomatous Disease Cooperative Study Group: A controlled trial of interferon gamma to prevent infection in chronic granulomatous disease. N Engl J Med 1991;324:509.

Rotrosen D, Gallin JI: Disorders of phagocyte function. Ann Rev Immunol 1987;5:127.

LYMPHOCYTOSIS

From the first week up to the fifth year of life, lymphocytes are the most numerous leukocytes in peripheral blood. After this time, the ratio reverses until the adult pattern of neutrophil predominance is reached. An absolute lymphocytosis in childhood is seen with acute or chronic viral infections, pertussis, syphilis, tuberculosis, and hyperthyroidism. Other noninfectious conditions, drugs, and hypersensitivity and serum sickness-like reactions cause lymphocytosis.

Clinical features, including fever, upper respiratory symptoms, gastrointestinal complaints, and rashes, are clues in distinguishing infectious from noninfectious causes. The presence of enlarged liver, spleen, or lymph nodes is crucial to the differential diagnosis, which includes acute leukemia and lymphoma. The majority of cases of infectious mononucleosis present with hepatosplenomegaly or adenopathy. The absence of anemia and thrombocytopenia will help differentiate these disorders. Evaluation of the morphology of lymphocytes on peripheral blood smear is also crucial. Infectious causes—particularly infectious mononucleosis—are associated with atypical features in the lymphocytes such as basophilic cytoplasm, vacuoles, finer and less dense chromatin, and an indented nucleus. These features are distinct from the characteristic morphology seen in lymphoblastic leukemia. Lymphocytosis in childhood is most commonly associated with infections and will resolve with recovery from the primary disease.

EOSINOPHILIA

Eosinophilia is defined as an increase in the absolute number of eosinophils greater than 300/µL in infants and children. Allergies are one of the primary causes of eosinophilia in children, and this condition is associated with asthma, hay fever, and atopic dermatitis. Eosinophilia is also a feature of drug reactions and tumors such as Hodgkin's and non-Hodgkin's lymphomas and brain tumors. Immunodeficiency states and histiocytosis syndromes may also exhibit eosinophilia. Increased eosinophil counts are a prominent feature of parasitic infections. Gastrointestinal disorders such as chronic hepatitis, ulcerative colitis, Crohn's disease, and milk precipitin disease may have eosinophilia as a clinical feature. Increased blood eosinophil counts have been identified in several families without association with any specific illness. Rare causes of eosinophilia include the hypereosinophilic syndrome, characterized by counts greater than 1500/µL and organ involvement and damage (hepatosplenomegaly, cardiopathy, pulmonary fibrosis, and central nervous system injury). This is a disorder of middle-aged adults and is rare in children. Eosinophilic leukemia has been described, but its existence as a distinct entity is controversial.

BLEEDING DISORDERS

Bleeding disorders may occur as a result of (1) quantitative and qualitative abnormalities of platelets, (2) quantitative and qualitative abnormalities in plasma coagulation factors, or (3) vascular abnormalities. The blood coagulation scheme is shown in Figure 28–4.

The initial laboratory workup for patients with possible bleeding disorders should include a careful history and physical examination and the following laboratory investigations:

(1) Bleeding time to test small vessel integrity and platelet function.

(2) Absolute platelet count or estimation of platelet number on blood smear.

(3) Partial thromboplastin time (PTT) to measure clotting activity of the following factors: high-molecular-weight kininogen (HMWK), prekallikrein (PK), XII, XI, IX, VIII, X, V, II, and fibrinogen.

(4) Prothrombin time (PT) to screen the tissue thromboplastin system of coagulation (factors VII, X, II, V, and fibrinogen).

(5) Thrombin time (TT) to measure the conversion of fibrinogen to fibrin as well as the antithrombin effect of fibrin split products or heparin.

(6) Fibrinogen level.

This battery of screening tests usually identifies the general area of the defect and helps guide the clinician to more specific tests that might be necessary for precise diagnosis.

Best tests for bleeding disorders. Emerg Med (Apr) 1989; 145.

Manno CS: Difficult pediatric diagnoses: Bruising and bleeding. Pediatr Clin North Am 1991;38:637.

ABNORMALITIES OF PLATELET NUMBER OR FUNCTION

1. IDIOPATHIC THROMBOCYTOPENIC PURPURA (ITP)

Essentials of Diagnosis
- Petechiae, ecchymoses.
- Decreased platelet count.
- Otherwise healthy child.

General Considerations
Acute idiopathic thrombocytopenic purpura is the most common bleeding disorder of childhood. It most frequently occurs in children 2–5 years of age and follows infection, classically infection with viruses such as rubella, varicella, measles, and Epstein-Barr. As a

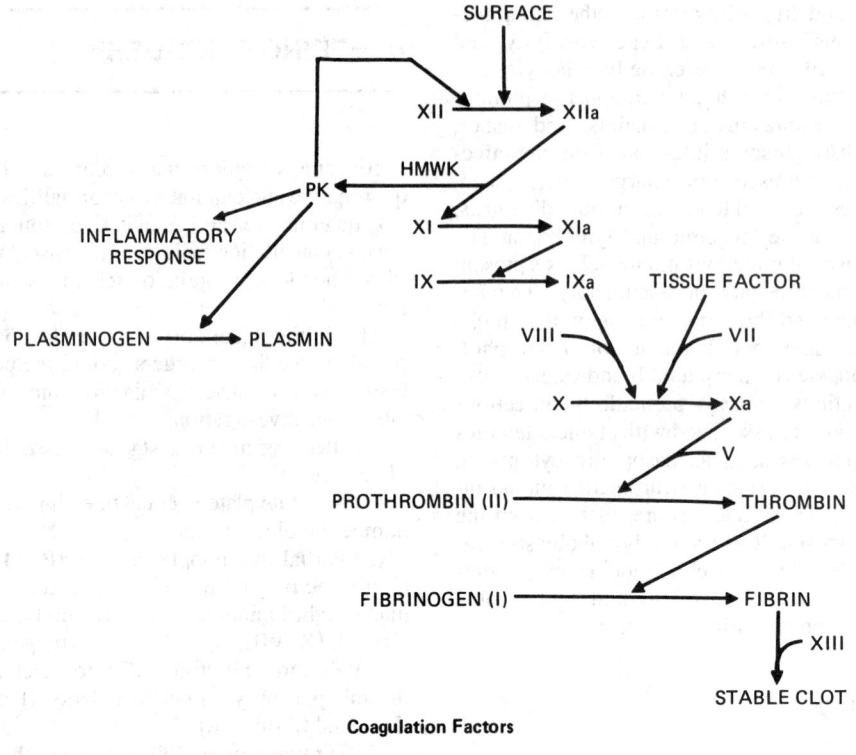

Figure 28–4. Blood coagulation scheme and terminology of coagulation factors.

Coagulation Factors

I	Fibrinogen	
II	Prothrombin	
V	Ac-globulin, proaccelerin, labile factor	
VII	Proconvertin, SPCA	
VIII	Antihemophilic factor (AHF)	
IX	Plasma thromboplastin component (PTC)	
	IXa Activated form	
X	Stuart-Prower factor	
	Xa Activated form	

XI	Plasma thromboplastin antecedent (PTA)
	XIa Activated form
XII	Hageman factor
	XIIa Activated form
XIII	Fibrin stabilizing factor, fibrinase
PK	Prekallikrein (Fletcher factor)
HMWK	High-molecular-weight kininogen

rule, it is self-limited; this is particularly true of the postinfectious type. The majority of such patients recover spontaneously within a few months and approximately 90% within a year after onset. Chronic idiopathic thrombocytopenia purpura (> 6 months' duration) occurs infrequently in childhood.

Idiopathic thrombocytopenia purpura is felt to be an immunologic disorder, and platelet-associated IgG or IgM can usually be demonstrated. The spleen plays a major role by forming antibodies and by sequestering damaged platelets.

Clinical Findings

A. Symptoms and Signs: The onset is usually acute, with the appearance of multiple ecchymoses. Petechiae are often present, especially on the lips and buccal mucosa, and epistaxis is common. There are generally no other physical findings. Rarely, concurrent infection with Epstein-Barr virus or cytomegalo-

virus may cause hepatosplenomegaly or lymphadenopathy simulating acute leukemia.

B. Laboratory Findings:

1. Blood–The platelet count is markedly reduced (usually < 50,000/μL and often < 10,000/μL), and platelets frequently are of larger size on peripheral blood smear. The white blood count and differential count are normal. Anemia is not present unless hemorrhage has occurred.

2. Bone marrow–An increased number of megakaryocytes is usually seen. Megakaryocytes may be larger than normal. Erythroid and myeloid cellularity is normal.

3. Other laboratory tests–The bleeding time is generally prolonged but less than would be expected solely from the platelet count. PTT and PT are normal. Platelet-associated IgG or IgM (or both) may be demonstrated on the platelets or in the serum (platelet antibody testing).

Differential Diagnosis

Causes of thrombocytopenia are shown in Table 28–9. Idiopathic thrombocytopenic purpura is a diagnosis of exclusion. Bone marrow examination is often indicated to exclude leukemia and aplastic anemia. Bone marrow examination should be performed if the history is atypical, if abnormalities other than purpura and petechiae are present on physical examination, if other cell lines are affected on CBC, or if steroid therapy is to be administered. Family history may be helpful in determining if thrombocytopenia is hereditary or familial.

Complications

Severe hemorrhage and bleeding into vital organs are the feared complications of idiopathic thrombocytopenic purpura. Intracranial hemorrhage is the most serious but rarely seen complication. The most important risk factor for hemorrhage is a platelet count less than 20,000/μL.

Treatment

A. General Measures: Many children require no therapy. Trauma should be avoided. Aspirin and aspirin-containing drugs should not be administered.

B. Corticosteroids: Patients with significant bleeding (ie, hematuria, hematochezia, epistaxis) or with a platelet count less than 10,000/μL are often treated with prednisone (2 mg/kg orally in divided daily doses) for a period of 2–4 weeks. The dosage is then tapered and stopped. No further prednisone is given regardless of the platelet count unless significant bleeding recurs, at which time the dosage of prednisone that should be used is the smallest that will give symptomatic relief (usually 2.5–5 mg twice daily). The patient is then followed until spontaneous remission occurs or until the patient is a candidate for further therapy.

C. Immune Globulin Intravenous (IGIV): As an alternative or adjunct to steroid treatment, IGIV has been shown to be effective in raising the platelet count in acute and chronic idiopathic thrombocytopenic purpura of childhood. IGIV may be effective even when the patient is resistant to steroids; responses are prompt and may last for several weeks. Most patients respond to 1 g/kg/d for 1–3 days.

D. Splenectomy: Splenectomy produces permanent remission in 70–90% of children with idiopathic thrombocytopenic purpura. It is usually reserved only for those who fail to remit over a period of 6 months to 1 year, since 90% of children will recover without surgical intervention within 1 year after onset. If symptoms are not controlled by medical management, splenectomy may be done earlier.

Although platelet transfusions are usually ineffective and bleeding is rarely a complication of splenectomy, platelet concentrates should be available for surgery. If the patient has been receiving corticosteroid therapy, the dose should be appropriately increased during and after surgery. Anticoagulant therapy is not indicated postoperatively even though the platelet count may rise to levels of approximately 1 million/μL.

The risk of overwhelming infection is increased after splenectomy, particularly in the young child. Therefore, the procedure should be postponed if possible until the child is at least 5 years of age. Administration of pneumococcal vaccine and possibly meningococcal vaccine prior to splenectomy is recommended. Prophylactic penicillin following splenectomy should be considered.

E. Other: Rh_o(D) immune globulin (RhoGAM) intravenously is an investigational treatment that appears equally as safe and as effective as IGIV in Rh-positive patients who have not been splenectomized. Remission of chronic ITP following therapy with chemotherapeutic agents or azathioprine has also been reported.

Table 28–9. Common causes of thrombocytopenia.

DESTRUCTIVE			REDUCED PRODUCTION	
Platelets Only	**Coagulopathy**	**Other Causes**	**Congenital**	**Acquired**
Antibody-mediated, as in idiopathic thrombocytopenic purpura, infection- or drug-induced, with autoimmune or lymphoproliferative diseases, neonatal alloimmune thrombocytopenia. **Nonimmunologic,** as in hemolytic uremic syndrome, thrombotic thrombocytopenic purpura, and with intravascular catheters and prostheses.	**Generalized,** as in disseminated intravascular coagulation. **Localized,** as in cavernous hemangiomas in the Kasabach-Merritt syndrome or with other localized coagulopathy.	Miscellaneous other causes, as in respiratory distress syndrome, preeclampsia, and sequestration in hypersplenism.	As in Fanconi's syndrome, Wiskott-Aldrich syndrome, thrombocytopenia with absent radii (TAR) syndrome, and other rare causes. In association with trisomy syndromes. With certain primary metabolic disorders.	Aplastic anemia, with marrow infiltration, secondary to drugs or radiation, secondary to folate or vitamin B_{12} deficiency.

Prognosis

Ninety percent of children with idiopathic thrombocytopenia purpura will have a spontaneous remission. Features associated with the development of chronic idiopathic thrombocytopenia purpura include female sex, age over 10 years at presentation, a more insidious onset of bruising, and the presence of other autoantibodies.

Bussel JB: Autoimmune thrombocytopenic purpura. Hematol Oncol Clin North Am 1990;4:179.

Bussel JB et al: Intravenous anti-D treatment of immune thrombocytopenic purpura: Analysis of efficacy, toxicity, and mechanism of effect. Blood 1991;77:1884.

2. THROMBOCYTOPENIA IN THE NEWBORN

Thrombocytopenia is one of the most common causes of purpura in the newborn and should be considered and investigated in any newborn with petechiae or a significant bleeding tendency. A platelet count less than 150,000/μL establishes a diagnosis of thrombocytopenia in the neonatal period. A number of specific entities may be responsible (Table 28–9). Infection and intravascular coagulation syndromes are the most common causes of thrombocytopenia in both sick term and preterm newborns. In the well-appearing newborn, antibody-mediated thrombocytopenia (alloimmune or maternal autoimmune), viral syndrome, hyperviscosity, or major vessel thrombosis are important causes. Management is directed toward alleviation of the specific cause; special situations are discussed below.

Thrombocytopenia Associated With Platelet Alloimmunization

An important cause of thrombocytopenia in the neonatal period is platelet alloimmunization. Alloimmunization occurs when a platelet antigen of the infant differs from that of the mother and when the mother is sensitized by a significant number of platelets that cross from the fetal to the maternal circulation. Platelet antibodies can usually be demonstrated. Petechiae or other bleeding manifestations are usually present shortly after birth. The bone marrow usually shows normal to increased megakaryocytes. The disease is self-limited; platelets usually rise spontaneously within 2 weeks, with complete recovery by 4–6 weeks. Severe intracranial bleeding can occur in utero or after delivery.

If severe alloimmunization occurs, platelet concentrate from the mother will be more effective in raising the platelet count than random donor platelets. Maternal platelets should be washed and irradiated. IGIV infusions have also been used successfully to raise the platelet count. If less severe, observation alone may be all that is required.

If alloimmunization has occurred with a previous pregnancy, ultrasound examination of the fetal brain to detect hemorrhage should be obtained at 20 weeks of gestation and repeated regularly. Percutaneous umbilical blood sampling can be performed at midgestation, and if the fetal platelet count is low, IGIV should be administered weekly to the mother. Delivery by elective cesarian section may be recommended, or induced vaginal delivery may be undertaken after in utero transfusion with maternal platelets.

Thrombocytopenia Associated With Idiopathic Thrombocytopenic Purpura in the Mother

Infants born to mothers with ITP or SLE may develop thrombocytopenia as a result of transfer of antibody from the mother to the infant. Prior to delivery, evaluation of the mother's platelet count and assay for platelet-bound IgG is indicated. If the mother is thrombocytopenic (or has undergone splenectomy) and platelet-associated IgG is present, elective cesarean section may be suggested, although controlled trials to prove its utility are lacking. Unfortunately, maternal platelet count, maternal anti-platelet antibody levels, and fetal scalp platelet counts are unreliable predictors of bleeding risk. Antenatal administration of either prednisone or IGIV to the mother has also been advocated, but again there are no controlled trials to support this approach.

Most neonates with thrombocytopenia secondary to passive transfer of maternal antibody do not bleed, and thus no specific treatment is indicated. However, if petechiae or puncture wound bleeding ensues in association with a platelet count less than 50,000/μL, a 1- to 2-week course of oral prednisone, 2 mg/kg/d, may be administered. If the platelet count remains consistently less than 25,000/μL or if severe hemorrhage is present, IGIV should be considered. Platelet transfusions may not be helpful without prior removal of antibody by exchange transfusion.

Neonatal Thrombocytopenia Associated With Infections

Thrombocytopenia is commonly associated with severe generalized infections during the newborn period, particularly those that develop in utero. Megakaryocytes are decreased and immature, and splenomegaly is often present. Intrauterine infections such as syphilis, toxoplasmosis, and cytomegalic inclusion disease are almost invariably associated with thrombocytopenia, and thrombocytopenia is frequently present with bacterial sepsis and with generalized infection with herpes simplex virus or other viruses.

In addition to specific treatment for the underlying disease if available, platelet transfusions may be indicated in severe cases. Platelet concentrates in the dosage of 10 mL/kg will raise the platelet count by about 75,000/μL.

Thrombocytopenia Associated With Giant Hemangiomas (Kasabach-Merritt Syndrome)

A rare but important cause of thrombocytopenic purpura in the newborn is giant hemangioma. Platelet sequestration in the lesion results in peripheral depletion of platelets. The bone marrow usually shows megakaryocytic hyperplasia. In the presence of massive hemangiomas, the thrombocytopenia may be associated with disseminated intravascular coagulation and result in fatal hemorrhage. Treatment is indicated if a serious coagulopathy is present or if the lesion exerts pressure on a vital structure (eg, trachea) or is cosmetically unacceptable (eg, facial).

Surgery is usually contraindicated because of the risk of hemorrhage. Prednisone therapy has been associated with marked regression of infantile hemangiomas. X-ray treatment has been beneficial. If disseminated intravascular coagulation is present, heparin or aminocaproic acid may be useful. Recently, alpha interferon has also been shown efficacious.

Bussell J et al: Recommendations for the evaluation and treatment of neonatal autoimmune and alloimmune thrombocytopenia. Thromb Haemost 1991;65:631.

Hathaway WE, Bonnar J: Bleeding disorders of the newborn infant. In: *Hemostatic Disorders of the Pregnant Woman and Newborn Infant.* Elsevier, 1987.

Samuels P et al: Estimation of the risk of thrombocytopenia in the offspring of pregnant women with presumed immune thrombocytopenic purpura. N Engl J Med 1990; 323:229.

White CW et al: Treatment of childhood angiomatous diseases with recombinant interferon alfa-2a. J Pediatr 1991;118:59.

3. DISORDERS OF PLATELET FUNCTION

The **hereditary** disorders of platelet function are characterized by a bleeding diathesis, usually associated with a prolonged bleeding time in spite of usually normal numbers of platelets. The findings in these diseases are summarized in Table 28–10.

Acquired disorders of platelet function include uremia, cirrhosis, disseminated intravascular coagulation, macroglobulinemias, systemic lupus erythematosus, myeloproliferative disorders, acyanotic congenital heart disease, and viral infections. Many pharmacologic agents decrease platelet function. Clinically, the most important of these and aspirin and synthetic penicillins.

Treatment

Many individuals with hereditary and acquired platelet function defects will respond to therapy with desmopressin acetate (DDAVP) at a dose of 0.3 µg/kg intravenously. If this is not effective, treatment with random donor platelets at a dose of one bag per 6 kg is indicated. Alternatively, calculations may be based on surface area, where one unit of platelet concentrate per meter squared is expected to raise the platelet count by 20,000/µL.

Rao AK: Congenital disorders of platelet function. Hematol Oncol Clin North Am 1990;4:65.

INHERITED ABNORMALITIES OF COAGULATION FACTORS

Normal values for coagulation factors are shown in Table 28–11. Inherited deficiencies of each factor have been described. The more common disorders are discussed here.

1. FACTOR VIII DEFICIENCY (Hemophilia A, Classic Hemophilia)

Essentials of Diagnosis

- Bruising, bleeding, and hemarthroses.
- Prolonged PTT.
- Reduced factor VIII activity.

General Considerations

Factor VIII deficiency is a bleeding disorder characterized by decreased activity of factor VIII. The disease occurs predominantly in males and is either inherited in an X-linked recessive manner or is caused by a new mutation. One-third of cases are due to a new mutation. All degrees of severity of the disease have been reported.

Clinical Findings

A. Symptoms and Signs: Patients with severe hemophilia, characterized by frequent spontaneous bleeding episodes involving skin, mucous membranes, joints, muscles, and viscera, have less than 1% circulating factor VIII activity. However, mild hemophilia is also recognized; these patients bleed only at times of trauma or surgery. They have 5–40% factor VIII activity. An intermediate group of patients with moderate symptoms (bleeding with trauma) have 1–5% factor VIII levels.

The most crippling aspect of hemophilia A is the tendency to develop chronic hemarthrosis, especially of knees and elbows, which leads to synovial thickening and joint contractures.

B. Laboratory Findings: In about 70% of families with this disease, the female carriers will have low levels of factor VIII (20–70%) and may occasionally be mildly symptomatic. Carriers of hemophilia can be detected in most instances by determination of the ratio of factor VIII to von Willebrand factor (vWF) or by molecular genetic techniques.

The partial thromboplastin time (PTT) is abnormal. The bleeding time and prothrombin time are usually

Table 28–10. Hereditary platelet function disorders.[1]

Category	Heredity	Morphology	Platelet-Rich Plasma Aggregation to:				Specific Defects
			ADP	Colla-gen	AA	Risto-cetin	
Glanzmann's thrombasthenia[2]	AR	Normal	–	–	–	+	Decreased membrane glycoprotein IIb–IIIa
Bernard-Soulier syndrome[2]	AR	Giant platelets	+	+	+	–	Decreased membrane glycoprotein Ib
Storage pool deficiency syndromes:[2] Dense body deficiency, Hermansky-Pudlak syndrome	AR	Electron micros-copy: de-creased to absent dense bodies	±	–	±	±	Decreased ADP-ATP, Ca^{2+}, serotonin storage and release
Dense body with α-granule deficiency[2]	AD	Electron micros-copy: de-creased dense bodies and α-granules	±	–	±	±	Decreased ADP, Ca^{2+}, serotonin, PF$_4$, fibrino-gen, βTG storage and release, decreased PDGF
α-Granule deficiency, gray platelet syndrome[2]	AR	Light gray plate-lets. Electron microscopy: de-creased α-granules	±	±	+	+	Decreased PF$_4$, βTG, fi-brinogen, decreased PDGF storage and re-lease
Wiskott-Aldrich syndrome[2]	X-linked	Tiny platelets; decreased or-ganelles	±	–	+	+	
Failure to release (aspirin-like defect)	Variable	Normal	±	–	–	±	Deficiency of cyclooxygenase or thromboxane synthetase
Isolated platelet factor V deficiency	AD	Normal	?	?	?	?	Decreased platelet fac-tor V function
Pseudo-von Willebrand's disease[2]	AD	Normal	+	+	+	Incr	Intrinsic platelet abnor-mality of increased reac-tion with vWF

[1]Modified and reproduced, with permission, from Hathaway WE, Bonnar J: *Hemostatic Disorders of the Pregnant Woman and Newborn Infant.* Elsevier, 1987. Copr © 1987 by Elsevier Science Publishing Co., Inc.
[2] Thrombocytopenia may be seen.

Key: + = yes: – = no; ± = partial or slight
AD = autosomal dominant; AR = autosomal recessive
AA = arachidonic acid; PF$_4$ = platelet factor 4; βTG = β-thromboglobulin; PDGF = platelet-derived growth factor

normal. The diagnosis is confirmed by finding a low level of factor VIII with a normal level of von Willebrand factor.

Complications

A serious complication of classic hemophilia is the development of an acquired circulating anticoagulant to factor VIII after exposure to administered factor VIII. Inhibitors or antibodies to factor VIII develop in 15–25% of factor VIII-deficient hemophiliacs. The inhibitor is an antibody that may be amenable to im-munosuppressive therapy. Factor IX or activated pro-thrombin complex concentrates (anti-inhibitor coag-ulant complex; Autoplex T, Feiba VH) may be of help in stopping hemorrhage. Recombinant factor VIIa is an alternative.

Other complications of hemophilia include chronic crippling arthritis due to repeated hemarthroses and

development of pseudotumors as a result of multiple bleeds in one site. Complications related to therapy include infection with hepatitis B or C. In addition, the majority of hemophilia patients exposed to factor concentrates before 1985 have contracted the human immunodeficiency virus (HIV). The use of virally in-activated, donor-screened products appears to have eliminated this risk; most current factor VIII con-centrates have been shown to be free of HIV and hepatitis.

Treatment

The basis of treatment of classic hemophilia is the administration of a factor VIII-containing concen-trates in order to achieve adequate hemostasis. Factor VIII is temperature and storage labile in biologic flu-ids. The in vitro half-life of infused factor VIII is about 12 hours.

Table 28–11. Coagulation factor and test values in normal pregnant women, and newborn infants.[1]

| Category | Fibrinogen (mg/dL) | Factors | | | | | | | | | | | | Platelet Count (per μL) | Euglobulin Lysis Time (minutes) | Partial Thromboplastin Time[2] (seconds) | Prothrombin Time (seconds) | Thrombin Time (seconds) |
		II (%)	V (%)	VII (%)	VIII (%)	IX (%)	X (%)	XI (%)	XII (%)	XIII (titer)							
Normal adult or child	190–420	100	100	100	100	100	100	100	100	1/16	200,000–450,000	90–300	37–50	12–14	8–10
Term pregnancy	483	92	108	170	196	130	130	69	…	1/16	290,000	278	44	13	8
Premature infant (1500–2500 g), cord blood	233	25	67	37	100	34	29	30	33	1/8	220,000	214	90	17 (12–21)	14 (11–17)
Term infant, cord blood	216	41	92	56	100	27	55	36	47	1/8	190,000	84	71	13.5 (12–16)	12 (10–16)
Term infant, 48 hours	210	46	105	20	100	↓	45	39	25	…	200,000	105	65	16 (12–21)	13 (10–16)

Note: All levels expressed as means or ranges.
[1]Modified and reproduced, with permission, from Hathaway WE: Coagulation problems in the newborn infant. Pediatr Clin North Am 1970;17:929.
[2]Kaolin PTT.

Although fresh frozen plasma (FFP) and cryopre- cipitate have been standard treatment, factor VIII concentrates that are administered in a lesser volume to achieve higher factor VIII levels and in which vi- ruses are inactivated are now the treatment of choice for moderate to severe hemophilia A. Virus is inacti- vated either by dry heat or treatment with organic sol- vents. Further means of purification include treat- ment with immunoaffinity columns to remove the factor VIII from extraneous proteins and contami- nants and then elution with monoclonal antibodies. These products appear free of both HIV and hepatitis virus. Recombinant factor VIII concentrates are now commercially available.

Independent of the specific factor VIII concentrate used, the dose can be calculated as follows:

Units of factor VIII = Weight in kg × Desired in vivo percentage × 0.5.

One unit of factor VIII per kg is expected to in- crease the factor VIII level by 2%. Treatment must be continued until adequate healing occurs, ie, 2–5 days for tooth extractions or epistaxis but 7–14 days for surgical wounds. The principle of therapy is to rap- idly achieve a hemostatic level of factor VIII (at least 40%) and to maintain this level until the lesion is ad- equately healed. For surgical procedures, levels of 60–80% are usually necessary. In mucous membrane bleeding or wounds (tongue, tooth socket), the dura- tion of factor VIII therapy can often be reduced to 1– 2 days if a fibrinolytic inhibitor (aminocaproic acid or tranexamic acid) is given orally until healing is com- plete. Major surgical procedures and central nervous system bleeding usually require levels of 80–100% for adequate hemostasis.

Bleeding in joints or soft tissue areas can often be controlled by a single infusion of factor VIII concen- trate to reach a peak of 40%. If bleeding is severe, this dose should be repeated in 12–24 hours. However, if the lesion is a dissecting hematoma that might threaten nerve function or endanger respiration or vi- sion, a level of at least 40% should be maintained for at least 48 hours.

Corticosteroids may be helpful in instances of re- current joint bleeding. Patients with renal bleeding have also benefited from corticosteroid therapy. Some patients with mild hemophilia may be treated with desmopressin acetate (DDAVP) (see p 853) in order to avoid the complications of concentrate therapy.

Prognosis

The prognosis for a normal life is good if care is taken to provide prophylaxis against injury, early treatment of bleeding episodes with virus-inactivated concentrate, careful orthopedic care of joint lesions, and attention to the emotional, social, and educa- tional adjustment of the individual.

Furie B, Furie B: The molecular basis of blood coagulation. Cell 1988;53:505.

Gill J: Therapy of factor VIII deficiency. Semin Thromb Hemost 1993;19:1.

Limentani SA et al: Recombinant blood clotting proteins for hemophilia therapy. Semin Throm Hemost 1993;19:62.

2. FACTOR IX DEFICIENCY (Hemophilia B, Christmas Disease)

The mode of inheritance and clinical manifesta- tions of factor IX deficiency are the same as those of factor VIII deficiency. Factor IX deficiency is 15– 20% as prevalent as factor VIII deficiency.

In hereditary factor IX deficiency, the PTT is pro- longed, but prothrombin time and thrombin time are normal. The patients present with bruising, bleeding, and hemarthroses. Diagnosis is confirmed by specific coagulation assays.

Although fresh frozen plasma has been used, factor IX concentrates are now recommended. Unlike factor VIII, approximately half of the administered dose of factor IX diffuses into the extravascular space. One unit of factor IX per kilogram is expected to increase the factor IX level by 1%. Factor IX has a half-life of 20–22 hours in vivo. Cryoprecipitates and factor VIII concentrates do not contain factor IX. Virus-inacti- vating techniques for factor IX concentrates appear effective in eradicating HIV and hepatitis C. As with factor VIII, monoclonally derived factor IX concen- trate is available, but in contrast with factor VIII, a recombinant concentrate has not yet been produced. The prognosis for individuals with factor IX defi- ciency is good.

Thompson A: Factor IX concentrates for clinical use. Semin Thromb Hemost 1993;19:25.

3. FACTOR XI DEFICIENCY (Hemophilia C)

Factor XI deficiency is a bleeding diathesis of mild to moderate severity. Inheritance is by the autosomal recessive mode. Heterozygotes may rarely show a mild bleeding tendency at surgery or following se- vere trauma. Homozygous patients may have spon- taneous hemorrhage (ecchymoses, epistaxis) in ad- dition to bleeding due to trauma. Only rarely do patients with hemophilia C have spontaneous hemar- throses. Hemophilia C has been found mainly in Ash- kenazi Jews and comprises less than 5% of all hemo- philia diseases.

The defect may be very mild, and a sensitive coag- ulation test is required to identify the deficiency. Bleeding usually requires intervention only at the time of surgery (eg, tooth extractions) or trauma. Treatment is therefore with FFP to the extent volume expansion is tolerated. Factor XI concentrate is in clinical trials.

The prognosis for an average life span is excellent.

Asakai R et al: Factor XI deficiency in Ashkenazi Jews in Israel. N Engl J Med 1991;325:153.

4. OTHER INHERITED COAGULATION FACTOR DEFECTS

Other hereditary single clotting factor deficiencies are rare. Transmission is generally autosomal. Homozygous individuals with a deficiency or structural abnormality of prothrombin, factor V, factor VII, or factor X may have excessive bleeding.

Individuals with dysfibrinogenemia (abnormal fibrinogen) are usually asymptomatic but may develop recurrent venous thromboembolic episodes or have a bleeding tendency. Immunologic determinations of fibrinogen are normal, but the thrombin and prothrombin times are often prolonged. Treatment is similar to that outlined for afibrinogenemia (absence of fibrinogen).

Afibrinogenemia resembles hemophilia clinically. However, the condition is inherited as an autosomal recessive and affects both sexes. The patients have persistent bleeding from small injuries, hematomas, ecchymoses, and hemarthroses. Fatal bleeding from the umbilical cord has been reported. Bleeding is generally similar to that found in individuals with moderate to severe hemophilia.

The principal laboratory finding in afibrinogenemia is complete absence of a fibrin clot by any of the usual clotting tests. Whole blood and plasma are incoagulable even upon the addition of optimal amounts of calcium, thromboplastin, and thrombin. The erythrocyte sedimentation rate is zero. There is an absence of precipitable fibrinogen upon heating of plasma to 56 °C for 10 minutes. Specific assays for other coagulation factors are normal. Hypofibrinogenemia (fibrinogen level < 100 mg/dL) is also rarely seen.

Transfusion with whole blood, fresh plasma, or cryoprecipitate generally controls the acute bleeding episodes. The minimal hemostatic level of circulating fibrinogen is about 60 mg/dL (normal, 250–450 mg/dL). The half-life of transfused fibrinogen is about 4 days. Therefore, 10–20 mL of plasma per kilogram of body weight or one bag of cryoprecipitate per 6 kg should achieve hemostasis. This dose may need to be repeated daily depending upon the type and severity of bleeding and the rate of healing.

Galanakis KK: Fibrinogen anomalies and disease: A clinical update. Hematol Oncol Clin North Am 1992;5:1171.

VON WILLEBRAND'S DISEASE

Essentials of Diagnosis

- History of easy bruising and epistaxis from early childhood.
- Bleeding time is usually prolonged, with a normal platelet count.
- Reduced levels or abnormal structure of von Willebrand factor.

General Considerations

Von Willebrand's disease is a familial bleeding disorder usually transmitted as an autosomal dominant trait. It is generally associated both with a prolonged bleeding time and with reduced levels of factor VIII and von Willebrand factor (vWF). The partial thromboplastin time is usually prolonged but may be normal.

Von Willebrand's disease and its variants are due to abnormalities of vWF. Normal vWF circulates in plasma as a multimeric complex with factor VIII. In classic von Willebrand's disease, both vWF and factor VIII are reduced. Variants of von Willebrand's disease are classified based on the identification of quantitative (decreased vWF antigen) or qualitative (functional; decreased ristocetin activity) abnormalities of vWF.

Clinical Findings

A. Symptoms and Signs: There is usually a history of increased bruising and excessive epistaxis. Increased bleeding will also occur with lacerations or at surgery. Menorrhagia is a problem in the adolescent female. Petechiae are usually not observed, and hemarthrosis is rare.

B. Laboratory Findings: A prolonged bleeding time is generally present, and the PTT is often prolonged. Platelet number and aggregations in platelet-rich plasma are normal except for decreased ristocetin-induced platelet aggregation. The ristocetin cofactor activity of plasma is reduced. Factor VIII and vWF antigen are decreased in classic (type I) von Willebrand's disease but may be normal in variants with dysfunctional vWF. Such variants are classified by multimeric analysis of vWF.

Treatment

All patients with von Willebrand's disease need additional normal von Willebrand factor (vWF) for treatment of bleeding or prevention of excess bleeding during surgical procedures. The treatment of choice for most individuals with mild to moderate von Willebrand's disease is desmopressin acetate (DDAVP) intravenously at a dose of 0.3 µg/kg in at least 20–30 mL of normal saline given over 20–30 minutes. DDAVP mediates the release of vWF from endothelial storage, and a twofold to threefold rise in vWF is expected. Efficacy is variable from patient to patient; bleeding time should be measured 30 minutes after infusion to ensure adequate effect. Since vWF storage is limited, tachyphylaxis is often seen. If further therapy is indicated 40 µg/kg of vWF-rich concentrate (currently Humate-P is such a product) or cryoprecipitate (one bag per 6 kg) is recommended to maintain vWF levels of 30–50%.

For individuals with type III (severe) or type IIB von Willebrand's disease, the treatment of choice is with Humate-P (or a similar vWF-enriched concentrate) or cryoprecipitate. DDAVP is ineffective therapy for individuals with severe von Willebrand's disease, and its administration to individuals with type IIB disease may evoke thrombocytopenia.

Supplemental antifibrinolytic drugs (aminocaproic acid or tranexamic acid) are indicated for any individual with von Willebrand's disease to preserve clots during oral, nasal, or vaginal bleeding.

Prognosis

Bleeding may cease spontaneously or may be controlled with the above measures. Life expectancy is normal.

Holmberg L, Nilsson IM: von Willebrand's disease. Eur J Haematol 1992;48:127.

Manucci PM: Desmopressin: A nontransfusional form of treatment for congenital and acquired bleeding disorders. New Engl J Med 1988;72:1449.

ACQUIRED ABNORMALITIES OF COAGULATION FACTORS

1. DISSEMINATED INTRAVASCULAR COAGULATION

Essentials of Diagnosis

- Presence of disorder known to trigger disseminated intravascular coagulation.
- Evidence for activation of coagulation (prolonged PTT, prothrombin time, or thrombin time; decreased fibrinogen or platelets).

General Considerations

Disseminated intravascular coagulation (DIC) is an acquired pathologic process characterized by activation of the coagulation system and leading to thrombin generation, intravascular fibrin deposition, and platelet consumption. Microthrombi, composed of fibrin and platelets, may produce ischemic tissue damage. The fibrinolytic system is also frequently activated, producing plasmin-mediated destruction of fibrin, fibrinogen, and other clotting factors (factor V, factor VIII). Degradation or split products of fibrin-fibrinogen are formed and function as anticoagulants and inhibitors of platelet function. Disseminated intravascular coagulation commonly accompanies disorders seen in critically ill infants and children. Con-

ditions known to trigger DIC include endothelial cell damage (endotoxin, virus), tissue destruction (necrosis, physical injuries), hypoxia (acidosis), ischemic and vascular changes (shock, hemangiomas), and release of tissue procoagulants (cancer, placental disorders).

Clinical Findings

A. Symptoms and Signs: Physical signs of the disorder may include (1) evidence of a diffuse bleeding tendency (hematuria, melena, purpura, petechiae, persistent oozing from needle punctures or other invasive procedures); (2) circulatory collapse, poor skin perfusion, early ischemic changes; and (3) evidence of thrombotic lesions (major vessel thrombosis, gangrene, purpura fulminans).

B. Laboratory Findings: Tests that are most sensitive, easiest to perform, and best reflect the hemostatic capacity of the patient are the prothrombin time, partial thromboplastin time, platelet count, fibrinogen level, and a test for fibrin-fibrinogen split products. A new test that measures the cross-linked fibrin degradation by-products called d-dimers may also be helpful in demonstrating activation of both coagulation and fibrinolysis. In general, the PT and PTT are prolonged and the platelet count and fibrinogen level are decreased. Levels of fibrin-fibrinogen split products and d-dimers are elevated. If these tests are normal or only slightly abnormal, clinically significant disseminated intravascular coagulation is not present.

The abnormalities associated with disseminated intravascular coagulation may be variable depending on the triggering event. Patients with infections may have primarily thrombocytopenia, with only slight prolongation of the PTT and PT and mild elevation of fibrin-fibrinogen split products; only platelets may be consumed in bacterial sepsis without any other evidence of activated coagulation. In contrast, asphyxia may produce significant consumption of fibrinogen and elevated fibrin-fibrinogen split products without depression of platelets.

Differential Diagnosis

Bleeding with liver disease, vitamin K deficiency, or uremia can mimic disseminated intravascular coagulation. Vitamin K deficiency can be easily diagnosed and treated, and uremia is not hard to recognize, but it may be more difficult to differentiate severe liver disease from disseminated intravascular coagulation. Patients with fulminant hepatitis or advanced cirrhosis often have evidence of both decreased production of liver factors and increased consumption of platelets and fibrinogen mimicking disseminated intravascular coagulation. Generally, factor VII levels are markedly decreased in liver disease as compared to mild to moderate decreases in disseminated intravascular coagulation. Factor VIII levels may be normal or even increased in liver disease as compared to decreased levels in disseminated intravascular coagulation.

Treatment

A. Therapy for Underlying Disorder: The most important aspect of therapy is identification and treatment of the triggering event, since deaths are usually related to failure to control the underlying disorder. If bacterial sepsis is present, antibiotic therapy and volume replacement for circulatory support are indicated. If respiratory compromise is present, oxygen must be provided and any metabolic derangements corrected. For hemorrhagic shock, blood must be promptly infused. If the precipitating event can be treated (eg, hypoxia, shock), often no other therapy is needed for the coagulopathy. Serial determination with coagulation tests will help in determining whether further therapy is indicated.

B. Replacement Therapy: Replacement of depleted coagulation factors and platelets may be necessary in severe DIC, especially with severe hemorrhage. Initial stabilization of children suspected of having DIC should be with fresh frozen plasma in order to replace depleted coagulation factors; 10–15 mL kg will raise the clotting factor levels by about 20%. Fibrinogen (and factor VIII) can be given as cryoprecipitate also; one bag of cryoprecipitate per 3 kg in infants or one bag of cryoprecipitate per 6 kg in older children will raise the fibrinogen level by 75–100 mg/dL. Platelets are replaced by use of platelet concentrate; in the neonate, 10 mL of platelet concentrate per kilogram will raise the platelet count by about 75,000–100,000/μL. In older children, one bag of platelet concentrate per 5–6 kg is the usual dose. An alternative formula is as follows: 1 unit/m^2 of platelet concentrate will increase the platelet count by approximately 20,000/μL. The minimal hemostatic levels are a platelet count greater than 30,000–50,000/μL, prothrombin time of less than 16 seconds, and fibrinogen level over 100 mg/dL.

C. Anticoagulant Therapy: Interruption of the clotting process with heparin may be necessary when the triggering event cannot be quickly treated and consumption coagulopathy or tissue necrosis is ongoing (eg, acute promyelocytic or monocytic leukemia, giant hemangioma, impending tissue necrosis or gangrene in septic shock, large vessel thrombosis, or purpura fulminans). In these instances, heparin will halt DIC or allow for more effective replacement therapy while the primary disease is being specifically treated. The most effective and safest method of giving heparin is by continuous intravenous administration. A loading dose of 50 units/kg is followed by 10–20 units/kg/h by continuous intravenous infusion. Unless there is significant tissue necrosis, such doses are usually effective, and improvement of coagulation screening tests should occur in 12–24 hours or sooner. Heparin should be administered to achieve a heparin level between 0.3 and 0.6 units/mL.

D. Management of DIC in Neonates: Premature and full-term neonates frequently develop generalized bleeding tendencies associated with other illnesses such as respiratory distress syndrome, cyanotic congenital heart disease, cerebral anoxia, and severe sepsis. Factors often present and possibly related to this bleeding syndrome are hypoxia, acidosis, vascular fragility, decreased platelet number and function, and increased fibrinolytic activity. Laboratory tests of bleeding and coagulation are difficult to interpret because results in affected patients overlap with those in normal infants. The values for these tests seen in "normal" full-term and premature neonates are shown in Table 28–11. The pathophysiologic mechanisms of these secondary bleeding syndromes (cerebral hemorrhage, pulmonary hemorrhage, generalized bleeding tendency) are related to increased consumption of clotting factors (due to pathologic proteolysis) and platelets or decreased synthesis of clotting factors (due to functional impairment of the liver).

Treatment consists of correcting the associated conditions and replacing clotting factors and platelets with doses of fresh frozen plasma and platelets. Occasionally, exchange transfusion or heparinization is indicated.

2. LIVER DISEASE

The liver is the major site of synthesis of the following clotting factors: high-molecular-weight kininogen (HMWK), XIII, XII, XI, X, IX, VII, V, prothrombin, and fibrinogen. Deficiency of factor V and the vitamin K-dependent factors (II, VII, IX, and X) is most often a problem as a result of decreased hepatic synthesis. Prolongation of the PT and PTT is usually seen. Extravascular loss and increased consumption of clotting factors may also contribute to prolongation of the PT and PTT. The amount of fibrinogen may be decreased, or an abnormal fibrinogen (dysfibrinogen) containing excess sialic acid residues may be synthesized. Dysfibrinogenemia is associated with prolongation of thrombin time (TT) and reptilase time. Increased fibrinolysis may further prolong the TT, reptilase time, PT, and PTT. Fibrin-fibrinogen degradation products and d-dimers may be present. Thrombocytopenia secondary to hypersplenism and qualitative platelet abnormalities may be seen. Treatment consists of replacement with fresh frozen plasma and platelets as needed. In cases where liver disease is associated with fat malabsorption, vitamin K (1–5 mg) should be given. Desmopressin acetate shortens the bleeding time and PTT in patients with chronic liver disease.

3. VITAMIN K DEFICIENCY

All newborns have physiologically depressed levels of the vitamin K-dependent factors (II, VII, IX, and X). If vitamin K is not administered at birth, these factor levels decrease even further in the next 48–72 hours and may cause a bleeding diathesis called hemorrhagic disease of the newborn. One of three patterns is seen in most affected infants.

(1) Early hemorrhagic disease of the newborn occurs within 24 hours of birth and is most often manifested by cephalhematoma, intracranial hemorrhage, or intra-abdominal bleeding. Although occasionally idiopathic, it is most often associated with maternal ingestion of drugs that interfere with vitamin K metabolism, eg, warfarin, phenytoin, isoniazid, and rifampin. This pattern of hemorrhagic disease is often life-threatening.

(2) Classic hemorrhagic disease of the newborn occurs at 24 hours to 7 days of age and usually is manifested as gastrointestinal, skin, or mucosal bleeding. Bleeding after circumcision may occur. Although occasionally associated with maternal drug usage, it most often occurs in well babies that do not receive vitamin K at birth and are solely breast-fed; breast milk has much less vitamin K than commercially prepared formulas.

(3) Late hemorrhagic disease occurs in infants 1–6 months of age. Manifestations are intracranial, gastrointestinal, or skin bleeding. Occasionally the disease is idiopathic, but usually it is secondary to chronic diarrhea, malabsorption syndromes, obstructive jaundice, or prolonged antibiotic therapy.

The diagnosis of vitamin K deficiency is based on the history, physical examination, and laboratory results. The prothrombin time is markedly prolonged. The PTT is prolonged. Thrombin time and platelet count are normal. The diagnosis is confirmed by the positive response to vitamin K treatment and by demonstration of noncarboxlyated protein in vitamin K absence (PIVKA). Treatment with vitamin K should be given immediately and not withheld awaiting test results.

4. UREMIA

Bleeding occurs in approximately 50% of patients with chronic renal failure. It is most often manifested as purpura, menorrhagia, or gastrointestinal bleeding. Decreased blood levels of factors XII, XI, and IX secondary to increased urinary losses result in prolongation of the PTT. An abnormality of von Willebrand factor may also occur, prolonging the bleeding time. Qualitative and quantitative platelet abnormalities may develop.

Bleeding is managed with infusion of desmopressin acetate or transfusion of cryoprecipitate.

Bick RL: Disseminated intravascular coagulation and related syndromes: A clinical review. Semin Thromb Hemost 1988;14:299.

Carvalho A: Acquired platelet dysfunction in patients with uremia. Hematol Oncol Clin North Am 1990;4:129.

Feinstein DI: Treatment of disseminated intravascular coagulation. Semin Thromb Hemost 1988;14:351.

Hathaway WE: New insights on vitamin K. Hematol Oncol Clin North Am 1987;1:367.

Shearer MJ: Vitamin K and vitamin K-dependent proteins. Br J Haematol 1990;75:156.

VASCULAR ABNORMALITIES ASSOCIATED WITH BLEEDING

1. HENOCH-SCHÖNLEIN PURPURA (Anaphylactoid Purpura)

Essentials of Diagnosis

- Purpuric cutaneous rash.
- Migratory polyarthritis or polyarthralgias.
- Colicky abdominal pain.
- Nephritis.

General Considerations

Patients with Henoch-Schönlein purpura have a characteristic purpuric skin rash plus all or some of the following: migratory polyarthralgias or polyarthritis, colicky abdominal pain, and nephritis. The disorder occurs primarily in males and most commonly in those 2–7 years of age. Occurrence is highest in the spring or fall. Two-thirds of affected children have a history of upper respiratory infection in the preceding 1–3 weeks.

Henoch-Schönlein purpura is characterized by vasculitis of the small vessels, particularly those of the skin, gastrointestinal tract, and kidney. Immune complexes (IgA with complement, IgG, or IgM) have been associated with blood vessel walls of the kidney, intestine, and skin. Suspected though not proved inciting antigens include group A β-hemolytic streptococci and other bacteria, viruses, drugs, foods, and insect bites.

Clinical Findings

A. Symptoms and Signs: The skin rash is often urticarial initially and then progresses to a macular-papular appearance that transforms into a diagnostic symmetric purpuric skin rash distributed on the ankles, buttocks, and elbows. Purpuric areas of a few millimeters in diameter are present and may progress to form larger hemorrhages ("palpable purpura"). Petechial lesions may occur, but the majority of hemorrhages are slightly larger. The rash usually begins on the lower extremities, but the entire body may be involved. New lesions may continue to appear for 2–4 weeks. Approximately two-thirds of patients develop migratory polyarthralgias or polyarthritis, primarily of the ankles and knees. Edema of the hands, feet, scalp, and periorbital regions may be noted. Abdominal colic—due to hemorrhage and edema primarily of the small intestine—occurs in about half of those affected; intussusception may ensue. Twenty-five to 50 percent of those affected develop renal involvement. This is most often manifested as hematuria, but proteinuria or nephrotic syndrome may be seen. Hematuria alone is never the presenting complaint for Henoch-Schönlein purpura but usually manifests in the second to third week of illness. Renal involvement occurs more commonly in males and in older patients. Testicular torsion may occur. Neurologic symptoms are possible.

B. Laboratory Findings: The platelet count, platelet function tests, and bleeding time are usually normal. The platelet count may even be elevated. Blood coagulation is normal. Urinalysis frequently reveals hematuria. Proteinuria may also be noted, but casts are uncommon. Stool analysis may be positive for blood even though melena is not observed. The ASO titer is frequently elevated or the throat culture positive for group A β-hemolytic streptococci. Serum IgA may be elevated.

Differential Diagnosis

Henoch-Schönlein purpura is differentiated from thrombocytopenic purpura in that the rash is raised and the platelet count is normal. The rash of septicemia (especially meningococcemia) may be very similar to that of Henoch-Schönlein purpura, though the distribution tends to be more generalized with meningococcemia. Blood culture may be necessary for final diagnosis. The possibility of child abuse should be considered in any child presenting with purpura.

Complications

Intussusception of the small bowel may occur in patients with intestinal manifestations. The most important serious complication derives from the renal involvement. About 15% of patients develop renal failure as a result of advancing proliferative glomerulonephritis with an associated mortality rate of 3%.

Treatment

There is no satisfactory treatment. Corticosteroid therapy may provide symptomatic relief for severe gastrointestinal or joint manifestations but does not alter skin or renal manifestations. Aspirin is useful for the arthritis, and sedatives may benefit the patient with gastrointestinal pain. If culture for group A β-hemolytic streptococci is positive or if the ASO titer is elevated, penicillin should be given in full therapeutic doses for 10 days.

Prognosis

The prognosis for recovery is generally good, though symptoms frequently (25–50%) recur over a period of several months. In patients who develop renal manifestations, microscopic hematuria may persist for years, and progression to renal failure occasionally occurs.

2. OTHER VASCULAR DISORDERS

Mild to life-threatening bleeding may occur with some types of Ehlers-Danlos syndrome, a connective tissue disorder. Bleeding time may be prolonged and manifested by easy bruising. Spontaneous rupture and dissection of aortic aneurysms has been reported.

Kontusaari S et al: Inheritance of an RNA splicing mutation (G+1 IVS20) in the type III procollagen gene (COL3A1) in a family having aortic aneurysms and easy bruisability: Phenotypic overlap between familial arterial aneurysms and Ehlers-Danlos syndrome type IV. Am J Hum Genet 1990;47:112.

Jones ME, Callen JP: Collagen vascular diseases in childhood. Ped Clin North Am 1991;38:1019.

Lanzkowsky S, Lanzkowsky L, Lanzkowsky P: Henoch-Schoenlein purpura. Pediatr Rev 1992;13:130.

THROMBOTIC DISORDERS

Children presenting with a thrombotic event may have either a congenital or an acquired hematologic disorder. Initial evaluation of such children must include a thorough history, family history, physical examination, and screening hematologic studies (CBC, platelet count, PT, and PTT). Specific assays of the procoagulant, anticoagulant, and fibrinolytic proteins are often warranted. Imaging studies to delineate the type (venous versus arterial) and extent of thrombosis are indicated.

CONGENITAL THROMBOTIC DISORDERS

The following features suggest the presence of a congenital rather than an acquired disorder: (1) thrombosis at an early age, (2) a family history of thrombotic disease, (3) thrombosis at an unusual site, or (4) recurrent thrombosis without precipitating events. If these features are present or if abnormalities are found on screening tests, a second tier of studies is indicated, including determination of the fibrinogen level, physiologic anticoagulant levels (protein C, protein S, and antithrombin III), and tests for lupus anticoagulant and anticardiolipin antibody. A third tier in the evaluation of a suspected congenital disorder would include investigating fibrinolytic activity by means of plasminogen, tissue plasminogen activator, and plasminogen activator inhibitor studies.

1. PROTEIN C DEFICIENCY

Protein C is a vitamin K-dependent protein that is normally activated by thrombin bound to thrombomodulin and inactivates activated factors V and VIII. In addition, it stimulates fibrinolysis. Two phenotypes of hereditary protein C deficiency are seen. Heterozygotes with autosomal dominant protein C deficiency typically present with venous thromboembolism as young adults, and require anticoagulation or fibrinolytic therapy. Homozygous or doubly heterozygous individuals generally present within the first 12 hours of life with purpura fulminans. Associated findings may include cerebral thrombosis or blindness. Immediate treatment of such neonates includes replacement of protein C by infusion of fresh frozen plasma approximately every 6 hours. Heparin therapy is generally not helpful. Subsequent management requires chronic anticoagulation with warfarin compounds. The long-term outlook is unknown. A human-derived protein C concentrate will soon be commercially available.

2. PROTEIN S DEFICIENCY

Protein S is a cofactor essential for the expression of activated protein C. Individuals with protein S deficiency usually present in the same way as those with heterozygous protein C deficiency. Current management with fresh frozen plasma is similar but will change when human-derived protein S concentrate, now in clinical trials, is commercially available.

3. ANTITHROMBIN III DEFICIENCY

Antithrombin III is the most important physiologic inhibitor of thrombin. In addition, it inhibits activated factors IX, X, XI, and XII. Antithrombin III deficiency is transmitted in an autosomal dominant pattern and is associated with venous thromboembolism. Symptoms before puberty are rare.

Initial management of a patient with thrombosis is with anticoagulant or fibrolytic therapy. Antithrombin III concentrate is available for replacement. Patients with recurrent venous thrombosis are maintained indefinitely on oral anticoagulants. Asymptomatic persons are generally not anticoagulated unless predisposing situations arise, ie, surgery, pregnancy, prolonged immobilization.

4. OTHER CONGENITAL THROMBOTIC DISORDERS

Qualitative abnormalities of fibrinogen (dysfibrinogenemias) are usually inherited in an autosomal dominant manner. Most individuals with dysfibrinogenemia are asymptomatic. Some have problems with bleeding, and others develop venous or arterial thrombosis.

Dysfunction of the fibrinolytic system may play a role in the development of thrombosis, but the association between defects in this system and thrombosis is less well documented than that between deficiencies of the physiologic anticoagulants and thrombosis. This may be due to the absence of sensitive laboratory tests to effectively diagnose fibrinolytic defects.

ACQUIRED THROMBOTIC DISORDERS

Individuals with the following medical problems are at increased risk for thrombosis: diabetes mellitus, nephrotic syndrome, congenital heart disease, liver disease, malignancy, and autoimmune diseases.

Thrombosis in autoimmune diseases may be related to the presence of a lupus anticoagulant. Lupus anticoagulants are immunoglobulins against phospholipid. Although first detected in a patient with lupus, they may develop with drug exposure, infection, or lymphoproliferative disorders. They may also be detected in well individuals. The presence of a lupus anticoagulant is often first suspected following detection of a prolonged PTT. Mixing patient plasma 1:1 with normal plasma does not correct the PTT into the normal range if a lupus inhibitor is present. Other tests used to diagnose a lupus inhibitor include the Russell's viper venom time and the platelet neutralization procedure. If a child with a lupus anticoagulant develops a thrombosis, then anticoagulant or fibrinolytic therapy is indicated. Therapy is generally not indicated for an asymptomatic child with a lupus anticoagulant.

Other conditions that predispose to thrombosis include shock, dehydration, hyperviscosity, polycythemia, and thrombocytosis, as do trauma and prolonged immobilization. Many of these conditions are associated with endothelial damage or vascular stasis, both of which have been implicated in the pathogenesis of clot formation. Similarly, foreign bodies such as Silastic catheters, ventriculojugular shunts, arteriovenous shunts, arterial grafts, and prosthetic heart valves increase the risk of thrombosis in normal individuals or especially in those with underlying thrombotic disorders.

Thrombosis is seen with purpura fulminans. Purpura fulminans may occur in association with hereditary homozygous protein C deficiency, may follow a bacterial or viral illness, or may be idiopathic. Central violaceous areas of thrombosis with advancing erythematous margins of hemorrhage are present in the skin. Gangrene may ensue with subsequent eschar formation and scarring. Heparin or replacement with fresh frozen plasma—or both measures—is usually indicated.

Dreyfuss M et al: Treatment of homozygous protein C deficiency and neonatal purpura fulminans with a purified protein C concentrate. N Engl J Med 1991;325:1565.

Francis R: Acquired purpura fulminans. Semin Thromb Hemost 1990;16:310.

Hathaway WE: Clinical aspects of antithrombin III deficiency. Semin Hematol 1991;28:19.

Marlar R et al: Diagnosis and treatment of homozygous protein C. J Pediatr 1989;114:528

Pegelow CH, et al: Severe protein S deficiency in a newborn. Pediatrics 1992;89:674.

Triplett D: Laboratory diagnosis of lupus anticoagulants. Semin Thromb Hemost 1990;16:182.

THE SPLEEN

SPLENOMEGALY & HYPERSPLENISM

The child with splenomegaly frequently presents a puzzling diagnostic problem. In the evaluation of chronic splenomegaly, the following categories of diseases should be considered: congestive spleno-megaly, chronic infections, leukemia and lymphomas, hemolytic anemias, reticuloendothelioses, and storage diseases. The clinical findings associated with these entities and some relevant diagnostic procedures are summarized in Table 28–12.

Splenomegaly due to any cause may be associated with hypersplenism and the excessive destruction of circulating red cells, white cells, and platelets. The degree of cytopenias is variable and in many instances is mild and requires no specific therapy. In other cases, the thrombocytopenia may cause life-threatening bleeding, particularly when the spleno-megaly is secondary to portal hypertension and associated with esophageal varices or the consequence of a storage disease. In such cases, treatment with surgical splenectomy or with splenic embolization may be warranted.

Kumpe DA et al: Partial splenic embolization in children with hypersplenism. Radiology 1985;155:357.

ASPLENIA & SPLENECTOMY

There is overwhelming evidence that children who lack normal splenic function are at risk for sepsis,

Table 28–12. Causes of chronic splenomegaly in children.

Cause	Associated Clinical Findings	Diagnostic Investigation
Congestive splenomegaly	History of umbilical vein catheter or neonatal omphalitis. Signs of portal hypertension (varices, hemorrhoids, dilated abdominal wall veins); pancytopenia, history of hepatitis or jaundice.	Complete blood count, platelet count, liver function tests, ultrasonography.
Chronic infections	History of exposure to tuberculosis, histoplasmosis, coccidioidomycosis, other fungal disease; chronic sepsis (foreign body in bloodstream; subacute infective endocarditis).	Appropriate cultures and skin tests, ie, blood cultures; PPD, histoplasmin, coccidioidin skin tests; chest film; HIV serology.
Infectious mononucleosis	Fever, fatigue, pharyngitis, rash, adenopathy, hepatomegaly.	Heterophil antibodies.
Leukemia, lymphoma, Hodgkin's disease	Evidence of systemic involvement with fever, bleeding tendencies, hepatomegaly, and lymphadenopathy; pancytopenia.	Blood smear, bone marrow examination, chest film, gallium scan, LDH, uric acid.
Hemolytic anemias	Anemia, jaundice; family history of anemia, jaundice, and gallbladder disease in young adults.	Reticulocyte count, Coombs test, blood smear, osmotic fragility test, hemoglobin electrophoresis.
Reticuloendothelioses (histiocytosis X)	Chronic otitis media, seborrheic or petechial skin rashes, anemia, infections, lymphadenopathy, hepatomegaly, bone lesions.	Skeletal x-rays for bone lesions; biopsy of bone, liver, bone marrow, or lymph node.
Storage diseases	Family history of similar disorders, neurologic involvement, evidence of macular degeneration, hepatomegaly.	Biopsy of rectal mucosa, liver, bone marrow, spleen, or brain in search for storage cells.
Splenic cyst	Evidence of other infections (postinfectious cyst) or congenital anomalies; peculiar shape of spleen.	Radionuclide scan, ultrasonography.
Splenic hemangioma	Other hemangiomas, consumptive coagulopathy.	Radionuclide scan, arteriography, platelet count, coagulation screen.

meningitis, and pneumonia due to encapsulated bacteria such as pneumococci and *Haemophilus influenzae*. Such infections are often fulminant and fatal because of inadequate antibody production and impaired phagocytosis of hematogenous bacteria.

Congenital asplenia is usually suspected in an infant born with abnormalities of abdominal viscera and complex cyanotic congenital heart disease. Howell-Jolly bodies are usually present on the peripheral blood smear, and the absence of splenic tissue is confirmed by technetium radionuclide scanning. The prognosis depends upon the underlying cardiac lesions, and many children die during the first few months. Prophylactic antibiotics, usually penicillin, and pneumococcal vaccine are recommended for those who survive.

The risk of overwhelming sepsis following surgical splenectomy is related to the child's age and to the underlying disorder. The risk is highest when the procedure is performed earlier in life, and for this reason splenectomy is usually postponed until after 5 years, if possible. The risk of postsplenectomy sepsis is also greater in children with malignancies, thalassemias, and reticuloendothelioses than in children whose splenectomy is performed for ITP, hereditary spherocytosis, or trauma.

Children with sickle cell anemia develop functional asplenia during the first year of life, and overwhelming sepsis is the leading cause of early deaths in this disease. Prophylactic penicillin has been shown to reduce the incidence of sepsis in this condition by 84%.

Gaston MH et al: Prophylaxis with oral penicillin in children with sickle cell anemia: A randomized trial. N Eng J Med 1986;314:1593.
Lortan JE: Clinical annotation: Management of asplenic patients. Br J Haematol 1993;84:566.

TRANSFUSION MEDICINE

DONOR SCREENING & BLOOD PROCESSING: RISK MANAGEMENT

Minimizing the risks of transfusion begins with the donor interview. During this process, questions that will protect the recipient from transmission of infectious agents as well as other risks of transfusions are asked of the donor. In addition, information defining high-risk groups whose behavior increases the possible transmission of AIDS, hepatitis, and other diseases is provided, with the request that these individuals not donate blood. After completion of the phlebotomy, the donor is given a final opportunity to

acknowledge previously undisclosed risk factors by confidentially indicating that his or her blood should not be used for transfusion.

Before blood components can be released for transfusion, a number of laboratory tests are completed (see Table 28–13). Assays routinely include screening studies for hepatitis B, hepatitis C, HIV (AIDS), human T cell lymphocytotropic virus (HTLV) I and II, and syphilis as well as surrogate tests for non-A, non-B hepatitis. For special clinical conditions, serologic screening for cytomegalovirus may also be completed to identify seronegative units for transfusion. Positive tests are repeated, and upon their confirmation the unit in question is destroyed and the donor placed in a deferral category. Many of the screening tests utilized are very sensitive and have a high rate of false-positive results. Because of this, confirmatory tests have been developed for a number of the screening assays. These confirm the initial screening results and separate the false positives from the true positives.

With these techniques, the risk of an infectious complication from blood components has been minimized, with the greatest risk being posttransfusion hepatitis (see sections on hepatitis C virus and non-A, non-B hepatitis elsewhere in this book). Because there is no absolute way to completely eliminate the risk of infection from homologous blood, the safest type of blood is obtained from autologous donation. Issues of donor size make the techniques of autologous donation difficult to apply to the pediatric population. Whenever possible, however, autologous donation should be considered.

STORAGE & PRESERVATION OF BLOOD & BLOOD COMPONENTS

The conditions for storage and biologic characteristics for various blood components are summarized in Table 28–13. The conditions provide the optimal environment to maintain appropriate recovery, survival, and function and are different for each blood component. Each unit of blood collected can be fractionated into packed red cells, platelets, and fresh frozen plasma or cryoprecipitate, allowing the most efficient preparation and utilization of blood resources.

As each component has its requirements for storage, special issues arise that are specific to that component. For example, red cells undergo dramatic metabolic changes during their 35-day storage. Included in this process is a dramatic decrease in 2,3-diphosphoglycerate (2,3-DPG) during the second week of storage, a decrease in ATP, and a gradual loss of intracellular potassium into the plasma. Fortunately, these changes are readily reversed within hours to days after the red cells are transfused. However, in certain clinical conditions, these effects may define the type of components used. For example,

Table 28–13. Transmission risks of infectious agents for which screening of blood products is routinely performed.

Disease Entity	Transmission	Screening and Processing Procedures	Approximate Risk of Transmission
Syphilis	Low risk that fresh blood drawn during spirochetemia can transmit infection. Organism not able to survive beyond 72 hours during storage at 4 °C.	Donor history. RPR or VDRL.	<1:100,000
Hepatitis A	Units drawn during prodrome could transmit virus. Because of brief viremia during acute phase, absence of asymptomatic carrier phase, and failure to detect transmission in multiple transfused individuals, infection by this agent is unlikely.	Donor history.	<1:100,000
Hepatitis B	Prolonged viremia during various phases of the disease and asymptomatic carrier state make HBV infection a significant risk of transfusion. Incidence has markedly decreased with screening strategies.	Donor history, education, and self-exclusion. Hepatitis B surface antigen (HBsAg). Surrogate tests for non-A, non-B hepatitis and screen for hepatitis C and retroviruses have helped screen out population at risk for transmitting hepatitis B virus.	1:200,000–1:5000
Hepatitis C	Over two-thirds of cases of non-A, non-B posttransfusion hepatitis may be due to this cause. The agent has characteristics similar to those of HBV which are responsible for the risk from transfusion. Infection may lead to a significant incidence of cirrhosis and end-stage liver disease.	Donor history. Surrogate tests: ALT and hepatitis B core antibody (anti-HBc), anti-HCV.	1:3000
Non-A, non-B hepatitis	Not a specific cause but a classification of agents other than HAV, HBV, HCV, Epstein-Barr virus, and cytomegalovirus, which can cause posttransfusion hepatitis.	Donor history. Surrogate tests: ALT and anti-HBc.	Undefined 1:3000
Human immunodeficiency virus (HIV-1) infection	Cytotoxic retrovirus spread by sexual contact, parenteral (including transfusion) and vertical routes. Resultant destruction of CD4-positive cells results in clinical manifestations of AIDS.	Donor history, education, and self-exclusion. Anti-HIV by EIA, screening test. Western blot confirmatory.	1:500,000–1:50,000
Human T cell lymphotropic virus I and II (HTLV-I and -II) infection	Transforming retroviruses spread by sexual contact, parenteral (including transfusion) and vertical. Over years to decades, infection with HTLV-I may cause lymphoid malignancies or myelopathy.	Donor history. Anti-HTLV-I and -II by enzyme immunoassay screening test. Western blot confirmatory.	<1:10,000–1:5000

blood less than 7–10 days old would be preferred for exchange transfusion or replacement of red cells in individuals with cardiopulmonary disease to ensure adequate oxygen-carrying capacity. However, storage time is not an issue when transfusing individuals with chronic anemia. Under certain conditions, where excessive potassium load is a problem, one has the option of using blood less than 10 days old, making packed cells out of an older unit of whole blood, or washing blood stored as packed cells. No matter what the age of the blood, over 70% of the red cells will circulate after transfusion and approximate a normal survival.

Platelets can be stored at 22 °C for a maximum of 3–5 days. At the extremes of storage, there should be at least a 60% recovery, a survival time that approximates turnover of fresh autologous platelets, and normalization of the bleeding time in proportion to the peak platelet count. Frozen components, red cells, fresh frozen plasma, and cryoprecipitate are outdated at 3 years, 1 year, and 1 year, respectively. Frozen red cells retain the same biochemical and functional characteristics as the day they were frozen. Fresh frozen plasma contains 80% or more of all of the clotting factors of fresh plasma. Factor VIII and fibrinogen are concentrated in cryoprecipitate.

PRETRANSFUSION TESTING

In addition to the screening tests previously noted, ABO and Rh(D) testing and a screen for auto- or alloantibodies are performed routinely on all donated blood. On a sample from the recipient, ABO, Rh(D), and antibody testing are also completed. The crossmatch is required on any component that contains red cells. In the major crossmatch, washed donor red cells are incubated with the serum from the patient, and agglutination is detected and graded. The antiglobulin phase of the test is then performed; Coombs reagent, which will detect the presence of IgG or complement on the surface of the red cells, is added to the mixture, and any possible reaction is evaluated. In the presence of a negative antibody screen in the recipient, a negative immediate spin or antiglobulin phase crossmatch confirms the compatibility of the blood. Further testing is required if the antibody screen or the crossmatch is positive, and blood should not be given until the nature of the reactivity is delineated. Two other tests similar to those described above are important tools for evaluating an incompatible crossmatch. The first is the direct antiglobulin or Coombs test, which detects the presence of IgG or complement on the surfaces of the patient's red cells. The other, the indirect antiglobulin test, evaluates the serum of the patient with respect to its ability to coat the surface of normal red cells with IgG or complement. These tests are the basis for defining the presence of red cell allo- or autoantibodies.

TRANSFUSION PRACTICE

General Rules

Several general rules should be followed in administering any blood component.

(1) In final preparation of the component, no solutions should be added to the bag or tubing set except for normal saline (0.9% sodium chloride for injection, USP), ABO-compatible plasma, or other expanders approved by the blood bank or the primary care physician. Hypotonic solutions will cause hemolysis of red cells and, if transfused, will result in a severe reaction in the recipient.

(2) Transfusion products should be protected from contact with any calcium-containing solution (such as lactated Ringer's); recalcification and reversal of the citrate effect will cause clotting of the blood component.

(3) Care must be taken when warming blood components to not heat the product to a temperature greater than 37 °C. If a component is incubated in a water bath, care should be taken to provide plastic overwraps and avoid contamination of entry ports.

(4) Whenever a blood bag is entered, the sterile integrity of the system is violated, and that unit should be discarded within 4 hours if left at room temperature or 24 hours if the temperature is between 1 and 4 °C.

(5) In general, transfusions of red cell-containing products should not exceed 4 hours. Blood components in excess of what can be infused during this time period should be stored in the blood bank until needed.

(6) Before transfusion, the blood component should be visually inspected for any unusual characteristics—such as the presence of flocculent material, hemolysis, or clumping of cells—and mixed thoroughly.

(7) The unit and the recipient should be properly identified.

(8) The administration set includes a standard 170–260 μm clot filter. Under certain clinical circumstances, an additional microaggregate filter may be used to eliminate small aggregates of fibrin, white cells, and platelets that will not be removed by the standard filter.

(9) The patient should be observed during the entire transfusion, but especially during the first 15 minutes. Any adverse symptoms or signs should be evaluated immediately and reactions to the transfusion reported promptly to the transfusion service.

(10) In the case where incompatible red cells or whole blood must be given to the patient, a test dose of 10% of the total volume (not to exceed 75 mL) should be administered over 15–20 minutes; the transfusion is then stopped and the patient evaluated for reaction. If no adverse effects are noted, the remainder of the volume can be carefully infused.

(11) Blood for exchange transfusion in the newborn period may be crossmatched with either infant's or mother's serum. If the exchange is for hemolysis, 500 mL of whole blood stored for less than 7 days will be adequate. If replacement of clotting factors is a key issue, packed red cells (< 7 days old) reconstituted with fresh frozen plasma may be considered. Based on posttransfusion platelet counts, platelet transfusion may be considered. Additional problems to anticipate include acid-base derangements, hyponatremia, hyperkalemia, hypocalcemia, hypoglycemia, hypothermia, and hyper- or hypovolemia.

Choice of Blood Component

In deciding on the need for blood transfusion, several principles should be considered. Indications for blood or blood components must be well defined, and the patient's medical condition and not just the laboratory numbers should be the basis for the decision. Specific deficiencies exhibited by the patient (eg, oxygen-carrying capacity, thrombocytopenia) should be treated with appropriate blood components and the use of whole blood minimized. Information about specific blood components is summarized in Table 28–14.

A. Whole Blood: Whole blood may be used in patients who require replacement of oxygen-carrying

Table 28–14. Characteristic of blood and blood components.

Component	Storage Conditions	Composition and Transfusion Characteristics	Indications	Risks and Precautions	Administration
Whole blood	4 °C for 35 days. RBC characteristics: • **Survival:** Recovery decreases during storage but is always > 70%. Cells that circulate approximate normal survival. • **Function:** 2,3-DPG levels fall to undetectable after second week of storage. This defect repaired within 24 hours of transfusion. • **Electrolytes:** With storage, potassium increases in plasma. This rises to high levels after 2 weeks of storage.	Contains RBCs and many plasma compounds of whole blood. Leukocytes and platelets lose activity or viability after a few days under these conditions. Procoagulant clotting factors (particularly VIII and V) deteriorate rapidly during storage. Each unit has about 500 mL volume and Hct 36–40%.	Oxygen-carrying capacity (anemia). Volume replacement (> 15–20%) for blood loss or severe shock.	Must be ABO-identical and crossmatch-compatible. Infectious diseases (see Table 28–12). Febrile or hemolytic transfusion reactions. Allo-immunization to RBC, WBC, or platelet antigens.	During acute blood loss, as rapidly as tolerated. In other settings, 2–4 hours. 10 mL/kg will raise Hct by 5% and support volume.
Packed red cells	Same as for whole blood.	Contains RBCs; plasma removed in preparation. Status of leukocytes, clotting factors, and platelets same as for whole blood. Hct about 70%, volume 200–250 mL. May request tighter pack to give Hct 80–90%.	Oxygen-carrying capacity. Acute trauma or bleeding, or situations requiring intensive cardiopulmonary support (Hct < 25–30%). Chronic anemia (Hct < 20%).	Same as for whole blood.	May be given as patient will tolerate based on cardiovascular status over 2–4 hours. Dose of 3 mL packed RBC/kg will raise the Hct by 3%. If cardiovascular status stable, give 10 mL/kg over 2–4 hours. If unstable, use smaller volume or do packed RBC exchange.
Washed or filtered red cells	When cells are washed, there is a 24-hour outdate. Up to that time, they have the same characteristics as packed red cells.	Same as packed red cells.	Same as packed red cells. Depending on technique used and extent of reduction of white blood cells, washed red cells may achieve the following: • Avoid febrile reactions. • Decreased the transmission of CMV. • Decreased the incidence of allo-immunization to white cell antigens.	Same as whole blood. Removal of white cells diminishes the risk of febrile reactions. Filtration with white cell filters may decrease rate of allo-immunization to white cell antigens and transmission of CMV.	Same as packed red cells.
Frozen red cells	Packed red cells frozen in 40% glycerol solution at under –65 °C. Can be stored 3 years. Retain the same biochemical characteristics, function, and capacity for survival as the day in storage they were frozen; when thawed, 24-hour outdate.	Same as packed red cells.	Same as packed red cells. Useful for avoiding febrile reactions, decreasing transmission of CMV, autologous blood donation, and developing an inventory of rare red cell blood groups.	Same as for whole blood. Risk of CMV transmission is less.	Same as packed red cells.

(continued)

Table 28–14. Characteristic of blood and blood components. (*continued*)

Fresh frozen plasma	Plasma from whole blood stored at under −18 °C for up to 1 year.	Contains > 80% of all procoagulant and anticoagulant plasma proteins.	Replacement of plasma procoagulant and anticoagulant plasma proteins. May provide "other" factors, eg, treatment of TTP.	Need not be crossmatched; should be type-compatible. Volume overload, infectious diseases, allergic reactions.	As rapidly as tolerated by patient but not > 4 hours. Dose: 10–15 mL/kg will increase level of all clotting factors by 10–20%.
Cryoprecipitate	Produced by freezing fresh plasma to under −65 °C, then allowing to thaw 18 hours at 4 °C. After centrifugation, cryoprecipitable proteins are separated. May be stored at −18 °C for up to 1 year.	Contains factor VIII, fibrinogen, and fibronectin at concentrations greater than those of plasma. Also contains factor XIII. VIII > 80 IU/pack, fibrinogen 100–350 mg/pack.	Treatment of acquired or congenital deficiencies of VIII, von Willebrand factor, and fibrinogen. Useful in making biologic glues that contain fibrinogen.	Same as for fresh frozen plasma. ABO agglutinogens may also be concentrated and can give positive direct agglutination test if not type-specific.	Cryoprecipitate can be given as a rapid infusion. Dose: ½ pack per kg body weight will increase factor VIII level by 80–100% and fibrinogen by 200–250 mg/dL.
Platelet concentrates (random donor units)	Separated from platelet-rich plasma and stored with gentle agitation at 22 °C for 3–5 days. Containers currently in use are plastic and allow for gas exchange, diffusion of CO_2 helps keep pH > 6.00, a major factor in keeping platelets viable and functional.	Each unit contains about 5 × 10^{10} platelets. Survival: Although there may be some loss with storage, 60–70% recovery should be achieved, with stored platelets correcting the bleeding time in proportion to the peak counts reached.	Treatment of thrombocytopenia or platelet function defects.	No crossmatch necessary. Should be type-specific. Other risks as for whole blood.	Can be given as rapid transfusion or as defined by cardiovascular status, not more than 4 hours. Dose: 10 mL/kg should increase platelet count by at least 50,000/μL.
Platelet concentrates by aphersis techniques	Same as random donor units.	Platelet content is equivalent to 6–10 units of random donor concentrates. Depending on technique used, these may be relatively free of leukocytes, a product useful in avoiding alloimmunization.	As above, particularly useful in treating patients who have insufficient production in whom alloisoimmunization is a potential problem.	Same as above.	As above.
Granulocytes	Although they may be stored stationary at 20–24 °C, transfuse as soon as possible after collection.	Contains at least 1 × 10^{10} granulocytes but also platelets and red cells.	Severely neutropenic individuals (< 500/μL) with poor marrow reserves and suspected bacterial or fungal infections not responding to 48–72 hours of parenteral antibiotics. Also in patients with neutrophil dysfunction.	Same as for platelets. Pulmonary leukostasis reactions. Severe febrile reactions.	Given in an infusion over 2–4 hours. Dose: 1 unit daily for newborns and infants, 1 × 10^9 granulocytes per kg.

capacity and volume. In particular, it may be considered when more than 15% of blood volume is lost. Doses will vary depending on volume considerations (see Table 28–14). In acute situations, the transfusion may be completed rapidly to support blood volume.

B. Packed Red Cells: Packed red cells (which include leukocyte-poor, filtered, or frozen deglycerolized products) prepared from whole blood by centrifugal techniques are the appropriate choice for almost all patients with deficient oxygen-carrying capacity. Exact indications will be defined by the clinical setting, the severity of the anemia, the acuity of the condition, and any other factors affecting oxygen transport.

C. Platelets: The decision to transfuse platelets depends upon the clinical condition of the patient, the status of plasma phase coagulation, the platelet count, the cause of the thrombocytopenia, and the functional ability of the patient's own platelets. With platelet counts less than 10,000–20,000/µL, the risk of severe, spontaneous bleeding is markedly increased, and—in the absence of antibody-mediated disease—transfusion should be considered. Under certain circumstances, especially with platelet dysfunction or

Table 28–15. Noninfectious complications of transfusions.

Event	Pathophysiology	Signs and Symptoms	Management
Acute hemolytic transfusion reaction	Preformed alloantibodies (most commonly to ABO) and occasionally autoantibodies cause rapid intravascular hemolysis of transfused cells with activation of clotting (DIC), activation of inflammatory mediators, and acute renal failure.	Fever, chills, nausea, chest pain, back pain, pain at transfusion site, hypotension, dyspnea, oliguria, dark urine.	The risk of this type of reaction overall is low (1:30,000), but the mortality rate is high (up to 40%). **Treatment:** Stop the transfusion; maintain renal output with intravenous fluids and diuretics (furosemide or mannitol); treat DIC with heparin; and institute other appropriate supportive measures.
Delayed hemolytic transfusion reaction	Formation of alloantibodies after transfusion and resultant destruction of transfused red cells, usually by extravascular hemolysis.	Fever, jaundice, anemia.	Detection, definition, and documentation (for future transfusions). Supportive care. Risk, 1:2500.
Bacterial contamination	Contamination of units results in growth of bacteria or production of clinically significant levels of endotoxin.	Chills, high fever, hypotension, other symptoms of sepsis or endotoxemia.	Stop transfusion; aggressive attempts to identify organism; vigorous supportive medical care.
Graft-versus-host disease	Lymphocytes from donor transfused in an immunoincompetent host.	Syndrome can present with a variety of organs involved, usually skin, liver, and bone marrow.	Preventive management: Irradiation (> 1500 cGy) of cellular blood components transfused to individuals with congenital or acquired immunodeficiency syndromes, intrauterine transfusion, severely premature infants, and when donors are first-degree relatives of the recipient.
Febrile reactions	Usually caused by leukoagglutinins in recipient.	Fever. May also have chills.	Supportive. Consider leukocyte-poor products for future. Risk, 1:200.
Allergic reactions	Most causes not identified. In IgA-deficient individuals, reaction occurs as a result of antibodies to IgA.	Itching, hives, occasionally chills and fever. In severe reactions, may see signs of anaphylaxis: dyspnea, pulmonary edema.	Mild to moderate reactions: diphenhydramine. More severe reactions: epinephrine SC and steroids IV. Risk for mild to moderate allergic reactions, 1:1000; severe anaphylactic reactions, 1:150,000.
Iron overload	There is no physiologic mechanism to excrete excess iron. Target organs include liver, heart, and endocrine organs. In patients receiving red cell transfusions over long periods of time, there is an increase in iron burden.	Signs and symptoms of dysfunctional organs affected by the iron.	Chronic administration of iron chelator such as deferoxamine.
Dilutional coagulopathy	Massive blood loss and transfusion with replacement with fluids or blood components and deficient clotting factors.	Bleeding.	Replacement of clotting factors or platelets with appropriate blood components.

treatment that inhibits the procoagulant system, transfusions at higher platelet counts may be necessary.

Transfused platelets are temporarily sequestered in the lungs and spleen before reaching their peak concentrations, 45–60 minutes after transfusion. A significant proportion of the transfused platelets never circulate but remain sequestered in the spleen. This phenomenon results in reduced recovery studies in which only 60–70% of the transfused platelets are counted when peripheral platelet count increments are used as a measure of response.

In addition to cessation of bleeding, two variables indicate the effectiveness of platelet transfusions. The first is platelet recovery, the measure of the maximum number of platelets circulating in response to transfusion. The practical measure is the platelet count at 1 hour after transfusion. In the absence of immune or nonimmune factors that markedly decrease platelet recovery, one would expect a 7000/μL increment for each random donor unit and a 40,000–70,000/μL increment for each single-donor apheresis unit in a large child or adolescent. For infants and small children, 10 mL/kg will increase the platelet count by at least 50,000/μL. The second variable is the survival of transfused platelets. Normally, transfused platelets have a half-life of 3–5 days. In the presence of immune or nonimmune destruction, the life span may be shortened to a few days or to a few hours. Frequent platelet transfusions may be required to maintain adequate hemostasis.

A particularly troublesome outcome in patients receiving long-term platelet transfusions is the development of a refractory state characterized by poor (< 30%) recovery or no response to platelet transfusion (as measured at 1 hour). Most (70–90%) of these refractory states result from the development of alloantibodies directed against HLA antigens on the platelet. A smaller proportion of these alloantibodies (10–30%) are directed against platelet-specific alloantigens. The most effective approach for the alloimmunized patient has been the provision of platelet transfusions from HLA-matched platelet donors. Recent reports have suggested that platelet crossmatching procedures using HLA-matched and unmatched donors may be helpful in quickly identifying platelet concentrates with the highest probability of resulting in a successful transfusion.

D. Fresh Frozen Plasma (FFP): The indication for fresh frozen plasma is the replacement of plasma coagulation factors in clinical situations where a deficiency of one or more clotting factors exists and there are associated bleeding manifestations. In some hereditary factor deficiencies such as factor VIII deficiency, commercially prepared concentrates contain these factors in higher concentrations and, because of specific preparation procedures, impose less infectious risk and are more appropriate than plasma.

E. Cryoprecipitate: This component may be used for acquired or congenital disorders of factor VIII activity, von Willebrand's disease, or hypo- or afibrinogenemia. The dose given will depend on the protein to be replaced. For example, one-half bag (one-half unit) of cryoprecipitate (40–50 units of factor VIII activity) for every kilogram of body weight will result in an approximately 80–100% increase in factor VIII activity. Cryoprecipitate can be given in a rapid transfusion over 30–60 minutes.

F. Granulocytes: With better supportive care over the past 10 years, the need for granulocytes in neutropenic patients with severe bacterial infections has decreased. Indications still remain for severe bacterial infections unresponsive to vigorous medical therapy in either newborns or older children with the presence of bone marrow failure.

Adverse Effects

The noninfectious complications of blood transfusions are outlined in Table 28–15. Most present a small but still significant risk to the recipient.

National Institutes of Health Consensus Conference: Fresh frozen plasma: Indications and risks. JAMA 1985;253: 551.

National Institutes of Health Consensus Conference: Platelet transfusion therapy. JAMA 1987;257:1777.

Rossi EC, Simon TL, Moss GS (editors): *Principles of Transfusion Medicine.* Williams & Wilkins, 1991.

Walker RH (editor): *Technical Manual of the American Association of Blood Banks.* American Association of Blood Banks, 1990.

Walker RH: Special report: Transfusion risks. Am J Clin Path 1987;88:374.

REFERENCES

Bunn HF, Forget BG: *Hemoglobin: Molecular, Genetic and Clinical Aspects.* Saunders, 1986.

Corrigan JJ Jr: *Hemorrhagic and Thrombotic Diseases in Childhood and Adolescence.* Churchill Livingstone, 1985.

Hathaway WE, Bonnar J: *Hemostatic Disorders of the Pregnant Woman and Newborn Infant.* Elsevier, 1987.

Hathaway WE, Goodnight SH: *Disorders of Hemostasis and Thrombosis: A Clinical Guide.* McGraw-Hill, 1993.

Mentzer WC, Wagner GM: *The Hereditary Hemolytic Anemias.* Churchill Livingstone, 1989.

Miller DR, Baehner RL: *Blood Diseases of Infancy and Childhood,* 6th ed. Mosby, 1989.

Nathan DG, Oski FA: *Hematology of Infancy and Childhood,* 4th ed. Saunders, 1993.

Oski FA (editor): Pediatric hematology. Hematol Oncol Clin North Am 1987;1:355.

Oski FA, Naiman JL: *Hematologic Problems in the Newborn,* 3rd ed. Saunders, 1982.

Petz LD, Garratty G: *Acquired Immune Hemolytic Anemias.* Churchill Livingstone, 1980.

Rossi EC, Simon TL, Moss GS: *Principles of Transfusion Medicine.* Williams & Wilkins, 1991.

Serjeant GR: *Sickle Cell Disease.* 2nd ed. Oxford Univ Press, 1993.

Stamatoyannopoulos G et al: *The Molecular Basis of Blood Diseases.* Saunders, 1987.

29

Immunodeficiency

Erwin W. Gelfand, MD, & Anthony R. Hayward, MD, PhD

Recurrent or severe infection is the commonest symptom of immunodeficiency, but most children with recurrent minor infections do not have an immunodeficiency that is definable by currently available tests. Protection from infection depends mainly on the exclusion of pathogens by intact surfaces, followed by decontamination of surfaces by mechanical and other nonspecific means. It is only after an organism gains access to the body that specific and nonspecific immune mechanisms are used to achieve its elimination. Specific immunity in this context consists of antibody and cell-mediated immunity (CMI). Nonspecific immune mechanisms include mechanical barriers, complement, phagocytes, and natural killer cells. Nonspecific mechanisms may be endowed with specificity by specific responses, such as the ability of antibody to direct killing by natural killer cells or to promote phagocytosis by opsonizing bacteria.

Before investigating a patient for a defined primary immunodeficiency (most of which are uncommon), one should exclude the commoner factors that increase local susceptibility to infection, such as cystic fibrosis and conditions that interfere with the integrity of the skin or the normal flora of mucous membranes (Table 29–1). Common causes of secondary immunodeficiency (HIV infection, drugs, protein loss) must also be excluded.

NONSPECIFIC FACTORS IN RESISTANCE TO INFECTION

DEFECTS OF COMPLEMENT

The complement series of proteins are activated by IgG or IgM antibody bound to surfaces. The split products of C3 and C5 activation attract neutrophils, and C3b bound to the surface of bacteria opsonizes for phagocytosis by neutrophils. Deficiencies of individual classic pathway factors (C1–C9) occur as au-

tosomal recessive traits and are rare. The commonest clinical association is with immune complex disorders, particularly systemic lupus erythematosus, chronic glomerulonephritis, dermatomyositis, and cutaneous vasculitis. Primary deficiency of C3 interferes with the opsonization of bacteria by the classic and alternative pathways of complement activation and results in recurrent bacterial infections similar to those seen in antibody deficiency. Treatment is mostly with antibiotics. Serum levels of C3 are occasionally low enough in membranoproliferative glomerulonephritis with nephritic factor to increase susceptibility to infection. Deficiency of two of the alternative pathway factors may also occasionally predispose to recurrent bacterial infection.

C5, C6, C7, C8, and C9 deficiencies are associated with dissemination of neisserial infections, resulting in an increased frequency of gonococcal arthritis in those with gonorrhea and recurrence of meningitis in the survivors of meningococcal meningitis. Complement function should be screened with a hemolytic assay in patients with recurrent meningitis.

The serum "opsonizing defect" associated with Leiner's disease and originally attributed to C5a deficiency has now been identified as a defect in the gene coding for "mannan-binding protein." The main clinical association is recurrent infections in infancy.

Recurrent angioedema without itching or wheals, usually beginning in late childhood, should lead one to suspect **hereditary angioedema.** This is a rare disorder resulting from C1 esterase inhibitor deficiency in which susceptibility to infection is not increased and attacks may not start until adolescence. Transmission is autosomal dominant. Affected individuals typically have recurrent episodes of edema lasting 48–72 hours affecting the face or a limb. Edema affecting the bowel can be very painful. Laryngeal edema is life-threatening. Diagnosis is by measurement of esterase inhibitor levels in serum; symptomatic individuals have levels below 30%. C4 levels are often low. Danazol, a synthetic androgen, prevents attacks by increasing C1 inhibitor levels. The diagnosis is suggested by decreased activity of whole complement, C4, and C2 and confirmed by direct assay of the C1 inhibitor.

Table 29–1. Host defense mechanisms and examples of nonspecific defects.

Protection by–	Example of Defect
Intact skin	Burns, eczema, sinus tracks, indwelling catheters
Drainage	Auditory tube obstruction, cystic fibrosis, foreign body, urinary obstruction
Normal flora	Antibiotic-induced diarrhea, postantibiotic candidiasis

Sumiya M et al: Molecular basis of opsonic defect in immunodeficient children. Lancet 1991;337:1569.

Wurzner R, Orren A, Lachmann PJ: Inherited deficiencies of the terminal components of human complement. Immunodefic Rev 1992;3:123.

Densen P: Complement deficiencies and meningococcal disease. Clin Exp Immunol 1991;86(Suppl 1):57.

DEFECTS OF PHAGOCYTE FUNCTION

1. CHEMOTAXIS DEFECTS

Useful phagocyte function requires the production of adequate numbers of neutrophils by the bone marrow and migration of these cells to sites of inflammation, followed by the ingestion and killing of bacteria. Defects may exist at one or more of these levels. Neutropenia is described in the section on hematology. Defects of chemotaxis may be due to abnormalities of the cell, either intrinsic or secondary; to a deficiency of complement-derived chemotactic factors; or to increased activity of cell-directed or chemotactic factor-directed inhibitors. Examples of primary cellular abnormalities are Chédiak-Higashi syndrome (see Chapter 28) and LFA-1 deficiency. Burns; infections such as HIV, rubella, and influenza; metabolic and nutritional disorders, including diabetes mellitus; the hypophosphatemia associated with hyperalimentation; uremia; and a wide variety of other conditions can be associated with depressed motility of phagocytic cells. The association of **impaired neutrophil chemotaxis with hyperimmunoglobulinemia E** (levels are usually > 2000 units IgE/mL), recurrent staphylococcal abscesses of the skin, eczema, and otitis media is clinically recognizable and sometimes described as Job's syndrome. The occurrence seems to be sporadic, and no cause is known. Treatment is symptomatic.

Other infections that occur in patients with chemotactic defects include furunculosis, subcutaneous abscesses, oral ulcers, gingivitis, and pneumonia. The pathogenesis of these associations is obscure. Familial chemotactic defects are reported. but these are the exception.

White CJ, Gallin JI: Phagocyte defects. Clin Immunol Immunopathol 1986;40:50.

van der Valk P, Herman CJ: Leukocyte functions. Lab Invest 1987;56:127.

2. BACTERIAL KILLING DEFECTS

Chronic granulomatous disease illustrates defects of bacterial killing by neutrophils. Patients have recurrent infections of skin with catalase-positive organism (mostly staphylococci, sometimes *Serratia, Nocardia,* or other opportunists), leading to abscesses in the draining lymph nodes. The patient's neutrophils fail to reduce nitroblue tetrazolium in the NBT test and fail to kill staphylococci in a bacterial killing test. X-linked recessive chronic granulomatous disease results from coding abnormalities of the gp91 membrane cytochrome b. Most autosomal recessive chronic granulomatous disease is due to abnormalities of the p47 or p67 proteins, which are functionally related to the cytochrome for electron transport.

Patients usually have staphylococcal infections in the first months of life and develop groin, cervical, or axillary abscesses requiring incision and drainage. The infections cause high neutrophil counts and fever and sometimes spread to cause osteomyelitis or liver abscess. Colitis, leading to diarrhea and slow growth, is common. The abscesses require drainage and appropriate antibiotics for lengthy courses (3 weeks or more). All forms of the disease appear to benefit from gamma interferon in doses of 0.1 mg/m$_2$ on 2 or more days per week. This does not correct the underlying defect. Long-term antibiotic treatment—either with trimethoprim-sulfamethoxazole or dicloxacillin—may be required, and good dental care is necessary because of the increased risk of gingivitis and periodontitis. Bacterial infections can usually be controlled by antibiotics. It is invasive fungal infections of lung and bone, especially by *Aspergillus,* that are most often fatal. Bone marrow transplantation has not been very successful because of difficulty in obtaining long-term engraftment of donor neutrophils. Patients with chronic granulomatous disease seem to have fewer abscesses as they grow older, so that the outlook for a working life is good for those who pass puberty.

Defective bacterial killing by neutrophils also results from deficiency of leukocyte glucose-6-phosphate dehydrogenase, glutathione dehydrogenase, and other metabolic defects. The severity is variable. A bacterial killing test should be used to screen for these abnormalities, since the NBT test is not always abnormal.

Baehner RL: Chronic granulomatous disease of childhood: Clinical, pathological, biochemical, molecular, and genetic aspects of the disease. Pediatr Pathol 1990;10;143.

Smith RM, Curnutte JT: Molecular basis of chronic granulomatous disease. Blood 1991 77;673.

3. LEUKOCYTE ADHESION DEFICIENCY

Leukocytes, monocytes, and some activated T cells normally express cell surface adhesion molecules that have a common beta subunit and cell-specific but related alpha subunits. Defects or deficiency of the beta subunit (encoded on chromosome 21 and called CD18) results in defective expression of this entire family of proteins: LFA-1 (CD11a), Mac-1 (CD11b), and p150,95 (CD11c).

The severity of the clinical presentation ranges from progressive, necrotic periumbilical infections with onset in infancy to recurrent surface infections starting in adult life, depending on the underlying defect. A range of organisms is isolated. The neutrophil count is high, but there is relatively little pus formation. In childhood, the infections are often around body orifices, but they also involve the skin, esophagus, and respiratory tract. Death in childhood is common. Other patients with a milder phenotype have survived for 20 or more years. Diagnosis is by phenotyping blood mononuclear cells for LFA-1 or Mac-1; this approach can also be used for antenatal diagnosis.

Treatment of infections is with antibiotics, and prophylactic antibiotics may suffice for the more mildly affected patients. Mixed but stable chimerism, sufficient to reduce the risk of infections, has followed bone marrow transplantation.

Harlan JM: Leukocyte adhesion deficiency syndrome: Insights into the molecular basis of leukocyte emigration. Clin Immunol Immunopathol 1993;67(3 Part 2):S16.

Wardlaw AJ et al: Distinct mutations in two patients with leukocyte adhesion deficiency and their functional correlates. J Exp Med 1990;172;335.

DEFICIENCIES OF SPECIFIC IMMUNITY

Defects of specific immunity are broadly subdivided into those affecting predominantly antibody formation, those affecting cellular immunity, and those in which both mechanisms are impaired. The classification in Table 29–2 is based on combinations of clinical and laboratory results and includes only the commoner conditions. Family studies in which a mode of inheritance can be shown are the most secure basis for classification, and in a few instances the underlying single gene defect is known, as in adenosine deaminase and purine nucleoside phosphorylase deficiencies. Occasionally, as in ataxia-telangiectasia, the phenotypic features are sufficiently characteristic to facilitate recognition. The fact that most cases of im-

Table 29–2. Classification of defects of specific immunity.

Deficiency of immunoglobulin	Deficiency of all Ig's = hypogamma-globulinemia Congenital (sometimes with high IgM) Acquired Unclassified (common variable hypogammaglobulinemia) Selective immunoglobulin deficiency IgA deficiency IgG subclass deficiencies IgM deficiency Antibody deficiency with immunoglobulins
Deficiency of cell-mediated immunity	Purine nucleoside phosphorylase DiGeorge syndrome Cartilage-hair hypoplasia Unclassified (common variable immunodeficiency affecting cell-mediated immunity)
Deficiency of both antibody and cell-mediated immunity	Severe combined immunodeficiency (various types) Ataxia-telangiectasia Wiskott-Aldrich syndrome

munodeficiency are still reported as "varied immunodeficiency, largely unclassified" indicates that major advances remain to be made.

Primary immunodeficiency diseases. Report of a WHO scientific group. Immunodefic Rev 1992;3:195.

IMMUNOGLOBULIN & ANTIBODY DEFICIENCY SYNDROME

1. HYPOGAMMAGLOBULINEMIA SYNDROMES

Congenital X-linked agammaglobulinemia occurs in about $1:10^5$ live births. Other types of hypogammaglobulinemia are a little commoner and may develop at any age. It is helpful to distinguish between the congenital X-linked and other forms of hypogammaglobulinemia for the sake of genetic counseling: The diagnosis, treatment, and complications are similar regardless of the type of antibody deficiency. The different types are summarized in Table 28–2. Diagnosis is based on low serum immunoglobulin levels for age with absence of serum isohemagglutinins and of antibody response to immunization. Causes of secondary hypogammaglobulinemia (nephrotic syndrome, HIV infection, and protein-losing enteropathy) should be excluded by measuring serum albumin.

Congenital X-Linked Agammaglobulinemia

The commonest symptoms arise from bacterial infection of the respiratory tract (sinusitis, otitis, pneumonia) or skin (cellulitis, abscesses), which, without antibiotic treatment, spread to cause septicemia and meningitis. Infections usually start after 4 months of age, when passively acquired maternal IgG levels have declined. The organisms responsible for the presenting infections are mostly encapsulated bacteria. Following courses of antibiotics, *Mycoplasma* strains such as *Ureaplasma* become important. A few boys have an asymmetric arthritis, mostly of the knee or ankle, at the time of diagnosis, which may resolve after adequate IgG replacement. There are no useful physical signs other than a paucity of tonsil and adenoid tissue. The severity of infections varies, so the diagnosis may not be made for many years.

These patients have an abnormal B progenitor tyrosine kinase and have few if any B cells in their blood, though they have normal blood counts and normal numbers of pre-B cells in their marrow. Carrier detection is available.

Thomas JD, Sideras P, Smith CIE: Co-localization of X-linked agammaglobulinemia and X linked immunodeficiency genes. Science 1993;261:355.

Immunodeficiency With High IgM Levels

This condition affects predominantly boys, who differ from those described above by having normal or high serum IgM levels, often with lymphadenopathy. The IgM does not have useful antibody activity, so the treatment is as for hypogammaglobulinemia. Impaired cell-mediated immunity with *Pneumocystis* infections, lymphomas, and neutropenia occur as complications. The disease results from abnormal expression of a T cell ligand for B cell help (the CD40 ligand, gp39).

Aruffo A, Farrington M, Hollenbaugh D: The CD40 ligand, gp39, is defective in activated T cells from patients with X-linked hyper-IgM syndrome. Cell 1993;72:291.

Common Variable Immunodeficiency Syndromes

Patients with congenital or acquired antibody deficiency syndromes not classified elsewhere are often included in this group, and they outnumber patients with all other types of antibody deficiency except selective IgA deficiency. Onset of the immunodeficiency may be at any age. Susceptibility to common variable immunodeficiency is inherited, linked with the same class III histocompatibility gene deletions (for C4 and 21-hydroxylase, on chromosome 6) as selective IgA deficiency, but the factors that precipitate expression of common variable immunodeficiency in susceptible individuals are not known. The circulating B cells of these patients are immature and do not generally differentiate normally in tissue culture, but the pathogenesis of these disorders is not understood.

Infections follow the patterns described for other types of antibody deficiency. Some patients have remarkably few infections despite long-standing, very low immunoglobulin levels. The laboratory findings are variable: Low levels of one or more immunoglobulin classes are associated with varying degrees of impairment of T cell proliferative responses. Autoantibody formation, raised IgE levels, and positive immediate hypersensitivity skin reactions occur. Almost all these patients have B cells in their blood, though their number may be low. Neutropenia and thrombocytopenia both occur in this syndrome. These varied syndromes are too heterogeneous for confident prognosis.

Jaffe JS et al: T-cell abnormalities in common variable immunodeficiency. Pediatr Res 1993;33(1 Suppl):S24. (See discussion on p S27.)

Sneller MC et al: NIH conference. New insights into common variable immunodeficiency. Ann Intern Med 1993; 118:720.

Shaffer FM et al: Individuals with IgA deficiency and common variable immunodeficiency share polymorphisms of major histocompatibility class III genes. Proc Natl Acad Sci USA 1989;86:8015.

Complications of Hypogammaglobulinemia

Many patients have B cell hyperplasia in the gut. About 10% of patients develop diarrhea and malabsorption that may be severe enough to resemble Crohn's disease. Infection is the likeliest cause of the diarrhea, and efforts should be made to exclude treatable agents such as *Giardia lamblia* or *Cryptosporidium*. In adult life, the patients often develop gastric atrophy with achlorhydria, sometimes followed by pernicious anemia. Affected boys occasionally develop optic atrophy or ataxia, evolving slowly or rapidly into fatal encephalitis. Echoviruses have sometimes been isolated from their cerebrospinal fluid or brains at biopsy or necropsy. A smaller proportion develop a dermatomyositis-like syndrome, with prominent peripheral cyanosis and myopathy but little heliotrope coloration. There is an impression that both of these complications are less commonly seen now that much higher immunoglobulin replacements are given. There are reports of an increased rate of cancer in patients with antibody deficiency. The association is predominantly with lymphoreticular proliferation and may sometimes result from EBV infection. Lymphoreticular proliferations in hypogammaglobulinemic patients are not always malignant.

Spickett GP, Misbah SA, Chapel HM: Primary antibody deficiency in adults. Lancet 1991;337:281.

Treatment

Patients with hypogammaglobulinemia should have serum IgG replaced to protect against infection. IgG is usually given by intravenous infusions of specially prepared deaggregated IgG (200–600 mg/kg every 4 weeks). If intravenous treatment is very difficult in young children, they may be temporarily managed on intramuscular injections of IgG concentrate (0.6 mL/kg every 2–3 weeks). The aim of treatment must be to avoid—or minimize progression of—chronic lung disease (bronchitis, bronchiectasis). Productive cough and purulent sputum or conjunctivitis must be taken seriously and antibiotics given until there has been radiologic and clinical resolution. *Mycoplasma* infections of the respiratory or urinary tract should be sought for and treated with doxycycline or other appropriate antibiotics.

Reactions to immunoglobulin infusions or injections are relatively common, especially with the initial infusion. They include headache, back and limb pain, anxiety, and tightness of the chest. Signs are tachycardia, shivering, fever, and, in severe cases, shock. Reactions are frequent in some patients and rare in others; their occurrence is sporadic and not generally due to hypersensitivity (anti-IgA reactions may be an exception). Skin tests are not helpful. When indicated, immunoglobulin replacement should be maintained for life and the severity of the reactions limited by premedication with acetaminophen, an antihistamine, or intravenous hydrocortisone immediately before the infusion. Alternative brands of IgG should be tried if reactions persist despite premedication.

2. OTHER TYPES OF HYPOGAMMAGLOBULINEMIA

Transient Hypogammaglobulinemia

Infants' IgG levels fall during the first 4–5 months of life while maternal IgG is diluted and catabolized. The physiologic trough that occurs before the infant's IgG production maintains adult levels is accentuated in premature and dysmature infants. IgG levels of 250–300 mg/dL lie within 2 SD of the mean at 3–4 months of age, and the diagnosis of transient hypogammaglobulinemia is often made in infants with infections and IgG levels in this range. Immunoglobulin levels should return to normal by 30 months of age, and the diagnosis can only be made retrospectively. The only diagnostic laboratory findings are of low IgG, with or without low IgA and IgM, and subsequent return to normal levels. Salivary IgA is generally detectable, and, despite the low immunoglobulin levels, antibody activity (isohemagglutinin or antidiphtheria or tetanus antibody) is present in serum. IgG antibody is generally made following immunization, and tests for cellular immunity are normal. No treatment is usually required for infants who make antibody following immunization other than appropriate antibiotics for bacterial infections. Infants with severe infection and hypogammaglobulinemia could rationally be given IgG injections, since maternal antibody to the infecting organism will be rapidly depleted, but this is rarely necessary. The prognosis for affected infants is (by definition)

excellent provided they do not succumb to infection before normal immunity is achieved.

Selective Immunoglobulin Deficiencies

A. IgA Deficiency: With a prevalence of 1:500 in Caucasian populations, this is by far the commonest defect of specific immunity. Susceptibility is linked to class III histocompatibility genes, but the factors determining expression of the deficiency are unknown. The histocompatibility gene association may mean that the failure of differentiation of IgA B lymphocytes which results in the failure of IgA production may be due to autoimmunity. Fifty percent or more of IgA-deficient subjects have no symptoms arising from the deficiency, perhaps because these individuals can protect their mucosa adequately with IgG and IgM antibodies. Failure of antibody responses in the IgG2 subclass is reported in many symptomatic patients. When symptoms are present, they are predominantly upper respiratory tract infections or to diarrhea. There are also strong associations with inflammatory bowel disease, allergy (mainly respiratory and gut), and autoimmune disorders (thyroiditis, arthritis, vitiligo, thrombocytopenia, and diabetes).

Arbitrary criteria for diagnosis are serum IgA less than 5 mg/dL, absent salivary IgA, normal IgM and IgG, and normal cellular immunity. The selective lack of IgA antibody responses and the presence of normal antibody responses in other immunoglobulin classes serve to distinguish IgA deficiency from unclassified variable immunodeficiency. IgA has a short half-life in serum, and replacement is impractical. It is conceivable but unproved that colostrum feeding could modify severe gut symptoms. Symptomatic IgA-deficient subjects who are also IgG2-deficient have sometimes been treated with IgG replacement. This approach has been both advocated and condemned on theoretical grounds but without controlled data. One concern is that immunization to IgA might lead to the production of anti-IgA antibodies. These are found in a subset of IgA-deficient patients and are an important cause of transfusion reactions. Most IgA-deficient patients manage reasonably well with antibiotics only; atopic or autoimmune symptoms should be treated conventionally.

B. Other Selective Subclass Deficiencies: The diagnosis of Immunoglobulin subclass deficiencies is controversial partly because measurement of subclass levels is not always reliable and there are also age- and drug-related variables. The IgG heavy chain genes are on chromosome 11, grouped with IgG1 close to IgG3 and IgG2 close to IgG4. Normally, IgG1 comprises over 60% of total IgG and IgG2 over 10%. IgG3 accounts for about 5%, and IgG4 may be undetectable in up to 20% of healthy individuals. When IgG1 is deficient, IgG2 and IgG3 are generally low also, giving the clinical picture of hypogammaglobulinemia. IgG1 and IgG2 contain much of the antibody to capsular polysaccharides. IgG2 (and IgG4) deficiency has been associated with IgA deficiency. IgG3 deficiency is less common but has been incriminated in subjects with antibody deficiency syndromes with normal total IgG or IgG1 subclass levels. The prevalence of IgG subclass deficiencies remains to be established, as does a link with upper respiratory tract infections and asthma. IgG replacement should be reserved for patients with defects of antibody production; many patients are managed with antibiotics alone.

Selective deficiencies of IgM, IgE, and kappa or lambda light chains have been described but are rare. IgM deficiency has been associated with marked susceptibility to septicemia. Since IgM replacement is impractical on a long-term basis, reliance is placed mainly on antibiotics.

Herrod HG: Management of the patient with IgG subclass deficiency and/or selective antibody deficiency. Ann Allergy 1993;70:3.

Mochizuki S et al: Systemic immunization against IgA in immunoglobulin deficiency. Clin Exp Immunol 1994;94:334.

Preud'homme JL, Hanson LA: IgG subclass deficiency. Immunodefic Rev 1990;2:129.

Schaffer FM et al: IgA deficiency. Immunodefic Rev 1991;3:15.

SELECTIVE DEFECTS OF CELL-MEDIATED IMMUNITY

Purine Nucleoside Phosphorylase Deficiency

Purine nucleoside phosphorylase deficiency causes a relatively selective CMI defect. It results in increased intracellular levels of deoxyguanosine triphosphate, which inhibit ribonucleotide reductase and interfere with DNA synthesis, especially in T cells. T cell help to B cells is not prevented, probably because it is not dependent on cell division. The structural locus for purine nucleoside phosphorylase is on chromosome 14, and transmission is recessive. Presenting features may be neurologic (developmental retardation, behavior disorders, and spasticity), with immunodeficiency (severe varicella, anemia, and failure to thrive) developing later. The age at presentation has ranged from 6 months to 7 years. Investigations show low blood uric acid, lymphopenia, absent delayed hypersensitivity skin responses, and low or absent lymphocyte responses to mitogens. Serum immunoglobulins and antibody responses to injected antigens may be normal. Several patients developed an autoimmune hemolytic anemia. Diagnosis depends on enzyme measurement, and all patients with severely impaired cellular immunity who make immunoglobulin should probably be tested. Antenatal diagnosis is possible. It has been difficult to achieve stable engraftment following bone marrow transplantation.

Markert ML: Purine nucleoside phosphorylase deficiency. Immunodefic Rev 1991;3:45.

Thymic hypoplasia (DiGeorge syndrome)

The diagnostic criteria for thymic hypoplasia are a small or absent thymus, lack of parathyroid glands, and major vessel abnormalities such as truncus arteriosus, anomalous pulmonary venous drainage, or right-sided aortic arch. Other features include a small jaw, low-set ears, and a short philtrum. A few cases are familial (some with deletions of C22), but a family history is exceptional, and environmental damage to the fetus, probably at 5–7 weeks of gestation, seems the most likely cause. The term "partial DiGeorge syndrome" is commonly applied to infants who have impaired rather than absent parathyroid or thymus function. Clinical presentation usually results from cardiac failure or, after 24–48 hours, from hypocalcemia, and the diagnosis is sometimes made during the course of cardiac surgery, when no thymus is found in the mediastinum. Postoperative hypocalcemia can be severe and persistent, requiring both calcium and vitamin D supplements. Despite receiving fresh blood transfusions during cardiopulmonary bypass, patients do not usually develop graft-versus-host disease. Their susceptibility to infection is variable—a few have died with septicemia, and some have had chronic candidiasis, but many appear to respond normally. This may reflect the tendency for the number of T cells in the patient's blood to rise spontaneously over the course of several years. The differential diagnosis includes hypocalcemia and a small or absent thymus on chest x-ray secondary to infection.

Treatment is primarily for the cardiac defects and correction of hypocalcemia. Blood for these patients should be irradiated. Grafting thymic hypoplasia patients with fetal thymus or thymic epithelial cells is often followed by rapid improvement in the lymphocyte response to mitogens. The improvement is so rapid that thymic humoral factors are thought to be responsible, but factors currently available for treatment have not been useful. Graft treatment is generally reserved for those who do not improve spontaneously and carries a risk for graft versus host disease.

Carey AH et al: Localization of 27 DNA markers to the region of human chromosome 22q11-pter deleted in patients with the DiGeorge syndrome and duplicated in the der22 syndrome. Genomics 1990;7:299.

Fibison WJ et al: Molecular studies of DiGeorge syndrome. Am J Hum Genet 1990;46:888.

Other Defects of Cell-Mediated Immunity

Many patients with the American (but not Finnish) type of **cartilage-hair hypoplasia** have a moderate degree of lymphopenia, low lymphocyte responses to mitogens, and higher than normal morbidity and mortality rates from herpesvirus and poxvirus infections. There is no established treatment. Short-limbed dwarfs who are immunodeficient should probably be tested for adenosine deaminase deficiency, since this is treatable. Other types of immunodeficiency affecting predominantly cellular immunity exist but are poorly classified. These are currently included in the "varied immunodeficiency" group. Their infections resemble those described above, with the frequent addition of chronic diarrhea and malabsorption and lung infections due to atypical mycobacteria, fungi, and *Pneumocystis carinii*. Treatment is experimental.

Brooks EG et al: Thymic hypoplasia and T-cell deficiency in ectodermal dysplasia: Case report and review of the literature. Clin Immunol Immunopathol 1994;71:44.
Fischer A et al: Bone marrow transplantation (BMT) in Europe for primary immunodeficiencies other than severe combined immunodeficiency: A report from the European Group for BMT and the European Group for Immunodeficiency. Blood 1994;83:1149.

COMBINED IMMUNODEFICIENCY DISORDERS

Severe combined immunodeficiency disease (SCID) comprises a heterogeneous group of conditions that have in common a primary severe impairment of both antibody- and cell-mediated immunity. The term SCID is usually restricted to infants with congenital immunodeficiency, but equally severe defects can be caused by AIDS or lymphocyte loss. The heterogeneity of the congenital forms reflects the range of underlying defects that may interfere with lymphocyte development at different stages and the varying degrees of engraftment with maternal lymphocytes that can occur during gestation or at birth. In an X-linked form of SCID, the abnormality has recently been identified as a defect of the IL-2 receptor γ chain.

Diarrhea, vomiting, and cough are common symptoms. The diarrhea causes failure to thrive, and though it may briefly remit after dietary changes, it recurs after a few days. The cough is usually persistent; it is often due to *P carinii* infection and can cause cyanosis. Skin rashes are common and frequently evanescent, except for rash following blood transfusion, which is due to graft-versus-host disease

(qv). A *Candida* diaper rash is usual. Findings initially include absence of tonsils or palpable lymph nodes; later, there is emaciation.

All patients with SCID have some degree of hypogammaglobulinemia and failure of antibody production (though maternal IgG will be present in infants). Lymphopenia is inconstant, but with the exception of zap 70 and HLA-DR-deficient SCID, all have very low or absent T (CD3) cells from blood, with normal numbers of NK (CD16) cells. B lymphocytes (with surface IgM) are usually present in blood. In vitro lymphocyte responses to mitogens are generally absent. Antigen-specific responses (T cell or antibody) are difficult to test for in infancy because of uncertainty about prior experience and because they are generally too time-consuming for clinical purposes. Antenatal diagnosis of X-linked SCID is possible by molecular methods. All other SCID syndromes may be detected by fetal blood sampling at 15 weeks of gestation and phenotyping the lymphocytes obtained.

Arpaia E et al: Defective T cell receptor signaling and CD8+ thymic selection in humans lacking zap-70 kinase. Cell 1994;76:947.
Fischer A: Severe combined immunodeficiencies. Immunodefic Rev 1992;3:83.
Taniguchi T, Minami Y: The IL-2/IL-2 receptor system: A current overview. Cell 1993;73:5.

Differential Diagnosis & Treatment

The combination of diarrhea and hypogammaglobulinemia in infancy is suggestive of SCID. The main differential is between severe varied immunodeficiency and secondary immunodeficiency due to HIV infection or severe gastrointestinal disease with loss of protein and cells. Some T cells are usually present in these secondary immunodeficiencies, with a weak lymphocyte response to phytohemagglutinin, and the serum albumin concentration may be low. Infants in whom the diagnosis is suspected should receive antibiotics for infection and IgG replacement. They should not be transfused with blood unless it has first been irradiated. With confirmation of the diagnosis, they may be started on trimethoprim-sulfamethoxazole for *Pneumocystis* prophylaxis. Bone marrow grafting offers the best hope for cure. If an HLA-matched sibling is available, there is a high chance of success; the treatment can be given without depleting the marrow of T cells or immunosuppressing the recipient. Most SCID patients do not have HLA-matched donors and are treated with grafts of parental bone marrow from which the T cells are removed by lectins or monoclonal antibodies. Pregraft suppression, with the attendant hazards of thrombocytopenia and neutropenia, may be required; reconstitution can take 4 months; and the overall rate of T cell engraftment is between 50% and 70%. Reconstitution for antibody responses may not occur even if B cells are produced.

Parkman R: The biology of bone marrow transplantation for severe combined immune deficiency. Adv Immunol 1991;49:381.

Filipovich AH: Bone marrow transplantation from unrelated donors for congenital immunodeficiencies. Bone Marrow Transplant 1993;11(Suppl)1:78.

VARIANTS OF SEVERE COMBINED IMMUNODEFICIENCY

1. ADENOSINE DEAMINASE DEFICIENCY

Adenosine deaminase converts adenosine and deoxyadenosine to inosine and deoxyinosine, respectively. Its structural locus is on chromosome 20, and individuals homozygous for a null gene account for about 20% of cases of SCID. Mechanisms by which lymphocyte function may be impaired in adenosine deaminase deficiency include (1) inhibition of ribonucleotide reductase (through raised deoxy-ATP levels), so that T lymphocytes are prevented from dividing; (2) increased DNA fragmentation; and (3) interference with methylation reactions. Affected infants may be near-normal at birth (presumably because their mothers keep deoxyadenosine levels down in utero). Their cellular immunity fails first; they then become antibody-deficient, though they may continue to make immunoglobulin for months or years. Diagnosis is by assay of adenosine deaminase in red cell lysates. A bone marrow graft from a matched normal sibling is the ideal treatment (see below). Transfection of blood lymphocytes and marrow cells is being evaluated for subjects who lack matched donors. Immune competence is also restored in parallel with erythrocyte deoxy-ATP levels by weekly infusions of polyethylene glycol-stabilized ADA enzyme conjugate.

Blaese RM: Development of gene therapy for immunodeficiency: Adenosine deaminase deficiency. Pediatr Res 1993;33(1 Suppl):S49.

Hershfield MS, Chaffee S, Sorensen RU: Enzyme replacement therapy with polyethylene glycol-adenosine deaminase in adenosine deaminase deficiency: Overview and case reports of three patients, including two now receiving gene therapy. Pediatr Res 1993;33(1 Suppl):S42. (See discussion on p S47.)

2. SCID WITH IMMUNOGLOBULINS (Nezelof's Syndrome)

Affected patients have severely impaired cellular immunity, and although they may make small or large amounts of immunoglobulin (usually IgM), they do not make useful antibodies. Their clinical course is therefore similar to that of patients with other types of SCID. The conditions is heterogeneous in that both X-linked and autosomal recessive forms exist.

3. SCID WITH RETICULO-ENDOTHELIOSIS (Omenn's Syndrome)

Omenn's syndrome is characterized by the combination of skin rash, lymphadenopathy, and splenomegaly with SCID. Some cases have been attributed to partial engraftment with sufficient maternal T cells to cause graft-versus-host disease in the infant with SCID. Immunosuppression and marrow ablation followed by bone marrow transplant has sometimes been successful under these conditions.

Melamed I, Cohen A, Roifman CM: Expansion of CD3+CD4−CD8− T-cell population expressing high levels of IL-5 in Omenn's syndrome. Clin Exp Immunol 1994;95:14.

4. SCID WITH LEUKOPENIA (Reticular Dysgenesis)

This disorder occurs in infants with SCID who also have severe neutropenia, often with reduced numbers of granulocyte precursors in the marrow. Only about 20 cases have been reported. There is a familial trend, but the severity of the neutropenia varies between affected siblings, so this may be a secondary feature.

Gasparetto C et al: Dyshematopoiesis in combined immune deficiency with congenital neutropenia. Am J Hematol 1994;45:63.

5. SCID WITH DEFECTIVE EXPRESSION OF HLA ANTIGENS

This is a difficult condition to diagnose because affected patients generally make immunoglobulins and have low to normal numbers of B and T cells in their blood, together with positive responses to phytohemagglutinin stimulation. Their clinical symptoms are nevertheless those of SCID. The defect is of HLA-D antigen expression, and the T cells do not make antigen-specific responses, so the patients remain antibody-deficient. Diagnosis is by phenotyping blood lymphocytes for HLA-DR antigen expression. A number of affected families has been of North African descent.

Casper JT et al: Successful treatment with an unrelated-donor bone marrow transplant in an HLA-deficient patient with severe combined immune deficiency ("bare lymphocyte syndrome"). J Pediatr 1990;116:262.

OTHER DISORDERS ASSOCIATED WITH IMMUNODEFICIENCY

WISKOTT-ALDRICH SYNDROME

The characteristics of Wiskott-Aldrich syndrome are thrombocytopenia, eczema, and recurrent infection (originally draining ears). Inheritance is X-linked recessive; the incidence is about 4 per million male births, and the gene has been localized to the p11 region of the X chromosome. The disorder is associated with deficient expression of a 115 kDa cell surface sialophorin identified as CD43. Common presenting symptoms are bloody diarrhea, cerebral hemorrhage, or septicemia followed by severe infections with polysaccharide-encapsulated bacteria. However, some patients have little if any eczema, while others have few infections. The main causes of death in infancy are bleeding and infections, but with increasing age lymphomas become increasingly common. Survival through the teens is rare in untreated patients, though partial syndromes are sometimes diagnosed in adults. The variability of the clinical picture makes diagnosis difficult in the absence of a family history. Laboratory tests which are helpful include a low platelet count, low or absent isohemagglutinins, and reduced antibody response to polysaccharides. Bone marrow transplantation with matched sibling marrow offers the best hope for long-term correction of the defect. Haploidentical T-depleted grafts may fail to take unless preceded by cyclophosphamide and busulfan conditioning. The platelet count generally rises following splenectomy, but this operation must be accompanied by antibiotic prophylaxis because of the increased risk of septicemia and sudden death. If the abnormal X chromosome in a family can be identified, then antenatal diagnosis should be possible either by restriction fragment length polymorphisms or by methylation protection analysis.

Goodship J et al: Carrier detection in Wiskott-Aldrich syndrome: Combined use of M27 beta for X-inactivation studies and as a linked probe. Blood 1991;77:2677.

Remold-O'Donnell E, & Rosen FS: Sialophorin (CD43) and the Wiskott-Aldrich syndrome. Immunodefic Rev 1990;2:151.

Rumelhart SL et al: Monoclonal antibody T-cell-depleted HLA-haploidentical bone marrow transplantation for Wiskott-Aldrich syndrome. Blood 1990;75:1031.

ATAXIA-TELANGIECTASIA

Ataxia-telangiectasia is characterized by cerebellar ataxia (due to degeneration of Purkinje cells) usually developing between 2 and 5 years of age and followed by the appearance of telangiectases, particularly on the conjunctiva and over exposed areas: the nose, ears, and shoulders. The disorder has an autosomal recessive inheritance pattern, but there are six or more different complementation groups. The abnormal gene is on chromosome 11—11q22–23 in one study—but its mechanism of action is unknown. Abnormal findings in ataxia-telangiectasia include raised serum alpha-fetoprotein levels (useful diagnostically), thymic hypoplasia, low or absent serum IgE, low IgA in 50%, abnormal carbohydrate tolerance, and defective ability to repair radiation-induced DNA fragmentation. Clinically, the most important symptom is the progressive loss of motor coordination, followed by weakness. Respiratory tract infections and many types of malignancy (including carcinomas) are the major causes of death. About 10% of patients develop lymphomas, the majority of which are T cell-derived. Many of the lymphomas have translocations or inversions at sites where T cell receptor genes are normally rearranged. Radiotherapy has been followed by skin breakdown, presumably the result of the DNA repair defect. The heterozygote frequency is 0.5–5%, depending on geographic and ethnic factors, and these individuals have an increased incidence of breast cancer.

Gatti RA et al: Ataxia-telangiectasia: An interdisciplinary approach to pathogenesis. Medicine 1991;70:99.

Taylor AM et al: Genetic and cellular features of ataxia telangiectasia. Int J Radiat Biol 1994;65:65.

CHRONIC MOCOCUTANEOUS CANDIDIASIS

Diagnostic criteria are chronic candidiasis, affecting skin or nails and mucous membranes, which is not attributable to antibiotic treatment or another defined immunodeficiency. Involvement of scalp and flexures is common, usually as erythema and scaling but occasionally as granulomas with skin hypertrophy. The recurrent candidiasis these patients experience points to an underlying immunodeficiency, but the faulty mechanism has not been identified. Affected patients make anti-*Candida* antibodies, and their in vitro lymphocyte responses may be positive even when *Candida* skin tests are negative. Evidence for the complexity of this form of immunodeficiency includes the frequent association with endocrinopathy, sometimes autoimmune (affecting parathyroid, thyroid, pituitary, or gonads), and, less commonly, susceptibility to staphylococcal infections with defective neutrophil mobility. There is usually some

control of the candidiasis with continuous ketoconazole treatment.

X-LINKED LYMPHOPROLIFERATIVE SYNDROME

This term is applied to boys who develop bone
marrow aplasia, hypogammaglobulinemia, or a
lymphoproliferative syndrome following Epstein-
Barr virus infection. The gene responsible has been
mapped to Xq2s, and antenatal diagnosis is possible
using polymorphisms at DXS42 and DXS37. Affected boys are immunologically normal prior to
EBV infection, and during acute mononucleosis they
make some antibody to the EBV. In most instances,
the EBV infection results in a lethal lymphoproliferative syndrome characterized by liver failure, disseminated intravascular coagulation, and multiple monoclonal serum IgM bands. Acyclovir is sometimes
beneficial, and alpha interferon and monoclonal anti-
B cell antibodies are being investigated as treatments.
Only 10–20% of affected boys who are infected with
EBV survive to develop hypogammaglobulinemia.

Purtilo DT et al: The X-linked lymphoproliferative disease:
From autopsy toward cloning the gene, 1975–1990. Pediatr Pathol 1991;11:685.

Graft-Versus-Host Disease

Graft-versus-host disease follows the transfusion
of immunocompetent but incompatible lymphocytes
into an individual incapable of rejecting them, such as
infants with SCID. It has been reported in infants receiving transfusions from HLA homozygous donors,
so blood products for infants should be irradiated. An
erythematous and then bullous skin rash is variably
followed by diarrhea, hepatitis, nephritis, pulmonary
infiltrates, and fever, while marrow damage results in
neutropenia and then thrombocytopenia. Many patients develop high IgE levels. Diagnosis is suspected
on the basis of an unirradiated blood or blood product
transfusion and is confirmed by skin biopsy. The disease is usually fatal in 1–3 weeks: it may be slowed
by high-dose steroids or cyclosporine and at least
temporarily halted by monoclonal anti-T cell antibodies.

Sanders MR, Graeber JE: Posttransfusion graft-versus-host
disease in infancy. J Pediatr 1990;117:159.
Parkman R: Human graft versus host disease. Immunodefic
Rev 1991;2:253.

BIOCHEMICAL DEFECTS SOMETIMES ASSOCIATED WITH IMMUNODEFICIENCY

Several primary errors of metabolism affect immunity adversely. Transcobalamin 2 deficiency causes a
megaloblastic anemia with impaired bacterial killing
by neutrophils and reduced serum immunoglobulins
of all classes. **Biotin-dependent decarboxylase
deficiencies** may be associated with convulsions,
alopecia, candidiasis, low serum IgA, and a reduced
number of T cells. Lymphopenia and impaired cell-
mediated immunity are reported in **hereditary orotic
aciduria,** which in one case has responded to oral
uridine replacement. Chromosomal instability syndromes impair cell-mediated immunity. In Bloom's
syndrome, this may be severe enough to cause malabsorption. An increased mortality rate from infection
suggests that Down's syndrome also impairs immunity.

Alvarado CS et al: Uridine-responsive hypogammaglobulinemia and congenital heart disease in a patient
with hereditary orotic aciduria. J Pediatr 1988;113:867.
Prigent C et al: Aberrant DNA repair and DNA replication
due to an inherited enzymatic defect in human DNA ligase I. Mol Cell Biol 1994;14:310.

SECONDARY IMMUNODEFICIENCY

Secondary immunodeficiency is a common cause
of pediatric illness. The mechanisms that may be impaired are summarized in Table 29–3, and the symptoms are generally those that would be anticipated
from the combination of the primary disorder and the
complicating immunodeficiency. Whenever possible,
treatment should be of the primary disorder. Occasionally, immunologic methods may help, eg, varicella-zoster immune globulin may prevent varicella
in patients with leukemia and intravenous IgG replacement might provide added protection where antibody production is diminished. IgG replacement is
unlikely to help when loss (as in nephrotic syndrome)
is responsible for hypogammaglobulinemia.

THERAPEUTIC IMMUNOSUPPRESSION

Therapeutic immunosuppression is increasingly
used in pediatrics for transplant recipients and for autoimmune disease. Modalities include monoclonal
CD3 antibody (OKT3), which clears antigen receptors off the T cell surface as well as depleting T cells;
cyclosporine and FK 506, which interfere with cytokine production and release; steroids, which alter
lymphocyte recirculation and interfere with cytokine
production; and antimitotic agents which block T cell
proliferation. The risks of immunosuppression include reactivation of latent herpesviruses (CMV,
HSV, VZV), though antiviral treatments have made

Table 29–3. Mechanisms of secondary immunodeficiency.

Mechanism	Example
Loss	
Immunoglobulin	Renal, in nephrotic syndrome
Immunoglobulin	Skin, from burns
Immunoglobulin and cells	Gut, in intestinal lymphangiectasia
Phagocytes	Following splenectomy
Malnutrition	Kwashiorkor
Zinc deficiency	Impaired cell-mediated immunity
Copper and iron deficiency	Impaired neutrophil function
Drugs	Steroids, cancer chemotherapy
	Specific immunosuppressants
	Phenytoin → IgA deficiency
Infections	HIV, EBV, CMV, measles, rubella, hepatitis, malaria

these less life-threatening. EBV reactivation is hazardous if it results in a lymphoproliferation with marrow phagocytosis of red and white cells. The appearance of serum oligoclonal immunoglobulin bands may give advance warning of this dangerous complication. Combined immunosuppression with agents having different modes of action tends to be much more potent, with a greater potential for opportunistic infections, than immunosuppression by single agents. The risk of infection is greatest when the neutrophil count is depressed by antimitotic agents at the same time as specific immunity is suppressed by steroids and cyclosporine.

Pinching AJ: Secondary immunodeficiency. Clin Immunol Allergy 1985;5:469.

ACQUIRED IMMUNODEFICIENCY SYNDROME (AIDS)

Secondary immunodeficiency caused by infection with human immunodeficiency virus (HIV) has become commoner than primary immunodeficiency syndromes. Most new cases now result from vertical transmission. Some subjects who were infected through blood products continue to come to medical attention because of the slow progression of the disease. Clinical findings common in HIV infections but less common in primary immunodeficiencies are lymphadenopathy, hepatosplenomegaly, and high IgG levels. The presence of serum antibodies to HIV antigens is useful for the diagnosis of HIV when passively acquired maternal antibody levels have fallen (by 15 months of age). In younger infants, or in infants thought to have defective antibody responses, the diagnosis depends on demonstrating virus, viral antigens, or viral genome in blood. Factors determining the rate of progression to AIDS (with failure to thrive, encephalopathy, recurrent or opportunistic infections, or lymphopenia) are unknown. Management of HIV infections is discussed in Chapter 35.

Cavelli TA, Rubinstein A: Pediatric HIV infection: A review. Immunodefic Rev 1990;2:83:128.

Childhood AIDS. Pediatr Clin North Am 1991;38:1.

INVESTIGATION OF IMMUNODEFICIENCY

Evaluation for a possible underlying immunodeficiency should begin with a thorough history, since this is useful diagnostically. Physical and anatomic defects are the commonest causes of recurrent infections, and recurrence at a single site should prompt a search for a local abnormality. The age at onset of infections may be an important clue. Infections associated with defects of phagocytes, C3, or cellular immunity commonly start in the first months of life, whereas maternal antibody protects infants with hypogammaglobulinemia for 3–6 months. Antibody, complement, and phagocyte defects predispose mainly to bacterial infections; superficial candidiasis and severe herpesvirus infections are typical of cellular immunodeficiency. A simple protocol for testing these mechanisms is presented in Table 29–4, and the level of investigation should reflect the frequency and severity of infections. A CBC and quantitative immunoglobulin measurement will identify 90% of *primary* immunodeficiency syndromes.

Phagocyte Function

Evaluation of phagocyte function should begin with white blood count and differential to rule out neutropenia. A blood film is useful to exclude the Howell-Jolly bodies of asplenia and to look for normal lysosomal granules in neutrophils. Chemotaxis is generally measured in migration chambers in the laboratory and can also be assessed by migration of cells from abraded skin onto a sterile coverslip. Results of

Table 29–4. Hierarchy of tests for investigation of primary immunodeficiency.

Test Level	Complement	Phagocytes	Antibody	CMI
Screening	CH_{50}	Count, morphology	Ig measurement	Skin tests
First level		NBT, LFA-1[1]	IHA,[2] TT	T cells counts[3]
Second level	Factor assays	Killing and chemotaxis	Immunize	In vitro tests

[1]Only where chronic granulomatous disease or LFA-1 deficiency is suspected.
[2]IHA = isohemagglutinins, after age 1; TT = tetanus toxoid.
[3]Identify all T cells with CD3, subsets with CD4, CD8. CD45RO for memory cells.

chemotaxis tests must be interpreted cautiously, since secondary and transient defects in chemotaxis are common. Quantitation of ingestion and microbicidal activity requires special techniques available chiefly in research laboratories. However, the chemical reduction of nitroblue tetrazolium by phagocytes requires normal oxidation metabolism, so this test screens for chronic granulomatous disease (the commonest bacterial killing defect) and for leukocyte glucose 6-phosphate dehydrogenase deficiency. Myeloperoxidase deficiency is excluded by histochemical stain available in most oncology laboratories.

Complement

Deficiency of a classic pathway component can be excluded by a normal hemolytic complement titer, for which the patient's serum must be separated within 30 minutes of collection and stored at –70 °C. Alternative pathway function is tested by lysis of rabbit red blood cells. There is little point in measuring individual complement component levels if the hemolytic titer is normal, unless it is to follow the activity of an immune complex-associated disease in which C4 and C3 may be low. The common form of opsonizing defect of yeast is now known to be due to deficiency of mannan-binding protein.

Antibodies & Immunoglobulins

In patients who are not blood group AB, isohemagglutinins are the most easily tested naturally occurring antibodies. They are of the IgM class, become detectable by 6 months of age, and reach adult levels about a year later. The importance of antibody tests is illustrated by the inverse correlation between isohemagglutinin titer and susceptibility to meningitis in patients with hypogammaglobulinemia, irrespective of their serum IgM levels. Tetanus and diphtheria antibody tests are widely available, as are antibodies to pneumococcal polysaccharide, rubella, and mumps. In practice, it is often easier to measure serum immunoglobulins as a screening procedure than to test for antibodies, but it should be appreciated that some patients with varied immunodeficiency syndromes and some infants with severely impaired cell-mediated immunity make immunoglobulin that does not have useful antibody activity. Properly performed immunoglobulin estimations are

reproducible to +10% for IgG and IgA and +20% for IgM, so small changes are of no significance. Measurement of serum IgD is not generally of diagnostic value in pediatrics. Immunoglobulin concentrations are lower in infants than in adults, and laboratories may erroneously report normal children's values as low. Comparisons of results from different laboratories may be difficult, because few commercial kit suppliers calibrate their control sera against the international standard. Simple protein electrophoresis is not sufficiently sensitive to make a confident diagnosis of hypogammaglobulinemia, though it is valuable for identifying the monoclonal excesses seen in macroglobulinemia, the oligoclonal gammopathy of EBV infections in X-linked lymphoproliferative syndrome, and in heavy chain diseases. Serum albumin should be measured at least once in patients with hypogammaglobulinemia to exclude secondary deficiencies due to loss. IgG or IgA subclass measurements may be abnormal in patients with varied immunodeficiency syndromes, but they are rarely helpful.

Cell-Mediated Immunity

Positive delayed hypersensitivity skin tests give good evidence for antigen-specific immunity. Only a positive response is interpretable—particularly in infancy, when prior immunization may not have been adequate to elicit good skin responses.

Extensive characterization of blood lymphocytes is now possible by immunofluorescence. Only small volumes of blood are required, and results are rapidly available. Some of the more useful antibodies—and common deviations from normal—are summarized in Table 29–5. When abnormalities are suspected, it is important to check absolute numbers of lymphocytes and their subsets. Tests of T cell proliferation in response to mitogens (PHA, ConA, or enterotoxins) are mainly useful to characterize immunodeficiency detected by simpler tests. It is possible to distinguish between defects of T cell activation, and lymphokine (IL-2) production and proliferation:effector function is measurable by lymphokine production and cytotoxicity testing.

Genetic Diagnosis

Molecular biology approaches are important for antenatal diagnosis, for carrier identification, and for

Table 29–5. Blood lymphocyte phenotyping.[1]

Antigen	Commercial Antibodies	Cells Stained	Normal Range and Changes Seen Clinically
CD2	OKT11	T, NK	70–90%. Falls to 10–20% when T cells absent.
CD3	OKT3, Leu4	All T	55–85%. Falls when T cell number reduced. Increases to 90% when B cells absent.
CD4	OKT4, Leu3	HLA-D restricted T cells, T cell, immature B cells	35–60%. Selectively reduced in HIV infections. Reduced with other T cells by steroids, defect of cell-mediated immunity.
CD5		T cells, immature B cells	55–85%. Falls when T cell number reduced. Increased with immature B cells.
CD8	OKT8, Leu2	HLA-A/B restricted T cells	25–50%. Selectively increased in response to some viral infections. Reduced with other T cell defects.
CD11	OKM1, Mac-1	Monocytes	Lacking in LFA-1 deficiency.
CD16	Leu11	NK cells	Increased by viral infections.
CD19		B cells	Increased when T cells lacking.
CD20		B cells	Increased when T cells lacking.
CD25		IL-2 receptor	Activated T cells. Increased in graft-versus-host disease.
CD45RO	UCHL1	T cells	Memory T cells, low in newborns.
CD56	NKH-1	NK cells	Raised in active viral infections.

[1]From Thompson RA (editor): Laboratory investigation of immunological disorders. Clin Immunol Allergy 1985;5:No. 3. See also Spickett GP, Matamoros N, Farrant J: Lymphocyte surface phenotype in common variable immunodeficiency. Dis Markers 1992;10:67.

characterizing an increasing number of primary immunodeficiencies. The X-linked defects have mostly been mapped, and others, such as adenosine deaminase deficiency, are well defined.

Di Santo JP et al: Prenatal diagnosis of X-linked hyper IgM syndrome. N Engl Med 1994;330:969.
Kinnon C, Levinsky R: The molecular basis of X-linked immunodeficiency disease. J Inherit Metab Dis 1992;15:674.
Hirschhorn R: Overview of biochemical abnormalities and molecular genetics of adenosine deaminase deficiency. Pediatr Res 1993;33(1 Suppl):S35.
Puck JM: Prenatal diagnosis and genetic analysis of X-linked immunodeficiency disorders. Pediatr Res 1993;33(1 Suppl):S29. (See discussion on p S33.)

Endocrine Disorders

30

Ronald W. Gotlin, MD. Michael Kappy, MD, PhD,
George Eisenbarth, MD, PhD & H. Peter Chase, MD

DISTURBANCES OF GROWTH & SEXUAL DEVELOPMENT

In the health care of children and adolescents, knowledge of the endocrine system is essential in order to differentiate disturbances in hormonal secretion and action from normal variations in the timing and pattern of development (ie, "constitutional" deviations from the average).

Disturbances of growth and development are the most common presenting complaints in the pediatric endocrine clinic. It is estimated that over 1 million children in the USA have abnormal short stature and that there are at least 10 million children whose growth is potentially abnormal.

Failure to thrive is a term usually reserved for infants who fail to gain weight and is most often due to undernutrition (see below).

Tall stature is currently an unusual presenting complaint in our society. Because of the preference for tallness in both males and females, the number of young people evaluated and treated for tall stature has decreased.

SHORT STATURE

Short stature is usually a normal variation of the usual pattern of growth. Influencing factors include sex, race, size of parents and other family members, nutrition, intrauterine growth pattern, timing of puberty, dysmorphism, the presence of systemic or chronic diseases, and psychosocial status. All must be considered in the total assessment of the child.

The causes of unusually short stature are listed in Table 30–1. The causes can generally be differentiated on the basis of the history, the physical examination, and the stage of skeletal maturation as assessed by radiography.

1. CONSTITUTIONAL SHORT STATURE

Many children have a constitutional delay in growth and skeletal maturation. In all other respects, they appear entirely normal. In children with constitutional short stature, birth weight and length are not affected, but typically the rate of growth is decreased during infancy. There is often a history of a similar pattern of growth in one of the parents or in other members of the family. Puberty is delayed ("late bloomer"), and these children characteristically reach normal adult height at a later than average age.

Treatment with anabolic agents or low dose-estrogen (girls) or testosterone (boys) may be useful in hastening the timing of puberty, but adult height is not enhanced. The future role (if any) of growth hormone for these normal children is unknown; ethical, economic, and social concerns have all appropriately been voiced.

2. GROWTH HORMONE & GROWTH HORMONE DEFICIENCY

Human growth hormone (hGH) is a 191-amino-acid peptide with two intramolecular disulfide bridges. The hGH gene is present on chromosome 17 in association with genes for human chorionic somatomammotropin. Human growth hormone has been synthesized recently in bacterial and mouse cell lines.

The recent biosynthesis of hGH employing recombinant DNA methods has made sufficient hormone available to treat all children with a deficiency state. Moreover, children with severe short stature and normal growth hormone secretion who may benefit from hGH in large doses can be evaluated in clinical trials. When rigid diagnostic criteria are employed, instances of hGH deficiency are found in approximately 1:4000 children. About two-thirds of cases are idiopathic (rarely familial): a deficiency or impairment in the hypothalamic secretion of hGH-releasing hormone is suspected. The remainder are secondary to pituitary or hypothalamic disease, infection,

Table 30–1. Causes of short stature.

Familial, racial, or genetic
Constitutional short stature and delayed adolescence
Endocrine disturbances
  Growth hormone deficiency
    Hereditary—gene deletion
    Idiopathic—deficiency of growth hormone or growth hormone releasing hormone (or both) with and without associated abnormalities of midline structures of the central nervous system
    Acquired
      Transient—eg, psychosocial short stature
      Organic—tumor, irradiation of the central nervous system, infection, or trauma
  Hypothyroidism
  Adrenal insufficiency
  Cushing's disease and Cushing's syndrome (including iatrogenic causes)
  Sexual precocity (androgen or estrogen excess)
  Diabetes mellitus (poorly controlled)
  Diabetes insipidus
  Hyperaldosteronism
Primordial short stature
  Intrauterine growth retardation
    Placental insufficiency
    Intrauterine infection
  Primordial dwarfism with premature aging
    Progeria (Hutchinson-Gilford syndrome)
    Progeroid syndrome
      Werner's syndrome
      Cachectic (Cockayne's syndrome)
  Short stature without dysmorphism
  Short stature with dysmorphism (eg, Seckel's bird-headed dwarfism, leprechaunism, Silver's syndrome, Bloom's syndrome, Cornelia de Lange syndrome, Hallerman-Streiff syndrome)
Inborn errors of metabolism
  Altered metabolism of calcium or phosphorus (eg, hypophosphatemic rickets, hypophosphatasia, infantile hypercalcemia, pseudohypoparathyroidism)
  Storage diseases
    Mucopolysaccharidoses (eg, Hurler's syndrome, Hunter's syndrome)
    Mucolipidoses (eg, generalized gangliosidosis, fucosidosis, mannosidosis)

Inborn errors of metabolism (cont'd)
    Sphingolipidoses (eg, Tay-Sachs disease, Niemann-Pick disease, Gaucher's disease)
    Miscellaneous (eg, cystinosis)
  Aminoacidemias and aminoacidurias
  Epithelial transport disorders (eg, renal tubular acidosis, cystic fibrosis, Bartter's syndrome, vasopressin-resistant diabetes insipidus, pseudohypoparathyroidism)
  Organic acidemias and acidurias (eg, methylmalonic aciduria, orotic aciduria, maple syrup urine disease, isovaleric acidemia)
  Metabolic anemias (eg, sickle cell disease, thalassemia, pyruvate kinase deficiency)
  Disorders of mineral metabolism (eg, Wilson's disease, magnesium malabsorption syndrome)
  Body defense disorders (eg, Bruton's agammaglobulinemia, thymic aplasia, chronic granulomatous disease)
Constitutional (intrinsic) diseases of bone
  Defects of growth of tubular bones or spine (eg, achondroplasia, metatropic dwarfism, diastrophic dwarfism, metaphyseal chondrodysplasia)
  Disorganized development of cartilage and fibrous components of the skeleton (eg, multiple cartilaginous exostoses, fibrous dysplasia with skin pigmentation, precocious puberty of McCune-Albright)
  Abnormalities of density of cortical diaphyseal structure or metaphyseal modeling (eg, osteogenesis imperfecta congenita, osteopetrosis, tubular stenosis)
Short stature associated with chromosomal defects
  Autosomal (eg, Down's syndrome, cri du chat syndrome, trisomy 18)
  Sex chromosomal (eg, Turner's syndrome-XO, penta X, XXXY)
Chronic systemic diseases, congenital defects, and cancers (eg, chronic infection and infestation, inflammatory bowel disease, hepatic disease, cardiovascular disease, hematologic disease, central nervous system disease, pulmonary disease, renal disease, malnutrition, cancers, collagen vascular disease)
Psychosocial short stature (deprivation dwarfism)
Miscellaneous syndromes (eg, arthrogryposis multiplex congenita, cerebrohepatorenal syndrome, Noonan's syndrome, Prader-Willi syndrome, Riley-Day syndrome)

trauma, reticuloendotheliosis, and craniopharyngioma or other tumors (eg, gliomas). The deficiency of hGH may be an isolated defect or may occur in combination with other pituitary hormone deficiencies. Idiopathic hGH deficiency affects both sexes equally.

At birth, affected children are of normal weight, but length may be reduced. The most characteristic clinical feature of the child with hGH deficiency is a linear growth rate as little as one-half that of the normal child. Growth retardation may begin during infancy or may be delayed until later childhood. Other findings include infantile fat distribution, youthful facial features, midfacial hypoplasia, and delayed sexual maturation. Epiphysial maturation ("bone age") is delayed. Headaches, visual field defects, polyuria, and polydipsia may precede or accompany the onset of growth failure in cases resulting from central nervous system disease. Abnormalities on skull radiography, CT, and MRI are common in organic hypopituitarism.

When results of growth hormone testing are equivocal, a trial of hGH treatment may be useful in determining whether an abnormally short child will benefit from growth hormone. Currently, the treatment of choice is synthetic hGH alone or in combination with other hormones. The dose of hGH is 0.15–0.3 mg/kg/wk administered subcutaneously; this dose is divided into six or seven equal daily doses. Results of clinical trials with hGH-releasing hormone (somatotropin-releasing hormone) have been encouraging, and this agent may be employed in the future in patients with hypothalamic hGH-releasing hormone deficiency. Protein anabolic agents may be effective in promoting linear growth but may cause undue acceleration of epiphysial closure, with a resultant lessening of adult height. Anabolic agents should ideally be used at the time of puberty and in combination with hGH.

The efficacy of hGH treatment for conditions associated with severe short stature and normal hGH secretion (eg, intrauterine growth retardation, chronic renal disease, steroid-dependent asthma) is currently under clinical investigation. In Turner's syndrome (see below), results over a 6-year study have been encouraging. Similarly, adults with hGH deficiency may benefit from continued therapy. The use of hGH in conditions other than definite deficiency states prompts scientific, social, and ethical questions. The greatest controversy surrounding hGH therapy is its role, if any, in management of a normal short child and as an anabolic agent in the elderly.

Physiologically, hGH is released from the anterior pituitary in response to a delicate interplay of hypothalamic releasing and inhibitory factors. Moreover, a variety of stimuli, including adrenergic and serotonergic agents, arginine, glucagon, and insulin-induced hypoglycemia, have been employed clinically to provoke hGH secretion. Physiologically, serum levels of hGH vary considerably; episodic surges occur in relation to nutrients, to activity, and particularly to natural sleep. The latter typically is associated with significant sustained elevation of hGH during the first 2 hours after the onset of sleep. Electroencephalographic monitoring during this interval reflects slow wave or "deep" sleep, suggesting a role for specific neurotransmitter influence.

Following secretion, hGH exerts its biologic effects following binding to specific receptors in a large variety of tissues. Actions are divided into direct and indirect. The latter division is used to designate actions, hormonal and paracrine, resulting from the activity of the somatomedin family (insulin-like growth factors; IGFs) generated in response to hGH.

3. HYPOTHYROIDISM

Hypothyroidism in childhood (discussed in a subsequent section) is invariably associated with poor growth and delayed epiphysial maturation. In occasional cases, short stature may be the principal finding.

4. INTRAUTERINE GROWTH RETARDATION (Primordial Short Stature)

Intrauterine growth retardation may occur in a number of disorders, including craniofacial disproportion (eg, Seckel's dwarfism, Silver's syndrome, Noonan's syndrome), some cases of progeria (eg, Hutchinson-Gilford syndrome), and cachectic dwarfism, or may occur in individuals with no accompanying significant dysmorphism. Children with these conditions are small at birth; both birth weight and length are below normal for gestational age. They grow parallel to but below the fifth percentile. Plasma hGH levels are usually normal but may be elevated.

In most instances, epiphysial maturation ("bone age") corresponds to chronologic age or is only mildly delayed, in contrast to the striking delay often present in children with hGH and thyroid deficiency.

There is no satisfactory long-term treatment for primordial short stature, though growth hormone in large doses may be efficacious and is being evaluated in clinical trials.

5. SHORT STATURE DUE TO EMOTIONAL FACTORS (Psychosocial Short Stature, Deprivation Dwarfism)

Psychologic deprivation with disturbances in motor and personality development may be associated with short stature. Although the growth retardation in some affected individuals is the result of undernutrition, in others undernutrition does not seem to be the major factor. In some instances, the child may have increased (often voracious) appetite; polydipsia and polyuria are sometimes present. These children are of normal size at birth and grow normally for a variable period of time before growth slows. A history of feeding problems in early infancy is common. Sleep is often restless. Emotional disturbances in the family are the rule. Skeletal maturation is delayed, and plasma hGH levels during sleep or in response to pharmacologic stimulation may be diminished.

Foster home placement or a change in the psychologic and emotional environment at home usually results in significantly improved growth, normalization of personality, appetite, and dietary intake, and return of normal hGH secretion.

DIFFERENTIAL DIAGNOSIS OF SHORT STATURE

Short stature may accompany or be caused by a large number of conditions (Table 30–1). When the etiology is not apparent from the history and physical examination, the following laboratory studies, in addition to bone age, are useful in detecting or categorizing the common causes of short stature:

(1) Complete blood count (to detect chronic anemia, infection, leukemia).

(2) Erythrocyte sedimentation rate (often elevated in collagen-vascular disease, cancer, chronic infection, inflammatory bowel disease).

(3) Urinalysis and microscopic examination (occult pyelonephritis, glomerulonephritis, renal tubular disease, etc).

(4) Stool examination for fat, occult blood, parasites, and parasite ova (inflammatory bowel disease, overwhelming parasitism).

(5) Serum electrolytes and phosphorus (mild adrenal insufficiency, renal tubular diseases, parathyroid

disease, rickets, etc); antigliadin antibody (for celiac disease).

(6) Blood urea nitrogen and serum creatinine (occult renal insufficiency).

(7) Karyotyping (should be performed in all short girls with delayed sexual maturation with or without phenotypic features of Turner's syndrome).

(8) Thyroid function assessment: total thyroxine (TT_4T_3RU), free thyroxine (FT_4), and thyroid-stimulating hormone (TSH) concentrations (short stature may be the only sign of hypothyroidism).

(9) Controversy persists concerning the diagnosis of hGH deficiency. The authors prefer a combination of physiologic assessments: hGH levels obtained during natural sleep and following administration of the provocative agents clonidine and arginine. Other provocative choices are discussed above.

Bugukgebiz A, Hindmarsh DC, Brooke CGD: Treatment of constitutional delay of growth and puberty with oxandrolone compared with growth hormone. Arch Dis Child 1990;65:448.

Cuttler L: Evaluation of growth disorders in children. Pediatrician 1987;14:109.

Grumbach MM: Growth hormone therapy and the short end of the stick. (Editorial.) N Engl J Med 1988;319:238.

Miller WL, Eberhardt NL: Structure and evolution of the growth hormone gene family. Endocr Rev 1983;4:97.

Saenger P: The current status of diagnosis and therapeutic intervention in Turner's syndrome. J Clin Endocrinol Metab 1993;77:297.

FAILURE TO THRIVE

Failure to thrive describes a reduction of growth from an established pattern or when the patient's weight plots consistently below the third percentile. (The term is best reserved for infants who for various reasons fail to gain weight.) Length and head circumference may also be affected; when this occurs, the underlying condition is generally more severe. Failure to thrive has many causes (see below and Table 30–1), of which inadequate caloric intake is the most common.

Currently, cases of failure to thrive due to HIV infection are not uncommon. Infants with lymphadenopathy, hepatosplenomegaly, parotitis, and unusual or opportunistic infections should be evaluated for HIV.

Classification & Etiologic Diagnosis

Failure to thrive is generally either organic (about 25% of cases, usually due to neurologic or gastrointestinal disease); nonorganic (50%); or mixed (25%); the distinction is usually apparent on the basis of the history and physical examination. When it is not, it is helpful to compare the patient's chronologic age with the height age (median age for the patient's height),

weight age, and head circumference. On the basis of these measurements, three principal patterns can be defined that provide a starting point in the diagnostic approach.

Group 1: (Most common type.) Normal head circumference; weight reduced out of proportion to height. In the majority of cases of failure to thrive, malnutrition is present as a result of either deficient caloric intake or malabsorption.

Group 2: Normal or increased head circumference; weight only moderately reduced, usually in proportion to height. Structural dystrophies, constitutional pattern short stature, endocrinopathies.

Group 3: Subnormal head circumference; weight reduced in proportion to height. Primary central nervous system deficit; intrauterine growth retardation.

An initial period of observed nutritional rehabilitation, usually in a hospital setting, is often helpful in the diagnosis. The child should be placed on a regular diet for age, and intake and weight should be carefully plotted for 1–2 weeks. If stools are abnormal, evaluate for carbohydrate intolerance and malabsorption. Caloric intake should be increased if weight gain does not occur but intake is well tolerated. The following three patterns are often noted during rehabilitation.

A. Pattern 1: (Most common type.) Intake adequate; weight gain satisfactory. Feeding technique or amount at fault. Disturbed infant-mother relationship leading to decreased caloric intake.

B. Pattern 2: Intake adequate; no weight gain. If weight gain is unsatisfactory after increasing the calories to an adequate level (based on the infant's ideal weight for height), malabsorption is the most likely diagnosis. A diencephalic tumor may also cause this pattern, with or without associated microcephaly or ocular abnormalities.

If malabsorption is present, it is usually necessary to differentiate pancreatic exocrine insufficiency (cystic fibrosis, Shwachman's syndrome) from abnormalities of intestinal mucosa (eg, celiac disease). In cystic fibrosis, growth velocity commonly declines from the time of birth, and appetite usually is voracious. In celiac disease, growth velocity is usually not reduced until 6–12 months of age, and inadequate caloric intake may be a prominent feature.

C. Pattern 3: Intake inadequate.

1. Sucking or swallowing difficulties–Central nervous system or neuromuscular disease; esophageal or oropharyngeal malformations.

2. Inability to eat large amounts–This is common in patients with cardiopulmonary disease or in anorexic children suffering from chronic infections, systemic diseases, inflammatory bowel disease, celiac disease, and endocrine problems (eg, hypothyroidism). Patients with celiac disease often have inadequate caloric intake in addition to malabsorption. Zinc deficiency may cause anorexia and resultant poor weight gain.

3. Vomiting, spitting up, or rumination–
Upper intestinal obstruction (eg, pyloric stenosis, hiatal hernia, chalasia), chronic metabolic aberrations and acidosis (eg, renal insufficiency, diabetes mellitus and insipidus, organic acidemias), aldosterone insufficiency, increased intracranial pressure, psychosocial abnormalities.

Laboratory Aids to Diagnosis

The laboratory may provide helpful corroborative diagnostic information; however, an exhaustive nonselective laboratory search is not a substitute for a thorough history and physical examination.

A. Initial: Initial laboratory investigations at the time of admission might be limited to the following:

1. Blood–Complete blood count, sedimentation rate, antigliadin antibody, electrolytes, BUN.

2. Urine–Urinalysis (including pH, microscopic examination of sediment) and culture.

3. Stool (if abnormal)–Culture, pH, reducing substances, examination for occult blood, fat, and parasites.

4. Other tests only if clinically indicated.

B. Definitive: The following laboratory investigations are recommended after the period of nutritional rehabilitation, when the patient has been classified in one of the three categories listed above.

1. Pattern 1–No further laboratory tests are indicated. Maternal (and family) social and psychologic evaluation may be indicated.

2. Pattern 2–

a. Evaluate for malabsorption (see Chapter 19) if stools are abnormal.

b. If stools are normal or malabsorption is excluded, consider cerebral imaging for diencephalic tumor.

3. Pattern 3–

a. With vomiting–

(1) Serum electrolytes, pH, glucose, creatinine, zinc, ammonia, and lactate or pyruvate; serum and urine osmolalities; serum and urine organic and amino acids.

(2) Upper gastrointestinal series and cine-esophagography.

(3) Cerebral imaging for causes of increased intracranial pressure (eg, subdural hematoma, hydrocephalus, tumor) or central vomiting.

b. Without vomiting–

(1) Sigmoidoscopy, rectal biopsy (ulcerative or granulomatous colitis).

(2) Barium enema (ulcerative colitis or Hirschsprung's disease).

(3) Upper gastrointestinal series and followthrough (regional enteritis, malrotations).

(4) Thyroid function tests.

C. Other Tests: Further testing (adrenal function tests, intravenous urograms, etc) may be indicated.

Treatment & Prognosis

Treatment varies according to the underlying disorder. Most patients will gain weight and thrive on an adequate caloric intake. Maternal counseling and support placement may be required.

The outcome is dependent on the underlying disorder. In general, infants whose length and, particularly, head circumference are affected along with weight have a less favorable prognosis.

Berwick DM: Nonorganic failure to thrive. Pediatr Rev 1980;1:265.
Edwards AGK et al: Recognizing failure to thrive in early childhood. Arch Dis Child 1990;65:1263.

TALL STATURE

Currently, tall stature is usually of concern only to adolescent and preadolescent girls. The upper limit of acceptable height in both sexes appears to be increasing, but there are occasions when the patient and her parents may wish to influence the pattern of growth. On the basis of the family history, previous pattern of growth, stage of physiologic development, assessment of epiphysial development ("bone age"), and standard growth data, the physician should make a tentative estimate of the patient's eventual height. Although there are several conditions (Table 30–2) that may produce tall stature, by far the most common cause is a constitutional or familial variation from the average.

Reassurance, counseling, and education are generally all that is required. If the predicted height appears to be excessive, hormonal therapy with estrogen (eg, ethinyl estradiol, 0.2–0.3 mg daily), cycled with a progestational agent for 7 out of 28 days, may be attempted. Treatment results in a disproportionate advancement in skeletal maturation—height gain—thus

Table 30–2. Causes of tall stature.

Constitutional (familial)
Endocrine causes
  Somatotropin excess (pituitary gigantism)
  Androgen excess (tall as children, short as adults)
    True sexual precocity
    Pseudosexual precocity
  Androgen deficiency (normal height as children, tall as adults)
    Klinefelter's syndrome
    Anorchia (infection, trauma, idiopathic)
  Hyperthyroidism
Genetic causes
  Klinefelter's syndrome
  Syndromes of XYY, XXYY (tall as adults)
Miscellaneous syndromes and entities
  Marfan's syndrome
  Cerebral gigantism (Sotos' syndrome)
  Total lipodystrophy
  Diencephalic syndrome
  Homocystinuria

shortening the interval of growth. Estrogens are of no proved value when the physiologic age (as determined by stage of sexual maturity and epiphysial development) has reached the 12-year-old level and may be of little value even when administered at earlier ages. Estrogens act to accelerate epiphysial closure and may be continued until fusion occurs. In the male, a short course of testosterone in supraphysiologic doses may be effective.

GIGANTISM & ACROMEGALY

While growth hormone treatment is being introduced for an increasing number of indications, endogenous hGH excess is rare in childhood. As with adults, hGH excess is the result of a pituitary adenoma, and the clinical presentation includes headaches and visual disturbance in most cases. Biochemical confirmation consists of an elevated somatomedin (IGF-1) and failure of blood hGH to be suppressed below 2 ng/mL during an oral glucose tolerance test.

Treatment consists of transsphenoidal surgery after localization by CT scanning or MRI. Somatostatin analogue or bromocriptine may be useful when resection is incomplete or there is a recurrence.

Frohman LA: Therapeutic options in acromegaly. J Clin Endocrinol Metab 1991;76:1175.
Hartman ML: The adverse systemic effects of growth hormone in acromegaly. Growth Genet Horm 1990;6:1.
Wettenhall HNB, Cahill C, Roche AF: Tall girls: A survey of 15 years of management and treatment. J Pediatr 1975;86:602.

THE POSTERIOR PITUITARY GLAND

The posterior pituitary (neurohypophysis) is an extension of the ventral hypothalamus. The two principal neurohormones of the posterior pituitary, oxytocin and vasopressin, are synthesized in the supraoptic and paraventricular nuclei. After synthesis, these neurohormones are packaged in granules with specific neurophysins and transported via the axons to their storage site in the neurohypophysis. Oxytocin is primarily important during parturition and breast feeding and is not discussed further.

Antidiuretic Hormone (Vasopressin)

Antidiuretic hormone (ADH) release is controlled by a complex system that under physiologic conditions modulates the effective osmotic pressure of plasma. Osmoreceptors in the anterolateral hypothalamus and baroreceptors in the cardiac atria respond to changes in osmolality and blood volume and pressure, respectively. Moreover, a large number of putative chemical mediators within the central nervous system, as well as nausea, vomiting, and a variety of drugs and hormones, influences the release of vasopressin. In the text, three important conditions involving abnormalities of ADH secretion and action are addressed: (1) central neurogenic diabetes insipidus (below), (2) nephrogenic diabetes insipidus (Chapter 21), and (3) syndrome of inappropriate antidiuretic hormone (SIADH) (Chapter 37).

DIABETES INSIPIDUS

Essentials of Diagnosis
- Polydipsia and polyuria (4–40 L/d).
- Urine specific gravity < 1.010; osmolality < 280 mOsm/kg.
- Inability to concentrate urine on fluid restriction.
- Hyperosmolality of plasma.
- Subnormal plasma ADH concentration.
- Vasopressin responsiveness.

General Considerations
Hypofunction of the hypothalamus or posterior pituitary with deficiency of ADH (neurogenic central diabetes insipidus) is usually due to loss of neurosecretory neurons in the neurohypophysis. The condition may be idiopathic, congenital, or acquired or may be associated with lesions of the posterior pituitary or hypothalamus (trauma, infections, suprasellar cysts, tumors, reticuloendotheliosis, or some developmental abnormality). Familial ADH deficiency may be transmitted as an autosomal dominant or X-linked recessive trait. When no specific cause of neurogenic diabetes insipidus can be determined, the search for an underlying lesion should be continued for many years.

In nephrogenic diabetes insipidus, the renal tubules fail to respond to physiologic or pharmacologic doses of vasopressin, and no lesion of the pituitary or hypothalamus can be demonstrated; this disease is believed to be X-linked with variable degrees of penetrance, with a milder variant present in carrier females (see Chapter 21).

Cerebral salt wasting polyuria results in an elevation of atrial natriuretic hormone (ANH) and urinary sodium loss. Unless the salt loss is replaced, hyponatremic dehydration ensues.

Clinical Findings
The onset is often sudden, with polyuria, intense thirst, constipation, fever, and dehydration, particularly in infants. A desire for very cold beverages is a common historical notation. The child who awakens at night to urinate, is very thirsty, and drinks copi-

ously is a typical presentation of this unusual condition. In young infants on an ordinary feeding regimen, polyuria may not be recognized as abnormal, and the infant may present with severe dehydration manifested by high fever, circulatory collapse, and convulsions. In long-standing cases, growth retardation, lack of sexual maturation, and central nervous system damage may occur. The inability to concentrate urine is reflected by serum osmolalities that may be elevated to 300 mOsm/kg or greater; urine osmolality remains below this level (usually < 280 mOsm/kg). Familial diabetes insipidus may have a more insidious onset and a progressive course.

Symptoms and signs of ADH deficiency may be absent in patients with panhypopituitarism. Treating these patients with adrenocorticosteroids may unmask their polyuria and polydipsia.

Differential Diagnosis

Diabetes insipidus may be differentiated from psychogenic polydipsia (compulsive water drinking, potomania) and polyuria by limiting the usual excessive intake of fluid for 2–3 days and then withholding water for 7 hours. The test should be terminated if distress is clinically notable or associated with a weight loss exceeding 3% of body weight. Patients with long-standing psychogenic polydipsia may be unable to concentrate urine initially. The preliminary fluid limitation is necessary because psychogenic polydipsia patients lose the ability to concentrate urine. This is recommended in view of the fact that the posterior pituitary "signal" (bright spot) may change over time. Normal children and those with psychogenic polydipsia respond to dehydration with urinary osmolality above 450 mOsm/kg (specific gravity 1.020). With neurogenic and nephrogenic diabetes insipidus, the urine osmolality usually does not increase above 280 mOsm/kg (specific gravity 1.010) even after the period of dehydration. The measurement of serum ADH concentration, vasopressin, and hypertonic saline tests may be employed to distinguish between the various forms and degrees of diabetes insipidus.

Decreased ability to concentrate urine may also occur with hypokalemia (eg, hyperaldosteronism) and with various forms of hypercalcemia (including hypervitaminosis D) and renal tubular abnormalities (eg, Fanconi's syndrome).

MRI may demonstrate anatomic abnormalities in central diabetes insipidus and may differentiate congenital from acquired (eg, posttraumatic) causes. Serial MRI should be useful in following posttraumatic diabetes insipidus.

Treatment

A. Medical Treatment: The treatment of choice for partial and total diabetes insipidus is desmopressin acetate administered intranasally. The dosage must be adjusted, but the duration of action is generally at least 12 hours and lessens or eliminates the inconvenience of nocturia.

Chlorpropamide has been found to have an antidiuretic action through its potentiation of endogenous ADH effect; hypotension and hypoglycemia are, however, uncommon side effects limiting its use.

B. Other Therapy: X-ray therapy, surgery, antitumor chemotherapy, or a combination of these is, of course, indicated in the treatment of known causative diseases (eg, reticuloendotheliosis).

Prognosis

In the absence of central nervous system damage in infancy resulting from severe dehydration and if there are no significant associated defects, life expectancy should be normal. Hydronephrosis and hydroureter are not uncommon sequelae of prolonged polyuria; patients should also be observed carefully for urinary tract infection.

Banon PL, Robinson AG: Central diabetes insipidus: Management in the postoperative period. The Endocrinologist 1991;1:180.
Ganong CA, Kappy MS: Cerebral salt wasting in children. Am J Dis Child 1993;147:167.

THE PINEAL GLAND

The pineal gland in animals other than humans may have parenchymal cells (pinealocytes) and is often assigned an endocrine function (eg, regulation of somatic growth, sexual maturation, body pigmentation, blood glucose regulation, and a day/night-sensitive neuroendocrine regulatory function). In humans, pineal tumors are rarely associated with sexual precocity in the male. Cases of gonadotropin-secreting choriocarcinomas of the pineal gland with secondary Leydig cell activation and resultant sexual precocity have been reported.

POLYENDOCRINE SYNDROMES

Two major syndromes associated with multiple endocrine autoimmune disorders can be distinguished: polyendocrine syndrome type I and polyendocrine type II syndrome. The type I syndrome usually presents in infancy. Characteristically affected individuals (often sibling pairs) have hypoparathyroidism, Addison's disease, or mucocutaneous candidiasis singly or in combination. It is rare for individuals with type II to have hypoparathyroidism or mucocutaneous candidiasis. Addison's disease is a prominent component of both syndromes. There are many other associated disorders (eg, type I diabetes, myasthenia gravis, celiac disease, vitiligo, pernicious anemia, and, for type I, hepatitis). Type I syndrome appears to be determined by an autosomal recessive gene without an HLA component, while the type II syndrome is strongly associated with HLA-DR3 and DR4. Disease susceptibility is inherited, and the precise disorders even in the same family cannot be predicted except for the observation that the more common the autoimmune disorder in the general population, the more likely it is that a family member will have the disease. All first-degree relatives of patients with rare disorders of these syndromes or the syndrome itself should be evaluated for associated morbid diseases. Prediction of type I diabetes in the type II syndrome is complicated by the presence of high-titer antibodies to glutamic acid decarboxylase which produce a "restricted" islet cell antibody pattern not usually associated with disease progression.

Gary S, Klingensmith GJ, Eisenbarth GS: Autoimmune polyendocrine syndromes. In: Type I Diabetes: Molecular and Cellular Immunology. Oxford Univ Press, 1994. [In press.]

THE THYROID GLAND

FETAL DEVELOPMENT OF THE THYROID

By the seventh week of intrauterine development, the thyroid gland has migrated to its ultimate location and the thyroglossal duct has atrophied. Cell differentiation and function progress over the next 7 weeks, and by the 14th week the thyroid is capable of hormone synthesis. At this stage, thyroid-stimulating hormone (TSH) is detectable in the fetal serum and pituitary gland.

Under normal conditions, neither TSH nor thyroid hormones cross the placenta in appreciable amounts, and the fetal pituitary-thyroid axis functions independently of the maternal pituitary-thyroid axis. Antithyroid drugs, including radioactive iodine, freely cross the placenta, and goitrous hypothyroid newborns may be born to hyperthyroid mothers who undergo treatment during pregnancy.

Although maternal TSH does not reach the fetus, pregnant hyperthyroid or previously hyperthyroid mothers may transmit human-specific thyroid stimulator immunoglobulin (HTSI) transplacentally, re-

sulting in thyrotoxic newborns who may develop goiter and exophthalmos. Because HTSI may be present in the serum of "controlled," previously hyperthyroid mothers, the possible transmission of HTSI should be considered in all mothers in whom hyperthyroidism is or has been present.

Physiology

Pituitary TSH stimulates the thyroid gland to take up iodine, synthesize mono- and diiodotyrosine, and release active thyroid hormones into the circulation.

The quantity released is regulated by a negative feedback mechanism involving pituitary TSH and "free" thyroid hormone (Figure 30–1).

Active hormone produced in excess of physiologic needs is stored within the thyroid follicles as colloid. Upon release into the circulation, T_4 and T_3 are bound to thyroid hormone-binding globulin (TBG), albumin, and prealbumin. The binding affinity of TBG for T_4 is approximately 20 times greater than that for T_3. A small percentage (1%) of T_3 and T_4 is not bound but is "free" and exists in equilibrium with the "bound" form. In the peripheral tissues, T_4 is deiodinated to either T_3 (active) or reverse T_3 (inactive), and the physiologic activity of thyroid hormone depends primarily on the amount of free T_3 presented to the cells. In the fetus, the majority of T_4 is converted to reverse T_3.

Synthesis, Release, Binding, & Transport of Thyroid Hormone & Its Function

The principal functions of the thyroid gland are to synthesize and store T_4 and T_3 and to release them in response to bodily needs. A number of chemical reactions are involved in thyroid hormone formation. The thyroid gland is regulated and stimulated by TSH; HTSI is important only in hyperthyroid states. TSH production may be inhibited by either endogenous or exogenous thyroid hormone. At birth, the T_4 approximates that of the mother. There is a rapid increase of

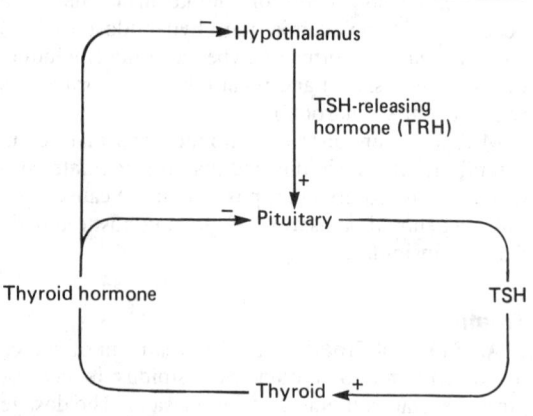

Figure 30–1. Pituitary-thyroid control.

T_4 during the second to fifth days of life in response to a TSH surge resulting from umbilical cord clamping and then a gradual decrease over several weeks or months.

The total T_4 is low in various forms of hypothyroidism and may be reduced in premature infants (particularly those with sepsis or respiratory distress), subacute and chronic thyroiditis, hypopituitarism, nephrosis, cirrhosis, hypoproteinemia, malnutrition, and following therapy with T_3. Prolonged administration of high doses of adrenocorticosteroids—as well as sulfonamides, testosterone, phenytoin, and salicylates—may also produce a decrease in total T_4. TSH and "free" T_4 levels remain in the normal range. The total T_3 and T_4 are high in hyperthyroidism and may be elevated in the acute forms of thyroiditis and acute hepatitis; in some types of inborn errors in the synthesis, release, or binding of thyroid hormone; following the administration of estrogens or clofibrate or during pregnancy; and following the administration of various iodine-containing globulins.

TBG is increased in pregnancy, after estrogen therapy (including oral contraceptives), occasionally as a genetic variation, in certain hepatic disorders, following administration of phenothiazines, and occasionally from an unknown cause. TBG is decreased in familial TBG deficiency; following the administration of glucocorticoids, androgens, or anabolic steroids; in nephrotic syndrome with marked hypoproteinemia; in some forms of hepatic disease; in patients receiving phenytoin; and as an idiopathic finding. T_3, which appears to be the active thyroid hormone, acts fairly rapidly and has a shorter duration of action. Receptors for T_3 are present in the cell membrane, mitochondria, and nucleus and within the cytosol; the physiologic action of thyroid hormone is complex.

HYPOTHYROIDISM
(Congenital & Acquired Hypothyroidism)

Essentials of Diagnosis

- Growth retardation, diminished physical activity, impaired tissue perfusion, constipation, thick tongue, poor muscle tone, hoarseness, anemia; intellectual retardation if hypothyroid untreated in infancy.
- Delayed dental and skeletal maturation.
- Thyroid function studies low (TT_4, FT_4, and T_3 resin uptake); TSH levels elevated in primary hypothyroidism.
- *Note:* The combination of physical findings in the newborn and early discharge from the nursery underscores the importance of the newborn screening procedure.

General Considerations

Thyroid hormone deficiency may be either congenital (with or without the physical features of cretinism) or acquired (juvenile hypothyroidism) and has many causes (see Tables 30–3 and 30–4). In the majority of these cases in childhood, particularly in the presence of a history of goiter, hypothyroidism is the result of chronic lymphocytic thyroiditis (see Thyroiditis, below).

Various types of enzymatic defects have been described (Table 30–4) that result from inborn errors of metabolism. With the exception of the defects associated with congenital nerve deafness (Pendred's syndrome), there are no distinguishing clinical features among the various types. In children who have enzymatic defects, thyroid enlargement may not be present in the newborn period but generally occurs within the first 2 decades of life. Enzymatic defects have a familial autosomal recessive inheritance pattern. Although thyroid function tests (including radioactive iodide uptake studies) may be helpful in diagnosis, final clarification of the defect generally requires chromatographic fractionation of iodinated compounds in the serum, urine, and thyroid tissue.

Several drugs and goitrogens taken during pregnancy (eg, cabbage, soybeans, aminosalicylic acid, thiourea derivatives, resorcinol, phenylbutazone, cobalt, and iodides in therapeutic doses for asthma—particularly in individuals who have also received adrenocortical steroids) have been reported to cause goiter and, in some instances, hypothyroidism. Because many of these agents cross the placenta freely, they should be used with great caution during preg-

Table 30–3. Physiologic disturbances of the thyroid gland may be due to the causes listed below, of which only the first is common:

(1) Decreased thyroid tissue: hypofunction may result from congenital aplasia or hypoplasia, destruction due to inflammatory disease (thyroiditis), neoplasm, thyroidectomy, or irradiation.

(2) Inborn errors in the synthesis of thyroid hormone: Defects may occur in any of the metabolic steps outlined in the text as well as the binding and release of T_4 and T_3 from thyroglobulin.

(3) Iodine deficiency.

(4) Inhibition of thyroidal iodide uptake and concentration by drugs (eg, thiocyanates, perchlorates, lithium nitrates).

(5) Interference with thyroid enzyme activity by antithyroid compounds. Antithyroid compounds include thiourea, thiouracil and its derivatives, cobalt, large doses of iodides, and certain foods such as cabbage, turnips, and soybeans. Iodides also interfere with the release of thyroid hormone.

(6) Disorders of the hypothalamus and pituitary gland that result in impairment of either thyrotropin-releasing hormone (TRH) or thyrotropin secretion.

(7) Defects in the peripheral tissue conversion of T_4 to T_3.

(8) Absence of or alteration in tissue receptors for thyroid hormones.

Table 30–4. Causes of hypothyroidism.

A. Congenital (cretinism):
  1. Aplasia, hypoplasia, or associated with maldescent of thyroid—
    a. Embryonic defect of development.
    b. Autoimmune disease (?).
  2. Familial iodine-induced goiter secondary to metabolic inborn errors—
    a. Iodide transport defect (defect 1).
    b. Organification defect (defect 2)—
      (1) Lack of iodine peroxidase.
      (2) Lack of iodine transferase: Pendred's syndrome, associated with congenital nerve deafness
    c. Coupling defect (defect 3).
    d. Iodotyrosine deiodinase defect (defect 4).
    e. Abnormal iodinated polypeptide (defects 5a and 5b)—
      (1) Resulting from defect in intrathyroidal proteolysis of thyroglobulin.
      (2) Abnormal plasma binding preventing use of T_4 by peripheral cells.
    f. Inability of tissues to convert T_4 to T_3.
  3. Maternal ingestion of medications during pregnancy—
    a. Maternal radioiodine.
    b. Goitrogens (propylthiouracil, methimazole).
    c. Iodides.
  4. Iodide deficiency (endemic cretinism).
  5. Idiopathic.
	B. Acquired (juvenile hypothyroidism):
	  1. Thyroidectomy of radioiodine therapy for—
	    a. Thyrotoxicosis.
	    b. Cancer.
	    c. Lingual thyroid.
	    d. Isolated midline thyroid.
	  2. Destruction by x-ray.
	  3. Thyrotropin deficiency—
	    a. Isolated.
	    b. Associated with other pituitary tropic hormone deficiencies.
	  4. TRH deficiency due to hypothalamic injury or disease.
	  5. Autoimmune disease (lymphocytic thyroiditis).
	  6. Chronic infections.
	  7. Medications—
	    a. Iodides—
	      (1) Prolonged, excessive ingestion.
	      (2) Deficiency.
	    b. Cobalt.
	  8. Idiopathic.

nancy. If these agents are taken by pregnant women, the goiter and decreased thyroid function that are produced in the newborn are generally transient and seldom a problem.

Several hundred patients with clinical and laboratory features of resistance to thyroid hormone have been described. These syndromes are generally familial and are classified on the basis of the site of the resistance (eg, generalized; pituitary or peripheral tissue [see Refetoff et al, 1993]).

Clinical Findings

The severity of the findings in cases of thyroid deficiency depends on the age at onset and the degree of deficiency of production of thyroid hormone.

A. Symptoms and Signs:

1. Functional changes–Even with congenital absence of the thyroid gland, the first finding may not appear for several days or weeks. Findings include physical and mental sluggishness; pale, gray, cool, or mottled skin; nonpitting myxedema; decreased intestinal activity (constipation); large tongue; poor muscle tone, giving rise to a protuberant abdomen, umbilical hernia, and lumbar lordosis; hypothermia; bradycardia; diminished sweating (variable); decreased pulse pressure; hoarse voice or cry; delayed transient deafness; and a slow relaxation component of deep tendon reflexes (best appreciated in the ankles). Nasal obstruction and discharge and persistent jaundice may be present in the neonatal period.

The skin may be dry, thick, scaly, and coarse, with a yellowish tinge due to excessive deposition of car-

otene. The hair is dry, coarse, and brittle (variable) and may be excessive. Lateral thinning of the eyebrows may occur. The axillary and supraclavicular fat pads may be prominent in infants. Muscular hypertrophy (Kocher-Debré-Semelaigne syndrome) is an unusual and poorly understood presentation.

2. Retardation of growth and development–Findings include shortness of stature; infantile skeletal proportions with relatively short extremities; infantile naso-orbital configuration (bridge of nose flat, broad, and underdeveloped; eyes seem to be widely spaced); delayed epiphysial development; delayed closure of fontanelles; and retarded dental eruption. Treatment of acquired hypothyroidism may not result in the predicted final adult target height. In hypothyroidism resulting from enzymatic defects, ingestion of goitrogens, or chronic lymphocytic thyroiditis, the thyroid gland may be enlarged. Thyroid enlargement in children is usually symmetric, and the gland is moderately firm and without nodularity. In chronic lymphocytic thyroiditis, however, a cobblestone surface frequently is present; size and shape are apparent on inspection in children. Slowing of mental responsiveness and retardation of development of the brain may occur in neonates and infants, and in many cases a coincidental congenital malformation of the brain is present also.

3. Alterations in sexual development (usually retardation, sometimes precocity)–Menometrorrhagia may be seen in older girls; galactorrhea has been reported.

B. Laboratory Findings: Total T_4 and FT_4 are

decreased. Radioiodine uptake is below 10% (normal: 10–50%).* The binding of T_3 by erythrocytes or resin in vitro (T_3RU test) is lowered. With primary hypothyroidism, the plasma TSH is elevated. A normocytic anemia is common, but microcytic or macrocytic anemia may occur because of decreased iron, folate, and cobalamin absorption. Serum cholesterol and carotene are usually elevated in childhood but may be low or normal in infants. Cessation of therapy in previously treated hypothyroid patients produces a marked rise in serum cholesterol levels in 6–8 weeks. Urinary creatine excretion is decreased, and urinary hydroxyproline is low. Serum alkaline phosphatase is occasionally reduced. Circulating autoantibodies to thyroid constituents may be present. Erythrocyte glucose-6-phosphate dehydrogenase activity is decreased. Plasma growth hormone may be decreased, with subnormal response to insulin-induced hypoglycemia and arginine stimulation.

C. Imaging: Epiphysial development ("bone age") is delayed. Centers of ossification, especially of the hip, may show multiple small centers or a single, stippled, porous, or fragmented center (epiphysial dysgenesis). Vertebrae may show anterior beaking. Cardiomegaly is common. Coxa vara and coxa plana may occur.

Screening Programs for Neonatal Hypothyroidism

Congenital hypothyroidism may be clinically recognized during the first month of life or may be so mild that it remains unrecognized clinically for months. Every effort should be made to establish the diagnosis of hypothyroidism as early as possible, because untreated hypothyroidism may be associated with irreversible damage to the central nervous system. Adequate treatment initiated prior to the second or third month of life is associated with a favorable prognosis. Mandatory screening programs for newborn infants facilitate prompt diagnosis (within 30–60 days after birth) and therapy of congenital hypothyroidism. Screening programs utilize either T_4 or TSH or both.

Differential Diagnosis

The various causes of primary hypothyroidism due to intrinsic defects of the thyroid gland must be differentiated from pituitary and hypothalamic failure with secondary thyroid insufficiency. As a practical matter, TSH and free T_4 levels are the most useful and are usually sufficient in directing treatment or the need for further investigations.

Down's syndrome, chondrodystrophy, generalized gangliosidosis, I-cell disease, Hurler's and Hunter's syndromes, and certain other causes of short stature and coarse features can all be readily distinguished by the clinical manifestations and by appropriate laboratory studies.

Treatment

Levothyroxine is the drug of choice in a dose of 100 $\mu g/m^2$ once daily. In newborns and infants, a dose of 10–12 $\mu g/kg$ is employed; a dose of 0.025 mg (25 μg) of levothyroxine is used initially and subsequently increased to the final dose in 1–2 weeks. Serum T_4 or free T_4 and TSH levels should be used as a guide to adequate therapy.

The hypothyroid patient may be quite responsive to thyroid and may be sensitive to slight excesses of thyroid hormone. After therapy is started, improvement in 7–21 days can be anticipated.

Triiodothyronine may be employed when a more rapid and short-lived effect is desired (eg, in the TSH suppression test) but probably is not as effective for maintenance therapy as levothyroxine. In the treatment of neonatal goiter with or without hypothyroidism resulting from drugs and goitrogens taken by the pregnant woman, temporary use of levothyroxine may be helpful in decreasing the size of the goiter.

Fisher DA: Management of congenital hypothyroidism. J Clin Endocrinol Metab 1991;72:523.

Glorieux J et al: Useful parameters to predict the eventual mental outcome of hypothyroid children. Pediatr Res 1988;24:6.

Rivkees SA, Bode HH, Crawford JD: Long-term growth in juvenile acquired hypothyroidism: The failure to achieve normal adult stature. N Engl J Med 1988;318:599.

Refetoff S, Weiss RE, Usala SJ: The syndrome of resistance to thyroid hormones. Endocr Rev 1993;14:348.

Sklar CA, Qazi R, David R: Juvenile autoimmune thyroiditis: Hormonal status at presentation after long-term follow-up. Am J Dis Child 1986;140:877.

THYROIDITIS

With the exception of chronic lymphocytic thyroiditis (Hashimoto's disease), the forms of thyroiditis listed in Table 30–5 are uncommon in childhood. In contrast, Hashimoto's disease is perhaps the most common endocrine condition in pediatric patients, particularly in adolescent females.

1. ACUTE SUPPURATIVE THYROIDITIS

Acute thyroiditis is rare and generally is thought to result from seeding of oropharyngeal organisms via a patent foramen cecum and thyroglossal duct track. As a result, the most common pathogens are group A streptococci, pneumococci, *Staphylococcus aureus,* and anaerobes. The patient is invariably toxic, and the thyroid gland is exquisitely tender. There may be ra-

---

*The presence of iodides in bread has resulted in a significant decrease in previous values of radioiodine uptake. The normal levels for any particular age group and area should be ascertained.

Table 30–5. Causes of thyroiditis.

I. Thyroiditis due to infectious agents.
  A. Acute bacterial thyroiditis (acute suppurative thyroiditis).
  B. Subacute viral thyroiditis (nonsuppurative, or De Quervain's, thyroiditis).
  C. Chronic or recurring thyroiditis.
II. Thyroiditis due to autoimmunity (chronic lymphocytic, or Hashimoto's, thyroiditis).
III. Thyroiditis due to physical agents.
  A. Radiation.
  B. Trauma.
IV. Thyroiditis of unknown etiology.
  A. Riedel's thyroiditis.

diation of pain to the ear or chest. There is usually no consistently associated endocrine disturbance. Specific antibiotic therapy should be administered.

2. SUBACUTE NONSUPPURATIVE THYROIDITIS

Subacute thyroiditis (de Quervain's thyroiditis) is rare in the USA. In most cases, the cause is a virus (mumps, influenza, echovirus, coxsackievirus, Epstein-Barr virus, or adenovirus). Presenting features are similar to those of acute thyroiditis: fever, malaise, sore throat, dysphagia, pain in the thyroid gland that may radiate to the ears, and mild and transient manifestations of hypermetabolism. In contrast to acute thyroiditis, the onset is generally insidious. The thyroid gland is firm, and the enlargement may be confined to one lobe. Radioiodine uptake is usually reduced, but thyroid hormone levels in the blood are normal or elevated. The differentiation from bacterial thyroiditis may be difficult, so antibiotic therapy may be necessary.

3. CHRONIC LYMPHOCYTIC THYROIDITIS
(Chronic Autoimmune Thyroiditis, Hashimoto's Thyroiditis, Lymphadenoid Goiter)

Essentials of Diagnosis

- Firm, freely movable, nontender, and diffusely enlarged goiter.
- T_4 generally normal but may be elevated or decreased, depending on the stage of the disease.

General Considerations

Chronic lymphocytic thyroiditis is being seen with increasing frequency in all age groups and currently is the most common cause of goiter and hypothyroidism in childhood. In children and adolescents, the incidence peaks between the ages of 8 and 15 years and occurs most commonly in females (4:1 ratio). The disease is the result of an autoimmune attack on the thyroid. Susceptibility to thyroid autoimmunity (and other endocrine autoimmune disorders, type I diabetes, etc) is associated with inheritance of certain histocompatibility alleles.

Clinical Findings

A. Symptoms and Signs: The goiter is characteristically firm, freely movable, nontender, "pebbly" in consistency, and diffusely enlarged, though it may be asymmetric. In long-standing cases, nodules and, rarely, malignant changes have been described. The onset is usually insidious. Most cases occur without clinical manifestations and are completely painless. Occasionally, a sensation of tracheal compression or fullness, hoarseness, and dysphagia are described by the patient. There are no local signs of inflammation and no evidence of systemic infection.

B. Laboratory Findings: Laboratory findings are variable. Levels of T_4, free T_4 and T_3 resin uptake are usually normal but may be elevated or depressed. TSH levels may be slightly elevated. Thyroid antibodies are usually present, though sometimes at low levels. A variety of abnormalities in radioactive iodide uptake studies have been described; thyroid scans usually show a diffuse or patchy pattern, and cold nodules have been reported. Thyroid scans and uptake studies add little to the diagnosis. Surgical or needle biopsy is diagnostic but seldom indicated.

Treatment

The treatment of choice for autoimmune thyroiditis is thyroid hormone in full therapeutic doses (levothyroxine, 100 $\mu g/m^2/d$). Approximately two-thirds of patients will have some decrease in the size of the goiter within 3 months. Hypothyroidism is believed to be a common end result of autoimmune thyroiditis in the second to third decades of life.

4. RIEDEL'S STRUMA
(Chronic Fibrous Thyroiditis, Woody Thyroiditis, Invasive Thyroiditis)

Riedel's struma is extremely rare in the USA, particularly in children. It is characterized by marked and invasive fibrosis that extends beyond the thyroid gland to involve the trachea, esophagus, blood vessels, nerves, and muscles of the neck, so that the gland becomes fixed to these tissues. Surgery is necessary to ascertain that carcinoma is not the cause and to relieve fibrotic obstruction or constriction of neighboring structures.

Mäenpää J et al: Natural course of juvenile autoimmune thyroiditis. J Pediatr 1985;10:898.

Rich EJ, Mendelman PM: Acute suppurative thyroiditis in pediatric patients. Pediatr Infect Dis J 1987;6:936.

Weetman AP, McGregor AM: Autoimmune thyroid disease: Developments in our understanding. Endocr Rev 1984;5:309.

HYPERTHYROIDISM

Essentials of Diagnosis

- Nervousness, irritability, emotional lability, tremor, excessive appetite, weight loss, smooth and warm skin, increased perspiration, and heat intolerance.
- Goiter, exophthalmos, tachycardia, increased pulse pressure.
- Thyroid function studies elevated (eg, TT_4, FT_4 T_3, radioiodine uptake). TSH level suppressed.

General Considerations

While the cause of hyperthyroidism has not been precisely determined; abnormalities in the immune system are operative in the pathophysiology. The association of hyperthyroidism and certain additional diseases that have an autoimmune basis and a familial pattern with a predilection for females supports the supposition that a heritable and autoimmune basis exists. Human-specific thyroid stimulator immunoglobulin (HTSI), an IgG antibody to thyroid receptors that stimulates thyroid hormone production, has been identified. Since HTSI is an IgG, it may cross the placenta from a thyrotoxic mother and affect the fetus and neonate. Transient congenital hyperthyroidism may occur in infants of thyrotoxic mothers. Hyperthyroidism may be associated with chronic thyroiditis, tumors of the thyroid, other tumors producing thyrotropin-like substances, and exogenous thyroid hormone excess.

Clinical Findings

A. Symptoms and Signs: Hyperthyroidism is five times as common in females as in males. The disease is most likely to appear in childhood at age 12–14 years; only 20% of cases present before 10 years of age. The course of hyperthyroidism tends to be cyclic, with spontaneous remissions and exacerbations. A deterioration in school performance is a common presenting feature. Findings include weakness, dyspnea, dysphagia, emotional instability, "nervousness," marked variability in mood, personality disturbances, and tremors and movements that may simulate chorea. The skin is warm and moist, the face is flushed. Palpitations, tachycardia, and systolic hypertension with increased pulse pressure are common. Proptosis and exophthalmos are common in hyperthyroid children. Goiter is present in more than 90% of cases and is characteristically diffuse and usually firm. A bruit and thrill may be present. Variable degrees of accelerated growth and development occur, and loss of weight is common despite polyphagia. (An occasional adolescent may gain weight.)

Amenorrhea may occur in adolescent girls. In neonatal hyperthyroidism, hepatosplenomegaly and thrombocytopenia with antiplatelet antibodies is common.

B. Laboratory Findings: The T_4, T_3 resin uptake, and free T_4 are elevated except in rare cases in which only the blood T_3 level is elevated ("T_3 thyrotoxicosis"). Radioiodine uptake is above 35–40% at 24 hours and suppressed less than 40% after administration of T_3 (25 μg three or four times daily for 7 days). The basal metabolic rate is elevated, but the BMR test is frequently unreliable and is seldom used. Serum cholesterol is low; glycosuria may occur. Agglutinating antibodies of thyroglobulin are found in most patients. Circulating TSH concentrations measured by very sensitive assays are depressed (< 0.5 μU/mL), and HTSI is often present in plasma.

C. Imaging: Epiphysial maturation assessed radiographically is advanced in younger children. In newborns, accelerated bony maturation may be associated with subsequent premature closure of the cranial sutures. Long-standing hyperthyroidism is associated with osteoporosis.

Differential Diagnosis

Although the well-established case of hyperthyroidism seldom presents a problem in diagnosis, the findings in the early stages of the disease may be confused with chorea or, more commonly, with euthyroid goiter. Typically, the patient is an adolescent with a recent decline in school performance, nervousness, emotional lability, and increased perspiration. Careful and sometimes repeated clinical and laboratory evaluation may be required before a definitive diagnosis is established. Various disease states associated with hypermetabolism (severe anemia, leukemia, chronic infections, pheochromocytoma, as well as muscle-wasting disease) may occasionally be confused with hyperthyroidism, but differentiation is readily made by the appropriate laboratory studies.

Treatment

The course of hyperthyroidism may exhibit fluctuations of improvement and remission. In some mild cases, therapy may not be required.

Both surgical and medical methods are available for treating the manifestations of hyperthyroidism.

A. General Measures: Bed rest is advisable only in severe cases, in preparation for surgery, or at the beginning of a medical regimen. The diet should be high in calories, carbohydrates, and vitamins (particularly vitamin B_1).

B. Medical Treatment: With medical treatment, clinical response may be noted in 2–3 weeks, and adequate control may be achieved in 2–3 months. The thyroid frequently increases in size after initiation of treatment but usually decreases in size within several months.

1. Propranolol–This β-adrenergic blocking agent may be useful in controlling symptoms of nervous instability and tachycardia. In mild cases, propranolol without other antithyroid treatment may be adequate. Propranolol may also be helpful in controlling life-threatening cardiac complications that may occur in thyroid storm (severe thyrotoxicosis, fever, and altered consciousness). In large doses, propranolol decreases the peripheral conversion of T_4 to T_3.

2. Propylthiouracil–This drug interferes with the intrathyroidal hormonogenesis and in large doses the peripheral conversion of T_4 to T_3. The correct dose must always be individually determined. Propylthiouracil is frequently used in the initial treatment of children with hyperthyroidism. Short-term therapy is occasionally successful, but treatment usually must be continued for at least 2–3 years with the smallest drug dosage that will produce a euthyroid state. If T_4 levels rise rapidly with reduction in drug dosage after 18–24 months of therapy, continued or alternative therapy will be necessary; relapses occur in 10–30% of cases, and severe cases may not respond. The safety of prolonged treatment has not been evaluated.

a. Initial dosage–Give 75–300 mg/d in three or four divided doses 6–8 hours apart until tests of thyroid function are normal and all signs and symptoms have subsided. Larger doses are frequently necessary.

b. Maintenance–Give 50–100 mg/d in two or three divided doses. Some authors recommend continuing the drug at higher levels until the euthyroid state is approached or reached and then, as the TSH level rises, adding thyroid hormone. If goiter develops or persists after 2–3 months with propylthiouracil therapy, T_4 and TSH levels should be obtained to determine whether the patient is becoming hypothyroid; thyroid hormone is added when indicated.

c. Toxicity–Granulocytopenia, fever, rash, and arthralgia may occur. The drug must be discontinued, and antibiotics and a short course of one of the adrenocorticosteroids should be prescribed if indicated.

3. Methimazole–This drug may be used in one-fifteenth to one-tenth the dosage of propylthiouracil and may be effective with a twice-daily dosage schedule. However, toxic reactions may be more common with methimazole than with propylthiouracil.

4. Iodide–Medical treatment with continuous iodide administration alone usually produces a rapid but brief response. Because the efficacy of iodide is short-lived, it is generally recommended only for acute management. A progressive increase in dosage is often required for satisfactory control, and toxic reactions to iodide are not uncommon.

C. Radiation Therapy: Radioactive iodide (^{131}I) is currently being used as initial therapy for children and adolescents. Reports do not support the fear of an increased incidence of thyroid cancer, particularly when an ablative dose of ^{131}I is employed. Therapy with thyroid hormone is necessary after thyroid ablation.

D. Surgical Measures: Subtotal thyroidectomy is considered by some to be the treatment of choice, especially when a close follow-up of the patient is difficult or impossible. In childhood, surgery should be employed in patients when medical treatment is impossible or has been unsuccessful. The patient should be prepared first with bed rest, diet, and propranolol (as above) and with iodide and propylthiouracil as follows: Propylthiouracil (as above) should be given for 2–4 weeks. Iodide (as saturated solution of potassium iodide) is added 10–21 days before surgery is scheduled. Iodides act by blocking the effect of TSH on the thyroid, with a resultant decrease in iodine trapping and reduction of vascularity, and by inhibiting the release of hormone, thus reducing the possibility of thyroid storm. Give 1–10 drops daily for 10–21 days. Continue the drug for 1 week after surgery.

Management of Congenital (Transient) Hyperthyroidism

Congenital hyperthyroidism has a significant death rate in the neonatal period, but the eventual prognosis in surviving infants is excellent. Temporary treatment of congenital hyperthyroidism may be necessary, in which case iodides appear to be the drug of choice. Reserpine or propranolol may be necessary to control cardiac arrhythmias. Transection of an enlarged thyroid isthmus may be of value if respiratory distress due to tracheal compression is present.

Course & Prognosis

Improvement may occur without therapy in as many as one-third of cases, but partial remissions and exacerbations may continue for several years. With medical treatment alone, prolonged remissions may be expected in one-half to two-thirds of cases. Surgical therapy yields similar results. Postoperative hypothyroidism is not uncommon, and hypoparathyroidism and other complications may occur. Because of the comparatively high incidence of carcinoma in nodular goiters of childhood, such glands should be removed routinely once the thyrotoxicosis is in remission. Progressive exophthalmos following surgery is uncommon in childhood.

Becker DV: Choice of therapy for Graves' hyperthyroidism. (Editorial.) N Engl J Med 1984;311:464.

Burros GN: Hyperthyroidism during pregnancy. N Engl J Med 1978;298:150.

Collen RJ et al: Remission rates of children and adolescents with thyrotoxicosis treated with antithyroid drugs. Pediatrics 1980;65:550.

Heshizume K et al: Administration of thyroxine in treated Graves' disease. N Engl J Med 1991;324:947.

Levy WJ, Schumacher OP, Gupta M: Treatment of childhood Graves' disease. Cleve Clin J Med 1988;55:373.

CARCINOMA OF THE THYROID

Carcinoma of the thyroid is uncommon in childhood. The presentation is usually with asymptomatic asymmetric thyroid enlargement. Neck discomfort, dysphagia, voice changes, and respiratory difficulty are unusual but may occur. Fifty percent of children have metastatic disease at the time of presentation, usually to regional lymph nodes. Pulmonary metastasis occurs in 5% of cases.

Thyroid function tests are normal. Thyroid carcinoma may elaborate thyroglobulin; if present, it is a useful tumor marker. A technetium or iodine scan of the thyroid shows a "cold" nodule and is the most definitive diagnostic test. Pulmonary metastases should be excluded by a CT scan of the chest.

Papillary carcinoma is the most common form in childhood, and the prognosis with treatment is relatively good, with a survival rate greater than 80% after 10–20 years. The treatment of choice is surgical extirpation of the entire gland and removal of all involved lymph nodes. Radical neck dissection is usually not indicated. If metastatic disease is not identified at surgery, replacement thyroid hormone is generally the only further therapy required. Follow-up thyroid scans every 2–5 years are recommended.

Other, less common malignant tumors of the thyroid include follicular, medullary, and undifferentiated carcinomas, lymphomas, and sarcomas. Medullary carcinoma of the thyroid may be familial (autosomal dominant), usually occurring as a component of type 2 multiple endocrine neoplasia. Thus, this condition may be associated with excessive elaboration of gastrin and calcitonin, with pheochromocytoma, parathyroid hyperplasia, "marfanoid habitus," and mucosal neuromas. The treatment and prognosis depend upon the cell type present, but the outcome is generally less favorable.

Gagel RF et al: Medullary thyroid carcinoma: Recent progress. J Clin Endocrinol Metab 1993;76:809.

Samuel AM, Sharma SM: Differentiated thyroid carcinomas in children and adolescents. Cancer 1991;67:2168.

DISORDERS OF CALCIUM HOMEOSTASIS

Parathyroid hormone (PTH) and vitamin D are the principal hormonal factors in the human that maintain calcium homeostasis. These agents exert their action primarily in bone, small intestine, and kidney. The integrated action of PTH and vitamin D maintains the serum calcium level within a narrow normal range and contributes to normal bone mineralization. Deficiencies and excesses of these agents—as well as abnormalities in their receptors or in the metabolic transformation of vitamin D—lead to the clinical disturbances described below and shown in Tables 30–6 and 30–7. Less important calciotropic factors (eg, calcitonin, magnesium, and phosphorus) also influence calcium homeostasis.

HYPOPARATHYROIDISM

Essentials of Diagnosis

- Tetany with numbness, tingling, cramps, spontaneous muscle contractures, carpopedal spasm, positive Trousseau and Chvostek signs, loss of consciousness, convulsions.
- Diarrhea, photophobia, prolongation of electrical systole (QT interval) and laryngospasm.
- Defective nails and teeth, cataracts, and calcific bodies in the subcutaneous tissues and basal ganglia.
- Serum and urine calcium normal or low; serum phosphorus high; urine phosphorus low; alkaline phosphatase normal or low; azotemia absent. Inappropriately low ratio of PTH to ionized calcium.

General Considerations

Bone and kidney are the target organs of PTH, and most of the hormonal effects are mediated by interaction with a plasma membrane-bound receptor and activation of the adenylyl cyclase complex—a complex consisting of at least three distinct proteins. Manifestations of PTH deficiency (Table 30–6) result either from an absolute deficiency in the hormone or from "resistant states" related to abnormalities of the receptor complex of the PTH molecule. Hypoparathyroidism may be idiopathic or may result from an autoimmune phenomenon or from parathyroidectomy. Hypoparathyroidism may develop following thyroidectomy, with either an acute or an insidious onset, and may be transient or permanent. Parathyroid deficiency has been reported following irradiation of the neck or the administration of therapeutic doses of radioactive iodine for carcinoma of the thyroid. Two types of transient hypoparathyroidism may be present in the newborn, both of which are due to a relative deficiency of PTH or hormone action. An early form occurs within the first 2 weeks of life in newborns with a history of birth asphyxia or those born to mothers with diabetes mellitus or hyperparathyroidism. Hypomagnesemia may also be seen in the early form and augments the severity of hypocalcemia. The more common later form occurs almost exclusively in infants fed a milk formula with a high phosphate:calcium ratio. In this group, episodes of tetany are often precipitated by febrile illnesses.

Autoimmune hypoparathyroidism with demonstrable antibodies to parathyroid tissue may be associated with candidal infection, Addison's disease, diabetes

Table 30-6. Parathyroid deficiency states.

Disease or Condition	Synonym	Inheritance Pattern	Major Clinical Features	Metabolic Features							
				Serum Concentration				Urinary Excretion			
								Basal Conditions		Response to Parathyroid Hormone[3]	
				Ca²⁺	P	Alk Ptase	PTH	Ca²⁺	P	P	Cyclic AMP
"Idiopathic" (spontaneous), surgical, or "autoimmune" hypoparathyroidism	Autoimmune polyendocrinopathy. Thyroiditis and hypoparathyroidism (Schmidt's syndrome). Absence of parathyroid glands and thymic aplasia (DiGeorge's syndrome)	Familial is autoimmune type and associated with certain HLA types	Tetany, seizures, photophobia, diarrhea, positive Chvostek and Trousseau signs, candidiasis. In autoimmune type, other autoimmune diseases (eg, adrenal insufficiency, thyroiditis, pernicious anemia, diabetes mellitus).	↓(N)	↑	↓(N)	↓	N(↑,↓)	↓	N	N
Pseudohypoparathyroidism and pseudopseudohypoparathyroidism	Albright's syndrome	X-linked dominant	Brachymetacarpal and metatarsal short stature; mental subnormality; ectopic calcification of lenses, basal ganglia, and subcutaneous tissue.	↓(N)	↑(N)	↓↑(N)	↑	↓(N)	↓	↓	↓
Pseudohypoparathyroidism type II	PTH unresponsiveness	Unknown	Seizures. Phenotype normal.	↓	↑		↑	↓	↓	↓	N
Pseudohypohyperparathyroidism with osteitis fibrosa[1]	Renal resistance to parathyroid hormone with osteitis fibrosa[1]	Probably familial	Clinical features of hypocalcemia. Phenotype normal.	↓	↓	↓	↓	N(↑)	↓(N)	↑	↑
Pseudoidiopathic hypoparathyroidism[2]			Clinical features of hypoparathyroidism. Phenotype normal.	↓	↑	↓↓	↓↓	↑	↑	↑	N

[1] The opposite (ie, skeletal unresponsiveness to PTH with normal renal responsiveness) has been described.
[2] Structural anomaly of PTH molecule has been proposed.
[3] Parathyroid hormone is not commercially available for testing.

Table 30–7. Rickets and disorders of calcium metabolism.[1]

Disease or Condition	Synonym	Inheritance Pattern	Clinical Features	Metabolic Features						Treatment
				Serum Concentrations				Urinary Excretion		
				Ca²⁺	P	Alk Ptase	PTH	Ca²⁺	P	
Hypoparathyroid states	See Table 30–6.			↓						Vitamin D and calcium
Transient tetany of the newborn			Tetany, focal seizures. More common in prematures and infants of diabetic mothers. Rarely described in association with maternal hyperparathyroidism.	↓	↓ (N)	↓ (N)	↓ (N)	↓ (N)	↑ (N)	Diet high in calcium, low in phosphate. Vitamin D may be necessary.
Malabsorption syndrome	Disease entities associated with malabsorption include cystic fibrosis, celiac disease, sprue, Shwachman syndrome; hypoplasia of cartilage and hair.	Generally familial with mode of inheritance related to specific disease	Steatorrhea, failure to thrive. Some forms associated with neutropenia, skeletal anomalies, immunologic deficiencies, and abnormalities of cartilage and hair.	↓ (N)	(N) ↓	↑ (N)	↑ (N)	↓	N (↑↓)	Vitamin D, calcium, and magnesium (hypomagnesemic states)
Chronic renal insufficiency			Growth failure, undernutrition, skeletal changes.	↓ (N)	↑	↑ (N)	↑	↓ (N)	↓	Diet high in calcium, low in phosphorus; vitamin D
Vitamin D-deficient rickets	Infantile rickets		Rickets.	↓ (N)	↓	↑	↑	↓	↓	Vitamin D and calcium
Familial hypophosphatemic vitamin D-resistant rickets[2]	(1) Hereditary vitamin D-resistant rickets (2) Phosphate diabetes (3) X-linked hypophosphatemia	X-linked dominant (occasionally autosomal dominant or sporadic)	Skeletal deformities, growth retardation.	N (↓)	↓	N	N (↑)	N	↑	Oral phosphate and vitamin D
Hereditary vitamin D-refractory rickets[3] Type I Type II	(1) Hypophosphatemic vitamin D-refractory rickets (2) Pseudo-vitamin D-deficiency rickets	Autosomal recessive	Severe rachitic bone changes; generalized aminoaciduria.	↓	↓ (N)	↑		↓	↑	Vitamin D (calciferol) in large doses or approximately physiologic doses of 1,25-dihydroxycholecalciferol

[1] Normal tubular reabsorption of phosphate (TRP) is 83–98%; the lower values are associated with higher serum levels of phosphorus. In hypoparathyroidism, TRP varies from 40 to 70%. Low values for TRP are also found in some forms of inherited renal tubular disease, eg, vitamin D-resistant rickets.

[2] A variety of diseases (cystinosis, galactosemia, tyrosinosis, Wilson's disease, hereditary fructose intolerance) are associated with renal tubular defects and should be considered in the differential diagnosis.

[3] Type I has been shown to be the result of defective renal 1α-hydroxylation of 25-hydroxycholecalciferol; type II is due to tissue unresponsiveness to normal levels of 1,25-dihydroxycholecalciferol; in this type, the vitamin D receptor complex fails to bind to DNA.

mellitus, pernicious anemia, alopecia, thyroiditis, hypogonadism, steatorrhea, and malabsorption. This form of hypoparathyroidism is often familial and is associated with certain HLA types. Infections resulting from lack of immune reaction to *Candida* (in spite of normal generalized T cell function) may lead to severe intractable cutaneous and gastrointestinal candidiasis. Because of the frequent association of adrenocortical insufficiency with parathyroid insufficiency, adrenocortical function should be tested repeatedly.

Congenital absence of the parathyroids may occur in association with congenital absence of the thymus (with resultant thymic-dependent immunologic deficiency) and cardiovascular (DiGeorge syndrome), cerebral, and ocular defects.

Clinical Findings

A. Symptoms and Signs: Prolonged hypocalcemia causes tetany (see below), photophobia, blepharospasm, and diarrhea. It may be associated with chronic conjunctivitis, cataracts, numbness of the extremities, poor dentition, skin rashes, alopecia, ectodermal dysplasias, candidal infections, "idiopathic" epilepsy, or symmetric punctate calcifications of basal ganglia. In early infancy, respiratory distress may be the presenting finding.

Tetany (hyperexcitability of the central and peripheral nervous system) is manifested by numbness, cramps, and twitchings of the extremities; carpopedal spasm and laryngospasm; a positive Chvostek sign (tapping of the face in front of the ear produces spasm of the facial muscles); a positive Trousseau sign (compression of the upper arm with a blood pressure cuff inflated to a pressure above systole for 2–4 minutes produces carpopedal spasm); unexplained bizarre behavior; irritability; loss of consciousness; convulsions; and retarded physical and mental development. Headache, vomiting, diarrhea, photophobia, increased intracranial pressure, papilledema, and pseudopapilledema may occur.

B. Laboratory Findings: (Table 30–6) Serum calcium is decreased, serum phosphorus increased, and serum alkaline phosphatase is usually low-normal. Urinary excretion of calcium and phosphorus is usually decreased but is influenced by the dietary intake. Renal clearance of phosphorus is decreased, and the maximum tubular reabsorption of phosphate falls by 12–30%. PTH levels are inappropriately reduced for the ionized calcium concentration.

C. Imaging: Soft tissue and basal ganglia calcification may occur in idiopathic hypoparathyroidism but is less common than in pseudohypoparathyroidism.

Differential Diagnosis

The differential diagnosis of hypoparathyroid states is outlined in Table 30–6. Convulsions suggest epilepsy and other chronic disorders of the central nervous system. The group of findings referable to the central nervous system (headache, vomiting, increased intracranial pressure, and convulsions) may make differentiation from brain tumor difficult.

Treatment

The objective of treatment is to maintain the serum calcium and phosphate at an approximately normal level.

A. Acute or Severe Tetany: Correct hypocalcemia immediately with calcium intravenously and orally.

Calcium lactate or carbonate is the treatment of choice for prolonged oral therapy both for raising serum calcium and lowering serum phosphate.

B. Maintenance Management of Hypoparathyroidism and Chronic Hypocalcemia:

1. Drugs–Give ergocalciferol, dihydrotachysterol, or calcitriol. Ergocalciferol may not reach its peak effect for 3–7 days, but activity of all vitamin D preparations persists for weeks or months. Careful control of dosage with frequent determinations of serum and urine calcium and of the ability to concentrate urine is essential to avoid hypercalcemia and the resultant nephrocalcinosis and potential renal damage.

2. Diet–Give a low-phosphate, high-calcium diet, with added calcium lactate or carbonate. The dose is 300–1200 mg of calcium lactate or carbonate three or four times daily with meals. Because calcium is efficiently absorbed, large doses of vitamin D are rarely necessary.

Course & Prognosis

Abnormal mineral concentrations in extracellular fluid are easily corrected, and most signs and symptoms can be ameliorated with conventional dietary and drug treatments. Central nervous system manifestations are usually reversible, and the prognosis for intellectual development is excellent. A major goal of therapy is avoidance of hypercalcemia and resultant renal damage; therefore, high doses of long-acting vitamin D preparations must be carefully monitored. Difficult therapeutic problems arise when manifestations are referable to other autoimmune diseases or when the immune defect gives rise to overgrowth of *Candida*.

Canalis E: The hormonal and local regulation of bone formation. Endocr Rev 1983;4:62.

Sanchez GJ et al: Hypercalcitonemia and hypocalcemia in acutely ill children: Studies in serum calcium, blood ionized calcium, and calcium-regulating hormones. J Pediatr 1989;114:952.

PSEUDOHYPOPARATHYROIDISM
(Albright's Syndrome
& Pseudopseudohypoparathyroidism)

Pseudohypoparathyroidism is an X-linked disease with a female:male ratio of approximately 2:1. Parathyroid hormone production is adequate, but there is a failure of response of the end organ (renal tubule, bone, or both) to the hormone. The failure of response is the result of an abnormality in the adenylyl cyclase complex, a complex consisting of at least three distinct proteins; specifically, there is a quantitative diminution in one of these units (the G unit), which is also low in other tissues. Hence, resistance to other hormones acting through the adenylyl cyclase complex (eg, ADH, TSH) has been described in pseudohypoparathyroidism.

Patients with pseudohypoparathyroidism may have the same signs and symptoms seen in hypocalcemia and the same chemical findings seen in idiopathic hypoparathyroidism (Table 30–6). In addition, these patients have round, full faces; irregularly shortened hands (with the index and third metacarpal often longer than the first, fourth, and fifth metacarpals); a short, thickset body; delayed and defective dentition; and mental retardation. The hair is dry and coarse, and nails and skin are thickened. Candidiasis has not been reported. X-ray films may show thickness of the long bones with limitation of growth at the metaphysial ends. There may be chondrodysplastic changes in the bones of the hands, demineralization of the bones, thickening of the cortices, and exostoses. Ectopic calcification of the basal ganglia and subcutaneous tissues may occur with or without abnormal serum calcium levels. Corneal and lenticular opacities may be present.

Treatment is the same as that for hypoparathyroidism.

Similar phenotypic findings may be found in **pseudopseudohypoparathyroidism,** a variant of pseudohypoparathyroidism in which the blood chemistry findings are normal. No treatment is necessary.

In both pseudo- and pseudopseudohypoparathyroidism, the parathyroid glands are hyperplastic, serum levels of PTH are elevated, and the kidneys are relatively unresponsive to PTH.

Patten JL et al: Mutation in the gene encoding the stimulatory G protein of adenylate cyclase in Albright's hereditary osteodystrophy. N Engl J Med 1990;322:1412.

Spiegel AM, Shenker A, Weinstein LS: Receptor-effector coupling by G-proteins: Implications for abnormal signal transduction. Endocr Rev 1992;13:536.

HYPERPARATHYROIDISM
& HYPERCALCEMIC STATES

Essentials of Diagnosis

- Elevated blood levels of PTH.
- Serum (and urine) ionized calcium elevated; urine phosphate high, with low or normal serum phosphate; alkaline phosphatase normal or elevated.
- Patients with short-term or mild hypercalcemia may be entirely asymptomatic; hypercalcemia is noted in laboratory screening.
- Abdominal pain, polyuria, polydipsia, hypertension, nephrocalcinosis, renal stones, intractable peptic ulcer, constipation, uremia, and pancreatitis.
- Bone pain and, rarely, pathologic fractures. X-ray film shows subperiosteal resorption, loss of the lamina dura of the teeth, renal parenchymal calcification or stones, and bone cysts or "brown tumors."
- Unusual (often bizarre) behavior and mood swings.

General Considerations

In children and adolescents, well over 80% of hypercalcemic patients have either hyperparathyroidism or a malignant tumor (Table 30–8). The latter condition is invariably associated with additional significant clinical features, and the diagnosis is readily established. Hyperparathyroidism is rare in childhood and may be primary or secondary. The most common cause of primary hyperparathyroidism is adenoma of the gland. Diffuse parathyroid hyperplasia or multiple adenoma has also been described in families. The

Table 30–8. Hypercalcemic states.

I. Primary hyperparathyroidism:
  A. Hyperplasia.
  B. Adenoma.
  C. Familial, including multiple endocrine neoplasia types I and II.
  D. Ectopic parathyroid hormone secretion.
II. Hypercalcemic states other than primary hyperparathyroidism associated with increased intestinal or renal absorption of calcium:
  A. Hypervitaminosis D (including idiopathic hypercalcemia of infancy).
  B. Familial hypercalciuric hypercalcemia.
  C. Lithium therapy.
  D. Sarcoidosis.
  E. Phosphate depletion.
  F. Aluminum intoxication.
III. Hypercalcemic states other than hyperparathyroidism associated with increased immobilization of bond mineral:
  A. Hyperthyroidism.
  B. Immobilization.
  C. Thiazides.
  D. Vitamin A intoxication.
  E. Malignant neoplasms.
    1. Ectopic parathyroid hormone secretion.
    2. Prostaglandin-secreting tumor and perhaps prostaglandin release from subcutaneous fat necrosis.
    3. Tumors metastatic to bone.
    4. Myeloma.

most common causes of the secondary form are chronic renal disease (glomerulonephritis, pyelonephritis), congenital anomalies of the genitourinary tract, or rickets. Familial hyperparathyroidism may be an isolated disease or may be associated with other endocrine neoplasias of type 1 and, rarely, type 2 multiple endocrine neoplasia (MEN) syndromes.

Clinical Findings

A. Symptoms and Signs:

1. Due to hypercalcemia–Findings include hypotonicity and weakness of muscles; apathy, mood swings, and bizarre behavior; nausea, vomiting, abdominal pain, constipation, and loss of weight; hyperextensibility of joints; and hypertension, cardiac irregularities, bradycardia, and shortening of the QT interval. Calcium deposits may occur in the cornea or conjunctiva ("band keratopathy"). Detection of this important finding may require slitlamp examination of the eye. Coma occurs rarely. Intractable peptic ulcer and pancreatitis occur in adults and rarely in children.

2. Due to increased calcium and phosphorus excretion–Findings include loss of renal concentrating ability, polyuria, polydipsia, precipitation of calcium phosphate in the renal parenchyma or as urinary calculi, and progressive renal damage.

3. Related to changes in the skeleton–There may be bone pain, osteitis fibrosa, subperiosteal absorption of phalanges, absence of lamina dura around the teeth, spontaneous fractures, and a "moth-eaten" appearance of the skull.

B. Imaging:
Bone changes may be subtle in children even when radiography shows nephrocalcinosis. When bone changes occur, the distal clavicle and middle phalanges are initially affected. Later, there is a generalized demineralization with a predilection for subperiosteal cortical bone.

Treatment

Treatment consists of complete removal of the tumor or subtotal removal of hyperplastic parathyroid glands. Preoperatively, intake of dietary calcium should be restricted and hypercalcemia controlled with normal saline infusion and nonthiazide diuretics. Postoperatively, one should observe carefully for evidence of hypocalcemic tetany; this may occur when the total serum calcium is within normal limits if a precipitous drop in calcium has occurred. The diet should be high in calcium and vitamin D.

Treatment of secondary hyperparathyroidism is directed at the underlying disease. Diminution in the absorption of phosphate with aluminum hydroxide orally is helpful. The hypocalcemia of severe renal disease (creatinine clearance < 15 mL/min) results from increased complexing with the elevated phosphate, metabolic acidosis, and impaired renal activation of vitamin D. Treatment with calcitriol has been useful in this disorder.

Course & Prognosis

The prognosis following removal of a single adenoma is excellent. The prognosis following subtotal parathyroidectomy and removal of multiple adenomas and diffuse hyperplasia or removal of an adenoma is usually good and depends on correction of the underlying defect. In patients with multiple sites of parathyroid adenoma or hyperplasia, the possibility of a familial disease (eg, multiple endocrine adenomatosis) must be considered. Because this may be either a sporadic or an autosomal dominant condition, other family members may be at risk, and genetic counseling is indicated.

A variety of drugs (excessive vitamin A or D, lithium, thiazide diuretics) may result in hypercalcemia; sarcoidosis, hyperthyroidism, and hypothyroidism are additional disease conditions associated with hypercalcemia.

Ross AJ: Parathyroid surgery in children. Prog Pediatr Surg 1991;26:48.

IDIOPATHIC FAMILIAL HYPOCALCIURIC HYPERCALCEMIA

As the name implies, this interesting condition is distinguished by low to normal urinary calcium in seemingly paradoxic association with hypercalcemia. The condition is usually familial (autosomal dominant). Patients are invariably asymptomatic, and treatment is unnecessary. The prognosis is excellent. PTH levels are mildly elevated. Since the renal response to PTH is calcium reabsorption, hypercalciuria is seen in hyperparathyroidism only when bone resorption exceeds renal calcium reabsorption. The condition appears explicable on the basis of mild hyperparathyroidism.

Page LA, Haddow JE: Self-limited neonatal hyperparathyroidism in familial hypocalciuric hypercalcemia. J Pediatr 1987;111:261.

HYPERVITAMINOSIS D

Exposure to sunlight and ingestion of vitamin D in a normal diet do not result in hypervitaminosis D and hypercalcemia, except possibly in sarcoidosis. Vitamin D intoxication is the result of ingestion of excessive amounts of vitamin D, some forms of which may be stored for months in adipose tissue.

Signs and symptoms of vitamin D-induced hypercalcemia are the same as those in other hypercalcemic states and include abdominal, renal, central nervous system, and bone findings. Renal insufficiency may be irreversible and is the result of renovascular effects of hypercalcemia and precipitation of calcium phosphate in the renal interstitial tissue. Ectopic calcification can occur in many other tissues, including the cornea and the gastric mucosa.

Treatment depends on the stage of hypercalcemic toxicity. Because of adipose tissue storage of vitamin D, several months of treatment may be necessary. Dietary intake of foods fortified with vitamin D (eg, milk) and calcium should be reduced or eliminated, if possible. Hypercalcemia can be treated with intravenous fluids and nonthiazide diuretics. Adrenocorticosteroids, salmon calcitonin, and the antineoplastic agent plicamycin have also been employed with success.

The central nervous system manifestations may be dramatic, and deaths have occurred during acute crises. Chronic brain damage in young infants has been reported. The insidious occult nature of the renal insult may result in renal insufficiency and failure by the time diagnosis is established.

IDIOPATHIC HYPERCALCEMIA OF INFANCY

Idiopathic hypercalcemia (Williams syndrome) is an uncommon disorder of infancy characterized in its severe form by peculiar ("elfin") facies (receding mandible, depressed bridge of nose, relatively large mouth, prominent eyes, occasional esotropia, and hypertelorism), failure to thrive, mental and motor retardation, cardiovascular abnormalities, irritability, purposeless movements, constipation, hypotonia, polyuria, polydipsia, and hypertension are common. Cardiac defects include supravalvular aortic stenosis, peripheral pulmonary stenosis, and aortic valve calcifications. Generalized osteosclerosis is common, and there may be premature craniosynostosis and nephrocalcinosis with evidence of urinary tract disease.

Clinical manifestations may not appear for several months after birth. Serum concentrations of 1,25-dihydroxycholecalciferol were frequently elevated in cases reported after World War II in England when excessive vitamin D was introduced into the diet. Currently, a defect in the metabolism of or responsiveness to vitamin D is postulated, rather than excessive dietary vitamin D intake and elevated serum 1,25-dihydroxycholecalciferol levels.

Treatment consists of rigid restriction of dietary calcium and vitamin D and, in severe, unresponsive cases, moderate doses of glucocorticoids.

IMMOBILIZATION HYPERCALCEMIA

Abrupt immobilization of a rapidly growing adolescent following an injury may lead to a rapid decrease in bone deposition with continued bone resorption, calcium mobilization, and hypercalcemia. For reasons that are not completely understood, immobilization may be associated with elevated parathyroid hormone levels in spite of elevated levels of ionized calcium.

HYPOPHOSPHATASIA

Hypophosphatasia is an uncommon inherited (autosomal recessive) condition characterized by a specific deficiency of alkaline phosphatase activity in serum, bone, and tissues. Radiographically, there is inadequate mineralization of epiphysial cartilage and osteoid, with localized areas of radiolucency. The disease is radiographically and histologically similar to rickets, but the lesions are not more severe in sites of rapid growth. The earlier the age at onset, the more severe the condition. Failure to thrive, feeding problems, dwarfing, hyperpyrexia, delayed dentition or premature loss of teeth, widening of the sutures, bulging fontanelles, convulsions, bony deformities indistinguishable from rickets, hyperpigmentation, conjunctival calcification, band keratopathy, and renal lesions have been reported. Premature closure of cranial sutures may occur. Calcium and phosphate concentrations in the extracellular fluid are usually normal; calcium levels, however, may be elevated. In the latter case, signs and symptoms may be similar to those of idiopathic hypercalcemia; late features include osteoporosis, osteopenia, and pseudofractures. The plasma and urine of patients and heterozygote carriers contain phosphoethanolamine in excessive amounts. In some cases, marked metaphysial irregularities may occur. A condition known as **pseudohypophosphatasia** has been described in which the clinical features of hypophosphatasia are seen in association with normal levels of alkaline phosphatase.

No specific treatment is available, but adrenocorticosteroids may be of value. The mortality rate is high in infancy. Adults are usually asymptomatic.

Russo AF et al: Characterization of the calcitonin/CGAP gene in Williams syndrome. Am J Med Genet 1991; 39:28.

THE GONADS (Ovaries & Testes)

DEVELOPMENT & PHYSIOLOGY

The gonads develop from a bipotential anlage in the genital ridge of the celomic cavity. The primordial germ cells, which will become the oocytes and spermatocytes, arise in the yolk sac and migrate to the genital ridge by the fourth week after conception, when the gonad is identifiable. Between the fourth and eighth weeks of gestation, differentiation into an ovary or testis occurs; by 7–9 weeks, the fetal testis begins to produce androgens, and granulosa cells can be identified in the ovary. Testicular androgen production at this time occurs in response to placental human chorionic gonadotropin (hCG) and is necessary for male sexual differentiation. Between 9 and 12 weeks of gestational age, the fetal pituitary starts to produce luteinizing hormone (LH) and follicle-stimulating hormone (FSH); these fetal pituitary hormones are important for gonadal development. In response to fetal gonadotropins, ovarian development proceeds, and at the time of birth, ovarian maturation has reached the follicular stage. In the testes, Leydig cell production of testosterone continues until several months after birth.

Throughout childhood, pulsatile secretion of FSH and LH occurs at 60- to 90-minute intervals and affects the output of gonadal hormones (Figure 30–2). As puberty approaches, the amplitude of the peaks increases, initially at night during sleep. As the basal LH levels rise, estrogen production from the ovaries or testosterone production from the testes increases toward adult levels.

SEXUAL DIFFERENTIATION

Normal Sexual Differentiation

For normal sexual differentiation to occur, a specific sequence of events must take place. The bipotential gonad requires at least two X chromosomes to develop into an ovary; in the absence of a second X chromosome, a fibrous streak develops along the genital ridge. In the presence of the testicular determining factor (TDF) gene located on the Y chromosome, a testis develops. Between the seventh and fourteenth weeks of gestation, testosterone produced by the fetal Leydig cells transforms wolffian ducts into the male

genital tract. In target tissues, the enzyme 5α-reductase converts testosterone to dihydrotestosterone (DHT), which virilizes the urogenital sinus and external genitalia. Tissue response to testosterone and DHT is dependent on androgen receptor activity. The gene coding for androgen receptors is located on the X chromosome; various point mutations and deletions have been described in patients with androgen insensitivity. Growth of the penis occurs mainly in the late second and third trimesters, requiring stimulation of the testis by fetal pituitary gonadotropins. Müllerian duct inhibiting factor, a glycoprotein produced by the Sertoli cells, causes regression of the internal female duct structures during the first 8 weeks of gestation. In the absence of this factor, the uterus and uterine (fallopian) tubes develop and mature.

Abnormal Sexual Differentiation

Abnormalities of sexual differentiation frequently result in ambiguous external genitalia. The causes of abnormal sexual differentiation may be divided into four major categories:

A. Abnormalities in Normal Gonadal Differentiation: These usually result from an unidentifiable abnormality of the sex chromosomes. Klinefelter's syndrome (see Chapter 29) with an XXY karyotype usually is associated with a male phenotype. Turner's syndrome (see Chapter 29) is usually associated with a female phenotype. Mosaic forms of gonadal dysgenesis that contain a Y-bearing cell line have an ambiguous phenotype and variable external phenotype. Idiopathic testicular failure prior to completion of sexual differentiation results in ambiguous genitalia. True hermaphroditism, with the presence of both spermatocytes and oocytes, is rare and produces external genitalia that range in type from fully masculine to almost completely feminine.

B. Abnormalities in Testosterone Synthesis or Action: These disorders cause male pseudohermaphroditism, frequently with ambiguous genitalia. The enzyme defects in testosterone synthesis may affect only testosterone synthesis, or they may also affect the synthesis of cortisol, as in variants of the adrenogenital syndrome. Defects in testosterone action result from either absent or defective end-organ receptors or a defect in peripheral testosterone metabolism to dihydrotestosterone due to 5α-reductase deficiency. The androgen receptor defect may be complete (testicular feminization) or incomplete (Reifenstein's syndrome and its variants).

C. Presence of Excessive Androgens in a Female Fetus: These disorders cause female pseudohermaphroditism and usually result in ambiguous genitalia. Excessive adrenal androgen production secondary to an adrenal enzyme defect in cortisol synthesis (ie, adrenal hyperplasia) is the cause of 95% of cases of XX patients with female pseudohermaphroditism and approximately half of all cases of patients with ambiguous genitalia. Occasionally, mater-

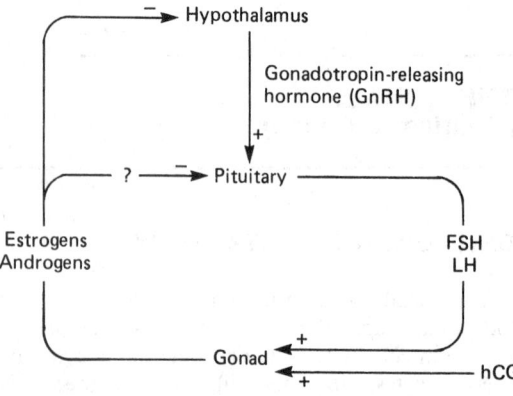

Figure 30–2. Hormonal regulation of gonadal function.

nally derived androgens (eg, maternal congenital adrenal hypoplasia, luteoma of pregnancy) may cause masculinization of the female fetus.

D. Miscellaneous Syndromes: These may be associated with multiple congenital anomalies, especially of the urinary tract and intestine. Occasionally, teratogenic agents may result in anomalous sexual development.

Saenger P: Abnormal sexual differentiation. J Pediatr 1984; 104:1.

ABNORMALITIES IN OVARIAN FUNCTION

The ovary is composed of follicles (germ cells surrounded by granulosa cells), theca cells immediately surrounding the follicle, and stromal or supporting tissue. The ovary produces several types of hormones, the most important of which are estrogens and progesterone. At least three natural estrogens have been identified: estrone, 17β-estradiol (the most potent), and estriol. Production of the major ovarian estrogen, estradiol, is stimulated by pituitary LH secretion (Figure 30–2). Significant quantities of estrogen are not produced until the onset of puberty. Estrogens stimulate the growth of the uterus, vagina, and breasts. They also appear to be essential for the adolescent growth spurt occurring in girls.

Most patients with significant ovarian abnormalities in childhood exhibit precocious puberty, delayed puberty (primary amenorrhea), or secondary amenorrhea.

1. PRECOCIOUS PUBERTY IN GIRLS

Puberty is considered precocious if the onset of secondary sexual characteristics occurs prior to 8 years of age. Recent studies in children with earlier onset suggest that these criteria may need to be decreased to 6 and 9 years of age in females and males, respectively. Precocious puberty is nine times more common in girls than in boys. True (complete; GNRH-dependent) precocious puberty refers to sexual maturation in response to hypothalamic-pituitary maturation; in pseudoprecocity, the etiology is elsewhere (eg, adrenal or gonadal tumor, exogenous hormones). GNRH-dependent precocious puberty is always isosexual and may progress to the production of mature ova. In pseudoprecocity, sexual characteristics may be isosexual or heterosexual; secondary sexual characteristics develop, but the hypothalamic-pituitary-gonadal axis (Figure 30–2) does not mature, and oocyte maturation does not occur.

Clinical Findings

A. Symptoms and Signs: Although the first sign of sexual development in girls is usually breast development, followed by pubic hair growth and vaginal bleeding, the pattern of development may be variable. The interval between breast development and menstruation (normally about 2 years) may be less than 1 year or more than 6 years. On careful abdominal examination of girls with ovarian or adrenal tumors, a mass may be palpated and then confirmed by ultrasonography. A growth spurt may precede or accompany the development of secondary sexual characteristics. A history of excessive mood changes and emotional lability frequently is obtained. Children with precocious puberty have accelerated growth and may be tall during childhood; because osseous maturation (bone age) advances at a more rapid rate than linear growth (particularly in the female), adult short stature may occur.

B. Laboratory Findings: In true precocious puberty, radioimmunoassays generally reveal that levels of serum or plasma gonadotropins are in the pubertal range. Early in the course of the disorder, random gonadotropin determinations may be within the prepubertal range. In these cases, further evaluation of serum LH and FSH levels during sleep and after stimulation with gonadotropin-releasing hormone (GnRH) is necessary (levels are obtained 30 and 60 minutes after intravenous stimulation with 100 μg of GnRH).

C. Imaging: Determination of epiphysial maturation at onset and then every 6–12 months is helpful in predicting the effect of the precocity on adult height.

Abdominal and pelvic ultrasonography can usually identify an ovarian mass, demonstrate an adrenal mass greater than 5 cm, and reveal the presence of follicular ovarian cysts. Serial examinations are useful in demonstrating significant changes. A cranial CT scan or MRI with special attention to the hypothalamic and pituitary regions will identify mass lesions and other structural abnormalities of the central nervous system. Some cases of precocious puberty are due to organic brain lesions and other structural abnormalities of the central nervous system. Some cases of precocious puberty due to organic brain lesions may produce no clinical manifestations for prolonged periods. When these conditions are suspected, examinations for central nervous system lesions should be performed periodically.

Differential Diagnosis

The causes of pseudo- and true precocious puberty are outlined in Table 30–9. Of girls with precocious puberty, 90% have true precocious puberty, and most of these have no definable abnormality on CT or MRI. With newer scanning techniques, static (presumably congenital) mass lesions in the hypothalamus, including benign hamartomas, can be seen in some subjects. A dysgerminoma in the hypothalamic region is the most common central nervous system

Table 30–9. Causes of isosexual precocious development.

True (complete) gonadotropin-dependent precocious puberty
  Constitutional (functional, idiopathic)
  Tumors producing destruction of the pineal (principally in males)
  Hypothalamic lesions (hamartomas, hyperplasia, congenital malformations, tumors)
  Dysgerminomas
  Internal hydrocephalus
  Cerebral and meningocerebral infections (postencephalitis, postmeningitis)
  Degenerative, possibly congenital encephalopathy
  Tuberous sclerosis
  Neurofibromatosis
Pseudoprecocious (incomplete) puberty
  Polyostotic fibrous dysplasia (McCune-Albright syndrome) (principally in females; often incomplete; usually infertile)
  Gonadotropin-independent precocious puberty (males; also known as testotoxicosis)
  Gonadal tumors
    Tumors of the ovary: Granulosa cell tumor (most common), theca cell tumor, teratoma, choriocarcinoma, dysgerminoma, luteoma
    Tumors of the testis: Interstitial (Leydig) cell tumor, teratoma
  Exogenous steroid administration
Premature pubarche (premature adrenarche) (both sexes)
Premature thelarche (premature gynarche) (females)
Unclassified causes
  With elevated gonadotropins
    Associated with hypothyroidism
    Presacral teratoma
    Primary liver cell tumors (hepatoma) (males only)
    Choriocarcinoma and seminoma of the testes
  Others
    Hyperinsulinism
    Primordial dwarfism
    Silver's syndrome (short stature, congenital asymmetry, and variations in the pattern of sexual development)

mass lesion causing precocious puberty, but any central nervous system lesion can be associated with abnormalities in pubertal timing. The most common cause of pseudoprecocious puberty is McCune-Albright syndrome. Clinical manifestations of this disorder include polyostotic fibrous dysplasia, café au lait lesions with irregular borders, and sexual precocity. Laboratory and x-ray findings helpful in differentiating true and pseudoprecocious puberty are discussed above.

Premature thelarche—benign early breast development—occurs most commonly between 12 and 36 months of age. It is most often bilateral but may begin or remain as unilateral breast enlargement. Breast enlargement generally occurs for 1–6 months, then remains at Tanner II–III. In the absence of other signs of pubertal development (ie, no change in growth rate, pubic hair, or vaginal maturation), no laboratory evaluation is necessary. Treatment consists of reassurance regarding the self-limited nature of the problem.

Premature adrenarche is benign early adrenal maturation, manifested by gradual increase in pubic and axillary hair, development of comedones, and body odor. The average age at onset is 5–6 years. Again, no increase in growth rate or other signs of virilization are present, and treatment consists of reassurance and expectant observation.

Treatment

Treatment of the underlying cause of pseudoprecocious puberty (removal of the tumor or correction of the adrenal enzyme disorder) usually results in cessation of abnormal pubertal development. Successful medical intervention in true precocious puberty is effective, but long-term safety has not been established. The most successful therapy employs analogues of gonadotropin-releasing hormone (GnRH agonists). The analogues given in sustained doses—either by daily injection or by means of depot sustained-release preparations—interrupt the physiologic pulsatile state described above. "Down-regulation" occurs, resulting in a block in pituitary LH synthesis and release and in the return of estrogen levels to prepubertal values. In most cases, menses cease, secondary sexual development stabilizes or regresses, and linear growth and bone maturation slow to prepubertal rates.

In patients with McCune-Albright syndrome, analogues of gonadotropin-releasing hormone are not initially helpful. Therapy with antiestrogens, agents that block estrogen synthesis (eg, ketoconazole), or both, may be effective.

Regardless of the cause of precocious puberty or the medical therapy selected, attention to the psychologic needs of the patient and family is essential.

Clemons RD et al: Long term effectiveness of depot gonadotropin releasing hormone analogue in the treatment of children with central sexual precocity. Am J Dis Child 1993;147:653.

Feuillan PP et al: Treatment of precocious puberty in the

McCune-Albright syndrome with the aromatase inhibitor testolactone. N Engl J Med 1986;315:1115.

Ibanez L et al: Natural history of premature pubarche: An auxological study. J Clin Endocrinol Metab 1992;74:254.

Manasco PK et al: Resumption of puberty after long term luteinizing hormone-releasing hormone agonist treatment of central precocious puberty. J Clin Endocrinol Metab 1988;67:368.

Perilongo G, Rigon R, Murgia A: Oncologic causes of precocious puberty. Pediatr Hematol Oncol 1989;6:33.

Siegel MJ: Pediatric gynecologic sonography. Radiology 1991;179:593.

Van Winter JL et al: Natural history of premature thelarche. J Pediatr 1990;116:278.

2. AMENORRHEA

Amenorrhea is the absence of menstruation in a female 14 years of age or older or in a female of any age who is over 2½–3 years postpubarche. Secondary amenorrhea is cessation of menses after an interval of time equal to at least 6 months postmenarche or three menstrual cycles. A history and physical examination (including pelvic examination) often identifies possible causes of amenorrhea (Table 30–10).

Primary Amenorrhea

The most common cause of primary amenorrhea is physiologic or constitutional delay. Turner's syndrome, chronic illness, and severe undernutrition or strenuous exercise are also common causes.

The term "pseudoamenorrhea" is used when the patient is menstruating but has a genital tract obstruction that prevents release of menstrual blood. Sexual development is usually at Tanner stage IV or V, and cyclic abdominal pain without menstruation is noted. Pelvic examination may reveal an imperforate hymen, transverse vaginal ridge, or other obstruction. Treatment is surgical.

Turner's syndrome (XO syndrome, gonadal dysgenesis) should be considered in patients with short stature and sexual infantilism or pubarche without normal pubertal progression. This is a form of hypergonadotropic hypogonadism in which the estrogen level is low (or absent), FSH and LH levels are elevated, bone maturation is usually delayed, buccal smear is sometimes chromatin-negative, and karyotype is abnormal. The phenotypic features of Turner's syndrome (described in Chapter 29) may be absent in 40–50% of girls with the syndrome. Current treatment for the short stature includes human growth hormone, anabolic steroids, and low doses of estrogens separately or in combination. At the time of adolescence, a combination of estrogen and progesterone in physiologic doses is indicated.

Mayer-Rokitansky-Küster-Hauser syndrome is characterized by congenital müllerian agenesis with normal ovaries, normal ovarian function, and normal breast development. Pelvic examination reveals an

Table 30–10. Causes of amenorrhea.

I. **With obstruction of outflow tract**
  A. Fusion or stenosis of labia, hymen (imperforate), vagina, or cervix.
  B. Müllerian agenesis (Mayer-Rokitansky-Küster-Hauser)
  C. Intrauterine synechia (Asherman's syndrome)
  D. After abortion infection, cesarean section, or hysterectomy
  E. XY female (complete androgen-resistant or testicular feminization syndrome)

II. **Secondary to estrogen deficiency**
  A. Primary ovarian failure
    1. Gonadal agenesis
    2. Gonadal dysgenesis
      a. Turner syndrome variants
      b. True gonadal dysgenesis
    3. Ovarian enzymatic deficiency
    4. Premature ovarian failure
      a. Autoimmune disease
      b. Galactosemia
      c. Surgery secondary to infection, radiation, or chemotherapy
      d. Idiopathic (premature menopause)
  B. Secondary ovarian failure
    1. Hypothalamic or pituitary tumor, infection, Langerhans cell disease, sarcoidosis, hemochromatosis, necrosis, and vascular lesion
    2. Kallman's syndrome
    3. Functional psychologic eating disorders (anorexia nervosa, bulimia), malnutrition, stress, excessive exercise, chronic systemic disease, thyroid disease

III. **Androgen excess**
  A. Polycystic ovary syndrome (PCOS), hyperthecosis
  B. Adrenal androgen excess (congenital adrenal hyperplasia, adrenal tumor, Cushing's syndrome

IV. **Ovarian tumors: Granulosa-theca cell, Brenner, teratoma**

absent vagina and various uterine abnormalities with or without additional renal and skeletal anomalies. Full evaluation is necessary, including karyotyping, intravenous pyelography, and laparoscopy. Therapy for this syndrome is surgical vaginoplasty.

Secondary Amenorrhea

Common causes of secondary amenorrhea include stress, pregnancy, major weight loss, polycystic ovary syndrome, and prolactin excess. Stress-induced amenorrhea is often noted in teenagers, but it should be diagnosed only after careful evaluation. Pregnancy is the most frequent cause of secondary amenorrhea in sexually active teenagers.

Irregular menses (oligomenorrhea) or amenorrhea may result from severe weight loss secondary to dieting, vigorous exercise (eg, in marathon runners), depression, anorexia nervosa, or chronic illness. In the normal ovulating female, it is believed that a major source of estrogen is aromatization of androgens in peripheral adipose tissue. When the proportion of body weight represented by fat falls below a critical level (15–25%), estrogen production is decreased.

This hypothesis has been advanced to explain amenorrhea in athletes and patients with anorexia nervosa.

In polycystic ovary syndrome (Stein-Leventhal syndrome), secondary amenorrhea is the result of chronic anovulation. Occasionally, dysfunctional uterine bleeding is the only finding; the full syndrome consists of obesity, hirsutism, secondary amenorrhea, bilaterally enlarged ovaries, and, in some cases, clitoromegaly. The results of tests of endocrine function reveal normal FSH concentrations, elevated LH levels, and borderline to elevated adrenal or ovarian androgen levels. The ratio of estrone to estradiol is often increased. Polycystic ovary syndrome may be idiopathic or secondary to adrenocortical hyperplasia or an adrenocortical neoplasm. Laparoscopy, ovarian biopsy, endometrial biopsy, or a combination of these procedures may be necessary for final diagnosis. Treatment consists of correction of the estrogen:androgen ratio and induction of ovulation in patients who wish to become pregnant. Agents with antiandrogen activity (eg, spironolactone) may be helpful in controlling the hirsutism.

Other causes of amenorrhea are shown in Table 30–10. Chronic illness and central nervous system disorders should always be considered. When galactorrhea and amenorrhea occur together, hyperprolactinemia, drug ingestion, hypothyroidism, stress, and hypothalamic injury should be considered.

Hall JG, Gilchrist DM: Turner syndrome and its variants. Pediatr Clin North Am 1990;37:1421.

Hurley DM et al: Induction of ovulation and fertility in amenorrheic women by pulsatile low-dose gonadotropin-releasing hormone. N Engl J Med 1984;310:1069.

Patton ML, Woolf PD: Hyperprolactinemia and delayed puberty: A report of three cases and their response to therapy. Pediatrics 1983;71:572.

Rosenfield RH: Puberty and its disorders in girls. Endocrinol Metab Clin North Am 1991;20:15.

Soules, MR: Adolescent amenorrhea. Pediatr Clin North Am 1987;34:1083.

OVARIAN TUMORS

Ovarian tumors are not rare in children. They may occur at any age and are usually large, benign, and unilateral. They may be estrogen-producing; ovarian tumors account for approximately 1% of cases of female sexual precocity. The most common estrogen-producing tumor is the granulosa cell tumor, but thecomas, luteomas, mixed types, and theca-lutein and follicular cysts have all been described in association with sexual precocity. An ovarian tumor is usually palpated on rectal examination and readily seen by ovarian ultrasonography.

Other ovarian tumors (teratomas, choriocarcinomas, and dysgerminomas) have been reported in association with sexual precocity.

Treatment is surgical removal. Recurrences are uncommon.

Mann JR et al: Results of United Kingdom Children's Cancer Study Group: Malignant germ cell tumor studies. Cancer 1989;63:1657.

ABNORMALITIES IN TESTICULAR FUNCTION

The major testicular hormone, testosterone, is produced by the Leydig (interstitial) cells. Production of testicular androgens is stimulated by LH secretion (Figure 30–2). Appreciable amounts of androgen usually begin to appear in boys at 12 years of age and are responsible, wholly or in part, for growth of internal and external genitalia and development of secondary sexual characteristics, including pubic, axillary, and facial hair. Androgens induce nitrogen retention, accelerate bone growth, and hasten the closure of bony epiphysial growth centers.

The seminiferous tubules are composed of germinal epithelium and Sertoli cells. Testicular androgens in combination with pituitary FSH stimulate the development and maturation of the germinal epithelium and thus promote spermatogenesis. The Sertoli cells provide mechanical support for the germinal epithelium.

Patients with abnormalities in testicular function may present with delayed or precocious sexual development, cryptorchidism, or gynecomastia.

1. PRECOCIOUS PUBERTY IN BOYS

Puberty is considered precocious in boys if secondary sexual characteristics appear prior to 9 years of age. Precocious puberty is much less common in boys than in girls. In boys presenting with sexual precocity, pseudoprecocious puberty is as common as true precocious puberty. In addition, boys with true precocious puberty are more likely to have an identifiable pathologic process (eg, tumor) rather than idiopathic precocious puberty.

Descriptions of a gonadotropin-independent form of precocious puberty have suggested that this may be the cause of male precocious puberty. In affected males, testicular production of testosterone is apparently independent of gonadotropin but is associated with Leydig cell hyperplasia.

Clinical Findings

A. Symptoms and Signs: In precocious development, increases in somatic growth and growth of pubic hair are the common presenting complaints. Testicular size may differentiate true precocity, in which the testes enlarge, from pseudoprecocity (most commonly due to adrenocortical hyperplasia), in which the testes usually remain small. There are some exceptions: In advanced cases of pseudoprecocity, for example, some testicular enlargement may occur, because seminiferous tubule elements may be stimulated by prolonged elevated testosterone levels. In the very young child with early true precocity, minimal increases of testosterone may result in dramatic increases in penis size and pubic hair growth, with very little testicular enlargement. Tumors of the testis present with asymmetric testicular enlargement.

B. Laboratory Findings: LH and FSH levels are elevated in boys with true sexual precocity. Sexual precocity caused by the adrenogenital syndrome is associated with abnormal levels of plasma dehydroepiandrosterone, androstenedione, 17α-hydroxyprogesterone, 11-deoxycortisol, or a combination of these steroids. The level of serum or plasma testosterone aids in the differentiation of true precocity and pseudoprecocity. Obtaining hCG levels to determine the presence of an hCG-producing tumor (eg, central nervous system dysgerminoma, hepatoma) may be necessary in boys with true sexual precocity.

C. Imaging: Diagnostic studies are similar to those used to evaluate sexual precocity in girls (see above). Ultrasonography may be useful in detection of hepatic, presacral, and testicular tumors.

Differential Diagnosis

The causes of sexual precocity are outlined in Table 30–9. In boys, it is particularly important to differentiate pseudoprecocity from true sexual precocity. Seventy percent of boys have pseudoprecocious puberty secondary to an adrenal enzyme abnormality. Of boys with true precocious puberty, 70% have benign central nervous system mass lesions. Premature adrenarche may occur in males as well as females.

Treatment

Specific therapy should be provided if the cause is known and treatable. Treatment of idiopathic true precocious puberty in boys is similar to that in girls (see above).

Treatment of familial gonadotropin-independent precocious puberty ("testotoxicosis") with agents that block steroid synthesis (eg, ketoconazole), antiandrogens (eg, spironolactone), or with a combination of both has been successful.

Holland FJ: Gonadotropin-independent precocious puberty. Endocrinol Metab Clin North Am 1991;29:191.

Oberfield SE et al: Adrenal steroidogenic function in a black and Hispanic population with precocious pubarche. J Clin Endocrinol Metab 1990;70:76.

Wheeler MD, Styne DM: Diagnosis and management of precocious puberty. Pediatr Clin North Am 1990;37:1255.

2. SEXUAL INFANTILISM (Primary & Secondary Testicular Failure)

Lack of development of secondary sexual characteristics after the age of 17 years suggests abnormal testicular maturation. While delay of puberty until 17 years of age may be physiologically normal, it is generally of concern to a boy if pubertal changes do not occur by 14–15 years of age, and evaluation should be initiated at that time.

Sexual infantilism may be difficult to differentiate from constitutionally delayed adolescence. Although the latter may be associated with a delay in testicular function, normal puberty occurs at a later date.

The differentiation of primary and secondary testicular failure is based on the cause of the disorder. In general, primary failure results from absence, malfunction, or destruction of testicular tissue; secondary failure results from pituitary or hypothalamic insufficiency.

Primary testicular failure may be due to anorchia, surgical castration, Klinefelter's syndrome or other sex chromosomal abnormalities, a genetic defect in testosterone synthesis or action, inflammation and destruction of the testes following infection or exposure to toxic agents (mumps, syphilis, gonorrhea, autoimmune disorders, irradiation), trauma, or tumor.

Causes of secondary testicular failure resulting from central nervous system or hypothalamic-pituitary dysfunction include panhypopituitarism, empty sella syndrome, Kallmann's syndrome, isolated LH deficiency, and isolated FSH deficiency. Destructive lesions in or near the anterior pituitary, especially craniopharyngiomas and gliomas, may result in hypothalamic or pituitary dysfunction, as can infection. These tumors may require irradiation to the central nervous system employing more than 3500 cGy. Prader-Willi syndrome and Laurence-Moon syndrome (Bardet-Biedl syndrome, Biemond syndrome II) are frequently associated with LH and FSH deficiency secondary to deficiency of hypothalamic gonadotropin-releasing hormone. Miscellaneous causes include chronic debilitating disease and hypothyroidism.

Clinical Findings

A. Symptoms and Signs: Physical examination may not be helpful in differentiating primary from secondary gonadal insufficiency. While cryptorchidism suggests primary testicular failure, hypothalamic or pituitary insufficiency as well as anatomic abnormalities may lead to failure of testicular descent.

B. Laboratory Findings: In primary testicular failure, the serum testosterone level is low, whereas LH and FSH values are elevated into the castrate range. In secondary testicular failure, levels of all three hormones are below the normal adult range. To establish the presence of the testes and their ability to respond to stimulation, the clinician may administer hCG; a dose of 2000 units/m^2 given intramuscularly every other day for two or three doses should result in a rise in the serum testosterone level to above 200 mg/dL 48 hours after the final dose. Determination of LH and FSH responses to exogenous GnRH may be useful.

Chromosomal karyotype should be determined in primary testicular failure of unknown cause.

C. Imaging: Skeletal maturation is usually delayed. A cranial CT scan or MRI should be performed in cases of secondary testicular failure.

Treatment

Specific therapy is indicated when the cause of testicular failure is known. Treatment with depot testosterone (eg, enanthate), beginning with 75–100 mg intramuscularly and increasing to 200 mg every 3–4 weeks, may be given until sexual maturity is reached. In patients with primary testicular failure, replacement therapy with testosterone, 300–400 mg every 3–4 weeks, may be continued indefinitely. Specific therapy (GnRH pulsations) may result in fertility in patients with hypothalamic-pituitary insufficiency.

Bourguignon JP et al: Hypopituitarism and idiopathic delayed puberty: A longitudinal study in an attempt to diagnose gonadotropin deficiency before puberty. J Clin Endocrinol Metab 1982;54:733.

Hoffman AR et al: Induction of puberty in men by long-term pulsatile administration of low-dose gonadotropin-releasing hormone. N Engl J Med 1982;307:1237.

Joss EE: Oxandrolone in constitutionally delayed growth: A longitudinal study of final height. J Clin Endocrinol Metab 1989;69:1109.

Lee PA, O'Dea LSLL: Primary and secondary testicular insufficiency. Pediatr Clin North Am 1990;37:1359.

Rosenfield RL: Low-dose testosterone effect on somatic growth. Pediatrics 1986;77:853.

3. CRYPTORCHIDISM

Cryptorchidism (undescended testes) is a common disorder in children. It may be unilateral or bilateral and may be classified as ectopic cryptorchidism or true cryptorchidism.

Approximately 3% of term male newborns and 30% of premature males have undescended testes at birth. In over half of these cases, the testes descend by the second month; by the age of 1 year, 80% of all undescended testes are in the scrotum. Further descent may occur through puberty, the latter perhaps stimulated by endogenous gonadotropin. If cryptorchidism persists into adult life, failure of spermatogenesis occurs, but testicular androgen production usually remains intact. The incidence of malignant neoplasm (usually seminoma) is appreciably greater in those testes which remain in the abdomen after puberty.

Ectopic testes are presumed to develop normally but are diverted as they descend through the inguinal canal. They are subclassified on the basis of their location; surgery is indicated once the diagnosis is established.

True cryptorchidism in most cases is thought to be the result of an abnormality in testicular development (dysgenesis). Cryptorchid testes frequently have a short spermatic artery, poor blood supply, or both. Although early scrotal positioning of these testes will obviate further damage related to intra-abdominal location, the testes generally remain abnormal, spermatogenesis is rare, and the risk of malignant neoplasm is increased. These testes should probably be removed if spermatogenesis does not occur after a reasonable period of observation.

Bilateral cryptorchidism is a common feature in prepubertal castrate syndrome (the vanishing testes syndrome), Noonan's syndrome, and disorders of androgen synthesis or action; it is seen less commonly with Klinefelter's syndrome, Sertoli-cell-only syndrome, and hypogonadotropin states.

Clinical Findings

Testosterone levels may be obtained after hCG stimulation to confirm the presence or absence of abdominal testes (see above). The child with bilaterally undescended testes should be evaluated for sex chromosome abnormalities; genetic sex should be determined by chromosome analysis (karyotyping) in the newborn period.

Differential Diagnosis

In palpating for the testes, the cremasteric reflex may be elicited, with a resultant ascent of the testes into the inguinal canal or abdomen (pseudocryptorchidism). To prevent this, the fingers first should be placed across the abdominal ring and the upper portion of the inguinal canal, obstructing ascent. Examination while the child is in the squatting position or a warm bath is also helpful. No treatment is necessary, and the prognosis for testicular descent and competence is excellent.

Treatment

The best age for medical or surgical treatment has not been determined, but there is a trend toward operation in infancy or early childhood. Surgical repair is indicated for cryptorchidism persisting beyond puberty.

Gonadotropin therapy (chorionic gonadotropin, 4000–5000 units intramuscularly three to five times a week for 2–3 weeks) is generally ineffective unless the child has retractive testes (pseudocryptorchidism) rather than cryptorchidism.

Androgen treatment (eg, depot testosterone enanthate; see above) is indicated as replacement therapy in the male beyond the normal age of puberty who has been shown to lack functional testes.

Rajfer J et al: Hormonal therapy of cryptorchidism: A randomized, double-blind study comparing human chorionic gonadotropin and gonadotropin-releasing hormone. N Engl J Med 1986;314:466.

4. GYNECOMASTIA

See Chapter 4.

TESTICULAR TUMORS

The primary malignant tumors of the testis are seminomas and teratomas. Seminomas are rare in childhood; they may be hormone-producing. The major hormone-producing tumor of the testis is the Leydig cell tumor. It is frequently associated with sexual precocity. Other testicular tumors (choriocarcinomas and dysgerminomas) have been reported in association with sexual precocity.

Treatment of testicular tumors is surgical removal; chemotherapy and radiation therapy are not employed in childhood unless there is a high-grade malignancy or metastasis. The prognosis in patients with Leydig cell tumors is generally good.

Leonard MP et al: Pediatric testicular tumors: The Johns Hopkins experience. Urology 1991;37:253.

ADRENAL CORTEX

The adrenal cortex develops from the dorsal celomic mesothelium between the fourth and sixth weeks of fetal life. By 8–9 weeks of gestation, the fetal adrenal cortex contains the enzymes necessary to produce cortisol from progesterone. At 7–9 weeks of gestation, the fetal pituitary seems capable of producing and releasing adrenocorticotropic hormone (ACTH) to provide regulation of adrenal hormone production.

The adult adrenal cortex is composed of three distinct zones. The glomerulosa is the outermost zone and seems to be the exclusive source of aldosterone, the major mineralocorticoid in humans. The zona fasciculata is the largest cortical zone and is the source of cortisol, the major glucocorticoid, as well as small amounts of mineralocorticoids. The zona reticularis is the innermost zone (adjacent to the adrenal medulla) and appears to produce mainly adrenal androgens and estrogens.

During fetal life, these zones comprise only a minor portion of the adrenal cortex. The predominant portion is the fetal zone, or provisional cortex, which is capable of producing glucocorticoids, mineralo-corticoids, androgens, and estrogens but is relatively deficient in production of 3β-hydroxydehydrogenase and Δ^5,Δ^4 isomerase (Figure 30–3). Therefore, placentally produced progesterone serves as the major precursor for fetal adrenal production of cortisol and aldosterone.

The adrenal cortex produces cortisol under the control of pituitary ACTH. The quantity of cortisol produced is regulated by a negative feedback mechanism involving the pituitary and hypothalamus (Figure 30–4). This negative feedback control is superimposed on a diurnal pattern of ACTH release. ACTH release is greatest during the early morning hours and least around midnight.

The actions of glucocorticoids are myriad and incompletely understood. Glucocorticoids are catabolic and antianabolic—ie, they promote the release of amino acids from muscle and increase gluconeogenesis while decreasing incorporation of amino acids into muscle protein. They also antagonize insulin action and permit lipogenesis. Glucocorticoids influence blood pressure through their "permissive effect" (norepinephrine enhancing cardiac inotrope tone and peripheral vascular tone) and by causing sodium and water retention.

Mineralocorticoids (primarily aldosterone in humans) promote sodium retention and permit potassium excretion. While ACTH can affect aldosterone production, the predominant regulators of aldosterone secretion are mediated via the renin-aldosterone system in response to changes in intravascular volume and serum sodium concentrations. Serum potassium concentrations also directly influence aldosterone release.

The zona reticularis of the adrenal cortex produces androgens (eg, dehydroepiandrosterone and androstenedione). In normal subjects, adrenal androgen production is insignificant; at pubarche, androgen production increases and may be an important factor in the initiation of puberty. The adrenal gland is the major source of androgen in the pubertal and adult female.

ADRENOCORTICAL INSUFFICIENCY
(Adrenal Crisis, Addison's Disease)

Essentials of Diagnosis

- Vomiting, dehydration, hypotension, circulatory collapse, small heart.
- Low serum sodium, high serum potassium, low glucose; eosinophilia.
- Low blood and urine adrenocorticosteroids.
- Weakness, fatigue, pallor; episodes of nausea, vomiting, and diarrhea; increased craving for salt.
- Increased pigmentation.

General Considerations

Adrenocortical hypofunction may be due to con-

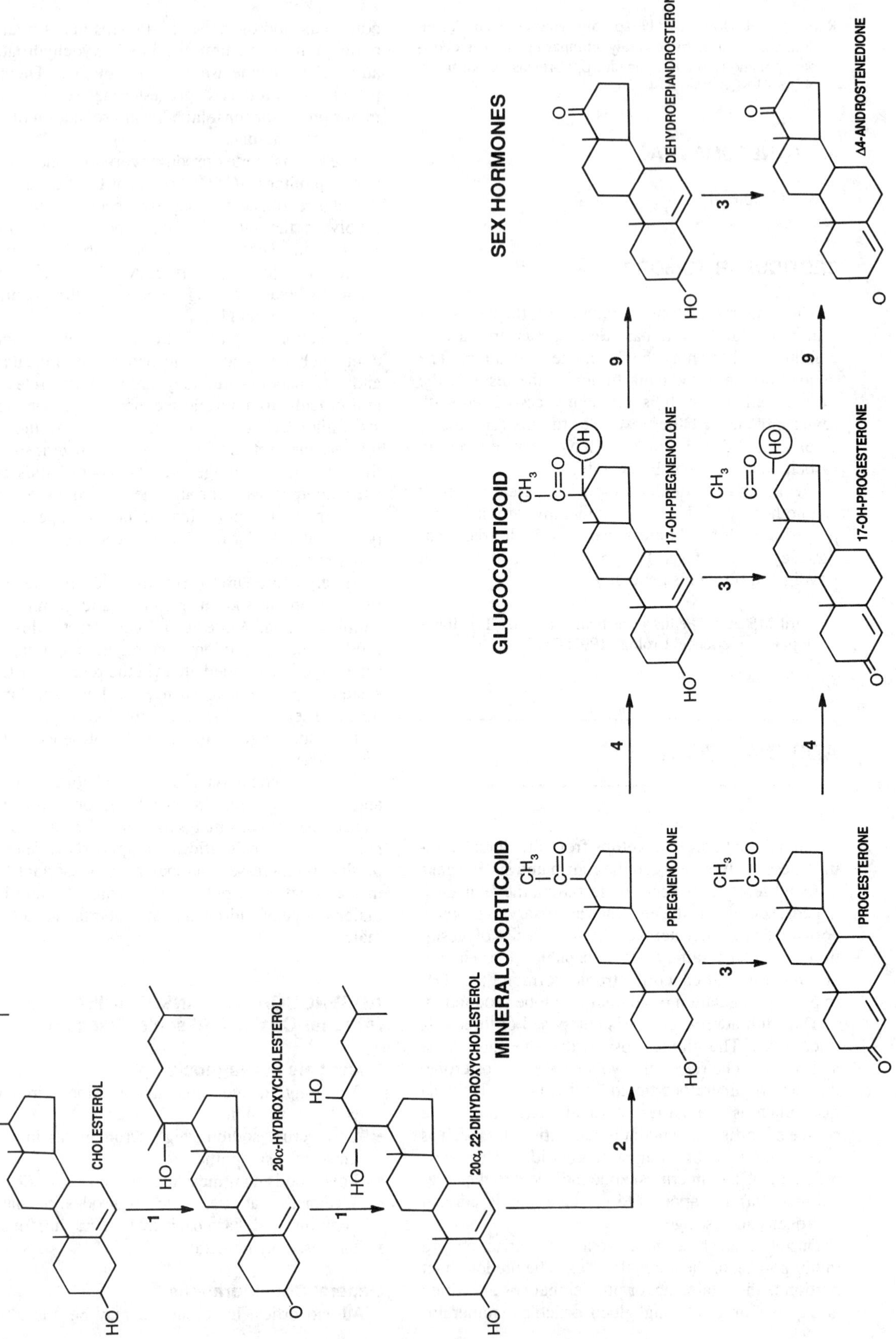

Figure 30-3. Adrenal steroid pathways.

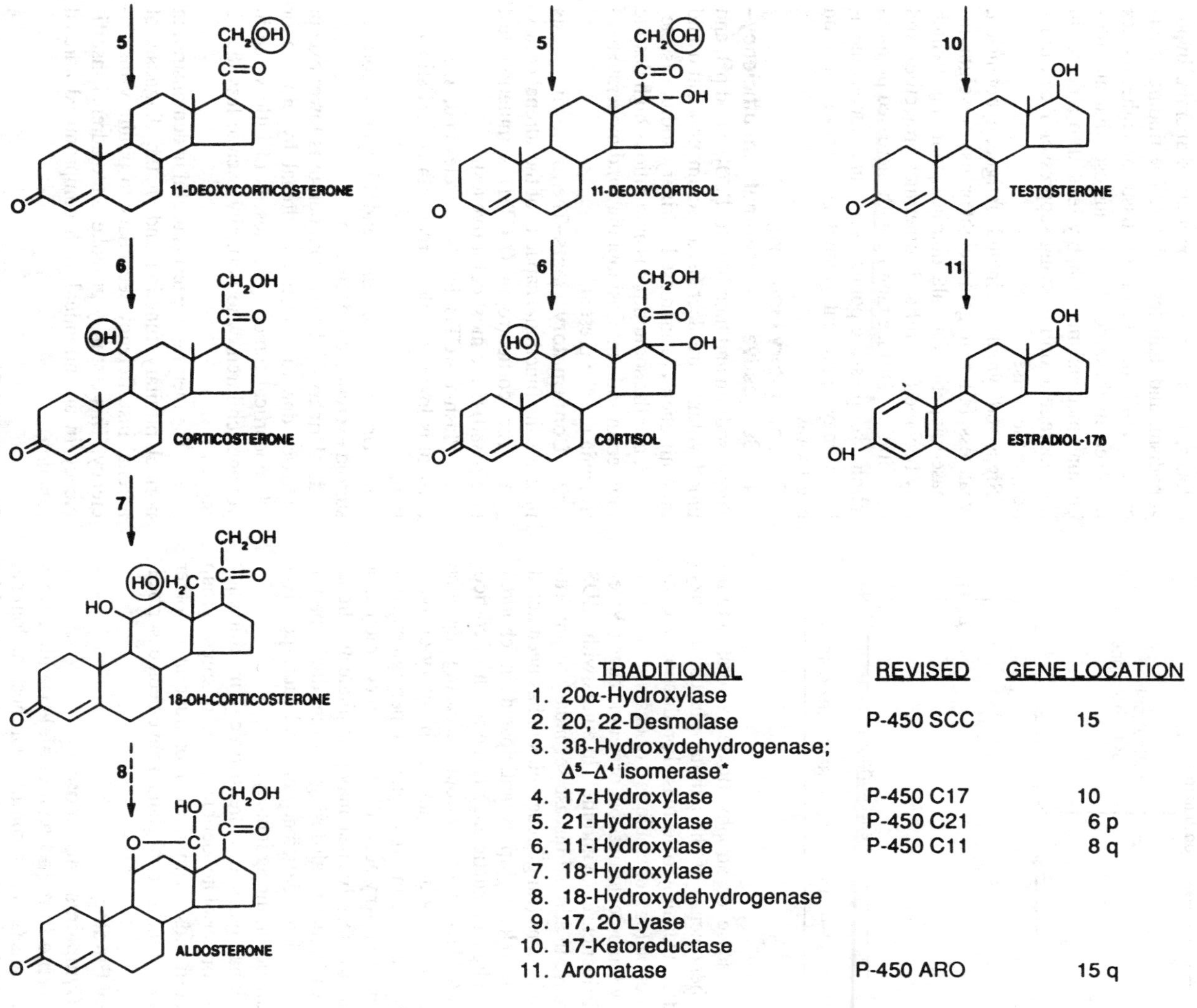

5
CH2OH
C=O
11-DEOXYCORTICOSTERONE
6
CH2OH
C=O
OH
CORTICOSTERONE
7
CH2OH
HOH2C
C=O
HO
18-OH-CORTICOSTERONE
8
HO
CH2OH
C=O
O
C
ALDOSTERONE
5
CH2OH
C=O
OH
11-DEOXYCORTISOL
6
CH2OH
C=O
HO
OH
CORTISOL
10
OH
TESTOSTERONE
11
OH
OH
ESTRADIOL-17B

TRADITIONAL	REVISED	GENE LOCATION
1. 20α-Hydroxylase		
2. 20, 22-Desmolase	P-450 SCC	15
3. 3β-Hydroxydehydrogenase; Δ^5–Δ^4 isomerase*		
4. 17-Hydroxylase	P-450 C17	10
5. 21-Hydroxylase	P-450 C21	6 p
6. 11-Hydroxylase	P-450 C11	8 q
7. 18-Hydroxylase		
8. 18-Hydroxydehydrogenase		
9. 17, 20 Lyase		
10. 17-Ketoreductase		
11. Aromatase	P-450 ARO	15 q

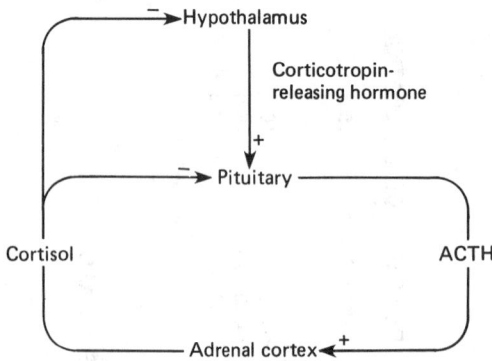

Figure 30–4. Pituitary-adrenal cortex control.

genital absence or atrophy (toxic factors, autoimmune phenomena) of the adrenal glands; an enzymatic defect leading to decreased production of cortisol; infection (eg, tuberculosis); or destruction of the gland by tumor, calcification, or hemorrhage (Waterhouse-Friderichsen syndrome). In adults with AIDS, an increase in adrenal disease secondary to opportunistic infections (fungi, tuberculosis) has been noted. A similar relationship is anticipated in children. Rarely, adrenal insufficiency is the result of corticotropin (ACTH) or corticotropin-releasing hormone (CRH) deficiency due to anterior pituitary or hypothalamic disease, in which case hyperpigmentation does not occur. Any acute illness, surgery, trauma, or exposure to excessive heat may precipitate an adrenal crisis. A temporary salt-losing disorder due to partial mineralocorticoid deficiency or renal subresponsiveness may occur during infancy.

Fractional types of adrenocortical insufficiency (relative or absolute deficiency of a single group [glucocorticoids] with normal production of other hormones of the adrenal glands) have been described.

Clinical Findings

A. Symptoms and Signs:

1. Acute form (adrenal crisis)–Manifestations include nausea and vomiting, diarrhea, abdominal pain, dehydration, fever (which may be followed by hypothermia), hypotension, circulatory collapse, and confusion or coma.

2. Chronic form (Addison's disease)–The leading causes of adrenal insufficiency today are hereditary enzymatic defects with congenital adrenal hyperplasia and idiopathic loss of adrenal function, the latter thought to be due to autoimmune mechanisms. Adrenal destruction may also occur secondary to infectious processes (eg, tuberculosis or fungal infection) and neoplasms. A rare form of familial Addison's disease may be seen in association with cerebral sclerosis and spastic paraplegia. Idiopathic Addison's disease may be familial and has been de-

scribed in association with hypoparathyroidism, candidiasis, hypothyroidism, pernicious anemia, hypogonadism, and diabetes mellitus. The finding of circulating antibodies to adrenal tissue and other tissues involved in these conditions suggests that an autoimmune mechanism, probably related to a defect in immunoregulation involving suppressor T cell function, is the cause.

Signs and symptoms include fatigue, hypotension, weakness, failure to gain weight or loss of weight, increased appetite for salt, diarrhea, vomiting (which may become forceful and sometimes projectile), and dehydration. Diffuse tanning with increased pigmentation over pressure points, scars, and mucous membranes may be present. A small heart may be seen on chest x-ray.

B. Laboratory Findings:

1. Suggestive of adrenal insufficiency–Serum sodium and bicarbonate, PCO_2, blood pH, and blood volume are decreased. Serum potassium and urea nitrogen are increased. Urinary sodium is elevated, and the sodium:potassium ratio is high despite low serum sodium. Eosinophilia* and moderate neutropenia may be present.

2. Confirmatory tests–The following tests measure the functional capacity of the adrenal cortex:

a. The corticotropin (ACTH) stimulation test (see p 880) is the most definitive test.

b. Plasma ACTH levels are elevated, whereas cortisol is low and fails to rise with ACTH stimulation.

c. Urinary free cortisol and 17-hydroxycorticosteroid excretion are decreased.

d. Urinary 17-ketosteroid output is lower except in cases due to congenital adrenal hyperplasia or adrenocortical tumor. (This test is of little value in younger children, who normally excrete less than 1 mg/d.)

e. The metyrapone test is useful in demonstrating normal pituitary function and in the diagnosis of adrenal insufficiency secondary to pituitary insufficiency. This test may provoke acute adrenal insufficiency in an individual with compromised adrenal function.

Differential Diagnosis

Acute adrenal insufficiency must be differentiated from severe acute infections, diabetic coma, various disturbances of the central nervous system, and acute poisoning. In the neonatal period, adrenal insufficiency may be clinically indistinguishable from respiratory distress, intracranial hemorrhage, or sepsis.

Chronic adrenocortical insufficiency must be differentiated from anorexia nervosa, certain muscular disorders (myasthenia gravis, etc), salt-losing nephri-

---

*A normal number of eosinophils during stress (eg, the day after operation or in the presence of a severe infection) is also suggestive of adrenocortical insufficiency.

tis, and chronic debilitating infections (tuberculosis, etc) and must be considered in cases of recurrent spontaneous hypoglycemia.

Treatment

A. Acute Form (Adrenal Crisis):

1. Replacement therapy–

a. Hydrocortisone sodium succinate, 2 mg/kg diluted in 2–10 mL of water intravenously, is given over 2–5 minutes, followed by an infusion of normal saline and 5–10% glucose, 100 mL/kg/24 h intravenously. Thereafter, hydrocortisone sodium succinate, 1.5 mg/kg in infants or 12.5 mg/m^2 in older children, is given intravenously every 4–6 hours until stabilization is achieved and oral therapy tolerated.

b. Fludrocortisone–When oral intake is tolerated, fludrocortisone, 0.1 mg daily, is started and continued as necessary every 12–24 hours.

c. Ten percent glucose in normal saline, 20 mL/kg intravenously in the first 2 hours, may be of value, particularly in infants with adrenal crisis who have congenital adrenal hyperplasia. Overtreatment must be avoided.

2. Hypotension–Specific treatment includes volume expansion (eg, normal saline solution, albumin) and hydrocortisone sodium succinate. Rarely, inotropic agents such as dopamine or dobutamine are needed.

3. Infections–Infections are treated with large doses of appropriate antibiotic or chemotherapeutic agents.

4. Waterhouse-Friderichsen syndrome with fulminant infections– The use of adrenocorticosteroids and norepinephrine in the treatment or "prophylaxis" of fulminant infections is still controversial; steroids may augment the generalized Shwartzman reaction in fatal cases of meningococcemia. However, corticosteroids should always be considered in the presence of adrenal insufficiency, particularly with hypotension and circulatory collapse.

5. Fluids and electrolytes–Ten percent glucose in saline, 20 mL/kg intravenously, is given over the first hour. *Caution:* Overtreatment must be avoided. Total parenteral fluid in the first 8 hours should not exceed the maintenance fluid requirement of the normal child (see Chapter 37).

B. Maintenance Therapy of Chronic Form (Addison's Disease):
Following initial stabilization, the most effective substitution therapy is hydrocortisone given with fludrocortisone. Overtreatment should be avoided, because it may result in obesity, growth retardation, and other cushingoid features.

Additional hydrocortisone, fludrocortisone, or sodium chloride, singly or in combination, may be necessary with acute illness, surgery, trauma, or other stress reactions.

Supportive adrenocortical therapy should be given whenever surgical operations are performed in patients who have at some time received prolonged therapy with adrenocorticosteroids. (See below.)

1. Glucocorticoids (hydrocortisone or equivalent)–The dosage of all glucocorticoids is increased to two to four times the usual dosage during intercurrent illness or times of stress.

a. Hydrocortisone–A dosage of 10–20 mg/m^2/d is given orally in three or four divided doses. For adrenal enzyme defects with excess ACTH, 25% of the dose is given in the morning and afternoon and 50% at night. For all other causes of adrenocortical insufficiency, 50% of the daily dose is given in the morning.

b. Prednisone–A dosage of 5–6 mg/m^2/d is given orally in two divided doses. Its potency may preclude necessary minor modulations in dosage.

2. Fludrocortisone–A dose of 0.05–0.2 mg is given orally once a day or in two divided doses. Periodic monitoring of blood pressure is recommended to avoid overdosing.

3. Salt–The child should be given ready access to table salt. Frequent blood pressure determinations in the recumbent position should be made to ensure that hypertension is avoided.

C. Corticosteroids in Patients With Adrenocortical Insufficiency Who Undergo Surgery:

1. Before operation–Hydrocortisone sodium succinate, 30 mg/m^2 intravenously, is given 1 hour before surgery.

2. During operation–Hydrocortisone sodium succinate, 25–100 mg intravenously, is administered with 5–10% glucose in saline throughout surgery.

3. During recovery–Hydrocortisone sodium succinate, 12.5 mg/m^2 intravenously, is given every 4–6 hours until oral doses are tolerated. The oral dose of three to five times the maintenance dose is gradually tapered to the maintenance dose as the patient recovers.

Course & Prognosis

A. Acute: The course of acute adrenal insufficiency is rapid, and death may occur within a few hours, particularly in infants, unless adequate treatment is given. Spontaneous recovery is unlikely. Patients who have received long-term treatment with adrenocorticosteroids may exhibit adrenal collapse if they undergo surgery or other acute stress. Pharmacologic doses of glucocorticoids during these episodes may be needed throughout life.

In all forms of acute adrenal insufficiency, the patient should be observed carefully once the crisis has passed and evaluated with laboratory tests to assess the degree of permanent adrenal insufficiency.

B. Chronic: Adequately treated chronic adrenocortical insufficiency is consistent with a relatively normal life. Patients on maintenance doses of glucocorticoids may require increases (twofold to threefold) during severe illnesses and operations.

CONGENITAL ADRENAL HYPERPLASIA (Adrenogenital Syndrome)

Essentials of Diagnosis

- Pseudohermaphroditism in females, with urogenital sinus, enlargement of clitoris, and other evidence of virilization.
- Isosexual precocity in males with infantile testes.
- Increased linear growth in young children; advancement of skeletal maturation.
- Urinary and plasma androgen elevation; plasma 17α-hydroxyprogesterone and urinary pregnanetriol concentrations increased in the common form.
- May be associated with electrolyte and water disturbances, particularly in the newborn period.

General Considerations

Congenital adrenal hyperplasia is most commonly the result of 21-hydroxylase deficiency (P450c21) resulting from inherited mutations of both 21-hydroxylase B genes, located adjacent to the C4B genes and between the HLA-B and HLA-DR genes of the HLA complex. In the severe form, excess adrenal androgen production beginning in the first trimester of fetal development results in virilization and life-threatening hypovolemic, hyponatremic shock (adrenal crisis). This form of the syndrome is the congenital familial (autosomal recessive) form, also known as adrenogenital syndrome, which affects males and females equally and is due to an inborn error of metabolism that has traditionally been equated with a deficiency in one of a number of distinct enzymes involved in adrenal steroidogenesis or sex hormone synthesis. Recent studies employing tools in molecular biology and protein chemistry have yielded evidence that has altered this view. It appears that the P450 group of oxidases are the operative enzymes, and four distinct multipurpose enzymes within the cytochrome P450 enzyme group are believed to be responsible for adrenal steroidogenesis. Within the text material and Table 30–11, the traditional terminology is retained to avoid confusion. In Figure 30–3, the new terminology is provided with the traditional terminology, and the presumed gene location for the enzymes is indicated.

Over 80% of cases are caused by a 21-hydroxylase enzyme deficiency, approximately 10% by an 11-hydroxylase enzyme deficiency, and the remainder by deficiencies of the other five enzymes (Figure 30–3). In some forms, the infant may appear normal at birth, with symptoms occurring later. In all forms except 17,20-desmolase deficiency, diminished secretion of cortisol results in excessive secretion of ACTH. ACTH excess results in adrenal hyperplasia with increased production of various adrenal hormone precursors and increased urinary excretion of their metabolites. Increased pigmentation, especially of the scrotum, labia majora, and nipples, frequently results from excessive ACTH secretion.

Studies in patients with 21-hydroxylase deficiency indicate that the clinical type (salt-wasting versus non-salt-wasting) is usually consistent within a family and that there is a close genetic linkage of the 21-hydroxylase gene to the HLA complex on chromosome 6. The latter finding has allowed more precise heterozygote detection and prenatal diagnosis. Population studies indicate that the defective gene is present in 1:100–50 people and that the incidence of the disorder is 1:15,000–5000. Hormonal evaluation of unaffected family members following ACTH stimulation allows detection of the heterozygote with a certainty of 80–90%, and a combination of hormonal and HLA studies can increase the number of cases de-

Table 30–11. Laboratory and clinical findings in adrenal enzyme defects resulting in adrenogenital syndrome.

Enzyme Deficiency[1]	Urinary 17-Ketosteroids	Elevated Plasma Metabolite	Plasma Androgens	Aldosterone	Hypertension/ Salt Loss	External Genitalia[2]
20,22-Desmolase (1)	↓↓↓		↓↓↓	↓↓↓	− / +	M: feminized F: normal
3β-Hydroxydehydrogenase (2)	↑↑ (DHEA)	Pregnenolone	↑ (DHEA)	↓↓↓	− / +	M: feminized F: masculinized
17-Hydroxylase (3)	↓↓↓	Progesterone	↓↓	↓↓ (↑ Deoxycorticosterone)	+ / −	M: feminized F: normal
21-Hydroxylase (simple) (4)	↑↑↑	17α-Hydroxyprogesterone	↑↑	↑	− / −	M: normal F: masculinized
21-Hydroxylase (salt-wasting) (4)	↑↑↑	17α-Hydroxyprogesterone	↑↑	↓↓	− / +	M: normal F: masculinized
11-Hydroxylase (5)	↑↑	11-Deoxycortisol	↑↑	↓↓ (↑ Deoxycorticosterone)	+ / −	M: normal F: masculinized
17,20-Desmolase (7)	↓↓↓		↓↓	Normal	− / −	M: feminized F: normal

[1]The numbers refer to the position of enzyme action as shown in Figure 30–3.
[2]M = male, F = female.

tected. HLA typing in combination with the measurement of 17α-hydroxyprogesterone and androstenedione in amniotic fluid has been used in the prenatal diagnosis of 21-hydroxylase deficiency. The potential for mass screening with a microfilter paper technique to evaluate 17α-hydroxyprogesterone is in progress in some centers.

Nonclassic presentations of 21-hydroxylase deficiency have been reported with increasing frequency. Affected individuals have a normal phenotype at birth and develop evidence of virilization during later childhood, adolescence, or early adulthood. In these cases, previously referred to as late-onset or acquired enzyme deficiencies, results of hormonal studies are characteristic of 21-hydroxylase deficiency. An asymptomatic form has also been identified in which individuals have none of the phenotypic features of the disorder but have hormonal study results identical to those in patients with nonclassic 21-hydroxylase deficiency. The nonclassic form appears to be less severe than the classic form. Because members of the same family may have classic, nonclassic, and asymptomatic forms, the disorders may be due to allelic variations of the same enzyme.

Pseudohermaphroditism can be caused by factors other than enzyme deficiencies. In females, these include virilizing maternal conditions or related hormones taken by the mother during the first trimester of pregnancy. In such cases, the condition does not progress after birth, and cortisol efficiency with abnormal steroidogenesis is not present. Pseudohermaphroditism occurs rarely with gonadal dysgenesis.

Adrenogenital syndrome may also result from tumors of the adrenal gland, ovary, or testis or from idiopathic adrenal hyperplasia later in life. Symptoms begin after birth and progress until treated.

Clinical Findings

A. Symptoms and Signs:

1. Adrenogenital syndrome in females–In the female with potentially normal ovaries and uterus, masculinization occurs, and sexual development is along heterosexual lines.

a. Congenital bilateral hyperplasia of the adrenal cortex secondary to enzyme deficiency (pseudohermaphroditism)– The abnormality of the external genitalia may vary from mild enlargement of the clitoris to complete fusion of the labioscrotal folds, forming a penile urethra, and enlargement of the clitoris to form a normal-sized phallus. When the defect is incomplete, signs of adrenal insufficiency may not occur; signs and symptoms of virilization predominate. In the complete form left untreated, growth in height and skeletal maturation are excessive, and patients become muscular. Pubic hair appears early (often before the second birthday); acne may be excessive; and the voice may deepen. Excessive pigmentation may develop. Dentition is normal or only slightly advanced for the chronologic age.

Similar abnormalities may be present in siblings and cousins. Signs of associated adrenal insufficiency may be present during the first days of life (typically in the first or second week). In some cases, adrenal insufficiency does not occur for months or years.

b. Postnatal adrenogenital syndrome (virilism)–This disorder may be due to adrenal hyperplasia or tumor or to arrhenoblastoma (extremely rare). Enlargement of the clitoris occurs, but other changes of the genitalia are not found. The family history is negative for similar abnormalities. If a tumor is present, it may be palpably enlarged. Other findings are similar to those of pseudohermaphroditism.

2. Adrenogenital syndrome in males (macrogenitosomia precox)– In males, sexual development proceeds along isosexual lines.

a. Congenital bilateral hyperplasia of the adrenal cortex due to enzyme deficiency–The infant may appear normal at birth, but during the first few months of life enlargement of the penis will be noted. There may be increased pigmentation resulting from excessive secretion of β-lipotropin and ACTH. Other symptoms and signs are similar to those of the congenital form in females. The testes are soft and not enlarged, except in the rare male in whom aberrant adrenal cells are present in the testes and produce unilateral or bilateral symmetric or asymmetric enlargement.

b. Tumor–The findings may be identical with those of congenital bilateral hyperplasia of the adrenal cortex, except that they appear at a later age. The tumor may be palpably enlarged. Rarely, an adrenal tumor in a male may produce feminization with gynecomastia.

B. Laboratory Findings:

1. Blood and urine–Hormonal studies are essential for accurate diagnosis. Findings characteristic of the enzyme deficiencies are shown in Table 30–11. With adrenal tumor, production and excretion of dehydroepiandrosterone are greatly elevated.

2. Genetic studies–When available, rapid chromosomal diagnosis should be obtained.

3. Dexamethasone suppression test–If lowdose dexamethasone, (eg, 2–4 mg/d in four divided doses for 7 days) reduces 17-ketosteroids to normal, hyperplasia rather than adenoma is the probable diagnosis.

C. Imaging: Adrenal ultrasonography, CT scanning, and MRI may be useful in defining pelvic anatomy or enlarged adrenals or in localizing an adrenal tumor. Vaginograms using contrast material may indicate the presence of a urogenital sinus and cervix; ultrasonography defines the pelvic contents with increasing accuracy.

Treatment

A. Congenital Hyperplasia of the Adrenal Cortex: Treatment goals consist of suppression of adrenal secretion through suppression of endogenous

ACTH and renin, restoration of physiologic gluco-corticoid and mineralocorticoid concentrations, and avoidance of the side effects of overtreatment (ie, Cushing's syndrome and hypertension).

1. Initially, hydrocortisone given in a dosage of 25–30 mg/m²/d orally suppresses abnormal adrenal steroidogenesis within 2 weeks. The maintenance dose is the same as that in Addison's disease. In congenital hyperplasia, 50% of the daily dose should be given in the late evening to suppress the early morning ACTH rise. Dosage is regulated to maintain a normal growth rate and a normal rate of osseous maturation; in cases of 21-hydroxylase deficiency, the plasma 17-hydroxyprogesterone and androstenedione levels should also be kept within the normal range. In adolescent females, menses are a sensitive index of the adequacy of therapy. Therapy should be continued throughout life in both males and females because of the possibility of malignant degeneration of the hyperplastic adrenal gland.

2. Other aspects of treatment are as for Addison's disease (eg, mineralocorticoid and glucocorticoid increases with stress; see p 872). Occasionally, inadequate mineralocorticoid therapy leads to increased renin levels and elevated 17α-hydroxyprogesterone production in the face of adequate or excessive glucocorticoid therapy.

3. Clitororecession is often indicated in the first year of life. Vaginoplasty for labial fusion should be performed in early childhood; it may be necessary during infancy if vaginal-urinary reflux and genitourinary tract infections occur. Partial clitoridectomy is occasionally indicated if the clitoris is abnormally large or sensitive.

B. Tumor: Because the malignant and benign lesions cannot be distinguished clinically, surgical removal is indicated whenever a tumor has been diagnosed. Preoperative and postoperative treatment is as for Cushing's syndrome due to tumor.

Course & Prognosis

When therapy is initiated in early infancy, abnormal metabolic effects are not observed, and masculinization does not progress. Unless adequately controlled, adrenal hyperplasia results in sexual precocity and masculinization throughout childhood. Affected individuals will be tall as children but short as adults. Treatment with the corticosteroids permits normal growth, development, and sexual maturation. If treatment is delayed until somatic development is over 12–14 years (as determined by bone age), true sexual precocity may occur in males and females.

Patient education stressing lifelong therapy is important to ensure compliance in adolescence and later life.

Female pseudohermaphrodites mistakenly raised as males for more than 3 years may have serious psychologic disturbances if their sex is "changed" after that time. Extensive psychologic evaluation is mandatory in determining the optimal course of action.

When adrenogenital syndrome is caused by a tumor, the progression of signs and symptoms ceases after surgical removal; however, evidence of masculinization, particularly deepening of the voice, may persist.

ADRENOCORTICAL HYPERFUNCTION (Cushing's Disease, Cushing's Syndrome)

Essentials of Diagnosis

- "Truncal type" adiposity with thin extremities, moon face, muscle wasting, weakness, plethora, easy bruisability, purplish striae, growth retardation.
- Hypertension, osteoporosis, glycosuria.
- Elevated serum and urine adrenocorticosteroids; low potassium; eosinopenia.

General Considerations

The principal findings in Cushing's syndrome in childhood result from excessive secretion of glucocorticoids and androgens. Depletion of body protein is typical. There may also be lesser degrees of overproduction of the mineralocorticoids. It has been suggested that in Cushing's disease with bilateral adrenal hyperplasia there is decreased responsiveness of the hypothalamic-pituitary feedback mechanism that regulates the release or production of ACTH. This may then result in a constant but only slightly excessive elevation in the secretion of ACTH or lead to qualitative or quantitative change in the diurnal variation.

Cushing's syndrome is more common in females. In children under 12, it is usually iatrogenic (secondary to therapeutic doses of corticotropin or one of the corticosteroids). It may rarely be due to an adrenal tumor or to adrenocortical hyperplasia, or associated with basophilic adenoma of the pituitary gland or, rarely, with an extrapituitary ACTH-producing tumor.

Clinical Findings

A. Symptoms and Signs:

1. Due to excessive secretion of the glucocorticoid hormones–Findings include "buffalo type" adiposity, most marked on the face, neck, and trunk (a fat pad in the interscapular area is characteristic); easy fatigability and weakness; plethoric facies; purplish striae; easy bruisability; ecchymoses; hirsutism; osteoporosis; hypertension; diabetes mellitus (usually latent); pain in the back; muscle wasting and weakness; and marked retardation of growth.

2. Due to excessive secretion of mineralocorticoids–Hypernatremia, increased blood volume, edema, and hypertension may be found.

3. Due to excessive secretion of androgens– Manifestations include hirsutism, acne, and varying degrees of excessive masculinization. Menstrual irregularities occur during puberty in older girls.

B. Laboratory Findings:

1. Blood–

a. Serum cortisol levels are elevated. There may be a loss of the normal diurnal variation.

b. Serum chloride and potassium may be lowered. Serum sodium and HCO_3^- concentrations may be elevated (metabolic alkalosis).

c. Plasma ACTH concentrations are slightly elevated with adrenal hyperplasia, decreased in cases of adrenal tumor, and greatly increased with ACTH-producing pituitary or extrapituitary tumors.

d. The leukocyte count shows polymorphonuclear leukocytosis with lymphopenia, and the eosinophil count is low ($< 50/\mu L$). The erythrocyte count may be elevated.

2. Urine–

a. Urinary free cortisol excretion is elevated. This is the most useful diagnostic test.

b. Urinary 17-hydroxycorticosteroid levels are elevated.

c. Urinary 17-ketosteroids are usually elevated in association with adrenal tumor.

d. Glycosuria may be present.

3. Response to corticotropin (ACTH) and corticosteroids– The response to corticotropin (ACTH) stimulation is excessive in patients with adrenal hyperplasia; a poor response is usually found in those with tumor. There is a diminished adrenal response to small doses (0.5 mg) of dexamethasone in the dexamethasone suppression test; larger doses cause suppression of adrenal activity when the disease is due to adrenal hyperplasia. Adenomas and adrenal carcinomas may rarely be suppressed by large doses of dexamethasone (4–16 mg/d in four divided doses).

C. Imaging: Pituitary imaging may demonstrate a pituitary adenoma. Adrenal imaging (eg, CT scan) demonstrates adenoma and may demonstrate bilateral hyperplasia. Radionuclide studies of the adrenals may be useful in complete cases. Urograms may be abnormal. Adrenal calcification may be present. Osteoporosis (evident first in the spine and pelvis) with compression fractures may be seen in advanced cases.

Differential Diagnosis

Children with obesity, particularly in the presence of striae and hypertension, are frequently suspected of having Cushing's syndrome. The growth rate is helpful in differentiating the two. Children with Cushing's syndrome have a poor growth rate and a delay in skeletal maturation, whereas those with exogenous obesity usually have a normal or slightly increased growth rate and advanced epiphysial maturation. In addition, the color of the striae (purplish in Cushing's syndrome, pink in obesity) and the distri-

bution of the obesity assist in the differentiation. The urinary free cortisol excretion is always normal in obesity.

Treatment

In all cases of primary hyperfunction due to tumor, surgical removal, if possible, is indicated. Corticotropin (ACTH) should be given preoperatively and postoperatively to stimulate the nontumorous adrenal cortex, which is generally atrophied. Adrenocorticosteroids should be administered during and after surgery until the patient is stable. Supplemental potassium, salt, and mineralocorticoids may be necessary. (See above for corticosteroid administration in surgical patients.)

Adrenal hyperplasia resulting from a pituitary microadenoma may respond to pituitary surgery, irradiation, or partial adrenalectomy. In some cases, total adrenalectomy is necessary. Substitution therapy is usually necessary after these measures.

The use of mitotane, a DDT derivative toxic to the adrenal cortex, and aminoglutethimide, an inhibitor of steroid synthesis, has been suggested, but the efficacy of these agents in children with adrenal tumors has not been determined.

Prognosis

If the tumor is malignant, the prognosis is poor; if benign, cure is to be expected following proper preparation and surgery.

Pituitary enlargement has been reported in some cases of Cushing's syndrome following both partial and complete adrenalectomy.

Cushing's syndrome (perhaps due to pituitary adenoma) may occasionally undergo spontaneous remission.

Although most of the changes resulting from adrenocorticosteroid excess disappear, hypertension, diabetes mellitus, and osteoporosis may persist, and the rate of growth may continue to be poor.

Aron DC et al: Cushing's syndrome: Problems in management. Endocr Rev 1982;3:229.

Drucker A, New M: Disorders of adrenal steroidogenesis. Pediatr Clin North Am 1987;34:1055.

Homoki J, Solyom J, Teller WM: Detection of late onset steroid 21-hydroxylase deficiency by capillary gas chromatographic profiling of urinary steroids in children and adolescents. Eur J Pediatr 1988;147:257.

Killean AA et al: Diagnosis of classical steroid 21-hydroxylase deficiency using an HLA-B locus-specific DNA-probe. Am J Med Genet 1988;29:703.

Krieger DT: Physiopathology of Cushing's disease. Endocr Rev 1983;4:22.

Miller WL, Levine LS: Molecular and clinical advances in congenital adrenal hyperplasia. J Pediatr 1987;111:1.

Streeten DH et al: Normal and abnormal function of the hypothalamic-pituitary-adrenocortical system in man. Endocr Rev 1984;5:371.

White PC, New MI, Dupont B: Congenital adrenal hyperplasia. (Two parts.) N Engl J Med 1987;316:1519, 1580.

PRIMARY HYPERALDOSTERONISM

Primary hyperaldosteronism may be caused by a benign adrenal tumor or by adrenal hyperplasia. It is characterized by paresthesias, tetany, weakness, polyuria (nocturnal enuresis is common in young children), periodic "paralysis," low serum potassium, elevated serum sodium, hypertension, metabolic alkalosis, and production of a large volume of alkaline urine with a low fixed specific gravity; the latter does not respond to vasopressin. Edema is rare. The glucose tolerance test is frequently abnormal. Plasma and urinary aldosterone are elevated, but other steroid levels are variable. Plasma renin levels are decreased (in contrast to increased levels in secondary hyperaldosteronism, eg, that due to renal vascular disease and Bartter's syndrome). In patients with tumor, the administration of ACTH may further increase the excretion of aldosterone. Marked decrease of aldosterone-induced hypokalemia, alkalosis, hypochloremia, or hypernatremia after the administration of a glucocorticoid or an aldosterone antagonist such a spironolactone, which blocks the action of aldosterone upon the renal tubule, may be of diagnostic value.

Treatment is with glucocorticoid administration, subtotal or total adrenalectomy for hyperplasia, and surgical removal of the tumor.

Findling JW, Adams AH, Raff H: Selective hypoaldosteronism due to an endogenous impairment in angiotensin II production. N Engl J Med 1987;316:1632.

USES OF ADRENOCORTICOSTEROIDS & CORTICOTROPIN (ACTH) IN TREATMENT OF NONENDOCRINE DISEASES

The adrenocorticosteroids and corticotropin are commonly employed for their anti-inflammatory and immunosuppressive properties in a variety of conditions in childhood. Pharmacologic doses are necessary to achieve these effects, and side effects are common. Numerous synthetic preparations possessing variable ratios of glucocorticoid to mineralocorticoid activity are available (Table 30–12).

Actions

The adrenocorticosteroids exert a direct or permissive effect on virtually every tissue of the body; major known effects include the following:

(1) Gluconeogenesis and glycogen synthesis in the liver.

(2) Stimulation of fat synthesis and redistribution of body fat.

(3) Catabolism of protein with an increase in nitrogen and phosphorus excretion.

(4) Decrease in lymphoid and thymic tissue, resulting in a decreased cellular response to inflammation and hypersensitivity.

(5) Alteration of central nervous system excitation.

(6) Retardation of connective tissue mitosis and migration, decreasing wound healing.

(7) Improved capillary tone and increased vascular compartment volume and pressure.

Table 30–12. Adrenocorticosteroids.

	Trade Names	Potency/mg Compared With Cortisol[1] (Glucocorticoid Effect)	Potency/mg Compared With Cortisol (Sodium-Retaining Effect)
Glucocorticoids Hydrocortisone (cortisol)	Cortef	1	1
Cortisone	Cortone Acetate	4/5	1
Prednisone	Meticorten, others	4–5	2/5
Methylprednisolone	Medrol, Meprolone	5–6	Minimal effect
Triamcinolone	Aristocort, Kenacort, Kenalog, Atolone	5–6	Minimal effect
Dexamethasone	Decadron, others	25–30	Minimal effect
Betamethasone	Celestone	25	
Mineralocorticoids Fludrocortisone	Florinef	15–20	300–400
Aldosterone	Not commercially available	30	500

[1]To convert hydrocortisone dosage to equivalent dosage in any of the other preparations listed, divide by the potency factors shown.

(8) In the case of mineralocorticoids, control of cation flux across membranes, with sodium retention and potassium excretion.

Uses

The adrenocorticosteroids and corticotropin are commonly employed in adrenal insufficiency and in the following nonendocrine deficiency states in childhood:

(1) Adrenogenital syndrome. (Corticotropin is not effective in these disorders.)

(2) Nephrotic syndrome.

(3) Ulcerative colitis and ileitis.

(4) Allergic disorders: Bronchial asthma (including status asthmaticus), intractable hay fever (pollinosis), urticaria, angioneurotic edema, serum sickness, atopic dermatitis, atopic eczema, exfoliative dermatitis.

(5) Inflammatory eye disease: Uveitis, chorioretinitis, sympathetic ophthalmia, iritis, iridocyclitis, retinitis centralis, herpes zoster (not herpes simplex) ophthalmicus, optic neuritis, retrobulbar neuritis.

(6) Collagen vascular diseases: Rheumatoid arthritis, acute rheumatic fever, disseminated lupus erythematosus, scleroderma, dermatomyositis.

(7) Neoplastic diseases (temporary remission): Pulmonary granulomatosis, lymphoma, Hodgkin's disease, acute leukemia.

(8) Blood dyscrasias: Idiopathic thrombocytopenic purpura, allergic purpura, aplastic anemia, acquired hemolytic anemia.

(9) Miscellaneous conditions: Idiopathic hypoglycemia, infantile cortical hyperostosis, reticuloendotheliosis, thymic enlargement, sarcoidosis, pulmonary fibrosis, transfusion reactions, contact dermatitis (including poison oak), drug reactions, neurodermatitis.

Contraindications

A. Absolute: Use is contraindicated in active, questionably healed, or suspected tuberculosis.

B. Relative: These drugs should be used with extreme caution in the presence of herpes simplex of the eye, osteoporosis, peptic ulcer, active infections, emotional instability, and thrombophlebitis.

Side Effects of Therapy

When pharmacologic doses or prolonged use of adrenocorticosteroids are necessary, clinical manifestations of Cushing's syndrome are common. Side effects may result either from the use of synthetic exogenous agents by any route, including inhalation and topical administration (inflamed skin), or from the use of corticotropin (ACTH), which stimulates excessive production of endogenous adrenocorticosteroids. Use of a large single dose of glucocorticoids given once every 48 hours (alternate-day therapy) lessens the incidence and severity of some of the side effects.

A. Endocrine Disorders:

1. Hyperglycemia and glycosuria (of particular significance in early chemical diabetes).

2. Cushing's syndrome.

3. Persistent suppression of pituitary-adrenal responsiveness to stress with resultant hypoadrenocorticism.

B. Electrolyte and Mineral Disorders:

1. Marked retention of sodium and water, producing edema, increased blood volume, and hypertension (more common in endogenous hyperadrenal states).

2. Potassium loss with symptoms of hypokalemia.

3. Hypocalcemia, tetany.

C. Protein and Skeletal Disorders:

1. Negative nitrogen balance, with loss of body protein and bone protein, resulting in osteoporosis, pathologic fractures, and aseptic bone necrosis.

2. Suppression of growth, retarded skeletal maturation.

3. Muscular weakness and wasting.

D. Effect on Gastrointestinal Tract:

1. Excessive appetite and intake of food.

2. Activation or production of peptic ulcer.

3. Gastrointestinal bleeding from ulceration or from unknown cause (particularly in children with hepatic disease).

4. Fatty liver with embolism, pancreatitis, nodular panniculitis.

E. Lowering of Resistance to Infectious Agents; Silent Infection; Decreased Inflammatory Reaction:

1. Susceptibility to acute pulmonary or disseminated fungal infections; intestinal parasitic infections.

2. Activation of tuberculosis; false-negative tuberculin reaction.

3. Stimulation of activity of herpes simplex virus.

F. Neuropsychiatric Disorders:

1. Euphoria, excitability, psychotic behavior, and status epilepticus with electroencephalographic changes.

2. Increased intracranial pressure with "pseudotumor cerebri" syndrome.

G. Hemorrhagic Disorders:

1. Bleeding into the skin as a result of increased capillary fragility.

2. Thrombosis, thrombophlebitis, cerebral hemorrhage.

H. Miscellaneous:

1. Myocarditis, pleuritis, and arteritis following abrupt cessation of therapy.

2. Cardiomegaly.

3. Nephrosclerosis, proteinuria.

4. Acne (in older children), hirsutism, amenorrhea or irregular menses.

5. Posterior subcapsular cataracts; glaucoma.

Tapering of Pharmacologic Doses of Steroids

Prolonged use of pharmacologic doses of glucocorticoids may result in suppression of ACTH and consequent adrenal atrophy; discontinuation of glucocorticoids may result in clinical adrenal insufficiency. A gradual reduction in the steroid dose may allow resumption of ACTH stimulation of the adrenal gland, thereby lessening the risk of adrenal insufficiency. ACTH elaboration will generally not occur until the administered steroid is given in subphysiologic doses. If glucocorticoid therapy is not considered necessary for more than 2 weeks, the drug can be discontinued abruptly because adrenal suppression is unlikely. Thus, pharmacologic doses of glucocorticoid employed for 2 weeks or less may be tapered and withdrawn as rapidly as the condition for which the glucocorticoid is prescribed allows. As a rule of thumb, a reduction of 25–50% every 2–7 days is sufficiently rapid to permit observation of clinical symptomatology. Moreover, withdrawal through use of an alternate-day schedule (eg, a single dose given every 48 hours) may allow for a 50% decrease in the total dosage while providing the desired pharmacologic effect.

Once a physiologic equivalent is achieved, the dose may be reduced by 25% every 5–7 days until a subphysiologic level is reached. At this point, assessment of endogenous adrenal activity is estimated by obtaining fasting plasma cortisol levels drawn prior to the morning steroid dose. When an alternate-day schedule is followed, a plasma cortisol level is drawn the morning prior to treatment. A cortisol level within the physiologic range (8–15 μg/dL) demonstrates return of basal physiologic adrenal function; exogenous steroids may then be discontinued. Once basal physiologic adrenal function returns, the adrenal reserve or capacity to respond to stress and infection is estimated by the ACTH stimulation test, in which 250 μg of synthetic ACTH is administered intravenously. Cortisol levels are obtained prior to the infusion, at the end of the infusion, and at 30 and 60 minutes after the infusion. A cortisol level above 20 μg/dL at 30 or 60 minutes indicates a satisfactory adrenal reserve. The ACTH test should be performed in all patients who have received pharmacologic doses of steroids for more than 2 weeks. Even if the results of the test are normal, however, patients who have received prolonged treatment with adrenocorticosteroids may exhibit signs and symptoms of adrenal insufficiency during acute stress, infection, or surgery for months to years after glucocorticoids have been withdrawn. Careful monitoring and (when necessary) the use of pharmacologic doses of glucocorticoids should be considered during severe illnesses and surgery for life.

Axelrod L: Corticosteroid therapy. In: *Principles and Practice of Endocrinology and Metabolism.* Becker KL (editor). Lippincott, 1990.

Chamberlain P, Meyer WJ: Management of pituitary-adrenal suppression secondary to corticosteroid therapy. Pediatrics 1981;67:245.

Messer J et al: Association of adrenocorticosteroid therapy and peptic ulcer disease. N Engl J Med 1983;309:21.

Schlagehecke R et al: The effect of long-term glucocorticoid therapy on pituitary-adrenal responses to exogenous corticotropin-releasing hormone. N Engl J Med 1992; 326:226.

ADRENAL MEDULLA

PHEOCHROMOCYTOMA (Chromaffinoma)

Pheochromocytoma is an uncommon tumor. Approximately 10% of the total number of cases occur in childhood. The tumor may be located wherever there is any chromaffin tissue (adrenal medulla, sympathetic ganglia, carotid body, etc). It may be multiple, familial (autosomal dominant, in which case a high prevalence of multiple endocrine neoplasia exists), recurrent, and (sometimes) malignant.

Although clinical manifestation of pheochromocytoma may result from physical expansion of lesions into surrounding tissue (eg, spinal cord), manifestations are generally due to excessive secretion of epinephrine or norepinephrine. Attacks of anxiety, unexplained perspiration, and headaches should arouse suspicion. Other findings are palpitation and tachycardia, dizziness, weakness, nausea and vomiting, diarrhea, dilated pupils with blurring of vision, abdominal and precordial pain, hypertension (usually persistent), postural hypotension, discomfort from heat, and vasomotor instability. The symptoms may be sustained, producing all of the above findings plus papilledema, retinopathy, and enlargement of the heart. There is an increased incidence of pheochromocytomas in patients and families with pheochromatoses, neurofibromatosis, and type 2 multiple endocrine neoplasia. Neuroblastomas, neurogangliomas, and other neural tumors may cause increased secretion of pressor amines and occasionally simulate the findings of pheochromocytoma. Carcinoid tumors may produce cardiovascular changes similar to those associated with pheochromocytoma.

Laboratory diagnosis is possible in over 90% of cases. Serum catecholamines are elevated, particularly while the patient is symptomatic, and urinary excretion of catecholamines parallels this elevation. Elevated levels are characteristically high enough to be diagnostic but may be limited to the period of a paroxysm. The 24-hour urine collection shows increased excretion of metanephrines and vanillylmandelic acid. Provocative tests employing histamine, tyramine, or glucagon and the phentolamine tests may be abnormal; the former are dangerous, however, and these agents are rarely necessary for diagnosis. Displacement of the kidney may be shown by routine x-ray and the tumor identified by CT scanning or MRI. Angiocatheterization and measurement of blood levels of catecholamines may be helpful in localizing the tumor prior to surgery.

Surgical removal of the tumor is the treatment of choice, though the procedure is dangerous and may cause sudden death. Oral phenoxybenzamine or intravenous phentolamine is used preoperatively. Profound hypotension may occur as the tumor is removed but may be controlled with an infusion of norepinephrine, which may have to be continued for 1–2 days.

Complete relief of symptoms is to be expected after recovery from removal of the nonmalignant tumor unless irreversible secondary vascular changes have occurred. If the disorder remains untreated, severe cardiac, renal, and cerebral damage may result.

Bravo EB, Gifford RW Jr: Pheochromocytoma: Diagnosis, localization and management. N Engl J Med 1984; 311:1298.

Cryer PE: Physiology and pathophysiology of the human sympathoadrenal neuroendocrine system. N Engl J Med 1980;303:436.

DIABETES MELLITUS

Essentials of Diagnosis

- Polyuria, polydipsia, and weight loss.
- Hyperglycemia and glycosuria with or without ketonuria.

General Considerations

Insulin-dependent (type I) diabetes mellitus (previously called juvenile-onset diabetes) is the most common type of diabetes in people under age 40 years. It is associated with diminished insulin production and a tendency to develop ketosis, though approximately 85% of people still make some insulin 1 year after diagnosis, and 42% still make small amounts of insulin 3 years after diagnosis. Type II (non-insulin-dependent) diabetes is commonest over age 40 and is not ketosis-prone. Type II patients are usually overweight and insulin-insensitive. Cases of type II diabetes are rare prior to 18 years of age but do occur in overweight teenagers and are referred to as maturity-onset diabetes in youth (MODY). Diet, exercise, and oral hypoglycemic agents are the main therapy for those patients. The remainder of this discussion will deal with type I diabetes.

Etiology

The development of type I diabetes is believed to require (1) a genetic predisposition; (2) environmental factors initiating islet cell damage; and (3) immunologic or lymphocyte-mediated damage. Type I diabetes develops gradually over months or years in most people, but the symptoms do not appear until about 90% of the pancreatic islets have been destroyed.

The importance of genetics is demonstrated by the observation that 35–50% of second identical twins develop diabetes after the first twin develops the disease. Approximately 6% of siblings or offspring of people with type I diabetes also develop diabetes (compared to the usual incidence of 2–3:1000). The condition is more frequent in Caucasian children but occurs in all other groups as well. There is an association with HLA groups DR3 and DR4, and approximately 95% of Caucasian diabetic children have at least one of these HLA types. Fifty-three percent have both one DR3 and one DR4 (one from each parent), compared with the presence of this combination in only 6% of the general population. The presence of aspartic acid on position 57 of the DQ beta chain of the HLA complex is associated with alleles which are protective (eg, DQβ0602) against type I diabetes, and, conversely, its absence provides a marker for susceptibility.

The etiologic importance of environmental factors is suggested by the observation that over half of second identical twins do not develop diabetes after diabetes has occurred in the first twin. If the condition were purely genetic, the second twin would always develop the disease. Important environmental factors may be viral diseases or chemicals in the diet. For example, 40% of infants with congenital rubella develop diabetes or an abnormal glucose tolerance test by 20 years of age, and the incidence of diabetes is high after ingestion of foods preserved with nitrates. The early introduction of cow's milk also has been suggested as a possible environmental factor.

The immunologic basis of the disease is demonstrated by the ability of a potent immunosuppressive agent, cyclosporine, to preserve islet tissue for 1–2 years when given to newly diagnosed patients. However, the renal damage from cyclosporine precludes its long-term use. White blood cells are found in the islets of newly diagnosed patients and may release toxic products (free radicals, interleukin-1, tumor necrosis factor) that injure the islets. Antibodies to islet cells, insulin, or glutamic acid decarboxylase are present in the serum of 80–90% of patients for months to years prior to diagnosis. It is likely that these antibodies are the effect rather than the cause of islet destruction. Many centers now screen for prediabetes using an islet cell antibody or other antibody test. An intravenous glucose tolerance test helps define those at highest risk so that they may enter prevention trials. Initial pilot data suggest a preventive role for nicotinamide, azathioprine, or early insulin administration. Intervention trials on antibody-positive first-degree relatives based on data from the pilot trials are about to start. European investigators will be doing a double-blind study of nicotinamide, while US centers will be doing a double-blind study of intravenous and subcutaneous insulin versus placebo (see Keller, 1993).

Diagnosis

The classic symptoms of polyuria and polydipsia are now so well recognized that friends or family members usually suspect the diagnosis of type I diabetes. Other cases may be detected by finding glycosuria on routine office urinalysis. Half of cases once presented in coma; most now present prior to development of severe ketonuria, ketonemia, and secondary acidosis. An oral glucose tolerance test is rarely necessary in children. A random blood glucose level above 300 mg/dL (16.6 mmol/L) or a fasting blood glucose above 200 mg/dL (11 mmol/L) is all that is needed to make the diagnosis. If the presentation is mild, hospitalization is usually not necessary. Good education for all family members is essential to help the family deal with the condition. All care-givers need to learn about diabetes, how to give insulin injections, and how to perform home blood glucose monitoring. There is also much stress for the family around the initial diagnosis, and the feelings of shock, denial, sadness, anger, fear, and guilt may be present in varying amounts. Meeting with a counselor to express these feelings at the time of diagnosis helps with long-term adaptation.

Treatment

The five major features of the treatment of type I diabetes are (1) insulin dosage, (2) diet, (3) exercise, (4) stress management, and (5) blood glucose and urine ketone monitoring. All of these must be considered in aiming for the best metabolic control that each family is able to achieve safely. Although teenagers can be taught to take responsibility for much of their own diabetes management from the outset, it must be remembered that teens do better when supportive (but not overly controlling) parents remain involved. Children under 10 or 11 years of age cannot reliably administer insulin without adult supervision, because they lack fine motor control and do not understand the importance of accuracy.

A. Insulin: The three most important functions of insulin are (1) to allow glucose to pass into the cell, (2) to decrease the body's (particularly liver and muscle) own production of glucose, and (3) to turn off ketone production.

If moderate or large ketonuria is present at the onset of type I diabetes and the child is adequately hydrated and has a normal venous blood pH (see ketonuria and ketoacidosis, below), it may be desirable to give one or two intramuscular injections of 0.1–0.2 unit of regular (short-lasting) insulin per kilogram of body weight approximately 1 hour apart to help shut down ketone production. If ketonuria is small or absent, this regimen is not necessary. When ketonuria is not present, the child is usually more sensitive to insulin, and a total daily dose of 0.25 unit/kg/24 h (by subcutaneous injection) can be used. The presence of ketonuria implies that the child does not produce much insulin and will require 0.5 unit/kg/24 h. These doses are then adjusted with each injection during the first week. Most physicians begin newly diagnosed children with synthetic human insulin. Approximately two-thirds of the total dose is usually given 30–60 minutes before breakfast and the other one-third 30–60 minutes before dinner. Children under age 4 years usually need 1 or 2 units of regular insulin to cover meals, and the remainder of the dosage is NPH insulin. Children 5–10 years of age may require up to 4 units of regular insulin to cover breakfast and dinner, whereas proportionately higher dosages (usually 4–10 units) of regular insulin are used for older children.

The total daily insulin dose may need to be gradually increased to 1 unit/kg body weight (especially if ketonuria was present at onset). When gluconeogenesis and glycolysis are suppressed by insulin, the honeymoon or "grace" period is often seen. This may occur 1–8 weeks after diagnosis in more than half of children. Continuing small doses of insulin at levels that do not cause frequent hypoglycemia may be important at this time to help preserve later β cell function.

Sliding scales for regular insulin, based on home blood glucose determinations, are acceptable. Once the initial correct dosage of NPH insulin is attained, daily adjustments of this long-acting insulin usually are not needed. However, small decreases may be made in anticipation of heavy activity (eg, afternoon sports or overnight social events). Many families gradually learn to make small (0.5–1 unit) weekly adjustments in a child's insulin dosage, based on home blood glucose testing results. Understanding the times of insulin activity is essential (Figure 30–5).

B. Diet: The mainstays of dietary management of diabetic children are as follows: (1) eat a well-balanced diet; (2) keep the day-to-day intake consistent; (3) eat meals and snacks at the same time each day; (4) use snacks to prevent insulin reactions (encourage solid protein at bedtime every night); (5) avoid pure sugar foods (candy, sodas, etc); (6) reduce cholesterol, total fat, and saturated fat intake; (7) maintain appropriate weight for height, and avoid becoming

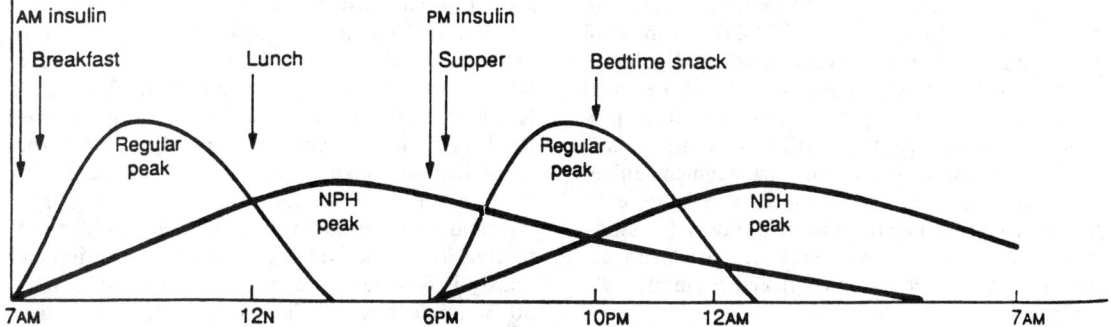

Figure 30–5. Patterns of insulin activity throughout the four periods of the day—breakfast to lunch, lunch to supper, supper to bedtime, and bedtime to morning—when two injections of regular and NPH insulin are given approximately 30 minutes before breakfast and supper.

overweight; (8) increase fiber intake; (9) avoid foods high in salt; and (10) avoid excessive protein intake. These recommendations are all discussed in detail in *Understanding Insulin Dependent Diabetes,* 7th ed (see references, below). Some families and children (particularly those with weight problems) find exchange diets helpful, at least initially when they are learning about categories of foods. Working with a knowledgeable dietitian is an important component of diabetes management.

C. Exercise: Regular aerobic exercise is important for children with diabetes because exercise fosters a sense of well-being; helps increase insulin sensitivity, maintain proper weight, blood pressure, and blood fat levels; and may help maintain normal peripheral circulation in later years.

D. Stress Management: The management of stress is important on a short-term basis because stress hormones increase blood glucose levels. Chronic emotional upsets may lead to missed injections or other compliance problems. When this happens, counseling becomes an important part of diabetes management.

E. Blood Glucose and Urine Ketone Measurements: All families must have the ability and materials to monitor blood glucose measurements at least twice daily, and more frequently for small infants or if there are problems with glucose control or with illness. They must also know when to do urine ketone checks. Blood glucose levels can be done using visual strips or by meter with accuracy of ± 10%. Blood glucose levels to aim for when no food has been eaten for 2 or more hours vary with the age of the child: 4 years and under, 100–200 mg/dL (5.5–11 mmol/L); 5–12 years, 80–180 mg/dL (4.6–10 mmol/L); and 13 years and older, 70–150 mg/dL (3.9–8.3 mmol/L).

Laboratory Evaluations

In addition to home measurements of blood glucose and urine ketone levels, it is now the accepted standard of care to measure the glycosylated hemoglobin every 3 months. This test reflects the frequency of elevated blood glucose levels over the previous 3 months. Normal values vary between laboratories but are usually below 6.2% (hemoglobin A_{1c}) or below 8% (total glycosylated hemoglobin). Using either method, longitudinal averages below 10% are associated with a much lower risk for the later renal and retinal complications of diabetes.

Acute Complications

Hypoglycemia and ketonuria or ketoacidosis are the acute complications of type I diabetes.

A. Hypoglycemia: The common symptoms of hypoglycemia (or "insulin reaction") are hunger, weakness, shakiness, sweating, drowsiness (at an unusual time), headache, and behavioral changes. If not treated immediately with simple sugar, the hypoglycemia may result in loss of consciousness or convulsions. If not treated for several hours, brain damage or death can occur. Consistency in the daily routine, correct insulin dosage, regular blood glucose monitoring, snacks, responsible patients and parents, and good education are all important in preventing severe hypoglycemia.

Among participating patients in the Diabetes Control and Complications Trial (DCCT), 10% of patients with standard management and 25% of patients with intensive insulin management (insulin pumps or four or more insulin shots per day) had one or more major hypoglycemic reactions each year. We thus advise all families to keep glucagon in the home. We suggest giving 0.3 mL (0.3 mg) if the patient is under 5 years old and 0.5 mL (0.5 mg) if over 5 years old by either subcutaneous or intramuscular injection. School personnel, sports coaches, and baby-sitters must be trained to recognize and treat hypoglycemia.

B. Ketonuria and Ketoacidosis: It is essential that families know how to check urine ketones during any illness (including vomiting even one time) or any time a blood glucose level is above 240 mg/dL (13.3

mmol/L). If moderate or large ketonuria is detected, the physician must be called and 10–20% of the total daily insulin dose given subcutaneously as regular insulin every 3 hours until the urine ketones are small or negative. This will prevent ketonuria from progression to ketoacidosis and will allow most cases to be treated at home by telephone management. Juices and other fluids are encouraged, and suppositories to prevent vomiting may be indicated. If deep breathing (Kussmaul respirations) or excessive weakness occurs, the patient should be evaluated promptly by a physician.

Acidosis (venous blood pH < 7.30) may develop in newly diagnosed children and with families who have not received good diabetes education or who are noncompliant and do not check for ketonuria and call the physician when moderate or large amounts of urine ketones are present. Repeated episodes of ketoacidosis usually are due to missed insulin injections and require that a responsible adult take over the diabetes management. If this adult participation is not forthcoming, a change in the child's living situation may be necessary.

The treatment of diabetic ketoacidosis is based on four physiologic principles: (1) restoration of fluid volume; (2) inhibition of lipolysis and return to glucose utilization; (3) replacement of body salts; and (4) correction of acidosis. Laboratory tests at the start of treatment should include a venous pH, a blood glucose, and an electrolyte panel. Mild diabetic ketoacidosis is defined as a venous pH of 7.20 or above; moderate ketoacidosis by a pH of 7.10–7.19; and severe ketoacidosis by a pH below 7.10. Patients with severe ketoacidosis should be hospitalized and not treated in a clinic or emergency room. More severe cases may benefit from determination of serum osmolality, calcium, phosphorus, and urea nitrogen levels. Severe and moderate episodes of diabetic ketoacidosis generally require hourly determinations of serum glucose, electrolytes, and venous blood pH levels, whereas these parameters can be measured every 2 hours if the pH level is between 7.20 and 7.30.

1. Restore fluid volume–Dehydration is judged by acute loss in body weight (if recent weight is known) as well as by dryness of oral mucous membranes, the low blood pressure, and the high heart rate. Initial treatment is with physiologic saline, 10–20 mL/kg during the first hour. If indicated, this is repeated during the second hour. Albumin, 10 mL/kg of 5% solution, can be given for 30 minutes if the patient is in shock. After initial reexpansion, half-physiologic (0.45%) saline usually is given at 1½ times the maintenance dosage.

2. Inhibit lipolysis and return to glucose utilization– Insulin turns off fat breakdown and ketone formation. Intravenous regular insulin usually is administered for the treatment of diabetic ketoacidosis at a dosage of 0.1 unit/kg/h. The insulin solution should be administered by pump and can be made by diluting 30 units of regular insulin in 150 mL of physiologic saline (1 unit/5 mL). If the glucose level falls below 250 mg/dL (13.9 mmol/L), 5% dextrose is added to the intravenous fluids. If the glucose level continues to decrease below 120 mg/dL (6.6 mmol/L), 10% dextrose can be added. If necessary, the insulin dose can be reduced to 0.05 unit/kg/h, but it should not be discontinued before venous blood pH reaches 7.30. The half-life of insulin given intravenously is 6 minutes, but subcutaneous insulin takes 30–60 minutes to act. Thus, it is often better to continue the intravenous insulin until the subcutaneous insulin can begin acting.

3. Replace body salts–Both sodium and potassium pass into the urine with the ketones and are depleted in diabetic ketoacidosis. Serum sodium concentrations may be falsely lowered by hyperglycemia, causing water to be drawn into the intravascular space, and by hyperlipemia if fat replaces some of the water in the serum used for electrolyte analysis. Sodium is usually replaced adequately by the use of physiologic and half-physiologic saline in the rehydration fluids as discussed above.

Serum potassium levels initially may be elevated owing to the inability of potassium to stay in the cell in the presence of acidosis (although the total body potassium is low). Potassium should not be given until the serum potassium level is known to be low or normal and the pH is above 7.10.

4. Correct the acidosis–Acidosis is corrected as the fluid volume and aerobic glycolysis are restored and as insulin is administered to inhibit ketogenesis. As noted earlier, measuring the venous pH (identical to the arterial pH) reveals the severity of acidosis. Bicarbonate is usually reserved for patients with a pH less than 7.00 and is given as 1–2 meq/kg body weight *over 1 or 2 hours*. The pH is monitored every hour and the bicarbonate discontinued when the pH reaches 7.10.

5. Management of cerebral edema–Some degree of cerebral edema has been shown by CT scan to be quite common in diabetic ketoacidosis. Associated clinical symptoms are rare, unpredictable, and often lethal. Cerebral edema may be related to overhydration with hypotonic fluids, though the cause is not well understood. The early neurologic signs may include headache, excessive drowsiness, and dilated pupils. Prompt initiation of therapy should include elevation of the head of the bed, hyperventilation, mannitol (1 g/kg body weight by intravenous bolus), and fluid restriction.

Chronic Complications

The Diabetes Control and Complications Trial (DCCT) showed that intensive diabetes management can delay the onset and slow the progression of retinopathy, nephropathy, and neuropathy. Approximately 30–40% of people with type I diabetes eventually develop renal failure or loss of vision. Factors that greatly reduce this likelihood include longitudinal HbA_1 levels in a good range, maintenance of blood pressure below the 90th percentile for age, and abstinence from smoking or chewing tobacco. Annual retinal examinations and urine microalbumin measurements are important for pubertal children who have had diabetes for 5 years or longer.

Baisch JM et al: Analysis of HLA-DQ genotypes and susceptibility in insulin-dependent diabetes mellitus. N Engl J Med 1990;322:1836.

Chase HP: *Understanding Insulin Dependent Diabetes,* 7th ed. Hirschfeld Press, 1992. (Available for $8.00 from The Children's Diabetes Foundation, 777 Grant Street, Suite 302, Denver, CO 80203.)

Chase HP, Garg SK, Jelley DH: Diabetic ketoacidosis in children and the role of outpatient management. Pediatr Rev 1990;11:297.

Chase HP et al: Cigarette smoking increases the risk of albu-minuria among subjects with type I diabetes. JAMA 1991;265:614.

Chase HP et al: Cyclosporine A for the treatment of new-onset insulin-dependent diabetes mellitus. Pediatrics 1990;85:241.

Chase HP et al: Glucose control and the renal and retinal complications of insulin-dependent diabetes. JAMA 1989;261:1155.

Chase HP et al: Prediction of the course of pre-type I diabetes. J Pediatr 1991;118:838.

The Diabetes Control and Complications Trial Research Group. The effect of intensive treatment of diabetes on the development and progression of long-term complications in insulin-dependent diabetes mellitus. N Engl J Med 1993;329:977.

Keller RJ, Eisenbarth GS, Jackson RA: Insulin prophylaxis in individuals at high risk of type I diabetes. Lancet 1993;341:927.

Krane EJ et al: Subclinical brain swelling in children during treatment of diabetic ketoacidosis. N Engl J Med 1985; 312:1147.

REFERENCES

DeGroot LJ et al (editors): *Endocrinology,* 2nd ed. 3 vols. Saunders, 1989.

Felig P et al: *Endocrinology and Metabolism,* 2nd ed. McGraw-Hill, 1987.

Greenspan FS, Baxter JD: *Basic and Clinical Endocrinology,* 4th ed. Appleton & Lange, 1994.

Hung W, August GP, Glasgow AM: *Pediatric Endocrinology.* Medical Examination, 1983.

Kappy MS, Blizzard RM, Migeon C: *The Diagnosis and Treatment of Endocrine Disorders in Childhood and Adolescence.* Thomas, 1994. [In press.]

Travis LB, Bronhard BH, Schreiner BJ: *Diabetes Mellitus in Children and Adolescents.* Saunders, 1987.

31

Inborn Errors of Metabolism

Carol L. Greene, MD, & Stephen I. Goodman, MD

Disorders in which defects of single genes cause clinically significant blocks in metabolic pathways are called **inborn errors of metabolism.** For many years after Garrod first described them in 1908, these conditions were considered esoteric and rare. The number of known inborn errors has increased rapidly in recent years, however, and they are now recognized as important causes of disease in the pediatric age group. Many of them can now be treated effectively. Even when treatment is not available, correct diagnosis permits couples to make informed decisions about future offspring.

Pathogenesis is almost always due to accumulation of enzyme substrate behind the metabolic block or to deficiency of the reaction product. In some cases, the accumulated enzyme substrate is diffusible and has an adverse effect on distant organs; in others, as in lysosomal storage diseases, the substrate accumulates only locally.

The clinical manifestations of inborn errors vary significantly; there are mild and severe forms of virtually every disorder, and many patients do not match the classical phenotype. In many cases, this is because the mutations in different patients, even though they are in the same gene, are not identical.

Strategies used to treat inborn errors include avoiding enzyme substrate in the diet (eg, low-phenylalanine diet for phenylketonuria), removing accumulated substrate by pharmacologic means (eg, glycine therapy for isovaleric acidemia), supplementing an inadequately produced metabolite (eg, arginine administration for urea cycle disorders), providing additional coenzyme (eg, vitamin B_{12} therapy for methylmalonic acidemia), and providing normal enzyme (eg, enzyme infusion in Gaucher's disease or liver transplantation for Wilson's disease). Gene replacement is a long-term goal, and trials of treatment of adenine deaminase deficiency began in 1990. However, problems of delivery to target organs and control of gene action make this an unrealistic option at present for most of these disorders.

Inborn errors can present at any time, affect virtually any organ system, and cause all but the most common pediatric problems. This chapter focuses first on when these conditions should be considered in the differential diagnosis of common pediatric problems. A few of the more important disorders are then discussed in detail.

DIAGNOSIS

Inborn errors must be considered in the differential diagnosis of the critically ill newborn and of the child with seizures, Reye-like syndromes, parenchymal liver disease, mental retardation or developmental delay, recurrent vomiting, unusual odor, unexplained acidosis, hyperammonemia, and hypoglycemia.

Inborn errors should be strongly suspected when (1) symptoms accompany changes in diet, (2) there is developmental slowing or regression, (3) there is a history of food preferences or aversions, or (4) there is a history of parental consanguinity or a history of problems that could be due to an inborn error, eg, retardation or unexplained death in sibs, cousins, or other relatives.

Physical findings that should always raise the suspicion of an inborn error include alopecia or abnormal hair, retinal cherry-red spot or retinitis pigmentosa, cataracts or corneal opacity, hepatomegaly or splenomegaly, coarse features, skeletal changes (including gibbus), and ataxia. Features that may be important, in combination with a suspicious history, include failure to thrive, microcephaly, rash, jaundice, hypotonia, and hypertonia.

Finding an immediate cause of symptoms does not rule out an underlying inborn error. For example, renal tubular acidosis and cirrhosis are often due to an underlying inborn error. Some inborn errors predispose to infection, eg, gram-negative septicemia in patients with galactosemia. In other inborn errors, acute crises may be brought on by intercurrent infections.

Table 31–1 lists common clinical and laboratory features of different groups of inborn errors. Table 31–2 lists laboratory tests used to diagnose these diseases and gives some comments about their use.

Laboratory studies are almost always needed for the diagnosis of inborn errors. Serum electrolytes and pH can be determined in any hospital laboratory and should be used to estimate anion gap as well as acid-base status. Analysis of serum lactate, pyruvate, and ammonia may be available in laboratories of large hospitals. Amino acid and organic acid studies must be performed at specialized facilities to ensure adequate analysis and interpretation. It is becoming possible to diagnose an increasing number of inborn errors with DNA probes. For most disorders, this requires an extensive genealogic chart or a knowledge of the precise mutation carried in the family.

The physician should know what conditions a test will detect and when it will detect them. For example, urine organic acids may be normal in patients with medium-chain acyl-CoA dehydrogenase deficiency or biotinidase deficiency, glycine may be elevated only in cerebrospinal fluid in patients with glycine encephalopathy, and a result that is normal in one physiologic state may be abnormal in another. For instance, the urine of a hypoglycemic child should be positive for ketones; in such children, a ketone-negative urine test may suggest the presence of a defect in fatty acid oxidation.

Samples used to diagnose metabolic disease may be obtained at autopsy. They may be analyzed directly or stored frozen until a particular analysis is justified by the results of postmortem examination, new clinical information, or new developments in the field. Studies of other family members may also help to establish the diagnosis in a deceased patient; these include demonstrating that the parents are heterozygous carriers of a particular disorder or showing that another sibling has the condition.

ACUTE PRESENTATION IN NEONATE—THE CHILD WITH "RULE OUT SEPSIS"

Acute metabolic disease in the newborn may be clinically indistinguishable from sepsis and is most often caused by disorders of protein or carbohydrate metabolism. Initial symptoms may include poor feeding or vomiting, altered mental status or tone, jitteriness or seizures, and jaundice. Acidosis or altered mental status out of proportion to systemic symptoms should increase suspicion of metabolic disorder. Laboratory studies should include determination of electrolytes, ammonia, glucose, urine pH, and urine ketones. Glycine in cerebrospinal fluid should be measured if glycine encephalopathy is suspected. Serum and urine to be used for amino and organic acid analysis should be collected before oral intake is stopped and sent for analysis if indicated by the results of initial studies.

VOMITING & ENCEPHALOPATHY IN THE INFANT OR OLDER CHILD

Even though vomiting and altered consciousness in the infant or child are more often due to infection and trauma than to an inborn error, the physician should order laboratory studies of electrolytes, ammonia, glucose, urine pH, urine-reducing substances, and urine ketones in all patients before the results are altered by treatment. Samples for amino and organic acid analysis should be obtained early and frozen pending the results of initial studies. An inborn error is even more likely when the presentation is judged "typical" of Reye's syndrome (vomiting, encephalopathy, and hepatomegaly), and amino and organic acids should be studied immediately. If there is hypoglycemia with inappropriately low urine or serum ketones, disorders of fatty acid oxidation should be considered.

MENTAL RETARDATION

Many inborn errors can cause mental retardation without other distinguishing characteristics. Laboratory studies of serum and urine amino acids should be obtained for every patient with nonspecific mental retardation. Because physical stigmas of certain mucopolysaccharidoses are subtle, urine screens for mucopolysacchariduria may also be useful. Electrolytes should be examined because the presence of a high anion gap or renal tubular acidosis significantly increases the chance of finding an underlying inborn error. If developmental regression or specific neurologic findings are present, the evaluation should be expanded accordingly.

HYPOGLYCEMIA

Studies of electrolytes, ammonia, uric acid, urine-reducing substances, and urine ketones should be performed, and urine should be obtained to measure levels of organic acids. Ketone body production is usually not efficient in the neonate, and ketonuria in a hypoglycemic neonate suggests an inborn error. In the older child, however, the absence of ketonuria suggests inborn error, particularly of fatty acid oxidation.

HYPERAMMONEMIA

Symptoms of hyperammonemia may appear and progress rapidly or insidiously. Decreased appetite and irritability usually appear first, with vomiting, lethargy, seizures, and coma appearing as ammonia levels increase. Tachypnea is caused by a direct effect on respiratory drive. Physical examination cannot ex-

Table 31–1. Presenting clinical and laboratory features of inborn errors.[1]

	Defects of Carbohydrate Metabolism	Defects of Amino Acid Metabolism[2]	Organic Acid Disorders[3]	Defects of Fatty Acid Oxidation	Defects of Purine Metabolism	Lysosomal Storage Diseases	Disorders of Peroxisomes
Neurodevelopmental							
Mental/developmental retardation	+++	+++	+++	+	++	+++	+++
Developmental regression	-	-	+	-	-	+++	+++
Acute encephalopathy	+++	+++	+++	+++	-	-	-
Seizures	++	+++	+++	+	-	+++	++
Ataxia/movement disorder	-	+	++	-	+++	-	-
Hypotonia	++	++	++	+++	-	+	+++
Hypertonia	-	++	+++	-	++	+	-
Abnormal behavior	-	++	++	-	++	+++	-
Growth							
Failure to thrive	+++	+++	+++	+	-	+	-
Short stature	++	-	+	-	-	++	-
Macrocephaly	-	-	+	-	-	+++	++
Microcephaly	+	++	+++	-	-	+	-
General							
Vomiting/anorexia	++	+++	+++	+++	-	-	++
Food aversion or craving	++	+++	+++	+++	-	-	-
Odor	-	++	++	-	-	-	-
Dysmorphic features	-	+	+	-	-	++	++
Congenital malformations	-	++	++	-	-	-	++

Organ specific							
Hepatomegaly	+++	−	++	+++	−	+++	+++
Liver disease/cirrhosis	++	+	−	+	−	−	+
Splenomegaly	−	−	−	−	−	++	+
Skeletal dysplasia	−	−	−	−	−	++	++
Cardiomyopathy	++	−	+	+++	−	++	−
Tachypnea/hyperpnea	++	++	++	++	−	−	−
Rash	−	++	++	−	−	−	−
Alopecia or abnormal hair	−	+	++	−	−	−	+
Cataracts or corneal opacity	++	−	−	−	−	++	−
Retinal abnormality	−	+	+	+	−	++	++
Frequent infections	++	−	++	−	++	−	−
Deafness	−	−	+	−	−	++	−
Laboratory - general							
Hypoglycemia	+++	+	++	++	−	−	−
Hyperammonemia	−	++	++	++	−	−	−
Metabolic acidosis	++	++	+++	+++	−	−	−
Respiratory alkalosis	−	++	−	−	−	−	−
Elevated lactate/pyruvate	++	−	+++	++	−	−	−
Elevated liver enzymes	++	++	++	+++	−	+	+
Neutropenia or thrombocytopenia	+	−	+	−	++	+	−
Ketosis	+++	++	+++	−	−	−	−
Hypoketosis	−	−	+	+++	−	−	−

[1] + + +, most conditions in group; + +, some; +, one or few; −, not found.
[2] Includes disorders of urea cycle but not maple syrup urine disease.
[3] Includes maple syrup urine disease and disorders of pyruvate oxidation.

Table 31–2. Obtaining and handling samples to diagnose inborn errors.

Test	Comments
Acid-base status	Accurate estimation of anion gap must be possible. Samples for blood gases should be kept on ice and analyzed immediately.
Blood ammonia	Sample should be collected without a tourniquet, kept on ice, and analyzed immediately.
Blood lactic acid and pyruvic acid	Sample should be collected without a tourniquet, kept on ice, and analyzed immediately. Reduction of pyruvic acid to lactic acid must be prevented. Normal literature values are for the fasting, rested state.
Amino acids	Blood and urine should be examined. CSF glycine should be measured if nonketotic hyperglycinemia is to be ruled out. Normal literature values are for the fasting state. Growth of bacteria in urine should be prevented. At autopsy: liver, kidney, or vitreous may be analyzed if urine is not available.
Organic acids	Urine preferred for analysis. At autopsy: liver, kidney, or vitreous may be analyzed if urine is not available.
Urine mucopolysaccharides	Variations in urine concentration may cause errors in screening tests. Diagnosis requires knowing which mucopolysaccharides are increased. Some patients with Morquio's disease do not have abnormal mucopolysacchariduria.
Enzyme assays	Specific assays must be requested. Exposure to heat may cause loss of enzyme activity. Enzyme activity in whole blood may become normal after transfusion or vitamin therapy. Leukocyte or fibroblast pellets should be kept frozen prior to assays. Fibroblasts may be grown from skin biopsies taken up to 72 hours after death. Tissues such as liver and kidney should be taken as soon as possible after death, frozen immediately, and kept at −70 °C until assayed.

clude the presence of hyperammonemia, and serum ammonia should be measured whenever hyperammonemia is possible.

Severe hyperammonemia may be due to urea cycle disorders, organic acidemias or, in the neonate, to transient hyperammonemia of the newborn. The cause can usually be ascertained by measuring citrulline and electrolytes in serum and measuring amino acids, organic acids, and orotic acid in urine. Respiratory alkalosis is usually present in transient hyperammonemia of the newborn and hyperammonemia due to a urea cycle defect, whereas metabolic acidosis is usually associated with hyperammonemia due to

organic acidemia. Urine organic acid analysis will demonstrate the cause if the condition is due to organic acidemia. Serum citrulline is usually low or undetectable in early urea cycle defects; normal or slightly high in transient hyperammonemia of the newborn; and very high in citrullinemia and argininosuccinic acidemia, and argininosuccinic acid is found in urine only in the latter. Of infants with early urea cycle defects, only those with hyperammonemia due to ornithine transcarbamoylase deficiency have increased urine orotic acid levels and (often) a family history of male newborn deaths due to defects that appear to be transmitted as an X-linked trait.

ACIDOSIS

Inborn errors may cause chronic or acute acidosis at any age, and with or without an increased anion gap. Inborn errors should be considered when acidosis occurs with recurrent emesis or hyperammonemia, and when acidosis is out of proportion to the clinical state of the patient. Acidosis due to an inborn error is usually, but not always, difficult to correct. The presence of renal tubular acidosis does not exclude an underlying inborn error.

Serum glucose and ammonia, and urine pH and ketones should always be examined. Samples for amino and organic acids should be obtained at once and sent to the laboratory or saved in the freezer depending on how strongly an inborn error is suspected. It is useful to test blood lactate and pyruvate levels in the chronically acidotic patient even if urine organic acid levels are normal. Lactate and pyruvate levels are difficult to interpret in the acutely ill patient, but in the absence of shock very high levels of lactic acid suggest primary lactic acidosis.

MANAGEMENT OF METABOLIC EMERGENCIES

Patients with severe acidosis, hypoglycemia, and hyperammonemia may be very ill; initially mild symptoms may worsen quickly, and coma and death may ensue within hours. With prompt and vigorous treatment, however, patients can recover completely, even from deep coma. All oral intake should be stopped. Glucose should be given intravenously in amounts sufficient to stop catabolic processes or to prevent development of catabolism in a patient with a known inborn error at risk for crisis. Most conditions respond favorably to glucose administration, and few (eg, primary lactic acidosis due to pyruvate dehydrogenase deficiency) do not. Severe or increasing hyperammonemia should be treated pharmacologically or with dialysis, and severe acidosis should be treated with bicarbonate administration. More specific measures can be instituted when a diagnosis is established.

NEWBORN SCREENING

Criteria used to decide whether or not to screen newborns for a disorder include its frequency, the significance of consequences if it is not treated, the availability and cost of screening and diagnostic tests, and the availability and cost of treatment. All states of the USA screen newborns for phenylketonuria and hypothyroidism, and many states also screen for galactosemia. Other metabolic disorders for which newborns are frequently screened include maple syrup urine disease, homocystinuria due to cystathionine synthase deficiency, and biotinidase deficiency.

Some screening tests measure a metabolite (eg, phenylalanine) that becomes abnormal only with time and exposure to diet, and in such instances the disease cannot be detected reliably until intake of the enzyme substrate has become established. Other tests (eg, for biotinidase deficiency) assay an enzyme and can be performed at any time; however, transfusions may cause false-negative results, and exposure of the sample to heat may cause false-positive results. Screening tests are not diagnostic, and diagnostic tests must be undertaken when an abnormal screening result is obtained. Also, because false-negative results are not unknown, a normal newborn screening test does not rule out a condition if symptoms develop.

The time of newborn screening recommended by the American Academy of Pediatrics is appropriate for the detection of phenylketonuria; hypothyroidism, for instance, can be missed when screening is carried out at this time.

Bickel H: Early diagnosis and treatment of inborn errors of metabolism. Enzyme 1987;38:14.

Buist NRM, Tuerck JM: The practitioner's role in newborn screening. Pediatr Clin North Am 1992;39:199.

Chaves-Carballo E: Detection of inherited neurometabolic disorders: A practical clinical approach. Pediatr Clin North Am 1992;39:801.

Childs B: Sir Archibald Garrod's conception of chemical individuality: A modern appreciation. N Engl J Med 1970; 282:71.

Cohn RM, Roth KS: *Metabolic Disease: A Guide to Early Recognition.* Saunders, 1983.

Coude MM et al: Organic acids in aqueous humour and plasma: Post mortem study in infants and diagnosis of enzymopathies. J Inherit Metab Dis 1991;14:668.

Emery JL et al: Investigation of inborn errors of metabolism in unexpected infant deaths. Lancet 1988;2:29.

Goodman SI, Greene CL: Inborn errors as causes of acute disease in infancy. Semin Perinatol 1991;15:31.

Greene CL, Blitzer MG, Shapira E: Inborn errors of metabolism and Reye syndrome: Differential diagnosis. J Pediatr 1988;113:156.

Ozand PT, Gascon GG: Organic acidurias: A review. Part 1. J Child Neurol 1991;6:196.

Phillip M et al: An algorithmic approach to diagnosis of hypoglycemia. J Pediatr 1987;110:387.

Rowe PC, Valle D, Brusilow SW: Inborn errors of metabolism in children referred with Reye's syndrome: A changing pattern. JAMA 1988;260:3167.

Shih VE: Detection of hereditary metabolic disorders involving amino acids and organic acids. Clin Biochem 1991;24:301.

Surtees R, Leonard JV: Acute metabolic encephalopathy: A review of causes, mechanism and treatment. J Inherit Metab Dis 1989;12:42.

Valle D: Treatment of genetic disease: Current status and prospects for the future. Semin Perinatol 1991;15:52.

Ward JC: Inborn errors of metabolism of acute onset in infancy. Pediatr Rev 1990;11:205.

DISORDERS OF CARBOHYDRATE METABOLISM

GLYCOGEN STORAGE DISEASES

Glycogen is a highly branched polymer of glucose that is stored in liver and muscle. Many different disorders of its biosynthesis and degradation have been described, and the enzyme defects responsible have been identified. The most common forms of glycogenosis are characterized by growth failure, hepatomegaly, and fasting hypoglycemia. Defects that cause these so-called hepatic forms of the disease include glucose-6-phosphatase (type I; von Gierke's disease), debrancher enzyme (type III), hepatic phosphorylase (type VI), and phosphorylase kinase (type IX), which normally regulates hepatic phosphorylase activity. Further, there are two forms of glucose-6-phosphatase deficiency; in one the enzyme defect can be demonstrated in fresh or frozen liver; in the other, the defect can be demonstrated only in fresh tissue.

Forms of the disease affecting primarily muscle include acid maltase deficiency (type II; Pompe's disease), which presents in infancy with cardiomegaly and macroglossia, and muscle phosphorylase (type V) and phosphofructokinase (type VII) deficiencies, in which the most striking features are easy fatigability and muscle weakness and stiffness.

Diagnosis

Precise diagnosis is by appropriate biochemical

tests, such as responsiveness of blood glucose to glucagon and epinephrine, and enzyme assays on leukocytes, liver, or muscle. Disorders that can be diagnosed using red or white blood cells include deficiencies of debrancher enzyme (type III) and phosphorylase kinase (IX). Pompe's disease can usually be diagnosed by assaying acid maltase in fibroblasts or peripheral leukocytes.

Treatment

In general, treatment is designed to prevent hypoglycemia while avoiding storage of even more glycogen in liver. In the most severe hepatic forms, this requires careful monitoring of specific diets, using restriction of free sugars and measured amounts of cornstarch, and some good results have been reported following continuous nighttime carbohydrate feeding.

Fernandes J et al: Glycogen storage disease: Recommendations for treatment. Eur J Pediatr 1988;147:226.
Greene HL et al: Type I glycogen storage disease: A metabolic basis for advances in treatment. Adv Pediatr 1979;26:63.
Hers HG et al: Glycogen storage diseases. In: *The Metabolic Basis of Inherited Disease,* 6th ed. Scriver CR et al (editors). McGraw-Hill, 1989.

GALACTOSEMIA

Classical galactosemia is caused by almost total deficiency of galactose-1-phosphate uridyltransferase. Accumulation of galactose-1-phosphate in liver, brain, and renal tubules causes hepatic parenchymal disease, mental retardation, and renal Fanconi's syndrome. Accumulation of galactitol (dulcitol) in the lens produces cataracts. With prompt institution of a galactose-free diet, the prognosis for life is excellent.

In the severe form of the disease, onset is marked by vomiting, jaundice, and hepatomegaly in the newborn period after milk feeding. Without treatment, death frequently occurs in the first month of life, often from *Escherichia coli* sepsis. Cataracts usually develop within 2 months in untreated cases, and hepatic cirrhosis is progressive. Some cases are not severe, however, as shown by the occasional recognition of undiagnosed patients in surveys of mental institutions. If untreated, galactosemia leads to seemingly irreversible mental retardation. Even when dietary restrictions are instituted early, patients with galactosemia are at increased risk for speech and language deficits and ovarian failure, and some patients develop progressive delay, tremor, and ataxia. Clinical and laboratory evidence of the disease abates gradually with effective treatment.

The disorder is inherited as an autosomal recessive trait with an incidence of approximately one in 40,000 live births. Because disease in infancy may be severe and difficult to diagnose, newborn screening is becoming increasingly common. Screening is accomplished either by demonstrating enzyme deficiency in red cells with the Beutler test or by demonstrating increased serum galactose. Prenatal diagnosis of fetal status can be made by enzyme assay of cultured amniotic cells or cells obtained by chorionic villus sampling.

Diagnosis

In infants receiving foods containing galactose, laboratory findings include galactosuria and hypergalactosemia together with proteinuria, aminoaciduria, and tyrosyluria. It is important not to exclude the diagnosis simply because the urine does not contain reducing substances. When the diagnosis is suspected, galactose-1-phosphate uridyltransferase should be assayed in erythrocytes; only blood transfusions will cause this test to be falsely negative, and only sample deterioration will cause it to be falsely positive.

Treatment

A galactose-free diet should be instituted as soon as the diagnosis is made, and compliance with the diet monitored. Avoidance of galactose should be lifelong in severe cases, although tolerance increases somewhat with age. Heterozygous and homozygous mothers are advised to follow a galactose-free diet during pregnancies.

Donnel G (editor): Galactosemia: New frontiers in research. NIH Publication No. 93-3438, 1993.
Gross KC, Acosta PB: Fruits and vegetables are a source of galactose: Implications in planning the diets of patients with galactosemia. J Inherit Metab Dis 1991;253.
Kaufman FR et al: Correlation of ovarian function with galactose-1-phosphate uridyl transferase levels in galactosemia. J Pediatr 1988;112:755.
Levy HL et al: Sepsis due to *Escherichia coli* in neonates with galactosemia. N Engl J Med 1977;297:823.
Lo W et al: Neurologic sequelae in galactosemia. Pediatrics 1984;73:309.
Sardharwalla IB, Wraith JE: Galactosemia. Nutr Health 1987;5:175.

HEREDITARY FRUCTOSE INTOLERANCE

Hereditary fructose intolerance is an autosomal recessive disorder in which deficient activity of fructose-1-phosphate aldolase causes hypoglycemia and tissue accumulation of fructose-1-phosphate on fructose ingestion. Other abnormalities include failure to thrive, vomiting, jaundice, hepatomegaly, proteinuria, generalized aminoaciduria, and tyrosyluria. The untreated condition can progress to death as a result of liver failure.

Diagnosis

The diagnosis is supported by the demonstration of fructosuria following an inpatient, closely monitored fructose load. The appearance of hypoglycemia and hypophosphatemia after fructose loading (200 mg/kg) is diagnostic, as is reduced activity of fructose-1-phosphate aldolase in liver. Some patients may be diagnosed by identification of one of the common mutations on DNA analysis.

Treatment

Treatment consists of eliminating cane sugar from the diet and is complicated by the fact that many proprietary drugs and vitamins are in a sucrose base. If the diet is subsequently relaxed, there may be retardation of physical growth, but growth will resume when more stringent dietary restrictions are instituted. If the disorder is recognized early enough, the prospects for normal development are good. As less severely affected individuals grow up, they may recognize the association of nausea and vomiting with fructose-containing foods and selectively avoid them.

Brooks CC, Tolan DR: Association of the widespread A149P hereditary fructose intolerance mutation with newly identified sequence polymorphisms in the aldolase B gene. Am J Hum Genet 1993;52:835.

Odierre M et al: Hereditary fructose intolerance in childhood: Diagnosis, management and course in 55 patients. Am J Dis Child 1978;132:605.

Steinmann B, Gitzelmann R: The diagnosis of hereditary fructose intolerance. Helv Paediatr Acta 1981;36:297.

PRIMARY LACTIC ACIDEMIAS

Primary lactic acidemia is a diagnosis made with increasing frequency and may be one of the more common causes of neurodevelopmental problems in children. Lactic acidemia is said to be primary when it is due to a defect in the metabolism of pyruvic acid and secondary when a change in cellular redox potential favors the reduction of pyruvate to lactate (as in shock). Some causes of primary lactic acidosis are shown in Table 31–3. In general, such disorders may present at any age with neurologic findings and, when the defect is in gluconeogenesis, with hypoglycemia. Patients with a defect in the E_1 component of the pyruvate dehydrogenase complex often show central nervous system malformations or mild facial dysmorphism.

Defects in the mitochondrial respiratory chain are also included in this category; these conditions may present with nonspecific findings such as hypotonia or renal tubular acidosis or with more specific features such as ophthalmoplegia. Ragged red fibers and mitochondrial abnormalities may be noted on histologic examination of muscle. These disorders may be progressive.

Table 31–3. Causes in primary lactic acidosis in childhood.

Defects of the pyruvate dehydrogenase complex
1. E_1 (pyruvate decarboxylase) deficiency
2. E_2 (dihydrolipoyl transacetylase) deficiency
3. E_3 (lipoamide dehydrogenase) deficiency
4. Pyruvate decarboxylase phosphate phosphatase deficiency

Abnormalities of gluconeogenesis
1. Pyruvate carboxylase deficiency
   a) Isolated
   b) Biotinidase deficiency
   c) Holocarboxylase synthetase deficiency
2. Fructose-1,6-diphosphatase deficiency
3. Glucose-6-phosphatase deficiency (von Gierke disease)

Defects in mitochondrial respiratory chain
1. Complex I deficiency
2. Complex IV deficiency (cytochrome C oxidase deficiency; frequent cause of Leigh disease)
3. ATPase deficiency (frequent cause of Leigh disease)
4. Other respiratory chain disorders

Diagnosis

Diagnosis of primary lactic acidemia may be based on (1) demonstrating significant elevations of blood lactic acid concentration (more than 2 mmol/L venous/fasting/resting/free flowing sample) or pyruvic acid in blood or spinal fluid and excluding secondary lactic acidemia; or (2) demonstration of classic features of mitochondrial disorder such as ragged red fibers. Primary lactic acidemia may be present even if blood lactic acid concentration is normal, since lactate levels may vary according to the state of the patient (eg, resting versus active; fasting versus fed). Unless a specific diagnosis is suggested by fructose intolerance or by the typical findings of von Gierke's disease or biotinidase deficiency, enzyme analysis of fibroblasts or skeletal muscle is often required. In many patients, the cause of the disorder cannot be defined.

Treatment

In some patients, defects in gluconeogenesis can be treated with glucose administration, fructose avoidance, or administration of pharmacologic amounts of biotin. Modified ketogenic diet has been reported to be useful in some cases of proved or presumed pyruvate dehydrogenase deficiency. Other treatments are of theoretic or empiric value but have not been extensively studied. Thiamine or lipoic acid can be tried in patients with pyruvate dehydrogenase complex deficiencies, and coenzyme Q has been reported to be helpful in some patients with respiratory chain defects.

Brown GK et al: "Cerebral" lactic acidosis: Defects in pyruvate metabolism with profound brain damage and minimal systemic acidosis. Eur J Pediatr 1988;147:10.

Clarke LA: Mitochondrial disorders in pediatrics: Clinical, biochemical and genetic implications. Pediatr Clin North Am 1992;39:319.

Kerr DS: Lactic acidosis and mitochondrial disorders. Clin Biochem 1991;24:33.

Hart Z, Chang C: A newborn infant with respiratory distress and persistent stridulous breathing. J Pediatr 1988;113:150.

Robinson BH et al: Variable clinical presentation in patients with defective E_1 component of pyruvate dehydrogenase complex. J Pediatr 1987;111:525.

Shoffner JM, Wallace DC: Mitochondrial genetics: Principles and practice. Am J Hum Genet 1992;51:1179.

Tulinius MH et al: Mitochondrial encephalomyopathies in childhood: I. Biochemical and morphologic investigations. J Pediatr 1991;119:242.

Tulinius MH et al: Mitochondrial encephalomyopathies in childhood: II. Clinical manifestations and syndromes. J Pediatr 1991;119 251.

DISORDERS OF AMINO ACID METABOLISM

DISORDERS OF THE UREA CYCLE

Ammonia is converted to an amino group in urea by enzymes of the urea cycle. Defects in early urea cycle enzymes, such as carbamoyl phosphate synthetase or ornithine transcarbamoylase, usually present in infancy with severe and rapidly fatal hyperammonemia, vomiting, and encephalopathy, but the course may also be milder, with vomiting and encephalopathy following protein ingestion or infections. Although defects in argininosuccinic acid synthetase (citrullinemia) and argininosuccinic acid lyase (argininosuccinic acidemia) may also present with severe hyperammonemia in infancy, a chronic course with mental retardation is more usual in these conditions.

Except for ornithine transcarbamoylase deficiency, which is X-linked, urea cycle disorders are inherited as autosomal recessive traits. Citrullinemia and argininosuccinic acidemia can be diagnosed in utero by appropriate enzyme assays on cultured amniotic cells or material obtained from chorionic villus sampling, but carbamoyl phosphate synthetase and ornithine transcarbamoylase deficiency states can be diagnosed in utero only by using specific gene probes, and then only in certain families.

Diagnosis

Blood ammonia levels should be measured in any newborn who is acutely ill without obvious cause. A urea cycle defect should be suspected when severe hyperammonemia is associated with respiratory alkalosis. Serum citrulline is low or undetectable in carbamoyl phosphate synthetase and ornithine transcarbamoylase deficiency, high in argininosuccinic acidemia, and very high in citrullinemia. Large amounts of argininosuccinic acid are found in the urine of patients with argininosuccinic acidemia. Urine orotic acid is increased in infants with ornithine transcarbamoylase deficiency, and there may also be a family history of male newborn deaths that appear to be transmitted as an X-linked trait.

Many female carriers of ornithine transcarbamoylase deficiency show protein intolerance; some develop migraine-like symptoms after protein loads and others develop potentially fatal episodes of vomiting and encephalopathy after ingesting protein or contracting infections. Trichorrhexis nodosa is common in patients with the chronic form of argininosuccinic acidemia.

Treatment

In the newborn, measures to reduce serum ammonia by hemodialysis, peritoneal dialysis, or double-volume exchange transfusion should be instituted as soon as hyperammonemia is documented. Protein intake should be stopped, and glucose should be given to reduce endogenous protein breakdown. Arginine should be given intravenously, both because it is an essential amino acid for patients with urea cycle defects and because it increases the excretion of waste nitrogen in patients with citrullinemia and argininosuccinic acidemia. Sodium benzoate, sodium phenylacetate, and sodium phenylbutyrate can also be given intravenously, and one or more of these drugs is needed intravenously for treatment of hyperammonemic coma.

Long-term treatment includes oral administration of arginine (or citrulline), adherence to a low-protein diet, and administration of sodium benzoate and sodium phenylacetate or sodium phenylbutyrate to increase excretion of nitrogen as hippuric acid and phenylacetylglutamine. Female ornithine transcarbamoylase-deficient heterozygotes who develop hyperammonemia should also receive such treatment.

The outcome of argininosuccinic acidemia and citrullinemia is better than that of ornithine transcarbamoylase and carbamoyl phosphate synthetase deficiency. Most patients with urea cycle defects, no matter what the enzyme defect, develop permanent neurologic and intellectual impairments, with cortical atrophy and ventricular dilatation seen on CT scan. The prognosis may be improved if the initial hyperammonemic episode is rapidly identified and treated.

Batshaw ML et al: Risk of serious illness in heterozygotes for ornithine transcarbamylase deficiency. J Pediatr 1986;108:236.

Brusilow SW et al: Treatment of episodic hyperammonemia in children with inborn errors of urea synthesis. N Engl J Med 1984;310:1630.

Cederbaum SD: The treatment of urea cycle disorders. Int Pediatr 1992;7:61.

Hudak ML, Jones MD, Brusilow SW: Differentiation of transient hyperammonemia of the newborn and urea cycle enzyme defects by clinical presentation. J Pediatr 1985;107:712.

Msall M et al: Neurologic outcome in children with inborn errors of urea synthesis: Outcome of urea cycle enzymopathies. N Engl J Med 1984;310:1500.

Nagata N et al: Retrospective survey of urea cycle disorders: Part 2. Neurological outcome in forty-nine Japanese patients with urea cycle enzymopathies. Am J Med Genet 1991;40:477.

PHENYLKETONURIA & THE HYPERPHENYLALANINEMIAS

Probably the best known disorder of amino acid metabolism is the classic form of phenylketonuria. It was first recognized in 1934 by Fölling in several retarded children who excreted phenylpyruvic acid in the urine. The disorder is due to decreased activity of phenylalanine hydroxylase, the enzyme that converts phenylalanine to tyrosine. Phenylketonuria is inherited as an autosomal recessive trait, with a frequency in Caucasians of approximately one in 10,000 live births. On normal phenylalanine intake, affected patients develop hyperphenylalaninemia and produce and excrete phenylpyruvic, phenyllactic, phenylacetic, and 2-hydroxyphenylacetic acid. The untreated patient shows severe mental retardation, hyperactivity, seizures, a light complexion, and eczema. The patient's urine has a "mouse-like" odor.

Clinicians had early success preventing severe mental retardation in phenylketonuric children by restricting phenylalanine from the diet starting in early infancy. This success led to the development of screening programs to detect the disease early. Since the outcome is best when treatment is begun in the first month of life, infants are usually screened during the first few days of life. A second test is necessary only when newborn screening is done before 24 hours of age, and in such cases the second test should be completed by the third week of life. Infants receiving hyperalimentation and premature infants should be screened at or near 7 days, and rescreened if they were transfused or not fed at the time of the initial test.

Enzymes involved with the interconversion of phenylalanine and tyrosine, and whose deficiencies can produce hyperphenylalaninemia, are shown in Figure 31–1. In classic phenylketonuria, there is little or no phenylalanine hydroxylase activity, but in the less severe hyperphenylalaninemias there is significant residual activity. Rare variants can be due to deficiency of dihydrobiopterin reductase or to defects in biopterin synthesis. All are inherited as autosomal recessive traits.

Prenatal diagnosis of phenylketonuria is often possible using DNA probes. Molecular approaches are replacing serum measurements of phenylalanine and tyrosine to determine carrier status. Prenatal diagnosis of defects in pterin metabolism can often be made

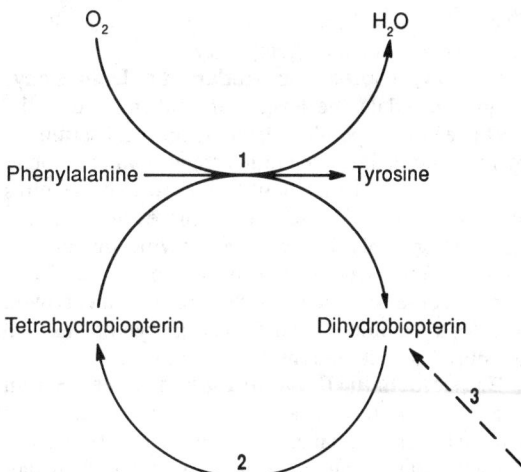

Figure 31–1. Oxidation of phenylalanine to tyrosine. **1.** Phenylalanine hydroxylase. **2.** Dihydropteridine reductase. **3.** Enzymes of biopterin biosynthesis.

by enzyme assay of amniocytes or by examination of pterin metabolites in amniotic fluid.

Diagnosis & Treatment

The diagnosis of phenylketonuria in a severely retarded older child with typical biochemical and physical characteristics is straightforward, but in the newborn period, especially when there is no family history, the condition must be differentiated from other forms of hyperphenylalaninemia. This is done by determining serum phenylalanine and tyrosine levels on a normal diet, and by examining pterins and metabolites of phenylalanine in urine. Oral phenylalanine loads and liver biopsy are almost never necessary.

A. Classic Phenylketonuria: Findings include persistently elevated serum levels of phenylalanine (> 20 mg/dL on a regular diet), normal or low serum levels of tyrosine, urinary excretion of phenylpyruvic and 2-hydroxyphenylacetic acids, and normal pterins. Poor phenylalanine tolerance persists throughout life, and serum tyrosine levels do not rise after a phenylalanine load. Restriction of dietary phenylalanine intake (see below) is indicated to lower serum phenylalanine, and a favorable outcome is the rule.

B. Persistent Hyperphenylalaninemia: In infants receiving a normal protein intake, serum phenylalanine levels are usually 4–20 mg/dL. The serum tyrosine level rises after a phenylalanine load, urine pterins are normal, and phenylketones are either not excreted or excreted only transiently. Phenylalanine restriction may or may not be indicated, depending on the phenylalanine tolerance.

C. Transient Hyperphenylalaninemia: Serum phenylalanine levels are elevated early but progressively decline toward normal. If required at all, dietary restriction is only temporary.

D. Dihydropteridine Reductase Deficiency: Serum phenylalanine levels vary but may be in the range seen in hyperphenylalaninemia, and serum tyrosine is normal. Urine pterins are normal in amount, but the pattern of metabolites is abnormal. Seizures and psychomotor regression occur even with diet therapy, probably because the enzyme defect also causes neuronal deficiency of serotonin and dopamine. These deficiencies require treatment with levodopa, carbidopa, and 5-hydroxytryptophan, and possibly also with tetrahydrobiopterin.

E. Defects in Biopterin Biosynthesis: Serum phenylalanine levels vary but may be in the range seen in hyperphenylalaninemia, and serum tyrosine is normal. Total pterins in urine are low, and their pattern may suggest the specific defect, which can be at several steps in the biosynthetic pathway. Clinical findings include myoclonus, tetraplegia, and other movement disorders. Treatment is the same as for dihydropteridine reductase deficiency, but in general is not as effective.

F. Tyrosinemia of the Newborn: Serum phenylalanine levels are lower than those seen in phenylketonuria and are accompanied by marked hypertyrosinemia. This usually occurs in premature infants and is due to immaturity of 4-hydroxyphenylpyruvic acid oxidase. The condition resolves spontaneously within 3 months, almost always without sequelae. If necessary, intramuscular injection of 100 mg ascorbic acid will normalize serum tyrosine (and phenylalanine) within 48 hours.

G. Maternal Phenylketonuria: Heterozygous offspring of phenylketonuric mothers have transient hyperphenylalaninemia at birth; in such cases diagnosis is made by determining the serum phenylalanine level of the mother. Nearly all such offspring are mentally retarded, most are microcephalic, and many are small and have congenital heart disease or other malformations. The risk to the fetus is considerably lessened if phenylalanine restriction is begun before conception and maintained throughout pregnancy.

Treatment of Classic Phenylketonuria

Treatment of classic phenylketonuria is to limit dietary phenylalanine intake to amounts that permit normal growth and development without marked hyperphenylalaninemia, and this can be done with several low-phenylalanine milk substitutes. Serum phenylalanine concentrations must be monitored frequently, while ensuring that growth, development, and nutrition are adequate. This monitoring is best done in clinics experienced in dealing with such problems. Although dietary treatment is most effective when initiated during the first months of life, it may also be of benefit in reversing behaviors such as hyperactivity, irritability, and distractibility when started later in life.

Phenylalanine restriction should continue throughout life, both because of subtle changes in IQ and behavior in individuals treated early who go off diet; and because of the risk of late development of potentially irreversible neurologic damage after stopping diet. Females with phenylketonuria merit special attention during the childbearing years. Counseling should be given during adolescence, and the woman's diet should be closely monitored prior to conception and throughout pregnancy.

Children with classic phenylketonuria who are treated promptly after birth and achieve phenylalanine and tyrosine homeostasis will develop well physically and can be expected to have normal or nearly normal intellectual development.

Blau N et al: Tetrahydrobiopterin deficiency: From phenotype to genotype. Pteridines 1993;4:1.

Koch R et al: The effects of diet discontinuation in children with phenylketonuria. Eur J Pediatr 1987;146(Suppl): A12.

Matalon R, Michals K: Phenylketonuria: Screening, treatment and maternal PKU. Clin Biochem 1991;24:337.

Niederwieser A, Ponzone A, Curtius H-Ch: Differential diagnosis of tetrahydrobiopterin deficiency. J Inherited Metab Dis 1985;8(Suppl 1):34.

O'Flynn ME: Newborn screening for phenylketonuria: Thirty years of progress. Curr Probl Pediatr 1992:159.

Okano Y et al: Molecular basis of phenotypic heterogeneity in phenylketonuria. N Engl J Med 1991;324:1232.

Soeters RP et al: Maternal phenylketonuria: Comparison of two treated full term pregnancies. Eur J Pediatr 1986; 145:221.

Thompson AJ et al: Neurologic deterioration in young adults with phenylketonuria. Lancet 1990;336:602.

Villasana D et al: Neurological deterioration in adult phenylketonuria. J Inherited Metab Dis 1989;12:451.

Williamson ML et al: Correlates of intelligence test results in treated phenylketonuric children. Pediatrics 1981; 68:161.

HEREDITARY TYROSINEMIA

Hereditary tyrosinemia is caused by deficiency of fumarylacetoacetase and is characterized by progressive hepatic parenchymal damage, renal tubular dystrophy with generalized aminoaciduria and hypophosphatemic rickets, hypermethioninemia, and tyrosine metabolites, succinylacetone, and δ-aminolevulinic acid in the urine. The course may be rapidly fatal in infancy or somewhat more chronic, with liver cell carcinoma almost invariable.

The condition is inherited as an autosomal recessive trait and is especially common in Scandinavia and in the Chicoutimi-Lac St Jean region of Quebec. Prenatal diagnosis can be established by demonstrating deficiency of fumarylacetoacetase in cultured amniocytes or increased concentrations of succinylacetone in amniotic fluid.

Diagnosis

Similar clinical and biochemical findings may occur in galactosemia and hereditary fructose intolerance, but increased succinylacetone occurs only in fumarylacetoacetase deficiency, and diagnosis is based on demonstrating this compound in urine. This may be done by gas chromatography-mass spectrometry or by demonstration that a urine extract can inhibit δ-aminolevulinic acid synthetase activity.

Treatment

A diet low in phenylalanine and tyrosine (50 mg each/kg/d) is indicated but not usually successful in preventing or reversing liver disease, and liver transplantation appears to be the only effective therapy for these children. Recent reports suggest that pharmacologic therapy to inhibit 4-hydroxyphenylpyruvate dehydrogenase holds promise.

Kvittingen EA et al: Prenatal diagnosis of hereditary tyrosinemia by determination of fumarylacetoacetase in cultured amniotic fluid cells. Pediatr Res 1985;19:334.
Lindstedt S et al: Treatment of hereditary tyrosinaemia type I by inhibition of 4-hydroxyphenylpyruvate dioxygenase. Lancet 1992;340:813.

MAPLE SYRUP URINE DISEASE (Branched-Chain Ketoaciduria)

Maple syrup urine disease is due to deficiency of the enzyme that catalyzes oxidative decarboxylation of the branched-chain keto acid derivatives of leucine, isoleucine, and valine. The accumulated keto acids of leucine and isoleucine cause the characteristic odor, while only the keto acid of leucine has been implicated in causing central nervous system dysfunction. Many variants of this disorder have been described, including mild, intermittent, and thiamine-dependent forms, and all are inherited as autosomal recessive traits. Fetal diagnosis of the disease is possible by demonstrating decreased branched-chain keto acid dehydrogenase activity in cultured amniotic cells.

Patients with classical maple syrup urine disease are normal at birth but soon develop the characteristic odor, lethargy, feeding difficulties, coma, and seizures. Unless diagnosis is made and dietary restriction of branched-chain amino acids is begun, most will die in the first month of life, but normal growth and development can be achieved if treatment is begun before about 10 days of age. The requirement for early diagnosis has made this disorder one of those screened for in the newborn period.

Diagnosis

Marked elevations of branched-chain amino acids, including alloisoleucine, in serum and urine are characteristic. Alloisoleucine, a transamination product of the keto acid of isoleucine, is almost pathognomonic. Branched-chain α-keto- and hydroxy acids are also present in the urine. The magnitude and consistency of amino and organic acid changes are altered in mild and intermittent forms of the disease.

Treatment

Products deficient in branched-chain amino acids but in other respects identical to milk are commercially available but must be supplemented with normal milk and other foods to supply enough branched-chain amino acids to permit normal growth and development. Serum levels of branched-chain amino acids must be monitored frequently, even at intervals of 1 or 2 days in the first months of life, to cope with changing protein requirements. Acute episodes must be aggressively treated to *prevent* catabolism and negative nitrogen balance.

Clow CL et al: Outcome of early and long-term management of classical maple syrup urine disease. Pediatrics 1981;68:856.
Nord A et al: Developmental profile of patients with maple syrup urine disease. J Inherit Metab Dis 1991;14:881.
Parini et al: Nasogastric drip feeding as the only treatment of neonatal maple syrup urine disease. Pediatrics 1993; 92:280.
Treacy E et al: Maple syrup urine disease: Interrelation between branched-chain amino, oxo, and hydroxy acids; implications for treatment; associations with CNS dysmyelination. J Inherit Metab Dis 1992;15:121.

HOMOCYSTINURIA

Homocystinuria is most often due to deficiency of cystathionine synthase, but it may also be due to deficiency of methylenetetrahydrofolate reductase or to defects in the biosynthesis of methyl-B_{12}, which is the coenzyme for N^5-methyltetrahydrofolate methyltransferase. All known inherited forms of homocystinuria are transmitted as autosomal recessive traits and can be diagnosed in the fetus by assaying appropriate enzymes in cultured amniotic cells.

About half of untreated patients with cystathionine synthase deficiency are retarded, and most have arachnodactyly, osteoporosis, and a tendency to develop dislocated lenses and thromboembolic phenomena. A relationship between risk of arteriosclerotic heart disease and carrier status for cystathionine synthase deficiency is suspected. Patients with remethylation defects usually show failure to thrive and a variety of neurologic symptoms, including microcephaly and seizures in infancy and early childhood.

Diagnosis

Diagnosis is made by demonstrating homocystinuria in a patient who is not severely deficient in vitamin B_{12}. Serum methionine levels are usually high in patients with cystathionine synthase deficiency and often low in patients with remethylation defects. When the remethylation defect is due to deficiency of methyl-B_{12}, megaloblastic anemia may be present, and an associated deficiency of adenosyl-B_{12} may cause methylmalonic aciduria. Studies of cultured fibroblasts may be necessary to make a specific diagnosis.

Treatment

About 50% of patients with cystathionine synthase deficiency respond to large oral doses of pyridoxine. Early treatment of pyridoxine nonresponders by dietary methionine restriction may prevent mental retardation and delay lens dislocations, perhaps justifying screening of newborn infants for the condition. Oral administration of betaine (250 mg/kg/d) will increase methylation of homocystine to methionine in patients with remethylation defects and may also improve neurologic function. Large doses of cobalamin, eg 1 mg hydroxy-B_{12} administered intramuscularly every other day, are indicated in some patients.

Bartholomew DW et al: Therapeutic approaches to cobalamin-C methylmalonic acidemia and homocystinuria. J Pediatr 1988;112:32.

Malinow MR: Hyperhomocyst(e)inemia: A common and easily reversible risk factor for occlusive atherosclerosis. Circulation 1990;81:2004.

Mitchell GA et al: Clinical heterogeneity in cobalamin C variant of combined homocystinuria and methylmalonic aciduria. J Pediatr 1986;108:410.

Mudd SH et al: The natural history of homocystinuria due to cystathionine β-synthase deficiency. Am J Hum Genet 1985;37:1.

Rosenblatt DS et al: Vitamin B_{12} responsive homocystinuria and megaloblastic anemia: Heterogeneity in methylcobalamin deficiency. Am J Med Genet 1987;26:377.

NONKETOTIC HYPERGLYCINEMIA

Inherited deficiency of various subunits of the glycine cleavage enzyme causes nonketotic hyperglycinemia. In its most severe form, also termed **glycine encephalopathy,** the condition presents in the newborn period with unremitting seizures, hypotonia, hiccups, a burst suppression pattern on EEG, and (usually) death in infancy. Forms that present with seizures later in infancy or with developmental delay in childhood are less common. All forms of the condition are inherited as autosomal recessive traits.

Diagnosis

This deficiency should be suspected in any infant with intractable seizures, especially when hiccupping, and is confirmed by demonstrating a large increase in glycine in cerebrospinal fluid, with the CSF:serum glycine ratio being abnormally high. Demonstrating the specific enzyme defect by liver bi-

opsy is necessary only if the couple is contemplating having more children, and prenatal diagnosis is possible only by assaying the enzyme in chorionic villus.

Treatment

Treatment is generally unsuccessful, although large doses of diazepam may be necessary to control seizures in some patients. Early efforts to use sodium benzoate therapy were thought to be without effect on long-term outcome, but recent studies suggest that this drug may be useful in seizure control.

Eyskens FJM et al: Neurologic sequelae in transient nonketotic hyperglycenemia of the neonate. J Pediatr 1992:121:620.

Hamogh et al: Dextromethorphan and high dose benzoate therapy for nonketotic hyperglycinemia in an infant. J Pediatr 1992;121:131.

Hayasaka K et al: Nonketotic hyperglycinemia: Analyses of glycine cleavage system in typical and atypical cases. J Pediatr 1987;110:873.

Tada K, Hayasaka K: Non-ketotic hyperglycinaemia: Clinical and biochemical aspects. Eur J Pediatr 1987;146:221.

MOLYBDENUM COFACTOR DEFICIENCY

Defects in the synthesis of a common molybdenum-containing pterin cofactor reduce the activities of sulfate oxidase, xanthine oxidase, and aldehyde dehydrogenase. Clinical features in the neonate include refractory tonic-clonic seizures and profound hypotonia, with the later development of lens dislocations and severe mental retardation in the few survivors. The disorder is transmitted as an autosomal recessive trait.

Diagnosis

Deficiency of xanthine oxidase causes low serum uric acid, the simplest diagnostic indicator, and deficiency of sulfite oxidase causes accumulation and urinary excretion of thiosulfate and S-sulfocysteine. The latter is demonstrable by the methods used to measure amino acids in serum and urine but is difficult to appreciate unless the laboratory is made aware that the diagnosis is being considered. Prenatal diagnosis is possible based on sulfite oxidase activity in amniocytes or chorionic villi, or increased S-sulfocysteine in amniotic fluid.

Treatment

There is no effective treatment.

Arnold GL et al: Molybdenum cofactor deficiency. J Pediatr 1993;123:595.

ORGANIC ACIDEMIAS

Organic acidemias are disorders of amino (and fatty) acid metabolism in which nonamino organic acids accumulate in serum and urine. These conditions are usually diagnosed by examining organic acids in urine, a complex procedure that requires considerable interpretive expertise and is usually performed only in specialized laboratories. Clinical features of organic acidemias are given in Table 31–4, together with the urine organic acid patterns typical of each. Additional details about some of the more important organic acidemias are provided below.

KETOTIC HYPERGLYCINEMIAS (Propionic and Methylmalonic Acidemia)

Idiopathic hyperglycinemia was first reported in 1961 as a syndrome of mental retardation and episodic ketoacidosis, neutropenia, thrombocytopenia, osteoporosis, and hyperglycinemia induced by protein intake or infection. It was then renamed ketotic hyperglycinemia to distinguish it from nonketotic hyperglycinemia, described above. It is now known that the syndrome is almost always due to propionic or methylmalonic acidemia.

The oxidation of threonine, valine, isoleucine, and methionine through propionyl- and L-methylmalonyl-CoA is shown in Figure 31–2. Propionic acidemia is due to a defect in the biotin-containing enzyme pro-

Table 31–4. Clinical and laboratory features of organic acidemias.

Disorder	Enzyme Defect	Clinical and Laboratory Features
Isovaleric acidemia	Isovaleryl-CoA dehydrogenase	Acidosis and "odor of sweaty feet" in infancy, or growth retardation and episodes of vomiting, lethargy, acidosis, and odor. Isovalerylglycine always present in urine, with 3-hydroxy-isovaleric acid during acute episodes.
3-Methylcrotonyl-CoA carboxylase deficiency	3-Methylcrotonyl-CoA carboxylase	Acidosis and feeding problems in infancy, or Reye-like episodes in older child. 3-Methylcrotonylglycine in urine, usually with 3-hydroxyisovaleric acid.
Combined carboxylase deficiency	Holocarboxylase synthetase	Hypotonia and lactic acidosis in infancy. 3-Hydroxyisovaleric acid in urine, often with small amounts of 3-hydroxypropionic and methylcitric acids. Often biotin responsive.
	Biotinidase	Alopecia, seborrheic rash, and ataxia in infancy or childhood. Urine organic acids as above. Usually biotin responsive.
3-Hydroxy-3-methylglutaric acidemia	Hydroxymethylglutaryl-CoA lyase	Hypoglycemia and acidosis in infancy; Reye-like episodes with nonketotic hypoglycemia in older children. 3-Hydroxy-3-methyl-glutaric, 3-methylglutaconic, and 3-hydroxyisovaleric acids in urine.
3-Ketothiolase deficiency	3-Ketothiolase	Ketotic hyperglycinemia syndrome in infancy, or developmental and growth retardation with episodes of vomiting, acidosis, and encephalopathy. 2-Methyl-3-hydroxybutyric and 2-methylacetoacetic acids and tiglylglycine in urine, especially after isoleucine load.
Propionic acidemia	Propionyl-CoA carboxylase	Hyperammonemia and metabolic acidosis in infancy; ketotic hyperglycinemia syndrome later. 3-Hydroxypropionic and methylcitric acids in urine, with 3-hydroxy- and 3-ketovaleric during ketotic episodes.
Methylmalonic acidemia	Methylmalonyl-CoA mutase	Clinical features same as propionic acidemia. Methylmalonic acid in urine, often with 3-hydroxypropionic and methylcitric acids.
	Defects in B_{12} biosynthesis	Clinical features same as above when only adenosyl-B_{12} synthesis is decreased; early neurological features prominent when accompanied by decreased synthesis of methyl-B_{12}. In latter instance, hypomethioninemia and homocystinuria accompany methylmalonic aciduria.
Pyroglutamic acidemia	Glutathione synthetase	Acidosis and hemolytic anemia in infancy; chronic acidosis later. Pyroglutamic acid in urine.
Glutaric acidemia type I	Glutaryl-CoA dehydrogenase	Progressive extrapyramidal movement disorder in childhood, with episodes of acidosis, vomiting, and encephalopathy. Glutaric acid in urine, usually with 3-hydroxyglutaric acid.
Glutaric acidemia type II	Electron transfer flavoprotein (ETF) ETF: ubiquinone oxidoreductase (ETF dehydrogenase)	Hypoglycemia, acidosis, hyperammonemia, and "smell of sweaty feet" in infancy, often with polycystic and dysplastic kidneys. Later onset may be with episodes of hypoketotic hypoglycemia, or slowly progressive skeletal myopathy. Glutaric, ethylmalonic, 3-hydroxy-isovaleric, isovalerylglycine, and 2-hydroxyglutaric acids in urine, often with sarcosine in serum and urine.
4-Hydroxybutyric acidemia	Succinic semialdehyde dehydrogenase	Seizures and developmental retardation. 4-Hydroxybutyric acid in urine.

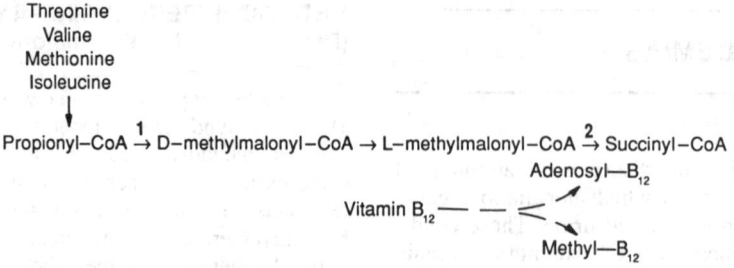

Figure 31–2. Oxidation of propionyl-CoA to succinyl-CoA. *1.* Propionyl-CoA carboxylase. *2.* Methylmalonyl-CoA mutase.

pionyl-CoA carboxylase, and methylmalonic acidemia is due to a defect in methylmalonyl-CoA mutase. In most cases the latter is due to a defect in the mutase apoenzyme, but in others it is due to a defect in the biosynthesis of its adenosyl-B_{12} coenzyme. In some of these defects only the synthesis of adenosyl-B_{12} is blocked; in others, the synthesis of methyl-B_{12} is also blocked.

Clinical symptoms in propionic and methylmalonic acidemia vary according to the location and severity of the enzyme block. Those with severe blocks present with acute, life-threatening metabolic acidemia and hyperammonemia early in infancy or with metabolic acidemia, vomiting, and failure to thrive during the first few months of life. Children with less severe blocks may show only mild or moderate mental retardation.

All known forms of propionic and methylmalonic acidemia are transmitted as autosomal recessive traits and can be diagnosed in utero by performing appropriate enzyme assays of cultured amniotic fluid cells or by demonstrating characteristic abnormalities of organic acids in amniotic fluid.

Diagnosis

Laboratory findings include hyperglycinemia and hyperglycinuria, a positive methylmalonic aciduria screening test, the presence of diagnostic changes on urine organic acid chromatography (Table 31–4) and, in certain blocks of B_{12} metabolism, hypomethioninemic homocystinuria.

Treatment

Patients with enzyme blocks in B_{12} metabolism usually respond to massive (1 mg/d) doses of vitamin B_{12}, given orally or intramuscularly, whereas nonresponders require amino acid restriction and correction of their rather constant metabolic acidemia. Secondary carnitine deficiency has been reported, and blood carnitine should be measured and supplemented if required.

Matsui SM et al: The natural history of the inherited methylmalonic acidemias. N Engl J Med 1983;308:857.
Werlin SL: *E. coli* sepsis as a presenting sign in neonatal propionic acidemia. Am J Med Genet 1993;46:455.

Shevell MI et al: Varying neurological phenotypes among mut° and mut⁻ patients with methylmalonyl-CoA mutase deficiency. Am J Med Genet 1993;45:619.
Shinnar S, Singer HS: Cobalamin C mutation (methylmalonic aciduria and homocystinuria) in adolescence: A treatable cause of dementia and myelopathy. N Engl J Med 1984;311:451.

ISOVALERIC ACIDEMIA

This condition, due to deficiency of isovaleryl-CoA dehydrogenase in the leucine oxidative pathway, was the first organic acidemia to be described in humans. It usually presents with poor feeding, metabolic acidosis, seizures, and an odor of "sweaty feet" during the first few days of life, with coma and death occurring if the condition is not recognized and appropriate therapy quickly begun. Other patients show a more chronic course, with episodes of vomiting, lethargy, and urine (and body) odor precipitated by intercurrent infections or increased protein intake. Therapy by dietary means of by providing glycine is very effective. The condition is inherited as an autosomal recessive trait, and fetal disease can be diagnosed by demonstrating enzyme deficiency in cultured amniotic cells or the presence of isovaleryl-glycine in urine.

Diagnosis

Isovaleric acidemia and glutaric acidemia type II are the only conditions in which the characteristic odor of "sweaty feet" occurs. Isovalerylglycine is consistently detected in the urine by organic acid chromatography. During infections or following the intake of large amounts of protein, 3-hydroxyisovaleric acid is also detected.

Treatment

Providing a low-protein diet or diets low in leucine or all three branched-chain amino acids is quite effective. Oral administration of glycine (250 mg/kg/d) appears to prevent complications during acute infections, but poses the risk of neurotoxicity due to severe hyperglycinemia. Oral administration of L-carnitine (40 mg/kg/d) may also be indicated.

Cohn RM et al: Isovaleric acidemia: Use of glycine therapy in neonates. N Engl J Med 1978;299:996.

de Sousa C et al: The response to L-carnitine and glycine therapy in isovaleric acidaemia. Eur J Pediatr 1986; 144:451.

COMBINED CARBOXYLASE DEFICIENCY

Holocarboxylase synthetase and biotinidase are two enzymes of biotin metabolism in mammals. Holocarboxylase synthetase covalently binds biotin to the apocarboxylases for pyruvate, 3-methylcrotonyl-CoA and propionyl-CoA; and biotinidase releases biotin from these proteins and from proteins in the diet. Recessively inherited deficiency of either enzyme causes deficiency of all three carboxylases, ie, multiple carboxylase deficiency. Holocarboxylase synthetase deficiency usually presents in the neonatal period with hypotonia, and biotinidase deficiency more often presents somewhat later with a syndrome of ataxia, seborrhea, and alopecia. Because many patients with biotinidase deficiency do not show typical symptoms but do develop neurologic sequelae, newborn screening for the condition may be justified.

Diagnosis

This diagnosis should be excluded in patients with typical symptoms or in those with primary lactic acidosis. Urine organic acids are usually, but not always, abnormal (Table 31–4). Diagnosis is usually by enzyme assay. Biotinidase can be assayed in serum; holocarboxylase synthetase, in leukocytes or fibroblasts.

Treatment

Oral administration of biotin in large doses, 10–20 mg/d, often reverses the organic aciduria within days and the clinical symptoms within days to weeks. Incidence of hearing loss is high, even in treated patients.

Burri BJ, Sweetman L, Nyhan WL: Heterogeneity of holocarboxylase synthetase in patients with biotin-responsive multiple carboxylase deficiency. Am J Hum Genet 1985;37:326.

McVoy JRS et al: Partial biotinidase deficiency: Clinical and biochemical features. J Pediatr 1990;116;78.

Wolf B, Heard GS: Screening for biotinidase deficiency in newborns: Worldwide experience. Pediatrics 1990;85: 512.

GLUTARIC ACIDEMIA TYPE I

Glutaric acidemia type I is due to deficiency of glutaryl-CoA dehydrogenase and causes a progressive extrapyramidal movement disorder in childhood, with dystonia and athetosis and neuronal degeneration in the caudate and putamen. Macrocephaly at birth is common. Death usually occurs during the first decade of life, but the clinical course is highly variable, and several patients have only mild neurologic abnormalities. The condition is inherited as an autosomal recessive trait.

Diagnosis

Glutaric acidemia type I should be suspected in any patient with progressive dystonia or athetosis. The diagnosis is confirmed by demonstration of glutaric and 3-hydroxyglutaric acids in urine by organic acid analysis. Deficiency of glutaryl-CoA dehydrogenase can be demonstrated in fibroblasts, leukocytes, and, for prenatal diagnosis, amniotic cells. Prenatal diagnosis is also possible by demonstrating increased glutaric acid in amniotic fluid.

Treatment

Restriction of dietary lysine and tryptophan are indicated but do not usually reverse or prevent symptoms. A variety of drugs that alter neurotransmitter levels, especially GABA, may be used to control dystonia. Studies suggest that early dietary treatment and aggressive management of intercurrent illness may prevent neurologic deterioration in some patients.

Goodman SI, Frerman FE: Organic acidemias due to defects in lysine oxidation: 2-ketoadipic acidemia and glutaric acidemia. In: *The Metabolic Basis of Inherited Disease,* 6th ed. Scriver CR et al (editors). McGraw-Hill, 1989.

Haworth JC et al: Phenotypic variability in glutaric aciduria type I: Report of fourteen cases in five Canadian Indian kindreds. J Pediatr 1991;118:52.

Hoffman GF et al: Glutaryl-coenzyme A dehydrogenase deficiency: A distinct encephalopathy. Pediatrics 1991;88: 1194.

Iafolla AK, Kahler SG: Megalencephaly in the neonatal period as the initial manifestation of glutaric aciduria type I. J Pediatr 1989;115:1004.

DISORDERS OF FATTY ACID OXIDATION & CARNITINE

LONG-CHAIN AND MEDIUM-CHAIN ACYL-CoA DEHYDROGENASE DEFICIENCIES

Deficiencies of long-chain and medium-chain acyl-CoA dehydrogenase (LCAD, MCAD), two enzymes of fatty acid β-oxidation, usually cause Reye-like episodes of hypoketotic hypoglycemia, mild hyperammonemia, hepatomegaly and encephalopathy, or less often, sudden death in infancy. The long- and medium-chain effects can usually be distinguished clinically, with the long-chain defect more often causing early severe hypotonia and cardiomyopathy. MCAD deficiency is by far the more common, occurring in perhaps 1:5000 live births. Although Reye-like episodes may be fatal, they tend to become less frequent and severe with time, and prolonged survival is not unusual in MCAD. In LCAD deficiency, cardiomyopathy is the direct result of the defect in the oxidation of long chain fatty acids. In MCAD deficiency, cardiomyopathy occurs possibly because the loss of octanoylcarnitine in the urine causes carnitine deficiency, which restricts entry of long-chain fatty acids into mitochondria. Both conditions are inherited as autosomal recessive traits.

Diagnosis

Suspicion should be aroused by the lack of an appropriate ketone response to fasting. Patients with MCAD deficiency excrete octanoylcarnitine phenylpropionylglycine and hexanoylglycine in the urine; octanoylcarnitine is excreted only when the patient is not carnitine-depleted. Assays of MCAD (and LCAD) activity in fibroblasts are necessary only when octanoylcarnitine, phenylpropionylglycine, and hexanoylglycine are not found. The finding of normal urine organic acids does not exclude these conditions, since excretion of dicarboxylic acids and other products of microsomal and peroxisomal oxidation of fatty acids can be intermittent.

Treatment

Acute management is directed toward preventing or reversing catabolism and hypoglycemia. Long-term measures include providing carbohydrate snacks before bedtime and vigorous treatment of intercurrent infections. Because cardiomyopathy and muscle weakness in MCAD deficiency may be due to secondary carnitine deficiency, oral administration of carnitine may be indicated. Medium-chain triglycerides are contraindicated in MCAD deficiency, because they may raise serum octanoic acid to rise to neurotoxic concentrations, but they may be a useful energy source for patients with LCAD deficiency.

Duran M et al: Sudden child death and "healthy" affected family members with medium-chain acyl-coenzyme A dehydrogenase deficiency. Pediatrics 1986;78:1052.

Hale DE, Bennett MJ: Fatty acid oxidation disorders: A new class of metabolic diseases. J Pediatr 1992;121:1.

Pollitt RJ: Disorders of mitochondrial β-oxidation: Prenatal and early postnatal diagnosis and their relevance to Reye's syndrome and sudden infant death. J Inherited Metab Dis 1989;12:215.

Rhead WJ: Inborn errors of fatty acid oxidation in man. Clin Biochem 1991;24:319.

Roe CR, Coates PM: Acyl-CoA dehydrogenase deficiencies. In: *The Metabolic Basis of Inherited Disease,* 6th ed. Scriver CR et al (editors). McGraw-Hill, 1989.

Taubman B, Hale DE, Kelley RI: Familial Reye-like syndrome: A presentation of medium-chain acyl-coenzyme A dehydrogenase deficiency. Pediatrics 1987;79:382.

GLUTARIC ACIDEMIA TYPE II

Glutaric acidemia type II (multiple acyl-CoA dehydrogenation deficiency) was first described in 1976 in a baby who died at 3 days of age with profound hypoglycemia, metabolic acidosis, and the "smell of sweaty feet." Since that time, many others have been diagnosed. Some have renal cysts and die in early infancy, and others have Reye-like episodes or skeletal muscle weakness (or both) beginning in childhood or adolescence. Some patients are deficient in electron transfer flavoprotein and others in ETF:ubiquinone oxidoreductase, proteins that transfer electrons from many flavin-containing enzymes of fatty- and amino acid oxidation into the respiratory chain. Both enzyme deficiencies are inherited as autosomal recessive traits, and the infantile form of the disease can be diagnosed in utero by demonstrating increased glutaric acid in the amniotic fluid.

Diagnosis

Diagnosis can be made by demonstrating derivatives of the substrates of mitochondrial flavin-containing dehydrogenases on organic acid analysis of urine (Table 31–4). Tissue assays of electron transfer flavoprotein and ETF:ubiquinone oxidoreductase are not usually necessary.

Treatment

Dietary measures (carbohydrate feedings before bedtime, provision of bicarbonate, and restriction of fat) are usually not effective, but administration of riboflavin and carnitine has shown promise, usually in older patients.

Frerman FE, Goodman SI. Glutaric acidemia type II and defects of the mitochondrial respiratory chain. In: *The Metabolic Basis of Inherited Disease,* 6th ed. Scriver CR et al (editors). McGraw-Hill, 1989.

Goodman SI, Loehr JP, Frerman FE: Clinical and biochemical aspects of glutaric acidemia Type II. In: *Fatty Acid Oxidation: Clinical Biochemical and Molecular Aspects.* Liss, 1990.

Jacobs C et al: Prenatal diagnosis of glutaric aciduria type II by direct chemical analysis of dicarboxylic acids in amniotic fluid. Eur J Pediatr 1984;141:153.

Mooy PD et al: Glutaric aciduria type II: Treatment with riboflavine, carnitine and insulin. Eur J Pediatr 1984;143:92.

CARNITINE

Carnitine is an essential nutrient that is found in highest concentrations in red meats. Its primary function is to transport long-chain fatty acids into mitochondria for oxidation. Primary defects of carnitine biosynthesis and transport exist and may present with Reye's syndrome, myoglobinuria, hypotonia, or cardiomyopathy. These disorders are exceedingly rare compared to secondary carnitine deficiency or insufficiency, which may be due to diet (especially hyperalimentation), renal losses, drug therapy (especially valproic acid), and other metabolic disorders (especially disorders of fatty acid oxidation and organic acidemias). The prognosis depends upon the cause of the carnitine abnormality.

Carnitine can be measured in blood. Unless the purpose is solely to monitor dietary deficiency, amounts of free and esterified carnitine should be determined. In some situations, muscle carnitine may be low despite normal blood levels. Free and esterified carnitine also can be measured in urine, and specialized laboratories can identify the specific ester present. If carnitine insufficiency is suspected, the patient should be evaluated to rule out disorders that might cause secondary carnitine deficiency.

Oral carnitine is used in carnitine deficiency or insufficiency in doses of 25–100 mg/kg/d or higher. Intravenous carnitine may be added to hyperalimentation, and high dose intravenous carnitine is available. Treatment is aimed at maintaining normal free carnitine levels. Carnitine supplementation in patients with disorders of fatty acid oxidation and organic acidosis may also augment excretion of accumulated metabolites, in addition to ameliorating carnitine insufficiency. Supplementation may not prevent metabolic crises in such patients, however, even when serum carnitine has been returned to normal.

DeVivo DC, Tein I: Primary and secondary disorders of carnitine metabolism. Int Pediatr 1990;5:134.

Kelly KJ et al: Fatal rhabdomyolysis following influenza infection in a girl with familial carnitine palmityl transferase deficiency. Pediatrics 1988;84:312.

Matsuda I et al: Carnitine deficiency and hyperammonemia with valproate therapy. J Pediatr 1986;109:131.

Moukarzel AA et al: Carnitine status of children receiving long-term total parenteral nutrition: A longitudinal prospective study. J Pediatr 1992;120:759.

Rinaldo P et al: Effect of treatment with glycine and L-carnitine in medium-chain acylcoenzyme A dehydrogenase deficiency. J Pediatr 1993;122:580.

Steenhout P et al: Carnitine deficiency with cardiomyopathy presenting as neonatal hydrops: Successful response to carnitine therapy. J Inherited Metab Dis 1990;13:69.

DISORDERS OF PURINE METABOLISM

HYPOXANTHINE-GUANINE PHOSPHORIBOSYLTRANSFERASE DEFICIENCY (Lesch-Nyhan Syndrome)

Hypoxanthine-guanine phosphoribosyltransferase (HPRT) is the enzyme that converts the purine bases hypoxanthine and guanine to inosine monophosphate (IMP) and guanosine monophosphate (GMP), respectively. The X-linked recessive disorder due to its complete deficiency is characterized by central nervous system dysfunction and purine overproduction with hyperuricemia and hyperuricuria. Depending on the residual activity of the mutant enzyme, male hemizygotes may be severely retarded and show choreoathetosis, spasticity, and compulsive, mutilating lip and finger biting, or they may present with only gouty arthritis and urate ureterolithiasis. The enzyme deficiency can be demonstrated in erythrocytes, fibroblasts, and cultured amniotic cells; this disorder can thus be diagnosed with certainty in utero.

Although the cause of the central nervous system dysfunction in Lesch-Nyhan syndrome remains obscure, the absent or less severe central nervous system manifestations of purine nucleoside phosphorylase deficiency (in which HPRT is functionally inactive because of lack of substrate) suggest that the problem relates to accumulation of substrate behind the block.

Diagnosis

Diagnosis is made by demonstrating elevated uric acid:creatinine ratio in urine, followed by demonstration of enzyme deficiency in red blood cells.

Treatment

Allopurinol and probenecid may be given to reduce hyperuricemia but do not affect neurologic status. Insertions of the HPRT gene into cultured cells from affected patients and into experimental animals have been effective and offer promise as models for human gene therapy in the future.

Silverman LJ, Kelley WN, Palella TD: Genetic analysis of human hypoxanthine-guanine phosphoribosyltransferase deficiency. Enzyme 1987;38:36.

LYSOSOMAL DISEASES

Lysosomes are cellular organelles in which complex macromolecules are degraded by specific acid hydrolases. Deficiency of a lysosomal enzyme causes its substrate to accumulate in lysosomes of tissues that degrade it, creating a characteristic clinical picture. These so-called storage disorders are classified as mucopolysaccharidoses, lipidoses, or mucolipidoses, depending on the nature of the stored material. Two additional disorders, cystinosis and Salla's disease, are caused by defects in lysosomal proteins that normally transport material from the lysosome to the cytoplasm.

Clinical and laboratory features of these conditions are shown in Table 31–5. Most are inherited as autosomal recessive traits, and all can be diagnosed in utero by enzyme assays of cultured amniotic cells.

The diagnosis of mucopolysaccharidosis is suggested by certain clinical and radiologic findings and confirmed by urine screening tests. Further tests are needed to determine which particular mucopolysaccharides are present. Diagnosis should be confirmed by enzyme assays of cultured fibroblasts or leukocytes; this is especially important when the parents are contemplating having more children.

When a lipidosis or mucolipidosis is suspected, diagnosis is made by appropriate enzyme assays of biopsy specimens, cultured skin fibroblasts, and peripheral leukocytes.

Most of these conditions cannot be treated effectively, although there is increasing evidence that bone marrow transplantation may affect the course of some lysosomal diseases. Gaucher's disease is treated effectively with infusions of natural enzyme modified to allow uptake of the enzyme by lysosomes.

Beutler E: Gaucher disease: New molecular approaches to diagnosis and treatment. Science 1992;256:794.

Muenzer J: Mucopolysaccharidoses. Acta Pediatr 1986; 33:269.

Sidransky E, Ginns EI: Clinical heterogeneity among patients with Gaucher's disease. JAMA 1993;269:1154.

Spranger J: Inborn errors of complex carbohydrate metabolism. Am J Med Genet 1987;28:489.

von Figura K et al: Mutations affecting transport and stability of lysosomal enzymes. Enzyme 1987;38:144.

Whitley CB et al: Long-term outcome of Hurler syndrome following bone marrow transplantation. Am J Med Genet 1993;46:209.

PEROXISOMAL DISEASES

Peroxisomes are intracellular organelles that contain a large number of enzymes, many of which are oxidases linked to catalase or peroxidase. Among the enzyme systems in peroxisomes is one for β-oxidation of very long chain fatty acids (which is analagous in many ways to the system for fatty acid oxidation in mitochondria) and another for plasmalogen biosynthesis. In addition, peroxisomes contain oxidases for D-and L-amino acids, pipecolic acid and phytanic acid, and an enzyme (alanine-glyoxylate aminotransferase) that effects transamination of glyoxylate to glycine.

In some peroxisomal diseases, many enzymes are deficient. Zellweger's (cerebrohepatorenal) syndrome, the best known among these, is probably due to a defect in organelle assembly. Patients present in infancy with seizures, hypotonia, characteristic facies with a large forehead, and hepatomegaly, and at autopsy show renal cysts and absent peroxisomes. Neonatal adrenoleukodystrophy and hyperpipecolic acidemia are similar conditions, with similar clinical and laboratory findings and multiple enzyme deficiencies in cultured fibroblasts, but peroxisomes are usually detected in tissues.

In other perixosomal diseases, only a single enzyme is deficient. Primary hyperoxaluria (alanine-glyoxalate aminotransferase deficiency), X-linked adrenoleukodystrophy and adrenomyeloneuropathy (very long chain acyl-CoA ligase deficiency), and adult Refsum's disease (phytanic acid oxidase deficiency) are disorders due to deficiency of single peroxisomal enzymes.

Except for childhood adrenoleukodystrophy, which is X-linked, all peroxisomal diseases are transmitted as autosomal recessive traits and can be diagnosed in utero by specific enzyme assays or by examining very long chain fatty acids in cultured amniotic cells. There is no treatment for most peroxisomal disorders, but dietary treatment may have some promise for female carriers of X-linked adrenomyeloneuropathy and is being studied in affected males as well.

Diagnosis

The best screening test for Zellweger's syndrome, hyperpipecolic acidemia, X-linked adrenoleukodystrophy, neonatal adrenoleukodystrophy, and infantile Refsum's disease is determination of very long chain fatty acids in serum or plasma; these acids are increased in all these conditions. Tissue biopsy may also be required to determine the presence and morphologic characteristics of peroxisomes.

Table 31–5. Clinical and laboratory features of lysosomal storage diseases.

Disorder	Enzyme Defect	Clinical and Laboratory Features
I. Mucopolysaccharidoses		
Hurler syndrome	α-Iduronidase	Autosomal recessive. Mental retardation, hepatosplenomegaly, umbilical hernia, coarse facies, corneal clouding, dorsolumbar gibbus, severe heart disease. Heparan sulfate and dermatan sulfate in urine.
Scheie syndrome	α-Iduronidase (incomplete)	Autosomal recessive. Corneal clouding, stiff joints, normal intellect. Clinical types intermediate between Hurler and Scheie common. Heparan sulfate and dermatan sulfate in urine.
Hunter syndrome	Sulfoiduronate sulfatase	X-linked recessive. Coarse facies, hepatosplenomegaly, mental retardation variable. Corneal clouding and gibbus not present. Heparan sulfate and dermatan sulfate in urine.

Sanfilippo syndrome:
  Type A
  Type B
 	
  Type C
 	
  Type D
	
	Sulfamidase
	α-N-Acetylglucos-
	  aminidase
	Acetyl-CoA: α-
	  glucosaminide-N-
	  acetyltransferase
	α-N-acetylglucosamine-
	  6-sulfatase
		Autosomal recessive. Severe mental retardation with comparatively mild skeletal changes, visceromegaly, and facial coarseness. Types cannot be differentiated clinically. Heparan sulfate in urine.

Morquio syndrome	N-Acetylgalactosamine- 6-sulfatase	Autosomal recessive. Severe skeletal changes, platyspondylisis, corneal clouding. Keratan sulfate in urine.
Maroteaux-Lamy syndrome	N-Acetylgalactosamine- 4-sulfatase	Autosomal recessive. Coarse facies, growth retardation, dorsolumbar gibbus, corneal clouding, hepatosplenomegaly, normal intellect. Dermatan sulfate in urine.
β-Glucuronidase deficiency	β-Glucuronidase	Autosomal recessive. Varies from mental retardation, dorsolumbar gibbus, corneal clouding, and hepatosplenomegaly to mild facial coarseness, retardation, and loose joints. Hearing loss common. Dermatan sulfate or heparan sulfate in urine.
II. Mucolipidoses		
Mannosidosis	α-Mannosidase	Autosomal recessive. Varies from severe mental retardation, coarse facies, short stature, skeletal changes, and hepatosplenomegaly to mild facial coarseness and loose joints. Hearing loss common. Abnormal oligosaccharides in urine.
Fucosidosis	α-Fucosidase	Autosomal recessive. Variable: coarse facies, skeletal changes, hepatosplenomegaly, occasional angiokeratoma corporis diffusum. Abnormal oligosaccharides in urine.
I-cell disease (mucolipidosis II)	N-Acetylglucosaminyl- phosphotransferase	Autosomal recessive; severe and mild forms known. Very short stature, mental retardation, early facial coarsening, clear cornea, stiffness of joints. Increased lysosomal enzymes in serum. Abnormal sialyl oligosaccharides in urine.
Sialidosis	N-Acetylneuraminidase (sialidase)	Autosomal recessive. Mental retardation, coarse facies, skeletal dysplasia, myoclonic seizures, cherry-red macular spot. Abnormal sialyl oligosaccharides in urine.
III. Lipidoses		
Niemann-Pick disease	Sphingomyelinase	Autosomal recessive. Acute and chronic forms known. Acute neuronopathic form common in eastern European Jews. Accumulation of sphingomyelin in lysosomes of RE system and CNS. Hepatosplenomegaly, developmental retardation, macular cherry-red spot. Death by 1–4 years.
Metachromatic leukodystrophy	Arylsulfatase A	Autosomal recessive. Late infantile form, with onset at 1–4 years, most common. Accumulation of sulfatide in white matter. Gait disturbances (ataxia), motor incoordination, and dementia. Death usually in first decade.
Krabbe disease (globoid cell leukodystrophy)	Galactocerebroside β-galactosidase	Autosomal recessive. Globoid cells in white matter. Onset at 3–6 months with seizures, irritability, and retardation. Death by 1–2 years. Juvenile and adult forms are rare.
Fabry disease	α-Galactosidase A	X-linked recessive. Storage of trihexosylceramide in endothelial cells. Pain in extremities, angiokeratoma corporis diffusum and (later) poor vision, hypertension, and renal failure.

(continued)

Table 31–5. Clinical and laboratory features of lysosomal storage diseases. (continued)

Disorder	Enzyme Defect	Clinical and Laboratory Features
Farber disease	Ceramidase	Autosomal recessive. Storage of ceramide in tissues. Subcutaneous nodules, arthropathy with deformed and painful joints, and poor growth and development. Death within first year.
Gaucher disease	Glucocerebroside β-glucosidase	Autosomal recessive. Acute neuronopathic form: Accumulation of glucocerebroside in lysosomes of RE system and CNS. Retardation, hepatosplenomegaly, macular cherry-red spot, and Gaucher cells in bone marrow. Death by 1–2 years. Chronic form common in eastern European Jews. Accumulation of spingomyelin in lysosomes of RE system. Hepatosplenomegaly and flask-shaped osteolytic bone lesions. Consistent with normal life expectancy.
G_{M1} gangliosidosis	GM_1 ganglioside β-galactosidase	Autosomal recessive. Accumulation of G_{M1} ganglioside in lysosomes of RE system and CNS. Infantile form: Abnormalities at birth with dysostosis multiplex, hepatosplenomegaly, macular cherry-red spot, and death by 2 years. Juvenile form: Normal development to 1 year of age, then ataxia, weakness, dementia, and death by 4–5 years. Occasional inferior beaking of vertebral bodies of L1 and L2.
G_{M2} gangliosidoses Tay-Sachs disease Sandhoff disease	β-*N*-Acetylhexosaminidase A β-*N*-Acetylhexosaminidase A & B	Autosomal recessive. Tay-Sachs disease common in eastern European Jews; Sandhoff disease is panethnic. Clinical phenotypes are identical, with accumulation of G_{M2} ganglioside in lysosomes of CNS. Onset at age 3–6 months, with hypotonia, hyperacusis, retardation, and macular cherry-red spot. Death by 2–3 years. Juvenile and adult onset forms of Tay-Sachs disease are rare.
Wolman disease	Acid lipase	Autosomal recessive. Accumulation of cholesterol esters and triglycerides in lysosomes of reticuloendothelial system. Onset in infancy with gastrointestinal symptoms and hepatosplenomegaly, and death by 3–6 months. Adrenals commonly enlarged and calcified.

Moser HW: Peroxisomal disorders. Clin Biochem 1991; 24:343.

Moser HW et al: Adrenoleukodystrophy: Phenotypic variability and implications for therapy. J Inherit Metab Dis 1992;15:645.

Sadeghi-Nejad A, Senior B: Adreno-myeloneuropathy presenting as Addison's disease in childhood. N Engl J Med 1990;322:13.

Wanders RJA et al: The inborn errors of metabolism: A review. J Inherit Metab Dis 1990;13:4.

REFERENCES

Cohn RM, Roth KS: *Metabolic Disease: A Guide to Early Recognition.* Saunders, 1983.

Fernandez J, Saudubray J-M, Tada K (editors): *Inborn Metabolic Diseases: Diagnosis and Treatment.* Springer-Verlag, 1990.

Goodman SI, Markey SP: *Diagnosis of Organic Acidemias by Gas Chromatography-Mass Spectrometry.* AR Liss, 1981.

Scriver CR et al (editors): *The Metabolic Basis of Inherited Diseases,* 6th ed. McGraw-Hill, 1989.

Genetics & Dysmorphology

32

Janet M. Stewart, MD, David K. Manchester, MD,
& Eva Sujansky, MD

New techniques in molecular biology and biochemistry have changed the way clinicians think about and approach birth defects. Scientific reports that advance the understanding of human genetics and development appear almost daily. Molecular approaches to clinical problems now support "reverse genetics," the characterization of human disorders at the level of the gene before their clinical biochemistry and pathophysiology are described. Worldwide, scientists have united to map the human genome.

The clinical implications of these advances are too numerous to discuss completely in this text. This chapter reviews human chromosomes and chromosome abnormalities, briefly describes diagnostic and therapeutic applications of recombinant DNA technology, and then outlines clinically important aspects of mendelian genetics, dysmorphology, and teratology. The chapter concludes with a review of the scope and approach of genetic counseling and some comments about fetal surgery. The reader is directed to the referenced publications for more comprehensive treatments of the rapidly expanding field of clinical genetics.

I. CHROMOSOMES & CELL DIVISIONS

Human chromosomes consist of deoxyribonucleic acid (DNA) and specific proteins. In a nondividing cell, chromosomes are tightly packaged in the nucleus. Chromosomes contain most of the genetic information necessary for growth and differentiation. Chromosome aberrations lead to physical and mental abnormalities. Documentation of chromosome abnormality is important for appropriate management of the affected child and for assessment of the risk of recurrence; sometimes this risk affects many family members.

Although the correct number of chromosomes was established in 1956, it was not until the early 1970s that newly developed cytogenetic techniques allowed recognition of the more detailed characteristics of chromosomes and identification of a whole array of chromosome abnormalities.

The nuclei of all normal human cells, with the exception of gametes, contain 46 chromosomes, consisting of 23 pairs (Figure 32–1). Of these, 22 pairs are called **autosomes.** They are numbered according to their size; chromosome 1 is the largest, and chromosome 22 is the smallest. In addition, there are two **sex chromosomes:** two X chromosomes in females and one X and one Y chromosome in males. The two members of a chromosome pair are called **homologous chromosomes.** One homologue of each chromosome pair is maternal in origin (from the egg); the second is paternal (from the sperm). The egg and sperm each contain 23 chromosomes (**haploid cells**). During the formation of the zygote, they fuse into a cell with 46 chromosomes (**diploid cell**). The subsequent prenatal and postnatal growth of the human organism is through somatic cell divisions, called mitosis.

Mitosis (Figure 32–2) is a cell division of somatic cells. The process has different stages, during which the DNA replication takes place and two daughter cells, genetically identical to the original parent cells, are formed. During **metaphase,** the phase following DNA replication but preceding cell division, individual chromosomes can be visualized. They consist of two arms, a short arm and a long arm separated by a centromere. Each arm consists of two identical parts, called **chromatids.** Chromatids of the same chromosome are called **sister chromatids.**

Meiosis (Figure 32–3), during which eggs and sperm are formed, is cell division limited to gametes. During meiosis, three unique processes take place:

(1) Crossing over of genetic material between two homologous chromosomes; this is preceded by the pairing of both members of each chromosome pair, thus facilitating the physical exchange of homologous genetic material between them.

(2) Random assortment of maternally and paternally derived homologous chromosomes into the daughter cells. The distribution of maternal or pater-

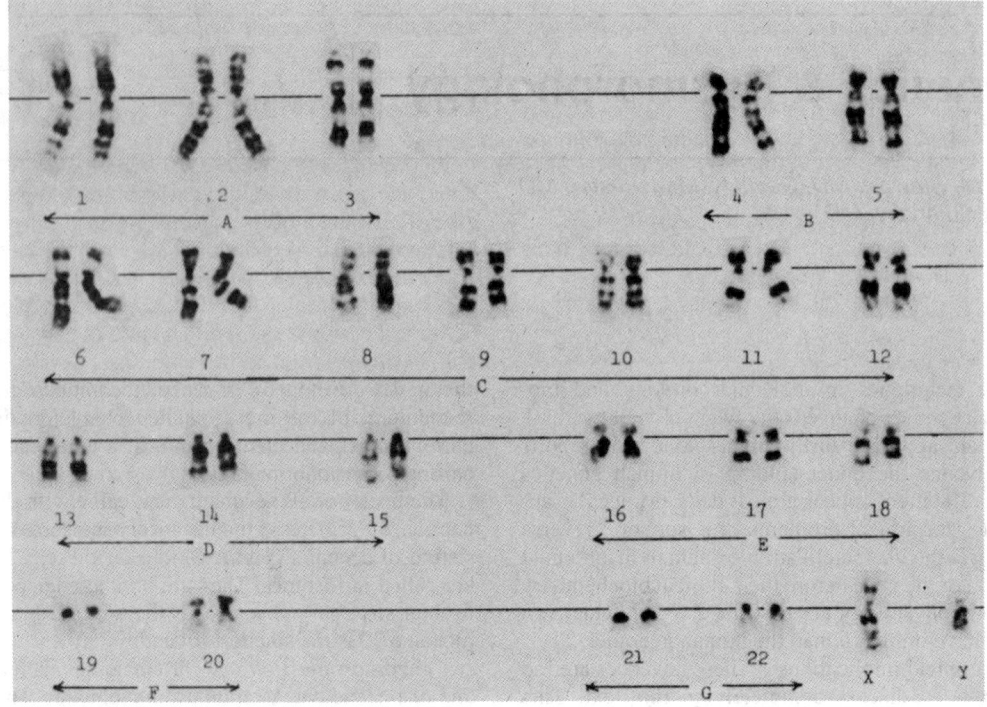

Figure 32–1. Normal male human karyotype.

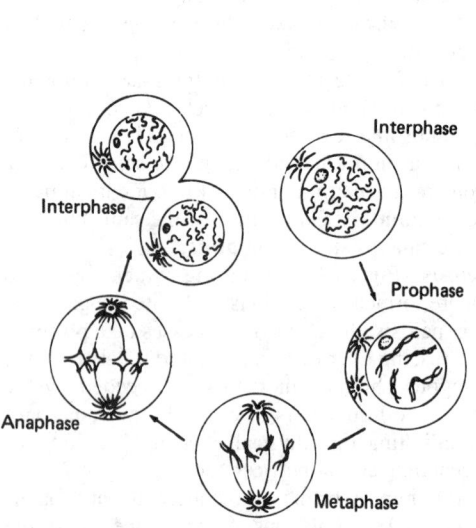

Figure 32–2. Diagram demonstrating the various stages of the mitotic cycle.

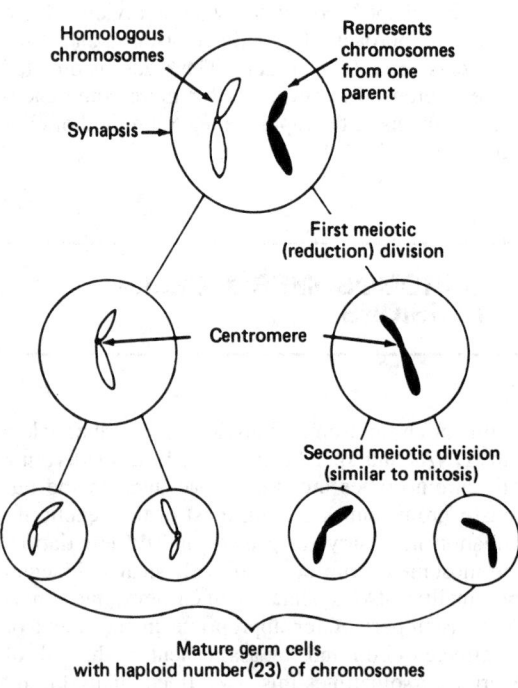

Figure 32–3. Diagram of meiosis, demonstrating the conversion from the diploid somatic cell to the haploid gamete.

nal chromosomes to a particular daughter cell is independent for each such cell.

(3) Two cell divisions, the first of which is a **reduction division,** ie, a parental cell with 46 chromosomes divides into two daughter cells with 23 chromosomes each.

CHROMOSOME PREPARATION & ANALYSIS

Because the structure of chromosomes can be visualized only during mitosis, the tissue obtained for chromosome analysis must contain many cells in a dividing state. This condition exists naturally only in bone marrow. Because bone marrow is not readily accessible, it is used for chromosome analysis only when immediate identification of a patient's chromosome constitution is necessary for appropriate management (eg, to rule out trisomy 13 in a newborn with a complex congenital heart disease requiring immediate intervention).

The peripheral blood lymphocytes are easy to obtain and are therefore most frequently used for chromosome analysis. Other tissues used for this purpose include skin or internal organs, such as thymus or gonads. Chorionic villi or amniocytes are used for prenatal diagnosis. If tissue other than bone marrow is used, the cells must be exposed to a mitogenic agent to increase the rate of mitosis.

Lymphocytes require 3 days' growth in a culture medium, and other tissues require 1–2 weeks' growth before enough mitoses are present to allow complete analysis. The chromosome preparation protocol calls for the processed cells to be placed on a glass slide and stained using new techniques that produce a light-and-dark band pattern across the arms of the chromosomes (see Figure 32–1). This band pattern is characteristic and reproducible for each chromosome, allowing the chromosomes to be arranged in homologous pairs and numeric and structural abnormalities to be identified. The layout of chromosomes on a sheet of paper in a predetermined order is called a **karyotype.**

In addition to the previously described routine chromosome analysis, the following specific studies can be requested:

(1) High-resolution chromosome analysis of more elongated chromosomes, allowing visualization of more detailed chromosome bands and detection of abnormalities in a smaller segment of chromosome.

(2) Fluorescent in situ hybridization (FISH). The technique involves the use of specific fluorescent-labeled DNA probes that hybridize to the corresponding regions of chromosomes, thus allowing their visu-alization under a fluorescent microscope. If a cocktail of probes from the same chromosome is used, the whole chromosome may be stained (chromosome painting). FISH can be used for the detection of sub-microscopic structural rearrangements, undetectable by classic cytogenetic techniques, or the identification of marker chromosomes in metaphase cells (Figure 32–12). In addition, it allows interphase cells (lymphocytes, amniocytes) to be screened for numerical abnormalities, such as trisomy 21. However, the study of interphase nuclei is not 100% accurate, and any abnormality must be confirmed by a conventional chromosome analysis.

(3) Fragile X study (see the section on fragile X syndrome, below).

(4) Assessment of chromosome breaks and sister chromatid exchanges requires special techniques that may lead to enhancement of the breaks or special staining that allows visualization of the exchanged chromatids.

CHROMOSOME NOMENCLATURE

A uniform nomenclature consisting of a simple system of symbols has been developed to describe normal and abnormal chromosome findings.

The symbols for normal male and female constitution are 46,XY and 46,XX, respectively. The signs (+) and (–) in front of the chromosome number indicate trisomy or monosomy, respectively, for that particular whole chromosome. For example, 47,XY,+21 designates a male with trisomy 21. The sign (+) or (–) after the chromosome number describes extra material or missing material, respectively, on one of the arms of the chromosome. The symbol for the short arm is p; for the long arm, q. Thus, 46,XX,8q– denotes a deletion on the long arm of chromosome 8. More detailed description of structural abnormalities includes break points in the rearrangement. For example, 46,XY,t(4:8)(q22;p21) means a reciprocal translocation (letter t) between the long arm of chromosome 4, at band 22, and the short arm of chromosome 8, at band 21. Other common symbols include *del* (deletion), *dup* (duplication), and *inv* (inversion).

CHROMOSOME ABNORMALITIES

Errors during cell division may result in numerical or structural abnormalities of chromosomes.

Numerical abnormalities are the result of unequal division, called **nondisjunction,** of chromosomes into the daughter cells. Any deviation from the normal diploid number of chromosomes is called **aneuploidy.** This most frequently involves the presence of an additional chromosome, called **trisomy** (eg, trisomy 21, Down syndrome) (Figure 32–4), or the presence of only a single copy of a chromosome, called **monosomy** (eg, monosomy X, Turner syndrome). Rarely, three copies **(triploidy)** of the whole set of 23 chromosomes are found. Four sets of chromosomes **(tetraploidy)** are not found in liveborns.

Structural abnormalities are the result of breaks in chromosomes, which join randomly to form new combinations. In contrast to the numerical abnormalities, which result in trisomy or monosomy of a whole chromosome, structural chromosome abnormalities result in trisomy or monosomy (or both) of only part of a chromosome. The number of possible chromosome abnormalities is infinite. The following types of chromosome rearrangements, according to the mechanism leading to the abnormality, are recognized (Figure 32–5): (1) **Deletion** is the absence of a part of a chromosome. The deletion is called **terminal** if the distal end of a chromosome arm is included and **interstitial** if it is not included in the deletion. A terminal deletion of both arms of a chromosome may result in reattachment of the remaining arms, leading to formation of a **ring chromosome.** (2) **Translocation** is detachment of a chromosome segment from its normal location and its attachment to another chromosome. The translocation is **balanced** if the cell contains two complete copies of all the chromosome material, although in a different order. In an **unbalanced** translocation, the rearrangement results in partial trisomy or monosomy.

Translocations can be reciprocal or Robertsonian. A **reciprocal** translocation involves exchange of segments between two chromosomes; eg, part of the short arm of chromosome 4 trades places with part of the long arm of chromosome 10. In **Robertsonian** translocations, two acrocentric chromosomes fuse at their centromeres. The most frequent Robertsonian translocation is formed between chromosomes 14 and 21.

(3) **Inversion** is the result of a double break in the same chromosome. The detached middle section turns upside down before reattaching. If both breaks are on the same side of the centromere, the inversion is **paracentric;** if the breaks are on the opposite arms of a chromosome, the inversion is **pericentric.**

MOSAICISM

Mosaicism is the presence of two or more different chromosome constitutions in different cells of the same individual. For example, a patient may have some cells with 47 chromosomes and others with 46 chromosomes; 46,XX/47,XX,+21 indicates mosaicism for trisomy 21; 45,X/46,XX/47,XXX indicates mosaicism for a monosomy and a trisomy X. Mosaicism should be suspected if clinical symptoms are milder than expected in a nonmosaic patient with the same chromosome abnormality. The prognosis is frequently better for a patient with mosaicism than one with a corresponding chromosome abnormality without mosaicism. In general, the smaller the proportion of the abnormal cell line, the better the prognosis. In the same patient, however, the proportion of normal and abnormal cells in various tissues, such as in skin and peripheral blood, may be significantly different. A prognosis frequently cannot be reliably assessed and should be made with caution or deferred. Mosaicism for structural abnormalities is very rare.

UNIPARENTAL DISOMY

Under normal circumstances, one member of each homologous pair of chromosomes is of maternal origin from the egg and the other is of paternal origin from the sperm (Figure 32–6A). In uniparental disomy, both copies of a particular chromosome pair originate from the same parent. If the uniparental disomy is caused by chromosome error in the first meiotic division, both homologous chromosomes of that parent will be present in the gamete. This is called **heterodisomy** (Figure 32–6B). If it is caused by an error in the second meiotic division, two copies of the same chromosome will be present. This is called **isodisomy** (Figure 32–6C). The union of a disomic gamete with a nullisomic gamete from the other parent will result in a zygote with a normal karyotype. Therefore, a uniparental disomy would not be detected by chromosome analysis. However, DNA analysis would reveal that the child inherited two copies of DNA of a particular chromosome from one parent without the contribution from the other parent. Uniparental disomy has been documented for human chromosomes 7, 11, 15, and X. It has been found in patients with Prader-Willi, Angelman, and Beckwith-Wiedemann syndromes. In addition, cystic fibrosis with only one carrier parent (due to maternal isodisomy) has been reported. Hemophilia A has been passed from father to son as a result of paternal heterodisomy of X and Y.

Uniparental disomy causes severe pre- and postnatal growth retardation. Furthermore it is suspected that uniparental disomy of some chromosomes is lethal. The possible mechanisms for the adverse effects of uniparental disomy include possible homozygosity for deleterious recessive genes and the consequences of imprinting. (See principles of imprinting in the section on dysmorphology, below.)

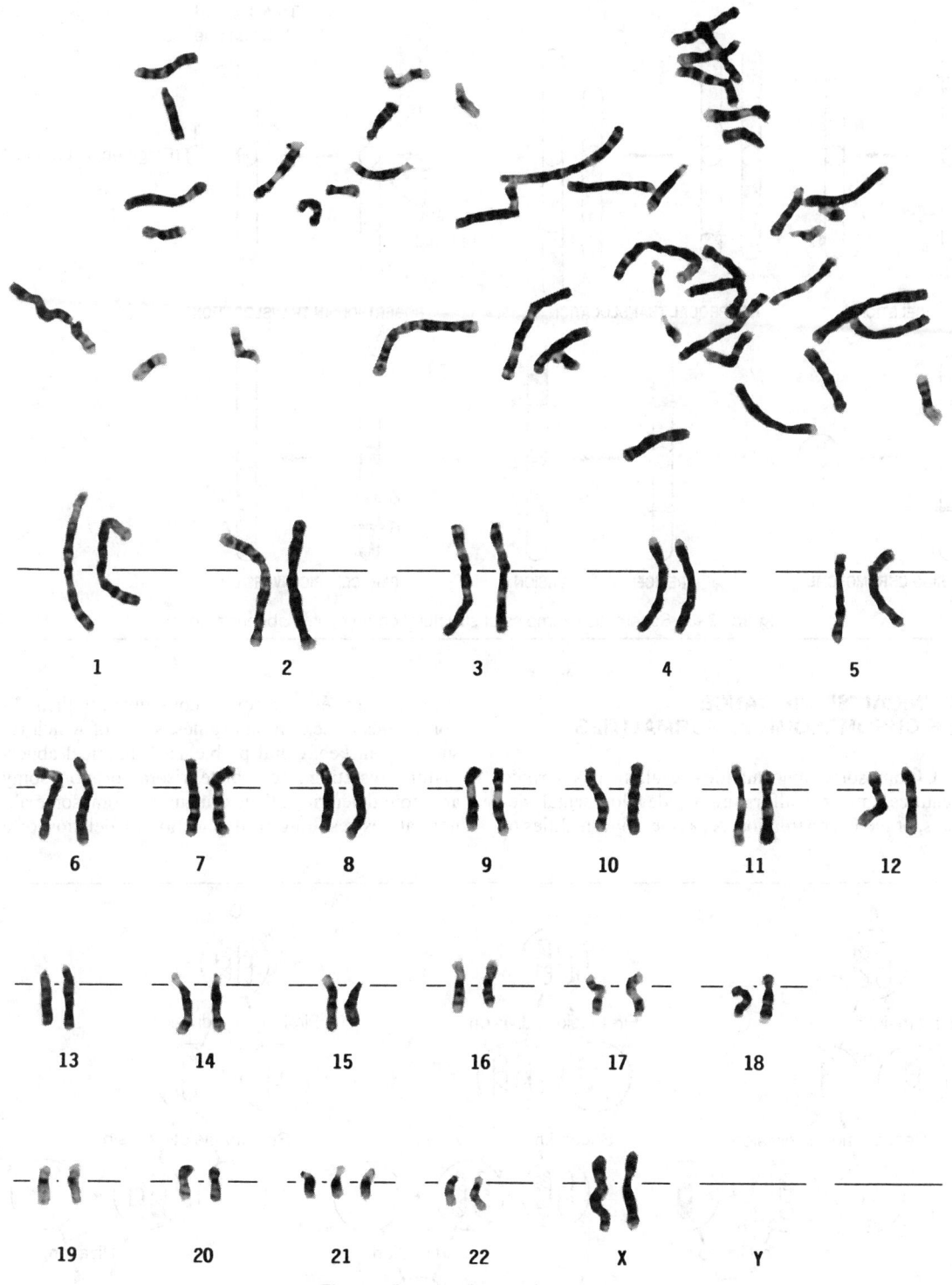

Figure 32–4. Karyotype of trisomy 21.

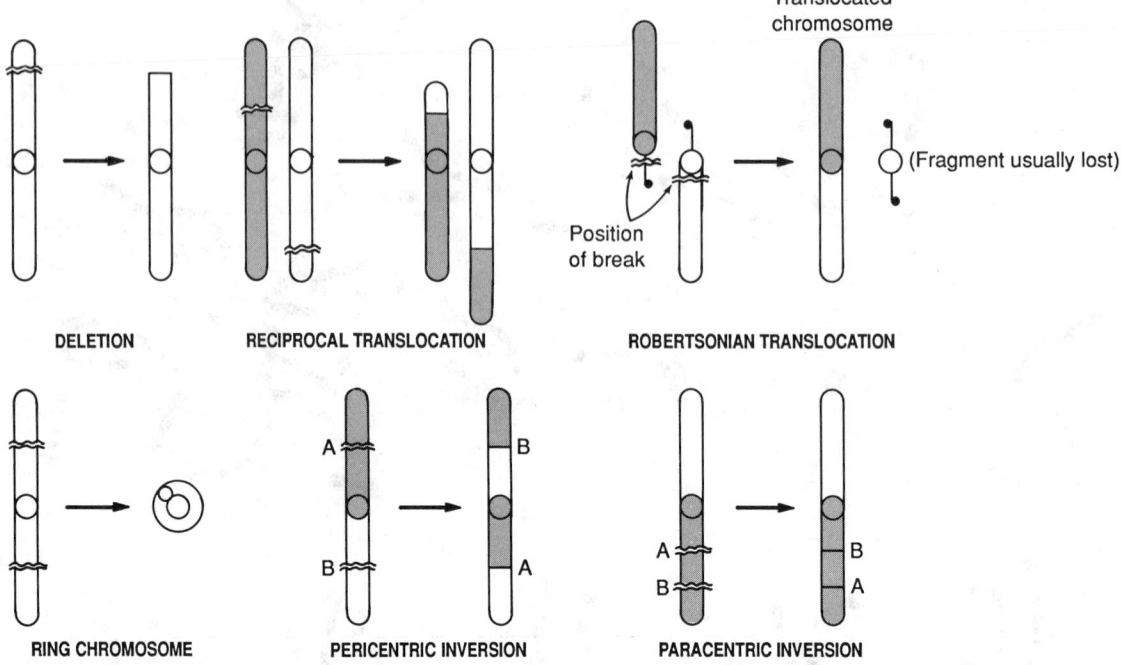

Figure 32–5. Schematic examples of structural chromosome abnormalities.

CLINICAL SIGNIFICANCE OF CHROMOSOME ABNORMALITIES

Chromosome abnormalities result in dysmorphic features, major malformations, developmental delays, or mental retardation. As a rule, abnormalities of autosomes have more severe consequences than abnormalities of sex chromosomes, some of which result only in behavioral problems. Numerical abnormalities resulting in complete trisomy or monosomy are more deleterious than structural chromosome abnormalities resulting in duplication or deletion of a

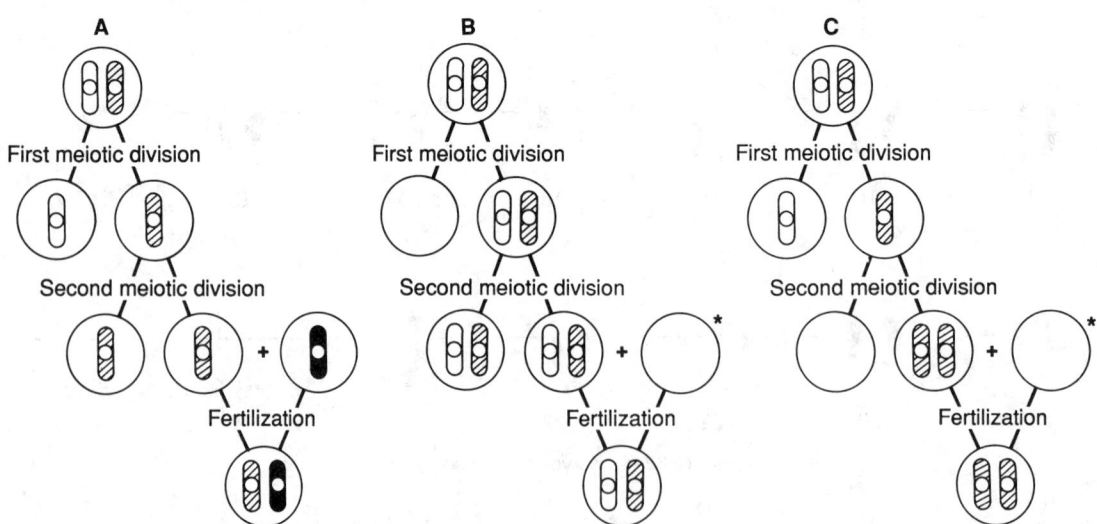

Figure 32–6. Diagram demonstrating the assortment of homologous chromosomes during normal gametogenesis and uniparental disomy. **A:** Fertilization of normal gametes. **B:** Heterodisomy. **C:** Isodisomy. The asterisks (*) in **B** and **C** indicate the nullisomic gametes from the other parent.

chromosome segment. Frequently, the smaller the duplicated or deleted segment, the milder the clinical symptoms. However, comparison of patients with duplications or deletions of different sizes in a particular chromosome indicates that involvement of a small specific segment sometimes has a disproportionately great effect on mortality and morbidity.

ABNORMALITIES OF AUTOSOMES

DOWN SYNDROME

The term *Down syndrome* is preferred to the previously used term *mongolism.* The most constant characteristic of the disease is mental retardation. IQs vary between 20 and 80, with the great majority between 45 and 55. Down syndrome occurs in about 1:600 newborns; however, the incidence is greater among children of mothers over 35 years of age. The mother's age at the time of conception and the nature of the chromosome abnormality are important in genetic counseling.

Clinical Findings

A. Symptoms and Signs: The principal findings are a small, brachycephalic head; flat nasal bridge; ruddy cheeks; dry lips; large, protruding "scrotal" tongue; small ears; upslanted palpebral fissures that narrow laterally; epicanthic folds; occasionally Brushfield spots; and a short, fleshy neck (Figure 32–7). About one-third of children with Down syndrome have congenital heart disease, most often an endocardial cushion defect or other septal defect. Patients tend to have short, stubby, spade-like hands with transverse palmar simian lines and abnormal dermatoglyphics. Generalized hypotonia is often present, as well as umbilical hernia. The distance between the big toe and second toe is often greater than usual. Sexual development is retarded, especially in males. The affected newborn is prone to have a third fontanelle, prolonged physiologic jaundice, polycythemia, and a transient leukemoid reaction. Cutis marmorata is often present. Later, there is an increased tendency for thyroid dysfunction, hearing loss, and atlanto-occipital instability. Leukemia is 20 times more common than in unaffected children. Susceptibility to intercurrent infections is increased. Patients with Down syndrome display an increased sensitivity to the mydriatic effects of atropine instilled into the conjunctiva.

B. Laboratory Findings: The chromosome abnormalities are pathognomonic. The great majority of cases (95%) have 47 chromosomes with trisomy of

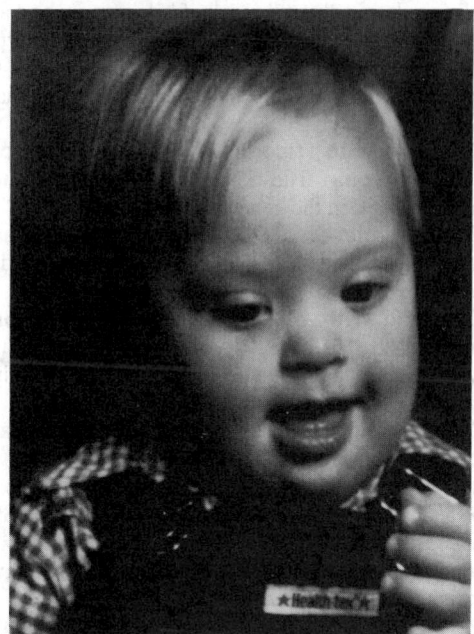

Figure 32–7. Child with Down syndrome.

21. However, about 4% of sporadic cases and about one-third of the familial cases have 46 chromosomes, including an abnormal translocated chromosome formed as the result of a centric fusion between two acrocentric chromosomes (Robertsonian translocation), one of which is chromosome 21. The translocation is found in 10% of patients whose mothers are younger but in only 3% of those with older mothers.

Mosaicism of the 46/47 type can also occur in persons with Down syndrome. These patients may have milder symptoms, especially higher than expected IQs. Occasionally, normal parents of affected children have inapparent mosaicism.

Only band q22 on the long arm of chromosome 21 need be trisomic for Down syndrome to occur. Some genes located near this band, eg, those for superoxide dismutase, the interferon receptor, and several enzymes involved in the pathway of de novo purine biosynthesis, do not seem to be the cause of Down syndrome.

Prevention

Down syndrome is sporadic in most families; however, the recurrence risk may be increased under certain circumstances. The risk of having a child affected with trisomy 21 varies with maternal age (1:2000 for mothers under 25 years of age; 1:50 for mothers 35–39 years of age; 1:20 for mothers over 40 years of age). These figures are different when one of the parents is a balanced translocation carrier.

In counseling parents who have one child with

Down syndrome about the risk of having a second affected child, the geneticist must study the karyotype of the affected child and sometimes the parents to achieve diagnostic accuracy. Several situations may occur.

A. Child With Trisomy 21, Parents With Normal Karyotypes: The risk is only slightly greater than for parents in the general population (1–2%).

B. Trisomic Child, One Parent With Mosaicism: The risk depends on the degree of gonadal mosaicism of the affected parent.

C. Child With 14/21 or 21/21 Translocation, Parents With Normal Karyotypes: The risks are unknown but should be considered only slightly increased.

D. Child With 14/21 Translocation, One Parent is a Balanced Translocation Carrier:

1. When the mother is the carrier, there is a 10–15% chance that the child will be affected, a 33% chance that the child will be a balanced translocation carrier, and a 43–48% chance that the child will have a normal karyotype.

2. When the father is the carrier, there is a 3–5% chance of having another affected child, and 50% of the apparently unaffected children may be carriers.

E. Child With 21/21 Translocation and One Parent With the Translocation: The recurrence risk is 100%.

Treatment

There is no convincing documentation of the merit of any of the forms of specific therapy that have been attempted, ranging from megadoses of vitamins to exercise programs proposed to overcome the physical and developmental abnormalities of the syndrome. Therapy is thus directed toward specific problems, eg, cardiac surgery or digitalis administration for heart problems, antibiotic administration for infections, tests of thyroid function, infant stimulation programs, special education, and occupational training. The goal of treatment is to help affected children develop to their full potential. Parents' participation in support groups should be encouraged.

TRISOMY 18 SYNDROME

The incidence of trisomy 18 syndrome is about 1:4000 live births, and the ratio of affected males to females is approximately 1:3. The mean maternal age is advanced. Affected babies frequently die in early infancy, though patients occasionally survive into childhood.

Clinical Findings

A. Symptoms and Signs: Trisomy 18 is characterized by prenatal and postnatal growth retardation, hypertonicity, prominent occiput, low-set and malformed ears, micrognathia, abnormal flexion of the fingers (index over third and fifth over fourth), equinovarus or "rocker-bottom" feet, short sternum and narrow pelvis, congenital heart disease (often ventricular septal defect or patent ductus arteriosus), and inguinal or umbilical hernias (Figure 32–8). There is an increased occurrence of single umbilical artery.

Dermatoglyphics show simple arches on fingers, a single flexion crease on the fifth finger, and transverse palmar lines. Surviving children show significant developmental delay and mental retardation.

B. Laboratory Findings: In place of uniform trisomy 18, chromosome analysis occasionally reveals mosaicism for trisomy 18 or an unbalanced translocation involving a third number 18 and other chromosome. Rarely, double trisomies have been found in which trisomy X or trisomy 21 is present in addition to trisomy 18.

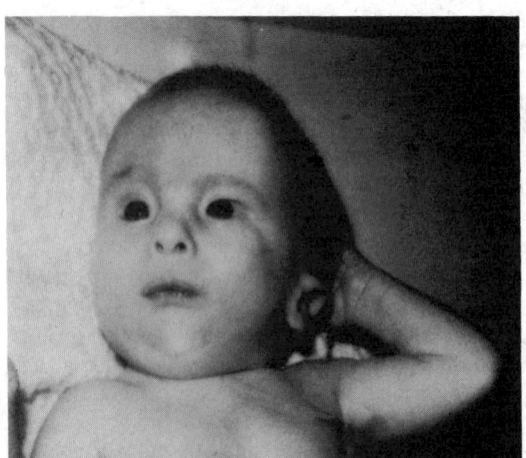 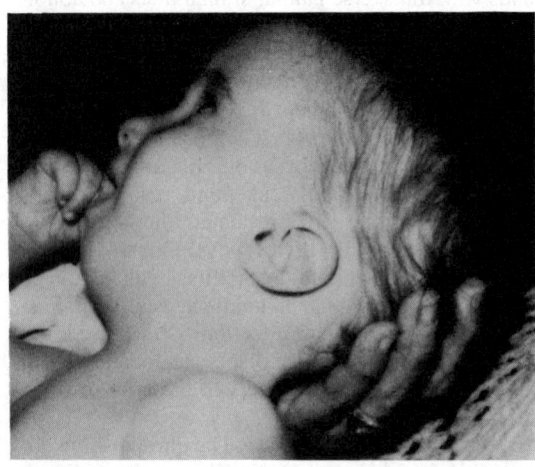

Figure 32–8. Child with trisomy 18.

Complications

Complications are related to associated lesions. Death is often due to heart failure or pneumonia.

Treatment & Prognosis

There is no treatment other than general supportive care. Death usually occurs in infancy or early childhood, though some patients have reached adulthood.

TRISOMY 13 SYNDROME

The incidence of trisomy 13 is about 1:12,000 live births, and 60% of the patients are female. The mean maternal age is increased. Death usually (but not always) occurs in infancy or by the second year of life, commonly as a result of heart failure or infection.

The symptoms and signs include prenatal and postnatal growth deficiency, arrhinencephaly, sloping forehead, eye malformations (anophthalmia, colobomas), low-set ears, cleft lip and palate, capillary hemangiomas, polydactyly or syndactyly, and congenital heart disease (usually ventricular septal defect). The facies of an infant with trisomy 13 is shown in Figure 32–9. Other abnormal findings may include hyperconvex, narrow fingernails; "rocker-bottom" feet; retroflexible thumbs; urinary tract anomalies; umbilical hernia; and cryptorchidism or bicornuate uterus. Surviving children demonstrate failure to thrive, developmental retardation, apneic spells, seizures, and deafness.

Treatment is supportive. Because it is sometimes necessary to decide immediately after birth how extensive therapy should be for a severely malformed infant, this diagnosis (as well as one of trisomy 18) can be immediately confirmed by direct examination

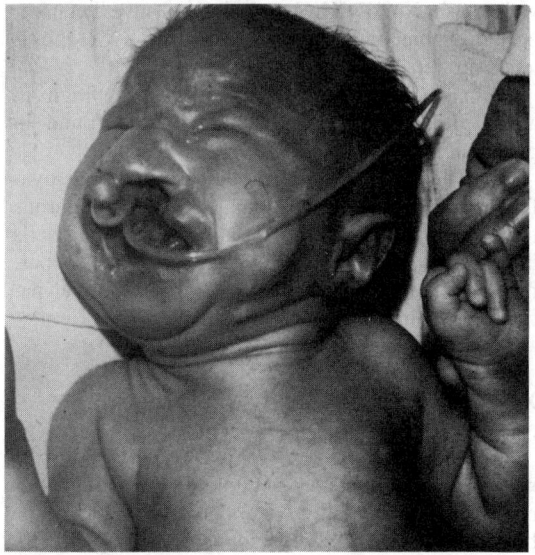

Figure 32–9. Child with trisomy 13.

of mitotic figures obtained from bone marrow. Prevention in the form of genetic counseling is indicated. Prenatal diagnosis is available. The recurrence risks are analogous to those of similar chromosome situations in Down syndrome.

ABNORMALITIES OF SEX CHROMOSOMES

TURNER SYNDROME

The incidence of Turner syndrome is 1:10,000 among females. However, it is estimated that 95% of conceptuses with monosomy X are miscarried and only 5% liveborn. Turner syndrome must be ruled out in all females with shortness of stature, webbing of the neck, coarctation of the aorta, or amenorrhea. The diagnosis is made by chromosome analysis. Patients with pseudohypoparathyroidism and Noonan syndrome have a similar phenotype with normal chromosomes.

Clinical Findings

A. Symptoms and Signs: In a newborn, Turner syndrome may be manifested by webbing of the neck, edema of the hands and feet, coarctation of the aorta, and a characteristic triangular face (Figure 32–10). Later symptoms include short stature, a shield chest with wide-set nipples, streak ovaries, amenorrhea, absence of secondary sex characteristics, and infertility. However, only short stature and amenorrhea and none of the other characteristics may be seen in some affected girls.

Complications relate primarily to the dangers of coarctation of the aorta, when present. Rarely, the dysgenetic gonads may become neoplastic (gonadoblastoma). The incidence of malformations of the urinary tract is increased. Sexual infantilism and the perceptual motor difficulties to which these patients are prone may pose psychologic hazards.

B. Laboratory Findings: Monosomy X (45,X) is found in a majority of patients with the Turner syndrome. Mosaicism 45,X/46,XX or 45,X/46,XX/47,XXX may be present. Occasionally, the patient has two X chromosomes, one of which has a structural abnormality, eg, a deletion or a translocation of part of one X to one of the autosomal chromosomes. Rarely, mosaicism 45,X/46,XY is found. The presence of a Y chromosome significantly increases the risk for gonadoblastoma.

Treatment & Prognosis

Treatment consists of identifying and treating perceptual problems before they become established. Es-

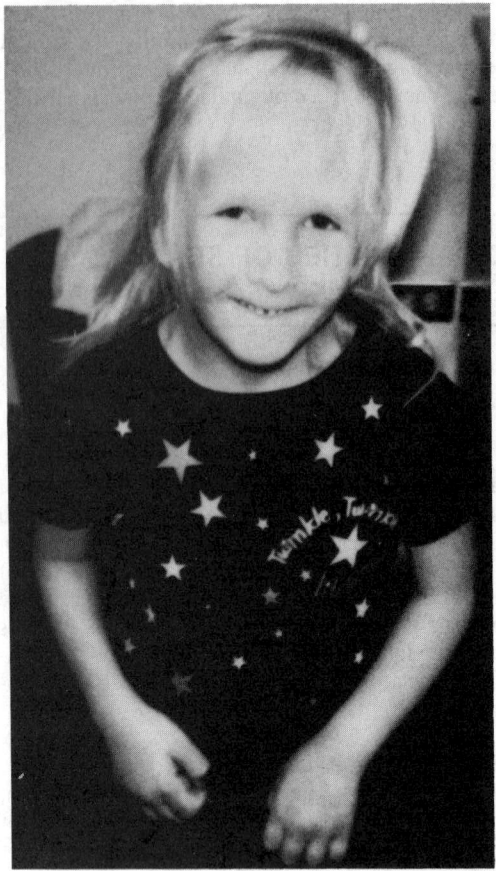

Figure 32–10. Child with Turner syndrome.

trogen replacement therapy will cause development of secondary sex characteristics, permit normal menstruation, and prevent development of osteoporosis. Teenage patients need counseling to cope with the stigma of their condition and to understand the need for hormone therapy. In recent years, growth hormone therapy has been used successfully to increase the height of affected girls. Females with 45,X or 45,X mosaicism have a low fertility rate, and those who become pregnant have been reported to have a high risk of fetal wastage (spontaneous miscarriage, approximately 30%; stillbirth, 6–10%). Furthermore, their liveborn offspring have an increased frequency of chromosome abnormalities involving either sex chromosomes or autosomes (14/102), and congenital malformations (19/102). Thus, prenatal ultrasound and chromosome analysis are indicated for females with sex chromosome abnormalities.

KLINEFELTER SYNDROME

The incidence of Klinefelter syndrome in the newborn population is roughly 1:500, but it is about 1% among mentally retarded males and about 3% among males seen at infertility clinics. The maternal age at birth is often advanced. The diagnosis is rarely made before puberty except as a result of prenatal diagnosis. Unlike gonadal dysgenesis, the Klinefelter syndrome is rarely the cause of spontaneous abortions.

Clinical Findings

A. Symptoms and Signs: The characteristic findings do not usually appear until after puberty. Therefore, it is improper to diagnose a child with a 47,XXY karyotype as having Klinefelter syndrome. The most that can be said is that such a child is at increased risk of developing the clinical signs of the syndrome during adolescence. Micro-orchidism associated with otherwise normal external genitals, azoospermia, and sterility are almost invariable in diagnosed cases. Gynecomastia, normal to borderline IQ, diminished facial hair, lack of libido and potency, and a tall, eunuchoid build are frequent features. In chromosome variants with three and four X chromosomes (XXXY and XXXXY), mental retardation may be severe, and radioulnar synostosis may be present as well as anomalies of the external genitalia and cryptorchidism. In the XXXXY cases, these findings are especially prominent, as well as microcephaly, hypertelorism, epicanthus, prognathism, short stature, and incurved fifth fingers.

The adult XXYY patient tends to be taller and more retarded than the average XXY patient.

In general, the physical and mental abnormalities associated with the Klinefelter syndrome increase as the number of sex chromosomes increases.

B. Laboratory Findings: The majority of cases have a 47,XXY constitution. Rare variants are 48,XXXY, 49,XXXXY, and 48,XXYY. A variety of mosaicisms containing combinations of the above, as well as 46,XY/47,XXY mosaicism, have been reported. Some patients with 46,XY/47,XXY mosaicism are fertile.

Urinary excretion of gonadotropins is high in adults. Levels are comparable to those found in postmenopausal women.

Histologic analysis of the adult testis reveals hyalinization and atrophy of the majority of seminiferous tubules, with large clumps of abnormal Leydig cells in between. A marked deficiency of germ cells (spermatogonia) has been found also in prepubertal patients (even in a 10-month-old child).

XYY SYNDROME

The incidence of the 47,XYY karyotype in the newborn population is as yet unknown, although current estimates are that it occurs in about 1:1000 male births. Affected newborns in general are perfectly normal and do not have the "XYY syndrome." This syndrome may be present in 10% of men over 6 feet tall who come into conflict with the law because of their aggressive personalities.

Affected individuals may on occasion exhibit an abnormal behavior pattern from early childhood and may be slightly retarded. Fertility may be normal.

There is no treatment. Many males with an XYY karyotype are normal. Long-term problems may relate to low IQ and environmental stress.

RECURRENCE RISKS

Most numerical chromosome abnormalities occur sporadically. However, occurrences in siblings or other relatives have been reported, suggesting a hereditary predisposition to nondisjunction in some kindreds. Attempts to identify a single cause have been unsuccessful. It is reasonable to assign parents of a child with aneuploidy an empirical recurrence risk of 1–2% and offer prenatal diagnosis for subsequent pregnancies. Determination of the recurrence risk in structural chromosome abnormalities requires chromosome analysis of the patient's parents to assess whether the abnormality was a de novo event in the patient or if a parental balanced rearrangement of chromosomes exists in one of the parents. If a balanced rearrangement is found, chromosome analysis of other family members must be attempted until all family members with the rearrangement are identified. This analysis is important because, although members of kindreds with normal chromosomes are not at increased risk of recurrence (except in a rare case of gonadal mosaicism), those with balanced structural rearrangements are. The specific risk varies according to the type of rearrangement and the chromosomes involved.

OTHER CHROMOSOME ABNORMALITIES

FRAGILE X SYNDROME

Fragile X syndrome, present in approximately 1:1000 males, accounts for 30–50% of cases of X-linked mental retardation. It is associated in a high proportion of gene carriers with a fragile site (a chromatin gap) on the long arm of the X chromosome (Xq27.3) (Figure 32–11). This fragile site is visible only when the tissue culture medium used for chromosome analysis is deficient in folate or thymidine. Thus, the laboratory performing chromosome analysis must be informed in advance that a fragile X study is desired. Even under optimal circumstances, the fragile site is not expressed in all cells. In affected males, 1–50% of cells are positive. In female carriers of the gene, the fragile site is usually expressed in a low percentage of cells. Furthermore, approximately 40% of carrier females and 20% of males who carry the gene do not express the fragile site at all.

Recently, direct DNA testing became available. The fragile X mental retardation-1 gene has been identified and named FMR-1. The gene was found to have unstable CGG repeats at the 5 end. Normal individuals have an up to 200-bp (base pair) fragment of cytidine phosphate guanosine dinucleotides. In asymptomatic carriers, this fragment is increased up to 500 bp (**premutation**) and in persons expressing the fragile X phenotype to over 600 bp (**full mutation**). Abnormal methylation of this region, found in the persons with full mutation, shuts off the expression of the adjacent genes. DNA analysis is more reliable in detecting fragile X than the cytogenetic study and should be used when fragile X is highly suspicious, especially in known fragile X families. However, in the case of isolated developmental delay or behavior problems, cytogenetic analysis is preferable as it may detect another chromosome abnormality.

Typically, the majority of males with fragile X syndrome present with mental retardation, oblong face with large ears, and large testicles, especially after puberty. Other physical signs include evidence of connective tissue disorder, eg, hyperextensible joints and mitral valve prolapse. The majority are hyperac-

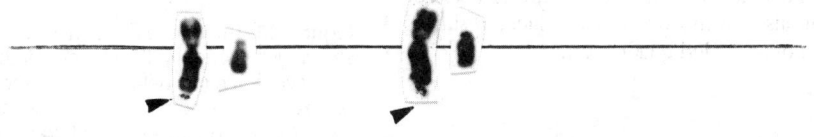

Figure 32–11. Partial karyotype showing fragile X and normal Y chromosomes. Arrow points to the fragile site.

tive and exhibit infantile autism or autistic-like be-havior. However, some males with the abnormal gene are of normal phenotype.

In contrast, only about one-third of females with the fragile X show some degree of mental retardation. Typical physical features and behavioral problems are also less common. There is a difference in the clinical expression of fragile X in male and female offspring depending on which parent is transmitting the gene. The premutation can change into the full mutation only when passed through a female. Persons with the premutation have minimal or no risk of retar-dation.

Genetic counseling in families with this disorder used to be difficult because the incomplete pene-trance of cytogenetic and clinical symptoms in both sexes precluded identification of all carriers of the gene. Identification of the abnormal DNA amplifica-tion by direct DNA analysis can detect nearly all asymptomatic gene carriers of both sexes. Therefore, it is a reliable text for prenatal and postnatal diagnosis of fragile X and facilitates genetic counseling.

SYNDROMES ASSOCIATED WITH CHROMOSOME FRAGILITY

It is well known that such environmental factors as exposure to radiation, certain chemicals, and viruses contribute to chromosome breaks and rearrange-ments. However, some well-defined autosomal re-cessive syndromes are associated with a greatly increased risk of chromosome aberrations. These in-clude **Bloom syndrome,** characterized by small stat-ure and development of telangiectasia upon exposure to sunlight; **Fanconi anemia,** frequently associated with a radial ray defect, pigmentary changes, hypo-gonadism, mild mental retardation, and development of pancytopenia; **ataxia telangiectasia** (Louis-Bar syndrome), characterized by telangiectasia of the skin and eyes, immunodeficiency, and progressive ataxia; **xeroderma pigmentosum,** resulting in the formation of skin lesions secondary to sun exposure; and **Wer-ner syndrome,** which is associated with premature senility.

The knowledge that specific chromosome aberra-tions are associated with these syndromes is fre-quently the basis for cytogenetic confirmation of their diagnosis. For example, Bloom syndrome is associated with an increased tendency to exchange segments between homologous chromosomes during mitosis; this tendency is called sister chromatid ex-change. In Fanconi anemia, translocations between nonhomologous chromosomes take place, resulting in formation of so-called quadriradii.

CONTIGUOUS GENE SYNDROMES

Syndromes are disorders with recognizable pat-terns of malformations. Some syndromes are caused by chromosome abnormalities; others, by single gene defects. In many syndromes, the cause is unknown. In some of these syndromes, which usually occur spo-radically but in uncommon instances are familial, high-resolution chromosome analysis can lead to the identification of small interstitial deletions. The dele-tion is visible under the microscope in the chromo-somes of some but not all affected individuals. It is postulated that the syndrome is caused by the absence of a cluster of genes located in the deleted segment. In some cases with normal karyotypes, the deletion is submicroscopic, subject to detection by FISH or DNA analysis. In other cases, other mechanisms in-terfere with the normal activity of the genes believed to be responsible for the syndrome. Uniparental dis-omy has been documented in some patients with Prader-Willi syndrome (short stature, obesity, hypo-gonadism, mental retardation), Angelman syndrome (happy puppet syndrome with mental retardation, in-appropriate laughter and hand flapping), Beckwith-Wiedemann syndrome (overgrowth, macroglossia, omphalocele, mental retardation) with normal high-

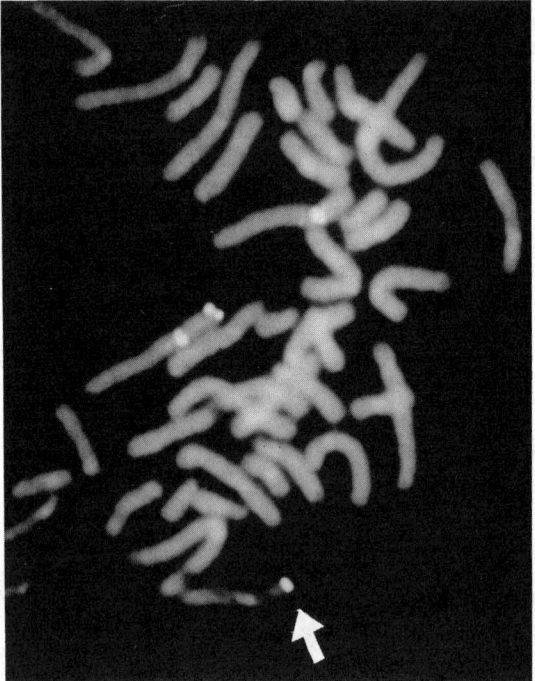

Figure 32–12. Fluorescent in situ hybridization (FISH) showing the brightly fluorescent probes of Wolf-Hirsch-horn syndrome (4p deletion syndrome). One probe is hy-bridized to the normal location on chromosome 4; the other (arrow) documents 4/11 translocation, which was not detectable by a classic cytogenetic analysis.

resolution chromosomes. Abnormal imprinting, caused by the uniparental origin of the responsible chromosome segment, is implicated in the etiology. (See the discussion on imprinting in the section on dysmorphology.) The group of genes causing the syndrome are related only through their linear placement on the same chromosome segments and do not influence each others' functions directly (thus the term "contiguous gene syndrome"). Table 32–1 lists examples of the currently known contiguous gene syndromes and their associated chromosome abnormalities.

CHROMOSOME ABNORMALITIES IN CANCER

Numerical and structural chromosome abnormalities have been identified in numerous hematopoietic and solid tumor malignancies of individuals with otherwise normal chromosomes. The cytogenetic abnormalities have been categorized as follows: In **primary abnormalities,** their presence is necessary for initiation of the malignancy. (*Example:* 13q– in retinoblastoma.) **Secondary abnormalities** appear only after the malignancy has developed. (*Example:* Philadelphia chromosome, t[9;22][q34;q11], in acute and chronic myeloid leukemia.) **Cytogenetic noise** is the term used to denote a variety of random chromosome abnormalities.

The primary and secondary chromosome abnormalities are specific for particular malignancies and can be utilized for diagnosis or prognosis. For example, the presence of Philadelphia chromosome is a good prognostic sign in CML and indicates a poor prognosis in ALL. The sites of chromosome breaks coincide with the known loci of oncogenes and anti-oncogenes.

Clarke A: Genetic imprinting in clinical genetics. Development 1990, Suppl 131.

Emanuel BS: Molecular cytogenetics: Toward dissection of the contiguous gene syndrome. (Invited editorial.) Am J Hum Genet 1988;43:575.

Table 32–1. Currently recognized contiguous gene syndromes.

Syndrome	Abnormal Chromosome Segment
Prader-Willi syndrome	del 15q11
DiGeorge syndrome	del 22q11
Langer-Gideon syndrome	del 8q24
Miller-Dieker syndrome	del 17p13
Retinoblastoma/mental retardation	del 13q14
Beckwith-Wiedemann syndrome	del 11p15
Wilms tumor with aniridia, genitourinary malformations, and mental retardation	del 11p13

Hagerman RJ, Cronister-Silverman A (editors): Fragile X syndrome. Johns Hopkins Univ Press, 1991.

Hall JG: How imprinting is relevant to human disease. Development 1990, Suppl 141.

Kaneko N, Kawagoe S, Hiroi M: Turner's Syndrome: Review of the literature with reference to a successful pregnancy outcome. Gynecol Obstet Invest 1990;29:81.

Mittleman F, Heim S: Chromosome abnormalities in cancer. Cancer Detect Prev 1990;14:527.

Rooney DE, Czepulkowski BH (editors): *Human Cytogenetics: A Practical Approach.* Oxford Univ Press, New York, 1986.

Rousseau F et al: Direct diagnosis by DNA analysis of the fragile X syndrome of mental retardation. N Engl J Med 1991;325:1673.

Smith AN, Scott JA (editors): *Genetic Applications: A Health Perspective.* Learner Managed Designs, 1988.

Spence JE et al: Uniparental disomy as a mechanism for human genetic disease. Am J Hum Genet 1988;42:217.

Tkachuk DC et al: Clinical applications of fluorescence in situ hybridization. Genet Anal Tech Appl 1991;8:67.

Trask BJ: Fluorescence in situ hybridization: Applications in cytogenetics and gene mapping. Trends Genet 1991; 7:149.

II. PRINCIPLES OF RECOMBINANT DNA

The revolutionary progress made in molecular biology during the past 2 decades has led to the development of recombinant DNA methods, which have greatly advanced our understanding of the structure and function of human genes. The recombinant DNA technology has major implications for all medical disciplines and especially for human genetics, since it allows location of genes on chromosomes, isolation and characterization of genes, and determination of DNA sequences and encoded protein sequences.

The development of recombinant DNA technology was based on the discovery of bacterial enzymes **(restriction enzymes).** These endonucleases cleave DNA at sites specific for each enzyme. Each restriction endonuclease recognizes a specific nucleotide sequence consisting of four, six, eight, or ten nucleotides and cleaves DNA within that sequence, thus producing DNA fragments. A difference in DNA sequence caused by a normal variation of DNA or by a gene mutation either produces or eliminates an endonuclease recognition site, resulting in a DNA fragment of a different size. Thus, the number and arrangement of restriction sites (called a "restriction map") are characteristic of a given DNA sequence. Mapping of DNA serves three purposes: (1) it is a signature, since each sequence has a unique map; (2) it is an aid to manipulation, such as subcloning and restriction fragment length polymorphism (RFLP) analysis; and (3) it is a prelude to nucleotide sequencing. Before a DNA fragment of interest can be analyzed, multiple copies of it must be produced. This can be achieved by incorporating the human DNA fragment into a **vector,** ie, a DNA segment containing the means of replication and selection in bacteria. The vector-containing human DNA insert is replicated, thus producing multiple copies of the segment of interest. The source of inserts can be **genomic DNA,** obtained directly from the cleaving of the target organism, or **complementary DNA** (cDNA), obtained by copying messenger RNA (mRNA) into DNA by reverse transcription.

A **genomic library** can be constructed by randomly fragmenting human genomic DNA with restriction enzymes and then inserting the fragments into a vector. Such a library contains large numbers of different DNA sequences. Some of these specific DNA fragments are used to manufacture human proteins (eg, insulin, growth hormone, interferon, and blood clotting factors) for pharmacologic applications; others are used as **probes,** which may be thought of as DNA segment-specific, radioactively labeled reagents for mapping and diagnosis.

Molecular genetics is most commonly used to look for changes in genomic DNA detected by Southern blot analysis, but a similar technique of Northern blot analysis is being used increasingly to look for mRNA abnormalities. **Southern blot analysis** (Figure 32–13) relies on the use of restriction endonucleases to cleave human genomic DNA at specific nucleotide sequences and to produce DNA fragments of different lengths. These DNA fragments are then separated by agarose gel electrophoresis, transferred to a membrane, and overlaid with a radioactive probe, which hybridizes only with a fragment having complementary DNA. This fragment is identified by autoradiography, and its size is determined.

In recent years, a gene amplification technique called **polymerase chain reaction** (PCR) has been developed. This technique is having a tremendous effect on the use of DNA probes in diagnosis, because it is simpler and less time-consuming than older methods. PCR substantially increases the amount of DNA sequence to be analyzed by easy enzymatic synthesis of 100,000–1,000,000 copies of the original DNA segment in a short time. Oligonucleotides, which usually consist of 120 bases and are complementary to the DNA flanking the target segment, are synthesized and used to prime DNA synthesis by DNA polymerase. Each cycle, consisting of denaturation of genomic DNA, primer annealing, and polymerase extension, produces new DNA strands complementary to the target DNA. During each cycle, the amount of amplified DNA doubles, accumulating rapidly in an exponential fashion. After 20 cycles, the DNA is amplified a millionfold.

The amplified DNA can be labeled with **synthetic oligonucleotide probes.** DNA sequence variation

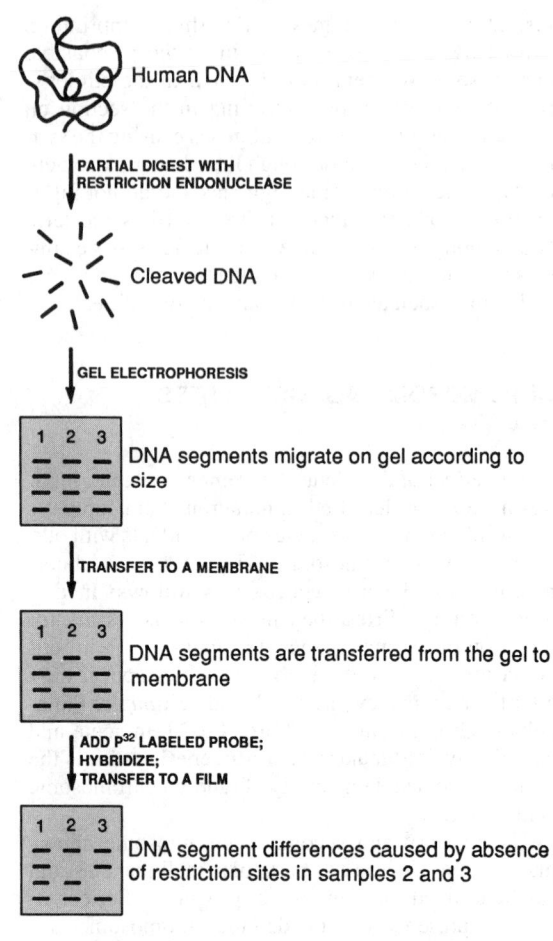

Human DNA

PARTIAL DIGEST WITH
RESTRICTION ENDONUCLEASE

Cleaved DNA

GEL ELECTROPHORESIS

1 2 3

DNA segments migrate on gel according to size

TRANSFER TO A MEMBRANE

1 2 3

DNA segments are transferred from the gel to membrane

ADD P32 LABELED PROBE;
HYBRIDIZE;
TRANSFER TO A FILM

1 2 3

DNA segment differences caused by absence of restriction sites in samples 2 and 3

Figure 32–13. Diagram of Southern blot.

can be analyzed in a crude cell lysate of less than 100 cells in a dot blot format. This method, therefore, eliminates the need for DNA purification, gel electrophoresis, and the use of radioactive probes. It can be performed on a small DNA sample in a short time. The disadvantage is that a small contamination with a foreign DNA can result in an incorrect diagnosis.

APPLICATION OF RECOMBINANT DNA TECHNOLOGIES IN CLINICAL GENETICS

GENETIC DIAGNOSIS

Genetic diagnosis can be performed by direct detection of a mutant gene or by indirect methods.

Direct detection of an abnormal gene is possible

only when the nature of the mutation is known. If the abnormal gene has a partial deletion, insertion, or rearrangement, restriction endonuclease analysis with the Southern blot technique is used. Cloned DNA fragments of the gene are used as molecular probes to label the gene, demonstrating the altered size of the gene in comparison with a normal control. Gene deletions have been found in α- and β-thalassemia, antithrombin III deficiency, congenital adrenal hyperplasia secondary to 21-hydroxylase deficiency, Duchenne muscular dystrophy, hemophilia A and B, Lesch-Nyhan syndrome, ornithine transcarbamoylase deficiency, neurofibromatosis, and other disorders.

An abnormal gene with a point mutation can be diagnosed by restriction analysis if the mutation either created or abolished a restriction recognition site, but a restriction recognition site is created or abolished in only 5–10% of point mutations. In the remainder, PCR can be used for DNA amplification, and the mutation can be documented by a mutant-specific oligonucleotide probe, which recognizes the mutant but not the normal alleles. In addition to point mutations, deletions, and insertions, a new phenomenon called **unstable expansion of trinucleotide repeats** was found to be responsible for human gene mutations. These repeats were found to be CGG in fragile X syndrome, CTG in myotonic dystrophy (autosomal dominant), and CAG in both Huntington disease (autosomal dominant) and spinobulbar muscular atrophy (Kennedy disease, X-linked). The repeats are found in the 3′ or 5′ region of the genes, and their size varies within the normal population. Mutations result in the increase in the number of repeats; the number of repeats frequently corresponds with the severity of the disorder. The tendency of the repeats to increase in number in each successive generation is the molecular basis for so called anticipation, ie, increased severity of the disorder in successive generations.

The advantage of a diagnostic study employing the direct detection of the mutant gene is that it requires the affected individual only and it need not involve other family members.

Indirect detection of abnormal genes is used (1) when the gene is known but there is extensive heterogeneity of the molecular defect between families, and (2) when the gene responsible for a disease is unknown but its chromosome location is known. In the former situation—the gene is known—it is not always necessary to know the exact molecular defect to determine the presence of the gene. It is, however, necessary to mark and trace the inheritance of the abnormal gene. This can be done on the basis of intragenic DNA polymorphism, which is characterized by the addition or removal of a restriction site and is thus identifiable by restriction fragment length polymorphism (RFLP) analysis. This DNA polymorphism, although it is intragenic, is not the mutation that causes the disorder—it simply marks and helps to differentiate the abnormal gene from the normal one. RFLP

cannot be used, however, unless both parents of the tested individual are heterozygous. Thus, a family study is necessary to determine the haplotypes of the chromosomes with and without the mutant gene. However, crossover and recombination are not a problem, because the polymorphism is intragenic or in very close proximity to the gene. Examples of disorders that can be screened by this method are phenylketonuria, hemophilia, β-thalassemia, and Fabry disease.

The latter situation—the abnormal gene is unknown—exists in the majority of single gene disorders. In this case, linkage analysis using a large number of DNA polymorphic markers may reveal a close link between one or more such markers and the presence of the clinical disorder. Such a linkage study localizes the gene of interest to a specific chromosome or to a specific region of a chromosome. Once the location of the gene is known, the same technique (using probes known to be linked to the gene locus of interest) can be used to trace the presence or absence of the gene through the family. This method assumes that the two loci—the locus of the gene and the locus of the DNA polymorphism used to mark the gene—are so close that they will not segregate independently but will be transmitted together. The presence of the marker, therefore, is a reliable indication of the presence of the gene of interest. Thus, the distance between the two loci is of utmost importance in determining the reliability of any linkage analysis, because crossing over and recombination between the gene and the marker during meiosis will result in an error in the diagnosis. To minimize the errors, multiple linked markers should be used in linkage analysis of any gene.

DETECTION OF GENETIC HETEROGENEITY

Genetic heterogeneity is occasionally suspected on the basis of clinical variability. In other instances, there is no clinical clue. For example, enzyme deficiencies may be caused by a number of different mutations, such as an abnormal active site in one case and an abnormal coenzyme in another. Alternatively, the phenotype may be caused in different families by different enzyme defects. Such heterogeneity cannot be suspected on a clinical basis; however, it can be detected using DNA technology.

PREVENTION

Recombinant DNA technology has the potential to prevent genetic disease by facilitating the detection of carriers of defective genes and permitting prenatal diagnosis. Family studies can also clarify the mode of inheritance, thus allowing more accurate determination of recurrence risks and appropriate options. For example, differentiation of a gonadal mosaicism from decreased penetrance of a dominant gene has important implications for genetic counseling.

In the past, the diagnosis of a genetic disease characterized by a late onset of symptoms, eg, Huntington disease, could not be made prior to the appearance of clinical symptoms. In some inborn errors of metabolism, diagnostic tests (eg, measurement of enzyme activities) could be conducted only on inaccessible tissues. Gene identification techniques can enormously enhance our ability to diagnose symptomatic and presymptomatic individuals, conduct prenatal diagnosis, and detect heterozygous carriers.

TREATMENT

Recombinant DNA technology could facilitate treatment in the following ways:

(1) By production of large amounts of therapeutic agents, eg, growth hormone and interferon, which are present naturally in small quantities and are therefore very expensive. This is already being done.

(2) By gene therapy—the introduction of a normal gene into an individual affected with a serious inherited disorder. In principle, genes could be introduced either during embryonic life (germ line therapy), in which case the gene could be transmitted to future generations; or the gene could be introduced only into somatic cells (somatic therapy), in which case it would be present only during the life of the recipient. Gene therapy through bone marrow transplantation thus far has been done experimentally on two patients with severe combined immunodeficiency and one patient with the nonneurologic form of Gaucher's disease.

Antonarakis SE: Diagnosis of genetic disorders at the DNA level. N Engl J Med 1989;320:153.
Mandel JL: Questions of expansion. Nature Genet 1993;4:8.
Nelson DL: Fragile X syndrome: Review and current status. Growth Genet Horm 1993;9:1.

III. MENDELIAN GENETICS

SINGLE GENE DEFECTS

A **gene** is the unit of inheritance that determines the genetic makeup of an individual. Genes occur in pairs at a single locus or site on specific chromosomes. These paired genes, called **alleles,** determine the genotype of an individual at that locus. If the genes at a specific locus are identical, the individual is **homozygous;** if they are different, **heterozygous.** During normal meiosis, these alleles separate, one going to each of the two gametes. An understanding of this process is necessary for an understanding of single gene inheritance.

Disorders due to an abnormality in a single gene are either autosomal or X-linked, depending upon the location of the gene on an autosome in the former and on the X chromosome in the latter. If the abnormality is present when the defective gene is in either the heterozygous or the homozygous state, it is dominantly inherited. If, however, it is present only when the gene involved is in the homozygous state, the disorder is recessively inherited.

AUTOSOMAL DOMINANT INHERITANCE

Autosomal dominant inheritance (AD) has the following characteristics:

(1) Individuals in the same family may show very different manifestations of the same disorder. This phenomenon is called **variable expressivity.** Typically, at least some persons who carry the gene are mildly affected, because an individual must be healthy enough and fertile enough to reproduce and pass on the trait. In some disorders, such as Huntington disease, manifestations do not appear until after the child-bearing years. In others, which tend to be more severe (eg, achondroplasia), there is a high mutation rate.

(2) Some persons who are obligatory carriers of the gene (ie, both their parent and their child are affected) may have no apparent manifestations. This phenomenon is called **nonpenetrance,** and the penetrance rate varies for each dominantly inherited condition.

(3) Males and females are equally affected, though the manifestations may vary according to sex. For example, baldness is a dominant trait but affects only males. In this case, the trait is said to be **sex-limited.** Both males and females can pass on the abnormality to children of either sex.

(4) Dominant inheritance is typically said to be "vertical," ie, the condition passes from one generation to the next in a vertical fashion (Figure 32–14).

(5) In some cases, the family history seems to be completely negative, and the affected individual appears to be the first abnormal case. This spontaneous appearance may be caused by a point mutation or a change in the structure of a specific gene. Such a change may be a deletion, a duplication, or an amino acid substitution. The mutation rate varies with each

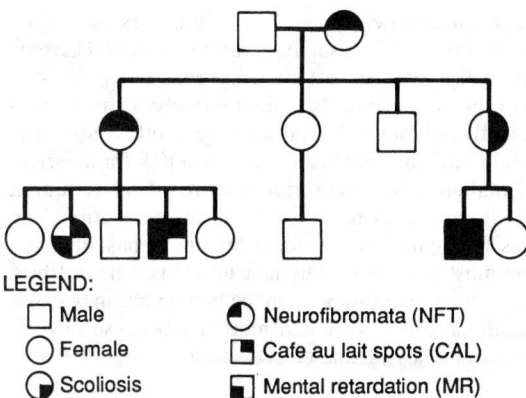

LEGEND:

☐	Male	◖ NFT symbol	Neurofibromata (NFT)
◯	Female	◨	Cafe au lait spots (CAL)
◒	Scoliosis	◪	Mental retardation (MR)

Figure 32–14. Autosomal dominant inheritance: Neurofibromatosis, showing variable expressivity.

---

dominant condition, and in some cases the mutation rate increases with advancing paternal age. There are, however, several other possible explanations for a negative family history:

(a) Nonpaternity.

(b) Decreased penetrance or mild manifestations in one of the parents. For this reason, both parents must be carefully examined and a thorough family history taken.

(c) Germ cell mosaicism. In rare cases, there may be mosaicism in the germ cell line of either parent, in which case the risk of recurrence increases. This is a proposed explanation for cases in which two children of completely normal parents are affected with a dominant condition. The best example of this is osteogenesis imperfecta. Earlier it was thought that there were two forms of the disorder—one autosomal dominant, milder and later in onset; and one autosomal recessive, perinatal in onset and severe (often lethal). The latter was felt to be recessive because of affected siblings born to clinically normal parents. However, newer studies have shown that only one of the paired collagen genes is abnormal in the severe form instead of two, as would be expected in a recessive disease. Recurrent cases, therefore, must be due to germ cell mosaicism and indeed, prenatal diagnosis has shown that the actual recurrence risk in this form of osteogenesis imperfecta is 7%.

It is not known how common germ cell mosaicism is, but it has been described in two X-linked disorders as well (Duchenne muscular dystrophy and hemophilia A). The incidence of germ cell mosaicism may depend upon many factors which are just beginning to be understood.

(d) The possibility that the abnormality is not truly an autosomal dominant condition. It may be a phenocopy, ie, a nongenetic condition that mimics a certain genotype, or it may be a similar but genetically different abnormality with a different mode of inheritance.

(6) As a general rule, dominant conditions are not

due to enzyme defects, since most biochemical defects are substrate-limited rather than enzyme-limited. Therefore, enzyme levels at 50% of the normal value are sufficient for normal function. There are exceptions, eg, acute intermittent porphyria. Dominant traits are more often related to structural abnormalities of protein, eg, as in the Marfan syndrome.

(7) The risk of any offspring carrying an abnormal dominant gene is 50%, or 1:2 for each pregnancy. This is true whether the gene is penetrant or not, and the severity in the offspring is not related to the severity in the affected parent but may be related to the sex of the parent transmitting the gene. For example, if the gene for myotonic dystrophy is passed through the mother, there is a 10–20% chance that the child (regardless of sex) may have a severe congenital form of the disease. Conversely, if the gene for Huntington disease is passed through the father, there is a 5–10% possibility that the offspring may have the severe, rigid juvenile form. This is independent of the severity of the condition in the transmitting parent. It has been attributed to imprinting, though we know in these two conditions that it is associated with an expansion of the repeat segment that causes the disease in question. There are certainly other mechanisms of imprinting in other conditions. If an abnormality represents a new mutation of a dominant trait, the parents of the affected individual run a low risk during subsequent pregnancies, but the risk for the offspring of the affected individual is 50%.

(8) Options available for future pregnancies include prenatal diagnosis in an increasing number of cases and artificial insemination or egg donation, depending upon which parent carries the abnormal gene.

NEUROFIBROMATOSIS

Essentials of Diagnosis (Neurofibromatosis 1)

Two or more of the following:

- Six or more café au lait macules, > 15 mm in diameter in postpubertal and > 5 mm in prepubertal individuals.
- Two or more neurofibromas of any type or one plexiform neurofibroma.
- Axillary or inguinal freckling.
- Two or more Lisch nodules (iris hamartomas).
- Distinctive bony lesions such as sphenoid dysplasia or pseudarthrosis.
- An affected first-degree relative.

General Considerations

Neurofibromatosis is one of the most common autosomal dominant disorders, occurring in 1:4000–1:3000 births and seen in all races and ethnic groups. It has a wide range of variability and can present in many ways. In general, however, the disorder is progressive, and new manifestations appear over time. There are at least two types of neurofibromatosis: Neurofibromatosis 1 is characterized by multiple skin findings; and neurofibromatosis 2 is characterized by bilateral acoustic neuromas, with minimal or no skin manifestations. A third category includes all of the atypical forms. Because neurofibromatosis 2 is less common and rarely presents before late adolescence, this discussion is limited to type 1.

Clinical Findings

Café au lait macules may be present at birth or may appear shortly thereafter, and most are apparent by 1 year of age. The typical skin lesion is 10–30 mm, ovoid, and smooth-bordered, but there is great variation. Neurofibromas are benign tumors consisting of Schwann cells, nerve fibers, and fibroblasts; they may be discrete or plexiform. Discrete tumors are more common and can occur at any age. They are well demarcated and can present in cutaneous, subcutaneous, or internal tissues. Plexiform neurofibromas are more diffuse and can invade normal tissue. They are congenital and are frequently detected during periods of rapid growth. If the face or a limb is involved, there may be associated hypertrophy or overgrowth. The incidence of Lisch nodules, which can be seen with a slitlamp, also increases with age. Common features of affected individuals include a large head (although only a small percentage have true hydrocephalus), bony abnormalities on x-ray studies, scoliosis, and a wide spectrum of developmental problems ranging from learning disabilities to true mental retardation. The most common problems in childhood are secondary to plexiform neurofibromas and learning disabilities. While the average IQ is within the normal range, it is lower than in unaffected family members. The learning problem seems to be quite specific and involves a visual-perceptual disability that could lead to difficulties in reading and writing or to behavioral impulsivity.

Differential Diagnosis

Areas of hyperpigmentation can be seen in other conditions (eg, the Albright, Noonan, and LEOPARD syndromes), but the lesions are either single or different in character. Isolated neurofibromas and familial café au lait spots (fewer than six and with no other manifestations of neurofibromatosis) have been described. The relationship of such cases to classic neurofibromatosis 1 is uncertain.

Complications

It is difficult to differentiate a complication from a rare manifestation of the underlying disorder. Seen in less than 25% of persons with neurofibromatosis are seizures, optic glioma, deafness, constipation, short stature, early puberty, and hypertension. Optic glioma seems to occur in about 15% of individuals with neurofibromatosis 1. While the tumor may be apparent at an early age, it rarely causes functional problems and is usually nonprogressive. There is some disagreement as to whether central nervous system imaging should be done routinely on an asymptomatic individual, but close clinical follow-up is certainly critical. There is an increased risk for a variety of malignancies. Neurofibrosarcoma is a rare tumor, but it may occur in up to 5% of this population. The risk for malignancy is about 5% above baseline, and the most common malignant tumor is a neurofibrosarcoma. Other tumors may be benign but may cause significant morbidity and mortality because of their location in a vital and closed space.

Treatment

Appropriate therapy should be initiated as each new manifestation arises. Neurofibromas can be removed, but removal is of limited help if they are multiple or in a vital area. The most important part of therapy is close, ongoing follow-up. Because this disorder is progressive, affected individuals should be seen at regular intervals and have regular eye examinations, hearing tests, and developmental screening, as well as other evaluations (eg, CT scans) as indicated.

Prognosis

Because there is such variability in neurofibromatosis, it is difficult to assess the prognosis. However, most affected persons have only skin lesions and few other problems. Severely affected individuals are rare in the pediatric age range, and close follow-up and early intervention may ameliorate some complications.

Genetic Counseling

The gene for neurofibromatosis-1 was localized to the long arm of chromosome 17 in 1987 and partially cloned in 1990. It is very long and actually includes three other "nested genes" whose significance is unknown. About 80% of the gene has been cloned at this time. It seems to code for a protein similar to a tumor suppressor factor. There are a variety of mutations in the gene for neurofibromatosis, including substitutions, deletions, and additions. In only 20% of the cases can the specific deletion be identified, most often when the Noonan phenotype coexists with neurofibromatosis. Fortunately, there are numerous informative, flanking DNA probes that can be used in a high percentage of families for linkage analysis to identify those carrying the gene, including affected fetuses through prenatal diagnosis.

Between 30% and 50% of all cases of neurofibromatosis are felt to be due to new mutations. Before attributing an individual case to a new mutation, however, both parents must be carefully evaluated, including a thorough examination of the skin and slitlamp examination to look for Lisch nodules. Recent evidence suggests that penetrance is quite high if individuals are carefully examined.

AUTOSOMAL RECESSIVE INHERITANCE

Autosomal recessive inheritance also has some distinctive characteristics:

(1) There is less variability among affected persons. Parents are carriers and are clinically normal. (There are exceptions to this rule, however. For example, sickle cell disease is considered recessive. Under normal circumstances, carriers—those with the sickle cell trait—are normal but may become symptomatic if they become hypoxic.)

(2) Both males and females are affected equally.

(3) Inheritance is horizontal; siblings may be affected, but both parents are normal (Figure 32–15).

(4) Recessive conditions are frequently rare; the rarer the condition, the more likely there is to be consanguinity. Conversely, if a child whose parents are related presents with an unrecognized abnormality, a recessive condition is likely.

(5) A negative family history is not unusual. In common conditions such as cystic fibrosis, there may be an affected second- or third-degree relative, but usually not. Because parents are clinically normal even though they are carriers, one must not be lulled into a false sense of security by the negative family history.

(6) Recessive conditions are frequently associated with enzyme defects. (See Chapter 28.)

(7) The recurrence risk is 25%, or 1:4 for each pregnancy. When there is a new partner, however, the risk drops and can be recalculated on the basis of the gene frequency in the population.

(8) In rare instances, a child with a recessive disorder and a normal karyotype may have inherited both copies of the abnormal gene from one parent and none from the other. This **uniparental disomy** (see p 910) was first described in a girl with cystic fibrosis and growth retardation. This phenomenon is of unknown frequency, but it is more likely to be present in a child with several autosomal recessive conditions or one who has some unexpected and seemingly unrelated abnormalities. Molecular testing can confirm the presence of uniparental disomy. The recurrence risk is obviously lower in such a situation, though it is not known what factors predispose to uniparental disomy.

(9) Options available for future pregnancies include prenatal diagnosis in many cases and artificial insemination.

CYSTIC FIBROSIS

The gene for cystic fibrosis is one of the most common abnormal genes in the Caucasian population. Approximately 1:22 persons is a carrier. Before 1980, there was no reliable prenatal diagnostic technique, and the risk of having a second affected child (25%) could not be reduced. Since that time, the accumulation of knowledge about this disease has been remarkable. In 1985, the cystic fibrosis gene was located on the long arm of chromosome 7, and numerous DNA probes have been identified that detect restriction fragment length polymorphisms (RFLP) tightly linked to the gene. At about the same time, it was noted that certain DNA polymorphisms with particular alleles were frequently associated with the cystic fibrosis gene, a phenomenon known as linkage disequilibrium. The combination of these tests greatly improved carrier detection and prenatal diagnosis. In 1989, the gene for cystic fibrosis was cloned, and it was discovered that a three-base deletion coding for phenylalanine was present in the majority of cases. Subsequent studies have shown that the incidence of this delta F508 mutation varies with ethnic background and is present in about 75% of patients in North America and the United Kingdom, 50% in Spain, 43% in Italy, and 30% of individuals with Ashkenazic ethnic backgrounds. This gene is called the cystic fibrosis transmembrane conductance regulator (CFTR), which codes for a protein that functions as a chloride channel important in secreting chloride from the cell. It has been shown that the introduction of

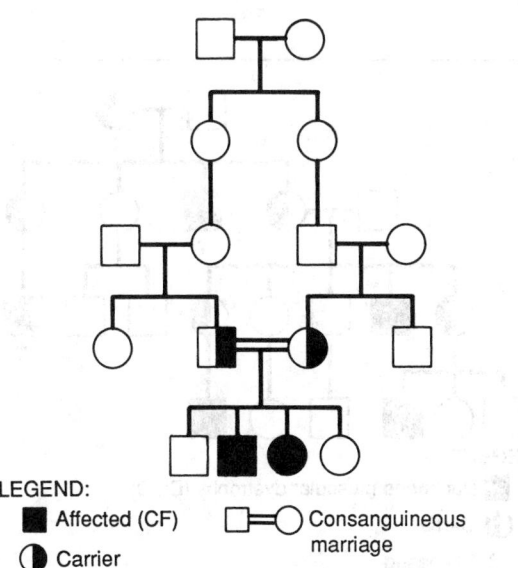

LEGEND:
■ Affected (CF)   ▭═○ Consanguineous marriage
◑ Carrier

Figure 32–15. Autosomal recessive inheritance: Cystic fibrosis.

normal CFTR into cells with the cystic fibrosis gene will correct the biologic abnormality, raising the possibility of gene therapy. Trials are beginning in which the gene will be attached to a vector and delivered to the respiratory epithelium via an aerosol. This therapy is directed at somatic cells and will in no way affect the cystic fibrosis gene in germ cells. While many unanswered questions remain, gene therapy for cystic fibrosis has exciting promise.

Cloning of the gene for cystic fibrosis and identification of the mutation in the majority of cases have completely changed genetic counseling and prenatal diagnosis for this disorder. Today, the affected child is studied using polymerase chain reaction (PCR) techniques to search for an identifiable mutation. If this is found, carriers can be identified and specific prenatal diagnosis performed, identifying both carriers and affected fetuses. If a mutation cannot be identified, then linkage analysis, DNA haplotyping, and amniotic fluid enzyme studies can be done. With continuing research, more mutations are being identified, but linkage analysis available today can achieve 90–99% accuracy.

The identification of the mutation in the cystic fibrosis gene has also raised the issue of mass screening because of the high frequency of this gene in the Caucasian population. While screening is definitely indicated in families with an affected member, mass population screening has not been recommended. Since all of the mutations have not yet been identified, a significant number of "negative" individuals would still carry a gene for cystic fibrosis. While a specific risk could be calculated for each couple, the high false-negative rate and the counseling required for each couple tested make the value and cost effectiveness of mass screening questionable at this time.

X-LINKED INHERITANCE

When a gene for a specific disorder is on the X chromosome, the condition is said to be X-linked, or sex-linked. Females may be either homozygous or heterozygous, since they have two X chromosomes. Males, by contrast, have only one, and an affected male is said to be hemizygous. The severity of any disorder is more consistent in males than in females (within a specific family). According to the Lyon hypothesis, since one of the two X chromosomes is inactivated and since this inactivation is random, the clinical picture in females depends on the percentage of mutant versus normal alleles inactivated. The X chromosome is not inactivated until about 14 days of gestation, and parts of the short arm remain active throughout life.

X-LINKED RECESSIVE INHERITANCE

The following features are characteristic of X-linked recessive inheritance:

(1) Males are affected, and heterozygous females are either normal or have mild manifestations.

(2) Inheritance is "diagonal" through the maternal side of the family (Figure 32–16).

(3) A female carrier has a 50% chance of having carrier daughters and a 50% chance of having affected sons.

(4) All of the daughters of an affected male are carriers, and none of his sons are affected. Since a father can give only his Y chromosome to his sons, male-to-male transmission excludes X-linked inheritance except in the rare case of uniparental disomy, where a son receives both the X and the Y from his father.

(5) The mutation rate is high in some X-linked disorders, particularly when the affected male is infertile. In such instances, the mutation is felt to occur in the propositus in one-third of cases, in the mother in one-third of cases, and in earlier generations in one-third of cases. For this reason, genetic counseling may be difficult in families with an isolated case.

(6) On rare occasions, a female may be fully affected. Several possible mechanisms may account for a fully affected female: (a) unfavorable lyonization, (b) 45,X karyotype, (c) homozygosity in the female, (d) an X-autosome translocation in which the X chromosome of normal structure is preferentially inactivated, and (e) uniparental disomy.

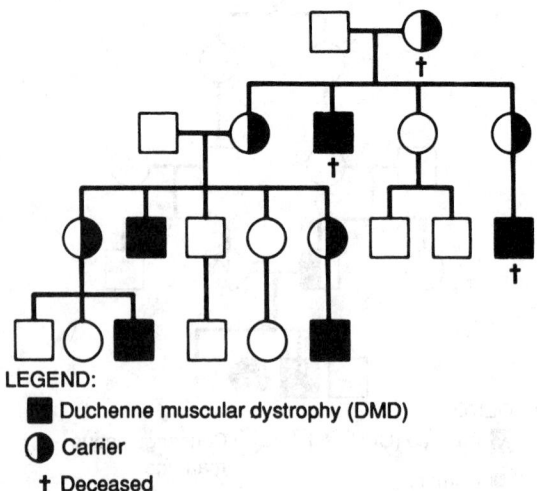

LEGEND:

◼ Duchenne muscular dystrophy (DMD)

◖ Carrier

† Deceased

Figure 32–16. X-linked recessive inheritance: Duchenne type muscular dystrophy.

DUCHENNE TYPE MUSCULAR DYSTROPHY

Duchenne type muscular dystrophy has been recognized as an X-linked recessive condition for many years. There is also a milder type, Becker muscular dystrophy, which is allelic. The gene, now known to be in band Xp21, is one of the largest genes in the human genome, which may explain its high mutation rate. About 60–65% of families have a deletion in the gene. In rare cases, this may be visible on cytogenetic analysis, but molecular studies are usually required. Because of the length of the gene, there are many available informative restriction fragment length polymorphisms (RFLP) both flanking and within the gene itself.This gene has been shown to encode mRNA for a protein called dystrophin, which is localized to the muscle surface membrane, the sarcolemma. Males with low or undetectable levels of dystrophin have Duchenne type muscular dystrophy, whereas those with nearly normal levels but dystrophin of an abnormal size have Becker muscular dystrophy. In addition to general supportive care, many children with Duchenne type muscular dystrophy are now being treated with prednisone. This is started when weakness becomes a functional problem and continued indefinitely or until complications require discontinuation. The exact mechanism of action is not understood, but the prednisone seems to delay the progression of the disease and may even result in improved strength. Because of the very significant side effects of long-term steroid therapy, all children should be treated as part of a protocol and closely monitored.

In the past, carrier detection has depended upon such nonspecific tests as serum creatine kinase, but newer molecular techniques have markedly improved the accuracy of this prediction. If a deletion is present, it is usually apparent in the female carrier as well, using gene dosage studies. If there is no deletion, linkage studies, combined with CK levels, help to predict female carriers in informative families with a high degree of probability. Negative studies in the mother, however, do not guarantee a negligible risk because of germ cell mosaicism. This may be present in 20–25% of the women, giving an actual recurrence risk of about 5–7% even with negative studies. Both deletion testing and linkage studies can be used to identify an affected fetus.

X-LINKED DOMINANT INHERITANCE

The X-linked dominant inheritance pattern is much less common than the X-linked recessive type. Examples include incontinentia pigmenti and hypophosphatemic or vitamin D-resistant rickets.

(1) The heterozygous female is symptomatic, and the disease is twice as common in females because they have two X chromosomes that can be affected.

(2) Clinical manifestations are more variable in females than in males.

(3) The risk for the offspring of heterozygous females is 50% regardless of sex.

(4) All of the daughters but none of the sons of affected males will have the disorder.

(5) Although a homozygous female is possible (particularly in an inbred population), she would be severely involved. All of her children would also be affected, but more mildly.

(6) Some disorders (eg, incontinentia pigmenti) are lethal in males (and in homozygous females). Affected women have twice as many daughters as sons and an increased incidence of miscarriages, because all affected males will be spontaneously aborted.

For more complete information about specific single gene defects, see the McKusick 1992 reference cited at the end of this chapter.

MITOCHONDRIAL INHERITANCE

Some unusual disorders seem to be transmitted only by female members of a family and affect a high proportion of offspring, both male and female. Examples include Leber hereditary optic neuropathy, Leigh disease, MELAS (mitochondrial encephalomyopathy, lactic acidosis, and stroke-like episodes), and MERRF (myoclonic epilepsy and ragged red fibers). It is now known that these diseases are due to mutations in mitochondrial DNA (mtDNA). Mitochondrial DNA is double-stranded, circular, and smaller than nuclear DNA and is found in the cytoplasm. It codes for enzymes involved in oxidative phosphorylation, which generates ATP.

There are several characteristics of mitochondrial disorders:

(1) All mitochondrial disorders show remarkable phenotypic variability.

(2) They are maternally inherited, since only the egg has any cytoplasmic material.

(3) All cells are heteroplasmic—ie, all cells contain both normal and mutated or abnormal mtDNA. The proportion of normal to abnormal mtDNA seems to determine the severity of the disease and the age at onset in most cases.

(4) Those tissues with the highest ATP requirements—specifically, central nervous system and skeletal muscle—seem to be most susceptible to mutations in mtDNA.

(5) There is an increase in somatic cell mtDNA mutations and a decline in oxidative phosphorylation

function with age. This explains the later onset of some of these disorders and may indeed be a clue to the whole aging process.

POLYGENIC DISEASE (Multifactorial Inheritance)

The inheritance of many common traits and abnormalities does not seem to be due to a single gene. In the past, multiple genes, each with a small effect, as well as a variety of environmental factors were felt to be important, and the terms polygenic and multifactorial inheritance have been used. It is now felt that there may be a smaller number of genes involved, with one or more major genes important in each condition. The terms oligogenic or multilocus have been used to denote this more limited concept. Inherited in this way are a variety of normal traits, eg, height, intelligence, and dermal ridge counts, as well as a variety of common abnormalities, eg, hypertension and allergies. It is important to realize that many of these conditions do not have a single cause and represent genetic heterogeneity or a group of diseases with common manifestations and different causes. In some conditions, there is an association with certain HLA types. For example, there is a high correlation between ankylosing spondylitis and HLA-B27. It is important to understand the difference between an association such as this and linkage of a certain disease with the HLA locus. In the latter instance, the gene for the disease is on chromosome 6, close to the HLA locus, but there is no association with a specific HLA type. Although the concept of polygenic inheritance has been questioned, many of the principles still hold true. The actual recurrence risks remain the same unless a broad category (such as coronary artery disease or diabetes) can be subdivided and the consultand identified as being in a higher or lower risk group. For these reasons, the earlier terminology will be used in this section.

Many common congenital abnormalities, eg, cleft lip and palate, neural tube defects, and some kinds of congenital heart disease, are inherited in a polygenic manner. If the combination of predisposing genes from both parents and certain environmental factors (mostly unknown) exceeds the "threshold," the abnormality then becomes manifest. Twin studies have been helpful in determining the relative importance of genetic versus environmental factors. If genetic factors are of little or no importance, then the concordance between monozygotic and dizygotic twins should be the same. (Dizygotic twins are no more genetically similar to each other than to other siblings.) If an abnormality is completely genetic, the concor-

dance between identical twins should be 100%. Most polygenic conditions are associated with concordance rates somewhere in between.

Polygenic or multifactorial inheritance has some distinctive characteristics:

(1) The risk for relatives of affected persons is increased, and the risk is higher for first-degree relatives (those who have 50% of their genes in common) and lower for more distant relations, although the risk for the latter is higher than for the general population (Table 32–2).

(2) The recurrence risk varies with the number of affected family members. For example, after one child is born with a neural tube defect, the recurrence risk is 2–3%. If a second affected child is born, the risk increases to 10–12%. This is in contrast to single gene disorders, where the risk is the same no matter how many family members are affected.

Table 32–2. Empiric risks for some congenital disorders.

Mental deficiency of unknown cause: Incidence 3:1000
  Risks for siblings
    Both parents normal: 5–13% retarded
    One parent retarded: 20% retarded
    Both parents retarded: 42% retarded
Anencephaly and spina bifida: Incidence (average) 1:1000
    One affected child: 2–3%
    Two affected children: 10–12%
    One affected parent: 2–3%
Hydrocephalus: Incidence 1:2000 newborns
    Occasional X-linked recessive
    Often associated with neural tube defect
    Some environmental etiologies, eg, toxoplasmosis
    Recurrence risk, one affected child
      Hydrocephalus: 1%
      Some CNS abnormality: 3%
Cleft Lip and/or palate: Incidence (average) 1:1000
    One affected child: 2–4%
    One affected parent: 2–4%
    Two affected children: 10%
    One affected parent, one affected child: 10–20%
Cleft palate: Incidence 1:2000
    One affected child: 2%
    Two affected children: 6–8%
    One affected parent: 4–6%
    One affected parent, one affected child: 15–20%
Congenital heart disease: Incidence 8:1000
    One affected child: 2–3%
    One affected parent, one affected child: 10%
Clubfoot: Incidence 1:1000 (male:female = 2:1)
    One affected child: 2–3%
Congenital dislocated hip: Incidence 1:1000
    (female>male), with marked regional variation
    One child affected: 2–14%
Pyloric stenosis: Incidence, males: 1:200; females: 1:1000
    Male index patient
      Brothers   3.2%
      Sons   6.8%
      Sisters   3.0%
      Daughters   1.2%
    Female index patient
      Brothers   13.2%
      Sons   20.5%
      Sisters   2.5%
      Daughters   11.1%

(3) The risk is higher if the defect is more severe. In Hirschsprung disease, another polygenic condition, the longer the aganglionic segment, the higher the recurrence risk.

(4) Sex ratios may not be equal. If there is a marked discrepancy, the recurrence risk is higher if a child of the less commonly affected sex has the disorder. This assumes that more genetic factors are required to raise the more resistant sex above the threshold than to raise the less resistant sex. For example, pyloric stenosis is more common in males. If the first affected child is a female, the recurrence risk is higher than if the child is a male.

(5) The risk for the offspring of an affected person is approximately the same as the risk for siblings, assuming that the spouse of the affected person has a negative family history.

Two common polygenic conditions are discussed in the following sections, which address genetic considerations as well as issues of management.

CLEFT LIP & CLEFT PALATE

From a genetic standpoint, cleft lip with or without cleft palate is distinct from isolated cleft palate. The former is more common in males, the latter in females. Although both can occur in a single family, particularly in association with certain syndromes, this pattern is unusual. There is racial variation in the incidence of facial clefting. Among Asians, whites, and blacks, the incidence is 1.61, 0.9, and 0.31, respectively, per 1000 live births.

Clinical Findings

A cleft lip may be unilateral or bilateral and complete or incomplete. It may occur with a cleft of the entire palate or just the primary (anterior and gingival ridge) or secondary (posterior) palate. An isolated cleft palate can involve only the soft palate or both the soft and hard palates. It can be a V-shaped or wide horseshoe cleft. A cleft associated with micrognathia and glossoptosis (a tongue that falls back and causes respiratory or feeding problems) is called Pierre Robin syndrome. Among individuals with facial clefts—more commonly those with isolated cleft palate—there is an increased incidence of other congenital abnormalities. The incidence of congenital heart disease, for example, is between 1% and 2%, but among those with Pierre Robin syndrome, it can be as high as 15%. Associated abnormalities should be identified in the period immediately after birth and before surgery.

Differential Diagnosis

It is important to remember that a facial cleft may occur in many different circumstances. It may be an isolated abnormality or part of a more generalized syndrome. Prognosis, management, and accurate determination of recurrence risks all depend on an accurate diagnosis. The following causes must be considered in individuals with cleft lip and cleft palate or isolated cleft palate:

(1) Environmental factors, eg, a history of use of anticonvulsants (especially phenytoin) by the mother, fetal alcohol syndrome, and amniotic band syndrome.

(2) Chromosome abnormalities, particularly trisomies 13 and 18 and 4p–.

(3) Single gene disorders, including van der Woude syndrome (an autosomal dominant condition characterized by lip pits and either cleft lip and palate or cleft palate). Treacher Collins syndrome (cleft palate), or Stickler syndrome (Pierre Robin syndrome with severe myopia, hearing loss, and arthropathies).

(4) Syndromes of unknown cause, eg, Möbius syndrome (cleft palate) or Cornelia de Lange syndrome (cleft palate).

(5) Nonsyndromic. In the past, nonsyndromic cleft lip or cleft palate has been considered a classic example of polygenic or multifactorial inheritance. More recently, however, this mode of inheritance has been questioned, and several studies have suggested one or more major autosomal loci, both recessive and dominant or codominant. Empirically, however, the recurrence risk is still in the range of 2–3% because of nonpenetrance or the presence of other contributing genes.

Complications

The most immediate and potentially life-threatening complication in the newborn period is difficulty with feeding. This may be secondary to inadequate suction or to poorly coordinated sucking and swallowing. The Pierre Robin complex may also be associated with respiratory distress. Special bottles and nipples and occasionally a palatal prosthesis may be needed for feeding, and special positioning and supplemental O_2 may be necessary for children with Pierre Robin syndrome. Breast feeding is not usually successful if the palate is involved. Rarely, gavage feedings and even a tracheostomy may be required. Later complications include recurrent serous otitis media and decreased or fluctuating hearing. The former is treated aggressively, because evidence suggests that serous otitis contributes to delayed speech and language. Although antihistamine and decongestant medications are commonly used, there is little evidence that they are effective. The recommended therapy continues to be antibiotics and the insertion of polyethylene ventilation tubes. Tonsillectomy or adenoidectomy should not be done without careful team evaluation because of the risk of producing hypernasality. Speech problems may also be the result of a short or poorly mobile palate or of multiple dental problems and malocclusion.

Treatment

The cleft lip is repaired surgically either shortly after birth or later, but in any case by 2–3 months of age; the cleft palate is repaired at 9–12 months. The trend is toward earlier surgical repair as advances are made in pediatric anesthesia and nursing care. At the time of the initial surgery, the ears should be examined and tubes inserted if fluid is present. Additional surgery is usually needed to improve the appearance of the lip, correct nasal deformities, and provide adequate palatal length for normal speech. Hearing should be closely monitored and polyethylene tubes replaced as needed. Most children with a cleft palate need speech therapy starting at age 2–3 years. They also need orthodontic treatment, sometimes as early as 8 or 9 years. Midfacial hypoplasia is commonly seen in children with facial clefts, and a midface advancement may be necessary at the end of the growth period. Because of the complexity of the management of these patients and the necessity for coordinated care, it is recommended that they be followed in a multidisciplinary cleft palate clinic.

Genetic Counseling

Accurate counseling depends on accurate diagnosis. A complete family history must be taken, and both parents must be examined. The choice of laboratory studies is guided by the presence of other abnormalities and clinical suspicions. They may include chromosome analysis, eye examination, and x-ray studies. Clefts of both the lip and the palate have been detected on ultrasound prenatally, but intrauterine diagnosis is most likely in syndromes where other, more serious abnormalities can be identified.

NEURAL TUBE DEFECTS

The term **neural tube defect** encompasses a variety of malformations, including anencephaly, spina bifida or myelomeningocele, sacral agenesis, sacral lipomas, and other spinal dysraphisms. Hydrocephalus associated with the Arnold-Chiari malformation is commonly seen with spina bifida at all levels. Sacral agenesis, also called the caudal regression syndrome, is seen more frequently in infants of diabetic mothers than in other infants.

Clinical Findings

At birth, neural tube defects can present as rachischisis at any level, as a fluid-filled sac that may or may not be leaking, or as a variety of skin-covered lesions associated with a fatty mass, a hemangioma, a tuft of hair, or asymmetric buttock creases. In the latter cases, CT or MRI studies should be conducted to look for bony and neural involvement. The extent of associated abnormalities depends on the level of the lesion and may include a variety of foot deformities, flexion contractures, dislocated hips, or total flaccid paralysis below the level of the lesion. Hydrocephalus may be apparent at birth, but more often there is an increase in head circumference, irritability, and poor feeding, with vomiting beginning shortly after the back has been closed. Neurogenic bladder and bowel may present as constant urinary dribbling, frequent stooling, and occasionally rectal or even vaginal prolapse. Urinary retention may also occur, particularly in the immediate postoperative period. There is also a higher incidence of unassociated abnormalities, particularly with higher lesions and anencephaly.

Differential Diagnosis

It is important to look for syndromes that may present as neural tube defects. Some chromosome abnormalities, congenital rubella, and the fetal valproic acid syndrome have been associated with neural tube defects.

Complications & Management

If the spinal defect is leaking or open at birth, the major concerns are infection and drying of the nerve roots, leading to further loss of function. For this reason, surgical closure is recommended as soon as possible. The infant should be closely monitored, and a shunt, usually ventriculoperitoneal, should be inserted as soon as signs of hydrocephalus become apparent. The shunt may need to be replaced if it becomes obstructed, infected, or separated, or it may need to be lengthened as the child grows. There has been much discussion about whether true shunt independence ever develops. The signs and symptoms of chronic shunt malfunction may be very insidious and consist only of slow deterioration of school performance or staring spells. Hydromyelia may develop and lead to progressive scoliosis; sudden death has also been ascribed to shunt malfunction in adults with spina bifida.

The child's ability to walk varies according to the level of the lesion. Children with low lumbar and sacral lesions walk with minimal support; those with high lumbar and thoracic lesions are rarely functional walkers; and those with midlumbar lesions vary. In any case, the child should receive physical therapy and assume the upright position at the appropriate developmental age. Orthopedic surgery may be necessary to get the child upright and ambulatory.

Concerns about the bladder begin at birth. The bladder may be small and spastic or large and hypotonic; the sphincter may be flaccid or tight. The child may therefore be constantly wet because the bladder holds little urine, or there may be incomplete emptying of the bladder and ureteral reflux. In the latter case, there is a high risk for urinary tract infections. In addition, there may be a problem called "bladder dyssynergy." Normally, when the bladder contracts, the sphincter relaxes, allowing for an unimpeded flow of urine. In a dyssynergic state, the sphincter also contracts, predisposing to urethral reflux. Management is guided by the results of early studies to determine the type of bladder present. If the bladder is emptying, nothing need be done immediately, though the Credé maneuver is usually recommended to assist in complete emptying. If there is retention or reflux, clean intermittent catheterization should be started immediately, and occasionally a temporary vesicostomy is needed. Continence can be achieved in a variety of ways. In most cases, medications are necessary, such as anticholinergic agents to relax the smooth muscle of the bladder or alpha-sympathomimetic drugs to increase bladder outlet resistance. The mother and ultimately the child are taught the technique for clean intermittent catheterization. If the child still cannot achieve continence, a surgical procedure may be required such as an artificial sphincter, bladder neck reconstruction or suspension, or collagen injection. If the bladder is small, with increased tone, augmentation using a portion of bowel may be necessary to prevent reflux and upper tract deterioration. These procedures improve urinary retention and decrease leakage, but they usually require intermittent catheterization as well to ensure complete emptying. Diversionary procedures are rarely done unless there is damage to the upper tracts. If a surgical diversion is indicated, a continent stoma can often be created, eliminating the need for a urinary collecting bag. Renal function should be monitored regularly and ultrasound examination performed annually. Cultures should also be obtained frequently, and symptomatic infections should be treated.

Bowel control can be more of a problem, because a lax sphincter and poor peristalsis predispose to constipation and poor emptying. The principles of management include increasing the bulk of the stool to facilitate spontaneous and more complete evacuation and at the same time keep the child as free from accidents as possible. This is done with a combination of a high-fiber diet, fluids, and suppositories. Enemas, digital stimulation or evacuation, and biofeedback training have been used as well.

Areas of skin anesthesia or hypesthesia roughly correlate to motor level. Skin breakdown in the foot and perineal regions is always a threat, and skin care must be meticulous. Wheelchairs should have appropriate cushions, and new braces should be used very cautiously until it is certain that they fit. If skin breakdown does occur, all pressure must be relieved, the wound kept clean, and an artificial skin dressing used to promote healing. Surgical closure is sometimes required. The advantages of prevention over treatment cannot be emphasized too strongly. Recently, it has become apparent that children with spina bifida and urinary tract anomalies have a significant risk for type I (IgE-mediated) allergic reactions to latex. Symptoms may vary from urticaria to anaphylaxis during surgery. Some but not all children will have a history of allergic reactions to rubber. It is difficult to predict

who has this sensitivity. Skin tests are poorly standardized and carry some risk. The IgE radioallergosorbent test (RAST) is helpful if positive, but it is not 100% sensitive. It has been predicted that up to 40% of children with spina bifida are latex sensitive, with the incidence increasing with age. Recognition of this problem and the avoidance of latex products is essential.

There is a wide range of intellectual capacity in children with neural tube defects, but most function at the low normal to borderline levels. Most children are now mainstreamed, but they have a higher incidence of fine motor and visual-perceptual problems. Because of early aggressive care, most children with neural tube defects now survive into adolescence, when different problems become apparent. The introduction of MRI has demonstrated that most individuals with spina bifida have tethered cords. Many are asymptomatic, but others develop back or leg pain, change in bladder function, change in motor or sensory level, spasticity, or scoliosis. These symptoms may develop at any age, and prompt surgical intervention is necessary as lost function may not be regained. Scoliosis may also become apparent in adolescence and may be associated with syringomyelia or a tethered cord. Neurologic evaluation is indicated before scoliosis surgery. Respiratory compromise and even sleep apnea may occur. A small percentage of patients have progressive loss of renal function secondary to chronic infection and stones despite aggressive treatment, and some develop renal failure. Problems with bowel management and skin breakdown increase as individuals become obese and less ambulatory. The major problems, however, are psychosocial. The transition into independent adulthood is very difficult because of poor social skills, limited social contacts, inferior education, and poor preparation for the competitive work world. Society must do more for these disabled young adults.

Individuals with closed spinal cord abnormalities (eg, sacral lipomas) have similar problems, though hydrocephalus is rarely seen and intelligence is usually normal. Early surgical treatment is important to preserve function and prevent further disability secondary to cord tethering. Because needs are ongoing and management approaches change with time, all children with spinal defects of any type should be followed in a multidisciplinary clinic.

Genetic Counseling

Recurrence risks vary according to etiology, but most neural tube defects are polygenic, with a recurrence risk of 2–3%. The risk for the offspring of an affected person is essentially the same. There would be a considerably higher risk if the anencephaly or encephalocele were associated with renal abnormalities or polydactyly as seen in Meckel-Gruber syndrome (see p 934). Prenatal diagnosis is available, and pregnancies can be monitored in a variety of ways. In fetuses with open neural tube defects, serum alpha-fetoprotein levels, measured at 16–18 weeks of gestation, are elevated. In countries such as Great Britain, where the incidence is particularly high, pregnant women are routinely screened. Routine screening has also been recommended by the American Academy of Obstetrics and Gynecology. Alpha-fetoprotein levels in amniotic fluid are also elevated, and amniocentesis combined with experienced ultrasound studies will detect more than 90% of neural tube defects. Recent studies have shown that the periconceptional use of folic acid can significantly lower the incidence of neural tube defects. It is now recommended that all women of childbearing age take 0.4 mg of folic acid daily. This can be achieved by dietary modification (see Table 11–8) or by taking a multivitamin capsule once daily that contains 0.4 mg of folic acid. For the woman at increased risk because of a previous child with a neural tube defect, the current recommendation is to increase folic acid intake to 4 mg when a pregnancy is planned. There is no evidence that the use of folic acid will prevent other midline defects or other types of anomalies.

Austin KD, Hall JG: Nontraditional inheritance. Pediatr Clin North Am 1992;39:335.

Carey JC: Health supervision and anticipatory guidance for children with genetic disorders (including specific recommendations for trisomy 21, trisomy 18, and neurofibromatosis 1). Pediatr Clin North Am 1992;39:25.

Collins FS: Cystic fibrosis: Molecular biology and therapeutic implications. Science 1992;256:774.

Crystal RG: Gene therapy strategies for pulmonary disease. Am J Med 1992;92(Suppl 6A):44S.

Darras BT: Molecular genetics of Duchenne and Becker muscular dystrophy. J Pediatr 1990;117:1.

Kernahan DAJ, Rosenstein SW (editors): *Cleft Lip and Palate: A System of Management.* Williams & Wilkins, 1990.

Listernick R, Charrow J: Neurofibromatosis type 1 in childhood. J Pediatr 1990;116:845.

Recommendations for use of folic acid to reduce number of spina bifida cases and other neural tube defects. JAMA 1993;269:1233.

Rekate HL (editor): Comprehensive Management of Spina Bifida. CRC Press, 1991.

Shoffner JM, Wallace DC: Mitochondrial genetics: Principles and practice. Am J Hum Genet 1992;51:1179.

IV. DYSMORPHOLOGY

Morphogenesis is the complex process by which developmentally regulated genes form the structures necessary for survival. Dysmorphology is the study of those processes that produce birth defects, ie, those abnormalities of morphogenesis that affect bodily function and integrity. Birth defects are evident in 2–3% of infants and up to 7% of persons later in life. They are now the leading cause of death in the first year of life. Since 20–30% of admissions to pediatric hospital beds are for genetic conditions and birth defects, dysmorphology has become an important component of pediatric practice.

Management of dysmorphic infants requires an understanding of pathophysiology and an organized approach to diagnosis. This discussion emphasizes mechanisms of teratogenesis—the process that produces birth defects—and outlines a general approach to diagnosis. Congenital abnormalities of specific organs are discussed in appropriate chapters throughout this book.

INTERACTING MECHANISMS IN TERATOGENESIS

There are multiple causes of congenital malformations, including chromosomal aberrations and single-gene mutations, mechanical stresses, and certain environmental agents (teratogens). Single etiologic factors are recognized in only about 30% of cases. Most birth defects occur because normal development has been altered by abnormal interactions between genetic and environmental factors.

GENETIC FACTORS

About 25% of birth defects can be directly attributed to single gene defects and chromosome aberrations. The phenotypes of several chromosome abnormalities are now recognized (see chromosome disorders and contiguous gene syndromes), and experimental biology is beginning to provide the tools to understand their pathogenesis.

Major advances in the understanding of morphogenesis have come through two major avenues: (1) the recognition that the genetic control of development is homologous across species; and (2) advances in experimental techniques, particularly through development of transgenic animals.

The major themes and patterns of embryology and the genes that regulate them have been conserved throughout evolution. For example, families of homeotic genes that regulate segmentation and axis formation in *Drosophila* serve similar functions in mammals. Another family of developmentally important regulatory genes, the *Pax* genes, have recently been discovered. These genes are highly conserved in evolution, and their products function as transcription factors that regulate expression of genes affecting tissue differentiation. Mutations in *Pax* genes have been found to produce birth defects in humans such as aniridia (maldevelopment of the iris and anterior chamber of the eye) and Waardenburg syndrome (a disorder in which maldevelopment of structures derived from neural crest cells results in hearing impairment, altered pigmentation of the hair, and characteristic facial features).

Perhaps the most powerful tool in the field of developmental biology is now the transgenic mouse. Briefly, mice are made chimeric at the blastocyst stage of development by addition of multipotential stem cells into which various exogenous genes (transgenes) have been incorporated. These chimeric animals are then bred, and their offspring that carry the experimental gene are referred to as "transgenic." Transgenic mice provide a powerful experimental model because, depending on how the addition of the transgene has been accomplished, its function during development can be studied by causing its overexpression or by knocking it out and then observing the effects.

Genes that contribute to multifactorial disorders, including birth defects, are also being isolated through linkage studies. Mapping and sequencing the human genome is making it possible to track the segregation of multiple loci through families in which genetic predisposition to multifactorial processes is evidenced in multiple affected members. This strategy will help to localize candidate genes whose products can then be evaluated for their roles in morphogenesis by taking advantage of homologies with experimental animals.

ENVIRONMENTAL FACTORS

Epidemiologic studies consistently indicate that certain environmental factors (eg, season, residence, occupation, socioeconomic status, and exposures to drugs, chemicals, and environmental contaminants) contribute to risks for congenital malformations, but few specific human teratogens have been identified. Among these are congenital infections (see Chapters 32–34), a dozen or so prescribed drugs, a growing list of abused substances, and a few well-documented environmental agents, including ionizing radiation in doses exceeding 10–50 cGy, methyl mercury, lead, and industrial products contaminated with dioxins.

Although animal studies have traditionally been used to assess reproductive risks, more recent applications attest to their greater value as models for investigation of teratogenic mechanisms. The following principles of reproductive toxicity were identified in animal models but are directly relevant to human birth defects:

(1) Most chemicals and drugs capable of being absorbed into the maternal circulation will also cross the placenta and equilibrate with the conceptus.

(2) Drug, toxins, and hazardous agents are teratogenic through dose-dependent mechanisms. Hence, the level of exposure is an important consideration in risk assessment. For prescribed and abused substances, transplacental levels are expected to be high enough to be pharmacologically active. For environmental contaminants, transplacental levels will also be exposure-dependent. Most exposures that do not produce maternal signs and symptoms will not achieve toxic concentrations in the conceptus. Exceptions such as lead and other heavy metals that are concentrated by placental mechanisms, however, demonstrate the need for continued toxicologic evaluations and surveillance.

(3) Extensive preclinical testing of pharmaceuticals and selection of agents with low reproductive toxicities is useful and provides some measure of reassurance, particularly in the context of over-the-counter agents. However, idiosyncratic reactions, ie, toxicities or hypersensitivities that occur in isolated individuals, can and probably do occur during development. It is anticipated that most idiosyncratic reactions will reflect genetically determined sensitivities.

(4) Genetic polymorphism for drug receptor-effector systems and for drug metabolism contributes significantly to risks for reproductive toxicity. Excellent examples of these effects are provided by animal models of facial clefting and spina bifida. Recent associations between birth defects and polymorphic drug metabolizing enzymes in animals and humans suggest that drug distribution also plays an important role in dysmorphogenesis.

DEVELOPMENTAL FACTORS

Embryonic and fetal development are classically understood in terms of morphogenetic stages during which individual organs pass through their critical periods (Figure 32–17). Using molecular genetic techniques, however, developmental biology has moved rapidly from a descriptive to an experimental science that is exploding into the field of clinical dysmorphology. Some familiarity with both developmental biology and human embryology is now essential for an understanding of human birth defects.

Data are accumulating too rapidly for there yet to have emerged any simple or unifying synthesis of molecular processes during development. Nonetheless, from a dysmorphologic perspective, a number of emerging concepts prove to be clinically relevant.

Development begins with the ordered expression of genes. Not only is the type of gene important but also its physical location and organization within the genome. The most dramatic example of this organization so far are the **homeotic genes** that were discovered in *Drosophila* but are now also known to be involved in organizing tissues during mammalian development. The physical ordering of these genes

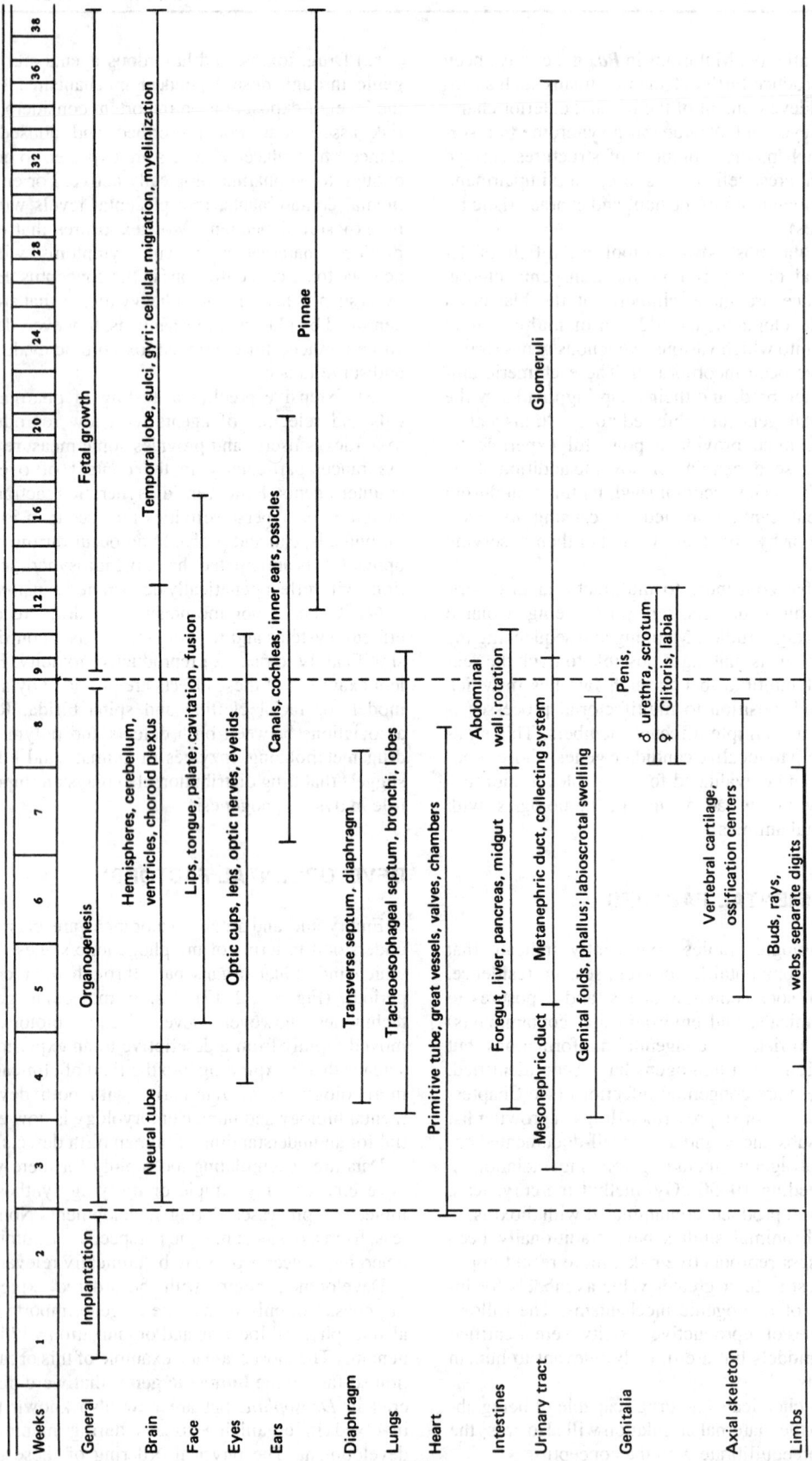

Figure 32–17. Critical periods in human gestation.

controls their expression along the anterior-posterior axis. Altered expression of homeotic genes produces a variety of birth defects.

Research into the regulation of gene expression during development has intensified following the discovery that epigenetic modification of DNA, called imprinting, is active during mammalian development. **Parental imprinting** is the term geneticists use to describe the process whereby the degree to which a gene is expressed depends upon the parent from which it is inherited. The phenomenon is readily demonstrated in transgenic mice where the expression of certain exogenous genes during embryogenesis can be shown to depend on whether they were derived from males or females. The molecular basis for these modifications is not entirely understood, but most evidence points to sex-dependent modification of DNA by addition of methyl groups (DNA methylation).

Parental imprinting is becoming an important clinical consideration. Examples include involvement of imprinting in the expression of the Angelman and Prader-Willi phenotypes, as discussed above, where the syndrome produced depends upon the respective loss of maternally or paternally inherited portions of chromosome 15. Imprinting also affects expression of the gene for insulin-like growth factor-2 (IGF-2), a potentially important determinant of morphogenesis. The gene for IGF-2 is located on chromosome 11, and it is the paternally derived allele that is expressed. Since partial duplication of this region of paternally derived chromosome 11 has been associated with Beckwith-Wiedemann syndrome (a syndrome of multiple congenital anomalies, including omphalocele, macroglossia, hemihypertrophy, and neonatal hypoglycemia that is associated with increased risk for development of Wilms tumor), IGF-2 has been proposed as a candidate gene for this disorder.

Expression of genes is also regulated during development through transduction of both chemical and physical signals to nuclei of embryonic cells. Within cells, molecules participating in these communications include cellular matrix and cytoskeleton, kinase enzymes, soluble proteins, and unknown numbers of protein complexes. Extracellular communications involve peptide and soluble hormones, collectively called **growth factors,** and molecules fixed in space within the **extracellular matrix.** These molecules control differentiation to a great extent, and abnormalities in their expression or structure are beginning to be recognized as associated with common birth defects such as cleft lip and cleft palate.

Embryonic cells must interact to form structures. They first differentiate into epithelial cells anchored against basement membranes, and some then further differentiate into mesenchymal cells that can migrate to distant sites. Much of differentiation is regulated by fixed signals that, in turn, find receptors on the surfaces of cells. Through homologous and heterologous binding, **cellular adhesion molecules** constrain the surfaces of contiguous cells so that they grow in patterns and form structures. Proteins secreted into the **extracellular matrix** provide local signals for further differentiation of migratory cells. Clearly, deficiencies or dysfunctions of proteins involved in morphogenetic cell interactions will produce birth defects. Developmental biologists predict that elucidation of both genetic disorders and environmental conditions that produce birth defects by disturbing their interactions is imminent.

Although the contributions of developmental biology to clinical dysmorphology are rapidly expanding, it remains practical to relate processes of maldevelopment to a descriptive division of gestation into five clinical phases.

The **first phase**—preconception—includes gametogenesis and fertilization, during which new mutations frequently occur. The **second phase**—implantation—begins with fertilization and is complete by 13–14 days. During this period, the blastocyst invades endometrium, and the placenta differentiates and begins to function. In humans, placentation precedes organogenesis. Although the trophoblastic tissues that separate maternal and embryonic circulation are readily permeable by most xenobiotics (compounds foreign to the biologic system), environmental exposures during this stage of development are not often associated with birth defects. The reason for this is unclear, but the phenomenon could be explained by spontaneous abortion during implantation. A final common pathway for pregnancy loss during this period may be trophoblast failure. Deficient or abnormal function of trophoblast during this period may present as threatened miscarriage.

The **third phase** of prenatal development is organogenesis, extending from the second to the eighth weeks following conception. Most critical periods of organ formation occur during this stage; thus, most structural abnormalities can be traced to these or preceding weeks. While considerations of teratogenic mechanisms necessarily concentrate on this stage of development, it should not be assumed that adverse effects of environmental agents or genetic disorders are limited to this period.

The **fourth phase**—fetal development (weeks 9–38)—is the longest phase of human gestation. During this stage, cytotoxicity is less likely to be expressed as a structural defect but is not necessarily less likely to occur. Although organs are formed by this time, functional differentiation and growth occur during these weeks. This is an especially important period for the brain. Investigators in the field of behavioral teratology, which concentrates on this period, are just beginning to study relationships between events in fetal life and later brain function.

The **fifth and final phase** of intrauterine development is the intrapartum period. Fetal presentation at the time of delivery as well as the route of delivery and any trauma sustained can affect morphologic features in the neonate. Many apparently abnormal findings are related to molding of the head or the position of the extremities and are transient in nature.

CLASSIFICATION OF DYSMORPHIC FEATURES

Accurate diagnosis is the key to prognosis and management of birth defects. Recognition of specific syndromes and patterns of maldevelopment can be extremely valuable but is often difficult in the neonatal period. A dysmorphologist should be consulted, if possible, but classification of defects by etiology can also be useful and requires less first-hand experience than does recognition of specific syndromes. The approach to classification taken here begins with an attempt to distinguish intrinsic from extrinsic causes on the basis of the history and physical examination. Each anomaly found is then assigned to one of the etiologic categories listed in Figure 32–18.

Malformations are the result of intrinsically abnormal processes of development. The conceptus is abnormal from the outset of gestation, and malformations are generally attributed to genetic processes. The characteristic morphologic features of Down syndrome and the hypoplastic thumbs and pancytopenia associated with Fanconi syndrome are classified as malformations.

Disruptions are the result of extrinsic processes. Development is perceived as proceeding normally

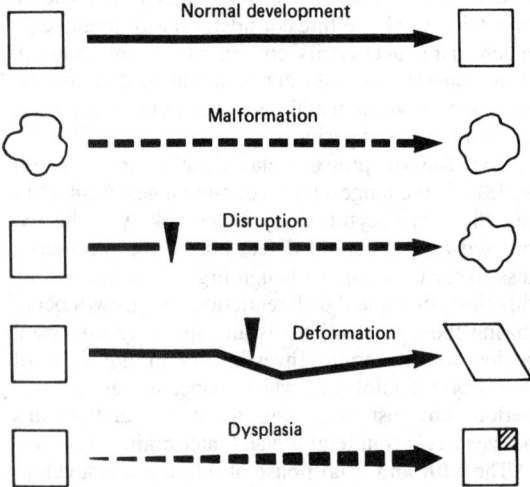

Figure 32–18. Etiologic classification of congenital anomalies.

when factors external to the conceptus interfere at a cellular level. Note that external factors need not be distributed in the general environment; they also include maternal factors. Drug-related embryopathies such as those associated with use of thalidomide are prototypical disruptions, but multifactorial processes such as neural tube defects are currently classified as disruptions despite their considerable genetic influence. The distinction between a disruption and a malformation may be difficult to discern on the basis of form alone. Careful histories—especially family histories and cytogenic studies—are useful in this case. It is easier to establish the classification of malformation on the basis of a positive family history or abnormal karyotype than it is to rule out a disruption. Disruptions, however, are far more common.

Deformations are the result of extrinsic mechanical forces. Deformations rarely involve internal organs but may range from minor malpositioning of limbs to major disturbances of the head and trunk. Intrauterine problems resulting in deformations include multiple pregnancies, abnormal uterine shape, fetal positioning, rupture of the amnion, and oligohydramnios caused by loss of or failure to produce fluid or by failure of the fetus to urinate. Deformations are characteristically asymmetric. Deforming processes may bend, cut, or fuse tissues.

Dysplasias occur as a result of abnormal tissue differentiation. In theory, extrinsic processes may be involved, but intrinsic, genetically determined factors are most often responsible. Dysplasias emphasize the link between cell function and morphogenesis. Examples include osteogenesis imperfecta (a disorder in which poorly ossified bone is easily fractured) and mucopolysaccharidoses (inborn errors of metabolism that result in growth deficiency, skeletal abnormalities, and unusual facies). Most dysplasias are the result of single gene mutations.

Pathogenetic categories imply prognoses. The presence of deformations, for instance, often means that the development and function of unaffected organs will be normal. When deformations are the result of neurologic abnormalities, however, the prognosis is poorer. Many dysplasias are not recognizable in the neonatal period. Those presenting at birth (eg, thanatophoric dwarfism) frequently have poor prognoses. Disruptions are probably the most common cause of birth defects and demonstrate the vulnerability of the developing human to extrinsic factors. Isolated disruptions, such as congenital heart defects, have excellent prognoses if repair is possible. Malformations are often multiple and, like dysplasias, often have poor prognoses.

Such categorization provides information about risks for recurrence. The highest risks are associated with single gene disorders, producing dysplasias and malformations. Most chromosomally mediated malformations occur sporadically, but careful cytogenetic analyses of family members may be required.

Risks for recurrence are higher if parents carry balanced translocations. Disruptions also tend to occur sporadically, but many are the result of multifactorial processes with substantial genetic input. Empirical data indicate higher than normal risks for recurrence in relatives of infants affected with disruptions. Isolated deformations that do not occur as a result of uterine abnormalities have a low risk for recurrence.

MULTIPLE MALFORMATIONS

Many dysmorphic infants have more than one abnormality. Recognition of relationships between multiple malformations also provides important clues to etiology and prognosis.

A "developmental field" is a region or a group of cells in an embryo that responds as a coordinated unit to intrinsic or extrinsic stimuli. The pathogenesis of developmental field defects may involve functional disturbances in primordial cells, interactions among tissues, or processes common to multiple tissues. Disturbances of rostral mesoderm, for instance, may lead to multiple anomalies of the head and face. Genital and cardiac abnormalities may be related through disturbances in other organs such as the hypothalamus or vascular structures.

A "sequence" is a pattern of anomalies caused by a single event. Renal agenesis, for instance, results in decreased amniotic fluid, fetal compression, pulmonary hypoplasia, and limb deformation. This same sequence may occur as a result of loss of amniotic fluid or urethral obstruction. The sequence of micrognathia, glossoptosis, and cleft soft palate (Pierre Robin syndrome) may begin with mandibular hypoplasia, which pushes the developing tongue posteriorly so that it interferes with movements of the posterior palatal shelves.

The term "association," when used to describe multiple anomalies, refers to their nonrandom occurrence outside any known developmental field. It denotes statistical but not necessarily causal relationships. The pathogenesis may involve both developmental field defects and sequences. Knowledge of associations is useful because it alerts the clinician to investigate other specific organs further if a defect is recognized in one.

The term "syndrome" is applied to patterns of multiple anomalies that recur with such regularity that they are considered to be pathogenetically related. Down syndrome and Turner syndrome are disorders with morphologic features found in individuals with specific chromosome abnormalities: trisomy 21 and 45,X karyotype, respectively.

DYSMORPHIC PATTERNS IN NEONATES

The following are examples of patterns of maldevelopment recognizable in the neonate. Numerous other patterns have been described in older children. Photographs of these entities are available in Jones KL: *Smith's Recognizable Patterns of Human Malformation.* Saunders, 1988.

It should be emphasized that many syndromes and conditions presenting in childhood are not recognizable in the neonate. Clinicians may frequently be forced to wait for infants to "grow into" recognizable syndromes.

Chromosome Abnormalities

Several chromosome abnormalities are recognizable in neonates. These include trisomies 21, 13, and 18 and monosomy X (Turner syndrome). Chromosome abnormalities should be considered in the evaluation of all infants with multiple anomalies.

The triad of intrauterine growth retardation, major or multiple minor malformations, and poor adaptation to extrauterine life should always be investigated cytogenetically. Note that breech presentation at term, polyhydramnios, and unexplained low Apgar scores may be important symptoms of central nervous system maldevelopment.

Of the numerous other conditions presenting in newborns, the following recognizable patterns are emphasized because they have important prognostic implications.

Cornelia de Lange Syndrome

Cornelia de Lange syndrome, a sporadically occurring constellation of congenital anomalies, has typical features that can be recognized in the newborn. Intrauterine growth retardation and characteristic facial features, including prominent eyebrows with central fusion (synophrys) and thin, downturned lips, are invariable. These infants are hirsute, and limb abnormalities occur in over 50%. Hypoplasia of the hand and feet is common, but major limb reductions occur in 30% and frequently involve the ulnar—rather than radial—ray. One affected infant in four has congenital heart disease. No specific chromosome abnormalities have been found. The immediate prognosis depends largely on the presence of congenital heart disease or respiratory failure. Subsequent failure to thrive and severe mental deficiency are the rule.

Meckel Syndrome (Meckel-Gruber Syndrome)

Meckel syndrome is rare and is inherited as an autosomal recessive trait. Infants with this syndrome have encephaloceles, polydactyly, renal cysts, and a characteristic pattern of hepatic fibrosis. The prognosis is generally poor, owing to central nervous system and renal dysfunction. Central nervous system anomalies are variably expressed and range from anencephaly and holoprosencephaly to small encephaloceles. Oligohydramnios due to renal hypoplasia may lead to a sequence that includes pulmonary hypoplasia and clubfoot. The renal cysts are bilateral and typically small and uniform. They must be distinguished from the more commonly occurring multicystic renal dysplasia, which may be associated with other anomalies. Meckel syndrome is often recognized only at autopsy.

VATER (VACTERL) Association

Vertebral anomalies and abnormalities of the heart, trachea, esophagus, kidneys, and limbs are found in association with each other and in association with anal atresia more often than would be expected by chance alone. The acronym VATER (*v*ertebral defects, imperforate *a*nus, *t*racheo*e*sophageal fistula, and *r*adial and *r*enal dysplasia) is sometimes written as VACTERL to include *c*ardiac and *l*imb anomalies. The limb defects seen are usually preaxial (radial or fibular). The association occurs sporadically. Although the anomalies themselves may be immediately or ultimately life-threatening, neurologic abnormalities are absent, and the prognosis for intellectual development is good if the VATER association is recognized early enough for proper treatment to be instituted.

CHARGE Association

The CHARGE association, *c*oloboma, *h*eart disease, choanal *a*tresia, *r*etarded growth, *g*enital anomalies, and *e*ar anomalies, was recognized through nonrandom association of facial anomalies. More recently, maldevelopment within a developmental field involving neural crest cells has been suggested. The importance of recognizing this condition is that the central nervous system is involved and that hypothalamic maldevelopment may affect secretion of pituitary trophic hormones.

Arthrogryposis Multiplex

Lack of movement in utero produces joint contractures. These may affect a single extremity, as in club foot, but are potentially much more ominous when they involve multiple joints. This phenotype is etiologically extremely heterogeneous. The differential diagnosis of multiple joint contractures in the neonate must carefully consider external causes (deformation), abnormalities of bones, joints, and connective tissue, maldevelopment or injury of the central nervous system, and myopathic processes. The prognosis in this condition is also extremely variable and usually cannot be determined without evaluation by multiple disciplines (neurology, clinical genetics, orthopedics, etc). Imaging and cytogenetic, biochemical, and electrophysiologic studies are frequently indicated. Muscle biopsy may also need to be considered.

Amnion Rupture Sequence

Rupture of the amniotic membrane in early gestation may lead to loss of fluid and entrapment of the developing conceptus. Early rupture is often associated with major structural abnormalities that are incompatible with life. Later rupture may lead to complex deformations of the head and limbs or to amputation of structures by constricting amniotic bands. It may be difficult to distinguish these deformations from malformations unless the placenta is carefully examined for the presence of amniotic bands. If the head has escaped significant deformation, neurologic development proceeds normally. The amniotic rupture sequence occurs sporadically, and its recognition allows counseling for low recurrence risks.

Twins

Multiple pregnancies are at high risk for abnormal development. Crowding may result in deformations in both identical and nonidentical twins. In one sense, monozygosity itself is a "birth defect," since it occurs after conception. Depending on the timing of division, placental circulations and amniotic sacs may or may not be shared. Division after day 13 of gestation results in conjoined twins. Despite genetic concordance, congenital abnormalities in monozygotes are frequently discordant. This observation demonstrates the role of environmental factors in multifactorial birth defects. Monochorionic twins are particularly at risk for abnormalities resulting from vascular accidents, since emboli are more likely to form in shared circulations.

Skeletal Dysplasias

Several distinct dysplasias of bone and cartilage produce a phenotype with short, curved, or malformed limbs. The head and trunk may appear normal in a few of these disorders, but more frequently there is a protuberant abdomen with or without ascites. Many of these dysplasias result in death due to pulmonary hypoplasia associated with small or poorly compliant chest walls. The differential diagnosis includes achondroplasia, achondrogenesis, osteogenesis imperfecta, camptomelic syndrome, asphyxiating thoracic dystrophy, thanatophoric dwarfism, and several other rare syndromes. Many are the result of new dominant mutations, but recessive inheritance must always be considered. Accurate diagnosis is extremely important and is best made radiographically. Films should include all extremities. A lateral view of the spine, which may be critical to the diagnosis, should be obtained as well. The immediate prognosis depends largely on the extent of pulmonary hypoplasia. Long-term prognoses are variable.

DYSMORPHIC PATTERNS IN CHILDREN

The reader is referred to the general references at the end of this chapter for detailed information about the large number of recurrent patterns of maldevelopment now recognized in older children. Recognition of these phenotypes (ie, physical, developmental, and behavioral characteristics) often requires direct experience with rare syndromes, making diagnosis difficult without consultation with experienced clinical geneticists. Even with experience, however, specific dysmorphologic diagnoses are made in only about 50% of cases on initial referral. Further investigation of undiagnosed cases is warranted and often includes specialized cytogenetic and biochemical analyses. Follow-up is also important, because syndromes may not become recognizable until children are older.

Many dysmorphologic diagnoses are "phenotypic"—ie, they are made in the absence of pathognomonic features and cannot be confirmed by biochemical or genetic testing. The four examples that follow are phenotypic diagnoses commonly suspected by general pediatric practitioners. They are presented to illustrate the approach taken by clinical geneticists to confirm diagnoses in referred cases.

Noonan syndrome is recognized in children who have short stature, low-set ears, characteristic facies with downslanting palpebral fissures, webbed neck, and congenital heart disease, typically atrial septal defects or abnormalities of the pulmonary outflow tract. Arrhythmias and abnormal conduction are frequent. The syndrome can be inherited as an autosomal dominant trait, but because its features change with age, affected parents or other older relatives may be difficult to recognize. Affected children are large for gestational age at birth and may have had mild subcutaneous edema recognized prenatally by ultrasound. The classic phenotype is usually present by school age, but by adulthood it may have further evolved in less predictable fashion, with variability in stature and associated findings such as hearing loss. The diagnosis may require follow-up of suspected cases over years with careful attention paid to ruling out other conditions.

Williams syndrome is also recognized by a phenotype that evolves over years. The classic pattern of findings includes supravalvular aortic or pulmonary stenosis, growth and developmental delays, blue eyes with stellate irides, and characteristic facies often described as elfin in young children but which tend to coarsen with age. An overly friendly, outgoing personality characteristically develops. The disorder is not typically familial. Disturbances of calcium metabolism with increased absorption and urinary excretion can sometimes be documented, but these findings appear to be transient in many cases. Since the phenotype evolves over time, it may not be suspected until after urinary calcium excretion has normalized. In the absence of biochemical evidence, the diagnosis is made on the basis of accumulating clinical findings and a predictable course after other disorders affecting growth and development have been ruled out. Follow-up of this diagnosis is particularly important because significant medical problems such as hypertension, renal complications, and degenerative spinal problems may develop in adults.

Disorders of connective tissue are frequently suspected in children with hyperextensible joints. Important diagnoses included in the differential for this finding are **Ehlers-Danlos syndrome** (for which 11 clinical subtypes have been described) and **Marfan syndrome,** an autosomal dominant disorder in which abnormal elastic tissue can lead to dislocation of lenses and development of aortic aneurysms. Most connective tissue disorders are dominantly inherited, in which case positive family histories and findings become important diagnostic criteria. Recessive forms of Ehlers-Danlos syndrome do occur, and both disorders are encountered as new mutations, in which case the diagnosis may again depend on evolution of the phenotype over years. Minimal criteria for Ehlers-Danlos syndrome include clinically apparent involvement of skin and, for subtype classification, changes in other structures such as joints and, teeth. Care must be taken to rule out conditions in which low muscle tone leads to hyperextensibility of joints. In Marfan syndrome, hyperextensibility of joints is accompanied by alterations in growth, especially of extremities. Lens dislocation, which can be pathognomonic, is inconsistently present and may not develop until late childhood or adulthood. Widening of the aortic root, another hallmark of the disorder, also may not develop for years.

DRUG-RELATED DISORDERS

Thalidomide is the classic example of a human teratogen producing a specific syndrome. The compounds discussed below are also associated with specific abnormalities. Regional teratogen information services can provide additional information.

Warfarin

The use of warfarin derivatives as anticoagulants during pregnancy was initially felt to be safe, but closer examination of exposed fetuses has shown untoward effects, including nasal hypoplasia, optic nerve hypoplasia, extraosseous calcification, and abnormalities of brain development and function. Central nervous system abnormalities can occur in fetuses exposed to warfarin during the second or third trimester of pregnancy, demonstrating the potential susceptibility of the brain to drug-related disorders during this period. Approximately one in three exposed fetuses may be affected. Mechanisms appear to involve transplacental anticoagulation and hemorrhage as well as direct effects on cartilage growth.

Anticonvulsants

There is now general agreement that exposure to anticonvulsant drugs increases risks for maldevelopment. Significant abnormalities may occur as frequently as once in every ten pregnancies in this population. Growth of the brain and mid face are consistently affected. A recognizable "fetal anticonvulsant syndrome," initially described in association with phenytoin use, has now also been reported in children exposed in utero to carbamazepine and valproic acid. Additional structural anomalies are also associated with exposures to individual agents. Maternal use of phenytoin has been associated with cleft lip and palate, hypoplasia of distal phalanges and nails, and sacral teratomas. Maternal use of trimethadione has also been associated with growth retardation, decreased mentation, and unusual facies (fetal trimethadione syndrome). An increased risk for neural tube defects has recently been linked to maternal use of valproic acid.

Isotretinoin

Excessive doses of vitamin A have long been recognized as teratogenic in animals. The potent vitamin A analogue isotretinoin (Accutane) was therefore considered a potential teratogen when it was introduced as treatment for acne. Despite warnings, some women have taken this drug during pregnancy, and several infants with multiple anomalies have been born. A specific syndrome that includes abnormalities of the central nervous system, ears, and great vessels along with hypoplasia of the thymus and parathyroid gland has been described. This condition is a phenocopy of the **DiGeorge sequence** that occurs as a contiguous gene syndrome related to microdeletions of chromosome 22. It is now clear that both isotretinoin and the deletion produce the same developmental field defect. The mechanism involves failure of cells to migrate normally from the neural crest to form structures in the head and neck.

Ethyl Alcohol

Admonitions against heavy use of alcohol during pregnancy have been given since ancient times. More recently, a specific syndrome has been recognized in the offspring of heavy drinkers. The fetal alcohol syndrome consists of intrauterine and postnatal growth retardation, microcephaly, significant mental dysfunction, and craniofacial changes including short palpebral fissures, short nose, and a long, smooth philtrum. A variety of other structural abnormalities has also been reported.

Although it is clear that high concentrations of alcohol are cytotoxic, the mechanisms of alcohol toxicity are poorly understood. The dose-response relationship is not entirely clear, but maternal alcohol intake exceeding 2–3 oz daily is considered toxic. The timing of fetal exposure to alcohol is important. Structural abnormalities occur with increased frequency in the offspring of chronic alcohol abusers, but neurologic abnormalities can be decreased if women stop drinking by 16–20 weeks of gestation. Approximately two-thirds of pregnancies in active alcoholics will have significant complications, including prematurity, growth retardation, and perinatal asphyxia. Fetal alcohol syndrome is seen in about one-third of offspring of active alcoholics.

Cocaine

As use of cocaine has increased, its effects on pregnancy have become more evident. Stimulation of the central and peripheral sympathetic nervous systems by cocaine can produce intense uterine vasoconstriction, leading to placental ischemia and abruption. Cocaine readily crosses the placenta and is active in the fetal circulation. Ischemic injury occurs in fetal limbs, intestines, and kidneys, and the central nervous system appears to be particularly vulnerable. Intracranial hemorrhage and porencephalic cysts have been reported in as many as one-third of infants born to women abusing "crack" cocaine in combination with alcohol and other substances.

Inhalants

Abuse of inhalants is widespread and includes sniffing glue, gasoline, spray paints, and other hydrocarbons. Toxic effects in users lead to a chronic organic brain syndrome and hepatotoxicity. These agents are absorbed into the maternal central circulation through pulmonary veins and delivered as highly concentrated boluses to the placenta and fetal circulation. It is now recognized that inhalant neurotoxicity in fetuses results in microcephaly and a syndrome of growth retardation similar to fetal alcohol syndrome.

CLINICAL APPROACH TO THE DYSMORPHIC INFANT

Physicians caring for neonates with birth defects must frequently provide care and make accurate diagnoses under conditions of great stress. The extent of an infant's abnormalities may not be immediately apparent, and parents who feel grief and guilt are often desperate for information. As with any medical problem, however, the history and physical examination provide most of the clues to diagnosis. Special aspects of these procedures are outlined below.

HISTORY

Environmental, family, and pregnancy histories may contain important clues to the diagnosis. In the postpartum period, frightened parents are attempting to cope with their grief and fears. Feelings of guilt are likely to be heightened during a review of the pregnancy history. Thus, the interviewer must be prepared to answer as well as ask questions.

Parental recall after delivery of an infant with an anomaly is better than recall after a normal birth. An obstetric wheel can help document gestational age and events of the first trimester: the last menstrual period, the onset of symptoms of pregnancy, the date of diagnosis of the pregnancy, the date of the first prenatal visit, and the physician's impressions of fetal growth at that time.

Next, it is important to investigate fetal growth and development. Prenatal visits should be noted and, with the aid of the obstetric wheel, a record should be made of the patterns of fetal growth, the onset of fetal movement (usually at 16 weeks), and the mother's perceptions of fetal movements. Normal fetal movement is usually strong enough to hurt the mother and be visible to the father. Abnormal fetal movement may indicate neuromuscular dysfunction or fetal constraint. These are particularly important when asphyxia accompanies the birth of a dysmorphic infant. A history of decreased fetal movement will often distinguish neuromuscular abnormalities (which result in a low Apgar score) from intrapartum events (which depress the infant).

Abnormal patterns of uterine growth may also provide clues to fetal function. Increased uterine size may indicate accumulation of amniotic fluid (hydramnios). Fluid may accumulate if the fetus fails to swallow as a result of a neuromuscular disorder, obstruction of the fetal esophagus or proximal small bowel, or fetal heart failure. Hydramnios is also associated with diabetes and high-output renal failure in the fetus. Lack or delay of uterine growth may reflect fetal growth directly or may indicate too little amniotic fluid (oligohydramnios). Amniotic fluid may be lost through premature rupture of membranes with or without formation of amniotic bands, or it may be the result of compromised function of fetal kidneys. The mother should be questioned about loss or leakage of amniotic fluid, which is often mistakenly perceived as a vaginal discharge. Information from prenatal ultrasound examination is often very helpful in distinguishing different entities associated with altered uterine growth.

The history should also include details about the onset and progression of labor. Breech presentation at term may indicate a uterine anomaly or abnormality of the fetal central nervous system.

Family histories, as described below, should always be included but may seem threatening to parents or relatives attempting to cope with strong feelings about birth defects. The interviewer should be prepared to respond to specific questions from family members.

Finally, an environmental history that includes parental habits and their work and home environments should be obtained. Maternal and paternal health, use of medications, and environmental exposures during the embryonic period should be reviewed. Questions should be considered carefully because of their emotional impact. Society is currently preoccupied with the roles of drugs, radiation, and chemical exposures in birth defects.

PHYSICAL EXAMINATION

Meticulous physical examination is crucial to accurate diagnosis in dysmorphic infants. Delivery of an affected infant may necessitate immediate attention to potentially life-threatening problems, but it is precisely because intensive support may be required that a complete examination becomes urgent. The examination should be performed as soon as possible.

In addition to the routine procedures described in Chapter 5, special attention should be paid to the neonate's physical measurements (Figure 32–19). Photographs are very helpful and should include a scale of measurements for reference. The placenta should also be examined.

Since most syndromes occur infrequently in the general population and patterns of abnormalities are therefore difficult to recognize, an experienced dysmorphologist and geneticist should be consulted if possible.

LABORATORY STUDIES

Radiologic and ultrasonographic examinations can be extremely helpful in the evaluation of dysmorphic infants. In general, films of infants with apparent limb or skeletal anomalies should include views of the skull and all of the long bones in addition to frontal and lateral views of the axial skeleton. Chest and abdominal films should be obtained when indicated. The pediatrician should consult a radiologist for further workup. Nuclear scans and imaging by CT, MRI, and ultrasound are all useful diagnostic tools, but their interpretation in the presence of birth defects may require considerable experience.

Cytogenetic analysis provides specific diagnoses in approximately 5% of dysmorphic infants who survive the newborn period. Chromosome abnormalities are recognized in 10–15% of infants who die. Karyotypes can be determined rapidly through analysis of cells in bone marrow. These allow limited interpretation and should always be accompanied by complete analysis of cultured cells. Any case requiring rapid diagnosis should be discussed with an experienced cytogeneticist. The clinician should not base decisions about further workup and management on the results of only one test. A normal karyotype does not rule out the presence of significant genetic disease.

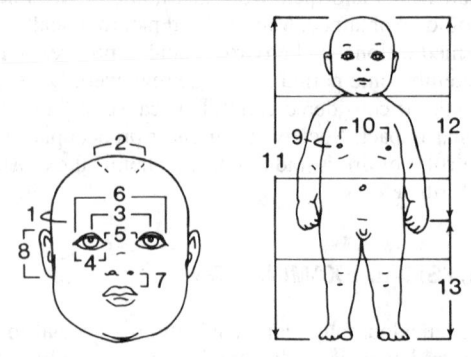

	Range (cm)	
Measurement	**Term** **(38—40 weeks)**	**Preterm** **(32—33 weeks)**
1 Head circumference	32—37	27—32
2 Anterior fontanelle $\left(\frac{L-W}{2}\right)$	0.7—3.7	. . .
3 Interpupillary distance	3.3—4.5	3.1—3.9
4 Palpebral fissure	1.5—2.1	1.3—1.6
5 Inner canthal distance	1.5—2.5	1.4—2.1
6 Outer canthal distance	5.3—7.3	3.9—5.1
7 Philtrum	0.6—1.2	0.5—0.9
8 Ear length	3—4.3	2.4—3.5
9 Chest circumference	28—38	23—29
10 Internipple distance*	6.5—10	5—6.5
11 Height	47—55	39—47
12 Ratio $\dfrac{\text{Upper body segment}}{\text{Lower body segment}}$ 13	1.7	. . .
14 Hand (palm to middle finger)	5.3—7.8	4.1—5.5
15 Ratio of middle finger to hand	0.38—0.48	0.38—0.5
16 Penis (pubic bone to tip of glans)	2.7—4.3	1.8—3.2

*Internipple distance should not exceed 25% of chest circumference.

Figure 32–19. Neonatal measurements.

PERINATAL AUTOPSY

When a dysmorphic infant dies, postmortem examination can provide important diagnostic information and should include sampling of tissue for cytogenetic analysis. The pediatrician and pathologist should consider whether samples of blood, urine, or tissue should be obtained for metabolic analyses. X-ray studies should be done whenever limb anomalies or disproportionate growth are present. Placental as well as fetal tissue can be used for viral culture. The pediatrician should discuss the case thoroughly with the pathologist, and photographs should always be taken.

IMMEDIATE MANAGEMENT OF THE DYSMORPHIC INFANT

Birth defects may be life-threatening. One physician should assume responsibility for overall care, but the skills of several other health professionals are usually required.

Vital functions should be supported until a thorough evaluation can be completed. When lethal or inoperable anomalies are recognized, humane and compassionate treatment directed at ensuring comfort should be provided. All neonates should be kept warm and given an opportunity to interact with their families.

DECISION MAKING

The birth of a dysmorphic infant is a highly emotional event and may give rise to difficult ethical and medical dilemmas. Modern medicine and technology now offer the potential to sustain life under extraordinary circumstances. Very often, the appropriate use of this capability is not immediately apparent. Society is currently agonizing over the dilemmas presented by infants with multiple anomalies, and it is clear that agreement on general principles does not always lead to agreement about what to do in individual cases. All decisions are best made in a supportive atmosphere by parents who are well informed and aware of the options open to them and who have been given clear medical recommendations. Most parents need both time and support from within their own community. A sense of the time available before a decision must be made should be given to the parents, and they should have an opportunity to discuss their feelings with supportive individuals. The infant's physician has an important role in this process but should not be the sole individual involved. Care of infants with birth defects requires access to medical, psychosocial, and ethical consultation.

Hall JG, Fnoster-Iskenium UG, Allanson JE: *Handbook of Normal Physical Measurements.* Oxford Univ Press, 1989.

Hall JG: Somatic mosaicism: Observations related to clinical genetics. Am J Hum Genet 1988;43:355.

Shepard TH: *Catalog of Teratogenic Agents,* 7th ed. Johns Hopkins Univ Press, 1992.

Spranger J et al: Errors of morphogenesis: Concepts and terms. Recommendations of an international working group. J Pediatr 1982;100:160.

Wynne-Davies R, Hall C, Apley A: *Atlas of Skeletal Dysplasias.* Churchill Livingstone, 1987.

V. GENETIC COUNSELING

ISSUES

Genetic counseling is more than just a communication process about the risk for recurrence of genetic disorders in a family. When families come for counseling, specific questions need to be addressed:

(1) What is the problem? An accurate *diagnosis* is the sine qua non of genetic counseling.

(2) What does it mean? For a family to make informed decisions concerning future pregnancies, they must understand the *prognosis* of the disorder. The birth of an infant with anencephaly is undoubtedly a traumatic experience, but caring for a child with a high myelomeningocele poses greater long-term stresses.

(3) What caused the abnormality? Determination of *etiology* is essential for correct counseling. The risk for recurrence of cleft lip and palate caused by amniotic bands is minimal, whereas the risk for recurrence of van der Woude syndrome could be 50%.

(4) Is it curable or treatable? Possible *therapy*—its success, burden, and expense—need to be discussed.

(5) Will the problem recur in future pregnancies? Only after the first four questions have been addressed can meaningful *recurrence risk figures* be given. At this time, it is often necessary to review with the family some basic genetic information, showing pictures of chromosomes, explaining the difference between chromosomes and genes, and diagramming the more common mechanisms of inheritance.

(6) Can the abnormality be prevented or anticipated in future pregnancies? This question brings up the issue of *prenatal diagnosis* and other options available to the couple.

This may appear to be a formidable list of questions for the counselor to address, and answers may come from other members of the genetic counseling team and appropriate consultants. In addition, ongoing psychologic support is essential throughout the counseling process.

PROCESS

History

The cornerstone of a genetic evaluation is a thorough history, both of any pregnancy that resulted in an abnormal infant and of the family in general. Issues to be addressed in the pregnancy history include problems conceiving, bleeding, maternal illnesses or exposures, medications, smoking, the use of alcohol or other recreational drugs, possible exposures to teratogens, and lifetime histories of both parents' exposure to x-rays. Information such as onset, intensity, and distribution of fetal activity may help to differentiate a prenatal from a postnatal problem. It is often helpful to ask if this pregnancy was "different" from others in any way. Information about the delivery should be obtained from birth records whenever possible. A family history should always be taken in a pedigree form. Parental ages, recurrent miscarriages, stillbirths, and infant deaths are all important. The possibility of consanguinity should be explored by asking for common family names and family origins. The general health and development of all first- and second-degree relatives should be ascertained. Information about ethnic background may be valuable. It is sometimes hard to know how extensive the family history should be. This depends to some extent on what may be suspected, but the major limiting factor is availability of information. Often, couples need to explore their family history in more depth and objective documentation should be assembled if that is possible.

Physical Examination

The type of examination done as part of a genetic evaluation differs from others in that minor abnormalities are stressed as well as more obvious defects. It may also be necessary to examine parents, siblings, and even more distant relatives to make or confirm a diagnosis. Photographs should be obtained when relatives cannot be examined.

Laboratory Tests

The need for specific laboratory tests varies with the situation. Because these tests are expensive, they should be ordered with care, but they should certainly be done when important information can be gained. Chromosome analysis is indicated in any child with multiple major or minor anomalies, particularly if associated with mental retardation or developmental delay. High-resolution analysis or parental chromosomes may also be appropriate. Fragile X testing should be done in instances of mental retardation of unknown cause. Molecular testing is not routine but may be of value in particular families.

COUNSELING

Much has been written about directive versus nondirective genetic counseling, but in the USA at least, the latter is recommended and more widely practiced. Although it is difficult to be totally objective, particularly if the geneticist is familiar with the long-term burden of a disorder, it is important to remember that the ultimate choice belongs to the parents. A geneticist may have concerns about society at large, but a counselor should be the advocate for the family and not for society. The timing of genetic counseling is also important. There is a fine line between counseling that is too early (because the family, still concerned about the welfare of the affected person, is emotionally unprepared) and counseling that is too late (because another at-risk fetus has already been conceived). The possibility of a genetic basis for the mishap should be mentioned early, but continuing contact is needed to refine the diagnosis and help the family understand the implications.

There are many ways to communicate information to the parents, but all explanations should be given in language that the family can understand and in a relaxed and unhurried atmosphere. The baseline risk for congenital abnormalities should be discussed and put into the perspective of the risk being quoted. The actual risk should be compared with the burden (or the parents' perception of the burden) of the abnormality in question. Examples can be helpful. The issues of guilt and blame must be addressed. This part of counseling can be difficult if one of the parents carries an abnormal gene or used a teratogenic substance, such as cocaine or alcohol. Ongoing psychologic counseling may be needed. It may be difficult for parents to understand how an isolated abnormality in a family can still be genetic and be associated with a significant recurrence risk; it may be necessary to review with them such concepts as phenocopy, new mutations, decreased penetrance, and variable expressivity.

All too often, no specific diagnosis can be made and no cause can be determined. In these cases, recurrence risks can only be estimated. It may be helpful for families to explore possible mechanisms and for the geneticist to discuss the implications for subsequent pregnancies. In any case, parents should consider their own emotional response to the birth of a second affected child.

Genetic counseling is not a static process. Families often continue to have questions. A letter explaining clearly and concisely the information covered in the counseling session is helpful. Although a geneticist cannot assume responsibility for all problems a family may have, appropriate referrals can be made. Continued contact is advisable to ensure adequate understanding and reopen counseling as new information and testing become available. A social worker, genetic nurse, or genetic associate who is a member of the counseling team is an ideal person to maintain contact.

A word should be said about responsibility to the extended family. As more genetic disorders become diagnosable by new molecular techniques, counseling needs to be expanded to the family at large. This requires both the cooperation of the consultand and collaboration between genetic units throughout the country. During counseling, it is necessary to educate families concerning this need and at the same time respect confidentiality.

OPTIONS

In situations of increased risk, families have a variety of options. They can have no further children or they can take the risk, but in many cases there are more and better choices. Some families for whom prenatal diagnosis is unacceptable or unavailable may prefer adoption. Artificial insemination is genetically appropriate if a disease is recessive or if the father is the carrier, and in vitro fertilization with donor ova if the mother is the carrier. Preimplantation diagnosis of an embryo obtained after in vitro fertilization with maternal eggs and paternal sperm is theoretically possible in many single-gene conditions. A successful pregnancy has followed this procedure done to rule out cystic fibrosis in the embryo. However, this is still experimental and is of limited availability. Even if it were more available, cost might be a determining factor in its application. Some families may consider sterilization, but they should realize that the risk for each of the parents may drop markedly if in the future the couple should separate and remarry. For most families, however, some type of prenatal diagnosis is requested and often available. All of these options are expensive. Prevention of an abnormality is of course the ideal. To date, the use of periconceptional folic acid is the only known effective preventive agent other than the avoidance of teratogenic substances such as alcohol and cocaine. Technology has outstripped society's responsiveness to the needs of these families. This problem must be addressed in the future.

PRENATAL DIAGNOSIS

It has been estimated that prenatal diagnosis is indicated in 7–8% of all pregnancies. As technology improves, the indications for and the accuracy of prenatal diagnosis can only increase. Today, a large proportion of pregnant women undergo at least one ultrasound study during pregnancy, and more congenital abnormalities are being detected prior to birth even in low-risk women. Prenatal diagnosis not only gives women the option to interrupt an abnormal pregnancy but also allows the physician to give optimal care during and immediately after delivery. As intrauterine therapy becomes feasible, prenatal diagnosis will become even more important.

METHODS

Prenatal diagnosis techniques may be divided into three broad categories: (1) testing of maternal blood,

(2) testing of fetal tissue, and (3) fetal visualization. There have been rapid advances in all of these areas.

Testing of Maternal Blood

The use of maternal serum alpha-fetoprotein as a screening test was originally introduced because elevated values were found in association with neural tube defects. It was also noted that women who carried a fetus with Down syndrome had a 25% lower value compared to those in whom the fetus was normal. Combining this test with maternal age enabled about 20% of fetuses with trisomy 21 to be detected in women under 35 years of age. Subsequent studies have shown that the addition of two other tests can raise the detection rate to 60%. Human chorionic gonadotropin is increased twofold and unconjugated estriol is decreased by 25% in maternal blood if the fetus has Down syndrome. The use of all three tests or the "triple test" is currently recommended. It is done at 16–18 weeks of gestation, though there is some evidence that the estriol value may be decreased earlier in pregnancy. These tests are all dependent upon gestational age and must be interpreted with care.

Fetal cells, including lymphocytes, trophoblasts, and nucleated red blood cells, are present in maternal circulation. There is hope, therefore, that abnormalities in fetal cells may be detected by sampling maternal blood. Polymerase chain reaction could be used to amplify an allele not present in maternal cells (as in cases where the fetus is heterozygous and the paternal allele could be amplified). Fluorescent in situ hybridization (FISH) could also be used to identify aneuploid cells in the maternal circulation. These techniques are still experimental.

Testing of Fetal Tissue

Amniocentesis has been available for many years. Its accuracy and safety are well established. Traditionally, fluid containing fetal cells is removed at 16–18 weeks of gestation. There is a trend today, however, to do the procedure earlier, at 13–14 weeks. These cells are then cultured, and when adequate cell growth has occurred, cytogenetic or biochemical tests (or both) can be done. Studies such as alpha-fetoprotein tests, predictive of neural tube defects, are done directly on the amniotic fluid. This is a safe procedure with a complication rate (primarily for miscarriage) of less than 1% in experienced hands. It is also readily available in many communities. There are two major disadvantages: (1) The test is not done until the second trimester, after fetal activity has been felt. The cells must be grown, which causes further delay before the results are available. This delay is emotionally difficult for the parents, particularly if they decide to abort the fetus. This problem may be partially alleviated by applying FISH to uncultured amniocytes. Region-specific probes are available for chromosomes 13, 18, 21, X, and Y. An abnormal number of signals in most cells would be highly suggestive of

an abnormality involving one of these five chromosomes. (No other chromosome abnormalities would be detected using FISH alone.) At the present time, this is done only in conjunction with traditional cytogenetic analysis, but it is of particular value where fetal abnormalities have been detected on ultrasonography or when the amniocentesis is done late in pregnancy. (2) It is difficult to obtain enough tissue for DNA studies.

Chorionic villus sampling is now available in many centers. This test may be done by a transcervical or transabdominal approach and is done late in the first trimester, which is an attractive feature. Since more tissue can be obtained by chorionic villus sampling, it is easier to do DNA studies with this test. The cells also can be examined or assayed directly, and results are available much sooner. However, direct preparations may be of poorer quality and may show mosaicism which is confined to the placenta and does not represent the fetal karyotype. Cultured preparations may be more accurate. Certainly, if an unusual cytogenetic picture is found on chorionic villus sampling, further studies should be considered before the pregnancy is interrupted. Numerous studies have been done comparing the safety of first-trimester chorionic villus sampling with amniocentesis. With one exception, safety rates are comparable in experienced hands. A study done in the United Kingdom did show a 2.9% increase in fetal loss rate. Of more concern lately has been the possible association of chorionic villus sampling with terminal transverse limb defects, perhaps secondary to vascular disruption. Although the actual incidence of limb defects may not be significantly increased, the type of abnormality is an unusual one and may be part of an oromandibular-limb hypogenesis syndrome. It does seem to be more common with early chorionic villus sampling, and for this reason the procedure is now usually done after 9, 10, or even 11 weeks of gestation. At the present time, chorionic villus sampling is probably still the procedure of choice if DNA testing is indicated or if the risk for an abnormal fetus is high. This gives the parents the option for earlier termination of pregnancy. This test should only be done by experienced persons because of the potentially higher complication rate.

Fetal Visualization

The most commonly used prenatal test is **ultrasound.** At 18 weeks of gestation, it is possible to view all major fetal organs, including the kidneys, heart, brain, spinal cord, bladder, and limbs. In addition, the finer structures of the eye, the vasculature, and digits are also visible. It is therefore possible to look for almost any genetic syndrome that is characterized by a structural defect. Although an abnormality could be missed and an unaffected child can never be guaranteed, many abnormalities are being detected by ultrasound in the second trimester. Routine ultrasound screening has demonstrated many unexpected abnormalities. Most of these are major defects, however, and minor anomalies are easily missed, especially if unexpected. In addition, procedures such as percutaneous umbilical blood sampling and skin biopsies can also be done under ultrasound guidance. An exciting new development is the use of first-trimester vaginal ultrasound probes. Using this technique, early fetal development is now being closely monitored, and some early abnormalities are being suspected if not actually diagnosed. Although this technique holds much potential, there are several caveats that must be considered at this time: (1) Visualization depends to a great extent upon the quality of the equipment and the experience of the interpreter. (2) All abnormalities may not be detectable in the first trimester. (3) All unusual findings may not be abnormal, and until normal developmental variation is better understood the results should be interpreted with caution. (4) Every attempt should be made to confirm an abnormality suspected in the first trimester.

X-ray studies of the fetus are rarely necessary because ultrasonography has improved so greatly. If a skeletal abnormality or bone dysplasia is suspected, however, x-ray films may be helpful.

INDICATIONS

Amniocentesis or chorionic villous sampling is indicated in the following instances:

(1) Maternal age over 35 years.

(2) Previous child with a chromosome abnormality.

(3) Either parent a translocation carrier. In this case, the risk for a fetus with an unbalanced chromosome abnormality depends upon the type of translocation.

(4) A history of any genetic disorder diagnosable by biochemical techniques or by DNA analysis. The list of such conditions changes daily, and a genetic center should be contacted for the most recent information.

(5) A request by the parents for fetal sexing because of a history of an X-linked disorder that is not diagnosable by current methods.

(6) Previous child or a parent with a neural tube defect. Unlike the indications listed above, for which either amniocentesis or chorionic villous sampling can be done, amniotic fluid is required in this case, and for that reason only amniocentesis is appropriate.

(7) An abnormality of any component of the triple test.

Fetal ultrasonography is indicated whenever an abnormality characterized by a structural defect is suspected. The defect may be suspected because of the family history, potential teratogenic exposure during pregnancy or questionable abnormalities noted on a routine ultrasound done in the obstetrician's office. In any case, the patient should be referred to a medical center experienced in fetal ultrasonography for further evaluation.

FETAL THERAPY

Since fetal ultrasonography has become almost routine in many places, many unsuspected birth defects are being detected prior to delivery. In some cases, the diagnosis is made in the second trimester, and it is possible to terminate an abnormal pregnancy. Often, however, the defect is not suspected until 30 or 32 weeks. Percutaneous blood sampling has become a low-risk procedure that is routine in many medical centers. This gives access to fetal blood not only for diagnostic but also for therapeutic purposes. The fetus can be transfused or given appropriate medical treatment as technology advances and specific therapies become available. Intrauterine diagnosis has led to the new field of fetal therapy, which may be defined as any intervention during gestation that improves eventual neonatal outcome. Surgical intervention for abnormalities such as hydrocephalus, diaphragmatic hernia, and bladder outlet obstruction has been disappointing. Medical intervention, on the other hand, holds considerable promise. Thyroid abnormalities and congenital adrenal hyperplasia may be dealt with in utero either by treating the fetus directly or by treating the mother and monitoring amniotic fluid levels. Awareness of a fetal abnormality can be important for perinatal care. A mother may be transferred to a larger delivery center, where surgery for the newborn can be performed immediately. The timing of delivery may be influenced by the progression of hydrocephalus or bladder distention. This is a very difficult time for parents, however, and adequate psychologic support is essential. It is important for physicians and parents to realize that prenatal diagnosis has much to offer and that treatment of the newborn can be improved even if an abnormal pregnancy is allowed to continue.

Aylsworth AS: Genetic counseling for patients with birth defects. Pediatr Clin North Am 1992;39:229.

D'Alton ME, DeCherney AH: Prenatal diagnosis. N Engl J Med 1993;328:114.

DiLiberti JH, Greenstein MA, Rosengren SS: Prenatal diagnosis. Pediatr Rev 1992;13:334.

Reece EA et al: *Medicine of the Fetus and Mother.* Lippincott, 1992.

Simpson, JL, Elias S (editors): *Essentials of Prenatal Diagnosis.* Churchill Livingstone, 1993.

REFERENCES

Buyse ML: *Birth Defects Encyclopedia.* Blackwell, 1990.

Childs B et al (editors): *Progress in Medical Genetics,* vol 7, 1988.

Emery AEH, Rimoin DL: *Principles and Practice of Medical Genetics,* 2nd ed. Churchill Livingstone, 1990.

Gorlin RJ, Cohen MM, Levin LS: *Syndromes of the Head and Neck,* 3rd ed. Oxford Univ Press, 1990.

Jones KL: *Smith's Recognizable Patterns of Human Malformation,* 4th ed. Saunders, 1988.

King RA, Rotter JI, Motulsky AG: *The Genetic Basis of Common Diseases.* Oxford Univ Press, 1993.

King RC, Stansfield WD:*A Dictionary of Genetics.* Oxford Univ Press, 1990.

McKusick VA: *Mendelian Inheritance in Man,* 10th ed. Johns Hopkins Univ Press, 1992.

Stevenson RE, Hall JG, Goodman RM (editors): *Human Malformations and Related Anomalies,* vols 1 and 2. Oxford Univ Press, 1993.

33

Allergic Disorders

David S. Pearlman, MD, & Carolyn R. Comer, MD

Allergic disorders include a variety of local and systemic manifestations that commonly are ultimate expressions of the union between antigen and antibody. Although this union triggers the chain of events that culminates in the clinical allergic reaction, nonimmunologic factors are important in modifying this chain of events. In some instances, nonimmunologic factors can be completely responsible for clinical reactions indistinguishable from immunologically induced reactions (eg, some forms of chronic urticaria).

Allergic reactivity is normal. The reaction that results from the transfusion of mismatched blood is an allergic reaction; the repeated injection of antitoxin in the form of foreign serum often leads to serum sickness; and contact with poison ivy frequently causes an allergic dermatitis. By definition, allergic reactions stem from an antigen-antibody interaction; identification of these participants is of prime importance both in the diagnosis and in the therapy of allergic disorders. It is often difficult to identify the antigens (allergens) responsible for a particular clinical disorder, but the most helpful procedure is a thorough and detailed history. Tests for the presence of a specific antibody that will implicate specific allergens are also helpful and may be necessary for diagnosis.

Some forms of allergic reactivity, however, occur only in certain members of the population. These disorders (allergic rhinitis, asthma, and atopic dermatitis) are called **atopic disorders,** a term signifying an unusual form of reactivity for which there is some unknown and probably genetic predisposition. An individual with such a disorder is sensitized to substances usually considered innocuous to other people. Animal danders, feathers, spores from indoor molds, and house dust mites are the most common perennial allergens. Animal danders and emanations of house dust mites (high in mattress flock) and of cockroaches (abundant in poor housing situations) are important factors contributing to the allergenicity of house dust. Many variants of tree, grass and weed pollens, and molds cause atopic disorders in a more or less seasonal incidence (trees in the spring; grasses in late spring and summer; weeds in late summer and fall; and outdoor molds in summer and fall). Foods and a number of other substances may contribute to perennial or seasonal problems. Atopic individuals commonly become sensitized to one or more of these substances.

It is important to remember that many atopic disorders, including many cases of asthma and atopic dermatitis, are due to or are influenced by causes other than allergic sensitization.

PRINCIPLES OF DIAGNOSIS

The diagnosis of allergic disease is based primarily on the clinical findings. Laboratory procedures (including allergy testing) can be very helpful, but results should be interpreted in the light of the history and physical findings. Arriving at a diagnosis of any or all atopic diseases requires a detailed history and complete physical examination. More than one atopic disease may be present, and a history of familial atopic disorders or of other past or present atopic symptoms is especially useful. The following is a guideline for the overall history, physical examination, and supplementary diagnostic procedures.

History
A. Chief complaint of patient.

B. History of Present Illness: Details of development of first episode and circumstances of subsequent and most recent episodes. Areas of inquiry include infection, change in environment (family move, acquisitions of pets or toys, different household furnishings, improvement or worsening in symptoms with travel to different regions), season of year, ingestion of "new" food, special occasions, emotional and social upheavals.

C. Other Allergic Diseases: Associated atopic or other allergic diseases (past or present), especially allergic rhinitis, bronchial asthma, "allergic cough," atopic dermatitis, food intolerance (eg, colic, vomiting, abdominal pain, abnormal stools, skin rashes), eczema, hives, and angioedema.

D. Infections: History of pneumonia, bronchitis, bronchiolitis, croup, recurrent ear infections, recurrent or chronic sinusitis, removal of tonsils and adenoids.

E. Past therapy and response to it.

F. Emotional and Social Factors and Habits:

Family structure; general attitudes and behavior; family, school, and social adjustments.

G. Family History: Of allergic rhinitis, asthma, eczema, hives.

H. Environmental History: House pets; exposure to cigarette smoke; type of heating and air conditioning (including the presence of a central humidifier and other forms of heating such as a wood-burning stove); use of a portable vaporizer or humidifier; presence of mold or mildew in the home; details of patient's bedroom, including location in the home, composition and age of mattress and pillows, type of bedding and window dressing, and floor covering (age and type of carpet); details regarding day-care center or baby-sitter's home, including amount of time spent weekly, number of children, and presence of animals or cigarette smoke.

Physical Examination

A complete physical examination is essential. The following signs deserve special emphasis:

A. General Appearance of Patient: State of nourishment and physical development, including weight and height; degree of activity; signs of fatigue; sneezing; cough and its character; dyspnea.

B. Attitudes: Responses and relationships of the patient to parents, physician, nurses, etc.

C. Vital Signs: Blood pressure, temperature, pulse rate, and character of respirations.

D. Skin: Rashes, pallor, cyanosis, temperature changes, sweating, degree of dryness.

E. Eyes: "Allergic shiners" (lower lid edema, eye shadowing), conjunctival injection, blebs, itching, cataracts (in severe, long-standing atopic dermatitis), blepharitis (from chronic rubbing), tearing.

F. Nose: Itching ("allergic salute," "bunny nose," nasal crease), excoriation of nares, hyperemia, mucosal edema, polypoid changes, purplish pallor, excessive serous or mucoid discharge.

G. Ears: Hearing loss, changes in drum (immobility, distortion, retraction, fullness, opacity, narrow and "chalky" malleus), evidence of fluid in middle ear.

H. Mouth: Palatal malformations, character of speech, "canker sores," changes in tongue (geographism, grooving).

I. Throat: Presence and appearance of tonsils and pharyngeal lymphoid tissue, appearance of mucosal epithelium (anterior pillars, soft palate, pharyngeal wall), character of secretions.

J. Chest: Configuration ("barrel chest," "pigeon breast," prominent Harrison's grooves—all may be present in long-standing asthma), evidence of hyperinflation, pattern of breathing, development and use of accessory muscles for respiration (eg, hypertrophy of pectorals, trapezii, sternocleidomastoids), retractions.

K. Lungs: Relationship to inspiratory-expiratory cycle of gross or auscultatory wheezes (including wheezing brought on after exercise and forced expiration), rhonchi, or rales; degree and equality of air exchange; level and movement of diaphragm.

L. Heart: Tachycardia, size, accentuation of pulmonic second sound (for evidence of pulmonary hypertension in asthma), arrhythmias, murmurs.

Supplementary Diagnostic Procedures

A. Allergy Tests: In all atopic disorders, reaginic or skin-sensitizing (IgE) antibody is important. Testing for the presence of IgE antibody is potentially useful in identifying allergens that may play a role in the disorder.

1. Skin tests—Prick/puncture testing should be done first, because it is less likely than intradermal testing to cause severe reactions in sensitive individuals. Intradermal testing is about 100 times more sensitive than prick/puncture testing. The tests are read at the peak of the reaction, usually within 15–20 minutes. If these tests are negative, intradermal tests (on an extremity) may be performed. Skin testing is potentially dangerous in highly sensitive individuals; for this reason, epinephrine and a tourniquet should always be at hand as well as additional preparations for treatment of anaphylaxis (Table 33–1).

A positive test reaction occurs when antigen combines with skin-sensitizing (IgE) antibody, thus producing erythema, wheal, and flare (triple response) from the liberation of histamine and other chemical mediators. In properly interpreting the skin tests and assessing their clinical significance, the following should be kept in mind: (1) Mild reactions are less likely to be clinically significant than more strongly positive reactions. (2) Strong (3–4+) reactions to foods are likely to be of clinical significance (in contrast to mild reactions), but negative reactions do not rule out nonallergic (nor completely rule out allergic) clinical sensitivity. (3) A positive skin test suggests only that antibody is present in the skin. It may reflect past, present, or potential clinical hypersensitivity, but it is not necessarily clinically significant. The patient may or may not develop an atopic disease due to the specific allergen. The clinical importance of positive skin tests should be interpreted in correlation with the clinical history.

2. Serologic tests—The use of immunoassays to measure serum IgE antibody is increasing. The best known is the radioallergosorbent test (RAST), a radioimmunoassay, but enzyme-linked immunoassays that eliminate the need for radioactive material are also available.

Results of RAST and similar tests correlate well with those of skin tests, although the former are somewhat less sensitive. They are advantageous because they allow for testing of individuals in whom skin testing would be difficult (eg, patients with extensive dermatitis) and because there is no risk of provoking a hypersensitivity reaction. These tests would

Table 33–1. Preparations and dosages of drugs commonly used in allergic disorders.

Agent	Route	Dosage
ADRENERGIC AGENTS		
Albuterol	PO[1]	Short-acting: 2–4 mg every 8 hours. Long-acting: 4 mg every 12 hours. Extended-release[4]: 4–8 mg every 12 hours.
	Inhaled	One or two inhalations from pressurized aerosol.[2] May use as often as every 4 hours, but *avoid excessive use.* *or* 0.25–0.5 mL of 0.5% inhalant solution[4] diluted with 2 mL of water or saline administered by hand- or compressor-driven nebulizer. May use every 2–4 hours. In an emergency room, may use 0.15 mg/kg up to 1 mL every 20 minutes for three doses, then hourly.
Bitolterol[4]	Inhaled	One or two inhalations from pressurized aerosol. May use as often as every 4 hours, but *avoid excessive use.*
Epinephrine Aqueous 1:1000	SC, IM	0.01 mL/kg up to 0.3 mL. (May repeat at intervals of 15–20 minutes for a total of three doses.)
Suspension 1:200	SC	0.005 mL/kg up to 0.15 mL. May repeat in 8–12 hours. (Shake well before administering.)
Isoetharine	Inhaled	One or two inhalations from pressurized aerosol. May use as often as every 4 hours, but *avoid excessive use.* *or* 0.15–0.5 mL of 1% inhalant solution diluted with 2 mL of water or saline and administered by hand- or compressor-driven nebulizer. May use every 2–4 hours.
Metaproterenol	PO[2]	10–20 mg every 6–8 hours.
	Inhaled	One or two inhalations from pressurized aerosol. May use as often as every 4 hours, but *avoid excessive use.* *or* 0.1–0.3 mL of 5% inhalant solution diluted with 2 mL of water or saline and administered by hand- or compressor-driven nebulizer. May use every 2–4 hours.
Pirbuterol[4]	Inhaled	One or two inhalations from pressurized aerosol. May use as often as every 4 hours, but *avoid excessive use.*
Salmeterol[4]	Inhaled	Two inhalations every 12 hours for maintenance therapy or nocturnal symptoms.
Terbutaline[4]	PO	2.5 mg every 8 hours.
	SC, IM	0.01 mL/kg up to 0.25 mL. May repeat once after 20 minutes.
	Inhaled	One or two inhalations from pressurized aerosol. May use as often as every 4 hours, but *avoid excessive use.*
ANTIHISTAMINES		
Astemizole[4]	PO	10 mg once daily.
Chlorpheniramine Short-acting	PO	0.1 mg/kg/dose (up to 50 kg) four times daily.
Long-acting	PO	0.1–0.2 mg/kg/dose (up to 50 kg) twice daily.
Injectable	IM, IV	4–8 mg (if IV, give slowly).
Clemastine fumarate	PO	6–12 years: Up to 3 mg/d in two or three divided doses. Over 12 years: Up to 6 mg/d in two or three divided doses.
Cyproheptadine[1]	PO	0.25 mg/kg/d in three or four divided doses, not to exceed 16 mg daily.
Diphenhydramine hydrochloride	PO IM, IV	1 mg/kg/dose (up to 50 kg) four times daily. 25–50 mg (if IV, give slowly).
Hydroxyzine hydrochloride	PO	0.2–0.5 mg/kg/dose (up to 50 kg) three times daily.
Loratadine[4]	PO	10 mg once daily.
Terfenadine[4]	PO	60 mg twice daily.

(continued)

Table 33–1. Preparations and dosages of drugs commonly used in allergic disorders. (continued)

Agent	Route	Dosage
SYSTEMIC CORTICOSTEROIDS		
Hydrocortisone, dexamethasone, prednisolone, methylprednisolone	IV, PO	Most rapid therapeutic effect follows intravenous or oral administration, but there may be no perceptible effect for hours. In acute situations, high doses of corticosteroids (eg, 1 mg/kg/dose of methylprednisolone every 4–6 hours) are generally employed the first day and the dose tapered as rapidly as possible to maintenance levels or withdrawn completely. **Approximate equivalents of activity:** 100 mg hydrocortisone = 4 mg dexamethasone = 25 mg prednisolone = 20 mg methylprednisolone.
TOPICAL CORTICOSTEROIDS FOR ASTHMA AND RHINITIS		
Beclomethasone[2]	Inhaled	6–12 years: Up to ten inhalations per day in two to four divided doses. Over 12 years: Up to 16 inhalations per day.
	Intranasal	One spray in each nostril up to three times a day, or two sprays in each nostril twice a day. Discontinue if nasal bleeding occurs.
Dexamethasone sodium phosphate	Intranasal	One or two sprays in each nostril twice a day. (Should be used for short periods only.) Discontinue if nasal bleeding occurs.
Flunisolide[2]	Inhaled	Two inhalations twice a day.
	Intranasal	One spray in each nostril three times a day, or two sprays in each nostril twice a day. Discontinue if nasal bleeding occurs.
Triamcinolone[2]	Inhaled	6–12 years: Up to 12 inhalations per day in two to four divided doses. Over 12 years: Up to 16 inhalations per day.
	Intranasal	One or two sprays in each nostril once daily; up to two sprays in each nostril twice daily, or one spray in each nostril three times daily. Discontinue if nasal bleeding occurs.
OTHER DRUGS USED IN ALLERGIC DISORDERS		
Cromolyn sodium	Inhaled	Two inhalations from pressurized aerosol or one ampule (20 mg/2 mL) by hand- or compressor-driven nebulizer three or four times a day. May also be used just prior to exercise or contact with asthma-precipitating agent (eg, animals).
	Intranasal	One or two sprays in each nostril every 3–4 hours.
Nedocromil sodium[4]	Inhaled	Two inhalations from pressurized aerosol four times a day initially. This may be reduced to three or two times a day as maintenance dosage.
Aminophylline, theophylline	IV	4–6 mg/kg[5] every 4–6 hours (infuse over 10–20 minutes) or 0.6–1 mg/kg/h[5] as constant infusion.
	PO	16–24 mg/kg/day[5] (use with extreme caution in children under 1 year of age). Short-acting: every 6 hours. Long-acting: every 8–12 hours.

[1]Safety and efficacy for children under 2 years of age has not been established.
[2]Safety and efficacy for children under 6 years of age has not been estalished.
[3]Safety and efficacy for children under 4 years of age has not been established.
[4]Safety and efficacy for children under 12 years of age has not been established.
[5]Refers to theophylline dose. See text for further discussion of dosage.

be especially useful in testing for severe hypersensitivity to drugs and stinging insects; however, at present, these tests are for the most part less sensitive than skin tests. The usefulness of RAST and similar tests for this purpose is therefore somewhat limited. The number of antigens available for testing is also limited; furthermore, the greater expense of these tests and the delay in obtaining results make skin testing much preferable at this time.

B. Measurement of IgE Immunoglobulin Levels: The radioimmunosorbent test (RIST) measures the concentration of IgE immunoglobulin in the blood. Elevated IgE levels as measured by RIST or PRIST (paper RIST) suggest an atopic disorder, but the correlation is so imperfect that this is not a generally useful screening procedure. Greatly elevated IgE levels in infancy (> 2 SD above the mean) are highly predictive of an atopic diathesis, and elevated IgE levels in bronchiolitis suggest the diagnosis of asthma. However, a normal or low level of IgE does not rule out an atopic disorder or allergic sensitization.

C. Provocative Testing: The suspicion of the clinical importance of an allergen may be confirmed by the use of a "provocative test," ie, challenging a given individual with the suspected allergen and observing the response. Provocative testing may be employed but is not recommended as a routine procedure for any potentially severe disorder such as asthma and ordinarily should not be performed with a substance suspected of causing a potentially life-threatening reaction. Provocative tests are most valuable in determining clinical sensitivity to foods. Elimination and subsequent challenge may be especially revealing if done properly but also can be misleading if an objective protocol for assessing the response is not followed. Direct provocative inhalant testing is potentially hazardous and is best performed by specialists in an appropriate medical setting.

D. Eosinophilia: Increased numbers of eosinophils in the blood or bodily secretions (nasal, gastrointestinal) are frequently present in a variety of allergic conditions, especially in atopic disorders; the presence of eosinophilia may strengthen a suspicion of allergic diathesis. Nasal eosinophilia (> 15%) is highly suggestive of allergic rhinitis, but eosinophilia can occur in the absence of clinical allergies. Conversely, the absence of eosinophilia does not rule out allergy, particularly because a variety of factors (eg, concurrent infection, use of intranasal steroid) may suppress eosinophilia. The degree of eosinophilia correlates inversely with the degree of control of allergic and nonallergic asthma. Nasal eosinophilia in infants up to 3 months of age may be normal.

E. Controversial Techniques for Diagnosis And Treatment: Intracutaneous end point titration, sublingual and serial intracutaneous *provocative* titration tests, cytotoxic tests, and sublingual desensitization all have been claimed by some to be of value in diagnosing and treating allergic disorders. Their merit is yet to be validated scientifically, and they remain techniques of unproved value that are not recommended.

GENERAL PRINCIPLES OF TREATMENT

Environmental Control of Exposure

Because the clinical allergic reaction stems from the union of antigen with antibody, avoidance of the offending antigen is the most effective means of therapy of all allergic disorders. Moreover, there is reason to believe that continued exposure to an allergen can heighten sensitivity to other unrelated allergens and nonallergic irritants; thus, avoidance therapy has additional therapeutic implications. In many instances, complete avoidance of identified allergens is impossible, but it is frequently feasible to reduce the incidence and severity of reactions by minimizing the contact. Many nonimmune factors can precipitate or aggravate atopic disorders (eg, irritating smoke; cold air in asthma), and avoidance of such known or suspected irritants is also important.

The following are sample directions for environmental control of common (mostly) indoor allergens. They pertain mainly to the patient's bedroom, but the principles are applicable to the rest of the house as well.

(1) House dust is a common offender as an irritant and allergen (especially from mites and insects, cats, and dogs). The accumulation of dust may be minimized by the avoidance of dust catchers and dust producers, such as wool (in rugs and blankets), flannel (in bedding and pajamas), upholstered furniture, toys stuffed with plant or animal products, chenille (bedspreads, drapes, and rugs), cotton quilts, stuffed cotton pads, venetian blinds and carpets.

(2) Rooms should be dusted daily with a damp or oiled cloth. The room should be cleaned thoroughly at least once a week—never with the patient present.

(3) All forced air ducts, which frequently contain dust and molds and tend to stir up room dust, should be sealed off. An electric radiator may be substituted as a source of heat, if necessary. If pollinosis is a problem, windows should be kept closed during the pollen seasons. Air cleaners (central or room) and refrigerated air conditioners may be useful. Automatic humidifiers with provision for humidity not to exceed 40% can be helpful in dry climates and with heating systems. Humidifiers should be kept as free of mold as possible. In humid climates where dust mite, and mold sensitivity are more of a problem, dehumidification may be appropriate.

(4) Plant products (kapok, cotton) and animal products sometimes used for pillows, stuffing of furniture, toys, bedding, and hair pads for rugs should be eliminated. Alternatively, all mattresses, box springs, and pillows in the bedroom should be completely enclosed in impermeable plastic or rubber casings. Inexpensive casings may be obtained from department stores; better quality casings may be obtained from Environtrol, PO Box 31313, St. Louis, MO 63131; or Aller-Guard, Inc., Southgate Office Park, 1645 S.W. 41st Street, Topeka, KA 66609. Plastic casings especially should be checked periodically for tears or punctures. Furniture and bedding stuffed solely with synthetic products or rubber are permissible; rubber or foam pillows, however, may harbor molds. Toys stuffed with old nylon stockings or synthetic foam and covered with plain, nonfuzzy cotton or synthetic materials are satisfactory.

(5) Cleaning equipment, wool, and fur coats should not be kept in or near the child's room or closet.

(6) Sensitization to animals develops so frequently in atopic individuals that close contact with animals of any sort is best avoided. Danders, saliva, and urine are the important sources of allergen. Depending on the degree of sensitivity, it may be important to rid the environment of animals altogether. As a less satisfactory alternative to eliminating a cat or dog from the home, the animal should be washed weekly and kept out of the patient's bedroom at all times; the carpet removed from the child's bedroom and replaced with a throw rug, linoleum, or wooden floor; and a high-efficiency particulate air (HEPA) or other room filter used in the bedroom.

Hyposensitization (Immunotherapy)

If avoidance of offensive allergens is not possible, specific hyposensitization is sometimes attempted. The value of hyposensitization is limited mainly to atopic disorders and to severe insect allergy. There are a variety of hyposensitization procedures, but the same general principle applies to all: Extremely small amounts of allergen are injected subcutaneously at frequent intervals and in increasing amounts until a "top dose" is reached; this is usually the highest tolerated dose of a given allergen extract or that amount which induces a state of clinical hyporeactivity to the allergen as demonstrated after natural contact. When perennial therapy is adopted, the top tolerated dose is used as a maintenance dose, with carefully regulated lengthening of intervals generally up to 4 weeks, as tolerated.

Most allergists agree that the majority of well-selected patients with pollen asthma or hay fever are significantly improved after 1–2 years of therapy. There is evidence to substantiate the effectiveness of therapy in perennial and seasonal allergic rhinitis and in allergic asthma. The effectiveness of therapy is dose-related. Repository therapy using alum-precipitated extracts (Allpyral, Center-Al) is useful mainly in increasing the antigen dosage in individuals who are extremely sensitive to small amounts of aqueous antigen. Theoretically, fewer injections of alum-precipitated material are required to reach a maintenance dose of antigen, and maintenance injections need to be given less frequently. The value of hyposensitization against house dust mites is substantiated; it is beneficial but is no substitute for good environmental control. Venom therapy for sensitivity to stinging insects is efficacious and essential for those patients who have experienced a life-threatening systemic reaction following an insect sting. The use of bacterial extracts appears to be of little value and has been largely abandoned. Hyposensitization to foods in general is nonefficacious. For anaphylactic sensitivity to foods, hyposensitization is especially dangerous; it may be lifesaving but should be considered experimental at this time.

Drug Therapy

Many drugs are effective in the treatment of allergic disorders (Table 33–1). The principal groups include adrenergic agents, antihistamines, methylxanthines, cromolyn sodium, nedocromil sodium, anticholinergic agents, expectorants, oxygen, and adrenocorticosteroids. The selection of drugs depends upon the pathologic processes involved.

A. Adrenergic Agents: As a group, adrenergic agents exhibit many different pharmacologic effects. Their usefulness in allergic disorders depends mainly on their ability to constrict blood vessels and relax other smooth muscle. The manifestation of many allergic reactions is due, at least in part, to chemical mediators, such as histamine and leukotrienes, that produce varying degrees of vasodilation, edema, and smooth muscle spasm. Adrenergic agents are the principal pharmacologic antagonists of these chemical mediators and at times may even reverse their effects completely. However, the pharmacologic properties of adrenergic drugs as a group are not shared uniformly by all members of the group, and these drugs cannot be used interchangeably to produce a given effect. In rhinitis, for example, phenylephrine, an effective vasoconstrictor but a poor smooth muscle dilator, is especially useful. Albuterol, on the other hand, although devoid of vasoconstrictor action, is an effective bronchodilator and is useful in asthma. In anaphylaxis—in which vasodilation, edema, and asthma may all be a problem—epinephrine, which is a potent antagonist of all of these effects, is the drug of choice.

Adrenergic drugs are not always effective in a given disorder and are not without undesirable effects. Epinephrine resistance may occur in severe asthma, for example, and the repeated use of the drug in such cases may actually aggravate the disorder by increasing the patient's anxiety and contributing to venous congestion and mucus plugging. The injection of epinephrine when severe hypoxemia and acidosis are present may produce cardiac dysrhythmia or arrest. Adrenergic aerosols can be extremely effective in acute asthma, but some (eg, isoproterenol) have been shown to severely aggravate asthma if used excessively. Aerosols containing newer β_2-adrenergic drugs appear to be safer, but there is an unsettled issue whether chronic routine use of β_2-adrenergic aerosols may be detrimental. Recently, β_2-adrenergic agents which have prolonged (12-hour) durations of action have been developed (eg, salmeterol) .

B. Antihistamines: The antihistamines act through competition with histamine for receptors, preventing histamine from exerting its activity. There are three classes of antihistamines: H_1 receptor inhibitors, the classic antihistamines used for many years in allergic disorders; H_2 receptor inhibitors, which are useful in inhibiting gastric acid secretion; and agents that affect a newly identified H_3 receptor. H_1 antihistamines are particularly useful in urticaria, anaphylaxis, and allergic rhinitis; however, their effectiveness is limited in many disorders because numerous mediators unrelated to histamine operate in most allergic conditions. In certain circumstances, such as chronic urticaria and anaphylaxis, the combination of H_1 and H_2 antihistamines is therapeutic when either alone is not sufficiently effective.

Although antihistamines may be useful in severe allergic disorders, they are not the drug of first choice in medical emergencies due to allergic reactions but may be administered after epinephrine has been given. Antihistamines have antipruritic properties and are useful in atopic dermatitis and in contact dermatitis, in which histamine may play a major role. The sedation that occurs as a side effect, although undesirable in many instances, may be an advantage in others. On the other hand, the potential central nervous system depressant properties of most antihistamines may interfere with normal functioning, overtly or subtly. A small number of nonsedating antihistamines are available. Some antihistamines possess atropine-like drying actions. Although considered for years to be potentially harmful in asthma, it is now generally agreed that their use is not contraindicated for other allergic disorders when asthma is present; in fact, there is evidence for a beneficial effect on asthma in many patients.

C. Methylxanthines: Theophylline and its ethylenediamine derivative, aminophylline, are effective bronchodilators that appear to act at a different point but in the same pathway through which epinephrine exerts its dilating effect on smooth muscle. The improper use of these agents has been associated with severe toxic reactions, in some cases resulting in death. Overdosage frequently occurs as a result of failure to appreciate the variability of rate and extent of absorption with different routes of administration. Toxic reactions include headache, palpitations, dizziness, stomachache, nausea and vomiting, excessive thirst, and hypotension. Nausea and stomachache may be related to local irritation but can also represent a central nervous system-mediated toxic effect of the drug when administered by any route. In recent years, more subtle but significant toxicity, including behavioral changes, has been recognized but appear to be a transient problem for the most part . When used properly, theophylline and aminophylline are valuable drugs with a potent bronchodilating effect. There is great individual variation in the metabolism of methylxanthines, and dosage must be highly individualized. Optimal therapeutic blood levels of theophylline are considered to be 10–20 μg/mL serum or plasma, with levels over 20 μg/mL more likely to be associated with drug toxicity. *However, side effects such as behavioral changes and effects on attention span and learning occasionally can occur, especially in young children, at significantly lower levels.* Also, levels below 10 μg/ml can be therapeutic. Average dosages likely to achieve blood levels of 10–20 μg/mL are 25 ± 5 mg/kg/d between ages 1 and 8, then 20 ± 5 mg/kg/d until about age 16; thereafter, average daily dose is closer to 12 ± 3 mg/kg/d. A single daily dose can be given, or the daily dosage can be divided into two to four doses (every 6–24 hours), depending on the preparation used. Safe peak blood levels appear to be those below 15 μg/mL, and it is wise to keep peak blood levels below this concentration for chronic therapy. *In early to mid infancy, metabolism is markedly diminished, and methylxanthines should be employed with particular caution.* These drugs can be used at bedtime only as well in order to control nocturnal asthma.

For chronic administration of methylxanthines, long-acting preparations given orally are preferred. Theophylline levels should be monitored periodically in patients on chronic therapy. Factors known to accelerate theophylline clearance include young age (1–16) years, high-protein diet, smoking (tobacco and marihuana) and anticonvulsant drugs (phenobarbital or phenytoin). Theophylline clearance is inhibited by extremes in age (neonates and > 50 years), high-carbohydrate diet, ciprofloxacin, erythromycin, cimetidine, viremia, and congestive heart failure.

D. Expectorants: Expectorants such as guaifenesin (glyceryl guaiacolate) are used mainly in bronchial asthma to liquefy thick, tenacious mucus, but it is not clear whether any therapeutic effectiveness of these agents is in fact due to their expectorant action. Iodides seem more effective than guaifenesin, but—especially with prolonged use—goiter, salivary gland inflammation, gastric irritation, skin eruptions, and acne may occur. *Note:* It is important to keep in mind that adequate hydration is essential to effective expectoration. Expectorant preparations containing narcotics should be used cautiously in asthma.

E. Corticosteroids: Adrenal glucocorticoids have been used in the treatment of all of the allergic disorders. Their effectiveness is apparently due to their anti-inflammatory actions. The untoward side effects of prolonged systemic corticosteroid administration (eg, growth suppression, myopathy, Cushing's syndrome, hypertension, peptic ulcer [controversial], diabetes, cataracts, and osteoporosis) limit their use mainly to those conditions that are refractory to other measures or are life-threatening. Even then, however, their slow onset of action (even when given intravenously) precludes first-choice administration of these drugs in acute allergic emergencies. Most allergic syndromes are amenable to other forms of therapy, and the long-term systemic use of the corticosteroids usually is unnecessary. When chronic use is necessary, alternate-day corticosteroid therapy with a short-acting preparation (eg, prednisone) in the early morning every other day should be attempted. However, the development of inhalational corticosteroids with high topical potency but which are readily (albeit incompletely) inactivated on absorption makes the topical route of administration a more attractive option in asthma and rhinitis. In fact, the recognition that chronic asthma is in large part an inflammatory disorder has prompted increased enthusiasm for chronic therapy with topical corticosteroids in even milder forms of chronic disease. Topical use retains the potential for inducing steroid side effects depending upon dosage, duration of therapy, and individual patient sensitivity.

The main indications for the use of systemic corticosteroids are anaphylaxis, acute severe asthma, and control of chronic severe disorders, such as asthma, that are refractory to other appropriate therapy. In some instances, administration of a short course of corticosteroids for self-limiting allergic disorders (eg, serum sickness) may be warranted.

Topical corticosteroids are also extremely effective anti-inflammatory agents in the control of allergic dermatitis (mainly contact dermatitis and atopic dermatitis). Topical application is the preferred route of administration in such disorders, keeping long-term use of the more potent preparations to a minimum.

F. Sedatives: Sedatives have been grossly misused in asthma and have been responsible for some deaths. Although the psyche undoubtedly exerts a significant influence on asthma and other allergic disorders, the anxiety associated with extreme asthma is more often a reflection of the severity of the respiratory distress than the main cause of it. Sedatives that suppress the respiratory center (as the barbiturates do) should not be used in the therapy of severe asthma.

G. Oxygen: Oxygen is extremely important in the treatment of severe asthma. Hypoxemia usually occurs early in the course of moderately severe or severe asthma, much in advance of any detectable cyanosis. Oxygen is potentially drying and should be humidified when administered. Excessively high concentrations of oxygen should be avoided because they can lead to atelectasis or perhaps lessening of respiratory drive.

H. Antibiotics: There are no special indications for the use of antibiotics in allergic disorders. Antibiotics should be used when evidence of bacterial infection exists. However, their excessive use in children with allergic disorders should be avoided to reduce the risk of sensitization to these drugs.

Erythromycin seems to be one of the least sensitizing antibiotics and offers good coverage against many respiratory pathogens. It should be noted, however, that erythromycins interfere with theophylline metabolism and can elevate theophylline levels.

I. Cromolyn Sodium: This drug is used in the management of asthma and noninfectious rhinitis. It is considered to have anti-inflammatory activity, though the exact mechanisms of action are unclear. In many children, cromolyn sodium and perhaps nedocromil sodium are interchangeable with theophylline as first-line therapy for chronic asthma therapy and appear to be among the safest of antiallergic drugs. However, cromolyn sodium and nedocromil sodium do not reverse tissue changes induced by chemical mediators and are therefore of no value in the treatment of acute asthmatic paroxysms. Theophylline, on the other hand, is not considered to be as anti-inflammatory. Cromolyn sodium and probably nedocromil sodium are useful in blocking exercise-induced asthma and irritant- and allergen-provoked asthma if used prior to anticipated exposure to irritating agents. These drugs should receive further consideration for chronic anti-inflammatory therapy in children with asthma.

J. Other Prospective Drugs: Major pharmacologic advances in the control of allergic diseases have occurred in recent years. Currently, various drugs—many with novel pharmacologic properties—are under investigation. Some already are marketed in other countries. Among the more interesting drugs that may soon become available in the USA are ceterizine (a nonsedating antihistamine), azelastine (an antiallergic agent), and fluticasone propionate (a topical nasal steroid).

Prophylaxis of Atopic Disorders

There is suggestive evidence that the avoidance of cow products, eggs, wheat, and chicken during the first 9 months of life significantly lessens the likelihood of developing allergic rhinitis and asthma. There is also some evidence that a diet excluding cow products, fish, and eggs for the first 6 months of life, coupled with general environmental precautions to minimize contact with house dust and animal dander, is associated with a diminished likelihood of developing atopic dermatitis, at least in the first year. It seems prudent, therefore, to institute the dietary and environmental restrictions mentioned above in the first few months of life in children with a strong family history of atopy.

Hamilton RG et al: House dust aeroallergen measurements in clinical practice: A guide to allergen-free home and work environments. Immunol Allergy Pract 1992;14:96.

Hendeles L, Weinberger M: Safety and efficacy of theophylline in children with asthma. J Pediatr 1992;120:177.

Janssens MM: Introduction: Second-generation antihistamines. Clin Rev Allergy 1993;11:1.

Johnstone DE: The natural history of allergic disease in children and its intervention. Pediatr Asthma Allergy Immunol 1989;3:161.

Kemp JP: Nedocromil sodium, a new bronchial anti-inflammatory agent. Today's Ther Trends 1992;10:39.

Ohman JL: Allergen immunotherapy: Review of efficacy and current practice. Med Clin North Am 1992;76:977.

Shapiro GG: Diagnostic methods for assessing the patient with possible allergic disease. In: *Allergic Disease from Infancy to Adulthood,* 2nd ed. Bierman CW, Pearlman DS (editors). Saunders, 1988.

Szefler SJ: Anti-inflammatory drugs in the treatment of allergic disease. Med Clin North Am 1992;76:953.

Terr AI: In vitro tests for immediate hypersensitivity. Ann Rev Med 1988;39:135.

MEDICAL EMERGENCIES DUE TO ALLERGIC REACTIONS

The most common causes of severe allergic reactions are skin testing, hyposensitization with allergen extracts, drugs, insect stings, and food sensitivity. Anaphylaxis related to strenuous exercise has been described. Also, latex sensitivity with anaphylaxis during surgical procedures has been reported with increasing frequency in recent years. Anaphylactic shock, angioedema, and bronchial obstruction, alone or in combination, are the principal life-threatening manifestations of severe allergic reactions. Light-headedness, paresthesias, sweating, flushing, palpitations, and urticaria may precede or accompany severe reactions.

Prevention

Prevention consists mainly of avoiding allergens known or believed to be responsible for allergic reactions. A history suggestive of a reaction to a given drug is an indication that an alternative and unrelated drug should be selected for therapeutic use.

Treatment

A. Emergency Measures: Immediate treatment is essential for management of these reactions.

1. Epinephrine–Epinephrine, 1:1000, 0.2–0.4 mL, should be injected intramuscularly without delay. This may be repeated at intervals of 15–20 minutes as necessary. If the reaction is due to the recent injection of a drug, serum, or other substance, a tourniquet should be applied proximal to the injection. If the offending substance has been injected intradermally or subcutaneously, absorption of the material may be delayed further by injecting epinephrine, 0.1 mL subcutaneously, near the site of injection. Subsequent therapy depends partly upon the response.

2. Antihistamines–Antihistamines (Table 33–1) should be given intramuscularly or intravenously. When intravenous infusions are used, they should be given over a period of 5–10 minutes because untoward reactions, particularly hypotension, have been induced by too rapid administration. A combination of H_1 antihistamines (eg, diphenhydramine, hydroxyzine, chlorpheniramine) and H_2 antihistamines (eg, cimetidine) is recommended.

3. Theophylline–Theophylline is useful when bronchospasm occurs. (See also p 949.)

4. Tracheostomy–Tracheostomy may be lifesaving in cases of profound laryngeal edema.

5. Fluids–Because anaphylactic shock is in part produced by hypovolemia secondary to massive exudation of intravascular fluid, maintenance of a proper volume by intravenous fluids (isotonic saline, 5% dextrose in water, or 5% dextrose in saline) is particularly important.

B. Follow-Up Measures: Adrenocorticosteroids should be given only after epinephrine and antihistamines have been administered. The onset of action of these drugs is slow (hours, even by intravenous administration).

The patient should be watched for 24 hours because a recurrence (delayed anaphylaxis) has been noted in some cases many hours after initial treatment.

C. Hyposensitization for Insect Stings: Children who have experienced life-threatening reactions following an insect sting should be hyposensitized. A large local reaction or generalized urticaria *without* respiratory or cardiovascular compromise is probably not an indication for hyposensitization. The main allergens responsible for severe allergic reactions are found in the venoms of Hymenoptera (bees, wasps, hornets, and fire ants). Venom antigens for diagnosis and treatment are much more efficacious than whole body extracts, and the latter should no longer be employed. Hyposensitization with venom antigens, however, is associated with a high incidence of significant reactions in the course of treatment; testing and therapy are therefore best left to physicians experienced in dealing with insect allergy. Treatment kits for anaphylactic reactions should be available for immediate use in individuals with insect hypersensitivity and should be kept in the home or taken along by a responsible person when the sensitive person travels in an area likely to be infested with the offensive insects. The single most important item in such a kit is epinephrine. The patient and parents should be instructed in proper use of the kit and in ways to avoid insects. The kits should also be available for patients with severe recurrent allergic reactions from any cause.

Bochner BS, Lichtenstein LM: Anaphylaxis. N Engl J Med 1991;324:1785.

Sampson H, Mendelson L, Rosen JP: Fatal and near fatal anaphylactic reactions to food in children and adolescents. N Engl J Med 1992;327:380.

Saryan JA, O'Loughlin JM: Anaphylaxis in children. Am J Asthma Allergy Pediatricians 1992;5:89.

Valentine MD et al: The value of immunotherapy with venom in children with allergy to insect sting. N Engl J Med 1990;323:1601.

BRONCHIAL ASTHMA ("Reactive Airways Disorder")

Essentials of Diagnosis

- Paroxysmal or chronically exacerbating dyspnea characterized by bilateral wheezing, prolongation of expiration, hyperinflation of the lungs, and cough (overt wheezing may not occur).
- Reversal of abnormal pulmonary function to (or significantly toward) normal by inhalation of adrenergic aerosols or other therapeutic measures (can also reverse spontaneously).

- Eosinophilia of sputum and blood (common).
- IgE antibody to provoking allergens (common but not necessary).

General Considerations

Bronchial asthma is a largely reversible obstructive process of the tracheobronchial tree caused by inflammation with epithelial denudation, mucosal edema, increased and unusually viscid secretions, and smooth muscle constriction. Especially in protracted asthmatic episodes, the obstructive pathologic changes may cause not only hypoxemia but also retention of CO_2 and respiratory acidosis.

The incidence of asthma is reportedly less than 5% of the total population, but in the authors' opinion, this figure is a gross underestimation. Before adolescence, boys are affected twice as frequently as girls. Onset in early childhood is common (but asthma frequently begins in adulthood). In the majority of cases in childhood, the onset occurs by the seventh year.

Evidence of sensitization to inhalant allergens is found eventually in the majority of children with asthma. However, in many patients, offensive allergens cannot be identified by history or suggested by allergy testing, and it is uncertain that IgE-mediated allergy is related to the pathogenesis of the disorder. Nevertheless, allergic sensitization probably plays a major role in the pathogenesis of asthma in many if not *most* children and in many adults. When allergens contribute to or are major precipitants of asthma, "allergy" rarely is the sole significant factor involved (see below). The most common allergens causing asthma in children are inhalants: house dust mites; cockroach allergens, particularly in inner city areas; indoor molds; epidermals (especially the saliva and danders of cats and dogs); airborne pollens (trees, grasses, weeds); and out-of-doors seasonal molds. Foods occasionally provoke asthma, especially in infants, but do so less commonly in later childhood. The same allergens that cause asthma frequently cause allergic rhinitis in the same patient; many children who initially present with hay fever subsequently develop asthma. Parental smoking also may be a risk factor for asthma.

An important pathogenic feature of asthma is a "nonspecific" hyperreactivity of the tracheobronchial tree to various chemical mediators (eg, acetylcholine, histamine, leukotrienes) and, in turn, to various insulting agents or events that cause their activation or liberation. Because of this feature, asthma is sometimes called "reactive airways disorder." (However, airway hyperreactivity is not always present in asthma.) In addition to allergic reactions, numerous factors trigger or aggravate asthma, principally upper and lower respiratory tract infections of *viral* origin. The role of bacterial organisms in the precipitation of asthma is a disputed question, although there is evidence indicating that acute and chronic sinusitis can exacerbate asthma. Other triggering factors are rapid changes in temperature or barometric pressure, the common air pollutants in cities, odors, smoke, paint fumes, cold air, and exercise. Psychologic factors appear to be important in some cases but are seldom the sole cause. Aspirin idiosyncrasy can be a cause of asthma in childhood as well as in adult life.

Clinical Findings

A. History: Onset may occur as early as the first few weeks of life. Particularly in infancy, the first attack usually is associated with a lower respiratory tract infection or bronchiolitis. As age increases, there is a progressively greater tendency for initial and subsequent episodes to be associated with inhalant allergens or irritants. The initial inciting event appears to render the tracheobronchial tree more susceptible to reactions to both similar and unrelated precipitants.

A history of atopic dermatitis or allergic rhinitis is often noted. A family history of atopic diseases (especially allergic rhinitis and bronchial asthma) is often present and may arouse suspicion of the diagnosis. Asthma can (and all too frequently does) occur in the *absence of overt wheezing,* and complaints may include "chest congestion," prolonged cough, exercise intolerance, dyspnea, and recurrent bronchitis or pneumonia. A careful physical examination, including chest auscultation on a forced expiratory maneuver rather than on simple tidal volume, can be revealing, especially when the patient is experiencing clinical discomfort.

Episodes of asthma associated with infections may have a sudden onset but are frequently insidious in onset and prolonged; those due to specific, identifiable allergens tend to be acute in onset and relatively brief if the causative agent is removed. However, chronic allergen exposure to mites, cockroach, and animal allergens, for instance, *may produce chronic disease without an obvious cause-and-effect association.* Chronic exposure to cigarette smoke, in addition, may predispose to, intensify, and prolong asthma.

Bronchial asthma in infants (under 2 years of age) deserves special comment. The first attack usually follows by a few days the onset of a respiratory infection; some degree of cough or wheezing may persist for prolonged periods and becomes worse with subsequent "colds." In infants, the predominant symptoms may be dyspnea, excessive secretions, noisy and rattly breathing, cough, and, in many cases, some intercostal and suprasternal retractions—rather than the typical pronounced expiratory wheezes that occur in older children. Initial and repeated diagnoses of these episodes are apt to be croup, bronchiolitis, and pneumonia. Infection (viral) is often present.

A syndrome of paroxysmal cough, presumably tracheal in origin ("irritable trachea," "allergic cough"), occurs and may be difficult to differentiate from true asthma, particularly because bronchodilator drugs are sometimes effective in this condition. In this condition, wheezing generally does not occur and signs of lower respiratory tract obstruction are absent. The condition frequently is provoked by a (viral) respiratory infection, and allergic factors may or may not play a role. This condition also may presage later asthma.

B. Physical Examination: The following may occur during an acute, severe, or prolonged attack:

1. Distressing cough, dyspnea, increasing prolongation of expirations, high-pitched rhonchi and wheezes throughout the chest (diminishing in intensity as the obstruction becomes more severe), secretions (variable), hyperinflation, retractions, use of accessory respiratory muscles, poor air exchange.

2. Restlessness, apprehension, fatigue, drowsiness, coma.

3. Increasing tachycardia; initially, perhaps mild hypertension; ultimately, hypotension; rarely, signs of cardiac failure; pulsus paradoxus.

4. Flushed, moist skin; pallid cyanosis; dry mucous membranes.

5. Initially good response to inhalant adrenergic drugs or epinephrine. If the attack is prolonged, the response to the above drugs may be poor.

C. Laboratory Findings: Eosinophil accumulations (eg, clumps of eosinophils on sputum smear) and blood eosinophilia are commonly found but are often absent in infection or when corticosteroids are given. Their presence tends to reflect disease activity and does not necessarily mean that allergic factors are involved.

Hematocrit can be elevated with dehydration, as in prolonged attacks, or in severe chronic disease.

In severe asthma, the first sign is hypoxemia with a normal or low CO_2 level . Moderately severe hypoxemia may occur with low CO_2 tension due to a combination of hyperventilation and ventilation-perfusion disturbances. Respiratory acidosis and increased CO_2 tension may ensue.

D. Imaging: Bilateral hyperinflation, bronchial thickening, peribronchial infiltration, and areas of densities (patchy atelectasis or associated bronchopneumonia) may be present. (Patchy atelectasis is common and often misread as pneumonitis.) The pulmonary arteries may also appear prominent.

E. Pulmonary Function Studies: (See Chapter 17.) Increased airway resistance occurs with a decrease in flow rates, decreased vital capacity (VC), and increased functional residual capacity (FRC) and residual volume (RV). The first three may be normal in asymptomatic intervals, but residual hyperinflation is frequently chronic.

F. Allergy Tests: IgE antibodies to allergens may be present.

G. Provocative Tests:

1. Food and drugs–Reactions occur within minutes to hours after ingestion in sensitive children.

2. Inhalants–A reaction usually occurs immediately after inhalation and may occur again 4–8 hours later ("late" reaction). Asthma may occasionally be provoked by skin testing in unusually sensitive children.

Differential Diagnosis

Bronchial asthma may be confused with middle and lower respiratory tract infections (eg, laryngotracheobronchitis, acute bronchiolitis, bronchopneumonia, and pertussis), especially in the very young. Immunodeficiency (primarily defects in immunoglobulin production or function) may have associated cough and wheezing due to chronic lower respiratory tract infection.

Nasal "wheezes" may be transmitted to the chest (especially in infants) from upper airway edema, increased secretions, or other obstructing factors such as allergic rhinitis, upper respiratory tract infections, adenoidal hypertrophy, foreign body, choanal stenosis, and nasal polyps (eg, in cystic fibrosis).

Congenital laryngeal stridor is usually associated with other anomalies. Vocal cord dysfunction can masquerade as asthma.

In cases of tracheal or bronchial foreign body, dyspnea or wheezing is usually of sudden onset; on auscultation, the wheezes are usually but not always unilateral. Characteristic x-ray findings are not always present.

The differentiation between bronchial asthma and cystic fibrosis is made on the basis of high sweat sodium and chloride, a history (often present) in cystic fibrosis of serious pulmonary infection since birth, a personal and family history of associated intestinal disturbances with profuse, bulky stools, and pancreatic enzyme deficiency. Chronic inflammatory changes seen on chest x-ray in cystic fibrosis also can be a helpful differential point. There is evidence for a significant reactive airway (asthmatic) component with or without allergic precipitants in many children with cystic fibrosis, and cystic fibrosis and asthma can coexist. In these children, asthma therapy is helpful.

Tracheal or bronchial compression by extramural forces may resemble asthma and may be due to foreign body in the esophagus, aortic ring, anomalous vessels, or inflammatory or neoplastic lymphadenopathy.

Wheezing may be present in immotile cilia syndrome, but chronic upper respiratory tract infections (sinusitis and otitis media) and recurrent pneumonias are usually more common manifestations because of the lack of mucociliary clearance.

Treatment of Mild & Moderate Asthma

A. Specific Measures: The patient should avoid contact with proved or suspected irritants and allergens as much as possible. (See Environmental Control of Exposure.) Hyposensitization therapy is for allergens that cannot be avoided (eg, pollens, seasonal molds, and house dust mites) when such allergens play a substantial role in the disorder.

B. General Measures: Depending upon the frequency and severity of asthma, some or all of the measures listed below may be used, either with the onset of an asthmatic attack or as a constant regimen—especially during the times of year when asthma is most severe.

1. Education–The parents (and patient, if old enough) must understand the asthmatic process. Complete understanding of all recommendations is essential. The educational process may also need to extend to school personnel and baby-sitters.

2. Liquefaction and expectoration of mucus–Maintain adequate hydration by encouraging oral fluid intake, or give intravenous fluids if necessary. The value of expectorants is dubious.

3. Bronchodilation–The major bronchodilating drugs are theophylline (aminophylline) and adrenergic drugs used alone or in combination with theophylline. Adrenergic aerosols are extremely useful but must not be abused. Adequate dosing and proper technique of administration are extremely important in therapy. Aerosolized agents can be as effective as injected drugs in reversing acute severe asthma and have fewer side effects.

4. Control of inflammation–Because of evidence of ongoing inflammation even in mild asthma, topical corticosteroids, cromolyn sodium, or nedocromil sodium should be an early consideration for long-term routine therapy combined with bronchodilators as needed to maximize lung function and minimize symptoms. In children with severe acute asthma or with chronic asthma unresponsive to other measures, including topical corticosteroids, systemic adrenal glucocorticoids may be indicated. If chronic use of oral corticosteroids is necessary for adequate control of asthma, prednisone or a short-acting equivalent given before 8:00 AM on alternate days should be attempted.

5. Antibiotics–If there is evidence of bacterial infection, give antibiotics. Leukocytosis up to 15,000/μL is common in acute severe asthma without any evidence of bacterial infection (even higher counts can be seen after epinephrine administration). Patchy atelectasis can be confused with pneumonitis on x-ray film.

6. Breathing and fitness exercise–In children with chronic or recurrent asthma, breathing and fitness exercises under the guidance of a properly trained physical therapist may help improve the patient's cardiopulmonary status, including muscular functions of the thoracic cage.

Exercise should be encouraged rather than restricted. Exercise-induced bronchospasm can be ameliorated, if necessary, by cromolyn sodium or nedocromil sodium or with adrenergic aerosol, or both, just prior to exercise; by theophylline given 1–2 hours before exercise; or by a combination of these.

7. Daily regimen for control of asthma–Children with frequent overt asthma attacks (eg, one or two per week) and evidence of more or less constant pulmonary obstruction should be on constant pharmacologic therapy. Theophylline (taken orally) and cromolyn sodium and nedocromil sodium (three or four times daily by inhalation) may be considered first-line drugs for chronic symptomatic asthma in addition to adrenergic drugs. The latter two drugs appear to be more anti-inflammatory and are particularly recommended for long-term therapy in children. Topical corticosteroids may be added or used in place of cromolyn, nedocromil, and particularly theophylline, which has relatively little anti-inflammatory activity. Anticholinergics may be useful for the patient with a strong cough or irritant component.

8. Airflow assessment–In instances when perception of the degree of airflow limitation may be poorly appreciated by the parents or patient, have the patient use a peak flow meter at home to assist in assessment of airflow. Peak flow meters can also be helpful in monitoring progress of patients who require around-the-clock therapy and assist in determining medication requirements.

Treatment of Acute Severe Asthma (Status Asthmaticus, Intractable Asthma)

This is a medical emergency!

A. Emergency Care: Aerosolized adrenergic drugs given by a compressed air device, preferably with oxygen, are the drugs of first choice. Aerosolized adrenergic drugs have been found to be as effective as epinephrine, at least in older children, and have the advantage of minimizing systemic side effects. These drugs can be used every 20–60 minutes. The more specific β_2 agonists such as albuterol are recommended. Dosages that do not induce jitteriness or tachycardia are used. In severe asthma unresponsive to initial aerosolized therapy, epinephrine (1:1000 solution) may be used, followed in 10–15 minutes by additional aerosolized treatments. The lack of therapeutic response to adrenergic drugs is sometimes used as the criterion for "status asthmaticus." Relative or apparently complete lack of responsiveness to these drugs may be due to hypoxemia and acidosis, bronchial obstruction with thick mucus plugs, pneumothorax, or simply severe asthma. Sensitivity to adrenergic drugs may improve after initiation of other therapy.

B. Hospital Care: If signs are relatively early, an overnight stay may suffice. Close follow-up after discharge from the hospital or emergency room is essential, however.

1. Give 5% dextrose solution with 0.2% saline intravenously at the first sign of resistance to adrenergic drugs or when there is poor fluid intake, vomiting, or dehydration. (Use maintenance requirements; *do not* *overhydrate.*) Particularly if corticosteroids are used, remember to add potassium (10–20 meq/L of intravenous fluid) after urination is established.

2. Give moisturized oxygen (by mask or nasal prongs–not by tent) at a flow rate of approximately 4 L/min. All patients with acute severe asthma will be hypoxemic, largely as a result of the ventilation-perfusion imbalance that is integral to asthma.

3. The effectiveness of aminophylline when given in addition to aggressive therapy with β_2-adrenergic agents is unclear. If aminophylline is used, give 4–6 mg/kg in intravenous tubing over a 10- to 20-minute period (if not already receiving theophylline the previous 4 hours) and repeat every 4–6 hours, or give as a constant infusion beginning with a loading dose of 4–6 mg/kg over 15 minutes and then 0.6–1 mg/kg/h.*

Age	Average Total Daily Dose ± SD
12 months to 8 years	25 ± 5 mg/kg
8–16 years	20 ± 5 mg/kg
Over 16 years	12 ± 3 mg/kg

4. Take an arterial blood sample for pH, PCO_2, and PO_2 determinations. Early in the course of an asthmatic paroxysm, the patient usually hyperventilates and blows off CO_2, with a resultant low $PaCO_2$. (A normal $PaCO_2$ in acute severe asthma, in other words, is an indication of impending respiratory failure.) Continued close monitoring of blood gases and pH is essential to proper management of severe asthma. (Determination of gases or pH on capillary blood generally is unreliable.) An ear oximeter can be used to measure oxygen saturation of the blood; this is a useful substitute for measurement of arterial blood oxygen only.

5. Attempt to correct acidosis (pH 7.3 or below) with sodium bicarbonate. With the increased work of breathing and hypoxemia, there may be metabolic acidosis due to lactic acid production. This may be compensated by a respiratory alkalosis due to hyperventilation. The appropriate bicarbonate dose may be calculated with the following formula:

Bicarbonate needed (meq) = Negative base excess
× 0.3 × Body weight (kg)

---

*In patients receiving chronic theophylline therapy, use the usual total daily maintenance dose infused over a 24-hour period. Theophylline blood levels of 10–20 µg/mL serum are considered "optimally therapeutic" for hospitalized patients, but levels should be on the low side of this range when theophylline is used on a long-term basis. Average total daily dosages of theophylline to achieve therapeutic levels are listed, but there is much individual variation in requirements. *Caution:* In the first few months of life, theophylline (aminophylline) is metabolized very slowly, and *this drug should be used (if at all) with extreme caution in patients at this age* .

The bicarbonate can be given rapidly by the intravenous route. (Sodium bicarbonate for injection may be obtained in ampules or multidose vials that contain approximately 1 meq/mL.) Arterial or venous pH should be redetermined 5–10 minutes later, and further correction of acidosis, using bicarbonate, should be considered at that time if necessary. In respiratory failure, in the absence of a pH determination, 2 meq/kg may be infused initially.

6. Give albuterol, 0.5% by inhalation, or other adrenergic aerosols every 1–4 hours or by continuous nebulization . (The proper use of aerosolized adrenergic agents early in the course of acute severe asthma may obviate the need for injected epinephrine or aminophylline.)

7. If the patient is already receiving corticosteroids, do not withdraw the medication; rather, increase the dose temporarily. Patients requiring hospitalization should receive corticosteroids promptly, even though patients may not realize the full benefit from the medication for 48 hours. The use of corticosteroids in status asthmaticus reduces the morbidity and mortality and accelerates the recovery by reducing inflammation and by potentiating the effectiveness of adrenergic drugs. (For dosage schedule, see Table 33–1.) As the symptoms are relieved, the dose should be decreased as rapidly as possible and maintained at the lowest dose that controls symptoms. (If the patient has not been on prolonged corticosteroid therapy within the past year, the corticosteroids can be discontinued abruptly rather than tapered. It is frequently feasible to use high doses of corticosteroids for 48 hours or less.)

8. Give antibiotics as indicated.

9. Mist tents are not beneficial and may actually increase bronchospasm because of an irritant effect.

10. Respiratory failure that does not respond to the above therapy may require assisted ventilation by a mechanical respirator. *Intubation and assisted ventilation should be performed only by medical personnel trained in such techniques.*

C. Precautions in Therapy:

1. Do not use narcotics or barbiturates. (They depress the respiratory center. Tranquilizers may do the same in the presence of severe hypoxemia.) Severe cough due to irritation may necessitate use of nondepressant doses of antitussives, however.

2. Do not use epinephrine excessively. (It tends to thicken secretions, deplete glycogen stores, and increase apprehension.)

D. Follow-Up Therapy:

1. Fluids–When the patient is improved and is able to take fluids or oral medications, give fluids orally in the form of fruit juices. Give no fluids that contain caffeine or chocolate if the patient is receiving theophylline . Give no milk or iced drinks.

2. Drugs–The following medications are of value at this stage:

a. Adrenergic aerosol every 4–6 hours.

b. Resume maintenance medications or start inhalational corticosteroids until outpatient recheck or asymptomatic with good peak flows.

c. If systemic corticosteroids have been started, withdraw after 72 hours or taper gradually and discontinue as soon as possible.

Prognosis

In the past 25–30 years, the morbidity and mortality rates in asthma have increased. Mortality statistics indicate that a high percentage of deaths have been due to underrecognition of asthma severity and *undertreatment,* particularly in labile asthmatics and asthmatics whose perception of pulmonary obstruction is poor. "Continuity" symptoms of night cough, breathlessness, and wheezing provoked by exercise or exposure to allergens or irritants usually indicate more serious disease than do occasional, spontaneous, and brief attacks due to recognizable allergens with symptom-free periods in between. Prolonged exposure of asthmatic children to cigarette smoke ("passive smoking") may be associated with an increased risk of irreversible small airway obstruction in adulthood.

There is no evidence that bronchial asthma can be cured, and there is evidence for ongoing inflammation even in asthmatics asymptomatic for prolonged periods. There also is evidence that the rate of decline of lung function in adulthood is abnormally high in many asthmatics and that there may be decreased growth of lung function in children with moderate to severe asthma . On the other hand, the prognosis for symptom-free control in childhood asthma is fairly good. The majority of asthmatic children have less symptomatic asthma in their teens, and some appear to achieve freedom from any asthmatic symptomatology, perhaps for life. Unfortunately, however, only a minority (probably < 30%) fall into this category, and it is usually the pediatrician rather than the disorder that the child outgrows. Many asthmatics have persistent, significant (though often unrecognized) chronic pulmonary obstruction, and others later redevelop symptomatic obstruction. Mild asthma is more likely to be outgrown than moder ate or severe asthma.

Asthma: A follow-up statement from an international paediatric asthma consensus group. Arch Dis Child 1992; 67:240.

Canny GJ, Levison H: Childhood asthma: A rational approach to treatment. Ann Allergy 1990;64:406.

Canny GJ: Silent asthma. Am J Asthma Allergy Pediatricians 1992;5:181.

Cross D, Nelson HS: The role of the peak flow meter in the diagnosis and management of asthma. J Allergy Clin Immunol 1991;87:1220.

Furukawa CI et al: The proper role of β_2 adrenergic agonists in the treatment of children with asthma. Pediatrics 1992;90:639.

Li JTC, Reed CE: What role for immunotherapy for allergic asthma. J Respir Dis 1992;13:1735.

McFadden ER Jr, Gilbert IA: Asthma. N Engl J Med 1992; 327:1928.

National Asthma Education Program: Guidelines for the diagnosis and management of asthma. Department of Health & Human Services Publication No. 91–3042, 1991.

Pearlman DS: Bronchial asthma: A perspective from childhood through adulthood: Update. Pediatr Asthma Allergy Immunol 1989;3:191.

Phelan P: The natural history of childhood asthma on adult life. Immunol Allergy Pract 1988;10:334.

Sears MR: Fatal asthma: A perspective. Immunol Allergy Pract 1988;10:259.

Strunk RS: Getting asthmatics out of the "I can't exercise" slump. J Respir Dis 1991;12:377.

Toogood JH: Making better—and safer—use of inhaled steroids. J Resp Dis 1993;14:221.

Van Bever HP, Stevens WJ: Pharmacotherapy of childhood asthma. An inflammatory disease. Drugs 1992;44:36.

ALLERGIC RHINITIS

Essentials of Diagnosis

- Chronic or recurrent nasal obstruction; itching and sneezing (frequently paroxysmal), with seromucoid discharge. There may be accompanying conjunctival injection and itching, with or without tearing.
- Mucosal hyperemia to purplish pallor and edema of nasal mucous membranes.
- Eosinophils of nasal secretions when symptomatic (frequent).
- Presence of IgE antibody to provoking allergens.

General Considerations

Allergic rhinitis is the most common atopic disease, perhaps because the nose is anatomically and physiologically vulnerable to inhalant allergens. The pathologic changes are chiefly hyperemia, edema, and increased serous and mucoid secretions due to mediator release, all of which lead to variable degrees of nasal obstruction, rhinorrhea, and pruritus. Inhalant allergens are principally responsible for symptoms, but food allergens on occasion may provoke rhinitis.

Classification

Allergic rhinitis may be classified as perennial, seasonal (hay fever), or episodic, but these entities frequently occur concomitantly. Children with allergic rhinitis seem to be more susceptible to upper respiratory infections, which in turn intensify the symptoms of existing allergic rhinitis.

A. Perennial Allergic Rhinitis: Perennial allergic rhinitis occurs to some degree all year long but may be more severe in winter. Nasal stuffiness, frequent sniffing, and constant rhinorrhea with evidence of mild to moderate itching (frequent nose rubbing) are often the dominant symptoms, although more severe symptoms, including paroxysmal sneezing, may occur. Sneezing is often most pronounced in the morning shortly after waking. Poor appetite, fatigue, and pharyngeal irritation from nasopharyngeal mucus drainage are frequent accompanying symptoms. Greater exposure to house dust allergens during the winter months is due to increased indoor activities and heating systems that raise, disperse, and circulate dust. The increased dryness of heated air and greater exposure to pets housed indoors may also add to the problem.

This disease frequently begins before the second year of life. It often accompanies bronchial asthma and may be provoked by the same allergens. Dental abnormalities, including disturbances in dental arch growth and malocclusion, have been attributed to long-standing perennial allergic rhinitis with nasal obstruction.

B. Seasonal Allergic Rhinitis (Hay Fever): Hay fever occurs seasonally as a result of exposure to specific wind-borne pollens. The major important pollen groups in the temperate zones are trees (late winter, early spring), grasses (spring to early summer), and weeds (late summer to early fall). Seasons may vary significantly in different parts of the country. Mold spores also cause seasonal allergic rhinitis, principally in the summer and fall.

The age of onset is generally later than that of perennial allergic rhinitis, usually after 2 years of age. Worsening or extension of pollen sensitivities over a period of several years after onset can be expected.

Clinical Findings

A. Symptoms and Signs: Nasal obstruction is manifested by mouth breathing, snoring, difficulty in nursing or eating, nasal speech, and inability to clear the nose with blowing. Nasal seromucoid secretions are increased, with anterior drainage, sniffling, "nasal stuffiness," postnasal drip, and loose cough. Nasal itching leads to nose rubbing ("allergic salute," "bunny nose"), nose picking, epistaxis, and sneezing. Eye manifestations consist of itching, tearing, conjunctival injection, lid and periorbital edema, and circumorbital cyanosis ("allergic shiners"). Palatal and pharyngeal irritation and frank fatigue often occur. In perennial rhinitis, nasal obstruction tends to be a predominant symptom; in seasonal rhinitis, there tends to be more intense itching, coryza, and sneezing.

Examination shows decreased patency of nasal airways and increased seromucoid discharge (usually more serous in seasonal rhinitis). The mucous membranes range from reddened with little edema to pale blue, swollen, and boggy, with dimpling in the turbinates. Increased pharyngeal lymphoid tissue from chronic pharyngeal drainage or enlarged tonsillar and adenoid tissue may be present. Bleeding points or ulceration may be seen on the anterior nasal septum. There may be a horizontal crease extending across the lower third of the nose, owing to frequent upward rubbing of the nose. Malocclusion (overbite), presumably due to chronic mouth-breathing and excess pressure of digit sucking to relieve palatal itching, may be seen in long-standing cases.

The florid conjunctival injection, coryza, intense itching of the eyes and nose, and violent sneezing experienced by older children and adults are not so commonly seen in young children. Paroxysmal sneezing, however, is frequent even in young children.

B. Laboratory Findings: Eosinophilia frequently can be demonstrated on smears of nasal secretions or blood. This is a frequent but not universal finding in allergic rhinitis and reflects mast cell or basophil mediator release. The presence of eosinophils, in addition to suggesting the probability of allergic mechanisms, indicates the likelihood that antiallergic medications will be helpful in therapy, whether or not allergic mechanisms are operative. Eosinophils in numbers consistently greater than 15% or in clusters on nasal smears are suggestive of this disorder.

C. Allergy Testing: Skin or serologic tests reveal IgE antibody to offending allergens.

D. Associated Conditions: Sinusitis may accompany allergic rhinitis and is frequently demonstrated on x-ray film (mucosal thickening, fluid levels, or complete opacification of sinuses). Vigorous treatment is indicated until there is resolution of x-ray as well as clinical findings.

Auditory tube dysfunction and chronic or recurrent serous or secretory otitis media can also be a complication of allergic rhinitis. The atopic young child seems particularly prone to the development of serous otitis media. The middle ear is rarely a "shock organ" for allergy per se; rather, otitis media is related to auditory tube dysfunction that can be associated with allergic rhinitis. There is little evidence that allergy-associated serous otitis media exists in the absence of allergic rhinitis.

Nasal polyps are unusual in children and generally are not caused by allergy. When polyps are present, cystic fibrosis should be considered.

Differential Diagnosis

The most common disorder which must be differentiated from allergic rhinitis is **vasomotor rhinitis** This nonallergic, noninfectious form of perennial rhinitis, which occurs in children and adults, masquerades as allergic rhinitis. Manifestations of the condition include variable degrees of serous or mucoid rhinorrhea and nasal stuffiness, often with pharyngeal drainage. Rarely, there may be nasal eosinophilia. Diagnosis depends upon ruling out an allergic or infectious cause.

Other disorders that must be differentiated from allergic rhinitis include the common cold, other infectious diseases (eg, purulent rhinitis and sinusitis), adenoidal hypertrophy, foreign bodies (usually unilateral), nasal polyposis associated with cystic fibrosis or aspirin idiosyncrasy (nasal polyposis is rarely due to allergy), choanal stenosis or atresia, nasopharyngeal neoplasms, and palatal malformations (eg, congenitally high arch, cleft palate).

Treatment

A. Specific Measures:

1. Avoid exposure to proved allergens to the extent reasonably possible.

2. Immunotherapy should be considered when symptoms are severe and other symptomatic measures have failed or when the disease is associated with complications such as chronic or recurrent sinusitis, recurrent serous otitis media, and hearing loss. There is controversial evidence that immunotherapy for hay fever may prevent the onset of asthma.

B. General Measures:

1. Give antihistamines with or without vasoconstricting adrenergic drugs by mouth. (See Table 33–1.)

2. Nasal cromolyn (Nasalcrom) may be used alone or in conjunction with the medications named in the first measure, above.

3. Treat associated infections.

4. Topical decongestants (eg, phenylephrine) can be used for no more than 5 days for severe episodes.

5. Topical corticosteroids can be used for nasal symptoms not controllable by other means, but care must be taken to prevent patient overuse or complications, including nasal bleeding and potential nasal septal perforation.

6. Surgical procedures (removal of nasal polyps, corrective surgery for maxillary sinusitis, insertion of ventilating tubes for chronic otitis media) should be considered only when medical therapy fails.

Prognosis

A. Perennial Allergic Rhinitis:
Unless specific allergens can be identified and eliminated from the environment or diet (unusual cases), this atopic disease tends to be very protracted. However, nasal obstruction may become less troublesome as the child grows and the nasal airway increases in caliber.

B. Seasonal Allergic Rhinitis:
Hay fever patients tend to suffer repeatedly from their seasonal symptoms if exposure to offending allergens is high. These symptoms are expected to be most severe from adolescence through early to mid adult life. On moving to a region devoid of problem allergens, patients may be free of seasonal allergic rhinitis for 1–3 years but frequently acquire new pollen hypersensitivities from airborne pollens in the areas to which they move.

Allansmith MR, Ross RN: Ocular allergy. Clin Allergy 1988;18:1.

Busse WW (Chairman): A comprehensive approach to managing allergic rhinitis and nasal congestion. J Respir Dis 1992;13(Suppl 8);1.

International Symposium on Allergy and Associated Disorders in Otolaryngology. J Allergy Clin Immunol 1988; 81(Part 2):1.

Druce HM: Allergic and nonallergic rhinitis. In: *Allergy Principles and Practice,* 4th ed. Middleton E Jr et al (editors), Mosby, 1993.

ATOPIC DERMATITIS*
(Infantile Eczema)

Essentials of Diagnosis

- Lesions varying from erythematous and papular to scaling, vesicular, and oozing; lichenification in more chronic forms.
- Predilection in infants for cheeks and extensor areas and in older children and adolescents for flexural creases.
- Pruritus, frequently intense.

General Considerations

Atopic dermatitis is considered to be an atopic disorder because of its frequent association with allergic rhinitis and asthma and the high incidence of IgE antibodies in children with this disorder. Children with atopic dermatitis have many immune aberrations, but the role of these immune defects is also unclear. The common denominator in all individuals with atopic dermatitis appears to be a lowered threshold for itching; atopic dermatitis has been called "an itch that rashes."

In some infants and children, IgE antibody to one or more foods can be demonstrated; ingestion of a food(s) to which IgE antibody is present has been shown to be a major cause of the eczema in many cases. The presence of IgE antibody to a food also may be of no clinical importance, however; it appears to be a necessary but not sufficient condition for food-induced eczema. Foods implicated most frequently in atopic dermatitis include egg white, milk, legumes (including peanut butter), wheat, and corn. Certain foods, especially citrus fruits and tomatoes, may induce facial erythema in children with atopic dermatitis but generally do not induce more extensive dermatitis. Inhalant allergens also can play an important and even critical role in the pathogenesis of atopic dermatitis, in some instances probably by direct skin contact (eg, animal allergens, house dust mites).

Scratching plays a major role in the occurrence and progression of dermatitis, predisposing the skin to infection. Factors that aggravate itching include dryness, sweating, and contact with rough materials and detergents. Psychologic factors may intensify itching and complicate management at home and at school.

---

*From the perspective of a pediatric allergist (see also Dermatitis, Chapter 16).

Clinical Findings

A. Symptoms and Signs: Although infantile eczema ordinarily begins in infancy, it can begin at almost any time in childhood. In infants, lesions typically appear after 2 months of age, beginning on the cheeks and forehead and spreading in a patchy or generalized distribution over the extremities and trunk. Initially, involvement of extremities is primarily on extensor surfaces, but after infancy, involvement of flexural creases (antecubital, popliteal, neck) predominates; frequently, the wrists, hands, feet, face, and eyelids are also involved. The lesions may vary from facial erythema and minimal scaling to frank oozing and "weeping." As the child grows older, the eczema tends to wax and wane, sometimes disappearing completely for months, and in many children abates altogether by age 3 years. The skin may be thickened and somewhat plaque-like (lichenified) because of long-standing irritation from scratching. Although scarring is unusual, hyperpigmentation and hypopigmentation may occur. Excessive skin dryness is a frequent concomitant finding in eczema, and a form of congenital ichthyosis often accompanies atopic dermatitis. Infection sometimes occurs; however, it is not usual, even though the concentration of staphylococci in and on the skin of children with atopic dermatitis tends to be much higher than normal.

B. Laboratory Findings: There are no practical tests for atopic dermatitis. IgE immunoglobulin levels are frequently elevated, and there may be specific IgE antibodies to various inhalant and food allergens. Evidence of IgE antibody to a food allergen may or may not be clinically relevant; therefore, a trial elimination and challenge to that food is recommended. IgE antibody to inhalants also suggests only the possibility of clinical relevance to the disease. Eosinophilia may occur.

Differential Diagnosis

Seborrheic dermatitis may be distinguished by a lack of significant pruritus, its predilection for the scalp ("cradle cap"), and its coarse, yellowish "potato chip" scales. Seborrheic dermatitis may occur in association with atopic dermatitis. Candidiasis occurs predominantly in the diaper region and is characteristically intensely red, with satellite lesions. Contact dermatitis is distinguished chiefly by the distribution of lesions (usually on extensor and exposed areas), generally with a greater demarcation of dermatitis than in atopic dermatitis. Nummular eczema is characterized by coin-shaped plaques, with minimal to sometimes intense eczema. Scabies is more papulovesicular and relatively nonerythematous, occurring chiefly in the interdigital and waistline areas, with itching that may be intense, particularly at night; because of scratching, an eczematous dermatitis may develop.

Various other disorders have associated skin eruptions that may resemble atopic dermatitis. These include Wiskott-Aldrich syndrome, X-linked agammaglobulinemia, ataxia-telangiectasia, severe combined immunodeficiency disease, phenylketonuria, Hurler syndrome, and Hartnup syndrome.

In Buckley's syndrome, there is marked elevation of IgE, with a dermatitis associated with increased susceptibility to infectious agents, especially staphylococci. The skin eruption is easily distinguishable from atopic dermatitis.

Complications & Sequelae

Bacterial skin infections, particularly those produced by staphylococcal and streptococcal organisms, occur with some frequency. Viral infections, mainly with herpesvirus (Kaposi's varicelliform eruption), can occur from exposure to individuals with herpetic lesions, and varicella can be unusually severe in children with atopic dermatitis, although this generally is not a problem.

Nutritional disturbances may result from unwarranted and unnecessarily vigorous dietary restrictions imposed by physicians and parents. Cataracts in late childhood or adulthood occur in a small percentage of cases, even when corticosteroids are not used in treatment. Temporary or chronic emotional disturbances may occur as a result of feelings of disfigurement, imposed restrictions, and unhealthy attitudes of parents toward a child with this disease. Poor academic performance and behavioral disturbances may be a result of uncontrolled intense or frequent itching.

Treatment

Good general skin care and vigorous specific dermatologic treatment are the most important aspects of treatment of atopic dermatitis. Any foods that have been shown to aggravate eczema should be eliminated, provided that the diet remains nutritionally adequate. Minimizing direct contact with irritants (wool and other rough materials, irritating soaps and detergents) and allergens (eg, animal emanations, house dust mites, molds), avoiding excessive sweating, and maintaining good skin hydration are important. Immunotherapy is generally of unclear value in atopic dermatitis.

A. General Skin Care: Provide good skin hydration and have the patient bathe at least once daily (even in dry climate), using a bath oil (Alpha Keri or Lubath) added halfway through the bath; superfatted and nonirritating soaps (Basis, Dove, Lowila, Neutrogena) should be used. The skin should be thoroughly rinsed. The skin may be patted partly dry, and areas that are ordinarily excessively dry can then be coated with a small amount of bland cream (eg, Eucerin) to help trap water in the skin.

B. Acute Weeping Stage: Apply Burow's solution (aluminum subacetate) soaks made up to 1:20 solution (Domeboro tablets or packets) for 20 minutes, using three layers of gauze or cloth thoroughly moistened with solution four times a day. Do not use for more than 3 days. Treat infection with a systemic antibiotic (eg, cephalexin, erythromycin). Antihistamines can be used as antipruritic agents but are of secondary importance to topical treatment in controlling pruritus. Hydroxyzine is of value.

C. Subacute and Chronic Stages: The liberal use of emollients along with the *cautious* use of corticosteroid topical agents to control inflammation is the mainstay of therapy. Encourage daily bathing followed by application of corticosteroid cream to allow for penetration of the corticosteroid through the skin barrier and to aid in trapping water in the skin. Although creams are generally preferred to ointments, ointments may be more effective in some situations, especially when the hands and feet are involved. Corticosteroids should be applied two or three times a day until inflammation is controlled. As active inflammation subsides, bland creams should be substituted. The choice of a corticosteroid preparation depends upon the degree of inflammation and, to some extent, the location of the lesions. Potent (fluorinated) topical agents are used for short periods of time to bring inflammation under control; with more chronic use, the weakest preparations compatible with control are used. (Hydrocortisone cream, 1%, is recommended.) Corticosteroid absorption from a potent agent used for a prolonged period and over large areas of inflamed skin (especially if used under occlusive dressing) can produce adrenal suppression and other complications of systemic corticosteroid therapy. Prolonged use of topical corticosteroids may also produce skin thinning. Potent topical corticosteroids should not be used with any frequency or duration on the face or periorbital areas.

An alternative approach to therapy (the Scholtz regimen) avoids bathing with water completely. A moist washcloth can be used to clean the groin and axillary areas. Cetaphil is applied liberally to other areas until it foams and is then gently wiped from the skin, so that a thin film of lotion is left on the skin. In the authors' experience, this regimen is of limited value in a dry climate. Topical ointments of any kind, with the exception of topical corticosteroid preparations in the form of creams or solutions, are avoided.

Prognosis

Many cases of atopic dermatitis resolve spontaneously by 3 years of age, but atopic dermatitis may persist through childhood and even into adult life. Emotional problems that stem from severe dermatitis may require special consideration. There is a high likelihood (up to 80% of children in some series) that a child with atopic dermatitis will develop allergic rhinitis, asthma, or both. Consequently, it seems wise to institute simple environmental control procedures in the homes of children with atopic dermatitis and to follow these children particularly closely for the development of these disorders.

Adinoff AD, Tellez P, Clark RAF: Atopic dermatitis and aeroallergen contact sensitivity. J Allergy Clin Immunol 1988;81:736.

Clark RAF, Nicol N, Adinoff AD: Atopic dermatitis: In: *Principles and Practice of Dermatology.* Sams WT, Lunch PJ (editors). Churchill Livingstone, 1990.

Sampson HA: Atopic dermatitis. Allergy 1992;69:469.

Sampson HA: The role of food allergy and mediator release in atopic dermatitis. J Allergy Clin Immunol 1988;81:635.

ADVERSE REACTIONS TO FOODS

Adverse reactions to foods occur quite frequently and can be classified on the basis of the mechanism of the reaction. Although these reactions are often diagnosed as "allergic," the majority of adverse reactions to foods are, in fact, caused by many other factors that are nonimmune in origin, such as pharmacologic or metabolic mechanisms and food "idiosyncrasy" (mechanism unknown), or by food toxins. (See Table 33–2.) Reactions can occur in all body tissues. A wide variety of signs and symptoms can be encountered, many of which may appear extremely vague. Serious allergic reactions include anaphylaxis, acute angioedema of the upper airway, and severe bronchial asthma. Such reactions usually occur from within minutes to 2 hours. Other symptom complexes of lesser consequence, both allergic and nonallergic, can also occur in response to a variety of common foods. These are more likely to appear after several hours.

Several factors may influence a patient's potential to react to food. First, heredity influences the risk of developing food allergy. The incidence of food allergy increases if one or both parents are allergic. Also, early introduction of cow's milk or solid foods may induce a risk of food allergy. In general, those

Table 33–2. Adverse reactions to foods.

Food hypersensitivity (true allergic reactions)
Classic "allergic" reactions due to IgE antibody and release of mediators.
Nonanaphylactic reactions due to IgG or IgM or delayed-type hypersensitivity and release of mediators.
Food intolerance (mechanism unknown)
Idiosyncrasy
    Dyes
    Preservatives
    Exercise (may be allergic in part, in some cases)
Metabolic mechanisms
    Carbohydrate enzyme deficiencies
    Gluten sensitivity (celiac disease)
    G6PD deficiency
    Phenylketonuria
    Ceruloplasmin deficiency (Wilson's disease)
Pharmacologic mechanisms
    Histamine intoxication (ingestion of contaminated scombroid fish, (eg, tuna and mackerel)
    Vasoactive amines occurring naturally in foods (strawberries, melons, cheese, chocolate, some wines and beers)
    Methylxanthines (caffeine)

foods that cause an allergic reaction during early childhood are less likely to be a problem as the child grows than are those food sensitivities that are acquired later in life. For example, 60–90% of children who develop a milk allergy in infancy are able to tolerate milk in the diet by the age of 4 years (even though skin tests and RAST may remain positive to milk). Finally, the potential for an allergic reaction to food is influenced by the rate and by the type of food particles that are absorbed across the intestinal mucosa. For example, infectious and toxic enteritis damages the mucosal lining, thereby permitting partially digested food allergens to be absorbed and increasing the potential for an allergic food reaction.

Syndromes Sometimes Associated With Food Sensitivity

A. Angioedema: Angioedema is often accompanied by urticaria. In mild cases, findings include periorbital and lip edema, a few hives, mild arthralgia, and malaise. In severe cases, there may be tongue, pharyngeal, and laryngotracheal edema and joint swelling. Death may occur from asphyxia. (See Medical Emergencies Due to Allergic Reactions.)

B. Anaphylaxis: Immediate reaction is characterized by light-headedness to syncope, flushing to pallor, paresthesias, generalized itching, palpitations, and tachycardia. There may be symptoms and signs of pulmonary edema, bronchial asthma, and vascular collapse. (See Medical Emergencies Due to Allergic Reactions.) Most often, food anaphylaxis results from the interaction of food allergen and IgE antibody with the release of histamine and other chemical mediators. There is, however, a reaction that is anaphylaxis-like in clinical appearance, termed an **anaphylactoid reaction.** This reaction results from nonimmune release of chemical mediators.

C. Gastrointestinal Intolerance: In mild cases, findings may include nausea, diarrhea, flatulence, bloating, and abdominal discomfort. In severe cases, there may be forceful vomiting, severe colic, bloody and mucoid diarrhea, and dehydration. Prolonged episodes of gastrointestinal intolerance can result in malnutrition and growth retardation. In many instances, food-associated symptoms are attributed to "allergy," but the mechanism upon which the reaction is based is unclear.

D. Perennial Allergic Rhinitis, Bronchial Asthma, Atopic Dermatitis, Urticaria: See elsewhere in this chapter.

E. Tension-Fatigue Syndrome: A combination of the following symptoms has been reported: fatigue, lassitude, irritability, sleeplessness, disturbed behavior, apathy, pallor, "shadowy" eyes with "allergic pleats", "run-down feeling", and sometimes a generalized headache with vague abdominal complaints. This syndrome is claimed to be associated in particular with foods commonly and abundantly eaten, eg, cow's milk, cereal grains, chocolate, eggs,

and pork. It is not clear that these symptoms (when they can be associated with the ingestion of a specific food) are mediated by an allergic mechanism. Similar symptoms have also been attributed to yeast allergy ("yeast connection"), but neither a relationship to ingestion of yeast nor an allergic mechanism has been established.

F. Hyperactivity: Claims that salicylates, dyes, sugar, and other food ingredients may contribute to hyperactivity in children with attention deficit disorder are controversial. In the occasional case in which a child appears to benefit from restricted diets (eg, the "Feingold diet"), there is no evidence of an allergic reaction to the foodstuffs involved.

G. Migraine: In addition to other causes, foods may precipitate a migrainous episode either on an allergic or nonallergic basis. Certain foods in which significant amounts of vasoactive amines have been found, such as chocolate, cheese, liver, and some wines and beers, have been demonstrated to precipitate migraine.

Clinical Findings

A. History; Symptoms and Signs: (Refer to the section on history in the discussion of atopic disorders; see also individual disorders). Often, a symptom diary kept for 7–14 days is helpful in establishing a baseline pattern for symptoms.

B. Laboratory Findings:

1. Eosinophilia of stool mucus may be present in cases of gastrointestinal allergy but may be a normal finding in the first 3 months of life; blood eosinophilia may occur.

2. Large positive reactions in skin tests (use puncture or prick tests only) are likely to be clinically relevant; mild (1–2+) reactions correlate poorly with clinical sensitivity. Interpretations of skin tests in the child of less than 2 years may vary slightly because of decreased skin reactivity. Negative reactions do not rule out a nonimmune clinical reaction or even an allergic reaction to some elements of food (eg, partially hydrolyzed product). The most common food allergens in young children are cow's milk, eggs, peanuts, soy, and wheat. In older children and adults, fish, shellfish, and nuts are most often involved in allergic reactions. Keep in mind, however, that severe reactions can occur to almost any food.

3. Serologic tests are in principle the same as skin tests. RAST scores of less than 3 usually are not associated with clinical sensitivity.

4. Provocative food tests are important in the less serious entities. Elimination, challenge, and rechallenge must be relied upon for definitive diagnosis. In very serious reactions such as angioedema, anaphylaxis, and bronchial asthma, the causative food is usually known by the patient or parents or can be identified by the physician with the aid of a history. Food challenges and food skin testing would be hazardous in these situations. In the less serious and more obscure symptom entities, the likely food is a common one (eg, milk); the suspected food should be withdrawn for 1 week before challenge.

Differential Diagnosis of Important Symptoms

A. Gastrointestinal Intolerance: Differentiate from cystic fibrosis, pyloric stenosis, celiac disease, acute or chronic intestinal infections, gastrointestinal malformations, carbohydrate enzyme deficiencies (eg, lactase), and irritable bowel syndrome.

B. Angioedema of the Upper Airway: Differentiate from acute epiglottitis and foreign body in the upper airway.

Treatment & Prognosis

Treatment consists of eliminating the offending food, but the physician must be careful to provide specific advice for ensuring the nutritional adequacy of the diet. If milk or a milk substitute is withdrawn from the diet for over 1 month, the daily maintenance requirement of calcium should be administered (see Chapter 8). *Note*: Especially in the growing child, the unnecessary and unjustified restriction of many foods over an indefinite period merely because they *might* be involved or because they happened to give a positive skin reaction is to be condemned. The majority of proved offending foods in young children can be tolerated as time passes and should be rechallenged at 6-month intervals (unless the symptoms have been life-threatening) until the food can be reintroduced without symptoms.

Treat specific signs or symptoms as indicated.

The prognosis is good if the offending food can be identified. In some of the vague chronic syndromes, identification may not be possible, in which case the patient will remain symptomatic. In the severe syndromes, the offending food is usually known and can be avoided.

Bahna SL: Diagnostic tests for food allergy. Clin Rev Allergy 1988;6:259.

Metcalfe DD, Sampson HA, Simon RA (editors): *Food Allergy: Adverse Reactions to Foods and Food Additives.* Blackwell, 1991.

Sampson HA: Food sensitivity in children. *Current Therapy in Allergy, Immunology, and Rheumatology 3.* Lichtenstein LM, Fauci AS (editors). BC Decker, 1988.

Weber RW: Food additives and allergy. Ann Allergy 1993;70:183.

Zeiger RS: Prevention of food allergy in infancy. Annals of Allergy 1990;64:430.

CONTACT DERMATITIS

Essentials of Diagnosis

- Erythematous, papular eruption that may progress to include vesiculation, bullae formation, and denudation.

- Pruritus, often intense.
- Eruption confined more or less to areas of direct skin contact with allergen.

General Considerations

Contact dermatitis is a delayed hypersensitivity reaction in the skin. The allergen is believed to conjugate locally within skin tissue elements. Sensitization after initial contact requires at least a few days, but an already sensitized individual may react to allergen contact in as little as 24 hours. Fur, leather and fabric dyes, formalin, dichromates (used in leather), nickel, rubber compounds, ethylenediamine (used in topical medications), neomycin, poison ivy, poison oak, and poison sumac are the most common offenders in contact dermatitis. Although most contact is local, dermatitis can be induced systemically in an already sensitized individual by ingestion of the antigen.

Clinical Findings

A. History: A history of contact with possible allergens corresponding to the distribution of the lesions, in conjunction with the appearance of the lesions, may be sufficient for the diagnosis or may serve only as a starting point for further investigation. Itching, frequently intense, is the rule and may precede the onset of observable lesions.

B. Physical Examination: The appearance and distribution of the lesions are the main criteria for diagnosis. Eruptions may be confined to areas of contact with the offending allergen, and inflammations may be sharply demarcated from normal skin. With more severe and chronic eruptions, however, dissemination may occur as a result of scratching and repeated contact with the allergen. If the eruption is mild, only erythema with some papulation may be present; more intense reactions include vesiculation with denudation of skin and frank weeping. Exfoliative dermatitis and secondary infection can also occur. There may be evidence of excoriation reflecting the pruritic nature of these lesions. With chronic dermatitis, skin thickening may be present.

C. Patch Testing: Patch testing with suspected allergens can be used to identify the contactants involved. In general, patch testing should not be performed when the dermatitis is active because this procedure may exacerbate the dermatitis.

Prevention

Sensitizing substances should be avoided. Inflamed skin is more susceptible to sensitization than normal skin, and virtually any substance applied to the skin is potentially sensitizing; only those topical agents considered necessary for treatment should be used.

Parenteral or oral hyposensitization is not generally successful and can induce serious reactions. Moreover, the striking beneficial effects of a brief course of local or systemic corticosteroid treatment virtually nullify justification for hyposensitization at the present time.

Treatment

A. Early Treatment:

1. Terminate exposure to the contactant.

2. Soaks with Burow's solution (Domeboro powder or tablet, 1 package or tablet to 1–2 pints of water) or with 1:6000 solution of potassium permanganate (0.3-g tablet plus 2 quarts of water) may be used in the early stage of treatment, especially if oozing is present, to diminish itching.

B. Mild Dermatitis: A short period of treatment with a mild adrenocorticosteroid cream or ointment is recommended.

C. Severe Dermatitis: Creams or ointments containing potent corticosteroids are helpful. These should be applied liberally and frequently so that the inflamed areas are covered at all times. In unusual circumstances, eg, when the dermatitis is extremely severe and extensive, systemic corticosteroids should be considered. A short course of systemic corticosteroids followed by topical corticosteroid administration is frequently helpful in controlling acute severe contact dermatitis (eg, poison ivy dermatitis). Pastes, ointments, and creams should not be applied to weeping skin.

D. General Measures:

1. Avoid all secondary irritants to the skin, eg, wool and detergents.

2. Treat infection, if present. Early in the course of the dermatitis, potassium permanganate solution can be employed instead of Burow's solution. This topical treatment may be sufficient; however, when the lesions are extensive, systemic antibiotic therapy must be used. Topical antibiotics should not be used, because they have potential for sensitization.

3. Give antihistamines orally for pruritus (hydroxyzine is recommended). Topical antihistamine creams or ointments should be avoided, since they may cause additional sensitization. Colloidal soaks, such as starch baths, may be employed when the dermatitis is extensive.

Belsito DV: Mechanisms of allergic contact dermatitis. Immunol Allergy Clin North Am 1989;9:579.

Fisher AA: *Contact Dermatitis,* 3rd ed. Lea & Febiger, 1986.

Parker F: Contact dermatitis. In: *Allergic Disease From Infancy to Adulthood,* 2nd ed. Bierman CW, Pearlman DS (editors). Saunders, 1988.

DRUG HYPERSENSITIVITY

Drugs are so widely used that drug reactions of one type or another are commonplace. It is helpful to categorize drug reactions according to the mechanism of the reaction. **Toxic drug reactions** are due to the inherent pharmacologic properties of the drug and are most frequently encountered after drug overdosage. Some individuals exhibit inordinate sensitivity to the recognized pharmacologic effects of a drug, however, and may therefore develop toxicity after administration of amounts that are usually nontoxic. **Drug idiosyncrasy** is an unusual response to the pharmacologic action of the drug (eg, hyperactivity rather than sedation following the administration of phenobarbital). **Allergic reactions to drugs** are independent of the drug's pharmacologic action and are the result of antigen-antibody interaction. This interaction may cause the release of histamine and other chemical mediators from mast cells (as in anaphylaxis) or may cause the production and deposition of immune complexes (as in serum sickness). The allergen may not be the drug administered but a metabolic derivative of it produced in the body. Although the immune reaction is highly specific, cross-reactions with chemically related drugs are not infrequent, for example, among the various kinds of penicillins. **Anaphylactoid (pseudoallergic) reactions** mimic true allergic reactions but are caused by nonspecific release of histamine or other vasoactive mediators from mast cells (eg, some reactions to iodinated radiocontrast dyes).

The manifestations of drug allergy are extremely varied, and virtually all allergic syndromes can be produced by drugs. The most common manifestations are skin eruptions and fever. In serum sickness, symptoms may occur 7–10 days after the first encounter with the substance (particularly penicillins and sulfonamides). Reexposure to the antigen in an already sensitized individual may result in symptoms as early as 12–36 hours. This disorder usually begins with a low-grade fever and malaise, which are followed to a variable extent by skin rash (90% of cases), lymphadenopathy, polyarthritis, and neurologic symptoms.

In recent years, various syndromes related to reactivity to aspirin have been recognized, predominantly in adults but also in children. The reactions appear to be nonallergic, based rather on some peculiar biochemical idiosyncrasy. A syndrome of nasal polyposis, severe aspirin-induced bronchospasm, and rhinitis with sinusitis has been well publicized, but a more subtle bronchospastic influence also has been documented in many children with asthma. Urticaria or angioedema also occurs in association with rhinitis and nasal polyposis, generally without bronchospasm in the urticarial forms.

Although any drug is a potential sensitizer, some (particularly penicillin and the sulfonamides) are more often associated with allergic reactions by repeated exposure. It is also probable that parenteral administration is more sensitizing than oral administration. Topical administration of drugs, especially over inflamed skin, is particularly sensitizing.

Exposure to sunlight may activate skin reactions to photosensitizing drugs such as sulfonamides, tetracycline antibiotics, and topically applied coal tar products.

In questioning a patient about drug reactions, remember that certain drugs such as penicillin G benzathine remain in the body for a long time. Reactions to a single depot injection of penicillin have been known to last for months.

With the exception of patch testing in contact dermatitis, allergy testing has usually been a disappointing procedure in identifying or predicting drug allergy. The reasons are many, and—in some cases at least—the allergic reaction is due to a metabolically altered form of the drug. In the case of penicillin, some of the offensive metabolites have been identified. When these substances are used in testing, prediction of allergic reactions on the basis of a test reaction is more successful. However, these reagents are not readily available, and until the exact allergens in other drugs are identified and preparations containing the appropriate allergens become widely available, skin and serologic testing for drug allergy cannot be considered a reliable procedure. The basis for "hypersensitivity" reactions to urographic or other radiocontrast material is unknown, and skin testing and other tests, including use of a smaller "test dose" of the material, cannot reliably predict reactivity to these agents.

The history of previous reactions to drugs remains the best means of diagnosing drug sensitivity. This is often difficult, however. For this reason, an alternative drug should be used (if possible) in any instance where a reaction to a drug is questionable. Furthermore, the patient should be advised to avoid the drug even though a definite drug allergy has not been established.

Treatment & Prognosis

Regardless of the manifestation, the treatment of drug allergy includes discontinuance of the offending drug at the first sign of an adverse reaction, the use of antihistamines with or without adrenergic drugs, and, in more severe and prolonged cases, administration of adrenocorticosteroids. Further contact with the drug is avoided. Small amounts of drugs to which a patient may be sensitive may be found in vaccines, foods, and other substances. Individuals with extreme hypersensitivity to a given drug should be warned, therefore, of other hidden sources of contact with the drug. Although desensitization has been used successfully, it is not recommended; it is better to substitute a chemically unrelated drug for the offending drug.

Symptomatic treatment is usually effective. If the possibility of a reaction to a radiocontrast dye is suspected, the patient should be pretreated with corticosteroids and antihistamines if the use of the dye is considered necessary.

The prognosis is good, especially when drug allergies are identified early.

Anderson JA: Allergic reactions to drugs and biological agents. JAMA 1992;268:2845.

Blaiss MS: Drug-induced pulmonary reactions in children. Respiratory Management 1991;21:10.

Kyung K, Evans R, Mahr TA: Drug allergy. Allergy Proc 1990;11:299.

Patterson R: Diagnosis and treatment of drug allergy. J Allergy Clin Immunol 1988;81:380.

Van Arsdel PP Jr: Drug Allergy. Immunol Allergy Clin North Am 1991;11;461.

URICARIA

Essentials of Diagnosis

- Multiple (occasionally single) macular lesions, consisting of localized edema (wheal) with surrounding erythema.
- Pruritus, frequently intense.

General Considerations

Urticaria is a vascular reaction of the upper dermis consisting mainly of vasodilation and perivascular transudation, resulting in the classic "hive" or wheal and flare. Lesions are characteristically pruritic. Ordinarily, this vascular reaction is due to the liberation of histamine, but other mediators may be involved.

Urticarial reactions are usually transient (hours) but can persist for months or more. They may be the sole allergic manifestation or may represent only a part of the clinical picture, as in serum sickness and erythema multiforme. They also may occur on a nonallergic basis. Emotional tension may be an aggravating factor. **Angioedema** is essentially an urticarial reaction of the lower parts of the dermis, resulting in the production of a more diffuse edema. **Hereditary angioedema** is a rare, nonallergic disorder characterized by periodic bouts of angioedema that are nonpruritic. It can be life-threatening.

There are various forms of urticaria and urticarial syndromes, with various classifications and etiologic origins (see Clinical Findings). Two deserve special attention because they can be life-threatening. **Cold-induced urticaria** is a syndrome in which exposure to cold air, cold water, or other cold objects induces localized urticaria or angioedema, sometimes in the rewarming phase. Death from sudden massive mediator release can occur, for example, from swimming in cold water. **Exercise-related urticaria** takes various forms. One form that appears to be "cholinergic" relates to overheating and is characterized by intense itching and small wheals with erythema. It rarely is life-threatening. However, a more generalized anaphylactic syndrome (with urticaria and angioedema) may occur with exercise and can be fatal.

Papular urticaria is a term given to a syndrome characterized by multiple papules from insect bites, found especially on the extremities. It is not true urticaria. Scabies also may present in papules secondary to infection and scratching.

Dermatographism is the appearance of a wheal and erythema on the skin when "written" on, ie, stroked with a fingernail, for example. Dermatographism can occur in allergic and nonallergic individuals. It generally is of no pathologic significance but may accompany chronic urticaria or urticaria pigmentosa (mastocytosis).

Clinical Findings

A. History: The history is of prime importance in ascertaining the possible cause. The most common causes of urticaria are categorized below. However, the cause most often is not identifiable, especially in chronic urticaria (urticaria lasting weeks to years).

1. Drugs (antibiotics, aspirin), hyposensitization extracts, vaccines, toxoids, and hormone preparations.

2. Infections, including bacterial (especially staphylococcal and group A β-hemolytic streptococcal), parasitic, fungal, and viral, including viral hepatitis, herpesvirus, and various other common viral pathogens.

3. Foods (especially eggs, milk, soy, shellfish, fish, berries, peanuts, and nuts); food dyes and other food additives may be infrequent causes.

4. Inhalants, pollens, and molds (sometimes by direct contact as well as inhalation).

5. Psychologic factors (probably overrated).

6. Physical factors (cold, heat, vibration, delayed pressure), exercise, histamine liberators, and dermatographism.

B. Symptoms and Signs: Urticarial lesions characteristically appear as erythematous areas with a pale center and usually occur in large numbers. Pruritus is the rule and is frequently intense; it may precede the appearance of the lesions. Pruritus is not, however, characteristic of angioneurotic edema, which occurs most often as a solitary lesion or together with multiple urticaria. When angioedema involves the laryngeal area, it may be a threat to life.

Dermatographism may be symptomatic and occurs in a small percentage of allergic and nonallergic patients.

C. Laboratory Findings: Diagnostic procedures may include drug elimination, dietary elimination and challenge of suspected foods, and a thorough search for infection elsewhere in the body. Allergy testing is occasionally of value.

Differential Diagnosis

Urticaria is a prominent feature of mastocytosis (urticaria pigmentosa) and may occur in systemic diseases such as lupus erythematosus, various liver diseases, lymphoma, leukemia, and carcinoma.

Treatment & Prognosis

Treatment consists mainly of the detection and elimination of the appropriate allergens, when possible. Aspirin should be avoided because it may sec-

ondarily aggravate the urticaria. Antihistamines are usually the most useful therapeutic agents in urticarial disorders, but adrenergic agents with vasoconstrictor properties can be a useful adjunct. Epinephrine is especially effective when rapid relief is needed. Hydroxyzine is among the most effective antihistamines, especially in treatment of chronic urticaria and dermatographism. In resistant cases, combining an H_1 antihistamine (eg, hydroxyzine) with an H_2 antihistamine (eg, cimetidine) may be helpful. Cyproheptadine hydrochloride is most effective in some patients with cold-induced urticaria. Mild sedation may also be indicated.

Adrenocorticosteroids are sometimes useful in the more chronic form of urticaria but are reserved for more refractory cases. Topical medications generally are not effective, and topical antihistamines may aggravate the problem by inducing contact sensitivity. Except for cases of life-threatening laryngeal edema, the prognosis is good. Identification of the offending agent is more important.

Fox RW, Russel DW: Drug therapy of chronic urticaria and angioedema. Immunol Allergy Clin North Am 1991; 11:45.

Kaplan AP: Urticaria and angioedema. In: *Allergy: Principles and Practice,* 4th ed. Middleton E Jr et al (editors). Mosby, 1993.

Stafford CS: Urticaria as a sign of systemic disease. Ann Allergy 1990;64:264.

Wanderer AA: Cold urticaria syndromes. J Allergy Clin Immunol 1990;85:965.

OTHER ALLERGIC PULMONARY DISORDERS

A syndrome thought to be related to cow's milk hypersensitivity has been described and consists of recurrent pulmonary infiltrates, wheezing, chronic cough, chronic or frequent otitis media and rhinorrhea, and iron deficiency anemia related to excessive gastrointestinal blood loss. Gastrointestinal symptoms (diarrhea, vomiting) and poor weight gain are also features of this disorder, which is seen in children chiefly in the first 2 years of life. Some of these children have evidence of pulmonary hemosiderosis, and blood eosinophilia is sometimes seen. Multiple precipitins to cow's milk can be demonstrated, but the significance of this finding is controversial. Dietary elimination of cow's milk is followed by improvement of the disorder, although symptoms also have been reported to subside spontaneously.

Hypersensitivity pneumonitis is an inflammatory reaction involving principally the alveoli and bronchioles and characterized clinically by malaise, fever, chills, cough, and dyspnea. Tissue damage stems from a hypersensitivity reaction to any of a variety of inhaled organic dusts or of fungi that may or may not also be infective. The disease is seen predominantly in adults as a result of occupational exposure to large concentrations of certain antigens (eg, thermophilic actinomycetes from hay, as in farmer's lung, or from contaminated air conditioners), but the disease can occur at any age. The onset may be insidious or acute. Symptoms of these disorders—particularly in the acute onset form—typically occur 4–8 hours after exposure to the offending antigen. In asthmatic individuals, wheezing also may be present, with involvement of IgE-mediated mechanisms.

Treatment consists mainly of avoiding the offensive inhalants. Glucocorticoids may be very helpful in minimizing the hypersensitivity reaction early in the disease.

Allergic bronchopulmonary aspergillosis, with or without tissue invasion by the organism, is seen with some frequency in Great Britain but is rare in the USA (especially in children). The syndrome occurs in allergic asthmatics and includes symptoms of asthma and recurrent pneumonitis. High levels of eosinophils in tissue and blood, high IgE levels, and the presence of IgE and precipitating antibody to *Aspergillus* are characteristic laboratory findings. *Aspergillus* may also be found on sputum smear or culture. Treatment includes use of corticosteroids and antifungal agents.

An association between tissue and blood eosinophilia and pulmonary infiltrates has been discovered in various disorders (eg, asthma, allergic bronchopulmonary aspergillosis, connective tissue diseases) and is thought to reflect an allergic mechanism in these disorders. A number of drugs (especially sulfonamides and nitrofurantoin), parasites (eg, *Ascaris*), and other antigens have been implicated at times in the production of this syndrome, but frequently no cause can be found.

Bierman CW, Pierson WE, Massie FS: Nonasthmatic allergic pulmonary disease. In: *Kendig's Disorders of the Respiratory Tract in Children,* 5th ed. Cherniak V (editor). Saunders, 1990.

Greenberger PA: Allergic bronchopulmonary aspergillosis. In: *Current Therapy in Allergy, Immunology and Rheumatology 3.* Lichtenstein LM, Fauci AS (editors). BC Decker, 1988.

Shellito JE: Hypersensitivity pneumonitis. Semin Respir Med 1991;12:196.

REFERENCES

References for Physicians

Bierman CW, Pearlman DS (editors): *Allergic Diseases from Infancy to Adulthood,* 2nd ed. Saunders, 1988.

Middleton E Jr et al (editors): *Allergy: Principles and Practice,* 4th ed. Mosby, 1993.

Naspitz CK, Tinkelman DG (editors): *Childhood Rhinitis and Sinusitis. Pathophysiology and Treatment.* Marcel Dekker, 1990.

Tinkelman DG, Naspitz CK (editors): *Childhood Asthma: Pathophysiology and Treatment,* 2nd ed. Marcel Dekker, 1992.

References for Parents & Patients

Feldman BR with Carroll D: *The Complete Book of Children's Allergies: A Guide for Parents.* Random House, 1986.

Hannaway PJ: *The Asthma Self-Help Book.* Lighthouse Press, 1989.

Plaut MF: *Children with Asthma: A Manual for Parents,* 2nd ed. Pediapress, 1988.

Young SH, Dobozin BS, Miner M: Allergies: *The Complete Guide to Diagnosis, Treatment and Daily Management.* Consumer Reports Books, New York, 1992.

Useful Organizations for Parents, Patients, & Physicians

Asthma and Allergy Foundation of America. National Headquarters: 1125 15th Sreet N.W., Suite 502, Washington, DC 20005. (Chapters in various states.)

Asthma and Allergy Network/Mothers of Asthmatics. 3554 Chain Bridge Rd., Suite 200, Fairfax, VA 22030. (1-703-385-4403.)

(These organizations provide information helpful for understanding and treating allergic problems.)

34

Antimicrobial Therapy of Pediatric Infections

James K. Todd, MD

PRINCIPLES OF ANTIMICROBIAL TREATMENT

The process of decision making related to choosing appropriate antimicrobial treatment is summarized in Table 34–1. Accurate clinical diagnosis of the suspected site of infection—based on the history, physical examination, and initial laboratory tests—leads to the appropriate consideration of common organisms usually associated with such infections and their probable patterns of susceptibility to antimicrobial agents. After obtaining cultures to identify the precise cause of potentially serious infections, the physician initiates empiric antimicrobial therapy, taking into account the above considerations as well as a knowledge of regimens that have proved successful in the past. Therapy is modified according to patient response and culture results.

Important considerations include the age of the child, the presence of any host defense deficiencies, a thorough understanding of unusual exposures (eg, via travel or direct contact with others), and the severity of the child's illness. Children who are severely ill (eg, with suspected meningitis) or who have infections known to progress rapidly to more severe illness (eg, bacteremia) should be evaluated quickly, hospitalized, and treated expeditiously with broad antimicrobial coverage until culture results allow a narrowing of therapy. Patients with milder illness (eg, otitis media without severe systemic symptoms) may be treated empirically with a single agent administered orally. If that initial therapy fails, a more extensive workup is then done.

In patients whose initial treatment is parenteral therapy, it is often desirable to change to oral therapy once symptoms are ameliorated and the causative agent is identified. As Table 34–2 shows, such a change in therapy cannot be made unless (1) an oral agent that results in sufficient blood levels is available; (2) the causative organism and its susceptibility patterns are known (or inferred from the response to single-agent parenteral therapy); (3) compliance with oral administration of antibiotic can be anticipated; and (4) appropriate blood levels can be ensured by either the pharmacology of the drug or measurement of blood levels or serum killing powers.

It is important to recognize that these principles are merely guidelines. The only accurate measure of the success of antimicrobial therapy is the response of the patient. Tables 34–3 to 34–7 give general information about selecting and prescribing antimicrobial agents. Table 34–3 is a summary of common infecting organisms and their usual patterns of susceptibility to antimicrobial agents. Table 34–4 provides general information on various groups of antibacterial agents and their common or unique adverse reactions. Table 34–5 gives dosages of commonly used parenteral antibiotics for children 1 month of age or older; Table 34–6 gives dosages for oral antibiotics; and Table 34–7 provides recommendations for use in the newborn. These tables are not comprehensive in that all possible information cannot be provided. For this reason, clinicians need to consult the specific chapter of this book related to the suspected disease and the more extensive dosage and side-effect information provided with the antibiotic package insert or available from other sources (see References). Clinicians must also learn to use a few drugs well rather than many different drugs infrequently. Using this strategy, the clinician can become familiar with various dosage forms of drugs, their palatability, their common as well as unusual side effects, and their cost. For initial therapy of many infections, the physician can usually choose among several different antibiotics, and it is reasonable to take cost into consideration if efficacy and side effects are comparable.

ANTIMICROBIAL SUSCEPTIBILITY TESTING

It is critically important to obtain cultures and other diagnostic material from patients prior to initiating antimicrobial therapy. Obtaining cultures is especially important when the patient has a serious infection, initial attempts at therapy have failed, or the use of multiple antimicrobial agents is anticipated. If

Table 34–1. Steps in decision making for use of antimicrobial agents.

Step	Action	Example
1	Determine diagnosis.	Septic arthritis
2	Consider age and preexisting condition.	Normal 2-year-old child
3	Consider common organisms.	*Staphylococus aureus, Haemophilus influenzae*
4	Consider organism susceptibility.	Penicillin- or ampicillin-resistant
5	Obtain proper cultures.[1]	Blood, joint fluid
6	Initiate empiric therapy based on above considerations and past experience (eg, personal, literature).	Nafcillin and cefotaxime
7	Modify therapy based on culture results and patient response.	*S aureus* isolated. Discontinue cefotaxime.
8	Follow clinical response.	

[1]Indicated for serious or unusual infections or those with unpredictable clinical response to empiric therapy; may use other tests such as antigen detection or Gram's stain.

these cultures identify the causative agent, therapy can be narrowed or optimized according to susceptibility results. Antimicrobial susceptibility testing should be done in a laboratory using carefully defined procedures (National Committee for Clinical Laboratory Standards). The use of nonstandard media, inoculum size, or growth conditions may give markedly different and undependable results.

There are several different ways to test antimicrobial susceptibility. The identification of an antibiotic-destroying enzyme (eg, β-lactamase) implies resistance to that group of antimicrobial agents. Tube or microtiter broth dilution techniques can be used to determine the minimum inhibitory concentration (MIC) of antibiotic, which is the amount of antibiotic (μg/mL) necessary to inhibit the organism under specific laboratory conditions. The physician who also has a knowledge of the clinical pharmacology of the antimicrobial agent can infer antibiotic susceptibility if the MIC is less then the antibiotic concentration achievable in the patient using appropriate antibi-

otic dosages. Disk susceptibility testing (again, only under carefully controlled conditions) yields similar results.

It should be remembered that, for the most part, clinical laboratories report antimicrobial susceptibility (susceptible, intermediate, resistant) as it relates to levels of that antibiotic achievable in the blood (or serum). In general, organisms are considered susceptible to an antibiotic if the MIC of the antibiotic for that organism is lower than levels of that antimicrobial agent achievable in the blood using appropriate parenteral dosages. This assumption of susceptibility should be reconsidered if the patient has a focus of infection (eg, meningitis, osteomyelitis, abscess) where poor antibiotic penetration might occur, since the levels of antibiotic might be lower than the MIC in such areas. Conversely, certain organisms may be reported as resistant to a certain antibiotic because sufficiently high blood concentrations cannot be achieved. However, urine concentrations may be much higher. If so, a urinary tract infection would respond to that antibiotic, whereas septicemia would not.

Thus, antimicrobial susceptibility testing, although a very important part of therapeutic decision making, reflects assumptions that the clinician must understand, especially for management of patients with serious infections. Ultimately, the true test of the efficacy of therapy is patient response. Patients who do not respond to seemingly appropriate therapy may require reassessment, including reculturing and repeat susceptibility testing, to determine whether resistant strains have evolved or superinfection with a resistant organism is present. In addition, antimicrobial therapy cannot be expected to cure all infections unless additional supportive treatment is undertaken. Some antibiotics are only marginally effective against certain organisms, and many sequestered infections require surgical drainage procedures as an adjunct to antimicrobial therapy.

Table 34–2. Steps in switching from parenteral to oral therapy for an initially serious infection.

Step	Action
1	Define infection.
2	Determine causative organisms and antimicrobial susceptibility.
3	Achieve a favorable response to parenteral therapy: (1) systemic (eg, afebrile) and (2) local (eg, decreased inflammation).
4	Determine if comparable blood levels can be achieved with an oral agent.
5	Assess patient compliance potential.
6	Initiate oral therapy.
7	Measure blood levels (eg, serum inhibitory powers).
8	Follow clinical response.

Table 34–3. Susceptibility of some common pathogenic microorganisms to various antimicrobial drugs.

Organism	Potentially Useful Antibiotics[1]
BACTERIA	
Anaerobic bacteria[2]	Cefoxitin, cefotetan, chloramphenicol, clindamycin, metronidazole, penicillins with or without β-lactamase inhibitor
Bordetella pertussis	Erythromycin, tetracyclines
Campylobacter spp	Erythromycin, furazolidone, tetracyclines
Clostridium spp	Clindamycin, penicillins, tetracyclines
Clostridium difficile	Bacitracin (PO), metronidazole, vancomycin (PO)
Corynebacterium diphtheriae	Erythromycin, penicillins
Enterobacteriaceae[3]	Aminoglycosides,[4] ampicillins, cephalosporins, imipenem, monobactams, trimethoprim-sulfamethoxazole, [quinolones][5]
Enterococcus	Ampicillin (with aminoglycoside), vancomycin
Haemophilus influenzae	Amoxicillin/clavulanate, ampicillins (if β-lactamase negative),[6] cephalosporins (II and III),[7] chloramphenicol, rifampin, trimethoprim-sulfamethoxazole
Listeria monocytogenes	Ampicillin, trimethoprim-sulfamethoxazole
Moraxella catarrhalis	Amoxicillin/clavulanate, ampicillins (if β-lactamase negative),[6] cephalosporins (III),[7] erythromycin, tetracycline, trimethoprim-sulfamethoxazole
Neisseria gonorrhoeae	Ampicillins, cephalosporins (II and III),[7] penicillins, spectinomycin, tetracyclines, trimethoprim-sulfamethoxazole, (quinolones)
Neisseria meningitidis	Ampicillins, cephalosporins (II and III),[7] chloramphenicol, penicillins, rifampin
Pasteurella multocida	Amoxicillin/clavulanate, ampicillins, chloramphenicol, penicillins, tetracyclines
Pseudomonas aeruginosa	Aminoglycosides,[4] antipseudomonas penicillins,[8] aztreonam, ceftazidime, imipenem, [quinolones][5]
Salmonella spp	Ampicillin, cephalosporins (III),[7] chloramphenicol, trimethoprim-sulfamethoxazole
Shigella spp	Ampicillin, cephalosporins (III), chloramphenicol, tetracyclines, trimethoprim-sulfamethoxazole
Staphylococcus aureus	Antistaphylococcal penicillins,[9] cephalosporins (I and II), clindamycin, erythromycin, rifampin, trimethoprim-sulfamethoxazole, vancomycin
Staphylococci (coagulase-negative)	Cephalosporins (I and II),[10] clindamycin, rifampin, vancomycin
Streptococci (most species)	Ampicillins, cephalosporins, clindamycin, erythromycin, penicillins, vancomycin
Streptococcus pneumoniae[11]	Ampicillins, cephalosporins, erythromycin, penicillin, vancomycin[11]
INTERMEDIATE ORGANISMS	
Chlamydia spp	Clarithromycin, erythromycin, (quinolones)[5] tetracyclines
Mycoplasma spp	Erythromycin, tetracyclines
Rickettsia spp	Chloramphenicol, tetracyclines
FUNGI	
Candida spp	Amphotericin B, fluconazole, flucytosine, ketoconazole, miconazole
Fungi, systemic	Amphotericin B, fluconazole, itraconazole,[12] ketoconazole, miconazole
Dermatophytes	Griseofulvin, topical antifungals
VIRUSES	
Herpes simplex	Acyclovir, vidarabine
Human immunodeficiency virus	Dideoxyinosine (ddI),[12] dideoxycytodine (ddC),[12] zidovudine (AZT)
Influenza A virus	Amantadine, ribavirin, rimantidine
Respiratory syncytial virus	Ribavirin
Varicella-zoster virus	Acyclovir, vidarabine
Cytomegalovirus	Foscarnet, ganciclovir

[1]In alphabetical order. Selection depends on patient's age, diagnosis, site of infection, severity of illness, antimicrobial susceptibility of suspected organism, and drug risk.

[2]Species-dependent.

[3]Includes *E coli*, *Klebsiella* spp, *Enterobacter* spp, and others; antimicrobial susceptibilities should always be measured.

[4]Amikacin, gentamicin, kanamycin, netilmicin, tobramycin

[5]Not recommended for use in children.

[6]Also applies to amoxicillin and related compounds.

[7]Refer to second- (II) or third- (III) generation cephalosporins.

[8]Carbenicillin, mezlocillin, piperacillin, ticarcillin.

[9]Cloxacillin, dicloxacillin, methicillin, nafcillin, oxacillin.

[10]Only if the coagulase-negative *Staphylococcus* is also methicillin- or oxacillin-sensitive.

[11]Because of increasing frequency of *S pneumoniae* strains resistant to penicillin and cephalosporins, therapy for presumed severe infections (eg, meningitis) is with vancomycin until susceptibility studies are available.

[12]Not yet approved for children.

Table 34–4. Groups of common antibacterial agents.

Group	Examples	Some Common Susceptible Organisms (Genus)[1]	Common Resistant Organisms (Genus)	Common or Unique Adverse Reactions
PENICILLIN GROUP				Rash, anaphylaxis, drug fever, bone marrow suppression
Penicillins	Penicillin G, V	*Streptococcus, Neisseria*	*Staphylococcus, Haemophilus,* enterobacteriaceae	
Ampicillins	Ampicillin, amoxicillin	(Same as penicillins), *Haemophilus* (β-lactamase negative), *Escherichia coli, Enterococcus*	*Staphylococcus,* many enterobacteriaceae	Diarrhea
Antistaphylococ-cal penicillins	Cloxacillin, dicloxacillin, methicillin, nafcillin, ox-acillin	*Streptococcus, Staphylococcus aureus*	Gram-negative, *Staphylococcus* (coagulase-negative), enterococci	Renal (interstitial nephritis)
Antipseudomonas penicillins	Azlocillin, carbenicillin, mezlocillin, piperacillin, ticarcillin	(Same as ampicillins), *Pseudomonas*	(Same as ampicillins)	Decreased platelet ad-hesiveness, hypokale-mia, hypernatremia
Penicillin/β-lactamase inhibitor combination	Amoxicillin/clavulanate, ampicillin/sulbactam, ticarcillin/clavulanate	Broad spectrum	Some enterobacteria-ceae, *Pseudomonas*	Diarrhea
Other β-lactams	Aztreonam, imipenem/cilastatin	Broad spectrum, gram-negative rods, *Pseu-domonas*	Gram-positive	CNS, seizures
CEPHALOSPORIN GROUP				Rash; anaphylaxis, drug fever
First generation (I)	Cefazolin, cephalexin, cephalothin, cephapi-rin, cephradine	Gram-positive	Gram-negative, enterococci, some staphylococci (coagulase-negative)	
Second generation (II)	Cefaclor, cefamandole, cefonicid, cefuroxime	Gram-positive, some *Haemophilus,* some enterobacteriaceae	*Enterococcus, Pseudomonas,* some staphylococci (coagulase-negative)	Serum sickness (cefaclor)
	Cefoxitin, cefotetan	Anaerobes		
Third generation (III)	Cefotaxime, ceftizox-ime, ceftriaxone, cefix-ime, moxalactam, cef-podoxine, loracarbef	*Streptococcus, Haemophilus,* Enterobacteriaceae, *Neisseria*	*Pseudomonas,* staphylococci	Increased prothrombin time (moxalactam), biliary sludging (ceftriaxone)
	Ceftazidime	(Same as other third-generation cephalosporins), *Pseudomonas*	Staphylococci	
OTHER DRUGS Clindamycin	Clindamycin	Gram-positive, anaerobes	Gram-negative, *Enterococcus*	Nausea, vomiting, hepatotoxicity
Vancomycins	Vancomycin	Gram-positive	Gram-negative	"Redman" Syndrome, shock, ototoxicity, renal
Erythromycins	Erythromycin, clarithro-mycin, azithromycin	Gram-negative, *Bordetella, mycoplasma, chlamydia*	Gram-negative	Nausea and vomiting
Quinolones[2]	Ciprofloxacin, norflox-acin	Broad spectrum	*Enterococcus*	Cartilage damage, GI, rash, CNS

(continued)

Table 34–4. Groups of common antibacterial agents. (continued)

Group	Examples	Some Common Susceptible Organisms (Genus)	Common Resistant Organisms (Genus)	Common or Unique Adverse Reactions
Tetracyclines	Chlortetracycline, tetra-cycline, doxycycline	Anaerobes, *Myco-plasma, Chlamydia*	Many enterobacteria-ceae, *Staphylococcus*	Teeth staining, rash, flora overgrowth, hepatotoxicity, pseudotumor cerebri
Chloramphenicol	Chloramphenicol	*S pneumoniae, H influenzae, Salmonella*	*Staphylococcus,* many enterobacteriaceae	Bone marrow, gray baby syndrome, neuritis
Sulfonamides	Many	Gram-negative (urine)	Gram-positive	Rash, renal, bone marrow suppression, Stevens-Johnson syndrome
Trimethoprim-sulfa-methoxazole	Trimethoprim-sulfa-methoxazole	*S aureus,* gram-nega-tive	*Streptococcus, Pseudomonas*	Rash, renal, bone marrow suppression, Stevens-Johnson syndrome
Rifampin	Rifampin	*Neisseria, Haemo-philus, Staphylococcus*	Resistance develops rapidly if used as sole agent	Rash, GI, hepatotoxic-ity, CNS, bone marrow suppression
Aminoglycosides	Amikacin, gentamicin, kanamycin, netilmicin, streptomycin, tobramycin	Gram-negative	Gram-positive, anaerobes, some pseudomonads	Renal, ototoxicity, potentiates neuromus-cular blocking agents

[1]Not all strains susceptible; always obtain antimicrobial susceptibility tests on significant isolates.
[2]Not recommended for children.

ALTERATION OF DOSE & MEASUREMENT OF BLOOD LEVELS

Certain antimicrobial agents have not been approved (and often not tested) for use in newborns. For those that have, it is important to recognize that both dose and frequency of administration may need to be altered (see Tables 34–5 and 34–6), especially in young ($\leq$ 7 days) or low birth weight ($\leq$ 2000 g) neonates.

Antimicrobial agents are excreted or metabolized through various physiologic mechanisms (eg, renal, hepatic). It is important to consider these routes of excretion and alter the antimicrobial dosage appropriately in any patient with some degree of organ dysfunction. As indicated in Table 34–5, an assessment of renal or hepatic function may be routinely necessary for patients receiving certain drugs (eg, renal function for aminoglycosides, hepatic function for chloramphenicol); otherwise, harmful levels may accumulate. If some degree of organ dysfunction is present, dosage modification may be necessary (see detailed description in individual drug information packet), and the measurement of drug levels may be indicated.

Serum levels of drugs posing a high risk of toxicity (eg, aminoglycosides, chloramphenicol, vancomycin) are ordinarily measured. For other drugs (eg, β-lactams) in certain circumstances, it is useful to know

the relative drug concentration as compared with the MIC of the organism (ie, the serum bacteriostatic assay). For certain infections, the target peak therapeutic levels are defined (eg, subacute infective endocarditis $\geq$ 1:64, osteomyelitis and septic arthritis $\geq$ 1:8). Appropriate levels for other infections are less well defined. Measurement of serum inhibitory powers can also be used to assess compliance with an oral therapeutic regimen for serious infections.

THE USE OF NEW ANTIMICROBIAL AGENTS

New antibiotics are introduced frequently, and manufacturers often claim unique features that distinguish these usually more expensive products from their predecessors. The true role that new antimicrobials will play can be determined only over time, during which new or previously unrecognized side effects are described and the clinical efficacy of the agent is established in large numbers of patients. Because this process may take many years, a conservative approach to the clinical introduction of new antibiotics seems appropriate, especially since the costs are often higher and appropriate antimicrobial choices for most common infections already exist. It is appropriate to ask if this new antimicrobial therapy has been proved to be as effective as (or more effec-

Table 34–5. Guidelines for use of common parenteral antibacterial agents[1] in children ≥ 1 month of age.

Agent	Route	Dose[2] (mg/kg/d)	Maximum Daily Dose	Interval (hours)	Adjust-ment[3]	Blood Levels[4] (μg/mL) Peak	Trough
Amikacin	IM, IV	15–22.5	1.5 g	8	R	15–30	5–10
Ampicillin	IM, IV	100–400	12 g	4–6	R		
Aztreonam	IM, IV	90–120	6 g	6–8	R		
Cefazolin	IM, IV	50–100	6 g	8	R		
Cefotaxime	IM, IV	100–200	12 g	6–8	R		
Cefoxitin	IM, IV	80–160	12 g	4–6	R		
Ceftazidime	IM, IV	100–225	6 g	8	R		
Ceftizoxime	IM, IV	150–200	12 g	6–8	R		
Ceftriaxone	IM, IV	50–100	4 g	12–24	R		
Cefuroxime	IM, IV	100–150	6 g	6–8	R		
Cephalothin	IM, IV	75–125	12 g	4–6	R		
Cephradine	IM, IV	50–100	8 g	6	R		
Chloramphenicol	IV	50–100	4 g	6	R, H	15–25	5–10
Clindamycin	IM, IV	25–40	4.8 g	6–8	R, H		
Gentamicin	IM, IV	3–7.5	300 mg	8	R	6–10	< 2.0
Kanamycin	IM, IV	15–30	1 g	8	R	15–30	5–10
Methicillin	IM, IV	150–200	12 g	6	R		
Metronidazole	(IV)[5]	(30)[5]	4 g	6	H		
Mezlocillin	IV	200–300	24 g	6	R		
Nafcillin	IM, IV	50–150	12 g	6	None		
Netilmicin	IM, IV	3–7.5	300 mg	8	R	6–12	0.5–2
Penicillin G	IV	100,000–200,000 units/kg	20 million units	4–6	H, R		
Penicillin G (benzathine)	IM	50,000 units/kg	2.4 million units	Single dose	None		
Penicillin G (procaine)	IM	25,000–50,000 units/kg	4.8 million units	12–24	R		
Tetracycline[6]	(IV)[5]	(20–30)[5]	2 g	12	R		
Ticarcillin	IV	200–300	24 g	4–6	R		
Tobramycin	IM, IV	3–6	300 mg	8	R	6–10	< 2
Vancomycin	IV	40–60	2 g	6	R	20–40	5–10

[1]Not including some newly released drugs, ones not recommended for use in chiildren, or ones not widely used.

[2]Always consult package insert for complete prescribing information. Dosage may differ for alternative routes, newborns (see Table 34–7), or patients with liver or renal failure (see Adjustment column) and may not be recommended for use in pregnant women or newborns. Maximum dosage may be indicated only in severe infections or by parenteral routes.

[3]Mode of excretion (R = renal, H = hepatic) of antimicrobial agent should be assessed at the onset of therapy and dosage modified or levels determined as indicated in package insert.

[4]Suggested levels to reduce toxicity.

[5]Parentheses indicate less common route and dosage.

[6]Not recommended in children 8 years of age and under.

tive than) the current drug of choice—and, if so, whether its side effects are comparable or less and its cost reasonable. The development of new antibiotics is important as a response to the emergence of organism resistance and for treatment of infections now difficult to treat (eg, viruses, fungi, and some resistant bacteria). Fortunately, these infections are either rare or (usually) self-limited in normal hosts, and for the most part we have reasonable initial therapies for treating common infections.

Table 34–6. Guidelines for use of common oral antibacterial agents in children ≥ 1 month of age.

| Agent[1] | Dose[2] (mg/kg/d) | Interval (hours) | Spectrum of Action | | | Other Considerations |
			Gram-Positive	Gram-Negative	Other	
Amoxicillin	40	8	+	+		GI side effects
Amoxicillin/clavulanate	40	8	++	++		GI side effects
Ampicillin	50	6	+	+		GI side effects
Cefaclor	40	8	++	+		Serum sickness-like illness
Cefadroxil	30	12	++	+		
Cefixime	8	12–24	+	++		
Cefpodoxime	10	12	++	++		Taste (suspension)
Cefprozil	30	12	++	+		GI side effects
Cefuroxime	30–40	12	++	++		GI side effects
Cephalexin	25–50	6	++	+		
Cephradine	25–50	6	++	+		
Chloramphenicol	See Table 34–5.		+	++	Rickettsia	Aplastic anemia
Clarithromycin	15	12	++	+	Mycoplasma, Chlamydia, B pertussis	GI side effects
Clindamycin	20–30	6	++	0	Anaerobes	GI side effects
Cloxacillin	50–100	6	++	0		
Dicloxacillin	12–25	6	++	0		
Doxycycline[3]	2–4[3]	12–24	0	+	Mycoplasma, Chlamydia, B pertussis	Teeth staining ≤ 8 years
Erythromycin	20–50[4]	6–12[4]	++	0	Mycoplasma, Chlamydia, B pertussis	GI side effects
Erythromycin/sulfisoxazole	40 (erythromycin)	6–8	++	+	Mycoplasma, Chlamydia, B pertussis	
Furazolidone	5–8	6	0	+	Giardia	
Loracarbef	15–30	12	++	++		
Metronidazole	15–35	8	0	0	Anaerobes	
Nitrofurantoin	5–7	6	(Urine)	(Urine)		
Oxacillin	50–100	6	++	0		
Penicillin V	25–50	6	+	+		Taste (suspension)
Rifampin	10–20	12–25	+	+		
Sulfisoxazole	120–150	6	(Urine)	(Urine)		
Tetracycline[3]	25–50[3]	6	0	+	Mycoplasma, Chlamydia, B pertussis, Rickettsia	Teeth staining ≤ 8 years
Trimethoprim-sulfamethoxazole	8–20 (TMP)	12	+	++		Stevens-Johnson syndrome

[1]Not including some newly released drugs, ones not recommended for use in children, or ones not widely used.
[2]Always consult package insert for complete prescribing information. Dosage may differ for alternative routes, newborns (see Table 34–7), or patients with liver or renal failure (see Adjustment column) and may not be recommended for use in pregnant women or newborns. Maximum dosage may be indicated only in severe infections or by parenteral routes.
[3]Not recomended in children 8 years of age and under.
[4]Preparation-dependent.

Table 34–7. Guidelines for use of selected antimicrobial agents in newborns.[1]

| Antibiotic Drug | Route | Body Wt (g) | Maximum Dosage (mg/kg/d) [Frequency] | | Blood Levels (μg/mL) | |
			< 7 Days	8–30 Days	Peak	Trough
Amikacin[2]	IV, IM	< 2000	15 [q12h]	20 [q8h]	15–30	5–10
		> 2000	20 [q12h]	30 [q8h]		
Ampicillin	IV, IM	< 2000	100 [q12h]	150 [q8h]		
		> 2000	150 [q8h]	200 [q6h]		
Cefotaxime	IV, IM		100 [q12h]	150 [q8h]		
Ceftazidime	IV, IM		100 [q12h]	150 [q8h]		
Chloramphenicol[3]	IV, PO	< 2000	25 [q24h]	25 [q24h]	15–25	5–10
		> 2000	25 [q24h]	50 [q12h]		
Clindamycin	IV, IM, PO	< 2000	10 [q12h]	15 [q8h]		
		> 2000	15 [q8h]	20 [q6h]		
Erythromycin	PO		20 [q12h]	30 [q8h]		
Gentamicin[2]	IV, IM		5 [q12h]	7.5 [q8h]	6–10	< 2
Methicillin	IV, IM	< 2000	100 [q12h]	150 [q8h]		
		> 2000	150 [q8h]	200 [q6h]		
Mezlocillin	IV, IM		150 [q12h]	225 [q8h]		
Nafcillin	IV	< 2000	50 [q12h]	75 [q8h]		
		> 2000	60 [q8h]	150 [q6h]		
Netilmicin[2]	IV, IM		5 [q8h]	7.5 [q8h]		
Oxacillin	IV, IM	< 2000	50 [q12h]	100 [q8h]		
		> 2000	75 [q8h]	150 [q6h]		
Penicillin G[4]	IV	< 2000	100,000[4] [q12h]	150,000[4] [q8h]		
		> 2000	150,000[4] [q8h]	200,000[4] [q6h]		
Ticarcillin	IV, IM	< 2000	150 [q12h]	225 [q8h]		
		> 2000	225 [q8h]	300 [q6h]		
Tobramycin[2]	IV, IM		4 [q12h]	6 [q8h]	6–10	< 2
Vancomycin	IV		20 [q12h]	30 [q8h]	20–40	5–10

[1]Adapted from Nelson JD: *Pocketbook of Pediatric Antimicrobial Therapy,* 9th ed. Williams & Wilkins, 1991.
[2]Neonates weighing < 1200 g may require even smaller doses. Antibiotic levels should be closely monitored.
[3]Chloramphenicol must be used with extreme caution. Levels should be measured in all patients to ensure proper dosing.
[4]Penicillin dosages are in units/kg/d. Other preparations (eg, benzathine penicillin) may be given IM. See specific diseases for dosage.

REFERENCES

Committee on Infectious Diseases: Report of the Committee on Infectious Diseases, 22nd ed. American Academy of Pediatrics, 1991.

McEvoy GK (editor): *AHFS Drug Information 1994: American Hospital Formulary Service.* American Society of Hospital Pharmacists, 1994.

Nelson JD: *Pocketbook of Pediatric Antimicrobial Therapy,* 10th ed. Williams & Wilkins, 1993.

Physicians' Desk Reference, 48th ed. Medical Economics, 1994.

Todd JK: Antimicrobial susceptibility testing in the office laboratory. Pediatr Infect Dis 1983;2:481.

35

Infections: Viral & Rickettsial

Myron J. Levin, MD, & Jose R. Romero, MD

I. VIRAL INFECTIONS

Viruses cause most pediatric infections. Although immunizations have made some viral infections rare, new viruses have been discovered. Mixed viral or viral-bacterial infections of the respiratory and intestinal tracts are rather common, as is prolonged, asymptomatic shedding of some viruses in childhood. Thus, the detection of a virus is not always proof that it is the cause of a given illness.

Diagnosis of many viral illnesses is now possible through antigen detection techniques, which are more rapid than isolation of viruses in tissue culture and in many cases almost as sensitive. Nucleic acid hybridization and polymerase chain reaction amplification of the viral genome permit recognition of previously undetectable infections. New diagnostic tests are changing many basic concepts about viral diseases and make diagnosis of viral infections an increasingly complex field. Only laboratories with excellent quality control procedures should be used, and the results of new tests must be interpreted cautiously. The availability of specific antiviral agents increases the value of early diagnosis in some serious viral infections. Table 35–1 lists some viral agents associated with common clinical signs, and Table 35–2 lists some diagnostic tests.

The local viral diagnostic laboratory should be contacted for details regarding specimen collection, handling, and shipping.

INFECTIONS DUE TO MYXOVIRUSES

INFLUENZA

Because young children have little prior experience with influenza, clinical infection is common.

Upper respiratory infection is typical. More severe disease may occur at any age, but lower respiratory tract symptoms are more common in children under age 5, especially with their first influenza infection. Spread is by respiratory secretions. Neonates are partially protected by maternal antibody.

Although only three main types (A/H1N1, A/H3N2, B) have been prevalent recently, antigenic shift and drift ensure a supply of susceptible hosts of all ages. Outbreaks occur in fall and winter. Each year's strain tends to be first seen in the Far East.

Clinical Findings

The incubation period is 2–7 days, similar to that of other respiratory viruses but shorter than that of *Mycoplasma pneumoniae* (10–20 days). An influenza epidemic is often present in the community.

A. Symptoms and Signs: Influenza in older children and adults is characterized by sudden onset of high fever, severe myalgia, headache, and chills. These overshadow the associated coryza, pharyngitis, and cough. Usually absent are rash, marked conjunctivitis, adenopathy, exudative pharyngitis, and dehydrating enteritis. Diarrhea, vomiting, and abdominal pain are common in young children. Chest examination is usually unremarkable. Unusual clinical findings or variants include croup (most severe with type A influenza), exacerbation of asthma, myositis (especially calf muscles), myocarditis, parotitis, encephalopathy (distinct from Reye's syndrome), nephritis, and a transient maculopapular rash.

Acute illness lasts 2–5 days. Cough and fatigue last several weeks.

B. Laboratory Findings: The leukocyte count is normal to low, with variable shift. The virus may be found in respiratory secretions by rapid fluorescent antibody staining or enzyme immunoassay (EIA). It can also be cultured within 3–5 days from pharyngeal swabs or throat washings. Some laboratories obtain positive cultures within 48 hours by centrifuging specimens onto cell layers and using antigen detection. Other body fluids or tissues (except lung) rarely yield the virus. Diagnosis may also be made with paired serology, using hemagglutination inhibition assays.

C. Imaging: The chest radiograph is nonspe-

Table 35–1. Common viral causes of clinical syndromes.

Rash
Enterovirus
Adenovirus
Measles
Rubella
Human herpes virus type 6[1]
Varicella
Parvovirus B19[2]
Epstein-Barr virus
Dengue

Fever
Enterovirus
Adenovirus
Epstein-Barr virus
Human herpes virus type 6[1]
Arbovirus
Colorado tick fever
Cytomegalovirus
Influenza
Rhinovirus
Many others

Conjuctivitis
Adenovirus
Enterovirus 70
Influenza
Measles
Herpes simplex[3]

Parotitis
Mumps
Parainfluenza
Enterovirus
Influenza
Cytomegalovirus
Epstein-Barr virus
Human immunodeficiency virus

Pharyngitis
Adenovirus
Enterovirus
Epstein-Barr virus
Herpes simplex virus[4]
Influenza

Adenopathy
Epstein-Barr virus
Cytomegalovirus
Rubella[5]
Human immunodeficiency virus

Croup
Parainfluenza
Influenza
Adenovirus
Measles

Bronchiolitis
Respiratory syncytial virus[6]
Adenovirus
Parainfluenza
Influenza

Pneumonia
Respiratory syncytial virus[7]
Adenovirus
Parainfluenza
Measles
Varicella[8]
Rhinovirus[7]
Cytomegalovirus[7, 10]

Enteritis
Rotavirus
Enteric adenovirus
Hepatitis A[9]
Enterovirus
Norwalk agent
Calicivirus

Hepatitis
Hepatitis[9] A, B, C, D, E
Epstein-Barr virus
Cytomegalovirus
Yellow fever

Arthritis
Parvovirus B19
Rubella
Hepatitis B
Arbovirus

Congenital infection
Cytomegalovirus
Hepatitis B
Rubella
Human immunodeficiency virus
Parvovirus B19
Enterovirus
Varicella
Herpes simplex virus

Meningoencephalitis
Enterovirus
Mumps
Arbovirus
Herpes simplex virus
Cytomegalovirus
Lymphocytic choriomeningitis virus
Measles
Varicella
Rabies
Adenovirus
Human immunodeficiency virus
Epstein-Barr virus

[1]Roseola agent.
[2]Erythema infectiosum agent.
[3]Conjunctivitis rare, only in primary infections; keratitis in older patients.
[4]May cause isolated pharyngeal vesicles at any age.
[5]May cause adenopathy without rash.
[6]Over 90% of cases.
[7]Usually only in young infants.
[8]Immunosuppressed, pregnant, rarely other adults.
[9]Anicteric cases more common in children; these may resemble viral gastroenteritis.
[10]Severely immunosuppressed at risk.

Table 35–2. Diagnostic tests for viral infections.

Agent	Rapid Antigen Detection (Specimen)	Tissue Culture Days to Positive (Mean, Range)	Serology		Polymerase Chain Reaction[1]	Comments
			Acute	Paired		
Adenovirus	+ (respiratory secretions)	+ 10 (1–21)	–	+		"Enteric" strains detected by culture on special cell line, electron microscopy, or antigen detection.
Arboviruses	–	–	+	+		Acute serum may diagnose many forms.
Astrovirus	–	–	–	–		Diagnosis by electron microscopy.
Calicivirus	–	–	–	–		Diagnosis by electron microscopy.
Colorado tick fever	–	–	–	+		Serologic diagnosis available through CDC.
Cytomegalovirus	+ (urine, tissue biopsy, blood, respiratory secretions)	+ 2	RL, CDC	+	+	EIA may be done on tissue culture.
Enterovirus	–	+ 4 (2–15)	–	+	+	Serology for coxsackie B viruses.
Epstein-Barr virus	–	–	+	+		Single serologic panel defines infection status; heterophil titer less sensitive.
Hantavirus	–	–	+	ND	+	Diagnosis by presence of IgM antibody.
Hepatitis A virus	–	–	+	ND		Diagnosis by presence of IgM antibody.
Hepatitis B virus	+ (blood)	–	+	ND		Diagnosis by presence of surface antigen or anti-core IgM antibody.
Herpes simplex virus	+ (skin, respiratory secretions, CSF, tissue biopsy)	+ 2	+	+	+	Serology rarely used for herpes simplex. IgM antibody used in selected cases. Tzanck preparation of vesicle easy, 70% sensitive.
Human herpesvirus-6	–	–	RL, CDC	RL, CDC		Roseola agent.
Human immunodeficiency virus	+ (blood) (acid dissociation of immune complexes)	+ 15 (5–28)	+	+	+	Antibody proves infection unless passively acquired (< age 15 months); culture not widely available.
Influenza virus	+ (respiratory secretions)	+ 3 (2–7)	–	+		Antigen detection 70–90% sensitive.
Lymphocytic choriomeningitis virus	–	Blood, CSF 7 (5–20)	–	+		Can be isolated in suckling mice.
Measles virus	+ (respiratory secretions)	+ (5–14)	+	+		Difficult to grow; IgM serology diagnostic.
Mumps virus	–	+ (> 5)	+	+		Complement fixation titers may allow single-specimen diagnosis.
Parvovirus B19	–	–	+	+	+	Erythema infectiosum agent; antigen detection not yet commercially available.
Parainfluenza virus	+ (respiratory secretions)	+ 5 (2–10)	–	+		
Rabies virus	+ (skin, conjunctiva, tissue biopsy)	–	–	+		Usually diagnosed by antigen detection.
Respiratory syncytial virus	+ (respiratory secretions)	+ 5 (3–14)	–	+		Rapid antigen detection; 85–90% sensitive.
Rhinovirus	–	+ 4 (2–7)	–	–		Too many types to diagnose serologically.
Rotavirus	+ (feces)	–	–	–		Electron microscopy useful for many enteric viruses.
Rubella virus	–	+ (> 10)	RL, CDC	+		Recommended that paired sera be tested simultaneously.
Varicella-zoster virus	+ (skin scraping, tissue biopsy)	+ 3	RL	+	+	Tzanck preparation 70% sensitive.

[1]Useful only when performed on selected specimens by qualified laboratories

Key: + = Commercially or widely available. *Note:* Results from some commercial laboratories are unreliable.
    – = Not available commercially.
RL, CDC = Specific antibody titers available by arrangement with individual research laboratories or the Centers for Disease Control and Prevention.
ND = Not done.

cific; it may show hyperaeration, peribronchial thickening, diffuse interstitial infiltrates, or bronchopneumonia in severe cases. Pneumothorax may occur. Hilar nodes are not enlarged. Pleural effusion is rare in uncomplicated influenza.

Differential Diagnosis

The following may be considered: all other respiratory viruses, *M pneumoniae* or *C pneumoniae* (longer incubation period, prolonged illness), streptococcal pharyngitis (pharyngeal exudate or petechiae, adenitis, no cough), bacterial sepsis (petechial or purpuric rash may occur), meningitis, toxic shock syndrome (rash, hypotension), arboviral infections (fewer respiratory symptoms, summer onset), and rickettsial infections (rash, different season, insect exposure).

Complications & Sequelae

Secondary bacterial infections (classically staphylococcal) of the middle ear, sinuses, or lungs are most common. Of the viral infections that precede Reye's syndrome, varicella and influenza (usually type B) are most notable. During an influenza outbreak, ill children who develop protracted vomiting or irrational behavior should be evaluated for Reye's syndrome (see Chapter 23). Influenza can also cause a viral or postviral encephalitis, with cerebral symptoms much more prominent than those of the accompanying respiratory infection. Although the myositis is usually mild and resolves promptly, severe rhabdomyolysis and renal failure have been reported.

Children with underlying cardiopulmonary, metabolic, neuromuscular, or immunosuppressive disease may develop severe viral pneumonia.

Prevention

Influenza vaccine is moderately protective in older children (see Chapter 10). Medical staff and family members should also be immunized to protect high-risk patients. Type A infections may be prevented by amantadine (3 mg/kg/dose orally twice daily; maximum, 200 mg/d) or rimantadine (5 mg/kg once daily; maximum 150 mg/d under age 10; 200 mg/d if older). The physician should consider administering chemoprophylaxis during an epidemic to high-risk children who cannot be immunized or who have not yet developed immunity (about 6 weeks after primary vaccination or 2 weeks after a booster dose). These agents are inactive against influenza B.

Treatment & Prognosis

Treatment consists of general support and management of pulmonary complications, especially bacterial superinfections. Amantadine and rimantadine are of some benefit against influenza A if begun within 48 hours after onset. Their value in compromised hosts or others with severe disease is uncertain. Ribavirin is active in vitro against influenza A and B. The efficacy of aerosolized ribavirin in humans is contro-

versial, but it may be tried in severe infections, especially in compromised hosts.

Recovery is usually complete unless severe cardiopulmonary or neurologic damage has occurred.

Christenson JC, San Joaquin VH: Influenza-associated rhabdomyolysis in a child. Pediatr Infect Dis J 1990;9: 60.

Douglas RG Jr: Prophylaxis and treatment of influenza. N Engl J Med 1990;322:443.

Kondos AK: The effects of influenza virus infection on FEV$_1$ in asthmatic children. Chest 1991;100:1235.

Liou Y et al: Children hospitalized with influenza B infection. Pediatr Infect Dis 1987;6:541.

Rimantadine for prevention and treatment of influenza. Med Lett Drugs Ther 1993;35:109.

Serwint JR, Hiller RM, Korsch BM: Influenza type A and B infections in hospitalized pediatric patients who should be immunized. Am J Dis Child 1991;145:623.

Sugaya N et al: Impact of influenza virus infection as a cause of pediatric hospitalization. J Infect Dis 1992;165: 373.

PARAINFLUENZA

Parainfluenza viruses (types 1–4) are the most important cause of croup. Most infants are infected with type 3 in the first 2 years of life; all types may cause outbreaks. Infection with types 1 and 2 are experienced gradually over the first 5 years of life. The season and extent vary by location and prior immunity. Most primary infections are symptomatic and frequently involve the lower respiratory tract. In many areas, extensive outbreaks occur every other fall.

Clinical Findings

A. Symptoms and Signs: Clinical diseases include febrile upper respiratory infection (especially in older children with reexposure), laryngitis, tracheobronchitis, croup, and bronchiolitis (second most common cause after respiratory syncytial virus). The relative incidence of these manifestations is type-specific. Croup is the most prominent manifestation in young children. Pneumonia occurs in infants and immunodeficient children. Onset is acute. Most children are febrile. Symptoms of upper respiratory tract infection often accompany croup.

B. Laboratory Findings: Diagnosis is often based on clinical findings in the correct season. These viruses can be identified by rapid culture techniques (48 hours) or antigen detection methods.

Differential Diagnosis

Parainfluenza-induced respiratory syndromes are difficult to distinguish from those caused by other respiratory viruses. Croup must be distinguished from epiglottitis caused by *H influenzae* (abrupt onset, toxicity, drooling, dyspnea, little cough, left shift of blood smear).

Therapy

There is no specific therapy or vaccine. Croup management is discussed in Chapter 20. Ribavirin is active in vitro and has been used in immunocompromised children, but its efficacy is unproved.

Heidemann SM: Clinical characteristics of parainfluenza virus infection in hospitalized children. Pediatr Pulmonol 1992;13:86.

Husby et al: Treatment of croup with nebulized steroid (budesonide): A double blind, placebo controlled study. Arch Dis Child 1993;68:352.

Singh-Naz N, Willy M, Riggs N: Outbreak of parainfluenza virus type 3 in a neonatal nursery. Pediatr Infect Dis J 1990;9:31.

Welliver RC et al: Parainfluenza virus bronchiolitis. Am J Dis Child 1986;140:34.

MUMPS

Essentials of Diagnosis

- No prior mumps vaccine; exposure 14–21 days previously.
- Parotid gland swelling.
- Aseptic meningitis with or without parotitis.
- Orchitis, pancreatitis, or oophoritis.

General Considerations

Mumps is one of the classic childhood infections; the virus spreads by the respiratory route and attacks almost all unimmunized children (asymptomatically in 30–40% of cases) and produces lifelong immunity. The vaccine is so efficacious that clinical disease is rare in immunized children. As a result of subclinical infections, 95% of adults—regardless of the history—are immune. The epidemiology of this illness is changing, however. The vaccine was not in broad use until 1977. Geographic differences in vaccine requirements for school also existed. Thus, there is a large group of adolescents and young adults who are not immune. Since 1986, mumps has been reported with increasing frequency. College outbreaks are notable.

Clinical Findings

A history of exposure to a child with parotitis is not proof of mumps exposure. In an adequately immunized individual, parotitis is usually due to another virus.

A. Symptoms and Signs:

1. Salivary gland disease–Tender swelling of one or more glands, variable fever, and facial lymphedema are typical. Parotid involvement is most common. The ear is displaced upward and outward; the mandibular angle is obliterated. Systemic toxicity is usually absent. Parotid stimulation with sour foods may be quite painful. The orifice of Stensen's duct may be red and swollen; yellow secretions may be expressed, but pus is absent.

2. Meningoencephalitis–Prior to widespread immunization, mumps was the most common cause of aseptic meningitis, which occurs in up to 50% of cases, usually manifested by mild headache or asymptomatic mononuclear pleocytosis. Cerebral symptoms do not correlate with parotid symptoms. Although neck stiffness, nausea, and vomiting can occur, encephalitic symptoms are rare (1:1000 cases of mumps); recovery in 3–10 days is the rule. Vaccine-related meningoencephalitis is also self-limited.

3. Pancreatitis–Abdominal pain may represent transient pancreatitis. Because salivary disease may elevate serum amylase, specific markers of pancreatic function (lipase, amylase isoenzymes) are required for assessing pancreatic involvement.

4. Orchitis, oophoritis–Involvement of the gonads is associated with fever, local tenderness, and swelling. Orchitis is unusual in children but occurs in up to a third of affected postpubertal males. Usually it is unilateral and resolves in 1–2 weeks. Although a third of infected testes atrophy, bilateral involvement and sterility are rare. Atrophic testes have rarely been reported to develop malignant tumors.

5. Other–Thyroiditis, mastitis (especially adolescent females), arthritis, and presternal edema (occasionally with dysphagia or hoarseness) may be seen.

B. Laboratory Findings: Peripheral blood leukocyte counts are usually normal. Up to 1000/μL (predominantly lymphocytes) may be present in the spinal fluid, with mildly elevated protein and normal to slightly decreased glucose. Viral culture of saliva, throat, urine, or spinal fluid may be positive. Spinal fluid often yields the vaccine strain in cases of meningitis following the Urabe vaccine. It is not easily distinguishable from the wild strain. Paired sera assayed by EIA are currently used for diagnosis. Complement-fixing antibody to the soluble antigen disappears in several months; its presence in a single specimen thus indicates recent infection.

Differential Diagnosis

Mumps parotitis may resemble the following: cervical adenitis (the jaw angle may be obliterated, but the ear does not usually protrude; Stensen's duct orifice is normal; leukocytosis and neutrophilia are observed), bacterial parotitis (pus in Stensen's duct, toxicity, exquisite tenderness); recurrent parotitis (idiopathic or associated with calculi), tumors, and tooth infections. Many viruses, including parainfluenza, enteroviruses, Epstein-Barr virus, CMV, HIV, and influenza, can cause parotitis.

Unless parotitis is present, mumps meningitis resembles that caused by enteroviruses or early bacterial infection. An elevated amylase is a useful clue in this situation. Isolated pancreatitis is not distinguishable from many other causes of epigastric pain and vomiting. Mumps is a classic cause of orchitis, but torsion, epididymitis, *Mycoplasma*, other viruses, hematomas, hernias, and tumors must also be considered.

Complications

The major neurologic complication is nerve deafness (usually unilateral), which may be transient and usually results in inability to hear high tones. It may occur without meningitis. Permanent damage is rare, occurring in less than 0.1% of cases of mumps. Aqueductal stenosis and hydrocephalus (especially following congenital infection), myocarditis, transverse myelitis, and facial paralysis are other rare complications.

Treatment & Prognosis

Treatment is supportive and includes provision of fluids, analgesics, and scrotal support for orchitis. Systemic steroids have been used for orchitis, but their value is anecdotal. Surgery is not recommended.

Brunell PA: Mumps. In: *Textbook of Pediatric Infectious Diseases*. 3rd ed. Feigin RD, Cherry JD (editors). Saunders, 1992.

Harel L et al: Mumps arthritis in children. Pediatr Infect Dis J 1990;9:928.

Hersh BS et al: Mumps outbreak in a highly vaccinated population. J Pediatr 1991;119:187.

Koskiniemi M et al: Clinical appearance and outcome in mumps encephalitis in children. Acta Paediatr Scand 1983;72:603.

Manson AL: Mumps orchitis. Urology 1990;36:355.

McDonald JC, Moore DL, Quennec P: Clinical and epidemiologic features of mumps meningoencephalitis and possible vaccine-related disease. Pediatr Infect Dis J 1989;8:751.

Sugiura A, Yamada A: Aseptic meningitis as a complication of mumps vaccination. Pediatr Infect Dis J 1991;10:209.

RESPIRATORY SYNCYTIAL VIRUS (RSV) DISEASE

Essentials of Diagnosis

- Diffuse wheezing and tachypnea following upper respiratory symptoms in an infant (bronchiolitis).
- Epidemics in late fall to early spring.
- Hyperinflation on chest radiograph.
- RSV antigen detected in nasal secretions

General Considerations

Respiratory syncytial virus is the most important cause of lower respiratory tract illness in young children, accounting for over 90% of cases of bronchiolitis and many cases of pneumonia. Winter outbreaks occur annually, and attack rates are high; most children are infected in the first year of life. During peak season, the clinical diagnosis of RSV infection in infants with bronchiolitis is as accurate as most laboratory tests. Despite the presence of serum antibody, reinfection is common. No vaccine is available. Immunosuppressed patients may develop progressive severe pneumonia. Children with congenital heart disease, chronic lung disease, and premature infants under 6 months of age are also at higher risk.

Clinical Findings

A. Symptoms and Signs: Initial symptoms are those of upper respiratory infection. Fever is common. The classic disease is bronchiolitis, characterized by diffuse wheezing, variable fever, cough, tachypnea, difficulty feeding, and cyanosis in severe cases. Hyperinflation ("barrel chest" appearance), rales, rhonchi, wheezing, and retractions are present. Rash and conjunctivitis are unusual. The liver and spleen may be palpable because of lung hyperinflation but are not enlarged. The disease usually lasts 3–7 days.

Apnea may be the presenting manifestation, especially in premature infants in the first few months of life; it usually resolves in the first day or so of illness, often being replaced by obvious signs of bronchiolitis. No explanation for the apnea has been found.

RSV infections in subsequent years are more likely to cause tracheobronchitis or upper respiratory tract infection except in compromised hosts, who may have additional attacks of severe pneumonitis.

B. Laboratory Findings: Routine tests are nonspecific. Rapid detection of RSV antigen in nasal or pulmonary secretions by fluorescent antibody staining or EIA is over 90% sensitive and specific. Rapid tissue culture methods take 48 hours and have comparable sensitivity.

C. Imaging: Diffuse hyperinflation and peribronchiolar thickening are most common; atelectasis and patchy infiltrates also occur in uncomplicated infection, but pleural effusions are rare. Consolidation occurs in 25% of children with lower tract disease, usually in conjunction with other abnormal findings.

Differential Diagnosis

Although almost all cases of bronchiolitis are due to RSV during an epidemic, other viruses cannot be excluded. Mixed infections with other viruses or bacteria are not uncommon. Wheezing may be due to asthma, a foreign body, or other airway obstruction. Respiratory syncytial virus may closely resemble *Chlamydia* pneumonitis when fine rales are present and fever and wheezing are not prominent. The two may also coexist. Cystic fibrosis may resemble RSV infection; a positive family history or failure to thrive associated with hyponatremia or hypoalbuminemia should prompt a sweat chloride test. Pertussis should also be considered in this age group, especially if cough is prominent and if the infant is under 6 months of age. A markedly elevated leukocyte count should suggest bacterial superinfection (neutrophilia) or pertussis (lymphocytosis).

Complications

Secondary bacterial infection of the middle ear or lung (usually due to pneumococci or *H influenzae*) is the most common complication. Sudden exacerbations of fever and leukocytosis should suggest bacterial infection. However, bacterial pneumonia occurs in only 0.5–1% of hospitalized cases. Respiratory failure or apnea may require mechanical ventilation. Cardiac failure may occur as a complication of pulmonary disease or myocarditis. Respiratory syncytial virus—as well as parainfluenza and influenza viruses—can cause acute exacerbations of asthma. Nosocomial infection is so common during outbreaks that elective hospitalization or surgery, especially for those with underlying illness, should be postponed.

Treatment

Children who are very hypoxic or cannot feed because of respiratory distress must be hospitalized and given humidified oxygen and tube or intravenous feedings. Antibiotics, decongestants, expectorants, and steroids are of no value in routine infections. The child should be kept in respiratory isolation. Cohorting ill infants in respiratory isolation during peak season (with or without rapid diagnostic attempts) and emphasizing good handwashing may greatly decrease nosocomial transmission.

Often a trial of bronchodilator therapy is given to determine if bronchospasm coexists. Terbutaline (0.01/mg/kg; up to 0.25 mg) may be administered with bronchodilator inhalation therapy. Discontinue these if there is no improvement. A minimal or equivocal clinical response does not usually justify the expense. If they do help, nebulized treatments (every 2–6 hours as needed) or oral albuterol or theophylline may be tried (see Chapter 20). Because of the possible toxicity of theophylline, especially in children under 1 year of age, inhaled bronchodilators are preferred.

Ribavirin is the only antiviral therapy for RSV infection in humans. It is given by continuous aerosolization (6 g in a 300 mL vial of water) by a special nebulizer (Small Particle Aerosol Generator, ICN Pharmaceuticals) for 12–18 hours of every day for 3–4 days. This agent has minimal effect on viral shedding and a measurable but very modest effect on disease severity in normal infants. It is more efficacious in high-risk infants. It is very expensive. It is teratogenic in animals, but the significance of that observation in humans is unknown. It should be used in a negative-pressure room, preferably fitted with additional respiratory care equipment capable of preventing contamination of room air. Caregivers should wear masks, and pregnant women should not be in a room when ribavirin is being administered.

Bronchospasm may be exacerbated by this drug. It should be used with extreme caution in ventilated patients and only by therapists expert in pediatric ventilator management. In general, it should be considered for use only for very young infants (≤ 8 weeks), former premature infants (< 35 weeks) who are under 6 months old, children with underlying cardiopulmonary or immunologic diseases, and normal infants with evidence of severe RSV pneumonitis (ventilated or with PO$_2$ < 65 mm Hg; PCO$_2$ rising).

Monthly administration of gamma-globulin containing high titers of anti-RSV antibody will prevent severe disease in high-risk patients during epidemic periods.

Prognosis

Although mild bronchiolitis does not produce long-term problems, 30–40% of patients hospitalized with this infection will wheeze later in childhood. Chronic restrictive lung disease and bronchiolitis obliterans are rare sequelae.

Groothuis JR, Gutierrez KM, Lauer BA: Respiratory syncytial virus infection in children with bronchopulmonary dysplasia. Pediatrics 1988;82:199.

Groothuis JR, Salbenblatt CK, Lauer BA: Severe respiratory syncytial virus infection in older children. Am J Dis Child 1990;144:346.

Hall CB et al: Risk of secondary bacterial infection in infants hospitalized with respiratory syncytial viral infection. J Pediatr 1988;113:266.

Isaacs D et al: Handwashing and cohorting in prevention of hospital acquired infections with respiratory syncytial virus. Arch Dis Child 1991;66:227.

La Via WV, Marks MI, Stutman HR: Respiratory syncytial virus puzzle: Clinical features, pathophysiology, treatment, and prevention. J Pediatr 1992;121:503

MacDonald NE et al: Respiratory syncytial viral infection in infants with congenital heart disease. N Engl J Med 1982;307:397.

Madge P et al: Prospective controlled study of four infection-control procedures to prevent nosocomial infection with respiratory syncytial virus. Lancet 1992;340:1079.

Smith DW et al: A controlled trial of aerosolized ribavirin in infants receiving mechanical ventilation for severe respiratory syncytial virus infection. N Engl J Med 1991;325:24.

MEASLES
(Rubeola)

Essentials of Diagnosis

- Exposure to measles 9–14 days previously.
- Prodrome of fever, cough, conjunctivitis, and coryza.
- Koplik's spots (few to countless small white papules on a diffusely red base on the buccal mucosa) 1–2 days prior to and after onset of rash.
- Maculopapular rash spreading down from the face and hairline over 3 days and later becoming confluent.
- Leukopenia.

General Considerations

Until 1989, this classic childhood exanthem had greatly decreased in incidence in the USA because of vaccination against it. The recent increase in cases is more the result of no or improper immunization than of vaccine failures. It is now recommended that all children be revaccinated once again upon entrance into primary or secondary school (Chapter 10). The attack rate in susceptibles is extremely high; spread is respiratory. Morbidity and mortality rates in the developing world are substantial because of underlying malnutrition and secondary infections. Immunity following natural disease is lifelong.

Clinical Findings

A history of contact with a suspected case is often obtainable during an epidemic. In temperate climates, measles is a winter-spring disease. Many suspected cases at other times are misdiagnoses of other viral infections. Since airborne spread is efficient and patients are quite contagious during the prodrome, no contact history may be obtained.

A. Symptoms and Signs: High fever and lethargy are prominent. Sneezing, eyelid edema, tearing, copious coryza, photophobia, and harsh cough ensue and worsen. Koplik's spots are almost pathognomonic for rubeola, though they may be absent. They have rarely been described with rubella and enteroviral infections.

The discrete maculopapular rash spreads quickly over the face and trunk, coalescing to a bright red. As it involves the extremities, it fades from the face and is completely gone within 6 days; fine desquamation may occur. Fever usually falls 2–3 days after the onset of the rash.

The use of killed-virus vaccine until 1967 resulted in partial immunity; upon exposure to wild virus, some vaccinees develop a severe atypical measles characterized by peripheral rash, pneumonia, headache, high fever, and abdominal pain. Koplik's spots are absent. Many adults who were not reimmunized with live-virus vaccines are still at risk for this atypical disease. Partial immunity may be seen in infants with residual maternal antibody, those given immune globulin in any form, and some who have been "appropriately" immunized. These individuals may develop mild cases of measles that can be easily missed because of a nonspecific rash or the absence of fever.

B. Laboratory Findings: Total leukocyte counts may fall to 1500/μL. Lymphopenia is characteristic. An experienced cytologist may see multinucleated giant cells in oral mucosal scrapings and in nasal secretions, but diagnosis is usually made by detection of measles IgM antibody in serum drawn at least 2 days after the onset of rash or by detection of a significant rise in antibody. Tissue culture may also be used, but it takes longer and is less sensitive in many laboratories. Direct detection of measles antigen by fluorescent antibody staining of nasopharyngeal cells is a useful rapid method.

C. Imaging: Chest radiographs often show hyperinflation, perihilar infiltrates, or parenchymal patchy, fluffy densities. Secondary bacterial infection produces consolidation or effusion.

Differential Diagnosis

Table 35–3 lists other illnesses that may resemble measles and some distinguishing features.

Complications & Sequelae

A. Respiratory Complications: These occur in up to 15% of cases. Bacterial superinfections of lung, middle ear, sinus, and cervical nodes are most common. Fever that persists after the third or fourth day of rash suggests such a complication, as does leukocytosis. Bronchospasm, severe croup, and progressive viral pneumonia or bronchiolitis (in infants) also occur. Immunosuppressed patients are at much greater risk of fatal pneumonia.

B. Cerebral Complications: Encephalitis occurs in 1:2000 cases. Onset is usually within a week after appearance of rash. Symptoms include combativeness, ataxia, vomiting, seizures, and coma. Lymphocytic pleocytosis and a mildly elevated protein are usual cerebrospinal fluid findings, but the fluid may be normal. Fifty percent of patients so affected die or are severely damaged.

Subacute sclerosing panencephalitis is a slow measles virus infection of the brain that becomes symptomatic years later in about 1:100,000 previously infected children. This progressive cerebral deterioration is associated with myoclonic jerks and a typical electroencephalographic pattern. It is fatal in 6–12 months. It may occur following administration of vaccine, with an estimated incidence of 1:1,000,000. High titers of measles antibody are present in serum and spinal fluid.

C. Other Complications: These include hemorrhagic or "black" measles (severe disease with multiorgan bleeding, fever, cerebral symptoms), thrombocytopenia, appendicitis, keratitis, myocarditis, optic neuritis, reactivation or progression of tuberculosis (including transient cutaneous anergy), and premature delivery or stillbirth.

Mild liver function test elevation has been detected in up to 50% of cases in young adults; frank jaundice may also occur.

Treatment, Prognosis, & Prevention

Recovery generally occurs 7–10 days after onset of symptoms. Therapy is supportive: eye care, cough relief (avoid narcotic suppressants in infants), and fever reduction (acetaminophen, lukewarm baths; avoid salicylates). Secondary bacterial infections should be treated promptly; antimicrobial prophylaxis is not in-

Table 35–3. Red rashes in children.

Disease	Incubation Period (Days)	Prodrome	Rash	Laboratory Tests	Comments, Other Diagnostic Features
Measles	9–14	Cough, rhinitis, conjunctivitis	Maculopapular; face to extremities; lasts 7–10 d; Koplik's spots in mouth	Leukopenia	Toxic. Bright red rash becomes confluent, may desquamate.
Rubella	14–21	Usually none	Mild maculopapular; rapid spread face to extremities; gone by day 4	Normal or leukopenia	Postauricular, occipital adenopathy common. Polyarthralgia in some older girls. Mild clinical illness.
Roseola (exanthem subitum)	10–14	Fever (3–4 d)	Pink, macular rash occurs at end of illness; transient	Normal	Fever often high, and dissappears when rash develops; child appears well. Usually occurs in children 6 m–2 y of age.
Erythema infectiosum	13–18	None	Erythematous "slapped" cheeks; then reticular rash on extremities, trunk	Normal (reticulocytopenia)	Rash may reappear over weeks, especially with exposure to heat, sunlight. May cause arthralgia/arthritis, usually in older children or adults. Red cell maturation arrest in children with chronic hemolysis can cause aplastic crisis.
Enterovirus	2–7	Variable fever, chills, myalgia, sore throat	Usually macular, maculopapular on trunk or palms, soles; vesicles, petechiae also seen	Variable	Varied rashes may resemble those of many other infections. Pharyngeal or hand-foot-mouth vesicles may occur.
Streptococcal scarlet fever	1–7	Fever, abdominal pain, headache, sore throat	Diffuse erythema, "sandpaper" texture; neck, axillae, inguinal areas; spreads to rest of body; desquamates 7–14 d	Leukocytosis; positive group A streptococcus culture of throat or wound	Strawberry tongue, red pharynx with or without exudate. Eyes, perioral and periorbital area, palms, and soles spared. Pastia's lines. Brief prodrome. Cervical adenopathy, mild variant, scarlatina. Usually occurs in children 2–10 y of age.
Staphylococcal scarlet fever	1–7	Variable fever	Diffuse erythroderma; resembles streptococcal scarlet fever except eyes may be hyperemic, no "strawberry" tongue, pharynx spared	Variable leukocytosis if infected	Focal *Staphylococcus aureus* infection usually present.

Staphylococcal scalded skin	Variable	Irritability, absent to low fever	Painful erythroderma, followed in 1–2 d by dry cracking around eyes, mouth; bullae form with friction (Nikolsky's sign)	Normal if colonized only by staph; leukocytosis and sometimes bacteremia if infected	Normal pharynx. Look for focal staph infection. Usually occurs in infants.
Toxic shock syndrome	Variable	Fever, myalgia, headache, diarrhea, vomiting	Nontender erythroderma; red eyes, palms, soles, pharynx, lips	Leukocytosis; abnormal liver enzymes, coagulation tests; proteinuria	*S aureus* infection, multiorgan involvement. Swollen hands, feet. Hypotension or shock.
Erythema multiforme	–	Usually none or related to underlying cause	Discrete, red maculopapular lesions; symmetric, distal, palms and soles; target lesions classic	Normal or eosinophilia	Reaction to drugs (especially sulfas), or infectious agents. Urticaria, arthralgia also seen.
Stevens-Johnson syndrome	–	Pharyngitis, conjunctivitis, fever, malaise	Bullous erythema multiforme; may slough in large areas; hemorrhagic lips; purulent conjunctivitis	Leukocytosis	Classic precipitants are drugs (especially sulfas), *Mycoplasma pneumoniae* and herpes simplex infections. Pneumonitis and urethritis also seen.
Drug allergy	–	None, fever alone, or fever, myalgia, pruritus	Macular, maculopapular, urticarial, or erythroderma	Leukopenia, eosinophilia	Rash variable. Severe reactions may resemble measles, scarlet fever; adenopathy, hepatosplenomegaly; marked toxicity possible.
Kawasaki disease	Unknown	Fever, cervical adenopathy, irritability	Polymorphous (may be erythroderma) on trunk and extremities; red palms and soles, lips, tongue, pharynx	Leukocytosis, thrombocytosis, elevated ESR; pyuria; negative cultures and streptococcal serology	Swollen hands, feet; prolonged illness; bulbar hyperemia; uveitis; aseptic meningitis; no response to antibiotics. Vasculitis and aneurysms of coronary and other arteries occur.
Leptospirosis	4–19	Fever, myalgia, chills	Variable erythroderma	Leukocytosis; hematuria, proteinuria; hyperbilirubinemia	Conjunctivitis; toxic. Hepatitis, aseptic meningitis may be seen. Rodent, dog contact.

dicated. Ribavirin is active in vitro and may be useful in infected immunocompromised children. In malnourished children, acute vitamin A supplementation will attenuate the illness.

The current two-dose active vaccination strategy is successful. Vaccine should not be withheld for concurrent mild acute illness, tuberculosis or positive PPD, breast feeding, or exposure to an immunodeficient contact.

Vaccination prevents the disease in susceptible exposed individuals if given within 72 hours (see Chapter 10). Immune globulin (0.25 mL/kg intramuscularly) will prevent or modify measles if given within 6 days. Suspected cases should be diagnosed promptly and reported to the local health department.

Fortenberry JD et al: Severe laryngotracheobronchitis complicating measles. Am J Dis Child 1992;146:1040.

Hussey GD, Klein M: Randomized, controlled trial of vitamin A in children with severe measles. N Engl J Med 1990;323:160.

Kaplan LJ et al: Severe measles in immunocompromised patients. JAMA 1992;267:1237.

Kipps A, Dick G, Moodie JW: Measles and the central nervous system. Lancet 1983;2:1406.

Mason WH et al: Epidemic measles in the postvaccine era: Evaluation of epidemiology, clinical presentation and complications during an urban outbreak. Pediatr Infect Dis J 1993;12:42.

The National Vaccine Advisory Committee: The measles epidemic: The problems, barriers, and recommendations. JAMA 1991;266:1549.

INFECTIONS DUE TO ENTEROVIRUSES & RHINOVIRUSES

Enteroviruses are a major cause of illness in children. They are physically and biochemically similar and may produce identical syndromes. The multiple types make vaccine development impractical and have hindered development of antigen-detection and serologic tests. However, common RNA sequences and group antigens have led to diagnostic tests for viral nucleic acid and proteins. Tissue culture is the commonly used diagnostic method for echoviruses, polioviruses, and coxsackie B viruses. Since cultures may turn positive in 2–4 days, they should be inoculated promptly and may be clinically useful, particularly in cases of meningoencephalitis. Many coxsackie A viruses fail to grow.

Transmission is fecal-oral. Multiple enteroviruses circulate in the community at any one time; summer-fall outbreaks are common in temperate climates, but illness is seen year-round. After poliovirus, coxsackie B virus is most virulent, followed by echovirus. Neu-

rologic, cardiac, and overwhelming neonatal infections are the severest forms of illness.

ACUTE FEBRILE ILLNESS

Accompanied by nonspecific upper respiratory or enteric symptoms, sudden onset of fever and irritability in infants or young children is often enteroviral in origin, especially in late summer and fall. Occasionally, a petechial rash is seen; more often, a diffuse maculopapular eruption (often prominent on palms and soles) occurs on the second to fourth days of fever. Purpura is rare and should suggest bacterial sepsis. Rapid recovery is the rule. Leukocyte counts are usually normal. Many types of coxsackievirus and echovirus infections present in this manner, which often prompts an evaluation for bacteremia or meningitis.

RESPIRATORY TRACT ILLNESSES

1. NONSPECIFIC, FEBRILE UPPER RESPIRATORY INFECTION WITH PHARYNGITIS

This syndrome is most common. Pneumonia or wheezing is unusual. Vesicles or papules may be seen in the pharynx. There is no exudate.

2. HERPANGINA

Herpangina is characterized by an acute onset of fever and posterior pharyngeal ulcers, often linearly arranged on the anterior fauces. Bilateral faucial ulcers may also be seen. Dysphagia, vomiting, and anorexia also occur and, rarely, parotitis or vaginal ulcers. Symptoms disappear in a week. The epidemic form is due to a variety of coxsackie A viruses; coxsackie B viruses and echoviruses cause sporadic cases.

The differential diagnosis includes primary herpes simplex gingivostomatitis (ulcers are more prominent anteriorly, and gingivitis is present), aphthous stomatitis (fever absent, recurrent episodes, anterior lesions), trauma, burns (usually not discrete), hand-foot-and-mouth disease (see below), and Vincent's angina (spreading painful gingivitis from the gum line, underlying dental disease).

3. ACUTE LYMPHONODULAR PHARYNGITIS

Coxsackievirus A10 has been associated with a febrile pharyngitis characterized by nonulcerating yellow-white posterior pharyngeal papules. The duration is 1–2 weeks; therapy is supportive.

4. PLEURODYNIA
(Bornholm Disease, Epidemic Myalgia)

Caused by coxsackie B virus (epidemic form) or many nonpolio enteroviruses (sporadic form), pleurodynia presents with an abrupt onset of unilateral pleuritic pain of variable intensity. Symptoms are episodic, and relapses occur. Associated symptoms include headache, fever, vomiting, myalgias, and abdominal and neck pain. Physical findings include fever, chest muscle tenderness, decreased thoracic excursion, and occasionally a friction rub. The chest radiograph is normal. Hematologic tests are nondiagnostic.

The differential diagnosis includes bacterial pneumonia, empyema, tuberculosis, and coccidioidomycosis (all excluded radiographically), costochondritis (no fever or other symptoms), and a variety of abdominal problems, especially those causing diaphragmatic irritation.

There is no specific therapy. Potent analgesic agents and chest splinting alleviate the pain.

RASHES

The rash may be macular, maculopapular, urticarial, scarlatiniform, petechial, or vesicular. One of the most characteristic is that of hand-foot-and-mouth disease (caused by coxsackievirus, especially types A5, A10, and A16), in which vesicles or red papules are found on the tongue, oral mucosa, hands, and feet. Associated fever and malaise are mild. The rash may appear when fever abates, simulating roseola.

CARDIAC INVOLVEMENT

Myocarditis and pericarditis may be caused by a number of nonpolio enteroviruses, particularly type B coxsackieviruses; disease may be mild or fatal. In infants, other organs may be involved at the same time; in older patients, cardiac disease is usually isolated (see Chapter 21 for therapy). Enteroviral genomes are present in cardiac tissue in some cases of dilated cardiomyopathy or myocarditis; the significance of this finding is not known.

SEVERE NEONATAL INFECTION

Sporadic and nosocomial nursery cases of severe systemic enteroviral disease occur. Clinical manifestations include combinations of fever, rash, pneumonitis, encephalitis, hepatitis, gastroenteritis, myocarditis, pancreatitis, and myositis. The infants may appear septic, with cyanosis and dyspnea. The differential diagnosis includes bacterial and herpes infections, necrotizing enterocolitis, other causes of heart or liver failure, and metabolic diseases. Diagnosis is suggested by the finding of cerebrospinal fluid mononuclear pleocytosis and confirmed by the isolation of virus from urine, stool, cerebrospinal fluid, or pharynx. Strict isolation is needed; therapy is supportive. Intravenous immunoglobulin is often administered, but its value is uncertain. Passively acquired maternal antibody may protect newborns from severe disease. For this reason, labor should not be induced in pregnant women near term with suspected enteroviral disease.

Abzug M, Levin MJ, Rotbart HA: Profile of enterovirus disease in the first two weeks of life. Pediatr Infect Dis J 1993;12:820.

Modlin JF: Perinatal echovirus and group B coxsackie infections. Clin Perinatol 1988;15:233.

CENTRAL NERVOUS SYSTEM ILLNESSES

1. POLIOMYELITIS

Essentials of Diagnosis

- Usually no prior immunization.
- Headache, fever, nausea, vomiting, muscle weakness.
- Asymmetric, flaccid paralysis; muscle tenderness; intact sensation; late atrophy.
- Aseptic meningitis.

General Considerations

Poliovirus infection is subclinical in 90–95% of cases; causes nonspecific febrile illness in about 5%; and causes aseptic meningitis or paralytic disease in 1–3%. In endemic areas, most older children and adults are immune because of prior inapparent infections. Occasional cases in the USA occur in patients who have traveled to foreign countries; most cases are in immunodeficient patients who receive the poliovirus vaccine. Severe poliovirus infections rarely follow oral poliovirus vaccination as a result of reversion of the vaccine virus. The incidence varies from 1:10,000,000 to 1:1,000,000, depending on virus type and the age of the vaccinee. The risk of this complication is much greater in immunodeficient children.

Clinical Findings

A. Symptoms and Signs: The initial symptoms are fever, myalgia, sore throat, and headache for 2–6 days. Several symptom-free days are followed by recurrent fever and signs of aseptic meningitis—headache, stiff neck, spinal rigidity, and nausea. Mild cases resolve completely. High fever, severe myalgia, and anxiety usually portend progression to loss of reflexes and subsequent flaccid paralysis. Sensation remains intact. The disease progression is variable, especially in infants.

Paralysis is usually asymmetric. Bulbar involvement affects swallowing, speech, and cardiorespiratory function and accounts for most deaths. Paralysis is usually complete by the time the temperature normalizes. Weakness often resolves completely. Atrophy is usually apparent by 4–8 weeks. Most of the improvement of muscle paralysis that is going to occur will take place within 6 months and the remainder over the next 12 months.

B. Laboratory Findings: In patients with meningeal symptoms, the cerebrospinal fluid shows up to several hundred leukocytes (mostly lymphocytes); glucose level is normal, and protein concentration is mildly elevated. Poliovirus is easy to grow in cell culture and can be readily differentiated from other enteroviruses. It may be isolated from spinal fluid for 3–5 days after meningitis is appreciated or from throat and stool for several weeks following infection. Paired serology is also diagnostic. Differentiation of wild from live attenuated vaccine strains requires expertise.

Differential Diagnosis

Aseptic meningitis due to poliovirus is indistinguishable from that due to other viruses. Paralytic disease in the USA is usually due to nonpolio enteroviruses. Polio may resemble Guillain-Barré syndrome (variable sensory loss, symmetric loss of function; minimal pleocytosis, high protein concentration in spinal fluid), polyneuritis (sensory loss), pseudoparalysis due to bone or joint problems (eg, trauma, infection), botulism, or tick paralysis.

Complications & Sequelae

Complications are the result of the acute and permanent effects of paralysis. Respiratory, pharyngeal, bladder, and bowel malfunction are most critical. Deaths are usually due to complications arising from respiratory dysfunction.

Treatment & Prognosis

Therapy is supportive. Bed rest, fever and pain control (heat therapy is helpful), and careful attention to progression of weakness (particularly of respiratory muscles) are important. Intubation or tracheostomy for secretion control and catheter drainage of the bladder may be needed. Assisted ventilation and enteral feeding may also be needed. Paralysis is mild in about 30%, permanent in 15%, and results in death in 5–10%. Disease is worse in adults and pregnant women than in children.

Agre JC, Rodriguez AA: Neuromuscular function in polio survivors at one-year follow-up. Arch Phys Med Rehabil 1991;72:7.

Hovi T et al: Outbreak of paralytic poliomyelitis in Finland: Widespread circulation of antigenically altered poliovirus type 3 in a vaccinated population. Lancet 1986;1: 1427.

Nikowane BM et al: Vaccine associated paralytic poliomyelitis. JAMA 1987;257:1335.

2. ASEPTIC MENINGITIS

Nonpolio enteroviruses cause over 80% of cases of aseptic meningitis at all ages. In the summer and fall, multiple cases may be seen associated with circulation of neurotropic strains. Nosocomial outbreaks also occur; severe disease and death may occur in neonates. Spread is fecal-oral.

Clinical Findings

The usual enteroviral incubation period is 4–6 days. Since enteroviral infections are often subclinical, a history of contact with a patient with meningitis is unusual. Neonates may acquire infection from maternal blood, vaginal secretions, or feces at birth; occasionally, the mother has had a febrile illness just prior to delivery.

A. Symptoms and Signs: Onset is usually acute with variable fever, marked irritability, and lethargy in infants. Incidence is much greater in children less than 1 year of age. Older children also describe frontal headache, photophobia, and myalgia. Abdominal pain, diarrhea, and vomiting may occur. The incidence of rash varies with the infecting strain. If rash occurs, it is usually seen after several days of illness and is diffuse, macular or maculopapular, occasionally petechial, but not purpuric. Oropharyngeal vesicles and rash on the palms and soles suggest an enteroviral cause. The anterior fontanelle may be full. In older children, it is easier to demonstrate meningeal signs. Seizures are unusual, and focal neurologic findings are so rare that they suggest another agent or diagnosis. Frank encephalitis is rare at all ages, though more common in neonates.

B. Laboratory Findings: Blood leukocyte counts are nonspecific and often within the normal range. The spinal fluid leukocyte count is 100–1000/μL. Early in the illness, polymorphonuclear cells predominate; a shift to mononuclear cells occurs within 8–36 hours. In about 95% of cases, spinal fluid parameters include a total leukocyte count less than 3000/μL, protein less than 80 mg/dL, and glucose more than 40% of serum values. Marked deviation from any of these findings should prompt consideration of another diagnosis (see below). The syndrome of inappropriate secretion of antidiuretic hormone may occur but is rarely clinically significant.

Culture of cerebrospinal fluid may yield an enterovirus within a few days; virus may be found in acellular spinal fluids. Isolation of an enterovirus from throat or stool suggests but does not prove enteroviral meningitis. Vaccine poliovirus present in feces in infants being evaluated for aseptic meningitis may confuse the diagnosis. It can usually be distinguished by growth characteristics from other enteroviruses. Rarely, vaccine poliovirus has caused ventriculoperitoneal shunt infections.

C. Imaging: Cerebral imaging is not often indicated; if done, it is usually normal; subdural effusions, infarcts, edema, or focal abnormalities seen in bacterial meningitis are absent.

Differential Diagnosis

In the prevaccine era, mumps and polio were leading causes of aseptic meningitis. Other viral agents include arbovirus and herpes simplex. In adolescents, herpesvirus type 2 may cause concomitant aseptic meningitis and genital infection. In neonates, early herpesvirus meningoencephalitis may mimic enteroviral disease (see the section on herpesviruses, below).

Other causes of aseptic meningitis that may resemble enteroviral infection include partially treated bacterial meningitis (recent antibiotic treatment; spinal fluid parameters resembling those seen in bacterial disease and bacterial antigen sometimes present); parameningeal foci of bacterial infection such as brain abscess, subdural empyema, mastoiditis (predisposing factors, glucose level in cerebrospinal fluid possibly lower, focal neurologic signs); tumors or cysts (malignant cells detected by cytologic examination, a history of neurologic symptoms, higher protein concentration or lower glucose level in cerebrospinal fluid); trauma (presence, without exception, of red blood cells, which are often assumed to be due to traumatic lumbar puncture but are crenated and fail to clear); vasculitis (other systemic or neurologic signs; older children); tuberculous or fungal meningitis (Chapters 36 and 37); cysticercosis; parainfectious encephalopathies (*Mycoplasma pneumoniae,* respiratory viruses); Lyme disease; leptospirosis; and rickettsial diseases.

Treatment & Prevention

There is no specific therapy. Infants are usually hospitalized, isolated, and treated with fluids and antipyretics. If they are moderately to severely ill, infants are given appropriate antibiotics for bacterial pathogens until cultures are negative for 48–72 hours. If patients—especially older children—are mildly ill, antibiotics may be withheld and the child observed. A repeat lumbar puncture in 8–12 hours may be helpful; with viral infection, the Gram stain is again negative, the cell count does not rise substantially, and there is a further shift to mononuclear cells. In these cases, children who are clinically stable may be closely observed in the hospital or at home. Adequate analgesia, including codeine compounds or other strong pain relievers, may be needed. C-reactive protein and lactate levels are usually low in the cerebrospinal fluid of children with viral meningitis; both may be elevated

with bacterial infection. With clinical deterioration, repeat lumbar puncture, cerebral imaging, neurologic consultation, and more aggressive diagnostic tests (eg, viral cultures, brain biopsy) should be considered. Herpesvirus encephalitis is of graver concern in such cases, particularly in infants under 1 month of age. Newborns may receive empiric acyclovir therapy until an etiologic diagnosis is made.

Measures to prevent enteroviral infection include good hygiene, scrupulous hand washing, and proper isolation in the hospital.

Prognosis

In general, enteroviral meningitis has no significant short-term neurologic or developmental sequelae. Developmental delay may follow infection in the first few months of life. Unlike mumps, enterovirus infections rarely cause hearing loss. Frank encephalitis may cause diffuse brain damage.

Cherry JD: Aseptic meningitis and viral meningitis. In: *Textbook of Pediatric Infectious Disease.* 3rd Edition Feigin RD, Cherry JD (editors). Saunders, 1992.

Dalton M, Newton RW: Aseptic meningitis. Dev Med Child Neurol 1991;33:446.

Modlin JF et al: Focal encephalitis with enterovirus infections. Pediatrics 1991;88:841.

Sumaya CV, Corman LI: Enteroviral meningitis in early infancy: Significance in community outbreaks. Pediatr Infect Dis J 1982;1:151.

Wilfert CM, Lehrman SN, Katz SL: Enteroviruses and meningitis. Pediatr Infect Dis J 1983;2:333.

RHINOVIRAL INFECTIONS

The many serotypes of rhinoviruses are best known as agents of the common cold. Profuse rhinorrhea, sneezing, cough, mild pharyngitis, and mild fever are typical. The viruses have been isolated from the lower respiratory tract in normal infants and children and in immunosuppressed patients. Therapy is supportive.

INFECTIONS DUE TO HERPESVIRUSES

HERPES SIMPLEX

Essentials of Diagnosis

- Grouped vesicles on an erythematous base.
- Tender regional adenopathy, especially with primary infection.
- Fever and malaise with primary infection.
- Recurrent episodes in many patients.

General Considerations

There are two types of herpes simplex viruses. Type 1 causes most oral, skin, and cerebral disease. Type 2 causes most (80–85%) genital and congenital infections. Latent infection in sensory ganglia routinely follows primary infection. Recurrences may be spontaneous, induced by external events (eg, fever, menstruation, or sunlight) or immunosuppression. Transmission is by direct contact with infected secretions. Herpes simplex viruses are very susceptible to antiviral drugs.

Primary infection usually occurs early in childhood, though many adults (20–50%) have never been infected. Primary infection with HSV-1 is subclinical in 80% of cases and causes gingivostomatitis in the remainder. Type 2 HSV is sexually transmitted and is also usually subclinical. Infection with one type usually precludes infection with other strains of the same type, but individuals can be infected with both type 1 and type 2 HSV. Recurrent episodes are due to reactivation of latent virus.

Clinical Findings

The source of primary infection is often an asymptomatic excretor; at any one time, 1–2% of normal seropositive adults excrete HSV-1 in the saliva or HSV-2 in genital secretions. Prior infection and subclinical disease are so common that the history is of little diagnostic value.

A. Symptoms and Signs:

1. Gingivostomatitis–High fever, irritability, and drooling are seen in infants. Multiple oral ulcers are seen on the tongue and on the buccal and gingival mucosa, occasionally extending to the pharynx. Pharyngeal ulcers may predominate in older children. Diffusely swollen red gums that are friable and bleed easily are typical. Cervical nodes are swollen and tender. Duration is 7–14 days. Herpangina, aphthous stomatitis, thrush, and Vincent's angina should be excluded.

2. Vulvovaginitis or urethritis–Genital herpes (especially type 2) in a prepubertal child should suggest sexual abuse. Vesicles or ulcers on the vulva, vagina, or penis and tender adenopathy are seen. Painful urination may cause retention. Primary infections last 10–21 days. Lesions may resemble trauma, syphilis, or chancroid in the adolescent and bullous impetigo, trauma, severe chemical irritation, and burns in younger children.

3. Cutaneous infections–Direct inoculation onto cuts (eg, herpetic whitlow on a thumb) or abrasions may produce localized or extensive vesicles or ulcers. A deeper HSV infection on the fingers may be mistaken for a bacterial felon or paronychia; surgical drainage is of no value and is contraindicated. Herpes simplex virus infection of eczematous skin may result in extensive areas of vesicles and shallow ulcers (eczema herpeticum), which may be mistaken for impetigo or varicella.

4. Recurrent cutaneous infection–Recurrent oral shedding is usually asymptomatic. Perioral recurrences often begin with a prodrome of tingling or burning limited to the vermilion border, followed by vesiculation, scabbing, and crusting around the lips over the next few days. Rarely, intraoral lesions recur. Fever, adenopathy, and other symptoms are absent. Recurrent cutaneous herpes most closely resembles impetigo; the latter is often outside the perinasal and perioral region, responds to antibiotics, and yields *Streptococcus pyogenes* or *Staphylococcus aureus* on culture.

5. Keratoconjunctivitis–Keratoconjunctivitis may be part of a primary infection due to spread from infected saliva. Most cases are caused by reactivation of virus latent in the ciliary ganglion. Keratoconjunctivitis produces photophobia, pain, and conjunctival irritation. With recurrences, dendritic corneal ulcers may be demonstrable with fluorescein staining. Stromal invasion may occur. Steroids should never be used without ophthalmologic consultation. Other causes of these symptoms include trauma and bacterial and viral infection (especially adenovirus if pharyngitis is present).

6. Encephalitis–Although unusual in infants outside the neonatal period, encephalitis may occur at any age, usually without cutaneous herpes lesions. In older children, HSV encephalitis often represents a reactivation of latent virus. Herpes simplex virus is probably the most common cause of sporadic severe encephalitis. Fever, headache, behavioral changes, and focal seizures occur (the latter as a result of the typical temporal lobe involvement). Early in infection, all studies may be normal. Later, mild mononuclear pleocytosis (often with erythrocytes) is present along with elevated protein concentration, which continues to rise on repeat lumbar punctures. Hypodense areas with a temporal lobe predilection are seen on CT scan, especially after 3–5 days. MRI is more sensitive and is positive sooner. Periodic focal epileptiform discharges are seen on EEGs but are not diagnostic of HSV infection. Viral cultures of spinal fluid are usually negative. The polymerase chain reaction to detect HSV DNA in spinal fluid is the most sensitive test short of biopsy. Without early antiviral therapy, the prognosis is very poor. The differential diagnosis includes mumps and arbovirus encephalitis, rabies, parainfectious encephalopathy, brain abscess, acute demyelinating syndromes, and bacterial meningoencephalitis.

7. Neonatal infections–The infection is acquired by ascending spread (5–10% of cases) prior to delivery or at the time of vaginal delivery of a mother with genital infection. Occasionally, the infection is acquired from oral secretions of family members or hospital personnel. A history of genital herpes in the mother is usually absent. Within a few days to weeks, skin vesicles (especially at sites of trauma, such as the sites where scalp monitors were placed) appear in about half of infected infants. Some infants are acutely ill, presenting with jaundice, shock, bleeding, or respiratory distress. Others appear well initially, but dissemination to brain or other organs usually occurs over the next week if the infection is untreated. Some infants present with only neurologic symptoms at 2–3 weeks after delivery: apnea, lethargy, fever, poor feeding, or persistent overt seizures. The brain infection in these children is often diffuse and is best appreciated by MRI. The skin lesions may resemble impetigo, bacterial scalp abscesses, trauma, or miliaria. The systemic signs are nonspecific.

B. Laboratory Findings: Routine tests are nonspecific. A finding of lymphocytic pleocytosis is the rule in aseptic meningitis or encephalitis. Virus may be cultured from infected epithelial sites (vesicles, ulcers, or corneal scrapings) and from infected tissue (skin, brain) obtained by biopsy. Cultures of spinal fluid are positive in about 50% of cases. Isolation from throat, eye, urine, or stool of a newborn is diagnostic. Vaginal culture of the mother may offer circumstantial evidence for the diagnosis.

Herpes simplex virus will be detected within 2 days in tissue culture. The value of serologic tests in older individuals is limited by the presence of antibody in all patients with latent infections, the lack of serologic rise during most reactivations, and cross-reactivity between type 1 and type 2 antibody.

Rapid diagnostic tests include cytology of scrapings from the base of vesicles or ulcers using chemical stains (Tzanck test) to look for characteristic multinucleated giant cells, immunofluorescent stains to detect viral antigen, or EIA.

Complications, Sequelae, & Prognosis

Gingivostomatitis may result in dehydration due to dysphagia; severe chronic oral disease and esophageal involvement may occur in immunosuppressed patients.

Primary vulvovaginitis may be associated with aseptic meningitis, paresthesias, autonomic dysfunction due to neuritis (urinary retention, constipation), and secondary candidal infection.

Extensive cutaneous disease (as in eczema) may be associated with dissemination, bacterial superinfection, and death.

Keratitis may result in corneal opacification or perforation.

Untreated encephalitis is fatal in 70% of patients and causes severe damage in most of the remainder. When acyclovir treatment is instituted early, 20% die and 40% are neurologically impaired.

Disseminated neonatal infection is often fatal in spite of therapy.

Treatment

A. Specific Measures: Herpes simplex virus is very sensitive to antiviral therapy. Topical antivirals are most effective for corneal disease and include 1% trifluridine, 3% acyclovir, and 3% vidarabine. Trifluridine appears superior; cure rates over 95% are reported. The dose is 1 drop every 2 hours while the patient is awake until the ulcer heals, then 1 drop every 4 hours for 7 more days. Vidarabine ointment requires fewer treatments and may be more practical for young children.

Mucocutaneous HSV infections respond to oral administration of acyclovir. The main indication is severe genital HSV infection in adolescents; acyclovir (200 mg orally five times a day for 5–10 days) is beneficial for primary disease when therapy is begun early. Recurrent disease rarely requires therapy. Frequent recurrences may be suppressed by oral administration of acyclovir (200 mg three times a day or 400 mg twice a day), but this regimen should be used sparingly. Other forms of severe cutaneous disease, such as eczema herpeticum and HSV infections in immunocompromised children, also respond. Intravenous therapy is often used in this setting (250 mg/m$_2$ every 8 hours). Oral acyclovir is also used for severe gingivostomatitis in infants (5–10 mg/kg per dose four times a day for 5–7 days).

The only two parenteral drugs of value are acyclovir and vidarabine. Acyclovir is superior; the dosage is 500 mg/m$_2$ every 8 hours intravenously for 14 days for encephalitis and 14–21 days for neonates.

Antiviral therapy does not alter the incidence or severity of recurrences of genital infection. Development of resistance to acyclovir is rare after standard courses but is increasingly reported in immunocompromised patients after prolonged therapy.

B. General Measures:

1. Gingivostomatitis–Gingivostomatitis is treated with pain relief and temperature control. Maintaining hydration is important because of the long duration of illness (7–14 days). Nonacidic, cool fluids are best. Topical anesthetic agents (such as viscous lidocaine or an equal mixture of Kaopectate, diphenhydramine, and viscous lidocaine) may be used as a mouthwash for older children who will not swallow it; ingested lidocaine may be toxic to infants. Antiviral therapy is not generally indicated in normal hosts, though it could be considered for those with severe disease. Antibiotics are not helpful.

2. Genital infections–Genital infections require pain relief, assistance with voiding (warm baths, topical anesthetics, rarely catheterization), and psychologic support. Lesions should be kept clean; drying decreases the potential for spread and may shorten the duration of infection. Sexual contact should be avoided during the interval from prodrome to crusting stages.

3. Cutaneous lesions–Skin lesions should be kept clean, dry, and covered if possible to prevent spread. Systemic analgesics may be helpful. Secondary bacterial infection is uncommon in patients with lesions on the mucosa or involving small areas. Secondary infection should be considered and treated if necessary (usually with an antistaphylococcal agent) in patients with more extensive lesions. *Candida* superinfection occurs in 10% of women with primary genital infections.

4. Recurrent cutaneous disease–Recurrent disease is usually milder than primary infection. Sun block lip balm helps prevent labial recurrences after intense sun exposure. There is no evidence that the many popular topical or vitamin therapies are efficacious.

5. Keratoconjunctivitis–An ophthalmologist should be consulted regarding the use of cycloplegics, anti-inflammatory agents, local debridement, and other therapies.

6. Encephalitis–See Chapter 25.

7. Neonatal infection–The affected infant should be isolated. Therapy is supportive. Cesarian section is indicated if there are obvious maternal cervical or vaginal lesions, especially if these represent primary infection. In women with a history of genital herpes infection, vaginal delivery with peripartum cultures of maternal cervix is the standard. Clinical follow-up is recommended when maternal cultures are positive. Repeated cervical cultures during pregnancy are not useful.

Arvin AM: Oral therapy with acyclovir in infants and children. Pediatr Infect Dis J 1987;6:56.

Arvin AM et al: Consensus management of the patient with herpes simplex encephalitis. Pediatr Infect Dis J 1987; 6:2.

Brown ZA et al: Neonatal herpes simplex virus infection in relation to asymptomatic maternal infection at the time of labor. N Engl J Med 1991;324:1247.

Corey L, Spear PG: Infections with herpes simplex viruses. (Two parts.) N Engl J Med 1986;314:686, 749.

Gasecki AP, Steg RE: Correlation of early MRI with CT scan, EEG, and CSF: Analyses in a case of biopsy-proven herpes simplex encephalitis. Eur Neurol 1991; 31:372.

Kimura H et al: Relapse of herpes simplex encephalitis in children. Pediatrics 1992;89:891.

Koskiniemi M et al: Neonatal herpes simplex virus infection: A report of 43 patients. Pediatr Infect Dis 1989; 8:30.

Kuzushima K et al: Clinical manifestations of primary herpes simplex type 1 infection in a closed community. Pediatrics 1991;87:152.

Toltzis P: Current issues in neonatal herpes simplex virus infections. Clin Perinatol 1991;18:193.

Troendle-Atkins J, Demmler GJ, Buffone GJ: Rapid diagnosis of herpes simplex virus encephalitis by using the polymerase chain reaction. J Pediatr 1993;123:376.

VARICELLA (Chickenpox) & HERPES ZOSTER (Shingles)

Essentials of Diagnosis

Varicella:
- Exposure to varicella or herpes zoster 10–20 days previously; no prior history of varicella.
- Widely scattered macules and papules rapidly progressing to clear vesicles, pustules, and then crusting, over 5–6 days. Variable fever and nonspecific systemic symptoms.

Herpes zoster:
- History of varicella.
- Local paresthesias and pain prior to eruption (more common in older children).
- Dermatomal distribution of grouped vesicles on an erythematous base.

General Considerations

Primary infection results in varicella, which almost always confers lifelong immunity; the virus remains latent in sensory ganglia and reappears in 10–15% of individuals as herpes zoster. The incidence of reactivation is increased in immunosuppressed patients. Spread from a contact with varicella during primary infection is by respiratory secretions, with a greater than 95% infection rate in susceptibles. Infection may also be caused by fomites from vesicles or pustules. Herpes zoster is about one-third as infectious. Over 95% of young adults with a history of varicella are immune, as are 90% of native-born Americans who are unaware of having had varicella. Many individuals from tropical or subtropical areas never have childhood exposure. Humans are the only reservoir.

Clinical Findings

Exposure to varicella has usually occurred 14–16 days previously (range, 10–21 days). Contact with a patient with herpes zoster or mild varicella may not have been recognized. Although varicella is the most distinctive childhood exanthem, inexperienced observers may mistake other diseases for varicella. A 1- to 3- day prodrome of fever and respiratory symptoms may occur, especially in older children. The preeruptive pain of herpes zoster may last several days and be mistaken for other illnesses.

A. Symptoms and Signs:

1. Varicella–The usual case consists of mild systemic symptoms followed by crops of red macules that rapidly become tiny vesicles with surrounding erythema ("dew drop on a rose petal"), form pustules, become crusted and then scab over, and leave no scar. The rash appears predominantly on the trunk and face. Lesions occur in the scalp, nose, mouth (where they are nonspecific ulcers), and intestine (usually asymptomatic). The magnitude of systemic symptoms usually parallels skin involvement. Up to five crops of lesions may be seen. New ones usually stop forming after 5–7 days. Pruritus is often intense. If varicella occurs in the first few months of life, it is often mild as a result of persisting maternal antibody. Once crusting begins, the patient is no longer contagious.

2. Herpes zoster–The eruption of shingles involves a single dermatome, usually truncal or cranial. The rash does not cross the midline. Ophthalmic zoster may be associated with corneal involvement. The closely grouped vesicles often coalesce. The duration is 7–10 days before crusting. Postherpetic neuralgia is rare in children. A few vesicles are occasionally seen outside the involved dermatome. This disease is a common problem in HIV-infected children.

B. Laboratory Findings: Leukocyte counts are normal or low. Leukocytosis suggests secondary bacterial infection. Multinucleated giant cells in a stained cytologic scraping from a vesicle base (Tzanck test) will indicate the presence of either a varicella-zoster virus or HSV infection. Further distinction is usually made on clinical grounds. The virus may also be identified by fluorescent antibody staining of a lesion smear. Rapid culture methods take 48 hours. Diagnosis may also be made with paired serology. Serum transaminase levels may be modestly elevated during normal varicella.

C. Imaging: Varicella pneumonia classically produces numerous bilateral nodular densities and hyperinflation. This is very rare in children. Abnormal chest radiographs can occur in young adults, but there are usually no symptoms.

Differential Diagnosis

Varicella is usually distinctive. Similar rashes include those of coxsackievirus infection (fewer lesions, lack of crusting), impetigo (fewer lesions, no classic vesicles, response to antimicrobial agents, perioral or peripheral lesions), papular urticaria (insect bite history, nonvesicular rash), scabies (burrows, no typical vesicles), parapsoriasis (rare in children under 10 years of age; chronic or recurrent; often a history of prior varicella), rickettsialpox (eschar where the mite bites, smaller lesions, no crusting), dermatitis herpetiformis (chronic, urticaria, residual pigmentation), and folliculitis.

Complications & Sequelae

Secondary bacterial infection with staphylococci or group A streptococci is most common, presenting as impetigo, cellulitis, abscesses, scarlet fever, or sepsis.

Protracted vomiting or a change in sensorium suggests Reye's syndrome or encephalitis. Since Reye's syndrome usually occurs in patients who are also using salicylates, this drug should be especially avoided in patients with varicella. Encephalitis occurs in less than 0.1% of cases, usually in the first week of illness. It is often limited to cerebellitis with ataxia and resolves completely. Diffuse encephalitis may result in some deaths (5%).

Varicella pneumonia usually afflicts immunocompromised, pregnant, or older patients and may be fatal. Cough, dyspnea, tachypnea, rales, and cyanosis occur several days after onset of rash.

Hemorrhagic varicella lesions may be seen without other complications. Usually due to autoimmune thrombocytopenia, hemorrhagic lesions can occasionally represent idiopathic disseminated intravascular coagulation (purpura fulminans).

Varicella may be life-threatening in immunosuppressed patients (especially those with leukemia or lymphoma or those receiving high doses of steroids). Their disease is complicated by severe pneumonitis, hepatitis, and encephalitis. Varicella exposure in such patients must be evaluated immediately (see Chapter 10).

Neonates born to mothers who develop varicella from 5 days before to 2 days after delivery are at high risk for severe or fatal (5%) disease and must be given varicella-zoster immune globulin and followed closely (see Chapter 10).

Unusual complications of varicella include optic neuritis, transverse myelitis, orchitis, and arthritis.

Complications of herpes zoster include secondary bacterial infection, motor or cranial nerve paralysis, encephalitis, keratitis, and dissemination in immunosuppressed patients. Prolonged pain does not occur in normal children.

Treatment

A. General Measures: Supportive measures include maintenance of hydration, administration of acetaminophen for discomfort, cool soaks or antipruritics for itching (diphenhydramine, 1.25 mg/kg every 6 hours; or hydroxyzine, 0.5 mg/kg every 6 hours), and observance of general hygiene measures (keep nails trimmed and skin clean). Topical or systemic antistaphylococcal antibiotics may be needed.

B. Specific Measures: Although acyclovir is more active against herpes simplex, it is the preferred drug for varicella and herpes zoster infections. Recommended parenteral acyclovir dosage for severe disease is 30 mg/kg/d intravenously in three divided doses, each infused over 1 hour. Parenteral therapy should be started early in immunosuppressed patients or high-risk infected neonates. Varicella-zoster immune globulin is of no value. The effect of oral acyclovir (80 mg/kg/d in four doses) on varicella in normal children was modestly beneficial and nontoxic but only when administered within 24 hour after the onset of varicella. This should be used selectively in normal children (intercurrent illness; possibly second attacks in the household or adolescent age—both of which are associated with more severe disease) and in children with underlying chronic illnesses.

Prevention

See Chapter 10 for a discussion of the live attenuated vaccine and the use of varicella-zoster immune globulin for prevention of varicella.

Prognosis

Except for secondary bacterial infections, serious complications are rare and recovery complete in normal hosts.

Abzug MJ, Cotton MF: Severe chickenpox after intranasal use of corticosteroids. J Pediatr 1993;123:577.

American Academy of Pediatrics Committee on Infectious Diseases: The use of oral acyclovir in otherwise healthy children with varicella. Pediatrics 1993;91:674.

Dunkle LM et al: A controlled trial of acyclovir for chickenpox in normal children. N Engl J Med 1991;325:1539.

Fleischer G et al: Life-threatening complications of varicella. Am J Dis Child 1981;135:896.

Jackson MA, Burry VF, Olson LC: Complications of varicella requiring hospitalization in previously healthy children. Pediatr Infect Dis J 1992;11:441.

Srugo I et al: Clinical manifestations of varicella-zoster virus infections in human immunodeficiency virus-infected children. Am J Dis Child 1993;147:742.

Wurzel CL et al: Prognosis of herpes zoster in healthy children. Am J Dis Child 1986;140:477.

ROSEOLA INFANTUM
(Exanthema Subitum)

Roseola infantum is a benign illness caused by human herpesvirus 6 (HHV-6). HHV-6 is a major cause of acute febrile illness in young children. Its significance is its ability to mimic more serious causes of high fever and its role in inciting febrile seizures.

Clinical Findings

The most prominent historical feature is the abrupt onset of fever, often reaching 40.6 °C, which lasts up to 8 days (mean, 4 days) in an otherwise mildly ill child. The fever then ceases abruptly, and a characteristic rash may appear. Roseola occurs predominantly in children 6 months to 4 years old, with 90% of cases occurring before the second year. It is the most common recognized cause of exanthematous rash in this age group.

A. Symptoms and Signs: Mild lethargy and irritability may be present, but generally there is a dissociation between systemic symptoms and the febrile course. The pharynx, tonsils, and tympanic membranes may be injected. Conjunctivitis, coryza, cough, and pharyngeal exudate are notably absent. Adenopathy of the head and neck often occurs. If rash appears (10–20% incidence), it begins on the trunk and spreads to the face, neck, and extremities. Rose-pink macules or maculopapules, 2–3 mm in diameter, are nonpruritic, tend to coalesce, and disappear in 1–2 days without pigmentation or desquamation. Rash may occur without fever.

B. Laboratory Findings: Early leukocytosis gives way to leukopenia and a relative lymphocytosis with atypical lymphocytes. Laboratory evidence of hepatitis occurs in some patients, especially adults.

Differential Diagnosis

The initial high fever may require exclusion of serious bacterial infection. However, the relative well-being of most children and the typical course and rash soon clarify the diagnosis. The erythrocyte sedimentation rate is normal. If the child has a febrile seizure, it is important to exclude bacterial meningitis. The cerebrospinal fluid is normal in children with roseola. In children who receive antibiotics or other medication at the beginning of the fever, the rash may be incorrectly attributed to a drug allergy.

Complications & Sequelae

Febrile seizures occur, but no more commonly than with other self-limited infections. There is some evidence that HHV-6 can directly infect the central nervous system, causing meningoencephalitis or aseptic meningitis. Multiorgan disease (pneumonia, hepatitis) may occur in immunocompromised patients.

Treatment & Prognosis

Fever is readily managed with acetaminophen and sponge baths. Fever control should be a major consideration in children with a history of febrile seizures. Roseola infantum is otherwise entirely benign.

Caserta MT and Hall CB: Human herpesvirus-6. Annu Rev Med 1993;44:377.

Leach CT, Sumaya CV, Brown NA: Human herpesvirus-6: Clinical implications of a recently discovered, ubiquitous agent. J Pediatr 1992;121:173.

Okada K et al: Exanthema subitum and human herpesvirus 6 infection: clinical observations in fifty-seven cases. Pediatr Infect Dis J 1993;12:204.

Pruksananonda P et al: Primary human herpesvirus 6 infection in young children. N Engl J Med 1992;326:1445.

Suga S et al: Clinical and virological analyses of 21 infants with exanthem subitum (roseola infantum) and central nervous system complications. Ann Neurol 1993;33:597.

CYTOMEGALOVIRUS (CMV) INFECTIONS

Cytomegalovirus is a ubiquitous human herpesvirus transmitted by many routes. It can be acquired following maternal viremia or from birth canal secretions and maternal milk. Young children are infected by the saliva of playmates; older individuals are infected by sexual partners (saliva, vaginal secretions, and semen). Transfused blood products and transplanted organs can be a source of CMV infection. Clinical illness is largely determined by the immune competence of the patient. Normal individuals usually develop a mild, self-limited illness, whereas immunocompromised children can develop severe, progressive, often multiorgan disease. In addition, in utero infection can be teratogenic.

1. IN UTERO CYTOMEGALOVIRUS INFECTION

Clinical Findings

Approximately 0.5–1.5% of children are born with CMV infections acquired during maternal viremia. Over 95% of them are asymptomatic and are usually born to mothers who had experienced reactivation of latent CMV infection during the pregnancy. Symptomatic infants are born to mothers with primary CMV infection. Even after primary maternal infection, less than 50% of fetuses are infected, and only 10% of those infected are symptomatic at birth. Primary infection in the first half of pregnancy poses the greatest risk for severe fetal damage.

A. Symptoms and Signs: Severely affected infants are born ill; they are often small for gestational age, floppy, and lethargic. They feed poorly and have poor temperature control. Hepatosplenomegaly, jaundice, petechiae, seizures, and microcephaly are often present. Characteristic signs are a distinctive chorioretinitis and periventricular calcification. A purpuric ("blueberry muffin") rash similar to that seen with congenital rubella may be present. The mortality rate is 20–30%. Survivors usually have significant sequelae. Less severely ill children are born with one or more of the above findings. Isolated hepatosplenomegaly or thrombocytopenia may occur. Even mildly affected children may subsequently manifest mental retardation and psychomotor delay. Most infected infants (90%) are born to mothers with preexisting immunity and have no clinical manifestations at birth. Of these, 10–15% develop sensorineural hearing loss, which is often bilateral.

B. Laboratory Findings: Anemia, thrombocytopenia, hyperbilirubinemia, and elevated aminotransferase levels are common. Lymphocytosis is occasionally seen. Pleocytosis and an elevated protein content are seen in cerebrospinal fluid. The diagnosis is readily confirmed by isolation of CMV from urine, saliva, cerebrospinal fluid, and stool. Urine and saliva isolates can often be obtained in 3 days by combining culture with enzyme immunoassay. The presence in the infant of IgM-specific CMV antibodies suggests the diagnosis. The commercial EIA kit is 90% sensitive and 98% specific.

C. Imaging: Skull radiographs show microcephaly and periventricular calcification. CT scan shows calcification and ventricular dilatation. Long bone films show the "celery stalk" pattern characteristic of congenital viral infections. Interstitial pneumonia may be present.

Differential Diagnosis

Cytomegalovirus infection should be considered in any newborn who is seriously ill shortly after birth, especially once bacterial sepsis, metabolic disease, intracranial bleeding, and cardiac disease have been excluded. Other congenital infections to be considered in the differential diagnosis include toxoplasmosis (serology, more diffuse calcification of the central nervous system, specific type of retinitis, macrocephaly), rubella (serology, specific type of retinitis, cardiac lesions, eye abnormalities), enteroviral infections (time of year, maternal illness, severe hepatitis), herpes simplex (skin lesions, cultures, severe hepatitis), and syphilis (serology for both infant and mother, skin lesions, bone involvement).

Treatment & Prevention

Support is rarely required for anemia and thrombocytopenia. The antiviral drug ganciclovir is under study in severely ill children. Most children with symptoms at birth have significant neurologic, intellectual, visual, or auditory impairment. Children who are asymptomatic at birth have a 5–15% incidence of hearing loss but few other sequelae. It is possible that the late sequelae of CMV infection—including abnormalities occurring in initially asymptomatic infants—may be ameliorated by ganciclovir use. Delayed development and hearing loss should be discovered and treated as soon as possible.

2. PERINATAL CYTOMEGALOVIRUS INFECTION

Cytomegalovirus infection can be acquired from birth canal secretions or shortly after birth from maternal milk. In some socioeconomic groups, 10–20% of infants are infected at birth and excrete CMV for many months. Infection can also be acquired in the postnatal period from unscreened transfused blood products.

Clinical Findings

A. Symptoms and Signs: Ninety percent of normal infants infected by their mothers at birth develop subclinical illness (ie, virus excretion only) or a minor illness within 1–3 months. The remainder develop an illness lasting several weeks which is characterized by hepatosplenomegaly, lymphadenopathy, and interstitial pneumonitis in various combinations. The severity of the pneumonitis may be increased by the simultaneous presence of *Chlamydia trachomatis*. Infants who receive blood products are often premature and immunologically impaired. If they are born to CMV-negative mothers and subsequently receive CMV-containing blood, they frequently develop severe infection and pneumonia after a 2- to 6-week incubation period.

B. Laboratory Findings: Lymphocytosis, atypical lymphocytes, anemia, and thrombocytopenia may be present, especially in premature infants. Liver function is abnormal. Cytomegalovirus can be isolated from urine and saliva. Secretions obtained at bronchoscopy contain CMV and epithelial cells bearing CMV antigens. Serum levels of CMV antibody rise significantly.

C. Imaging: Chest films show a diffuse interstitial pneumonitis.

Differential Diagnosis

Cytomegalovirus infection should be considered as a cause of any prolonged illness in early infancy, especially if hepatosplenomegaly, lymphadenopathy, or atypical lymphocytosis is present. This must be distinguished from granulomatous or malignant diseases and from congenital infections (syphilis, toxoplasmosis, hepatitis B) not previously appreciated. Other viruses (Epstein-Barr virus, HIV, adenovirus) can cause this syndrome. Cytomegalovirus is a recognized cause of viral pneumonia in this age group. However, since asymptomatic CMV excretion is common in early infancy, care must be taken to establish the diagnosis and to rule out concomitant pathogens such as *Chlamydia* and RSV.

Treatment & Prevention

The self-limited disease of normal infants requires no therapy. Severe pneumonitis in premature infants requires oxygen administration and often intubation. Very ill infants should receive ganciclovir (5 mg/kg every 12 hours). Cytomegalovirus infection acquired by transfusion can be prevented by excluding CMV-seropositive blood donors. Milk donors should also be screened for prior CMV infection. It is likely that high-risk infants receiving large doses of intravenous immune globulin for other reasons will be protected against severe CMV disease.

3. CYTOMEGALOVIRUS INFECTION ACQUIRED IN CHILDHOOD & ADOLESCENCE

Young children are readily infected by playmates, especially since CMV continues to be excreted in saliva and urine for many months after infection. The annual incidence of CMV excretion by children in day care centers exceeds 75%. In fact, young children in a family are often the source of primary CMV infection of the mother during subsequent pregnancies. An additional peak of CMV infection occurs in sexually active individuals. Blood transfusion represents another source of CMV infection.

Clinical Findings

A. Symptoms and Signs: The large majority of young children acquiring CMV are asymptomatic or have a minor febrile illness, occasionally with adenopathy. They provide the reservoir of virus shedders that facilitate spread of CMV. Occasionally, a child may have a prolonged fever with hepatosplenomegaly and adenopathy. Older children and adults are more likely to be symptomatic in this fashion and can present with a syndrome that mimics the infectious mononucleosis syndrome which follows infection by Epstein-Barr virus (1–2 weeks of fever, malaise, anorexia, splenomegaly, and some adenopathy). This syndrome can also occur 2–4 weeks after transfusion of CMV-infected blood.

B. Laboratory Findings: In the CMV mononucleosis syndrome, lymphocytosis and atypical lymphocytes are common, as is a mild rise in aminotransferase levels. Cytomegalovirus is present in saliva and urine, and diagnosis is made as above.

Differential Diagnosis

In older children, CMV infection should be included as a possible cause of fever of unknown origin, especially when lymphocytosis and atypical lymphocytes are present. Cytomegalovirus infection is distinguished from Epstein-Barr virus infection by the absence of pharyngitis, the relatively minor adenopathy, and the absence of serologic evidence of acute Epstein-Barr virus infection. Mononucleosis syndromes are also caused by *Toxoplasma gondii*, rubella virus, adenovirus, hepatitis A virus, and HIV.

Prevention

Screening of transfused blood would prevent cases related to this source.

4. CYTOMEGALOVIRUS INFECTION IN IMMUNOCOMPROMISED CHILDREN

Cytomegalovirus infection in this setting can be acquired from infused blood products or transplanted tissue as well as from playmates. In addition, reactivation of latent CMV can cause symptomatic disease. This is clearly seen in children with AIDS or congenital immunodeficiencies. However, in most other immunocompromised patients, primary infection is much more likely to cause severe symptoms than is reactivation disease. The severity of the resulting disease is generally proportionate to the degree of immunosuppression.

Clinical Findings

A. Symptoms and Signs: A mild febrile illness with myalgia, malaise, and arthralgia may occur, especially with reactivation disease. Severe disease often includes subacute onset of dyspnea and cyanosis as manifestations of an interstitial pneumonitis. Auscultation reveals only coarse breath sounds and scattered rales. A rapid respiratory rate may precede clinical or x-ray evidence of pneumonia. Hepatitis without jaundice or hepatomegaly is common. Diarrhea, which can be severe, occurs with CMV colitis, and CMV can cause esophagitis with symptoms of odynophagia or dysphagia. These enteropathies are most common in AIDS, as is the presence of a retinitis that often progresses to blindness.

B. Laboratory Findings: Neutropenia and thrombocytopenia are common. Atypical lymphocytosis is not frequent. Serum aminotransferase levels are often elevated. The stools may contain occult blood if enteropathy is present. Cytomegalovirus is readily isolated from saliva, urine, buffy coat, and bronchial secretions. Results are available in 48 hours.

C. Imaging: Bilateral interstitial pneumonitis is present on chest radiographs.

Differential Diagnosis

The initial febrile illness must be distinguished from treatable bacterial and fungal infection. Similarly, the pulmonary disease must be distinguished from intrapulmonary hemorrhage, drug-induced or radiation pneumonitis, pulmonary edema, and bacterial, fungal, and parasitic infection in this population. In this regard, it is noteworthy that CMV infection is bilateral and interstitial on x-ray films of the chest, cough is nonproductive, chest pain is absent, and the patient is not usually toxic. *Pneumocystis carinii* infection may present in a similar manner. Polymicrobial disease may be present in these patients. It is suspected that bacterial and fungal infections are enhanced by the neutropenia that can accompany CMV infection. Infection of the gastrointestinal tract is diagnosed by endoscopy, mainly to exclude candidal and herpes simplex infections.

Treatment & Prognosis

Blood donors should be screened to exclude those with prior CMV infection. Ideally, seronegative transplant recipients should receive organs from seronegative donors. Severe symptoms, most commonly pneumonitis, often respond to early therapy with intravenous ganciclovir (5 mg/kg every 12 hours for 14–21 days). Neutropenia is a frequent side effect of this therapy. Prophylactic use of oral acyclovir or intravenous ganciclovir may prevent this problem in organ transplant recipients.

Boppana SB et al: Symptomatic congenital cytomegalovirus infection: Neonatal morbidity and mortality. Pediatr Infect Dis J 1992;11:93.

Demmler GJ: Infectious Diseases Society of America and Centers for Disease Control. Summary of a workshop on surveillance for congenital cytomegalovirus disease. Rev Infect Dis 1991;13:315.

Jordan CJ et al: Spontaneous cytomegalovirus mononucleosis. Ann Intern Med 1973;79:153.

Kumar ML et al: Postnatally acquired cytomegalovirus infections in infants of CMV-excreting mothers. J Pediatr 1984;104:669.

Lynch L et al: Prenatal diagnosis of fetal cytomegalovirus infection. Am J Obstet Gynecol 1991;165:714.

Stagno S, Whitley RJ: Herpesvirus infections of pregnancy: Part 1. Cytomegalovirus and Epstein-Barr virus infections. N Engl J Med 1985;313:1270.

INFECTIOUS MONONUCLEOSIS

Mononucleosis is the most characteristic syndrome produced by infection with the Epstein-Barr virus (EBV). Its elements are fever, pharyngitis, lymphadenopathy, splenomegaly, atypical lymphocytosis, and the production of heterophil antibodies. Young children infected with EBV have either no symptoms or a mild nonspecific febrile illness. As the age of the host increases, EBV infection is more likely to produce the mononucleosis syndrome, occurring in 20–25% of infected adolescents. Epstein-Barr virus is readily acquired from asymptomatic carriers (15–20% of whom excrete the virus on any given day) and from recently ill patients, who excrete virus for many months. Young children are infected from the saliva of playmates and family members. Adolescents may be infected through sexual activity. Epstein-Barr virus can also be transmitted by blood transfusion and organ transplantation.

Clinical Findings

A. Symptoms and Signs: After an incubation period of 1–2 months, a 2- to 3-day prodrome of malaise and anorexia yields, abruptly or insidiously, to a febrile illness with temperatures exceeding 39 °C. The major complaint is pharyngitis, which is often (50%) exudative. Lymph nodes are enlarged, firm, and mildly tender. Any area may be affected, but posterior and anterior cervical nodes are almost always enlarged. Splenomegaly is present in 50–75% of patients. Hepatomegaly is common (30%), and the liver is frequently tender. Five percent of patients have a rash, which can be macular, scarlatiniform, or urticarial. Rash is almost universal in patients taking penicillin or ampicillin. Soft palate petechiae and eyelid edema are also observed.

B. Laboratory Findings:

1. Peripheral blood–Leukopenia may occur early, but an atypical lymphocytosis (comprising over 10% of the total leukocytes at some time in the illness) is most notable. Hematologic changes may not be seen until the third week of illness and may be entirely absent in some EBV syndromes, eg, neurologic ones.

2. Heterophil antibodies–These nonspecific antibodies appear in over 90% of older patients with mononucleosis but in fewer than 50% of children under age 5. They may not be detectable until the second week of illness and may persist for up to 12 months after recovery. Rapid screening tests (slide agglutination) are usually positive if the titer is significant; a positive result strongly suggests but does not prove EBV infection.

3. Anti-EBV antibodies–It may be necessary to

measure specific antibody titers when heterophil antibodies fail to appear, as in young children. Epstein-Barr virus infection is established by detecting IgM antibody to the viral capsid antigen (VCA); by detecting a rise over several weeks of IgG antibody to the VCA antigen; or by detecting IgG-VCA antibody in the absence of antibody to the Epstein-Barr nuclear antigen (EBNA), which appears late in the illness. Seroconversion of antibody to EBNA confirms the above indicators.

4. Aminotransferase, γ-glutamyl transferase, and bilirubin levels–Aminotransferase and γ-glutamyl transferase levels are mildly elevated in 80% of patients; bilirubin is mildly elevated in 25%.

Differential Diagnosis

Severe pharyngitis may suggest group A streptococcal infection. Enlargement of only anterior cervical lymph nodes, a neutrophilic leukocytosis, and the absence of splenomegaly suggest bacterial infection. Although a child with a positive throat culture usually requires therapy, up to 10% of children with mononucleosis are asymptomatic carriers. In this group, penicillin therapy is unnecessary and often causes a rash. Severe primary herpes simplex pharyngitis, occurring in adolescence, may also mimic infectious mononucleosis. In this type of pharyngitis, some anterior mouth ulcerations should suggest the correct diagnosis. Epstein-Barr virus infection should be considered in the differential diagnosis of any perplexing prolonged febrile illness. Some similar illnesses that produce atypical lymphocytosis include rubella (pharyngitis not prominent, shorter illness, less adenopathy and splenomegaly), adenovirus (upper respiratory infection symptoms and cough, conjunctivitis, less adenopathy, fewer atypical lymphocytes), hepatitis (more severe liver function abnormalities, no pharyngitis or splenomegaly), and toxoplasmosis (negative heterophil test and less pharyngitis). Serum sickness-like drug reactions and leukemia (smear morphology is important) may be confused with infectious mononucleosis. Cytomegalovirus mononucleosis is a close mimic except for minimal pharyngitis and less adenopathy; it is much less common. Serologic tests for EBV and cytomegalovirus should clarify the correct diagnosis. The primary manifestation of HIV infection is a mononucleosis-like syndrome in some children.

Complications

Splenic rupture is a very rare complication, which usually follows significant trauma. Hematologic complications, including hemolytic anemia, thrombocytopenia, or neutropenia, are more common. Neurologic involvement can include aseptic meningitis, encephalitis, isolated neuropathy such as Bell's palsy, and Guillain-Barré syndrome. Any of these may appear prior to or in the absence of the more typical signs and symptoms of infectious mononucleo-sis. Rare complications include myocarditis, pericarditis, and atypical pneumonia. Very rarely, EBV infection becomes a progressive lymphoproliferative disorder characterized by persistent fever, multiple organ involvement, neutropenia or pancytopenia, and agammaglobulinemia. Hemocytophagia is often present in the bone marrow. An X-linked genetic defect in immune response has been inferred for some patients (Duncan's syndrome, X-linked lymphoproliferative disorder). Children with other congenital immunodeficiencies or chemotherapy-induced immunosuppression can also develop progressive EBV infection or EBV-induced lymphomas.

Treatment & Prognosis

Bed rest may be necessary in severe cases. Acetaminophen controls high fever. Potential airway obstruction due to swollen pharyngeal lymphoid tissue responds rapidly to systemic steroids. Steroids may also be given for hematologic and neurologic complications, though no controlled trials have proved their efficacy in these conditions. Fever and pharyngitis disappear by 10–14 days. Adenopathy and splenomegaly can persist several weeks longer. Some patients complain of fatigue, malaise, or lack of well being for several months. Although steroids may shorten the duration of fatigue and malaise, their long-term effects on this potentially oncogenic viral infection are unknown, and indiscriminate use is discouraged. Patients with splenic enlargement should avoid contact sports for 6–8 weeks.

Alpert G, Fleisher GR: Complications of infection with Epstein-Barr virus during childhood: A study of children admitted to the hospital. Pediatr Infect Dis 1984;3:304.

Chetham MM, Roberts KB: Infectious mononucleosis in adolescents. Pediatr Ann 1991;20:206.

Schuster V, Kreth HW: Epstein-Barr virus infection and associated diseases in children: II. Diagnostic and therapeutic strategies. Eur J Pediatr 1992;151:794.

Sumaya CV: Epstein-Barr virus serologic testing: Diagnostic indications and interpretations. Pediatr Infect Dis J 1986;5:337.

INFECTIONS DUE TO ARBOVIRUSES (Table 35–4)

Goodpasture HC et al: Colorado tick fever: Clinical, epidemiologic, and laboratory aspects of 228 cases in Colorado in 1973–74. Ann Intern Med 1978;88:303.

Hayes EB, Gubler DJ: Dengue and dengue hemorrhagic fever. Pediatr Infect Dis J 1992;11:311.

Tsai TF: Arboviral diseases of North America. In: Textbook of Pediatric Infections Diseases, 3rd ed. Feigin RD, Cherry, JD (editors). Saunders, 1992.

Table 35–4. Arboviral diseases.

Disease	Natural Reservoir (Vector)	Geographic Distribution	Incubation Period	Clinical Presentation	Laboratory Findings	Complications, Sequelae	Diagnosis, Therapy, Comments[1]
St. Louis encephalitis (SLE)	Birds (*Culex* mosquitoes)	Southern Canada, Central USA, South America	2–5 days (up to 3 weeks)	Abrupt onset of fever, chills, headache, nausea, vomiting; may develop generalized weakness, seizures, coma, paralysis; aseptic meningitis is common in children.	Modest leukocytosis, neutrophilia. CSF: 100–200 wbc/μL (PMNs predominate early).	Mortality rate 2–5% in children (especially <age 5). Neurologic sequelae in 1–20%.	Most important arbovirus in USA: 20–500 cases a year, < 20% symptomatic. (Worse in elderly.) Therapy: supportive. Diagnosis: serology. Specific antibody often present within 5 days.
California encephalitis (LaCrosse, Jamestown Canyon, 3 others)	Chipmunks and other small mammals (*Aedes* mosquitoes)	Northern and mid Central USA, southern Canada	2–5 days	Similar to SLE; focal neurologic signs in up to 25%.	Variable white counts. CSF: 30–200 (up to 600) wbc/μL; variable PMNs; protein often normal.	Mortality rate < 1%. Seizure disorder if this appeared during acute illness.	About 50–150 cases a year in USA, 5% symptomatic. Therapy: supportive. Diagnosis: serology. Up to 90% have specific IgM antibody in first week; 25% of population has IgG antibody.
Western equine encephalitis	Birds (*Culex* mosquitoes)	Canada, USA, and Mexico west of Mississippi River longitude; South America	2–5 days	Similar to that of SLE. Most infections are subclinical.	Variable white counts. CSF: 10–300 wbc/μL.	Permanent brain damage, 10% overall; 30% in infants < 1 year of age.	About 10–150 cases a year in USA. Worse in infants. Equine illness precedes human outbreaks. Therapy: supportive. Diagnosis: serology. Often IgM antibody in first week.
Eastern equine encephalitis	Birds (*Culex*, *Aedes* mosquitoes)	Eastern seaboard USA; Caribbean, South America	2–5 days	Similar to that of SLE but more severe. Progresses rapidly in one-third to coma and death.	Leukocytosis with neutrophilia. CSF: 500–2000 wbc/μL; PMNs predominate early.	Mortality rate 20–70%; neurologic sequelae in over 50% of children.	Most severe arboviral encephalitis in USA. Fewer than 20 cases a year. Only 3–10% of cases are symptomatic. Therapy: supportive. Diagnosis: serology. Background seropositivity very low. Titers often positive in first week.
Colorado tick fever[2]	Small mammals (Dermacentor andersoni, or wood tick)	Rocky Mountain region of USA and Canada	3–34 days (range, 1–14 days)	Fever, myalgia, conjunctivitis, headache, retro-orbital pain; rash in < 10%. No respiratory symptoms. Biphasic in 50%.	Leukopenia (maximum at 4–6 days), mild thrombocytopenia.	Rare encephalitis, coagulopathy.	Patient may have no known tick bite. Acute illness lasts 7 days; prolonged fatigue in adults. Therapy: supportive. Diagnosis: serology.
Dengue (4 types)	Humans (*Aedes* mosquitoes)	Asia, Africa, Central and South America, Caribbean; rarely in southern USA	2–7 days	Fever, headache, myalgia, retro-ocular pain, pharyngitis, cough; maculopapular or petechial rash in 20%; adenopathy.	Leukopenia, thrombocytopenia.	Hemorrhagic fever, shock syndrome, prolonged weakness.	High infection rate. Biphasic course may occur. Therapy: supportive. Ribavirin is experimental. Diagnosis: serology.
Yellow fever	Humans, monkeys (*Aedes* mosquitoes)	Africa, South America	3–7 days (up to 13 days)	Abrupt onset of fever, headache, vomiting; may progress to jaundice, gastrointestinal bleeding, hepatitis, death.	Leukopenia, abnormal liver function tests, proteinuria, elevated creatinine.	Severe in 10–20% with 50% mortality rate in this group. Milder in children.	May be biphasic. Liver biopsy: characteristic midzonal necrosis, eosinophilic inclusions. Therapy: supportive. Diagnosis: paired serology; mouse inoculation with blood, liver tissue.

[1] Vaccine available only for yellow fever.

[2] Not classic arbovirus but similar clinical picture in some patients, and seasonally.

INFECTIONS DUE TO ADENOVIRUSES

There are over 40 types of adenoviruses, which account for 2–10% of all respiratory illnesses. In addition, enteric adenoviruses are an important cause of childhood diarrhea. Adenoviral infections are common early in life. Epidemic disease occurs in the winter and spring, especially in closed environments, such as day care and institutions. Because of latent infection in lymphoid tissue, asymptomatic shedding from the respiratory or intestinal tract is common.

Diagnosis is by culture of conjunctival, respiratory, or stool specimens. Several days to weeks are required for growth in conventional cultures. Rapid culture using the shell vial technique detects virus in 48 hours. Special cells are needed to isolate enteric adenoviruses. Respiratory adenovirus infections can be detected by serology using acute and convalescent serum. Detection of enteric adenoviruses in diarrheal specimens can now be done rapidly with EIA.

Specific Adenoviral Syndromes

A. Pharyngitis: The most common adenoviral disease in children. Fever and adenopathy are common. Tonsillitis may be exudative. An influenza-like systemic illness may be present. Laryngotracheitis or bronchitis may accompany pharyngitis.

B. Follicular Conjunctivitis: This form of conjunctivitis may be prolonged and associated with preauricular adenopathy and corneal damage. Association with fever and pharyngitis is called "pharyngoconjunctival fever."

C. Epidemic Keratoconjunctivitis: Severe conjunctivitis with punctate keratitis and occasionally visual impairment. Preauricular adenopathy is common.

D. Pneumonia: Severe pneumonia may occur at all ages. It is especially common in young children (< 3 years). Chest radiographs show bilateral peribronchial and interstitial infiltrates. Symptoms persist for 2–4 weeks. This adenoviral pneumonia is necrotizing and can cause permanent lung damage.

E. Rash: A diffuse morbilliform (rarely petechial) rash resembling measles, rubella, or roseola. Koplik's spots are absent.

F. Diarrhea: Enteric adenoviruses (types 40 and 41) are the second most common cause of short-lived diarrhea in an afebrile child.

G. Mesenteric Lymphadenitis: Fever and abdominal pain may mimic appendicitis. Pharyngitis is often associated. Adenovirus-induced adenopathy may be a factor in appendicitis and intussusception.

H. Other: Immunosuppressed patients, including neonates, may develop severe or fatal pulmonary or gastrointestinal infections or multisystem disease. Other rare complications include hemorrhagic cystitis, encephalitis, hepatitis, and myocarditis.

Treatment

There is no specific treatment. Intravenous immune globulin may be tried in immunocompromised patients with severe pneumonia.

Abzug MJ, Levin MJ: Neonatal adenovirus infection: Four patients and a review of the literature. Pediatrics 1991; 87:890.

Krajden M et al: Clinical features of adenoviral enteritis: A review of 127 proven cases. Pediatr Infect Dis J 1990;9: 636.

Krilov LR et al: Disseminated adenovirus infection with hepatic necrosis in patients with human immunodeficiency virus infection and other immunodeficiency states. Rev Infect Dis 1990;12:303.

INFECTIONS DUE TO MISCELLANEOUS VIRUSES

ERYTHEMA INFECTIOSUM

This benign exanthematous illness of school-age children is caused by a human parvovirus designated B19. It is not related to the canine parvoviruses. Spread is respiratory, occurring in winter-spring epidemics. A nonspecific mild flu-like illness may occur during the initial viremia at 7–10 days; the characteristic rash occurring at 10–14 days actually represents an immune response. The patient is viremic and contagious prior to—but not after—the onset of rash. Springtime outbreaks are typical. The disease is mildly contagious; only about half of susceptible household contacts are infected.

Approximately one-half of infected individuals have a subclinical illness. Most cases (70%) occur in children between the ages of 5 and 15, with an additional 20% occurring later in life. Forty percent of adults are seronegative. Rare complications of parvovirus infection include aplastic crises in children with chronic hemolytic anemia, occasionally hydrops fetalis when susceptible pregnant women are infected, and persistent anemia or pancytopenia in immunocompromised patients.

Clinical Findings

Owing to the nonspecific nature of the exanthem and the many subclinical cases, a history of contact with an infected individual is often absent or unreliable. Recognition of the illness is easier during outbreaks.

A. Symptoms and Signs: Typically, the first sign of illness is the rash, which begins as raised maculopapular lesions on the cheeks that coalesce to give a "slapped cheek" appearance. The lesions are warm, nontender, and sometimes pruritic. They may be scattered on the forehead, chin, and postauricular areas, but the circumoral region is spared. Within 1–2 days, similar lesions appear on the proximal extensor surfaces of the extremities and spread distally in a symmetric fashion. Palms and soles are usually spared. The trunk, neck, and buttocks are also commonly involved. Central clearing of confluent lesions produces a characteristic lace-like pattern. The rash fades in several days to several weeks but frequently reappears in response to local irritation, heat (bathing), sunlight, and stress. Almost one-half of infected children have some rash remaining (or recurring) for 10 days. Fine desquamation may be present.

Mild systemic symptoms occur in up to 50% of children during outbreaks. These include low-grade fever (38–38.5 °C) mild malaise, sore throat, and coryza. They appear for 2–3 days and are followed by a week-long asymptomatic phase before the rash appears.

B. Laboratory Findings: A mild leukopenia occurs early in some patients, followed by leukocytosis and lymphocytosis. Serum IgM and IgG antibody tests are available and preferred. Antigen and nucleic acid detection tests are available. The disease is not diagnosed by routine viral culture.

Differential Diagnosis

The characteristic rash and the mild nature of the illness distinguish erythema infectiosum from other childhood exanthems. It lacks the prodromal symptoms of measles and the lymphadenopathy of rubella. Systemic symptoms and pharyngitis are more prominent with enteroviral infections and scarlet fever.

Complications & Sequelae

A. Arthritis: This occurs in older patients, beginning with late adolescence. Pain and stiffness occur symmetrically in the peripheral joints. Arthritis usually follows the rash and may persist for 2–4 weeks but resolves without permanent damage in most patients.

B. Aplastic Crisis: Parvovirus B19 replicates primarily in erythroid progenitor cells. Consequently, reticulocytopenia occurs for approximately 1 week during the illness. This goes unnoticed in normal individuals but results in severe anemia in patients with chronic hemolytic anemia. The rash of erythema infectiosum follows the hemolysis in these patients.

Pure red cell aplasia, chronic pancytopenia, idiopathic thrombocytopenic purpura, and a hemophagocytic syndrome have also been described. Patients with AIDS may develop prolonged anemia or pancytopenia. Patients with hemolytic anemia and aplastic crisis or immunosuppressed patients may still be contagious and should be isolated in the hospital.

C. In Utero Infections: Infection of susceptible pregnant women may produce fetal infection with hydrops fetalis; fetal death occurs in about 6%, with most fatalities occurring in the first 20 weeks—compared with a fetal loss of 3.5% in controls. The risk of fetal infection is not known. Congenital anomalies have not been associated with parvovirus B19 infection during pregnancy.

Treatment & Prognosis

Erythema infectiosum is a benign illness for normal individuals. Patients with aplastic crisis may require blood transfusions. It is unlikely that this complication can be prevented by quarantine measures, since acute parvovirus infection in contacts is often unrecognized and is most contagious prior to the rash. Pregnant women who are exposed to erythema infectiosum or who work in a setting where an epidemic occurs should be tested for evidence of prior infection if a reliable serologic test is available. Susceptible pregnant women should then be followed for evidence of parvovirus infection. If maternal infection occurs, the fetus should be followed for evidence of hydrops and distress. In utero transfusion or early delivery may salvage some fetuses. Pregnancies should not be terminated because of parvovirus infection.

Standard immune globulin is not protective. High-dose intravenous immune globulin has stopped viremia and led to marrow recovery in some cases of prolonged aplasia. Its role in normal patients and pregnant women is unknown.

Koch WC et al: Manifestations and treatment of human parvovirus B19 infections in immunocompromised patients. J Pediatr 1990;116:355.

Kumar ML: Human parvovirus B19 and its associated diseases. Clin Perinatol 1991;18:209.

Plotkin SA et al: Parvovirus, erythema infectiosum, and pregnancy: Report of the Committee on Infectious Diseases of the American Academy of Pediatrics. Pediatrics 1990;85:131.

Rodis J et al: Management and outcome of pregnancies complicated by human B19 parvovirus infection: A prospective study. Am J Obstet Gynecol 1990;163:1168.

Torok TJ: Human parvovirus B19 infection in pregnancy. Pediatr Infect Dis J 1990;9:772.

HANTAVIRUS INFECTION

Essentials of Diagnosis

- Influenza-like prodrome (fever, myalgia, headache, cough).
- Rapid onset of unexplained pulmonary edema (ARDS).
- Residence or travel in epidemic area; exposure to aerosols from deer mouse droppings or secretions.
- Confirmation by serology.

General Considerations

A new severe viral disease appeared in an epidemic cluster in the Southwestern USA in 1993. This unique viral illness is the first native bunyavirus epidemic in this country. Hantavirus disease is distinctly different in mode of spread (no arthropod vector) and clinical picture from other bunyavirus diseases.

Clinical Findings

The essential feature is travel to an area where New Mexico, Colorado, Utah, and Arizona are contiguous and potential exposure to the habitat of the reservoir, ie, the deer mouse. This rodent lives in many other locales, and small numbers of cases have been suspected in 20 other states west of the Mississippi River and in Louisiana.

A. Symptoms and Signs: Onset is sudden, with a nonspecific virus-like prodrome: fever; back, hip, and leg pain; chills; headache, dry cough, and nausea and vomiting. Abdominal pain may be present. Sore throat, conjunctivitis, rash, and adenopathy are absent. After 1–10 days (usually 4–5), dyspnea, tachypnea, and evidence of a pulmonary capillary leak syndrome appear. This often progresses rapidly over a period of hours.

B. Laboratory Findings: The hemogram is significant for leukocytosis with a prominent left shift and hemoconcentration. LDH is elevated, as are liver function tests; serum albumin is low. Urinalysis is normal. A serum IgM ELISA test is positive early in the illness. Otherwise the diagnosis is made by specific staining of tissue, usually at autopsy.

C. Imaging: Initial chest x-rays are normal. This is followed by bilateral interstitial infiltrates with the typical butterfly pattern of acute pulmonary edema. Significant pleural effusions are often present.

Differential Diagnosis

In the same area, plague and tularemia are possibilities (absence of exposure to the reservoir associated with these; no adenopathy; no primary lesion). Viral respiratory pathogens and *Mycoplasma* have a slower tempo, do not elevate the LDH, and do not cause the hematologic changes. Q fever, toxin exposure, *Legionella,* and fungi are possibilities, but the history and tempo of the illness should be distinguishing features.

Treatment & Prognosis

Intravenous ribavirin is effective when given early for other bunyavirus infections. A trial of this therapy for hantavirus is under way. The virus is not spread by person-to-person contact. No isolation is required. Thus far, the case-fatality rate is approximately 50%.

LeDuc JW et al: Hantaan (Korean hemorrhagic fever) and related rodent zoonoses. In: *Emerging Viruses.* Krause RM (editor). Oxford Univ Press, 1993.

Outbreak of hantavirus infection—southwestern United States, 1993. MMWR Morb Mortal Wkly Rep 1993; 42:495.

HUMAN IMMUNODEFICIENCY VIRUS (HIV) INFECTIONS (Acquired Immune Deficiency Syndrome [AIDS])

Essentials of Diagnosis

Children > 15 months:
- Presence of HIV in blood or tissue determined by culture, antigen detection, or nucleic acid detection.

or

- Presence of HIV antibody determined by repeated screening tests and confirmatory test.

or

- Symptoms of AIDS (multiple infections, opportunistic infections, lymphoid interstitial pneumonitis, encephalopathy, Kaposi's sarcoma, other; see CDC case definition).

Children < 15 months:
- HIV in blood or tissue (as above).

or

- Symptoms of AIDS (as above).

or

- HIV antibody *and* evidence of cellular and humoral immunodeficiency (without an obvious cause) *and* symptoms compatible with HIV infection (eg, weight loss, hepatosplenomegaly, generalized adenopathy, chronic thrush, diarrhea, lymphoid interstitial pneumonitis, progressive developmental delay, unexplained fevers, or recurrent bacterial or opportunistic infections).

General Considerations

HIV is the most common cause of acquired immunodeficiency in children. It is a retrovirus that infects helper T cells, monocytes, macrophages, neural cells, and other cell types. The destruction of helper T cells profoundly affects B cell function and cell-mediated immunity and results in progressive generalized immune incompetence. Among prepubertal pediatric AIDS cases, 90% are now acquired perinatally (transplacentally or at birth); the remainder follow transfusion or hemophilia therapy. Prior to the introduction of screening of donors, children were more frequently infected from blood products. Of hemophiliacs who received blood products prior to 1985, when screening began, 65–90% are infected. Sexual activity and contaminated needles account for most infections after puberty.

About 90% of infected women are of childbearing age; 40% are intravenous drug abusers, and most of the remainder are sexual partners of infected men. The number of women who are unknowingly exposed by heterosexual contact is increasing. Women represent the fastest-growing subset of HIV-infected adults. About 15–30% of infants born to these women will be infected.

The incubation period for primary infection is 2–4 weeks. Primary infection is nonspecific ("flu" or mild mononucleosis-like illness) and often subclinical. Approximately 20% of HIV-infected infants develop an AIDS-defining illness by 1 year, have a rapidly progressive course, and die before age 2. In the remainder, who develop AIDS at a rate of 8% per year, the disease progresses at a slower rate. The latent period is longer for transfusion-acquired and sexually acquired infections (median of 7–10 years). Almost every child infected with HIV will eventually develop symptomatic immunodeficiency.

Risk factors for HIV infection include exposure to blood products from 1978 to the spring of 1985; parenteral illicit drug use; multiple heterosexual or homosexual contacts; and a heterosexual partner or mother with one of the above risk factors. Casual, classroom, or household contact with an HIV-infected person poses no risk.

Clinical Findings

A. Symptoms and Signs: Frequent illness is a typical historical feature, including recurrent otitis media, sinusitis, poor weight gain, chronic cough, chronic diarrhea or candidal infection, developmental delay, or unexplained fevers.

1. Nonspecific–See above. These are the most common and earliest findings and may be present for years in an otherwise well child.

2. Infections–Recurrent or severe infections include sepsis, pneumonia, abscesses, meningitis, bone and joint infections, and cellulitis. Organisms include *Haemophilus influenzae,* pneumococci, *Staphylococcus aureus, Salmonella,* and opportunistic pathogens (*Candida* esophagitis, severe varicella-zoster infections, and CMV retinitis are common).

3. Pulmonary–Lymphoid interstitial pneumonitis is seen in almost half of children with AIDS. Histologically, it is characterized by a diffuse peribronchial and interstitial infiltrate composed of lymphocytes and plasma cells. It may be asymptomatic or associated with dry cough, hypoxemia, and dyspnea or wheezing on exertion. Children with this disorder frequently have increased immunoglobulin levels, clubbing of the digits, enlargement of the parotid glands, and generalized lymphadenopathy. Auscultatory findings may be few. *Pneumocystis carinii* pneumonia is also common (40%), but it is a more acute illness presenting with fever, retractions, progressive hypoxemia, and elevated LDH (See chapter 34).

4. Encephalopathy–This is rather common as a late sequela and consists of acquired microcephaly, retardation, progressive motor deficit, ataxia, pseudobulbar palsy, and failure to attain (or surrender of previously attained) developmental milestones. The course is variable but usually not acute; seizures are uncommon.

5. Other–Other findings include hepatomegaly, splenomegaly, and lymphadenopathy. Chronic parotid enlargement, thrombocytopenia, hepatitis, cardiomyopathy, nephritis, pancreatitis, and Bell's palsy have also been described. Malignancy is AIDS-defining in 1% of children.

B. Laboratory Findings: Routine tests are often nonspecific and reflect inflammation in the affected organs. The lymphocyte and helper T cell counts fall. Since these are normally higher in infants than in older children, values for this laboratory test must be age-adjusted. Helper T cells become very low and helper/suppressor T cell ratios reversed. The sedimentation rate is often elevated. Anemia and thrombocytopenia may occur. Hypergammaglobulinemia is characteristic: Some children fail to make specific antibody to antigens (eg, tetanus, *Haemophilus influenzae* type b, pneumococcus). This failure contributes to subsequent infections. With brain involvement, the protein level in cerebrospinal fluid may be elevated, and a mononuclear pleocytosis may be present. Serum LDH levels are high in children with *P carinii* infection.

In children older than 15 months, HIV antibody is positive, both by the EIA and confirmatory blot test. Rarely (< 1%), an infected child may fail to make antibody. However, they are usually obviously ill, and tests for virus or viral antigens are positive. No reliable IgM antibody test is available. Diagnosis of infection in infants requires culture of the virus (usually from blood), demonstration of viral antigen or nucleic acid in blood or tissue, or evidence of immunodeficiency with no other explanation in a child with signs of AIDS. Using a combination of HIV culture, polymerase chain reaction, and p24 antigen detection, approximately 80% of infected infants can be identified at birth or soon after and more than 95% by 3–6 months of age. Infants who are antibody-positive after 15 months are probably infected even if clinically well, though in rare cases maternal antibody may persist for up to 18 months in an uninfected infant.

C. Imaging: Chest radiographs of children with lymphoid interstitial pneumonitis show a diffuse interstitial reticulonodular infiltrate, occasionally with hilar adenopathy. Cerebral images demonstrate atrophy and calcification in the basal ganglia and frontal lobes in patients with brain infection. Infection with other opportunistic pathogens usually results in x-ray findings typical of each agent. The more severe the immunodeficiency, however, the more atypical these presentations can be.

Differential Diagnosis

In children older than 18 months, the diagnosis of infection can be quickly made by serologic tests. In younger children, a negative result usually excludes HIV infection but a positive result must be followed by careful confirmatory testing. In these children, other congenital immunodeficiencies, congenital infections (CMV infection, toxoplasmosis, syphilis), and many other illnesses may cause similar presenting clinical signs.

Complications & Sequelae

These result from direct viral invasion (brain, lung, heart, kidney), secondary malignancies (less common than in adults; Kaposi's sarcoma, lymphomas, and polyclonal B cell lymphoproliferative syndromes), and infections with a multitude of agents (eg, *P carinii, Candida albicans,* herpes simplex, CMV, measles, varicella-zoster virus, *Toxoplasma gondii, Cryptosporidium, Isospora belli, Mycobacterium avium-intracellulare, Cryptococcus neoformans, Nocardia,* and *Histoplasma capsulatum.*)

Prevention

Awareness of modes of transmission is crucial for prevention. Caregivers should encourage AIDS education for children entering puberty. Heterosexual spread is becoming an important route. Condom use is imperative.

All medical equipment that can penetrate skin should be sterile. Infected blood and secretions should be handled according to the recommendations made by the Centers for Disease Control (see below).

Perinatal or in utero transmission can be substantially (65%) prevented by antiretroviral therapy of the mother and early prophylaxis of the newborn. It is recommended that HIV-infected women not become pregnant. Since breast milk can carry the virus, breast feeding by HIV-positive mothers is contraindicated.

Therapy

A. Specific Measures: Zidovudine (azidothymidine; AZT), an orally absorbed nucleoside analogue that prevents viral DNA synthesis and secondarily inhibits replication, is the best-studied antiretroviral drug. Since it is virostatic, it must be taken for life. The major toxicities are anemia, neutropenia, headache, myalgia, and insomnia. A suspension is available for use in children. An alternative drug, didanosine (dideoxyinosine; ddI) is available for patients who cannot tolerate or no longer respond to zidovudine. A solution may be prepared from powder packets, and side effects include pancreatitis and peripheral retinal depigmentation. For adolescents and adults, zalcitabine (dideoxycytidine; ddC) is available for use in combination with zidovudine. In adults, peripheral neuropathy is seen in up to one-third of patients receiving this agent. Clinical trials in children are under way. Whenever possible, children should be enrolled in collaborative treatment studies. Current information on clinical trials may be obtained by calling the AIDS Clinical Trials Group (1-800 TRIALS-A) or the Pediatric Branch, National Cancer Institute (301-402-0696). Currently, antiretroviral therapy is indicated in children with a definitive diagnosis of HIV infection who demonstrate evidence of significant immunodeficiency or HIV-associated symptoms. Recommendations for therapy change rapidly; consultation must be obtained.

B. General Measures:

1. Immunizations–Combined diphtheria-tetanus-pertussis (DTP), conjugated *Haemophilus influenzae* type b (HIB), hepatitis B, pneumococcal, and influenza vaccines should be given at the recommended times. Because of the possibility of development of vaccine-associated polio in the patient or in the patient's immunodeficient contacts after administration of oral poliovaccine, the inactivated poliovaccine is recommended both for patients and for well children in their households (see Chapter 10). The risk of measles is considered greater than the potential risk of the vaccine in asymptomatic children; thus, measles-mumps-rubella vaccine should be given at the usual time. Varicella or measles may be fatal; prophylaxis with immune globulin (for measles) or varicella-zoster immune globulin (for varicella) should be given to all unimmunized HIV-infected children after each exposure to these infections.

2. Infections–Bacterial infections should be diagnosed and treated aggressively. Antibiotic prophylaxis for *P carinii* pneumonia is recommended for children with low (for age) helper cell numbers. Rifabutin has recently been approved for use as prophylaxis for *Mycobacterium avium* complex disease in adults. No data are available as to its efficacy in children. Unusual infections may require invasive diagnostic techniques such as biopsy or bronchoscopy. Agents such as *M avium* complex, CMV, and *Cryptosporidium* are often impossible to eradicate.

CMV-seropositive children with CD4 counts less than $100/\mu L$ should have ophthalmologic examinations every 3–6 months for early detection of retinitis. Periodic intravenous immune globulin (IGIV) was effective in reducing the number of bacterial infections and hospitalizations in some HIV-infected children who were not receiving *Pneumocystis* prophylaxis with trimethoprim-sulfamethoxazole. No rigid criteria for the routine use of IGIV have been defined. Appropriate candidates might include children with hypogammaglobulinemia, poor functional antibody development, and serious recurrent infections.

3. Lymphoid interstitial pneumonitis–This may respond to steroid therapy. The long-term toxicity of steroids in patients with HIV-infection is unknown.

4. General support–Attention must be paid to psychosocial needs and nutrition. Ideally, care should be coordinated by a team of caregivers familiar with this disease, the newest therapies, and community support systems available. Transfusions may be needed; CMV seronegative blood is preferred.

Prognosis

Poor prognosis is associated with perinatal infection, encephalopathy, infection with *P carinii,* and early development of AIDS. Some children, especially those infected by blood products, may live many years. The presence of lymphoid interstitial pneumonitis is a relatively good indicator (median survival over 7 years). Owing to the great variability in individual response to infection and treatment, definite statements regarding the prognosis for life expectancy or quality of life should not be made.

Public Health Issues

In general, the child who is well enough to attend school should be educated no differently from any other child. Although health care providers and the teacher and nurse need to be aware of the underlying diagnosis, it should otherwise remain confidential. The social consequences of HIV infection often overshadow the medical problems.

Saliva, tears, urine, and stool are not considered contagious in routine living situations. The virus in blood or serum is easily neutralized by a variety of agents, including household bleach (1:10 dilution), some commercial disinfectants (eg, Lysol), and 70% isopropyl alcohol.

Belman AL: AIDS and pediatric neurology. Neurol Clin 1990;8:571.

Classification system for human immunodeficiency virus (HIV) infection in children under 13 years of age. MMWR Morb Mortal Wkly Rep 1987;36:225.

European Collaborative Study: Children born to women with HIV-1 infection: natural history and risk of transmission. Lancet 1991;337:253.

Guidelines for prophylaxis against *Pneumocystis carinii* pneumonia for children infected with human immunodeficiency virus. MMWR Morb Mortal Wkly Rep 1991; 40(RR-2):1.

Immunization of children infected with human immunodeficiency virus: Supplemental ACIP statement. MMWR Morb Mortal Wkly Rep 1988;37:181.

McKinney RE et al: Safety and tolerance of intermittent intravenous and oral zidovudine therapy in human immunodeficiency virus-infected pediatric patients. J Pediatr 1990;116:640.

The NICHD Intravenous Globulin Study Group: Intravenous immune globulin for the prevention of bacterial infections in children with symptomatic human immunodeficiency virus infection. N Engl J Med 1991;325:73.

Petrou A et al: Reliability of polymerase chain reaction in the detection of human immunodeficiency virus infection in children. Pediatr Infect Dis J 1992;11:30.

Prober CG, Gershon AA: Medical management of newborns and infants born to human immunodeficiency virus-seropositive mothers. Pediatr Infect Dis J 1991; 10:684.

Thomas P et al: Trends in survival for children reported with maternally transmitted acquired immunodeficiency syndrome in New York City, 1982–1989. Pediatr Infect Dis J 1992;11:34.

The Working Group on Antiretroviral Therapy: National Pediatric HIV Resource Center: Antiretroviral therapy and medical management of the human immunodeficiency virus-infected child. Pediatr Infect Dis J 1993; 12:513.

RABIES

Essentials of Diagnosis

- History of animal bite 10 days to 1 year previously.
- Paresthesias or hyperesthesia in bite area.
- Irritability followed by fever, confusion, combativeness, muscle spasms (especially pharyngeal with swallowing).
- Progressive symptoms, death.
- Rabies antigen detected in corneal scrapings or tissue obtained by brain or skin biopsy; Negri bodies seen in brain tissue.

General Considerations

Rabies remains a serious public health problem wherever animal immunization is not widely practiced. Although infection does not always follow a bite by a rabid animal (about 40% infection rate following rabid dog bites), infection is fatal. Any warmblooded animal may be infected, but susceptibility and transmissibility vary with different species. Bats may be well yet carry and excrete the virus in saliva or feces for prolonged periods. Dogs and cats are usually clinically ill within 10 days after becoming contagious (the standard quarantine period for suspect animals). Valid quarantine periods or signs of illness are not fully known for many species. Rodents rarely transmit infection. Animal vaccines are only partially immunogenic; a single inoculation may fail to produce immunity in up to 20% of dogs.

Clinical Findings

The risk is assessed according to the type of animal (bats always considered rabid); the animal's behavior (unprovoked bite or unusual behavior); wound extent and location (infection more common after head or arm bites, or if wounds have extensive salivary contamination or are not quickly and thoroughly cleaned); geographic area (urban rabies rare to nonexistent in many United States cities; rural rabies always possible, especially outside USA); and animal vaccination history (risk low if documented). Owing partially to the long incubation period, a bite history is not always obtained. Aerosolized virus in caves inhabited by bats has caused infection.

A. Symptoms and Signs: Paresthesias at the bite site are usually the first symptom. Nonspecific anxiety and excitability follow, then muscle spasms, drooling, hydrophobia, delirium, and lethargy. Swallowing or even the sensation of air blown on the face may cause pharyngeal spasms. Seizures, fever, coma, and death follow within a week after onset.

B. Laboratory Findings: Leukocytosis is common. The spinal fluid may be normal or may show elevation of protein and mononuclear cells. Cerebral imaging and electroencephalography are not diagnostic.

Infection in an animal may be determined by use of the fluorescent antibody test to examine brain tissue for antigen.

Rabies virus is excreted in the saliva of infected humans, but the diagnosis is usually made by antigen detection in scrapings or tissue samples of richly innervated epithelium, eg, the cornea or hairline of the neck. Classic Negri cytoplasmic inclusion bodies in brain tissue are not always present.

Seroconversion occurs after 7–10 days.

Differential Diagnosis

Failure to elicit the bite history in areas where rabies is rare may delay diagnosis. Other disorders to be considered include pseudorabies (hysterical belief that one has the disease); parainfectious encephalopathy; encephalitis due to herpes simplex, arboviruses, enteroviruses, and lymphocytic choriomeningitis virus; and Guillain-Barré syndrome.

Prevention

See Chapter 10 for information regarding vaccination and postexposure prophylaxis. The development of human immune globulin and diploid cell vaccine has made prophylaxis more effective and minimally toxic. Since rabies is almost always fatal, presumed exposures must be managed carefully.

Treatment & Prognosis

Survival is rare but has been reported in patients receiving meticulous intensive care. No antiviral preparations are of proved benefit.

Baevsky RH, Bartfield JM: Human rabies: A review. Am J Emerg Med 1993;11:279.

Fishbein DB, Robinson LE: Rabies. N Engl J Med 1993;329:1632.

Mann JM: Systematic decision-making in rabies prophylaxis. Pediatr Infect Dis 1983;2:162.

Shah U, Jaswal GS: Victims of a rabid wolf in India: Effect of severity and location of bites on development of rabies. J Infect Dis 1976;134:25.

RUBELLA

Essentials of Diagnosis

- History of rubella vaccination usually absent.
- Prodromal nonspecific respiratory symptoms and adenopathy (postauricular and occipital).

- Maculopapular rash beginning on face, rapidly spreading to entire body, and disappearing by fourth day.
- Few systemic symptoms.

Congenital infection:
- Retarded growth, development.
- Cataracts, retinopathy.
- Purpuric "blueberry muffin" rash at birth, jaundice, thrombocytopenia.
- Deafness.
- Congenital heart defect.

General Considerations

If it were not teratogenic, rubella would be of little clinical importance. Clinical diagnosis is difficult in some cases because of its variable expression. In one study, over 80% of infections were subclinical. Because of inadequate vaccination, many outbreaks now occur in adolescents or adults.

The number of reported rubella cases in the USA decreased until 1989, when a resurgence was noted. Congenital rubella, both in infants of unimmunized women and in some who have apparently been reinfected in pregnancy, is also increasing.

Clinical Findings

The incubation period is 14–21 days. The nondistinctive signs may make exposure history unreliable. A history of immunization makes rubella unlikely but still possible.

Congenital rubella usually follows maternal infection in the first trimester.

A. Symptoms and Signs:

1. Infection in children–Young children may only have rash. Older patients often have a nonspecific prodrome of low-grade fever, ocular pain, sore throat, and myalgia. Postauricular and suboccipital adenopathy (sometimes generalized) is characteristic. This often precedes the rash or may occur without rash. The rash consists of discrete maculopapules beginning on the face. A "slapped cheek" appearance or pruritus may occur. The rash quickly spreads to the trunk and extremities after it fades from the face; it is gone by the fourth day. Enanthem is usually absent.

2. Congenital infection–Over 80% of women infected in the first 4 months of gestation deliver affected infants; less than 10% of those infected later in pregnancy do so. Later infections can result in isolated defects, eg, deafness. The main manifestations are as follows:

a. Growth retardation–Fifty to 85 percent are small at birth and remain so.

b. Cardiac anomalies–Pulmonary artery stenosis, patent ductus arteriosus, ventricular septal defect.

c. Ocular anomalies–Cataracts, microphthalmia, glaucoma, retinitis.

d. Deafness.

e. Cerebral disorders–Chronic encephalitis.

f. Hematologic disorders–Thrombocytopenia,

dermal nests of extramedullary hematopoiesis or purpura ("blueberry muffin" spots), lymphopenia.

g. Others–Hepatitis, osteomyelitis, immune disorders, malabsorption, diabetes.

B. Laboratory Findings: Leukopenia is common, and platelet counts may be low. Congenital infection is associated with low platelet counts, abnormal liver function tests, hemolytic anemia, pleocytosis, and very high rubella IgM antibody titers. Total serum IgM is elevated, and IgA and IgG levels may be depressed.

C. Imaging: Pneumonitis and bone metaphysial longitudinal lucencies may be present in films of children with congenital infection.

Diagnosis

Virus may be isolated from throat or urine from 1 week before to 2 weeks after onset of rash. Children with congenital infection are infectious for months. The virus laboratory must be notified that rubella is suspected. Serologic diagnosis is best made by demonstrating a fourfold rise in antibody titer between specimens drawn 1–2 weeks apart. The first should be drawn promptly, since titers increase rapidly after onset of rash. Both specimens must be tested simultaneously by a single laboratory. Specific IgM titers are used, but specificity and sensitivity vary with the testing site diagnosing disease. Because the decision to terminate a pregnancy is usually based on serologic results, testing must be done carefully.

Differential Diagnosis

Rubella may resemble infections due to enterovirus, adenovirus, measles, Epstein-Barr virus, roseola, parvovirus (erythema infectiosum), and *Toxoplasma gondii*. Because public health implications are great, sporadic suspected cases should be serologically or virologically confirmed.

Congenital rubella must be differentiated from congenital CMV infection, toxoplasmosis, and syphilis.

Complications & Sequelae

A. Arthralgia and Arthritis: Both occur more often in adult women. Polyarticular involvement (fingers, knees, wrists), lasting a few days to weeks, is typical. Frank arthritis occurs in a small percentage. It may resemble acute rheumatoid arthritis.

B. Encephalitis: With an incidence of about 1:6000, this is a nonspecific parainfectious encephalitis associated with a low mortality rate. A syndrome resembling subacute sclerosing panencephalitis (see rubeola) has also been described in congenital rubella.

C. Rubella in Pregnancy: Infection in the mother is self-limited and not severe (see above for sequelae).

Prevention

See Chapter 10 for the indications for and efficacy of rubella vaccine. Standard prenatal care in many areas includes rubella antibody testing. Seropositive mothers are at no risk; seronegative mothers are vaccinated after delivery.

A pregnant woman possibly exposed to rubella should be tested immediately; if seropositive, she is immune and need not worry. If she is seronegative, a second specimen should be drawn in 4–6 weeks, and both specimens should be tested simultaneously. Seroconversion in the first trimester suggests high fetal risk; such women require counseling regarding therapeutic abortion.

When pregnancy termination is not an option, some experts recommend intramuscular administration of 20 mL of standard immune globulin within 72 hours after exposure in an attempt to prevent infection. (This negates the value of subsequent antibody testing.) The efficacy of this practice is unknown.

Treatment & Prognosis

Symptomatic therapy is sufficient. Arthritis may improve with administration of anti-inflammatory agents. The prognosis is excellent in those with acquired disease but poor in congenitally infected infants, in whom most defects are irreversible or progressive. The severe cognitive defects seem to correlate closely in these infants with the degree of growth failure.

Chantler JK et al: Persistent rubella virus infection associated with chronic arthritis in children. N Engl J Med 1985;313:1117.

Freij BJ, South MA, Sever JL: Maternal rubella and the congenital rubella syndrome. Clin Perinatol 1988;15:247.

Increase in rubella and congenital rubella syndrome: United States, 1988–1990. MMWR Morb Mortal Wkly Rep 1991;40:93.

Kaplan KM et al: A profile of mothers giving birth to infants with congenital rubella syndrome: An assessment of risk factors. Am J Dis Child 1990;144:118.

Weber B et al: Congenital rubella syndrome after maternal reinfection. Infection 1993;21:118.

II. RICKETTSIAL INFECTIONS

The rickettsiae are pleomorphic, gram-negative coccobacilli which are obligate intracellular parasites. Rickettsial diseases are often included in the differential diagnosis of febrile rashes, though some are not characterized by rash. Severe headache is a prominent symptom. The endothelium is the primary target tissue, and the ensuing vasculitis is responsible for severe illness.

All rickettsioses except Q fever are transmitted by cutaneous arthropod contact, either by bite or fecal contamination of skin breaks. Evidence of such contact by history or physical examination may be completely lacking, especially in young children. The geographic distribution of the vector is often the primary determinant for suspicion of these infections.

Diagnosis is by serologic testing; elevation of antibodies to *Proteus* strains (OX19, OX2, OXK, the classic Weil-Felix test) is easily measured but less sensitive and specific than many other tests now available. Therapy must often be empirical. Most new broad-spectrum antimicrobials are inactive against these cell wall-deficient organisms; chloramphenicol and tetracycline are usually effective.

HUMAN EHRLICHIOSIS

Ehrlichia species are responsible for febrile pancytopenia in animals. In humans, *Ehrlichia sennetsu* is responsible for a mononucleosis-like syndrome seen in Japan and Malaysia. The agent of North American human ehrlichiosis has been identified as a new species, *Ehrlichia chaffeensis*. The reservoir is currently unknown; ticks are the presumed vectors. Most cases in the United States are reported in the south central and mid to southern Atlantic states. Almost all cases occur between March and October. Recent evidence suggests that human ehrlichiosis is underrecognized; in one study, 10% of adults suspected of having Rocky Mountain spotted fever had serologic evidence of human ehrlichiosis.

Clinical Findings

In approximately three-fourths of cases, a history of tick bite can be elicited. The majority of the remaining patients report having been in a tick-infested area. The incubation period ranges from 1 to 21 days.

A. Symptoms and Signs: Fever is universally present in children. Gastrointestinal symptoms (anorexia, nausea and vomiting) are reported in 70% of pediatric cases. Headache, myalgia, and rash are seen in over half. The rash may be erythematous, macular, papular, vesicular, petechial, scarlatiniform, or vasculitic. Several cases of meningitis have occurred in children. The physical examination, except for rash, is usually normal. Conjunctival injection, mild cervical adenopathy, and organomegaly have been described but are usually absent.

B. Laboratory Findings: Laboratory abnormalities include leukopenia, lymphopenia, thrombocytopenia, and elevated aminotransferase levels. Anemia is seen in one-third of cases.

The diagnosis is made serologically. The CDC uses *E chaffeensis* as the antigen in an immunofluorescent antibody test. Morulae may occasionally be observed in mononuclear and polymorphonuclear cells from the peripheral blood, bone marrow, or cerebrospinal fluid.

Differential Diagnosis

The differential diagnosis includes other rickettsial infections, Colorado tick fever, leptospirosis, Epstein-Barr virus infection, cytomegalovirus infection, hepatitis, other viral infections, systemic lupus erythematosus, and leukemia.

Treatment & Prognosis

Children have an excellent prognosis. Although the disease may last several weeks, it is usually self-limited. In vitro and in vivo evidence suggest that tetracycline is effective. While clinical reports of therapeutic success using chloramphenicol exist, a study that evaluated the in vitro effectiveness of that agent found that *E chaffeensis* was resistant.

Anderson BE et al: *Ehrlichia chaffeensis*, a new species associated with human ehrlichiosis. J Clin Microbiol 1991;29:2838.

Barton LL et al: Infection with *Ehrlichia* in childhood. J Pediatr 1992;120:998.

Harkness JR: Ehrlichiosis. Infect Dis Clin North Am 1991;5:37.

Rohrbach BW et al: Epidemiologic and clinical characteristics of persons with serologic evidence of *E canis* infection. Am J Public Health 1990;80:442.

RICKETTSIALPOX

Rickettsia akari is transmitted by mites on infected house mice. Infection is rarely diagnosed; most cases in the USA have occurred in northeastern cities, particularly New York. The bite site becomes a papule, then a pustule; it ulcerates and then scabs at about the time fever develops at 9–14 days. Local adenopathy is the rule. Headache, myalgia, and photophobia are followed in 2–4 days by a generalized, central, and discrete papular rash. Vesicles develop on the papules and form crusts. The fever lasts about a week.

The differential diagnosis includes varicella, enteroviral infections, the other rickettsial spotted fevers, meningococcemia, and gonococcemia. Mild cases require no therapy. The Weil-Felix test is negative.

Brettman LK et al: Rickettsialpox: Report of an outbreak and contemporary review. South Afr Med J 1981;60:363.

ROCKY MOUNTAIN SPOTTED FEVER

Rickettsia rickettsii infection causes one of many similar tick-borne illnesses characterized by fever and a rash. Most are named for their geographic area: Siberian, Queensland, Kenyan, etc. In all except Rocky Mountain spotted fever, there is a characteristic eschar at the bite site, the "tache noire." Dogs and rodents are reservoirs of *R rickettsii*.

Rocky Mountain spotted fever is the most severe of these infections and the most important in the USA. It occurs predominantly in the eastern half of the country and in Arkansas, Texas, and Oklahoma—rarely in the West. Most cases occur in children exposed in rural areas in the spring and summer. Since tick attachment lasting 4 hours or longer is needed, frequent tick removal is a preventive measure.

Clinical Findings

A. Symptoms and Signs: After the incubation period of 2–8 days, there is high fever (over 40 °C, often hectic) of abrupt onset, myalgia, severe and persistent headache (less obvious in infants), general toxicity, vomiting, and diarrhea. The characteristic rash occurs in over 95% of patients and appears 2–6 days after fever onset as macules on the palms, soles, and extremities, becoming petechial and spreading centrally. Conjunctivitis, splenomegaly, muscle tenderness, edema, and meningismus may be seen.

B. Laboratory Findings: Laboratory findings are nonspecific and reflect diffuse vasculitis: thrombocytopenia, hyponatremia, early mild leukopenia, proteinuria, and hematuria. Cerebrospinal fluid pleocytosis is common. Serologic diagnosis is achieved with indirect fluorescent or indirect hemagglutination antibody methods.

Differential Diagnosis

The differential diagnosis includes meningococcemia, measles, meningitis, staphylococcal sepsis, enteroviral infection, leptospirosis, Colorado tick fever or infection by other arboviruses, streptococcal pharyngitis, and ehrlichiosis.

Treatment & Prognosis

To be effective, therapy must be started early and is often based on a presumptive diagnosis in endemic areas prior to rash onset. It is important to remember that atypical presentations often lead to delay in appropriate therapy. Chloramphenicol is the agent of choice for children under 8 years of age; a tetracycline may be used for older children. Treatment should be continued for 2 or 3 days after the temperature has returned to normal for a full day. A minimum of 10 days of therapy is recommended.

Complications and death result from severe vasculitis, especially in the brain, heart, and lung. The mortality rate is 5–7%.

Kirk JL et al: Rocky Mountain spotted fever: A clinical review based on 48 confirmed cases. Medicine 1990;69:35.

Sexton DJ, Corey CR: Rocky Mountain "spotless" and "almost spotless" fever: A wolf in sheep's clothing. Clin Infect Dis 1992;15:439.

Weber DJ, Walker DH: Rocky Mountain spotted fever. Infect Dis Clin North Am 1991;5:19.

ENDEMIC TYPHUS (Murine Typhus)

Endemic typhus is present in the USA mainly in southern Texas. The disease is transmitted by fleas from infected rodents. A recent study suggested that domestic cats and opposums may play a role in the transmission of suburban cases. There is no eschar at the bite, which may go unnoticed. The incubation period is 6–14 days. Headache, myalgia, and chills slowly worsen. Fever may last 10–14 days. After 3–8 days, a rash appears. Truncal macules spread to the extremities but spare the palms and soles; the rash may become petechial. Intestinal and respiratory symptoms may occur. The illness is usually self-limited and milder than epidemic typhus. More prolonged neurologic symptoms have been described. Therapy is not usually needed. Diagnosis is by serologic testing.

Samra Y, Shaked Y, Maier MK: Delayed neurologic toxicity in murine typhus: Report of two cases. Arch Intern Med 1989;149:949.

Sorvillo FJ et al: A suburban focus of endemic typhus in Los Angeles county: Association with seropositive domestic cats and opossums. Am J Trop Med Hyg 1993;48:269.

REFERENCES

Feigin RD, Cherry JD (editors): *Textbook of Pediatric Infectious Diseases,* 3rd ed. Saunders, 1992.

Galasso GH, Merigan TC, Buchanan RA (editors): *Antiviral Agents and Viral Diseases of Man,* 32nd ed. Raven Press, 1990.

Moffett HL: *Pediatric Infectious Diseases,* 3rd ed. Lippincott, 1989.

Remington JS, Klein JO: *Infectious Disease of the Fetus and Newborn Infant.* Saunders, 1990.

Zuckerman AJ, Banatvala JE, Pattison JR: *Principles and Practice of Clinical Virology.* Wiley, 1987.

Infections: Bacterial & Spirochetal

John W. Ogle, MD

BACTERIAL INFECTIONS

GROUP A STREPTOCOCCAL INFECTIONS

Essentials of Diagnosis

Streptococcal pharyngitis:
- Clinical diagnosis based entirely on symptoms; signs and physical examination unreliable.
- Throat culture or rapid antigen detection test positive for group A streptococci.

Impetigo:
- Rapidly spreading, highly infectious skin rash.
- Erythematous denuded areas and honey-colored crusts.
- On culture, group A streptococci are grown in most (not all) cases.

General Considerations

Group A streptococci are common gram-positive bacteria capable of producing a wide variety of clinical illnesses. Prominent among these are acute pharyngitis; impetigo; cellulitis; and scarlet fever, the generalized illness caused by strains that elaborate erythrogenic toxin. Group A streptococci can also cause pneumonia, septic arthritis, osteomyelitis, meningitis, and numerous other less common infections. Group A streptococcal infections may also produce nonsuppurative sequelae (rheumatic fever or acute glomerulonephritis).

The cell walls of streptococci contain both carbohydrate and protein antigens. The C-carbohydrate antigen determines the *group,* and the M- or T-protein antigens determine the specific *type*. In most strains, the M protein appears to confer virulence, and antibodies developed against the M protein are protective against reinfection with that type.

Group A streptococci are almost all β-hemolytic. These organisms may be carried asymptomatically on the skin and in the pharynx, rectum, and vagina. Ten to 15 percent of school children in some studies are asymptomatic pharyngeal carriers of group A strepto-cocci. Streptococcal carriers are asymptomatic individuals who do not mount an immune response to the organism and are therefore believed to be at low risk for nonsuppurative sequelae. Unfortunately, there are no accepted criteria for identification of streptococcal carriers.

All group A streptococci are sensitive to penicillin. Resistance to erythromycin is common in some countries and has increased in the USA.

Clinical Findings

A. Symptoms and Signs:

1. Respiratory infections–

a. Infancy and early childhood (under 3 years of age)–The onset of infection is insidious, with mild symptoms, eg, low-grade fever, serous nasal discharge, and pallor. Otitis media is common. Pharyngitis with exudate and cervical adenitis are uncommon in this age group.

b. Childhood type–Onset is sudden, with fever and marked malaise and often with repeated vomiting. The pharynx is sore and edematous, and the tonsillar area generally shows exudate. Anterior cervical lymph nodes are tender and enlarged. Small petechiae are frequently seen on the soft palate. Fine discrete petechiae occasionally appear also on the upper abdomen and trunk. In scarlet fever, the skin is diffusely erythematous and appears sunburned and roughened (sandpaper rash). The rash is most intense in the axillas and groin and on the abdomen and trunk. It blanches on pressure except in the skin folds, which do not blanch and are pigmented (Pastia's sign). The rash usually appears 24 hours after the onset of fever and rapidly spreads over the next 1–2 days. Desquamation begins on the face at the end of the first week and becomes generalized by the third week. Early, the surface of the tongue is coated white, with the papillae enlarged and bright red ("white strawberry tongue"). Subsequently, desquamation occurs, and the tongue appears beefy red ("red strawberry tongue"). The face generally shows circumoral pallor. Petechiae may be seen on all mucosal surfaces.

c. Adult type–The adult type is characterized by exudative or nonexudative tonsillitis with fewer systemic manifestations, lower fever, and no vomiting. Scarlet fever is uncommon in this age group.

2. Impetigo–Streptococcal impetigo begins as a papule that vesiculates and then breaks, leaving a denuded area covered by a honey-colored crust. Both *Staphylococcus aureus* and group A streptococci are isolated in some cases. The lesions spread readily and diffusely. Local lymph nodes may become swollen and inflamed. Although the affected child often lacks systemic symptoms, occasionally a high fever and toxicity are present. If flaccid bullae are present, the disease is called bullous impetigo and is caused by an epidermolytic toxin-producing strain of *S aureus*.

3. Cellulitis–The portal of entry is often an insect bite or superficial abrasion on an extremity. There is a diffuse and rapidly spreading cellulitis that involves the subcutaneous tissues and extends along the lymphatic pathways with only minimal local suppuration. Local acute lymphadenitis occurs. The child is usually acutely ill, with fever and malaise. In classic erysipelas, the involved area is bright red, swollen, warm, and very tender. The infection may extend rapidly from the lymphatics to the bloodstream.

Streptococcal perianal cellulitis is an entity peculiar to young children. Pain with defecation often leads to constipation, which may be the presenting complaint. The child is afebrile and otherwise well. Perianal erythema and tenderness and painful rectal examination are the only abnormal physical findings. Culture of a perianal swab specimen usually yields a heavy growth of group A streptococcus. Any of the antimicrobial regimens for streptococcal infection is usually effective. A variant of this syndrome is streptococcal vaginitis in prepubertal girls. Symptoms are dysuria and pain; marked erythema and tenderness of the introitus and blood-tinged discharge are seen.

4. Necrotizing fasciitis–Formerly called streptococcal gangrene, this is an uncommon but dangerous entity. Only 20–40% of cases are due to group A streptococci. About 30–40% are due to *S aureus* and the rest to mixed bacterial infections. The disease is characterized by extensive necrosis of superficial fasciae, with undermining of surrounding tissue and extreme systemic toxicity. Initially, the skin overlying the infection is pale red without distinct borders, resembling subcutaneous cellulitis. Blisters or bullae may appear. The color deepens to a distinct purple. The involved area may develop mild to massive edema. Early recognition and aggressive debridement of necrotic tissue are essential.

5. Group A streptococcal infections in newborn nurseries–Group A streptococcal epidemics still occasionally occur in nurseries. The organism may be introduced into the nursery from the vaginal tract of a mother or from the throat or nose of a mother or member of the staff. The organism then spreads from infant to infant. The umbilical stump is colonized while the infant is in the nursery. As is true also in staphylococcal infections, there may be no or few clinical manifestations while infants are still in the nursery; most often, a colonized infant develops a chronic, oozing omphalitis days later at home. The organism may spread from the infant to other family members. More serious and even fatal infections may develop, including sepsis, meningitis, empyema, septic arthritis, and peritonitis.

6. Streptococcal sepsis–Serious illness from group A streptococcal sepsis is now more common both in children and in adults. Rash and scarlet fever may be present; prostration and shock result in high mortality rates. Pharyngitis is uncommon as an antecedent illness. Underlying disease is a predisposing factor. Some authors hypothesize that a more virulent clone of group A streptococci is responsible for the increase in cases of streptococcal sepsis.

B. Laboratory Findings: Leukocytosis with a marked shift to the left is seen early. Eosinophilia regularly appears during convalescence. β-Hemolytic streptococci are cultured with ease from the throat. The organism may be cultured from the skin and by needle aspiration from subcutaneous tissues and other involved sites, such as infected nodes. Occasionally, blood cultures are positive. Group A streptococci may be identified most easily by demonstrable sensitivity to bacitracin. Grouping by immunofluorescence or coagglutination studies correlates best with the original precipitin reactions described by Lancefield. Typing is not routinely done.

Rapid antigen detection tests are 60–95% sensitive and over 95% specific for detecting group A streptococci in throat swabs. The predictive value of negative tests is about 80%, meaning that one in five patients with a positive throat culture will have a negative rapid antigen test. Rapid tests may be useful when early antibiotic therapy is considered, but because the currently available tests lack sensitivity, a standard culture should be done on specimens testing negative. Rapid detection tests with improved sensitivity are entering the market and may improve the utility of rapid tests.

Antistreptolysin O (ASO) titers rise about 150 units within 2 weeks after an acute infection. Elevated ASO and anti-DNase B titers are useful in documenting prior throat infections in cases of acute rheumatic fever. However, elevated anti-DNase B and antihyaluronidase titers are most useful in associating pyoderma and acute glomerulonephritis. The streptozyme test is a useful 2-minute slide test that detects antibodies to streptolysin O, hyaluronidase, streptokinase, DNase B, and NADase. It is somewhat more sensitive than the measurement of ASO titers.

Proteinuria, cylindruria, and minimal hematuria may be seen early in children with streptococcal infection. More commonly, true poststreptococcal glomerulonephritis is seen 1–4 weeks after the respiratory infection.

Differential Diagnosis

Streptococcosis of the early childhood type must be differentiated from adenovirus and other respiratory virus infections.

Adenoviruses, coxsackieviruses (both A and B), echoviruses, Epstein-Barr virus (infectious mononucleosis), and many other respiratory viruses can produce pharyngitis. The pharyngitis in herpangina (coxsackie A viruses) is vesicular or ulcerative. Herpes simplex also causes ulcerative lesions, which most commonly involve the anterior pharynx, tongue, and gums. With other viruses (coxsackieviruses and echoviruses), rashes are common. In infectious mononucleosis, the pharyngitis is often exudative, but generalized lymphadenopathy is also present, and laboratory findings are often diagnostic (atypical lymphocytes, elevated liver enzymes, and a positive heterophil or other serologic test for mononucleosis). Uncomplicated streptococcal pharyngitis improves within 24–48 hours if penicillin is given and by 72–96 hours without antimicrobials.

Group G and group C streptococci are uncommon causes of pharyngitis but have been implicated in epidemics of sore throat in college students. Acute rheumatic fever does not occur following group G or C infection, though acute glomerulonephritis is a complication.

Arcanobacterium hemolyticum is also a cause of pharyngitis. Scarlatinal or maculopapular truncal rashes may be been seen.

In diphtheria, systemic symptoms, vomiting, and fever are less marked; the pseudomembrane is confluent and adherent; the throat is less red; and cervical adenopathy is prominent.

Pharyngeal tularemia causes white rather than yellow exudate. There is little erythema, and cultures for β-hemolytic streptococci are negative. A history of exposure to rabbits and a failure to respond to antimicrobials may suggest a diagnosis of tularemia. Response to specific antibiotic therapy is prompt.

Leukemia and agranulocytosis may present with pharyngitis and are diagnosed by bone marrow examination.

Scarlet fever must be differentiated from other exanthematous diseases, principally rubella. Erythema due to sunburn, drug reactions, fever, Kawasaki disease, toxic shock syndrome, and staphylococcal scalded skin syndrome must at times be considered. (See also Table 35–3.)

Complications

The most common suppurative complications of group A streptococcal infections are purulent or serous rhinitis, sinusitis, otitis, mastoiditis, cervical lymphadenitis, pneumonia, empyema, septic arthritis, and meningitis. Spread of streptococcal infection from the throat to other sites—principally the skin (impetigo) and vagina—is common also and should be considered in every instance of chronic vaginal discharge or chronic skin infection, such as that complicating childhood eczema.

Both acute rheumatic fever and acute glomerulonephritis are nonsuppurative complications of group A streptococcal infections.

A. Acute Rheumatic Fever: See Chapter 21.

B. Acute Glomerulonephritis: Acute nephritis can follow streptococcal infections of either the pharynx or the skin—in contrast to rheumatic fever, which follows pharyngeal infection only. Glomerulonephritis may occur at any age, including infancy. In most reported series of acute glomerulonephritis, males predominate by a ratio of 2:1, whereas acute rheumatic fever occurs with equal frequency in both sexes.

Certain M types are strongly associated with poststreptococcal glomerulonephritis ("nephritogenic types"). Moreover, the serotypes resident on or producing disease on the skin often differ from those found in the pharynx. Pharyngeal infections leading to glomerulonephritis include M types 1, 4, 12, and 18, with limited evidence for 3, 6, and 25. Skin M types leading to nephritis include 2, 31, 49, 52–55, 57, and 60.

The incidence of acute glomerulonephritis after streptococcal infection is variable and has ranged from nil to 28%. Several outbreaks of acute glomerulonephritis in families have involved 50–75% of siblings of affected patients in 1- to 7-week periods. Second attacks of glomerulonephritis are rare. The median latent period between infection and the development of glomerulonephritis is 10 days. This contrasts with acute rheumatic fever, which occurs after a median latent period of 18 days.

Treatment

A. Specific Measures: Treatment is directed not only toward eradication of acute infection but also toward the prevention of rheumatic fever. In patients with pharyngitis, antibiotics should be started early to relieve symptoms and should be continued for 10 days to prevent rheumatic fever. Although early therapy has not been shown to prevent glomerulonephritis, it seems advisable to promptly treat impetigo in sibling contacts of patients with poststreptococcal nephritis. Neither sulfonamides nor trimethoprim-sulfamethoxazole is effective in the treatment of streptococcal infections.

Although topical therapy for impetigo with antimicrobial ointments (eg, bacitracin, mupiricin) is as effective as systemic therapy, it does not eradicate pharyngeal carriage and is less practical for extensive disease.

1. Penicillin–A single dose of benzathine penicillin G given intramuscularly (0.6 million units for children weighing < 60 lb and 1.2 million units for children weighing > 60 lb) is preferred for treatment of pharyngitis and impetigo. Phenoxymethyl penicillin (penicillin V) (250 mg for children weighing < 40 lb and 500 mg for children weighing > 40 lb) administered orally three or four times daily between meals for 10 days is successful in about 90% of cases. Giving penicillin V (250 mg) twice daily is as effective as more frequent oral administration or intramuscular therapy and may achieve better compliance, but a single daily dose results in a higher failure rate. Parenteral therapy is indicated if there is vomiting or sepsis. Mild cellulitis may be similarly treated. Cellulitis requiring hospitalization should be treated with aqueous penicillin G (150,000 units/kg/d intravenously in four to six divided doses) or procaine penicillin (50,000 units/kg intramuscularly once or twice a day) until there is marked improvement. Penicillin V, 125–250 mg every 6 hours, may then be given orally to complete a 10-day course. Acute cervical lymphadenitis may require incision and drainage. Treatment of necrotizing fasciitis requires emergency surgical debridement followed by high-dose parenteral antibiotics appropriate to the organisms cultured.

2. Other antibiotics–For pharyngitis or impetigo, erythromycin estolate (20–40 mg/kg/d in two to four divided doses) should be given for 10 days. Erythromycin ethyl succinate (40–50 mg/kg/d) is best tolerated if given in four divided doses. Both erythromycin preparations are best absorbed and tolerated when taken with food. Clindamycin, cephalexin, cefuroxime, cefaclor, loracarbef, cefprozil, cefpodoxime, cefixime, and cefadroxil are also effective oral antimicrobials. Cefixime and cefadroxil may be given once daily, while cefuroxime, loracarbef, cefprozil, and cefaclor may be used twice daily. In most studies, bacteriologic failures after cephalosporin therapy are less frequent than failures following penicillin. However, cephalosporins are far more expensive than penicillin, and penicillin currently remains the agent of choice. The dosage of clindamycin is 10–20 mg/kg/d in four divided doses. Each of these drugs should be given for 10 days. Many strains are resistant to tetracycline. For serious or life-threatening infections in patients with known penicillin allergy, cefazolin (100–150 mg/kg/d intravenously or intramuscularly in three divided doses), clindamycin (25–40 mg/kg/d intravenously in four divided doses), or vancomycin (40 mg/kg/d intravenously in four divided doses) should be given.

3. Treatment failure–Even when compliance is perfect, organisms will be found in 5–15% of children cultured after cessation of therapy. Reculture is indicated only in the patient with pharyngitis who has a personal or family history of rheumatic fever. Retreatment at least once with an oral cephalosporin is indicated in patients with recurrent culture positive pharyngitis.

4. Prevention of recurrences in rheumatic individuals– The preferred prophylaxis for rheumatic individuals is benzathine penicillin G, 1.2 million units intramuscularly once every 3 weeks. One of the following alternative oral prophylactic regimens may be used: sulfadiazine, 0.5–1 g daily; penicillin G, 200,000 units twice daily; or erythromycin, 250 mg twice daily. Most authorities feel that lifelong prophylaxis is indicated, particularly in the presence of rheumatic heart disease. A similar approach to the prevention of recurrences of glomerulonephritis is debatable but may be indicated during childhood when there is a suspicion that repeated streptococcal infections coincide with flare-ups of acute glomerulonephritis.

B. General Measures: Analgesic lozenges or gargles with 30% glucose or warm saline solution may be used for relief of sore throat. A soft, bland diet that includes noncarbonated high-glucose drinks (such as apple, grape, and pear juice) and iced milk or sherbet is helpful. Acetaminophen is useful for pain or fever.

With impetigo, local treatment may promote earlier healing. Crusts should first be soaked off; areas beneath the crusts should then be washed with soap daily.

C. Treatment of Complications: Acute complications are best treated with penicillin. Rheumatic fever is best prevented by early and adequate penicillin treatment of the streptococcal infection (see above).

D. Treatment of Carriers: Identification and management of group A streptococcal carriers is difficult. There are no established clinical or serologic criteria for differentiating carriers from the truly infected. Some children receive multiple courses of antimicrobials, with persistence of group A streptococci in the throat, leading to a "streptococcal neurosis" on the part of families.

Clindamycin (20 mg/kg/d in four divided doses) given orally or a combination of rifampin (20 mg/kg/d for 4 days) given orally and penicillin in standard dosage given orally has been used to improve bacteriologic cure rates after streptococcal pharyngitis and may be useful in selected streptococcal carriers.

Prognosis

Death is rare except in infants or young children with sepsis or pneumonia. The febrile course is shortened and complications eliminated by early and adequate treatment with penicillin.

Bisno AL: Group A streptococcal infections and acute rheumatic fever. N Engl J Med 1991;325:783.

Chaudhary S et al: Penicillin V and rifampin for the treatment of group A streptococcal pharyngitis: A randomized trial of 10 days penicillin vs 10 days penicillin with rifampin during the final 4 days of therapy. J Pediatr 1985;106:481.

Gerber MA, Randolph MF, Mayo DR: The group A streptococcal carrier state. Am J Dis Child 1988;142:562.

Karn KC et al: *Arcanobacterium hemolyticum* infection: Confused with scarlet fever and diphtheria. J Emerg Med 1991;9:33.

Kellogg JA: Suitability of throat culture procedures for detection of group A streptococci and as reference standards for evaluation of streptococcal antigen detection kits. J Clin Microbiol 1990;28:165.

Peter G: Streptococcal pharyngitis: Current therapy and criteria for evaluation of new agents. Clin Infect Dis 1992; 14(Suppl 2):S218.

Pichichero ME: Cephalosporins are superior to penicillin for treatment of streptococcal tonsillopharyngitis: Is the difference worth it? Pediatr Infect Dis J 1993;12:268.

Randolph MF et al: Effect of antibiotic therapy on the clinical course of streptococcal pharyngitis. J Pediatr 1985; 106:870.

Rathore MH, Barton LL, Kaplan EL: Suppurative group A beta-hemolytic streptococcal infections in children. Pediatrics 92;89:743.

Seppälä H et al: Resistance to erythromycin in group A streptococci. N Engl J Med 1992;326:292.

Wheeler M et al: Outbreak of group A streptococcus septicemia in children: Clinical, epidemiological, and microbiological correlates. JAMA 1991;266:533.

GROUP B STREPTOCOCCAL INFECTIONS

Essentials of Diagnosis

Early-onset neonatal sepsis or meningitis:
- Newborn infant, age birth to 5 days, with rapidly progressing overwhelming sepsis, with or without meningitis.
- Pneumonia with respiratory failure frequently present; chest x-ray resembles that seen in hyaline membrane disease.
- Leukopenia with a shift to the left.
- Blood or spinal fluid cultures growing group B streptococci.

Late-onset neonatal sepsis or meningitis:
- Meningitis in a child 1–16 weeks old with spinal fluid or blood cultures growing group B streptococci.

General Considerations

Although most patients with group B streptococcal disease are infants under 3 months of age, cases are seen in infants 4–5 months of age. Serious infection also occurs in women with puerperal sepsis, in immunocompromised patients, in patients with cirrhosis and spontaneous peritonitis, and in diabetics with cellulitis. Group B streptococcal infections occur as frequently as gram-negative infections in the newborn period. Two distinct clinical syndromes distinguished by differing perinatal events, age at onset, and serotype of the infecting strain have been described in these infants.

Clinical Findings

Early-onset illness is observed in newborns less than 7 days old. The onset of symptoms in the majority of these infants occurs in the first 48 hours of life, and most are ill within 6 hours. Apnea is often the first sign. There is a high incidence of associated maternal obstetric complications, especially premature labor and prolonged rupture of the membranes. Newborns with early-onset disease are severely ill at the time of diagnosis, and the mortality rate is more than 50%. Although the majority of infants with early-onset infections are full term, premature infants are at increased risk for the disease. Newborns with early-onset infection acquire group B streptococci from the maternal genital tract in utero or during passage through the birth canal. When early-onset infection is complicated by meningitis, as occurs in approximately 30% of cases, more than 80% of the bacterial isolates belong to serotype III. Postmortem examination of infants with early-onset disease almost always reveals pulmonary inflammatory infiltrates and hyaline membranes containing large numbers of group B streptococci.

Late-onset infection occurs in infants between 7 days and 4 months of age; the median age at onset is about 4 weeks. Maternal obstetric complications are infrequently associated with late-onset infection. These infants are usually not as severely ill at the time of diagnosis as those with early-onset disease, and the mortality rate is significantly lower. In recent series, about 37% of patients have meningitis and 46% have sepsis. Other clinical manifestations, eg, septic arthritis and osteomyelitis, "occult" bacteremia, otitis media, ethmoiditis, conjunctivitis, cellulitis (particularly of the face or submandibular area), lymphadenitis, breast abscess, empyema, and impetigo, have been described. Strains of group B streptococci possessing the capsular type III polysaccharide antigen are isolated from more than 95% of infants with late-onset disease, regardless of clinical manifestations. The exact mode of transmission of the organisms is not well defined.

Type III group B streptococci that cause neonatal disease are genetically closely related. Dissemination of a clone of high virulence in neonates is responsible for the increase in cases of disease reported from many nurseries in the 1970s and 1980s.

Prevention

Many women of childbearing age possess circulating antibody to the polysaccharide antigen of type III group B streptococci. This antibody is transferred to the newborn via the placental circulation. Carriers delivering healthy infants have significant serum levels of IgG antibody to this antigen. In contrast, women delivering infants who develop type III group B streptococcal disease of either the early- or late-onset type rarely have detectable antibody in their sera. Similar findings have recently been described for type Ia infections.

A vaccine prepared with type III polysaccharide has been evaluated in pregnant women. Although the vaccine is not optimally immunogenic, 63% of mothers produced IgG antibody.

The American Academy of Pediatrics recommends screening all pregnant women for group B streptococcus at 26–28 weeks of gestation by cultures obtained from both the rectum and the lower vagina using a selective broth medium. Women with positive cultures or rapid antigen tests who also have one or more risk factors should receive ampicillin intravenously intrapartum. The risk factors are (1) preterm labor at less than 37 weeks of gestation, (2) premature rupture of membranes at less than 37 weeks of gestation, (3) fever during labor, (4) multiple births, and (5) rupture of membranes beyond 18 hours at any gestation. Mothers who deliver an infant infected with group B streptococci should receive intrapartum antibiotic chemoprophylaxis with each subsequent delivery. Application of these guidelines would significantly reduce early-onset disease, but the practice is controversial because they are difficult and expensive to implement.

Diagnosis

Culture of group B streptococci from a normally sterile site such as blood or cerebrospinal fluid provides proof of diagnosis. Group B streptococcal antigen may be detected in concentrated urine samples using commercially available kits.

Treatment

Penicillin G is the drug of choice. Group B streptococci are less susceptible than other streptococci to penicillin, and high doses are recommended, especially for meningitis (at least 250,000 units/kg/d, given in three doses per day to infants less than 1 week old and in four doses per day to older infants). Aminoglycosides act synergistically with penicillin in vitro; for this reason, both penicillin and gentamicin should be used for meningitis and other serious infections. Penicillin dosage for nonmeningeal infections is 50,000 units/kg/d (in divided doses every 12 hours) for infants less than 1 week old and 75,000–100,000 units/kg/d (in divided doses every 8 hours) for older infants. Duration of therapy is 3 weeks for meningitis, at least 4 weeks for osteomyelitis or endocarditis, and 10–14 days for other infections. Therapy does not eradicate carriage of the organism. Ceftriaxone is active in vitro against group B streptococci, and because of its long serum half-life it may be given once or twice daily intramuscularly or intravenously. Ceftriaxone is sometimes used to complete a course of therapy when intravenous access has become difficult.

American Academy of Pediatrics Committee on Infectious Diseases: Guidelines for prevention of group B streptococcal (GBS) infection by chemoprophylaxis. Pediatrics 1992;90:775.

Baker CJ et al: Immunization of pregnant women with a polysaccharide vaccine of group B streptococcus. N Engl J Med 1988;319:1180.

Dillon HC, Khare S, Gray BM: Group B streptococcal carriage and disease: A 6-year prospective study. J Pediatr 1987;110:31.

Edwards MS et al: Long-term sequelae of group B streptococcal meningitis in infants. J Pediatr 1985;106:717.

Fischer GW: Immunoglobulin therapy of neonatal group B streptococcal infections: An overview. Pediatr Infect Dis J 1988;7(Suppl):13.

Gibbs RS et al: Consensus: Perinatal prophylaxis for group B streptococcal infection. Pediatr Infect Dis J 1992; 11:179.

Hachey WE, Wiswell TE: Limitations in the usefulness of urine latex particle agglutination tests and hematologic measurements in diagnosing neonatal sepsis during the first week of life. J Perinatol 1992;12:240.

Noya FJ, Baker CJ: Prevention of group B streptococcal infection. Infect Dis Clin North Am 1992;6:41.

Sanchez PJ et al: Significance of a positive urine group B streptococcal latex agglutination test in neonates. J Pediatr 1990;116:601.

Yagupsky P, Menegus MA, Powell KR: The changing spectrum of group B streptococcal disease in infants: An eleven-year experience in a tertiary care hospital. Pediatr Infect Dis J 1991;10:801.

STREPTOCOCCAL INFECTIONS WITH ORGANISMS OTHER THAN GROUP A OR B

Streptococci of groups other than A and B are part of the normal flora of humans and can cause disease. Group C or G organisms occasionally produce pharyngitis (with an ASO rise) but without risk of subsequent rheumatic fever, though acute glomerulonephritis may occasionally occur. Group D streptococci and *Enterococcus* are normal inhabitants of the gastrointestinal tract and may produce urinary tract infections, meningitis and sepsis in the newborn, and endocarditis. Nosocomial infections caused by *Enterococcus* are frequent in neonatal and oncology units. Nonhemolytic aerobic streptococci and α-hemolytic streptococci are normal flora of the mouth. They are involved in the production of dental plaque and probably dental caries and are the most common cause of subacute infective endocarditis. Finally, there are numerous anaerobic and microaerophilic streptococci, normal flora of the mouth, skin, and gastrointestinal tract, which alone or in combination with other bacteria may cause sinusitis, dental abscesses, brain abscesses, and intra-abdominal or lung abscesses.

Treatment

A. Enterococcal Infections: Urinary tract infections can be treated with oral amoxicillin alone. Sepsis or meningitis in the newborn should be treated intravenously with a combination of ampicillin (100–200 mg/kg/d in three divided doses) and gentamicin (6–7.5 mg/kg/d in three divided doses). Endocarditis requires at least 30 days of intravenous treatment. Penicillin G (250,000 units/kg/d in six to eight divided doses) plus streptomycin (30 mg/kg/d) or gentamicin (6–7.5 mg/kg/d in three divided doses) is most often used. Third-generation cephalosporins are not effective. Ampicillin-resistant enterococci are usually susceptible to vancomycin (40–60 mg/kg/d in four divided doses). Careful monitoring of aminoglycoside levels is required, both to avoid toxicity and to ensure therapeutic levels.

Whenever endocarditis is being treated, peak and trough serum killing powers should be obtained. A bactericidal level of 1:8 or greater immediately before the next penicillin dose should be maintained.

High-level resistance to aminoglycosides (MIC > 1000 µg/mL) is an increasing problem in many hospitals. Vancomycin resistance has also increased. Patients with serious enterococcal infections require consultation with infectious disease experts and with the clinical microbiology laboratory to determine the optimal combination of antimicrobials.

B. Viridans Streptococcal Infections (Subacute Infective Endocarditis): It is important to determine the penicillin sensitivity of the infecting strain as early as possible in the treatment of viridans streptococcal endocarditis. Resistant organisms are most commonly seen in patients receiving chronic penicillin prophylaxis for rheumatic heart disease. Strains sensitive to penicillin G (MIC < 0.1 µg/mL) may be treated for 4 weeks with penicillin, 150,000–200,000 units/kg/d intravenously, with gentamicin added during the first 2 weeks. If the MIC is 0.5 µg/mL or higher, longer therapy and higher doses of penicillin G must be used (200,000–300,000 units/kg/d intravenously in combination with streptomycin or gentamicin for 4–6 weeks). If the MIC is 0.1–0.5 µg/mL, penicillin G at the higher dose for a minimum of 4 weeks is recommended, with gentamicin added for the first 2 weeks. Vancomycin, 40 mg/kg/d, is usually preferred for resistant strains and patients allergic to penicillin.

Bisno AL et al: Antimicrobial treatment of infective endocarditis due to viridans streptococci, enterococci, and staphylococci. JAMA 1989;261:1471.

Boulanger JM, Ford-Jones EL, Matlow AG: Enterococcal bacteremia in a pediatric institution: A four-year review. Rev Infect Dis 1991;13:847.

Frieden TR et al: Emergence of vancomycin-resistant enterococci in New York City. Lancet 1993;342:76.

Moellering RC: Emergency of *Enterococcus* as a significant pathogen. Clin Infect Dis 1992;14:1173.

Rhinehart E et al: Rapid dissemination of β-lactamase-producing aminoglycoside-resistant *Enterococcus faecalis* among patients and staff on an infant-toddler surgical ward. N Engl J Med 1990;323:814.

Simon RM, Dobson MB, Baker CJ: Enterococcal sepsis in neonates: Features by age at onset and occurrence of focal infection. Pediatrics 1990;85:165.

PNEUMOCOCCAL INFECTIONS

Essentials of Diagnosis

Bacteremia:
- High fever (≥ 39.4 °C).
- Leukocytosis (≥ 15,000/µL).
- Age 6–24 months.

Pneumonia:
- Fever, leukocytosis, and cough.
- Localized chest pain.
- Localized or diffuse rales. Chest x-ray may show lobar infiltrate (with effusion).

Meningitis:
- Fever, leukocytosis.
- Bulging fontanelle, neck stiffness.
- Irritability and lethargy.

All types:
- Diagnosis confirmed by cultures of blood, spinal fluid, pleural fluid, or other body fluid or by detection of pneumococcal antigen in urine or spinal fluid.

General Considerations

Pneumococcal sepsis, sinusitis, otitis media, pneumonitis, meningitis, osteomyelitis, cellulitis, arthritis, vaginitis, and peritonitis are all part of a spectrum of pneumococcal infection. Clinical findings that correlate with occult bacteremia in ambulatory patients include age (6–24 months), degree of temperature elevation (≥ 39.4 °C), and leukocytosis (≥ 15,000/µL). Although each of these findings is in itself nonspecific, a combination of them should arouse suspicion. This constellation of findings in a child who has no focus of infection may be an indication for blood cultures and antibiotic therapy. The cause of two-thirds of such bacteremic episodes is pneumococci. *Haemophilus influenzae* type b is the second most frequent cause in the unimmunized child.

Streptococcus pneumoniae is the most common cause of acute purulent otitis media.

Pneumococci are the organisms responsible for most cases of acute bacterial pneumonia in children. The disease is indistinguishable on clinical grounds from other bacterial pneumonias. Effusions are common, though frank empyema is less common. Abscesses also occasionally occur.

Pneumococcal meningitis is now more common than H influenzae type b meningitis because of widespread vaccination. Pneumococcal meningitis, sometimes recurrent, may complicate serious head trauma, particularly if there is persistent leakage of cerebrospinal fluid. This has led some physicians to recommend the prophylactic administration of penicillin or other antimicrobials in such cases.

Children with sickle cell disease, other hemoglobinopathies, congenital or acquired asplenia, and some immunoglobulin and complement deficiencies are unusually susceptible to overwhelming pneumococcal sepsis and meningitis. These children often have a catastrophic illness with shock and disseminated intravascular coagulation. Even with excellent supportive care, the mortality rate is 20–50%. The spleen is important in the control of pneumococcal infection by clearing organisms from the blood and producing an opsonin that enhances phagocytosis. Autosplenectomy may explain why children with sickle cell disease are at increased risk for developing serious pneumococcal infections.

S pneumoniae rarely causes serious disease in the neonate. Although *S pneumoniae* does not normally colonize the vagina, transient colonization does occur. Serious neonatal disease—including pneumonia, sepsis, and meningitis—and maternal infection may occur and clinically are similar to group B streptococcal infection.

For more than 30 years, penicillin has been the agent of choice for pneumococcal infections. Most strains are still highly susceptible to penicillin; however, during the last 10 years, there have been increasing reports of pneumococci with moderately increased resistance to penicillin and reports of treatment failure, particularly in meningitis. The prevalence of these relatively penicillin-resistant strains in North America is about 3–15%. An outbreak of infections due to markedly penicillin-resistant pneumococci has been reported from South Africa, and similar strains including strains with multiple antimicrobial resistances are now recognized throughout the world. Pneumococci from normally sterile body fluids should be screened routinely for susceptibility to penicillin as well as other drugs.

Pneumococci have been classified into 83 serotypes based on capsular polysaccharide antigens. Serotypes 6, 14, 18, 19, and 23 cause most pneumococcal infections in children. The frequency distribution of serotypes varies at different times, in different geographic areas, and with different sites of infection. The most recently developed polyvalent pneumococcal vaccine contains capsular polysaccharides of 23 serotypes and is discussed in Chapter 10. Specific antibody induced by the vaccine protects only against the serotypes included in the vaccine. Children under age 18–24 months generally do not have a good antibody response to this vaccine, and the protective efficacy of the vaccine in older children is controversial. Despite these limitations, the vaccine is recommended for high-risk children over 2 years of age. The successful development of conjugate vaccines that protect against *H influenzae* type b has spurred interest in the development of protein-polysaccharide conjugates to protect against pneumococci.

Clinical Findings

A. Symptoms and Signs: In pneumococcal sepsis, fever usually appears abruptly, often accompanied by chills. There may be no respiratory symptoms. In pneumococcal sinusitis, mucopurulent nasal discharge may occur. In infants and young children with pneumonia, cough and diffuse rales are found more often than the lobar distribution characteristic of adult forms of pneumococcal pneumonia. Respiratory distress is manifested by flaring of the alae nasi, chest retractions, and tachypnea. Abdominal pain is common. In older children, the adult form of pneumococcal pneumonia with signs of lobar consolidation may occur, but sputum is rarely bloody. Thoracic pain resulting from pleural involvement is sometimes present, but less often in children than in adults. With involvement of the right hemidiaphragm, pain may be referred to the right lower quadrant, suggesting appendicitis. Vomiting is common at onset but seldom persists. Convulsions are relatively common at onset in infants.

Meningitis is characterized by fever, irritability, convulsions, and neck stiffness. The most important sign in very young infants is a tense, bulging anterior fontanelle. In older children, fever, chills, headache, and vomiting are common symptoms. Classic signs are nuchal rigidity associated with positive Brudzinski and Kernig signs. With progression of untreated disease, the child may develop opisthotonos, stupor, and coma.

B. Laboratory Findings: Leukocytosis is often pronounced (20,000–45,000/μL), with 80–90% polymorphonuclear neutrophils. Neutropenia may be seen early in very serious infections. The presence of pneumococci in the nasopharynx is not a helpful finding, because up to 40% of normal children carry pneumococci in the upper respiratory tract. Large numbers of organisms seen on gram-stained smears of endotracheal aspirate are seen with pneumonia. Needle aspiration of the lung rarely is indicated. In meningitis, cerebrospinal fluid usually shows an elevated white cell count of several thousand, chiefly polymorphonuclear neutrophils, with decreased glucose and elevated protein levels. Gram-positive diplococci are seen on stained smears of cerebrospinal fluid sediment in 70–90% of cases. Antigen detection in cerebrospinal fluid, pleural fluid, serum, or joint fluid may also be helpful in selected cases. Testing urine for pneumococcal antigen is generally not helpful; this test lacks sensitivity, presumably because the antigen is degraded and only small molecular-size fragments are found in the urine.

Differential Diagnosis

There are many causes of high fever and leukocytosis in young infants; 80–90% of children presenting with these signs have a disease other than pneumococcal bacteremia, such as enteroviral or other viral infection, urinary tract infection, unrecognized focal infection elsewhere in the body, roseola infantum, or early acute shigellosis (diarrhea will appear later).

Infants with upper respiratory tract infection who subsequently develop signs of lower respiratory disease are most likely to be infected with a respiratory virus. Hoarseness or wheezing is often present. X-ray of the chest typically shows perihilar infiltrates and increased bronchovascular markings. It must be remembered, however, that viral respiratory infection often precedes pneumococcal pneumonia and that the clinical picture may be mixed.

Staphylococcal pneumonia frequently causes cavities and empyema, but it may be indistinguishable early in its course from pneumococcal pneumonia. It is most common in infants.

In primary pulmonary tuberculosis, children are not toxic, and x-rays show a primary focus associated with hilar adenopathy and often with signs of pleurisy. Miliary tuberculosis presents a classic x-ray appearance.

Pneumonia caused by *Mycoplasma pneumoniae* is most common in children 5 years of age and older. Onset is insidious, with infrequent chills, low-grade fever, prominent headache and malaise, cough, and, often, striking x-ray changes. Marked leukocytosis (eg, > 18,000/µL) is unusual.

Pneumococcal meningitis is diagnosed by lumbar puncture. Without a gram-stained smear and culture of spinal fluid, it is not distinguishable from other types of acute bacterial meningitis.

Complications

Complications of sepsis include meningitis and osteomyelitis; complications of pneumonia include empyema, parapneumonic effusion, and, rarely, lung abscess. Mastoiditis and meningitis may follow untreated pneumococcal otitis media. Both pneumococcal meningitis and peritonitis are more likely to occur independently without coexisting pneumonia. Shock, disseminated intravascular coagulation, and Waterhouse-Friderichsen syndrome resembling meningococcemia are occasionally seen in pneumococcal sepsis, particularly in asplenic patients.

Treatment

A. Specific Measures: Penicillin is the drug of choice, but erythromycin and cephalosporins are also effective. All significant *S pneumoniae* isolates should be confirmed as susceptible to penicillin. Both relatively resistant and absolutely penicillin-resistant *S pneumoniae* are reported. Absolutely resistant and multiply resistant *S pneumoniae* are currently uncommon in the USA.

1. Sepsis–All children with blood cultures that grow pneumococci must be reexamined as soon as possible. The child who has a focal infection such as pneumonia or meningitis or who appears septic should be admitted to the hospital and should receive parenteral antimicrobials. Only if the child is afebrile and appears well should management on an ambulatory basis be considered. If the physician is assured of close follow-up, lumbar puncture is not mandatory; penicillin V (50–100 mg/kg/d orally for 10 days) is prescribed, and the initial dose is given at once. Some

children may be intermittently afebrile yet still progress to meningitis.

2. Pneumonia–For infants, severely ill patients, and immunocompromised hosts, aqueous penicillin G (150,000–200,000 units/kg/d intravenously in four to six divided doses) is given. Mild pneumonia may be treated with phenoxymethyl penicillin (50 mg/kg/d orally in four divided doses for 7–10 days). Erythromycin (40–50 mg/kg/d orally in two to four divided doses) is given to patients allergic to penicillin. Oral cephalosporins may be used.

3. Otitis media–Treat with oral ampicillin, amoxicillin, trimethoprim-sulfamethoxazole, or erythromycin for 10 days.

4. Meningitis–Until bacteriologic confirmation and susceptibility testing are completed, vancomycin (60 mg/kg/d intravenously if four divided doses) should be given. After bacteriologic confirmation of susceptibility, aqueous penicillin G (300,000 units/kg/d intravenously in six divided doses for 10–14 days) should be given. Third-generation cephalosporins are acceptable if in vitro testing shows the isolate is susceptible, but uncommon resistant strains are associated with clinical failures.

B. General Measures: Supportive and symptomatic care is required.

Prognosis

In children, case fatality rates of less than 1% should be achieved except in meningitis, in which rates of 5–20% still prevail. The presence of large numbers of organisms without a prominent cerebrospinal fluid inflammatory response or of meningitis due to a penicillin-resistant strain indicates a poor prognosis. Serious neurologic sequelae, particularly hearing loss, are more frequent following pneumococcal meningitis than following meningococcal or *H influenzae* type b meningitis.

Baraff LJ et al: Practice guideline for management of infants and children 0 to 36 months of age with fever without source. Pediatrics 1993;92:1.

Brieman RF et al: Pneumococcal bacteremia in Charleston County, South Carolina: A decade later. Arch Intern Med 1990;150:1401.

Burman LA, Norrby R, Trollfors B: Invasive pneumococcal infections: Incidence, predisposing factors, and prognosis. Rev Infect Dis 1985;7:133.

Davies AJ, Kumaratne DS: The continuing problem of pneumococcal infection. J Antimicrob Chemother 1988; 21(4):387.

Friedland IR, Istre GR: Management of penicillin-resistant pneumococcal infections. Pediatr Infect Dis J 1992;11:433.

Friedland IR et al: Dilemmas in diagnosis and management of cephalosporin-resistant *Streptococcus pneumoniae* meningitis. Pediatr Infect Dis J 1993;12:196.

Gorensek MJ, Lebel MH, Nelson JD: Peritonitis in children with nephrotic syndrome. Pediatrics 1988;81:849.

Gray BM, Dillon HC Jr: Epidemiological studies of *Streptococcus pneumoniae* in infants: Antibody to types 3, 6, 14, and 23 in the first two years of life. J Infect Dis 1988; 158:948.

Jacobs NM: Pneumococcal osteomyelitis and arthritis in children: A hospital series and literature review. Am J Dis Child 1991;145:70.

Murdoch IA, Dos Anjos R: Continued need for pneumococcal prophylaxis after splenectomy. Arch Dis Child 1991; 65:1268.

Rauch AM et al: Invasive disease due to multiply resistant *Streptococcus pneumoniae* in a Houston, Texas, day-care center. Am J Dis Child 1990;144:923.

STAPHYLOCOCCAL INFECTIONS

Staphylococcal infections are common and important in childhood. Staphylococcal skin infections range from minor furuncles to the varied syndromes now collected under the encompassing term "scalded skin syndrome." Staphylococci are the major cause of osteomyelitis and, in older children, of septic arthritis. They are an uncommon but important cause of bacterial pneumonia. A toxin produced by certain strains causes staphylococcal food poisoning. Staphylococci are now responsible for most infections of artificial heart valves. They cause toxic shock syndrome (see below). Finally, they are found in infections at all ages and in multiple sites, particularly when infection is introduced from the skin or upper respiratory tract or when closed compartments become infected (pericarditis, sinusitis, cervical adenitis, surgical wounds, abscesses in the liver or brain, and abscesses elsewhere in the body).

Staphylococci, which do not produce the enzyme coagulase, are termed coagulase-negative but are seldom speciated in the clinical microbiology laboratory. Most *Staphylococcus aureus* strains produce coagulase. S aureus and coagulase-negative staphylococci are normal flora of the skin and respiratory tract. The latter rarely causes disease except in compromised hosts, the newborn, or patients with plastic prostheses in place, where coagulase-negative staphylococci infection occurs frequently.

Most strains of *S aureus* elaborate a β-lactamase that confers penicillin resistance. This can be overcome in clinical practice by the use of a nonpenicillin antibiotic, a cephalosporin, or a penicillinase-resistant penicillin such as methicillin, oxacillin, nafcillin, cloxacillin, or dicloxacillin. Methicillin-resistant strains are found worldwide and are now common in certain hospitals and areas in the USA. Most of these strains retain β-lactamase production, and many are resistant to other antibiotics as well. Methicillin-resistant strains are also resistant in vivo to all of the penicillinase-resistant penicillins and cephalosporins.

S aureus produces a variety of exotoxins, most of which are of uncertain importance. Two toxins are recognized as playing a central role in specific diseases: exfoliatin and staphylococcal enterotoxin. The former is largely responsible for the various clinical presentations of the scalded skin syndrome. Most strains that elaborate exfoliatin are of phage group II. Enterotoxin causes staphylococcal food poisoning. The exoprotein toxin most commonly associated with toxic shock syndrome has been termed TSST-1. However, *S aureus* strains isolated from patients with toxic shock syndrome who have focal infections do not produce detectable TSST-1. Their organisms have been found to produce enterotoxins B or C, suggesting that the syndrome may be caused by more than one *S aureus* exoprotein.

Clinical Findings
A. Symptoms and Signs:
1. Staphylococcal skin diseases–Dermal infection with *S aureus* causes furuncles or cellulitis. *S aureus* are often found along with streptococci in impetigo. If the strains produce exfoliatin, localized lesions become bullous (bullous impetigo).

Generalized exfoliative disease (scalded skin syndrome) occurs as a result of more generalized involvement with exfoliatin-producing strains. The infection may begin at any site but appears to be introduced through the respiratory tract in most cases. There is a prodromal phase of erythema, often beginning around the mouth, accompanied by fever and irritability. The involved skin becomes tender, and a sick infant will cry when picked up or touched. A day or so later, exfoliation begins, usually around the mouth. The inside of the mouth is red, and a peeling rash is present around the lips, often in a radial pattern resembling rhagades. Generalized, painful peeling may follow, involving the limbs and trunk but often sparing the feet. More commonly, peeling is confined to areas around body orifices. If erythematous but unpeeled skin is rubbed sideways, superficial epidermal layers separate from deeper ones and sloughs (Nikolsky's sign). In the newborn, the disease is termed **Ritter's disease** and may be fulminant. If there is tender erythema but not exfoliation, the disease is termed nonstreptococcal scarlet fever. The scarlatiniform rash is sandpaper-like, but strawberry tongue is not seen, and cultures grow *S aureus* rather than streptococci.

2. Osteomyelitis and septic arthritis–See Chapter 26.

3. Staphylococcal pneumonia–Staphylococcal pneumonia in infancy is characterized by abdominal distention, high fever, respiratory distress, and toxemia. It often occurs without predisposing factors or after minor skin infections. The organism is necrotizing, producing bronchoalveolar destruction. Pneumatoceles, pyopneumothorax, and empyema are frequently encountered. Rapid progression of disease is characteristic. Frequent chest x-rays to monitor the progress of disease are indicated and may be lifesaving. Presenting symptoms may be typical of paralytic ileus, suggestive of an abdominal catastrophe. When this is suspected, the abdominal films should always be accompanied by a chest film to rule out staphylococcal pneumonitis.

Staphylococcal pneumonia usually is peribronchial and diffuse and begins with a focal infiltrative lesion progressing to patchy consolidation. Most often only one lung is involved (80%), more often the right. Purulent pericarditis occurs by direct extension in about 10% of cases, with or without empyema.

4. Staphylococcal food poisoning–Staphylococcal food poisoning is produced by enterotoxin. The most common source is poorly refrigerated and contaminated food. The disease is characterized by vomiting, prostration, and diarrhea occurring 2–6 hours after ingestion of contaminated foods.

5. Staphylococcal endocarditis–*S aureus* may produce infection of normal heart valves, of valves or endocardium in children with congenital or rheumatic heart disease, or of artificial valves. In large recent series, about 25% of all cases of endocarditis are due to *S aureus*. The great majority of artificial heart valve infections involve either *S aureus* or coagulase-negative staphylococci. Infection usually begins in an extracardiac focus, often the skin. Involvement of the endocardium must be suspected in every case of *S aureus* bacteremia regardless of the presence of signs. Suspicion must be highest in the presence of congenital heart disease, particularly ventricular septal defects with aortic insufficiency, but also simple ventricular septal defect, patent ductus arteriosus, and tetralogy of Fallot.

Clinical presentation in staphylococcal endocarditis is with fever, weight loss, weakness, muscle pain or diffuse skeletal pain, poor feeding, pallor, and cardiac decompensation. Signs include splenomegaly, cardiomegaly, petechiae, hematuria, and a new or changing murmur. The course of *S aureus* endocarditis is commonly rapid, though subacute disease is occasionally seen. Peripheral septic embolization and uncontrollable cardiac failure are not uncommon, even when optimal antibiotic therapy is administered, and may be indications for surgical intervention (see below).

6. Nursery infections–*S aureus* colonizes the umbilicus and respiratory tract of a highly variable proportion of newborn infants (10–90%) during their nursery stay. The source of colonization is the skin and anterior nares of those handling the infants. Under normal circumstances, such colonization is harmless, since the bacterial strains involved are of low virulence. However, if a virulent strain is introduced (usually from an infected lesion), the proportion of sick to colonized infants can rise from less than 1% to over 50%. Such outbreaks may begin insidiously, since infants usually do not develop symptoms (furuncles, omphalitis, mastitis, impetigo, with occasional more serious disease) until after discharge. Thus, the occurrence of even a single case of staphylococcal disease in a nursery is an indication for epidemiologic surveillance of infants recently resident in that nursery, with possible subsequent institution of control measures.

7. Toxic shock syndrome–Toxic shock syndrome is characterized by fever, blanching erythroderma, diarrhea, vomiting, myalgia, prostration, hypotension, and multiple organ involvement associated with cultures of *S aureus*. Bacteremia does not occur.

Large numbers of cases have been described in menstruating adolescents and young women using vaginal tampons. Toxic shock syndrome has also been seen in both boys and girls with focal staphylococcal infections as well as in individuals with postoperative wound infections due to *S aureus*. Additional clinical features include sudden onset; conjunctival suffusion; mucosal hyperemia; desquamation of skin on the palms, soles, fingers, and toes during convalescence; disseminated intravascular coagulation in severe cases; renal and hepatic functional abnormalities; and evidence of myolysis. The mortality rate is now about 2%. Recurrences were seen during subsequent menstrual periods in as many as 60% of untreated women who continued to use tampons. Recurrences were reported in up to 15% of those who were treated with antistaphylococcal antibiotics and stopped using tampons. The disease is caused by strains of *S aureus* that produce TSST-1 or one of the related enterotoxins.

8. *S epidermidis* infections–Localized and systemic coagulase-negative staphylococci infections occur primarily in immunocompromised patients, high-risk newborns, and patients with plastic prostheses or catheters. In low-birth-weight infants, coagulase-negative staphylococci have emerged as the commonest nosocomial pathogen in nurseries in the USA. Intravenous administration of lipid emulsions and indwelling central venous catheters are risk factors contributing to coagulase-negative staphylococcal bacteremia in newborn infants. In patients with an artificial heart valve, Dacron patch, ventriculoperitoneal shunt for hydrocephalus, or a Hickman or Broviac vascular catheter, coagulase-negative staphylococci are one of the common causes of sepsis or catheter infection, often necessitating removal of the foreign material and prolonged antibiotic therapy. Because blood cultures are frequently contaminated by this organism, diagnosis of genuine localized or systemic infection is often difficult and sometimes uncertain.

B. Laboratory Findings: Moderate leukocytosis (15,000–20,000/μL) with a shift to the left is occasionally found, although normal counts are common, particularly in infants. The sedimentation rate is elevated. Blood cultures are frequently positive in systemic staphylococcal disease and should always be obtained when it is suspected. Similarly, pus from sites of infection should always be aspirated or obtained surgically, examined with Gram's stain, and cultured both aerobically and anaerobically.

There are no useful serologic tests for staphylococcal disease.

Differential Diagnosis

Staphylococcal skin disease has many morphologic forms and therefore many differential diagnoses. Bullous impetigo must be differentiated from chemical or thermal burns, from drug reactions, and, in the very young, from the various congenital epidermolytic syndromes or even herpes simplex infections. Staphylococcal scalded skin syndrome resembles scarlet fever in some instances and in others appears similar to Kawasaki disease, Stevens-Johnson syndrome, erythema multiforme, and other drug reactions. A skin biopsy may be critical in establishing the correct diagnosis. The skin lesions of varicella may become superinfected with exfoliatin-producing staphylococci and produce a combination of the two diseases (bullous varicella).

Osteomyelitis of the long bones and septic arthritis must often be differentiated (see Chapter 26).

Severe, rapidly progressing pneumonia, including ileus, is typical of *S aureus* infection but may occasionally be produced by pneumococci. Abscesses and pneumatoceles may be seen in pneumonia due to pneumococci, *Haemophilus influenzae,* and group A streptococci. Empyema formation occurs with all bacterial pneumonias.

Staphylococcal food poisoning is often epidemic. It is differentiated from other common-source gastroenteritis syndromes *(Salmonella, Clostridium perfringens, Vibrio parahaemolyticus)* by the short incubation period (2–6 hours), the prominence of vomiting (as opposed to diarrhea), and the general absence of fever.

Endocarditis must be suspected in any instance of *S aureus* bacteremia, particularly when there is a significant heart murmur or preexisting cardiac disease (see Chapter 21).

Newborn infections with *S aureus* can resemble infections with streptococci and a variety of gram-negative organisms. Umbilical and respiratory tract colonization occurs with a variety of pathogenic organisms (group B streptococci, *Escherichia coli, Klebsiella*), and both skin and systemic infections occur with virtually all of these.

Toxic shock syndrome must be differentiated from Rocky Mountain spotted fever, leptospirosis, Kawasaki disease, drug reactions, and measles. (See also Table 35–3.)

Treatment

A. Specific Measures: Since 85% of *S aureus* strains are penicillin-resistant, it is important to use a β-lactamase-resistant penicillin as the first drug in treatment. In serious systemic disease, in osteomyelitis, and in the treatment of large abscesses, intravenous therapy is indicated initially (oxacillin or nafcillin, 100–200 mg/kg/d in four divided doses, or

methicillin, 200–300 mg/kg/d in four divided doses). When high doses over a long period are required, it is preferable not to use methicillin, because of the frequency with which interstitial nephritis is seen. In life-threatening illness, an aminoglycoside antibiotic (gentamicin or tobramycin) may be used in addition for its possible synergistic action.

In those instances where *S aureus* is penicillin-sensitive, penicillin G may be used for treatment.

When children with established penicillin sensitivity are treated, cephalosporins may be used (cefazolin, 100–150 mg/kg/d intravenously in three divided doses; or cephalexin, 50–100 mg/kg/d orally in four divided doses). The third-generation cephalosporins should not generally be used for staphylococcal infections.

For methicillin-resistant infections, vancomycin (40 mg/kg/d intravenously in three or four divided doses) should be used. Infections due to methicillin-resistant staphylococci frequently do not respond to cephalosporins despite in vitro testing that suggests susceptibility. Combinations including rifampin may be either synergistic or antagonistic.

1. Skin Infections–See Chapter 16.

2. Osteomyelitis and septic arthritis–Treatment should be begun intravenously, with antibiotics selected to cover the most likely organisms (staphylococci in hematogenous osteomyelitis; *H influenzae,* meningococci, pneumococci, staphylococci in children with septic arthritis under the age of 3 years; staphylococci and gonococci in arthritis in older children). Antibiotic levels should be kept high at all times, with monitoring by serum killing powers at least once and at suitable intervals if dosage or route of administration is changed.

In osteomyelitis, clinical studies support the use of intravenous treatment until fever and local symptoms and signs have subsided—usually after at least 1 week—followed by oral therapy (dicloxacillin, 100–150 mg/kg/d in four divided doses; or cephalexin, 100–150 mg/kg/d in four divided doses) for at least 3 additional weeks. Longer treatment may be required, particularly when x-rays show extensive involvement. In arthritis, where drug diffusion into synovial fluid is good, intravenous therapy need be given only for a few days, followed by adequate oral therapy for at least 3 weeks. In all instances, oral therapy should be administered under careful supervision, either in the hospital or, in some instances, at home with frequent support and reinforcement from physicians or visiting nurses.

Surgical drainage of osteomyelitis or septic arthritis is often required (see Chapter 26).

3. Staphylococcal pneumonia–Antibiotic therapy should consist of a parenteral penicillinase-resistant penicillin with or without an aminoglycoside. Empyema or pyopneumothorax require chest tube drainage. The tube should be removed as soon as drainage has become clinically insignificant.

If staphylococcal pneumonia is promptly treated and empyema promptly drained, resolution in children is almost always complete—in spite of evidence of widespread parenchymal destruction and the persistence of bullae, blebs, and even pockets of empyema or abscess fluid well into convalescence. Surgical decortication or segmental resection is usually not required.

4. Staphylococcal food poisoning–Therapy is supportive and usually not required except in severe cases or for small infants with marked dehydration.

5. Staphylococcal endocarditis–As outlined above, high-dose, prolonged, parenteral treatment with oxacillin, nafcillin, or methicillin plus gentamicin or tobramycin is indicated. In penicillin-allergic patients, vancomycin should be used. With penicillin-sensitive organisms, penicillin G is the drug of choice. Therapy lasts in all instances for at least 6 weeks.

In some patients, medical treatment may fail. Signs of this are (1) recurrent fever without apparent treatable other cause (eg, thrombophlebitis, incidental respiratory or urinary tract infection, drug fever), (2) persistently positive blood cultures, (3) intractable and progressive congestive heart failure, and (4) recurrent (septic) embolization. In such circumstances—particularly (2), (3), and (4)—valve replacement becomes necessary. Antibiotics are continued for at least another 4 weeks. Persistent or recurrent infection may require a second surgical procedure.

6. Nursery infections–(See also Chapter 2.) Methods available to stop a nursery epidemic include the following:

a. Emphasis and reemphasis on the first principle of infection control: thorough washing of hands with soap, an iodophore, or other antiseptic agent between handling of infants.

b. Prompt and adequate management of known infections.

c. Prevention of colonization of newborns with epidemic strains by the following means:

(1) Treatment of the umbilical cord with triple dye immediately after birth.

(2) Removal and treatment of personnel carrying the epidemic strain.

(3) Segregation of infants according to age; discharge as soon as medically safe.

(4) Cohorting of nursing personnel.

(5) Restriction of visitors to the nursery area.

(6) Complete cleansing and disinfection of nurseries after discharge of colonized and infected infants.

7. Toxic shock syndrome–Treatment is first with volume expansion and inotropic agents and later with oxacillin, nafcillin, or cephalosporins. If a tampon is in place, it should be removed. All focal staphylococcal infections should be drained aggressively.

Some experts feel that corticosteroid therapy may be effective if given to patients with severe illness early in the course of their disease. Antibiotic treatment reduces risk of recurrence.

8. Coagulase-negative staphylococcal infections–Bacteremia and other serious coagulase-negative staphylococcal infections are treated initially with vancomycin. Coagulase-negative staphylococci are uncommonly resistant to vancomycin. (see Chapter 34 for dosing) Strains susceptible to penicillin or oxacillin are treated with those agents.

B. General Measures: Localized pus should be drained. Oxygen, intravenous fluids, and other supportive care are indicated in staphylococcal pneumonia and other systemic infections. Blood transfusion may be indicated if the patient is severely anemic.

Prognosis

Septicemia, endocarditis, and widespread pneumonitis in infancy all have a serious prognosis. Infants and children who recover from serious staphylococcal pneumonia have a good long-term prognosis without development of chronic respiratory disease. Osteomyelitis is now never fatal if promptly treated.

Baltimore RS: Infective endocarditis in children. Pediatr Infect Dis J 1992;11:907.

Choux M et al: Shunt implantation: Reducing the incidence of shunt infection. J Neurosurg 1992;77:875.

Dagan R: Management of acute hematogenous osteomyelitis and septic arthritis in the pediatric patient. Pediatr Infect Dis J 1993;12:88.

Ferguson MA, Todd JK: Toxic shock syndrome associated with *Staphylococcus aureus* sinusitis in children. J Infect Dis 1990;161:953.

Freeman J et al: Association of intravenous lipid emulsion and coagulase negative staphylococcal bacteremia in neonatal intensive care units. N Engl J Med 1990;2:30.

Freeman J et al: Extra hospital stay and antibiotic usage with nosocomial coagulase-negative staphylococcal bacteremia in two neonatal intensive care unit populations. Am J Dis Child 1990;144:324.

Givner LB, Kaplan SL: Meningitis due to *Staphylococcus aureus* in children. Clin Infect Dis 1993;16:766.

Hieber JP, Nelson AJ, McCracken GH: Acute disseminated staphylococcal disease in childhood. Am J Dis Child 1977;131:181.

Low DE et al: An endemic strain of *Staphylococcus haemolyticus* colonizing and causing bacteremia in neonatal intensive care unit patients. Pediatrics 1992;89:696.

MacDonald KL et al: Toxic shock syndrome: A newly recognized complication of influenza and influenza-like illness. JAMA 1987;257:1053.

Raad II, Sabbagh MF: Optimal duration of therapy for catheter-related *Staphylococcus aureus* bacteremia: A study of 35 cases and review. Clin Infect Dis 1992;14:75.

Ribner BS: Endemic, multiply resistant *Staphylococcus aureus* in a pediatric population. Am J Dis Child 1987;141:1183.

Schwalbe RS, Stapleton JT, Gilligan PH: Emergence of vancomycin resistance in coagulase-negative staphylococci. N Engl J Med 1987;316:927.

Shulman ST, Ayoub EM: Severe staphylococcal sepsis in adolescents. Pediatrics 1976;58:59.

Todd JKT: Toxic shock syndrome. Clin Microbiol Rev 1988;1:432.

Todd JKT: Staphylococcal toxin syndromes. Ann Rev Med 1985;36:337.

Tolan RW Jr et al: Operative intervention in active endocarditis in children: Report of a series of cases and review. Clin Infect Dis 1992;14:852.

MENINGOCOCCAL INFECTIONS

Essentials of Diagnosis

- Fever, headache, vomiting, convulsions, shock (meningitis).
- Fever, shock, petechial or purpuric skin rash (meningococcemia).
- Diagnosis confirmed by culture or detection of meningococcal antigen in normally sterile body fluids.

General Considerations

Meningococci may be carried asymptomatically for many months in the upper respiratory tract. Fewer than 1% of carriers develop disease. Meningitis and sepsis are the two commonest forms of illness, but septic arthritis, pericarditis, pneumonia, chronic meningococcemia, otitis media, conjunctivitis, and vaginitis also occur. The highest attack rate for meningococcal meningitis is in the first year of life. The incidence in the USA is about 1.2 cases per 100,000 people.

Meningococci are classified serologically into groups A, B, C, D, X, Y, Z, 29-E, and W-135. The serologic groups serve as specific markers for studying outbreaks and transmission of disease. Major epidemics of meningococcal disease in the USA prior to 1950 were caused by group A strains. In recent years, however, group A organisms have accounted for only about 2% of meningococcal isolates. Group B, the most common serogroup, accounts for about 40%; group C, for 30%; and group Y, for 20%. Sulfonamide resistance is common in non-group A strains. *N meningitidis* resistant to penicillin G are reported from South Africa and Spain but not in the USA. Resistant isolates are susceptible to third-generation cephalosporins. Few isolates are resistant to rifampin. Pathogenic strains differ in their virulence and in their potential for epidemic spread. Serogroup A meningococci have the greatest propensity to cause widespread outbreaks.

Children develop immunity from asymptomatic carriage of meningococci (usually nontypable, nonpathogenic strains) or other cross-reacting bacteria. Patients deficient in one of the late components of complement (C6, C7, or C8) are uniquely susceptible to meningococcal infection, particularly group A meningococci. Deficiencies of early and alternate pathway complement components are also reported.

Meningococci are gram-negative organisms containing endotoxin in their cell walls. Endotoxins may damage the walls of blood vessels and may also cause disseminated intravascular coagulation. The development of irreversible shock with multiple organ failure is a significant factor in the fatal outcome of acute meningococcal infections.

Vaccines prepared from purified meningococcal polysaccharides (A, C, Y, and W-135) are available for controlling outbreaks and preventing spread in special high-risk groups such as household contacts and military recruits. Unfortunately, the vaccines, except for the A component, are ineffective in children under 2 years of age (see Chapter 10).

Clinical Findings

A. Symptoms and Signs: Many children with clinical meningococcemia also have meningitis, and some may have other foci of infection. All children with suspected meningococcemia should have a lumbar puncture.

1. Meningococcemia–A prodrome of upper respiratory infection is followed by high fever, headache, nausea, marked toxicity, and hypotension. Purpura, petechiae, and occasionally bright pink, tender macules or papules over the extremities and trunk are seen. The rash usually progresses rapidly.

Fulminant meningococcemia (Waterhouse-Friderichsen syndrome) progresses rapidly and is characterized by disseminated intravascular coagulation, massive skin and mucosal hemorrhages, and shock. This syndrome also may be due to *Haemophilus influenzae, Streptococcus pneumoniae,* or other bacteria.

Chronic meningococcemia is characterized by periodic bouts of fever, arthralgia or arthritis, and recurrent petechiae. Splenomegaly is often present. The patient may be free of symptoms between bouts. Chronic meningococcemia occurs primarily in adults and mimics Henoch-Schönlein purpura.

2. Meningitis–In many children, meningococcemia is followed within a few hours by symptoms and signs of acute purulent meningitis, with severe headache, stiff neck, nausea, vomiting, and stupor. Children with meningitis and meningococcemia generally fare better than children with meningococcemia alone.

B. Laboratory Findings: The peripheral white blood cell count may be either low or elevated. Thrombocytopenia may be present with or without disseminated intravascular coagulation (see Chapter 28). If petechial or hemorrhagic lesions are present, meningococci can sometimes be demonstrated on smear by puncturing the lesions and expressing a drop of tissue fluid. Organisms may be demonstrated by Gram's stain of buffy coat preparations of blood. The spinal fluid is generally cloudy and contains more than 1000 white cells per microliter, with many polymorphonuclear cells and gram-negative intracellular diplococci.

Meningococcal polysaccharide antigen of some types may be detected in body fluids, but the available tests are much less sensitive than tests for other bacterial antigens and therefore are not often useful.

A total hemolytic complement assay may reveal absence of late components as an underlying cause.

Differential Diagnosis

The lesions of meningococcemia may be mistaken for those seen in sepsis, infections due to *H influenzae* or pneumococci, enterovirus infection, endocarditis, leptospirosis, Rocky Mountain spotted fever, other rickettsial diseases, Henoch-Schönlein purpura, and blood dyscrasias. Other causes of sepsis and meningitis are distinguished by appropriate Gram's stain and cultures.

Complications

Meningitis may lead to permanent central nervous system damage, with deafness, convulsions, paralysis, or impairment of intellectual function. Hydrocephalus may develop and requires ventriculo-peritoneal shunt. Subdural collections of fluid are common but usually resolve spontaneously. Extensive skin necrosis, loss of digits or extremities, intestinal hemorrhage, and late adrenal insufficiency may complicate fulminant meningococcemia.

Prevention

Household contacts, day-care center contacts, and hospital personnel directly exposed to the respiratory secretions of patients are at increased risk of developing meningococcal infection and should be given chemoprophylaxis with rifampin. The secondary attack rate among household members is 1–5% during epidemics and less than 1% in nonepidemic situations. Children 3 months to 2 years of age are at the greatest risk, presumably because they lack protective antibodies. Secondary cases are reported in day-care centers, but school classroom outbreaks are rare. Hospital personnel are not at increased risk unless they have had contact with a patient's oral secretions, eg, during mouth-to-mouth resuscitation, intubation, or suctioning procedures. Approximately 50% of secondary cases in households have their onset within 24 hours of identification of the index case. Exposed children should be examined promptly. If they are febrile, they should be fully evaluated and treated with high doses of penicillin or another effective antimicrobial pending the results of blood cultures.

All intimate contacts should be given chemoprophylaxis with rifampin given orally in the following dosages twice daily for 2 days: 600 mg for adults, 10 mg/kg for children 1 month to 12 years of age, and 5 mg/kg for infants under 1 month of age. An alternate dosing schedule for rifampin, which is also effective chemoprophylaxis for *H influenzae* type b, is 20 mg/kg/d (maximum adult dose 600 mg/d) once daily for 4 days. If the organism is sensitive to sulfonamides, sulfadiazine may be used. Penicillin and most other antibiotics (even with parenteral administration) are not effective chemoprophylactic agents, since they do not eradicate upper respiratory tract carriage of meningococci. Cephalosporins such as ceftriaxone intramuscularly or cefixime orally are effective for prophylaxis. Ciprofloxacin has been used to eradicate nasopharyngeal carriage in adults but is not approved for use in children. In some situations, meningococcal polysaccharide vaccine should be given to contacts in addition to chemoprophylaxis. Throat cultures to identify carriers are not useful.

Treatment

Blood cultures should be obtained for all children with fever and purpura or other signs of meningococcemia, and antibiotics should be administered immediately as an emergency procedure. There is a good correlation between survival rates and initiation of prompt antibiotic therapy. Purpura and fever should be considered a medical emergency.

Children with meningococcemia or meningococcal meningitis should be managed as though shock were imminent even if their vital signs are stable when they are first seen. If hypotension already is present, supportive measures should be aggressive, because the prognosis is grave in such situations. It is optimal to initiate treatment in an intensive care setting. Treatment should not be delayed for the sake of transporting the patient. Shock may worsen following antimicrobial therapy due to endotoxin release. To minimize the risk of nosocomial transmission, patients should be treated in respiratory isolation for the first 24 hours of antibiotic treatment.

A. Specific Measures: Antibiotics should be begun promptly. Since other bacteria, especially *H influenzae,* can cause identical syndromes in young children, initial therapy should be effective against that organism until the diagnosis is made. Cefotaxime, ceftriaxone, or ampicillin and chloramphenicol are alternatives (see Chapter 34 for dosages). When the diagnosis is confirmed, penicillin G (250,000 units/kg/d in six doses) intravenously for seven days is the drug of choice.

B. General Measures:

1. Cardiovascular–See Chapter 14 for management of septic shock. Recent evidence suggests that corticosteroids are not beneficial. Sympathetic blockade has been used to improve limb perfusion. Topically applied nitroglycerin has been used locally to improve perfusion.

2. Hematologic–Since hypercoagulability is frequently present in patients with meningococcemia, administration of heparin should be considered for patients with disseminated intravascular coagulation. A loading dose of 100 units/kg is followed by 15 units/kg/h as a continuous drip for 48 hours. The patient is monitored by following the partial thromboplastin time. See Chapter 28 for the management of disseminated intravascular coagulation.

Prognosis

Unfavorable prognostic features include shock, disseminated intravascular coagulation, and extensive skin lesions. The case fatality rate in fulminant meningococcemia is very high—over 50%. In uncomplicated meningococcal meningitis, the fatality rate is much lower—generally 10–20%.

Algren JT et al: Predictors of outcome in acute meningococcal infection in children. Crit Care Med 1993;21:447.

Boyer D, Gordon RC, Baker T: Lack of clinical usefulness of a positive latex agglutination test for *Neisseria meningitidis/Escherichia coli* antigens in the urine. Pediatr Infect Dis J 1993;12:779.

Dashefsky B, Teele DW, Klein JO: Unsuspected meningococcemia. J Pediatr 1983;102:69.

Edwards MS, Baker CJ: Complications and sequelae of meningococcal infections in children. J Pediatr 1981; 99:540.

Griffiss JM et al: Immune response of infants and children to disseminated infections with *Neisseria meningitidis.* J Infect Dis 1984;150:71.

Leggiadro RJ, Winkelstein JA: Prevalence of complement deficiencies in children with systemic meningococcal infections. Pediatr Infect Dis J 1987;6:75.

Lennon D et al: Successful intervention in a group A meningococcal outbreak in Auckland, New Zealand. Pediatr Infect Dis J 1992;11:617.

Mayatepek E et al: Deafness, complement deficiencies and immunoglobulin status in patients with meningococcal diseases due to uncommon serogroups. Pediatr Infect Dis J 1993;12:808.

Nguyen QV, Nguyen EA, Weiner LB: Incidence of invasive bacterial disease in children with fever and petechiae. Pediatrics 1984;74:77.

Perez-Trallero E et al: Meningococci with increased resistance to penicillin. Lancet 1990;335:1096.

Pinner et al: Meningococcal disease in the U.S.—1986. J Infect Dis 1991;164:568.

Waage A, Halstensen A, Espevik T: Association between tumor necrosis factor in serum and fatal outcome in patients with meningococcal disease. Lancet 1987;1:355.

Wong VK et al: Meningococcal infections in children: A review of 100 cases. Pediatr Infect Dis J 1989;8:224.

GONOCOCCAL INFECTIONS

Essentials of Diagnosis

- Purulent urethral discharge showing intracellular gram-negative diplococci on smear in male patient (usually adolescent).
- Purulent, edematous, sometimes hemorrhagic conjunctivitis showing intracellular gram-negative diplococci on smear in infant 2–4 days of age.
- Fever, arthritis (often polyarticular) or tenosynovitis, and maculopapular peripheral rash that may be vesiculopustular or hemorrhagic.

- Positive culture of blood or pharyngeal or genital secretions.

General Considerations

Gonorrhea is the most commonly reported communicable disease. *Neisseria gonorrhoeae* is a gram-negative diplococcus. Although morphologically similar to other neisseriae, it differs in its ability to grow on selective media and to ferment only glucose. The cell wall of *N gonorrhoeae* contains endotoxin, which is liberated when the organism dies and is responsible for the production of a cellular exudate. The incubation period is short, usually 2–5 days.

Antimicrobial-resistant gonococci are now a serious problem. Nationally, 2% of *N gonorrhoeae* are highly resistant as a result of plasmid-encoded penicillinase; 1% are highly resistant as a result of plasmid-encoded resistance to tetracycline; and 16% have chromosomal resistance to penicillin, tetracycline, or cefoxitin.

Gonococcal disease in children may be transmitted sexually or nonsexually. Prepubertal girls usually manifest gonococcal vulvovaginitis because of the neutral-alkaline pH of the vagina and thin vaginal mucosa.

Prepubertal gonococcal infection outside the neonatal period should be considered presumptive evidence of sexual contact or child abuse. In the adolescent or adult, the workup of every case of gonorrhea should include a careful and accurate inquiry into sexual practices, since pharyngeal infection must be detected if present and may be difficult to eradicate. In addition, efforts should be made to identify and treat all sexual contacts. When prepubertal children are infected, all family members should be cultured, and epidemiologic investigation should be thorough.

Clinical Findings

A. Symptoms and Signs:

1. Asymptomatic gonorrhea–The ratio of asymptomatic to symptomatic gonorrheal infections in adolescents and adults is probably 3–4:1 in women and 0.5–1:1 in men. Asymptomatic infections are considered as infectious as symptomatic ones.

2. Uncomplicated genital gonorrhea–

a. Male with urethritis–Urethral discharge is sometimes painful and bloody and may be white, yellow, or green. There may be associated dysuria. The patient is usually afebrile.

b. Prepubertal female with vaginitis–The only clinical findings initially may be dysuria and polymorphonuclear neutrophils in the urine. Vulvitis characterized by erythema, edema, and excoriation accompanied by a purulent discharge may follow.

c. Postpubertal female with cervicitis–Symptomatic disease is characterized by a purulent discharge, dysuria, and, occasionally, dyspareunia. Lower abdominal pain is absent. Physical examination reveals an afebrile patient with a yellow, foul-smelling discharge. The cervix is frequently hyperemic and tender when touched by the examining finger. This tenderness is not worsened by moving the cervix, nor are the adnexa tender to palpation.

d. Rectal gonorrhea–Rectal gonorrhea is often asymptomatic. There may be purulent discharge, edema, and pain during evacuation.

3. Pharyngeal gonorrhea–Pharyngeal involvement is usually asymptomatic. There may be some sore throat and, rarely, acute exudative tonsillitis with bilateral cervical lymphadenopathy and fever.

4. Conjunctivitis and iridocyclitis–In the adolescent or adult eye, infection probably is spread from infected genital secretions by the fingers.

5. Pelvic inflammatory disease (salpingitis)–The interval between initiation of genital infection and its ascent to the uterine tubes is variable and may range from days to months, with menses frequently the initiating factor. With the onset of a menstrual period, gonococci invade the endometrium, causing transient endometritis. Subsequently, salpingitis may occur, resulting in pyosalpinx or hydrosalpinx; rarely, it leads to peritonitis or perihepatitis. Gonococcal salpingitis occurs in an acute, subacute, or chronic form. All three forms have in common tenderness on gentle movement of the cervix and bilateral tubal tenderness during pelvic examination.

Not all pelvic inflammatory disease is due to gonococci. In many instances, gonococci may be an initial cause of infection, but the predominant intrapelvic organisms may be enteric bacilli, *Bacteroides fragilis,* or other anaerobes. In other cases, *Chlamydia trachomatis* may be the triggering or sole cause. Nongonococcal salpingitis is sometimes seen in girls or women with intrauterine devices.

6. Gonococcal perihepatitis (Fitz-Hugh and Curtis syndrome)–In the typical clinical pattern, there is right upper quadrant tenderness in association with signs of acute or subacute salpingitis. Pain may be pleuritic and referred to the shoulder. Hepatic friction rub is a valuable but inconstant sign.

7. Disseminated gonorrhea–Dissemination follows asymptomatic more often than symptomatic genital infection and often results from gonococcal pharyngitis or anorectal gonorrhea. The most common form of disseminated gonorrhea is polyarthritis or polytenosynovitis, with or without dermatitis. Monarticular arthritis is less common, and gonococcal endocarditis and meningitis are fortunately rare.

a. Polyarthritis–Disease usually begins with the simultaneous onset of low-grade fever, polyarthralgia, and general malaise. After a day or so, the joint symptoms become acute, and swelling, redness, and tenderness occur, frequently over the wrists, ankles, and knees but also in the fingers, feet, and other peripheral joints. Skin lesions may be noted at the same time: individual, tender, evolving 5- to 8-mm maculopapular lesions that may become vesicular, pustular, and then hemorrhagic. They are noted on the fingers, palms, feet, and other distal surfaces and may be single or multiple. In patients with this form of the disease, blood cultures are often positive, but joint fluids rarely yield organisms. Skin lesions often are positive by Gram's stain but rarely by culture. Genital, rectal, and pharyngeal cultures must always be performed.

b. Monarticular arthritis–In this somewhat less common form of disseminated gonorrhea, fever is often absent. Arthritis evolves in a single joint. Dermatitis usually does not occur. Systemic symptoms are minimal. Blood cultures are negative, but joint aspirates may yield gonococci on smear and culture. Genital, rectal, and pharyngeal cultures must always be performed.

B. Laboratory Findings: Demonstration of gram-negative, kidney bean-shaped diplococci on smears of urethral exudate in males is presumptive evidence of gonorrhea. Positive culture confirms the diagnosis. Negative smears do not rule out gonorrhea. Gram-stained smears of cervical or vaginal discharge in girls are more difficult to interpret because of normal gram-negative flora, but they may be useful when technical personnel are experienced. In girls with suspected gonorrhea, both the cervical os and the anus should be cultured. Gonococcal pharyngitis requires culture for diagnosis.

Cultures for *N gonorrhoeae* are plated on a selective chocolate agar containing antibiotics (eg, Thayer-Martin agar) to suppress normal flora. If bacteriologic diagnosis is critical, suspected material should be cultured on chocolate agar as well. Since gonococci are labile, agar plates should be inoculated immediately and placed without delay in an atmosphere containing CO_2 (candle jar). When transportation is necessary, material should be directly inoculated into Transgrow medium prior to shipment to an appropriate laboratory. In cases of possible sexual molestation, notify the laboratory that definite speciation is needed, since nongonococcal *Neisseria* spp can grow on the selective media.

All children or adolescents with a suspected or established diagnosis of gonorrhea should have a serologic test for syphilis.

Differential Diagnosis

Urethritis in the male may be gonococcal or "nonspecific." The latter is a syndrome characterized by discharge (rarely painful), mild dysuria, and a subacute course. The discharge is usually scant or moderate in amount but may be profuse. The responsible microorganisms cannot all be identified, but about half of cases are due to *C trachomatis*. The remainder are probably due to *Ureaplasma,* trichomonads, or other as yet unknown agents. Most cases respond to tetracycline therapy (500 mg orally four times a day for 7 days in adolescents). *C trachomatis* has been shown to cause epididymitis in males and salpingitis in females.

Vulvovaginitis in a prepubertal female may be due to infection caused by miscellaneous bacteria, including *Shigella* sp and group A streptococci, *Candida,* and herpes simplex; discharges may be caused by trichomonads, *Enterobius vermicularis* (pinworm), or foreign bodies. Symptom-free discharge (leukorrhea) normally accompanies rising estrogen levels.

Cervicitis in a postpubertal female, alone or in association with urethritis and involvement of Skene's and Bartholin's glands, may be due to infection caused by *Candida,* herpes simplex, *Trichomonas,* or discharge resulting from inflammation caused by foreign bodies (usually some form of contraceptive device). Leukorrhea may be associated with birth control pills.

Salpingitis may be due to infection with other organisms. The symptoms must be differentiated from those of appendicitis, urinary tract infection, ectopic pregnancy, endometriosis, or ovarian cysts or torsion.

Disseminated gonorrhea presents a wide differential diagnosis that must include meningococcemia, acute rheumatic fever, Henoch-Schönlein purpura, juvenile rheumatoid arthritis, lupus erythematosus, leptospirosis, secondary syphilis, certain viral infections (particularly rubella, but also enteroviruses and parvovirus), serum sickness, type B hepatitis (in the prodromal phase), infective endocarditis, and even acute leukemia and other types of cancer. The fully evolved skin lesions of disseminated gonorrhea are remarkably specific, and genital, rectal, or pharyngeal cultures, plus cultures of blood and joint fluid, usually yield gonococci from at least one source.

Prevention

Prevention of gonorrhea is principally a problem of sex education and treatment of contacts.

Treatment

A. Uncomplicated Urethral, Endocervical, or Rectal Gonococcal Infections in Adolescents:

Due to increasing penicillin resistance, current recommended therapy is ceftriaxone (125 mg or 250 mg intramuscularly once) plus, for concurrent *Chlamydia trachomatis* infection, doxycycline (100 mg orally twice daily for 7 days). Erythromycin base (500 mg orally four times daily for 7 days) should be substituted for the doxycycline in pregnant patients. An alternative regimen is spectinomycin (2 g intramuscularly once) plus the same doxycycline regimen. Alternatives to ceftriaxone include cefixime 400 mg orally, ciprofloxacin 500 mg orally, or ofloxacin 400 mg orally, each given in one dose. Quinolone antibiotics should not be used in pregnant women or children. If the contact's infecting strain was proved susceptible to penicillin, the patient may be treated orally with amoxicillin, 50 mg/kg to a maximum of 3 g, and probenecid, 25 mg/kg to a maximum of 1 g, taken together as a single dose. A "test of cure" culture is not necessary after the ceftriaxone/doxycycline regimen; repeat screening in 1–2 months is preferable.

B. Pharyngeal Gonococcal Infection: Ceftri-
axone (125 mg or 250 mg intramuscularly once) should be used; ciprofloxacin (0.5 g orally once) is an alternative. Neither spectinomycin nor amoxicillin is recommended. A repeat culture is recommended 4–7 days after therapy.

C. Disseminated Gonorrhea: Recommended
regimens include ceftriaxone (1 g intramuscularly or intravenously once daily) or cefotaxime (1 g intravenously every 8 hours). Proved penicillin-sensitive organisms may be treated with ampicillin (1 g intravenously every 6 hours) or an equivalent penicillin regimen. Oral therapy may follow parenteral therapy after clinical resolution. Recommended regimens include cefixime (400 mg orally twice daily) or ciprofloxacin (0.5 g twice daily; not used for pregnant patients) to complete 7 days therapy. If concurrent infection with *Chlamydia* is present or has not been excluded, a course of doxycycline or erythromycin should also be prescribed.

Total duration of therapy is 7 days for disseminated infections.

D. Prepubertal Gonococcal Infections:

1. Uncomplicated genitourinary, rectal, or pharyngeal infections–These infections may be treated with ceftriaxone (25–50 mg/kg/d to a maximum of 125 mg intramuscularly once). Children over 8 years of age should also receive doxycycline (100 mg orally twice daily for 7 days). The physician should evaluate all children for evidence of sexual abuse and coinfection with syphilis and *Chlamydia.*

2. Disseminated gonorrhea–This should be treated with ceftriaxone (50 mg/kg once daily parenterally).

Alexander ER: Misidentification of sexually transmitted organisms in children: Medicolegal implications. Pediatr Infect Dis J 1988;7:1.

Sexually transmitted diseases: Treatment guidelines MMWR Morb Mortal Wkly Rep 1989;38(Suppl):8.

Gorwitz RJ et al: Sentinel surveillance for antimicrobial resistance in *Neisseria gonorrhoeae*–United States, 1988–1991. The Gonococcal Isolate Surveillance Project Study Group. MMWR Morb Mortal Wkly Rep 1993;42:29.

Hammerschlag MR et al: Efficacy of neonatal ocular prophylaxis for the prevention of chlamydial and gonococcal conjunctivitis. N Engl J Med 1989;320:769.

Handsfield HH et al: A comparison of single-dose cefixime with ceftriaxone as treatment for uncomplicated gonorrhea. N Engl J Med 1991;325:1337.

Ingram D et al: Sexual contact in children with gonorrhea. Am J Dis Child 1982;136:994.

Moran JS, Zenilman JM: Therapy for gonococcal infections: Options in 1989. Rev Infect Dis 1990;12(Suppl 6): S633.

Schwarcz SK et al: National surveillance of antimicrobial resistance in *Neisseria gonorrhoeae.* JAMA 1990;264: 1413.

Whittington WL et al: Incorrect identification of *Neisseria gonorrhoeae* from infants and children. Pediatr Infect Dis J 1988;7:3.

BOTULISM

Essentials of Diagnosis

- Dry mucous membranes.
- Nausea and vomiting.
- Diplopia; dilated, unreactive pupils.
- Descending paralysis.
- Difficulty in swallowing and speech occurring within 12–36 hours after ingestion of toxin contaminated home-canned food.
- Multiple cases in a family or group.
- Hypotonia and constipation in infants.
- Diagnosis by clinical findings and identification of toxin in blood, stool, or implicated food.

General Considerations

Botulism is a paralytic disease caused by *Clostridium botulinum,* an anaerobic, gram-positive, spore-forming bacillus normally found in soil. The organism produces an extremely potent neurotoxin. Of the seven types of toxin (A–G), types A, B, and E cause most human disease, and types C and D cause outbreaks of botulism in birds and mammals. The toxin, a polypeptide, is so potent that 0.1 μg is lethal for humans.

Food-borne botulism usually results from ingestion of toxin-containing food. Preformed toxin is absorbed from the gut and produces paralysis by preventing acetylcholine release from cholinergic fibers at myoneural junctions.

In the USA, home-canned vegetables are usually the cause. Commercially canned foods rarely are responsible. Virtually any food will support the growth of *C botulinum* spores into vegetative toxin-producing bacilli if an anaerobic, nonacid environment is provided. The food may not appear or taste spoiled. The toxin is heat-labile, but the spores are heat-resistant. Inadequate heating during processing (temperature < 115 °C) allows the spores to survive and later resume toxin production. Boiling of foods for 10 minutes or heating at 80 °C for 30 minutes before eating will destroy the toxin.

Infant botulism is seen in infants less than 6 months of age. It usually presents as constipation and severe hypotonia at a median age of 10 weeks. Uncommonly, infants less than 2 weeks of age develop botulism. The toxin appears to be produced by *C botulinum* organisms residing in the gastrointestinal tract. In some instances, honey has been the source of spores. Clinical findings include constipation, weak suck and cry, pooled oral secretions, cranial nerve deficits, generalized weakness, and, on occasion, sudden apnea. A characteristic electromyographic pattern termed "brief, small, abundant motor-unit action potentials" (BSAP) is observed.

Clinical Findings

A. Symptoms and Signs: The incubation period for food-borne botulism is 8–36 hours. Initially, there is lassitude or fatigue, generally with headache. This is followed by double vision, dilated pupils, ptosis, and, within a few hours, difficulty in swallowing and in speech. Pharyngeal paralysis occurs in some cases, and food may be regurgitated. The mucous membranes often are very dry. Descending skeletal muscle paralysis may be seen. The sensorium is clear, and the temperature normal. Death usually results from respiratory failure.

B. Laboratory Findings: Feces, vomitus, serum, and suspect food should be examined for the presence of toxin by injection into mice. The organism also may be cultured from feces or the suspect food. Laboratory findings, including cerebrospinal fluid examination, are usually normal. Electromyography (EMG) suggests the diagnosis if the characteristic abnormalities—small amplitude, brief polyphasic potentials with an incremental response to repeated stimuli—are seen.

A nondiagnostic EMG does not exclude the diagnosis and should be repeated.

Differential Diagnosis

Carbon monoxide poisoning causes unconsciousness without cranial nerve paralysis, and carboxyhemoglobin can be detected in blood. Guillain-Barré syndrome is characterized by ascending paralysis, sensory deficits, and elevated cerebrospinal fluid protein without pleocytosis.

Other illnesses that should be considered include poliomyelitis, postdiphtheritic polyneuritis, certain chemical intoxications, tick paralysis, and myasthenia gravis. The history and elevated cerebrospinal fluid protein characterize postdiphtheritic polyneuritis.

Poisoning with methyl alcohol, organic phosphorus compounds, methyl chloride, sodium fluoride, or atropine may have to be ruled out.

Tick paralysis is characterized by a flaccid ascending motor paralysis that begins in the legs. An attached tick should be sought.

Myasthenia gravis usually occurs in adolescent girls. It is characterized by ocular and bulbar symptoms, with normal pupils, fluctuating weakness, the absence of other neurologic signs, and clinical response to cholinesterase inhibitors.

Complications

Difficulty in swallowing leads to aspiration pneumonia. Serious respiratory paralysis may be fatal despite assisted ventilation and modern intensive supportive measures.

Treatment

A. Specific Measures: Equine botulism antitoxin is of probable value in the treatment of botulism. Trivalent antitoxin (types A, B, and E) should be given intramuscularly as soon as the diagnosis is made after skin testing for horse serum sensitivity. The antitoxin, 24-hour diagnostic consultation, epidemic assistance, and laboratory testing services are available from the Centers for Disease Control. Botulism immune globulin is available from the Massachusetts Public Health Biologic Laboratory (510-540-2646). A clinical trial is under way to evaluate this product. Guanidine hydrochloride, 15–35 mg/kg/d orally in three doses, may reverse the neuromuscular block, but its efficacy is questionable.

B. General Measures: General and supportive therapy consists of bed rest, ventilatory support (if necessary), fluid therapy, and administration of purgatives and high enemas. In cases of infant botulism, some authorities recommend penicillin to eliminate organisms continuing to produce toxin within the gastrointestinal tract. Aminoglycoside antimicrobials may exacerbate neuromuscular blockage and should be avoided.

Prognosis

The mortality rate is about 25% and is lower in children than adults. In nonfatal cases, symptoms subside over 2–3 months and recovery is eventually complete. The availability of antitoxin and modern respiratory support affects the prognosis.

Dowell VR Jr: Botulism and tetanus: Selected epidemiologic and microbiologic aspects. Rev Infect Dis 1984; 6(Suppl 1):S202.

Graf WD et al: Electrodiagnosis reliability in the diagnosis of infant botulism. J Pediatr 1992;120:747.

Mills DC, Arnon SS: The large intestine as the site of *Clostridium botulinum* colonization in human infant botulism. J Infect Dis 1987;156:997.

Schreiner MS et al: Infant botulism: A review of 12 years experience at the Children's Hospital of Philadelphia. Pediatrics 1991;87:159.

Schwartz PJ, Arnon SS: Botulism immune globulin for infant botulism arrives: One year and a Gulf war later. West J Med 1992;156:197.

Thilo EH, Townsend SF: Infant botulism at 1 week of age: Report of two cases. Pediatrics 1993;92:151.

Wainwright RB et al: Food-borne botulism in Alaska, 1947–1985: Epidemiology and clinical findings. J Infect Dis 1988;157:158.

Wilcox P et al: Long-term follow-up of symptoms, pulmonary function, respiratory muscle strength, and exercise performance after botulism. Am Rev Respir Dis 1989; 139:157.

TETANUS

Essentials of Diagnosis

- Unimmunized or partially immunized patient.
- History of skin wound.
- Spasms of jaw muscles (trismus).
- Stiffness of neck, back, and abdominal muscles, with hyperirritability and hyperreflexia.
- Episodic, generalized muscle contractions.
- Diagnosis is based on clinical findings and the immunization history.

General Considerations

Tetanus is caused by *Clostridium tetani,* an anaerobic, gram-positive bacillus that produces a potent neurotoxin. In unimmunized or incompletely immunized individuals, infection follows contamination of a wound by soil containing clostridial spores from animal manure. The toxin reaches the central nervous system by retrograde axon transport, is bound to cerebral gangliosides, and is thought to increase reflex excitability in neurons of the spinal cord by blocking function of inhibitory synapses. Intense muscle spasms result. Two-thirds of cases in the USA follow minor puncture wounds of the hands or feet. In many cases, no history of a wound can be obtained. In the newborn, infection usually results from contamination of the umbilical cord. The incubation period typically is 4–14 days but may be longer.

There are an estimated 500,000 deaths yearly from tetanus worldwide. The World Health Organization estimates that about 1% of newborns in developing countries die of tetanus.

Clinical Findings

A. Symptoms and Signs: In children and adults, the first symptom is often minimal pain at the site of inoculation, followed by hypertonicity and spasm of the regional muscles. Characteristically, difficulty in opening the mouth (trismus) is evident within 48 hours. In newborns, the first signs are irritability and inability to suck at the breast. The disease may then progress to stiffness of the jaw and neck, increasing dysphagia, and generalized hyperreflexia with extreme rigidity and spasms of all muscles of the abdomen and back (opisthotonos). The facial distortion resembles a grimace (risus sardonicus). Difficulty in swallowing and convulsions triggered by minimal stimuli such as sound, light, or movement may occur. Individual spasms may last seconds or minutes. Recurrent spasms are seen several times each hour, or they may be almost continuous. In most cases, the temperature is normal or only mildly elevated. A high or subnormal temperature is a bad prognostic sign. Patients are fully conscious and lucid. A profound circulatory disturbance associated with sympathetic overactivity may occur on the second to fourth day, which may contribute to the mortality rate. This is characterized by elevated blood pressure, increased cardiac output, tachycardia (> 120 beats/min), and dysrhythmia.

B. Laboratory Findings: The diagnosis is made on clinical grounds. There may be a mild polymorphonuclear leukocytosis. The cerebrospinal fluid is normal with the exception of some elevation of pressure. Serum muscle enzymes may be elevated. Transient electrocardiographic and electroencephalographic abnormalities may occur. Anaerobic culture and microscopic examination of pus from the wound can be helpful, but *C tetani* is difficult to grow, and the drumstick-shaped gram-positive bacilli often cannot be found.

Differential Diagnosis

In areas where tetanus is rarely seen, physicians may not recognize the infection until classic findings are present. Poliomyelitis is characterized by asymmetric paralysis in an incompletely immunized child. The history of an animal bite, absence of trismus, and pleocytosis suggest rabies. Local infections of the throat and jaw should be easily recognized. In strychnine poisoning, spasms of the jaw muscles are not common, and periods of complete relaxation between spasms are more obvious. Bacterial meningitis, phenothiazine reactions, decerebrate posturing, narcotic withdrawal, spondylitis, and hypocalcemic tetany may be confused with tetanus.

Complications

Complications include sepsis, malnutrition, pneumonia, atelectasis, asphyxial spasms, decubitus ulcers, and fractures of the spine due to intense contractions. They can be prevented in part by skilled supportive care.

Prevention

A. Tetanus Toxoid: Active immunization with tetanus toxoid is the cornerstone of prevention of tetanus (see Chapter 10) and almost always is achieved after the third dose of vaccine. A booster at the time of injury is needed if none has been given in the past 10 years—or within 5 years in case of a heavily contaminated wound. Nearly all cases of tetanus (99%) in the USA are in unimmunized or incompletely immunized individuals.

B. Tetanus Antitoxin: Human tetanus immune globulin (TIG) should be used in nonimmunized individuals with soil-contaminated wounds. For children who have had no or one tetanus toxoid immunization, 250–500 units should be given intramuscularly. Tetanus toxoid and TIG should be administered concurrently at different sites using different syringes.

C. Treatment of Wounds: Proper surgical cleansing and debridement of contaminated wounds will decrease the risk of tetanus.

D. Prophylactic Antimicrobials: Prophylactic antimicrobials are useful if the child is unimmunized and TIG is not available.

Treatment

A. Specific Measures: Serotherapy lowers the mortality rate from tetanus, but not dramatically. TIG, 500 units intramuscularly for newborns and 3000–6000 units intramuscularly for children and adults, is preferred to horse serum. Surgical debridement of wounds is indicated, but more extensive surgery or amputation to eliminate the site of infection is not necessary. Penicillin G is given in a dosage of 150,000 units/kg/d intravenously for 10–14 days.

Cephalosporins may be substituted in penicillin-sensitive children.

B. General Measures: The patient is kept in a quiet room with minimal stimulation. Control of spasms and prevention of hypoxic episodes are crucial. Diazepam is useful (0.6–1.2 mg/kg/d intravenously in six divided doses). In the newborn, two or three divided doses should be given. Large doses (up to 25 mg/kg/d) may be required for older children. Diazepam is given intravenously until muscular spasms become infrequent and the generalized muscular rigidity much less prominent. The drug may then be given orally and the dose reduced as the child improves. Barbiturates, chlorpromazine, and paraldehyde may also be useful.

Mechanical ventilation and muscle paralysis are necessary in severe cases.

Prognosis

The fatality rate in newborns and heroin addicts is high (70–90%). The overall mortality rate in the USA is 65%. In a recent series of 44 neonates treated in Mexico City, the mortality rate was 25%. The fatality rate depends primarily on the quality of supportive care. Many deaths are due to pneumonia or respiratory failure. If the patient survives 1 week, recovery is likely.

Bleck TP: Tetanus: Pathophysiology, management and prophylaxis. Dis Mon (Sept) 1991;37:545.

Bowen V et al: Tetanus: A continuing problem in minor injuries. Can J Surg 1988;31:7.

Simental PS et al: Neonatal tetanus experience at the National Institute of Pediatrics in Mexico City. Pediatr Infect Dis J 1993;12:722.

Stanfield JP, Galazka A: Neonatal tetanus in the world today. Bull WHO 1984;62:647.

Sutton DN: Management of autonomic dysfunction in severe tetanus: The use of magnesium sulphate and clonidine. Intensive Care Med 1990;16:75.

GAS GANGRENE

Essentials of Diagnosis

- Contamination of a wound with soil or feces.
- Massive edema, skin discoloration, bleb formation, and pain in an area of trauma.
- Serosanguineous exudate from wound.
- Crepitation of subcutaneous tissue.
- Rapid progression of signs and symptoms.
- Clostridia cultured or seen on stained smears.

General Considerations

Gas gangrene (clostridial myonecrosis) is a necrotizing infection that follows trauma or surgery and is caused by several anaerobic, gram-positive, spore-forming bacilli of the genus *Clostridium*. These are soil, genital tract (female), and fecal organisms. In devitalized tissue, the spores germinate into vegetative bacilli that proliferate and produce toxins causing thrombosis, hemolysis, and tissue necrosis. *Clostridium perfringens,* the species causing approximately 80% of cases of gas gangrene, produces at least 8 such toxins. The areas involved most often are the extremities, abdomen, and uterus. *Clostridium septicum* may also cause myonecrosis and causes septicemia in patients with neutropenia. Nonclostridial infections with gas formation can mimic clostridial infections and are more common.

Clinical Findings

A. Symptoms and Signs: The onset is sudden, usually 1–20 days (mean 3–4 days) after trauma or surgery. The skin around the wound becomes discolored, with hemorrhagic bullae, serosanguineous exudate, and crepitation in the subcutaneous tissues. Pain and swelling are usually intense. Systemic illness appears early and progresses rapidly to intravascular hemolysis, jaundice, shock, toxic delirium, and renal failure.

B. Laboratory Findings: Isolation of the organism requires anaerobic culture. Gram-stained smears may demonstrate many gram-positive rods and few inflammatory cells.

C. Imaging: X-ray films may demonstrate gas in tissues, but this is a late finding and is also seen in infections with other gas-forming organisms or may be due to air introduced into tissues during trauma or surgery.

D. Surgical Findings: Direct visualization of the muscle at surgery may be necessary to diagnose gas gangrene. Early, the muscle is pale and edematous and does not contract normally; later, the muscle may be frankly gangrenous.

Differential Diagnosis

Gangrene and cellulitis caused by other organisms and clostridial cellulitis (not myonecrosis) must be distinguished. Necrotizing fasciitis may resemble gas gangrene.

Prevention

Gas gangrene can be prevented by the adequate cleansing and debridement of all wounds. It is essential that foreign bodies and dead tissue be removed. A clean wound does not provide a suitable anaerobic environment for the growth of clostridial species.

Treatment

A. Specific Measures: Penicillin G (300,000–400,000 units/kg/d intravenously in six divided doses) should be given.

B. Surgical Measures: Surgery should be prompt and extensive, with removal of all necrotic tissue.

C. Hyperbaric Oxygen: Hyperbaric oxygen therapy has been shown to be effective, but it is not a substitute for surgery. A patient may be exposed to 2–3 atm in pure oxygen for 1- to 2-hour periods for as many sessions as necessary until there is clinical remission.

Prognosis

Clostridial myonecrosis is fatal if untreated. With early diagnosis, antibiotics, and surgery, the mortality rate is about 20–60%. Involvement of the abdominal wall, leukopenia, intravascular hemolysis, renal failure, and shock are ominous prognostic findings.

Bessman AN, Wagner W: Nonclostridial gas gangrene: Report of 48 cases and review of the literature. *Clostridium septicum* JAMA 1975;233:958.

Bratton SL et al: Clostridium septicum infections in children. Pediatr Infect Dis J 1992;11:569.

Hart GB et al: Gas gangrene. J Trauma 1983;23:991.

Rudge FW: The role of hyperbaric oxygen in the treatment of clostridial myonecrosis. Mil Med 1993;158:80.

Stevens DL et al: Comparison of clindamycin, rifampin, tetracycline, metronidazole, and penicillin for efficacy in prevention of experimental gas gangrene due to *Clostridium perfringens.* J Infect Dis 1987;155:220.

DIPHTHERIA

Essentials of Diagnosis

- A gray, adherent pseudomembrane, most often in the pharynx but also in the nasopharynx or trachea.
- Sore throat, serosanguineous nasal discharge, hoarseness, and fever in a nonimmunized child.
- Peripheral neuritis or myocarditis.
- Positive culture.
- Treatment should *not* be withheld pending culture results.

General Considerations

Diphtheria is an acute infection of the upper respiratory tract or skin caused by toxin-producing *Corynebacterium diphtheriae.* Five or fewer cases per year are reported in the USA, but significant numbers of elderly adults and unimmunized children are susceptible to infection. Corynebacteria are gram-positive club-shaped rods with a beaded appearance on Gram's stain.

The capacity to produce exotoxin is conferred by a lysogenic bacteriophage and is not present in all strains of *C diphtheriae.* In immunized communities, infection probably occurs through spread of the phage among carriers of susceptible bacteria rather than through spread of phage-containing bacteria themselves. Diphtheria toxin kills susceptible cells by irreversible inhibition of protein synthesis.

The toxin is absorbed into the mucous membranes and causes destruction of epithelium and a superficial inflammatory response. The necrotic epithelium becomes embedded in exuding fibrin and red and white cells, forming a grayish "pseudomembrane" commonly present over the tonsils, pharynx, or larynx.

Any attempt to remove the membrane exposes and tears the capillaries, resulting in bleeding. The diphtheria bacilli within the membrane continue to produce toxin, which is absorbed and may result in toxic injury to heart muscle, liver, kidneys, and adrenals, and is sometimes accompanied by hemorrhage. The toxin also produces neuritis, resulting in paralysis of the soft palate, eye muscles, or extremities. Death may occur as a result of respiratory obstruction or acute toxemia and circulatory collapse. The patient may succumb after a somewhat longer time as a result of cardiac damage. The incubation period is 1–6 days.

Clinical Findings

A. Symptoms and Signs:

1. Pharyngeal diphtheria–Early manifestations of diphtheritic pharyngitis are mild sore throat, moderate fever, and malaise, followed fairly rapidly by severe prostration and circulatory collapse. The pulse is more rapid than the fever would seem to justify. A pharyngeal membrane forms and may spread into the nasopharynx or the trachea, producing respiratory obstruction. The membrane is tenacious and gray and is surrounded by a narrow zone of erythema and a broader zone of edema. The cervical lymph nodes become swollen, and swelling is associated with brawny edema of the neck ("bull neck"). Laryngeal diphtheria presents with stridor, which can lead to obstruction of the airway.

2. Other forms–Cutaneous, vaginal diphtheria and wound diphtheria currently account for as many as 33% of cases and are characterized by ulcerative lesions with membrane formation.

B. Laboratory Findings:
Diagnosis is clinical. Direct smears are unreliable. Material is first obtained from the nose, throat, or skin lesions, if present, for culture on Loeffler's and tellurite agar. Sixteen to 48 hours are required before identification of the organism is possible. A toxigenicity test is then performed. Cultures may be negative in individuals who have received antibiotics. The white blood cell count is usually normal, but hemolytic anemia and thrombocytopenia are frequent. The red blood cell count may show evidence of rapid destruction of erythrocytes. Thrombocytopenia due to peripheral destruction is frequent.

Differential Diagnosis

Pharyngeal diphtheria resembles acute streptococcal pharyngitis, mononucleosis, and occasionally, other viral pharyngitis. Nasal diphtheria may be mimicked by a foreign body or purulent sinusitis. Other causes of laryngeal obstruction are epiglottitis and viral croup. Neuropathy may be a manifestation of Guillain-Barré syndrome, poliomyelitis, or acute poisoning.

Complications

A. Myocarditis: Diphtheritic myocarditis is characterized by a rapid, thready pulse; indistinct heart sounds, ST–T wave changes, conduction abnormalities, dysrhythmias, or cardiac failure; hepatomegaly; and fluid retention. Myocardial dysfunction may occur from 2 to 40 days after the onset of pharyngitis.

B. Polyneuritis: Neuritis of the nerves innervating the palate and pharyngeal muscles occurs during the first or second week. Nasal speech and regurgitation of food through the nose are seen. Diplopia and strabismus occur during the third week or later. Neuritis may also involve peripheral motor nerves supplying the intercostal muscles and diaphragm and other muscle groups. Generalized paresis usually occurs after the fourth week.

C. Bronchopneumonia: Secondary pneumonia is common in fatal cases.

Prevention

A. Immunization: Immunization with diphtheria toxoid combined with pertussis and tetanus toxoids (DTP) should be used routinely for infants and children (see Chapter 10).

B. Care of Exposed Susceptibles: Children exposed to diphtheria should be examined, and nose and throat cultures obtained. If signs and symptoms of early diphtheria are found, treatment should be as for diphtheria. Immunized asymptomatic individuals should receive diphtheria toxoid if a booster has not been received within 5 years. Unimmunized close contacts should receive either erythromycin orally (40 mg/kg/d in four divided doses) for 7 days or benzathine penicillin G intramuscularly (25,000 units/kg), active immunization with diphtheria toxoid and be observed daily.

Treatment

A. Specific Measures:

1. Antitoxin–Diphtheria antitoxin should be administered within 48 hours to be effective (see Chapter 10).

2. Antibiotics–Penicillin G (150,000 units/kg/d intravenously) should be given for 10 days. For the patient allergic to penicillin, erythromycin, 40 mg/kg/d, is given orally for 10 days.

B. General Measures:
Bed rest in the hospital for 10–14 days is usually required. All patients must be strictly isolated for 1–7 days until respiratory secretions are noncontagious. Isolation may be discontinued when 3 successive nose and throat cultures at 24-hour intervals are negative. These cultures should not be taken until at least 24 hours have elapsed since the cessation of antibiotic treatment.

C. Treatment of Carriers:
All carriers should be treated. Erythromycin (40 mg/kg/d orally in three or four divided doses), penicillin V potassium (50 mg/kg/d for 10 days), or benzathine penicillin G

(600,000–1,200,000 units intramuscularly) should be given. All carriers must be confined at home. Before they can be released, carriers must have three negative cultures of both the nose and the throat taken 24 hours apart and obtained at least 24 hours after the cessation of antibiotic therapy.

Prognosis

Mortality rates vary from 3% to 25% and are particularly high in the presence of early myocarditis. Neuritis is reversible; it is fatal only if an intact airway and adequate respiration cannot be maintained. Permanent damage due to myocarditis occurs rarely.

Chen RT et al: Diphtheria in the United States, 1971–1981. Am J Pub Health 1985;75:1393.

English PC: Diphtheria and theories of infectious disease: Centennial appreciation of the critical role of diphtheria in the history of medicine. Pediatrics 1985;76:1.

Pappenheimer AM Jr, Murphy JR: Studies on the molecular epidemiology of diphtheria. Lancet 1983;2:923.

Thisyakorn USA, Wongvanich J, Kumpeng V: Failure of corticosteroid therapy to prevent diphtheritic myocarditis or neuritis. Pediatr Infect Dis J 1984;3:126.

INFECTIONS DUE TO ENTEROBACTERIACEAE

Essentials of Diagnosis

- Diarrhea by several different mechanisms due to *Escherichia coli.*
- Neonatal sepsis or meningitis.
- Urinary tract infection.
- Opportunistic infections.
- Diagnosis confirmed by culture.

General Considerations

Enterobacteriaceae are a family of gram-negative bacilli that are part of the normal flora of the gastrointestinal tract and are also found in water and soil. They cause gastroenteritis, urinary tract infections, neonatal sepsis and meningitis, opportunistic infections, and, occasionally, other infections. *Escherichia coli* is the organism in this family that most commonly causes infection in children, but *Klebsiella, Morganella, Enterobacter, Serratia, Proteus,* and other genera are also important, particularly in the compromised host. *Shigella* and *Salmonella* are discussed in separate sections.

E coli strains capable of causing diarrhea were originally termed enteropathogenic and were recognized by serotype. It is now known that *E coli* may cause diarrhea by several distinct mechanisms. The mechanisms responsible for diarrhea in the originally described EPEC strains are not known. Enterotoxigenic *E coli* cause a secretory, watery diarrhea. ETEC adhere to enterocytes and secrete one or more plasmid-encoded enterotoxins. One of these toxins resembles cholera toxin in structure, function, and mechanism of action. Enteroinvasive *E coli* are very similar to *Shigella* in pathogenetic mechanism. Enterohemorrhagic *E coli* (EHEC) are the cause of hemorrhagic colitis and the hemolytic uremic syndrome. The most common enterohemorrhagic serotype is O157:H7, though several other serotypes cause the same syndrome. These strains elaborate a toxin, closely related to Shiga toxin produced by *S dysenteriae,* and termed verotoxin or Shiga-like toxin. Several outbreaks of hemolytic uremic syndrome associated with EHEC have followed consumption of inadequately cooked ground beef. Thorough heating to 68–71 °C is necessary.

Eighty percent of *E coli* strains causing neonatal meningitis possess specific capsular polysaccharide (K1 antigen), which, alone or in association with specific somatic antigens, confers virulence. K1 antigen is also present on approximately 40% of strains causing neonatal septicemia. The *E coli* K1 organisms do not appear to cause gastrointestinal disease.

Approximately 90% of urinary tract infections in children are caused by *E coli. E coli* bind to the uroepithelium by P-fimbria, which are present in greater than 90% of *E coli* that cause pyelonephritis. Other bacterial cell-surface structures, such as O and K antigens, and host factors are also important in the pathogenesis of urinary tract infections.

Klebsiella, Enterobacter, Serratia, and *Morganella* are normally found in the gastrointestinal tract and in soil and water. *Klebsiella* may cause a bronchopneumonia with cavity formation. *Klebsiella, Enterobacter,* and *Serratia* are often opportunists associated with antibiotic usage, debilitating states, and chronic respiratory conditions. They frequently cause urinary tract infection or sepsis. In many newborn nurseries, nosocomial outbreaks caused by aminoglycoside-resistant *Klebsiella pneumoniae* are a major problem.

Many of these infections are difficult to treat because of antibiotic resistance. Antibiotic susceptibility tests are necessary. Parenteral third-generation cephalosporins are usually more active than ampicillin, but resistance due to high level production of chromosomal cephalosporinase may occur. Aminoglycoside antibiotics (gentamicin, tobramycin, amikacin) are usually effective but require monitoring of serum levels to assure therapeutic, non-toxic levels.

Clinical Findings

A. Symptoms and Signs:

1. *E coli* gastroenteritis–*E coli* may cause diarrhea of varying type and severity. Enterotoxigenic *E coli* usually produce mild, self-limiting illness without significant fever or systemic toxicity, often known as traveler's diarrhea. However, diarrhea may be severe in newborns and infants, and occasionally an older child or adult will have a cholera-like syndrome. Enteroinvasive strains cause a shigellosis-like illness characterized by fever, systemic symptoms, blood and mucus in the stool, and leukocytosis, but currently are uncommon in the USA. Enterohemorrhagic strains cause hemorrhagic colitis. Diarrhea is initially watery, and fever is usually absent. Abdominal pain and cramping occur, and diarrhea progresses to blood streaking or grossly bloody stools. Hemolytic uremic syndrome occurs within a few days of diarrhea in 2–5% of children and is characterized by microangiopathic hemolytic anemia, thrombocytopenia, and renal failure (Chapter 24).

E coli are transmitted from person to person and in food and water. Undercooked meat may transmit enterohemorrhagic *E coli*.

2. Neonatal sepsis–Findings include jaundice, hepatosplenomegaly, fever, temperature lability, apneic spells, irritability, and failure to suck vigorously. Meningitis is associated with sepsis in 25–40% of cases. Other metastatic foci of infection may be present, including pneumonia and pyelonephritis. Sepsis may lead to severe metabolic acidosis, shock, disseminated intravascular coagulation, and death.

3. Neonatal meningitis–Findings include high fever, full fontanelles, vomiting, coma, convulsions, pareses or paralyses, poor or absent Moro reflex, opisthotonos, and, occasionally, hyper- or hypotonia. Sepsis coexists or precedes meningitis in most cases. Thus, signs of sepsis often accompany those of meningitis. Cerebrospinal fluid usually shows a cell count of over 1000/µL, mostly polymorphonuclear neutrophils, and bacteria on Gram's stain. Cerebrospinal fluid glucose concentration is low (usually less than half that of blood), and the protein is elevated above the levels normally seen in newborns and premature infants (> 150 mg/dL).

4. Acute urinary tract infection–Symptoms include dysuria, increased urinary frequency, and fever in the older child. Nonspecific symptoms such as anorexia, vomiting, irritability, failure to thrive, and unexplained fever are seen in children under 2 years of age. Young infants may present with jaundice. As many as 1% of girls of school age and 0.05% of boys have asymptomatic bacteriuria.

B. Laboratory Findings: Because *E coli* are normal flora in the stool, a positive stool culture alone does not prove that the *E coli* in the stool are causing disease. Serotyping, tests for enterotoxin production or invasiveness, and tests for P-fimbria are performed in research laboratories, but these tests are not available in most laboratories. MacConkey's agar with sorbitol substituted for lactose (SMAC agar) is useful to screen stool for enterohemorrhagic *E coli*. Serotyping and testing for enterotoxin are available at many state health departments. Blood cultures are positive in neonatal sepsis. Cultures of cerebrospinal fluid and urine should also be obtained. The diagnosis of urinary tract infections is discussed in Chapter 24.

Differential Diagnosis

The clinical picture of enteropathogenic *E coli* infection may resemble that of salmonellosis, shigellosis, or viral gastroenteritis.

Neonatal sepsis and meningitis caused by *E coli* can be differentiated from other causes of neonatal infection only by blood and cerebrospinal fluid culture.

Treatment

A. Specific Measures:

1. *E coli* gastroenteritis–Gastroenteritis due to enteropathogenic *E coli* seldom requires antimicrobial treatment. Fluid and electrolyte therapy ,preferably given orally, may be required to avoid dehydration. Bismuth subsalicylate reduces stool volume by about one-third in infants with watery diarrhea probably including toxigenic *E coli*. In nursery outbreaks, infants have been treated with neomycin (100/mg/kg/d orally in three divided doses for 5 days) or colistin (10–15 mg/kg/d orally in three divided doses for 5 days). Clinical efficacy is not established. Trimethoprim-sulfamethoxazole may be used in older children. It is not clear whether the risk of hemolytic uremic syndrome increases or decreases following treatment of enterohemorrhagic colitis, but many experts withhold antimicrobials in this setting.

2. *E coli* sepsis, pneumonia, or pyelonephritis–The drugs of choice are ampicillin (150–200 mg/kg/d intravenously or intramuscularly in divided doses every 4–6 hours), cefotaxime (150–200 mg/kg/d intravenously or intramuscularly in divided doses every 6–8 hours), ceftriaxone (50–100 mg/kg/d intramuscularly as single dose or in two divided doses), or gentamicin (5–7.5 mg/kg/d intramuscularly or intravenously in divided doses every 8 hours). Treatment is for 10–14 days. Amikacin or tobramycin may be used instead of gentamicin if the strain is susceptible. Third-generation cephalosporins are often an attractive alternative as single-drug therapy and do not require monitoring for toxicity.

3. *E coli* meningitis–Third-generation cephalosporins such as cefotaxime (200 mg/kg/d intravenously in four divided doses) are given for a minimum of 3 weeks. Ampicillin (200–300 mg/kg/d intravenously in four to six divided doses) and gentamicin (5–7.5 mg/kg/d intramuscularly or intravenously in three divided doses) are also effective. Treatment with intrathecal and intraventricular aminoglycosides does not improve outcome. Newborns treated with aminoglycosides or chloramphenicol must have serum levels monitored.

4. Acute urinary tract infection–See Chapter 24.

Prognosis

Death due to gastroenteritis can be prevented by early fluid and electrolyte therapy. Neonatal sepsis with meningitis is still associated with a mortality rate of over 50%. Most children with recurrent urinary tract infections do well if they have no serious underlying anatomic defects. The mortality rate in opportunistic infections usually depends on the severity of infection and the underlying condition.

Belongia EA et al: An outbreak of *Escherichia coli* O157:H7 colitis associated with consumption of pre-cooked meat patties. J Infect Dis 1991;164:338.

Bonadio WA et al: *Escherichia coli* bacteremia in children: A review of 91 cases in 10 years. Am J Dis Child 1991; 145:671.

Cohen MB, Giannella RA: Hemorrhagic colitis associated with *Escherichia coli* O157:H7. Adv Intern Med 1992; 37:173.

Durbin WA, Peter G: Management of urinary tract infections in infants and children. Pediatr Infect Dis 1984;3: 564.

Ericsson CD, DuPont HL: Travelers' diarrhea: Approaches to prevention and treatment. Clin Infect Dis 1993;16:616.

Figueroa-Quintanilla D et al: A controlled trial of bismuth subsalicylate in infants with acute watery diarrheal disease. N Engl J Med 1993;328:1654.

Gallagher PG: *Enterobacter* bacteremia in pediatric patients. Rev Infect Dis 1990;12:808.

Levine MM: *Escherichia coli* that cause diarrhea: Enterotoxigenic, enteropathogenic, enteroinvasive, enterohemorrhagic, and enteroadherent. J Infect Dis 1987;155:377.

MacDonald KL et al: *Escherichia coli* O157:H7, an emerging gastrointestinal pathogen. JAMA 1988;259:3567.

Martin DL et al: The epidemiological and clinical aspects of the hemolytic uremic syndrome in Minnesota. N Engl J Med 1991;323:1161.

Siitonen A et al: Invasive *Escherichia coli* infections in children: bacterial characteristics in different age groups and clinical entities. Pediatr Infect Dis J 1993;12:606.

Stull TL: Epidemiology and natural history of urinary tract infections in children. Med Clin North Am 1991;75:287.

PSEUDOMONAS INFECTIONS

Essentials of Diagnosis

- Opportunistic infection.
- Confirmed by cultures.

General Considerations

Pseudomonas aeruginosa is an important cause of infection in children with cystic fibrosis, neoplastic disease, neutropenia, or extensive burns and in those receiving antibiotic therapy. Infections of the urinary and respiratory tracts, ears, mastoids, paranasal sinuses, eyes, skin, meninges, and bones are seen. *Pseudomonas* pneumonia is a common nosocomial infection in patients receiving assisted ventilation. *P aeruginosa* sepsis may be accompanied by characteristic peripheral lesions called ecthyma gangrenosum. *P aeruginosa* is an infrequent cause of sepsis in previously healthy infants, and may be the initial sign of underlying medical problems. *P aeruginosa* osteomyelitis sometimes complicates puncture wounds of the feet. *P aeruginosa* is a frequent cause of malignant external otitis media and of chronic suppurative otitis media. Outbreaks of vesiculopustular skin rash have been associated with exposure to contaminated water in whirlpool baths and hot tubs.

P aeruginosa is an aerobic gram-negative rod with versatile metabolic requirements. *P aeruginosa* may grow in distilled water and in commonly used disinfectants, complicating the problem of infection control. *P aeruginosa* is both invasive and destructive to tissue, and toxigenic due to secreted exotoxins, which contribute to virulence. Other *Pseudomonas* species occasionally cause nosocomial infections. *Xanthomonas maltophilia* (previously *P maltophilia*) and *Birkholderhea cepacia* (previously P cepacia) are the most frequent.

P aeruginosa infects the tracheobronchial tree of nearly all patients with cystic fibrosis. Mucoid exopolysaccharide, an exuberant capsule, is characteristically overproduced by isolates from patients with cystic fibrosis. Although bacteremia seldom occurs, patients with cystic fibrosis ultimately succumb to chronic lung infection with *P aeruginosa*. Infection due to *B cepacia* has caused a rapidly progressive pulmonary disease in some colonized patients and may be spread by close personal contact.

Clinical Findings

The clinical findings depend on the site of infection and the patient's underlying disease. Sepsis with these organisms resembles gram-negative sepsis with other organisms, though the presence of ecythema gangrenosa suggests the diagnosis. The diagnosis is made by culture. *Pseudomonas* infection should be suspected in neonates and neutropenic patients with clinical sepsis.

A severe necrotizing pneumonia occurs in patients on ventilators.

Patients with cystic fibrosis have a persistent bronchitis which progresses to bronchiectasis and ultimately to respiratory failure. During exacerbations of illness, cough and sputum production increase with low grade fever, malaise, and diminished energy.

The purulent aural drainage without fever in patients with chronic suppurative otitis media is not distinguishable from that due to other cause.

Prevention

A. Infections in Debilitated Patients: Colonization of extensive second- and third-degree burns by *P aeruginosa* can lead to fatal septicemia. Aggressive debridement and topical treatment with 0.5% silver nitrate solution, 10% mafenide cream, or gentamicin ointment will greatly inhibit *P aeruginosa* contamination of burns. (See Chapter 14 for a discussion of burn wound infections and prevention.)

B. Nosocomial Infections: Faucet aerators, communal soap dispensers, disinfectants, improperly cleaned inhalation therapy equipment, infant incubators, and back rub lotions have all been associated with *Pseudomonas* epidemics. Infant-to-infant transmission by nursery personnel carrying *Pseudomonas* on the hands is frequent in neonatal units. Careful maintenance of equipment and enforcement of infection control procedures are essential to minimize nosocomial transmission.

C. Patients With Cystic Fibrosis: Chronic infection of the lower respiratory tract occurs in nearly all patients with cystic fibrosis. The infecting organism is seldom cleared from the respiratory tract, even with intensive antimicrobial therapy, and the resultant injury to the lung eventually leads to pulmonary insufficiency. Treatment is aimed at controlling signs and symptoms of the infection.

Treatment

P aeruginosa is inherently resistant to many antimicrobials and may develop resistance during therapy. Mortality rates in hospitalized patients exceed 50%, due both to the severity of underlying illnesses in patients predisposed to *Pseudomonas* infection and to the limitations of therapy. Aminoglycoside antimicrobials; expanded-spectrum cephalosporins, such as ceftazidime; imipenem; and the fluoroquinolones are active against most *P aeruginosa* strains, as well as other enteric gram-negative rods. However, antimicrobial susceptibility patterns vary from area to area, and resistance tends to appear as new drugs become popular. Treatment of infections is best guided by clinical response and susceptibility tests.

Use of gentamicin or tobramycin (5–7.5 mg/kg/d intramuscularly or intravenously in three divided doses) or amikacin (15–22 mg/kg/d in two or three divided doses) in combination with ticarcillin (200–300 mg/kg/d intravenously in six divided doses) or with another anti-*Pseudomonas* β-lactam antibiotic is recommended for treatment of serious *Pseudomonas* infections. Ceftazidime (150-200 mg/kg/d in four divided doses) is a third-generation cephalosporin with excellent activity against *P aeruginosa*. Treatment should be continued for 10–14 days. Treatment with two active drugs is recommended for all serious infections.

Pseudomonas osteomyelitis requires surgical debridement and antimicrobial therapy for 2 weeks. *Pseudomonas* folliculitis does not require antibiotic therapy.

Chronic suppurative otitis media responds to intravenous ceftazidime (150–200 mg/kg/d in three or four divided doses) given until the drainage has ceased for 3 days. Twice-daily ceftazidime with aural debridement and cleaning given on an outpatient basis has also been successful. Oral ciprofloxacin is also effective but is not FDA-approved in children because of concerns about skeletal toxicity.

Swimmer's ear may be caused by *P aeruginosa* and responds well to topical drying agents (alcohol, vinegar mix) and cleansing.

Prognosis

Because debilitated patients are most frequently affected, the mortality rate is high. These infections may have a protracted course, and eradication of the organisms may be difficult.

Bodey GP et al: Infections caused by *Pseudomonas aeruginosa*. Rev Infect Dis 1983;5:279.

Dagan R et al: Outpatient management of chronic suppurative otitis media without cholesteatoma in children. Pediatr Infect Dis J 1992;11:542.

Fiel SB: Clinical management of pulmonary disease in cystic fibrosis. Lancet 1993;341:1070.

Fisher MC et al: Sneakers as a source of *Pseudomonas aeruginosa* in children with osteomyelitis following puncture wounds. J Pediatr 1985;106:607.

Flores G, Stavola JJ, Noel GJ: Bacteremia due to *Pseudomonas aeruginosa* in children with AIDS. Clin Infect Dis 1993;16:706.

Govan JRW et al: Evidence for transmission of *Pseudomonas cepacia* by social contact in cystic fibrosis. Lancet 1993;342:15.

Grundmann H et al: *Pseudomonas aeruginosa* in a neonatal intensive care unit: Reservoirs and ecology of the nosocomial pathogen. J Infect Dis 1993;168:943.

Gustafson TL et al: *Pseudomonas* folliculitis: An outbreak and review. Rev Infect Dis 1983;5:1.

Jackson MA, Wong KY, Lampkin B: *Pseudomonas aeruginosa* septicemia in childhood cancer patients. Pediatr Infect Dis J 1982;1:239.

Martin-Ancel A, Borque C, del Castillo F: *Pseudomonas* sepsis in children without previous medical problems. Pediatr Infect Dis J 1993;12:258.

Ruvalo C, Bauer CR: Intrauterinely acquired *Pseudomonas* infection in the neonate. Clin Pediatr 1982;21:664.

SALMONELLA GASTROENTERITIS

Essentials of Diagnosis

- Nausea, vomiting, headache, meningismus.
- Fever, diarrhea, abdominal pain.
- Culture or organism from stool, blood, or other specimens.

General Considerations

Salmonellae are gram-negative rods that frequently cause food-borne gastroenteritis and occasionally bacteremic infection of bone, meninges, and other foci. Three species—*Salmonella typhi, Salmonella choleraesuis,* and *Salmonella enteritidis*—and approximately 2000 serotypes are recognized. *S typhimurium* is the most frequently isolated serotype in most parts of the world. Approximately 50,000 cases of salmonellosis are reported annually in the USA, but many cases are either not reported or not recognized.

Salmonellae are able to penetrate the mucin layer of the small bowel and attach to epithelial cells. Organisms penetrate the epithelial cells and multiply in the submucosa. Infection results in fever, vomiting, watery diarrhea, and occasionally, mucus with some polymorphonuclear leukocytes in the stool. Although the small intestine is generally regarded as the principal site of infection, colitis also occurs. *S typhimurium* frequently involves the large bowel.

Salmonella infections in childhood occur in two major forms: (1) gastroenteritis (including food poisoning), which may be complicated by sepsis and focal suppurative complications; and (2) enteric fever (typhoid fever and paratyphoid fever). (See next section.) Although the incidence of typhoid fever has decreased in the USA, the incidence of *Salmonella* gastroenteritis has greatly increased in the past 15–20 years. The highest attack rates occur in children under 6 years of age, with a peak in the age group from 6 months to 2 years old.

Salmonellae are widespread in nature, infecting domestic and wild animals. Fowl and reptiles have a particularly high carriage rate. Transmission results primarily from ingestion of contaminated food. Transmission from human to human occurs by the fecal-oral route via contaminated food, water, and fomites. Numerous foods are associated with outbreaks including meats, milk, cheese, ice cream, chocolate and other foods. Contaminated egg powder and frozen whole egg preparations used to make ice cream, custards, and mayonnaise are responsible for outbreaks. Eggs with contaminated shells that are consumed raw or undercooked have been incriminated in outbreaks and sporadic cases.

Salmonellae are susceptible to gastric acidity and, therefore, the elderly, infants, and patients treated with antacids or H-2 blocking drugs are at increased risk of infection. Most cases of *Salmonella* meningitis (80%) and bacteremia occur in infancy. Newborns may acquire the infection from their mothers during delivery and may precipitate outbreaks in nurseries. Newborns are at special risk of developing meningitis.

Clinical Findings

A. Symptoms and Signs: Infants usually develop fever, vomiting, and diarrhea. The older child may also complain of headache, nausea, and abdominal pain. Stools are often watery or may contain mucus and, in some instances, blood, suggesting shigellosis. Drowsiness and disorientation may be associated with meningismus. Convulsions occur less frequently than with shigellosis. Splenomegaly is occasionally noted. In the usual case, diarrhea is moderate and subsides after 4–5 days, but it may be protracted.

B. Laboratory Findings: Diagnosis is made by isolation of the organism from stool, blood, or, in some cases, from urine, cerebrospinal fluid, or pus from a suppurative lesion. The white blood cell count usually shows a polymorphonuclear leukocytosis but may show leukopenia. Typing of isolates is done with specific antisera. *Salmonella* isolates should be re-

ported to public health authorities for epidemiologic purposes.

Differential Diagnosis

In staphylococcal food poisoning, the incubation period is shorter (2–4 hours) than in *Salmonella* food poisoning (12–24 hours). Fever is absent, and vomiting rather than diarrhea is the main symptom. In shigellosis, many pus cells are likely to be seen on a stained smear of stool, and there is more likely to be a marked shift to the left in the peripheral white count, although some cases of salmonellosis are indistinguishable from shigellosis. *Campylobacter* gastroenteritis commonly resembles salmonellosis clinically. (Organisms previously classified as *Arizona* are considered *Salmonella* and cause a similar illness.) Culture of the stools is necessary to distinguish the causes of bacterial gastroenteritis.

Complications

Unlike most types of infectious diarrhea, salmonellosis is frequently accompanied by bacteremia, especially in newborns and infants. Septicemia with extraintestinal infection is seen, most commonly with *S choleraesuis* but also with *S enteritidis, S typhimurium,* and *S paratyphi* B and C. The organism may localize in any tissue and may cause arthritis, osteomyelitis, cholecystitis, endocarditis, meningitis, pericarditis, pneumonia, or pyelonephritis. In patients with sickle cell anemia or other hemoglobinopathies, there is a predilection for osteomyelitis to develop. Severe dehydration and shock are more likely to occur with shigellosis but may occur with *Salmonella* gastroenteritis.

Prevention

Measures for the prevention of *Salmonella* infections include thorough cooking of foodstuffs derived from potentially infected sources; proper refrigeration during storage; and recognition and control of infection among domestic animals, combined with proper meat and poultry inspections. Raw and undercooked fresh eggs should be avoided. Adults with salmonellosis who are food handlers or who have occupations involving care of young children should have three negative stool cultures before resuming work.

Treatment

A. Specific Measures: In uncomplicated *Salmonella* gastroenteritis antibiotic treatment does not shorten the course of the clinical illness and may prolong convalescent carriage of the organism. Colitis due to *Salmonella* may improve with antibiotic therapy.

However, to prevent sepsis and focal disease, antibiotic treatment is recommended for newborns and infants less than 3 months of age, for severely ill children, and for children with sickle cell disease, liver disease, recent gastrointestinal surgery, cancer, depressed immunity, and chronic renal or cardiac disease. Infants with positive stool cultures or suspected salmonellosis at less than 3 months of age should be admitted to hospital, evaluated for focal infection including blood culture and cerebrospinal fluid examination, and treated intravenously. Ampicillin (150–200 mg/kg/d intravenously in four divided doses for 5–10 days), or trimethoprim-sulfamethoxazole is recommended. Older patients developing bacteremia during the course of gastroenteritis should receive parenteral treatment initially, and a careful search should be made for additional foci of infection. After signs and symptoms subside, these patients should receive oral medication. Parenteral and oral treatment should last a total of 7–10 days. Longer treatment is indicated for specific complications. If susceptibility tests indicate resistance to ampicillin, chloramphenicol, third-generation cephalosporins or trimethoprim-sulfamethoxazole should be given. Fluoroquinolones also are efficacious but are not FDA-approved for administration to children.

Salmonella meningitis is best treated with a combination of chloramphenicol (100 mg/kg/d intravenously in four divided doses) and ampicillin (200–300 mg/kg/d intravenously in four to six divided doses) for 3 weeks or a third-generation cephalosporin (cefotaxime, ceftriaxone) for 3 weeks. If the child improves rapidly and the cerebrospinal fluid is sterile, treatment may be completed with a single drug, the choice guided by results of susceptibility tests.

Outbreaks on pediatric wards are difficult to control. Strict hand washing, cohorting of patients and personnel, and ultimate closure of the unit may be necessary.

B. Treatment of the Carrier States: About half of patients are still infectious after 4 weeks. Infants tend to remain convalescent carriers for up to a year. Antibiotic treatment of carriers is not effective.

C. General Measures: Careful attention must be given to maintaining fluid and electrolyte balance, especially in infants.

Prognosis

In gastroenteritis, the prognosis is good. In sepsis with focal suppurative complications, the prognosis is more guarded.

The case fatality rate of *Salmonella* meningitis is high in infants. There is a strong tendency to relapse if treatment is not prolonged.

Blaser MJ, Newman LS: A review of human salmonellosis: I. Infective dose. Rev Infect Dis 1982;4:1096.

Buchwald DS, Balser MJ: A review of human salmonellosis: II. Duration of excretion following infection with nontyphi *Salmonella.* Rev Infect Dis 1984;6:345.

Chalker RB, Blaser MJ: A review of human salmonellosis: III. Magnitude of *Salmonella* infection in the United States. Rev Infect Dis 1988;10:111.

Hedberg CW et al: A multistate outbreak of *Salmonella javiana* and *Salmonella oranienburg* infections due to consumption of contaminated cheese. JAMA 1992;268:3203.

Ryan CA et al: Massive outbreak of antimicrobial-resistant salmonellosis traced to pasteurized milk. JAMA 1987;258:3269.

Rennels MB, Leving MM: Classical bacterial diarrhea: Perspectives and update—*Salmonella, Shigella, Escherichia coli, Aeromonas,* and *Plesiomonas.* Pediatr Infect Dis J 1986;5(Suppl):21.

Salmonella enteritidis infections and shell eggs: Update, US 1990. MMWR Morb Mortal Wkly Rep 1990;50:909.

St Geme JW III et al: Consensus: management of *Salmonella* infection in the first year of life. Pediatr Infect Dis J 1988;7:615.

TYPHOID FEVER & PARATYPHOID FEVER

Essentials of Diagnosis

- Insidious or acute onset of headache, anorexia, vomiting, constipation or diarrhea, ileus, and high fever.
- Meningismus, splenomegaly, and rose spots.
- Leukopenia; positive blood, stool, bone marrow, and urine cultures.

General Considerations

Typhoid fever is caused by the gram-negative bacillus *Salmonella typhi;* paratyphoid fevers, which are usually milder but may be clinically indistinguishable, are caused by *Salmonella paratyphi* A, *Salmonella schottmülleri,* or *Salmonella hirschfeldi* (formerly *Salmonella paratyphi* A, B, and C). Children have a shorter incubation period than do adults (usually 5–8 days instead of 8–14 days). The organism enters the body through the walls of the intestinal tract and, following a transient bacteremia, multiplies in the reticuloendothelial cells of the liver and spleen. Persistent bacteremia and symptoms then follow. Reinfection of the intestine occurs as organisms are excreted in the bile. Bacterial emboli produce the characteristic skin lesions (rose spots). Symptoms in children may be mild or severe, but children younger than age 5 uncommonly have clinically severe typhoid fever.

Chloramphenicol-resistant typhoid fever has been reported in Southeast Asia, India, and South America, and ampicillin- and chloramphenicol-resistant strains are seen in Latin America and elsewhere.

Typhoid fever is transmitted by the fecal-oral route and by contamination of food or water. Unlike other *Salmonella* species, there are no animal reservoirs of *S typhi;* each case is the result of direct or indirect contact with the organism or with an individual who is actively infected or a chronic carrier. Laboratory-acquired infections are common.

About 500 cases per year are reported in the USA, 60% of which are acquired during foreign travel.

Clinical Findings

A. Symptoms and Signs: In children, the onset is apt to be sudden rather than insidious, with malaise, headache, crampy abdominal pains and distention, and sometimes constipation followed within 48 hours by diarrhea, high fever, and toxemia. An encephalopathy may be seen with irritability, confusion, delirium, and stupor. Vomiting and meningismus may be prominent in the young. The classic prolonged three-stage disease seen in adult patients is often shortened in children. The prodrome may be only 2–4 days; the toxic stage may last only 2–3 days; and the defervescence stage may last 1–2 weeks.

During the prodromal stage, physical findings may be absent, or there may merely be some abdominal distention and tenderness, meningismus, mild hepatomegaly, and minimal splenomegaly. The typical typhoidal rash (rose spots) is present in 10–15% of children. It appears during the second week of the disease and may erupt in crops for the succeeding 10–14 days. Rose spots are erythematous maculopapular lesions 2–3 mm in diameter that fade on pressure. They are found principally on the trunk and chest, and they generally disappear within 3–4 days. The lesions usually number less than 20.

B. Laboratory Findings: Typhoid bacilli can be isolated from many sites, including blood, stool, urine, and bone marrow. Blood cultures are positive in 50–80% of cases during the first week and less often later in the illness. Stool cultures are positive in about 50% of cases after the first week. Urine and bone marrow cultures are also valuable. Most patients will have negative cultures (including stool) by the end of a 6-week period. Serologic tests (Widal reaction) are not as useful as cultures because both false-positive and false-negative results occur. A fourfold rise in titer of O (somatic) agglutinins is suggestive but not diagnostic of infection.

Leukopenia is common in the second week of the disease, but in the first week, leukocytosis may be seen. Proteinuria, mild elevation of liver enzymes, thrombocytopenia, and disseminated intravascular coagulation are common.

Differential Diagnosis

Typhoid and paratyphoid fevers must be distinguished from other serious prolonged fevers. These include typhus, brucellosis, tularemia, miliary tuberculosis, psittacosis, vasculitis, lymphoma, mononucleosis, and Kawasaki disease.

The diagnosis of typhoid fever if often made clinically in developing countries. In developed countries, where typhoid fever is uncommon and physicians are unfamiliar with the clinical picture, the diagnosis is often not suspected until late. Positive cultures confirm the diagnosis.

Complications

The most important complications of typhoid fever are gastrointestinal hemorrhage (2–10%) and perforation (1–3%). They occur toward the end of the second week or during the third week of the disease.

Intestinal perforation is one of the principal causes of death. The site of perforation generally is the terminal ileum or cecum. The clinical manifestations are indistinguishable from those of acute appendicitis, with pain, tenderness, and rigidity in the right lower quadrant. The x-ray finding of free air in the peritoneal cavity is diagnostic.

Bacterial pneumonia, meningitis, septic arthritis, abscesses, and osteomyelitis are uncommon complications, particularly if specific treatment is given promptly. Shock and electrolyte disturbances may lead to death.

About 1–3% of patients become chronic carriers of *S typhi*. Chronic carriage is defined as excretion of typhoid bacilli for more than a year, but carriage is often lifelong. Adults with underlying biliary or urinary tract disease are much more likely than children to become chronic carriers.

Prevention

Routine typhoid vaccine is not recommended in the USA but should be considered for some foreign travel to endemic areas. A heat- and phenol-killed vaccine is available, but its efficacy is only fair. An attenuated oral typhoid vaccine produced from strain Ty21a has better efficacy and causes minimal side effects but is not approved for children under 6 years (see Chapter 10).

Treatment

A. Specific Measures: Equally effective regimens for susceptible strains include the following: chloramphenicol (50–100 mg/kg/d orally or intravenously in four doses), trimethoprim-sulfamethoxazole (10 mg/kg trimethoprim and 50 mg/kg sulfamethoxazole per day orally in two or three divided doses), amoxicillin (100 mg/kg/d orally in four divided doses), and ampicillin (100–200 mg/kg/d intravenously in four divided doses). Aminoglycosides and first- and second-generation cephalosporins are clinically ineffective regardless of in vitro susceptibility results. Ceftriaxone and cefotaxime also are effective; one of these drugs should be used initially in infections caused by strains with proved or suspected resistance to the standard agents.

Treatment duration is 14–21 days. Patients remain febrile for 3–5 days even on appropriate therapy.

B. General Measures: General support of the patient is exceedingly important and includes rest, good nutrition, and careful observation, with particular regard to evidence of intestinal bleeding or perforation. Blood transfusions may be needed even in the absence of frank hemorrhage.

Prognosis

A prolonged convalescent carrier stage in children often continues 3–6 months. This does not require re-treatment with antibiotics or exclusion from school or other activities.

With early antibiotic therapy, the prognosis is excellent. With early treatment, the mortality rate is less than 1%. Relapse occurs 1–3 weeks later in 10–20% of cases despite appropriate antibiotic treatment.

Bitar R, Tarpley J: Intestinal perforation in typhoid fever: A historical and state-of-the-art review. Rev Infect Dis 1985;7:257.

Butler T et al: Patterns of morbidity and mortality in typhoid fever dependent on age and gender: Review of 552 hospitalized patients with diarrhea. Rev Infect Dis 1991; 13:85.

Ferreccio C et al: Comparative efficacy of two, three, or four doses of Ty21, a live oral typhoid vaccine in enteric coated capsules: a field trial in an endemic area. J Infect Dis 1989;159:766.

Hoffman SL et al: Reduction of mortality in chloramphenicol-treated severe typhoid fever by high-dose dexamethasone. N Engl J Med 1984;310:82.

Mahle WT, Levine MM: Salmonella typhi infection in children younger than five years of age. Pediatr Infect Dis J 1993;12:627.

Mandal BK: Modern treatment of typhoid fever. J Infect 1991;22:1.

Meloni T et al: Ceftriaxone treatment of Salmonella enteric fever. Pediatr Infect Dis J 1988;7:734.

Scully RE, Mark EJ, McNeely BU: Fever of unknown origin after a visit to India. (Case records of the Massachusetts General Hospital.) N Engl J Med 1983;309:600.

Thisyakorn U, Mansuwan P, Taylor DN: Typhoid and paratyphoid fever in 192 hospitalized children in Thailand. Am J Dis Child 1987;141:862.

Woodruff BA, Pavia AT, Blake PA: A new look at typhoid vaccination. JAMA 1991;265:756.

SHIGELLOSIS
(Bacillary Dysentery)

Essentials of Diagnosis

- Cramps and bloody diarrhea.
- High fever, malaise, convulsions.
- Pus and blood in diarrheal stools examined microscopically.
- Diagnosis confirmed by stool culture.

General Considerations

Shigellae are nonmotile gram-negative rods of the family Enterobacteriaceae and are closely related to *Escherichia coli.* The genus *Shigella* is divided into four major groups, A–D: *Shigella dysenteriae, Shigella flexneri, Shigella boydii,* and *Shigella sonnei.* Approximately 20,000 cases of shigellosis are reported each year in the USA. *S sonnei* followed by *S flexneri* are the most common isolates. *S dysenteriae,* which causes the most severe diarrhea of all species

and the greatest number of extraintestinal complications, accounts for fewer than 1% of all *Shigella* infections in the USA.

Shigellosis is often a serious disease, particularly in children under 2 years of age, and without supportive treatment there is an appreciable mortality rate. In older children and adults, the disease tends to be self-limited and milder. Shigellosis is unusual in infants under 3 months of age, although in rare cases shigellae may be transmitted from the mother to the newborn during delivery. Diarrhea and refusal to take feedings are the most common symptoms in neonatal shigellosis, and bloody diarrhea and fever occur less frequently. Vomiting, convulsions, or high fever is almost never encountered.

Shigella is usually transmitted by the fecal-oral route. Food- and water-borne outbreaks occur but are less important overall than person-to-person transmission. The disease is very communicable; as few as 200 bacteria can produce illness in an adult. The secondary attack rate in families is high, and shigellosis is a serious problem in day-care centers and custodial institutions. *Shigella* organisms produce disease by invading the colonic mucosa, causing mucosal ulcerations and microabscesses. A plasmid-encoded gene is required for enterotoxin production, chromosomal genes are required for invasiveness, and smooth lipopolysaccharide are required for virulence.

Clinical Findings

A. Symptoms and Signs: The incubation period usually is 2–4 days. Onset is abrupt, with abdominal cramps, urgency, tenesmus, chills, fever, malaise, and diarrhea. In severe forms, blood and mucus are seen in small volume in the watery stool (dysentery), and meningismus and convulsions may occur. In older children, the disease may be mild and may be characterized by watery diarrhea without blood. In young children, a fever of 39.4–40 °C is common. Rarely, there is rectal prolapse. Symptoms generally last 3–7 days.

B. Laboratory Findings: The total white blood cell count varies, but often there is a marked shift to the left. The stool may contain gross blood and mucus, and many neutrophils are seen if mucus from the stool is examined microscopically. Stool cultures usually are positive; however, they may be negative because the organism is somewhat fragile and present in small numbers late in the disease, and because laboratory techniques are suboptimal for the recovery of shigellae.

Differential Diagnosis

Diarrhea due to rotavirus infection is a winter rather than a summer disease, usually children are not as febrile or toxic, and stool does not contain gross blood or neutrophils. Intestinal infections caused by *Salmonella* or *Campylobacter* are differentiated by culture. Amebic dysentery is diagnosed by microscopic examination of fresh stools or sigmoidoscopy specimens; intussusception is characterized by an abdominal mass, "currant jelly" stools without leukocytes, and absence of fever. Mild shigellosis is not distinguishable clinically from other forms of infectious diarrhea.

Complications

Dehydration, acidosis, shock, and renal failure are the major complications. In some cases, a chronic form of dysentery occurs, characterized by mucoid stools and poor nutrition. Bacteremia and metastatic infections are rare but serious complications. Febrile seizures are common. Fulminating fatal dysentery (Ikari syndrome) and hemolytic uremic syndrome occur rarely.

Treatment

A. Specific Measures: Trimethoprim-sulfamethoxazole (10 mg/kg/d trimethoprim and 50 mg/kg/d sulfamethoxazole, in two divided doses orally for 5 days) is the treatment of choice. Amoxicillin is not effective. Ampicillin (100 mg/kg/d in four divided doses) is also efficacious if the strain is sensitive. Ciprofloxacin, 500 mg twice daily for 5 days, is efficacious in adults but is not approved in children. Successful treatment results in reduced duration of fever, cramping, and diarrhea and in termination of fecal excretion of *Shigella*. Strains resistant to ampicillin and trimethoprim-sulfamethoxazole are common in Mexico and underdeveloped countries and increasingly in the USA. In the USA, 7% of isolates are resistant to trimethoprim-sulfamethoxazole and one-third are resistant to ampicillin. Recent foreign travel is the best predictor of resistance. Tetracycline and chloramphenicol are also effective, but resistance may be seen. Third-generation cephalosporins and quinolones are active in vitro against resistant strains, but clinical experience is limited. Presumptive therapy should be based on the susceptibility pattern of recent local isolates.

B. General Measures: In severe cases, immediate rehydration is critical. A mild form of chronic malabsorption syndrome may supervene and require prolonged dietary control.

Prognosis

The prognosis is excellent if vascular collapse is treated promptly by adequate fluid therapy. The mortality rate is high in very young, malnourished infants who do not receive fluid and electrolyte therapy. Convalescent fecal excretion of *Shigella* lasts 1–4 weeks in patients not receiving antimicrobial therapy. Long-term carriers are rare.

Ashkenazi S et al: Convulsions in shigellosis: Evaluation of possible risk factors. Am J Dis Child 1983;137:985.
Bennish ML: Potentially lethal complications of shigellosis. Rev Infect Dis 1991;13:5319.
Bennish ML et al: Therapy for shigellosis: II. Randomized, double-blind comparison of ciprofloxacin and ampicillin. J Infect Dis 1990;162:711.
Blaser MJ et al: *Shigella* infections in the United States, 1974–1980. J Infect Dis 1983;147:771.
DeWitt TG, Humphrey KF, McParthy P: Clinical predictors of acute bacterial diarrhea in young children. Pediatrics 1985;76:551.
Dupont HL, Nornick RB: Adverse effects of Lomotil therapy in shigellosis. JAMA 1973;226:1525.
Kagalwalla AF et al: Childhood shigellosis in Saudi Arabia. Pediatr Infect Dis J 1992;11:215.
Martin T, Habbick BF, Nyssen J: Shigellosis with bacteremia: A report of two cases and a review of the literature. Pediatr Infect Dis 1983;2:21.
O'Brien AD, Holmes RK: Shiga and Shiga-like toxins. Microbiol Rev 1987;51:206.
Tacket CO, Cohen ML: Shigellosis in day-care centers: Use of plasmid analysis to assess control measures. Pediatr Infect Dis 1983;2:127.
Tauxe RV et al: Antimicrobial resistance of *Shigella* isolates in the USA: The importance of international travelers. J Infect Dis 1990;162:1107.

CHOLERA

Essentials of Diagnosis

- Sudden onset of severe watery diarrhea.
- Persistent vomiting without nausea or fever.
- Extreme and rapid dehydration and electrolyte loss, with rapid development of vascular collapse.
- Contact with a case of cholera, with shellfish, or the presence of cholera in the community.
- Diagnosis confirmed by stool culture.

General Considerations

Cholera is an acute diarrheal disease caused by the gram-negative organism *Vibrio cholerae*. It is transmitted by contaminated water or food, especially contaminated shellfish. The disease is generally so dramatic that in endemic areas the diagnosis is obvious. Individuals with mild illness and young children may play an important role in transmission of the infection.

Asymptomatic infection is far more common than clinical disease. In endemic areas, rising titers of vibriocidal antibody are seen with increasing age; infection occurs in individuals with low titers. The age-specific attack rate is highest in children under 5 years and declines with age. Cholera is unusual in infancy.

Cholera toxin is a protein enterotoxin that is primarily responsible for symptoms. Cholera toxin binds to a regulatory subunit of adenylyl cyclase in enterocytes, causing increased cyclic adenosine monophosphate and an outpouring of NaCl and water into the lumen of the small bowel.

Nutritional status is an important factor determining the severity of the diarrhea. Duration of diarrhea is prolonged in adults and children suffering from severe malnutrition.

Cholera is endemic in India and southern and Southeast Asia and in parts of Africa. Seven major pandemics have occurred since 1817. The most recent pandemic, caused by the El Tor biotype of *Vibrio cholerae* 01, began in 1961 in Indonesia. In 1982, 37 countries were affected and 54,000 cases reported. An epidemic of cholera began in Peru in 1991 and spread throughout South and Central America. More than 300,000 cases occurred. Cases in the USA occurred in the course of foreign travel or as a result of consumption of contaminated imported food. Cholera is increasingly recognized to be associated with consumption of shellfish. Interstate shipments of oysters have resulted in cholera in several inland states.

Several recent studies provide evidence that *V cholerae* is a natural inhabitant of shellfish and copepods in estuarine environments. Seasonal multiplication of *V cholerae* may provide a source for outbreaks in endemic areas. Chronic cholera carriers are rare. The incubation period is short, usually 1–3 days.

Clinical Findings

A. Symptoms and Signs: Many patients infected with *V cholerae* have mild disease, with 1–2% developing severe diarrhea. During severe cholera, there is a sudden onset of massive, frequent, watery stools, generally light gray in color ("rice water") and containing some mucus but no pus. Vomiting may be projectile and is not accompanied by nausea. Within 2–3 hours, the tremendous loss of fluids results in severe and life-threatening dehydration, hypochloremia, and hypokalemia, with marked weakness and collapse. Renal failure with uremia and irreversible peripheral vascular collapse will occur if fluid therapy is not administered. The illness lasts 1–7 days and is shortened by appropriate antibiotic therapy.

B. Laboratory Findings: Markedly elevated hemoglobin (20 g/dL) and marked acidosis, hypochloremia, and hyponatremia are seen, and marked acidosis may complicate isotonic dehydration.

Cultural confirmation using thiosulfate-citrate-bile-salt-sucrose (TCBS) agar takes 16–18 hours for a presumptive diagnosis and 36–48 hours for a definitive bacteriologic diagnosis.

Prevention

Cholera vaccine is available in the USA and provides 50% efficacy. Protection lasts 3–6 months. Cholera vaccine is not generally recommended for travelers. In endemic areas, all water and milk must be boiled, food protected from flies, and sanitary precautions observed. Thorough cooking of shellfish prevents transmission. All patients with cholera should be isolated.

Chemoprophylaxis is indicated for household and other close contacts of cholera patients. It should be initiated as soon as possible after the onset of the disease in the index patient. Tetracycline (500 mg daily for 5 days) is effective in preventing infection.

Trimethoprim-sulfamethoxazole may be substituted in children.

Tourists visiting endemic areas are at little risk if they exercise common sense in what they eat and drink and maintain good personal hygiene.

Treatment

Physiologic saline or lactated Ringer's solution should be administered intravenously in large amounts to restore blood volume and urine output and to prevent irreversible shock. Potassium supplements are required. Sodium bicarbonate, given intravenously, may also be needed initially to overcome profound acidosis. Moderate dehydration and acidosis can be corrected in 3–6 hours by oral therapy alone, because the active glucose transport system of the small bowel is normally functional. The optimal composition of the oral solution (in meq/L) is as follows: Na^+ 90, Cl^- 80, and K^+ 20—with glucose, 110 mmol/L.

Treatment of children with tetracycline (50 mg/kg/d orally in four divided doses for 2–5 days) shortens the duration of the disease and prevents clinical relapse but is not as important as fluid and electrolyte therapy. Tetracycline resistance occurs in some regions. Trimethoprim-sulfamethoxazole should be used in children under 9 years of age.

Prognosis

With early and rapid replacement of fluids and electrolytes, the case fatality rate is 1–2% in children. If significant symptoms appear and no treatment is given, the mortality rate is over 50%.

Carpenter CC: The treatment of cholera: Clinical science at the bedside. J Infect Dis 1992;166:2.

Finkelstein RA et al: Epitopes of the cholera family of enterotoxins. Rev Infect Dis 1987;9:544.

Johnston JM et al: Cholera on a Gulf Coast oil rig. N Engl J Med 1983;309:523.

Kaper JB et al: Molecular epidemiology of *Vibrio cholerae* in the U.S. Gulf Coast. J Clin Microbiol 1982;16:129.

Kelly MT: Cholera: A worldwide perspective. Pediatr Infect Dis 1986;5(Suppl):101.

Swerdlow DL, Ries AA: Cholera in the Americas: Guidelines for the clinician. JAMA 1992;267:1495.

Tauxe RV, Blake PA: Epidemic cholera in Latin America. JAMA 1992;267:1388.

CAMPYLOBACTER INFECTION

Essentials of Diagnosis

- Fever, vomiting, abdominal pain, diarrhea.
- Blood, mucus, pus in stools (dysentery).
- Presumptive diagnosis by darkfield or phase contrast microscopy of stool wet mount or modified Gram stain.
- Definitive diagnosis by stool culture.

General Considerations

Campylobacter species (formerly grouped with vibrios and known as *Vibrio fetus*) are small, gram-negative, curved or spiral bacilli that are commensals or pathogens in many animals. *Campylobacter jejuni* frequently causes acute enteritis in humans, and *Campylobacter fetus* causes bacteremia and meningitis in immunocompromised patients. *Campylobacter fetus* may cause maternal fever, abortion, stillbirth, and severe neonatal infection. *Helicobacter pylori* (previously called *Campylobacter pylori*) has been associated with gastritis and peptic ulcer disease in both adults and children (see Chapter 22).

In the past decade, *C jejuni* has been responsible for 3–11% of cases of acute gastroenteritis in North America and Europe; in many areas, enteritis due to *C jejuni* is more common than that due to *Salmonella* or *Shigella*.

Campylobacter colonizes domestic and wild animals, especially poultry. Numerous cases have been associated with sick puppies or other animal contacts. Contaminated food and water, improperly cooked poultry, and person-to-person spread by the fecal-oral route are important in transmission. Outbreaks associated with day-care centers, contaminated water supplies, and raw milk have been reported. Raw milk consumption, often during visits to dairy farms, was responsible for 20 outbreaks involving nearly 500 children from 1981 to 1990. Newborns may acquire the organism from their mothers at delivery.

Clinical Findings

A. Symptoms and Signs: *C jejuni* enteritis can be mild or severe. In tropical countries, asymptomatic stool carriage is common. The incubation period is usually 1–7 days. The disease usually begins with sudden onset of high fever, malaise, headache, abdominal cramps, nausea, and vomiting. Diarrhea follows and may be watery or bile-stained, mucoid, and bloody. Passage of up to 20 stools per day is not uncommon. The illness is self-limiting, lasting 2–7 days, but relapses occur in 15–25% of cases. Without antimicrobial treatment, the organism remains in the stool for 1–6 weeks.

B. Laboratory Findings: The peripheral white blood cell count generally is elevated, with many band forms. Microscopic examination of stool reveals erythrocytes and pus cells, and darkfield or phase contrast microscopic examination of wet mounts may reveal darting bacilli characteristic of *Campylobacter*. Other bacteria, particularly *Vibrio* species, may exhibit similar motility, but in areas where cholera and *Vibrio parahaemolyticus* diarrhea are rare, a positive darkfield examination has a predictive value of about 90%. Isolation of *C jejuni* from stool is not difficult but requires selective agar, incubation at 42 °C, rather than 35 °C, and incubation in an atmosphere of about 5% oxygen and 5% CO_2 (candle jar is satisfactory).

Differential Diagnosis

Campylobacter enteritis may resemble viral gastroenteritis, salmonellosis, shigellosis, amebiasis, or other infectious diarrheas. Because it also mimics ulcerative colitis, Crohn's disease, intussusception, and appendicitis, mistaken diagnosis can lead to unnecessary surgery.

Complications

The most important complications are dehydration and inappropriate treatment due to misdiagnosis as inflammatory bowel disease. Other complications are uncommon but include erythema nodosum, convulsions, reactive arthritis, bacteremia, urinary tract infection, and cholecystitis.

Prevention

No vaccine is yet available. Hand washing and adherence to basic food sanitation practices help prevent disease. Handwashing and cleaning kitchen utensils after contact with raw poultry are important.

Treatment

Treatment of fluid and electrolyte disturbances is most important. Antimicrobial treatment with erythromycin in children (30–50 mg/kg/d orally in four divided doses for 5 days) or with tetracycline in adults terminates fecal excretion and may prevent relapses, but antimicrobial treatment does not shorten or modify the illness unless given early in the disease. Antimicrobials used for shigellosis, such as trimethoprim-sulfamethoxazole and ampicillin, are inactive against *Campylobacter*. Supportive therapy is sufficient in most cases.

Prognosis

The outlook is excellent if dehydration is corrected and misdiagnosis does not lead to inappropriate diagnostic or surgical procedures.

Anders BJ et al: Double-blind placebo controlled trial of erythromycin for treatment of *Campylobacter* enteritis. Lancet 1982;1:131.

Blaser MJ, Reller LB: *Campylobacter* enteritis. N Engl J Med 1981;305:1444.

Paisley JW et al: Dark-field microscopy of human feces for presumptive diagnosis of *Campylobacter fetus* subsp *jejuni* enteritis. J Clin Microbiol 1982;15:61.

Schwartz RH et al: Experience with the microbiologic diagnosis of *Campylobacter* enteritis in an office laboratory. Pediatr Infect Dis 1983;2:298.

Wong S-N et al: *Campylobacter* infection in the neonate: Case report and review of the literature. Pediatr Inf Dis J 1990;9:665.

Wood RC et al: Campylobacter enteritis outbreaks associated with drinking raw milk during youth activities. JAMA 1992;268:3228.

TULAREMIA

Essentials of Diagnosis

- A cutaneous or mucous membrane lesion at the site of inoculation and regional lymph node enlargement.
- Sudden onset of fever, chills, and prostration.
- History of contact with infected animals, principally wild rabbits, or history of tick exposure.
- Positive culture or immunofluorescence of mucocutaneous ulcer or regional lymph nodes.
- High serum antibody titer.

General Considerations

Tularemia is caused by *Francisella tularensis,* a gram-negative organism usually acquired from infected animals, principally wild rabbits; occasionally from infected domestic dogs or cats; by contamination of the skin or mucous membranes with infected blood or tissues; by inhalation of infected material; by bites of ticks, fleas, or deerflies that have been in contact with infected animals; or by ingestion of contaminated meat or water. Strains of high virulence for humans and rabbits (Jellison type A) and strains with lowered virulence (Jellison type B) for humans, which are avirulent in rabbits, are present throughout the USA. The incubation period is short, usually 3–7 days, but may vary from 2 to 25 days.

Ticks are the most important vector. Rabbits are the classic vectors of tularemia. It is important to seek a history of rabbit hunting, skinning, or food preparation in any patient who has a febrile illness with tender lymphadenopathy, often in the region of a draining skin ulcer.

Clinical Findings

A. Symptoms and Signs: Several clinical types are seen in children. Sixty percent of infections are of the ulceroglandular form and start as a reddened papule that may be pruritic, quickly ulcerates, and is not very painful. Shortly thereafter, the regional lymph nodes become large and tender. Fluctuance quickly follows. At the same time, there may be marked systemic manifestations, including high fever, chills, weakness, and vomiting. Pneumonitis occasionally accompanies the ulceroglandular form or may be seen as the sole manifestation of infection (pneumonic form). A detectable skin lesion is occasionally absent, and localized lymphoid enlargement exists alone (glandular form). Oculoglandular and oropharyngeal forms also occur in children. The latter is characterized by tonsillitis, often with membrane formation, cervical adenopathy, and high fever. In the absence of any primary ulcer or localized lymphadenitis, a prolonged febrile disease reminiscent of typhoid fever can be seen (typhoidal form). Splenomegaly is common in all forms.

B. Laboratory Findings: *F tularensis* can be recovered from ulcers, regional lymph nodes, and sputum of patients with the pneumonic form. However, the organism grows only on an enriched medium (blood-cystine-glucose agar), and laboratory handling is dangerous owing to the risk of airborne transmission to laboratory personnel. Immunofluorescent staining of biopsy material or aspirates of involved lymph nodes is diagnostic, though it is not widely available.

The white blood cell count is not remarkable. Agglutinins are present after the second week of illness, and in the absence of a positive culture their development confirms the diagnosis. An agglutination titer of 1:160 or higher is considered positive.

Differential Diagnosis

The typhoidal form of tularemia may mimic typhoid, brucellosis, miliary tuberculosis, Rocky Mountain spotted fever, and infectious mononucleosis. Pneumonic tularemia resembles atypical and mycotic pneumonitis. The ulceroglandular type of tularemia resembles pyoderma caused by staphylococci or streptococci, rat-bite fever, plague, anthrax, and cat-scratch fever. The oropharyngeal type must be distinguished from streptococcal or diphtheritic pharyngitis, infectious mononucleosis, herpangina, or other viral pharyngitides.

Prevention

Reasonable attempts should be made to protect children from bites of insects, principally ticks, fleas, and deerflies, by the use of proper clothing and repellents. Since rabbits are the source of most human infections, the dressing and handling of such game should be performed with great care. If contact occurs, thorough washing with soap and water is indicated.

Treatment

A. Specific Measures: Streptomycin (30 mg/kg/d intramuscularly in two divided doses for 8–10 days) is the drug of choice, though commercial availability has sometimes been a problem. The maximum daily dose is 1 g. Gentamicin has been used in individual cases and is probably effective. The tetracyclines and chloramphenicol are also effective, but the organism is not eradicated, and relapses occur.

B. General Measures: Antipyretics and analgesics may be given as necessary. Skin lesions are best left open. Glandular lesions occasionally require incision and drainage.

Prognosis

The prognosis is excellent with appropriate therapy in patients recognized early.

Jacobs RF, Condrey YM, Yamauchi T: Tularemia in adults and children: A changing presentation. Pediatrics 1985;76:818.

Liles WC, Burger RJ: Tularemia from domestic cats. West J Med 1993;158:619.

Markowitz LE et al: Tick-borne tularemia. JAMA 1985; 254:292.

Rohrbach BW et al: Epidemiological and clinical characteristics of tularemia in Oklahoma, 1979 to 1985. South Med J 1991;84:1091.

Spach DH et al: Tick-borne diseases in the United States. N Engl J Med 1993;329:936.

Uhari M, Syrjälä H, Salminen A: Tularemia in children caused by *Francisella tularensis* biovar *palaearctica*. Pediatr Infect Dis J 1990;9:80.

PLAGUE

Essentials of Diagnosis

- Sudden onset of fever, chills, and prostration.
- Regional lymph node tender; lymphadenitis with suppuration of nodes (bubonic form).
- Hemorrhages into skin and mucous membranes and shock (septicemia).
- Cough, dyspnea, cyanosis, and hemoptysis (pneumonia).
- History of exposure to infected animals.

General Considerations

Plague is an extremely serious, acute infection caused by a gram-negative bacillus, *Yersinia pestis*. It is a disease of rodents that is transmitted to humans by the bites of fleas. Plague bacilli have been isolated from rodents in 15 of the western states in the USA. Direct contact with rodents, rabbits, or domestic cats may transmit fleas infected with plague bacilli. During the 1980s, a mean of 18 cases per year was reported in the USA, primarily from the southwestern region. Most cases occur from June through September.

Human plague in the USA appears to occur in cycles that reflect comparable cycles in wild animal reservoirs of infection.

Clinical Findings

A. Symptoms and Signs: The disease assumes several different clinical forms, the two most common being bubonic and septicemic. Pneumonic plague, the form that occurs when organisms enter the body through the respiratory tract, is now very uncommon.

1. Bubonic plague—Bubonic plague begins after an incubation period of 2–6 days with a sudden onset of high fever, chills, headache, vomiting, and marked delirium or clouding of consciousness. A less severe form also exists, with a less precipitous onset but with progression over several days to severe symptoms. Although the flea bite is rarely seen, the regional lymph node, usually inguinal and unilateral, is painful and tender, 1–5 cm in diameter. The node usually suppurates and drains spontaneously after 1

week. The plague bacillus is known to produce an endotoxin that causes vascular necrosis. Bacilli may overwhelm regional lymph nodes and enter the circulation to produce septicemia. Severe vascular necrosis results in widely disseminated hemorrhages in skin, mucous membranes, liver, and spleen. Myocarditis and circulatory collapse may result from damage by the endotoxin.

A septicemic form of bubonic plague also exists that begins with fever, delirium, and bacteremia, with regional lymphadenopathy and bubo formation occurring after 3–5 days.

Plague meningitis or pneumonia may occur secondarily following bacteremic spread from an infected lymph node.

2. Septicemic plague—The septicemic form is defined as any case of plague without evidence of lymphadenopathy. This form is less common than bubonic plague but carries a worse prognosis, largely because it is less likely to be recognized and treated early. Patients may present initially with a nonspecific febrile illness characterized by fever, myalgia, chills, and anorexia. It is frequently complicated by pneumonia.

B. Laboratory Findings: Aspiration of a bubo leads to visualization of bipolar staining gram-negative bacilli on a stained smear. Pus, sputum, and blood all yield the organism, although laboratory infections are common enough to make isolation dangerous. A buffy coat Gram's stain may reveal the organism, and blood-agar cultures yield positive results in 48 hours. The white blood cell count is markedly elevated, with a shift to the left.

Sera obtained during disease and convalescence should be collected and stored for use in confirming the diagnosis in cases where the organism may not be recovered.

Differential Diagnosis

The septic phase of the disease may be confused with such illnesses as meningococcemia, sepsis, and rickettsioses. The bubonic form resembles tularemia, anthrax, cat-scratch fever, streptococcal adenitis, and cellulitis. Primary gastroenteritis and appendicitis may have to be distinguished.

Prevention

Proper disposal of household and commercial wastes and chemical control of rats are basic for control of plague. Flea control is instituted and maintained with the liberal use of insecticides. Children vacationing in remote camping areas should be warned not to handle dead or dying animals. Travelers to wild areas in the enzootic western states are at low risk of infection, and immunization of visitors to these areas is not recommended.

Vaccination is recommended for those traveling or living in areas of high incidence (see Chapter 10).

Treatment

A. Specific Measures: Streptomycin is the drug of choice in a dosage of 20–40 mg/kg intramuscularly in three divided doses for 5–7 days. For patients not requiring parenteral therapy, tetracycline, 20-30 mg/kg/d in four divided doses, or chloramphenicol (75–100 mg/kg/d intravenously or orally in four divided doses) may be given for 10–14 days. Tetracycline is not recommended for children under 9 years of age.

In septicemia and pneumonic plague, specific antibiotic treatment must be started in the first 15–24 hours of the disease if survival is to be expected. Treatment with streptomycin started 36–48 hours after onset of the disease may result in death due to liberation of plague toxin.

Bubonic plague is not highly contagious. Every effort is made to effect resolution of buboes without resorting to surgery. Pus from draining lymph nodes should be handled with gloves.

B. General Measures: Pneumonic plague is highly infectious, and strict isolation is required. All contacts should receive prophylaxis with sulfadiazine (100–200 mg/kg/d orally in four divided doses for 7 days) or tetracycline (30 mg/kg/d in four divided doses for 7 days).

Prognosis

The mortality rate in untreated bubonic plague is about 50%; it is 90% in the septicemic form and nearly 100% in the pneumonic form. Recent mortality rates in New Mexico were 3% for bubonic plague and 71% for the septicemic form.

Craven BB, Barnes AM: Plague and tularemia. Infect Dis Clin North Am 1991;5:165.

Crook LD: Plague: A clinical review of 27 cases. Arch Intern Med 1992;152:1253.

Hull HF, Montes JM, Mann JM: Septicemic plague in New Mexico. J Infect Dis 1987;155(1):113.

Human plague—United States, 1988. MMWR Morb Mortal Wkly Rep 1988;37:653.

Mann JM, Shandler L, Cushing AH: Pediatric plague. Pediatrics 1982;69:762.

HAEMOPHILUS INFLUENZAE TYPE b INFECTIONS

Essentials of Diagnosis

- Purulent meningitis in children under age 4 years with direct smears of cerebrospinal fluid showing gram-negative pleomorphic rods.
- Acute epiglottitis: High fever, drooling, dysphagia, aphonia, and croup. White blood cell count over 20,000/μL.
- Septic arthritis: Fever, local redness, swelling, heat, and pain with active or passive motion of the involved joint in a child 4 months to 4 years of age.
- Cellulitis: Sudden onset of fever and distinctive cellulitis in an infant, often involving the cheek or periorbital area, and starting as a mild swelling with central erythema that rapidly progresses to a lesion without a distinct border with central reddish discoloration, surrounded by and merging into purplish areas that fade peripherally.
- In all cases, a positive culture from the blood, cerebrospinal fluid, or aspirated pus confirm the diagnosis.

General Considerations

Haemophilus influenzae type b (HIB) is rapidly decreasing in incidence as a result of widespread immunization beginning in early infancy. The 95% reduction in disease seen in many parts of the USA is due to high rates of vaccine coverage and reduced nasopharyngeal carriage after vaccination. Although the incidence is reduced, the disease remains important because of its potential for serious invasive pathogenicity. It causes meningitis, bacteremia, epiglottitis (supraglottic croup), septic arthritis, periorbital and facial cellulitis, pneumonia, and pericarditis. HIB infections occur most frequently in the age group from 4 months to 4 years (epiglottitis: 2–5 years). Recognition and prompt therapy of the many serious manifestations of HIB infection will become more challenging as physicians encounter fewer infections.

Antibody to the HIB capsular polysaccharide, polyribose-phosphate (PRP) is protective against invasive disease. PRP is a poor immunogen, particularly in infants less than 2 years old. Vaccines consisting of PRP chemically conjugated to protein are far more immunogenic and raise protective levels of antibody in infants beginning at age 2 months. Four separate PRP protein conjugate vaccines are available (see Chapter 10).

Disease due to encapsulated *H influenzae* types A, C, D, E, or F is uncommonly seen but now comprises a larger proportion of positive cultures. Ampicillin-resistant HIB were first reported in 1974. Resistance is due to the production of plasmid-encoded β-lactamase in most cases. Currently, 25–40% of HIB strains in the USA are ampicillin-resistant. HIB resistant to chloramphenicol—or resistant to both ampicillin and chloramphenicol—are uncommon in the USA. Third-generation cephalosporins are preferred for initial therapy of suspected HIB infections. Resistance of HIB to the third-generation cephalosporins has not been reported, and the cephalosporins lack the hematologic toxicity of chloramphenicol. Ampicillin is adequate for culture-proved HIB where susceptibility to ampicillin has been proved by the microbiology laboratory.

Unencapsulated, nontypable *H influenzae* frequently colonize the mucous membranes and cause otitis media, sinusitis, bronchitis, and pneumonia in both children and adults. Bacteremia is uncommon but does occur. Neonatal sepsis similar to early onset group B streptococci is recognized. Obstetric complications of chorioamnionitis and bacteremia are associated with these neonatal cases.

Ampicillin resistance occurs in 25–40% of nontypable *H influenzae*.

Clinical Findings

A. Symptoms and Signs:

1. Meningitis–In the USA, HIB is responsible for about 80% of cases of bacterial meningitis in children after the neonatal period who have not received the HIB vaccine. In many other countries, this percentage is lower. Infants usually present with fever, irritability, lethargy, poor feeding with or without vomiting, and a high-pitched cry. Signs of localized disease elsewhere should be looked for carefully, including otitis, cellulitis, arthritis, and pneumonia.

2. Acute epiglottitis–The most useful clinical finding in the early diagnosis of HIB epiglottitis is evidence of dysphagia characterized by a refusal to eat or swallow saliva and by drooling. This finding, plus the presence of a high fever in a "toxic" child—even in the absence of cherry-red epiglottis on direct examination of the epiglottis—should strongly suggest the diagnosis and lead to prompt intubation. Stridor is a late sign. (See Chapter 19 for details.)

3. Septic arthritis–HIB is a common cause of bacterial septic arthritis in unimmunized children under 4 years of age in the USA. Disease may involve multiple joints and is complicated by osteomyelitis in about 20% of cases. The child is febrile and refuses to move the involved joint and limb because of pain. Examination reveals swelling, warmth, redness, tenderness on palpation, and severe pain on attempted movement of the joint.

4. Cellulitis–Cellulitis due to HIB occurs almost exclusively in the 3-month to 4-year age group. Fever is usually noted at the same time as the cellulitis, and many infants appear toxic. The cheek or periorbital (preseptal) area is usually involved. There is mild swelling with central erythema, rapidly progressing to a lesion without a distinct border that exhibits central reddish discoloration surrounded by a purplish area. Superficial trauma is characteristically absent. Bacteremia is frequent.

Periorbital cellulitis due to HIB must be distinguished from two other similar entities. The first is periorbital (preseptal) cellulitis caused by other bacteria. This frequently presents with evidence of a primary local infection nearby (conjunctivitis, sinusitis) or trauma to the skin. Staphylococci, streptococci, or a combination of the two is usually involved. Bacteremia is rare. The second is true orbital cellulitis. This disease is rare and occurs primarily in older children with ethmoid or sphenoid sinusitis. HIB is usually not involved.

5. Pneumonia–Pneumonia due to HIB usually presents clinically in much the same fashion as pneumonia due to the pneumococcus. Disease is most common in the age group from 3 months to 4 years, just as it is with *H influenzae* meningitis. Most cases are segmental or lobar in distribution, but diffuse bronchopneumonia or interstitial involvement is occasionally seen. Both empyema and lung abscesses occur. HIB involvement of other organs (meningitis, epiglottitis, otitis media) may be present.

The true incidence of HIB pneumonia is not known. Pneumonia due to unencapsulated *H influenzae* is difficult to diagnose because a small percentage have positive blood cultures.

6. Bacteremia–Acutely ill children 4–36 months of age, with temperatures higher than 39 °C and nonspecific symptoms associated with an elevated white blood cell count, may have HIB bacteremia. This syndrome is associated most frequently with pneumococcal bacteremia and next most frequently with HIB bacteremia.

B. Laboratory Findings:
The white blood cell count in HIB infections may be high or normal with a shift to the left. Blood culture is frequently positive. Positive culture of aspirated pus or fluid from the involved site or nearby proves the diagnosis.

In meningitis (before treatment), spinal fluid smear may show the characteristic pleomorphic gram-negative rods.

The diagnosis of HIB pneumonia depends on isolation of the organism from blood, lung tissue, or empyema fluid. A positive culture from the upper respiratory tract is not diagnostic. Detection of antigen in body fluids, including urine, may be helpful. Latex agglutination can be used to detect PRP, the capsular antigen of HIB in cerebrospinal fluid, joint fluid, urine, sputum, and serum. The test is particularly useful in the diagnosis of patients with meningitis or arthritis who have received antibiotic therapy and have negative cultures. Antigenemia may last from days to weeks in certain infants. PRP antigen may be detected in the urine for several days after immunization, and in two case reports it was detected for up to 21 days in cerebrospinal fluid.

C. Imaging:
A lateral view of the neck in suspected acute epiglottitis may be helpful but should not delay intubation. Haziness of maxillary and ethmoid sinuses occurs with orbital cellulitis.

Differential Diagnosis

A. Meningitis:
Meningitis must be differentiated from head injury, brain abscess, tumor, lead encephalopathy, and other forms of meningoencephalitis, including tuberculous meningitis, due to viral, fungal, and bacterial agents.

B. Acute Epiglottitis:
In croup caused by viral agents (parainfluenza 1, 2, and 3, respiratory syncytial virus, influenza A, adenovirus), the child has more definite upper respiratory symptoms, cough, hoarseness, slower progression of obstructive signs, and only low-grade fever. Spasmodic croup occurs typically at night in a child with a history of previous

attacks; these attacks may be of allergic origin. A history of sudden onset of choking and paroxysmal coughing suggests aspiration of a foreign body. Occasionally, retropharyngeal abscess or laryngeal diphtheria may have to be differentiated from epiglottitis.

C. Septic Arthritis: Differential diagnosis includes acute osteomyelitis, prepatellar bursitis, cellulitis, rheumatic fever, and fractures and sprains.

D. Cellulitis: Erysipelas, streptococcal cellulitis, insect bites, and trauma (including Popsicle panniculitis or other types of freezing injury) may occur. Periorbital cellulitis must be differentiated from paranasal sinus disease without cellulitis, allergic inflammatory disease of the lids, conjunctivitis, and herpes zoster infection.

E. Pneumonia: See Chapter 20.

F. Bacteremia: Sepsis due to other bacteria, including *S pneumoniae* and *N meningitidis,* must be differentiated by blood culture.

Complications

A. Meningitis: See Chapter 25.

B. Acute Epiglottitis: Mediastinal emphysema and pneumothorax may occur.

C. Septic Arthritis: Septic arthritis may result in rapid destruction of cartilage and ankylosis if diagnosis and treatment are delayed. Even with early treatment, the incidence of residual damage and disability after septic arthritis in weight-bearing joints may be as high as 25%.

D. Cellulitis: Bacteremia may lead to metastatic meningitis or pyarthrosis.

E. Pneumonia: Complications include empyema and, rarely, pneumatocele and pneumothorax.

F. Bacteremia: Meningitis, pneumonia, or other infected foci may develop. Children with HIB bacteremia should be evaluated thoroughly (including lumbar puncture) for infected foci. Inpatient management with intravenous antimicrobials is indicated until the child is afebrile and appears to be well.

Prevention

Epidemiologic studies have demonstrated that families and close contacts of patients with HIB infections are at increased risk of acquiring infection. The index case and all household contacts should be given rifampin, 20 mg/kg/d (maximum adult dose 600 mg/d), orally for 4 successive days. There is controversy regarding a recommendation for chemoprophylaxis for day-care-center contacts. Some authorities recommend rifampin chemoprophylaxis for young contacts (especially children age 2 or less) of a case who regularly attended a day-care center. Other authorities believe that the risk to day-care-center contacts is low and do not recommend prophylaxis unless two cases of systemic HIB disease have occurred in children in the day-care center within a 60-day period. Rifampin, if used, should be given to children in the same classroom as the index case and to adults working in that classroom.

Treatment

For comments regarding the problem of ampicillin-resistant strains of HIB, see General Considerations (above). All bacteremic or potentially bacteremic HIB diseases require hospitalization for treatment. The drugs of choice in hospitalized cases are a third-generation cephalosporin (cefotaxime or ceftriaxone) until the sensitivity of the organism is known.

Second-generation cephalosporins (cefuroxime, cefamandole, cefoxitin, and cefaclor) should not be used for any HIB infection in which meningitis is a possibility, since these drugs do not reach cerebrospinal fluid in concentrations adequate to treat or prevent infection. Cefuroxime is effective for nonmeningeal infections. Ceftriaxone or cefotaxime is preferred for meningitis because of more rapid and reliable sterilization of cerebrospinal fluid. Oral therapy with amoxicillin is preferred for susceptible strains. Several agents may be used for ampicillin-resistant strains or for those of unknown susceptibility. These include trimethoprim-sulfamethoxazole, erythromycin-sulfonamide combinations, cefaclor, amoxicillin-clavulanic acid, cefixime, loracarbef, cefpodoxime, and cefprozil. Penicillin, erythromycin alone, and first-generation cephalosporins are not reliable. Oral chloramphenicol is very effective but is less commonly used, since there are many other oral agents that do not pose the hematologic risk.

A. Meningitis: Therapy is begun as soon as bacterial meningitis has been identified and cerebrospinal fluid, blood, and other appropriate cultures have been obtained. Therapy is begun with cefotaxime (50 mg/kg intravenously every 6 hours) or ceftriaxone (50 mg/kg intravenously every 12 hours). If the organism is sensitive to ampicillin, it is the drug of choice. Therapy should preferably be given intravenously for the entire course; chloramphenicol may be given orally when tolerated (if it is used levels must be monitored), and ceftriaxone may be given intramuscularly if venous access becomes difficult.

Duration of therapy is 10 days. Although a 7-day regimen appears effective in most uncomplicated cases, it has not been studied in children who have also been treated with steroids to prevent hearing loss (see below). Longer treatment is reserved for those children who respond slowly or in whom septic complications have occurred. Antibiotics can be discontinued after 10 days in a febrile child if the clinical response was rapid and satisfactory, but the source of prolonged or recurrent fevers must always be sought with great care. The most common causes for recurrence of fever or persistence of fever beyond 6 days are the following: phlebitis, hospital-acquired viral or bacterial superinfection, metastatic disease requiring drainage (eg, subdural empyema, septic pericarditis, arthritis), drug fever, and subdural effusions. Fever commonly recurs after steroids are discontinued.

Repeated lumbar taps are usually not necessary in HIB meningitis. They should be obtained in the following circumstances: unsatisfactory or questionable clinical response, seizure occurring after several days of therapy, and prolonged (7 days) or recurrent fever if the neurologic examination is abnormal or difficult to evaluate. Routine lumbar tap at the end of therapy is not recommended. (See Chapter 25 for additional information.)

Supportive therapy with intravenous fluids and oxygen, should be given as required. Patients should be observed carefully for development of the syndrome of inappropriate ADH secretion (SIADH). Dexamethasone given immediately after diagnosis and continued for a period of 4 days may reduce the incidence of hearing loss in children with HIB meningitis. The use of dexamethasone is controversial, but when it is used, the dose is 0.6 mg/kg/d in four divided doses for 4 days. Therapy for longer than 4 days, for neonates, or for viral meningitis is not recommended. In animal models, it is important to give the dexamethasone prior to beginning antimicrobials; this maximally blocks formation of inflammatory mediators (interleukin-1β and tumor necrosis factor) thought responsible for eighth nerve damage.

B. Acute Epiglottitis: See Chapter 19.

C. Septic Arthritis: Initial therapy should include nafcillin (or another effective antistaphylococcal antibiotic), 150 mg/kg/d in four divided doses, and cefotaxime or ceftriaxone (dosage as for meningitis). If the isolate is sensitive to ampicillin, it is given in a dosage 200–300 mg/kg/d intravenously in four divided doses. This may be followed by oral amoxicillin (75–100 mg/kg/d in four divided doses every 6 hours) administered under careful supervision to complete a 2-week course. Oral agents for ampicillin-resistant organisms include chloramphenicol, cefaclor, trimethoprim-sulfamethoxazole, amoxicillin-clavulanic acid, and cefixime. Ideally, susceptibility to these agents should be proved prior to use. Drainage of infected joint fluid is an essential part of treatment. In joints other than the hip, this can often be accomplished by one or more needle aspirations. In hip infections—and in arthritis of other joints where treatment is delayed or clinical response is slow—open surgical drainage is advised. Local instillation of antibiotics is not necessary and may be injurious.

The joint should be immobilized. Antipyretics and analgesics are given as required, and adequate hydration is maintained.

D. Cellulitis and Orbital Cellulitis: Initial therapy should include an agent effective against staphylococci in combination with cefotaxime or ceftriaxone. Ampicillin may be used if the isolate is shown to be susceptible. Therapy is given parenterally for 3–7 days, followed by oral treatment as for septic arthritis,

and supportive and symptomatic treatment as required. There is usually marked improvement after 72 hours of treatment. Antibiotics should be given for 10–14 days.

E. Pneumonia: Initial therapy is with cefotaxime, ceftriaxone, or cefuroxime. In seriously ill children with pneumatocele or empyema, initial therapy should include nafcillin, 150–200 mg/kg/d in four divided doses, until *Staphylococcus* is proved not to be the cause. Ampicillin may be used if the HIB isolate is shown to be susceptible. Oxygen, intravenous fluids, and supportive care are given as needed. Treatment lasts 3 weeks. Empyema should be treated by placement of one or more chest tubes into the pleural space. When possible, a chest tube should be removed after 4 or 5 days.

Prognosis

The case fatality rate for HIB meningitis is less than 5%. Young infants have the highest mortality rate. Neurologic sequelae should be watched for but are appreciably reduced with prompt antibiotic treatment. One of the most common neurologic sequelae, which develops in approximately 5–10% of patients with HIB meningitis, is significant sensory neural hearing loss. All patients with HIB meningitis should have their hearing checked at some time during the course of the illness or shortly after recovery.

The case fatality rate in acute epiglottitis is 2–5%; deaths are associated with bacteremia and the rapid development of airway obstruction.

The prognosis for the other diseases requiring hospitalization is good with the institution of early and adequate antibiotic therapy.

Black SB, Shinefield HR: Immunization with oligosaccharide conjugate *Haemophilus influenzae* type b (HbOC) vaccine on a large health maintenance organization population: Extended follow-up and impact on *Haemophilus influenzae* disease epidemiology. Pediatr Infect Dis J 1992;11:610.

Black SB et al: Efficacy in infancy of oligosaccharide conjugate *Haemophilus influenzae* type b (HBOC) vaccine in a United States population of 61,080 children. Pediatr Infect Dis J 1991;10:99.

Cortese MM et al: Children with *Haemophilus influenzae* bacteremia initially treated as outpatients: Outcome in 85 American Indian children. Pediatr Infect Dis J 1992; 11:521.

Falla TJ et al: Population-based study of non-typable *Haemophilus influenzae* invasive disease in children and neonates. Lancet 1993;341:851.

Farley MM et al: Invasive *Haemophilus influenzae* disease in adults. Ann Int Med 1992;116:806.

Ginsburg CM et al: Report of 65 cases of *Haemophilus influenzae* b pneumonia. Pediatrics 1979;64:283.

Kinney JS et al: Early onset *Haemophilus influenzae* sepsis in the newborn infant. Pediatr Infect Dis J 1993;12:739.

Korones DN, Marshall GS, Shapiro ED: Outcome of children with occult bacteremia caused by *Haemophilus influenzae* type b. Pediatr Infect Dis J 1992;11:516.

Lebel MH, Freij BJ, Syrogiannopoulos GA: Dexamethasone therapy for bacterial meningitis: Results of two double-blind, placebo-controlled trials. N Engl J Med 1988;319:964.

Makintubee S, Istre GR, Ward JI: Transmission of invasive *Haemophilus influenzae* type b disease in day care settings. J Pediatr 1987;111:180.

Molteni RA: Epiglottitis. Incidence of extraepiglottic infection: Report of 72 cases and review of the literature. Pediatrics 1976;58:526.

Perkins M: False positive latex agglutination test in cerebrospinal fluid after immunization for *Haemophilus influenzae* type b. Pediatr Infect Dis J 1993;12:614.

Rotbart HA, Glode MP: *Haemophilus influenzae* type b septic arthritis in children; Report of 23 cases. Pediatrics 1985;75:254.

Takala AK et al: Vaccination with *Haemophilus influenzae* type b meningococcal protein conjugate vaccine reduces oropharyngeal carriage of *Haemophilus influenzae* type b among American Indian children. Pediatr Infect Dis J 1993;12:593.

Taylor HG et al: The sequelae of *Haemophilus influenzae* meningitis in school-age children. N Engl J Med 1990; 323:1657.

PERTUSSIS
(Whooping Cough)

Essentials of Diagnosis

- Prodromal catarrhal stage (1–3 weeks) characterized by mild cough, coryza, and fever.
- Persistent staccato, paroxysmal cough ending with a high-pitched inspiratory "whoop."
- Leukocytosis with absolute lymphocytosis.
- Diagnosis confirmed by fluorescent stain or culture of nasopharyngeal secretions.

General Considerations

Pertussis is an acute, highly communicable infection of the respiratory tract caused by *Bordetella pertussis* and characterized by severe bronchitis. Children usually acquire the disease from symptomatic family contacts. Adults who have mild respiratory illness, not recognized as pertussis, frequently are the source of infection. Asymptomatic carriage of *B pertussis* is not documented. Infectivity is greatest during the catarrhal and early paroxysmal cough stage (for about 4 weeks after onset).

The disease is most common and most severe in early infancy. Of 5500 reported cases in the USA in 1984 and 1985, 48% were in children less than one year of age, and 37% were in children less than 6 months of age. Seventy-four percent of infants aged 6 months or less were hospitalized; 20% had pneumonia, 2.6% had seizures, 0.8% had encephalopathy, and 1% died. In recent years, 3000–4000 cases were reported, but underreporting is likely.

Active immunity follows natural pertussis. Reinfections occur years to decades later but are usually mild. Immunity following immunization wanes in 5–10 years. The majority of young adults in the USA are susceptible to pertussis infection and disease is probably common but unrecognized.

Bordetella parapertussis causes a similar but milder syndrome and is reported frequently in central Europe.

B pertussis organisms attach to the ciliated respiratory epithelium and multiply there; deeper invasion does not occur. Disease is due to several bacterial toxins; the most potent is pertussis toxin, which is responsible for lymphocytosis and many of the symptoms of pertussis.

Clinical Findings

A. Symptoms and Signs: The onset of pertussis is insidious, with catarrhal upper respiratory tract symptoms (rhinitis, sneezing, and an irritating cough). Slight fever may be present; temperature greater than 38.3 °C suggests bacterial superinfection or another cause of respiratory tract infection. After about 2 weeks, cough becomes paroxysmal, characterized by 10–30 forceful coughs ending with a loud inspiration (the "whoop"). Infants and adults with otherwise typical, severe pertussis often lack characteristic whooping. Vomiting commonly follows a paroxysm. Coughing is accompanied by cyanosis, sweating, prostration, and exhaustion. This stage lasts for 2–4 weeks, with gradual improvement. Cough suggestive of chronic bronchitis lasts for another 2–3 weeks. Paroxysmal coughing may continue for some months in the absence of any infection and may worsen with intercurrent viral respiratory infection. In adults, older children, and partially immunized individuals, symptoms may consist only of low-grade fever and irritating cough lasting 1–2 weeks. In the younger unimmunized child, symptoms of pertussis last about 8 weeks or longer.

B. Laboratory Findings: White blood cell counts of 20,000–30,000/μL with 70–80% lymphocytes typically appear near the end of the catarrhal stage. Many older children and adults with mild infections never demonstrate lymphocytosis. The blood picture may resemble lymphocytic leukemia or leukemoid reactions. Identification of *B pertussis* by culture from nasopharyngeal swabs or nasal wash specimens proves the diagnosis. The organism may be found in the respiratory tract in diminishing numbers beginning in the catarrhal stage and ending about 2 weeks after the beginning of the paroxysmal stage. After 4–5 weeks of symptoms, cultures and fluorescent antibody tests are almost always negative. Fresh Bordet-Gengou agar or charcoal agar containing an antimicrobial should be inoculated as soon as possible; *B pertussis* does not tolerate drying nor prolonged transport. Serum agglutinins appear late in the infection and are of little value in diagnosis. Enzyme-linked immunosorbent assays for detection of antibody to pertussis toxin or filamentous hemagglutinin may be useful for diagnosis but are currently not widely available. The chest x-ray reveals thickened bronchi and sometimes shows a "shaggy" heart border, indicating bronchopneumonia and patchy atelectasis.

Differential Diagnosis

The differential diagnosis of pertussis includes bacterial, tuberculous, chlamydial, and viral pneumonia. Cystic fibrosis and foreign body aspiration may be considerations.

Adenoviruses and respiratory syncytial virus may cause paroxysmal coughing with an associated elevation of lymphocytes in the peripheral blood, mimicking pertussis.

Complications

Bronchopneumonia due to superinfection is the most common serious complication. It is characterized by abrupt clinical deterioration during the paroxysmal stage, accompanied by high fever and sometimes a striking leukemoid reaction with a shift to predominantly polymorphonuclear leukocytes. Atelectasis is a second common pulmonary complication. Atelectasis may be patchy or extensive and may shift rapidly to involve different areas of lung. Intercurrent viral respiratory infection is also a common complication and may provoke worsening or recurrence of paroxysmal coughing. Otitis media is common. Residual chronic bronchiectasis is infrequent despite the severity of the illness. Apnea and sudden death may occur during a particularly severe paroxysm. A diffuse encephalopathy of uncertain cause may complicate severe cases and frequently is fatal. It is unclear whether anoxic brain damage, cerebral hemorrhage, or pertussis neurotoxins are to blame, but anoxia is most likely the cause. Epistaxis and subconjunctival hemorrhages are common.

Prevention

Active immunization (see Chapter 10) with pertussis vaccine in combination with diphtheria and tetanus toxoids (DTP) should be given in early infancy. Acellular pertussis vaccines cause less fever and fewer local and febrile systemic reactions, but they are recommended only for the fourth and fifth doses. Pertussis cases have increased recently, probably due in part to the large number of children who are not adequately immunized and in part due to an increased incidence of the disease in adults.

Chemoprophylaxis with erythromycin should be given to exposed family and hospital contacts, particularly those under age 2 years, for 14 days. Hospitalized children with pertussis should be isolated because of the great risk of transmission to patients and staff. Several large hospital outbreaks have been reported in the last decade.

Treatment

A. Specific Measures: Antibiotics may ameliorate early infections but not those in the paroxysmal stage. Erythromycin is the drug of choice since it promptly terminates respiratory tract carriage of *B pertussis*. Patients should be treated with erythromycin estolate (40–50 mg/kg/24 h in four divided doses for 14 days). Erythromycin ethylsuccinate is efficacious, but the higher dose recommended causes considerable gastrointestinal intolerance. There is no clinical experience with clarithromycin or azithromycin. Ampicillin 100 mg/kg/d divided in four doses may be used for erythromycin-intolerant patients. Household or other close contacts such as in day care centers should be treated with erythromycin to reduce secondary transmission. This prophylaxis should be used regardless of age or immunization status.

Corticosteroids reduce the severity of disease but may mask signs of bacterial superinfection. Albuterol, 0.3–0.5 mg/kg/d in 4 doses, has reduced severity of illness, but tachycardia is common when the drug is given orally, and aerosol administration may precipitate paroxysms.

B. General Measures: Nutritional support during the paroxysmal phase is very important. Frequent small feedings, tube feeding, or parenteral fluid supplementation may be needed. Minimizing stimuli that trigger paroxysms is probably the best way of controlling cough. In general, cough suppressants are of little benefit.

C. Treatment of Complications: Respiratory insufficiency due to pneumonia or other pulmonary complications should be treated with oxygen and assisted ventilation if necessary. Convulsions are treated with oxygen and anticonvulsants. Bacterial pneumonia or otitis media may require additional antibiotics.

Prognosis

The prognosis for patients with pertussis has improved in recent years because of adequate nursing care, treatment of complications, nutrition, and modern intensive care. However, the disease is still very serious in infants under 1 year of age; most deaths occur in this age group. Children with encephalopathy have a poor prognosis.

Edwards KM: Acellular pertussis vaccines: A solution to the pertussis problem? J Infect Dis 1993;168:15.

Etkind P et al: Pertussis outbreaks in groups claiming religious exemptions to vaccinations. Am J Dis Child 1992;146:173.

Gan VN, Murphy TV: Pertussis in hospitalized children. Am J Dis Child 1990;144:1130.

Hoppe JE: Comparison of erythromycin estolate and erythromycin ethylsuccinate for treatment of pertussis. Pediatr Infect Dis J 1992;11:189.

Long SS et al: Widespread silent transmission of pertussis in families: Antibody correlates of infection and symptomatology. J Infect Dis 1990;161:480.

Nkowane BM et al: Pertussis epidemic in Oklahoma. Am J Dis Child 1986;140:433.

Placebo-controlled trial of two acellular pertussis vaccines in Sweden: Protective efficacy and adverse events. Lancet 1988;1:954.

Report of the Task Force on Pertussis and Pertussis Immunization: 1988. Pediatrics 1988;81.

Roberts I, Gavin R, Lennon D: Randomized controlled trial of steroids in pertussis. Pediatr Infect Dis J 1992;11:982.

Sutter RW, Cochi SL: Pertussis hospitalizations and mortality in the United States, 1985–1988. JAMA 1992:267:386.

LISTERIOSIS

Essentials of Diagnosis

Early-onset of neonatal disease:
• Signs of sepsis a few hours after birth in an infant born with fetal distress; hepatosplenomegaly. Maternal fever.

Late-onset neonatal disease:
• Meningitis, sometimes with monocytes in the cerebrospinal fluid and peripheral blood. Onset at 9–30 days of age.

General Considerations

Listeria monocytogenes is a gram-positive, non-spore-forming aerobic rod distributed widely in the animal kingdom and in food, dust, and soil. It causes systemic infections in newborn infants and immunosuppressed older children. In pregnant women, infection is relatively mild, with fever, aches, and chills, but it is accompanied by bacteremia and sometimes results in intrauterine or perinatal infection with grave consequences for the fetus or newborn. In 1986, 1700 cases and 450 deaths due to *L monocytogenes* are estimated to have occurred. One-fourth of the cases occurred in pregnant women, and 20% of these perinatal cases resulted in stillbirth or neonatal death. *Listeria* is present in the stool of approximately 10% of the normal population. Persons in contact with animals seem to be at particular risk. Recent large food-borne outbreaks have been traced to contaminated cabbage in coleslaw, contaminated soft cheese, and milk. The role of contaminated food in sporadic listeriosis is now recognized.

Like group B streptococcal infections, *Listeria* infections in the newborn can be divided into early and late forms. Early infections are more common and are frequently severe and generalized, sometimes leading to granulomatosis infantiseptica, a severe congenital form of infection. Later infections are often characterized by meningitis.

Clinical Findings

A. Symptoms and Signs: In the early neonatal form, symptoms usually appear on the first day of life and always by the third day. Infants are frequently premature and have signs of fetal distress. Respiratory distress, diarrhea, and fever occur. On examination, hepatosplenomegaly and a papular rash are found. A history of maternal fever is common. Meningitis may accompany the septic course.

The late neonatal form usually occurs after 9 days of age and can occur as late as 5 weeks. Meningitis is common, characterized by irritability, fever, and poor feeding.

Listeria infections occur rarely in older children, usually in those with animal contact or those who are immunosuppressed. Signs and symptoms are those of meningitis, usually with insidious onset.

B. Laboratory Findings: In all patients except those receiving white cell depressant drugs, the white blood cell count is elevated, with 10–20% monocytes. When meningitis is found, the characteristic cell count is high (> 500/μL) with a predominance of polymorphonuclear leukocytes in 70% of cases; monocytes predominate in up to 30%. The chief pathologic feature in severe neonatal sepsis is miliary granulomatosis with microabscesses in liver, spleen, central nervous system, lung, and bowel.

In meningitis, gram-stained smears of cerebrospinal fluid are usually negative, but the short gram-positive rods may be seen.

Cultures are frequently positive from multiple sites, including blood in the infant and the mother. The organisms form small, weakly hemolytic colonies on blood agar and may be mistaken for streptococci.

Differential Diagnosis

Early-onset neonatal disease resembles hemolytic disease of the newborn, group B streptococcal sepsis or severe cytomegalovirus infection, rubella, or toxoplasmosis. Late-onset disease must be differentiated from meningitis due to echovirus and coxsackievirus, group B streptococci, and gram-negative enteric bacteria.

Prevention

Immunosuppressed, pregnant, and elderly patients can decrease the risk of *Listeria* infection by avoiding soft cheeses and by thoroughly reheated or avoiding ready-to-eat foods. These recommendations include avoiding raw meat and milk, and thorough washing of vegetables by all persons.

Treatment

Ampicillin (150–300 mg/kg/d every 6 hours intravenously) is the drug of choice in most cases. Gentamicin (2.5 mg/kg every 8 hours intravenously) should also be given, since it has a synergistic effect with ampicillin in vitro. If ampicillin cannot be used, trimethoprim-sulfamethoxazole is also effective. Cephalosporins are not effective. Treatment of severe disease should continue for at least 2 weeks.

Prognosis

In a recent outbreak of early-onset neonatal disease, the mortality rate was 27% despite aggressive and appropriate management. Meningitis in older infants has quite a good prognosis. In immunosuppressed children, prognosis depends to a great extent on that of the underlying illness.

Cherubin CE et al: Epidemiological spectrum and current treatment of listeriosis. Rev Infect Dis 1991;13:1108.

Foodborne listeriosis, United States 1988–1990: Update. MMWR Morb Mortal Wkly Rep 1992:41:251.

Gellin BG et al: The epidemiology of listeriosis in the United States—1986. Listeriosis Study Group. Am J Epidemiol 1991;133:392.

Lennon D et al: Epidemic perinatal listeriosis. Pediatr Infect Dis J 1984;3:30.

Linnan MJ et al: Epidemic listeriosis associated with Mexican-style cheese. N Engl J Med 1988;319:823.

Schlech WF III et al: Epidemic listeriosis: Evidence for transmission by food. N Engl J Med 1983;308:203.

Schuchat A et al: Role of foods in sporadic listeriosis. I. Case-control study of dietary risk factors. JAMA 1992; 267:2041.

Visintine AM, Oleske JM, Nahmias AJ: *Listeria monocytogenes.* Infection in infants and children. Am J Dis Child 1977;131:393.

TUBERCULOSIS

Essentials of Diagnosis

- All types: Positive tuberculin test in patient or members of household, suspicious chest x-ray, history of contact, and demonstration of organism by stain and culture.
- Pulmonary: Fatigue, irritability, and undernutrition, with or without fever and cough.
- Glandular: Chronic cervical adenitis.
- Miliary: Classic "snowstorm" appearance of chest x-ray; choroidal tubercles.
- Meningitis: Fever and manifestations of meningeal irritation and increased intracranial pressure. Characteristic cerebrospinal fluid.

General Considerations

Tuberculosis is a granulomatous disease caused by *Mycobacterium tuberculosis.* It remains a leading cause of death throughout the world. Children under 3 years of age are most susceptible, and lymphohematogenous dissemination through the lungs and spread to extrapulmonary sites, including the brain and meninges, eyes, bones and joints, lymph nodes, kidneys, intestines, larynx, and skin, are more likely to occur in infants. Increased susceptibility occurs again in adolescence, particularly in girls within 2 years of menarche. Tuberculosis in the USA has increased substantially since 1986 following 3 decades of decline. In 1990, 25,071 cases were reported. Certain high-risk groups are identified, including ethnic minorities, foreign-born persons, prisoners, residents of nursing homes, indigents, migrant workers, and health care providers. HIV infection is an important

risk factor both for development and spread of disease. Pediatric tuberculosis is also increasing, with 1596 cases in children under age 15 reported in 1990. Exposure to an adult at risk for tuberculosis is the most common risk factor in children. The primary complex in infancy and childhood consists of a small parenchymal lesion in any area of the lung with caseation of regional nodes and calcification. Postprimary tuberculosis in adolescents and adults occurs in the apexes of the lungs and is likely to cause chronic, progressive cavitary pulmonary disease with less tendency for hematogenous dissemination.

Clinical Findings

A. Symptoms and Signs:

1. Pulmonary–See Chapter 20.

2. Miliary–Diagnosis is made on the basis of a classic snowstorm or millet seed appearance of lung fields on x-ray, though early in the course of disseminated tuberculosis the chest x-ray may show no or only subtle abnormalities. The majority also have a fresh primary complex and pleural effusion. Choroidal tubercles are sometimes seen on funduscopic examination. Other lesions may be present and produce osteomyelitis, arthritis, meningitis, tuberculomas of the brain, enteritis, or infection of the kidneys and liver.

3. Meningitis–Symptoms include fever, vomiting, headache, lethargy, and irritability, with signs of meningeal irritation and increased intracranial pressure, including cranial nerve palsies, convulsions, and coma. Choroidal tubercles are pathognomonic when associated with these signs and symptoms. Otorrhea or acute otitis media may be seen.

4. Glandular–The primary complex may be associated with a skin lesion drained by regional nodes or chronic cervical node enlargement and infection of the tonsils. Involved nodes may become fixed to the overlying skin and suppurative, and they may drain.

B. Laboratory Findings: The Mantoux test (0.1 mL of intermediate strength PPD [5 TU] inoculated intradermally) is read as positive at 48–72 hours if there is significant induration (Table 36–1). False-negative results are seen in malnourished patients, those with overwhelming disease, and in a few percent of children with isolated pulmonary disease. Temporary suppression of tuberculin reactivity may also be seen with viral infections (eg, measles, influenza, varicella, mumps), after live virus immunization, and when corticosteroids or other immunosuppressive drugs are present. The two commercially available reagents for Mantoux testing give discrepant results in some cases. For this reason, every Mantoux test should be accompanied by intradermal injection of control antigens (such as *Candida albicans* or tetanus toxoid) that are usually positive in persons with normal immune response. When tuberculosis is suspected and the child is anergic, household members and adult contacts (eg, teachers) should also be

Table 36–1. Interpretation of tuberculin skin test reactions.[1]

Degree of Risk	Risk Factors	Positive Reaction
High	Recent close contact with a case of active tuberculosis. Chest radiograph compatible with tuberculosis. Immunocompromise. Patients with HIV infection.	≥ 5 mm induration
Medium	Current or previous residence in high-prevalence area (Asia, Africa, Latin America). Recent skin test converters within 2 years. Intravenous drug use. Homelessness, or residence in a correctional institution. Recent weight loss or malnutrition. Leukemia, Hodgkin's disease, diabetes mellitus.	≥ 10 mm induration
Low	All others	≥ 15 mm induration

[1]Standard intradermal Mantoux test, 5 test units.

tested immediately. Multiple puncture tests (tine tests) are associated with false-negative and false-positive reactions. Furthermore, a positive tine test is not sufficient for diagnosis, necessitating a Mantoux test. The subsequent Mantoux test may lead to "boosting" and a false-positive reaction. Because of these problems, tine tests should not be used.

The erythrocyte sedimentation rate is usually elevated. Cultures of pooled early morning gastric aspirates from three successive days will yield *M tuberculosis* in about 40% of cases. Biopsy may be necessary to establish the diagnosis in some cases. Therapy should not be delayed in suspected cases. The cerebrospinal fluid in tuberculous meningitis shows slight to moderate pleocytosis (50–300 white blood cells, predominantly lymphocytes), decreased glucose, and increased protein.

The direct detection of mycobacteria in body fluids or discharges is best done by staining specimens with auramine O and examining them with blue-light fluorescence microscopy; this is superior to the Ziehl-Neelsen method.

C. Imaging: Chest x-ray should be obtained in all children with suspicion of tuberculosis at any site or with a positive skin test. Segmental consolidation with some volume loss and hilar adenopathy are common findings in children. Pleural effusion also occurs with primary infection. Cavities and apical disease are unusual.

Differential Diagnosis

Pulmonary tuberculosis must be differentiated from fungal, parasitic, mycoplasmal, and bacterial pneumonias; lung abscess; foreign body aspiration; lipoid pneumonia; sarcoidosis; and mediastinal cancer. Cervical lymphadenitis is most apt to be due to streptococcal or staphylococcal infections. Cat-scratch fever and infection with atypical mycobacte-

ria may need to be distinguished from tuberculous lymphadenitis also. Viral meningoencephalitis, head trauma (battered child), lead poisoning, brain abscess, acute bacterial meningitis, brain tumor, and disseminated fungal infections must be excluded in tuberculous meningitis. The skin test in the patient or family contacts is frequently valuable in differentiation of these conditions from tuberculosis.

Prevention

A. BCG Vaccine: BCG vaccines are live attenuated strains of *M bovis*. Although this BCG is often routinely given to infants and children in countries with a high prevalence of tuberculosis, protective efficacy varies greatly with vaccine potency and method of delivery. In the USA, BCG vaccination is considered only for tuberculin-negative children and neonates in high-risk situations who are unlikely to receive isoniazid (INH) prophylaxis or close follow-up , or who are at high risk of exposure to persons infected with *M tuberculosis* resistant to isoniazid and rifampin (see Chapter 10).

B. Isoniazid (INH) Chemoprophylaxis: Daily administration of isoniazid (10 mg/kg/d orally; maximum 300 mg) is advised for children who cannot avoid intimate household contact with adolescents or adults with active disease. Isoniazid is given until 3 months after last contact. At the end of this time, a Mantoux test should be done, and therapy should be continued for 9 months if it is positive. BCG is not recommended during the period of isoniazid chemoprophylaxis.

C. Other Measures: Tuberculosis in infants and young children is evidence of recent exposure to active infection in an adult. The source contact (index case) should be identified, isolated, and treated to prevent other secondary cases. Reporting cases to local health departments is essential for contact tracing. Exposed tuberculin-negative children should be skin-tested every 2 months for 6 months after contact has been terminated. Routine tuberculin skin testing is advised at 12–15 months of age, prior to school entry, and again in adolescence. Yearly testing of school children is recommended in high-risk populations, including children from socioeconomically deprived neighborhoods and those from high-risk foreign countries.

Treatment

A. Specific Measures: Most children in the USA are hospitalized initially. If the infecting organism has not been isolated for susceptibility testing from the presumed contact, reasonable attempts should be made to obtain it from the child using gastric aspirates, sputum induction, bronchoscopy, thoracentesis, etc. Cooperation with outpatient therapy must be assured.

All children with positive skin tests (see Table 36–1) without overt disease should receive 9 months of isoniazid (10 mg/kg/d orally, maximum 300 mg) therapy. In children with overt pulmonary disease, therapy for 6–9 months using isoniazid (10 mg/kg/d), rifampin (15 mg/kg/d), and pyrazinamide (25–30 mg/kg/d) in a single daily oral dose for 2 months, followed by isoniazid plus rifampin (either in a daily or twice-weekly regimen) for 4 months appears effective for isoniazid-susceptible organisms. For more severe disease, such as miliary or central nervous system infection, duration is increased to 12 months or more, and a fourth drug (streptomycin or ethambutol) is added for the first 2 months.

1. Isoniazid–The hepatotoxicity seen in adults and some adolescents is rare in children. Transient elevation of transaminases (up to three times normal) may be seen at 6–12 weeks, but therapy is continued unless clinical illness occurs. Routine monitoring of liver function tests is unnecessary. Peripheral neuropathy associated with pyridoxine deficiency is rare in children, and it is not necessary to add pyridoxine unless significant malnutrition coexists.

2. Rifampin–Although an excellent bactericidal agent, rifampin is never used alone due to rapid development of resistance. Hepatotoxicity may be seen but rarely with recommended doses. The orange discoloration of secretions is benign.

3. Pyrazinamide–This excellent sterilizing agent has most effect during the first 2 months of therapy; with the recommended duration and dosing, it is well tolerated. Although it elevates the uric acid level, it rarely causes symptoms of hyperuricemia in children. Use of this drug is now common for tuberculous disease in children; resistance is almost unknown. Oral acceptance and central nervous system penetration are good.

4. Ethambutol–Since color blindness and optic neuritis are the major side effects, ethambutol is usually given only to children who can be reliably vision tested every 2 months. This complication occurs in a few percent of patients, usually those receiving more than the recommended dosage of 15 mg/kg/d.

5. Streptomycin–Streptomycin, 20–30 mg/kg/d intramuscularly in one or two doses) should be given in severe disease. Hearing should be tested periodically during use.

B. Chemotherapy for Drug-Resistant Tuberculosis: The incidence of drug resistance is increasing and nationally averages 5–10%. Transmission of multiply resistant strains to contacts have resulted in some epidemics. In areas with high rates of resistance, it may be necessary to begin therapy with four drugs pending susceptibility testing. Consultation of local laboratories or experts in treating tuberculosis is important. Therapy should continue for 12 months or longer.

C. General Measures:

1. Corticosteroids–These drugs may be used for suppressing inflammatory reactions in meningeal, pleural, and pericardial tuberculosis and for the relief of bronchial obstruction due to hilar adenopathy. Prednisone is given orally, 1 mg/kg/d for 6–8 weeks, with gradual withdrawal at the end of that time.

2. Bed rest–Rest in bed is indicated only while the child feels ill. Isolation is necessary only for children with draining lesions or renal disease and those with chronic pulmonary tuberculosis. Most children with tuberculosis are noninfectious and can attend school while being treated.

Prognosis

If bacteria are sensitive and treatment is completed, most patients make lasting recovery. Re-treatment is more difficult and less successful. With antituberculosis chemotherapy (especially isoniazid), there should now be nearly 100% recovery in miliary tuberculosis. Without treatment, the mortality rate in both miliary tuberculosis and tuberculous meningitis is almost 100%. In the latter form, about two-thirds of treated patients survive. There may be a high incidence of neurologic abnormalities among survivors if treatment is started late.

Biddulph J, Kokoha V, Sharma S: Short course chemotherapy in childhood tuberculosis. J Trop Pediatr 1988;34:20.

Grossman M et al: Consensus: Management of tuberculin-positive children without evidence of disease. Pediatr Infect Dis J 1988;7:243.

Iseman MD: Treatment of multidrug-resistant tuberculosis. N Engl J Med 1993;329:784.

Jacobs RF et al: Intensive short course chemotherapy for tuberculous meningitis. Pediatr Infect Dis J 1992;11:194.

Lifson AR et al: Discrepancies in tuberculin skin test results with two commercial products in a population of intravenous drug users. J Infect Dis 1993;168:1048.

Nemir RL, Krasinski K: Tuberculosis in children and adolescents in the 1980's. Pediatr Infect Dis J 1988;7:375.

Nemir RL, O'Hare D: Tuberculosis in children 10 years of age and younger: Three decades of experience during the chemotherapeutic era. Pediatrics 1991;88:236.

Reis FJ et al: Six-month isoniazid-rifampin treatment for pulmonary tuberculosis in children. Am Rev Respir Dis 1990;142:996.

Screening for tuberculosis and tuberculous infection in high risk populations and the use of preventive therapy for tuberculous infection in the United States. MMWR 1990; 39:1.

Starke JR: Childhood tuberculosis in the 1990's. Pediatric Annals 1993;22:550.

Visudhiphan P, Chiemchanya S: Tuberculous meningitis in children: Treatment with isoniazid and rifampicin for twelve months. J Pediatr 1989;114:875.

INFECTIONS WITH NONTUBERCULOUS MYCOBACTERIA

Essentials of Diagnosis

- Chronic unilateral cervical lymphadenitis.
- Granulomas of the skin.

- Chronic bone lesion with draining sinus (chronic osteomyelitis).
- Reaction to PPD-S (standard) of 5–8 mm, negative chest x-ray, and negative history of contact with tuberculosis.
- Positive skin reaction to a specific atypical antigen.
- Diagnosis by positive acid-fast stain or culture.
- Disseminated infection in patients with AIDS.

General Considerations

Various species of acid-fast mycobacteria other than *Mycobacterium tuberculosis* may cause subclinical infections and, occasionally, clinical disease closely simulating tuberculosis. Strains of nontuberculous mycobacteria are common in soil, food and water. Organisms enter the host by small abrasions in skin, oral mucosa, or gastrointestinal mucosa. Strain cross-reactivity with *M tuberculosis* can be demonstrated by simultaneous skin testing (Mantoux) with PPD-S (standard) and PPD prepared from one of the atypical antigens (available from the CDC). The larger skin reaction suggests infection with the homologous strain.

The Runyon classification of mycobacteria includes the following:

Group I: Photochromogens (PPD-Y): Yellow color develops upon exposure to light in previously white colony grown 2–4 weeks in the dark. Group 1 includes *Mycobacterium kansasii* and *Mycobacterium marinum.*

Group II: Scotochromogens (PPD-G): Colonies are definitely yellow-orange after incubation in the dark. Organisms may be found in small numbers in the normal flora of some human saliva and gastric contents. Subclinical infection is widespread in the USA, but clinical disease appears rarely. Group II includes *Mycobacterium scrofulaceum.*

Group III: Nonphotochromogens (PPD-B): "Battey avian-swine group" grows as small white colonies after incubation in the dark, with no significant development of pigment upon exposure to light. Infection with *Mycobacterium avium* complex is prevalent on the East Coast of the USA, particularly the Southeast. Patients with acquired immunodeficiency syndrome (AIDS) commonly are infected.

Group IV: "Rapid growers": *Mycobacterium fortuitum* and *Mycobacterium chelonei* are the recognized pathogens. Within 1 week after inoculation, they form colonies closely resembling *M tuberculosis* morphologically.

Clinical Findings

A. Symptoms and Signs:

1. Lymphadenitis–In children, the commonest form of infection due to mycobacteria other than tuberculosis is cervical lymphadenitis. *M scrofulaceum* or *M avium* complex is almost always the cause. A submandibular node swells slowly and is firm and usually nontender. Over time, the node suppurates and may drain chronically. Nodes in other areas of the head and neck and elsewhere are sometimes involved. There is no fever or toxicity.

2. Pulmonary disease–In the western USA, this is usually due to *M kansasii;* in the eastern USA, it may be due to *M avium* complex. In other countries, disease is usually caused by *M avium* complex. In adults, there is usually underlying chronic pulmonary disease, but in children, this is often not the case. Immunologic deficiency may be present. Presentation is clinically indistinguishable from that of tuberculosis. Patients with cystic fibrosis may be infected with nontuberculous mycobacteria. It may be difficult to differentiate infection from colonization in these patients with chronic symptoms.

3. Swimming pool granuloma–This is due to *M marinum.* A solitary chronic granulomatous lesion, frequently on the elbow, develops after minor trauma in infected swimming pools. Minor trauma in home aquariums or other aquatic environments also may lead to infection.

4. Chronic osteomyelitis–Osteomyelitis is caused by *M kansasii, M scrofulaceum,* or "rapid growers." Findings include swelling and pain over a distal extremity, radiolucent defects in bone, fever, and clinical and x-ray evidence of bronchopneumonia. Such cases are rare.

5. Meningitis–Disease is due to *M kansasii* and may be indistinguishable from tuberculous meningitis.

6. Disseminated infection–Rarely apparently immunologically normal children develop disseminated infection due to nontuberculous mycobacteria. Children are ill, with fever and hepatosplenomegaly, and organisms are demonstrated in bone lesions, lymph nodes, or liver. Chest x-rays are usually normal. Sixty to 80 percent of AIDS patients will acquire *M avium* complex infection characterized by fever, night sweats, weight loss, and diarrhea. Infection usually indicates severe immune dysfunction and is associated with low CD4 lymphocyte counts.

B. Laboratory Findings:
In most cases, there is a small reaction (< 10 mm) when Mantoux testing is done with PPD-S. Larger reactions may be seen. The chest x-ray is negative, and there is no history of contact with tuberculosis. Needle aspiration of the node excludes bacterial infection and may yield acid-fast bacilli on stain or culture. Fistulization should not be a problem because total excision follows if the infection is due to atypical mycobacteria. If other organisms are found, formal excision may be avoided. Excision is usually required if aspiration is nondiagnostic and the clinical findings support the diagnosis. If performed, simultaneous tuberculin testing with the infecting atypical antigen (PPD-Y,-G, or -B) will usually give a reaction greater than the reaction to PPD-S.

Cultures of any normally sterile body site will yield *M avium* complex in immunocompromised patients with disseminated disease. Blood cultures are positive, with a large density of bacteria.

Differential Diagnosis

See section on differential diagnosis in the discussion of tuberculosis above and in Chapter 20.

Treatment

A. Specific Measures: The usual treatment of lymphadenitis is complete surgical excision. Chemotherapy is neither necessary nor sufficient for cure. Occasionally, resolution of the adenopathy is under way when the diagnosis is made. In these cases, careful follow-up is adequate.

Response of extensive adenopathy or other forms of infection varies according to the infecting species and susceptibility. Recent data suggest that isoniazid, rifampin, and streptomycin with or without ethambutol (depending on sensitivity to isoniazid) will result in a favorable response in almost all patients with *M kansasii* infection. Chemotherapeutic treatment of *M avium* complex is much less satisfactory as resistance to isoniazid, rifampin, and pyrazinamide is usual. Susceptibility testing is necessary to optimize therapy. Most authors favor surgical excision of involved tissue if possible and treatment with at least three drugs to which the organism has been shown to be sensitive. Disseminated disease in patients with AIDS calls for a combination of three or more active drugs. Effective drugs may include ethionamide, capreomycin, amikacin, clofazimine, rifabutin, ciprofloxacin, and cycloserine. New macrolides such as clarithromycin and azithromycin are very promising. *M fortuitum* and *M chelonei* are usually susceptible to amikacin plus erythromycin or doxycycline and may be successfully treated with such combinations. Swimming pool granuloma due to *M marinum* is usually self-limited but may be treated either with drugs or by surgical excision with good results.

B. General Measures: Isolation of the patient is usually not necessary. General supportive care is indicated for the child with disseminated disease.

Prognosis

The prognosis is good for localized disease, though fatalities occur in immunocompromised children with disseminated disease.

Benjamin DR: Granulomatous lymphadenitis in children. Arch Pathol Lab Med 1987;111:750.

Contreras MA et al: Pulmonary infection with nontuberculous mycobacteria. Am Rev Respir Dis 1988;137:149.

Gill MJ, Fanning EA, Chomyc S: Childhood lymphadenitis in a harsh northern climate due to atypical mycobacteria. Scand J Infect Dis 1987;19:77.

Horsburgh CR Jr: *Mycobacterium avium* complex infection in the acquired immunodeficiency syndrome. N Engl J Med 1991;324:1332.

Levin RH, Bolinger AM: Treatment of nontuberculous my-

cobacterial infections in pediatric patients. Clin Pharm 1988;7:545.

Lowry PW et al: *Mycobacterium chelonei* causing otitis media in an ear-nose-and-throat practice. N Engl J Med 1988;319:978.

Margileth AM: Management of nontuberculous (atypical) mycobacterial infections in children and adolescents. Pediatr Infect Dis J 1985;4:119.

Street ML et al: Nontuberculous mycobacterial infections of the skin. Report of 14 cases and a review of the literature. J Am Acad Dermatol 1991;24:208.

Woods GL, Washington JA: Mycobacteria other than *Mycobacterium tuberculosis:* Review of microbiologic and clinical aspects. Rev Infect Dis J 1987;9:275.

LEGIONELLA INFECTION

Essentials of Diagnosis

- Severe progressive pneumonia in a child with compromised immunity.
- Diarrhea and neurologic signs are common.
- Positive culture requires buffered charcoal yeast extract media and proves infection.
- Direct fluorescent antibody staining of respiratory secretions proves infection.

General Considerations

Legionella pneumophila is an ubiquitous gramnegative bacillus that causes two distinct clinical syndromes: Legionnaires' disease and Pontiac fever. Legionnaires' disease is an acute, severe pneumonia that is frequently fatal in immunocompromised patients. Pontiac fever is a mild, nonpneumonic, flu-like illness characterized by fever, headache, myalgia, and arthralgia. The disease is self-limited and is described in outbreaks in otherwise healthy adults.

Twenty-two different species of *Legionella* have been discovered. *Legionella* is present in many natural water sources as well as domestic water supplies (faucets, showers). Contaminated cooling towers and heat exchangers have been implicated in several large institutional outbreaks. Sporadic, community-acquired cases also occur, and the source of infection is not usually clear. Person-to-person transmission has not been documented.

Few cases of Legionnaires' disease have been reported in children. Most have been children with compromised cellular immunity or children receiving steroids. In adults, risk factors include smoking, underlying cardiopulmonary or renal disease, alcoholism, and diabetes.

L pneumophila is thought to be acquired by inhalation of a contaminated aerosol. The bacteria are phagocytosed but proliferate within macrophages. Cell-mediated immunity is necessary to activate macrophages to kill intracellular bacteria.

Clinical Findings

A. Signs and Symptoms: Onset of fever,

chills, anorexia, and headache is abrupt. Pulmonary symptoms occur within 2–3 days but progress rapidly. The cough is nonproductive early on. Purulent sputum occurs late. Hemoptysis, diarrhea, and neurologic signs (including lethargy, irritability, tremors, and delirium) are seen.

B. Laboratory Findings: White blood count is usually elevated. Chest radiographs show rapidly progressive, patchy consolidation. Cavitation and large pleural effusions are uncommon. Cultures from sputum, tracheal aspirates, or bronchoscopic specimens, when grown on buffered yeast charcoal extract media, are positive in 50–70% of patients at 3–7 days. Direct fluorescent antibody staining of sputum or other respiratory specimens is only 70–75% sensitive but 95% specific. As such, a negative culture or direct fluorescent antibody staining of sputum or tracheal secretions does not rule out Legionnaires' disease. Serologic tests are available and aid in diagnosis, but a maximum rise in titer may require 6–8 weeks.

Differential diagnosis

Legionnaires' disease is usually a rapidly progressive pneumonia in a patient who appears very ill with unremitting fevers. Other bacterial pneumonias, viral pneumonias, *Mycoplasma* pneumonia, and fungal disease are all possibilities and may be difficult to differentiate on clinical grounds in an immunocompromised patient.

Complications

In sporadic untreated cases, mortality rates are 5–25%. In untreated immunocompromised patients, mortality approaches 80%. Hematogenous dissemination may result in extrapulmonary foci of infection, including pericardium, myocardium, and renal involvement. *Legionella* may present as "culture-negative" endocarditis.

Prevention

No vaccine is available. Hyperchlorination and periodic superheating of water supplies in hospitals have been shown to reduce the number of organisms and the frequency of cases.

Treatment

Erythromycin (40–50 mg/kg/d in four divided doses, orally or intravenously) results in clinical improvement in 48–72 hours. Rifampin (20 mg/kg/d divided in two doses) is very active in vitro and is also given to gravely ill patients. Therapy is continued for 21 days to reduce the likelihood of relapse.

Prognosis

Mortality is frequent if Legionnaires' disease is not recognized and appropriately treated. Malaise, problems with memory, and fatigue are common problems in patients after recovery.

Carlson NC et al: Legionellosis in children: An expanding spectrum. Pediatr Infect Dis J 1990;9:133.

Esposito AL, Gantz NM: Legionnaires' disease: The distance travelled since Philadelphia. Pediatr Infect Dis J 1986;5:163.

Greene KA et al: Fatal postoperative *Legionella* pneumonia in a newborn. J Perinatol 1990;10:183.

Helms CM et al: Legionnaires' disease associated with a hospital water system. JAMA 1988;259:2423.

Hervas JA, Alomar P: Multiple organ system failure in an infant with *Legionella* infection. Pediatr Infect Dis J 1988;7:671.

Lowry PW et al: A cluster of *Legionella* sternal wound infection due to postoperative topical exposure to contaminated tap water. N Engl J Med 1991;324:109.

Meyer RD: *Legionella* infections: A review of five years of research. Rev Infect Dis 1983;5:258.

Tompkins LS: *Legionella* prosthetic-valve endocarditis. N Engl J Med 1988;318:530.

PSITTACOSIS (ORNITHOSIS) & *CHLAMYDIA PNEUMONIAE* INFECTION

Essentials of Diagnosis

- Fever, cough, malaise, chills, headache.
- Diffuse rales; no consolidation.
- Long-lasting x-ray findings of bronchopneumonia.
- Isolation of the organism or rising titer of complement-fixing antibodies.
- Exposure to infected birds.

General Considerations

Psittacosis is caused by *Chlamydia psittaci.* When the agent is transmitted to humans from psittacine birds (parrots, parakeets, cockatoos, and budgerigars), the disease is often called **psittacosis** or **parrot fever.** However, other avian genera (pigeons, turkeys) are common sources of infection in the USA, and the general term **ornithosis** is often used. About 100 cases per year are reported in the USA. The agent is an obligatory intracellular parasite. Human-to-human spread occurs rarely. The incubation period is 5–21 days with a mean of 15 days. The bird from whom the disease was transmitted may not be clinically ill.

Recently, a new strain of *Chlamydia,* designated the TWAR agent or *C pneumoniae,* has been found to cause an atypical pneumonia in previously well individuals. Transmission is by respiratory spread. Infection appears to become prevalent during the second decade; half of surveyed adults are seropositive. Only a small percentage of infections result in clinical pneumonia. The disease may be more common than atypical pneumonia due to *M pneumoniae.* Lower respiratory tract infection due to *C pneumoniae* is uncommon in infants and young children.

Clinical Findings

A. Symptoms and Signs:

1. *C psittaci*–The disease is extremely variable but tends to be mild in children. The onset is rapid or insidious, with fever, chills, headache, backache, malaise, myalgia, and dry cough. Signs include those of pneumonitis, alteration of percussion note and breath sounds, and rales. Pulmonary findings may be absent early. Splenomegaly, epistaxis, prostration, and meningismus are occasionally seen. Delirium, constipation or diarrhea, and abdominal distress may occur. Dyspnea and cyanosis may occur later.

2. *C pneumoniae*–Clinically, *C pneumoniae* infection is very similar to *M pneumoniae* infection. Most are mild upper respiratory infections. Lower tract infection is characterized by fever, sore throat (perhaps more severe with *C pneumoniae*), cough, and bilateral pulmonary findings and infiltrates. Prolonged symptoms in some patients suggest that therapy with erythromycin or tetracycline may have to be more prolonged than that usually given for *Mycoplasma*.

B. Laboratory Findings: In psittacosis, the white blood cell count is normal or decreased, often with a shift to the left. Proteinuria is frequently present. *C psittaci* is present in the blood and sputum during the first 2 weeks of illness and can be isolated by inoculation of clinical specimens into mice or embryonated hens' eggs, but culture is available only in research laboratories. Complement-fixing antibodies appear during or after the second week, and a fourfold rise or a single titer ≥ 1:32 suggests the diagnosis. The rise in titer may be minimized or delayed by early chemotherapy. Infection with C pneumoniae may lead to diagnostic confusion because cross-reactive antibody may cause falsely positive C psittaci titers. Serologic tests for *C pneumoniae* are now available in reference laboratories.

C. Imaging: The x-ray findings in psittacosis are those of central pneumonia, which later becomes widespread or migratory. Psittacosis is indistinguishable from viral pneumonias by x-ray. Signs of pneumonitis may appear by x-ray in the absence of clinical suspicion of pulmonary involvement.

Differential Diagnosis

Psittacosis can be differentiated from acute viral pneumonias only by the history of contact with potentially infected birds. In severe or prolonged cases with extrapulmonary involvement, the differential diagnosis includes a wide spectrum of diseases such as typhoid fever, brucellosis, rheumatic fever, etc.

Complications

Complications of psittacosis include myocarditis, endocarditis, hepatitis, pancreatitis, and secondary bacterial pneumonia. *C pneumoniae* infection may be prolonged or recur.

Treatment

For psittacosis, tetracyclines in full doses should be given for 14 days. Erythromycin is an alternative for children under 9 years of age. Supportive oxygen may be needed. The patient should be kept in isolation. The role of the expanded-spectrum macrolides is not yet clear. *C pneumoniae* responds to either erythromycin or tetracycline.

Aldous MB, Grayston JT, Wang SP: Seroepidemiology of *Chlamydia pneumoniae* TWAR infection in Seattle families, 1966–1979. J Infect Dis 1992;166:646.

Byrom NP, Wells J, Mair HJ: Fulminant psittacosis. Lancet 1979;1:353.

Crosse BA: Psittacosis: A clinical review. J Infect 1990; 21:251.

Hammerschlag MR et al: Persistent infection with *Chlamydia pneumoniae* following acute respiratory illness. Clin Infect Dis 1992;14:178.

Ozanne G, Lefebvre J: Specificity of the microimmunofluorescence assay for the serodiagnosis of *Chlamydia pneumoniae* infections. Can J Microbiol 1992;38:1185.

Thom DH et al: *Chlamydia pneumoniae* strain TWAR, *Mycoplasma pneumoniae,* and viral infections in acute respiratory disease in a University student health clinic population. Am J Epidemiol 1990;132:248.

CAT-SCRATCH DISEASE

Essentials of Diagnosis

- History of a cat scratch or cat contact.
- Primary lesion (papule, pustule, conjunctivitis) at site of inoculation.
- Acute or subacute regional lymphadenopathy.
- Aspiration of sterile pus from a node.
- Laboratory studies excluding other causes.
- Biopsy of node or papule showing histopathologic findings consistent with cat-scratch disease and occasionally characteristic bacilli on Warthin-Starry stain.
- Positive cat-scratch serology (antibody to *Rochalimaea henselae*).

General Considerations

Cat-scratch disease is a benign, self-limiting form of lymphadenitis. Patients often report a cat scratch (67%) or contact with a cat or kitten (90%). The cat almost invariably is healthy. The clinical picture is that of a regional lymphadenitis associated with an erythematous papular skin lesion without intervening lymphangitis. The disease occurs worldwide and is more common in the fall and winter. It is estimated that more than 20,000 cases per year occur in the USA. The most common systemic complication is encephalitis.

After some years of controversy and vacillation, the etiologic agent of cat-scratch disease has now been identified as *Bartonella henselae,* a gram-negative bacillus that also causes bacillary angiomatosis.

Clinical Findings

A. Symptoms and Signs: About 50% of patients develop a primary lesion at the site of inoculation, though some authors report a much higher percentage. The lesion usually is a papule or pustule and is located most often on the arm or hand (50%), head or leg (30%), or trunk or neck (10%). The lesion may be conjunctival (10%). Regional lymphadenopathy appears 10–30 days later and may be accompanied by mild malaise, lassitude, headache, and fever. Multiple sites are seen in about 10% of cases. Involved nodes may be hard or soft and 1–6 cm in diameter. They are usually tender, and about 25% of them suppurate. The overlying skin may or may not be inflamed. Lymphadenopathy usually resolves in about 2 months, but it may persist for up to 8 months.

Unusual manifestations include nonpruritic maculopapular rash, erythema multiforme or nodosum, purpura, conjunctivitis (Parinaud's oculoglandular fever), parotid swelling, pneumonia, chronic sinus drainage, osteolytic lesions, mesenteric and mediastinal adenitis, peripheral neuritis, hepatosplenomegaly, and encephalitis.

B. Laboratory Findings: Antigens prepared from pus aspirated from nodes of infected individuals have been used for skin testing. Because they are poorly standardized antigens and are not available commercially, their use is discouraged. The skin test is positive in more than 90% of patients thought to have cat-scratch disease and 5% of normal controls.

Histopathologic examination of involved nodes shows characteristic changes that are nondiagnostic unless the organism is demonstrated. The lymph node architecture is distorted by multiple areas of central necrosis with acidophilic staining. These areas are surrounded by foci of epithelioid cells and scattered giant cells of the Langhans type. There is usually some elevation in the sedimentation rate. In cases with central nervous system involvement, the cerebrospinal fluid is usually normal but may show a slight pleocytosis and modest elevation of protein. All routine cultures, including anaerobic, fungal, and mycobacterial culture, are negative.

A serologic test for *R henselae* is now available and appears to be diagnostically useful.

Differential Diagnosis

Cat-scratch disease must be distinguished from pyogenic adenitis, tuberculosis (typical and atypical), tularemia, plague, brucellosis, Hodgkin's disease, lymphoma, rat-bite fever, primary toxoplasmosis, infectious mononucleosis, lymphogranuloma venereum, and fungal infections.

Treatment

The best therapy is reassurance that the adenopathy is benign and will subside spontaneously within 4–8 weeks in most cases. In cases of suppuration, node aspiration under local anesthesia with an 18- to 19-gauge needle relieves the pain. Excision of the involved node is indicated in cases of chronic adenitis. Antimicrobial therapy has not been proved to alter the course of illness; gentamicin and ciprofloxacin have been useful anecdotally in a few severe infections, and trimethoprim-sulfamethoxazole has also been useful in some cases.

Prognosis

The prognosis is good if complications do not occur.

Bogue CW et al: Antibiotic therapy for cat scratch disease. JAMA 1989;262:813.

Carithers HA: Cat-scratch disease: An overview based on a study of 1200 patients. Am J Dis Child 1985;139:1124.

Collipp PJ: Cat-scratch disease: therapy with trimethoprim-sulfamethoxazole. Am J Dis Child 1992;146:397.

Holley HP Jr: Successful treatment of cat-scratch disease with ciprofloxacin. JAMA 1991;265:1563.

Malatack JJ, Jaffe R: Granulomatous hepatitis in three children due to cat-scratch disease without peripheral adenopathy: An unrecognized cause of fever of unknown origin. Am J Dis Child 1993;147:949.

Margileth AM, Hayden GF: Cat scratch disease. N Engl J Med 1993;329:53.

Margileth AM, Wear DJ, English CK: Systemic cat scratch disease: Report of 23 patients with prolonged or recurrent severe bacterial infection. J Infect Dis 1987;155:390.

Relman DA et al: The agent of bacillary angiomatosis: An approach to the identification of uncultured pathogens. N Engl J Med 1990;323:1573.

Shinall EA: Cat scratch disease: a review of the literature. Pediatr Dermatol 1990;7:11.

Zangwill KM et al: Cat scratch disease in Connecticut. N Engl J Med 1993;329:8.

SPIROCHETAL INFECTIONS

SYPHILIS

Essentials of Diagnosis

Congenital:

- All types: History of untreated maternal syphilis, a positive serologic test, and a positive darkfield examination.
- Newborn: Hepatosplenomegaly, characteristic x-ray bone changes, anemia, increased nucleated red cells, thrombocytopenia, abnormal spinal fluid, jaundice, edema.
- Young infant (3–12 weeks): Snuffles, maculopapular skin rash, mucocutaneous lesions, pseudoparalysis (in addition to x-ray bone changes).
- Children: Stigmas of early congenital syphilis

(saddle nose, Hutchinson's teeth, etc), interstitial keratitis, saber shins, gummas of nose and palate.

Acquired:

- Chancre of genitals, lip, or anus in child or adolescent. History of sexual contact.

General Considerations

Syphilis is a chronic, generalized infectious disease caused by a slender spirochete, *Treponema pallidum.* In the acquired form, the disease is transmitted by sexual contact. Primary syphilis is characterized by the presence of an indurated painless chancre, which heals in 7–10 days. A secondary eruption involving the skin and mucous membranes appears in 4–6 weeks. After a long latency period, late lesions of tertiary syphilis involve the eyes, skin, bones, viscera, central nervous system, and cardiovascular system.

Congenital syphilis results from transplacental infection. Characteristic disease occurs after the fourth month of gestation and may result in stillbirth or manifest illness in the newborn, in early infancy, or later in childhood. First-trimester fetal infection has been found in the products of conception in therapeutic abortions. Syphilis occurring in the newborn and young infant is comparable to secondary disease in the adult but is more severe and life-threatening. Late congenital syphilis (developing in childhood) is comparable to tertiary disease.

Congenital syphilis is increasing in the USA due to increasing primary and secondary syphilis in women of childbearing age, and perhaps due to inadequate diagnosis and treatment of syphilis in prenatal care programs. Prostitution in women addicted to crack cocaine has been associated with a more than 500% increase in congenital syphilis in New York City.

Clinical Findings

A. Symptoms and Signs:

1. Congenital syphilis–

a. Newborns–Most newborns with congenital syphilis are asymptomatic. If not detected and treated, symptoms develop within several weeks to months. When clinical signs are present, they usually consist of jaundice, anemia with or without thrombocytopenia, increase in nucleated red blood cells, hepatosplenomegaly, and edema. There may be overt signs of meningitis (bulging fontanelle, opisthotonos), but subclinical infection with cerebrospinal fluid abnormalities is more likely.

b. Young infants (3–12 weeks)–The infant may appear normal for the first few weeks of life only to develop "snuffles," a syphilitic skin eruption, mucocutaneous lesions, and pseudoparalysis of the arms or legs. Shotty lymphadenopathy may sometimes be felt. Hepatomegaly is universal, with splenomegaly in 50%. Other signs of disease seen in the newborn may be present. Anemia has been reported as the only presenting manifestation of congenital syphilis in this age group. "Snuffles" (rhinitis) is characterized by a profuse mucopurulent discharge that excoriates the upper lip and is present in 25%. A syphilitic rash is common on the palms and soles but may occur anywhere on the body; it consists of bright red, raised maculopapular lesions that gradually fade. Moist lesions occur at the mucocutaneous junctions (nose, mouth, anus, genitals) and lead to fissuring and bleeding.

Syphilis in the young infant may lead to stigmas recognizable in later childhood, such as rhagades (scars) around the mouth or nose, a "saddle" nose, and a high forehead (secondary to mild hydrocephalus associated with low-grade meningitis and frontal periostitis). The permanent upper central incisors may be peg-shaped with a central notch (Hutchinson's teeth), and the cusps of the sixth-year molars may have a lobulated mulberry appearance.

c. Children–Bilateral interstitial keratitis (at 6–12 years) is characterized by photophobia, increased lacrimation, and vascularization of the cornea associated with exudation. Chorioretinitis and optic atrophy may also be seen. Meningovascular syphilis (at 2–10 years) is usually slowly progressive, with mental retardation, spasticity, abnormal pupil response, speech defects, and abnormal spinal fluid. Deafness sometimes occurs. Thickening of the periosteum of the anterior tibias produces saber shins. A bilateral effusion into the knee joints (Clutton's joints) may occur but is not associated with sequelae. Gummas may develop in the nasal septum, palate, long bones, and subcutaneous tissues.

2. Acquired syphilis–The primary chancre of the genitals, mouth, or anus may occur as a result of intimate sexual contact. If the chancre is missed, signs of secondary syphilis , such as rash, fever, headache and malaise, may be the first manifestation of the disease.

B. Laboratory Findings:

1. Darkfield microscopy–Treponemes can be seen in scrapings from a chancre and from moist lesions.

2. Serologic tests for syphilis (STS)–There are two general types of serologic tests for syphilis: treponemal and nontreponemal. The latter (Venereal Disease Research Laboratory, or VDRL) is useful for screening and follow-up of known cases. A rapid test (the rapid plasma reagin, or RPR) is useful for screening, but positive sera should be further examined by quantitative nontreponemal and treponemal tests. Positive nontreponemal tests are confirmed with more specific fluorescent treponemal antibody absorption, or FTA-ABS test. False-positive FTA-ABS tests are uncommon except with other spirochetal disease.

One or 2 weeks after the onset of primary syphilis (chancre), the FTA-ABS test becomes positive. The VDRL or a similar nontreponemal test usually turns positive a few days later. By the time the secondary stage has arrived, virtually all patients show both positive FTA-ABS and positive nontreponemal tests. During latent and tertiary syphilis, the VDRL may become negative, but the FTA-ABS test usually remains positive. The quantitative VDRL or a similar nontreponemal test should be used to follow treated cases (see below).

Positive serologic tests in cord sera may represent passively transferred antibody rather than congenital infection and therefore must be supplemented by a combination of clinical and laboratory data. Elevated total cord IgM is a helpful but nonspecific finding. A specific IgM-FTA-ABS is available, but negative results are not conclusive and should not be relied upon. Demonstration of characteristic treponemes by darkfield examination of material from a moist lesion (skin, nasal or other mucous membranes) is definitive. Serial measurement of quantitative VDRL is also very useful, since passively transferred antibody in the absence of active infection should decay with a normal half-life of about 18 days.

In one study, 15% of infants with congenital syphilis had negative cord blood serology, presumably due to maternal infection late in pregnancy.

C. Imaging: Radiographic abnormalities are present in 90% of infants with symptoms of congenital syphilis and 20% of asymptomatic infants. Metaphysial lucent bands, periostitis, and a widened zone of provisional calcification may be present. Bilateral symmetric osteomyelitis with pathologic fractures of the medial tibial metaphyses (Wimberger's sign) is almost pathognomonic.

Differential Diagnosis
A. Congenital Syphilis:

1. Newborns–Sepsis, congestive heart failure, congenital rubella, toxoplasmosis, disseminated herpes simplex, cytomegalovirus infection, and hemolytic disease of the newborn have to be differentiated. Positive Coombs test and blood group incompatibility distinguish hemolytic disease.

2. Young infants–Pseudoparalysis (a flaccid paralysis) occurs in poliomyelitis. Signs of scurvy do not appear until the latter half of the first year of life. Injury to the brachial plexus, acute osteomyelitis, and septic arthritis must be differentiated from pseudoparalysis. Coryza due to viral infection will often respond to symptomatic treatment. Rash (ammoniacal diaper rash) and scabies may be confused with a syphilitic eruption.

3. Children–Interstitial keratitis and bone lesions of tuberculosis are distinguished by positive tuberculin reaction and chest x-ray. Arthritis associated with syphilis is unaccompanied by systemic signs, and joints are not tender. Mental retardation, spasticity, and hyperactivity are shown to be of syphilitic origin by strongly positive serologic tests.

B. Acquired Syphilis: Herpes genitalis, traumatic lesions, and other venereal diseases must be differentiated.

Prevention
A serologic test for syphilis should be performed at the initiation of prenatal care and repeated once during pregnancy. In mothers at high risk of syphilis, repeated tests may be necessary. Serologic tests for syphilis may be negative on both the mother and the baby at the time of birth if the mother acquired syphilis near term. Adequate treatment of mothers with secondary syphilis before the last month of pregnancy reduces the incidence of congenital syphilis from 90% to less than 2%. Examination and serology of sexual partners and siblings should also be done.

Treatment
A. Specific Measures: Penicillin is the drug of choice for *T pallidum*. If the patient is allergic to penicillin, erythromycin or one of the tetracyclines may be used.

1. Congenital syphilis–Infants with positive serology should be fully evaluated: history of maternal disease and therapy, CBC, liver function tests, long bone radiographs, cerebrospinal fluid examination, and quantitative serologic tests.

Treatment is indicated for infants with physical signs, abnormal radiographs, elevated cerebrospinal fluid protein or cell counts, or reactive cerebrospinal fluid VDRL. In addition, infants born to inadequately treated mothers or mothers treated with nonpenicillin drugs should be treated. If there are no clinical or laboratory signs of syphilis, the infant may be followed at monthly intervals with quantitative serologic tests and physical examinations if follow-up is ensured. Rising titers or clinical signs usually occur within 4 months in infants with infection. Infants with suspected congenital syphilis should have roentenography of the long bones and a cerebrospinal fluid examination.

Infants with proved or suspected congenital syphilis should receive either of the following: (1) aqueous crystalline penicillin G, 50,000 units/kg/dose intramuscularly or intravenously every 12 hours (if < 1 week old) or every 8 hours (if between 1 and 4 weeks of age) for 10–14 days; or (2) aqueous procaine penicillin G, 50,000 units/kg/d intramuscularly for a minimum of 10 days. All infants diagnosed after 4 weeks of age should receive 50,000 units/kg/dose intramuscularly or intravenously every 6 hours for 10–14 days. Because treatment failures in early congenital syphilis may be due to low levels of benzathine penicillin in the cerebrospinal fluid and the eye—and because cerebrospinal fluid serology may fail to detect central nervous system infection—benzathine penicillin is no longer recommended for proved or strongly suspected congenital syphilis. Asymptomatic seropositive infants with normal cerebrospinal fluid born to adequately treated mothers may be given benzathine penicillin G (50,000 units/kg intramuscularly in a single dose) with follow-up serologic examinations at 1, 2, 3, 6, and 12 months. For larger children, the total dose of penicillin need not exceed the dosage used in adult syphilis of more than 1 year's duration.

Follow-up quantitative VDRL or RPR tests should be performed at 2, 4, 6, and 12 months after the end of therapy or should be repeated until they become nonreactive. Repeat cerebrospinal fluid examination every 6 months for 3 years is indicated for infants with a positive cerebrospinal fluid VDRL reaction. Titers decline with treatment and are usually negative by 12 months. Re-treatment is indicated for rising titers or stable titers that do not decline.

2. Acquired syphilis–Benzathine penicillin G, 50,000 units/kg up to a maximum of 2.4 million units to adolescents with primary, secondary, or latent disease less than 1 year's duration. Late latent disease and neurosyphilis require weekly therapy for 3 weeks.

B. General Measures: Care should be given to the maintenance of adequate nutrition.

Penicillin treatment of early congenital or secondary syphilis may result in a febrile Jarisch-Herxheimer reaction. Treatment is symptomatic, with careful follow-up and aspirin or acetaminophen, although transfusion may be necessary in infants with severe hemolytic anemia.

Prognosis

Severe disease, if unexpected, may be fatal in the newborn. Complete cure can be expected if the young infant is treated with penicillin. Serologic reversal usually occurs within 1 year. Treatment of primary syphilis with penicillin is curative. Permanent neurologic sequelae may be seen with meningovascular syphilis.

Beck-Sague C, Alexander ER: Failure of benzathine penicillin G treatment in early congenital syphilis. Pediatr Infect Dis J 1987;6:1061.

Dunn RA, Zenker PN: Why radiographs are useful in evaluation of neonates suspected of having congenital syphilis. Radiology 1992;182:639.

Dorfman DH, Glaser JH: Congenital syphilis presenting in infants after the newborn period. N Engl J Med 1990; 323:1299.

Hook EW III, Marra CM: Acquired syphilis in adults. (Medical Progress.) N Engl J Med 1992;326:1060.

Johns DR, Tierney M, Felsenstein D: Alteration in the natural history of neurosyphilis by concurrent infection with the human immunodeficiency virus. N Engl J Med 1987; 316:1569.

Ricci JM, Fojaco RM, O'Sullivan MJ: Congenital syphilis: The University of Miami/Jacksonville Memorial Medical Experience—1986–1988. Obstet Gynecol 1989;74: 687.

Sanchez PJ: Congenital syphilis. Adv Pediatr Infect Dis 1992;7:161.

Wright MS, Tecklenburg FW: Critical illness in congenital syphilis after the newborn period. Clin Pediatr 1992; 31:247.

Zenker PN, Berman FM: Congenital syphilis: Trends and recommendations for valuation and management. Pediatr Infect Dis J 1991;10:516.

RELAPSING FEVER

Essentials of Diagnosis

- Episodes of fever, chills, malaise.
- Occasional rash, arthritis, cough, hepatosplenomegaly, conjunctivitis.
- Diagnosis confirmed by direct microscopic identification of spirochetes in smears of peripheral blood.

General Considerations

Relapsing fever is a vector-borne disease caused by spirochetes of the genus *Borrelia*. Epidemic relapsing fever is transmitted to humans by body lice *(Pediculus humanus)* and endemic relapsing fever by soft-bodied ticks (genus *Ornithodoros*).

Tick-borne relapsing fever is endemic in the western USA. Transmission usually takes place during the warm months, when ticks are active and recreation or work brings people into contact with *Ornithodoros* ticks. Mountain camping areas and cabins are sites where infection often is acquired. The ticks are nocturnal feeders and remain attached for only 5–20 minutes. Consequently, the patient seldom remembers a tick bite.

Rarely, neonatal relapsing fever results from transplacental transmission of *Borrelia*. Both louse-borne and tick-borne relapsing fever may be acquired during foreign travel.

Clinical Findings

A. Symptoms and Signs: The incubation period is 4–18 days. The attack is sudden, with high fever, chills, tachycardia, nausea and vomiting, headache, myalgia, arthralgia, bronchitis, and a dry, nonproductive cough. Hepatomegaly and splenomegaly appear later. Meningeal irritation may be present. An erythematous rash may be seen over the trunk and extremities, and petechiae may be present. After 3–10 days, the fever falls by crisis. Jaundice, iritis, conjunctivitis, cranial nerve palsies, and hemorrhage are more common during relapses.

The disease is characterized by relapses lasting 3–5 days, occurring at intervals of 1–2 weeks, with interim asymptomatic periods. The relapses duplicate the initial attack but become progressively less severe. In louse-borne relapsing fever, there is usually a single relapse; in tick-borne infection, there are two to six relapses.

B. Laboratory Findings: During febrile episodes, the urine contains protein, casts, and, occasionally, erythrocytes; there is a marked polymorphonuclear leukocytosis and, in about one-fourth of cases, a false-positive serologic test for syphilis. Spirochetes can be found in the peripheral blood by direct microscopy in approximately 70% of cases by darkfield examination or by Wright, Giemsa, or acridine orange staining of thick and thin smears. They are not found during afebrile periods. The blood may be injected into young mice and the spirochetes found 1–14 days later in the tail blood. OXK agglutinin titers in serum may be positive.

Differential Diagnosis

Relapsing fever may be confused with malaria, leptospirosis, dengue, yellow fever, typhus, rat-bite fever, Colorado tick fever, Rocky Mountain spotted fever, collagen vascular disease, or any fever of unknown origin.

Complications

Complications include facial paralysis, iridocyclitis, optic atrophy, hypochromic anemia, pneumonia, nephritis, myocarditis, endocarditis, and seizures. Central nervous system involvement is seen in 10–30% of cases.

Treatment

For children under 7 years of age with tick-borne relapsing fever, erythromycin (40–50 mg/kg/d orally in divided doses every 6 hours for 10 days) should be given. Older children may be given tetracycline instead. Penicillin and chloramphenicol are also efficacious.

In louse-borne relapsing fever, a single dose of tetracycline or erythromycin has been effective.

Severely ill patients should be hospitalized. Antibiotic treatment should be started after the fever has dropped; this will lessen the risk of severe or even fatal Jarisch-Herxheimer reaction. Isolation precautions are not necessary.

Prognosis

The mortality rate in treated cases is very low, except in debilitated or very young children. With treatment, the initial attack is shortened and relapses prevented. The response to antimicrobial therapy is dramatic.

Le CT: Tick-borne relapsing fever in children. Pediatrics 1980;66:963.

Outbreak of relapsing fever—Grand Canyon National Park, Arizona, 1990. MMWR Morb Mortal Wkly Rep 1991; 40:296.

Perine PL, Teklu B: Antibiotic treatment of louse-borne relapsing fever in Ethiopia: A report of 377 cases. Am J Trop Med Hyg 1983;32:1096.

Relapsing fever: New lessons about antibiotic action. (Editorial.) Ann Intern Med 1985;102:397.

Sciotto CG et al: Detection of *Borrelia* in acridine orange–stained blood smears by fluorescence microscopy. Arch Pathol Lab Med 1983;107:384.

Spach DH et al: Tick-borne diseases in the United States. N Engl J Med 1993;329:936.

LEPTOSPIROSIS

Essentials of Diagnosis

- Biphasic course lasting 2 or 3 weeks.
- Initial phase: high fever, headache, myalgia, and conjunctivitis.
- Apparent recovery for 2–3 days.
- Return of fever associated with meningitis.
- Jaundice, hemorrhages, and renal insufficiency (severe cases).
- Culture of organism from blood and cerebrospinal fluid (early) and from urine (later), or direct microscopy of urine or cerebrospinal fluid.
- Positive leptospiral agglutination test.

General Considerations

Leptospirosis is a zoonosis caused by many antigenically distinct but morphologically similar spirochetes. The organism enters through the skin or respiratory tract. Classically, the severe form—Weil's disease, with jaundice and a high mortality rate—was associated with infection with *Leptospira icterohaemorrhagiae* following immersion in water contaminated with rat urine. It is now known that a variety of animals (dogs, rats, cattle, etc) may serve as reservoirs for pathogenic *Leptospira,* that a given serogroup may have multiple animal species as hosts, and that severe disease may be caused by many different serogroups other than *L icterohaemorrhagiae.*

In the USA, leptospirosis occurs in children, students, and housewives due to contact with dogs. Cattle, swine, or rodents may transmit the organism. Sewer workers, farmers, abattoir workers, animal handlers, and soldiers are at risk of occupational exposure. Outbreaks have resulted from swimming in contaminated streams and harvesting field crops.

In the USA, about 100 cases are reported yearly, and about one-third are in children.

Clinical Findings

A. Symptoms and Signs:

1. Initial phase–The incubation period is 4–19 days, with a mean of 10 days. Chills, fever, headache, myalgia, conjunctivitis (episcleral injection), photophobia, cervical lymphadenopathy, and pharyngitis occur commonly. This leptospiremic phase lasts for 3–7 days.

2. Phase of apparent recovery–Symptoms typically (but not always) subside for 2–3 days.

3. Systemic phase–Fever reappears and is associated with headache, muscular pain and tenderness in the abdomen and back, and nausea and vomiting. Lung, heart, and joint involvement occasionally occurs. These manifestations are due to extensive vasculitis.

a. Central nervous system involvement–The central nervous system is involved in 50–90% of cases. Severe headache and mild nuchal rigidity are usual, but delirium, coma, and focal neurologic signs may be seen.

b. Renal and hepatic involvement–In about 50% of cases, the kidney or liver or both are affected. Gross hematuria and oliguria or anuria are sometimes seen. Jaundice may be associated with an enlarged and tender liver.

c. Gallbladder involvement–Leptospirosis may cause acalculous cholecystitis in children. An abdominal ultrasound study may reveal a dilated, nonfunctioning gallbladder. Pancreatitis is unusual.

d. Hemorrhage–Petechiae, ecchymoses, and gastrointestinal bleeding may be severe.

e. Rash–A rash is seen in 10–30% of cases. It may be maculopapular and generalized or may be petechial or purpuric. Occasionally, erythema nodosum is seen. Peripheral desquamation of the rash may occur. Gangrenous areas are sometimes noted over the distal extremities. In such cases, skin biopsy demonstrates the presence of severe vasculitis involving both the arterial and the venous circulations.

B. Laboratory Findings: Leptospires are present in the blood and cerebrospinal fluid only during the first 10 days of illness. They appear in the urine during the second week, where they may persist for 30 days or longer. The organism can be isolated from blood inoculated into Fletcher's semisolid medium or EMJH semisolid medium, but culture techniques are slow (7–10 days), difficult, and not generally available.

The white blood cell count often is elevated, especially when there is liver involvement. Serum bilirubin levels usually remain below 20 mg/dL. Other liver function tests may be abnormal, although the AST usually shows only slight elevation. An elevated serum creatinine phosphokinase is frequently found. Cerebrospinal fluid shows moderate pleocytosis ($< 500/\mu L$) predominantly mononuclear cells, increased protein (50–100 mg/dL), and normal glucose. Urine often shows microscopic pyuria, hematuria, and, less often, proteinuria (++ or greater). The erythrocyte sedimentation rate is markedly elevated. Chest x-ray may show pneumonitis.

The serologic test of choice is a microscopic agglutination test using live organisms (performed at the Centers for Disease Control and Prevention, Atlanta, GA 30333). Leptospiral agglutinins generally reach peak levels by the third to fourth week. A 1:100 titer is considered suspicious; a fourfold or greater rise is diagnostic.

Differential Diagnosis

Fever and myalgia associated with the characteristic conjunctival (episcleral) injection should suggest leptospirosis. During the prodrome, malaria, typhoid fever, typhus, rheumatoid arthritis, brucellosis, and influenza may be suspected. Later, depending on the organ systems involved, a variety of other diseases need to be distinguished, including encephalitis, viral or tuberculous meningitis, viral hepatitis, glomerulonephritis, viral or bacterial pneumonia, rheumatic fever, subacute infective endocarditis, acute surgical abdomen, and Kawasaki disease (see Table 35–3).

Prevention

Preventive measures include the avoidance of contaminated water and soil, the use of rodent control, immunization of dogs and other domestic animals, and good sanitation. Immunization or antimicrobial prophylaxis with doxycycline may be of value to certain high-risk occupational groups.

Treatment

A. Specific Measures: Aqueous penicillin G (150,000 units/kg/d in four to six divided doses intravenously for 7–10 days) should be given when the diagnosis is suspected. Recent studies in severely ill patients indicate a benefit even if started 4 days into the illness. A Jarisch-Herxheimer reaction may be seen. Tetracycline (40–50 mg/kg/d) may be used for mildly ill patients.

B. General Measures: Symptomatic and supportive care is indicated, particularly for renal and hepatic failure and hemorrhage.

Prognosis

Leptospirosis generally is anicteric and self-limiting. The disease usually lasts 1–3 weeks but may be more prolonged. Relapse may occur.

There are usually no permanent sequelae associated with central nervous system infection, though headache may persist. The mortality rate in reported cases in the USA is 5%, usually from renal failure. The mortality rate may reach 20% or more in elderly patients who have severe kidney and hepatic involvement.

Gollop JH et al: Rat-bite leptospirosis. West J Med 1993; 159:76.

Lecour H et al: Human leptospirosis: A review of 50 cases. Infection 1989;17:8.

Peter G: Leptospirosis: A zoonosis of protean manifestations. Pediatr Infect Dis 1982;1:282.

Schmidt DR et al: Leptospirosis. Epidemiological features of a sporadic case. Arch Int Med 1989;149:1878.

Takafuji ET et al: An efficacy trial of doxycycline chemoprophylaxis against leptospirosis. N Engl J Med 1984; 310:497.

Watt G et al: Placebo-controlled trial of intravenous penicillin for severe and late leptospirosis. Lancet 1988;1:433.

Watt G et al: Limulus lysate positivity and Herxheimer-like reactions in leptospirosis: A placebo controlled study. J Infect Dis 1990;162:564.

LYME DISEASE

Essentials of Diagnosis

- Presence of skin lesion (erythema migrans) 3–30 days after tick bite.
- Arthritis, usually pauciarticular, occurring about 4 weeks after appearance of skin lesion. Headache, chills, and fever.
- Residence or travel in an endemic area during the late spring, summer, or early fall.

General Considerations

Lyme disease is a subacute or chronic spirochetal infection caused by *Borrelia burgdorferi* and transmitted by the bite of an infected deer tick (*Ixodes* spp). The disease was known in Europe for many years as tick-borne encephalomyelitis, often associated with a characteristic rash (erythema migrans). Discovery of the agent and vector followed investigation of an outbreak of pauciarticular arthritis in Lyme, Connecticut, in 1977.

Although cases are reported from many countries and states, endemic areas include the Northeast, upper Midwest, and West Coast in the US and the northern European countries. The disease is increasingly recognized and appears to be spreading due to increased infection in and distribution of the tick vector. Most cases with rash are recognized in spring and summer, when most tick bites occur. Since the incubation period for joint and neurologic disease may be months, however, cases may present at any time. Ixodes ticks are very small, and the infecting bite is often unrecognized.

Clinical Findings

A. Symptoms and Signs: Erythema migrans is the most characteristic feature of the disease and develops in 60–80% of patients. Three to 30 days after the bite, a ring of erythema develops at the site and spreads over days. It may attain a diameter of 20 cm. The center of the lesion may clear (resembling tinea corporis), remain red, or become raised (suggesting a chemical or infectious cellulitis). Many patients are otherwise asymptomatic; some have fever (usually low-grade), headache, and myalgias. Multiple satellite skin lesions, urticaria or diffuse erythema may occur. Untreated, the rash lasts days to 3 weeks and eventually disappears.

In up to 50% of patients, arthritis develops several weeks to months after the bite. Recurrent attacks of migratory, mono- or pauciarticular arthritis involving the knees and other large joints are seen. Each attack lasts for days to a few weeks. Fever is common and may be high. Complete resolution between attacks is typical. Chronic arthritis develops in less than 10%, more often in those with the DR4 haplotype.

Neurologic manifestations develop in up to 20% of cases and usually consist of Bell's palsy, aseptic meningitis (which may be indistinguishable from viral meningitis), or polyradiculitis. Peripheral neuritis, Guillain-Barré syndrome, encephalitis, ataxia, chorea and other cranial neuropathies are less common. Seizures suggest another diagnosis. Untreated, the neurologic symptoms are usually self-limited but may be chronic or permanent. Although the fatigue and nonspecific neurologic symptoms may be prolonged in a few patients, Lyme disease is not usually proved as a cause of the chronic fatigue syndrome.

Self-limited heart-block or myocardial dysfunction occur in about 5% of patients.

B. Laboratory Findings: Most patients with only rash have no abnormal laboratory tests. Children with arthritis may have moderately elevated sedimentation rates and white blood cell counts; the ANA and rheumatoid factor are negative or non-specific; streptococcal antibodies are not usually elevated. Circulating IgM cryoglobulins may be present. Joint fluid may show up to 100,000 cells with a polymorphonuclear predominance, normal glucose, elevated protein and immune complexes; the Gram stain and culture are negative. In patients with central nervous system involvement, the spinal fluid may show lymphocytic pleocytosis and elevated protein; the glucose and all cultures and stains are normal or negative. Abnormal nerve conduction may be present with peripheral neuropathy.

Diagnosis

Lyme disease is a clinical diagnosis. History, physical examination, and laboratory features are important to consider. The causative organism is difficult to culture. Serologic testing may support the clinical diagnosis. Antibody testing should be performed in experienced laboratories: The enzyme immunoassay is currently the most accurate test, and confirmation of positives by Western blot should be considered, especially with unusual clinical syndromes. Serologic tests are positive in only 30–60% of patients with early disease. Therapy early in disease may blunt antibody titers. Recent studies have shown considerable intralaboratory and interlaboratory variability in titers reported. Overdiagnosis of Lyme disease based on atypical symptoms and "positive" serology appears to be common. Sera from patients with syphilis, HIV, and leptospirosis may give false-positive results for Lyme disease. Diagnosis of central nervous system disease requires both objective abnormalities of the neurologic examination, laboratory or radiographic studies, and consistent positive serology.

Differential Diagnosis

Aside from the disorders already mentioned, the rash may resemble pityriasis, erythema multiforme, a drug eruption, or erythema nodosum. Erythema migrans is nonscaly, minimally or nontender, and persists longer in the same place than many of the more common childhood erythematous rashes. The arthritis may resemble juvenile rheumatoid arthritis, reactive arthritis, septic arthritis, reactive effusion from a contiguous osteomyelitis, rheumatic fever, leukemic arthritis, lupus, and Henoch-Schönlein purpura. Spontaneous resolution in a few days to weeks helps differentiate it from juvenile rheumatoid arthritis, in which arthritis lasting a minimum of 6 weeks is required for diagnosis. The neurologic signs may suggest idiopathic Bell's palsy, viral or parainfectious meningitis or meningoencephalitis, lead poisoning, psychosomatic illness, and many other conditions.

Treatment

Although antimicrobial therapy is beneficial in most cases, it is most effective if started early; prolonged treatment is important for all forms. Relapses are seen with all regimens in some patients.

A. Rash, Other Early Infections: Amoxicillin (40 mg/kg/d) orally in three divided doses, or penicillin V potassium, 25–50 mg/kg/d in three divided doses—some experts add probenecid, 10 mg/kg/dose—for 2–3 weeks. Use erythromycin (30 mg/kg/d) in penicillin-allergic children, though it may be less effective. Doxycycline (100 mg orally twice a day) or tetracycline (250 mg four times daily) may be used in children over age 9.

B. Arthritis: Use the amoxicillin or doxycycline regimen (same dosage as above), but treat for 4 weeks. Parenteral ceftriaxone, 75–100 mg/kg once daily, or penicillin G, 300,000 units/kg/d in four divided doses for 2–3 weeks, is used for persistent arthritis.

C. Bell's Palsy: The same oral drug regimens may be used for 4 weeks.

D. Other Neurologic Disease or Cardiac Disease: Parenteral therapy for 2 weeks is recommended with either ceftriaxone, 75–100 kg/d in one daily dose; or penicillin G, 300,000 units/kg/d in four divided doses.

Prevention

Prevention consists of avoidance of endemic areas, wearing long sleeves and pants, frequent "tick checks," and applications of tick repellents. Permethrin sprayed on clothing decreases tick attachment. Repellents containing high concentrations of deet may be neurotoxic and should be used cautiously and washed off when tick exposure ends. Prophylactic antibiotics should not be used.

Dattwyler RJ et al: Treatment of late Lyme borreliosis: Randomized comparison of ceftriaxone and penicillin. Lancet 1988;1:1191.

Eichenfield AH, Athreye BH: Lyme disease: Of ticks and titers. J Pediatr 1989;114:328.

Luft EJ et al: Invasion of the central nervous system by *Borrelia burgdorferi* in acute disseminated infection. JAMA 1992;267:1364.

Malane MS et al: Diagnosis of Lyme disease based on dermatologic manifestations. Ann Intern Med 1991;144:490.

Millner MM et al: Lyme borreliosis of the central nervous system in children: A diagnostic challenge. Infection 1991;19:273.

Pfister HW et al: Randomized comparison of ceftriaxone and cefotaxime in Lyme neuroborreliosis. J Infect Dis 1991;163:311.

Rahn DW et al: Lyme disease: Recommendations for diagnosis and treatment. Ann Intern Med 1991;114:472.

Shapiro ED et al: A controlled trial of antimicrobial prophylaxis for Lyme disease after deer-tick bites. N Engl J Med 1992;327:1769.

Steere AC et al: The overdiagnosis of Lyme disease. JAMA 1993;269:1812.

Szer IL et al: The long term course of Lyme arthritis in children. N Engl J Med 1991;325:159.

Williams CL et al: Lyme disease in childhood: Clinical and epidemiologic features of 90 cases. Pediatr Infect Dis J 1990;9:10.

REFERENCES

Committee on Infectious Diseases: *Report,* 22nd ed. American Academy of Pediatrics, 1991.

Feigin RD, Cherry JD (editors): *Textbook of Pediatric Infectious Disease,* 3rd ed. Saunders, 1993.

37 Infections: Parasitic & Mycotic

Harley A. Rotbart, MD, & Myron J. Levin, MD

I. INFECTIONS: PARASITIC

Parasitic diseases are common and may present clinically in a variety of ways (Table 37–1). Although travel to endemic areas suggests particular infections, many are acquired from contact with human carriers and can occur anywhere. The most common infections acquired abroad are giardiasis and malaria—at home, giardiasis, toxoplasmosis, and cryptosporidiosis. A list of antiparasitic agents is presented in Table 37–2.

Some of the less common parasitic infections and those seen primarily in the developing world are presented in abbreviated form in Table 37–3.

Selection of Patients for Evaluation

The incidence of parasitic infection varies greatly with geographic area. Children who have traveled or lived in endemic areas are at risk of infection with a variety of intestinal and tissue parasites. Children who have resided only in developed countries, however, are usually free of tissue parasites (except perhaps *Toxoplasma*). Although they may have a variety of intestinal parasites, searching for them is expensive for the patient and time-consuming for the laboratory. Over 90% of ovum and parasite examinations done in most hospital laboratories in the USA are negative; many have been ordered inappropriately. An approach to determining which children with diarrhea need such examinations is presented in Figure 37–1.

Children with underlying immunodeficiency, in both developed and developing countries, are uniquely susceptible to parasites, particularly protozoan intestinal infections. In these patients, normally commensal infestations may become debilitating infections, and multiple simultaneous pathogens are frequently identified. The yield for diagnostic testing in compromised hosts is higher and the threshold for ordering tests must be lower.

Specimen Processing

For tissue parasites, contact the laboratory for proper collection procedure. Diarrheal stools may contain trophozoites that rapidly die during transport. The specimen should either be examined immediately or placed in a stool fixative such as polyvinyl alcohol. Several types of commercial vials containing fixatives are available and may be sent home with the child for outpatient specimen collection. Since they may contain toxic compounds, the vials should be safely stored until use. Once fixed, the specimens are stable at room temperature. Formed stools usually contain cysts that are more stable. It is best to fix these also after collection, but they may be reliably examined after room temperature transport.

Eosinophilia & Parasitic Infections

Although parasites commonly cause eosinophilia, in developed countries other causes are much more common and include allergies, drugs, and other infections. Heavy intestinal nematode infections cause eosinophilia; they are easily detected on a single ovum and parasite examination. Light nematode infections and common protozoan infections—giardiasis, cryptosporidiosis, and amebiasis—rarely cause eosinophilia. Eosinophilia is also unusual or minimal in more serious infections such as amebic liver abscess, cysticercosis, toxoplasmosis, and malaria.

The most common parasitic infection in the USA that causes significant eosinophilia with negative stool examination is toxocariasis. In a young child with eosinophilia and a negative stool examination, a serologic test for *Toxocara* may be the next appropriate test. Trichinosis may cause marked eosinophilia, but it is rare; strongyloidiasis may also be difficult to diagnose with stool examinations. Patients with eosinophilia who have lived in or traveled to developing regions of the world have a much broader differential diagnosis.

Table 37–1. Symptoms of parasitic infection.

Sign	Agent	Comments*
Abdominal pain	Anisakis	Shortly after raw fish ingestion.
	Ascaris	Heavy infection; may obstruct bowel, biliary tract.
	Clonorchis	Heavy, early infection. Hepatomegaly later.
	Entamoeba histolytica	Hematochezia, variable fever, diarrhea.
	Fasciola hepatica	Diarrhea, vomiting.
	Hookworm	Heavy infection. Iron deficiency anemia.
	Strongyloides	Eosinophilia, pruritus. May resemble peptic disease.
	Trichinella	Myalgia, periorbital edema, eosinophilia.
	Trichuris	Heavy infection; diarrhea, dysentery.
Cough	Ascaris	Wheezing, eosinophilia. During migration phase.
	Paragonimus westermani	Hemoptysis; chronic. May mimic tuberculosis.
	Strongyloides	Wheezing, pruritus, eosinophilia during migration or dissemination.
	Toxocara	Affects ages 1–5; hepatosplenomegaly; eosinophilia.
	Tropical eosinophilia	Pulmonary infiltrates, eosinophilia.
Diarrhea	Blastocystis	Possibly with heavy infection in immunosuppressed or normal individuals.
	Cryptosporidium	Watery; prolonged in normals, chronic in immunosuppressed.
	Dientamoeba fragilis	Heavy infection.
	Entamoeba histolytica	Hematochezia, variable fever; no eosinophilia.
	Giardia	Afebrile, chronic; anorexia; no hematochezia or eosinophilia.
	Schistosoma	Chronic; hepatosplenomegaly.
	Strongyloides	Abdominal pain; eosinophilia.
	Trichinella	Myalgia, periorbital edema, eosinophilia.
	Trichuris	Heavy infection.
Dysentery	Balantidium coli	Swine contact.
	Entamoeba histolytica	Few to no leukocytes in stool; fever; hematochezia
	Schistosoma	During acute infections.
	Trichuris	Heavy infection.
Dysuria	Enterobius	Usually girls with worms in urethra, bladder; nocturnal, perianal pruritus.
	Schistosoma	Hematuria. Exclude bacteriuria, stones.
Headache (and other cerebral symptoms)	Angiostrongylus	Eosinophilic meningitis.
	Naegleria	Fresh-water swimming; rapidly progressive meningoencephalitis.
	Plasmodium	Fever, chills, jaundice, splenomegaly. Cerebral ischemia (with P falciparum).
	Taenia solium	Cysticercosis. Focal seizures, deficits; hydrocephalus, aseptic meningitis.
	Toxoplasma	Meningoencephalitis (especially in the immunosuppressed); hydrocephalus in infants.
	Trypanosoma	African forms. Chronic lethargy (sleeping sickness).
Pruritus	Ancylostoma braziliense	Creeping eruption; dermal serpiginous burrow.
	Enterobius	Perianal, nocturnal.
	Filaria	Variable; seen in many filarial diseases.
	Hookworm	Local at penetration site in heavy exposure.
	Strongyloides	Diffuse with migration; may be recurrent.
	Trypanosoma	African forms; one of many nonspecific symptoms.

(continued)

Table 37–1. Symptoms of parasitic infection. (continued)

Sign	Agent	Comments*
Fever	*Entamoeba histolytica*	With acute dysentery or liver abscess.
	Leishmania donovani	Hepatosplenomegaly, anemia, leukopenia.
	Plasmodium	Chills, headache, jaundice; periodic.
	Toxocara	Cough, hepatosplenomegaly, eosinophilia.
	Toxoplasma	Generalized adenopathy; splenomegaly.
	Trichinella	Myalgia, periorbital edema, eosinophilia.
	Trypanosoma	Early stage, African forms; lymphadenopathy.
Anemia	*Diphyllobothrium*	Megaloblastic due to B_{12} deficiency; rare.
	Hookworm	Iron deficiency.
	Leishmania donovani	Fever, hepatosplenomegaly, leukopenia (kala-azar).
	Plasmodium	Hemolysis.
	Trichuris	Heavy infection, due to iron loss.
Eosinophilia	*Angiostrongylus*	Eosinophilic meningitis.
	Fasciola	Abdominal pain.
	Filaria	Microfilariae in blood. Lymphadenopathy.
	Onchocerca	Nodules, keratitis.
	Schistosoma	Chronic; intestinal or genitourinary symptoms.
	Strongyloides	Abdominal pain, diarrhea.
	Toxocara	Hepatosplenomegaly, cough; affects ages 1–5.
	Trichinella	Myalgia, periorbital edema.
	Tropical eosinophilia	Unknown filarial agent. Cough.
Hematuria	*Schistosoma*	*S haematobium*. Bladder, urethral granulomas. Exclude stones, bacteriuria.
Hemoptysis	*Paragonimus westermani*	Lung fluke. Variable chest pain; chronic.
Hepatomegaly	*Clonorchis*	Heavy infection. Tenderness early; cirrhosis late.
	Echinococcus	Chronic; cysts.
	Entamoeba histolytica	Toxic hepatitis or abscess. No eosinophilia.
	Leishmania donovani	Kala-azar. Splenomegaly, fever, anemia.
	Schistosoma	Chronic; cirrhosis, splenomegaly.
	Toxocara	Splenomegaly, eosinophilia, cough; no adenopathy.
Splenomegaly	*Leishmania donovani*	Kala-azar. Hepatomegaly, fever, anemia.
	Plasmodium	Fever, chills, jaundice, headache.
	Schistosoma	Hepatomegaly.
	Toxocara	Eosinophilia, hepatomegaly.
	Toxoplasma	Lymphadenopathy, other symptoms.
Lymphadenopathy	Filaria	Inguinal typical; chronic.
	Leishmania donovani	Hepatosplenomegaly, leukopenia, anemia, fever (kala-azar).
	Toxoplasma	Cervical common; may involve single site; splenomegaly.
	Trypanosoma	Localized near bite (Chagas' disease); generalized (especially posterior cervical) in African forms.

*Symptoms usually related to degree of infestation. Infestation with small numbers of organisms are often asymptomatic.

Table 37–2. Some parasitic infections seen less commonly in developed regions.

Agent (Disease)	Geographic Region	Vector	Symptoms and Signs	Laboratory Findings	Diagnosis	Therapy and Comments
Trypanosoma cruzi (Chagas' disease)	South and Central America, Mexico	Reduviid bug	Early: Painful red nodule at bite site, conjunctivitis, periorbital edema (Romaña's sign), fever, local adenitis. Late: Myocarditis, megaesophagus, encephalitis.	Mononuclear leukocytosis	Organisms in peripheral blood during febrile phase. Organisms in bone marrow, liver, spleen. Positive serology.	Nifurtimox may help early. No therapy for late disease. May be transmitted by blood transfusion or congenitally.
Trypanosoma brucei (sleeping sickness)	Africa	Tsetse fly	Hepatosplenomegaly, adenopathy. Nodule at bite site (resolves). Recurrent fever, headache, myalgia, progressive encephalitis.	Elevated ESR, anemia, CSF pleocytosis	Organisms in blood, CSF, marrow, nodes. Positive serology.	Suramin for non-CNS disease. Eflornithine promising.
Leishmania donovani (kala-azar)	Mideast, India, Mediterranean, South and Central America	Sandfly	Fever, generalized adenopathy, hepatosplenomegaly weeks to months after infection.	Pancytopenia, hypergammaglobulinemia	Organisms in marrow, nodes, spleen. Positive serology.	Sodium stibogluconate or meglumine antimonate.
Leishmania tropica (Oriental sore)	Asia, India, North Africa	Sandfly	Papule at bite site (usually on face, limbs) develops after weeks to months, then ulcerates and scars.	. . .	Organisms in skin biopsy. Positive skin test, serology.	Same as for *L donovani*.
Leishmania braziliensis, L mexicana (chiclero ulcer)	South America	Sandfly	Painful mucocutaneous ulcers or granulomas. Nasolabial lesions common.	. . .	Skin biopsy. Positive skin test, serology.	Same as for *L donovani*.
Wucherichia, Brugia (filariasis)	Tropics, subtropics	Mosquito	Chronic adenopathy, often inguinal. Obstructive edema.	Eosinophilia	Concentrated blood smears for larvae. Positive serology.	Ivermectin, diethylcarbamazine kill larvae. Surgery for lymphatic obstruction.
Angiostrongylus cantonensis (eosinophilic meningitis)	Hawaii, Asia, Pacific Islands	Snails, slugs	Ingestion (usually inadvertent) followed in 1–4 weeks by meningitis of variable severity. Paresthesias.	Eosinophils in CSF and blood	Positive serology. Larvae may be present in CSF.	Fever absent or low. No focal lesions on CNS imaging. No specific therapy. Steroids may be beneficial. Mebendazole may help.
Naegleria fowleri (amebic meningoencephalitis)	Worldwide	Fresh water (ponds, lakes)	Swimming (usually in warm, fresh water) followed in 7 days by rhinitis, altered sense of taste or smell, fever, headache, meningismus, coma.	CSF pleocytosis. Negative Gram stain.	Amebas in CSF by direct examination or cytologic stain. Cultures are positive.	Free-living amebas; may resemble leukocytes in CSF. Amphotericin B may be helpful. Usually fatal.
Paragonimus westermani (lung fluke infection)	Asia, South America, Africa	Raw crabs, crustaceans	Cough, hemoptysis. Rarely seizures, other CNS signs if migration to brain occurs.	. . .	Large ova in concentrated specimens, feces. Cystic nodular lesions on chest x-ray or CNS imaging.	Resembles pulmonary tuberculosis. Praziquantel very effective.
Clonorchis sinensis (liver fluke infection)	Asia	Raw fish	Adult flukes obstruct biliary tree. Acute: Hepatomegaly, fever, jaundice, urticaria. Late: Cirrhosis, carcinoma.	Variable liver function test abnormalities	Ova in feces.	Praziquantel. Advanced disease not treatable. Liver transplant.

Berman JD: Chemotherapy for leishmaniasis: Biochemical mechanisms, clinical efficacy, and future strategies. Rev Infect Dis 1988;10:560.

Evans T et al: American visceral leishmaniasis (kala-azar). West J Med 1985;142:777.

Grimaldi G JR, Tesh RB, McMahon-Pratt D: A review of the geographic distribution and epidemiology of leishmaniasis in the New World. Am J Trop Med Hyg 1989;41:687.

Kirchoff LV, Gam AA, Gilliam FC: American trypanosomiasis (Chagas' disease) in Central American immigrants. Am J Med 1987;82:915.

Koo J, Pien R, Klinks MM: *Angiostrongylus (Parastrongylus)* eosinophilic meningitis. Rev Infect Dis 1988;10:1155.

Leiguarda R et al: Acute CNS infection by *Trypanosoma cruzi* (Chagas' disease) in immunosuppressed patients. Neurology 1990;30:850.

Marsden PD: American trypanosomiasis. BMJ 1989;299:969.

Ottesen EA: Filariasis now. Am J Trop Med Hyg 1989;41S:9.

Ottesen EA et al: A controlled trial of ivermectin and diethylcarbamazine in lymphatic filariasis. N Engl J Med 1990;322:1113.

Olness K et al: Loiasis in an expatriate American child: Diagnostic and treatment difficulties. Pediatrics 1987;80:943.

Rees PG et al: The treatment of kala-azar: A review with comments drawn from experience in Kenya. Trop Georgr Med 1985;37:37.

Simon MW, Wilson HD: The amebic meningoencephalitides. Pediatr Infect Dis J 1986;5:562.

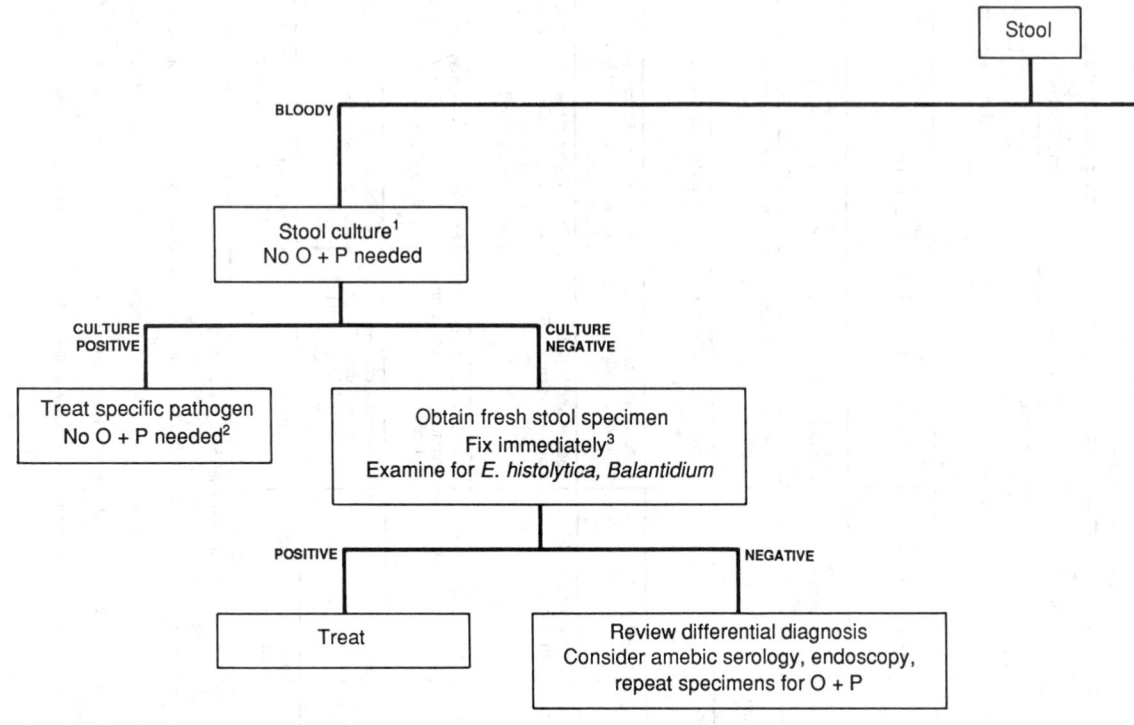

O + P = Ova and parasite examination.
1. *Shigella, Salmonella, Campylobacter, E coli (Escherichia coli)* 0157, *Yersinia*; assay for *Clostridium difficile* toxin if recent antimicrobial use.
2. Unless critically ill, from endemic area for amebiasis, or unresponsive to standard therapy.
3. In stool fixative, eg, polyvinyl alcohol.
4. If symptoms typical; especially if history of ingestion of potentially contaminated water or food or contact with day care center attendees and no underlying gastrointestinal illness.
5. Include examination for *Cryptosporidium*; immediate stool fixation needed if stool is diarrheal.

Figure 37–1. Parasitologic evaluation of acute diarrhea.

PROTOZOAL INFECTIONS

MALARIA

Essentials of Diagnosis

- Residence in or travel to an endemic area.
- High fever, chills, headache, jaundice, vomiting, diarrhea.
- Splenomegaly, anemia.
- Seizures, coma.
- Malaria parasites in blood smear.

General Considerations

Malaria kills a million children worldwide each year and is undergoing resurgence in areas where it was previously controlled. Imported cases diagnosed in the United States each year number approximately 1000. The female anopheline mosquito transmits the parasites—*Plasmodium vivax* (most common), *Plasmodium falciparum* (most virulent), *Plasmodium ovale* (similar to *P vivax*), and *Plasmodium malariae*. The gametocytes ingested from an infected human form sporozoites in the mosquito; when inoculated into a susceptible host, these sporozoites infect hepatocytes. Antibody—but not drug therapy—decreases sporozoite infectivity. The preerythrocytic phase (hepatic) is about 1-2 weeks for all but *P malariae* infection (3–5 weeks), but the initial symptoms may be delayed for up to a year in *P falciparum,* 4 years in *P vivax,* and decades in *P malariae* infections. Merozoites released into the circulation from hepatocytes infect red cells (young cells by *P vivax and P ovale*, old cells by *P malariae,* and all cells by *P falciparum*) and begin the synchronous erythrocytic cycles—rupturing the infected cells at intervals of 48 hours for all but *P malariae*, which has a 72-hour cycle. Asynchronous cycles causing daily fevers are not uncommon. Survival is associated with a progressive decrease in intensity of cycles; relapses years later may occur as a result of hepatic infection, which persists

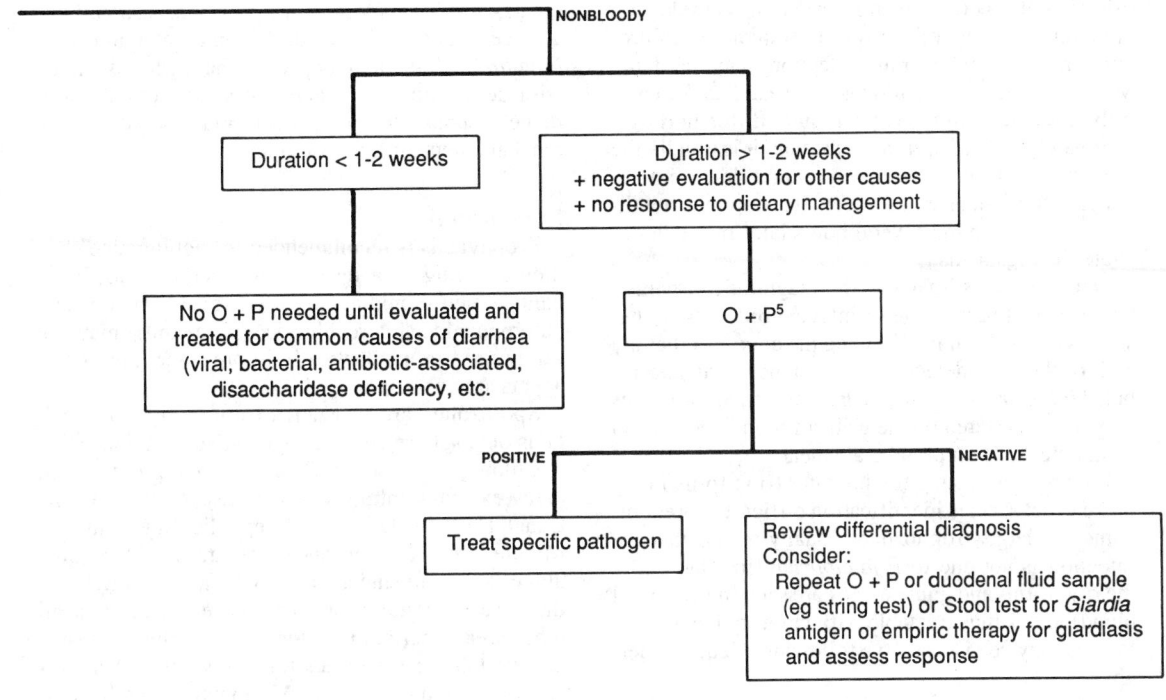

Figure 37–1. Parasitologic evaluation of acute diarrhea. (*continued*)

in all but *P falciparum* infections. Infection acquired congenitally or from transfusions or needle sticks does not result in a hepatic phase.

Susceptibility varies genetically; certain red cell phenotypes are partially resistant to infection (hemoglobin S, hemoglobin F, thalassemia, G6PD deficiency). The worldwide distribution of the four species is determined, to some extent, by host genetic factors. The absence of *P.vivax* from Africa reflects the lack of specific Duffy blood group substances among most native Africans. Recurrent infections result in some natural species-specific immunity; this does not prevent sporozoite infection but does decrease parasitemia and symptoms. Maternal immunity protects the neonate despite the placental infection seen in active infection in pregnancy.

Clinical Findings

A. Symptoms and Signs: Clinical manifestations vary according to species, strain, and host immunity. The child presents with recurrent bouts of fever, irritability, poor feeding, vomiting, jaundice, and splenomegaly. Enanthem, rash, cough, and significant dehydration are usually absent in malaria and help distinguish it from many viral infections with similar symptoms. Symptoms are similar in older children, with headache, backache, chills, myalgia, and fatigue more easily elicited. Fever may be periodic (every other day for all but *P malariae* infection, in which it occurs every third day), daily, or irregularly. Between attacks, patients may look quite well. If the disease is untreated, relapses cease within a year in *P falciparum* and within several years in *P vivax* infections, but may recur decades later in *P malariae* infection. Infection during pregnancy often causes intrauterine growth retardation or premature delivery but rarely true fetal infection.

Physical examination in uncomplicated cases may be normal or show only mild jaundice or hepatosplenomegaly.

B. Laboratory Findings: Most cases in the USA are diagnosed by a Wright-stain preparation of thin blood smears, occasionally in the course of another investigation. To exclude malaria completely, multiple thick smears must be obtained frequently (every 8–12 hours for several days), properly made and examined by experienced personnel. Giemsa's stain of thin smears is preferable for the correct identification of species, which is critical in the selection of therapy. Improper therapy of misdiagnosed chloroquine-resistant falciparum infection may be fatal. Multiple infections should also be searched for carefully, because each type may require different drugs; fortunately, if *P falciparum* is present, it is usually the predominant form seen. Rarely, blood drawn immediately after synchronous merozoite rupture is not diagnostic; resampling several hours later may demonstrate the organism.

Quantitative estimates of the magnitude of parasitemia (actual percentage of infected red cells in thin smears) are helpful in following the course of therapy and for the early detection of resistance in all species but *P falciparum*. *P falciparum*-infected erythrocytes may be sequestered on the walls of blood vessels and be undetectable on peripheral smear.

Finding only young trophozoites (ring forms) may make exact species identification difficult; a predominance of larger trophozoites usually means that the infection is not due to *P falciparum* (in which only the ring forms and gametocytes are seen in peripheral blood) and is thus treatable with chloroquine. Gametocytes may persist for days following adequate therapy.

Laboratory findings include a mild normocytic, normochromic anemia, leukopenia or leukocytosis, normal to low platelet count, reticulocytosis, elevation of direct and indirect bilirubin, mild transaminase elevation, low C3 level, and hyperglobulinemia; occasionally, a positive rheumatoid factor and falsely elevated non-treponemal syphilis, antinuclear, and heterophil titers are present.

Differential Diagnosis

Relapsing fever may be seen with borreliosis, brucellosis, sequential common infections, Hodgkin's disease, juvenile rheumatoid arthritis, rat-bite fever, or one of the idiopathic periodic fevers. Other common causes of high fever and headache include influenza, *Mycoplasma pneumoniae* or enteroviral infection, sinusitis, meningitis, enteric fever, tuberculosis, juvenile rheumatoid arthritis, occult pneumonia, or bacteremia. Malaria may also coexist with other diseases.

Complications & Sequelae

Severe complications are usually limited to *P falciparum* infections. Chronic infections due to the other species may result in anemia, debilitation, and massive splenomegaly (with potential rupture). Erythrocytes infected with *P falciparum* stick to capillary endothelium, causing microthrombosis and ischemia of any organ; involvement of the intestinal tract (bleeding, enteritis), lung (pneumonitis, ARDS), and

brain (diffuse edema, seizures, encephalopathy) are most common. Severe hemolysis with hemoglobinuria (blackwater fever) is an unusual complication of *P falciparum* infection. Erythrocyte destruction is greatest in *P falciparum* infection, because cells of all ages may be infected. Chronic infection with *P malariae,* but not other species, has been associated with development of nephrotic syndrome. The immune response to *Plasmodium* plays a role in the renal and hematologic complications.

Prevention

Prophylaxis is recommended for nonimmune children traveling to or residing in endemic areas. Pregnant women should avoid exposure; chloroquine and chloroguanide hydrochloride (proguanil) may be safely used prophylactically in pregnancy, but other agents are contraindicated.

Sporozoites are resistant to drugs; thus, prophylaxis only suppresses schizogony and symptoms.

Chloroquine-resistant *P falciparum* is present in all areas except Central America west of the Panama Canal, Haiti, the Dominican Republic, Egypt, and the Middle East. In resistance-free areas, chloroquine alone is recommended for prophylaxis (5 mg/kg of the base [maximum, 300 mg] once a week). In all other areas, mefloquine alone is recommended (one 250 mg tablet once a week for adults; lower doses for children based on weight). Mefloquine is not recommended for children under 15 kg, however; they may be given chloroquine prophylaxis and closely observed and treated for possible resistant *P falciparum* infection if symptoms occur. Doxycycline is an alternative regimen for prophylaxis in areas of resistance, but should not be given to children under 8 years of age. Proguanil may also be given to children, though it is not available in the USA. Chloroquine prophylaxis is begun 2 weeks before travel and continued for 4 weeks after return; mefloquine is started 1 week prior to potential exposure and continued for 4 weeks after leaving the malarious area. Some experts recommend 2 weeks of primaquine at the end of prophylaxis to eradicate any hepatic malarial infection.

For the most current details of prophylaxis, a 24-hour computer-assisted telephone information service is available through the Centers for Disease Control (1-404-332-4555).

Mosquitoes feed from dusk to dawn, and for that reason personal protective measures should be emphasized during those hours. Insect repellents containing 35% or less of Deet (diethyltoluamide), permethrin-impregnated mosquito netting, aerosolized insecticides, and electric coil insect repellents are important preventive measures.

Treatment

Malaria should always be excluded in children with fever or unexplained coma who have traveled to an endemic area. Blood transfusion and illicit intravenous drug use also put them at risk.

One must be careful to calculate drug dosages by weight and formulation (base versus salt).

A. Specific Measures: Chloroquine phosphate is the drug of choice for nonresistant *P falciparum* infections and for most infections due to other species. (A few chloroquine-resistant *P vivax* strains have recently been recognized in Indonesia and New Guinea.) Three days of therapy completely eradicates the erythrocytic phase (Table 37–3). Chloroquine may be given parenterally if necessary. Slow administration is important.

For proven *P vivax* or *P ovale* infections, primaquine phosphate should be given for 2 weeks following chloroquine completion; patients should be screened for G6PD deficiency before receiving primaquine. Quinidine gluconate is the parenteral agent of choice (Table 37–3).

B. General Measures:

1. For uncomplicated malaria, hydration and fever control are emphasized. Hypoglycemia is a common complication and must be monitored for. Blood and needle precautions are indicated. Hospitalization should be considered if the patient is vomiting, severely ill, or nonimmune and infected with *P falciparum.* Tests for incidental hepatitis B carrier states are indicated in high-risk groups (illicit drug users, native Orientals). Iron and folate levels may be low as a consequence of preexisting deficiency and exacerbated by hemolysis. Anemia may require transfusions.

2. For suspected cerebral malaria, other causes must be ruled out. Anticonvulsants and management appropriate for ischemic cerebral edema are needed. Corticosteroids are detrimental and should not be used.

3. For blackwater fever, parasitemia must be treated and renal failure managed; dialysis may be lifesaving.

Drugs for parasitic infections. Med Lett Drugs Ther 1993; 35:111.

Lynk A, Gold R: Review of 40 children with imported malaria. Pediatr Infect Dis J 1989;8:745.

Pender E, Newman J: Malaria in children. Pediatr Emerg Care 1990;6:40.

Phillips RE, Solomon T: Cerebral malaria in children. Lancet 1990;336:1355.

Randall G, Seidel JS: Malaria. Pediatr Clin North Am 1985;32:893.

WHO Malaria Action Programme: Severe and complicated malaria. Trans R Soc Trop Med Hyg 1986;80(Suppl):1.

Wyler DJ: Malaria chemoprophylaxis for the traveler. N Engl J Med 1993;329:31-37.

Wyler DJ: Malaria: Overview and update. Clin Infect Dis 1993;16:449-458.

AMEBIASIS

Essentials of Diagnosis

- Acute dysentery: Evidence of colitis (diarrhea with blood and mucus, pain, tenderness).
- Chronic dysentery: Recurrent diarrhea and abdominal pain.
- Hepatic amebiasis: Tender hepatomegaly.
- Amebas or cysts in stools or abscesses.

General Considerations

Amebiasis, due to *Entamoeba histolytica* is a common problem in endemic areas of poor hygiene. It is estimated that 12% of the world's population is infected by *E histolytica.* Amebiasis should be suspected in patients with a history of travel to such areas or of contact with individuals from endemic areas who may be asymptomatic carriers. In the USA, amebiasis may be seen in homes for the retarded or handicapped, where poor hygiene fosters the spread of enteric pathogens. *E histolytica* has been found in the stools of as many as 30% of gay men, in whom nonpathogenic variants of the organism may predominate. Individuals of any age may be infected. Transmission is usually fecal-oral, often from asymptomatic carriers who pass cysts. Trophozoites are killed by stomach acid and are not infectious. *Entamoeba coli* is a nonpathogenic commensal, as are *Entamoeba hartmanni, Entamoeba gingivalis,* and *Entamoeba moshkovskii.* Only 10% of *E histolytica* infections result in gastrointestinal or other symptoms, but as many as 100,000 people die of their infections each year.

Clinical Findings

A. Symptoms and Signs: Clinical symptoms may be unrelated to the presence of stool cysts; indeed, few cysts may be passed during acute dysentery compared with chronic diarrheal and asymptomatic states. A response to specific therapy and a positive serologic test support a causative association.

The incubation period varies from days to months. Severity, acuteness of onset, degree of fever or abdominal pain (usually present over the cecum or sigmoid), and degree of dehydration are also quite variable. Stools usually contain blood and mucus. Chronic or recurrent symptoms may occur—an atypical finding in most bacterial enteritides. Fulminant colitis is rare but occurs more frequently in children than adults; colonic perforations are common with this presentation, as is hepatic abscess. Ameboma, an intestinal mass, occurs in 1% of patients with gastrointestinal symptoms.

B. Laboratory Findings: In cases of colitis, a freshly passed stool specimen should be examined immediately for trophozoites and preserved in polyvinyl alcohol. Trophozoite motility, an important diagnostic characteristic, is rapidly lost with cooling or staining. Expert technologic help is mandatory; mis-

Table 37–3. Malaria treatment.

Indication	Drug	Dosage
All *Plasmodium* infections except chloroquine-resistant *P falciparum*[1]	**Oral:** Chloroquine phosphate[2]	10 mg base/kg (maximum 600 mg base), then 5 mg/kg 6 hours, 24 hours, and 48 hours later.
	Parenteral: Quinidine gluconate	10 mg base/kg (maximum 600 mg base) over 1–2 hours, then 0.02 mg base/kg/min as continuous infusion
Chloroquine-resistant *P falciparum*	**Oral:** Quinine sulfate	8 mg/kg/dose every 8 hours for 3–7 days,[3]
	Plus	
	Pyrimethamine-sulfadoxine (Fansidar)	< 1 years: ¼ tablet[4] 1–3 years: ½ tablet 4–8 years: 1 tablet 9–14 years: 2 tablets
	Or	
	Quinine sulfate	Same as above
	Plus	
	Tetracycline	5mg/kg 4 times daily for 7 days in children > 8 years of age.
	Or	
	Quinine sulfate	Same as above
	Plus	
	Clindamycin	20–40 mg/kg/d in three doses for 3 days
	Parenteral: Quinidine gluconate	10 mg base/kg (maximum 600 mg base) over 1–2 hours followed by 0.02 mg base/kg/min as continuous infusion until oral therapy can be started
Prevention of *P vivax* or *P ovale* relapses	Primaquine phosphate	0.3 mg base/kg/d orally (maximum, 15 mg) for 14 days (screen for G6PD deficiency first)

[1]Rare chloroquine-resistant *P vivax* in Indonesia.
[2]Chloroquine phosphate contains 60% base by weight; quinidine gluconate contains 66% base; quinine sulfate contains 83% base; primaquine phosphate contains 57% base.
[3]Seven days may be required for Southeast Asian strains, in which relative resistance to quinine is increasing.
[4]Pyrimethamine sulfadoxine tablets contain 25 mg pyrimethamine and 500 mg sulfadoxine.

taking leukocytes (usually absent in amebiasis) for trophozoites has resulted in many false diagnoses. Colonoscopy may reveal the classic "buttonhole" ulcers and provide biopsy diagnosis; biopsy specimens should be obtained from the edge of the ulcer.

In chronic infections, several stools collected over a period of days should be examined for the characteristic tetranucleated cysts; because cysts are stable at room temperature, special handling is not needed. Cysts less than 10 μm in diameter are classified as the nonpathogenic *E hartmanni*. Oral cathartics, barium, and antibiotics may temporarily stop cyst shedding. Routine laboratory tests are nondiagnostic. Leukocytosis may be present with acute colitis. Eosinophilia is absent.

A barium enema may demonstrate colitis but is not specific for amebiasis and may increase the risk of colonic perforation.

Specific antibodies measured by indirect hemagglutination are present in the blood of 95% of patients with active amebic dysentery or abscess but in less than 10% of asymptomatic carriers or noninfected individuals.

Differential Diagnosis

Bacterial dysentery is usually more abrupt in onset. Very high fever, seizures, encephalopathy, and leukopenia with many immature neutrophils are characteristic of shigellosis and are unusual in amebiasis. Fecal leukocytes suggest bacterial or inflammatory colitis; colitis can also be associated with antibiotic therapy, allergies, hemolytic-uremic syndrome, ulcerative colitis, Crohn's disease, and *Balantidium coli* infection. Other intestinal parasites do not cause dysentery. The differential diagnosis for chronic amebiasis is even longer (see Chapter 23).

Complications & Sequelae

These may result from failure to consider the diagnosis in patients with colitis who have negative cultures for bacterial pathogens and negative assays for *C difficile* toxin.

Intestinal complications include perforation, peritonitis, granulomatous proliferation (producing a mass or ameboma, which is rare in children), hemorrhage, intussusception, fistulization to bladder or skin, and late colonic strictures. Hepatic complications include hepatitis and abscess. The former is associated with dysentery and is characterized by tender hepatomegaly and mildly abnormal liver function tests without abscess formation. It is considered a form of toxic hepatitis and resolves with therapy. The diagnosis and management of amebic liver abscess are discussed in Chapter 23.

Treatment

A. Specific Measures: Although several drugs are available, none are unfailingly curative.

1. Asymptomatic intestinal infection is best eradicated with a luminal amebicide such as diloxanide furoate (7 mg/kg three times daily for 10 days; available only from the CDC (phone 404-639-3670) or iodoquinol (10 mg/kg three times daily for 20 days). Paromomycin (8 mg/kg three times daily for 7 days) is an alternative.

2. Mild to moderate intestinal disease is treated with metronidazole (15 mg/kg [maximum, 750 mg] three times daily for 10 days), followed by a luminal amebicide (because metronidazole may fail to eradicate cysts) such as diloxanide furoate or iodoquinol (see above).

3. Severe intestinal disease or liver abscess is treated with oral metronidazole (see above regimen) or intravenous metronidazole. An alternative regimen is dehydroemetine (0.5 mg/kg twice daily intramuscularly for 5 days [maximum, 90 mg/d]). Chloroquine is effective for abscesses but not intestinal disease. Dehydroemetine is cardiotoxic. Luminal amebicides should also be given when tolerated.

B. General Measures: Enteric isolation is advised. Adequate hydration and repeated evaluations should be done to detect complications. For follow-up (particularly in cases where diloxanide has not been given), examination of three stool specimens on alternate days determines whether the infection has been eradicated.

Bruckner DA: Amebiasis. Clin Microbiol Rev 1992;5:356.
Merritt RJ et al: Spectrum of amebiasis in children. Am J Dis Child 1982;136:785.
Ravdin JI: Amebiasis now. Am J Trop Med Hyg 1989; 41:40.
Reed SL: Amebiasis: An update. Clin Infect Dis 1992; 14:385.
Rustgi AK, Richter JM: Pyogenic and amebic liver abscess. Med Clin North Am 1989;73:847.

DIARRHEA ASSOCIATED WITH *BLASTOCYSTIS HOMINIS*

The role of this protozoan in causing enteritis is controversial. Although it may be found in asymptomatic children, many investigators believe that it can cause acute enteritis in normal individuals and acute or chronic diarrhea in immunocompromised children. The clinical presentation is nonspecific. The organism is usually detected by routine examination of feces for the presence of ova and parasites; it is reported, if present, in large numbers. There are no characteristic laboratory findings or serologic diagnostic tests. If therapy is considered because of severity of the symptoms and lack of another cause, either metronidazole (15 mg/kg orally three times a day for 10 days) or iodoquinol (10 mg/kg orally three times a day for 20 days) may be effective.

Doyle PW et al: Epidemiology and pathogenicity of *Blastocystis hominis.* J Clin Microbiol 1990;28:116
O'Gorman MA et al: Prevalence and characteristics of *Blastocystis hominis* infection in children. Clin Pediatr 1993;91.
Senay H, MacPherson D: *Blastocystis hominis:* Epidemiology and natural history. J Infect Dis 1990;162:987.
Zierdt CH: *Blastocystis hominis:* Past and future. Clin Microbiol Rev 1991;4:61.

DIARRHEA ASSOCIATED WITH *DIENTAMOEBA FRAGILIS*

The pathogenicity of *Dientamoeba fragilis* is controversial, and even a presumptive diagnosis requires exclusion of other enteric pathogens. Purported symptoms include abdominal pain, diarrhea, nausea, anorexia, vomiting, and fatigue. Iodoquinol, 40 mg/kg/d in three divided doses for 20 days, has been used with success. Paromomycin (25 mg/kg/d in three divided doses for 10 days) and tetracycline (40 mg/kg/d in four divided doses for 10 days; maximum 2 g/d; only for children > 8 years old) are alternatives. Given the potential toxicity of therapy, the usual mild nature of symptoms, and the organism's questionable pathogenicity, *D fragilis* infection should not be routinely treated.

Spencer MJ, Garcia LS, Chapin MR: *Dientamoeba fragilis:* An intestinal pathogen in children? Am J Dis Child 1979;133:390.
Turner JA: Giardiasis and infections with *Dientamoeba fragilis.* Pediatr Clin North Am 1985;32:865.

GIARDIASIS

Essentials of Diagnosis

- Chronic or relapsing diarrhea, flatulence, bloating, anorexia, poor weight gain.

- Absence of fever and hematochezia.
- Presence of trophozoites in loose stools or duodenal contents; cysts in formed stools.

General Considerations

Giardiasis is the most common intestinal protozoal infection in children in the USA and in most areas around the world. It is caused by *Giardia lamblia*. Endemic worldwide, it is classically associated with drinking contaminated water, either in rural areas or in areas with faulty purification systems. Acquisition in swimming pools has occurred. Because even ostensibly clean urban water supplies can be intermittently contaminated, giardiasis can be acquired by almost any traveler. Fecal-oral contamination allows person-to-person spread. Recently, day care centers have been recognized as major sources, with an incidence of up to 50% reported in some centers. Asymptomatic infections are the rule and facilitate spread to household contacts. Food-borne outbreaks have also occurred. Although infection is rare in neonates, it may occur at any age.

Clinical Findings

A. Symptoms and Signs: Following cyst ingestion, liberated trophozoites live noninvasively in the small bowel. Symptoms develop in 1–2 weeks and include nausea, anorexia, low-grade fever, and chills. Diarrheal, soft, or steatorrheal stools with mucus—but no blood or leukocytes—are passed. Abdominal cramps, vomiting, flatulence, and weight loss may occur. Rash and high fever are absent. The illness may last days to months and may relapse. Rarely, intermittent diarrhea over years may occur. Failure to thrive may be diagnosed in these children.

B. Laboratory Findings: Routine blood tests are normal; there is no eosinophilia. Examination of several stool specimens usually reveals the pear-shaped trophozoites (2–15 μm) (in fresh loose stools) or the oval cysts. Immediate fixation of loose stools with subsequent trichrome staining to look for trophozoites is recommended. If results are negative despite multiple repeat examinations over many days, samples can be taken directly from the duodenum by aspiration, biopsy, or the string test (Entero-Test). Because only trophozoites are present in the duodenum, rapid processing is necessary. Cyst shedding is intermittent, and multiple stools may be negative in infected patients. Tests for *Giardia* antigen in stools are promising, as are experimental applications of the polymerase chain reaction, and could prove more cost-effective than multiple stool examinations. Serologic studies are not yet commercially available.

Differential Diagnosis

Many other causes of steatorrhea and chronic diarrhea should be considered, including cryptosporidiosis and chronic amebiasis. (See Chapter 23.)

Prevention

Spread is usually fecal-oral. Untreated water or potentially contaminated foods (fresh fruit, vegetables from areas with poor sanitation facilities or water supplies) should be avoided; good handwashing is important. Although animals may carry *Giardia* and have been implicated in contamination of water supplies, they are not considered important vectors for human cases and do not have to be tested. Identification and treatment of asymptomatic human carriers may be needed.

Treatment

Ideally, the diagnosis is made prior to treatment, though many clinicians use a single empiric course of therapy before resorting to invasive diagnostic tests.

Failures and reinfections occur with all regimens and can frustrate attempts at eradication. Symptomatic children in day care centers and their contacts should be evaluated and treated if infected. Asymptomatic children should probably not be tested unless there are multiple or recurrent cases. Eradicating every cyst from a large group of infants is a monumental task, and treatment of asymptomatic cyst passers is controversial.

The only available stable suspension (making it particularly useful for infants and small children) active against *Giardia* is furazolidone (50 mg/15 mL); the dosage is 1.5 mg/kg four times daily for 7–10 days. Children able to take tablets may be treated with quinacrine hydrochloride, 2 mg/kg three times daily (maximum, 300 mg/d) for 5 days. Gastrointestinal upset, yellow skin, and other troublesome side effects have tempered enthusiasm for this drug despite the fact that it is the most effective agent against *Giardia* available in the USA. Metronidazole, 5 mg/kg three times daily for 5 days, may also be used. A single dose of tinidazole (50 mg/kg [maximum, 2 g]) is also highly effective, but the drug is not available in the USA.

Giardia excretion is self-limited; if symptoms resolve with therapy, repeated stool examinations may not be necessary.

Secondary lactase deficiency may also occur; a secondary invasion of giardiasis should be considered in patients who have diarrhea with cystic fibrosis, chronic pancreatitis, or achlorhydria. In hypogammaglobulinemic patients, relapses are common.

Addiss DG, Juranek DD, Spencer HC: Treatment of children with asymptomatic and non-diarrheal *Giardia* infection. Pediatr Infect Dis J 1991;10:843.

Dupont JL, Sullivan PS: Giardiasis: The clinical spectrum, diagnosis and therapy. Pediatr Infect Dis J 1986; 5(Suppl):131.

Kavousi S: Giardiasis in infancy and childhood: A prospective study of 160 cases with comparison of quinacrine (Atabrine) and metronidazole (Flagyl). Am J Trop Med Hyg 1979;28:19.

Wolfe MS: Giardiasis. Clin Microbiol Rev 1992; 5:93.

CRYPTOSPORIDIOSIS

The protozoan *Cryptosporidium* belongs to the same family as *Toxoplasma* and *Isospora*. It is distributed worldwide. The parasite lines the villi of the small bowel and is noninvasive; it has been found in the biliary and respiratory tracts as well; biliary obstruction may result. *Cryptosporidium* is found in many animals and is a prominent cause of diarrhea in calves; intractable, watery diarrhea and inanition may occur in immunocompromised patients, particularly those with HIV infection. Symptoms may improve with better immune function following antiviral therapy. A similar but self-limited (up to several weeks) diarrheal illness may occur in normal individuals of all ages. Other symptoms include vomiting, fever, and cramps; stools may be positive for occult blood but are usually free of leukocytes. Outbreaks in day care centers and cases in travelers and handlers of large animals are noteworthy. Recently, citywide water-borne outbreaks have been reported in the USA. Diagnosis is by intestinal biopsy or fecal examination for the characteristic 3-µm round cysts. Optimal detection requires an additional laboratory procedure, such as a modified acid-fast stain, which may not be part of the routine parasitologic examination. Cyst excretion lasts 1–4 weeks in patients with normal immune systems, and therapy is not necessary. In immunocompromised patients, cholera-like diarrhea may be fatal. Octreotide may control the diarrhea but does not cure the infection. Paromomycin and azithromycin have separately been shown to be effective in some adult patients. Spiramycin is of questionable benefit.

Current WL, Garcia LS: Cryptosporidiosis. Clin Microbiol Rev 1991; 4:325.
Drugs for parasitic infections. Med Lett Drugs Ther 1993; 35:111.
Egger M et al: Symptoms and transmission of intestinal cryptosporidiosis. Arch Dis Child 1990;65:445.
Janoff EN, Reller LB: *Cryptosporidium* species: A protean protozoan. J Clin Microbiol 1987;25:967.
Petersen C: Cryptosporidiosis in patients infected with the human immunodeficiency virus. Clin Infect Dis 1992; 15:903.
Saez-Llorens et al: Spiramycin vs. placebo for treatment of acute diarrhea caused by *Cryptosporidium*. Pediatr Infect Dis J 1989;8:136.
Vuorio AF, Jokipii AM, Jokipii L: *Cryptosporidium* in asymptomatic children. Rev Infect Dis 1991;13:261.

TRICHOMONIASIS

Trichomonas vaginalis lives on vaginal squamous epithelial cells and in the urethra, prostate, and Skene's glands. It is a common cause of vaginitis, usually in sexually active girls and rarely in prepubertal children as a result of sexual abuse. Nonsexual transmission to prepubertal children may also occur, since the organism may survive on damp clothing for hours. However, finding *Trichomonas* in prepubertal children should always suggest sexual molestation.

Half of infected women and 90% of infected men are asymptomatic. The organism does not cause pelvic inflammatory disease. Some neonates who acquire it during vaginal delivery develop vaginitis or urinary tract infection.

Clinical findings in females include pruritus, dysuria, frothy leukorrhea, and vaginal erythema and edema. Males may have urethritis. Diagnosis by wet prep examination of vaginal or urethral specimens is usually attempted. This technique may miss 10–50% of cases that can be diagnosed by culture. Immunofluorescent and latex agglutination tests are promising for rapid diagnosis. Other sexually transmitted pathogens may also be present in these patients.

Metronidazole is most often prescribed (a single oral dose of 2 g for teenagers is usually effective; 5 mg/kg three times daily for 7 days is an alternative). Refractory cases may respond to higher doses for up to 14 days. Intravaginal clotrimazole is a less effective choice but should be used in early pregnancy, because metronidazole is contraindicated.

Sexual partners should be treated concomitantly. Detecting the organism in males is difficult, and empiric therapy is advised if they are sexual contacts of known cases.

Lossick JG: Treatment of sexually transmitted vaginosis/vaginitis. Rev Infect Dis 1990;12:S665.
Thomason JL, Gelbart SM: *Trichomonas vaginalis*. Obstet Gynecol 1988;74:536.

TOXOPLASMOSIS

Essentials of Diagnosis

- Congenital toxoplasmosis: Hepatosplenomegaly, chorioretinitis, hydrocephalus or microcephaly with cortical calcification, rash, and mental retardation.
- Acquired toxoplasmosis: Fever, rash, lymphadenopathy, chorioretinitis, encephalitis, and myocarditis.
- Demonstration of *Toxoplasma gondii* in tissue or serologic evidence of infection is required for confirmation.

General Considerations

Toxoplasma gondii is a protozoal parasite of humans and some animals. The cat family is the definitive host; 1% of cattle and up to 25% of sheep and pigs in the USA are infected. The proliferative form, or tachyzoite, is crescentic, 4–7 µm long, and has a single nucleus. True cysts containing large numbers of bradyzoites form in tissues, including brain, eye, myocardium, skeletal muscle, and others, where they may persist for life. The normal immune response—

especially via macrophages and gamma interferon—maintains cyst dormancy. Affected individuals are usually asymptomatic. Reactivation and symptomatic infection may occur years later, with immunosuppression. About one-fourth of HIV-infected adults who are seropositive for *T gondii* will develop cerebral toxoplasmosis.

Congenital toxoplasmosis is acquired in utero during a primary maternal infection, the incidence of which is approximately 0.5% of pregnancies in the USA. The 50% transmission rate results in an incidence of 0.2% of all live births. Reactivation of prior infection in an immunocompromised pregnant woman may rarely lead to congenital transmission.

Infection may be acquired by consumption of raw or undercooked infected meat or by inadvertent oral contamination with oocysts from infected cat feces in litter boxes or soil. Oocysts become infectious in 1–21 days and may remain so for over a year in moist conditions. Oocyst survival is decreased by drying; this may explain the low incidence of infection in dry climates.

Oocyst-contaminated water and vegetables have caused small outbreaks of disease.

Ingested oocysts or tissue cysts release the sporozoites, which penetrate the intestine and spread within the host.

The prevalence of infection is 0–20% in children under 10 years of age in the USA, depending on geographic location. Colder and dryer climates have lower prevalence than warm, moist areas of the country, probably reflecting oocyst survivability in various soil conditions.

Clinical Findings

A. Symptoms and Signs:

1. Congenital toxoplasmosis–Clinical abnormalities are more common following infection in early gestation, though transmission is more frequent in late gestation. Maternal infections are frequently asymptomatic. More overt findings typify the classic congenital toxoplasmosis syndrome, including hepatosplenomegaly, jaundice, rash, thrombocytopenia, a characteristic chorioretinitis, and encephalitis, with widely scattered calcifications, hydrocephalus, microcephaly, and mental retardation. This severe form is found in only about 10% of infected infants; 15% have milder disease, and 75% are asymptomatic. Subtle ocular or neurologic abnormalities may be found on careful examination of otherwise asymptomatic babies. Late-onset abnormalities also develop in some asymptomatic babies, including chorioretinitis, strabismus, hydrocephalus, mental retardation, and seizures. Cardiac, pulmonary, bone, or lens abnormalities are not common; their presence suggests rubella, syphilis, or infection with cytomegalovirus.

2. Acquired toxoplasmosis–Acquired toxoplasmosis occurs at any age and is usually asymptom-

atic. The most common clinical manifestation is adenopathy, usually cervical. Single groups of enlarged nodes are common, including axillary, inguinal, and abdominal. They do not suppurate. Other manifestations include fever, hepatomegaly, myalgias, maculopapular rash, encephalitis, myocarditis, pericarditis, retinitis, and pneumonia. About 1% of mononucleosis-like syndromes are due to toxoplasmosis. Chorioretinitis may develop, but is usually thought to represent a late manifestation of congenital infection.

3. Immunocompromised hosts–Patients with lymphoma, leukemia, cardiac transplantation, and HIV infection are especially prone to reactivation of toxoplasmosis, with severe involvement of brain, eye, heart, or lung.

B. Laboratory Findings: Visualization or culture of organisms in spinal fluid or biopsy material is diagnostic. Serologic tests should be performed carefully; commercial kits may be very inaccurate. Other serologic tests, including the Sabin-Feldman dye test, are more sensitive than indirect fluorescent antibody (IFA) titers. An acute specific IgG titer over 1:1000 by IFA, a positive specific IgM titer, or a two-dilution rise suggests acute infection. IgM antibody may persist for years. A negative IgM titer essentially excludes active infection; a low titer is compatible with prior infection; a high titer suggests acute infection. Detection of toxoplasmal DNA in amniotic fluid by polymerase chain reaction is a promising technique for rapid diagnosis of in utero infection. Other laboratory tests are nonspecific. The retinal abnormalities are very characteristic—as are cranial imaging findings—in congenital infection. The cerebral findings in acquired disease may closely resemble those of bacterial abscess or tumor. Histologically, *Toxoplasma* lymph node infection may closely resemble lymphoma.

Differential Diagnosis

Congenital infection may resemble that due to cytomegalovirus, syphilis, herpes, or other agents. Acquired infection mimics a number of viral or lymphoproliferative diseases.

Prevention

Pregnant women should wash hands thoroughly after handling raw meat. Cook meat to 66 °C or greater, wash fruits and vegetables before consumption, and avoid contact with cat feces.

Treatment

Although therapy does not alter established central nervous system damage, it does markedly decrease late sequelae. A year of treatment is recommended for all congenitally infected infants; symptomatic patients receive 6 months of pyrimethamine and sulfadiazine, followed by alternating spiramycin and pyrimethamine-sulfadiazine monthly for the next 6 months. Subclinical infection is treated with pyrimethamine and sulfadiazine for 6 weeks, followed by alternating spiramycin for 6 weeks with pyrimethamine-sulfadiazine for 4 weeks.

Pyrimethamine is given orally at a dosage of 1 mg/kg/d (maximum, 25 mg); gastrointestinal upset, leukopenia, thrombocytopenia, and, rarely, agranulocytosis are side effects. Frequent blood counts should be performed and the drug stopped if the counts fall very low. Leucovorin calcium (folinic acid), 5 mg intramuscularly every 3 days, should be given to decrease the myelotoxicity. The dosage of sulfadiazine or trisulfapyrimidines is 40–45 mg/kg twice a day orally (maximum, 8 g/d). Clindamycin is used for chorioretinitis and encephalitis, especially if sulfonamides are not tolerated.

Therapy of congenital infection may result in normal developmental, neurologic, and eye findings despite apparently severe initial disease. Because acquired infection is usually self-limited, the potentially toxic therapy should be prescribed with discretion, usually only if the illness is complicated.

In chorioretinitis, especially in the acquired form, or if there is evidence of inflammatory central nervous system or systemic disease, a course of corticosteroids (eg, prednisone, 1 mg/kg orally initially and then tapered over 3–4 weeks) is often given along with the antimicrobial agents. Antimicrobial therapy is continued until the eye disease has improved or stabilized. For recurrence of retinitis, steroids may be given alone.

Therapy of primary infection in pregnancy decreases infection in the infant by about 50%. Spiramycin should be started immediately; pyrimethamine plus sulfadiazine are used when spiramycin is not available. Alternating these two regimens during pregnancy is also promising.

Freij BG, Sever HL: Toxoplasmosis. Pediatr Rev 1991;12: 227.

Frenkel JK: Toxoplasmosis. Pediatr Clin North Am 1985; 32:917.

Hohlfeld P et al: Fetal toxoplasmosis: Outcome of pregnancy and infant follow-up after in utero treatment. J Pediatr 1989;115:765.

McAuley J et al: Early and longitudinal evaluations of treated infants and children and untreated historical patients with congenital toxoplasmosis: the Chicago collaborative treatment trial. Clin Infect Dis 1994;18:38.

McCabe RE et al: Clinical spectrum in 107 cases of toxoplasmic lymphadenopathy. Rev Infect Dis 1987;9:754.

Wilson CB: Treatment of congenital toxoplasmosis during pregnancy. J Pediatr 1990;116:1003.

METAZOAL INFECTIONS

NEMATODE INFECTIONS

1. ENTEROBIASIS (Pinworms)

Essentials of Diagnosis

- Nocturnal anal pruritus.
- Worms in the stool or eggs on perianal skin.

General Considerations

This worldwide infection is caused by *Enterobius vermicularis*. The adult worms are about 5–10 mm long and live in the colon; females deposit eggs on the perianal area, primarily at night, causing intense pruritus. Scratching contaminates the fingers and allows transmission back to the host (autoinfection) or to contacts.

Clinical Findings

A. Symptoms and Signs: Although blamed for a myriad of symptoms, pinworms are definitely associated only with localized pruritus. Adult worms may migrate within the colon or up the urethra or vagina in girls. They can be found within the bowel wall, in the lumen of the appendix (usually an incidental finding by the pathologist), in the bladder, and even the peritoneal cavity of girls. The granulomatous reaction that may be present around these ectopic worms is usually asymptomatic. Worm eradication may correspond with the cure of recurrent urinary tract infections in some young girls.

B. Laboratory Findings: The usual diagnostic test consists of pressing a piece of transparent tape on the child's anus in the morning prior to bathing, then placing it on a drop of xylene on a slide. Microscopic examination under low power usually demonstrates the ova. Occasionally, eggs or adult worms are seen in fecal specimens. Parents may also notice adult worms.

Differential Diagnosis

Nonspecific irritation or vaginitis, streptococcal perianal cellulitis (usually painful), and vaginal or urinary bacterial infections may at times resemble pinworm infection, although the symptoms of pinworms are often so suggestive that a therapeutic trial is justified without a confirmed diagnosis.

Treatment

A. Specific Measures: Treat all household members at the same time to prevent reinfections. Since the drugs are not active against the eggs, therapy should be repeated after 2 weeks to kill the recently hatched adults.

1. Pyrantel pamoate–This drug is given as a single dose (11 mg/kg [maximum, 1 g]); it is safe and very effective.

2. Mebendazole–Mebendazole is also highly effective for this infection as well as for most of the other common nematodes. A single oral dose of 100 mg is used for all ages. It should not be given to pregnant women, nor has it been well studied in children under age 2.

B. General Measures: Personal hygiene must be emphasized. Nails should be kept short and clean. Children should wear undergarments to bed to diminish contamination of fingers; bedclothes should be laundered frequently. Although eggs may be widely dispersed in the house and multiple family members infected, the disease is mild and treatable. Avoid creating "pinworm psychosis" in the parents.

Tornieporth NG et al: Ectopic enterobiasis: A case report and review. J Infect 1992;24:87.

2. ASCARIASIS

Essentials of Diagnosis

- Abdominal cramps and discomfort.
- Large, white, round worms or ova in the feces.

General Considerations

Ascaris lumbricoides is a worldwide human parasite. Ova passed by carriers may remain viable for months under the proper soil conditions. The ova contaminate food or fingers and are subsequently ingested by a new host. The larvae hatch, penetrate the intestinal wall, enter the venous system, reach the alveoli, are coughed up, and return to the small intestine, where they mature. The female lays thousands of eggs daily.

Clinical Findings

A. Symptoms and Signs: Infections usually remain asymptomatic; severe cases, however, can be associated with pain, weight loss, anorexia, diarrhea, or vomiting. Adult worms may be seen in feces or vomitus. Rarely, they perforate or obstruct the small bowel, biliary system, or appendix.

Large numbers of larvae migrating through the lungs may cause an acute, transient eosinophilic pneumonia (Löffler's syndrome). Otitis media has been occasionally reported.

B. Laboratory Findings: The diagnosis is made by observing the large, round worms in the stool or by microscopic detection of the ova.

Treatment

Because the adult worms live less than a year, asymptomatic infection need not be treated. Meben-

dazole (100 mg twice daily for 3 days for children over 2 years old) or pyrantel pamoate (a single dose of 11 mg/kg [maximum, 1 g]) is the drug of choice. If there are large numbers of worms, intestinal obstruction may result from the mass of paralyzed parasites. Surgical removal is sometimes needed.

Fagan JJ, Prescott CA: Ascariasis in acute otitis media. Int J Pediatr Otorhinolaryngol 1993; 26:67.
Sasaki J, Seidel JS: Ascariasis mimicking an acute abdomen. Ann Emerg Med 1992; 21:217.

3. TRICHURIASIS (Whipworm)

Trichuris trichiura is a widespread human and animal parasite common in poor children living in warm, humid areas conducive to survival of the ova. The adult worms live in the cecum and colon; the ova are passed and become infectious after several weeks in the soil. Ingested infective eggs hatch in the upper small intestine. Unlike *Ascaris, Trichuris* does not have a migratory tissue phase. No symptoms are usually present unless the infection is severe, in which case it can cause pain, diarrhea, and mild abdominal distention. Massive infections may also cause rectal prolapse and dysentery. Detecting the characteristic barrel-shaped ova in the feces makes the diagnosis. Adult worms may be seen in the prolapsed rectum or at proctoscopy; their thin heads are buried in the mucosa, and the thicker posterior portions extrude. Mild to moderate eosinophilia may be present.

Mebendazole is the drug of choice (100 mg orally twice daily for 3 days for children over 2 years). Treatment improves gastrointestinal symptoms as well as having constitutional effects such as improving school attendance and performance among heavily infected children in endemic areas.

Nokes C et al: Parasitic helminth infection and cognitive function in school children. Proc R Soc Lond [Biol] 1992;247:77.
Robertson LJ et al: *Trichuris trichiura* and the growth of primary school children in Panama. Trans R Soc Trop Med Hyg 1992;86:656.

4. HOOKWORM

Essentials of Diagnosis

- Iron deficiency anemia.
- Hematochezia.
- Abdominal discomfort, weight loss.
- Ova in the feces.

General Considerations

The common human hookworms are *Ancylostoma duodenale* and *Necator americanus*. Both are widespread in the tropics and subtropics. The larger *Ancylostoma* is more pathogenic because it consumes more blood, up to 0.5 mL per worm per day.

The adults live in the jejunum. Eggs are passed in the feces and develop and hatch into infective larvae in warm, damp soil within 2 weeks. The larvae penetrate human skin on contact, enter the blood, reach the alveoli, are coughed up and swallowed, and develop into adults in the intestine. The adult worms attach with their mouth parts to the mucosa from which they suck blood. Blood loss is the major sequel of infection. Infection rates reach 90% in areas without sanitation.

A separate species, *Ancylostoma braziliense* (the dog or cat hookworm), causes creeping eruption (cutaneous larva migrans). This disease is seen mainly on the warm-water American coasts.

Clinical Findings

A. Symptoms and Signs: The larvae usually penetrate the skin of the feet and cause intense local itching ("ground itch"). This subsides as the larvae continue their migration. In creeping eruption, the nonhuman larvae migrate blindly in the skin before dying, creating serpiginous burrows.

Mild infections produce no symptoms. Severe infections may cause pain, loose stools, iron deficiency anemia, and malnutrition.

B. Laboratory Findings: The large ova of both species of hookworm are found in feces and are indistinguishable. Microcytic anemia, folate deficiency, hypoalbuminemia, eosinophilia, and hematochezia are seen in severe cases.

Prevention

Fecal contamination of soil should be prevented; skin contact with potentially contaminated soil should also be avoided.

Treatment

A. Specific Measures: Mebendazole (100 mg orally twice daily for 3 days) is the drug of choice. It is also active against a number of other nematodes that may coexist with hookworm. Pyrantel pamoate (11 mg/kg [maximum, 1 g], daily for 3 days) is an alternative. Topical thiabendazole and albendazole and oral thiabendazole are useful for creeping eruption.

B. General Measures: Iron therapy may be more important than worm eradication. Parenteral iron or transfusions may be needed in severe cases.

Prognosis

The outcome is usually excellent.

Hotez PJ: Hookworm disease in children. Pediatr Infect Dis J 1989;8:516.

5. STRONGYLOIDIASIS

Essentials of Diagnosis

- Cough and hemoptysis.
- Abdominal pain, diarrhea.
- Eosinophilia, malnutrition.
- Larvae in stools and duodenal aspirates.

General Considerations

The responsible parasite, *Strongyloides stercoralis,* is unique in having both parasitic and free-living forms; the latter can survive in the soil for several generations. The parasite is found in most tropical and subtropical regions of the world. The adults live in the submucosal tissue of the duodenum and occasionally in the whole intestine. Eggs deposited in the mucosa hatch rapidly; the first-stage (rhabditiform) larvae, therefore, are the predominant form found in duodenal aspirates and feces. The larvae rapidly mature to the tissue-penetrating filariform stage and initiate internal autoinfection. The filariform larvae also inhabit the soil and can penetrate the skin of another host, subsequently migrating into veins and alveoli and reaching the intestine when coughed up and swallowed.

Older children and adults are more often infected than young children. Even low worm burden can result in significant clinical symptoms. Infestations due to poor sanitation and hygiene in homes for the retarded are noteworthy. Immunosuppressed patients may develop fatal disseminated strongyloidiasis, known as the hyperinfective cycle.

Clinical Findings

A. Symptoms and Signs: At the site of the skin penetration, there may be a pruritic rash. Large numbers of migrating larvae can cause wheezing, cough, and hemoptysis. Most intestinal infections are asymptomatic. Symptoms may include abdominal pain, distention, diarrhea, and (sometimes) vomiting. Because the upper bowel is involved, a high obstruction or peptic disease may be simulated.

B. Laboratory Findings: Finding larvae in the feces or in duodenal aspirates is diagnostic. Because even multiple stools may be negative, duodenal aspirates or use of the string test (Entero-Test) should be considered. Marked eosinophilia is common.

C. Imaging: Patchy pulmonary infiltrates may be seen during the migration phase; later, inflammation or narrowing of the duodenum on a barium study is typical.

Differential Diagnosis

Strongyloidiasis should be differentiated from peptic disease, celiac disease, regional or tuberculous enteritis, hookworm infection, and other causes of intestinal symptoms or malabsorption. The pulmonary phase may mimic asthma or bronchopneumonia. Severe infection can present as an acute abdomen.

Complications & Sequelae

Chronic diarrhea and malabsorption can lead to malnutrition. Overwhelming strongyloidiasis is an opportunistic infection in heavily immunosuppressed patients, usually those who have resided in or traveled to endemic areas. Suspect the diagnosis if bilateral pulmonary infiltrates and paralytic ileus are seen on radiographs. In these patients, larvae are usually easily found in many body fluids, including cerebrospinal fluid and secondary bacteremia occurs with coliforms.

Treatment

A. Specific Measures: Thiabendazole (25 mg/kg orally twice daily for 2 days [maximum, 3 g/d]) is the drug of choice. Ivermectin is also effective. Relapses are common.

B. General Measures: Fluid and nutritional support is needed.

Berk SL et al: Clinical and epidemiologic features of strongyloidiasis: A prospective study in rural Tennessee. Arch Intern Med 1987;147:1256.

Davidson RA, Fletcher RH, Chapman LE: Risk factors for strongyloidiasis: A case control study. Arch Intern Med 1984;144:321.

Neva FA: Biology and immunology of human strongyloidiasis. J Infect Dis 1986;153:397.

6. VISCERAL LARVA MIGRANS (Toxocariasis)

Essentials of Diagnosis

- Hepatosplenomegaly and marked eosinophilia in young children with pica.
- Hyperglobulinemia; elevated isohemagglutinin titers.
- Positive serology or demonstration of larvae on liver biopsy.

General Considerations

Visceral larva migrans is a worldwide disease. The agent is the cosmopolitan intestinal ascarid of dogs and cats, *Toxocara canis* or *Toxocara cati.* The eggs passed by infected animals contaminate parks and other areas that young children frequent. After an incubation period, the ova become infectious and may be inadvertently ingested. Children with pica are more at risk. Even urban areas may be contaminated; up to 30% of playground soils may contain eggs. Recent surveys have found 5% of New York City children and about 25% of rural Appalachian kindergarten children to be seropositive. Ingested eggs hatch and penetrate the intestinal wall, then migrate to the liver, lungs, and other organs, where they die and incite a granulomatous inflammatory reaction. The rodent whipworm, *Capillaria hepatica,* can cause a similar syndrome.

Clinical Findings

A. Symptoms and Signs: Presenting symptoms include anorexia, fever, pallor, abdominal distention, abdominal pain, and cough. Hepatomegaly is common, and splenomegaly is not unusual. Adenopathy is absent. Seizures and blindness are unusual manifestations. A recently described syndrome of "covert toxocariasis" includes fever, fatigue, and anorexia without typical visceral or ocular involvement.

B. Laboratory Findings: Marked leukocytosis (with 30–90% eosinophils) is typical of severe infections. Anemia, hypergammaglobulinemia, and elevated isohemagglutinins and ceruloplasmin are common. The diagnosis is confirmed by finding larvae in the liver, granulomatous lesions, muscle, or brain. Positive serology and the exclusion of other causes of hypereosinophilia allow a presumptive diagnosis to be made in typical cases. Milder cases may have slight or no eosinophilia; they may be asymptomatic or have vague abdominal complaints or recurrent pruritic cutaneous eruptions.

Differential Diagnosis

Diseases with hypereosinophilia must be considered. These include trichinosis (large liver and spleen not usually seen, muscle tenderness), eosinophilic leukemia (rare in children; eosinophils are abnormal in appearance), collagen vascular disease (those associated with eosinophilia are rare in young children), strongyloidiasis (no organomegaly; enteric symptoms are common), early ascariasis, and tropical eosinophilia (seen mainly in India), allergies, and hypersensitivity syndromes.

Complications & Sequelae

Myocarditis, retinitis, and encephalitis occur. A retinal mass resembling retinoblastoma may be the only manifestation in some children.

Treatment

A. Specific Measures: The clinical benefit of specific anthelmintic therapy is not defined. Thiabendazole has been used most often (25 mg/kg [maximum, 3 g/d] orally twice a day for 5–7 days). Diethylcarbamazine may also be used (2 mg/kg three times a day orally for 7–10 days). Albendazole and mebendazole are also alternatives. Significant lung involvement is one indication for specific therapy.

B. General Measures: Because the disease is usually self-limited, therapy is supportive and emphasizes prevention of reinfection. Treating any cause of pica, such as iron deficiency, is important. Corticosteroids are used for marked inflammation of lung, eye, or other organs. Pets should be dewormed routinely.

Other children in the household may be infected. Mild eosinophilia and positive serologic tests may be the only clue to their infection. Therapy is not necessary for these patients. "Covert" disease has been treated with good results reported.

Marmor M et al: *Toxocara canis* infection of children: Epidemiologic and neuropsychologic findings. Am J Pub Health 1987;77:554.

Nathwani D, Laing RB, Currie PF: Covert toxocariasis: A cause of recurrent abdominal pain in childhood. Br J Clin Pract 1992;46:271.

Rasmussen LN, Dirdal M, Birkebaek NH: "Covert toxocariasis" in a child treated with low-dose diethylcarbamazine. Acta Pediatr 1993;82:116.

Taylor MR et al: The expanded spectrum of toxocaral disease. Lancet 1988;1:692.

7. TRICHINOSIS

Essentials of Diagnosis

- Vomiting, diarrhea, and pain within 48 hours of eating infected meat.
- Fever, periorbital edema, myalgia, and marked eosinophilia.
- *Trichinella spiralis* larvae in muscle biopsy.

General Considerations

Trichinella spiralis is a small roundworm. The adults inhabit the intestines of hogs and several other meat-eating animals. The cycle begins when the larvae in the muscle of hogs, bear, walrus, and other animals are ingested; they then enter the bowel mucosa, develop into adults, reemerge into the intestine, mate, and reenter the mucosa. The hundreds of larvae produced by each female over the next weeks enter the bloodstream and encyst in the striated muscle. Their migration causes marked inflammation. Humans are usually infected by eating undercooked pork. Smoking, salting, or drying the meat does not kill the larvae. Machines used to grind infected pork may contaminate other meat, such as beef.

Clinical Findings

A. Symptoms and Signs: The initial bowel penetration may cause nausea, vomiting, diarrhea, and cramps. Patients may have mild or no symptoms. Two clinical syndromes have been described. The classic or myopathic form consists of fever, edema (primarily of the face and eyelids), myalgia, and weakness. A second form has been seen in the Arctic with primarily chronic intestinal complaints. Many organs may be infected by the migrating larvae—diaphragm, heart, lungs, kidneys, spleen, skin, and brain. Severe cerebral involvement may be fatal. Myocarditis may also be severe or fatal. Symptoms may last months.

B. Laboratory Findings: Marked eosinophilia is the rule.

Differential Diagnosis

The classic symptoms are quite pathognomonic if one is aware of this disease. It sometimes mimics typhoid fever. The L-tryptophan-associated eosinophilia-myalgia syndrome also resembles trichinosis.

Prevention

Because a microscopic exam must be done, meat in the USA is not inspected for trichinosis. Although all states require the cooking of hog swill, hog-to-hog or hog-to-rat cycles may continue. All pork and sylvatic meat (such as bear or walrus) should be heated to at least 65 °C. Freezing meat to at least –15 °C for 3 weeks may also prevent transmission.

Animals used for food should not be fed or allowed access to raw meat.

Treatment

Mebendazole has activity against the intestinal, circulating, and tissue stages of infection. The adult dose is 200–400 mg three times daily for 3 days followed by 400–500 mg three times daily for 10 days. Pediatric dosing has not been standardized. Concurrent corticosteroids are used in attempt to prevent the Herxheimer reaction associated with treatment.

Prognosis

Death may occur within the first weeks, but most infections are self-limited.

MacLean JD et al: Trichinosis in the Canadian Arctic: Report of five outbreaks and a new clinical syndrome. J Infect Dis 1989;160:513.

Santos Duran-Ortiz J et al: Trichinosis with severe myopathic involvement mimicking polymyositis. Report of a family outbreak. J Rheumatol 1992;19:310.

CESTODE INFECTIONS (Flukes)

1. TAENIASIS & CYSTICERCOSIS

Essentials of Diagnosis

- Abdominal discomfort, diarrhea (taeniasis).
- Focal seizures, headaches (neurocysticercosis).
- Passage of worm segments (proglottids) and eggs in feces.
- Cysticerci present in biopsy specimens, on plain films (as calcified masses), or on CT or MRI.

General Considerations

Both the beef tapeworm (*Taenia saginata*) and the pork (*Taenia solium*) tapeworm cause taeniasis. The adults live in the intestines of humans; the egg-laden distal segments, or proglottids, break off and are passed in feces, disintegrating and releasing the ova in the soil. After ingestion in food or water by cattle or pigs, the eggs hatch and the larvae migrate to and encyst in skeletal muscle. When ingested by humans, these larvae mature into adults.

Humans can be an intermediate host for *T solium* (but not *T saginata*), and the larvae released from ingested eggs encyst in a variety of tissues, especially muscle and brain. Full larval maturation occurs in 2 months, but the cysts cause little inflammation until they die months to years later. Inflammatory edema ensues with calcification or disappearance of the cyst. A slowly expanding mass of sterile cysts at the base of the brain may cause obstructive hydrocephalus (racemose cysticercosis).

Both parasites are distributed worldwide. Contamination of foods by eggs in human feces allows infection without exposure to meat or travel to endemic areas. Asymptomatic cases are common, but neurocysticercosis is a leading cause of seizures in endemic areas.

Person-person spread may occur, resulting in infection of individuals with no exposure to infected meat.

Clinical Findings

A. Symptoms and Signs:

1. Taeniasis–In most tapeworm infections, the only clinical manifestation is the passage of fecal proglottids—white, motile bodies 1 × 2 cm in size. They occasionally crawl out onto the skin and down the leg, especially the larger *T saginata*.

Children may harbor the adult worm for years and complain of abdominal pain, anorexia, and diarrhea. A more severe infection may be associated with more symptoms.

2. Cysticercosis–Most cases are asymptomatic. Subcutaneous nodules of 1–2 cm may be the only sign. After several years, the cysticerci calcify and appear as radiographic opacities. Brain cysts may remain silent or cause seizures, headache, hydrocephalus, and basilar meningitis. Rarely, the spinal cord is involved. Neurocysticercosis becomes manifest an average of 5 years after exposure but may cause symptoms in the first year of life. In the eye, cysts cause bleeding, retinal detachment, and uveitis. Definitive diagnosis requires histologic demonstration of larvae or cyst membrane. Presumptive diagnosis is often made by the characteristics of the cysts seen on CT or MRI studies; the differential diagnosis may include tuberculoma, brain abscess, arachnoid cyst, and tumor. The presence of *T solium* eggs in feces is uncommon but supports the diagnosis.

B. Laboratory Findings:
Eggs or proglottids may be found in feces or on the perianal skin (using the tape method employed for pinworms). Eggs of both *Taenia* species are identical. The species are identified by examination of proglottids; more than 18 lateral uterine branches are present in *T saginata*, less than 12 branches in *T solium*.

Peripheral eosinophilia is minimal or absent. Spinal fluid eosinophilia is seen in 10–75% of cases of neurocysticercosis; its presence supports an otherwise presumptive diagnosis.

Enzyme immunoassay (EIA) antibody titers are eventually positive in up to 98% of serum specimens and over 75% of cerebrospinal fluid specimens from patients with neurocysticercosis. Solitary cysts are less often associated with seropositivity than are multiple cysts. High titers tend to correlate with more severe disease. Cerebrospinal fluid titers are higher if cysts are near the meninges.

Treatment

A. Taeniasis: Niclosamide is effective and relatively nontoxic. It is given as a single dose of 1 g (two tablets) for children 11–34 kg and 1.5 g for heavier children. The adult dose is 2 g. Tablets should be crushed or chewed well before swallowing. Praziquantel (5–10 mg/kg once) is also effective. Feces free of segments or ova for 3 months suggest cure.

B. Cysticercosis: Medical treatment has traditionally been reserved for patients symptomatic with meningitis or increased intracranial pressure. Recently, adult patients with seizures as their only manifestation of neurocysticercosis have been shown to benefit by antiparasitic therapy. Praziquantel and albendazole cause disappearance of noninflamed cysts. The recommended dose of praziquantel is 50 mg/kg/d in three divided doses for 2 weeks; that for albendazole is 15 mg/kg divided into three doses daily for 28 days. Albendazole is more effective than praziquantel. Larval death may result in clinical worsening due to inflammatory edema. A short course of dexamethasone may decrease these symptoms, but it should not be used prophylactically because it may lower serum praziquantel levels. The clinical significance of lower praziquantel levels is unknown, and dose adjustment is not recommended if steroids are used. Once cyst inflammation is demonstrated by imaging (ring enhancement), resolution usually occurs, and therapy may not be of further benefit. Patients with multiple active (noninflamed) cysts should be treated. The racemose cysts contain no viable larvae and do not respond to medical therapy. Follow-up scans every several months help assess the response to therapy.

Prevention

The incidence in the USA is low, because beef and pork are inspected for taeniasis. Prevention requires proper cooking of meat, careful washing of raw vegetables and fruits, treatment of intestinal carriers, avoiding the use of human excrement for fertilizer, and providing proper sanitary facilities.

Prognosis

The prognosis is good in intestinal taeniasis. Symptoms associated with a few cerebral cysts may disappear in a few months; heavy infections may cause death or chronic neurologic impairment.

Del Brutto OH, Sotelo J: Neurocysticercosis: An update. Rev Infect Dis 1988;10:1975.

Mitchell WG, Crawford TO: Intraparenchymal cerebral cysticercosis in children: Diagnosis and treatment. Pediatrics 1988;82:76.

Schantz PM et al: Neurocysticercosis in an Orthodox Jewish community in New York City. N Engl J Med 1992; 327:692.

Sorvillo FJ et al: Cysticercosis surveillance: locally acquired and travel-related infections and detection of intestinal tapeworm carriers in Los Angeles County. Am J Trop Med Hyg 1992;47:365.

Sotelo J et al: Comparison of therapeutic regimens of anti-cysticercal drugs for parenchymal brain cysticercosis. J Neurol 1990;237:69.

St. Geme III JW et al: Consensus: Diagnosis and management of neurocysticercosis in children. Pediatr Infect Dis J 1993;12:455.

Takayanagui OM, Jardim E: Therapy for neurocysticercosis. Comparison between albendazole and praziquantel. Arch Neurol 1992;49:290.

2. HYMENOLEPIASIS

Hymenolepis nana, the cosmopolitan human tapeworm, is a common parasite of children; *Hymenolepis diminuta,* the rat tapeworm, is rare. The former is capable of causing autoinfection, because the entire life cycle may take place in the human intestine. The larvae hatched from the ingested eggs penetrate the intestinal wall and then reenter the lumen to mature into adults. Their eggs are immediately infectious for the same or a new host. The adult is only a few centimeters long. Finding the characteristic eggs in feces is diagnostic.

H diminuta has an intermediate stage in rat fleas and other insects; children are infected when they ingest these insects.

Light infections with either tapeworm are usually asymptomatic; heavy infection can cause diarrhea and abdominal pain. Therapy is with praziquantel (25 mg/kg once) or niclosamide (11–34 kg: 1 g on the first day of treatment followed by 0.5 g/d for 6 days; > 34 kg: 1.5 g on the first day, then 1 g/d for 6 days).

Drugs for parasitic infections. Med Lett Drugs Ther 1993; 35:111.

Jones WE: Niclosamide as a treatment for *Hymenolepis diminuta* and *Dipylidium caninum* infection in man. Am J Trop Med Hyg 1979;28:300.

3. ECHINOCOCCOSIS

Essentials of Diagnosis

- Cystic tumors of liver, lung, kidney, bone, brain, and other organs.
- Eosinophilia.
- Urticaria and pruritus if cysts rupture.
- Protoscoleces or daughter cysts in the primary cyst.
- Positive serology.

General Considerations

Dogs, cats, and other carnivores are the hosts for *Echinococcus granulosus.* Endemic areas include Australia, New Zealand, and southwestern USA, including Native American reservations where sheepherding is practiced. The adult tapeworm lives in the intestine, and eggs are passed in the animals' feces. When ingested by a child, the eggs hatch, and the larvae penetrate the intestinal mucosa and disseminate in the bloodstream. The larvae produce cysts; the primary sites of involvement are the liver (60–70%) and the lungs (20–25%). A unilocular cyst is most common. Over years, it may reach 25 cm in diameter, although most are much smaller. The cysts of *Echinococcus multilocularis* are multilocular and demonstrate more rapid growth.

Clinical Findings

A. Symptoms and Signs: Clinical disease is due to pressure from the enlarging cysts, vessel erosion, and sensitization to cyst or worm antigens. Liver cysts present as slowly expanding tumors that may cause biliary obstruction. Most are in the right lobe and extend inferiorly; one-fourth are on the upper surface and may be asymptomatic for years. Omental torsion or hemorrhage from vessel erosion may occur.

Rupture of a pulmonary cyst causes coughing, dyspnea, wheezing, urticaria, chest pain, and hemoptysis; cyst and worm remnants are found in sputum. Brain cysts may cause focal neurologic signs and convulsions; renal cysts cause pain and hematuria; bone cysts cause pain.

B. Laboratory Findings: Presumptive diagnosis is made by a combination of radiographic, cytologic, and serologic findings. The appropriate body fluid (tracheal aspirate, ascitic or pleural fluid, spinal fluid, or urine, depending on the site of the cyst) should be examined for protoscoleces. Passing a large amount of fluid through a 5 µm filter and then looking for protoscoleces with an acid-fast stain or other stain has been found to be a sensitive method.

Eosinophilia is variable and may be absent. Serologic tests are useful for diagnosis and follow-up of therapy.

Diagnostic titers vary among laboratories. The bentonite flocculation test is positive at a titer of 1:5, and the indirect hemagglutination test is positive at 1:128. Titers are much higher in secondary echinococcosis (due to cyst rupture). Titers remain high at least a year after surgery. They are usually negative by 10 years. Persistently elevated titers suggest persistent infection.

The skin test for echinococcosis (Casoni test) should not be used. It has never been standardized, and many false-positive results are seen.

C. Imaging: Pulmonary or bone cysts may be

visible on plain films. Other imaging techniques are preferred for cysts in other organs. Visualization of daughter cysts is highly suggestive of echinococcosis.

Differential Diagnosis

Tumors, bacterial or amebic abscess, and tuberculosis (pulmonary) must be considered.

Complications

Sudden cyst rupture with anaphylaxis and death is the worst complication. If the patient survives, secondary infections from seeding of daughter cysts may occur. Segmental lung collapse, secondary bacterial infections, effects of increased intracranial pressure, and severe renal damage due to renal cysts are other potential complications.

Treatment

Definitive therapy of *E multilocularis* requires meticulous surgical removal of the cysts, preceded by careful injection of the cyst with formalin or an iodine solution to sterilize infectious protoscoleces. Freezing the cyst wall and injecting silver nitrate prior to removal is another technique. A surgeon familiar with this disease should be consulted. Medical therapy (see below) may be of some benefit. If the cyst leaks or ruptures, the allergic symptoms must be managed immediately.

Albendazole (15 mg/kg/d for 28 days with repeat courses as necessary following a 14-day "rest period") is effective in many, but not all, cases of *E granulosus* infection (hydatid disease).

Prognosis

Large liver cysts may be asymptomatic for years. Surgery is often curative for lung and liver cysts but not always for cysts in other locations. Secondary disease has a much worse prognosis; about 15% of patients with this disease die.

Ersahin Y, Mutluer S, Guzelbag E: Intracranial hydatid cysts in children. Neurosurgery 1993;33:219.

Force L et al: Evaluation of eight serological tests in the diagnosis of human echinococcosis and follow-up. Clin Infect Dis 1992;15:473.

Morris DL et al: Albendazole: Objective evidence of response in human hydatid disease. JAMA 1985;253:2053.

TREMATODE INFECTIONS

1. SCHISTOSOMIASIS

Essentials of Diagnosis

- Transient pruritic rash after exposure to fresh water.
- Fever, urticaria, arthralgias, cough, lymphadenitis, and eosinophilia.
- Weight loss, anorexia, diarrhea.
- Hematuria, dysuria.
- Eggs in stool, urine, or rectal biopsy specimens.

General Considerations

One of the most common serious parasitic diseases, schistosomiasis is caused by several species of *Schistosoma* flukes; *Schistosoma japonicum, Schistosoma mekongi,* and *Schistosoma mansoni* involve the intestines, and *Schistosoma haematobium* the urinary tract. The first two are found in East and Southeast Asia; *S mansoni* in tropical Africa, the Caribbean, and parts of South America; and *S haematobium* in northern Africa.

Infection is caused by free-swimming larvae (cercariae), which emerge from the intermediate hosts, certain species of fresh-water snails. The cercariae penetrate human skin, migrate to the liver, and mature into adults, which then migrate through the portal vein to lodge in the bladder veins (*S haematobium*), superior mesenteric veins (*S mekongi, S japonicum*), or inferior mesenteric veins (*S mansoni*). Clinical disease results primarily from the inflammation caused by the many eggs that are laid in the perivascular tissues or embolize to the liver. Escape of ova into bowel or bladder lumen allows microscopic visualization and diagnosis from stool or urine specimens, as well as contamination of fresh water and infection of the snail hosts that ingest them.

Clinical Findings

Much of the population in endemic areas is infected but asymptomatic. Only heavy infections produce symptoms.

A. Symptoms and Signs: The cercarial penetration may cause a pruritic rash; larval migration may cause fever, urticaria, and cough; the maturation phase may cause tender hepatosplenomegaly followed by days to weeks of fever and malaise as the worms migrate to their final destination. Bladder infection results in dysuria, hematuria, reflux, stones, and incontinence. Secondary pyelonephritis and ureteral obstruction may occur. Intestinal infection causes pain, diarrhea (often with blood), and, finally, cirrhosis, splenomegaly, and ascites due to the chronic inflammation caused by the thousands of eggs embolized to the liver.

B. Laboratory Findings: The diagnosis is made by finding the species-specific eggs in feces (*S japonicum, S mekongi, S mansoni,* and occasionally *S haematobium*), urine (*S haematobium,* occasionally *S mansoni*). A rectal biopsy may reveal *S mansoni* and should be done if other specimens are negative. Peripheral eosinophilia is common, and eosinophils may be seen in urine.

Complications & Sequelae

The chronic inflammation in the urinary tract associated with *S haematobium* infections may result in obstructive uropathy, stones, infection, bladder cancer, fistulas, and anemia due to chronic hematuria. Spinal cord granulomas and paraplegia due to egg embolization into Batson's plexus have been seen.

The intestinal schistosomes cause cirrhosis. Intestinal perforation and stricture are uncommon.

Prevention

The best prevention is to avoid contact with contaminated fresh water in endemic areas. Efforts to destroy the snail hosts have not been successful.

Treatment

A. Specific Measures: Praziquantel is the drug of choice for schistosomiasis. A dose of 40 mg/kg/d divided in two divided doses (*S mansoni* or *S haematobium*) or 20 mg/kg three times in 1 day (*S japonicum* or *S mekongi*) is very effective and nontoxic.

B. General Measures: Medical therapy of nutritional deficiency or secondary bacterial infections may be needed. The urinary tract should be carefully evaluated in *S haematobium* infections; reconstructive surgery may be needed. Cirrhosis is treated supportively and with portal shunting if needed.

Prognosis

Medical therapy decreases the worm infection and liver size, despite continued exposure in endemic areas. Early disease responds well to therapy, but once significant scarring or severe inflammation has occurred, eradication of the parasites is of little benefit.

McGarvey ST et al: Child growth and schistosomiasis japonica in northeastern Leyte, the Philippines: Cross-sectional results. Am J Trop Med Hyg 1992; 46:571.

Novato-Silva E, Gazzinelli G, Colley DG: Immune responses during human schistosomiasis mansoni. XVIII. Immunologic status of pregnant women and their neonates. Scand J Immunol 1992;35:429.

II. INFECTIONS: MYCOTIC

The three major categories of fungal infections are shown in Table 37–4. Systemic disease in normal hosts is commonly caused by three organisms—*Coccidioides, Histoplasma,* and *Blastomyces*—which are restricted to certain geographic areas. Prior residence in or travel to these areas, even for a brief time, is a prerequisite for inclusion in a differential diagnosis. Of these three, *Histoplasma* most often relapses years later in patients who are immunosuppressed.

Immunosuppression, foreign bodies (eg, central catheters), ulceration of gastrointestinal and respiratory mucosae, and broad-spectrum antimicrobial therapy are major risk factors for opportunistic fungal disease.

Laboratory diagnosis may be difficult because of the small number of fungi present in some lesions, the slow growth of the organism, and difficulty in distinguishing colonization of mucosal surfaces from infection. A tissue biopsy with fungal stains and culture is the best method for diagnosing systemic disease. Repeat blood cultures may be negative even in the

Table 37–4. Pediatric fungal infections.

Type	Agents	Incidence	Diagnosis	Diagnostic Tests	Therapy	Prognosis
Superficial	Candida Dermatophytes Sporothrix Malassezia	Very common	Simple, accurate[1]	KOH prep	Topical[2]	Good
Systemic: Normal host	Coccidioides Histoplasma Blastomyces	Common: regional	Often presumptive	Chest x-ray Skin tests Serology Culture examination of body fluids or tissue	None[3] or systemic	Good
Systemic: Opportunistic infection	Candida Pneumocystis[4] Aspergillus Malassezia Pseudallescheria Zygomycetes Cryptococcus	Uncommon	Difficult[5]	Tissue biopsy, culture	Systemic, prolonged	Poor if therapy delayed

[1]Sporotrichosis may require biopsy for diagnosis and is treated with systemic therapy.
[2]These fungi in immunocompromised patients cause severe, rapidly progressive disease.
[3]Often self-limited in normal host.
[4]Now considered a yeast. May infect many normal individuals.
[5]Except *Cryptococcus,* which is often diagnosed by antigen detection.

presence of intravascular infections. Tests for antibody and antigen are currently too insensitive to diagnose many systemic infections, but serology is useful for coccidioidomycosis and histoplasmosis.

The risk of empiric treatment is greater for fungal than for bacterial infections because of the toxicity of some antifungals, the frequent need for prolonged parenteral administration, and the limited data available for choosing the best dose or regimen. Delay in treating systemic disease, however, may prove fatal.

Susceptibility testing of fungi is not well standardized, and the correlation of in vitro susceptibility to clinical response is not well defined.

Several less common fungal infections, are presented in Table 37–5.

BLASTOMYCOSIS

The causative fungus, *Blastomyces dermatitidis* is a soil organism found primarily in the Mississippi and Ohio River Valleys. Transmission is by inhalation of spores. Outbreaks associated with construction have occurred. Severe disease is much more common in adults and males.

Primary infection is usually pulmonary. Acute symptoms include cough, chest pain, headache, weight loss, and fever occurring several weeks to months after inoculation. They are usually self-limited in normal patients. Progressive pulmonary disease may occur. Radiographic consolidation is typical; effusions, nodules, hilar nodes, and cavities are less common. Chronic disease can develop in the upper lobes, with cavities and fibronodular infiltrations similar to that seen in tuberculosis.

Cutaneous lesions usually represent disseminated

Table 37–5. Unusual fungal infections in children.

Organism	Predisposing Factors	Route of Infection	Clinical Disease	Diagnostic Tests	Therapy and Comments
Aspergillus species	None	Inhalation of spores	Allergic bronchopulmonary aspergillosis; wheezing, migratory infiltrates.	Organisms in sputum; positive skin test; specific IgE antibody.	Hypersensitivity to fungal antigens. Use steroids. No antifungals needed.
	Immuno-suppression	Inhalation of spores	Progressive pulmonary disease: Consolidation, nodules, abscesses. Sinusitis Disseminated disease: Usually lung, brain; occasionally intestine, kidney, heart, bone.	Demonstrate organs in tissues by stain or culture	Amphotericin B for 4–6 weeks.
Malassezia furfur; M pachydermatis	Central venous catheter, lipid infusion	Line infection from skin colonization	Sepsis; pneumonitis, thrombocytopenia.	Culture of catheter tip or catheter blood specimen on lipid-enriched media (for *M furfur; M pachydermatis* does not need lipid).	Discontinuation of lipid may be sufficient. Remove catheter. Short-term amphotericin B may be added. Organism ubiquitous on normal skin; requires long-chain fatty acids for growth.
Pseudallescheria boydii	Immuno-suppression	Inhalation	Disseminated abscesses (lung, brain, liver, spleen, other).	Culture of pus or tissue.	Surgical drainage; itraconazole. Poor prognosis.
	Minor trauma	Cutaneous	Mycetoma (most common).	Yelow-white granules in pus. Culture.	Aggressive surgery. Amputation may be needed.
Sporothrix schenkii	Minor trauma (thorns, splinters)	Cutaneous	Chronic skin ulcers, subcutaneous nodules along lymphatics. Pneumonia, osteomyelitis, or arthritis.	Gram or fungal stain of pus or tissue may show "hockey stick" organisms. Culture of pus, tissue.	1. Potassium iodide (oral). 2. Itraconazole, drainage, debridement; amphotericin B may offer no advantage.
Zygomycetes (*Mucor, Rhizopus*)	Immunosuppression, diabetic acidosis	Inhalation, mucosal colonization, invasion of vessels or tissue	Rhinocerebral: sinus, nose, necrotizing vasculitis; central nervous system spread. Pulmonary. Disseminated: Any organ	Broad aseptate hyphae on tissue stains. Culture: rapidly growing, fluffy fungus.	Amphotericin B, surgical debridement; itraconazole may be alternative or a second agent for combined therapy. Poor prognosis.

disease, although local primary inoculation is possible. Slowly progressive ulcerating nodules are typical. Verrucous lesions may be seen. Bone disease resembles other forms of chronic osteomyelitis. Skull lesions in children and spinal involvement in adults are typical. A total body radiographic examination is advisable when blastomycosis is diagnosed.

The genitourinary tract involvement characteristic of dissemination in adults is rare in prepubertal children. Lymph nodes, brain, and kidneys may be involved.

Diagnosis requires isolation or visualization of the fungus. Pulmonary specimens (sputum, tracheal aspirates, lung biopsy) may be positive with conventional stains or fungal cell wall stains. Microscopically, the budding yeasts are large and very distinctive. Sputum specimens are positive in 50–80% of cases; skin lesions are positive in 80–100%. The fungus can be grown readily in most laboratories. The blastomycin skin test is neither sensitive nor specific. Antibody titers measured by enzyme immunoassay is most sensitive for detecting infection.

Recommended therapy for life-threatening or central nervous system infections is amphotericin B (30 mg/kg total dose; see Chapter 34). Itraconazole is suggested therapy for other forms of blastomycosis. Surgical debridement of infected tissue is also important.

Bosso JA: Fungal infections in pediatric patients. Pharmacotherapy 1990;10:1505.

Brown LR et al: Roentgenographic features of pulmonary blastomycosis. Mayo Clin Proc 1991;66:29.

Dismukes ED et al: Itraconazole therapy for blastomycosis and histoplasmosis. Am J Med 1992;93:489

Klein BS et al: Two outbreaks of blastomycosis along rivers in Wisconsin: Isolation of *Blastomyces dermatitidis* from riverbank soil and evaluation of its transmission along waterways. Am Rev Resp Dis 1987;136:1333.

Steele RW, Abernathy RS: Systemic blastomycosis in children. Pediatr Infect Dis J 1983;2:304.

CANDIDIASIS

Essentials of Diagnosis

- Superficial infections in normal or immunosuppressed individuals: Oral thrush or ulcerations; vulvovaginitis; erythematous intertriginous rash with satellite lesions.
- Systemic infection in the immunosuppressed: Renal, hepatic, splenic, pulmonary, or cerebral abscesses; "cotton-wool" retinal lesions; cutaneous nodules.
- Budding yeast and pseudohyphae seen in biopsy specimens, fluid, or scrapings of lesions; positive culture.

General Considerations

Disease due to *Candida* is usually caused by *Candida albicans;* similar systemic infection may be due to *Candida tropicalis,* other *Candida* species, or the closely related *Torulopsis.* In tissue, pseudohyphae are seen as well as the budding yeast phase. *Candida* grows on routine media more slowly than bacteria; growth is usually evident on agar after 2–3 days and in blood culture media in 2–7 days.

C albicans is ubiquitous and often present in small numbers on skin, mucous membranes, or in the intestinal tract. Normal bacterial flora, intact epithelial barriers, neutrophils in conjunction with antibody, and normal lymphocyte function (manifested by skin test reactivity) are all factors in preventing invasion. Disseminated infection is almost always preceded by prolonged broad-spectrum antibiotic therapy, instrumentation, or immunosuppression. Patients with diabetes mellitus are especially prone to *Candida* infection; thrush and vaginitis are most common.

Clinical Findings

A. Symptoms and Signs:

1. Oral candidiasis (thrush)–Adherent white plaques with mucosal ulceration are seen. Lesions may be few and asymptomatic, or they may be extensive, extending into the esophagus. Thrush is very common in otherwise normal infants in the first weeks of life; it may last weeks despite topical therapy. Spontaneous thrush in older children is unusual unless they have recently received antimicrobials. Steroid inhalation for asthma predisposes patients to thrush. Infection with human immunodeficiency virus should be considered if there is no other reason for oral thrush, or if it is persistent or recurrent.

2. Skin infection–

a. Diaper dermatitis is often due entirely or partly to *Candida.* Pronounced erythema with a sharply defined margin, and satellite lesions is typical. Pustules, vesicles, papules, or scales may be seen. Eroded lesions with a scalloped border are common. Any moist area, such as axillae or neck folds, may be involved.

b. Congenital skin lesions may be seen in infants born to women with *Candida* amnionitis. A red maculopapular or pustular rash is seen. Dissemination may occur.

c. Vulvovaginitis is seen in sexually active girls or diabetics, and occurs at any age in girls receiving antibiotics. Thick, cheesy discharge with intense pruritus is typical.

d. Scattered red papules or nodules may represent cutaneous dissemination.

e. Chronic mucocutaneous candidiasis may be associated with a specific lack of T cell response to *Candida.*

f. Paronychia and onychomycosis occur in normal children, but are often associated with immunosuppression, hypoparathyroidism, and adrenal insufficiency.

3. Enteric infection–Esophageal involvement in immunosuppressed patients is the most common enteric manifestation. It is manifested by substernal pain, dysphagia, painful swallowing, and anorexia. Only half of these patients have thrush. Stomach or intestinal ulcers also occur. A syndrome of mild diarrhea in normal individuals who have predominant *Candida* on stool culture has also been described, though *Candida* is not considered a true enteric pathogen. Its presence more often reflects recent antimicrobial therapy.

4. Pulmonary infection–Although the organism is occasionally found in respiratory secretions, demonstration of tissue invasion is needed to diagnose true *Candida* pneumonia or tracheitis. The infection may cause fever, cough, abscesses, nodular infiltrates, and effusion, but is rare and seen in immunosuppressed patients and patients intubated for long periods.

5. Renal infection–Candiduria may be the only manifestation of disseminated disease. More often, candiduria is associated with instrumentation or anatomic abnormality of the urinary tract. Masses of *Candida* may obstruct ureters and cause obstructive nephropathy.

6. Other infections–Endocarditis, myocarditis, meningitis, and osteomyelitis are usually only seen in compromised patients or neonates.

7. Disseminated candidiasis–Mucosal colonization precedes but does not predict dissemination. Too often, dissemination mimics bacterial sepsis; it fails to respond to antimicrobials. A careful search should be carried out for lesions highly suggestive of disseminated *Candida* (retinal "cotton-wool" spots or nodular dermal abscesses). If these findings are absent, diagnosis is often presumptively based on the presence of a compatible disease in a compromised patient who has no other cause for the symptoms; who fails to respond to antimicrobials; and who usually has *Candida* colonization of mucosal surfaces. This approach is necessary because candidemia is not appreciated antemortem in many such patients.

Hepatosplenic candidiasis is increasingly recognized in immunosuppressed patients. The typical case consists of a severely neutropenic patient who develops chronic fever and variable abdominal pain. No bacteria are isolated, and there is no response to antimicrobials. Symptoms persist even when neutrophils return. Ultrasound or CT scan of the liver and spleen demonstrates multiple round lesions. Biopsy is needed to confirm the diagnosis.

B. Laboratory Findings: Budding yeast cells are easily seen in scrapings or other samples. The presence of pseudohyphae is suggestive of tissue invasion. Culture is definitive. Blood cultures may take 3 or more days to yield positive results, or they may remain negative, even with disseminated disease or endocarditis. *Candida* should never be considered a contaminant in cultures from normally sterile sites. *Candida* in any number in the urine may represent true infection.

Candida antigen tests are not sensitive or specific enough for clinical use. Antibody tests are not useful.

Differential Diagnosis

Thrush may resemble formula (which can be easily wiped away with a tongue blade or swab, revealing normal mucosa), other types of ulcers, (including herpes), or burns. Skin lesions may resemble contact, allergic, chemical, or bacterial dermatitis, miliaria, folliculitis, or eczema. Systemic infection may resemble that due to bacteria, herpes simplex, cytomegalovirus, toxoplasmosis, and other fungi.

Complications

Failure to recognize disseminated disease while it is still treatable is the greatest complication. Osteoarthritis and meningitis occur more often than older children. Blindness from retinitis, massive emboli from large vegetations of endocarditis, intestinal perforation, and abscesses in any organ are other complications; the greater the length or degree of immunosuppression, the more complications are seen.

Treatment

A. Oral Candidiasis: In infants, oral nystatin suspension (100,000 units four to six times a day until resolution) usually suffices. It must come in contact with the lesions because it is not systemically absorbed. Older children may use it as a mouthwash (200,000–500,000 units four times a day), though it is poorly tolerated due to taste. Clotrimazole troches (10 mg) are an alternative in older children. Prolonged therapy with either agent and more frequent dosing may be needed. Painting the lesions with a cotton swab dipped in gentian violet (0.5–1%) is visually dramatic and messy but may help refractory cases. Eradication of *Candida* from pacifiers, bottle nipples, toys, or the mother's breasts (if the infant is breast-feeding and there is candidal infection of the nipples) may be helpful.

Oral azoles—ketoconazole (100–200 mg for 5–7 days) or fluconazole (100–200 mg)—are effective in older children with candidal infection refractory to nystatin. These drugs have not been evaluated in infants.

Discontinuation of antibiotics or steroids is advised.

B. Skin Infection: Cutaneous infection usually responds to a cream containing nystatin or an imidazole. Associated inflammation, such as severe diaper dermatitis, is also helped by concurrent use of a topical mild corticosteroid cream, such as 1% hydrocortisone. Covering the medicated areas with a thick coat of an occlusive ointment such as zinc oxide seems to promote healing and allows normal diapering.

Another approach is to keep the involved area dry; a heat lamp and nystatin powder may be used. Cornstarch is a yeast nutrient and should not be used as a drying agent.

Suppression of intestinal *Candida* and eradicating thrush may help prevent recurrence of the diaper dermatitis.

Vaginal infection is treated with clotrimazole, miconazole, or nystatin (cheapest if generic is used) suppositories or creams, usually applied once nightly for 7–14 days. *Candida* balanitis in sexual partners should be treated. Oral azole therapy is equally effective.

C. Renal Infection: Local candiduria may be treated with amphotericin B bladder irrigation (if a catheter is already in place), or a short course of oral flucytosine or fluconazole. Renal abscesses or ureteral fungus balls require amphotericin B therapy and surgical debridement in many cases. Amphotericin B may improve poor renal function due to renal candidiasis, even though the drug is nephrotoxic.

D. Systemic Infection: Systemic infection is dangerous and resistant to therapy. Surgical drainage of abscesses and removal of all infected tissue (such as a heart valve) are required for cure. Hepatosplenic candidiasis is never considered cured, and fungi may remain viable for life. Systemic infection is optimally treated with amphotericin B at 0.5–1 mg/kg/d, infused over 2–4 hours. It is continued for at least 4 weeks, depending on disease response. Correcting predisposing factors is important (eg, discontinuing antibiotics and immunosuppressives, and improving control of diabetes). Addition of flucytosine (100 mg/kg/d orally in four doses; keep serum levels below 75 μg/mL) may help. Unlike amphotericin B, it penetrates tissue well; it is also synergistic with amphotericin B against many organisms. It should not be used as a single agent in serious infections because resistance develops rapidly. Infected central venous lines must be removed immediately; this alone often is curative. Persistent fever and candidemia suggest infected thrombus or endocarditis. Ten to 14 days of an antifungal such as amphotericin B or fluconazole following line removal is recommended in compromised patients and fluconazole should be considered in all patients because of the late occurrence of focal *Candida* infection in some cases.

Fluconazole, is well absorbed (oral and intravenous therapy are equivalent), reasonably nontoxic, and effective for a variety of *Candida* infections. It is the drug of choice if amphotericin B is not tolerated. The dosage is 3–6 mg/kg/d in a single daily dose, depending on severity of infection. A loading dose which is twice as large may be desirable. Experience in children and systemic infections is accumulating.

Occasionally, specific immune defects may be treatable (eg, transfer factor for chronic cutaneous candidiasis), and this treatment secondarily improves the *Candida* infection.

Prognosis

Superficial disease in normal hosts has a good prognosis; in abnormal hosts, it may be quite refractory to therapy. Early therapy of systemic disease is often curative if the underlying immune response is adequate. The outcome is poor when therapy is delayed or when host response is inadequate.

Chun CS, Turner, RB: The outcome of candiduria in pediatric patients. Diagn Microbiol Infect Dis 1991;14:119.

Faix RG: Invasive neonatal candidiasis: comparison of albicans and parapsilosis infection. Pediatr Infect Dis J 1992;11:88.

Hughes WT: Systemic candidiasis: A study of 109 fatal cases. Pediatr Infect Dis J 1982;1:11.

Komshian SV et al: Fungemia caused by *Candida* species and *Torulopsis glabrata* in the hospitalized patient. Rev Infect Dis 1989;11:379.

Robinson PA, Knirsch AK, Joseph JA: Fluconazole for life-threatening fungal infections in patients who cannot be treated with conventional antifungal agents. Rev Infect Dis 1990;12:5349.

Thaler M et al: Hepatic candidiasis in cancer patients: The evolving picture of the syndrome. Ann Intern Med 1988;108:88.

Turner RB, Donowitz LG, Hendley JO: Consequences of candidemia for pediatric patients. Am J Dis Child 1985;139:178.

COCCIDIOIDOMYCOSIS

Essentials of Diagnosis

- Travel to an endemic area.
- Primary pulmonary form: Fever, chest pain, cough, anorexia, weight loss, and occasionally a macular rash or erythema nodosum or multiforme.
- Extrapulmonary form: Trauma followed in 1–3 weeks by an ulcer and regional adenopathy.
- Spherules seen in pus, sputum, cerebrospinal fluid, etc; positive culture.
- Positive coccidioidin skin test.
- Appearance of precipitating and complement-fixing antibodies.

General Considerations

This disease is caused by the dimorphic fungus *Coccidioides immitis,* which is endemic in the southwestern USA (Sonoran Desert areas of western Texas, New Mexico, Arizona, and California), Mexico, and South America. Infection results from inhalation or inoculation of arthrospores (highly contagious and readily airborne in the dry climate). Even brief travel in or through an endemic area, especially during windy seasons, may allow infection. Human-to-human transmission does not occur. About half of all infections are asymptomatic. Dissemination occurs in less than 1% of cases; the risk is much higher in Filipinos or blacks, especially in older males.

Clinical Findings

A. Symptoms and Signs:

1. Primary disease–The incubation period is 10–16 days (range, 7–28 days). Symptoms vary from those of a mild fever and arthralgia to severe influenza-like illness with high fever, cough, pleurisy, myalgias, arthralgias, headache, and anorexia. True upper respiratory tract signs are not common. Severe pleuritic chest pain suggests this diagnosis. Signs vary from none to rash, rales, pleural rubs, hilar adenopathy and signs of pulmonary consolidation. Weight loss may occur.

2. Skin disease–Up to 10% of children develop erythema nodosum or multiforme. Less specific maculopapular eruptions occur in a larger number of children. These imply a favorable host response to the organism. Primary skin inoculation sites develop indurated ulcers with local adenopathy. Contiguous involvement of skin from deep infection in nodes or bone also occurs.

3. Chronic pulmonary disease–This may be asymptomatic or associated with chronic cough (occasionally with hemoptysis), weight loss, pulmonary consolidation, effusion, cavitation, or pneumothorax.

4. Disseminated disease–This is less common in children than adults. It is more common in infants, neonates, pregnant women (especially during the third trimester), blacks, and Filipinos—or with any type of immunosuppression. One or more organs may be involved. The most common sites involved are bone or joint (subacute or chronic swelling, pain, redness), node, brain (slowly progressive meningeal signs, ataxia, vomiting, headache, cranial neuropathies), and kidney (dysuria, urinary frequency). As with most fungal diseases, the evolution of the illness is usually slow.

B. Laboratory Findings: Direct examination of respiratory secretions, pus, spinal fluid, or tissue may reveal the large spherules (30–60 μm). Phase-contrast microscopy is useful for demonstrating these refractile bodies; Gram or methylene blue stains are not helpful, but fungal stains are. Negative stains do not exclude the diagnosis.

The fluffy, gray-white colonies grow within 2–5 days on routine fungal or other media. They are highly infectious.

Routine laboratory tests are nonspecific. The sedimentation rate is usually elevated. Eosinophilia may occur, particularly prior to dissemination and is more common in coccidioidomycosis than in many other conditions with similar symptoms. Meningitis causes a mononuclear pleocytosis with elevated protein and mild hypoglycorrhachia.

Within 2–21 days, most patients develop a delayed hypersensitivity reaction to skin test antigen (coccidioidin 1:100 strength, or spherulin 0.1 mL, intradermally, should produce 5 mm induration at 48 hours). Erythema nodosum predicts strong reactivity; when this is present the antigen should be diluted 10–100 times before use. The skin test may be negative in compromised patients or those with disseminated disease. Positive reactions may remain for years and do not prove active infection.

Antibodies consist of precipitins (usually measurable by 1–3 weeks and gone by 6 weeks) and complement-fixing antibodies (elevated by several weeks and gone by 8 months, unless dissemination occurs, in which case persistent high titers may be seen). Antibodies can also be demonstrated by immunodiffusion. Serum precipitins usually indicate acute infection. The presence of antibody in spinal fluid indicates central nervous system infection.

C. Imaging: Pulmonary consolidation, hilar adenopathy, effusion, thin-walled cavities, or solitary granulomas (coin lesions) may be seen. Unlike reactivation tuberculosis, apical disease is not prominent. Bone infection causes osteolysis that enhances with technetium. Cerebral imaging may show hydrocephalus and meningitis; abscesses and calcifications are unusual. Radiographic evolution of all lesions is slow.

Differential Diagnosis

Primary pulmonary infection resembles acute viral, bacterial, or mycoplasmal infections or psittacosis; subacute presentation mimics tuberculosis, histoplasmosis and blastomycosis. Chronic pulmonary or disseminated disease must be differentiated from cancer, tuberculosis, or other fungal infections.

Complications

Dissemination of primary pulmonary disease is associated with ethnic background, prolonged fever (> 1 month), a negative skin test, high complement fixation antibody titer, and marked hilar adenopathy. Local pulmonary complications include effusion, empyema, and pneumothorax. Cerebral infection can cause noncommunicating hydrocephalus due to aqueductal obstruction.

Treatment

A. Specific Measures: Mild pulmonary infections require no therapy. Amphotericin B is the drug of choice for severe pulmonary disease (prolonged fever, pneumonitis > 4–6 weeks and mediastinal adenopathy), any form of disseminated disease, or in immunocompromised children. Fluconazole is superior for mild to moderate infections without central nervous system involvement and may be an alternative for coccidioidal meningitis.

Meningitis is best treated with parenteral amphotericin B. Prolonged intrathecal or intraventricular amphotericin B therapy is often required. It is the most effective and best-studied regimen in adults but carries a risk of adhesive arachnoiditis. This complication is more likely in children.

Duration of therapy is based on clinical response, normalization of laboratory values, sterilization of cultures, and antibody titer decline (in serum and cerebrospinal fluid). Outpatient therapy with parenteral amphotericin B and intraventricular therapy once or twice weekly may have to be continued for years.

B. General Measures: Most pulmonary infections require only symptomatic therapy, self-limited activity, and good nutrition. They are not contagious. Secondary bacterial infection is unusual.

C. Surgical Measures: Excision of pulmonary cavities or abscesses may be needed. Infected nodes, sinus tracts, and bone are other operable lesions. Amphotericin B should be given prior to surgery to prevent dissemination; it is continued for 4 weeks arbitrarily or until other criteria for cure are met.

Prognosis

Most patients recover. Even with amphotericin B, however, disseminated disease may be fatal, especially in those racially predisposed to severe disease. Reversion of the skin test to negative or a rising complement-fixing antibody titer is an ominous sign. Meningitis may require lifetime therapy to prevent progression or relapse.

Ampel NM, Wieden MA, Galgiani JN: Coccidioidomycosis: Clinical update. Rev Infect Dis 1989;11:897.

Child DC et al: Radiologic findings of pulmonary coccidioidomycosis in neonates and infants. Am J Radiol 1989;145:261.

Galgiani JN, Grace GM, Lundergan LL: New serologic tests for early detection of coccidioidomycosis. J Infect Dis 1991;163:671.

Galgiani JN et al: Fluconazole therapy for coccidioidal meningitis. Ann Int Med 1993;119:28.

Hedges E, Miller S: Coccidioidomycosis: Office diagnosis and treatment. Am Fam Phys 1990;41:1499.

Kafka JA, Catanzaro A: Disseminated coccidioidomycosis in children. J Pediatr 1981;98:355.

CRYPTOCOCCOSIS

Essentials of Diagnosis

- Mainly a problem for immunosuppressed individuals.
- Meningitis: headache, vomiting, cranial nerve palsies, meningeal signs; mononuclear cell pleocytosis.
- Cryptococcal antigen detected in cerebrospinal fluid; also in serum and urine in some patients.
- Readily isolated on routine media.

General Considerations

Cryptococcus neoformans is a ubiquitous soil yeast. It appears to survive better in soil contaminated with bird excrement, especially that of pigeons. However, most human cases are not associated with a history of significant contact with birds. Inhalation is the presumed route of inoculation. Infections in children are quite rare, even in heavily immunocompromised patients such as those with HIV infection. It is much more common in compromised adults. Normal individuals can also be infected. Asymptomatic carriage is not seen.

Clinical Findings

A. Symptoms and Signs:

1. Meningitis–The most common clinical disease is meningitis, following hematogenous spread from a pulmonary focus. Symptoms of headache, vomiting, and fever occur over days to months. Meningeal signs and papilledema are common. Cranial nerve palsies and seizures may occur.

2. Pulmonary disease–Pulmonary infection is the next most common infection and may coexist with cerebral involvement. Symptoms are nonspecific and subacute—cough, weight loss, and fatigue. Radiographic findings are usually lower lobe infiltrates or nodular densities, less often effusions, and rarely cavitation, hilar adenopathy, or calcification.

3. Other forms–Cutaneous forms are usually secondary to dissemination. Papules, pustules, and ulcerating nodules are typical. Bones (rarely joints) may be infected; osteolytic areas are seen, and the process may resemble osteosarcoma. Many other organs can be involved with dissemination.

B. Laboratory Findings: The spinal fluid usually has a lymphocytic pleocytosis; it may be completely normal in immunosuppressed patients with cryptococcal meningitis. Direct microscopy may reveal organisms in sputum, spinal fluid, or other specimens. The India ink stain demonstrates the capsules nicely, but it is insensitive; artifacts may give false-positive results. The capsular antigen can be detected by a latex agglutination test, which is both sensitive (> 90%) and specific. Serum, spinal fluid, and urine may be tested. False-negative cerebrospinal fluid tests have occurred. The organism grows well after several days on many routine media; for optimal culture, collecting and concentrating a large amount of spinal fluid (up to 10 mL) is recommended, because the number of organisms may be low.

Differential Diagnosis

Cryptococcal meningitis may mimic tuberculosis, viral meningoencephalitis, or a space-occupying central nervous system lesion.

Complications

Hydrocephalus may occur from chronic basilar meningitis. Significant pulmonary or osseous disease may accompany the primary infection or dissemination.

Treatment

Amphotericin B (0.3 mg/kg) and flucytosine (100 mg/kg/d) are used for most systemic infections, including meningitis. The combination is synergistic and allows lower doses of amphotericin B to be used. Therapy is usually 6 weeks for cerebral infections (or for 1 month after sterilization) and 8 weeks for osteomyelitis. Fluconazole is not as effective in some AIDS patients. However, fluconazole (200 mg/d) is the preferred maintenance therapy to prevent relapses in high-risk patients. Relapses occur in up to 25–50% of meningitis cases, especially with continued immunosuppression. Antigen levels should be followed every few weeks to assess the response.

Prognosis

Treatment failure, including death, is common in immunosuppressed patients, especially those with AIDS. Lifelong maintenance therapy is required in these patients. Poor prognostic signs are the presence of extrameningeal disease; fewer than 20 cells/μL of initial cerebrospinal fluid; initial cerebrospinal fluid antigen titer greater than 1:32.

Dismukes WE et al: Treatment of cryptococcal meningitis with combination amphotericin B and flucytosine for 4 as compared to 6 weeks. N Engl J Med 1987;317:334.

Leggiadro RJ, Barrett FF, Hughes WT: Extrapulmonary cryptococcosis in immunocompromised infants and children. Pediatr Infect Dis J 1992;11:43.

Sugar AM et al: Overview: Treatment of cryptococcal meningitis. Rev Infect Dis 1990; 12:S338.

Ting SF, Glader BE, Prober CG: Cryptococcal infection in a nine year old child with hemophilia and the acquired immunodeficiency syndrome. Pediatr Infect Dis J 1991; 10:76.

HISTOPLASMOSIS

Essentials of Diagnosis

- Residence in or travel to endemic areas.
- Pulmonary calcification.
- Hepatosplenomegaly, anemia, leukopenia.
- Positive skin test.
- Detection of the organism in smears or tissue or by culture.

General Considerations

The dimorphic fungus, *Histoplasma capsulatum*, is found in the central and eastern USA (Ohio and Mississippi River Valleys). The small yeast form (2–4 μm) is seen in tissue, especially within macrophages; the mycelial form is a slowly growing, fluffy, gray-white fungus. Endemic infections are very common at all ages and are usually asymptomatic. Over two-thirds of children are infected in endemic areas. Reactivation is very rare in children; it may occur years later, usually due to significant immunosuppression. Infection is acquired by the respiratory route. Soil contamination is enhanced by the presence of bat or bird feces.

Clinical Findings

Because human-to-human transmission does not occur, infection requires exposure to the endemic area—usually within the past weeks or months. Congenital infection is not seen.

A. Symptoms and Signs:

1. Asymptomatic infection (50% of infections)—This is usually diagnosed by the presence of scattered calcifications in lungs or spleen and a positive skin test. The calcification may resemble that due to tuberculosis but may be more extensive than the usual Ghon complex.

2. Pneumonia—Approximately 45% of patients have mild to moderate disease. Acute pulmonary disease may resemble influenza, with fever, myalgia, arthralgia, and cough occurring 1–3 weeks after exposure; the subacute form resembles infections such as tuberculosis, with weight loss, night sweats, and pleurisy. Chronic disease is unusual in children. Physical examination may be normal, or rales may be heard. Mediastinal nodes may be greatly enlarged. Effusion is uncommon. The usual duration of the disease is less than 2 weeks, followed by complete resolution. Symptoms may last several months and still resolve without antifungal therapy.

3. Disseminated infection (5% of infections)—Fungemia during primary infection is probably common; transient hepatosplenomegaly may occur, but resolution is the rule in normal individuals. Heavy infection, severe pulmonary disease, and immunosuppression may be followed by progressive reticuloendothelial cell infection, with anemia, fever, weight loss, organomegaly, bone marrow involvement, and death. Dissemination may occur in otherwise normal children; usually they are less than 2 years of age.

4. Other—Ocular involvement consists of multifocal choroiditis. This is usually seen in normal adults with other evidence of disseminated disease. Brain, heart valve, intestine, and skin (oral ulcers, nodules) are other involved sites. Adrenal gland involvement is common with systemic disease.

B. Laboratory Findings:
Routine tests are normal or nonspecific in the benign forms. Pancytopenia is present in many cases of dissemination. Definitive diagnosis usually requires demonstration of the organism by histology or culture. Tissue yeast forms are small and may be mistaken for artifact. They are usually found in macrophages, occasionally in peripheral blood leukocytes in severe disease, but rarely in sputum, urine, or spinal fluid. Cultures of infected fluids or tissues may yield the organism after 1–6 weeks of incubation on fungal media, but even cultures of bronchoalveolar lavage or transbronchial biopsy specimens in immunocompromised patients are often negative. Thus, bone marrow and tissue specimens are needed.

Antibodies may be detected by immunodiffusion, complement fixation, and precipitation; the latter two rise in the first few weeks of illness and fall unless dissemination occurs. A single high titer or rising titer indicates highly likely disease. Skin test antigen from the yeast phase is more sensitive. It is not useful in endemic disease, and patients with disseminated disease often have a negative test. Some antigens may induce a serologic response that may invalidate the use of serology for diagnosis. Thus, skin tests play no role in the management of individual cases.

C. Imaging: Scattered pulmonary calcifications in a well child is typical of past infection. Bronchopneumonia occurs with acute disease, often with hilar adenopathy, occasionally with nodules, but seldom with effusion or cavity formation.

Differential Diagnosis

Pulmonary disease resembles viral infection, tuberculosis, coccidioidomycosis, and blastomycosis. Systemic disease resembles disseminated fungal or mycobacterial infection or leukemia, histiocytosis, or cancer.

Treatment

Mild infections do not require therapy. Disseminated disease in infants may respond to as little as 10 days of amphotericin B, the drug of choice, although 4–6 weeks (or 30 mg/kg total dose) is usually recommended for this and other severe forms of infection. Surgical excision of local pulmonary disease may be useful. Fluconazole and itraconazole may be equivalent to amphotericin B therapy. With chronic pulmonary or disseminated disease therapy may be required for 6 months or more.

Prognosis

Mild infections do well. With early diagnosis and treatment, infants with disseminated disease usually recover; the prognosis worsens if immune response is poor.

Dismukes WE et al: Itraconazole therapy for blastomycosis and histoplasmosis. Am J Med 1992;93:489.

Kirchner SG et al: Imaging of pediatric mediastinal histoplasmosis. Radiographics 1991;11:365.

Leggiadro RJ, Barrett FF, Hughes WT: Disseminated histoplasmosis of infancy. Pediatr Infect Dis J 1988;7:799.

Weinberg GA et al: Unusual manifestations of histoplasmosis in childhood. Pediatrics 1983;72:99.

Wheat LJ et al: *Histoplasma capsulatum* infection of the central nervous system: A clinical review. Medicine 1990;69:244.

PNEUMOCYSTIS CARINII INFECTION

Essentials of Diagnosis

- Significant immunosuppression
- Fever, tachypnea, cough, dyspnea
- Hypoxemia; diffuse interstitial infiltrates

General Considerations

Although now classified as a fungus on the basis of structural and nucleic acid characteristics, *Pneumocystis* responds readily to antiprotozoal drugs. It is

a ubiquitous pathogen. Infection is presumed to occur via inhalation in most cases. With normal immune function, there is usually no recognized clinical disease. A syndrome of afebrile pneumonia similar to that caused by *Chlamydia trachomatis* in normal infants has been described but is rarely diagnosed. Organisms dormant in the lung may be reactivated in heavily immunosuppressed children, chiefly those with abnormal T cell function such as occur with HIV infection and hematologic malignancies. Prolonged, high-dose corticosteroid therapy is also a risk factor; onset of illness as steroids are tapered is a typical presentation. Severely malnourished infants with no underlying illness may also develop this infection, as can those with congenital or acquired humoral or cellular immune deficiency. The incubation period is usually at least a month after onset of immunosuppression.

Pneumocystis pneumonia is a common complication of advanced HIV infection and is one of the diseases that defines AIDS. Careful prophylaxis may prevent this infection (see Chapter 35).

Infection is generally limited to the lower respiratory tract. In advanced disease, spread to other organs has occurred.

Clinical Findings:

A. Symptoms and Signs: There is often a gradual onset of fever, tachypnea, dyspnea, and mild cough over 1–4 weeks. Initially, the chest is clear, although retractions and nasal flaring are present. At this stage, the illness is nonspecific. Hypoxemia out of proportion to the clinical and radiographic signs is an early finding, however, and even minimally decreased arterial PO$_2$ values should suggest this diagnosis in immunosuppressed children. Tachypnea, nonproductive cough, and dyspnea progress. Respiratory failure and death are common if not treated. In very immunosuppressed children the onset may be abrupt and progression more rapid.

The general examination is unremarkable. There are no upper respiratory signs, conjunctivitis, organomegaly, enanthem, or rash.

B. Laboratory Findings: These reflect each child's underlying illness and are not specific. Serum lactate dehydrogenase may be markedly elevated from pulmonary damage.

C. Imaging: Early chest radiographs are normal. The classic pattern is that of bilateral, interstitial, lower lobe infiltrates without effusion, consolidation, or hilar adenopathy. Older HIV-infected patients may present with other patterns, including nodular infiltrates, lobar pneumonia, cavities, and upper lobe infiltrates—especially those receiving aerosolized pentamidine for prophylaxis.

Diagnosis

Diagnosis requires finding the round (6–8 μm) cysts in a lung biopsy specimen, bronchial brushings or alveolar washings, sputum, or tracheal aspirates. The latter specimens are less sensitive but are more rapidly and easily obtained. They are more often negative in children with leukemia compared to those with HIV infection; presumably, greater immunosuppression results in larger numbers of organisms. Since immunosuppressed patients may have many causes of pneumonia, negative results from tracheal secretions should prompt more aggressive diagnostic attempts. Bronchial washing using fiberoptic bronchoscopy is usually well tolerated and rapidly performed.

Several rapid stains—as well as the standard methenamine silver stain—are useful. All require competent laboratory evaluation, because few organisms may be present and there are many artifacts.

There are no commercially available clinically useful tests for antigen or antibody detection.

Differential Diagnosis

In normal infants, *Chlamydia* and cytomegalovirus pneumonia are the most common causes of the afebrile pneumonia syndrome described for *Pneumocystis*. In older immunocompromised children, the differential diagnosis includes influenza, respiratory syncytial virus, adenovirus, and other viral infections; bacterial and fungal pneumonia; pulmonary emboli; congestive heart failure; and *Chlamydia pneumoniae* and *Mycoplasma* pneumonia. Lymphoid interstitial pneumonitis is seen in older infants with HIV infection and is more indolent (see Chapter 35). *Pneumocystis* pneumonia is uncommon in children currently (> 4 weeks) on appropriate prophylactic regimens.

Prevention

Children at high risk of developing *Pneumocystis* infection should receive prophylactic therapy immediately. This includes all those with hematologic malignancies or other reasons for receiving chemotherapy and many children with organ transplants or HIV infection (see Chapter 35).

The drug of choice is trimethoprim-sulfamethoxazole (5 mg/kg/d of trimethoprim and 25 mg/kg/d of sulfamethoxazole) once daily orally; the same dose for 3 days of each week is also effective.

Many patients with HIV infection have rashes and other adverse reactions that preclude use of sulfonamides. Intravenous pentamidine every 2–4 weeks is a substitute. Aerosolized pentamidine (300 mg per dose via a Respirgard II or equivalent jet nebulizer) every 4 weeks is a less toxic alternative in older children. It is a lung irritant in some children. Breakthrough infections, particularly in the upper lobes, are seen much more commonly than with trimethoprim-sulfamethoxazole prophylaxis. Dapsone and atovaquone are under study as alternative prophylaxis.

Treatment

A. General Measures: Supplemental oxygen and nutritional support may be needed. Bronchodilators may be tried but are usually not helpful. The patient should be in respiratory isolation, since hospital-acquired infections of other immunosuppressed patients have occurred.

B. Specific Measures: Trimethoprim-sulfamethoxazole (20 mg/kg/d of trimethoprim and 100 mg/kg of sulfamethoxazole in four divided doses intravenously or orally if well tolerated) is the drug of choice. It should be started immediately, since improvement may not be seen for 3–5 days. Duration of treatment is 2–3 weeks. Monitoring serum levels ensures delivery and may allow decreased dosage with less toxicity. Methylprednisolone (2–4 mg/kg/d in four divided doses intravenously) should also be given to HIV-infected patients with severe infection. If trimethoprim-sulfamethoxazole is not tolerated or there is no clinical response in 5 days, pentamidine isethionate (4 mg/kg once daily by slow intravenous infusion) should be given. Clinical efficacy is similar with pentamidine, but adverse reactions more common. These include dysglycemias, nephrotoxicity, and leukopenia.

Prognosis

The mortality rate is high in immunosuppressed patients who are treated late in the illness.

Bartlett MS, Smith JW: *Pneumocystis carinii:* An opportunist in immunocompromised patients. Clin Microbiol Rev 1991;4:137.

Guidelines for prophylaxis against *Pneumocystis carinii* pneumonia for children infected with human immunodeficiency virus. MMWR Morb Mortal Wkly Rep 1991;40 RR-2):1.

Masur H: Prevention and treatment of pneumocystis pneumonia. N Engl J Med 1992;327:1853.

Peters SG, Prakash UB: *Pneumocystis carinii* pneumonia: Review of 53 cases. Am J Med 1987;82:73.

Guidelines for prophylaxis against *Pneumocystis carinii* pneumonia for children infected with human immunodeficiency virus. MMWR Morb Mortal Wkly Rep 1991;40 RR-2):1.

Pneumocystis carinii pneumonia. Antimicrob Agents Chemother 1990;34:499.

Sattler FR et al: Trimethoprim-sulfamethoxazole compared with pentamidine for treatment of *Pneumocystis carinii* pneumonia in the acquired immunodeficiency syndrome: A prospective, noncrossover study. Ann Intern Med 1988;109:280.

Simonds RJ: *Pneumocystis carinii* pneumonia among US children with perinatally acquired HIV infection. JAMA 1993; 270:470.

Sleasman JW et al: Corticosteroids improve survival of children with AIDS and *Pneumocystis carinii* pneumonia. Am J Dis Child 1993; 147(1):30-34.

REFERENCES

Parasitic Infections

Balows A et al (editors): *Laboratory Diagnosis of Infectious Diseases: Principles and Practice.* Springer-Verlag, 1988.

Binford CH, Connor DH (editors): *Pathology of Tropical and Extraordinary Diseases.* Vols 1 and 2. Armed Forces Institute of Pathology, 1976.

Drugs for parasitic infections. Med Lett Drugs Ther 1993;35:11.

MacLeod CL (editor): *Parasitic Infections in Pregnancy and the Newborn.* Oxford Univ. Press, 1988.

Warren KS, Mahmoud AAF (editors): *Tropical and Geographic Medicine.* McGraw-Hill, 1989.

Mycotic Infections

Anaissie E et al: New spectrum of fungal infection in patients with cancer. Rev Infect Dis 1989;11:369.

Bailey EM, Krakovsky DJ, Rybak MJ: The triazole antifungal agents: A review of itraconazole and fluconazole. Pharmacotherapy 1990;10:146.

Denning DW, Stevens DA: Antifungal and surgical treatment of invasive aspergillosis: Review of 2121 published cases. Rev Infect Dis 1990;12:1147.

Gallis HA et al: Amphotericin B: 30 years of clinical experience. Rev Infect Dis 1990;12:329.

Hostetler JS, Denning DW, Stevens DA: US experience with itraconazole in *Aspergillus, Cryptococcus* and *Histoplasma* infections in the immunocompromised host. Chemotherapy 1992;38(Suppl 1):12.

Marcon MJ, Powell DA: Human infections due to *Malassezia* spp. Clin Microbiol Rev 1992;5:101.

Rippon JW: *Medical Mycology,* 3rd ed. Saunders, 1988.

Systemic antifungal drugs. Med Lett Drugs Ther 1994;36:11.

Terrell CL, Hughes CE: Antifungal agents used for deep-seated mycotic infections. Mayo Clin Porc 1992;67:69.

Sexually Transmitted Diseases

Kathleen A. Mammel, MD

The 15- to 24-year-old age group has the highest incidence of sexually transmitted diseases (STD) as a result of multiple sexual partners, failure to use barrier methods of contraception, and delay in seeking treatment. Their inexperience in communicating with each other about sexual matters further contributes to high rates when one partner develops symptoms of an STD. The use of alcohol or other substances in sexual situations may reduce the chance of practicing preventive behaviors, and substance use may contribute to multiple partners or the exchange of sex for drugs.

Chlamydia, an obligate intracellular organism half the size of the gonococcus, is the most common cause of STD, with 2–3 million new cases per year in the USA and a peak incidence in 15- to 20-year-olds. One-fourth to one-half of those infected are asymptomatic, and one-fourth to one-half are coinfected with gonorrhea. Forty-two percent of the cases of nongonococcal urethritis (NGU) in one study were caused by *Chlamydia,* and that organism accounts for 20–30% of the 170,000 cases of pelvic inflammatory disease (PID) per year and more than 60% of PID cases in women under 20 years of age. *Chlamydia* should always be excluded during any STD examination, since it is often present when another STD is diagnosed.

Gonorrhea is the second most common STD, with a peak incidence in the 15- to 25-year-old age group. Five to 25 percent of cases of gonorrhea are associated with another STD, and more than 50% of those infected are asymptomatic. Although syphilis is less prevalent than gonorrhea and chlamydial infection, its peak incidence is in 15- to 35-year-olds, and the prevalence has been increasing. Sexually transmitted viruses are also prevalent in the adolescent population—the 1970s saw a dramatic rise in the number of cases of herpes simplex infection.

In view of the prevalence of STDs in the adolescent population and the reluctance of teenagers to talk about them, the clinician must routinely ask adolescents about sexual activity, number of partners, and symptoms of STD when they present for routine physical examinations or sexually related symptoms (dysuria, penile or vaginal discharge, genital lesions, or abdominal pain). The history should be obtained in a fashion that is neutral to sexual orientation: "Have you had sexual contact with men, women, or both?" "Has your sexual contact involved genital, oral, or anal contact?" This will enable the caregiver to assess the risk level for STDs, obtain appropriate culture samples, and provide prevention services. The routine physical examination is an opportune time to provide anticipatory guidance to all adolescents about sexual decision-making and STD and pregnancy prevention. Because females with STDs are frequently asymptomatic, obtaining specimens for wet preparation, gonorrhea culture, and *Chlamydia* testing at the time of the annual Papanicolaou smear in sexually active females is advised. Although males are usually symptomatic, a significant number of those with chlamydial infections are asymptomatic. Furthermore, symptoms of gonorrhea may resolve, and the male adolescent may fail to seek treatment.

When an STD is diagnosed, the adolescent and his or her sexual partners should be treated simultaneously with the appropriate antibiotic or antiviral regimen. Close follow-up is important, because poor compliance with treatment is common in this age group. Serologic tests will need to be repeated in patients with syphilis. It is essential to emphasize abstinence until both partners complete treatment to avoid reinfection or spread and to advise use of barrier methods of contraception to prevent future infections.

Possible complications and the implications of recurrent infections with regard to fertility and ectopic pregnancy should also be discussed. Adolescents should also be made aware of transmission of STDs to a fetus.

URETHRITIS

Urethritis may be caused by gonorrhea, *Chlamydia, Ureaplasma, Mycoplasma,* and *Trichomonas.*

Clinical Findings

A. Symptoms and Signs: Females may develop urethritis, most often in association with cervicitis (see below), and may complain of dysuria. The male genital examination may be normal, or there may be dysuria and a clear, white, or purulent penile discharge. A clear or white discharge is more frequently found in nongonococcal urethritis (NGU), and a purulent discharge in gonorrhea; however, appearance is not diagnostic.

B. Laboratory Findings: Urinalysis may show a moderate amount of white blood cells without bacteriuria. A moderate pyuria with a negative urine culture, with or without symptoms of urethritis or cervicitis, suggests this diagnosis and the need for appropriate pelvic examination and cultures. Gram staining of the penile discharge shows polymorphonuclear white blood cells and may show gram-negative intracellular diplococci when gonorrhea is the cause. The penile discharge should be cultured for gonorrhea on chocolate agar or Thayer-Martin medium, and a diagnostic test for *Chlamydia* (culture, enzyme-linked immunoassay, or monoclonal antibody immunofluorescence test) should be performed.

Complications

Urethritis caused by gonorrhea or *Chlamydia* may cause nontender penile edema or ascend to result in prostatitis, epididymitis, or orchitis.

Treatment

See Table 38–1.

CERVICITIS

Cervicitis may be caused by *Chlamydia* or *Neisseria gonorrhoeae*. There may also be involvement of the cervix with *Trichomonas* vaginitis. Herpes simplex virus may cause characteristic cervical ulcerations. The adolescent cervix is particularly vulnerable because the transition zone between columnar and squamous epithelium has not yet receded into the cervical os. The columnar epithelium is the primary site of invasion by chlamydiae and gonococci.

Clinical Findings

A. Symptoms and Signs: Most females with uncomplicated gonococcal or chlamydial cervicitis are asymptomatic, but about one-third note a vaginal discharge. Dysuria may be present if there is an associated urethritis.

In typical cases of gonococcal cervicitis, the cervical os is erythematous and produces a mucopurulent discharge. Cervical abnormalities may be subtle in patients with chlamydial cervicitis. Although 19–32% of females with chlamydial cervicitis have hypertrophic cervicitis (marked by an intensely erythematous, irregular, raised surface that is friable or bleeds easily when touched) and 40% have a mucopurulent or purulent cervical discharge, 20% have a completely normal cervical examination. The findings in 90% of women with cervicitis and positive culture for herpesvirus are typically diffuse friability, occasionally frank ulcers, or necrosis. *Trichomonas*

Table 38–1. Treatment of urethritis or cervicitis in adolescents.[1]

	Drugs of Choice	Alternative Drugs
Neisseria gonorrhoeae	Ceftriaxone, 125–250 mg IM once, *followed by* treatment for chalamydial infection (below)	Cefixime, 400 mg orally once, *or* Ciprofloxacin,[2] 500 mg orally once, *or* Ofloxacin,[2] 400 mg orally once *or* Spectinomycin, 2 g IM once *Plus* treatment for chlamydial infection (below)
Chlamydia trachomatis	Doxycycline,[3] 100 mg orally twice daily for 7 days, *or* Erythromycin,[4] 500 mg orally four times daily for 7 days	Erythromycin, 500 mg orally four times daily for 7 days

[1]Modified and reproduced, with permission, from: Drugs for sexually transmitted diseases. Med Lett Drugs Ther 1991; 33:119.
[2]Quinolones, such as ciprofloxacin, are contraindicated during pregnancy and in children 16 or under.
[3]Contraindicated during pregnancy.
[4]Erythromycin estolate is contraindicated during pregnancy.

may cause petechiae of the cervix and upper vaginal vault, the so-called flea-bitten appearance.

B. Laboratory Findings: A wet preparation of the vaginal discharge reveals more than ten white blood cells per high-power field. There tend to be greater numbers of white blood cells with gonorrhea than with *Chlamydia;* however, this finding is not diagnostic. While Gram-negative intracellular diplococci may be seen on the Gram-stained smear, they are not specific for gonorrhea in females. Definitive diagnosis is provided by growth of *N gonorrhoeae* on culture of the cervical discharge plated on Thayer-Martin medium or chocolate agar. A *Chlamydia* culture or direct antigen detection test should also be performed.

Complications

Cervicitis caused by *Chlamydia* or gonorrhea may progress to pelvic inflammatory disease with its attendant complications. Infection of Bartholin's glands is also a potential consequence.

Treatment

See Table 38–1.

VAGINITIS

While candidal vulvovaginitis is not usually sexually transmitted, consideration should be given to simultaneous treatment of the sexual partners of patients with recurrent or persistent episodes. Likewise, bacterial vaginosis is most often caused by indigenous vaginal flora, though it is more prevalent in those who have had sexual intercourse. (See Vulvovaginitis in Chapter 4.)

PELVIC INFLAMMATORY DISEASE

Acute pelvic inflammatory disease (PID), or salpingitis, is the most common serious infection occurring in young women. The adolescent age group, with the most reproductive years at risk, has the highest rate of PID, with an annual rate of 1.5% of females aged 15–19 years. PID results from mucosal spread of sexually transmitted organisms from the cervix, through the uterus (where a transient endometritis may occur), to the uterine tube. Adolescents may be more vulnerable to the development of PID because of persistence of the columnar epithelial cells (for which *N gonorrhoeae* and *C trachomatis* have an affinity) on the ectocervix and perhaps an "inexperienced" reproductive tract immune system.

Gonorrhea and *Chlamydia* account for more than 75% of cases of PID; however, normal vaginal aerobic and anaerobic flora have also been recovered from tubal infections and are felt to be secondary invaders. Whereas gonococcal infection may be limited to the tubal mucosa, *Chlamydia* and other organisms may invade the basement membrane and involve the subepithelial connective tissue and muscularis and serosal surfaces in the inflammatory process, thereby producing greater tubal damage. Organisms recovered from the cervix are not necessarily predictive of those causing infection in the tube, since gonorrhea becomes more difficult to isolate later in the disease and since *Chlamydia* has been isolated from the uterine tubes of women with or without this organism in the cervix.

Risk factors for PID include sexual activity, multiple partners (five times greater risk than for one partner), age less than 25, presence of an intrauterine device (two to four times greater risk than for nonusers), nulliparity, prior history of PID (two times greater risk), prior history of uncomplicated STD, and prior induced abortion.

Clinical Findings

A. Symptoms and Signs: Abdominal pain is the most common complaint with PID, though 3% have no pain despite laparoscopic verification, and half of those with tubal occlusion from PID may report minimal pain. In patients with gonococcal PID, pain often begins with menses. Seventy-five percent report vaginal discharge of recent onset; 40% have excessive menstrual bleeding or intermenstrual spotting; 40% have fever; and 15% experience dysuria. In patients with chlamydial PID, the duration of pain is typically longer; but pain is less intense, and there is less fever and a higher sedimentation rate.

Only one-third of patients with laparoscopically confirmed salpingitis will have fever above 38 °C. Many have lower abdominal tenderness or uterine, adnexal, or cervical motion tenderness on pelvic examination. Only half have a grossly abnormal cervical discharge, but many have excessive white blood cells on wet preparation.

B. Laboratory Findings: In one large series of patients with laparoscopically confirmed salpingitis, only 45% had a white blood count over 7900/(m)L and only 75% had a sedimentation rate above 15 mm/h. Although the Gram-stained smear is positive for gonorrhea in only 67% of cases in which the cervical culture is positive, it may be helpful if positive. Cervical cultures for both gonorrhea and *Chlamydia* should be obtained; cultures for other flora are not helpful. Culdocentesis may be helpful if it yields white blood cells or nonclotting blood (indicating peritonitis from salpingitis or other causes—eg, appendicitis—versus ectopic pregnancy or ruptured ovarian cyst), but it is of no help if negative.

Differential Diagnosis

Diagnostic criteria for PID are set forth in Table 38–2. Gynecologic consultation for evaluation or laparoscopy is indicated in doubtful cases. Laparoscopy remains the best method for diagnosis of salpingitis and emphasizes the difficulty in making an accurate

Table 38–2. Criteria for the diagnosis of acute salpingitis.[1]

All three must be present:
1. History of lower abdominal pain and the presence of lower abdominal tenderness, with or without evidence of rebound.
2. Cervical motion tenderness.
3. Adnexal tenderness.

Plus

One of the following must be present:
1. Temperature of > 38 °C.
2. Leukocytosis of > 10,500/μL.
3. Culdocentesis that yields peritoneal fluid containing white blood cells and bacteria.
4. Presence of an inflammatory mass noted on pelvic examination or sonography.
5. Elevated erythrocyte sedimentation rate.
6. Gram stain from the endocervix revealing gram-negative intracellular diplococci suggestive of *Neisseria gonorrhoeae* or a smear from endocervical secretions revealing *chlamydia trachomatis* by fluorescence microscopy.
7. Presence of > 5 white blood cells per oil immersion field on Gram's stain of endocervical discharge.

[1]Modified and reproduced, with permission, from Sweet RL: Pelvic inflammatory disease. Sex Transm Dis 1986;13(Suppl 3):192.

clinical diagnosis. Adherence to rigid diagnostic criteria results in diagnosis of only the most overt cases. The diagnosis of acute salpingitis was confirmed by laparoscopy in only 65% of patients felt to have it prior to the procedure; however, other diagnoses were established in 15%, including benign ovarian cysts, ectopic pregnancy, appendicitis, and endometriosis (Table 38–3). Nonetheless, if only women with moderate to severe symptoms are considered, most women with tubal occlusion will be missed.

Pelvic ultrasonography may be helpful in diagnosing tubo-ovarian abscess before it is clinically apparent, and increased adnexal volume on ultrasound may suggest the diagnosis of PID.

Complications

The sequelae of acute PID are significant—thus the importance of prudent use of antibiotics. Tubo-ovarian abscess is not uncommon. Twenty to 25 percent of patients develop subsequent unrelated episodes of PID. Thirteen percent of women with acute PID have chronic abdominal pain felt to be related to adhesions around the uterine tubes.

The Fitz-Hugh and Curtis syndrome, or perihepatitis, which is found in 5–10% of women with salpingitis, is due to direct hematogenous or lymphatic spread of bacteria from the uterine tubes to the liver surface. The woman may experience right upper quadrant pain and hepatic tenderness without liver enlargement and usually has normal liver function tests. A friction rub may be present, and on laparoscopy a fibrinous or purulent exudate may be seen over the liver capsule and later result in adhesions between the liver capsule and the abdominal wall.

Occlusion of the uterine tubes after salpingitis accounts for 30–40% of cases of female infertility and half of cases of ectopic pregnancy. Twelve percent of women with one episode, 35% with two episodes, and over 73% with three or more episodes of PID are infertile because of tubal occlusion. Age is inversely related to risk of infertility resulting from tubal occlusion after PID. The risk of ectopic pregnancy is seven to ten times greater for women who have had salpingitis than for those who have not, and 5% who have

had one or more episodes of PID will have an ectopic pregnancy.

Treatment

Culture samples should be taken from the cervix, and gynecologic consultation or laparoscopy should be considered. The patient should be hospitalized if she exhibits significant fever or toxicity, is unable to tolerate oral medication and fluids, has not responded to outpatient therapy or is unlikely to comply with it, is a younger adolescent, or is ill enough to arouse concern but has no clear diagnosis. Furthermore, if the patient is pregnant, if a tubo-ovarian abscess is suspected, or if an IUD is in place, the patient should be hospitalized. If there is the slightest concern that PID may be present, the patient should be treated with appropriate antibiotics to cover *Chlamydia, N gonorrhoeae,* and anaerobes while cultures are pending (Table 38–4). The patient should be reevaluated in 48–72 hours and hospitalized if there is no improvement. Appropriate management includes treatment of the male partners regardless of whether urethritis is present.

Table 38–4. Treatment of pelvic inflammatory disease.[1]

	Drugs of Choice	Alternative Drugs
Hospitalized patients	Cefoxitin, 2 g IV every 6 hours, *or* Cefotetan, 2 g IV every 12 hours *(either one) plus* Doxycycline, 100 mg IV every 12 hours until improved, *followed by* Doxycycline, 100 mg orally twice daily to complete 14 days of therapy	Clindamycin, 900 mg IV every 8 hours, *plus* Gentamicin, 2 mg/kg IV once followed by 1.5 mg/kg every 8 hours until improved, *followed by* Doxycycline, 100 mg orally twice daily to complete 14 days of therapy
Outpatients	Cefoxitin, 2 g IM once, *plus* Probenecid, 1 g orally once, *or* Ceftriaxone, 250 mg IM once, *(either one) followed by* Doxycycline, 100 mg orally twice daily for 14 days	

[1]Modified and reproduced, with permission, from: Drugs for sexually transmitted diseases. Med Lett Drugs Ther 1991;33: 119.

Table 38–3. Differential diagnosis of pelvic inflammatory disease.

Acute appendicitis
Mesenteric lymphadenitis
Cholecystitis
Ectopic pregnancy
Intrauterine pregnancy
Septic abortion
Threatened abortion
Ovarian cyst
Ovarian tumor
Endometriosis
Urinary tract infection
Renal calculus

GENITAL LESIONS

Infectious causes of genital lesions in adolescents include condylomata acuminata, herpes simplex virus, and syphilis.

Condylomata Acuminata

Condylomata acuminata, or genital warts, are caused by human papillomavirus (HPV). The peak age incidence is from 18 to 24 years. Transmission may occur to 30–60% of sexual partners, with an incubation period of 1–8 months. Warts typically occur at the site of minute skin trauma, with 50% occurring on the glans penis or corona in males and 75% at the posterior introitus in females. Diagnosis is based on the clinical appearance of a verrucous skin lesion, which shows no organisms on darkfield examination.

Condylomata on the cervix or the penis, however, may be indiscernible to the unaided eye. Colposcopy is valuable in such circumstances and should be performed whenever HPV effects are noted on Papanicolaou smear and perhaps in any patient with condylomas. It is now accepted that HPV is the most important etiologic agent in the development of cervical intraepithelial neoplasia and invasive cervical cancers. It also appears to be associated with penile cancer. Types 6, 11, and 42 are the most common strains found in condylomas. Types 16, 18, 31, 33, 35, and 39 are associated with neoplasia. The developmental persistence of the transition zone (from columnar to squamous epithelium) onto the face of the cervix may make adolescents more susceptible to cytologic changes when HPV is encountered.

Treatment is by application to the wart of 20–25% podophyllum resin in tincture of benzoin after petroleum jelly is applied to the surrounding normal skin; the solution is washed off in 4 hours. Reapplication at weekly intervals may be necessary. Podophyllum resin should not be applied to vaginal or anal mucosa, both because it may cause a chemical burn and because the vascularity of these areas increases the risk of hematologic or neurologic toxicity. It should not be used in pregnant patients. Liquid nitrogen, preferred over podophyllum resin by some authorities, may be applied to mucosal and nonmucosal warts at similar intervals. Alternative therapies include laser therapy, topical trichloroacetic acid, fluorouracil, surgical excision, electrocauterization, and alpha interferon. Abnormalities detected on colposcopy are biopsied. Laser removal is often the treatment of choice for warts on the cervix, because there is minimal tissue damage. It is unlikely that HPV can be eliminated entirely from the genital tract. Repeated treatments will be necessary over time, and the patient should be counseled to use condoms.

Herpes Simplex Virus

Eighty to 90 percent of cases of genital herpes are due to herpes simplex virus type 2 (HSV-2); the remainder are due to HSV-1. More than 50% of new infections may be asymptomatic. The primary episode is generally more symptomatic and prolonged (14–21 days) than recurrent episodes and is characterized by systemic symptoms such as fever, headache, malaise, and myalgias as well as a cluster of painful papules that progress to vesicles, pustules, ulcers, and finally crusts. HSV remains dormant in the dorsal root ganglia between episodes and migrates down the axon to the same dermatome to cause recurrences. Recurrences may be preceded by prodromal tingling of the skin. Lesions last about 5–7 days.

If acyclovir (200 mg orally five times a day or 400 mg three times a day for 7–10 days) is initiated within 3 days after onset of the primary episode, the mean duration of the illness is shortened by 3–5 days, and systemic symptoms are reduced. Acyclovir does not reduce the risk, rate, or severity of recurrences. Minimal benefit can be expected from treating recurrences with acyclovir (200 mg orally five times a day, or 400 mg three times a day, for 5 days), instituted at the time of prodromal symptoms. Chronic suppressive therapy with 400 mg of acyclovir twice a day for up to 12 months should be considered for patients with severe, frequent recurrences or for psychosocial reasons. Suppressive therapy has been used safely for 3–5 years.

A primary episode of genital herpes in a pregnant woman may increase the risk of spontaneous abortion, prematurity, and congenital infection. With recurrent episodes, however, there is probably no greater risk of miscarriage or prematurity, and only a slight risk of congenital herpes.

Syphilis

Primary syphilis, caused by *Treponema pallidum,* typically presents with a painless chancre that starts as a clean ulcer with an erythematous, indurated border after an average incubation period of 3 weeks (range 10–90 days). While chancres most commonly occur on the genitalia, they can occur on any mucous membrane or skin surface; on the cervix, they may go undiagnosed because of their asymptomatic nature. The chancre is generally self-limited. Systemic signs and symptoms are absent. Regional adenopathy is common, but these nodes are nontender. The painless nature of the chancre distinguishes it from herpes simplex and chancroid. The nodes of herpes simplex are often tender, as are those of chancroid, which also tend to be fluctuant. The most certain diagnosis is by darkfield examination of a slide that has been pressed to the base of the lesion. The lesion is prepared by removing any crust, cleansing the surface with a moistened gauze sponge, and gently abrading the base with a dry gauze bandage. A coverslip is placed on the slide, which should be examined immediately. Aspirates of regional lymph nodes are another source for darkfield samples, and in secondary syphilis nonoral mucous patches or condylomata lata are positive.

The Venereal Disease Research Laboratory (VDRL) slide test is reactive in 60–75% of patients with primary syphilis, and the fluorescent treponemal antibody absorption (FTA-ABS) test in 80–90%.

After a latency period of 4–6 weeks, the disease may resurface in its secondary stage, characterized by a diffuse, nonpruritic, papulosquamous rash that often includes the palms and soles; mucous patches on the mucosal surfaces; generalized lymphadenopathy; constitutional symptoms; and the presence of condylomata lata (broad-based, flat, mucoid lesions) on the genitals. Transient proteinuria, hemorrhagic nephritis, hepatitis, arthritis, and iritis may also develop during secondary syphilis. At this stage, virtually all serologic tests for syphilis are positive. If the diagnosis is made with a qualitative nontreponemal test (such as VDRL or rapid plasma reagin [RPR] test), a quantitative titer should be obtained, and the same quantitative nontreponemal test followed over time. Treponemal tests (eg, FTA-ABS) may be reserved for patients with atypical presentations and a positive screening test.

The tertiary stage, unlikely to be seen in adolescents, is divided into early latent (first 4 years) and late latent. During the late period, symptoms of tertiary syphilis may include the cardiovascular and central nervous system complications of dissection of the ascending aorta, seizures, stroke, optic atrophy, and tabes dorsalis.

All stages may be treated with penicillin (Table 38–5). Quantitative serology should be repeated with the same test prior to and at 3, 6, and 12 months after treatment. Any patient with disease for longer than 1 year should have a cerebrospinal fluid examination for neurosyphilis. Because the VDRL will return to negative during the 2 years after treatment, a subsequent rise in the VDRL titer (or failure to fall) should be interpreted as a treatment failure or reinfection. The FTA-ABS test remains positive for life unless syphilis is treated very early.

TRICHOMONIASIS

Trichomonas vaginalis

Trichomonas vaginalis causes vaginitis in females and urethritis in males. Females may be asymptomatic or may complain of a pruritic vaginal discharge. Diagnosis is by examination of a vaginal wet preparation in females—or of a centrifuged urine sample in males—for the motile trichomonad. The organism is about the size of a white blood cell but is pointed at its flagellated end. It may be missed in a full field of white blood cells unless one looks carefully for the beating motion of the flagellum jolting the neighboring cells. Metronidazole (2 g orally once or 500 mg orally twice a day for 7 days) is the treatment of choice. Patients should not drink alcohol during treatment. In pregnant patients, clotrimazole (100 mg intravaginally at bedtime for 7 days) may reduce symptoms and produce some cures. Metronidazole is

Table 38–5. Treatment of syphilis.[1]

Stage	Drug of Choice	Dosage	Alternative Treatments
Early (primary, secondary, or latent less than 1 year)	Pencillin G benzathine	2.4 million units IM once	Doxycycline,[2,3] 100 mg orally twice daily for 14 days. Ceftriaxone, 250 mg IM once daily for 10 days if compliance is assured.
Late (more than 1 year's duration, cardiovascular)	Penicillin G benzathine	2.4 million units IM weekly for 3 weeks	Doxycycline,[2,3] 100 mg orally twice daily for 4 weeks.
Neurosyphilis	Penicillin G	2–4 million units IV every 4 hours for 10–14 days	No proved effective alternative; allergic patients should be desensitized.
	or		
	Penicillin G procaine	2.4 million units IM daily	
	plus		
	Probenecid	500 mg four times daily orally for 10–14 days	
Congenital	Penicillin G	50,000 units/kg IM or 100,000 units/kg IV twice daily for 10–14 days	
	or		
	Penicillin G procaine	50,000 units/kg IM daily for 10–14 days	

[1]Modified and reproduced, with permission, from: Drugs for sexually transmitted diseases. Med Lett Drugs Ther 1991;33:119.
[2]Contraindicated during pregnancy.
[3]Or tetracycline, 500 mg orally four times daily.

contraindicated in the first trimester of pregnancy, but many authorities use it thereafter.

ARTHROPOD INFESTATIONS

Pthirus pubis, the crab louse, lives a sedentary, 45-day life cycle on the pubic hair and is transmitted during intimate contact. The patient experiences a pruritic rash, and on physical examination the opalescent nits (eggs) are found securely anchored to the pubic hairs.

Sarcoptes scabiei, which causes scabies, is a round, flat, motile organism. The females embed themselves in the skin and deposit two or three eggs per day. Scabies also results in an intensely pruritic rash, which is located on the groin, thighs, or abdomen in the case of sexual transmission. Findings on physical examination are the scabietic burrows and an erythematous maculopapular rash with some scaliness and the tendency to impetiginize.

Treatment in either case is with topical application from neck to toe of lindane, which should remain on the skin for 8 hours, or application on two separate occasions of crotamiton at bedtime, remaining on the skin for 24 hours. (Lindane should not be applied to infants or pregnant or breast-feeding women.) The patient is no longer contagious 24 hours after treatment; however, symptoms of scabies may not abate for 2 weeks. Close contacts also need to be treated and fomites properly removed to prevent recurrences.

HEPATITIS B

Approximately 300,000 cases of hepatitis B infection occur annually in the USA. Sexual transmission accounts for at least 30% of reported cases of acute hepatitis B. While in the past homosexual transmission was responsible for the bulk of sexually transmitted cases, in recent years heterosexual transmission has increased and accounts for approximately 25% of cases.

See Chapter 23 for clinical presentation, prevention, and treatment.

HIV INFECTION

The human immunodeficiency virus (HIV), the cause of acquired immunodeficiency syndrome (AIDS), is transmitted in blood and semen—and potentially other body fluids—through sexual contact and sharing of needles. As of December 1992, the CDC reported 3058 adolescents 13–21 years old with AIDS. Many more acquire HIV infection in their teens, since the average latency period from HIV infection to AIDS is 11 years and 20% of all cases of AIDS occur among people in their twenties. About 75% of AIDS cases in the USA have occurred in homosexual or bisexual men and 15% in intravenous substance abusers. A greater percentage of adolescents than adults with AIDS are female (26% versus 10%), black or Latino (56% versus 44%), and are infected through heterosexual contact (14% versus 5%). Although to date few cases have occurred in adolescents, they are at significant potential risk from risk-taking behaviors such as their propensity for multiple sexual partners and their limited use of barrier contraceptives as well as the use of drugs by some. The management of HIV infection is discussed in Chapter 35. Adolescents with risk behaviors and tuberculosis should be screened for HIV infection.

Preventive measures need to be taken to ensure that adolescents have the necessary knowledge to protect themselves from HIV infection in current and future relationships and to eliminate hysteria. They need to be instructed in risk factors for HIV infection, modes of transmission, means of protection, and availability of confidential testing. The safer sex practices (Table 38–6) promoted as a result of HIV infection can reduce the rate of all kinds of STD. Adolescence is an ideal time to promote these practices, because it is at this time that intimate relationships are beginning and sexual decisions become important.

SEXUAL ABUSE & SEXUALLY TRANSMITTED DISEASE

Up to 20% of the 250,000–300,000 sexually abused children in the USA each year may have a sexually transmitted infection. Diagnosis is critical both to ensure proper treatment and for medicolegal documentation. To this end, examination by skilled personnel who obtain appropriate cultures, send them to credible laboratories, and follow chain-of-evidence guidelines is necessary. While routine STD screening of all suspected sexually abused children is not recommended, appropriate serologic tests and

Table 38–6. Safer sex practices.

1. Abstinence: greatest protection against HIV infection
2. Sexual activity without intercourse: hugging, massaging, masturbation
3. Sexual activity only in the context of a monogamous relationship
4. Limiting the number of sexual partners
5. Using condoms and spermicide for each sexual encounter, including oral and anal intercourse. (Hold rim of condom closed during withdrawal to prevent spilling semen.)
6. Refraining from anal intercourse
7. Refraining from oral sex when mouth sores or open wounds are present
8. Refraining from vaginal or oral sex during menstruation or when vaginal or vulvar sores or infection exist
9. Avoiding alcohol or drug use in sexual situations

cultures should be obtained if oral, genital, or anal contact is suggested by history or physical findings. Such studies might include wet preparations for *Trichomonas vaginalis,* gonorrhea and chlamydial cultures from the pharynx, vagina, urethra, and rectum, viral cultures if lesions suspicious for herpes simplex exist, and serologic tests for syphilis, HIV, and hepatitis B antigen if these cannot be ruled out in the alleged perpetrator. Repeat testing 3 months after the abuse must be done to fully evaluate the likelihood of STD transmission. Culture isolates must be saved for medicolegal purposes. Table 38-7 estimates the likelihood that sexual abuse has occurred for specific isolates.

Table 38–7. Implications of commonly encountered sexually transmitted diseases for the diagnosis and reporting of sexual abuse of prepubertal infants and children.[1]

STD Confirmed	Sexual Abuse	Suggested Action
Gonorrhea[2]	Certain	Report[3]
Syphilis[2]	Certain	Report
Chlamydia[2]	Probable[4]	Report
Condylomata acuminata[2]	Probable	Report
Trichomonas vaginalis	Probable	Report
Herpes 1 (in genital area)	Possible	Report[5]
Herpes 2	Probable	Report
Bacterial vaginosis	Uncertain	Medical follow-up
Candida albicans	Unlikely	Medical follow-up

[1]Reproduced, with permission, from: Guidelines for the evaluation of sexual abuse of children. Pediatrics 1991;87:254. Prepared by the AAP Committee on Child Abuse and Neglect.
[2]If not perinatally acquired.
[3]To agency mandated in community to receive reports of suspected sexual abuse.
[4]Culture is the only reliable diagnostic method.
[5]Unless there is a clear history of autoinoculation.

REFERENCES

AAP Committee on Child Abuse and Neglect: Guidelines for the evaluation of sexual abuse of children. Pediatrics 1991;87:254.

Alter MJ, Margolis HS: The emergence of hepatitis B as a sexually transmitted disease. Med Clin North Am 1990; 74:1529.

Bell TA: *Chlamydia trachomatis* infections in adolescents. Med Clin North Am 1990;74:1225.

Boyer CB: Psychosocial, behavioral, and educational factors in preventing sexually transmitted diseases. Adolescent Medicine: State of the Art Reviews 1990;1:597.

Davis AJ, Emans SJ: Human papilloma virus infection in the pediatric and adolescent patient. J Pediatr 1989; 115:1.

Drugs for sexually transmitted diseases. Med Lett Drugs Ther 1991;33:119.

Futterman D, Hein K, Kunins H: Teens and AIDS: Identifying and testing those at risk. Contemp Pediatr 1993; 10:68.

Holmes KK et al (editors): *Sexually Transmitted Diseases,* 2nd ed. McGraw-Hill, 1990.

Kunins H et al: Guide to adolescent HIV/AIDS program development. J Adol Health 1993;14(5 Suppl):1.

Judson FN: Gonorrhea. Med Clin North Am 1990;74:1353.

Manoff SB et al: Acquired immunodeficiency syndrome in adolescents: Epidemiology, prevention and public health issues. Pediatr Infect Dis J 1989;8:309.

Martin DH (editor): Sexually transmitted diseases. Med Clin North Am 1990;74:6.

Mertz GJ: Genital herpes simplex virus infections. Med Clin North Am 1990;74:1433.

Remafedi G: Sexually transmitted diseases in homosexual youth. AM:STARS 1990;1:565.

Shafer MA, Sweet RL: Pelvic inflammatory disease in adolescent females. AM:STARS 1990;1:545.

Wolner-Hanssen P et al: Clinical manifestations of vaginal trichomoniasis. JAMA 1989;261:571.

Neoplastic Disease

Edythe A. Albano, MD, Brian S. Greffe, MD,
Lorrie F. Odom, MD, & Linda C. Stork, MD

Cure of cancer in children is occurring with ever-increasing numbers. Combined-modality therapy (surgery, chemotherapy, radiation therapy) has improved survival dramatically, with the result that the overall cure rate of pediatric malignancies is now 60%. It is estimated that by the year 2000, one in 1000 adults will be a survivor of childhood cancer.

Therapeutic advances continue to be made. Because of the rare nature of pediatric malignancies, the cooperative clinical trial has become the mainstay of treatment planning. Studies such as those sponsored by the Children's Cancer Group (CCG) or Pediatric Oncology Group (POG) offer the most current therapeutic options and answer important therapeutic questions in a timely manner. For progress in treatment to continue, a newly diagnosed child with cancer should be enrolled in a cooperative clinical trial whenever possible. However, because many protocols are associated with significant toxicities, morbidity, and potential mortality, the supervision of a pediatric patient on such a treatment regimen should be by a pediatric oncologist familiar with all the inherent hazards of treatment.

Advances in molecular genetics, cell biology, and tumor immunology have contributed to our greater knowledge and understanding of pediatric malignancies; these in turn have also lead to advances in treatment and cure. However, these scientific breakthroughs also add greatly to the responsibility of the physician caring for a child with a suspected malignancy. Because these studies have therapeutic and prognostic implications, it is critically important that pathologic material submitted for evaluation of a suspected malignancy be handled by a pathologist who is familiar with these ancillary studies and will be able to arrive at an accurate diagnosis in a timely manner.

Research in supportive care areas such as pain management, emesis control, and infection prevention and treatment has contributed to improved survival as well as an improved quality of life for children undergoing cancer treatment. Long-term follow-up of childhood cancer survivors is yielding information that will provide a rational for modifying future treatment regimens to decrease morbidity.

A pediatric oncology center where all critically important adjunctive services are available is the ideal setting for pediatric cancer patients. It is no longer possible for one physician to diagnose and provide all the care needed for a child with cancer. Modern cancer therapy requires a blend of skills from various disciplines and specialties. A multidisciplinary approach to care is imperative. At a minimum, the team must include an oncologist, a surgeon, a pathologist, a radiologist, a nurse, a social worker, and a radiation oncologist. The team will often have additional members also such as a nutritionist, home health care personnel, physical and occupational therapists, a psychologist, a pain management team, and various pediatric subspecialists.

ACUTE LYMPHOBLASTIC LEUKEMIA

Essentials of Diagnosis

- Pallor, petechiae, purpura (50%), bone pain (25%).
- Hepatosplenomegaly (60%), lymphadenopathy (50%).
- Single or multiple cytopenias: neutropenia, thrombocytopenia, anemia.
- Leukopenia or leukocytosis, often with leukemic leukocytes identifiable on blood smear.
- Diagnosis confirmed by bone marrow examination.

General Considerations

Acute lymphoblastic leukemia (ALL) is the most common malignancy of childhood, accounting for about 25% of all cancer diagnoses under the age of 15 years. The worldwide incidence of ALL is about 1:25,000 children per year, including 2500 children per year in the United States. The peak age at onset is 4 years, with 85% of patients diagnosed between the ages of 2 and 10 years. Before the advent of chemotherapy, this disease was fatal, usually within 3–4 months, with virtually no survivors 1 year after diagnosis. ALL results from uncontrolled proliferation of immature lymphocytes; its cause is unknown, and genetic factors may play a role. Leukemia is defined by the presence of more than 25% malignant hematopoietic cells (blasts) on bone marrow aspirate. Leukemic blasts from the majority of cases of childhood ALL have an antigen on the cell surface called the common ALL antigen (CALLA). These blasts derive from B cell precursors early in their development. Less commonly, lymphoblasts are of T cell origin or of mature B cell origin. Current estimates are that over 70% of children receiving aggressive combination chemotherapy and early central nervous system prophylaxis are cured of ALL. In general, children diagnosed with ALL between 2 and 9 years of age who have a white blood cell count < 50,000/μL at diagnosis have the best chance of cure.

Clinical Findings

A. Symptoms and Signs: Presenting complaints of patients with ALL include those related to decreased bone marrow production of red cells, white cells, and platelets and to leukemic infiltration of extramedullary (outside bone marrow) sites. Intermittent fevers are common, either as a result of cytokines induced by the leukemia itself or of infections secondary to leukopenia. About 25% of patients experience bone pain, especially in the pelvis, vertebral bodies, and legs. Physical examination at diagnosis ranges from virtually normal to highly abnormal. Signs related to bone marrow infiltration by leukemia include pallor, petechiae, and purpura. Hepatomegaly or splenomegaly occurs in over 60% of cases. Lymphadenopathy is common, either localized or generalized to cervical, axillary, and inguinal regions. The testes may be unilaterally or bilaterally enlarged secondary to leukemic infiltration. Superior vena caval syndrome is manifest by a prominent venous pattern over the upper chest resulting from collateral vein enlargement. The neck may feel full owing to venous engorgement. The face may appear plethoric, and the periorbital area may be edematous.

Tachypnea, orthopnea, and respiratory distress may be apparent. Leukemic infiltration of cranial nerves may result in cranial nerve palsies along with mild nuchal rigidity. Funduscopic examination may show exudates representing leukemic infiltration and may also show hemorrhage from thrombocytopenia. Rarely, retinal detachment occurs secondary to hemorrhage. The cardiac examination often reveals a flow murmur and tachycardia due to anemia; rarely, signs of congestive heart failure are present. Bone and joint pain may be appreciated on examination, particularly in the pelvis, lower spine, and femurs. In addition, signs of infection may be found on physical examination. Infections may include otitis media, sinusitis, pharyngitis, pneumonia, cellulitis, or skin pustules from bacteremia.

B. Laboratory Findings: The CBC and differential is the most useful initial laboratory test for determining if a child has ALL. Ninety-five percent of patients have a decrease in at least one cell type (single cytopenia): neutropenia, thrombocytopenia, or

anemia. Most patients have decreases in at least two blood cell lines. The white count is low or normal (< 10,000/μL) in 50% of patients, but the differential often shows neutropenia (absolute neutrophil count < 1000/μL) along with a small percentage of blasts amid normal lymphocytes. In 30% of patients, the white count is between 10,000 and 50,000/μL, and in 20% of cases it is > 50,000/μL, occasionally higher than 300,000/μL. Blasts are usually readily identifiable on peripheral smears in patients with elevated white counts. Most patients with ALL have decreased platelet counts (< 150,000/μL) and decreased hemoglobin (< 11 g/dL) at diagnosis, though cases with normal platelet counts and hemoglobin do occur. Less than 1% of patients diagnosed with ALL have entirely normal CBCs and blood smears but have symptoms of bone pain that lead to bone marrow examination. Serum chemistries—particularly uric acid and lactate dehydrogenase (LDH)—are often elevated at diagnosis. Uric acid and LDH are intracellular products released after cell breakdown. Serum phosphorus is occasionally elevated at diagnosis as well. Liver function tests may also be mildly abnormal.

The diagnosis of ALL is established by bone marrow examination, which shows a homogeneous infiltration of leukemic blasts replacing normal marrow elements. The morphology of blasts on bone marrow aspirate can usually distinguish ALL from acute non-lymphocytic leukemia (ANLL). Lymphoblasts are typically small, with cell diameters equal to that of approximately two erythrocytes. Lymphoblasts have scant cytoplasm, usually without granules. The nucleus typically contains no nucleoli or one small indistinct nucleolus. Immunophenotyping of ALL blasts helps distinguish precursor B cell ALL from T cell ALL. Histochemical stains specific for myeloblastic and monoblastic leukemias (myeloperoxidase and nonspecific esterase) distinguish ALL from ANLL. Between 5% and 10% of patients present with central nervous system leukemia, which is defined as a cerebrospinal fluid white cell count > 5/μL with blasts apparent on cytocentrifuged specimen.

C. Imaging: Chest x-ray may show mediastinal widening or mediastinal mass and tracheal compression secondary to lymphadenopathy. Abdominal ultrasound may show kidney enlargement from leukemic infiltration or uric acid nephropathy and intra-abdominal adenopathy. Plain films of the long bones and spine may show demineralization and compression of vertebral bodies.

Differential Diagnosis

The differential diagnosis, based on the history and physical examination, includes chronic infections such as those caused by Epstein-Barr virus and cytomegalovirus, giving rise to lymphadenopathy, hepatosplenomegaly, fevers, and anemia. Prominent petechiae and purpura suggest a diagnosis of immune thrombocytopenic purpura. Significant pallor brings to mind diagnoses such as transient erythroblastopenia of childhood, autoimmune hemolytic anemias, and aplastic anemia. Fevers and joint pains, with or without hepatosplenomegaly and lymphadenopathy, suggest juvenile rheumatoid arthritis. The diagnosis of leukemia usually becomes straightforward once the CBC reveals multiple cytopenias and leukemic blasts. Serum LDH levels appear helpful in distinguishing juvenile rheumatoid arthritis from leukemia, since LDH is usually normal at diagnosis in juvenile rheumatoid arthritis but often elevated in patients presenting with leukemia and significant bone pain. An elevated white count with lymphocytosis is typical of pertussis infection; however, the lymphocytes are mature, and neutropenia is rarely associated.

Treatment & Prognosis

Specific treatment is determined by prognostic features recorded at diagnosis and is generally divided into three phases. The first month of therapy consists of **induction,** at the end of which over 95% of patients exhibit remission on bone marrow aspirates. The drugs most commonly used in induction include oral prednisone, intravenous vincristine, intramuscular asparaginase, intrathecal methotrexate, and intravenous daunorubicin. For T cell ALL, intravenous cyclophosphamide is often given during induction as well.

Consolidation is the second phase of treatment, during which intrathecal chemotherapy and sometimes cranial irradiation are given to treat lymphoblasts that may be present in the meninges.

Maintenance therapy is the third phase of treatment and usually is associated with fewer acute side effects than the first two phases. Drugs used in maintenance include daily oral mercaptopurine, weekly oral or intramuscular methotrexate, and monthly pulses of intravenous vincristine and oral prednisone. Intrathecal chemotherapy, either with methotrexate alone or combined with cytarabine and hydrocortisone, is usually administered every 2–3 months. Short courses of intensive chemotherapy may be interspersed within the maintenance chemotherapy phase of treatment.

All these drugs have significant potential side effects. Patients need to be closely monitored to prevent drug toxicities and to ensure early treatment of complications. Most patients are treated on protocols designed by the national Children's Cancer Group or Pediatric Oncology Group. The duration of treatment is between 2 and 3½ years.

The chance of cure depends on specific prognostic features present at diagnosis of ALL. The two most important features are white count and age. In the 1970s, it became clear that children with white counts under 50,000/μL had a much better chance of cure than did children with counts over 50,000/μL receiving the same chemotherapy. Children between ages 2 and 9 years have a better chance of cure than do younger and older patients. Certain chromosomal abnormalities present in the leukemic blasts at diagnosis also have prognostic significance. Patients with a translocation between chromosomes 9 and 22—t(9;22)—have a very poor chance of cure even with intensive therapy. Patients with a translocation between chromosomes 4 and 11—t(4;11)—generally have a poorer chance of cure than do other patients with ALL. On the other hand, patients whose blasts are hyperdiploid (contain over 50 chromosomes instead of the normal 46) have a better chance of cure than children without hyperdiploidy.

Treatment for ALL currently is tailored to prognostic groups. A child between the ages of 2 and 9 years with a white count under 50,000/μL at diagnosis and without t(9;22) or t(4;11) would be treated with less intensive therapy than a patient with a white count over 50,000/μL or a patient older than 10 years. This treatment approach has significantly increased the cure rate among patients with less favorable prognostic features while minimizing treatment-related toxicities in those with favorable prognostic features. The overall chance of cure for ALL is now at least 70%.

Bone marrow relapse is usually heralded by an abnormal CBC. Once a patient has completed the entire course of chemotherapy, the chance of relapse is about 10% in the next 2 years and much less after that time. CBCs are obtained monthly during the first year following completion of treatment and less often thereafter.

The central nervous system and testes are sanctuary sites of extramedullary leukemia. Systemic chemotherapy does not penetrate these tissues as well as it penetrates most organs. "Prophylactic" intrathecal chemotherapy is a critical part of ALL treatment protocols to prevent leukemic relapse in the central nervous system. Before the institution of such therapy in the 1970s, the central nervous system was a major site of initial leukemic relapse. Relapses isolated to the central nervous system now occur in only 10% of patients either during treatment or after treatment is completed. Symptoms suggestive of central nervous system recurrence include headache, nausea and vomiting, irritability, nuchal rigidity, photophobia, and cranial nerve palsies. Previously, up to 15% of boys relapsed in their testes following completion of chemotherapy. The presentation of testicular relapse is usually unilateral painless testicular enlargement. The incidence of testicular relapse has decreased significantly as treatment for ALL has intensified. Routine follow-up of boys both on and off treatment includes examination of the testes.

Bone marrow transplant is rarely used as initial treatment following induction of remission for ALL since the majority of patients are cured with chemotherapy alone. However, patients with certain chromosomal abnormalities in their leukemic blasts, such as t(9;22), appear to have a much better cure rate with early bone marrow transplant from an HLA-DR-matched sibling donor than with intensive chemotherapy alone. Bone marrow transplant does play a role in patients who have relapsed with ALL, particularly if the relapse is during the course of treatment or within about 6 months after completion of chemotherapy. For these patients, virtually the only chance of cure is with bone marrow transplant.

Supportive Care

At the start of induction treatment, tumor lysis syndrome should be anticipated. Hydration, alkalinization of urine, and oral allopurinol should be instituted. If superior vena caval syndrome is present, general anesthesia may be temporarily contraindicated owing to tracheal and airway compression. If hyperleukocytosis (> 100,000/μL) is present along with mental status changes, leukapheresis may be indicated to rapidly reduce the number of circulating blasts and minimize the potential thrombotic or hemorrhagic central nervous system complications. Severe anemia at diagnosis can usually be corrected with a number of small red blood cell transfusions and intravenous furosemide. During induction and throughout the course of treatment, all transfused blood and platelet products should be irradiated in order to prevent graft-versus-host disease from the transfused lymphocytes. Whenever possible, blood products should be leukodepleted as well. The white cells may harbor cytomegalovirus and are also responsible for transfusion reactions and platelet refractoriness.

Fever at diagnosis needs to be treated with broad-spectrum antibiotics for several days until blood and other culture sites are negative and the patient has been afebrile for 48 hours. During the course of treatment, fever (temperature > 38.3 °C) and neutropenia (absolute neutrophil count < 500/μL) need to be treated with empiric broad-spectrum antibiotics. All patients receiving ALL treatment must receive prophylaxis against *Pneumocystis carinii*. Trimethoprim-sulfamethoxazole is the drug of choice, currently recommended to be given on 3 consecutive days per week, twice each day. For patients allergic to this preparation, intravenous pentamidine every 3 weeks is effective *Pneumocystis* prophylaxis. Patients who have not had chickenpox are at risk of very serious and perhaps fatal infection if exposed to varicella. Such patients should receive varicella-zoster immune globulin (VZIG) within 72 hours after exposure. The management of a patient on chemotherapy for ALL is very complex because of the potential infectious complications and potential toxicities of chemotherapy. Treatment of patients with ALL should be guided by physicians and nurses who are specifically trained in pediatric oncology.

Bleyer WA: Acute lymphoblastic leukemia in children: Advances and prospective. Cancer 1990;65:689.

Gaynon PS: Primary treatment of childhood ALL of non-T all lineage (including infants). Hematol Oncol Clin North Am 1990;4:915.

Pui CH, Christ WM: Biology and treatment of acute lymphoblastic leukemia. 1994;124:491.

Rivera GK et al: Treatment of ALL: 30 years' experience at St. Jude's Research Hospital. N Engl J Med 1993; 329:1289.

Rubin CM, LeBeau MM: Cytogenetics abnormalities in childhood acute lymphoblastic leukemia. Am J Pediatr Hematol Oncol 1991;13:202.

ACUTE NONLYMPHOCYTIC LEUKEMIA

Acute nonlymphocytic leukemia (ANLL) is one-fifth as common in childhood as acute lymphoblastic leukemia (ALL). There are 500 new cases per year in the United States. Ionizing radiation, cytotoxic chemotherapeutic agents, benzene exposure, Down's syndrome, and chromosomal instability syndromes are known to be predisposing factors, but most children have none. Cytogenetic clonal abnormalities occur in 80% of patients with ANLL and are often predictive of outcome.

ANLL is broken down into seven subgroups based primarily on morphology and histochemical staining of the leukemic cells (French-American-British [FAB] classification). These subsets can have characteristic cytogenetic abnormalities, clinical features at presentation, and responses to treatment (Table 39–1).

Clinical presentation is usually related to symptoms of decreased hematopoiesis: anemia (44%), thrombocytopenia (33%), and neutropenia (69%). Symptoms can be few and innocuous or may be life-threatening. The median hemoglobin at diagnosis is 7 g/dL; platelets are usually less than 50,000/μL; and the absolute neutrophil count is under 1000/μL. The total white blood cell count is over 100,000/μL in one-fourth of children diagnosed with ANLL. Hyperleukocytosis is associated with life-threatening complications from venous stasis and sludging of blasts in small vessels causing hypoxia, hemorrhage, and infarction, most notably in the lung and central nervous system. This is a medical emergency requiring rapid intervention to decrease the leukocyte count. Central nervous system leukemia is present in 5–15% of patients at diagnosis, which is a much higher rate of involvement than in ALL.

Treatment is more difficult than in ALL and requires more intensive administration of chemotherapeutic drugs, particularly anthracyclines and cytarabine. Toxicities from therapy are common and likely to be life-threatening. Only 70–85% of children achieve remission (versus 98% in ALL); the long-term disease-free survival is 33–49%. Retinoic acid (all-*trans*) can cause differentiation of promyelocytic leukemia cells

Table 39–1. FAB subtypes of ANLL.

FAB Classification	Common Name	Distribution in Childhood		Cytogenetic Associations	Clinical Features
		< 2 Years	> 2 Years		
M_1	Acute myeloblastic leukemia without maturation	17%	25%	16q abnormalities	
M_2	Acute myeloblastic leukemia with maturation		26%	18;21, inv 16, del 16q	Myeloblastomas
M_3	Acute promyelocytic leukemia		4%	t15;17 (90% of cases)	DIC
M_4	Acute myelomonocytic leukemia	30%	26%	t3;3, inv 3, inv 16, del 16q, t11/del 11q	Hyperleukocytosis, CNS involvement, skin and gum infiltration
M_5	Acute monocytic leukemia	52%	16%	t9;11	Hyperleukocytosis, CNS involvement, skin and gum infiltration
M_6	Erythroleukemia		2%		
M_7	Acute megakaryocytic leukemia		5%	t1;21, t3;3, inv 3	Down's syndrome

and induce remission. Its role in the treatment of acute promyelocytic leukemia (M_3) is under investigation. Allogeneic bone marrow transplant during first remission may offer a survival advantage over chemotherapy alone. Published results from various centers show a 55–70% survival at 5 years. For patients relapsing following conventional chemotherapy, bone marrow transplant is a potentially curative option.

Grier HE et al: Acute myelogenous leukemia. In: *Principles and Practice of Pediatric Oncology.* Pizzo PA, Poplack DG (editors). Lippincott, 1993.

Kalwinsky DK et al: Prognostic importance of cytogenetic subgroups in de novo pediatric acute nonlymphocytic leukemia. J Clin Oncol 1990;8:75.

Sartori PCE et al: Treatment of childhood acute myeloid leukemia using the BFM-83 protocol. Med Pediatr Oncol 1993;21:8.

Warrell RP et al: Differentiation therapy of acute promyelocytic leukemia with tretinoin (all-*trans*-retinoic acid). N Engl J Med 1991;324:1385.

CHRONIC MYELOCYTIC LEUKEMIA

Chronic myelocytic leukemia (CML) accounts for less than 5% of the childhood leukemias. Two childhood variants are recognized: the Philadelphia chromosome t(9;22)-positive form, which is essentially identical to that occurring in adults, and the juvenile form (Table 39–2).

Adult CML can be palliated with single-drug chemotherapy (hydroxyurea or busulfan). The disease inexorably progresses from the chronic phase, usually within 3 years, to an accelerated phase and then to a blast crisis. The accelerated and blast phases are refractory to therapy. Bone marrow transplantation is the only known cure. The 4-year survival for patients

under 20 years of age transplanted in the chronic phase is 75%. Unfortunately, only one-third of patients have related, matched donors available. Consequently related mismatched, unrelated matched, autologous, and peripheral stem cell bone marrow transplants are being investigated. Alpha interferon has shown promising results in clinical trials by reducing or eliminating the Philadelphia chromosome-positive malignant clone. The long-term results are not yet known.

Juvenile CML accounts for one-third of chronic leukemias in childhood. Compared with the adult form it is a much more fulminant disease that occurs

Table 39–2. Comparison of juvenile and adult chronic myelogenous leukemia.

	Juvenile CML	Adult CML
Age at onset	< 2 years old	> 3 years old
Clinical presentation	Abrupt onset; eczematoid skin rash, marked lymphadenopathy, bleeding diathesis, moderate hepatosplenomegaly.	Nonspecific constitutional complaints, massive splenomegaly, variable hepatomegaly.
Chromosomal alterations	Absent.	t(9;22) present in 90% of cases.
Laboratory features	Moderate leukocytosis (< 100,000/μL), thrombocytopenia, monocytosis, elevated fetal hemoglobin, normal to diminished leukocyte alkaline phosphatase, elevated muramidase, elevated immunoglobulins.	Marked leukocytosis (> 100,000/μL), normal to elevated platelet count, decreased to absent leukocyte alkaline phosphatase, usually normal muramidase.

in infants and very young children. Survival is less than 9 months. Bone marrow transplant has been used successfully.

Altman A: Chronic leukemias of childhood. In: *Principles and Practice of Pediatric Oncology.* Pizzo PA, Poplack DG (editors). Lippincott, 1993.

Delage R et al: The evolving role of bone marrow transplantation in the treatment of chronic myelogenous leukemia. Hematol Oncol Clin North Am 1990;4:369.

Dow LW et at: Response to alpha-interferon in children with Philadelphia chromosome-positive chronic myelocytic leukemia. Cancer 1991;68:1678.

BRAIN TUMORS

Essentials of Diagnosis

- Cranial nerve palsies, dysarthria, ataxia, hemiplegia, papilledema, hyperreflexia, macrocephaly, cracked pot sign.
- Headache, vomiting, personality change, seizures, blurred vision, diplopia, weakness, decreased coordination, precocious or delayed puberty.

General Considerations

Brain tumors are the most common solid tumor of childhood, accounting for 1500–2000 new malignancies in children each year in the United States and for 25–30% of all childhood cancers. In general, children with brain tumors have a better prognosis than adults. Favorable outcome occurs most commonly with low-grade and fully resectable tumors. Unfortunately, cranial irradiation in young children is usually associated with significant neuropsychologic, intellectual, and endocrinologic sequelae.

Brain tumors in childhood are biologically and histologically heterogeneous, ranging from low-grade, localized lesions to high-grade tumors with neuraxis dissemination. High-dose systemic chemotherapy is being used more frequently, especially in young children with high-grade tumors, in an effort to delay, decrease or to completely avoid cranial irradiation. Such intensive treatment may be accompanied by autologous bone marrow transplantation or peripheral stem cell reconstitution.

The causes of pediatric brain tumors remain unknown. The risk of developing astrocytomas is increased in children with neurofibromatosis or tuberous sclerosis. Several studies show that some childhood brain tumors occur in families with increased genetic susceptibility to childhood cancers in general, brain tumors, or leukemia and lymphoma. An excess of seizures in relatives of children with astrocytoma has been observed. Certain pediatric brain tumors such as ependymoma have been linked to polyomavirus, but the exact relationship remains to be elucidated. The risk of developing a brain tumor is increased also in children who received cranial irradiation at a young age for treatment of presymptomatic meningeal leukemia.

Because pediatric brain tumors are rare, they are often misdiagnosed or diagnosed late; most pediatricians see no more than two children with brain tumors during their careers. Every effort must be made to enroll as many children as possible in therapeutic trials both to optimize the child's treatment and to systematically improve treatment outcomes in the future.

Clinical Findings

A. Symptoms and Signs: Clinical findings at presentation vary depending upon the age of the child and the location of the tumor. Children under 2 years of age more commonly have infratentorial tumors. They usually present with nonspecific symptoms such as vomiting, unsteadiness, lethargy, and irritability and signs such as macrocephaly, ataxia, hyperreflexia, and cranial nerve palsies. They may also present with extreme weight loss and emaciation with paradoxical alertness and euphoria (diencephalic syndrome) related to a tumor in the hypothalamic region. Eye findings and apparent visual disturbances such as difficulty tracking can be seen in optic pathway tumors such as optic glioma. Optic glioma occurring in a young child is usually associated with neurofibromatosis.

Older children more commonly have supratentorial tumors, which present with headache, visual symptoms, seizures, and focal neurologic deficits. Seizures secondary to frontal lobe tumors may begin with a focal motor onset or may be generalized. Seizures secondary to temporal lobe tumors are typically associated with behaviors such as staring spells and automatic movements. Frontal lobe tumors also affect personality and movement; parietal lobe tumors may affect reading and awareness of the contralateral extremities; temporal lobe tumors may cause fluent aphasias; and occipital lobe tumors may cause visual field deficits. Optic chiasm tumors cause visual field deficits and, if large, symptoms of hydrocephalus. Other supratentorial midline tumors such as craniopharyngiomas may cause short stature, delayed onset of puberty or hormonal insufficiencies, and visual field deficits.

Infratentorial tumors in older children characteristically present with symptoms and signs of hydrocephalus, which include progressively worsening morning headache and vomiting, gait unsteadiness, double vision, and papilledema. Cerebellar astrocytomas enlarge slowly, and symptoms may worsen over several months. Morning vomiting may be the only symptom of posterior fossa ependymomas, which originate in the floor of the fourth ventricle near the vomiting center. Brain stem tumors may present with facial and extraocular muscle palsies, ataxia, and hemiparesis; hydrocephalus occurs in approximately 25% of these patients at diagnosis.

B. Staging: In addition to the tumor biopsy, neuraxis imaging studies are obtained to determine if neuraxis dissemination is present. It is unusual for brain tumors in children and adolescents to disseminate outside of the central nervous system. However, it is generally recommended that bone marrow aspirates and biopsies be analyzed in a patient with newly diagnosed medulloblastoma or primitive neuroectodermal tumor, particularly if neuraxis spread is present.

MRI has become the preferred diagnostic study for pediatric brain tumors. MRI provides better definition of the tumor and delineates indolent gliomas that may not be seen on CT scan. On the other hand, a CT scan can be done in 15 minutes as opposed to 45 minutes for MRI and is still useful if an urgent diagnostic study is necessary or if there is a desire to demonstrate calcium. Both scans are generally done with and without contrast enhancement. Contrast enhances regions where the blood-brain barrier is disrupted. Postoperative scans obtained to document the extent of tumor resection should be obtained within 48 hours after surgery to avoid postsurgical enhancement. This usually develops 4–14 days postoperatively and can be confused with residual tumor.

Imaging of the entire neuraxis and cerebrospinal fluid cytologic examination should be part of the diagnostic evaluation for patients with tumors such as medulloblastoma, ependymoma, and pineal region tumors. Diagnosis of neuraxis "drop metastases" can be accomplished by conventional myelography or, more recently and less invasively, by gadolinium-enhanced MRI incorporating sagittal and axial views. Levels of biomarkers in the cerebrospinal fluid such as human chorionic gonadotropin (hCG) and alpha-fetoprotein (AFP) may be helpful for serial follow-up of patients with central nervous system germ cell tumors.

C. Classification: About half of the common pediatric brain tumors occur above the tentorium and half in the posterior fossa. Most childhood brain tumors can be divided by the cell of origin into glial tumors (astrocytomas and ependymomas) or nonglial tumors such as medulloblastoma and other primitive neuroectodermal tumors. Some tumors contain both glial and neural elements (eg, ganglioglioma). There are also a group of less common central nervous system tumors that do not fit into this classification (craniopharyngiomas, germ cell tumors, choroid plexus tumors, and meningiomas). Low-grade and high-grade tumors are found in most categories. Table 39–3 sets forth the location and frequency of the common pediatric brain tumors.

Astrocytoma is the most common brain tumor of childhood. The majority of astrocytomas in children are low-grade tumors found in the posterior fossa. These low-grade tumors have a bland cellular morphology, few or no mitotic figures, and tend to grow

Table 39–3. Location and frequency of common pediatric brain tumors.

Location	Frequency of Occurrence
Hemispheric	**37%**
Low-grade astrocytoma	23%
High-grade astrocytoma	11%
Other	3%
Posterior fossa	**49%**
Medulloblastoma	15%
Cerebellar astrocytoma	15%
Brain stem glioma	15%
Ependymoma	4%
Midline	**14%**
Craniopharyngioma	8%
Chiasmal glioma	4%
Pineal region tumor	2%

very slowly. Low-grade astrocytomas are in many cases curable by complete surgical excision alone.

Medulloblastoma and related primitive neuroectodermal tumors are the most common high-grade brain tumors in children. These tumors usually occur in the first decade of life, with a peak incidence between 5 and 10 years of age and a 2.1:1.3 female-to-male ratio. These tumors typically arise in the midline cerebellar vermis, with variable extension into the fourth ventricle. Reports of neuraxis dissemination at diagnosis range from 10% to 46% of patients. The presence of hyperdiploidy in medulloblastoma cells appears to be a favorable prognostic indicator, while the presence of an isochromosome for the long arm of chromosome 17 appears to be unfavorable. Other more traditional prognostic factors are outlined in Table 39–4.

Brain stem tumors are third in frequency of occurrence in children. This tumor is frequently of astrocytic origin and is high-grade. The tumors that diffusely infiltrate the brain stem and primarily involve the pons have a long-term survival rate of less than 15%. Brain stem tumors that occur above or below the pons and grow in an eccentric or cystic manner have a somewhat better outcome. Exophytic tumors in this location may be amenable to biopsy. Generally, brain stem tumors are treated without a tissue diagnosis.

Table 39–4. Prognostic factors in children with medulloblastoma.

Factor	Favorable	Unfavorable
Extent of disease	Nondisseminated	Disseminated
Size of primary tumor after surgery	≤ 3 cm (completely resected)	> 3 cm
Histologic features	Undifferentiated	Foci of glial, ependymal, or neuronal differentiation
Age	≥ 4 years	< 4 years

Other brain tumors such as ependymomas, germ cell tumors, choroid plexus tumors, and craniopharyngiomas are less common and each is associated with unique diagnostic and therapeutic challenges.

Treatment

A. Supportive Care: Dexamethasone should be started if there is evidence of edema impairing neurologic function or if subsequent surgery is likely to cause this situation (0.5–1 mg/kg initially, then 0.25–0.5 mg/kg/d in four divided doses). Anticonvulsants (usually phenytoin, 4–8 mg/kg/d) should be started if the child has had a seizure or if the surgical approach is likely to induce seizures. As postoperative treatment of young children with high-grade brain tumors incorporates increasingly more intensive systemic chemotherapy, consideration should also be given to the use of prophylaxis for prevention of oral candidiasis and *Pneumocystis* infection, especially when dexamethasone is part of the overall therapeutic approach.

Optimum care for the pediatric brain tumor patient requires a multidisciplinary team including subspecialists in pediatric neurosurgery, neuro-oncology, neurology, endocrinology, neuropsychology, radiation therapy, and rehabilitation medicine as well as highly specialized nurses, social workers, and staff in physical therapy, occupational therapy, and speech and language science.

B. Specific Therapy: The goal of treatment is to eradicate the tumor with the least short- and long-term morbidity. Long-term neuropsychologic morbidity becomes an especially important issue related to deficits caused by the tumor itself and the sequelae of treatment—in particular, conventional irradiation to the developing brain. Meticulous surgical removal of as much tumor as possible is generally the preferred initial approach. Technologic advances such as the magnification and illumination provided by the operating microscope, the gentleness of the ultrasonic tissue aspirator and CO_2 laser (the latter less commonly employed in pediatric brain tumor surgery), the accuracy of computerized stereotactic resection, and intraoperative monitoring techniques such as evoked potentials and electrocorticography have increased the feasibility and safety of surgical resection of many pediatric brain tumors.

If a tumor is not totally or subtotally resectable, open or stereotactic biopsy should be undertaken unless the tumor cannot be well localized by CT or MRI, or the treatment will not be influenced by biopsy results. Certain chiasmal and brain stem gliomas most commonly meet the criteria for not obtaining a biopsy.

Radiation therapy for pediatric brain tumors is in a state of evolution. Radiation therapy portals are made as small as possible (eg, to the tumor as localized on MRI plus a margin of 1–2 cm). Approaches to the delivery of radiation to minimize the adverse effects on normal brain are being explored and include hyperfractionation, stereotactic radiation such as the "gamma knife," implantation of interstitial seeds, and use of three-dimensional treatment planning.

The role of chemotherapy is increasing. Its effectiveness in treating malignant astrocytomas, medulloblastomas, and ependymomas has been confirmed. There is now general agreement that brain tumors in children under 5 years of age should be treated by extensive surgical resection and followed by intensive chemotherapy in order to delay irradiation for as many years as possible. In some cases, irradiation is being eliminated altogether. This approach to treatment of young children has clinical and scientific rationale, but it must be regarded as investigational and should be done in a study setting.

In the older child with malignant glioma, the present approach would be surgical resection of the tumor and combined modality treatment with irradiation and intensive chemotherapy. In selected patients with minimal residual glioblastoma, the use of high-dose chemotherapy and autologous bone marrow or peripheral stem cell reconstitution is being studied. Surgery is not indicated for diffuse brain stem gliomas. Traditional treatment of these tumors has been local irradiation. Hyperfractionation to increase the dose from the conventional 54 Gy to 72 to 78 Gy unfortunately shows no apparent benefit in a recent Children's Cancer Group study. New approaches are needed for this prognostically poor tumor.

The treatment of low-grade astrocytomas is also evolving. Increasing numbers of young children are treated with antitumor chemotherapeutic agents such as carboplatin and vincristine after incomplete resection of these tumors. The role of irradiation after subtotal resection even in the older child is being questioned. A combined CCG/POG study is currently evaluating the efficacy of irradiation and the natural history of this disease following subtotal resection only. Management of axial low-grade astrocytomas presents a particular challenge. In part related to the technologic advances, near-total resection of these lesions has cautiously been pioneered at New York University Medical Center. Preliminary results indicate an encouraging outcome.

Prognosis

Despite improvements in surgery and radiation therapy techniques, the outlook for cure or preservation of a normal life-style remains poor for children with high-grade brain tumors. The benefit of chemotherapy consisting of lomustine, vincristine, and prednisone in addition to irradiation for children with malignant gliomas was demonstrated conclusively in a CCG study. The 5-year event-free survival rate (EFS) was 46% when both modalities were employed versus 18% for children treated with irradiation alone. Additionally, extent of resection appeared to correlate positively with prognosis, with a 3-year EFS of 17% for biopsy-only patients, 29–32% for partially or subtotally resected patients, and 54% for those with greater than 90% resections.

Conventional craniospinal irradiation for children with low-stage medulloblastoma (< 1.5 cm^2 residual tumor and no evidence of spinal dissemination) results in 5-year survival rates of 80–90%. For children with high-stage medulloblastoma, 5-year progression-free survival rates have ranged from 25% to 40%. However, preliminary analysis of a limited institution study in which vincristine, lomustine, and cisplatin were incorporated in addition to conventional irradiation showed a 96% 2-year disease-free survival rate.

Numerous trials are currently under way to further improve the outlook for children with malignant brain tumors. These studies are investigating areas such as new chemotherapeutic agents with better penetration into the central nervous system, autologous bone marrow transplantation, or peripheral stem cell reconstitution to allow increased intensity of chemotherapy delivery and alternative methods of irradiation delivery.

Albright AL: Pediatric brain tumors. CA Cancer J Clin 1993;43:272.

Duffner PK et al: Postoperative chemotherapy and delayed radiation in children less than three years of age with malignant brain tumors. N Engl J Med 1993;328:1725.

Kuijten RR et al: Family history of cancer and seizures in young children with brain tumors: A report from the Childrens Cancer Group (United States and Canada). Cancer Causes Control 1993;4:455.

Occurring E et al: Brain tumors under the age of three: The price of survival. Acta Neurochir (Wien) 1990;106:93.

Schneider JH Jr, Raffel D, McComb JG: Benign cerebellar astrocytomas of childhood. Neurosurgery 1992;30:58.

Wisoff JH et al: Neurosurgical management and influence of extent of resection on survival in pediatric high-grade astrocytomas: A report on CCG-945. J Neurosurg 1993; 78:344A.

LYMPHOMAS

1. HODGKIN'S DISEASE

Essentials of Diagnosis

- Painless cervical (70–80%) or supraclavicular (25%) adenopathy; mediastinal mass (50%)
- Fatigue, anorexia, weight loss, fever, night sweats, pruritus, cough

General Considerations

Children with Hodgkin's disease have a better response to treatment than do adults, with a 75% overall survival at more than 20 years' follow-up. While "adult" therapies are applicable, the management of Hodgkin's disease in children under 16 years of age frequently differs. Because excellent disease control can result from several different therapeutic approaches, selection of staging procedures and treatment are often based on the potential long-term toxicity associated with the intervention.

Although Hodgkin's disease represents half of the lymphomas of childhood, only 15% of all cases occur in children 16 years of age or younger. Children less than 5 years of age account for 3% of childhood cases, while 60% occur in the age group from 10 to 16 years of age. There is a 4:1 male predominance in the first decade.

Hodgkin's disease is diagnosed by finding the Reed-Sternberg cell or variant in the appropriate histologic milieu. Hodgkin's disease is unique in that the bulk of the tumor is composed of normal cells while the malignant Reed-Sternberg cells are relatively scanty. The origin of the malignant cell remains elusive. The cause also remains unknown though a variety of environmental, infectious (particularly the Epstein-Barr virus) and genetic possibilities have been explored.

Hodgkin's disease is subdivided into four histologic groups, and the distribution parallels that of adults: lymphocyte-predominant (10–20%); nodular sclerosing (40–60%) (increases with age); mixed cellularity (20–40%); and lymphocyte-depleted (5–10%). Prognosis is independent of subclassification, with appropriate therapy based on stage.

Clinical Findings

A. Symptoms and Signs: Painless cervical adenopathy is the usual presentation of Hodgkin's disease. As Hodgkin's disease nearly always arises in lymph nodes and spreads to contiguous nodal groups, a detailed examination of all nodal sites is mandatory. The lymph nodes often feel firmer than inflammatory nodes and have a rubbery texture. They may be discrete or matted together and are not fixed to surrounding tissue. The growth rate is variable, and involved nodes may wax and wane in size over weeks to months.

As lymphadenopathy is common in general pediatric practice, the decision to biopsy is often difficult or delayed for a prolonged period. Indications for early lymph node biopsy include lack of identifiable infection in the region drained by the enlarged node, a node greater than 2 cm in size, supraclavicular adenopathy or abnormal chest x-ray, and lymphadenopathy increasing in size after 2 weeks or failing to resolve within 4–8 weeks.

Constitutional symptoms occur in about one-third of children at presentation. Symptoms of fever over 38 °C, weight loss of 10%, and drenching night sweats are defined by the Ann Arbor staging criteria (Table 39–5) as "B" symptoms. The "A" designation refers to the absence of these symptoms. "B" symptoms are of prognostic value, and more aggressive therapy is usually required for cure. Generalized pruritus and pain with alcohol ingestion may also occur.

Table 39–5. Ann Arbor staging classification
for Hodgkin's disease.

Stage I:	Involvement of a single lymph node or region of a single extralymphatic organ or site.
Stage II:	Involvement of two or more lymph node regions on the same side of the diaphragm or localized involvement of an extralymphatic organ or site.
Stage III:	Involvement of lymph node regions on both sides of the diaphragm or localized involvement of an extralymphatic organ or spleen.
Stage IV:	Diffuse or disseminated involvement of one or more extralymphatic organs with or without associated lymph node involvement.

A = asymptomatic
B = fever, sweats, weight loss > 10% of body weight

Half of patients have asymptomatic mediastinal disease (adenopathy or anterior mediastinal mass), though symptoms due to compression of vital structures in the thorax may occur. It is imperative to obtain a chest radiograph as soon as Hodgkin's disease is considered. Airway competency must be thoroughly evaluated before any surgical procedure is undertaken to avoid airway obstruction during anesthesia and possible death.

Splenomegaly and hepatomegaly (either or both) are generally associated with advanced disease; involvement of these organs can only be definitively established surgically.

B. Laboratory Findings: The blood count is usually normal, though anemia, neutrophilia, eosinophilia, and thrombocytosis may be present. The erythrocyte sedimentation rate and other acute-phase reactants are often elevated and can serve as markers of disease activity. Immunologic abnormalities occur, particularly in cell-mediated immunity, and anergy is common in advanced-stage disease at diagnosis. Autoantibody phenomenon such as hemolytic anemia and an idiopathic thrombocytopenic purpura-like picture have been reported.

C. Staging: Staging involves a systematic search for detectable disease using a variety of techniques. Classification is based on the Ann Arbor staging system (Table 39–5). Ultimately, staging determines the nature and duration of treatment.

Imaging studies for thoracic disease include chest radiography and computed tomography. CT adds significantly to the appreciation of mediastinal disease. Assessment of abdominal and pelvic disease is usually accomplished by CT, though lymphangiography may be more accurate. The lack of retroperitoneal fat in young children compromises the adequacy of CT imaging. Lymphangiography in children is variably successful depending on the skill and tenacity of the examiner.

Bilateral bone marrow aspirates and biopsies are performed. Technetium bone scanning may show bony involvement and is usually reserved for patients with bone pain or an elevated alkaline phosphatase,

since bone involvement is rare. Gallium scanning defines gallium-avid tumors and is most useful in detecting residual mediastinal disease at the completion of treatment.

Clinical staging may be followed by pathologic staging involving laparotomy with multiple lymph node samplings, liver biopsy, and splenectomy. Although controversial, the staging laparotomy is less important now than it once was. It is performed only if radiotherapy is the preferred treatment and the detection of abdominal disease would alter therapy. Excellent disease control with radiotherapy can be achieved in laparotomy-staged children, but this option must be weighed against the toxicities of high-dose, extended field radiation in prepubertal children and the complications of laparotomy, including postsplenectomy sepsis. Reports linking splenectomy with secondary acute myelogenous leukemia following Hodgkin's disease therapy are particularly disturbing.

Treatment & Prognosis

Optimal therapy involves a multidisciplinary approach with decisions made in collaboration by the pediatric oncologist, radiation oncologist, diagnostic radiologist, pediatric surgeon, and pathologist.

Both radiation therapy and combination chemotherapy are effective in treating Hodgkin's disease. The principles of therapy are to achieve long-term disease-free survival while minimizing the toxicities of therapy. Consequently, treatment of childhood Hodgkin's disease is evolving toward increased use of chemotherapy, even in stage I and stage II disease, with a corresponding reduction in radiotherapy.

Several combinations of chemotherapeutic agents are effective, but the most commonly used are MOPP (mechlorethamine, Oncovin [vincristine], procarbazine, and prednisone) and ABVD (Adriamycin [doxorubicin], bleomycin, vinblastine, and dacarbazine). These regimens are felt to be non-cross-resistant. When administered in an alternating schedule, exposure to an individual drug is decreased, and the toxicities associated with cumulative doses are in this way minimized.

Radiation continues to play a role in the treatment of childhood Hodgkin's disease, particularly in the control of bulky disease and residual disease following chemotherapy. The benefit of combined-modality therapy is that the cure rate appears to be increased. The most efficacious chemotherapy regimen and radiation schema with the least long-term toxicities awaits further clinical trials.

With current therapeutic approaches, it is expected that children with stage I and stage II Hodgkin's disease will have at least a 90% disease-free survival 5 years from diagnosis. Since two-thirds of all relapses occur within 2 years after diagnosis and since relapse rarely occurs beyond 4 years, 5-year disease-free survival generally equates with cure. In more advanced disease (stage III and stage IV), 5-year event-free survival ranges from over 60% to 90% depending on the treatment given.

Treatment of relapsed Hodgkin's disease involves radiotherapy in combination with chemotherapy. An alternative is autologous or allogeneic bone marrow transplantation. Although salvage therapy for Hodgkin's disease is relatively successful, this should not be a consideration in planning primary treatment.

Late Effects of Hodgkin's Disease

The most devastating consequence of Hodgkin's disease therapy is a second malignant neoplasm. Acute nonlymphocytic leukemia, lymphomas, and solid tumors are all reported to occur with increased frequency. The risk depends on treatment and certain patient-related factors.

AML may occur in up to 4% of Hodgkin's disease patients. Alkylating agents in particular are leukemogenic; prolonged chemotherapy, splenectomy, and extensive radiotherapy add substantially to the risk. The risk of developing leukemia seems to plateau at 10 years; unfortunately, no plateau has been seen in solid tumors. Basal cell carcinoma, thyroid cancer, breast cancer, melanoma, and sarcomas have all been observed.

Soft-tissue and bone growth impairment are complications of radiation. Clinical and biochemical hypothyroidism is noted in more than two-thirds of children 6 years following mantle irradiation. Both chemotherapy and irradiation can induce infertility. Cardiopulmonary complications can be seen following either radiation or chemotherapy; combined-modality therapy may increase damage to the heart and lungs.

Clearly, children treated for Hodgkin's disease require long-term follow-up by an experienced physician to monitor for and correct any potential sequelae of therapy.

De Vita VT et al: Hodgkin's disease. N Engl J Med 1993; 328:560.

Donaldson SS et al: Hodgkin's disease: Treatment of the young child. Pediatr Clin North Am 1991;38:457.

Kaldor jm et al: Leukemia following Hodgkin's disease. N Engl J Med 1990;322:7.

Leventhal BG et al: Hodgkin's disease. In: *Principles and Practice of Pediatric Oncology.* Pizzo PA, Poplack DG (editors). Lippincott, 1993.

Often J et al: Hodgkin's disease. N Engl J Med 1992;326: 678.

Tura S et al: Splenectomy and the increasing risk of secondary acute leukemia in Hodgkin's disease. J Clin Oncol 1993;11:925.

2. NON-HODGKIN'S LYMPHOMA

Essentials of Diagnosis

- Cough, dyspnea, swelling of the face; abdominal pain, abdominal distention, vomiting, constipation.

- Lymphadenopathy, mediastinal mass, pleural effusion, abdominal mass, ascites, hepatosplenomegaly.

General Considerations

Non-Hodgkin's lymphomas are a diverse group of malignancies of lymphatic tissue. In North America, non-Hodgkin's lymphoma constitutes 7–13% of malignancies in children less than 15 years of age. In equatorial Africa, non-Hodgkin's lymphoma represents almost 50% of pediatric malignancies. Approximately 390 new cases of non-Hodgkin's lymphoma are seen annually in the United States. The incidence of non-Hodgkin's lymphoma increases with age. Children 15 years of age or younger account for only 3% of all cases of non-Hodgkin's lymphoma; it is uncommon before 5 years of age. There is a marked male predominance, with the male:female ratio approximately 3:1.

Children with congenital or acquired immune deficiencies (eg, Wiscott-Aldrich syndrome, severe combined immunodeficiency syndrome, X-linked lymphoproliferative syndrome, HIV infection, immunosuppressive therapy following solid organ or marrow transplantation) have an increased risk of developing non-Hodgkin's lymphoma. It has been estimated that the risk is 100–10,000 times that of age-matched controls.

Most children who develop non-Hodgkin's lymphoma have no detectable immune defect. The pathogenesis of non-Hodgkin's lymphoma is under intense investigation. Animal models support a role for a viral origin. In equatorial Africa, 95% of Burkitt's lymphomas contain Epstein-Barr viral (EBV) DNA, further supporting a viral role in tumor development. However, in North America, less than 20% of Burkitt's tumors contain the EBV genome. Disturbances in host immunologic defenses, perhaps as a consequence of viral infection, chronic immunostimulation, and specific chromosomal rearrangements, are all under investigation as potential triggers in the development of non-Hodgkin's lymphoma.

In pediatrics, three major histologic classifications are sufficient for categorization: lymphoblastic lymphoma, small non-cleaved cell lymphoma (endemic or sporadic Burkitt's lymphoma), and large cell lymphoma (Table 39–6). Malignant lymphoma cells retain features similar to those of the lymphoid lineage cell from which they are derived. Cell membrane markers can therefore help clarify the origins of these cancers and serve as an adjunct to histologic classification. Typically, lymphoblastic lymphoma is associated with T cell surface markers, while small non-cleaved cell lymphomas have B cell phenotype such as surface immunoglobulins. The large cell lymphomas, which comprise less than 15% of pediatric non-Hodgkin's lymphomas, may show T cell, B cell, or histiocytic lineage.

Unlike adult non-Hodgkin's lymphoma, virtually

Table 39–6. Comparison of pediatric non-Hodgkin's lymphomas.

	Lymphoblastic Lymphoma	Small Non-Cleaved Cell Lymphoma	Large Cell Lymphoma
Incidence	30–40%	40–50%	≤ 15%
Histopathologic features	Indistinguishable from ALL lymphoblasts.	Large nucleus with prominent nucleoli surrounded by very basophilic cytoplasm that contains lipid vacuoles.	Large cells with cleaved or noncleaved nuclei.
Immunophenotype	Immature T cell	B cell	B cell, T cell, or histiocyte
Cytogenetic markers	Translocations involving chromosome 14q11 and chromosome 7; interstitial deletions of chromosome 1.	t(8;14), t(8;22), t(2;8)	t(2;5)
Clinical presentation	Intrathoracic tumor, mediastinal mass (50–70%), lymphadenopathy above diaphragm (50–80%).	Intra-abdominal tumor (90%), jaw involvement (10–20% sporadic Burkitt's, 70% epidemic Burkitt's). Bone marrow involvement.	Abdominal tumor most common; unusual sites: lung, face, brain, skin, testes, muscle.
Treatment	Similar to therapy for ALL 15–18 months' duration.	Intensive administration of alkylating agents and intermediate- to high-dose methotrexate; intensive CNS prophylaxis; 6–9 months' duration.	Similar to therapy for small non-cleaved cell lymphomas.

all childhood non-Hodgkin's lymphomas are rapidly proliferating, diffuse malignancies arising from extranodal tissue. These tumors exhibit aggressive behavior but are quite responsive to treatment.

Clinical Findings

A. Symptoms and Signs: Childhood non-Hodgkin's lymphomas can arise in any site of lymphoid tissue. including lymph nodes, Waldeyer's ring, Peyer's patches, thymus, liver, and spleen. Common sites of extralymphatic involvement include bone, bone marrow, the central nervous system, skin, and testis. Signs and symptoms at presentation usually relate to the tissue predominantly involved and the degree of dissemination. Because non-Hodgkin's lymphoma usually progresses very rapidly, the duration of symptoms is quite brief—from days to a few weeks. Despite the innumerable sites that can give rise to non-Hodgkin's lymphoma, children present with a limited number of syndromes, most of which correlate well with cell type.

Lymphoblastic lymphoma typically presents with symptoms of airway compression (cough, dyspnea, orthopnea) or superior venal caval obstruction (facial edema, chemosis, plethora, venous engorgement) which are a result of mediastinal disease. These symptoms are a true emergency necessitating rapid diagnosis and treatment. Pleural effusions may further compromise the patient's respiratory status. Central nervous system and bone marrow involvement are not common at diagnosis. When bone marrow contains more than 25% lymphoblasts, patients are considered to have acute lymphoblastic leukemia.

Ninety percent of small non-cleaved cell lymphomas present with abdominal disease. Abdominal pain, distention, a right lower quadrant mass, or intussusception in a child older than 5 years of age all

suggest the diagnosis of small non-cleaved cell lymphoma (Burkitt's lymphoma). Bone marrow involvement is frequent (up to 65% of patients). Burkitt's lymphoma is the most rapidly proliferating tumor known and has a high rate of spontaneous cell death as it outgrows its blood supply. Consequently, children with massive abdominal disease frequently have metabolic abnormalities, including hyperuricemia, hyperphosphatemia, and hyperkalemia. Impaired renal function because of tumor infiltration, urinary obstruction by tumor, or urate nephropathy further worsen the biochemical derangements of this life-threatening syndrome of acute tumor lysis. Although similar histologically, there are numerous differences between cases of Burkitt's lymphoma occurring in endemic areas of equatorial Africa and the sporadic cases of North America (Table 39–7).

Large cell lymphomas are similar clinically to the small non-cleaved cell lymphomas, though unusual sites of involvement are more common.

B. Diagnostic Evaluation: A biopsy at a facility capable of performing histopathologic examina-

Table 39–7. Comparison of endemic and sporadic Burkitt's lymphoma.

	Endemic	Sporadic
Incidence	10 per 100,000	0.9 per 100,000
Cytogenetics	Chromosome 8 breakpoint upstream of c-*myc* locus	Chromosome 8 breakpoint within c-*myc* locus
EBV association	≥ 95%	≤ 20%
Disease sites at presentation	Jaw (58%), abdomen (58%), CNS (19%), orbit (11%), marrow (7%)	Jaw (7%), abdomen (91%), CNS (14%), orbit (1%), marrow (20%)

tions, immunophenotyping, and cytogenetic studies is essential to establish the diagnosis. In the setting of mediastinal disease, it is imperative to avoid general anesthesia if the airway is compromised by tumor. Samples of pleural or ascitic fluid, bone marrow, or peripheral nodes obtained under local anesthesia may provide the diagnosis. Following the diagnosis of non-Hodgkin's lymphoma, studies should be obtained to determine the extent of disease. The rapid growth of these tumors and the life-threatening complications demand that studies be done expeditiously. Initiation of specific therapy should not be delayed by untimely investigations.

After a thorough physical examination, a CBC and liver and renal function tests plus a biochemical profile (electrolytes, calcium, phosphorus, uric acid) should be obtained. The lactic dehydrogenase (LDH) concentration reflects tumor burden and can serve as a marker of disease activity as well as prognosis. Imaging studies should include a chest radiograph and chest CT scan if the plain films are abnormal, an abdominal ultrasound or CT scan, and a radionuclide bone scan. Bone marrow and cerebrospinal fluid examinations are also essential parts of staging. Lymphangiography and staging laparotomy are not indicated.

Treatment

A. Supportive Care: The management of life-threatening problems at presentation is critical. The most common complications are the superior mediastinal syndrome and the acute tumor lysis syndrome. Patients with airway compromise require prompt initiation of specific therapy. Because of the risk of general anesthesia in these patients—and if a specific diagnosis cannot be made from peripheral studies—it is occasionally necessary to initiate steroids or, rarely, low-dose radiation until the mass is small enough for a biopsy to be undertaken safely. Response to steroids is usually prompt (12–24 hours).

The tumor lysis syndrome should be anticipated in all non-Hodgkin's lymphoma patients with extensive disease. Maintaining a brisk urine output (> 3 mL/kg/h) with intravenous fluids and diuretics is the key to management. Allopurinol will reduce serum uric acid, and alkalinization of urine will increase its solubility. Because phosphate precipitates in an alkaline urine, alkali administration should be discontinued if hyperphosphatemia occurs. Renal dialysis may be necessary to control metabolic abnormalities. Every attempt should be made to correct or minimize metabolic abnormalities before initiating chemotherapy. However, this period of stabilization should not exceed 24–48 hours.

B. Specific Therapy: Chemotherapy is the bulwark of therapy for non-Hodgkin's lymphoma. Surgery has little to offer beyond biopsy unless the entire tumor can be resected. There is no role for partial resection or debulking surgery. Radiotherapy likewise has little to offer. There is good evidence that radiation adds no therapeutic benefits but does increase both short- and long-term toxicities. Its use is confined to exceptional circumstances.

Therapy for lymphoblastic lymphoma is generally based on treatment protocols designed for ALL. Anthracyclines are usually an integral agent in effective treatment regimens for lymphoblastic lymphoma; cytarabine and podophyllotoxin derivatives (etoposide, teniposide) are emerging as promising agents. Duration of therapy is determined by disease extent. Localized disease is treated for 6 months, while extensive disease is treated for 15 months.

Small non-cleaved cell lymphomas do not respond well to therapy based on ALL protocols even when bone marrow is involved. Protocols using alkylating agents and intermediate- to high-dose methotrexate administered on an intensive schedule produce the highest cure rates. Large cell lymphomas are treated similarly.

All non-Hodgkin's lymphoma patients require central nervous system prophylaxis. Intensive administration of intrathecal chemotherapy is effective for this purpose.

Prognosis

A major predictor of outcome in non-Hodgkin's lymphoma is the extent of disease at diagnosis. For patients with localized disease, 90% of patients can expect long-term disease-free survival, while patients with extensive disease on both sides of the diaphragm, central nervous system involvement, or bone marrow involvement in addition to a primary site have a 70–80% failure-free survival. Relapses occur early in non-Hodgkin's lymphoma; patients with lymphoblastic lymphoma rarely have recurrences after 30 months from diagnosis, while patients with small non-cleaved cell lymphomas essentially never have recurrences beyond 1 year.

For patients who experience relapse, autologous or allogeneic bone marrow transplant may offer the possibility of cure.

Blay J Y et al: Management of pediatric non-Hodgkin's lymphoma. Blood Rev 1991;5:90.

Kurtzberg J et al: Non-Hodgkin's lymphoma: Biological classification and implication for therapy. Pediatr Clin North Am 1991;38:443.

Magrath I: Malignant non-Hodgkin's lymphomas in children. In: *Principles and Practice of Pediatric Oncology.* Pizzo PA, Poplack DG (editors). Lippincott, 1993.

Patte C et al: Results of the LMT81 protocol, a modified LSA$_2$L$_2$ protocol with high dose methotrexate, on 84 children with non-B-cell (lymphoblastic) lymphoma. Med Pediatr Oncol 1992;20:105.

Toogood IRG et al: Effective multi-agent chemotherapy for advanced abdominal lymphoma and FAB L3 leukemia of childhood. Pediatr Oncol 1993;21:103.

NEUROBLASTOMA

Essentials of Diagnosis

- Bone pain, abdominal pain, anorexia, weight loss, fatigue, fever, irritability.
- Abdominal mass (65%), adenopathy, proptosis, periorbital ecchymosis, skull masses, subcutaneous nodules, hepatomegaly, spinal cord compression.

General Considerations

Neuroblastoma is a tumor arising from neural crest tissue of the sympathetic ganglia or adrenal medulla. It is composed of small, fairly uniform cells with little cytoplasm and hyperchromatic nuclei that may form rosette patterns. Pathologic diagnosis is not always easy, and neuroblastoma must be differentiated from the other "small, round, blue cell" malignancies of childhood (Ewing's sarcoma, rhabdomyosarcoma, peripheral neuroepithelioma, lymphoma).

Predominantly a tumor of early childhood, 50% of neuroblastomas are diagnosed in the first 2 years of life and 90% before age 5. Neuroblastoma represents 7–10% of pediatric malignancies and is the most common solid neoplasm outside the central nervous system.

The biologic diversity of neuroblastoma makes this a fascinating tumor for study. Spontaneous regression in stage IV-S disease and spontaneous or induced differentiation to a benign neoplasm are examples of the unique behavior of this tumor. Unfortunately, neuroblastoma is also an extremely malignant neoplasm, and the overall survival in advanced disease has changed little in 20 years despite significant advances in our understanding of this tumor at a cellular and molecular level.

Clinical Findings

A. Symptoms and Signs: Clinical manifestations vary with the primary site of metastatic disease and the neuroendocrine function of the tumor. Many children present with constitutional symptoms such as fever, weight loss, and irritability. Bone pain suggests metastatic disease, which is present in 70% of children older than 1 year at diagnosis. Physical examination may reveal a firm, fixed, irregularly shaped mass that extends beyond the midline. The margins are often poorly defined. While the majority of children have an abdominal primary (40% adrenal gland, 25% paraspinal ganglion), neuroblastoma can arise wherever there is sympathetic tissue. In the posterior mediastinum, it is usually asymptomatic and discovered on a chest x-ray obtained for other reasons. Cervical neuroblastoma presents with a neck mass, often misdiagnosed as infection. Horner's syndrome or heterochromia iridis may accompany cervical neuroblastoma. Paraspinal tumors can extend through the spinal foramina, causing cord compression. Patients may present with paresis, paralysis, and bowel or bladder dysfunction.

The most common sites of metastases are bone, bone marrow, lymph nodes (regional as well as disseminated), liver, and subcutaneous tissue. Neuroblastoma has a predilection for metastasis to the skull, in particular the sphenoid bone and retrobulbar tissue. This causes orbital ecchymosis and proptosis. Liver metastasis, particularly in the newborn, can be massive. Subcutaneous nodules are bluish in color and associated with an erythematous flush followed by blanching when compressed, probably secondary to catecholamine release.

Neuroblastoma may also have unusual paraneoplastic manifestations. Examples include chronic watery diarrhea associated with tumor secretion of vasoactive intestinal peptides and opsoclonus-myoclonus (dancing eyes and dancing feet). It is postulated that the neurologic manifestations are secondary to cross-reacting antibodies.

B. Laboratory Findings: Anemia is present in 60% of children with neuroblastoma and can be due to "chronic disease" or marrow infiltration. Thrombocytopenia may be present, but thrombocytosis is more common, even with metastatic disease in the marrow.

Quantifying tumor markers has both prognostic significance and provides parameters for follow-up. LDH and ferritin can be elevated at diagnosis. Neuron-specific enolase, a cytoplasmic protein associated with neural cells, and serum ganglioside (GD2) are other serum markers for neuroblastoma. Urinary catecholamines (vanilmandelic acid, homovanillic acid) are elevated in at least 90% of patients at diagnosis and should be measured prior to surgery. Screening of infants is accomplished using this technique, though the cost-effectiveness remains to be established.

C. Imaging: Plain films or CT of the primary tumor may show stippled calcifications. CT scanning can evaluate the extent of the primary tumor, its effects on surrounding structures, and the presence of liver and lymph node metastases. Classically, in primaries originating from the adrenal, the kidney is displaced inferolaterally, which helps to differentiate neuroblastoma from Wilms' tumor. MRI is useful to evaluate for the presence of spinal cord involvement in tumors that appear to invade neural foramina.

Both skeletal survey (skull and long bones) and radionuclide bone scanning are obtained in the evaluation of bone metastases. On plain films, lesions are usually symmetric and appear irregular and lytic. Periosteal reaction and pathologic fractures may also be seen.

D. Staging: First a tissue diagnosis must be established and then the disease extent determined. In addition to the previously mentioned studies, bilateral bone marrow aspirates and biopsies are essential in evaluating for metastatic disease, even if the CBC is normal. The appearance of neuroblastoma in the bone marrow may simulate the appearance of acute lymphoblastic leukemia; however, monoclonal antibodies to cell surface antigens are able to resolve ambiguities.

Biologic parameters are essential in evaluating patients with neuroblastoma. They supplement clinical staging and aid in treatment planning. Amplification of the N-*myc* proto-oncogene or its gene product can be detected in tumor tissue. Rapid disease progression is associated with N-*myc* amplification and necessitates aggressive therapy. Tumor DNA content is determined by flow cytometry. Hyperdiploidy is a favorable finding, while near-diploid DNA content is associated with advanced disease and a poor outcome. Double-minute chromosomes and homogenous staining regions of DNA, manifestations of gene amplification, along with deletion of the short arm of chromosome 1, are cytogenetic characteristics of neuroblastoma.

Following completion of these studies and possible surgical resection of the primary tumor, patients are assigned a stage that further defines therapy. Various staging systems have been used in neuroblastoma. Although similar, these systems have made comparison of studies difficult. An International Neuroblastoma Staging System (INSS) has been formulated that allows for uniformity in staging patients with neuroblastoma for clinical trials and biologic studies (Table 39–8).

Treatment & Prognosis

As prognosis is independently influenced by age at diagnosis and stage of disease, both factors are taken into consideration when deciding a treatment plan. Infants less than 1 year of age with stage 4S disease may need little if any therapy to effect a cure, though treatment may be initiated because of bulky disease causing mechanical complications.

Therapy is usually multimodal and involves surgery, radiotherapy, and chemotherapy. Bone marrow transplant is being investigated as a therapeutic modality to improve the currently poor outcome for advanced neuroblastoma. Initial surgical efforts are aimed at resecting the primary tumor when feasible. The usually massive size of the tumor and the presence of widely metastatic disease often makes primary resection impossible. Under these circumstances, only a biopsy may be performed. Following chemotherapy, a second surgical procedure may allow for resection of the primary tumor. Radiation may be given intraoperatively at the time of resection or postoperatively by external beam radiotherapy.

Active chemotherapeutic agents in the treatment of neuroblastoma include cyclophosphamide, doxorubicin, etoposide, cisplatin, and vincristine. There is a clear dose-response relationship in neuroblastoma. About 80% of patients achieve complete or partial remission, though in advanced disease this is seldom durable. A current Children's Cancer Study Group (CCSG) treatment protocol compares aggressive conventional chemotherapy with chemotherapy plus autologous bone marrow transplantation. Although the early results from bone marrow transplant appear superior to conventional chemotherapy, late recurrences are occurring. Clinical trials using radioactive monoclonal antibodies against neuroblastoma cells such as ^{131}I-meta-iodobenzylguanidine (MIBG) and [131]I-3F8 (a murine IgG antibody specific for ganglioside GD2, the predominant antigen on neuroblastoma cells) are also under way. In another promising area of research, attempts are being made to manipulate the patient's immune system to eradicate residual disease. Agents such as interleukin-2 are being investigated as biologic response modifiers.

For children with stage 1, 2, or 4S disease, the 5-year survival is 70–90%. Infants under 1 year of age who have stage 4 disease have a greater than 60% likelihood of long-term survival. Children over 1 year of age with stage 3 disease have an intermediate prognosis (approximately 40–70%), and those with stage 4 disease have a poor prognosis (5–20% survival 5 years from diagnosis).

Table 39–8. The International Neuroblastoma Staging System.

Stage 1:	Localized tumor confined to the area of origin, complete gross excision, with or without microscopic residual disease; identifiable lymph nodes negative microscopically.
Stage 2:	Unilateral tumor with incomplete gross excision; identifiable lymph nodes negative microscopically.
Stage 3:	Unilateral tumor with complete or incomplete gross excision; with positive ipsilateral regional lymph nodes; identifiable contralateral lymph nodes negative microscopically.
Stage 4:	Dissemination of the tumor to distant lymph nodes, bone, bone marrow, liver, or other organs (except as defined in stage 4S).
Stage 4S:	Localized primary tumor as defined for stage 1 or 2 with dissemination limited to liver, skin, or bone marrow.

Brodeur GM et al: Molecular basis of clinical heterogeneity in neuroblastoma. Am J Pediatr Hematol Oncol 1992; 14:111.

Brodeur GM et al: Neuroblastoma. In: *Principles and Practice of Pediatric Oncology.* Pizzo PA, Poplack DG: (editors). JB Lippincott, 1993.

Brodeur GM et al: Neuroblastoma: Effect of genetic factors on prognosis and treatment. Cancer 1992;70:1685.

Cheung NK: Immunotherapy: Neuroblastoma as a model. Pediatr Clin North Am 1991;38:425.

Philip T: Overview of current treatment of neuroblastoma. Am J Pediatr Hematol Oncol 1992;14:97.

WILMS' TUMOR
(Nephroblastoma)

Essentials of Diagnosis

- Asymptomatic abdominal mass or swelling (83%).
- Fever (23%), hematuria (21%).
- Hypertension (25%), genitourinary malformations (6%), aniridia, hemihypertrophy.

General Considerations

Approximately 460 new cases of Wilms' tumor occur annually in the United States, representing 5–6% of cancers in children under 15 years of age. This is the second most common abdominal tumor in children following neuroblastoma. The tumor arises from kidney and is usually composed of three elements: blastema, epithelium, and stroma. The majority of Wilms' tumor are sporadically occurring malignancies. There are several important malformations, syndromes, and cytogenetic associations, including aniridia, hemihypertrophy, genitourinary malformations (eg, cryptorchidism, hypospadias, gonadal dysgenesis, pseudohermaphroditism, horseshoe kidney), Beckwith-Wiedemann syndrome, Drash syndrome, and WAGR (Wilms', aniridia, ambiguous genitalia, mental retardation) syndrome. Although most patients with Wilms' tumor are karyotypically normal, those with sporadic aniridia frequently have a constitutional deletion at the 11p13 locus. This deletion has also been found in the tumor cells of Wilms' patients without aniridia and who are karyotypically normal.

The median age at diagnosis is related both to gender and laterality, with bilateral tumors presenting at a younger age than unilateral tumors and males being diagnosed earlier than females. Wilms' tumor occurs most commonly between 2 and 5 years of age; it is unusual after 6 years of age. The mean age at diagnosis is 3 years.

Clinical Findings

A. Symptoms and Signs: The great majority of children with Wilms' tumor present with an increasing size of the abdomen or an abdominal mass incidentally discovered by a parent. The mass is usually smooth and firm, well-demarcated, and rarely crosses the midline, though it can extend inferiorly into the pelvis. Gross hematuria is an uncommon presentation, though microscopic hematuria is found in approximately 25% of cases.

B. Laboratory Findings: The CBC is usually normal, though some patients have anemia secondary to hemorrhage into the tumor; consequently, the LDH may be elevated. BUN and serum creatinine are usually normal. Urinalysis may show some blood or leukocytes.

C. Staging: Ultrasonography or CT of the abdomen should establish the presence of an intrarenal mass. It is also essential to evaluate the contralateral kidney for presence and function as well as synchro-

nous Wilms' tumor. The inferior vena cava needs to be evaluated for the presence and extent of tumor propagation. The liver should be imaged for the presence or absence of metastatic disease. A plain chest radiograph (four views) should be obtained to determine if pulmonary metastases are present. Approximately 10% of patients will have metastatic disease at diagnosis. Of these, 80% will have pulmonary disease, and 15% will have liver metastases. Bone and brain metastases are very unusual and associated with certain unfavorable histologic types; hence, bone and brain scans are not routinely performed.

The clinical stage is ultimately decided upon by the surgeon in the operating room and confirmed by the pathologist (Table 39–9).

Treatment & Prognosis

In the United States, treatment begins with surgical exploration of the abdomen. The contralateral kidney is inspected and palpated for tumor involvement (one-third of patients with bilateral disease have no evidence of this on preoperative studies). The liver and lymph nodes are inspected and suspicious areas biopsied or excised. An en bloc resection of tumor is performed. Every attempt is made to avoid tumor spillage at surgery. Because therapy is tailored to tumor stage, it is imperative that operation be done by a surgeon familiar with the staging requirements.

In addition to the staging, the histologic type has implications for therapy and prognosis. Favorable histology (FH; see below) refers to the class triphasic Wilms' tumor and its variants. Unfavorable histology (UH) refers to anaplasia, clear cell sarcoma of the kidney, and rhabdoid tumor of the kidney and is present in 10–12% of cases. Although clear cell sarcoma and rhabdoid tumor are no longer felt to be Wilms tumor variants, these histologic types were identified in early Wilms' tumor studies as being associated with a markedly worse outcome when compared with favorable histology tumors. Anaplasia is defined by extreme nuclear atypia. Only a few small foci of ana-

Table 39–9. Staging classification for Wilms' tumor.

Stage I:	Tumor limited to the kidney and completely excised.
Stage II:	Tumor extends beyond the kidney but is completely excised. There is no residual tumor beyond the margins of excision.
Stage III:	Residual nonhematogenous tumor confined to the abdomen. a. Lymph nodes are found to be involved. b. Diffuse peritoneal contamination by tumor. c. Peritoneal implants are found. d. Tumor beyond surgical margins (microscopic or gross). e. Unresectable tumor infiltrating into vital structures.
Stage IV:	Hematogenous metastases (eg, lung, liver).
Stage V:	Bilateral renal involvement at diagnosis

plasia in a Wilms' tumor is sufficient to impart a worse prognosis to stage II, III, or IV patients. Following excision and pathologic examination, the patient is assigned a stage that further defines therapy.

The progress and success in the treatment of Wilms' tumor is a result of the cooperative clinical trials of the National Wilms' Tumor Study (NWTS). Clinical trials that began in 1969 have resulted in an overall cure rate of approximately 90%. The current NWTS-IV seeks to further improve survival rate by intensifying therapy during the initial treatment phase while shortening treatment duration (6 versus 15 months of treatment). It is the first study of a pediatric population to evaluate the economic impact of two different treatment approaches, one of which requires fewer clinic visits.

Vincristine and dactinomycin are used in the treatment of all Wilms' tumor patients; doxorubicin is also administered to stage III and stage IV patients. NWTS-III showed that stage II Wilms' tumor patients did not benefit from flank irradiation while stage III children had similar outcomes whether they received 1000 or 2000 cGy. Chemotherapy is optimally begun within five days after surgery, while radiotherapy should be started within 10 days.

Using these approaches, survival at 4 years from diagnosis for patients treated on NWTS-III are as follows: stage I FH, 96.5%; stage II FH, 92.2%; stage III FH, 86.9%; and stage IV FH, 82.5%. Patients with unfavorable histology (UH) have only a 55–68% 4-year survival, depending on stage. Patients with recurrent Wilms' tumor have approximately a 50% salvage rate with surgery, radiotherapy, and chemotherapy (singly or in combination). Clearly, there is a need for more effective treatments in patients with UH and recurrent disease.

Late Effects of Wilms' Tumor

Because of the excellent prognosis for the majority of children with Wilms' tumor, consideration of late effects is essential in planning therapy and long-term follow-up for survivors. Musculoskeletal abnormalities (eg, scoliosis, atrophy) in patients who received radiation, cardiovascular abnormalities in doxorubicin-treated patients, and second malignant neoplasms are reported as the more common late effects of treatment. Liver toxicity occurs from radiotherapy, and renal impairment can be the result of inadequate remaining kidney tissue, hyperfiltration injury, or radiation damage.

Future Considerations

Although progress in the treatment of Wilms' tumor has been extraordinary, important questions remain to be answered. Results of previous NWTS and International Society of Pediatric Oncology (SIOP) trials suggest that not all stage I Wilms' tumor patients need chemotherapy and that some might be adequately treated with surgery alone. Many questions are being raised about the role of prenephrectomy chemotherapy in the treatment of Wilms' tumor. Presurgical chemotherapy seems to decrease tumor rupture at resection but may unfavorably affect outcome by changing staging. Whether pulmonary radiation can be eliminated in metastatic pulmonary disease is also being investigated.

Evans AE et al: Late effects of treatment for Wilms' tumor: A report from the National Wilms' Tumor Study group. Cancer 1991;67:331.

Green DM et al: Remaining problems in the treatment of patients with Wilms' tumor. Pediatr Clin North Am 1991;38:475.

Green DM et al: Wilms' tumor (nephroblastoma, renal embryoma). In: *Principles and Practice of Pediatric Oncology.* Pizzo PA, Poplack DG (editors). Lippincott, 1993.

National Wilms' Tumor Study Committee: Wilms' tumor: Status report, 1990. J Clin Oncol 1991;9:877.

Pinkerton CR et al: Response rates in relapsed Wilms' tumor: A need for new effective agents. Cancer 1991; 67:567.

BONE TUMORS

Primary malignant bone tumors are uncommon in childhood. Osteosarcoma accounts for 60% of cases and is seen primarily in adolescents and young adults. Ewing's sarcoma is the second most frequent malignant tumor of bony origin. Both tumors have a male predominance.

The cardinal signs of bone tumor are pain at the site of involvement, often following slight trauma; mass formation; and fracture through an area of cortical bone destruction.

1. OSTEOSARCOMA

While osteosarcoma is the sixth most common malignancy in childhood, it ranks third among adolescents and young adults. This peak occurrence during the adolescent growth spurt suggests a causal relationship between rapid bone growth and malignant transformation. Further evidence for this relationship is found in epidemiologic data showing patients with osteosarcoma to be taller than their peers, osteosarcoma occurring most frequently at sites where the greatest increase in length and size of bone occurs, and osteosarcoma occurring at an earlier age in girls than boys, corresponding to their earlier growth spurt. Long tubular bones are primarily affected. The distal femur accounts for more than 40% of cases, with the proximal tibia, proximal humerus, and mid and proximal femur following in frequency. Typically, osteosarcoma arises in an eccentric metaphysial location.

Radiographic findings show a permeative destruction of the normal bony trabecular pattern with indistinct margins. Additionally, periosteal new bone formation and lifting of the bony cortex may create a Codman triangle. A soft tissue mass plus calcifications in a radial or "sunburst" pattern are frequently noted. Despite this rather characteristic radiographic appearance, a tissue sample is needed to confirm the diagnosis. Further radiographic studies to better define the extent of the primary tumor include CT scan or MRI (or both). A bone scan is useful for detecting "skip" lesions as well as distant bony metastasis (present in 10% of newly diagnosed patients). A chest CT scan is essential to asses the lung for metastatic nodules. Pulmonary metastasis is present in as many as 20% of patients at diagnosis and imply a poor prognosis.

Placement of the incision for biopsy of a bone tumor is of critical importance. A misplaced incision could preclude a limb salvage procedure and necessitate amputation. Biopsy is best performed by the surgeon who would carry out the definitive surgical procedure. Histologically, osteosarcoma is characterized by the presence of malignant sarcomatous stroma associated with the production of tumor osteoid.

Once the diagnosis is established, treatment can begin. Surgery alone cures a maximum of 20% of patients with osteosarcoma. Over 70% of patients treated with surgery alone develop pulmonary metastases within 6 months after surgery. This suggests that micrometastatic disease is present at diagnosis though not detectable radiographically. Adjuvant chemotherapy trials have shown disease-free survival of 55–85% after 3–10 years of follow-up. Clearly, a substantial improvement in survival has been achieved with the use of chemotherapy.

Chemotherapy will often be administered prior to definitive surgery (neoadjuvant chemotherapy). This allows for an early attack on micrometastatic disease. Presurgical chemotherapy may also shrink the tumor, facilitating a limb salvage procedure. Preoperative chemotherapy allows for detailed histologic evaluation of tumor response to the preoperative chemotherapeutic agents. If there is a poor histologic response, postoperative chemotherapy can be changed on a more rational basis. Chemotherapy may be administered intra-arterially or intravenously. Agents having efficacy in the treatment of osteosarcoma include doxorubicin, cisplatin, high-dose methotrexate, and ifosfamide. A multi-agent regimen is most frequently employed.

Amputation and limb salvage are equally effective in achieving local control of osteosarcoma. Contraindications to limb-sparing surgery include major involvement of the neurovascular bundle by tumor; immature skeletal age, particularly for lower extremity tumors; infection in the region of the tumor; inappropriate biopsy site; and extensive muscle involvement that would result in a poor functional outcome.

Postsurgical chemotherapy is generally continued until the patient has received 1 year of treatment from the time of diagnosis. Relapses are rare beyond 3 years. Histologic response to neoadjuvant chemotherapy is an excellent predictor of outcome. Patients having 90% tumor necrosis have a 70-90% long-term disease free survival.

2. EWING'S SARCOMA

Ewing's sarcoma accounts for only 10% of primary malignant bone tumors; there are fewer than 200 new cases a year in the United States. It is a disease primarily of white males and almost never affects blacks.

The radiographic appearance of Ewing's sarcoma overlaps with osteosarcoma, though Ewing's sarcoma usually involves the diaphyses (versus the metaphyses in osteosarcoma) of long bones. The central axial skeleton gives rise to 40% of Ewing tumors.

Ewing's sarcoma is a "small, round, blue cell" malignancy. Although most commonly a tumor of bone, it may also occur in soft tissue (extraosseous Ewing's sarcoma). Histologically, it consists of sheets of undifferentiated cells with hyperchromatic nuclei, well-defined cell borders, and scanty cytoplasm. Necrosis is common. The differential diagnosis includes rhabdomyosarcoma, lymphoma, and neuroblastoma. In addition to light microscopy, electron microscopy, immunocytochemistry, and cytogenetics may be necessary to confirm the diagnosis. A generous tissue biopsy is often necessary for diagnosis. It is imperative, however, to avoid a surgical procedure that would result in a delay in initiation of chemotherapy or that would complicate local control.

A consistent cytogenetic abnormality (t11;22) has been identified in Ewing's sarcoma. This same abnormality is seen in peripheral neuroepitheliomas (primitive neuroectodermal tumor, Askin's tumor) and suggests that these tumors represent a spectrum of a single biologic entity. Both tumors also express the proto-oncogene c-*myc*. Research suggests that both of these tumors arise from postganglionic parasympathetic cholinergic neurons.

Evaluation of a patient diagnosed with Ewing's sarcoma should include CT or MRI (or both) of the primary lesion to define the extent of local disease as precisely as possible. This is imperative for planning future surgical procedures or radiation therapy. Metastatic disease is present in 25% of patients at diagnosis. The lung (38%), bone (particularly the spine) (31%), and the bone marrow (11%) are the most common sites for metastasis. CT of the chest, bone scanning, and bilateral bone marrow aspirates and biopsies are all essential to the staging work-up.

Therapy usually commences with the administration of chemotherapy (neoadjuvant) and is followed by local control measures. Depending on many factors, including the primary site of the tumor and response to chemotherapy, local control could be achieved by surgery, radiotherapy, or a combination of these methods. Following local control, chemotherapy continues for a total duration of 1 year. Agents that have been shown to have efficacy in the treatment of Ewing's sarcoma include dactinomycin, vincristine, doxorubicin, and cyclophosphamide. Etoposide and ifosfamide also appear promising. Modern therapy uses combinations of these drugs. With the availability of hematopoietic growth factors, more intensive dosing is being explored in an effort to improve the outcome of patients with this disease. Whenever possible, patients should be treated on a clinical research protocol.

Patients with small localized primaries can expect a 50–70% long-term disease-free survival. For patients with metastatic disease and large pelvic primaries, survival is poor. Autologous bone marrow transplant is being investigated for the management of these high risk patients.

Horowitz ME et al: Ewing's sarcoma family of tumors: Ewing's sarcoma of bone and soft tissue and the peripheral primitive neuroectodermal tumors. In: *Principles and Practice of Pediatric Oncology.* Pizzo PA, Poplack DG (editors). Lippincott, 1993.

Horowitz ME et al: Ewing's sarcoma: Radiotherapy versus surgery for local control. Pediatr Clin North Am 1991; 38:365.

Link MP et al: Osteosarcoma. In: *Principles and Practice of Pediatric Oncology.* Pizzo PA, Poplack DG (editors). Lippincott, 1993.

Marina NM: Improved prognosis of children with osteosarcoma metastatic to the lung(s) at the time of diagnosis. Cancer 1992;70:2722.

Meyer WH et al: Osteosarcoma: Clinical features and evolving surgical and chemotherapeutic strategies. Pediatr Clin North Am 1991;38:317.

RHABDOMYOSARCOMA

Essentials of Diagnosis

- Painless, progressively enlarging mass; proptosis; chronic drainage (nasal, aural, sinus, vaginal); cranial nerve palsies.
- Urinary obstruction, constipation, hematuria.

General Considerations

Rhabdomyosarcoma is the most common soft tissue sarcoma occurring in pediatrics and accounts for 10% of solid tumors in childhood. The peak incidence occurs between 2 and 5 years of age, with 70% of children diagnosed before 10 years of age. A second smaller peak is seen in adolescents with extremity tumors. Males are affected more commonly than females (1.4:1).

Arising from embryonic mesenchymal cells, rhabdomyosarcoma can occur anywhere in the body. Normally, mesenchymal cells give rise to various connective tissues. Rhabdomyosarcoma imitates striated muscle, and when cross-striations are seen by light microscopy the diagnosis is straightforward. Unfortunately, the diagnosis can be extremely difficult. Immunocytochemistry, electron microscopy, and chromosomal analysis can all be necessary before the diagnosis is established. Rhabdomyosarcoma is further classified into subtypes based on pathologic features: embryonal (63%), of which botryoid is a variant; alveolar (19%); pleomorphic, which is seen in adults (1%); undifferentiated sarcoma (10%); and other (7%). These subtypes occur in characteristic locations and have different metastatic potentials and outcomes (Table 39–10).

Although the pathogenesis of rhabdomyosarcoma is unknown, in rare cases a genetic predisposition has been determined. The Li-Fraumeni syndrome is an

Table 39–10. Characteristics of rhabdomyosarcoma.

Primary Site	Frequency	Symptoms and Signs	Three-Year Disease-Free Survival (Based on IRS-II)[1]	Predominant Pathologic Subtype
Head and neck	**40%**			Embryonal
Orbit	10%	Proptosis	93%	
Parameningeal	20%	Cranial nerve palsies; aural or sinus obstruction with or without drainage	71%	
Other	10%	Painless, progressively enlarging mass	69%	
Genitourinary	**20%**			Embryonal (botryoid variant in bladder and vagina)
Bladder and prostate	12%	Hematuria, urinary obstruction	64–80%	
Vagina and uterus	2%	Pelvic mass, vaginal discharge	60–80%	
Paratesticular	6%	Painless mass	64–80%	
Extremities	**20%**	Adolescents, swelling of affected body part	56%	Alveolar (50%), undifferentiated
Trunk	**10%**	Mass	57%	Alveolar, undifferentiated

[1]IRS = Intergroup Rhabdomyosarcoma Study.

inherited mutation of the p53 tumor-suppressor gene that results in a high risk of bone and soft tissue sarcomas in childhood plus breast cancer and other malignant neoplasms before age 45. Recent studies have extended the categories of patients that may harbor the p53 germline mutation and be predisposed to the development of cancer. A characteristic chromosomal translocation (t2;13) has been described in alveolar rhabdomyosarcoma, which may also shed light on the biology of this tumor.

Clinical Findings

A. Symptoms and Signs: The presenting signs and symptoms of rhabdomyosarcoma depend on the location of disease. Symptoms are usually from a mass lesion or result from disturbances of normal body function due to tumor growth. For example, orbital rhabdomyosarcoma presents as proptosis, while rhabdomyosarcoma of the bladder can present with hematuria, urinary frequency, or a pelvic mass. Typical symptoms for a given location are presented in Table 39–10.

B. Imaging: A plain film as well as a CT scan or MRI should be obtained to determine the exact extent of the primary tumor and to assess regional lymph nodes. A lung CT is obtained to rule out pulmonary metastasis, the most common site of metastatic disease at diagnosis. A skeletal survey and a bone scan are obtained to determine if bony metastasis is present. Bilateral bone marrow biopsies and aspirates are obtained to rule out bone marrow infiltration. Additional studies may be warranted in certain sites. For example, in parameningeal primaries, a lumbar puncture is performed to evaluate cerebrospinal fluid for tumor cells. Ultrasound examination is particularly useful in pelvic primaries.

C. Staging: Children diagnosed with rhabdomyosarcoma are staged according to both the Intergroup Rhabdomyosarcoma Study (IRS) clinical grouping classification (Table 39–11) and the TNM (tumor, nodes, metastases) system. The IRS system is

Table 39–11. Intergroup rhabdomyosarcoma study clinical grouping system.

Clinical Group	Definition
I	A. Localized, completely resected, confined to site of origin B. Localized, completely resected, infiltrated beyond site of origin
II	A. Localized, grossly resected, microscopic residual B. Regional disease, involved lymph nodes, completely resected.
III	A. Local or regional grossly visible disease after biopsy only B. Grossly visible disease after ≥ 50% resection of primary tumor
IV	Distant metastases present at diagnosis

a postsurgical system, whereas the TNM classification is a pretreatment schema that is not dependent on the local availability or skills of a surgeon. It is in wide use in Europe.

Treatment

Optimal management and treatment of children with rhabdomyosarcoma is complex. There can be no one single approach to a tumor that can occur at any site and at any age. Therefore, it is imperative for a multidisciplinary team to be involved in planning therapy from the outset. Whenever possible, it is in the patient's best interests to be enrolled in a cooperative study. The IRS group was initiated in 1972, and more than 2200 children have been enrolled and treated on protocol. Analysis of these studies shows a statistically significant increase in survival with each successive study. The current IRS-IV involves more than 60 institutions in the United States, Canada, and Europe.

The therapeutic approach to rhabdomyosarcoma involves combined-modality therapy. When feasible, primary surgical excision of the tumor should be accomplished. Unfortunately, because of site of origin and size of tumor, this is seldom possible. When only partial tumor resection is feasible, the operative procedure is usually limited to biopsy and sampling of lymph nodes. The role of debulking of unresectable tumor is unclear. Chemotherapy can often convert an inoperable tumor to a resectable one. A second-look procedure to remove residual disease and confirm the clinical response to chemotherapy and radiotherapy is generally performed around week 20 of therapy.

Radiation therapy is an effective method of local tumor control for both microscopic as well as gross residual disease. It is generally administered to all patients, the only exception being group I nonalveolar rhabdomyosarcoma. The dose administered is dependent on the extent of residual disease.

Chemotherapy is administered to all patients with rhabdomyosarcoma, even when their tumor is fully resected at diagnosis. The exact regimen and duration of chemotherapy is determined by primary site, group, and TNM classification. Vincristine, dactinomycin, and cyclophosphamide have shown the greatest efficacy in the treatment of rhabdomyosarcoma. Currently the IRS-IV is evaluating etoposide, ifosfamide, and melphalan in the treatment of rhabdomyosarcoma.

Prognosis

Several variables are related to outcome in rhabdomyosarcoma: the extent of disease at diagnosis, the primary site, pathologic subtype, and response to treatment all influence long-term disease-free survival from the time of diagnosis. Children with localized disease in a favorable site have a 93% 3-year disease-free survival rate, while children with metastatic disease at presentation (group IV) have a poor outcome (Table 39–10).

Newer treatment strategies include different drug combinations and dosing schedules, hematopoietic growth factor support, hyperfractionated radiotherapy, and autologous bone marrow transplantation for high risk patients.

Houghton PJ et al: Rhabdomyosarcoma: From the laboratory to the clinic. Pediatr Clin North Am 1991;38:349.

Levine AJ: The p53 tumor-suppressor gene. N Engl J Med 1992;326:1350.

Mandell LR: Ongoing progress in the treatment of childhood rhabdomyosarcoma. Oncology 1993;7:71.

Maurer HM: The intergroup rhabdomyosarcoma study-II. Cancer 1993;71:1904.

Raney RB et al: Rhabdomyosarcoma and the undifferentiated sarcomas. In: *Principles and Practice of Pediatric Oncology*. Pizzo PA, Poplack DG (editors). Lippincott, 1993.

RETINOBLASTOMA

Retinoblastoma is a neuroectodermal malignancy arising from embryonic retinal cells and accounts for 3% of malignant disease in children under 15 years of age. It is the most common intraocular tumor in pediatrics and causes 5% of cases of childhood blindness. There are 200–300 new cases per year in the United States. This is a malignancy of early childhood, with 90% of tumors diagnosed before 5 years of age. Bilateral disease typically presents at a younger age (median age 14 months) than unilateral disease (median age 23 months).

Retinoblastoma is the prototype of hereditary cancers. The pathogenesis of retinoblastoma is understood at a molecular level. Researchers have identified and cloned the retinoblastoma gene (RB1), which is located on the long arm of chromosome 13 (13q14). This gene is a tumor-suppressor gene or anti-oncogene. Normally, the function of this gene is to control cellular growth. When the gene is inactivated, cellular growth is uncontrolled. Uncontrolled cell growth leads to tumor formation. Inactivation of both RB1 alleles within the same cell are required for tumor formation.

Retinoblastoma is known to arise in heritable and nonheritable forms. Based on the different clinical characteristics of two forms, Knudson proposed a two-mutation hypothesis for retinoblastoma tumor development. He postulated that two independent events were necessary for a cell to acquire tumor potential. Mutations at the RB1 locus can be inherited or arise spontaneously. In heritable cases, the first mutation arises during gametogenesis, either spontaneously (90%) or transmitted from a parent (10%). This mutation is present in every retinal cell as well as all other somatic and germ cells. Ninety percent of persons who carry this germline mutation will develop retinoblastoma. For tumor formation, the loss of the second RB1 allele within a cell must occur; loss of only one allele is insufficient for tumor formation. The second mutation occurs in a somatic (retinal) cell. In nonheritable cases (60%), both mutations arise in a somatic cell after gametogenesis has taken place.

Clinical Findings

A. Symptoms and Signs: In the United States, children with retinoblastoma generally come to medical attention while the tumor is still confined to the globe. Although congenital, retinoblastoma in not usually detected until it has grown to a considerable size. Leukocoria (white pupillary reflex) is the most common manifestation (60% of cases). Parents may note an unusual appearance of the eye or an asymmetry of the eyes in a photograph. The differential diagnosis of leukocoria includes *Toxocara canis* granuloma, astrocytic hamartoma, retinopathy of prematurity, Coats's disease, and persistent hyperplastic primary vitreous. Strabismus (20% of cases) is seen when tumor involves the macula and central vision is lost. Rarely (7% of cases), a painful red eye with glaucoma, a hyphema, or proptosis is the initial manifestation. A single focus or multiple foci of tumor may be seen in one or both eyes at diagnosis. Bilateral involvement occurs in 20–30% of children.

B. Evaluation: A child suspected of retinoblastoma must have a detailed ophthalmologic examination under anesthesia. An ophthalmologist makes the diagnosis of retinoblastoma by the appearance of the tumor within the eye without pathologic confirmation. A white to creamy pink mass protruding into the vitreous suggests the diagnosis; intraocular calcifications and vitreous seeding are virtually pathognomonic for retinoblastoma. Supportive studies such as ultrasonography and CT are obtained. A CT of the orbits and head detects intraocular calcification, evaluates the optic nerve for tumor infiltration, and detects

Table 39–12. Reese-Ellsworth staging classification of retinoblastoma.

Group I: Very favorable
 (a) Solitary tumor, < 6 mm in size, at or behind the equator.
 (b) Multiple tumors, none > 6 mm in size, at or behind the equator.

Group II: Favorable
 (a) Solitary tumor, 6–15 mm in size, at or behind the equator.
 (b) Multiple tumors, 6–15 mm in size, behind the equator.

Group III: Doubtful
 (a) Any lesion anterior to the equator.
 (b) Solitary tumors > 15 mm in size, behind the equator.

Group IV: Unfavorable
 (a) Multiple tumors, some > 15 mm.
 (b) Any lesion extending anteriorly to the ora serrata.

Group V: Very unfavorable
 (a) Massive tumors involving over half the retina.
 (b) Vitreous seeding.

extraocular extension of tumor. Metastatic disease of the marrow and meninges can be ruled out with a bone marrow aspirate and biopsy plus cerebrospinal fluid cytology. Under some circumstances, a bone scan or CT of the liver are indicated.

Each eye is individually classified according to the Reese-Ellsworth staging system (Table 39–12). This schema predicts success for tumor control with external beam radiation; it does not predict the likelihood of useful vision or long term survival.

Treatment

Each eye is treated according to the potential for useful vision, and every attempt is made to preserve vision. The choice of therapy depends on the size, location, and number of intraocular lesions. Absolute indications for enucleation include no vision, neovascular glaucoma, inability to examine the treated eye, and inability to control tumor growth with conservative treatment. External beam irradiation is the mainstay of therapy. A total dose of 350–450 cGy is administered. Cryotherapy, photocoagulation, and radioactive plaques can be used for local tumor control. Patients with metastatic disease also receive chemotherapy. Agents that have activity against retinoblastoma include cyclophosphamide, doxorubicin, vincristine, cisplatin, and etoposide.

Children with retinoblastoma confined to the retina (whether unilateral or bilateral) have an excellent prognosis, with 5-year survival rates greater than 90%. Mortality is directly correlated with extent of optic nerve involvement, orbital extension of tumor, and massive choroid invasion. Patients who have disease in the optic nerve beyond the lamina cribrosa have only a 40% 5-year survival rate. Patients with meningeal or metastatic spread rarely survive, though intensive chemotherapy and autologous bone marrow transplants have produced long-term survivors.

Patients with the germinal mutation (heritable form) have a markedly increase risk for developing second malignant neoplasms. Second tumors develop within as well as outside the field of radiation. Tumors also develop in patients who have received no radiation therapy. Sarcomas are the most commonly occurring second malignant neoplasm, with osteosarcoma accounting for 40% of such tumors. The risk for a second neoplasm is 10% at 10 years from diagnosis in patients who did not receive radiation therapy and 20% in patients who received external beam radiation therapy. The risk continues to increase over time. Although radiation contributes to the risk, it is the presence of the retinoblastoma gene itself that is primarily responsible for the development of nonocular tumors in these patients.

Donaldson SS et al: Retinoblastoma. In: *Principles and Practice of Pediatric Oncology*. Pizzo PA, Poplack DG (editors). Lippincott, 1993.
Gallie BL et al: The genetics of retinoblastoma: Relevance to the patient. Pediatr Clin North Am 1991;38:299.

HEPATIC TUMORS

The majority (57%) of liver tumors found in childhood are malignant. Ninety percent of hepatic malignancies are either hepatoblastoma or hepatocellular carcinoma. Hepatoblastomas are somewhat more frequent than hepatocellular carcinomas (51% versus 39%). A comparison of the features of these hepatic malignancies is found in Table 39–13. Of the benign tumors, 60% are hamartomas or vascular tumors such as hemangiomas.

Children with hepatic tumors usually come to medical attention because of an enlarging abdomen. Approximately 10% of hepatoblastomas are first discovered on a routine examination. Anorexia, weight loss, vomiting, and abdominal pain are seen more commonly in hepatocellular carcinoma. Serum alpha-

Table 39–13. Comparison of hepatoblastoma and hepatocellular carcinoma in childhood.

	Hepatoblastoma	Hepatocellular Carcinoma
Median age at presentation	1 year (0–3 years)	12 years (5–18 years)
Male:female ratio	1.7:1	1.4:1
Associated conditions	Hemihypertrophy, Beckwith-Wiedemann syndrome	Hepatitis B virus infection, hereditary tyrosinemia, biliary cirrhosis, α_1-antitrypsin deficiency
Pathologic features	Fetal or embryonal cells; mesenchymal component (30%)	Large pleomorphic tumor cells and tumor giant cells
Solitary hepatic lesion	80%	20–50%
Unique features at diagnosis	Osteopenia (20–30%), isosexual precocity (3%)	Hemoperitoneum, polycythemia

Laboratory features
  Hyperbilirubinemia
  Elevated AFP
  Abnormal liver function tests
	5%
	60–70%
	15–30%
		25%
		50%
		30–50%

fetoprotein is often elevated and is an excellent indicator for following response to treatment.

Imaging studies should include an abdominal ultrasound as well as an abdominal CT scan or MRI. Malignant tumors have a diffuse hyperechoic pattern on ultrasonography, while benign tumors are usually poorly echoic. Vascular lesions contain areas with varying degrees of echogenicity. Ultrasound is also useful for imaging the hepatic veins, portal veins, and inferior vena cava. CT scanning and in particular MRI are important for defining the extent of tumor within the liver. CT scanning of the chest and bone scan should be obtained to evaluate for metastatic spread.

The prognosis for children with hepatic malignancies depends on the tumor type and the resectability of the tumor. Complete resectability is essential for survival. Chemotherapy can decrease the size of most hepatic malignancies. Following biopsy of the lesion, neoadjuvant chemotherapy is administered prior to attempting a complete surgical resection. Chemotherapy can often convert an inoperable tumor to a completely resectable one as well as eradicate metastatic disease. Approximately 50–60% of hepatoblastomas are fully resectable, while only one-third of hepatocellular carcinomas can be completely removed. Even with complete resection, only one-third of patients with hepatocellular carcinoma are long-term survivors. Continuous infusion doxorubicin over 96 hours and cisplatin have been shown to be effective agents for hepatic malignancies. Other drugs that have demonstrated benefit include fluorouracil and cyclophosphamide. Etoposide, carboplatin, and ifosfamide are under investigation. Liver transplantation is being investigated for patients whose tumors cannot be completely resected following chemotherapy.

Greenberg M et al: Hepatic tumors. In: *Principles and Practice of Pediatric Oncology*. Pizzo PA, Poplack DG: (editors). Lippincott, 1993.

Ni Y-H et al: Hepatocellular carcinoma in childhood: Clinical manifestations and prognosis. Cancer 1991;68:1737.

Ninane J et al: Effectiveness and toxicity of cisplatin and doxorubicin (PLADO) in childhood hepatoblastoma and hepatocellular carcinoma: A SIOP pilot study. Med Pediatr Oncol 1991;19:208.

LANGERHANS CELL HISTIOCYTOSIS

Langerhans cell histiocytosis (formerly called histiocytosis X) is a rare and poorly understood spectrum of disorders. It can occur as an isolated lesion or as widespread systemic disease involving virtually any body site. Eosinophilic granuloma, Hand-Schüller-Christian disease, and Letterer-Siwe disease are all syndromes encompassed by this disorder. Langerhans cell histiocytosis is not a true malignancy but a reactive proliferation of normal histiocytic cells, perhaps resulting from an immunoregulatory defect.

The distinctive pathologic feature is proliferation of histiocytic cells beyond what would be seen in a normal inflammatory process. Langerhans histiocytes have typical features: On light microscopy, the nuclei are deeply indented ("coffee-bean" shaped) and elongate, and the cytoplasm is pale, distinct, and abundant. Additional diagnostic characteristics include Birbeck granules on electron microscopy, expression of CD1 on the cell surface, and positive immunostaining for S-100 protein.

Clinical Findings

Because Langerhans cell histiocytosis encompasses a broad spectrum of diseases, its presentation can be quite variable, from a single asymptomatic lesion to widely disseminated disease. Although it is clearly a continuum of disease, patients tend to present in distinct ways. Some present primarily with lesions limited to bone. Occasionally found incidentally on radiographs obtained for other reasons, these lesions are well-demarcated and frequently found in the skull, clavicles, ribs, and vertebrae. Lesions can be painful. Lesions are often solitary, but patients may develop other bone lesions and even visceral involvement.

Bony lesions, fever, weight loss, otitis media, exophthalmos, and diabetes insipidus are seen in a small number of children with the disease. Formerly called Hand-Schüller-Christian disease, this multifocal disease commonly presents with generalized symptoms and organ dysfunction.

Disseminated Langerhans cell histiocytosis (formerly referred to as Letterer-Siwe disease) typically presents in children under 2 years of age with a seborrheic skin rash, fever, weight loss, lymphadenopathy, hepatosplenomegaly, and hematologic abnormalities.

Treatment and Prognosis

The outcome of Langerhans cell histiocytosis is extremely variable, but the process usually resolves spontaneously.

Isolated lesions may need no therapy at all. However intralesional steroids, curettage, or low-dose radiation therapy are useful local treatment measures for symptomatic lesions.

Multifocal disease is often treated with systemic chemotherapy. Prednisone, vinblastine. or etoposide, singly or in combination, can be given repeatedly or continuously until lesions heal and then is reduced and finally stopped. Single-agent therapy is as effective as multiagent therapy.

Patients with localized disease have an excellent prognosis. Multifocal disease is less predictable, but most cases resolve without sequelae. Age and degree of organ involvement are the most important prognostic factors. Infants with disseminated disease tend to do poorly, with mortality rates approaching 50%. New treatment approaches should be considered in this patient group. Cyclosporine is promising for this purpose.

Gonzales CL et al: The histiocytoses: Clinical presentation and differential diagnosis. Oncology 1990;4:47.

Komp DM: Concepts in staging and clinical studies for treatment of Langerhans' cell histiocytosis. Semin Oncol 1991;18:18.

Ladisch S et al: The histiocytoses. *Principles and Practice of Pediatric Oncology.* Pizzo PA, Poplack DG (editors). Lippincott, 1993.

LATE EFFECTS OF PEDIATRIC CANCER THERAPY

Late effects of treatment by surgery, radiation, and chemotherapy have been identified in survivors of pediatric cancer. In some studies, up to 40% of survivors of pediatric cancer will have some disability secondary to treatment.

Virtually any organ system can demonstrate sequelae related to previous cancer therapy. This has necessitated the creation of specialized oncology clinics whose function it is to identify and treat these patients.

The following sections discuss in greater detail the late effects of cancer therapy in specific organ systems. Guidelines for following those patients at risk are also presented.

Growth Complications

Growth complications of cancer therapy in the pediatric survivor are secondary to direct damage of tissues, as is seen in radiation therapy to the hypothalamic-pituitary axis. Children with acute lymphoblastic leukemia (ALL), brain tumors, orbital tumors, and nasopharyngeal cancers who have received radiation and chemotherapy are at particularly high risk.

Up to 90% of patients who receive greater than 3000 cGy of radiation to the central nervous system will show evidence of growth hormone deficiency within 2 years. Approximately 50% of children receiving 2400 cGy will have growth hormone problems. It is important to note that the effects of cranial radiation appear to be age-related, with children under 5 years at the time of therapy being particularly vulnerable. These patients may benefit from growth hormone therapy. There is currently no evidence that such therapy will induce a relapse in cancer.

Spinal radiation has also been shown to inhibit vertebral body growth. In 30% of such individuals, standing heights may be less than the fifth percentile. Asymmetric exposure of the spine to radiation may result in scoliosis; this is seen in patients who have been treated for Wilms' tumor or neuroblastoma.

Chemotherapy alone may result in an attenuation of linear growth. This, however, is usually temporary, as a period of catch-up occurs when the drugs are discontinued.

Growth should be monitored closely. Follow-up studies should include height, weight, growth velocity, scoliosis examination, and, if indicated, growth hormone testing.

Endocrine Complications

In addition to growth hormone deficiency, prepubertal children given cranial radiation may experience early puberty secondary to premature activation of the hypothalamic-pituitary-gonadal axis. This results in premature closure of the epiphyses, with decreased growth and height. This sequela appears to be more common in girls. Luteinizing hormone analogue along with growth hormone is used to halt early puberty and facilitate continued growth.

Thyroid dysfunction is common in children receiving radiation therapy to the neck and those with brain tumors who receive greater than 3000 cGy. Up to 65–90% of patients receiving more than 2500–3000 cGy to the neck region will develop hypothyroidism. The average time to develop thyroid dysfunction is 12 months after exposure, but dysfunction can occur as early as 6 months or as late as 7 years following radiation. While signs and symptoms of hypothyroidism may be present, many patients will have a normal T_4 level with elevated TSH. These individuals should be considered for thyroid hormone replacement since persistent stimulation of the thyroid from an elevated TSH may predispose to the development of thyroid nodules and carcinomas.

Gonadal dysfunction in males is usually the result of radiation to the testes, which can damage the germinal epithelium, producing azoospermia; individuals receiving 600 cGy or more usually suffer irreversible damage. Radiation to the testes can also produce Leydig cell damage with subsequent low testosterone levels and delayed sexual development. Patients who receive testicular radiation as part of their therapy for ALL, abdominal radiation for Hodgkin's disease, or total body irradiation in bone marrow transplant are at highest risk. In prepubescent boys, alkylating agents such as mechlorethamine and cyclophosphamide can also interfere with male gonadal function, resulting in oligospermia or azoospermia and low testosterone levels. Determination of testicular size, semen analysis, and measurement of testosterone, FSH, and LH levels will help identify abnormalities in patients at risk.

Exposure of the ovaries during abdominal radiation may result in failure to undergo menarche, increased FSH and LH levels, and low estrogen levels. Girls who undergo bone marrow transplantation incorporating total body irradiation in the preparative regimen are at particularly high risk. Girls receiving craniospinal radiation for ALL (1800–2400 cGy) may also develop delayed menses and are at risk for early menopause. In patients at highest risk for development of gonadal complications, a detailed menstrual history should be obtained, and FSH, LH, and estrogen levels should be monitored if indicated.

There is no study to date which confirms an increased risk of miscarriage or spontaneous abortion, stillbirths or premature births, and major and minor congenital malformations in offspring of childhood cancer survivors. Women who have received abdominal radiation and who develop uterine vascular insufficiency or fibrosis of the abdominal and pelvic musculature or uterus may have an increased risk of perinatal death or low-birth-weight premature infants and should be considered high-risk pregnancies.

Cardiopulmonary Complications

Several chemotherapeutic agents are known to cause pulmonary dysfunction as a late effect: bleomycin, the nitrosoureas, cyclophosphamide, methotrexate, and busulfan. Bleomycin has been implicated most frequently in chemotherapy-related lung injury. Ten percent of patients who receive greater than 400 units (cumulative dose) of this drug will have pulmonary toxicity, which takes the form of pulmonary fibrosis. Pulmonary function tests in patients with chemotherapy-induced toxicity will show restrictive lung disease, with decreased carbon monoxide diffusion and small lung volumes. Individuals exposed to this drug may benefit from routine pulmonary function testing and should be counseled to refrain from smoking and to give proper notification of the drug history if they should require general anesthesia.

Patients who have been treated for Hodgkin's disease using thoracic radiation and bleomycin are at high risk for pulmonary abnormalities. Chest radiation for other malignancies such as Wilms' tumor, neuroblastoma, or non-Hodgkin's lymphoma can result in pulmonary dysfunction and in the very young child may result in abnormal chest wall growth.

Cardiac complications are usually due to anthracycline exposure (daunorubicin, doxorubicin), which destroys myocytes and leads to inadequate myocardial growth as the child ages. Inadequate left ventricular mass with increased afterload and decreased function can occur. Long-term survivors can present with arrhythmias or congestive heart failure. The latter is seen in at least 5% of patients who have received greater than 550 mg/m_2 of anthracyclines (cumulative dose). In a recent study, complications from these agents were shown to become manifest 4–20 years following administration of the drugs. Pregnant women who have received anthracyclines should be followed closely for signs and symptoms of congestive heart failure, since pregnancy is associated with an increase in intravascular volume.

Radiation therapy to the mediastinal region, which is common as part of therapy for Hodgkin's disease, has been linked to an increase risk of coronary artery disease. Chronic restrictive pericarditis may also occur in these patients.

Current recommendations include an echocardiogram and electrocardiogram every 2–3 years in patients who have received anthracyclines. Closer follow-up may be indicated for those who have received more than 500 mg/m^2 of these drugs. Holter monitoring, exercise testing, or gated radionuclide angiography is indicated in patients who have received large cumulative doses, have a history of cardiac dysfunction, have had mediastinal radiation, or who were treated with anthracyclines under 4 years of age.

Renal Complications

Most of the renal long-term side effects stem from the use of chemotherapeutic agents. Patients who have received cisplatin therapy may develop an abnormal GFR and persistent tubular dysfunction with hypomagnesemia. Alkylating agents such as cyclophosphamide and ifosfamide can cause hemorrhagic cystitis, which may continue after chemotherapy has been terminated. Ifosfamide can also cause Fanconi's syndrome (proteinuria, glycosuria, phosphaturia with hypophosphatemia, aminoaciduria, and hyposthenuria), which may result in clinical rickets if adequate phosphate replacement is not given. Finally, carcinoma of the bladder has been reported in patients (mainly adults) who have received large cumulative doses of cyclophosphamide (250–300 g). Patients with a history of hemorrhagic cystitis may also be at risk for bladder carcinoma.

Patients who are seen in long-term follow-up and who have received nephrotoxic agents should be monitored with urinalysis, appropriate electrolyte profiles, and blood pressure. Urine collection for creatinine clearance or renal ultrasound may be indicated in individuals with suspected renal toxicity. Cystoscopy and cytologic study of urine sediment are recommended in patients with suspected malignancy.

Gastrointestinal & Hepatic Complications

Pediatric cancer patients who have received radiation to any site along the gastrointestinal tract can develop fibrosis and enteritis. The incidence of fibrosis is 5% for patients who have received 4000–5000 cGy and up to 36% for patients who have received over 6000 cGy. Gastric or duodenal ulcers may also occur. Intestinal fibrosis usually develops within 5 years.

Hepatic damage following chemotherapy is most commonly seen in patients who have received mercaptopurine and methotrexate with daily low-dose therapy, as is given in ALL maintenance. In one study, portal fibrosis was identified in 4–8% of children treated for ALL. Hepatotoxicity may also develop secondary to hepatitis B and C acquired via blood product transfusions. Off-therapy patients who have received hepatotoxic drugs should be followed with liver enzyme profiles as needed.

Neuropsychologic & Psychosocial Complications

Pediatric cancer survivors who have received cranial radiation for ALL or brain tumors appear to be at greatest risk for neuropsychologic problems. The severity of cranial radiation effects will vary among individual patients and depends on the dose and dose schedule, the size and location of the radiation field, the amount of time elapsed after treatment, the age of the child when the radiation was administered, and the gender of the child. Girls may be more susceptible than boys to central nervous system toxicity, since they have more rapid brain growth and development during childhood.

The main effects of central nervous system radiation appear to be related to nonverbal tasks such as visual processing speed, visual motor integration, sequencing ability, and short-term memory.

Psychosocial dysfunction can be traced to absenteeism from school, which is seen frequently in pediatric cancer patients. One recent study found that leukemia survivors were perceived as having more behavior problems and as being less socially competent than the sibling control group.

Four risk factors have been identified in patients with low social competence and behavioral problems: functional and physical limitations, cranial radiation, an older age at evaluation, and single-parent family. Adolescent survivors of cancer demonstrate an increased sense of physical fragility and vulnerability which manifests itself as hypochondriasis or counterphobic behaviors.

Pediatric cancer survivors may require ongoing counseling or other psychologic interventions once they have completed therapy. Children who have received central nervous system radiation may also require learning assistance in school, particularly in mathematics.

Second Malignancies

Approximately 3–12% of children treated for cancer will develop a new cancer within 20 years after their first diagnosis. This is a tenfold increased incidence when compared with age-matched controls. Exposure to alkylating agents and radiation therapy are risk factors in the majority of second malignan-

cies. There are also genetic and familial conditions which are associated with an increased risk of second malignancies. These include Li-Fraumeni syndrome, retinoblastoma, neurofibromatosis, nevoid basal cell carcinoma, and having a sibling with cancer.

In a report from the Late Effects Study Group, the most common primary tumors in individuals developing a second malignancy were retinoblastoma, Hodgkin's disease, soft tissue sarcomas, Wilms' tumor, brain tumors, and neuroblastoma. Sarcomas are the most common second malignant neoplasm in patients with hereditary retinoblastoma. Children treated for Hodgkin's disease have an increased risk of secondary leukemias (as a result of receiving alkylating agents such as mechlorethamine) and solid tumors (usually developing in the field of radiation).

Recently, acute nonlymphocytic leukemia has been reported as a second malignancy in patients treated with mitotic inhibitors such as etoposide and teniposide for ALL. It appears that the frequency of administration of the drug and the total dose may be important factors in the development of this secondary leukemia.

Children receiving radiation therapy as part of treatment for ALL appear to be at an increased risk to develop brain tumors as a secondary malignancy. The population at highest risk appear to be those patients who were 5 years old or less at the time of diagnosis.

Blatt J, Copeland DR, Bleyer WA: Late effects of childhood cancer and its treatment. In: *Principles and Practice of Pediatric Oncology.* Pizzo PA, Poplack DG (editors). Lippincott, 1993.

Copeland DR: Neuropyschological and psychosocial effects of childhood leukemia and its treatment. CA Cancer J Clin 1992;42:283.

Cousens P et al: Cognitive effects of childhood leukemia therapy: A case for four specific deficits. J Pediatr Psychol 1991;16:475.

Delaat CA, Lampkin BC: Long-term survivors of childhood cancer: Evaluation and identification of treatment. CA Cancer J Clin 1992;42:263.

Meadows AT et al: Second malignant neoplasms in children: An update from the late effects study group. J Clin Oncol 1985;3:532.

Neglia JP et al: Second neoplasms after acute lymphoblastic leukemia in childhood. N Engl J Med 1991;325:1330.

40 Fluid & Electrolyte Therapy

James V. Lustig, MD

BODY FLUIDS

In term infants, the total body water (TBW) accounts for approximately 70–75% of the body weight. Following the normal postnatal fluid adjustment with its attendant weight loss, the TBW represents about 65% of the total body weight. This fraction remains constant until puberty, when the TBW decreases to 55–60% of the body weight. Approximately two-thirds of the TBW is intracellular water (ICW), and one-third is extracellular water (ECW). The ECW is further divided into plasma volume and interstitial fluid (Figure 40–1).

The intracellular and extracellular fluids are separated by the cell membranes of the body. For the purposes of discussing clinical disorders of hydration, these membranes may be conceptualized as one aggregate cell membrane that is water-permeable. Furthermore, the cell membrane facilitates the passage into and the maintenance of sodium (Na^+) concentration in the ECW, whereas potassium (K^+) is moved into and maintained in the intracellular environment via a membrane-associated "pump."

Because the cell membrane is water-permeable and particles are dissolved in the water on each side of the cell membrane, shifts of water would occur if the number of particles dissolved on each side of the cell membrane were not the same. Normally the volumes of the ECW and ICW do not change, because the concentration of dissolved particles is identical on each side of the membrane. If this relationship were not maintained, there would be fluid shifts from one compartment to the other owing to the permeable nature of the membrane. The actual number of dissolved particles per unit of water is seldom computed. In clinical situations, the concept of osmolality is used. (Osmolality is usually expressed as mosm/L of water, which is equivalent to mmol/L times the number of particles formed when a molecule dissociates, eg, two particles for NaCl; one particle for glucose.) Osmolality represents the osmolar concentration of a dissolved substance multiplied by the number of particles produced by dissociation of a molecule of the substance.

Osmolality is the same throughout the body water. Normally, the osmolality of body water is approximately 285 mosm/L. Solutions with this osmolality are said to be "normal," because they are isosmolal or isotonic. Solutions of less than 285 mosm/L are hyposmolal or hypotonic, whereas those containing more than 285 mosm/L are hypertonic.

Conceptualizing osmotic shifts between the ECW and ICW is fundamental to understanding disorders of hydration. The "membrane" separating the extracellular and intracellular space must be freely permeable to water. Shifts occur only if there is an inequality on each side of the membrane in the concentration of solutes that cannot permeate the membrane. Normally Na^+, Cl^-, and HCO_3^- are primarily excluded from most cellular environments, whereas K^+ is maintained within cells.

In addition to the isosmolality maintained between fluid compartments, electroneutrality is maintained within body fluids so that the concentration of cations equals the concentration of anions within a body fluid.

The extracellular fluid (ECF) is the only fluid compartment that can be readily monitored and that its composition reflects interactions between the ECF and intracellular fluid (ICF). Therapeutically it is generally desirable to maintain a normal osmolality (285 mosm/L).

FLUID COMPARTMENTS

Although the majority of body water is intracellular, direct measurement and characterization of ICF remains difficult. Clinically, the status of ICF is inferred from analysis of plasma and the condition of the patient. This is obviously imprecise and frustrating because one cannot appreciate the early effects of hydration disorders upon the cell and its organelles.

The ECF is subdivided into the (1) plasma, (2) interstitial fluid (ISF), (3) transcellular fluid, and (4) bone fluid.

The connective tissue and bone fluid compartment has little role in the development of symptoms in disorders of hydration.

Transcellular fluids reside in a specific location as a result of a transport process through cells. These fluids include cerebrospinal fluid, bile, gastrointesti-

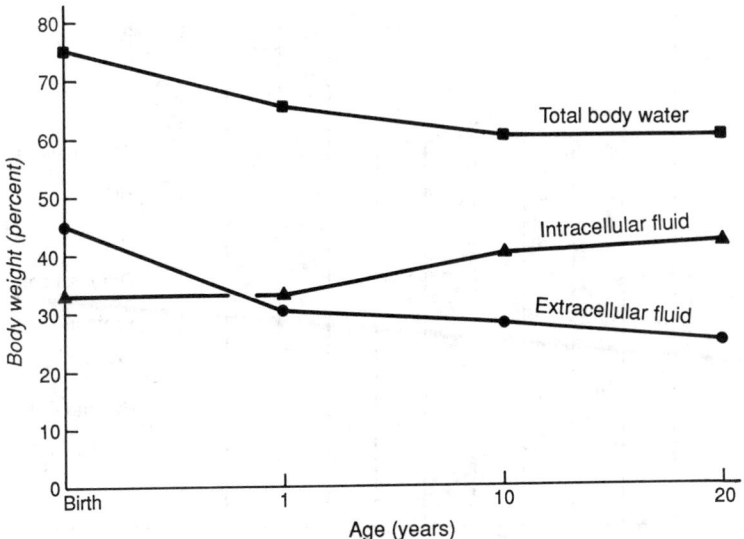

Figure 40–1. Body water compartments related to age.

nal fluid, humors of the eye, and fluids from the pancreas, salivary glands, and sweat gland ducts. These fluids normally account for a very small percentage of the TBW. The volume of gastrointestinal fluid can expand vastly, creating a fluid pool of great size and clinical significance. The elimination of or redistribution of this fluid into another fluid compartment such as the ECF may pose a significant clinical problem.

The ISF represents a large compartment of body fluid. The size of the ISF allows it to withstand rapid change so that it "buffers" change occurring in the significantly smaller plasma compartment. ISF surrounds and bathes the cells.

The electrolyte composition of the ISF is similar to that of plasma. The concentrations of Na^+, K^+, Cl^-, and HCO_3^- in the ISF closely resemble the concentrations found in the plasma. Clinically, plasma electrolyte analysis can be said to reflect the composition of the ISF.

When the volume of the ISF is depleted, poor skin turgor, depressed fontanelles, and sunken eyes result, whereas an expanded ISF volume results in edema. Although it accounts for only about one-fifth of the ECF volume, plasma plays a critical role in the assessment of the status of the body's fluid compartments. Plasma is in contact with the gastrointestinal tract, kidney, and skin. The plasma is separated from the ISF by the endothelium lining blood vessels. The endothelium permits very rapid passage of water and ions but inhibits movement of protein molecules, confining most albumin and globulin to the intravascular compartment. The inhibition of movement of protein molecules is presumably due to their size. Plasma proteins consist primarily of albumin, which has a molecular weight of about 60,000, and globulins, whose molecular weight ranges from 180,000 to over 1,000,000. Albumin molecules are more numerous than globulin molecules and exert three-fourths of the osmotic pressure exerted by plasma proteins. The protein osmotic pressure is referred to as colloid osmotic pressure. Although colloid osmotic pressure seems negligible compared to the osmotic pressure exerted by the low molecular weight electrolyte molecules, it is important in maintaining plasma volume.

As in other body fluids, electroneutrality is maintained in the plasma. As the previous discussion suggests, the majority of extracellular protein resides in the plasma. Alterations in plasma composition reflect the interaction of external forces on the internal environment. Figure 40–2 is a schematic depiction of the composition and distribution of the body fluids.

CONTROL OF THE ECF

Multiple mechanisms control the volume and content of the ECF. Among the more important control mechanisms are thirst, aldosterone, and antidiuretic hormone (ADH).

Aldosterone, from the adrenal cortex, enhances the tubular reabsorption of Na^+ in the kidney. As a constant osmolality is maintained, retention of Na^+ leads to increased ECF volume.

Thirst controls the need to drink and reflects changes in the volume of ECF. Thirst provides precise control over a wide range of fluid volumes and can even be a response to an inhibition or absence of ADH with its attendant copious, dilute urine. However, thirst acts to maintain volume even at the expense of osmolality. An individual who cannot perceive thirst rapidly develops a significant problem with fluid balance. Neurologically impaired children or children who cannot respond to thirst pose serious management problems.

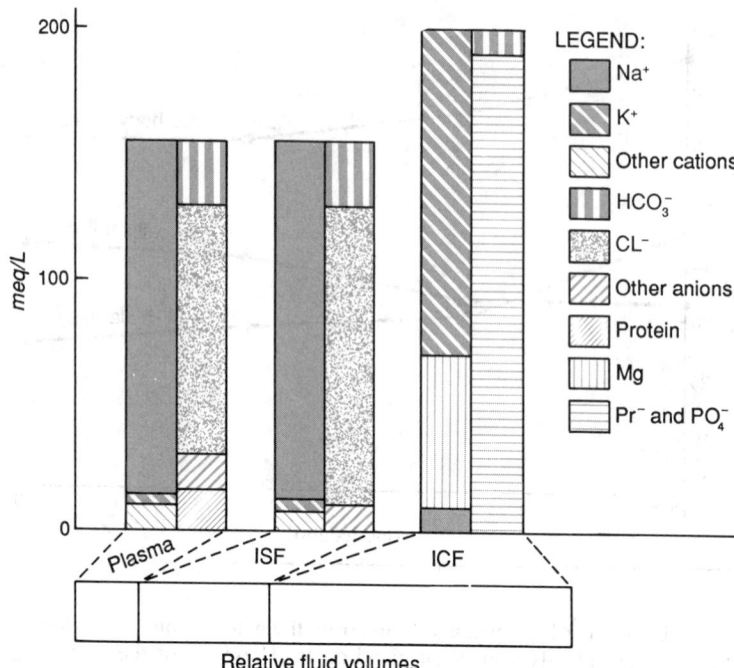

Figure 40–2. Composition of body fluids.

Relative fluid volumes

Under normal physiologic conditions, plasma osmolality, as opposed to plasma volume, is the variable primarily regulated. Plasma osmolality and volume are maintained through the interaction of thirst and ADH. Thirst controls fluid intake, whereas ADH controls the volume of urine output.

After being produced in the anterior hypothalamus, ADH is secreted from the posterior pituitary. ADH enhances the reabsorption of water in the kidney. Urine subsequently produced is low in volume and hypertonic relative to plasma. A small change in plasma osmolality precipitates a significant ADH response. ADH is secreted in response to a decrease in plasma ECF volume, an increase in osmolality, exercise, stress, and the ingestion of some drugs. Drugs that enhance ADH secretion include epinephrine, acetylcholine, histamine, morphine, barbiturates, and nicotine. Inhibition of ADH secretion results from decreased plasma osmolality, distention of the left atrium, and ethanol ingestion or administration.

Age also plays a role in regulating fluid volumes within the body, as the changes in the fluid compartments at birth and puberty demonstrate. In addition, growth necessitates a slight positive balance to accommodate the demands of the growing child.

ACID-BASE EQUILIBRIUM

The acidity of arterial blood is maintained within very narrow limits. The acidity is usually expressed in pH units, which represent

$$\log \frac{1}{[H^+]}$$

Normally, the pH is 7.40 ± 0.02 except in infants, in whom it ranges from 7.35 to 7.45. Acids dissociate into cations (C^+) and anions (A^-). The stronger the acid, the more complete the dissociation. The acidity of a solution is proportionate to the concentration of hydrogen ions.

Buffers, which act to inhibit changes in the acidity of a solution, consist of a weak acid and its conjugate base. In the body, the primary role of buffers in maintaining pH is enhanced by physiologic mechanisms in the lung and kidney. The carbonic acid buffering system is perhaps the best known, but there are nonbicarbonate buffers, which include plasma proteins, ammonium, phosphates, and erythrocyte hemoglobin. Over 50% of the blood's buffering capacity is in the bicarbonate system. The action of buffers is strengthened by the lung's effect on carbonic acid and the alkalinization or acidification of urine, which alters the concentration and amount of bicarbonate in the blood.

One can understand a buffer system's action by quantifying the system's reactions. Acid-base relationships are governed by the Henderson-Hasselbalch equation:

$$pH = pK' + \log \frac{[\text{conjugate base}]}{[\text{weak acid}]}$$

where pK' is a constant specific to the specific buffer system. In the carbonic acid system, whose pK' is 6.1,

H_2CO_3 dissociates to H^+ and HCO_3^-. Knowing that the normal concentration of HCO_3^- is 24 meq/L and the normal concentration of H_2CO_3 is 1.2 mmol/L, one can rewrite the Henderson-Hasselbalch equation as follows:

$$pH = pK' + \log \frac{[HCO^{-3}]}{[H_2CO_3]}$$

$$pH = 6.1 + \log \frac{[24 \text{ meq/L}]}{[1.2 \text{ mmol/L}]}$$

The equation can be rewritten in a number of equivalent forms. A clinically important form of the equation is based on the fact that blood in the pulmonary capillaries is in equilibrium with alveolar air. Therefore, the denominator of the log can be expressed as $PCO_2 \times S$ (S = solubility coefficient = 0.03 mmol/L/mm Hg). Given a normal PCO_2 of 40 mm Hg, the denominator is again 1.2 mmol/L. The equation is then–

$$pH = pK + \log \frac{[HCO_3^-]}{S \times PCO_2} = 6.1 + \log \frac{[HCO_3^-]}{1.2 \text{ mmol/L}}$$

To solve the equation, one must know two of the three variables (ie, pH, $[HCO_3^-]$, PCO_2).

The bicarbonate system can interact with the non-bicarbonate system. Such interaction may be represented by the equation $H_2CO_3 + Hb^- \leftrightarrow HCO_3^- + H$ Prot. The equation is shifted to the right by a increase of H_2CO_3 or PCO_2. Although this shift would increase $[HCO_3^-]$ and decrease $[Hb^-]$, the sum of $[HCO_3^-]$ + $[Hb^-]$ remains constant, and so the total buffer base remains the same. The total buffer base is normally 45–50 meq/L.

Both the lung and kidney can act to alter or stabilize pH. In respiratory alkalosis there is effective alveolar hyperventilation. Therefore, the denominator of the equation for pH–

$$\left(pH = pK' + \log \frac{[HCO_3^-]}{S \times PCO_2} \right)$$

decreases, and the pH increases.

In metabolic acidosis, which results from an increase of a strong acid or loss of bicarbonate, the respiratory center increases respiratory drive, CO_2 is exhaled, and PCO_2 decreases so that the ratio of–

$$\frac{[HCO_3^-]}{S \times PCO_2}$$

tends to be maintained and there is a compensatory shift in pH toward normal.

Renal regulation of acid-base status primarily alters HCO_3^- concentration. Unwanted acid or base can be excreted in the urine, and subsequently the HCO_3^- concentration can be altered throughout the entire ECF. Bicarbonate can be altered in two ways via the kidneys, since the urine may be either alkalinized or acidified. When the urine is alkalinized, HCO_3^- enters the kidney and is ultimately lost in the urine. This alkalinization of the urine can occur at any time that there is a relative or absolute excess of bicarbonate. This mechanism does not function if there is a deficiency of Na^+ or K^+, because the body could not maintain electroneutrality in this situation. A chloride deficiency also inhibits this mechanism.

If there is a relative or absolute decrease in HCO_3^-, the urine can be acidified. In this situation, water and CO_2 combine in the tubular cell to form carbonic acid, which then dissociates. H^+ is exchanged for Na^+, and the sodium bicarbonate gains access to the peritubular plasma and the ECF. This reaction facilitates the excretion of significant amounts of H^+. The reaction is limited by salt depletion or dehydration. Some of the processes controlling pH are illustrated schematically in Figure 40–3.

PRINCIPLES OF FLUID & ELECTROLYTE MANAGEMENT

The therapy for any disorder of fluids, and electrolytes is predicated on providing the patient with maintenance requirements of fluids and electrolytes, replacing any previous losses, and replenishing ongoing abnormal losses. In planning therapy, these three components should be addressed individually so that no basic needs are overlooked. In addition, therapy should be phased in order to (1) maintain adequate perfusion, (2) restore fluid and electrolyte deficits

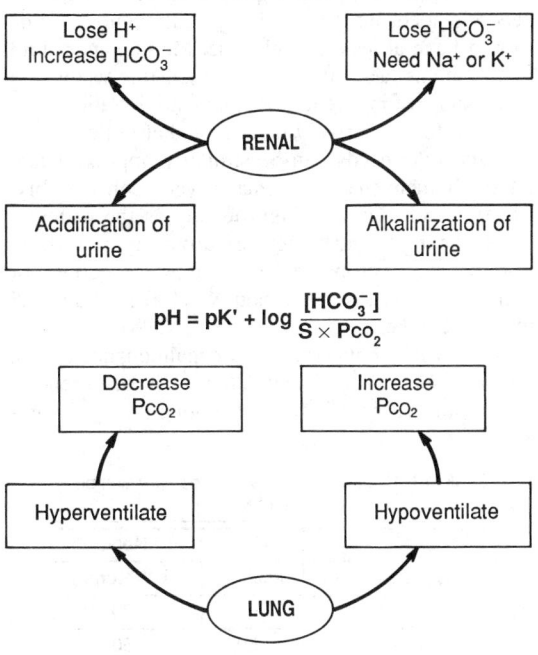

Figure 40–3. Composition of body fluids.

while correcting acid-base defects, and (3) meet nutritional needs.

The cornerstone of therapy is understanding maintenance requirements. The phrase "maintenance requirements" means enough water and electrolytes to prevent deterioration of body stores. When short-term (2–3 days) parenteral therapy is given, enough calories are given to blunt hunger and inhibit protein breakdown and ketosis. However, the amount given is usually little more than 20% of the patient's true caloric needs.

Different models have been devised to calculate maintenance fluid needs based on body weight, surface area, or caloric expenditures. A system based on caloric expenditures is helpful since we know that 1 mL of water is needed every 24 hours for each calorie expended and that metabolic needs, not size, determine the use of body stores.

Calories consumed per unit of body weight (metabolic rate) decrease as size and age increase. The schema presented, which is based on caloric needs, is applicable to youngsters weighing over 3 kg (see Table 40–1). The information presented in the table correlates well with the metabolic rate data presented in Figure 40–4.

As Table 40–1 shows, a child weighing 25 kg would need 1600 kcal daily and 1600 mL of water. If the child were admitted to the hospital for an elective procedure and received fluids intravenously for 2 days, the fluid would probably contain 5% glucose, which would provide 320 kcal/d, or about 20% of the maintenance needs. For short-term parenteral maintenance therapy in patients without preexisting nutritional deficits, 5% glucose providing 20% of caloric needs is adequate. In general, all intravenous fluids should have at least 5% glucose. Maintenance fluid requirements take into account insensible water loss and water lost in sweat, urine, and stool. Patients are assumed to be relatively inactive and afebrile.

Electrolyte needs can be similarly approximated, although maintenance estimates vary considerably. Electrolyte losses vary significantly as the patient's output changes, and therefore no one figure reflects true needs. Reasonable initial approximations for maintenance needs are 3 meq $Na^+/100$ kcal and 2.5 meq $K^+/100$ kcal.

Altered metabolic states alter maintenance needs. Allowances must be made for such occurrences. Fever and hyperventilation are among the most com-

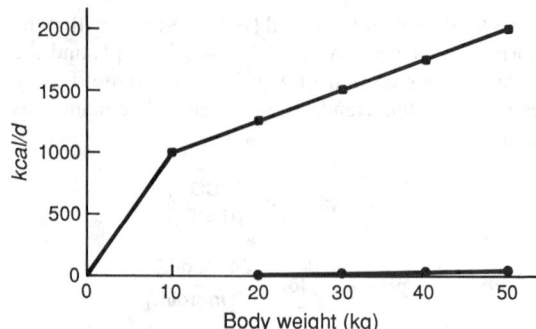

Figure 40–4. Estimate of caloric needs per day. For each calorie expended, 1 mL of water is needed. (Adapted from Holliday MA, Segar WE: Pediatrics 1957;19:823.)

monly encountered of these conditions. For every degree (centigrade) of body temperature, fluid needs increase by 12.5%. Corrections are made for temperatures above 38 °C. A fever of 39 °C would require maintenance fluid to be increased by 25%. Table 40–2 lists factors commonly altering fluid requirements.

Normally one need not measure individual components of output to ensure appropriate fluid balance. It is useful to monitor the patient's weight, urinary output, fluid input, and urine specific gravity. If there is an alteration of fluid or electrolyte balance, determination of electrolyte concentrations, urine osmolality, and pH may be necessary. Unless one is dealing with an osmotic diuresis, such as is seen in diabetic ketoacidosis, a urine osmolality between 200 and 600 mosm/L indicates adequate fluid intake. These measurements help the physician monitor the efficacy of therapy. In patients with significant burns, anuria, oliguria, or abnormal ongoing losses (eg, from a stoma), it is important to measure output and its fractions so that appropriate replacement can be instituted.

DEHYDRATION

Depletion of body fluids—dehydration—is one of the most commonly encountered problems in pediatrics. Dehydration, most often associated with gastro-

Table 40–1. Caloric and water needs per unit body weight.

| Body weight in kg | Maintenance Needs | |
	kcal/kg	mL Water/kg
3–10	100	100
11–20	50	50
> 20 kg	20	20

Table 40–2. Alterations of maintenance fluid requirements.

Factor	Altered Requirement
Fever	12% per °C[1]
Hyperventilation	10–60 mL/100 kcal
Sweating	10–25 mL/100 kcal
Hyperthyroidism	Variable: 25–50%
Gastrointestinal loss and renal disease	Monitor and analyze output. Adjust therapy accordingly.

[1]Do not correct for 38 °C; correct 24% for 39 °C.

enteritis, remained a major cause of death in the United States until well into this century and is still a major cause of morbidity and mortality in developing nations. The problems associated with dehydration remain common not only because of the frequency of gastroenteritis in young children but also because infants and young children often decrease their intake when ill. Furthermore, renal function in the first year of life does not maximally conserve water, the infant's high ratio of surface area to volume promotes evaporative fluid losses, and fever significantly increases fluid needs. Caregivers who treat both children and adults should remember that young children and adults have significant differences among compartments of body water as well as differences in total body water content. As a result, perfusion is compromised at a lower percentage of dehydration in adults than in children, but children require a greater proportionate deficit replacement when they are dehydrated.

Dehydration results in protean changes in the body, leading to cellular dysfunction. The clinical effects of dehydration are proportionate both to the degree of dehydration and to the relative ratio of salt to water lost. Briefly, dehydration decreases the extracellular volume, leading to decreased tissue perfusion. The decreased volume results in compensatory increases in pulse rate as the heart attempts to increase output in the face of decreased stroke volume. The decreased tissue perfusion also impairs renal function, leading to acidosis and uremia. Decreased oxygen delivery due to dehydration may lead to lactic acidosis. If there is an associated decrease in caloric intake or an inability to metabolize ingested calories, ketoacidosis may ensue. These changes are illustrated in Figures 40–5 and 40–6.

The clinical sequelae of dehydration reflect the amount of fluid depletion. A number of clinical profiles have been suggested as a way to correlate the appearance of symptoms and physical signs with the degree of dehydration. Such a system is illustrated in Table 40–3. However, such schema are imprecise at best. The primary utility of such systems is to remind the physician to estimate the degree of dehydration (because treatment varies with the degree of dehydration) and, more importantly, to assess the adequacy of perfusion. They also serve as a reminder that the more physical signs present, the more likely it is that the dehydration is profound. Simple measures—eg, checking the patient's last recorded weight and comparing it to the present weight; carefully assessing blood pressure, capillary refill, and orthostatic blood pressure changes; and meticulously reviewing the history of fluids ingested and frequency of output— are often most helpful. Physicians dealing with growing children must remember the fluid shift that occurs around the time of puberty. Young children may not suffer shock until the degree of dehydration is approximately 15%. However, after the fluid shift at puberty, shock may occur when the degree of dehydration is 9–10%. The significance of this shift underscores the need to constantly assess the adequacy of perfusion and the patient's response to treatment.

Dehydration is further characterized by the electrolyte composition of the plasma. When body salts are lost in proportion to water, the electrolyte readings yield normal values, and the dehydration is said to be isotonic. If relatively more solute than water is lost, the sodium concentration falls, and hyponatremic dehydration ($[Na^+] < 130$ meq/L) results. This finding is important because the hypotonicity of the plasma results in further volume loss from the ECF, and perfusion is therefore more significantly impaired for a given degree of hyponatremic dehydration than for the same degree of isotonic or hypertonic dehydration. Hypernatremic dehydration ($[Na^+] > 150$ meq/L) occurs when relatively less solute than body water is lost. It is important to remember that significant solute losses do occur in hypernatremic dehydration. Because plasma volume is protected, this might appear to be the least dangerous form of dehydration, but it poses the risk of an underestimation of the severity of dehydration. Further, if the hypertonicity is corrected too rapidly (a drop in $[Na^+]$ of $> 0.5–1$ meq/L in 1 hour) cerebral edema, seizures, and severe

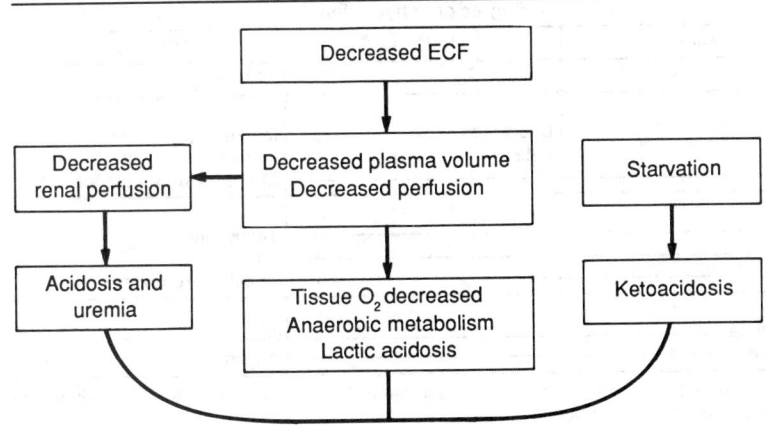

Figure 40–5. Sequelae of dehydration.

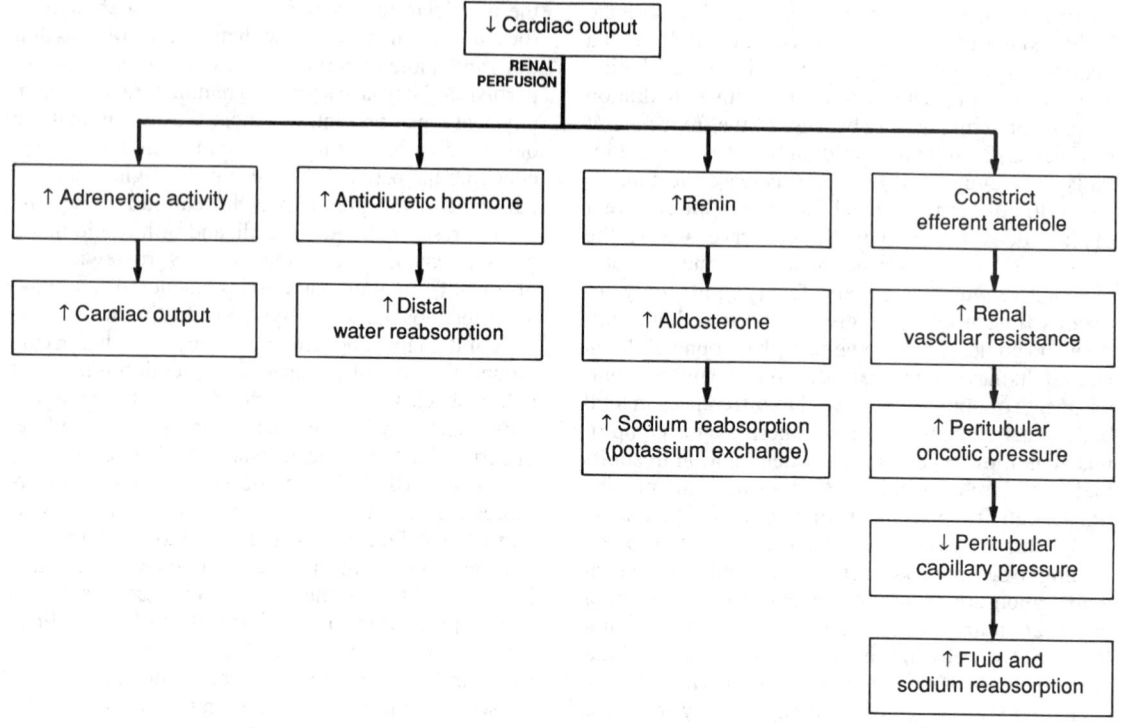

Figure 40–6. Pathophysiologic responses to decreased ECF.

central nervous system injury may occur. Typical electrolyte losses associated with each form of dehydration are listed in Table 40–4.

METABOLIC DERANGEMENTS

1. METABOLIC ACIDOSIS

Metabolic acidosis results from either increased abnormal production of a strong acid or loss of a buffer base, such as bicarbonate. Acids produced include ketone bodies, lactic acid, or, in the presence of renal impairment, phosphoric or sulfuric acids. Ketone body production is increased in starvation, diabetic ketoacidosis, and salicylism. Lactic acidosis usually reflects poor tissue perfusion or hypoxia, although primary lactic acidosis may rarely occur.

Loss of bicarbonate is most often associated with loss of alkaline fluid from the small intestine. Such losses often accompany diarrheal disease, the use of suction to remove fluid from the intestine, or a small

Table 40–3. Clinical manifestations of dehydration.[1]

Clinical Signs	Degree of Dehydration		
	Mild	Moderate	Severe
Decrease in body weight	3–5%	8–10%	12–15%
Skin			
Turgor	Normal (+/−)	Decreased	Markedly decreased
Color	Normal	Pale	Markedly decreased
Mucous membranes	Dry ————————————————————→		Mottled or gray; parched
Hemodynamic			
Pulse	Normal ————————————————————→		Tachycardia
Blood pressure	Normal ————————————————————→		Low
Perfusion	Normal ————————————————————→		Circulatory collapse
Fluid loss			
Urinary output	Mild oliguria ————————————————————→		Anuria
Tears	Decreased ————————————————————→		Absent

[1]The manifestations of dehydration reflect the ECF in general and the plasma in particular. Therefore, hypotonic dehydration is clinically more apparent, and hypertonic dehydration is less apparent.

Table 40–4. Estimated water and electrolyte deficits in dehydration (moderate to severe).[1]

Type of Dehydration	H₂O (mL/kg)	Na⁺ (meq/kg)	K⁺ (meq/kg)	Cl⁻ and HCO₃⁻ (meq/kg)
Isotonic	100–150	8–10	8–10	16–20
Hypotonic	50–100	10–14	10–14	20–28
Hypertonic	120–180	2–5	2–5	4–10

[1]Adapted from Winters RW: *Principles of Pediatric Fluid Therapy.* Little, Brown, 1982.

bowel fistula. Diarrheal stool is often acidic. The question arises as to how this occurs if the fluid from the small intestine is alkaline. The acidic pH reflects the bacterial fermentation of the intestinal fluid, which results in the production of organic acids. The stool has an anion gap. The stool of patients with cholera is usually alkaline as a result of the rapid transit time associated with this disorder. If a patient's stool is alkaline, the transit time may be assumed to be brief. Loss of bicarbonate is also seen in renal tubular acidosis.

Metabolic acidosis is associated with a significant negative base excess and compensatory hyperventilation. Effective treatment depends on treating the underlying disorder. Bicarbonate may be used to ameliorate severe acidosis. Normalization of pH which is too rapid or too aggressive may have serious deleterious sequelae. Therefore, only severe acidosis should be treated. In general, one need not attempt to correct the pH if it is greater than 7.10, and one need not correct to values greater than 7.25 with bicarbonate. The dose of sodium bicarbonate used to correct pH is given by the following formula:

Dose (in meq) = 0.3 × body weight (kg) × base excess

If sodium bicarbonate is given, the amount of sodium administered in maintenance fluids should be adjusted.

Many physicians rely on determination of the anion gap to detect cases of metabolic acidosis due to the production of strong acid. The anion gap may be calculated from either of the following formulas:

$$\text{Anion gap} = ([Na^+]) - ([Cl^-] + [HCO^{-3}])$$

or

$$\text{Anion gap} = ([Na^+] + [K^+]) - ([Cl^-] + [HCO_3^-])$$

This calculation approximates the sum of the undetermined anions (proteinates, lactate, phosphate, sulfate beta-hydroxybutyrate). Normal values depend on the formula used and on laboratory protocol. Small variations are not significant, and the anion gap determinations should not be overinterpreted. The anion gap

should be abnormal if a strong acid (not hydrochloric acid) is added, because the anion of the acid will appear in the undetermined fraction and increase the anion gap. The anion gap tends to be normal in diarrhea with its attendant hyperchloremic acidosis and bicarbonate loss. However, if azotemia ensues due to dehydration, the increase in phosphate and sulfate may increase the anion gap. The anion gap should always be positive. An anion gap of zero or less indicates a laboratory error. Clinical situations in which an exaggerated anion gap is encountered include diabetic ketoacidosis uremia, salicylate intoxication, lactic acidosis, hypokalemia, hypocalcemia, methanol intoxication, ethylene glycol, or other causes of metabolic acidosis. Therapy with various antibiotics, including carbenicillin and large doses of sodium penicillin, can also elevate the anion gap. A low anion gap is associated with hypoalbuminemia, dilution, hyperkalemia, hypercalcemia, and lithium intoxication. Hyperviscosity may lead to laboratory error in determining the anion gap.

2. METABOLIC ALKALOSIS

Metabolic alkalosis is the result of gaining buffer base or losing strong acid, most commonly due to the loss of gastric juice from vomiting or nasogastric suctioning. Pyloric stenosis is the prototypical situation leading to the development of metabolic alkalosis. Other situations that may lead to metabolic alkalosis include chronic diarrhea, the administration of diuretics, and the use of silver nitrate in the treatment of burns. Metabolic anomalies in which sodium is conserved without chloride, such as 11β-hydroxylase deficiency, predispose patients to the development of metabolic alkalosis.

The laboratory profile of metabolic alkalosis includes, in addition to an elevated pH, a positive base excess and a normal or mildly elevated P_{co2}.

The treatment of metabolic alkalosis includes, in addition to the treatment of the underlying disorder, the administration of chloride. Chloride may be supplied by a number of salts.

3. RESPIRATORY ACIDOSIS

Respiratory acidosis denotes a decrease in alveolar ventilation with an attendant increase in PO_2 (both in the alveoli and in plasma). In acute respiratory acidosis, CO_2 is retained. In addition to a drop in pH and an increase in PO_2, patients are likely to demonstrate an increased level of bicarbonate and a decreased level of chloride, which is lost as the urine is acidified. Clinically these patients are air hungry, and their respiration is characterized by retractions and the use of accessory muscles. Cyanosis may be present. This scenario may be seen in upper or lower airway obstruction, ventilation/perfusion disturbances, inadequate perfusion, or respiratory failure. The goal of treatment is to provide adequate ventilation. HCO_3^- therapy is not efficacious because the elevated PCO_2 inhibits the shifting of the equation $H^+ + HCO_3^- \leftrightarrow H_2CO_3$ to the right.

Chronic respiratory acidosis is characterized by gradual development of alveolar hypoventilation. A number of clinical entities, including primary lung problems, chest wall abnormalities, and neurologic problems, are associated with this disorder. Chronic respiratory acidosis is associated with kyphoscoliosis, chest wall deformities, osteogenesis imperfecta, rickets, polymyositis, cystic fibrosis, myasthenia gravis, muscular dystrophy, and poliomyelitis. Although respiratory acidosis has been seen in severe chronic asthma, such an occurrence should be very rare with present treatment modalities. Again, the goal of treatment is to control the underlying disorder and promote adequate ventilation.

4. RESPIRATORY ALKALOSIS

Respiratory alkalosis occurs when hyperventilation results in a decrease in PO_2. Patients describe tingling in the extremities, paresthesia, dizziness, and palpitations. Syncope may occur, and very occasionally tetany associated with hypocalcemia or even seizures may be seen. The hyperventilation is the result of central nervous system stimulation. Causes of respiratory alkalosis include hysteria, central nervous system irritation from meningitis or encephalitis, and salicylism. Treatment varies from providing a paper bag to facilitate rebreathing by the hysterical patient to increasing the dead space in a patient with a central nervous system anomaly who requires ventilation.

POTASSIUM DISORDERS

Potassium is the primary intracellular cation. Only about 2% of the body's K^+ is extracellular. The intracellular concentration of K^+ is over 40 times that found in the ECF. Skeletal muscle, which contains about 60% of the body's potassium, has an intracellular concentration of 150–160 meq/L, whereas the plasma concentration is only 4–5 meq/L. Over 90% of the potassium in the body is freely exchangeable. Maintenance of the appropriate potassium distribution and size of the body pool is maintained by the Na^+-K^+ pump at the cell membrane and by the kidney. Potassium is filtered by the glomerulus, reabsorbed in the proximal tubule, and excreted in the distal tubule. The kidney can either excrete or conserve K^+ readily, but secretion of potassium occurs via the mechanism that results in acidification of the urine. Therefore, potassium secretion depends on the body's Na^+ level and pH. When Na^+ is reabsorbed in

the tubular cell, it is exchanged for either H^+ or K^+. If an alkaline urine is to be excreted, K^+ is secreted preferentially. By contrast, acidification of the urine results in loss of H^+ and conservation of K^+. The kidney cannot conserve K^+ on short notice. In addition to the body's Na^+ load, the size of the body's potassium pool and steroids also affect K^+ balance. If K^+ is depleted, the urine is acidified, and systemic alkalosis ensues. Adrenal corticosteroids promote Na^+ retention, whereas Addison's disease results in Na^+ loss and K^+ retention. The concentration of K^+ in the ECF is increased by acidemia, whereas alkalosis, hypochloremia, and glycogen deposition result in decreased levels of K^+ in the ECF. Alkalosis promotes the entry of K^+ into cells, whereas acidemia results in K^+ leaving cells and entering the ECF. Treatment of a diabetic in ketoacidosis results in a decrease in the $[K^+]_s$ as the pH rises, and insulin administration results in glycogen deposition.

Potassium excretion continues for a significant period even if the intake of K^+ is decreased. By the time that a lowered urinary $[K^+]$ occurs, the body's K^+ pool has already been significantly depleted.

Diuretics, especially thiazides, acetazolamide, and mercurials, enhance the secretion of K^+. Aberrations in the concentration of potassium in the ECF alter myocardial contractility and can cause death from arrhythmia or cardiac standstill. When hypokalemia occurs with a loss of 10–20% of the body's potassium stores, apathy and muscle weakness occur. Occasionally paresthesias are reported, and tetany may be seen. Further, losses may result in flaccid paralysis and decreased respiration. Electrocardiographic changes associated with hypokalemia include T-wave depression, the appearance of U waves, ST segment depression and arrhythmia (see Figure 40–7). Arrhythmias associated with hypokalemia include premature ventricular contractions, atrial or nodal tachycardia, and ventricular tachycardia or fibrillation. Hypokalemia also heightens responsiveness to digitalis and may precipitate digitalis toxicity.

The first priority in the treatment of hypokalemia is maintaining an adequate concentration of K^+ in the serum. The magnitude of the total K^+ loss cannot be readily calculated because the vast majority of the body's K^+ is located intracellularly. Providing maintenance amounts of K^+ is usually sufficient to prevent problems. In those situations in which $[K^+]_s$ is dangerously low and K^+ must be administered intravenously, it is imperative that the patient have a cardiac monitor, and the physician must be prepared to treat any arrhythmias. Potassium should not be administered at a rate exceeding 0.5 meq/kg/h, and administration of this much K^+ should be done in an intensive care unit with adequate monitoring. Once the $[K^+]_s$ is stabilized, the body's K^+ deficit may be replaced by providing foods rich in potassium.

Hyperkalemia is characterized by muscle weakness, occasional paresthesias and tetany, and ascend-

HYPOKALEMIA	HYPERKALEMIA
Apathy, muscle weakness, paresthesias, tetany	Ascending paralysis; occasional tetany and paresthesias, muscle weakness
Depressed T wave, U wave; ST segment depression	Peaked T wave, prolonged PR interval, ST segment depression, wide QRS complex
Arrhythmias	Arrhythmias
Premature beats	Sinus bradycardia
Atrial or nodal tachycardia	Atrioventricular block
Ventricular tachycardia or fibrillation	Idioventricular tachycardia or fibrillation
	Cardiac arrest

Figure 40–7. Clinical sequelae of hypokalemia and hyperkalemia.

ing paralysis. Electrocardiographic changes associated with hyperkalemia include heightened T waves, widening of the QRS complex, and arrhythmias. The arrhythmias seen with hyperkalemia include sinus bradycardia or sinus arrest, AV block, nodal or idioventricular rhythms, and ventricular tachycardia or fibrillation. The clinical severity of hyperkalemia depends on the electrocardiographic changes, the status of the other electrolytes, and the progression of the underlying disorder. If the $[K^+]_s$ is less than 6.5 meq/L, one seldom need do anything more than discontinue the administration of potassium. If potentiating factors (eg, hyponatremia, a brisk rise in $[K^+]_s$, alkalemia, digitalis toxicity, or renal failure) are present, one needs to be more aggressive. Any suggestions of a dysrhythmia must be evaluated and treated aggressively. A rhythm strip should be obtained immediately whenever significant hyperkalemia is suspected. If electrocardiographic changes or arrhythmias are present, treatment must be promptly initiated. Intravenous Ca^{2+}, usually administered as 10% calcium gluconate (0.2–0.5 mL/kg over 2–10 minutes), will briefly ameliorate depolarization. The calcium should be administered with a cardiac monitor in place and should be discontinued immediately if bradycardia occurs. Administering Na^+ and increasing the pH with bicarbonate therapy will cause K^+ to move from the extracellular to intracellular environment. The administration of insulin will result in glycogen deposition and a shift of K^+ to the intracellular environment. Insulin (0.1 unit/kg per hour) must be accompanied by glucose (approximately 3.5 g/unit of insulin) to prevent hypoglycemia. Potassium may be removed by ion exchange resins, such as sodium polystyrene sulfonate (Kayexalate), which may be given orally or as a retention enema (0.2 g/kg orally or 1 g/kg as an enema). Because ion exchange is not rapid, other measures must be employed simultaneously. Dialysis is efficacious, although it is costly and poses its own risks.

HYPERNATREMIA & HYPONATREMIA

The presence of hypernatremia indicates a loss of proportionately less solute than water. Because of the relative water deficit, hyperosmolality should be anticipated. Severe hypernatremia may precipitate central nervous system injury, seizures, intracerebral bleeding, retardation, and even death. Causes of hypernatremia include inadequate water intake, salt overloading, extrarenal water loss, defective osmoregulation, and water loss with simultaneous gain of solute.

Unconscious patients, patients who cannot swallow or drink, and retarded patients who cannot express thirst are at risk for the development of hypernatremic dehydration.

Salt overloading may occur if formula is mixed incorrectly or if a fluid with a high solute load is ingested. Salt overloading may be a form of child abuse.

Extrarenal water loss is seen in a variety of clinical situations, including prolonged fever, the presence of a tracheostomy, prolonged respiratory distress, heat stroke, and burns, or it may accompany the hyperpnea seen in metabolic disorders, such as diabetic ketoacidosis or salicylism. Anticipating such occurrences may prevent the sequelae.

Defective osmoregulation is uncommonly seen in children. Tumors of the cerebral aqueduct, third ventricle, or anterior hypothalamus may lead to this disorder. Diabetes insipidus in its various forms may be associated with defective osmoregulation, which may be exacerbated by water deprivation or salt loading. Resistance to ADH may be present if there is chronic hypokalemia or hypercalciuria.

Water loss and simultaneous solute gain are associated with a variety of disorders. In straightforward infantile diarrhea, hypernatremia may ensue if the child's diet is high in sodium. Similarly, tube feeding protein-rich foods to an unconscious patient or to an infant may precipitate an osmotic diuresis in which salt is conserved in greater proportion than water. A poorly controlled diabetic with chronic glycosuria may develop osmotic diuresis, attended by sodium conservation and the development of hypernatremia.

Patients with hypernatremia may be lethargic, confused, stuporous, or even comatose. Twitching, seizures, or irregular respirations may be present. The thirst reported in hypernatremic states is profound. Fever may occur due to an inability to sweat. Because there is a relative water deficit in the ECF, body fluids flow from the ICF to the ECF. This shift preserves the extracellular space, and occasionally patients with hypernatremic dehydration lose over 20% of body weight before experiencing vascular collapse. Blood pressure is maintained. Often the severity of hypernatremic dehydration is underestimated due to the maintenance of the vascular space. The skin of a patient with hypernatremic dehydration is doughy or yielding but inelastic.

Extreme care is required to treat hypernatremic dehydration successfully. The cellular space of the brain cannot equilibrate as rapidly as the ECF. If the $[Na^+]_s$ decreases too rapidly, the osmolality of the ECF drops more rapidly than that of the brain. As a result, water leaves the ECF and enters the brain to maintain osmotic neutrality. This shift can lead to cerebral edema, seizures, and death. To prevent this, the $[Na^+]_s$ should not drop more than about 15 meq/L in 24 hours. A drop in $[Na^+]_s > 1$ meq/L/h should be avoided. To affect this gradual decrease in $[Na^+]_s$, the physician should order isotonic solutions to restore deficits in ECW. Electrolyte concentrations and serum osmolality must be monitored frequently. If metabolic acidosis is present, it must be corrected gradually to avoid central nervous system irritability. If hypernatremia has developed gradually and the ECF and BUN are not significantly compromised, hypotonic solutions may be used for rehydration. However, the rate of fall of the serum sodium must not be greater than indicated above. This method involves very gradual administration of fluid and may not be of use if the degree of dehydration is significant. Alterations of blood glucose levels and BUN may contribute to the hyperosmolar state. Hyperglycemia is often seen in hypernatremic dehydration. Hyperglycemia should be monitored closely, since it may contribute significantly to the osmolal disequilibrium.

Hyponatremia may occur with a decrease or increase in the ECF volume. Hyponatremia with a decrease in the volume of ECF is the more typical picture and may be present in association with gastroenteritis, diabetic ketoacidosis, vomiting, renal salt-losing disorders, or adrenal insufficiency.

The typical symptoms and signs of dehydration are present in patients with hyponatremic dehydration. This form of dehydration brings the patient to medical attention rapidly because, in contrast to hyperna-tremic dehydration, the vascular space is selectively compromised as water leaves the vascular space to maintain osmotic neutrality.

The treatment of hyponatremic dehydration is straightforward. The magnitude of the sodium loss may be calculated by the following formula:

$$Na^+_{\text{deficit}} = [Na^+]_{\text{desired}} - [Na^+]_{\text{observed}} \times BW \times V_d$$

where BW = body weight in kilograms and V_d = volume of distribution.

Similar formulas exist for calculating chloride and bicarbonate deficits.

The presence of hyponatremia without a deficit in the ECF is troublesome because it implies a change in osmotic regulation. This picture is usually seen in conjunction with an underlying problem such as renal failure, liver disease, heart disease, or central nervous system damage. In these situations, water restriction and treatment of the underlying defect are the primary keys to therapy.

Whenever there is a rapid decrease in serum osmolality, the central nervous system is at risk. Fluid shifts out of the vascular space and into the central nervous system may occur with intravenous water overload, overly rapid dialysis, or in the treatment of diabetic ketoacidosis if glucose levels are allowed to drop precipitously. Nausea, vomiting, headaches, irritability, twitchiness, or neurologic changes should alert the physician to the possible presence of this disequilibrium syndrome, and steps should be taken to prevent central nervous system injury.

Although most patients tolerate a water load easily, patients with compromised renal function or an obstructive uropathy cannot. In response to a water load, such patients may develop hyponatremia, hyposmolality, and central nervous system insult. Such patients require fluid restriction in addition to treatment of the primary problem.

The syndrome of inappropriate secretion of ADH (SIADH) is also characterized by hyponatremia. SIADH may be seen in wide variety of clinical settings, including meningitis, head injury, pneumonia, cystic fibrosis, intracranial tumors, stress, drugs (barbiturates and opiates), severe pain, and surgery. Patients with this syndrome pass small volumes of concentrated urine and experience thirst. For this reason, water is retained and $[Na^+]_s$ is decreased. Aldosterone secretion is eventually inhibited by the expansion of the ECF. The clinical manifestations of SIADH depend not only on the magnitude of the hyponatremia but also on the rapidity with which the syndrome evolved. The more rapid the change in $[Na^+]_s$, the more significant the clinical sequelae. If the hyponatremia develops gradually, patients do not usually experience symptoms unless the $[Na^+]_s$ is less than 120 meq/L. The effective treatment of SIADH depends on fluid restriction. Administration of isotonic or hypertonic saline elicits a brief, rapid response, but unfortunately this precipitates a saline diuresis and exacerbates the problem.

In cases of severe water intoxication a solution of 3% NaCl may be administered intravenously in the face of frank neurologic disturbances. This should be done to elevate the sodium only to a level at which seizures will not occur.

REHYDRATION

Due to the high worldwide incidence of dehydration caused by infantile diarrhea, the development of effective, inexpensive, technologically independent rehydration fluid has been a major priority. The demonstration of effective oral rehydration in developing countries has led to the introduction of easily administered oral rehydration solutions in developed nations.

The first solutions endorsed by the World Health Organization contained 90 meq/L of Na^+. This concentration was reasonable in areas with a high incidence of cholera, but such solutions may cause hypernatremia in patients who lose less Na^+ or who live in cooler areas, where insensible losses are not as great. In the United States today, a typical effective solution for oral rehydration of patients with mild-to-moderate dehydration contains 50–60 meq/L of Na^+, 20–30 meq/L of K^+, 30 meq/L of HCO_3^-, and enough chloride to provide electroneutrality. Glucose in a concentration of 2–3% provides adequate calories for the short term and facilitates absorption of electrolytes. Some companies offer another oral rehydration formula with greater concentrations of sodium and chloride for more severe cases of dehydration.

In more severe cases of dehydration, especially in patients with intractable vomiting, parenteral (usually intravenous) therapy is necessary to correct dehydration. As mentioned previously, the initial goal of therapy is to provide adequate perfusion. Once perfusion is ensured, acid-base defects may be corrected and deficits of body electrolytes may be replaced. Finally, nutritional deficiencies should be corrected. Unless hypernatremia is present, deficits of water and electrolytes are typically replaced in 24 hours, although potassium replacement generally takes longer.

The physician's first job is to assess the magnitude of dehydration. If previous records are available, comparing the last recorded body weight with the present weight is very helpful. A reliable history enables the physician to estimate fluid losses and intake. The physician should be especially alert for any suggestion in the history or physical that anything other than isotonic dehydration exists. The physician must not only assess the degree of dehydration but also assess and treat factors that affect maintenance fluid requirement, such as respiratory distress or fever.

By separating fluid therapy into three compo-

nents—previous losses, maintenance fluid needs, and ongoing loss—the physician can avoid many problems. Assessing previous losses allows the physician to anticipate the adequacy of perfusion and the type of dehydration that is likely to exist. If abnormal losses, eg, those associated with a stoma, nasogastric suction, or burns, have been present, the appropriate fluid can be analyzed and deficits replaced. The physician calculating maintenance needs must also take into account those metabolic factors that alter needs. In the vast majority of cases, abnormal losses stop once parenteral therapy is initiated. However, by addressing this issue directly, the physician will not overlook abnormal ongoing losses, eg, those associated with a fistula or tracheostomy.

Compromised perfusion (as evidenced by inadequate capillary refill, poor color, increased pulse, decreased urine output, or low blood pressure) constitutes an emergency that must be addressed at once. A 20 mL/kg bolus of fluid should be given intravenously as rapidly as possible. Either colloid or crystalloid may be used. The fluid may be administered intraosseously (the marrow space of the tibia is accessible) or even intraperitoneally if no intravenous site is available. If there is no response to the first bolus, a second may be given. It is important to document urine formation and output. Hypotonic solutions may create a problem unless it is known that hypernatremia is not present.

The magnitude of electrolyte deficit may be estimated from tables such as those previously presented or calculated from the formula (shown in the section on hyponatremic states) in hypotonic dehydration.

$$\frac{\text{Deficit}}{\text{(meq)}} = \frac{\text{(Desired concentration}}{\text{– Observed concentration)}} \times BW \times V_d$$

where BW = body weight (kg) and V_d = volume of distribution.

Potassium defects must be estimated, since deficits cannot be calculated because of the primarily intracellular location of potassium.

Typically, one-half the previous deficits are administered in the first 8 hours of therapy, and the remainder are given over the next 16 hours. Maintenance needs are provided at a steady rate. Ongoing losses are analyzed as needed and replaced at a steady rate as well. If the patient is unable to eat for a prolonged period, nutritional needs must be anticipated and met either through enteral nutrition or hyperalimentation.

It is unfortunately fashionable simply to provide twice the maintenance fluids needed and to assume that time will cure the problem that precipitated the dehydration. This prevents early detection of secondary problems, such as fluid shifts or deficits caused by ongoing losses. By calculating deficits and needs, the physician can monitor the efficacy of therapy as the patient is being treated.

41

Drug Therapy

Cynthia R. Gelman, BS Pharm, Robert G. Peterson, MD, PhD,
& Barry H. Rumack, MD

MANAGEMENT ISSUES IN DRUG THERAPY

Precautions

(1) Older children should never be given a dose greater than the adult dose. In the following pages, adult dosages are noted for the purpose of indicating the maximum dosage in older children when the dosage is calculated on the basis of weight. It must be recognized that on a milligram per kilogram basis, adult dosages are reached at 50 kg, not 70 kg.

(2) All drugs should be used with caution in children, and dosage should be individualized, based on age as well as weight.

(3) Once out of the neonatal period, children usually have more rapid hepatic metabolism than adults. Dosage may have to be adjusted downward for cases of kidney and liver disease, which may impair elimination of certain substances, and for individual metabolic capacities.

(4) The dosage recommendations on the following pages should be regarded only as estimates; careful clinical observations and the use of pertinent laboratory aids are necessary.

(5) Established drugs should be used in preference to newer and less familiar drugs, particularly because pediatric data are rarely submitted for new drugs.

(6) Drugs should be used in early infancy only for significant disorders. In both full-term and premature infants, metabolizing enzymes may be deficient or absent; renal function relatively inefficient; and the blood-brain barrier and protein binding altered.

(7) Dosages for newborn infants have not been determined as accurately as those for older children.

(8) At any age, oliguria requires a reduction of dosage of drugs excreted via the urine.

(9) Whenever possible, reference should also be made to the printed literature supplied by the manufacturer or to the recommendations of the American Academy of Pediatrics Committee on Drugs.

Determination of Drug Dosage

Dosage rules based on proportions of the adult dose are not satisfactory despite their wide use in the past. Dosage based on surface area is probably the most accurate method of estimating the dose for a child if extrapolated adult doses are ever used. Surface area in children can be estimated using Figure 41–1.

Administration of Drugs

A. Route of Administration:

1. Oral–Tablets may be crushed between spoons and given with chocolate, honey, jam, or maple or corn syrup. Many regularly prescribed drugs are commercially available in special pediatric preparations. The parent should be warned that the attractively flavored drug must be kept out of reach of children in the home. Avoid administering drugs with food. Attempt to administer the entire dose in one spoonful.

2. Parenteral–Parenteral administration of certain drugs is necessary, especially in the hospital. Its use as a matter of convenience should be evaluated in the light of the emotional trauma that may result.

3. Rectal–Rectal administration is often very useful, especially for home use. The physician must make certain, however, that rectal absorption is predictable before depending upon this route for a specific drug. Many drugs are prepared in suppository form, but pediatric dose forms are mandatory. It is not good practice to cut an adult suppository.

B. Flavoring Agents for Drugs: Drugs for children should not be so flavorful that they are sought out as "candy." Syrups are more useful as flavoring agents than alcoholic elixirs, because the ethanol content of the latter may produce toxicity.

Refusal of Medications

The administration of a drug to a child requires tact and skill. The parent or nurse should proceed as if protest is not anticipated. Persuasion before it is necessary sets the stage for struggle. The child must understand that the drug will be given despite protest, but great care should be exercised to avoid aspiration in a struggling child.

SPECIAL CONSIDERATIONS IN PEDIATRIC DRUG DOSAGE

The pediatrician must not only be aware of the correct drug dosage and indication but must also take

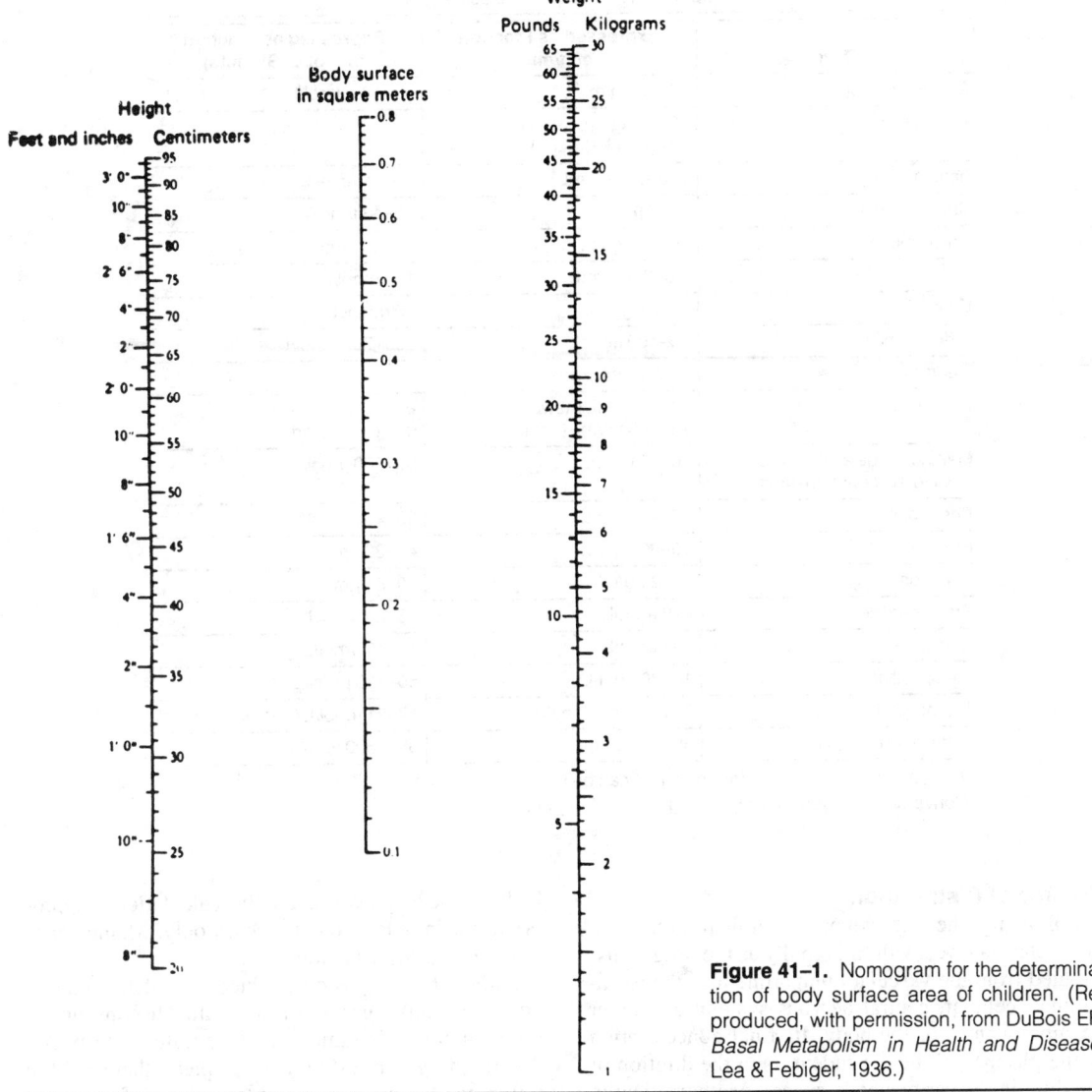

Weight

Pounds   Kilograms

Body surface in square meters

Height

Feet and inches   Centimeters

Figure 41–1. Nomogram for the determination of body surface area of children. (Reproduced, with permission, from DuBois EF: *Basal Metabolism in Health and Disease.* Lea & Febiger, 1936.)

into account optimal frequency of administration as well as rates of absorption, metabolism, and elimination, which may vary widely at different ages and under different conditions. The following approach to rational drug administration in the pediatric age group takes into account various states of renal function, liver metabolism, and body size that affect drug dosage in children.

Therapeutic Range

Determination of plasma levels of drugs can be extremely useful in monitoring therapy. For some drugs (eg, digoxin, theophylline, phenobarbital), the plasma level is well correlated with the drug's physiologic effect and is easier to quantify than the physiologic effect itself. For other classes of drugs (eg, antibiotics, anticoagulants, insulin), it is more important to measure the physiologic effect: serum bactericidal level, prothrombin time, blood glucose, etc.

The therapeutic range is defined as the range of plasma levels for any given drug at which the majority of a treated population will receive the drug's intended therapeutic benefit without experiencing serious toxic side effects. Table 41–1 lists the therapeutic ranges for some drugs commonly used in pediatric practice. Drug toxicity can be expected when plasma levels exceed the therapeutic range.

To obtain a therapeutic level for a particular drug, one must take into account the distribution of the drug throughout the body, whereas maintenance of a therapeutic level requires consideration of elimination processes.

Table 41–1. Therapeutic blood levels.[1]

Drug	Expressed as Fraction of g/mL	Expressed as Fraction of mol/L (SI Units)
Acetaminophen	10–20 µg/mL[2]	65–130 µmol/L
Amikacin	15–30 µg/mL (peak) < 5 µg/mL (trough)	. . .
Aspirin	150–300 µg/mL	1–2.2 mmol/L
Carbamazepine	4–12 µg/mL	16–48 µmol/L
Chloramphenicol	15–30 µg/mL	40–90 µmol/L
Digoxin	0.9–2.4 ng/mL	1–2 nmol/L
Ethanol	1000 µg/mL	20 mmol/L
Ethosuximide	40–100 µg/mL	280–700 µmol/L
Gentamicin	8–10 µg/mL (peak)	. . .
Lidocaine	< 100 ng/mL (newborn) 1.5–2.5 µg/mL (adult)	< 0.4 µmol/L (newborn) 6–9 µmol/L (adult)
Methsuximide as the metabolite of N-des-methsuximide	10–40 µg/mL	50–200 µmol/L
Phenobarbital	15–40 µg/mL	60–160 µmol/L
Phenytoin	10–20 µg/mL	40–80 µmol/L
Primidone	4–12 µg/mL	20–55 µmol/L
Procainamide	4–6 µg/mL	15–20 µmol/L
Quinidine	3–5 µg/mL	10–15 µmol/L
Theophylline	10–20 µg/mL	55–110 µmol/L
Tobramycin	8–10 µg/mL (peak)	17–21 µmol/L (peak)
Valproic acid	50–120 µg/mL	350–800 µmol/L

[1]Therapeutic level or range for drugs that can be routinely analyzed.
[2]Conversions: 1µg/mL = 1 mg/L; 1µg/mL = 0.1 mg/dL.

Volume of Distribution

Following the intravenous administration of a drug, plasma levels will fall rapidly as the drug is distributed from the vascular compartment to the extracellular, cellular, central nervous system, and other "compartments" of the body. Its final concentration in the plasma will be dependent upon the dilution of the drug in the various body spaces. Mathematically, this is expressed as–

$$\text{Plasma level} = \frac{\text{Dose}}{\text{Volume of distribution}}$$

Because different drugs have differing solubilities in the body fluids or bind to tissues to varying degrees, the volume of distribution (V_d) will vary from drug to drug. Table 41–2 gives the V_d values for a number of commonly used drugs. With the therapeutic level (from Table 41–1) and the volume of distribution (from Table 41–2), one can calculate the appropriate loading dose for a number of drugs as follows:

$$\text{Dose (mg/kg)} = \text{Plasma level (mg/L)} \times V_d \text{ (L/kg)}$$

It should be emphasized that this calculation is appropriate for initial or loading doses only. Maintenance doses are discussed below.

Although the V_d is determined from data gathered after intravenous use, it is also a valuable constant for use with oral or intramuscular preparations. Provided that the drug's absorption is complete, there is little difference between a slow intravenous infusion and an intramuscular injection. In an instance where an immediate effect is desired but intramuscular absorption is poor (eg, digoxin, phenytoin, diazepam), the slow intravenous route is preferred.

Renal Elimination

Maintenance of a therapeutic level requires that drugs be administered in amounts equivalent to their elimination. Charged or polar drugs (eg, penicillins, aminoglycosides) are directly excreted by the kidneys, and there is little danger of drug accumulation unless the drug is given more frequently than every half-life. Thus, the recommendation for dosage interval for this type of drug is approximately every one to two half-lives. When drugs are eliminated by renal processes alone, a steady state will be reached after approximately five half-lives, and the plasma level

Table 41–2. Approximate volumes of distribution (V_d) in L/kg.

Acetaminophen	1.0
Amobarbital	1.1
Secobarbital	1.5
Phenobarbital	0.75 (1.0)[1]
Pentobarbital	1.0
Phenytoin	0.75 (1.0)
Amphetamine	0.6
Caffeine	0.9
Salicylate[2]	0.2 (therapeutic doses)
	0.6 (toxic doses)
Furosemide	0.2
Phenothiazines	> 30
Theophylline	0.46 (0.69)
Narcotics	> 5
Penicillins	0.2–0.3
Digoxin	7.5
Local anesthetics	1.0–1.5
Aminoglycosides	0.3–0.5
Benzodiazepines	> 10

[1]Values in parentheses are for newborns.
[2]The V_d of salicylate increases with increasing dose owing to saturation of plasma protein binding.

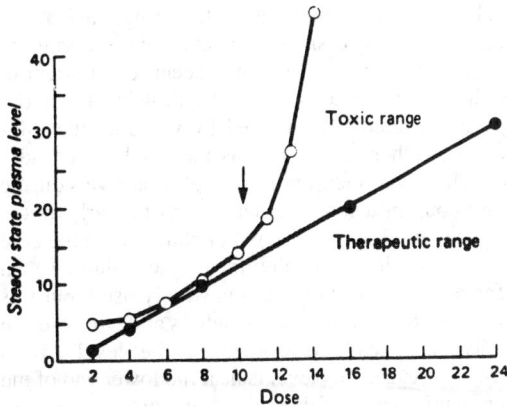

Figure 41–2. Plot (O—O) represents plasma level as a function of increasing dosage of any drug eliminated by hepatic metabolism. Arrow indicates dose at which rapid accumulation of drug occurs. This quantity of administered drug equals capacity of liver metabolism. Dosages above this level cause further rapid increase in plasma level. Plot (●—●) shows data observed with drugs eliminated directly by the kidney without metabolism; observe the difference.

will depend upon the dose and volume of distribution of the drug (see above).

Recommendations for dose and frequency of administration of a large number of medications are given in Average Drug Dosages for Children (below).

Hepatic Elimination

Nonpolar drugs are first metabolized in the liver to make them polar and are then excreted by the kidneys. A steady-state plasma level will be achieved only when the dose given is equivalent to the amount of drug metabolized in the interval between doses.

In deciding on dosages of drugs metabolized in the liver, care must be exercised to make certain that an amount of drug given at a particular frequency does not overwhelm the liver's capacity to metabolize it during the prescribed interval. Figure 41–2 demonstrates the effect of increasing dosage for a drug such as phenytoin upon the plasma level of the drug. As can be observed, one can determine a safe maximum dose (indicated by arrow) above which drug accumulation rapidly occurs. This dose approximates the maximum capacity of the liver for metabolism of this drug.

Drug toxicity can occur rapidly with drugs requiring hepatic elimination. When plasma levels in the upper portion of the therapeutic range are required, frequent plasma determinations should be utilized to avoid drug accumulation.

An example is as follows: A 20-kg child receiving phenytoin (V_d = 0.75 L/kg; see Table 41–2) has a plasma level of 18 µg/mL 4 hours following a daily oral dose. Just prior to the next dose (given at 24-hour intervals), a plasma level is 10 µg/mL. One can estimate the amount metabolized by this child and, therefore, the appropriate maintenance dose by means of the following equations:

$$\text{Fall in plasma level} = 8 \text{ mg/L}$$
$$V_d = 20 \text{ kg} \times 0.75 \text{ L/kg} = 15 \text{ L}$$
$$\text{Dose} = 15 \text{ L} \times 8 \text{ mg/L} = 120 \text{ mg}$$

In 20 hours, 120 mg was eliminated, or 144 mg would be eliminated in 24 hours. The appropriate dose of phenytoin for this child is 144 mg, or 7.2 mg/kg, given every 24 hours.

Table 41–3 outlines examples of drugs that are eliminated by the two routes discussed above.

Continuous Intravenous Infusions

Traditionally, several drugs have been administered by continuous intravenous infusion. Examples are theophylline, insulin, tolazoline, nitroprusside, lidocaine, and dopamine. Continuous intravenous infusion provides a constant amount of drug in the plasma and avoids the "peaks" and "troughs" in plasma lev-

Table 41–3. Principal routes of drug elimination.

Renal	Liver
Aminoglycosides	Acetaminophen[1]
Digoxin	Alcohol
Furosemide	Caffeine
Penicillins	Digitoxin (75%)
Phenobarbital (25%)	Phenobarbital (75%)
	Phenytoin
	Salicylates
	Theophylline

[1]Liver metabolism is rapid, and kinetics appear to be similar to those of drugs excreted by primary renal elimination.

els. For several of the shorter-acting drugs such as dopamine or nitroprusside, it has not been important to measure an actual plasma level because the effect of the drug is readily apparent to the clinician and toxicity can be rapidly terminated by stopping the infusion. For other drugs such as theophylline or lidocaine, however, measurement of plasma levels during continuous infusion is essential, particularly if the drugs are used aggressively. For example, in the case of aminophylline (theophylline ethylenediamine), an infusion rate of 0.9 mg/kg/h is widely used, but this infusion rate is correct only in adults and will result in an average steady-state theophylline level of 10 μg/mL. Because this level is near the lower end of the therapeutic range (Table 41–1), many asthmatics in status asthmaticus will not be adequately treated with this infusion rate. A useful calculation in estimating the infusion rate required to obtain a higher steady-state continuous plasma level is as follows:

$$\text{Infusion rate (mg/kg/h)} = \text{Plasma level (mg/L)} \times \text{Plasma clearance (L/kg/h)}$$

The utility of this formula is that the clinician who has decided on the therapeutic plasma level that is appropriate for an asthmatic patient (low [10 μg/mL], middle [15 μg/mL], or high [20 μg/mL]) can then estimate an appropriate infusion rate. The plasma level in the formula is in mg/L for the sake of equality in the units, but 1 mg/L = 1 μg/mL. The additional value necessary for this estimation, the plasma clearance, is given in Table 41–4. Note that there are distinct differences in plasma clearance in different age groups; the greater theophylline clearance in younger children requires a larger rate of infusion than used in adults.

If one wishes to estimate the theophylline infusion rate necessary to maintain a plasma level of 15 μg/mL in a 5-year-old child, the calculation would be:

$$\text{Rate (mg/kg/h)} = 15 \text{ (mg/L)} \times 0.1 \text{ (L/kg/h)}$$
$$= 1.5 \text{ (mg/kg/h)}$$

A continuous infusion should be initiated following a loading dose of theophylline based upon the V_d calculation to give an initial plasma level of 15 μg/mL.

These calculations do not take the place of laboratory monitoring of theophylline levels but provide a reference point to aid in dosage recommendations. In the case of theophylline, the use of a higher molecular weight dosage form, ie, aminophylline, will require an increment to be made in the dose administered. Also, theophylline elimination may not be linear at higher infusion rates. Drug accumulation should always be assessed by plasma levels.

Summary

The therapeutic ranges for a number of drugs are presented in Table 41–1. The measurement of plasma levels during therapy will facilitate the regulation of dosage to produce therapeutic effects without toxicity. Drugs whose elimination is dependent chiefly upon hepatic metabolism require special surveillance. Average Drug Dosages for Children (below) lists a number of drugs used in pediatric patients along with the appropriate dose and frequency for each.

DRUGS & BREAST FEEDING

Most drugs are excreted to some degree in breast milk, but this is not a pharmacologically important route for maternal drug elimination. Toxic quantities are rarely delivered to the infant by this route, and levels of drugs in breast milk rarely exceed levels in maternal plasma. In those cases where levels in milk have been reported to exceed the plasma level, the ratio is seldom greater than 1.5:1; ratios above 10:1 have not been reported for therapeutic agents. Quantitative drug overdose of the infant via breast milk is virtually never a problem.

Before administering a drug to a lactating woman, the following questions should be answered:

(1) Is the maternal drug therapy really necessary?

(2) Is this the least toxic drug that is effective?

(3) Can the dosing schedule be arranged to minimize delivery of the drug to the infant?

(4) Would this drug be given directly to the infant if the infant had an appropriate pediatric illness?

(5) In those instances where parenteral medications are given to the mother, is the drug absorbed by the oral route as it is delivered to the infant?

(6) Are idiosyncratic or allergic reactions a particular concern for this infant?

(7) Are there side effects? Will they be easily recognized (eg, drowsiness, rash, etc)?

(8) Does the infant have a known medical problem (eg, hepatic disease or renal disease) that would diminish the drug's excretion and thereby allow it to accumulate in the infant?

(9) Does the infant have a suspected medical problem (eg, suspected infection masked by low-dose antibiotic delivery via milk) whose eventual diagnosis might be delayed by subtherapeutic doses of the maternal drug?

(10) Will the amount of drug delivered via breast milk come close to approaching a therapeutic dose in the infant?

Table 41–4. Plasma theophylline clearance.

Age	Clearance (L/kg/h)
Newborn	0.018
Children (1–10 years)	0.10
Adults	0.07

The answers to these questions usually will give the health care provider the information needed to know whether a drug should be given to the mother.

Quantitative drug overdose of the infant via breast milk is virtually never an issue, but idiosyncratic or allergic reactions to drugs are often not dose-related, and this aspect of drug administration should be kept in mind.

Some drugs are relatively safe in the adult (eg, radioactive iodine) but are associated with higher toxicity rates in children. These drugs, as well as other radiolabeled compounds, many cancer chemotherapeutic agents, and organ-selective toxic substances, should not be given to the mother if breast feeding is to be continued.

AVERAGE DRUG DOSAGES FOR CHILDREN*

Acetaminophen: Dose based on weight is 10–15 mg/kg orally. Dose based on age is generally as follows: 0–3 months, 40 mg; 4–11 months, 80 mg; 12–23 months, 120 mg; 2–3 years, 160 mg; 4–5 years, 180 mg; 6–8 years, 320 mg; 9–10 years, 400 mg; 11–12 years, 480 mg. May be repeated up to 5 times in 24 hours.

Acetazolamide: 5–30 mg/kg/d orally every 6–8 hours (Adult = 5 mg/kg/d.) For hydrocephalus, 20–55 mg/kg/d orally in two or three divided doses. For anticonvulsant use, see Table 25–15.

Acetylcysteine: For acetaminophen antidote, use 20% solution diluted 3:1 with juice, water, or carbonated beverage, 140 mg/kg orally (loading dose) followed by 17 doses of 70 mg/kg orally every 4 hours.

ACTH (adrenocorticotropic hormone, corticotropin): For infantile spasms, usually 20–40 units/d or (in gel form) 80 units every other day intramuscularly. For anticonvulsant use, see Seizure Disorders in Chapter 25.

Acyclovir: For mucocutaneous HSV infection, 15 mg/kg/24 h intravenously every 8 hours for 5–10 days. For HSV encephalitis, 30 mg/kg/24 h intravenously every 8 hours for 10 days. For varicella-zoster infection 10–20 mg/kg/dose orally four times a day (maximum dose = 800 mg).

Albumin, human 25%: 0.5–1 g/kg intravenously as 25 g/dL solution. Maximum, up to 25 g per dose, as required.

Albuterol: For children 2–6 years, 0.1 mg/kg orally to a maximum of 4 mg/dose three times

daily. For children 6–12 years, 2 mg orally three or four times daily. Inhaler, for children < 12 years, one or two inhalations (90 μg/spray) four times a day, using tube spacer.

Alprostadil (prostaglandin E₁): To maintain patency of ductus arteriosus in patients with congenital heart lesions, 0.05–0.1 μg/kg/min by continuous infusion.

Aluminum hydroxide gel: 5–15 mL orally with meals.

Amantadine hydrochloride: 4.4–8.8 mg/kg/d orally.

Aminocaproic acid: 200 mg/kg orally, then 100 mg/kg/dose orally every 6 hours for 3–7 days (adult maximum = 30 g/24 h).

Aminophylline: For neonatal apnea, 4–6 mg/kg intravenously (see Special Considerations in Pediatric Drug Dosage, above). Intramuscular or rectal administration is not recommended.

Ammonium chloride: For urinary acidification, 75 mg/kg/d orally in four divided doses.

Aspirin: Not recommended for routine analgesic or antipyretic use in children. For rheumatoid arthritis, 80–100 mg/kg/d to maintain a blood level of 20–30 mg/dL. (Adult maximum = 6–8 g/d.) Monitor plasma levels and liver function during therapy.

Atropine sulfate: 0.01–0.03 mg/kg subcutaneously, intravenously, or endotracheally. Maximum = 0.04 mg/kg or 2 mg. For cardiac arrest, use intravenous or endotracheal route. For breath-holding spells, see Seizure Disorders in Chapter 25. *Caution.*

Azathioprine: 3–5 mg/kg/d orally initially, followed by 1–3 mg/kg/d.

Beclomethasone dipropionate: For reactive airway disease, one or two puffs every 6–8 hours. Metered aerosol delivers 42 μg per puff.

Benzoyl peroxide: Apply one to three times daily after washing face.

Benztropine mesylate: For drug-induced extrapyramidal reaction, 0.02–0.05 mg/kg/dose 1–2 times daily in children > 3 years of age. For parkinsonism, 0.5–1 mg/dose every 12 hours or daily.

Bethanechol chloride: Orally, 0.6 mg/kg/d in three divided doses. (Adult = 10–30 mg three or four times daily.) Subcutaneously, 0.15–0.2 mg/kg/d. (Adult = 2.5–5 mg/d.)

Bisacodyl: 5 mg orally or rectally. Children over 2 years, up to 10 mg rectally.

Bretylium tosylate: For ventricular arrhythmias, 5 mg/kg/dose every 6 hours intramuscularly or diluted in 5% dextrose in water or in normal saline over 10–30 minutes.

Brompheniramine: For children under 6 years, 0.5 mg/kg/d orally. For children over 6 years, 4 mg three or four times daily. (Adult = 4–8 mg three or four times daily.)

---

*For drugs discussed in other chapters, consult the index.

Busulfan: 0.06–0.12 mg/kg/d orally. (Adult = 4–8 mg daily.)

Calcium chloride (27% calcium): For newborns and infants, 0.2 g/kg/d orally as a 2% solution. For children, 0.3 g/kg/d. (Adult = 2–4 g three times daily.) *Caution.*

Calcium glubionate (6% calcium): 600–2000 mg/kg/d given in four doses. (Adult = 6–18 g/d.)

Calcium gluconate (9% calcium): For neonates, 200–400 mg/kg/24 h by continuous intravenous infusion. For infants and children, 200–1000 mg/kg/24 h by continuous intravenous infusion. (Adult = 2–15 g/24 h.) *Caution.*

Calcium lactate (13% calcium): 0.5 g/kg/d orally in divided doses as dilute solution. (Adult = 4–8 g three times daily.)

Captopril: For neonates, 0.05–0.1 mg/kg/dose every 8–24 hours initially; titrate to 0.5 mg/kg/dose every 6–24 hours. For infants, 0.15–0.3 mg/kg/dose initially; titrate to maximum of 6 mg/kg/d. For children, 0.5 mg/kg/dose initially; titrate to maximum of 6 mg/kg/d in 2–4 divided doses.

Charcoal, activated: 1–2 g/kg mixed in water and given orally or by orogastric tube. 20–30 g should be diluted in 8 oz of water.

Chloral hydrate: As hypnotic, 12.5–50 mg/kg (up to 1 g) orally or rectally. (Adult = 0.5–2 g.) As sedative, 4–20 mg/kg (up to 1 g) orally or rectally. (Adult = 0.25–1 g.) May be repeated in 1 hour to obtain desired effect, and then may be repeated every 6–8 hours.

Chlorambucil: 0.1–0.2 mg/kg/d orally. (Adult = 0.2 mg/kg/d.)

Chlordiazepoxide: For children over 6 years, 0.5 mg/kg/d orally in three or four divided doses.

Chlorothiazide: For children under 6 months, 30 mg/kg/d orally in two divided doses. For older children, 20 mg/kg/d. (Adult = 0.5–1 g once or twice daily.)

Chlorpheniramine: 0.35 mg/kg/d orally in four divided doses or subcutaneously. (Adult = 2–4 mg three or four times daily; long-acting, 8–12 mg two or three times daily.)

Chlorpromazine: Orally, 0.25–6 mg/kg/d in four to six divided doses. (Adult maximum = 1–2 g/d.) Intramuscularly, for children up to 5 years, 0.5 mg/kg every 6–8 hours as necessary but not over 40 mg/d; for children 5–12 years, not over 75 mg/d. (Adult = 25–100 mg per dose.) Rectally, 1 mg/kg per dose. (Adult = 10–50 mg per dose.)

Cholestyramine: 240 mg/kg/24 h in three divided doses. (*Note:* FDA warns that the dosage for children has not been established and the effects of long-term use are not known.) (Adult = 3–4 g three or four times daily.)

Cimetidine: For neonates, 5–10 mg/kg/d orally intramuscularly or intravenously in two or three divided doses. For infants, 10–20 mg/kg/d in two to four divided doses. For children, 20–30 mg/kg/d in four divided doses. (Adult = 300 mg four times daily.)

Ciprofloxacin: 20–30 mg/kg/d in two divided doses. (Maximum = 1.5 g/d.) (*Note:* Ciprofloxacin is not approved by FDA for use in children.)

Citrovorum factor (leucovorin calcium): 2–15 mg/d orally.

Clonazepam: 0.01 mg/kg/d orally in divided doses every 8 hours to start. Increase slowly to 0.1–0.2 mg/kg/d. See also Table 25–15.

Clonidine hydrochloride: For hypertension, 1–5 μg/kg/dose every 6 hours orally or as transdermal patch, 0.1–0.3 mg/24 hours. *Caution:* Rebound hypertension on discontinuation.

Cocaine: Topical, maximum dose = 1 mg/kg.

Codeine phosphate: Orally, 0.8–1.5 mg/kg as a single sedative or analgesic dose. (Adult = 8–60 mg every 4–6 hours.) Subcutaneously, 0.8 mg/kg. (Adult = 30 mg.) For cough, 0.2 mg/kg every 4–6 hours.

Corticotropin (adrenocorticotropic hormone, ACTH): For infantile spasms, usually 20–40 units/d or (in gel form) 80 units every other day intramuscularly. For anticonvulsant use, see Seizure Disorders in Chapter 25.

Co-Trimoxazole: See Trimethoprim and sulfamethoxazole, below.

Cromolyn sodium: One 20 mg capsule inhaled with a Spinhaler four times daily or two inhalations from a metered-dose dispenser. *Caution:* Should not be used during asthmatic attack.

Cyclizine: For children 6–10 years, 3 mg/kg/d orally in three divided doses. For adolescents, 50 mg every 4–6 hours as necessary (same as adult dose).

Cyclophosphamide: 2–8 mg/kg/d orally or intravenously for 7 or more days or 15–50 mg/kg once a week.

Cyclosporine: Initially, 5–6 mg/kg/d intravenously in divided doses every 12–24 h or 14–18 mg/kg/dose orally. Maintenance, 5–10 mg/kg/d orally.

Cyproheptadine hydrochloride: 0.25 mg/kg/d orally in three or four divided doses. (Adult = 12–16 mg/d.)

Cytarabine (cytosine arabinoside): 200 mg/m²/d intravenously for 5 days every 2 weeks.

Dactinomycin: 0.015 mg/kg/d intravenously for 5 days (same as adult dose).

Dantrolene sodium: For malignant hyperthermia prophylaxis, 1–2 mg/kg orally every 8 hours, starting 24–48 hours prior to anesthesia. For malignant hyperthermia treatment, 1 mg/kg intravenously as initial dose, and then increase by 0.5–1 mg/kg as required. Maximum dose = 10 mg/kg.

Deferoxamine mesylate: Intramuscularly, 90 mg/kg (up to 1 g) every 8 hours. Intravenously,

15 mg/kg/h by continuous infusion. *Caution:* Hypotension.

Dextroamphetamine: For children 3–5 years, 2.5 mg daily increased by 2.5 mg at weekly intervals; for children 6 years and older, 5–10 mg/d increased by 5 mg at weekly intervals. For anticonvulsant use, see Table 25–15.

Dextromethorphan hydrobromide: 1 mg/kg/d orally in divided doses.

Diazepam: Orally, 0.12–0.8 mg/kg/d in four divided doses. (Adult = 5–10 mg per dose.) Intravenously, 0.04–0.2 mg/kg slowly as a single dose. (Adult = 5–10 mg per dose.) See also Table 25–15.

Diazoxide: For hypertensive crisis, 3–5 mg/kg intravenously as bolus into peripheral vein within 30 seconds (maximum dose = 150 mg). May repeat in 5–15 minutes and then 4–24 hours. *Caution:* Monitor for sodium retention and hyperglycemia.

Dicyclomine hydrochloride: For infants, 5 mg orally (as syrup) three or four times daily. For children, 10 mg three or four times daily. (Adult = 10–20 mg three or four times daily.)

Digoxin: Digitalizing dose: 30 μg/kg over 24 hours as 15 μg/kg, then 7.5 μg/kg at 8- to 12-hour intervals orally or intravenously. Intramuscular administration not recommended. Maintenance: 10–15 μg/kg/24 h orally in one or two doses.

Dihydrotachysterol: Initially, 0.1–0.5 mg orally daily. (Adult = 0.5–1 mg/d.)

Dimenhydrinate: 1–1.5 mg/kg orally every 6 hours as needed. (Adult = 50–100 mg every 6 hours as needed.)

Dimercaprol (BAL): 2.5–3 mg/kg intramuscularly every 4 hours for 2 days, four times per day on day 3, then twice a day for 10 days.

Diphenhydramine hydrochloride: Orally, 4–6 mg/kg/d in three or four divided doses. (Adult = 100–200 mg/d.)

Diphenoxylate hydrochloride with atropine: Contraindicated in children under 2 years. Dose based on weight is 0.3–0.4 mg/kg administered in four divided doses. Dose based on age is generally as follows: 2–5 years, 2 mg three times a day; 5–8 years, 2 mg four times a day; 8–12 years, 2 mg five times a day.

Dobutamine: 2.5–15 μg/kg/min by continuous infusion. Incompatible with sodium bicarbonate in same line.

Docusate: Infants and children under 3 years, 10–40 mg/d orally; children 3–6 years, 20–60 mg/d orally; children 6–12 years, 40–120 mg/d orally. (Adults = 50–200 mg/d.)

Dopamine: 5–20 μg/kg/min by continuous intravenous infusion.

Doxylamine succinate: 2 mg/kg/d orally.

Edrophonium chloride: As test dose for infant, 0.2 mg/kg intravenously. Give only one-fifth of dose slowly initially; if tolerated, give remainder. (Adult = 5–10 mg.) For myasthenia gravis, see Chapter 25. *Caution:* Atropine should be available as antidote.

EDTA (calcium disodium salt, calcium EDTA, edetate calcium disodium): 50–75 mg/kg/d intravenously or intramuscularly in solution containing procaine, 0.5–1.5%.

Ephedrine sulfate: Intravenously, 0.8–1.2 mg/kg/d in four divided doses.

Epinephrine solution, 1:10,000 aqueous: 0.01 mg/kg (0.1 mL/kg) intravenously or via endotracheal tube. Dilute endotracheal doses with 1–2 mL normal saline.

Epinephrine solution, 1:1000 aqueous: Subcutaneously, 0.01–0.025 mL/kg. Maximum = 0.5 mL. (Adult = 0.5–1 mL.) For cardiac arrest, 0.01 mL/kg intravenously or via endotracheal tube.

Epinephrine solution, 1:200 aqueous: 0.004–0.005 mL/kg subcutaneously. Maximum = 0.15 mL every 8–12 hours.

Ergocalciferol (vitamin D$_2$): For renal osteodystrophy, 25,000–200,000 units/d orally. For hypoparathyroidism, 2000 IU/d (50 μg/kg/d) orally.

Estradiol valerate: For teenage girls, 10 mg/month intramuscularly. (Adult = 10–20 mg every 2–3 weeks.)

Ethosuximide: For children 3–6 years, 250 mg/d orally as starting dose. For children over 6 years, 250 mg twice daily as starting dose. See also Table 25–15.

Ferrous salts (medicinal iron): Elemental iron, 6–9 mg/kg/d orally in three divided doses. For iron deficiency anemia, see Chapter 28.

Filgrastim: 5–10 μg/kg/d for up to 14 days.

Fluorouracil: 12 mg/kg intravenously (up to 800 mg/d) for 4 successive days. If no toxicity is observed, give 6 mg/kg on the sixth, eighth, tenth, and twelfth days. If toxicity has not been a problem, the course of therapy may be repeated beginning 30 days after the last day of the previous course.

Flurazepam hydrochloride: Not recommended for children under 15 years. For adolescents and adults, 15–30 mg orally at bedtime for sleep.

Folic acid: 0.2–1 mg/d orally. (Adult = 1–3 mg/d.)

Folinic acid: See Leucovorin calcium.

Furazolidone: For children over 1 month of age, 5–8.8 mg/kg/d in four divided doses (maximum = 400 mg/d).

Furosemide: 1 mg/kg intravenously or intramuscularly, or 2 mg/kg orally. (Adult = 40–80 mg intravenously, intramuscularly, or orally in the morning for diuresis or 40 mg orally twice daily for hypertension.) For altered states of consciousness, see Chapter 25.

Glucagon: For newborns, 0.025–0.1 mg/kg intravenously as a single dose. Try smaller dose first. May repeat in 30 minutes. For older children,

0.25–1 mg subcutaneously, intramuscularly, or intravenously as a single dose. Maximum = 1 mg.

Gold sodium thiomalate: 1 mg/kg/wk intramuscularly.

Guanethidine: 0.2 mg/kg/d orally as a single dose. Increase dose at weekly intervals by same amount. (Adult = 10 mg/d; larger doses possible for hospitalized adults.) *Caution.*

Haloperidol: Children 3–12 years, 0.05–0.15 mg/kg/d in two or three doses (maximum = 6 mg/d). (Adult = 1–2 mg orally two or three times daily initially and then 1–2 mg three or four times daily for maintenance; maximum = 15 mg/d.)

Heparin: 50–100 units/kg intravenously as loading dose. May be followed by continuous infusion of 10–25 units/kg/h or by 40–100 units/kg subcutaneously every 4 hours. Control dosage with clotting times, and follow partial thromboplastin time. May prolong clotting for 24 hours.

Histamine: For provocative test, 0.0275 mg/kg subcutaneously. *Caution:* Phentolamine should be available.

Hydralazine hydrochloride: Orally, 0.75–1 mg/kg/d divided in 2–4 doses (maximum = 25 mg/dose). (Adult = 100 mg as single oral dose.) Intravenously or intramuscularly, 1.5–3.5 mg/kg/d in four to six divided doses. (Adult = 20–40 mg as initial parenteral dose.)

Hydrochlorothiazide: For children under 6 months, 2–3 mg/kg/d in two divided doses. For older children, 2 mg/kg/d as a single dose or in two divided doses. (Adult = 25–200 mg/d.)

Hydroxyzine: Orally, 1–2 mg/kg/d in three divided doses. (Adult = 25–50 mg three times daily.) Intramuscularly for preoperative use, 1 mg/kg/dose every 6 hours.

Ibuprofen: As an antipyretic in children 6 months to 12 years of age, 5–10 mg/kg/dose every 6–8 hours (maximum = 40 mg/kg/d). As analgesic, 4–10 mg/kg/dose every 6–8 hours.

Imipramine hydrochloride: Not generally recommended for children under 6 years. For older children, 25 mg/d orally as initial dose; may increase according to response and tolerance. For adolescents, generally not more than 75 mg/d. (Adult = 75 mg initially, increased to up to 150 mg/d.) *Caution.*

Indomethacin: For closure of patent ductus arteriosus, 0.2 mg/kg initially followed with two doses of 0.1 mg/kg at 12–24 hour intervals if less than 48 hours of age at first dose. *Caution:* Monitor vital signs and urinary output.

Ipecac syrup: 15–20 mL orally initially. (Adult = 30 mL.) Give water. Ambulate. Repeat in 20 minutes if necessary. *Caution:* Never use fluidextract of ipecac as emetic.

Isoproterenol: One or two metered doses up to five times per day. Nebulization, 0.01 mL/kg

(minimum = 0.1 mL; maximum = 0.5 mL). (Adult = 5 mg sublingually four times daily.) For hypotension, 0.05–2 µg/kg/min by continuous intravenous infusion.

Kaolin with pectin: For children 3–6 years, 15–30 mL. For children 6–12 years, 30–60 mL.

Ketoconazole: 5–10 mg/kg/d in one or two divided doses. Topically, 2% cream once daily for 2–4 weeks.

Leucovorin calcium (citrovorum factor): 2–15 mg/d orally.

Levothyroxine sodium (L-thyroxine): 0.1 mg of levothyroxine sodium = 65 mg of thyroid USP = 25–30 µg of triiodothyronine. For hypothyroidism, see Chapter 27.

Lidocaine: For ventricular ectopy, 0.5–1 mg/kg intravenously slowly. May repeat after 5–10 minutes for additional control. Give continuous intravenous infusion of 20–50 µg/kg/min following loading dose. Measure plasma levels during infusions. For seizures, 0.2–0.5 mg/kg as loading dose, followed by 5–15 µg/kg/min by continuous intravenous infusion. See Table 22–15. (Adult = 50–100 mg.) Local infiltration, 7 mg/kg with epinephrine; 4.5 mg/kg without epinephrine. Topically, 3 mg/kg. *Caution:* Do not repeat within 2 hours.

Lindane: For scabies, 1% lotion, applied to entire body. Wash carefully after 6 hours. Not for use in infants. *Caution:* Toxic with long or repeated contact.

Loperamide: For acute diarrhea: 2–5 years, 1 mg three times daily; 6–8 years, 2 mg twice daily; 8–12 years, 2 mg three times daily. For chronic diarrhea: 0.08–0.24 mg/kg/d in two or three divided doses.

Lorazepam: For seizures, 0.03–0.05 mg/kg slowly intravenously. See Table 25–15. (Adult maximum = 2.5–10 mg.) Repeat once in 15 minutes if required.

Lypressin (8-lysine vasopressin): One or two sprays into each nostril four times a day.

Magnesium hydroxide (milk of magnesia): 0.5–1 mL/kg orally. (Adult = 30–60 mL.)

Magnesium sulfate: As cathartic, 250 mg/kg orally. As anticonvulsant for hypertension, use 20% solution, 20–40 mg/kg intramuscularly every 4–6 hours. *Caution:* Check blood pressure carefully, and have calcium gluconate available.

Mannitol: As test dose for oliguria, 0.75 g/kg intravenously. For cerebral edema, 1–3 g/kg over a period of 30 minutes to 6 hours. For altered states of consciousness, see Chapter 25.

Mebendazole: For pinworm, 100 mg as a single oral dose; repeat after 2 weeks; for hookworm or roundworm, 100 mg twice a day for 3 days.

Mechlorethamine (nitrogen mustard): 0.1 mg/kg/d intravenously for 4 days (same as adult dose). Dilute and inject slowly.

Menadiol sodium diphosphate: For newborns, see Phytonadione. For older infants and children, 5–10 mg intramuscularly. (Adult = 5–15 mg.)

Meperidine hydrochloride (pethidine hydrochloride): 0.6–1.5 mg/kg intramuscularly, intravenously, or orally as a single analgesic dose. Maximum = 6 mg/kg/d. (Adult = 50–100 mg intramuscularly, intravenously, or orally every 4–6 hours.)

Mephenytoin: 3–15 mg/kg/d orally. Start with smaller dose and gradually increase. (Adult = 0.2–0.6 g daily.) See also Table 25–15.

Mercaptopurine (6-MP): 2.5 mg/kg/d orally (same as adult dose). *Caution.*

Metaraminol: Subcutaneously or intramuscularly, 0.1 mg/kg. Intravenously, 0.01 mg/kg. Titrate by effect or by blood pressure readings. (Adult = 2–10 mg intramuscularly or 0.5–5 mg intravenously.)

Methadone hydrochloride: For analgesia, 0.7 mg/kg/d orally in two divided doses.

Methimazole: Initially, 0.5–0.7 mg/kg/d orally in three divided doses. Maximum = 30 mg/d. For maintenance, half of initial dose. (Adult = 30 mg/d.)

Methionine: 200–300 mg/d orally in three or four divided doses. (Adult dose to acidify urine = 12–15 g/d orally.)

Methocarbamol: For tetanus, 15 mg/kg intravenously every 6 hours.

Methotrexate: For juvenile rheumatoid arthritis, 5–15 mg/m²/wk as a single oral dose or as three divided doses given 12 hours apart.

Methyldopa: Intravenously, 5–10 mg/kg every 6–8 hours to a total of 65 mg/kg/d. Dilute in 50–100 mL of fluid and infuse over 30–60 minutes. Orally, 10 mg/kg/d in divided doses every 6 hours, increasing at 2-day or greater intervals to 65 mg/kg/d. (Adult = 250 mg orally three times daily initially, adjusted at 2- to 7-day intervals.) *Caution.*

Methylene blue: 1% solution, 0.1–0.2 mL/kg (1–2 mg/kg) slowly intravenously. (Adult = 100–150 mg per dose.)

Methylphenidate hydrochloride: 0.2 mg/kg dose given orally with breakfast and lunch. (Adult = 10 mg three times daily.) Not recommended for children under 6 years of age. For attention deficit disorder, see Chapter 6.

Methyltestosterone: 10–50 mg daily orally; 5–25 mg daily buccally.

Metoclopramide hydrochloride: 0.1 mg/kg orally intramuscularly, intravenously up to four times daily. Total daily dose not to exceed 0.5 mg/kg. For chemotherapy-induced emesis, 1–2 mg/kg intravenously.

Midazolam: For anesthesia induction, 0.035 mg/kg/dose intravenously, repeated over several minutes as required up to a total dose of 0.1–0.2 mg/kg. For conscious sedation, 0.1–0.4 mg/kg (maximum 15 mg).

Mineral oil (liquid paraffin, liquid petrolatum): 10–20 mL twice daily. (Adult = 15–30 mL.)

Morphine sulfate: Orally, 0.2–0.5 mg/kg/dose every 4–6 hours. Intravenously or intramuscularly, 0.1–0.2 mg/kg/dose (maximum = 15 mg/kg/dose). (Adult = 10–15 mg.)

Muromonab-CD/3: For children < 30 kg, 2.5 mg/d intravenously for 10–14 days.

Naloxone hydrochloride: Usual dose is 0.01 mg/kg intravenously. In patients who are significantly depressed, the first dose should be 0.4 mg for those under 5 years and 0.8 mg for those over 5 years. If patient is still unresponsive, 2–4 mg may be given once intravenously to rule out opiate overdose.

Neostigmine: Orally, 7.5–15 mg three or four times daily. (Adult = 15 mg three times a day.) For myasthenia test, 0.025–0.04 mg/kg intramuscularly (see also Chapter 22). *Caution:* Atropine should be available.

Nifedipine: For hypertensive emergencies, 0.25–0.5 mg/kg/dose.

Nitroprusside: For hypertensive emergencies, 0.5–10 µg/kg/min as a continuous intravenous infusion. Start with lowest dose, and titrate blood pressure by increasing infusion by 0.3 µg/kg/min every 5 minutes.

Norepinephrine (levarterenol): Start at 0.1 µg/kg/min intravenously and titrate rate by blood pressure. For adrenal crisis, see Chapter 30.

Oxymetazoline hydrochloride: For children 2–5 years, 2–3 drops of a 0.025% solution in each nostril twice daily. For children over 6 years, 2 or 3 drops in each nostril twice daily. *Caution:* Do not use for more than 3 days.

Pancrelipase (pancreatic replacement): Three to twelve capsules or one to four teaspoonfuls of powder with each meal.

Paraldehyde: For sedation, 0.3 mL/kg orally or rectally. (Adult = 5–10 mL.) As hypnotic, 0.3 mL/kg. (Adult = 10–30 mL.) For rectal solutions, mix paraldehyde in one or two parts of vegetable oil. Do not use plastic equipment.

Paregoric (opium tincture, camphorated): Morphine content is 0.4 mg/mL. For newborns, 0.2–0.5 mL (0.08–0.2 mg morphine equivalents) orally every 3–4 hours until symptoms of withdrawal are controlled. For children, 0.25–0.5 mL/kg (not to exceed 10 mL) up to 4 times daily for diarrhea.

Penicillamine (D-isomer penicillamine): For arsenic poisoning, for infants over 6 months, 100 mg/kg/d orally in four divided doses. Maximum = 1 g/d. For Wilson's disease in infants, 250–500 mg daily.

Pentamidine: For treatment (intramuscularly and intravenously), 4 mg/kg/d as single dose for

14–21 days. For prevention (intramuscularly and intravenously), 4 mg/kg monthly or biweekly. Inhalation (children ≥ 5 years), 300 mg/dose given every 3 weeks or monthly.

Pentobarbital: 2–6 mg/kg orally. Intravenously, 3–5 mg/kg. (Adult = 100 mg.)

Phenobarbital: As sedative, 0.5–2 mg/kg orally every 4–6 hours. As anticonvulsant loading dose, 5–10 mg/kg intramuscularly (to receive 20 mg/kg in 24 hours). For maintenance, 5 mg/kg/d in two or three divided doses. See also Table 25–15.

Phentolamine: For hypertensive crisis, 0.05–0.1 mg/kg intravenously every 5 minutes until blood pressure is controlled. *Caution:* Avoid hypotension.

Phenytoin: For loading dose, 10–20 mg/kg intravenously slowly, not to exceed 1 mg/kg/min. (Adult = 500–1000 mg per dose.) For maintenance, 5–10 mg/kg/d orally as a single dose or in two divided doses. (Adult = 0.3–0.5 g/d.) See also Table 25–15.

Phytonadione (vitamin K₁): For prophylactic dose, 0.5–1 mg intramuscularly. For therapeutic dose, 1–2 mg intramuscularly, subcutaneously, or orally. (Mephyton for oral use; others for parenteral use.)

Pilocarpine: 0.25%, 0.5%, 1%, and 2% as eye drops.

Polyethylene glycol electrolyte solution: 25–40 mL/kg/h.

Potassium iodide: Saturated solution, 0.1–0.3 mL/d in two or three doses orally in cold milk or fruit juice. (Adult = 0.3 mL.)

Pralidoxime: 5% solution, 25–50 mg/kg intravenously.

Prednisolone: For acute asthma, 1–2 mg/kg/24 h orally once or twice a day for 3–5 days.

Primidone: 10–25 mg/kg/d orally. For children under 8 years, start with 125 mg daily; for those over 8 years, start with 250 mg daily. Increase dose slowly as necessary. (Adult = 250 mg as initial dose.) See also Table 22–15.

Probenecid: 25 mg/kg orally as initial dose and then 10 mg/kg every 6 hours. (Adult = 1–2 g as initial dose and then 0.5 g every 6 hours.)

Procainamide hydrochloride: Orally, 3–10 mg/kg every 4–6 hours. Intramuscularly, 6 mg/kg every 4–6 hours. Intravenously, for emergency use only, 2 mg/kg slowly over a 4- to 20-minute period. *Caution:* Monitor by continuous electrocardiography and blood pressure recording every minute.

Procarbazine hydrochloride: 50 mg/d orally as initial dose. *Caution.*

Prochlorperazine: For children greater than 10 kg, 0.4 mg/kg/d in three or four divided doses orally or rectally. (Adult = 25 mg rectally twice daily or 5 mg orally three or four times daily.)

Intramuscularly, 0.1–0.15 mg/kg/dose. *Caution:* Avoid overdosage; irritant to tissue.

Promethazine hydrochloride: As antihistaminic, 0.5 mg/kg orally at bedtime; 0.1 mg/kg orally three times daily. For nausea and vomiting, 0.25–0.5 mg/kg rectally or intramuscularly. For sedation, 0.5–1 mg/kg intramuscularly.

Propantheline bromide: 1–3 mg/kg/d orally in four divided doses after meals. (Adult = 15–30 mg three or four times daily.)

Propranolol: Intravenously, 0.01–0.15 mg/kg as slow push; tetralogy spells may require up to 0.25 mg/kg intravenously. Orally, 0.5–4 mg/kg/d given every 6–8 hours. For headaches, see Chapter 22.

Propylthiouracil: For children 6–10 years, 50–150 mg/d; for children older than 10 years, 150–300 mg/d.

Prostaglandin E₁ (alprostadil): To maintain patency of ductus arteriosus in patients with congenital heart lesions, 0.05–0.1 μg/kg/min by continuous infusion.

Protamine sulfate: 1 mg per 100 units of administered heparin.

Pseudoephedrine hydrochloride: 4 mg/kg/d orally in 4 divided doses. (Adult = 30–60 mg every 6–8 hours.)

Pyridostigmine bromide: 7 mg/kg/d orally in four to six divided doses. Increase as necessary. (Adult = 600 mg/d as average dose.) For myasthenia gravis, see Chapter 22.

Pyrimethamine: Children less than 10 kg, 6.25 mg/d for 3 days; children 10–20 kg, 12.5 mg/d for 3 days; children 20–40 kg, 25 mg/d for 3 days.

Quinidine: For test dose, 2 mg/kg orally. If tolerated, give 3–6 mg/kg every 2–3 hours. For therapeutic dose, 30 mg/kg/d orally in four or five divided doses.

Reserpine: Orally, 0.005–0.03 mg/kg/d in four divided doses. (Adult = 0.1–0.5 mg/d.)

Rifampin: 20 mg/kg/d in divided doses.

Secobarbital sodium: Orally, 2–6 mg/kg as a single sedative or light hypnotic dose. (Adult = 100 mg.) Rectally, 6 mg/kg as a minimal hypnotic dose. (Adult = 200 mg.)

Sodium polystyrene sulfonate: 1 meq of potassium per gram of resin. Calculate dose on basis of desired exchange. Instill rectally in 10% glucose. May be administered every 6 hours. Usual dose is approximately 1 g/kg orally every 6 hours or rectally every 2–6 hours.

Spironolactone: For edema and ascites, 1.7–3.3 mg/kg/d orally in divided doses. Start with small dose. (Adult = 25 mg three to six times daily.) *Caution.*

Sulfasalazine: 40–75 mg/kg/d orally in three to six divided doses (maximum = 6 g/d). (Adult = 1 g four to six times daily.)

Terfenadine: For children 3–6 years, 15 mg twice a day. For children 6–12 years, 30 mg twice a day.

Theophylline: 10–20 mg/kg/d orally in four divided doses. See Aminophylline for intravenous use.

Thiopental sodium: For general anesthesia, 1–2 mg/kg intravenously, slowly.

Thioridazine hydrochloride: For children under 2 years, do not use. For behavior disorder in children 2–12 years, 0.5–3 mg/kg/d (maximum) orally; for older children 20–40 mg/d. (Adult = 200–800 mg/d for psychosis.)

Tolazoline hydrochloride: For newborns, 1–2 mg/kg intravenously, followed by 1–2 mg/kg/h by continuous intravenous infusion. *Caution:* potent vasodilator.

Triiodothyronine (liothyronine): 25–30 μg of triiodothyronine = 65 mg of thyroid USP = 0.1 mg of levothyroxine sodium.

Trimethaphan camsylate: 50–150 μg/kg/min intravenously. (Adult = begin at 0.5–1 mg/min and titrate rate by blood pressure.) *Caution:* Hypotension, including orthostatic hypotension.

Trimethoprim and sulfamethoxazole (co-trimoxazole): For mild to moderate infection, 6–12 mg TMP/kg/d divided every 12 hours. For Pneumocystis infection, 15–20 mg TMP/kg/d divided every 6 hours. For Pneumocystis prophylaxis, 5–10 mg TMP/kg/d divided every 12 hours 3 days per week (maximum = 320 mg TMP).

Tubocurarine (curare): Initially, 0.2–0.4 mg/kg intravenously. Subsequently, 0.04–0.2 mg/kg as needed to maintain paralysis. *Caution.*

Valproic acid: 15 mg/kg/d as a single dose or in two or three divided doses. May increase by 5 mg/kg/d every 1–2 weeks. Maximum = 60 mg/kg/d. See also Table 22–15.

Vasopressin injection: 0.125–0.5 mL (20 units/mL) intramuscularly. Short duration. (Adult = 0.25–0.5 mL.)

Vasopressin tannate injection: 0.2–1 mL (5 units/mL in oil) intramuscularly every 2–4 days as necessary. Start with smaller dose and increase. Effective 1–3 days. (Adult = 0.3–1 mL per dose.)

Verapamil: For supraventricular tachycardia, 0.1 mg/kg intravenously over 30 seconds (repeat once if required) or 4–10 mg/kg/d orally in divided doses every 12 hours. *Caution:* Transient hypotension.

Vinblastine sulfate: 2.5 mg/m^2 intravenously as a single dose. (Adult = 3.7 mg/m^2 as a single dose.)

Zidovudine: For children 3 months to 2 years, 90–180 mg/m^2/dose orally every 6 hours by intermittent intravenous infusion.

REFERENCES

Benitz WE, Tatro DS: *Pediatric Drug Handbook,* 2nd ed. Year Book, 1988.

Gelman CR, Rumack BH (editors): *DRUGDEX® Information System.* Micromedex, 1993.

Physicians' Desk Reference, 47th ed. Medical Economics, 1993.

Roberts RJ (editor): *Drug Therapy in Infants: Pharmacologic Principles and Clinical Experience.* Saunders, 1984.

Normal Biochemical & Hematologic Values

42

Keith B. Hammond, MS, FIMLS

Pediatricians and other health professionals caring for children have the responsibility to insist on accurate, rapid, and comprehensive laboratory testing. Collecting large blood samples for biochemical assay is not suitable for the proper care of children—especially for premature infants or older children in intensive care, where repetitive sampling may be essential. Technology for performing biochemical assays on blood samples of 100 µL or less has been available for 30 years or more. Most of the earlier automated systems for assay were better adapted to larger samples. However, the newest automated systems have the capacity to work with small volumes.

In infants and young children, blood samples taken by heel-prick are better collected by laboratory personnel than by physicians or nurses.

INTERPRETATION OF LABORATORY VALUES

Accreditation by the College of American Pathologists and by state or federal agencies has done much to ensure standardized laboratory performance. Methods employed in various laboratories differ, as do normal values for the methods. Normal range is, of course, a combination of biologic variation and of intrinsic laboratory variation; thus, an acceptable range of normal values should ideally be composed of data developed within the laboratory for the population it serves. Any laboratory should be able to provide information on the coefficient of variation and standard deviation applicable to each test performed in that laboratory. Each laboratory should maintain a rigorous procedure of checks with daily standards and control specimens. Errors may still occur but can usually be detected by retesting before a questionable result is reported. Fortunately, errors occur much less commonly today than in the past.

The clinical value of a test is related to its sensitivity and specificity. Sensitivity is an expression of the incidence of positive test results in those who have the disease. Specificity is an expression of the incidence of negative test results in those free of the disease. Sensitivity and specificity are calculated as follows:

$$\text{Sensitivity \%} = \frac{TP}{TP + FN} \times 100$$

(ie, how many TP are missed)

$$\text{Specificity \%} = \frac{TN}{TN + FP} \times 100$$

(ie, how many TN are missed)

where TP = true-positive result; FP = false-positive result; TN = true-negative result; and FN = false-negative result.

Screening tests must be interpreted with appreciation of sensitivity and specificity. These expressions are illustrated in Figure 42–1 in terms of a screening test for phenylketonuria in newborns. The figures are not strictly correct but serve the purpose of illustration. According to Figure 42–1, a blood phenylalanine level of 4 mg/dL is the discriminating point above which all infants are presumed to have the disease and below which they are presumed to be normal. However, no test is ever quite that exact. Some normal infants will have levels above 4 mg/dL; the test results in these will be false positive. Some abnormal infants will have levels below 4 mg/dL; the test results in these will be false-negative. The discriminating point is a compromise between sensitivity and specificity. Moving the point to 2 mg/dL would effect 100% sensitivity, but there would be a large increase in the number of false-positive results. Moving it to 6 mg/dL would make it very specific, but this would increase the number of false-negative responses, which would result in failure to detect phenylketonuria in a much larger proportion of affected children.

These concepts can be viewed in yet another way. Suppose this test were set at a specificity of 99.9%. This would mean that in a sample of 10,000 tests, there would be ten false-positive results. In a rare condition like phenylketonuria, however, the true incidence of the disease may be only one in 12,000. The ratio of true- to false-positive results is thus 1:12; this

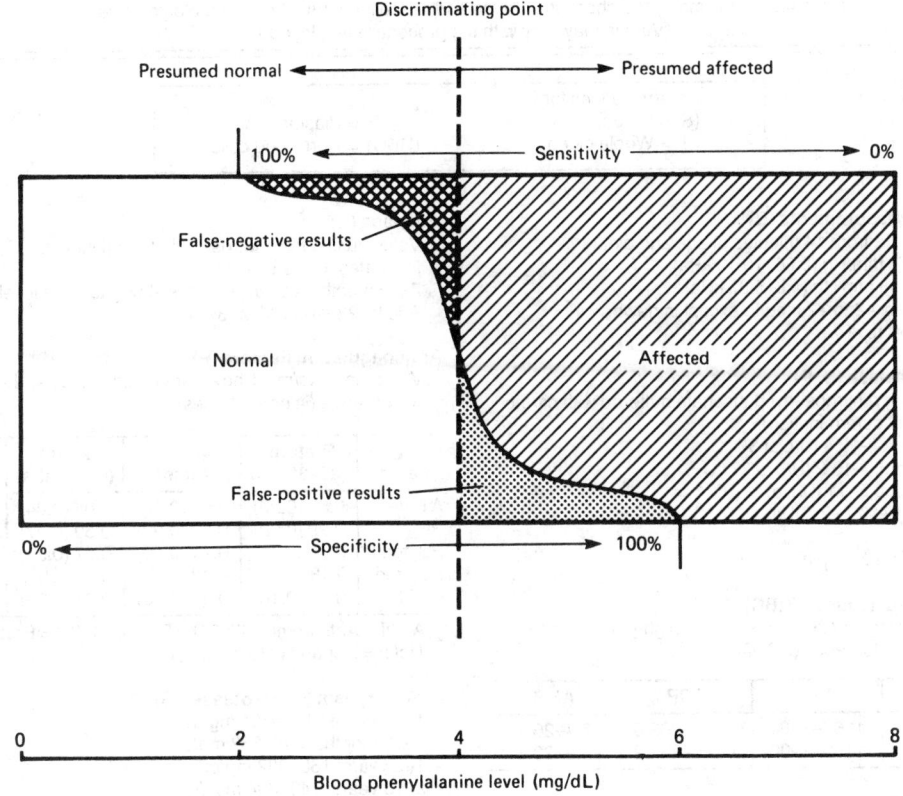

Figure 42–1. Screening test for phenylketonuria in newborns. Data have been simplified to illustrate the concepts of sensitivity and specificity (see text).

is a reflection of the low incidence of the disease and the relatively high incidence of false-positive results due to the nature of the assay. These considerations, of course, apply to the interpretation of all laboratory tests.

LABORATORY VALUES

Normal blood chemistry values and miscellaneous other laboratory values are shown in Tables 42–1 and 42–2.

Table 42–1. Normal blood chemistry values and miscellaneous other hematologic values.[1]
(Values may vary with the procedure employed.)

Determinations for		
(S) = Serum	(P)	= Plasma
(B) = Whole blood	(RBC)	= Red blood cells

Acid-Base Measurements (B)
pH: 7.38–7.42 from 14 minutes of age and older.
Pao_2: 65–76 mm Hg (8.66–10.13 kPa).
$Paco_2$: 36–38 mm Hg (4.8–5.07 kPa).
Base excess: –2 to +2 meq/L, except in newborns
(range, –4 to –0).

Acid Phosphatase (S, P)
Values using p-nitrophenyl phosphate buffered with citrate
(end-point determination).
Newborns: 7.4–19.4 IU/L at 37 °C.
2–13 years: 6.4–15.2 IU/L at 37 °C.
Adult males: 0.5–11 IU/L at 37 °C.
Adult females: 0.2–9.5 IU/L at 37 °C.

ACTH: See Corticotropin.

Adenosine Nucleotides (RBC)
Values in mmol/L RBC, measured by high-performance
liquid chromatography (HPLC).

	ATP	ADP	AMP
Newborns:	1168–1864	104.3–203.0	7.4–26.1
Adults:	1160–1900	116.5–255.2	8.9–23.3

Alanine Aminotransferase (ALT, SGPT) (S)
Newborns (1–3 days): 1–25 IU/L at 37 °C.
Adult males: 7–46 IU/L at 37 °C.
Adult females: 4–35 IU/L at 37 °C.

Aldolase (S)
Newborns: 17.5–47.8 IU/L at 37 °C.
Children: 8.8–23.9 IU/L at 37 °C.
Adults: 4.4–12 IU/L at 37 °C.

Aldosterone (P)
First year: 25–140 ng/dL.
Second year: 9–25 ng/dL.

Alkaline Phosphatase (S)
Values in IU/L at 37 °C using p-nitrophenol phosphate
buffered with AMP (kinetic).

Group	Males	Females
Newborns (1–3 days)	95–368	95–368
2–24 months	115–460	115–460
2–5 years	115–391	115–391
6–7 years	115–460	115–460
8–9 years	115–345	115–345
10–11 years	115–336	115–437
12–13 years	127–403	92–336
14–15 years	79–446	78–212
16–18 years	58–331	35–124
Adults	41–137	39–118

Ammonia (P)
Newborns: 90–150 µg/dL (53–88 µmol/L); higher in
premature and jaundiced infants.
Thereafter: 0–60 µg/dL (0–35 µmol/L) when blood is
drawn with proper precautions.

Amylase (S)
Values using maltotetrose substrate (kinetic).
Neonates: Undetectable.
2–12 months: Levels increase slowly to adult levels.
Adults: 28–108 IU/L at 37 °C.

Anticoagulation Factors (P)
Values in units/mL. Shown are mean values and –2 SD or
lower range (in parentheses).

Factor	Preterm (25–32 wk)	Term Infant	Infant (6 months)	Adult
AT III	0.35 (0.20)	0.56 (0.32)	1.04 (0.84)	1.0 (0.8)
PC	0.29 (0.20)	0.50 (0.30)	0.59 (0.37)	1.0 (0.6)
PS, total	...	0.24 (0.10)	0.87 (0.55)	1.0 (0.6)
PS, free	0.48	0.42	...	1.0 (0.5)
HcF II	0.25 (0.10)	0.49 (0.36)	0.97 (0.59)	1.0 (0.7)

AT III = Antithrombin III; PC = Protein C; PS = Protein S;
Hcf II = Heparin cofactor II

α_1-Antitrypsin (antiprotease) (S)
1–3 months: 127–404 mg/dL.
3–12 months: 145–362 mg/dL.
1–2 years: 160–382 mg/dL.
2–15 years: 148–394 mg/dL.

Ascorbic Acid: See Vitamin C.

Aspartate Aminotransferase (AST, SGOT) (S)
Newborns (1–3 days): 16–74 IU/L at 37 °C.
Adult males: 8–46 IU/L at 37 °C.
Adult females: 7–34 IU/L at 37 °C.

Base Excess: See Acid-Base Measurements.

Bicarbonate, Actual (P)
Calculated from pH and $Paco_2$
Newborns: 17.2–23.6 mmol/L.
2 months–2 years: 19–24 mmol/L.
Children: 18–25 mmol/L.
Adult males: 20.1–28.9 mmol/L.
Adult females: 18.4–28.8 mmol/L.

Bilirubin (S)
Values in mg/dL (µmol/L)
Levels after 1 month are as follows:
Conjugated: 0–0.3 mg/dL (0–5 µmol/L).
Unconjugated: 0.1–0.7 mg/dL (2–12 µmol/L).

Peak Newborn Level	Percentage of Newborns (Birth Weight) Exceeding Peak Level		
	< 2001 g	2001–2500 g	> 2500 g
20 (342)	8.2%	2.6%	0.8%
18 (308)	13.5%	4.6%	1.5%
16 (274)	20.3%	7.6%	2.6%
14 (239)	33.0%	12.0%	4.4%
11 (188)	53.8%	23.0%	9.3%
8 (137)	77.0%	45.4%	26.1%

(continued)

Table 42–1. Normal blood chemistry values and miscellaneous other hematologic values.[1]
(Values may vary with the procedure employed.) (continued)

Bleeding Time (Simplate)
2–9 minutes.

Blood Volume
Premature infants: 98 mL/kg.
At 1 year: 86 mL/kg (range, 69–112 mL/kg).
Older children: 70 mL/kg (range, 51–86 mL/kg).

BUN: See Urea Nitrogen.

C Peptide (S)
5–15 years (8:00 AM fasting): 1–4 ng/mL.
Adults (8:00 AM fasting): < 4 ng/mL.
Adults (nonfasting): < 8 ng/mL.

C-Reactive protein (S)
3–16 years: 0.1–1.5 mg/dL

Calcium (S)
Premature infants (first week) 3.5–4.5 meq/L
  1.7–2.3 mmol/L).
Full-term infants (first week): 4–5 meq/L (2–2.5 mmol/L).
Thereafter: 4.4–5.3 meq/L (2.2–2.7 mmol/L).

Carbon Dioxide, Total (S, P)
Cord blood: 15–20.2 mmol/L.
Children: 18–27 mmol/L.
Adults: 24–35 mmol/L.

Carboxyhemoglobin (B)
5% of total hemoglobin (0.05 mol/mol).

Carnitine (P)
Values in μmol/L, measured by an enzymatic radioisotopic method.

Age	Total Carnitine	Free Carnitine	Acylcarnitine	AC/FC ratio
1 day	23.3–67.9	11.5–36.0	7.0–36.6	0.37–1.68
2–7 d	17.4–40.6	10.1–21.0	2.9–23.8	0.15–1.44
8–28d	18.5–58.7	12.3–46.2	4.1–14.5	0.11–0.65
1m–1y	38.1–68.0	26.9–49.0	7.4–19.0	0.23–0.50
1–6y	34.6–83.6	24.3–62.5	4.0–28.3	0.11–0.83
6–10y	27.8–82.9	21.7–66.4	3.1–32.1	0.08–0.87
10–17y	33.7–77.0	21.6–64.5	3.7–29.2	0.09–0.88
22–60y	33.8–77.5	25.4–54.1	5.4–30.1	0.11–0.78

Carotene (S, P)
0–6 months: 0–40 μg/dL (0–0.75 μmol/L).
Children: 50–100 μg/dL (0.93–1.9 μmol/L).
Adults: 100–150 μg/dL (1.9–2.8 μmol/L).

Cation-Anion Gap (S, P)
5–15 mmol/L.

Ceruloplasmin (Copper Oxidase) (S, P)
21–43 mg/dL (1.3–2.7 μmol/L).

Chloride (S, P)
Premature infants: 95–110 mmol/L.
Full-term infants: 96–116 mmol/L.
Children: 98–105 mmol/L.
Adults: 98–108 mmol/L.

Cholesterol, Total (S, P)
Values in mg/dL (mmol/L)

Group	Males	Females
6–7 years	115–197 (2.97–5.09)	126–199 (3.25–5.14)
8–9 years	112–199 (2.89–5.14)	124–208 (3.20–5.37)
10–11 years	108–220 (2.79–5.68)	115–208 (2.97–5.37)
12–13 years	117–202 (3.02–5.21)	114–207 (2.94–5.34)
14–15 years	103–207 (2.66–5.34)	102–208 (2.63–5.37)
16–17 years	107–198 (2.76–5.11)	106–213 (2.73–5.50)

Cholinesterase (S, RBC)
2.5–5 μmol/min/mL of serum (pseudocholinesterase).
2.3–4 μmol/min/mL of red cells.

Coagulation Factors (P)
Values in units/mL. Shown are mean values and –2 SD or lower range (in parentheses).

Factor	Preterm (25–32 wk)	Term Infant	Infant (6 months)	Adult
II	0.32 (0.18)	0.52 (0.25)	0.88 (0.60)	1.0 (0.7)
V	0.80 (0.43)	1.00 (0.54)	0.91 (0.55)	1.0 (0.6)
VII	0.37 (0.24)	0.57 (0.35)	0.87 (0.50)	1.0 (0.6)
VIII	0.75 (0.40)	1.50 (0.55)	0.90 (0.50)	1.0 (0.6)
vWf	1.50 (0.90)	1.60 (0.84)	1.07 (0.60)	1.0 (0.6)
IX	0.22 (0.17)	0.35 (0.15)	0.86 (0.36)	1.0 (0.5)
X	0.38 (0.20)	0.45 (0.30)	0.78 (0.38)	1.0 (0.6)
XI	0.20 (0.12)	0.42 (0.20)	0.86 (0.38)	1.0 (0.6)
XII	0.22 (0.09)	0.44 (0.16)	0.77 (0.39)	1.0 (0.6)
XIII	. . .	0.61 (0.36)	1.04 (0.50)	1.0 (0.6)
PreK	0.26 (0.14)	0.35 (0.16)	0.86 (0.56)	1.1 (0.6)

vWf = von Willlebrand factor; PreK = prekallikrein

Complement (S)
C3: 96–195 mg/dL.
C4: 15–20 mg/dL.

Copper (S)
Cord blood: 26–32 μg/dL (4.1–5.2 μmol/L).
Newborns: 26–32 μg/dL (4.1–5.2 μmol/L).
1 month: 73–93 μg/dL (11.5–14.6 μmol/L).
2 months: 59–69 μg/dL (9.3–10.9 μmol/L).
6 months–5 years: 27–153 μg/dL (4.2–24.1 μmol/L).
5–17 years: 94–234 μg/dL (14.8–36.8 μmol/L).
Adults: 70–118 μg/dL (11–18.6 μmol/L).

Copper Oxidase: See Ceruloplasmin.

Corticotropin (ACTH) (P)
Morning (8:00 AM): 20–100 pg/mL (4.4–22 pmol/L).

Cortisol (S, P)
Morning (8:00 AM): 5–25 μg/dL (0.14–0.68 μmol/L).
Evening: 5–15 μg/dL (0.14–0.41 μmol/L).

Creatine (S, P)
0.2–0.8 mg/dL (15.2–61 mmol/L).

Creatine Kinase (S, P)
Newborns (1–3 days): 40–474 IU/L at 37 °C.
Adult males: 30–210 IU/L at 37 °C.
Adult females: 20–128 IU/L at 37 °C.

(*continued*)

Table 42-1. Normal blood chemistry values and miscellaneous other hematologic values.[1]
(Values may vary with the procedure employed.) (continued)

Creatinine (S, P)
Values in mg/dL (μmol/L).

Group	Males	Females
Newborns (1–3 days)[1]	0.2–1.0 (17.7–88.4)	0.2–1.0 (17.7–88.4)
1 year	0.2–0.6 (17.7–53.0)	0.2–0.5 (17.7–44.2)
2–3 years	0.2–0.7 (17.7–61.9)	0.3–0.6 (26.5–53.0)
4–7 years	0.2–0.8 (17.7–70.7)	0.2–0.7 (17.7–61.9)
8–10 years	0.3–0.9 (26.5–79.6)	0.3–0.8 (26.5–70.7)
11–12 years	0.3–1.0 (26.5–88.4)	0.3–0.9 (26.5–79.6)
13–17 years	0.3–1.2 (26.5–106.1)	0.3–1.1 (26.5–97.2)
18–20 years	0.5–1.3 (44.2–115.0)	0.3–1.1 (26.5–97.2)

[1]Values may be higher in premature newborns.

Creatinine Clearance
Values show great variability and depend on specificity of analytical methods used.
Newborns (1 day): 5–50 mL/min/1.73 m (mean, 18 mL/min/1.73 m).
Newborns (6 days): 15–90 mL/min/1.73 m² (mean, 36 mL/min/1.73 m²).
Adult males: 85–125 mL/min/1.73 m².
Adult females: 75–115 mL/min/1.73 m².

2,3-Diphosphoglycerate (B)
Values vary with method employed and with altitude.
4.5–6 mmol/L.

Factor: See Anticoagulation Factors and Coagulation Factors.

Fatty Acids, "Free" (P)
Newborns: 435–1375 μeq/L.
4 months–10 years (14-hour fast): 500–900 μeq/L.
4 months–10 years (19-hour fast): 730–1200 μeq/L.
Adults (14-hour fast) 310–590 μeq/L.
Adults (19-hour fast): 405–720 μeq/L.

Fatty Acids, Total Esterified (P, RBC)
Values in mg/dL.

Fatty Acid[1]	Plasma		Erythrocytes	
	mg/dL	% of Total	mg/dL	% of Total
16:0	29.4–55.8	20.7–28.3	24.8–49.0	18.5–28.3
16:1	1.4–6.8	1.1–2.5	0.0–9.4	0.0–4.9
18:0	11.2–28.6	6.9–16.1	13.7–47.3	13.1–26.5
18:1	21.9–51.1	16.9–24.5	11.6–46.8	12.7–23.3
18:2	24.5–78.5	19.5–39.1	0.7–47.9	6.1–22.1
20:3	0.0–8.0	0.0–4.9	0.8–7.6	0.8–4.4
20:4	5.5–26.9	3.2–15.6	14.2–46.2	12.5–26.3

[1]Ratio of number of carbons to number of unsaturated bonds.

Ferritin (S)
Newborns: 20–200 ng/ml (mean, 117 ng/mL).
1 month: 60–550 ng/mL (mean, 350 ng/mL).
1–15 years: 7–140 ng/mL (mean, 31 ng/mL).
Adult males: 50–225 ng/mL (mean, 140 ng/mL).
Adult females: 10–150 ng/mL (mean, 40 ng/mL).

Fibrinogen (P)
200–500 mg/dL (5.9–14.7 μmol/L).

Folate (S)
Values in ng/mL (nmol/L), measured by radioimmunoassay.

Group	Males		Females	
0–1 years	7.2–22.4	(16.3–50.8)	6.3–22.7	(14.3–51.5)
2–3 years	2.5–15.0	(5.7–34.0)	1.7–15.7	(3.9–35.6)
4–6 years	0.5–13.0	(1.1–29.4)	2.7–14.1	(6.1–31.9)
7–9 years	2.3–11.9	(5.2–27.0)	2.4–13.4	(5.4–30.4)
10–12 years	1.5–10.8	(3.4–24.5)	1.0–10.2	(2.3–23.1)
13–18 years	1.2– 8.8	(2.7–19.9)	1.2– 7.2	(2.7–16.3)

Galactose (S, P)
1.1–2.1 mg/dL (0.06–0.12 mmol/L).

Galactose 1-Phosphate (RBC)
Normal: 1 mg/dL of packed erythrocyte lysate; slightly higher in cord blood.
Infants with congenital galactosemia on a milk-free diet: < 2 mg/dL.
Infants with congenital galactosemia taking milk: 9–20 mg/dL.

Galactose-1-Phosphate Uridyl Transferase (RBC)
Normal: 308–475 mIU/g of hemoglobin.
Heterozygous for Duarte variant: 225–308 mIU/g of hemoglobin.
Homozygous for Duarte variant: 142–225 mIU/g of hemoglobin.
Heterozygous for congenital galactosemia: 142–225 mIU/g of hemoglobin.
Homozygous for congenital galactosemia: < 8 mIU/g of hemoglobin.

Gastrin (S)
Newborns (1–7 days): 20–300 pg/mL.
Children (8- to 12-hour overnight fast): < 10–125 pg/mL.
Adults (8- to 12-hour overnight fast): < 10–100 pg/mL.

Glomerular Filtration Rate
Newborns: About 50% of values for older children and adults.
Older children and adults: 75–165 mL/min/1.73 m² (levels reached by about 6 months).

Glucose (S, P)
Premature infants: 20–80 mg/dL (1.11–4.44 mmol/L).
Full-term infants: 30–100 mg/dL (1.67–5.56 mmol/L).
Children and adults (fasting): 60–105 mg/dL (3.33–5.88 mmol/L).

Glucose 6-Phosphate Dehydrogenase (RBC)
150–215 units/dL.

Glucose Tolerance Test (S)
(See Table, p 1207.)

λ-Glutamyl Transpeptidase (S)
0–1 month: 12–271 IU/L at 37 °C (kinetic).
1–2 months: 9–159 IU/L at 37 °C (kinetic).
2–4 months: 7–98 IU/L at 37 °C (kinetic).
4–7 months: 5–45 IU/L at 37 °C (kinetic).
7–12 months: 4–27 IU/L at 37 °C (kinetic).
1–15 years: 3–30 IU/L at 37 °C (kinetic).
Adult males: 9–69 IU/L at 37 °C (kinetic).
Adult females: 3–33 IU/L at 37 °C (kinetic).

(continued)

Table 42–1. Normal blood chemistry values and miscellaneous other hematologic values.[1]
(Values may vary with the procedure employed.) (continued)

Glucose tolerance test results in serum.

Normal levels based on results in 13 normal children given glucose.
1.75 g/kg orally in one dose, after 2 weeks on a high-carbohydrate diet.

Time	Glucose mg/dL	Glucose mmol/L	Insulin μU/mL	Insulin pmol/L	Phosphorus mg/dL	Phosphorus mmol/L
Fasting	59–96	3.11–5.33	5–40	36–287	3.2–4.9	1.03–1.58
30 minutes	91–185	5.05–10.27	36–110	258–789	2.0–4.4	0.64–1.42
60 minutes	66–164	3.66–9.10	22–124	158–890	1.8–3.6	0.58–1.16
90 minutes	68–148	3.77–8.22	17–105	122–753	1.8–3.6	0.58–1.16
2 hours	66–122	3.66–6.77	6–84	43–603	1.8–4.2	0.58–1.36
3 hours	47–99	2.61–5.49	2–46	14–330	2.0–4.6	0.64–1.48
4 hours	61–93	3.39–5.16	3–32	21–230	2.7–4.3	0.87–1.39
5 hours	63–86	3.50–4.77	5–37	36–265	2.9–4.4	0.94–1.42

Glycogen (RBC)
Cord blood: 10–338 μg/g of hemoglobin.
4½–19 hours: 48–361 μg/g of hemoglobin.
2–12 months: 32–134 μg/g of hemoglobin.
1–12 years: 22–109 μg/g of hemoglobin.
Adults: 20–105 μg/g of hemoglobin.

Glycohemoglobin (hemoglobin A_{1c}) (B)
Normal: 6.3–8.2% of total hemoglobin.
Diabetic patients in good control of their condition
ordinarily have levels < 10%.
Values tend to be lower during pregnancy; they also vary
with technique.

Growth Hormone (GH) (S)
After infancy (fasting specimen): 0–5 ng/mL.
In response to natural and artificial provocation (eg, sleep,
arginine, insulin, hypoglycemia): > 8 ng/mL.
During the newborn period (fasting specimen); GH levels
are high (15–40 ng/mL) and responses to provocation
variable.

Haptoglobin (S)
50–150 mg/dL has hemoglobin-binding capacity.

Hematocrit (B)
At birth: 44–64%.
14–90 days: 35–49%.
6 months–1 year: 30–40%.
4–10 years: 31–43%.

Hemoglobin (P)
No more than 0.5 mg/dL (0.3 μmol/L).

Hemoglobin A_{1c}: See Glycohemoglobin.

Hemoglobin Electrophoresis (B)
A_1 hemoglobin: 96–98.5% of total hemoglobin.
A_2 hemoglobin: 1.5–4% of total hemoglobin.

Hemoglobin, Fetal (B)
At birth: 50–85% of total hemoglobin.
At 1 year: < 15% of total hemoglobin.
Up to 2 years: Up to 5% of total hemoglobin.
Thereafter: < 2% of total hemoglobin.

Immunoglobulins (S)
Values in mg/dL.

Group	IgG	IgA	IgM
Cord blood	766–1693	0.04–9	4–26
2 weeks–3 months	299–852	3–66	15–149
3–6 months	142–988	4–90	18–118
6–12 months	418–1142	14–95	43–223
1–2 years	356–1204	13–118	37–239
2–3 years	492–1269	23–137	49–204
3–6 years	564–1381	35–209	51–214
6–9 years	658–1535	29–384	50–228
9–12 years	625–1598	60–294	64–278
12–16 years	660–1548	81–252	45–256

Insulin: See Glucose Tolerance Test and Table (top of page).

Inulin Clearance
< 1 month: 29–88 mL/min/1.73 m².
1–6 months: 40–112 mL/min/1.73 m².
6–12 months: 62–121 mL/min/1.73 m².
< 1 year: 78–164 mL/min/1.73 m².

Iron (S, P)
Newborns: 20–157 μg/dL (3.6–28.1 μmol/L).
6 weeks–3 years: 20–115 μg/dL (3.6–20.6 μmol/L).
3–9 years: 20–141 μg/dL (3.6–25.2 μmol/L).
9–14 years: 21–151 μg/dL (3.8–27 μmol/L).
14–16 years: 20–181 μg/dL (3.6–32.4 μmol/L).
Adults: 44–196 μg/dL (7.2–31.3 μmol/L).

Iron-Binding Capacity (S, P)
Newborns: 59–175 μg/dL (10.6–31.3 μmol/L).
Children and adults: 275–458 μg/dL (45–72 μmol/L).

Lactate (B)
Venous blood: 5–18 mg/dL (0.5–2 mmol/L).
Arterial blood: 3–7 mg/dL (0.3–0.8 mmol/L).

Lactate Dehydrogenase (LDH) (S, P)
Values using lactate substrate (kinetic).
Newborns (1–3 days): 40–348 IU/L at 37 °C.
1 month–5 years: 150–360 IU/L at 37 °C.
5–8 years: 150–300 IU/L at 37 °C.
8–12 years: 130–300 IU/L at 37 °C.
12–14 years: 130–280 IU/L at 37 °C.
14–16 years: 130–230 IU/L at 37 °C.
Adult males: 70–178 IU/L at 37 °C.
Adult females: 42–166 IU/L at 37 °C.

(continued)

Table 42–1. Normal blood chemistry values and miscellaneous other hematologic values.[1]
(Values may vary with the procedure employed.) (continued)

Lactate Dehydrogenase Isoenzymes (S)
LDH$_1$ (heart): 24–34%.
LDH$_2$ (heart, red cells): 35–45%.
LDH$_3$ (muscle): 15–25%.
LDH$_4$ (liver [trace], muscle): 4–10%.
LDH$_5$ (liver, muscle): 1–9%.

LDH: See Lactate Dehydrogenase.

Lead (B)
< 10 µg/dL (< 0.48 µmol/L)

When a large proportion of a population of children have blood lead levels in the range of 10–19 µg/dL (0.48–0.92 µmol/L), communitywide childhood lead poisoning activities are warranted.

Levels > 20 µg/dL (> 0.97 µmol/L) indicate the need for medical and environmental evaluation and possible pharmalogic intervention.

Levels > 70 µg/dL (> 3.38 µmol/L) indicate the immediate need for medical and environmental management.

Lipase (S, P)
20–136 IU/L based on 4-hour incubation.

Lipoprotein Cholesterol, High-Density (HDL) (S)
Values in mg/dL (mmol/L).

Group	Males	Females
6–7 years	35–77 (0.90–1.98)	24–76 (0.62–1.96)
8–9 years	31–80 (0.80–2.06)	34–77 (0.87–1.98)
10–11 years	34–81 (0.87–1.09)	30–74 (0.77–1.91)
12–13 years	30–82 (0.77–2.11)	33–73 (0.85–1.88)
14–15 years	26–72 (0.67–1.86)	29–73 (0.74–1.88)
16–17 years	25–66 (0.72–1.70)	27–78 (0.69–2.01)

Lipoprotein Cholesterol, Low-Density (LDL) (S)
Values in mg/dL (mmol/L).

Group	Males	Females
6–7 years	56–134 (1.44–3.46)	52–149 (1.34–3.85)
8–9 years	52–129 (1.34–3.33)	57–143 (1.47–3.69)
10–11 years	45–149 (1.16–3.85)	56–140 (1.44–3.61)
12–13 years	55–135 (1.42–3.48)	58–138 (1.49–3.56)
14–15 years	48–143 (1.24–3.69)	47–140 (1.21–3.61)
16–17 years	53–134 (1.36–3.36)	44–147 (1.13–3.79)

Magnesium (RBC)
3.92–5.28 meq/L (1.96–2.64 mmol/L).

Magnesium (S, P)
Newborns: 1.5–2.3 meq/L (0.75–1.15 mmol/L).
Adults: 1.4–2 meq/L (0.7–1 mmol/L).

Manganese (S)
Newborns: 2.4–9.6 µg/dL (0.44–1.75 µmol/L).
2–18 years: 0.8–1.2 µg/dL (0.15–0.38 µmol/L).

Methemoglobin (B)
0–0.3 g/dL (0–186 µmol/L).

NAD/NADH: (See Pyridine Coenzymes)

Osmolality (S, P)
270–290 mosm/kg.

Oxygen Capacity (B)
1.34 mL/g of hemoglobin.

Oxygen Saturation (B)
Newborns: 30–80% (0.3–0.8 mol/mol of venous blood).
Thereafter: 65–85% (0.65–0.85 mol/mol of venous blood).

Paco$_2$: See Acid-Base Measurements.

Pao$_2$: See Acid-Base Measurements.

Partial Thromboplastin Time (P)
Children: 42–54 seconds.

pH: See Acid-Base Measurements.

Phenylalanine (S, P)
0.7–3.5 mg/dL (0.04–0.21 mmol/L).

Phosphatase: See Acid Phosphatase and Alkaline Phosphatase.

Phospholipid (S)
Cord blood: 48–160 mg/dL (0.62–2.07 mmol/L).
2–13 years: 166–247 mg/dL (2.14–3.19 mmol/L).
13–20 years: 193–338 mg/dL (2.49–4.37 mmol/L).

Phosphorus, Inorganic (S, P)
Premature infants:
At birth: 5.6–8 mg/dL (1.81–2.58 mmol/L).
6–10 days: 6.1–11.7 mg/dL (1.97–3.78 mmol/L).
20–25 days: 6.6–9.4 mg/dL (2.13–3.04 mmol/L).
Full-term infants:
At birth: 5–7.8 mg/dL (1.61–2.52 mmol/L).
3 days: 5.8–9 mg/dL (1.87–2.91 mmol/L).
6–12 days: 4.9–8.9 mg/dL (1.58–2.87 mmol/L).
Children:
1 year: 3.8–6.2 mg/dL (1.23–2 mmol/L).
10 years: 3.6–5.6 mg/dL (1.16–1.81 mmol/L).
Adults: 3.1–5.1 mg/dL (1–1.65 mmol/L).
(See also Glucose Tolerance Test.)

Potassium (RBC)
87.2–97.6 mmol/L.

Potassium (S, P)
Premature infants: 4.5–7.2 mmol/L.
Full-term infants: 3.7–5.2 mmol/L.
Children: 3.5–5.8 mmol/L.
Adults: 3.5–5.5 mmol/L.

Prealbumin: See Transthyretin.

Prostaglandin E (P)
Newborns: 1000–1730 pg/mL.
2–3 days: 60–150 pg/mL.
1–6 years: 125–200 pg/mL.
6–14 years: 160–340 pg/mL.
Adults: 450–550 pg/mL.

Proteins (S)
(See Table, top of page 1209).

Prothrombin Time (P)
Children: 11–15 seconds.

(continued)

Table 42–1. Normal blood chemistry values and miscellaneous other hematologic values.[1]
(Values may vary with the procedure employed.) (continued)

Proteins in serum.

Values are for cellulose acetate electrophoresis and are
in g/dL. SI conversion factor: g/dL × 10 = g/L.

Group	Total Protein	Albumin	α_1-Globulin	α_2-Globulin	β-Globulin	λ-Globulin
At birth	4.6–7.0	3.2–4.8	0.1–0.3	0.2–0.3	0.3–0.6	0.6–1.2
3 months	4.5–6.5	3.2–4.8	0.1–0.3	0.3–0.7	0.3–0.7	0.2–0.7
1 year	5.4–7.5	3.7–5.7	0.1–0.3	0.5–1.1	0.4–1.0	0.2–0.9
> 4 years	5.9–8.0	3.8–5.4	0.1–0.3	0.4–0.8	0.5–1.0	0.4–1.3

Protoporphyrin, "Free" (FEP, ZPP) (B)
Values for free erythrocyte protoporphyrin (FEP) and zinc
protoporphyrin (ZPP) are 1.2–2.7 µg/g of hemoglobin.

Pseudocholinesterase (S)
2.5–5 µmol/mL/min.

Pyridine Coenzymes (RBC)
Values in mmol/L RBC, measured by high performance
liquid chromatography (HPLC).

	Newborns	Adults
NAD	31.75–74.25	33.14–61.48
NADH	0.61–4.48	1.42–3.93
NADP	19.49–44.89	11.82–35.26
NADPH	3.24–16.96	6.91–20.16
NAD/NADH Ratio	11.82–80.64	12.18–32.46
NADP/NADPH Ratio	1.35–8.18	0.80–2.84
NAD/NADP Ratio	1.12–2.22	1.16–3.04

Pyruvate (B)
Resting adult males (arterial blood); 50.5–60.1 µmol/L.
Adults (venous blood): 34–102 µmol/L.

Pyruvate Kinase (RBC)
7.4–15.7 units/g of hemoglobin.

Renin Activity (P)
3–6 days: 8–14 ng/mL/h.
0–3 years: 3–6 ng/mL/h.
Children: 1.3–2.6 ng/mL/h.

Retinol-binding protein (S)

3–5 years:	1.0–5.0 mg/dL
6–8 years:	1.5–5.9 mg/dL
9–11 years:	1.5–6.5 mg/dL
12–16 years:	1.5–7.0 mg/dL

Sedimentation Rate (Micro) (B)
< 2 years: 1–5 mm/h.
> 2 years: 1–8 mm/h.

Serotonin (S, P)
Children: 127–187 ng/mL.
Adults: 119–171 ng/mL.

SGOT: See Aspartate Aminotransferase.

SGPT: See Alanine Aminotransferase.

Sodium (S, P)
Children and adults: 135–148 mmol/L.

Sugar: See Glucose.

T_3: See Triiodothyronine.

T_4: See Thyroxine.

TBG: See Thyroxine-Binding Globulin.

Thrombin Time (P)
Children: 12–16 seconds.

Thyroid-Stimulating Hormone (TSH) (S)
Values in µIU/mL.

	Males	Females
1–30 days	0.52–16.0	0.72–13.1
1 month–5 years	0.55–7.1	0.46–8.1
6–18 years	0.37–6.0	0.36–5.8

Thyroxine (T_4) (S)
1–2 days: 11.4–25.5 µg/dL (147–328 nmol/L).
3–4 days: 9.8–25.2 µg/dL (126–324 nmol/L).
1–6 years: 5–15.2 µg/dL (64–196 nmol/L).
11–13 years: 4–13 µg/dL (51–167 nmol/L).
> 18 years: 4.7–11 µg/dL (60–142 nmol/L).

Thyroxine, "Free" (Free T_4) (S)
1–2.3 ng/dL.

Thyroxine-Binding Globulin (TBG) (S)
1–7 months: 2.9–6 mg/dL.
7–12 months: 2.1–5.9 mg/dL.
Prepubertal children: 2–5.3 mg/dL.
Pubertal children and adults: 1.8–4.2 mg/dL.

α-Tocopherol: See Vitamin E.

Transaminase: See Alanine Aminotransferase and
Aspartate Aminotransferase.

Transthyretin (S, P)
2–5 months: 14–33 mg/dL
6–11 months: 12–27 mg/dL
12–17 months: 11–26 mg/dL
18–23 months: 14–24 mg/dL
24–36 months: 11–26 mg/dL
3–5 years: 9.1–33.0 mg/dL
6–8 years: 15.3–45.5 mg/dL
9–11 years: 16.0–47.6 mg/dL
12–16 years: 19.0–50.0 mg/dL

(continued)

Table 42-1. Normal blood chemistry values and miscellaneous other hematologic values.[1]
(Values may vary with the procedure employed.) (continued)

Triglyceride (S, P)
Fasting (> 12 hour) values in mg/mL (mmol/L)

Group	Males	Females
6–7 years	32–79 (0.36–0.89)	24–128 (0.27–1.44)
8–9 years	28–105 (0.31–1.18)	34–115 (0.38–1.29)
10–11 years	30–115 (0.33–1.29)	39–131 (0.44–1.48)
12–13 years	33–112 (0.37–1.26)	36–125 (0.40–1.41)
14–15 years	35–136 (0.39–1.53)	36–122 (0.40–1.37)
16–17 years	38–167 (0.42–1.88)	34–136 (0.38–1.53)

Note: Lower values represent 5th percentile, whereas upper values are calculated from mean + 2 SD.

Triiodothyronine (T₃) (S)

1–3 days: 89–405 ng/dL.
1 week: 91–300 ng/dL.
1–12 months: 85–250 ng/dL.
Prepubertal children: 119–218 ng/dL.
Pubertal children and adults: 55–170 ng/dL.

TSH: See Thyroid-Stimulating Hormone.

Tyrosine (S, P)
Premature infants: 3–30.2 mg/dL (0.17–1.67 mmol/L).
Full-term infants: 1.7–4.7 mg/dL (0.09–0.26 mmol/L).
1–12 years: 1.4–3.4 mg/dL (0.08–0.19 mmol/L).
Adults: 0.6–1.6 mg/dL (0.03–0.09 mmol/L).

Urea Clearance
Premature infants: 3.5–17.3 mL/min/1.73 m^2.
Newborns: 8.7–33 mL/min/1.73 m^2.
2–12 months: 40–95 mL/min/1.73 m^2.
≥ 2 years: > 52 mL/min/1.73 m^2.

Urea Nitrogen (S, P)
1–2 years: 5–15 mg/dL (1.8–5.4 mmol/L).
Thereafter: 10–20 mg/dL (3.5–7.1 mmol/L).

Uric Acid (S, P)
Males:
  0–14 years: 2–7 mg/dL (119–416 μmol/L).
  > 14 years: 3–8 mg/dL (178–476 μmol/L).
Females:
  0–14 years: 2–7 mg/dL (119–416 μmol/L).
  > 14 years: 2–7 mg/dL (119–416 μmol/L).

Vitamin A (S, P)
Total vitamin A: 19–81 μg/dL (0.66–2.82 μmol/L).
Retinol: 19–77 μg/dL (0.66–2.68 μmol/L).
Retinyl esters: 0.1–4.7 μg/dL (0.01–0.16 μmol/L).

Vitamin B₁₂ (S, P)

Values in pg/mL (pmol/L), measured by radioimmunoassay.

Group	Males		Females	
0–1 years	291–1207	(216–891)	228–1513	(168–1117)
2–3 years	264–1215	(195–897)	416–1209	(307–892)
4–6 years	245–1077	(181–795)	313–1406	(231–1038)
7–9 years	271–1169	(200–863)	247–1173	(182–866)
10–12 years	182–1088	(135–803)	196–1019	(145–752)
13–18 years	214–864	(158–638)	182–820	(134–605)

Vitamin C (Ascorbic Acid) (S, P)
0.2–2 mg/dL (11–114 μmol/L).

Vitamin D (S)
1,25-Dihydroxycholecalciferol:
  Normal: 37 ± 12 pg/mL.
  X-linked vitamin D-resistant disease: 16 ± 8 pg/mL.
  Vitamin D dependency: 9.5 ± 3 pg/mL in type I. Normal in type II.
  Hypophosphatemic bone disease: 30 ± 6 pg/mL.
  Lead poisoning: 20 ± 1 pg/mL.
25-Hydroxycholecalciferol:
  Normal: 26–31 ng/mL.

Vitamin E (Tocopherol) (S, P)
Alpha-tocopherol:
  < 12 y 3.8–15.5 μg/mL (9.1–37.2 μmol/L).
  > 12 y 4.7–203 μg/mL (11.3–48.7 μmol/L).
Gamma-tocopherol:
  The gamma isomer contributes 10–20% of the total tocopherols in plasma but is only 10% as active as the alpha form in vivo.
Vitamin E status is best assessed by performing chromatographic separation of the isomers and determining both alpha and gamma tocopherol levels. Levels should be expressed in terms of vitamin E/total lipid ratio:
  < 12 y > 0.6 mg/g (> 1.4 μmol/g)
  > 12 y > 0.8 mg/g (> 1.9 μmol/g)

Volume (B)
Premature infants: 98 mL/kg (mean).
Full-term infants: 75–100 mL/kg.
1 year: 69–112 mL/kg (mean, 86 mL/kg).
Older children: 51–86 mL/kg (mean, 70 mL/kg).

Volume (P)
Full-term neonates: 39–77 mL/kg.
Infants: 40–50 mL/kg.
Older children: 30–54 mL/kg.

Water (B, S, RBC)
Whole blood: 79–81 g/dL.
Serum: 91–92 g/dL.
Red blood cells: 64–65 g/dL.

Xylose Absorption Test (B)
Following a 5-g loading dose, the laboratory will report the D-xylose concentration of the baseline and 60-minute samples in mg/dL. The difference between these 2 values should be corrected to a constant surface area of 1.73 m^2 according to the formula shown below.
The actual surface area can be derived from a number of available nomograms using the patient's weight and height.
Normal corrected blood values:[1] 9.8–20 mg/dL.
Effect of age and sex: No significant differences between males and females. No significant differences in ages 14–92.

Zinc (S)
Males: 83–88 μg/dL (12.7–13.5 μmol/L).
Females: 85–91 μg/dL (13–13.9 μmol/L).
Females taking oral contraceptives: 86–93 μg/dL (13.2–14.2 μmol/L).
At 16 weeks of gestation: 66–70 μg/dL (10.1–10.7 μmol/L).
At 38 weeks of gestation: 54–58 μg/dL (8.3–8.9 μmol/L).

$$^{1}\text{Corrected blood value} = \frac{(\text{Value}_{60\text{ min}} - \text{Value}_{\text{baseline}}) \times \text{Actual surface area}}{1.73}$$

[1]Adapted from Meites S (editor): *Pediatric Clinical Chemistry*, 2nd ed. American Association for Clinical Chemistry, 1982, and many other sources.

Table 42–2. Normal values: Urine, duodenal fluid, feces, sweat, and miscellaneous.[1]

URINE

Acidity, Titratable
20–50 meq/d.

Addis Count
Red cells (12-hour specimen): < 1 million.
White cells (12-hour specimen): < 2 million.
Casts (12-hour specimen): < 10,000.
Protein (12-hour specimen): < 55 mg.

Albumin
First month: 1–100 mg/L.
Second month: 0.2–34 mg/L.
2–12 months: 0.5–19 mg/L.

Aldosterone
Newborns: 0.5–5 μg/24 h (20–140 μg/g of creatinine).
Prepubertal children: 1–8 μg/24 h (4–22 μg/g of creatinine).
Adults: 3–19 μg/24 h (1.5–20 μg/g of creatinine).

δ-Aminolevulinic Acid: See Porphyrins.

Ammonia
2–12 months: 4–20 μeq/min/m^2.
1–16 years: 6–16 μeq/min/m^2.

Calcium
4–12 years: 4–8 meq/L (2–4 mmol/L).

Catecholamines (Norepinephrine, Epinephrine)
Values in μg/24 in (nmol/24 h).
(See Table, bottom of page.)

Chloride
Infants: 1.7–8.5 mmol/24 h.
Children: 17–34 mmol/24 h.
Adults: 140–240 mmol/24 h.

Copper
0–30 μg/24 h.

Coproporphyrin: See Porphyrins.

Corticosteroids (17-Hydroxycorticosteroids)
0–2 years: 2–4 mg/24 h (5.5–11 μmol).
2–6 years: 3–6 mg/24 h (8.3–16.6 μmol).
6–10 years: 6–8 mg/24 h (16.6–22.1 μmol).
10–14 years: 8–10 mg/24 h (22.1–27.6 μmol).

Creatine
18–58 mg/L (1.37–4.42 mmol/L).

Creatinine
Newborns: 7–10 mg/kg/24 h.
Children: 20–30 mg/kg/24 h.
Adult males: 21–26 mg/kg/24 h.
Adult females: 16–22 mg/kg/24 h.

Epinephrine: See Catecholamines.

Homovanillic Acid
Children: 3–16 μg/mg of creatinine.
Adults: 2–4 μg/mg of creatinine.

17-Hydroxycorticosteroids: See Corticosteroids.

5-Hydroxyindoleacetic Acid
0.11–0.61 μmol/kg/7 h, based on results in 15 well-nourished, apparently healthy, mentally defective children on a tryptophan load.

Hydroxyproline, Total
5–14 years: 38–126 mg/24 h (290–961 μmol/24 h).

Mercury
< 50 μg/24 h (249 nmol/24 h).

Metanephrine and Normetanephrine
< 2 years: < 4.6 μg/mg of creatinine (23.3 nmol).
2–10 years: < 3 μg/mg of creatinine (15.2 nmol).
10–15 years: < 2 μg/mg of creatinine (10.3 nmol).
> 15 years: < 1 μg/mg of creatinine (5.1 nmol).

Mucopolysaccharides
Acid mucopolysaccharide screen should yield negative results. Positive results after dialysis of the urine should be followed up with a thin-layer chromatogram for evaluation of the acid mucopolysaccharide excretion pattern.

Norepinephrine: See Catecholamines.

Normetanephrine: See Metanephrine and Normetanephrine.

Osmolality
Infants: 50–600 mosm/L.
Older children: 50–1400 mosm/L.

Phosphorus, Tubular Reabsorption
78–97%.

Porphobilinogen: See Porphyrins.

Porphyrins
δ-Aminolevulinic acid: 0–7 mg/24 h (0–53.4 μmol/24 h).
Porphobilinogen: 0–2 mg/24 h (0–8.8 μmol/24 h).
Coproporphyrin: 0–160 μg/24 h (0–244 nmol/24 h).
Uroporphyrin: 0–26 μg/24 h (0–31 nmol/24 h).

Potassium
26–123 mmol/L.

Pregnanetriol
2 weeks–2 years: 0–0.2 mg/24 h (0–0.59 μmol/24 h).
2–16 years: 0.3–1.1 mg/24 h (0.89–3.27 μmol/24 h).

Sodium
Infants: 0.3–3.5 mmol/24 h (6–10 mmol/m^2).
Children and adults: 5.6–17 mmol/24 h.

Catecholamines in urine.

Group	Total Catecholamines	Norepinephrine	Epinephrine
< 1 year	20	5.4–15.9 (32–94)	0.1–4.3 (0.5–23.5)
1–5 years	40	8.1–30.8 (48–182)	0.8–9.1 (4.4–49.7)
6–15 years	80	19.0–71.1 (112–421)	1.3–10.5 (7.1–57.3)
> 15 years	100	34.4–87.0 (203–514)	3.5–13.2 (19.1–72.1)

(continued)

Testosterone
Prepubertal children: 0.2–2.3 µg/24 h (0.3–5 µg/g of creatinine.
Adult males: 40–130 µg/24 h.
Adult females: 2–11 µg/24 h.

Urobilinogen
< 3 mg/24 h (< 5.1 µmol/24 h).

Uroporphyrin: See Porphyrins.

Vanilmandelic Acid (VMA)
Because of the difficulty in obtaining an accurately timed 24-hour collection, values based on microgram per milligram of creatinine are the most reliable indications of VMA excretion in young children.
1–12 months: 1–35 µg/mg of creatinine (31–135 µg/kg/24 h).
1–2 years: 1–30 µg/mg of creatinine.
2–5 years: 1–15 µg/mg of creatinine.
5–10 years: 1–14 µg/mg of creatinine.
10–15 years: 1–10g/mg of creatinine (1–7 mg/24 h; 5–35 µmol/24 h).
Adults: 1–7 µg/mg of creatinine (1–7 mg/24 h; 5–35 µmol/24 h).

VMA: See Vanilmandelic Acid.

Xylose Absorption Test
Mean 5-hour excretion expressed as percentage of ingested load.
< 6 months: 11–30%.
6–12 months: 20–32%.
1–3 years: 20–42%.
3–10 years: 25–45%.
> 10 years: 25–50%.
Or: % excretion > (0.2 × age in months) + 12.

DUODENAL FLUID VALUE

Enzymes
Amylase: (Anderson).
0–2 months: 0–10 units/mL.
2–6 months: 10–20 units/mL.
6–12 months: 40–150 units/mL.
1–2 years: 100–225 units/mL.
2–5 years: 125–275 units/mL.
Carboxypeptidase:
0.4–1 unit (Ravin).
Chymotrypsin:
11–65 units (Ravin).
Protease:
18–70 units (Free-Meyers).
Trypsin: (Anderson or as noted).
0–2 months: 110–160 units/mL.
2–6 months: 115–160 units/mL.
6–12 months: 120–290 units/mL; 3–10 units (Nothman et al).
1–2 years: 200–300 units/mL.
2–5 years: 200–275 units/mL.

pH
6–8.4.

Viscosity
< 3 minutes (Shwachman).

FECES

Chymotrypsin
3–14 mg/kg 72 h.

Fat, Percentage of Dry Weight
2–6 months: 5–43%.
6 months–6 years: 6–26%.

Fat, Total
2–6 months: 0.3–1.3 g/d.
6 months–1 year: < 4 g/d.
Children: < 3 g/d.
Adolescents: < 5 g/d.
Adults: < 7 g/d.

Lipids, Split Fat
Adults: > 40% of total lipids.

Lipids, Total
Adults: Up to 7 g/d on normal diet, 10–27% of dry weight.

Nitrogen
Infants: < 1 g/d.
Children: < 1.2 g/d.
Adults: < 3 g/d.

Urobilinogen
2–12 months: 0.03–14 mg/d.
5–10 years: 2.7–39 mg/d.
10–14 years: 7.3–99 mg/d.

SWEAT

Electrolytes
Values for chloride. Elevated values in the presence of a family history or clinical findings of cystic fibrosis are diagnostic of cystic fibrosis.
Normal: < 40 mmol/L.
Borderline: 40–60 mmol/L.
Elevated: > 60 mmol/L.

MISCELLANEOUS

Amylo-1,6-Glucosidase Debrancher (Liver)
> 1 µmol/min/g of wet tissue.

Chloride
Breast milk: 2.5–30 mmol/L.
Cow's milk: 20–80 mmol/L.
Muscle: 20–26 mmol/kg of wet-free tissue.
Spinal fluid: 120–128 mmol/L.

Copper (Liver)
< 20 µg/g of wet tissue.

Glucose 6-Phosphatase (Liver)
> 5 µmol/min/g of wet tissue.

Lactate Dehydrogenase (LDH) (CSF)
17–59 IU/L at 37 °C.

Potassium
Breast milk: 12–17 mmol/L.
Cow's milk: 20–45 mmol/L.
Muscle: 160–180 mmol/kg of wet fat-free tissue.

Proteins (CSF)
Total proteins:
Newborn: 40–120 mg/dL (0.4–1.2 g/L).
1 month: 20–70 mg/dL (0.2–0.7 g/L).
Thereafter: 15–40 mg/dL (0.15–0.4 g/L).
Gamma globulin:
Children: Up to 9% of total.
Adults: Up to 14% of total.

Sodium
Breast milk: 4.7–8.3 mmol/L.
Cow's milk: 22–26 mmol/L.
Muscle: 33–43 mmol/kg of wet fat-free tissue.

[1]Adapted from Meites S (editor): *Pediatric Clinical Chemistry,* 2nd ed. American Association for Clinical Chemistry, 1982, and many other sources.

Index

NOTE: Page numbers in bold face type indicate a major discussion. A *t* following a page number indicates tabular material and an *i* following a page number indicates an illustration. Drugs are listed under their generic names. When a drug trade name is listed, the reader is referred to the generic name.

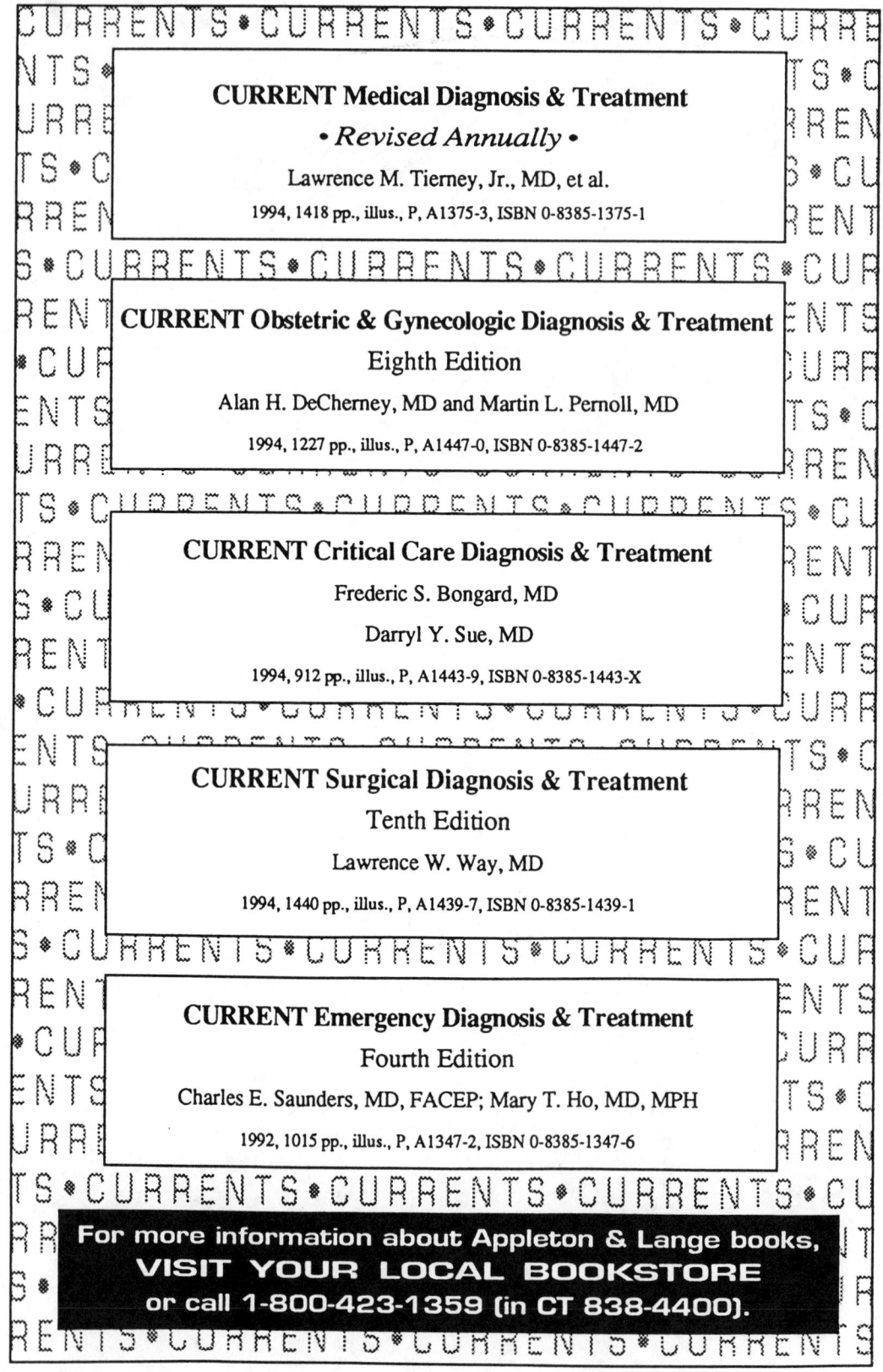